A companion to medical studies

Editorial board

FIRST PUBLISHED AUGUST 1968
REPRINTED JUNE 1969
REVISED PRINTING JULY 1971
REPRINTED OCTOBER 1973
SECOND EDITION 1976

SPANISH EDITION 1971
PORTUGESE EDITION 1974
ITALIAN EDITION IN PREPARATION
JAPANESE EDITION IN PREPARATION

ISBN
0 632 00308 1 Cloth
0 632 00288 3 Limp

Distributed in the United States of America by
J.B. LIPPINCOTT COMPANY, PHILADELPHIA
and in Canada by
J.B. LIPPINCOTT COMPANY OF CANADA LTD, TORONTO

Printed and bound in Great Britain by
WILLIAM CLOWES & SONS LTD, LONDON, BECCLES AND COLCHESTER

A companion to medical studies

IN THREE VOLUMES

Volume 1

Anatomy, biochemistry, physiology
and related subjects

EDITORS-IN-CHIEF

R. PASSMORE

J. S. ROBSON

SECOND EDITION

BLACKWELL SCIENTIFIC PUBLICATIONS

OXFORD LONDON EDINBURGH MELBOURNE

Contents

v

STRUCTURE AND FUNCTION OF TISSUES

STRUCTURE AND FUNCTION OF THE SYSTEMS

MAN IN HIS ENVIRONMENT

Colour illustrations

Volume 3

Medicine, surgery, systemic pathology, obstetrics, psychiatry, paediatrics, and community medicine

Contributors to volume 1

E. ASMUSSEN *Universitetets Gymnastikteoretiske Laboratorium, Copenhagen, Denmark*

JOYCE D. BAIRD *Department of Medicine, University of Edinburgh*

G.S. BOYD *Department of Biochemistry, University of Edinburgh*

J. CHALMERS *Department of Orthopaedic Surgery, University of Edinburgh*

S.H. DAVIES *Department of Haematology, University of Edinburgh*

P.R. DAVIS *Department of Biological Studies, University of Surrey*

A.N. DAVISON *Department of Neurochemistry, Institute of Neurology, London*

M.H. DRAPER *British Council, London*

O.G. EDHOLM *School of Environmental Studies, University College, London*

HAMAD ELNEIL *World Health Organization, Brazzaville, People's Republic of Congo*

R.B.L. EWART *University of Wisconsin, U.S.A.*

R.B. FISHER *Department of Biochemistry, University of Edinburgh*

D.C. FLENLEY *Department of Medicine, University of Edinburgh*

S. FLETCHER *Department of Pathology, University of Edinburgh*

J.M. FORRESTER *Department of Physiology, University of Edinburgh*

B.L. GINSBORG *Department of Pharmacology, University of Edinburgh*

T.W. GLENISTER *Department of Anatomy, Charing Cross Hospital Medical School, London*

J.A. HABESHAW *Department of Pathology, University of Edinburgh*

A.D. HALLY *Department of Anatomy, University of Newcastle*

D.G. HARNDEN *Department of Cancer Studies, University of Birmingham*

E.A. HARRIS *Clinical Physiology Department, Green Lane Hospital, Auckland, New Zealand*

E.R. HITCHCOCK *Department of Surgical Neurology, University of Edinburgh*

D.J. HITCHINGS *Department of Physiology, University of Edinburgh*

F.E. HYTTEN *Division of Perinatal Medicine, Clinical Research Centre, Harrow*

W.J. IRVINE *Department of Therapeutics, University of Edinburgh*

R.J. JOHNSTON *Department of Physiology, University of Edinburgh*

A.W.S. KERR *Department of Anatomy, University of Edinburgh*

M.G. KERR *Department of Obstetrics and Gynaecology, University of Edinburgh*

A.H. KITCHIN *Department of Medicine, University of Edinburgh*

K. KUCZYNSKI *Department of Anatomy, University of Edinburgh*

ANNE T. LAMBIE *Department of Therapeutics, University of Edinburgh*

T.R. LEE *Department of Psychology, University of Surrey*

SYBIL M. LLOYD *Department of Physiology, University of Edinburgh*

A. McGHIE *Department of Psychology, Queen's University, Kingston, Canada*

G.J.R. McHARDY *Department of Respiratory Diseases, University of Edinburgh*

I.B. MACLEOD *Department of Clinical Surgery, University of Edinburgh*

J.N. MILLS *Department of Physiology, University of Manchester*

J.A. MILNE *Department of Dermatology, University of Glasgow*

The late A.R. MUIR *Department of Veterinary Anatomy, University of Edinburgh*

P.R. MYERSCOUGH *Department of Obstetrics and Gynaecology, University of Edinburgh*

J.E. NEWSAM *Department of Urological Surgery, University of Edinburgh*

J.H. OTTAWAY *Department of Biochemistry, University of Edinburgh*

R. PASSMORE *Department of Physiology, University of Edinburgh*

A. PETERS *Department of Anatomy, Boston University, U.S.A.*

L. MARY PICKFORD *late of the Department of Physiology, University of Edinburgh*

W.N.M. RAMSAY *Department of Veterinary Biochemistry, University of Edinburgh*

J. RICHMOND *Department of Medicine, University of Sheffield*

M.H. RICHMOND *Department of Bacteriology, University of Bristol*

J.S. ROBSON *Department of Medicine, University of Edinburgh*

A.P. RYLE *Department of Biochemistry, University of Edinburgh*

R.J. SCOTHORNE *Department of Anatomy, University of Glasgow*

T. SCRATCHERD *Department of Physiology, University of Sheffield*

D.C. SINCLAIR *Department of Postgraduate Medical Education, Perth, Australia*

J.W. SMITH *Department of Anatomy, University of St Andrews*

WINIFRED L. STAFFORD *Department of Biochemistry, University of Edinburgh*

R.A. STOCKWELL *Department of Anatomy, University of Edinburgh*

A.D. TOFT *Department of Therapeutics, University of Edinburgh*

D.E.M. TAYLOR *Institute of Basic Medical Sciences, London*

L.G. WHITBY *Department of Clinical Chemistry, University of Edinburgh*

I. MAUREEN YOUNG *Department of Gynaecology, St Thomas's Hospital Medical School, London*

My object has been to express the leading facts of the science in as few words as possible, leaving them to be amplified, or freed from obscurity, by the reflection of the reader or the expository powers of the lecturer.

Mapother E.D. (1864) *A Manual of Physiology*

Preface

The editors of the Companion set out with the aim of giving undergraduates and graduate students an interesting, intelligent and exciting account of modern medicine and medical sciences. The task was completed in three volumes published in 1968, 1970 and 1974. Over 50 000 copies of volume 1 have been sold and sales of volumes 2 and 3 are approaching this figure; it is gratifying that our attempt has been so widely appreciated. In spite of several revised printings the passage of time now makes a second edition necessary.

The publication of a new edition of volume 1 has made possible a complete revision of its contents; many chapters have been completely rewritten, most of the others have been extensively revised and advances in knowledge accommodated. New chapters have been prepared to cover control of metabolism (14) and visual and auditory systems (26). Printing by lithography has permitted the freer use of EM and histological photomicrographs; many new line drawings have been added and others redrawn. We are again indebted to our authors for their patience in allowing us to adjust their manuscripts in order to interrelate contents, and to achieve a uniform English style and usage.

The Companion provides an opportunity to see all of the several facets of medicine related to each other in a single sequence. The publication of volumes 2 and 3 has enabled us to put into the new edition of volume 1 many forward references to clinical matters. These should help undergraduates to see more clearly the clinical relevance of their studies of the basic medical sciences and to achieve an overall perspective of medicine.

Many of the excellent advanced texts in all fields of medicine are listed in the Further Reading given at the end of each chapter. All students should be encouraged to read more deeply in selected subjects, but it is unrealistic to expect an undergraduate to have the time to study all subjects in depth or the money to purchase a comprehensive set of reference books. The three volumes of the Companion provide information for an understanding of medical science, and a rational basis for medical practice.

Many teachers and practising doctors may feel that justice has not been done to the subject in which their interests lie and where they have special knowledge. It is hoped that they will use and enjoy other parts of the book. After graduating it is difficult for all of us to keep up with the changing outlooks and new information in the diverse fields of medicine, and it is important to be able to carry on an intelligent conversation with experts in different fields.

As in the first edition, we are concerned with the precise use of the language of medicine, which continually grows and changes. There have been important changes in chemical nomenclature since the first edition was published, particularly in regard to enzymes and macromolecules containing protein, carbohydrate and lipid components. S.I. units, *Le Système International d'Unités*, have been used throughout, except in one or two instances, e.g. for blood pressure, where the old unit still appears more appropriate.

In the preparation of this edition we are greatly indebted to Dr D. Langslow for checking the biochemical formulae and also to Miss J.B. Gardner for her editorial help. We are indebted to the artists for drawing and redrawing many of the illustrations, and also Mrs Anne McCarthy for revising the index.

We continue to depend on and receive the enthusiastic support of our publishers, Per Saugman and Nigel Palmer.

Edinburgh   R. Passmore
May 1976   J. S. Robson

Acknowledgements

We wish to thank all publishers, editors and authors who have allowed us to reproduce illustrations but especially Professor Romanes and the Oxford University Press for the use of *Cunningham's Textbook of Anatomy* on which many of our anatomical illustrations are based. Others include Academic Press Inc; American Chemical Society; American Physiological Society; American Society of Biological Chemists Inc; Appleton-Century-Crofts; Edward Arnold (Publishers) Ltd; Athlone Press; Baillière Tindall; Blackwell Scientific Publications Ltd; Butterworth & Co. (Publishers) Ltd; Cambridge University Press; Chatto & Windus Ltd; Chemical Society; Churchill Livingstone; CIBA; G. Doin; Elsevier Scientific Publishing Co; J.R. Geigy S.A; Grune & Stratton; Harper & Row Publishers Inc; W. Heffer & Sons Ltd; William Heinemann Medical Books Ltd; Johns Hopkins Press; Henry Kimpton Ltd; Lange Medical Publications; H. K. Lewis & Co. Ltd; H.M. Stationery Office; J.B. Lippincott Co; Little, Brown & Co; Longman Group Ltd; McGraw-Hill Book Co; Macmillan Publishers Ltd; Josiah Macy Jr. Foundation; C.V. Mosby Co; Munksgaard Ltd; National Coal Board; New York Academy of Sciences; Oxford University Press; Pitman Medical & Scientific Publishing Co. Ltd; Prentice-Hall Inc; Princeton University Press; W.B. Saunders Co; Scientific American Inc; Society for Endocrinology; Charles C. Thomas; University of Chicago Press; John Wiley & Sons Inc; Williams & Wilkins Co; Yale University Press; *Acta Pathologica et Microbiologica Scandinavica; Acta Physiologica Scandinavica; American Heart Journal; American Journal of Medicine; American Journal of Obstetrics and Gynecology; American Journal of Physiology; Annals of the New York Academy of Sciences; Biochemical Journal; Biochemistry; Biochimica et Biophysica Acta; Brain; British Medical Bulletin; British Medical Journal; Bulletin of the Johns Hopkins Hospital; Clinical Science and Molecular Medicine; Cold Spring Harbor Symposia on Quantitative Biology; Contributions to Embryology; Developmental Medicine and Child Neurology; Diabetes; Endocrinology; Experimental Neurology; Journal of the American Medical Association; Journal of the American Oil Chemists Society; Journal of Applied Physiology; Journal of Biological Chemistry; Journal of Clinical Endocrinology and Metabolism; Journal of Clinical Investigation; Journal of Endocrinology; Journal of General Physiology; Journal of Histochemistry and Cytochemistry; Journal of Laboratory and Clinical Medicine; Journal of Neurology, Neurosurgery and Psychiatry; Journal of Neurophysiology; Journal of Obstetrics and Gynaecology of the British Commonwealth; Journal of Pediatrics; Journal of Physiology; Lancet; Nature; New England Journal of Medicine; Nutrition Today; Physiological Reviews; Proceedings of the Nutrition Society; Proceedings of the Royal Society; Progress in Cardiovascular Diseases; Quarterly Journal of Experimental Physiology; Recent Progress in Hormone Research; Science; Scientific American; Veterinary Record.*

Finally, we would like to acknowledge our indebtedness to other publications if through inadvertence this list is incomplete.

Chapter 1
Man and his environment

A struggle in which all,
The elderly, the amorous, the young, the handy and the
  thoughtful,
Those to whom feeling is a science, those to whom study
Of all that can be added and compared is a consuming love,
In cities, deserts, ships, in lodgings near the port,
Discovering the past of strangers in a library,
Creating their own future on a bed, each with his treasure,
Self-confident among the laughter and the *petits verres*,
Or motionless and lonely like a moping cormorant,
In all their living are profoundly implicated.

External environment, which is always changing

Thus W.H. Auden reports the struggle which the human biologist must analyse in detail. Man is a tough and ubiquitous animal. He can be found in little colonies in the polar regions or living as a nomad in arid deserts. He may inhabit small villages in the rarefied air of the higher ranges of the Andes or huge towns in the humid heat on the sea coast of southern Asia. He is capable of exploring outer space. He must come to terms with a great variety of other animals of all sizes. He may be both hunter and hunted. He is engaged in a constant struggle with viruses, bacteria, protozoa and worms, many species of which may become his parasites. With the majority of these a *modus vivendi* is established, but not a few can seriously incapacitate or even kill him. Man is also a social animal, normally utterly dependent on other men and women for his simplest necessities, and harmonious relations with our fellows are always difficult to achieve.

The essence of human biology is the study of adaptive processes made necessary by struggles with an ever-changing environment. The doctor is particularly concerned with the responses to parasites, social maladjustments and violence, often the result of motor, industrial and home accidents. He must know the effects of unsuitable or defective diets. Nowadays he is more and more concerned with the responses to new chemicals to which man is being exposed for the first time. Many of these chemicals are essential features of the environment in a modern industrial civilization. Others have been introduced as drugs for their healing properties. The doctor is concerned also with the adaptive changes that occur in the mother during pregnancy and with the effects of a great variety of degenerative diseases, the consequence of the wearing out of parts of the mechanisms of the body with increasing age.

On account of its continuous exposure to a changing environment, the human body must be considered as an **open system**. This distinguishes it from most of the chemical reactions and the physical behaviour of matter, which can be studied as a **closed system** in a fixed and constant environment. The behaviour of a closed system is more susceptible to scientific study and can often be described in terms of the limits imposed by precise natural laws. The student will already be familiar with many such laws, for instance, those associated with the names of Avogadro, Boyle, Dalton, Gay-Lussac, Henry, Hooke, Joule, Newton and Ohm. Fewer biologists have had their names perpetuated in a similar manner.

Internal environment, which is relatively constant

Perhaps the best known physiological principle is that first set out in 1857 by Claude Bernard in a lecture at the Sorbonne in Paris: 'All the vital mechanisms, however varied they may be, have always but one end, that of preserving the constancy of the conditions of life in the internal environment'.

The blood and the lymph which bathe the cells are conceived of as an internal environment, which protects the cells of the organs of the body from variations in the external environment. The American physiologist Cannon, in 1929, introduced the term **homeostasis** to describe this principle. *Homoios* is a Greek word meaning the like or the same. Homeostatic processes are those physiological reactions which tend to restore the internal environment to a steady or resting state; here are four examples. Heavy physical exercise raises the temperature of the blood and also its acidity. A meal raises the concentration of blood glucose, and drinking water lowers its osmolality. Exercise, food and drink each initiate responses which cause the blood to return to the normal state.

EXERCISE AND BLOOD TEMPERATURE

The normal temperature of the blood is around 37–38°C. A man running for 20 min produces some 800 kilojoules (kJ) or 190 kilocalories (kcal) of heat. The specific heat of the body is 3·47 kJ. So this heat is sufficient to raise the temperature of a 65 kg man by

$$\frac{800}{65 \times 3 \cdot 47} = 3 \cdot 5°C$$

Whilst running, the man starts to perspire and may lose 200 g of sweat; as the latent heat of evaporation of water is 2·43 kJ (0·580 kcal)/g this is equivalent to 485 kJ (116 kcal) of heat. The sweating reduces the rise in body temperature and helps to return it to the normal level soon after the end of the run. Sweating is a physiological cooling mechanism that is brought into action rapidly as soon as the body temperature rises.

EXERCISE AND THE ACIDITY OF THE BLOOD

The blood is normally slightly alkaline. The hydrogen ion concentration is about 40 ng/l (1 nanogram = 10^{-9} g), corresponding to a pH value of 7·40. During exercise the muscles produce carbon dioxide, which is an acid in solution. During a 20 min run, 40 litres of CO_2 may be produced. This is equivalent to 1·8 moles of carbonic acid. However, the acidity of the blood rises only slightly during exercise and the pH seldom falls by more than 0·05. This is partly due to the buffering power of the blood (p. 6.4), but also to the fact that as soon as exercise starts, the rate and depth of breathing are increased so that the carbon dioxide is blown off almost as rapidly as it is formed. Panting at the end of the run returns the pH of the blood to normal in a few minutes.

FASTING AND THE GLUCOSE CONCENTRATION IN BLOOD

The blood glucose of a fasting man is about 4 mmol/l (70 mg/100 ml). This glucose is utilized continuously by the tissues and the level is normally maintained by the absorption of dietary carbohydrate from the intestines. After a meal the blood glucose may rise to 8–9 mmol/l (140–160 mg/100 ml). This excess is stored temporarily as glycogen in the liver and muscles, a process which requires insulin, a hormone secreted by the pancreas. Yet a man may fast for two or three weeks or even longer and his blood glucose is well maintained and will probably not fall below 3 mmol/l (55 mg/100 ml). During this time glucose is still being used; the brain alone requires 80 g/day. The concentration in the blood is kept constant by the formation of glucose (gluconeogenesis) from protein and glycerol derived from fat. The liver has a predominant role in this adaptive reaction.

DRINKING AND THE OSMOLALITY OF BLOOD

Most of us drink much more fluid than is needed to excrete the urea and other waste products in the urine.

When an excess of water is drunk, the osmolality of the plasma (normally about 285 mosmol/l) falls slightly. This fall is immediately sensed by osmoreceptors in the brain. From a controlling centre in the hypothalamus, the secretion of a pituitary hormone, vasopressin, is regulated. The level of this hormone in the blood determines the rate at which the kidneys excrete water. The excretion of water in the urine is almost as rapid as the water absorption from the intestines. This mechanism controls the osmolality of the plasma so that in health it fluctuates only over a narrow range.

These four examples of homeostasis illustrate how the internal environment of the body is kept constant, despite the imposition of considerable external stresses. The effector organs in these examples are the sweat glands, lungs, liver and kidneys. The mechanisms by which these organs are brought into play involve elaborate control systems both chemical and nervous in nature.

In various disease states homeostasis may break down. The temperature may rise to 41°C as a result of infection by parasitic organisms; the acidity of the blood may rise to pH 7·10 in disease of the lungs preventing the normal excretion of CO_2; the blood glucose may fall to below 2 mmol/l (35 mg/100 ml) in patients with insulin-producing tumours of the pancreas. Under each of these conditions the patient is seriously ill and, unless they are remedied rapidly, may die.

Composition of the body and the size of the internal environment

The body can be considered as composed of three compartments. Firstly there is the **cell mass**, comprising all the cells of the body where most of the chemical work of the body is done; this compartment is sometimes referred to as the active mass. Secondly there is the **supporting tissue**. This includes the **extracellular fluid** in the blood and the fluid surrounding the cells in the various organs. This fluid makes up the **internal environment** of the cells. The supporting tissue also includes the minerals in the skeleton and the protein in connective tissue fibres. The third compartment is the **energy reserve**, composed largely of fat held mainly in the cells of adipose tissue beneath the skin and surrounding the principal internal organs.

It is, of course, impossible to separate out these compartments by physical dissection. There are, however, indirect ways of measuring the size of each. In a healthy young man, the body weight is divided approximately: 55 per cent cell mass, 30 per cent supporting tissue and 15 per cent energy reserve. In a young woman the energy reserve is usually almost twice as large.

The **dilution principle** is one of the means that are used to measure the size of the compartments of the body.

Suppose you want to measure the volume of water in a small ornamental fishpond in a garden. It would be tedious and difficult to empty it into measuring cylinders. A simpler procedure is to add to the pond a small quantity (Q) of a water-soluble dye. After a short interval, to allow the dye to diffuse throughout the pond, a sample of the water is taken and the concentration (C) of the dye determined. The volume (V) of water in the pond is then given by

$$V = \frac{Q}{C}$$

A variety of substances, deuterium oxide or heavy water, tritiated water, the drugs antipyrine and amino-antipyrine, and also ethyl alcohol, appear to diffuse evenly throughout the water in all the tissues of the body. They can be used to measure **total body water** by the dilution technique. A known amount of the substance is given either by mouth or by intravenous injection; after an interval to allow for absorption and diffusion, a sample of venous blood is taken and the concentration of the substance in the plasma determined. Then the volume of fluid in which the substance is dispersed can be calculated. This then equals the total body water, provided the assumption that the diffusion of the substance throughout the total body water is uniform is correct and corrections are made for losses in excretion or metabolism.

Another group of substances, including the polysaccharide inulin, sucrose and mannitol, sodium thiocyanate and the ions $^{35}SO_4^{--}$, $^{82}Br^-$ and $^{24}Na^+$, if injected into the body, occupy about the same volume, which is much smaller than the deuterium volume. These substances either do not cross the membranes of the cell walls or are extruded as a result of active processes within the cells. In consequence they can be used to measure the space occupied by extracellular fluids. The measurement of the extracellular water is not as precise as the measurement of total body water, because none of the substances used completely meet the requirements of the test. They are either found in the cells in small amounts (Na thiocyanate) or do not diffuse evenly throughout all the extracellular water (inulin).

In a healthy man weighing 65 kg, a normal value for the total body water is 40 litres and for the extracellular water is 15 litres. These figures are convenient to remember. They correspond to about two-thirds and one-fifth of the body weight. These proportions are higher in thin people and much less in the obese.

The extracellular water can be further subdivided into the **plasma water**, in the circulating blood, and the **interstitial water**, in the tissue spaces surrounding the cells. The plasma volume can be determined by the dilution technique, using the dye Evans blue or serum albumin labelled with radioactive iodine as an indicator. A normal value is 3 litres. This leaves 12 litres of fluid actually surrounding the tissue cells and forming the internal environment which determines their behaviour (table 1.1). The **cell water** can be determined only by difference, and in our example of a healthy man it amounts to 25 litres.

TABLE 1.1. The distribution of water in the body of a healthy man weighing 65 kg (in litres).

Interstitial water	12		
Plasma water	3	Extracellular water 15	
Intracellular water	25		Total body water 40

The water content of the various types of cells differs and is not always easily determined. Muscle cells are 75 per cent water, but the water content of red blood cells is less than 70 per cent, as also is probably the water content of connective tissue cells. If the cells are assumed to be on average 70 per cent water, then

$$\text{cell mass} = \text{cell water} \times \frac{100}{70}$$

The size of the energy reserve, the fat in the body, can be determined by density measurements (p. 4.7). A normal figure for a man is 9 kg. Women of course are usually fatter (p. 4.8).

We can now divide our normal man quantitatively into his three compartments (table 1.2). There is no method

TABLE 1.2. The compartments of a normal man.

	kg
Active tissue	
Cell mass	36
Supporting tissue	
Internal environment or extracellular fluid	15
Bone minerals and extracellular proteins	5
Energy reserve	
Fat	9
Body weight	65

as yet for determining the mass of the bone minerals and the extracellular proteins in life. The value of 5 kg in the table is obtained by difference.

The measurement of the body weight is frequently made in physiological studies and in clinical practice. Changes in body weight are rightly considered of great importance in assessing the progress of many diseases but the weighing-machine may not reflect accurately what is happening. Thus our man might be suffering from a wasting disease and his cell mass diminish by 2 kg and his energy reserve by 4 kg during a month. At the same time fluid may accumulate in the body (oedema) and his extracellular water increase by 6 kg. He would then still weigh 65 kg, although seriously wasted.

It is frequently necessary to make corrections for the great variations in size of human beings. Thus in therapeutics the dose of drugs may be given as so many mg/kg body weight. This is sound provided the distribution of the body weight amongst the three compartments is approximately normal. Such a system of dosage is unreliable for very thin or fat people or in infancy.

The measurement of the size of the various compartments of the body demands laboratory skills and equipment. It is an important part of clinical science and is leading to a new understanding of how the body works in health and in disease. It is not an essential in routine hospital practice. Yet every doctor makes frequent use of a weighing-machine. It must be remembered that what goes on the scales is not a uniform mass. Body weight is a measure of the sum of the size of three compartments of the body, each with very different functions.

The size of the internal environment is reduced when there is insufficient water to drink or if there are excessive water losses due to sweating. Diarrhoea and vomiting lead to losses of water and electrolytes and a reduced internal environment. This is important, especially in babies and young children. A significant increase probably never occurs in health in response to any stress from the external environment, but increased extracellular water giving rise to oedema is a common feature of many diseases (vol. 2, p. 26.10). It is found in starvation and other nutritional disorders and is characteristic of many cardiac, renal and liver diseases.

The size of the internal environment is regulated but not with great precision. If you weigh yourself every morning immediately after waking and emptying the bladder, you will often find a variation of up to 1 kg from day to day and occasionally greater. This is largely due to variations in extracellular fluid. How the control of the size of this volume is effected is only partially understood and is further discussed on p. 35.22.

Composition of the internal environment

This is relatively easy to determine. The capillaries of the circulation allow, for the most part, a free exchange between the electrolytes and crystalloid substances in the blood and interstitial fluid. Thus an analysis of a sample of blood plasma gives a good indication of the composition of the internal environment. Proteins do not pass readily across the capillary barrier and, whereas the plasma contains 50–80 g/l of protein, the concentration in the interstitial fluids is very small. Table 1.3 sets out the normal values for the electrolyte content of the extracellular fluid, based on analyses of plasma. For comparison, figures for the intracellular fluid are also given. It is, of course, difficult to obtain cell water for analysis: the figures given are estimates based on

analyses of whole tissues from which values for the extracellular electrolytes are subtracted.

TABLE 1.3. A normal distribution of ions in intracellular and extracellular fluids.

	Intracellular (mEq/l)	Extracellular (mEq/l)
Cations		
Na^+	10	140
K^+	150	5
Ca^{++}	2	3
Mg^{++}	15	2
	177	150
Anions		
Cl^-	5	100
HCO_3^-	10	25
Organic acids		6
PO_4^{---}	120	2
Proteins	42	17
	177	150

The concentrations of extracellular cations and anions add up to 300 mEq/l, but the osmolality of plasma, as measured by depression of the freezing point, is slightly less and about 285 mosmol/l. This is because in a solution of electrolytes in water interionic and electrostatic charges modify the osmotic effect of the ionized particles.

Sodium is the principal cation in the extracellular water and potassium in the intracellular water. The ability of cells to survive and to respond to nervous and chemical stimulation depends on ionic gradients across the cell wall. In the plasma the principal anions are Cl^- and HCO_3^-. In the cells phosphate and protein provide the chief anions for maintaining the electrochemical balance with the K^+ ions. The amount of HCO_3^- in the plasma is altered by changing the rate and depth of breathing. These determine the gaseous CO_2 output. Respiration in this way influences the HCO_3^- content of the extracellular fluid and is a fine adjustment in the control of the pH of the internal environment. Measurements of plasma bicarbonate are of great value in investigating disturbances of the acid-base balance. These occur in health during exercise, as already mentioned, and in acclimatization to high altitude; they are a common feature of many diseases, especially those associated with failure of the lungs and kidney.

The fact that the internal environment is primarily a solution of sodium chloride may be a reflection of the marine origin of mammals in the remote evolutionary past. In most parts of the oceans, the sea water contains about 3 per cent NaCl, corresponding to 500 mmol/litre of Na, more than three times the amount in the internal environment. Such a load of sodium is beyond the capacity of the kidneys, which are the guardians of the internal environment and accurately maintain its chemical composition. For this reason castaways on the ocean should not drink sea water, which will only exaggerate their thirst and accelerate their death (p. 44.3).

Stability of the internal environment

Few men have submitted their bodies to severe environmental stress in the interests of physiology as frequently as did Sir Joseph Barcroft. In his Cambridge laboratory there was a small room in which the chemical composition and pressure of the atmosphere could be varied experimentally. Barcroft once spent 14 days in this room in an atmosphere equivalent to that on the higher slopes of Everest. He pointed out that many, perhaps most, essential functions of the body can proceed over a fairly wide range of conditions, but the mental processes are much more restricted. He described how a small change of hydrogen ion concentration in the blood over a short period can affect the higher nervous system causing inability to concentrate, which may last for two or three days. Most of us are aware of how a trivial degree of fever can seriously impair mental effort. Perhaps the development of an accurate control over the internal environment has been a necessary prerequisite for the development of the higher nervous functions, which are characteristic of man. To quote Barcroft:

'The chemical and physical processes associated with the working of the mind are of so delicate a character that beside them the changes measured by the thermometer or the hydrogen electrode must be catastrophic—overwhelming. Processes (probably rhythmic) of such delicacy must surely require a medium of great constancy in which to attain ordered development. How often have I watched the ripples on the surface of a still lake made by a passing boat, noted their regularity and admired the patterns formed when two ripple-systems meet, but the lake must be perfectly calm, just as the atmosphere must be free from atmospherics if you are to find beauty in the subtle passages of a symphony. To look for high intellectual development in a *milieu* whose properties have not become stabilized is to seek music amongst the crashings of a rudimentary wireless or the ripple patterns on the surface of the stormy Atlantic.'

Levels of organization

A complex organization is necessary to make the adaptive changes in a system open to a constantly changing environment. Enzymes are the catalysts that determine the rate and course of all the organic chemical reactions in the body; in composition they are proteins. When studied in aqueous solution in test tubes, the behaviour of enzymic reactions is described by a well-defined set of laws. Enzymic kinetics is a precise and elegant branch of science. However, the behaviour of enzymes is not always readily explained by these rules, because their activity within the cell is influenced by many other concurrent chemical reactions as indicated on p. 7.17. Although most important chemical reactions in the body are in themselves relatively simple, they are interlocked in an elaborate manner. A particular compound may be able to take part in one of several reactions and in this way modifications of cell behaviour arise which can be controlled in relation to varying rates of biological function. Many of the hormones secreted by the endocrine glands modify the activity of cell enzymes (p. 14.12) and in this way control the rates of chemical reactions within the cells. Reactions of the cells appear more complex than those of the enzyme systems of which they are composed. Similarly the function of each of the organs of the body cannot be fully described in terms of the functions of the cells, of which they are composed. The behaviour of a whole man is more adaptable than that of the individual organs; the whole body possesses the ability to co-ordinate the individual organs. Finally, a human society becomes a powerful and effective unit when it is able to co-ordinate the behaviour of its individuals (chap. 41). The great physiologist J.S. Haldane stressed the importance of the different levels of organization in living systems. He taught that:

'The life of an organism must be regarded as an objective active unity which embraces its environment, and manifests itself not merely in the mutual relations between parts of the organism itself, but also between the organism and its environment. The use of this conception in biology separates it from the physical sciences.'

J. Barcroft and J.S. Haldane in England and L.J. Henderson and W.B. Cannon in the United States were four great physiologists, who in the first quarter of the twentieth century developed Bernard's conception of the stability of the internal environment. It is the most important theoretical generalization within the medical sciences. No student will regret spending a few evenings browsing through one or more of the books by these masters, which are listed at the end of this chapter.

Physiology and biochemistry are difficult subjects. Unfortunately pathology and the clinical sciences are no easier. The difficulty arises because you cannot understand how the whole body works, in either health or disease, unless you first have some knowledge of the function of its component systems. Yet a detailed study of the parts easily obscures the whole. It is difficult to know where to begin. In pre-medical courses, it is possible to set out concisely and dogmatically the essentials of physics and chemistry. The student starting physiology will soon realize that the human body is a complex mechanism about which we know much, but understand little. In these respects the human mind is no better. Whatever branch of medicine the student chooses for his final career, he will have to make important decisions, which may affect the health and even the lives of people, lacking a full understanding of what he is doing. The difficulties of the medical sciences will present a challenge that lasts a life time. The recurring glimpses of understanding are the intellectual rewards.

FURTHER READING

BARCROFT J. (1934) *Features in the Architecture of Physiological Function.* London: Cambridge University Press.

CANNON W.B. (1932) *The Wisdom of the Body.* New York: Norton.

HALDANE J.S. & PRIESTLEY J.G. (1935) *Respiration.* New Haven: Yale University Press.

HENDERSON L.J. (1928) *Blood—a Study in General Physiology.* Oxford: Clarendon Press.

MOORE F.D. *et al.* (1963) *The Body Cell Mass and its Supporting Environment.* Philadelphia: Saunders.

OLMSTED J.M.D. (1939) *Claude Bernard.* (An excellent short account of Bernard's life and work.) London: Cassell.

PASSMORE R. & DRAPER M.H. (1970) The chemical anatomy of the human body. In *Biochemical Disorders in Human Disease*, 3rd Edition, pp. 1–14, ed. Thompson R.H.S. & Wootton I.D.P. London: Churchill Livingstone.

Chapter 2
Control theory and systems

Chapter 1 outlined how life depends on the stability of certain features of the internal environment. All living organisms contain control systems which stabilize such features, by detecting deviations, or even by anticipating them, and applying the necessary correcting responses. Thus within our bodies there are many control systems, which appear to be independent of each other but may often interact. Such systems control, for example, body temperature, cardiac output, respiration, pupillary diameter and posture. During exercise the first three of these interact to provide the necessary oxygen and prevent overheating. In hot weather we dress more lightly and show other responses (p. 43.5) which allow us to face high environmental temperatures with safety.

Control systems can fail. For instance, if the temperature-regulating system fails, body temperature drifts up and down with the environmental temperature in an unstable and perilous fashion. If a more fundamental understanding of the way in which the system is organized could be achieved, it should be possible to determine the reasons for the breakdown of the system during disease. In this way more logical treatment should become practicable.

Engineers have over many years developed an ever-increasing complexity of control systems, and thus relieved mankind of the tedium of repetitive tasks, which are now done with a speed and efficiency impossible for a human operator. The steam engine governor, invented in 1775 by James Watt, was one of the first control devices. It was analysed in 1868 in a classic paper, *On Governors*, by James Clerk Maxwell, who was schooled in Edinburgh. The problem was to adjust the amount of steam delivered to the engine to keep a constant speed under a variable load. By linking the throttle to the engine speed, the amount of power was adjusted to overcome any departure from the desired speed. But it was not until 1934 with Hazen's paper, *Theory of Servomechanisms*, that the general study of control systems started. World War II provided the impetus to develop complex control systems, the zenith of achievement being automatic aiming of anti-aircraft guns guided by radar.

As man-made systems grew more complex, it became difficult to design a system to meet a specific requirement.

A new branch of mathematics was developed, and is still being improved. This is known as control theory and systems analysis. Through it the dynamic behaviour of any system can be predicted before it is actually produced. The engineer builds mathematical models and then computer models of the system which he needs. The reaction of the system to various inputs and constraints is then determined, using control theory analysis on the mathematical model or placing the actual inputs and constraints on the computer-simulated model.

Since physiological systems are controlled, it is logical to apply engineering principles for their analysis and to produce mathematical and computer models of them. The production of a model does not necessarily show how the real system works, but it does show how the components may interact to produce the response that occurs. New experiments can be developed from knowledge of the basic model to obtain more information about the system and thus improve the model. With an accurate model one can determine which parts of the system must go wrong to produce the responses found in a disorder of the real physiological system. Hence in theory the area of the system which needs medical or surgical attention can be defined. A good model also enables research workers to experiment upon it in a way which would not be possible with the human system. But the task of the biologist necessarily differs from that of the engineer. The engineer devises his own system to meet known requirements. The biologist studies systems already developed, most of which are more complex than the most elaborate yet proposed by man.

Control system analysis and modelling

When designing a control system an engineer tries to simplify it and the equations which describe it as much as possible, whilst preserving the standards of performance that are set. Almost all control systems can be simplified to the form shown in fig. 2.1.

In the first place it is necessary to measure the variable being controlled by a device shown as B. In order that the system may handle only one type of signal, the desired input quantity is measured with a device A, producing a signal in similar form. These signals are nearly always

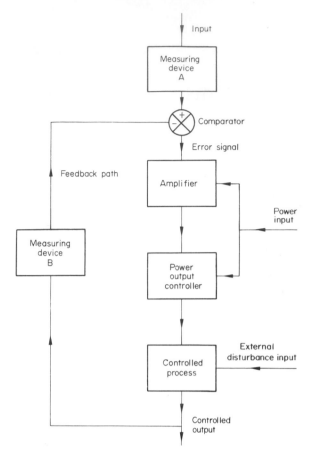

FIG. 2.1. Block diagram of a feedback control system.

in the form of varying electrical quantities, and many devices exist to change output quantities such as temperature, pressure, humidity, position, angular velocity and other into electrical signals. Electrical quantities are not invariably used, however, and outputs may be transformed into mechanical signals such as hydraulic pressures, lengths of rods or cables, rotation of shafts and many others. The two signals, representing present output and desired input, are compared in a comparator and the difference is used to give an **error signal.** This is then amplified in the error amplifier and used to drive an effector or output controller to change the output in such a way as to reduce the error. The concept of comparing the desired input with the actual output, i.e. of measuring the error, and then using this error to show what action is needed to eliminate the error, is the basis of control systems. A second essential feature is the amplification of the error signal to enable it to drive large outputs. This often is the main purpose of a control system, for example the steering mechanism of a large ship enables a man to move a rudder weighing many tons with fingertip control. The third essential feature is the closing of the loop from the output to the input by a feedback element which allows the output to be

added to or subtracted from the input in the comparator. This permits the system to provide complete automatic closed loop working of which homeostasis is an example.

In summary, a feedback control system is actuated by an error signal, possesses power amplification, and operates automatically in a closed loop.

We can now consider the methods for producing a model of a particular system. Take as an example the system for the control of the pupil. One of the functions of the system is to regulate the intensity of light falling on the retina for a wide range of ambient lighting conditions. Anatomical, observational and some basic experimental knowledge can all help in producing a simple pathway diagram of the system. There are two muscles associated with the control of the pupil diameter, the radial dilator and the sphincter. These muscles are antagonistic in operation, but it is assumed that the sphincter is most concerned with control of the pupil size. Although the neural pathways of both eyes can be shown to be coupled together, this fact is ignored for the moment in the interest of simplicity.

We can now draw fig. 2.2. Incident light passes through the pupil and falls on the retina. The retinal flux density

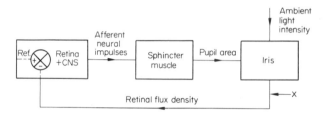

FIG. 2.2. Simplified block diagram of the pupil control system.

is compared with a reference level within the retina or central nervous system (CNS). The CNS processes the difference between the input and the reference level and uses this information to activate the sphincter muscle which contracts or dilates the iris, thus allowing less or more light to fall on the retina.

This simple block diagram only becomes a model of the system when the mathematical or graphical relationship of input to output of each block is known. It may not be feasible to define this relationship for each block in a biological system. In this case it may be necessary to lump some of the blocks together to avoid including pathways whose nature and behaviour cannot be determined. Later, the number of pathways and system components in the light of further anatomical and experimental findings could be increased.

The engineer has certain mathematical and experimental tools at his disposal in system analysis. All of these use the application of a well-defined input to the system and relate this input to the output produced by the system. In this way clues are obtained as to the nature of the various components and pathways in the system. It is therefore necessary to apply an external input to the biological system and to monitor an output at a known point in the system.

The output of the system to a fixed level of input gives information about the system which does not include the dynamic portion of the system's response. This is known as the steady state response. In the pupil control system, the pupil area can be plotted against incident light intensity; this gives data which help in relating the retinal flux density to incident light intensity. The relationship is logarithmic in form over a wide range of incident light intensities.

To determine information about the dynamic behaviour of a closed loop system, the engineer applies inputs to the system which have a dynamic relationship with time. Mathematical correlation of this input to the output of the system helps in determining the dynamic form of the system. Such inputs are transient steps, sinusoidal and random in form. This has been done with the pupil control system and has shown that the response of the pupil to sudden darkening is slower than its response to increased light and that the various system blocks are non-linear in form.

Another method that can be used in system analysis is to measure the response of the system to a particular input with any one of the information paths of the system opened. This is known as the open loop response. By using mathematics developed for the purpose it is possible to produce a clearer picture of the system under investigation. This is a difficult procedure to perform with closed internal physiological systems; animal experiments can be helpful in this respect. However in studies concerned with the eye it can be done. Since the pupil has a finite minimum diameter it is possible to shine through the pupil a beam of light of variable intensity and of a smaller diameter than the minimum pupil diameter. In fig. 2.2 this represents a break in the communication channel from the iris at point X; the pupil can no longer influence the amount of light entering the eye. Disease conditions in man can produce lesions which open one of the pathways in a closed loop system. An example of this is the Argyll Robertson pupil which fails to react to light but responds to convergence and accommodation (vol. 3, p. 34.60). Study of a person with this condition could be helpful in piecing together a more comprehensive picture of man's pupil control system.

Mathematical models and analog computing

In the preceding section some of the methods which could be used to define the nature of a biological control system were discussed. If it were possible to define the mathematical relationship of input and output for each of the component blocks in a system, then a mathematical model of that system could be produced. These individual relationships can be lumped together mathematically to produce a single mathematical relationship between the input and output of the system. Often with a complex system, where the component parts and their inter-relationship cannot be experimentally separated, this is the only relationship that can be produced. The mathematical definition of each component within such a system from this single equation is very difficult. If it is the only relationship that can be produced for a given system, it must be the starting point in producing experimental methods which will aid in obtaining such information.

There is another approach in defining a mathematical model for a system. Well-defined physical laws related to the mode of working of the system can be utilized, with experimental data, in producing a model. This will be demonstrated with the human thermoregulation system.

The possession of a good mathematical model of a particular system allows the experimenter to model that system on a computer. This gives him a simulation of his real system which reacts to input disturbances and constraints in exactly the same way as the real system. The use of such a model helps the experimenter to understand the dynamic relationship of the constituent parts of the real system. It also aids in devising new experiments which could be used in testing the real system to produce new knowledge about that system. The analog computer is most used in this type of modelling.

Analog computers work by simulating accurately physical quantities in terms of varying electrical signals which can be more easily and quickly manipulated and measured. In essence, the elements of an analog computer may be used to produce electrical models of the differential equations which describe the mathematical models of control systems.

The computer contains devices (simulators) to do all the mathematical operations, such as integration, differentiation, multiplication (amplification) or division, addition and subtraction, sign changing and many others. In each of these devices constants, representing the constants of the various elements of the system, can be inserted or altered at will. A flow diagram is compiled from the differential equations of the system to be analysed and each block in the diagram then represents a simulation element of the computer. These elements are connected together in the same way as in the flow diagram, with the appropriate constants inserted as desired, and then represent an electrical model of the system being studied. If an electrical input similar in form to an actual input to the system is applied, then the output of the computer is related, in an exactly similar way, to the actual output of the system.

For example, if the computer is set up to represent the motion of a bouncing ball and the output of an oscilloscope and the ball studied together, then the output will bounce and decay with the ball's motion, and its magnitude is proportional to the bounce of the ball at any time.

The input for the system model in the computer is usually derived from a **function generator**, a device which can provide inputs such as sine, square or triangular waves, continuously increasing or decreasing quantities (ramp functions) or sudden increases and decreases (step functions), trains of pulses and many others. Inputs derived from the environment of the real system can also be utilized. The reaction of the suspension system of a car to road surface variations can be studied by feeding into the computer model of the system a tape recording of the undulations of a representative road surface.

The output may be displayed on an oscilloscope as mentioned, and observed or photographed, or it may be recorded directly on tape or paper chart recorders. A major advantage of analog computers is that the solution need not only be presented at the rate at which it naturally occurs in real time, as in the ball example, but may be condensed in the time scale for rapidity and economy, or expanded for detailed study of a transient phenomenon. A further advantage is that following any alteration of the constants of the system the changed response appears almost at once and therefore the effect of a wide range of variation of constants can be quickly seen.

By comparison the digital computer deals directly with numbers and is essentially an arithmetic machine for the solution of problems which can be resolved into sequences of numerical operations. It can only solve differential equations by approximate step by step methods. By making these steps as small as one wishes and using many places of decimals these solutions may, in fact, be more accurate than those of an analog machine but lack the continuous nature of the other's solution.

As an example of a physiological problem to which the method of analysis might be applied, let us take only one simple stage of the complex control system which regulates the temperature of the human body. Heat is produced by metabolic processes, or gained by ingesting food or fluid at temperatures above that of the body. In addition, industrial workers may be exposed for intervals of time to external temperatures higher than that of the skin; under such circumstances they may gain heat from their surroundings. On the other hand, heat loss results from sweating, from conduction, convection and radiation of heat from the body to cooler surroundings, from respiration as the inspired air is warmed by the body before it is expired, and in urine and faeces. A few of these processes are immediately susceptible to mathematical analysis; for example the heat loss in the urine is (mass of urine) × (specific heat of urine) × (body temperature). But the complex gain or loss of heat by someone working under conditions where there is no external control of tem-

perature or humidity cannot be written in any simple mathematical form. At a physiological level this process is extremely complicated and is discussed on p. 43.3.

Newton's law of cooling can be used as a starting point in the modelling process. This states that the rate of transfer of heat between two compartments is proportional to the temperature difference between the two compartments. This can be expressed mathematically by the equation:

$$\frac{dQ}{dt} = -k_1(T_1 - T_2)$$

where dQ/dt is the rate of heat flow to or from the compartment of temperature T_1, T_2 is the temperature of the second compartment and k_1 is the constant of heat transfer between the two compartments. Thus if $T_1 > T_2$, dQ/dt will be negative and indicate a loss of heat from the compartment of temperature T_1. This equation can be related to the physiological temperature regulation system by making the two compartments the body core and skin.

Let $\quad T_1 = T_c = $ body core temperature
and $\quad T_2 = T_s = $ skin temperature

$$\therefore \quad \frac{dQ}{dt} = -k_1 (T_c - T_s)$$

k_1, the heat transfer constant, can now be considered to be a variable which changes with the core to skin blood flow. To simplify the model the only internal heat source will be considered to be the heat of metabolism. Let this heat source produce heat at a rate M in the same units as dQ/dt. The heat lost or gained by the body core will now be

$$M + \frac{dQ}{dt}$$

Thus $M - k_1 (T_c - T_s) = $ rate of heat loss or gain from body core. But the rate of heat loss or gain = mass × specific heat × rate of change of temperature. Therefore if m represents the body core mass and S its specific heat

$$M - k_1 (T_c - T_s) = mS\frac{dT_c}{dt} = k_2 \frac{dT_c}{dt}$$

assuming that M and S are constant. The equation

$$M - k_1 (T_c - T_s) = k_2 \frac{dT_c}{dt}$$

is known as a first order differential equation and gives a dynamic mathematical relationship of the variables in the system. To maintain the core temperature at a desired value when metabolic heat input and skin temperature could be changing, the factor that can be varied in this simple model is the thermal conductivity between core and skin. As mentioned earlier this can be considered as a variation in the core to skin blood flow. The control system will therefore monitor core temperature and compare this with a reference level. Physiologically this process is achieved by the hypothalamus. If the core temperature rises above this reference level the blood flow increases (k_1 increases) and vice versa. A diagram of this system is as shown in fig. 2.3. Taking the above equation and integrating both sides with respect to time

$$\int_0^T [M - k_1 (T_c - T_s)]dt = \int_0^T \left[k_2 \frac{dT_c}{dt} \right] dt$$

$$\therefore \quad \int_0^T [M - k_1 (T_c - T_s)]dt = k_2 T_c$$

at time t.

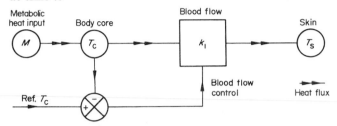

Fig. 2.3. Basic body core temperature control system.

This form of the equation can now be modelled by an analog computer as shown in fig. 2.4. This is known as

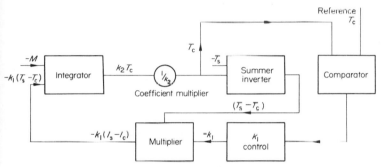

Fig. 2.4. Diagrammatic representation of the analog computer simulation of the simple temperature control model.

a closed loop simulation, since the value T_c that is being computed forms one of the inputs in its own computation. With this simple analog model the variables T_s and M can be changed and hence the reaction of the model compared to the real system response in similar circumstances. It can also be extended by placing constraints on the blood flow factor k_1 and the metabolic heat rate M, as in the human system. The change of skin temperature

due to the effects of clothing, sweating and radiation can be related to the ambient temperature and modelled in a similar way. This new model can be added to the simple model described and a more comprehensive model produced.

The approach described above is valid as a first approximation to the real system, although it is necessarily a very simple approach. The reader is referred to the bibliography to obtain a more detailed knowledge of more complex approaches to the same system.

Although for at least 30 years the fundamental anatomical pathways and physiological control regions have been known, it has always been difficult to define such central processes in a quantitative way. It is now appreciated that few biological problems can be stated even approximately by linear differential equations. Obviously this introduces immense difficulties in tackling physiological problems mathematically. Because of this the introduction of computers to the world of medicine has been of great importance. They can model complex systems and perform mathematical computations with speed and accuracy. Rapid feedback of information may lead to a research programme being moved quickly, in weeks rather than years, into its most productive channel. Computers already play a big part in the planning of many aspects of Health Services (vol. 3, chap. 67) and are beginning to be used in prediction of the outcome of treatments and in diagnosis (vol. 3, chap. 60).

FURTHER READING

FENDER D.H. (1964) Control Mechanisms of the Eye. *Scientific American* **211**, July, 24–33.

MILHORN H.T. (1966) *The Application of Control Theory to Physiological Systems*. Philadelphia: Saunders.

MILSUM J.H. (1966) *Biological Control Systems Analysis*. New York: McGraw-Hill.

WHITBY L.G. & LUTZ W. (1971) *Principles and Practice of Medical Computing*. Edinburgh: Churchill Livingstone.

Chapter 3
Biological variation and its measurement

Statistical techniques are used in every branch of medicine. As all may use the same techniques, illustrative examples of their application may be drawn from any branch of preclinical or clinical study. Perhaps the most frequent use of statistical methods is made by pharmacologists and by workers in social science and public health. For this reason some of the examples given in this chapter are taken, not from anatomy, physiology or biochemistry, but from subjects which the student will encounter in later studies.

It is not possible to provide, in the space of a single chapter, more than a very short account of actual methods. The aim is to provide enough to lead to some understanding of the potential and the limitations of statistical techniques. Those who find it necessary to apply the techniques should consult a statistician before starting their experiments, since he may give invaluable advice not only on the ultimate calculation but, prospectively, on the design of the experiments themselves.

Errors of measurement

Scientific work depends upon measurement, and all measurements are subject to error. Some of the sources of error are common to all sciences. There is the error associated with measuring instruments. Thus if we measure length with a good ruler graduated in millimetres we would expect to get a figure correct at least to the nearest millimetre, i.e. our measurement has an error of ± 0.5 mm. If, on the other hand, we measure length with a micrometer gauge the error may be reduced to ± 0.005 mm; however accurate our instruments, there is still a finite error. This is often overlooked since people who use complicated measuring instruments may be unaware of the error associated with the apparently precise readings on the dials of the machine. There is also the error associated with the operator. This may result from boredom or fatigue; for example it arises in those who have to watch a panel of instruments for long periods such as radar operators and also in people who use calculating machines, who make a predictable number of mistakes in entering figures. Errors may also arise from conscious or unconscious bias in that one individual may consistently overestimate and another consistently underestimate the end point of a titration. All of these sources of error arise in chemistry and physics as well as in biology.

Biological variation

In biology there is a further source of uncertainty which is so large that it overshadows all errors. This is called **biological variation** and stems from the fact that no two men or muscle cells or amoebae or bacteria or virus particles can be regarded as identical. The more complex the biological individual, the more variable the population is likely to be. This variability between individuals means that measurements made on any **sample** of individuals do not necessarily reflect the measurements of any other sample drawn from the same **population.** This is perfectly obvious but is often forgotten. If we draw a sample of one nail from a bag of nails bought from the ironmonger, measure it with a ruler and find that it is 2·5 cm long, it is a fair inference that all the other nails have the same length. Of course, if a micrometer gauge is used the nails will be found to vary in size a little; on the other hand, if we measure one medical student and find that his height is 178 cm it is not a fair inference, even if only a ruler is used, that all other medical students will appear to be of the same height. Strictly speaking, in statistics the words 'population' and 'sample' refer to values rather than to objects or people. Thus if height is being considered, the population or sample is a collection of values in cm or feet and inches. Fortunately, it is usually clear when the words are being used in their strict sense.

Purposes of measurement

Measurements are made for two main reasons. The first is to make inferences about the population of things in which we are interested. For example, what is the mean blood pressure of healthy men of 40? We could measure the blood pressure of one such man and infer that this value represents the value for the population. Common sense warns us that our inference might well be wrong. In other words our **estimate** of the true value in the population is subject to error. Common sense also tells us that if we want to decrease the error and have a better chance of drawing the right inference, the size of the sample should be increased. The second reason for making measurements is to discover whether the individual on whom we made the measurement is normal or abnormal. This presupposes that the normal measurements are already known. In this case the individual is compared with previously acquired knowledge and the appropriate inferences drawn. Such inferences may be right or wrong; all that can be done is to assess the **probability** of the inference being right. Much of statistics is concerned with such assessments.

We must also define the conditions of measurement very precisely. If we measure the blood pressures of a sample of healthy 40-year-old men when they are recumbent, any inference drawn can apply only to a population of healthy recumbent 40-year-old men. To make any inference about the same men when they are running in a marathon is obviously fallacious. Thus inferences must be limited to conditions identical to those under which sample measurements are made.

Measurements of central tendency

The most usual question asked about measurements is of the form: 'What is the blood pressure of a healthy 40-year-old man?' Since we know that individuals vary the only answer available is some sort of **average value** or, in other words, a measurement of the **central tendency** of all the values in the population. The most usual of these measurements is the **arithmetic mean**, usually called the **mean**. Other measurements such as the most commonly occurring value, the **mode**, or the middle value that separates the sample into two equal parts, the **median**, may be used. One other measure of central tendency is of especial importance in medical biology; for reasons, some of which are discussed later, it is often convenient to use the average of the logarithms of the measurements. This is the **logarithmic mean.**

In a sample of n values of a measurement y, we can express the mean, usually written as $\bar{y}$, algebraically as follows:

$$\bar{y} = \frac{\sum y}{n} \tag{1}$$

where $\sum y$ signifies the sum of all the values of y.

Measurements of scatter

Just as individual values in a sample show a central tendency, they also show a tendency to dispersal or scatter, depending on the degree of variability. Once again this tendency can be expressed in various ways. The simplest is to state the lowest and highest individual values, i.e. the **range** of the measurements. Another way is to measure the difference between each individual value and the mean value; this difference is usually called the **deviation** from the mean. However, the average value of the deviation is of no use as a measure of scatter because it always has the same value, i.e. zero. In fact this is another way of defining the mean. Algebraically this can be expressed as follows:

$$\sum (y - \bar{y}) = \sum y - \sum \bar{y}$$
$$= \sum y - n.\bar{y}$$
$$= \sum y - n.\frac{\sum y}{n}$$
$$= \sum y - \sum y$$
$$= 0$$

Since the sum of the deviations is always zero, then the mean deviation must also be zero.

This difficulty can be avoided in two ways. Firstly we can calculate the sum of the deviations ignoring the sign, and dividing this sum by n gives a **mean deviation**.

$$\text{Mean deviation} = \frac{\sum |(y - \bar{y})|}{n}$$

Alternatively the sign can be eliminated by squaring each individual deviation, thus making all the values positive. The sum of these values is called the **sum of squares**. The **mean square deviation** can then be reduced to the original scale by extracting its square root. This value, which, for reasons discussed below, has other major advantages, is the most commonly used measure of scatter and is called the **standard deviation** (s). It is calculated algebraically:

$$s = \sqrt{\frac{\sum (y - \bar{y})^2}{n - 1}} \tag{2}$$

For large samples, i.e. when n is big, the expression reduces to

$$s = \sqrt{\frac{\sum (y - \bar{y})^2}{n}} \tag{3}$$

With large samples the difference in the estimate of s using equations 2 and 3 is negligible, but with small samples it may be considerable. Thus nothing is lost by using equation 2 on all occasions.

CALCULATION OF SUM OF SQUARES

When using a desk machine one can calculate $\sum (y - \bar{y})^2$ without doing any tedious subtraction from the following equation:

$$\sum (y - \bar{y})^2 = \sum y^2 - \frac{(\sum y)^2}{n} \tag{4}$$

This equation is derived as follows:

$$\sum (y - \bar{y})^2 = \sum y^2 - 2 \sum y . \bar{y} + \sum \bar{y}^2$$

$$= \sum y^2 - 2 \sum y . \frac{\sum y}{n} + n . \bar{y}^2$$

$$= \sum y^2 - 2 \frac{(\sum y)^2}{n} + n . \frac{(\sum y)^2}{n^2}$$

$$= \sum y^2 - 2 \frac{(\sum y)^2}{n} + \frac{(\sum y)^2}{n}$$

$$= \sum y^2 - \frac{(\sum y)^2}{n}$$

The square of the standard deviation, s^2, is referred to as the **variance** (V).

DISTRIBUTIONS

If we measure the systolic blood pressure of 100 healthy 40-year-old men a series of values is obtained from which the measurements of central tendency and of scatter may be calculated (table 3.1a). The instrumental and operator

TABLE 3.1a. Systolic blood pressures (mmHg) measured on 100 healthy 40-year-old men

112	134	164	104	142	121	150	133	134	157
140	119	126	151	135	110	108	112	147	127
95	124	128	117	128	117	128	125	127	124
127	130	131	125	117	129	127	136	132	128
136	125	118	130	114	114	140	130	91	126
123	98	130	136	129	127	133	123	126	120
132	127	138	130	123	126	111	154	128	130
134	126	127	116	122	101	132	136	129	145
137	152	134	133	124	156	116	113	160	131
123	119	133	121	132	126	124	115	111	132

Mean	= 127·48	($\sum y/n$)
Median	= 127·5	(50 of the 100 men had blood pressures less than or equal to this value)
Mode	= 127	(Commonest value, occurring seven times)
Range	= 91–164	
Mid-range	=½(91 + 164)=127·5	
Mean deviation	= 9	
Standard deviation	= 13	*Calculations*

$\sum y$	= 12 748
$\sum y^2$	= 1 641 874
$(\sum y)^2/n$	= 1 625 115
$\sum (y - \bar{y})^2$	= 16 759
V	= 169
s	= 13
$\bar{y}$	= 127·48

errors are so small in relation to the biological variation that they do not need to be considered. The first thing to note is that the mean, median and mode, which are defined in the table, all lie close to the mid-range value. Table 3.1b gives the marks obtained in an examination by 100 medical students. These have been adjusted so that

the mean and standard deviations are the same as those for the blood pressure values. In this case, however, the

TABLE 3.1b. Marks obtained in class examination by 100 medical students (maximum mark = 242)

124	126	117	126	121	117	185	120	126	124
139	118	125	124	121	123	123	123	121	126
122	122	123	119	122	120	127	128	120	124
134	130	117	123	123	122	119	123	125	122
122	121	124	127	160	123	126	142	128	123
119	122	158	122	127	122	124	127	154	136
130	146	127	116	125	166	124	118	124	125
121	169	120	119	175	128	121	125	122	125
121	118	130	124	126	124	128	125	126	120
127	124	117	172	127	119	125	126	123	120

Mean	= 127·48	*Calculations*
Median	= 124	$\sum y$ = 12 748
Mode	= 124	$\sum y^2$ = 1 641 922
Range	= 116–185	$(\sum y)^2/n$ = 1 625 115
Mid-range	= 150·5	$\sum (y - \bar{y})^2$ = 16 807
Mean deviation	= 7·8	V = 169
Standard deviation	= 13	s = 13
		$\bar{y}$ = 127·48

mean and the median differ by more and are very different from the mid-range value. How can the differences between the two series of values be shown? One obvious way is to draw a diagram or graph to illustrate the **distribution** of the values. The simplest form of diagram is a **histogram**. The figures are arranged in groups and the **frequency** of the occurrence of values in each group is plotted against the range of that group, as shown in fig.

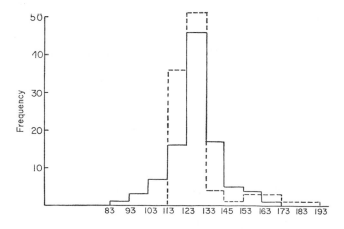

FIG. 3.1. Histograms of distributions in tables 3.1a & b. Systolic blood pressures (mmHg), solid line; examination marks, broken line.

3.1. It is clear that, despite the fact that both distributions have the same mean and standard deviation, they are very different in shape. In the case of the values for blood pressure the distribution is roughly symmetrical about the mean. If the samples are made bigger and the range of each group made narrower, a smoother set of narrower blocks is obtained; ultimately, with an infinite sample and

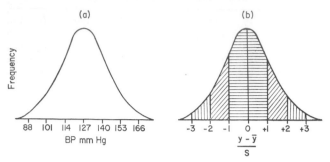

FIG. 3.2. Frequency distribution of population of systolic blood pressure (BP) of healthy 40-year-old men. Abscissa, (a) BP in mmHg; (b) BP in units of standard deviation (*s*) from mean.

an infinitely small range for each group, a curve called the **frequency distribution curve** may be drawn (fig. 3.2). In many biological measurements, the shape of this curve approximates closely to the so-called **normal distribution** or **Gaussian distribution** after the man who first described it mathematically. On the other hand the distribution of examination marks (fig. 3.1) is not normal; it is asymmetric and is said to be **skew.**

These are essentially empiric findings although various theoretical arguments have been advanced to account for them. The equation for the normal distribution is, of course, known and contains only two variables, the mean and the standard deviation. One of the reasons for using them as common descriptions of central tendency and of scatter is their appearance in the equation which has provided the basis of many statistical tests.

It is tacitly assumed, whenever statistical methods based on the normal distribution are used, that the measurements being examined have been drawn from a normal distribution of such measurements. Certain tests of the validity of this assumption are available, but usually they are not carried out. Although many statistical tests based on the normal distribution work quite well when applied to distributions which are not normal, a growing point in statistics is the development and application of methods which do not depend on the assumption of normality. These are called 'non-parametric', and they are discussed in the first two references given at the end of the chapter.

RELATIONSHIP OF THE NORMAL DISTRIBUTION TO THE MEAN AND THE STANDARD DEVIATION
Fig. 3.2a shows the normal frequency distribution curve; this is the distribution which is being assumed for the whole population of individuals from which a sample is drawn. The mode and the median both coincide with the mean of the distribution, i.e. the distribution is symmetrical about the mean. This is characteristic of the normal distribution and is clearly not true for skew distributions. The abscissa in fig. 3.2a is the actual value of the blood pressure. Now that the mean and the standard deviation are known we can redraw the distribution using for the abscissa a scale of standard deviations on either side of the mean (fig. 3.2b). If the area under the curve is now taken as unity, we can calculate, on the basis of the equation for the normal distribution curve, the proportion of the area under the curve that lies within the range ± 1 standard deviation or ± 2 standard deviations from the mean and so on for any number of standard deviations we wish to choose. Tables of these integrals are published and can be found in standard works.

In fig. 3.2b the areas of the normal curve enclosed are roughly:

mean ± 1 standard deviation
$\quad = 66$ per cent (horizontal shading)
mean ± 2 standard deviations
$\quad = 95$ per cent (horizontal plus diagonal shading)
mean ± 3 standard deviations
$\quad = 99$ per cent (horizontal, diagonal and vertical shading).

The value of this exercise should now be obvious. If the mean and the standard deviation of the population are known, then, for a sample of one individual, there is only one chance in a hundred that, if he is really a member of the population, his value will deviate from the mean by more than three times the standard deviation. Thus if a 40-year-old man has a blood pressure of 170 mmHg, which lies more than three times the standard deviation away from the mean, we would be tempted to assume that he is not a member of the population of healthy 40-year-old men; i.e. his blood pressure is abnormal. Even so this assumption would be wrong once in every hundred times that it was made and the possibility of an error of this type is unavoidable although we can set any **chance** we like. The levels of probability of being wrong that are usually chosen are 1 in 20 or 1 in 100.

While all this seems plain sailing, we must remember two points.

(1) The mean and standard deviation of a population are seldom known. We usually are obliged to estimate them from previous samples and these estimates may be wrong.

(2) If too high a standard is set for excluding a value from the population, then values which really are not part of the population will appear to belong to it. Thus if we say that a blood pressure is only abnormal or unhealthy if it is more than 166 mmHg, we may accept many blood pressure values of less than 166 mmHg as healthy when they are not. Failure to spot an abnormality may be as

dangerous as to regard a normal individual as abnormal. For these reasons it is difficult to lay down the normal ranges for any measurement with any real precision.

Design of experiments

One of the simplest forms of experimental design consists of choosing two comparable samples of individuals from the same population and then applying to one of the two samples some form of treatment. Treatment is used here to mean any change imposed upon the sample and does not necessarily mean a form of medical treatment. This sounds easy but is actually, in many circumstances, very difficult. The main problems are to ensure, firstly that the two samples are comparable and, secondly, that all the individuals in both samples are members of the same population throughout the experiment with the single exception of the treatment applied to the one sample.

It may suffice to give two examples. The result of a laboratory experiment on two samples of ten mice could be invalidated if, from a box of twenty mice, ten are picked out by hand and put in another box. By this technique one would tend to catch the least active mice in making the transfer, so that the two groups would not be comparable in this respect. One could improve on this by catching and putting the mice successively into two boxes, but it is better to allocate them in a truly **random fashion**. This can be accomplished by identifying each animal, e.g. with a colour code, numbering each and allocating each to one or other sample by using a table of random numbers. This is a time-consuming exercise but is worth the trouble since any individual mouse has the same chance of ending up in the first sample as in the second. This technique of **random sampling** is adequate if all the mice in the original box are to be regarded as members of the same population. If they are all males then an imbalance of the sexes in the two samples cannot arise; if they are of mixed sex then random sampling may give samples that are not comparable in that one sample may have a preponderance of one sex.

The second example is the selection of human subjects to form two comparable samples. Let us consider the problem of finding out if a particular drug is effective in preventing seasickness. If the subjects are allocated to the two samples completely at random, then imbalances may easily arise in such factors as sex, age, previous experience of sea voyages and so on. In these circumstances they can be regarded as members of the same population only in that they are all exposed to the same stress but not in respect of these other features. The usual answer to this problem is to impose some restraints upon the random sampling process. Thus men and women might be dealt with as separate groups allocating the members of each group at random to the two

samples. The problem is that the more restraints that are imposed, the less certain is it that two unbiased samples have been obtained, even if the two samples are balanced in respect of the restraints imposed. We are often obliged to compromise between these two competing features in designing experiments.

The two samples are then kept under identical conditions throughout the experiment, save that the treatment is given to one of the samples. This, too, raises problems. If a drug is given to one sample, and not to the other, we not only apply the action of the drug, we also apply a psychological stimulus so that the individuals may feel they are being looked after and cared for and may respond to this stimulus even if the drug is inactive. This is an extremely potent and well-recognized stimulus. Giving inert tablets of lactose (an inert medicine is usually called a placebo) causes improvement in the subjective feelings or symptoms in a large proportion of patients. Such people are called **placebo reactors**. Subjective effects may also appear to improve physical performance. The history of athletic training is full of accounts of special diets, vitamins, tonics and nowadays more dangerous drugs recommended by trainers and coaches. These are nearly always based on the subjective reports of athletes and not on their records.

It is therefore necessary to give the untreated sample the same apparent treatment as the treated sample, thus limiting the treatment to the actual action of the drug or other treatment.

Furthermore, the experimenter or the doctor, who is assessing the results of the experiment, is often swayed or biased in his judgement if he knows which subjects or patients have been treated. This unconscious bias becomes an operator error which may invalidate the experiments when the final assessment is made. Nowadays experiments are often designed to ensure that the operator does not know which individuals are in the treated group. This situation, where neither the individuals (the patients) nor the operator (the doctor) knows which individual is in which sample, is called a **double-blind trial.** Where patients are severely ill there may be ethical objections to such a design; but if it is not used, great care must be exercised in interpreting the results. The design of clinical trials is discussed in vol. 3, p. 61.16.

Analysis of results

When a properly designed experiment is completed, the measurement, whatever it may be, is made on all the individuals in both samples. How can the results be assessed? The fundamental basis of examining the data is called the **null hypothesis**; this is an hypothesis that the treatment applied to the one sample has had no effect. In this case both samples may be regarded as random samples of individuals from the same normally distributed population. The true values of the mean and the standard deviation of this population are unknown but estimates of these can be made from data on one or both samples. On the basis of these estimates the probability that both samples are drawn from the same population may be calculated. This calculation was developed by Gosset who wrote under the pseudonym of *Student*. He worked for the brewing firm of Guinness and was one of the pioneers of statistical theory. The test depends upon the distribution of the statistic *t*. When the sample size is infinitely large, then, for any given value of the integral of the normal distribution, *t* is the corresponding value of the abscissa expressed in terms of the standard deviation. Thus on p. 3.4 we made the approximate statement that 95 per cent of all values lay 'within the range of the mean ±2 standard deviations'. The accurate statement would be: 'within the range of the mean ±1·96 standard deviations', 1·96 being the value of *t* corresponding to a probability or frequency of 0·95 when the sample size is infinite or equals the population. Values for *t* have been calculated and tabulated for various sample sizes and for various probabilities.

Standard error of the mean

Before continuing with the main problem of comparing treated and untreated samples, it is necessary to know how representative they are. How close for example is the mean of a sample to that of its parent population? The answer is that it depends on the size of the sample and the standard deviation. We would certainly expect that bigger samples stood a better chance of closer estimates. On the other hand since larger standard deviations denote more variable populations we should expect smaller values to go together with better estimates for a given size of sample. This is easy to appreciate by going to the limit of a standard deviation of zero. For such a population, since all the members are identical, even a sample of one would give a mean without error.

The most useful way we can consider the precision of our sample mean in quantitative terms is to imagine drawing an infinite number of samples of *n* individuals from the population. Provided that this does not differ too greatly from a normal distribution it turns out that our sample means will themselves be normally distributed about the true value for the population. The standard deviation of these means is known as the **standard error of the mean**

$$s_{\bar{y}} = \frac{s}{\sqrt{n}} \qquad (5)$$

where *s* is the standard deviation of the population. As the sample gets bigger the standard error of the mean gets smaller. In the case where a population is of infinite size, then as the sample size approaches infinity, the standard error of the mean approaches zero; in other

words the mean is known without error. We are now in a position to calculate three statistics from the information obtained by drawing a single sample. Thus:

$$\text{Mean} \quad \bar{y} = \frac{\sum y}{n} \qquad (1)$$

$$\text{Standard deviation} \quad s = \sqrt{\frac{\sum (y - \bar{y})^2}{n - 1}} \qquad (2)$$

$$\text{Standard error of the mean} \quad s_{\bar{y}} = \frac{s}{\sqrt{n}} \qquad (5)$$

or

$$s_{\bar{y}} = \sqrt{\frac{\sum (y - \bar{y})^2}{n(n - 1)}} \qquad (5a)$$

Difference between two means

We can now return to the problem that faced *Student* in designing his *t* test to compare the means of two different samples. It is possible to measure the probability that any one sample mean deviates from the true mean by any given number of standard errors of that mean, but the true mean and the true standard error of the mean are unknown. We can only compare the estimates of the mean derived from two samples and use as the standard error an estimate based on the standard errors calculated for each sample. *Student* thus gave the following equation for calculating *t* from such data:

$$t = \frac{\bar{y}_1 - \bar{y}_2}{s_{(\bar{y}_1 - \bar{y}_2)}} \qquad (6)$$

where $s_{(\bar{y}_1 - \bar{y}_2)}$ is the standard error of the difference between the two means (see below). Having calculated the value of *t*, the probability that, if the two samples had been drawn from the same population, this value would be reached or exceeded, can be obtained from a table of *t*, entering the table for the value of $n = n_1 + n_2 - 2$. If the value found for the probability is less than 0.05 then there is less than one chance in twenty that the samples are drawn from the same population, or less than one chance in twenty that the treatment applied to one sample has had no effect.

The reason why the table of *t* is entered for the value corresponding to $n = n_1 + n_2 - 2$ is that this is the number of **degrees of freedom** associated with the comparison being made. The concept of degrees of freedom is used widely in statistics and is at first difficult to follow. If, however, we were told that the mean height of a sample of sixteen medical students was 170 cm we could create our own hypothetical series of sixteen individual heights with freedom to choose our own values for the first fifteen students, but the sixteenth value would be fixed for us since the mean was given. We can be said to have only fifteen degrees of freedom in this exercise. Thus if we assigned a hypothetical height of 180 cm to fifteen students our last student must be only 20 cm tall. This follows from the fact that:

$$\bar{y} = \frac{\sum y}{n}$$

$$\therefore 170 = \frac{\sum y}{16}$$

$$\therefore \sum y = 16 \times 170$$

$$= 2720 \text{ cm}$$

and

$$\sum y \text{ for 15 students} = 15 \times 180$$

$$= 2700 \text{ cm}$$

Thus, once we have calculated the mean of a sample of n values, only $(n-1)$ degrees of freedom are left; and in comparing two means the sum of the degrees of freedom associated with each, i.e. $(n_1 - 1)$ and $(n_2 - 1)$ is $n_1 + n_2 - 2$.

The **standard error of the difference between two means** may be calculated in the following way. For any two independent measurements, the variance of their difference (or sum) is equal to the sum of their variances. In our case, the samples are supposed to be drawn randomly so that the sample means should be independent.

Thus:

$$V(\bar{y}_1 - \bar{y}_2) = V(\bar{y}_1) + V(\bar{y}_2)$$

$$= s_{\bar{y}_1}^2 + s_{\bar{y}_2}^2$$

Since the null hypothesis requires that both samples are drawn from the same population, the variance is calculated from both samples combined together. First we calculate the population variance $V(y)$. The best estimate can be shown to be:

$$V(y) = \frac{\sum (y_1 - \bar{y}_1)^2 + \sum (y_2 - \bar{y}_2)^2}{n_1 + n_2 - 2}$$

Hence

$$V(\bar{y}_1) = \frac{V(y)}{n_1}$$

$$V(\bar{y}_2) = \frac{V(y)}{n_2}$$

so that, summing the variances of the two means

$$V(\bar{y}_1 - \bar{y}_2) = \frac{V(y)}{n_1} + \frac{V(y)}{n_2}$$

$$= \frac{n_1 + n_2}{n_1 n_2} \cdot V(y)$$

Where $n_1 = n_2 = n$, this becomes

$$\frac{2n}{n^2} V(y) = \frac{2V(y)}{n}$$

Analysis of variance

The t test is a method of comparing two samples. It cannot be used for more than two samples without making separate analyses for each pair of samples. R.A. Fisher developed a different technique for coping with the problem of examining the differences between a number of samples, and it is instructive to examine this technique in relation to the simple case of two samples at this stage.

Fisher's technique consists of examining not the differences between means but the ratio between variances. The null hypothesis is that the samples are drawn from the same normal population; the combined samples give an estimate of both the population mean and its variance. Another estimate of the population variance is given by the scatter of the sample means. The discrepancy between the two estimates may be taken as a test of the likeliness of the samples having been drawn from populations with the same mean. The arithmetic is done on 'sums of squares', short for the sum of squares of deviations from the mean, which can be partitioned into additive components. Let us consider the heights of two samples of sixteen medical students (table 3.2a). On the basis that all the individuals in both samples are members of the same population we can calculate an overall mean for the thirty-two values and an overall sum of squares:

$$\bar{\bar{y}} = \frac{\sum y_1 + \sum y_2}{n_1 + n_2} = \frac{\sum y}{32}$$

$$SS = \sum (y - \bar{\bar{y}})^2$$

There are thirty-one degrees of freedom associated with the overall sum of squares. When we consider each sample separately we get:

$$\bar{y}_1 = \frac{\sum y_1}{n_1} = \frac{\sum y_1}{16}$$

and

$$SS_1 = \sum (y_1 - \bar{y}_1)^2$$

Similarly,

$$SS_2 = \sum (y_2 - \bar{y}_2)^2$$

There are $(n_1 - 1)$ and $(n_2 - 1)$ degrees of freedom associated with the sample sum of squares i.e. in this case thirty. We thus have a component associated with the individual samples with thirty degrees of freedom, and a total associated with thirty-one degrees of freedom. The remaining degree of freedom is associated with the scatter of the two sample means about the overall mean. Thus we can write:

$$SS \text{ between samples} = \sum (\bar{y} - \bar{\bar{y}})^2$$

The separate sums of squares can be shown to be additive in the following way:

$$\sum (y - \bar{\bar{y}})^2 = \sum (y_1 - \bar{y}_1)^2 \\ + \sum (y_2 - \bar{y}_2)^2 + \sum n.(\bar{y} - \bar{\bar{y}})^2 \quad (7)$$

We can regard the last term as a source of variation 'between samples'. Since the mean of each sample represents n values its squared deviation is multiplied by n to bring it into line with the other sources of variation which are to be regarded as 'within samples'.

Fisher went on to compare the variances derived from the separate components of the overall sum of squares. This gave rise to the descriptive term **analysis of variance**. If the variance 'between samples' is large compared to the variance 'within samples', as in the example (table 3.2b), then it is improbable that the samples have been drawn from the same population, even though the values for the combined data on all thirty-two students look like a homogeneous normal population. The test is based on a statistic called the **variance ratio**, usually written F, and the calculated probabilities of getting various values of F with different sample sizes. Tables of F are available just as are tables of t. The general form of expressing an analysis of variance of the kind of data we have been describing is in table 3.3. Since within any one sample the individuals have been treated in exactly the same way, the within samples variance depends only on the essential biological variation between individuals. We can regard

TABLE 3.2a. Heights of thirty-two medical students. The heights are arranged as two samples from sixteen students. Each individual height in the table is represented by a dot.

Height in cm	All 32 students	Sample 1	Sample 2
182	·	·	
179	···	···	
176	····	····	
173	·····	····	·
170	······	···	···
167	·····	·	····
164	····		····
161	···		···
158	·		·

TABLE 3.2b. Analysis of variance.

Source of variation	Sum of squares	Degrees of freedom (d.f.)	V	F
Between samples	648	1	648	39
Within samples	504	30	16·8	—
Total	1152	31		

this inescapable minimum variation as basic to any experimental situation. Thus the within samples variance is often called the **error variance** and is used to calculate the significance of the other estimates of variance, in this case the variance between samples. The simple example given here is really a form of the t test. The technique is, however, very much more versatile as we shall see.

PAIRED DATA

Sometimes in experiments to compare two treatments, the variability of the individuals within the samples is so great that it may require very large samples to show up a difference. In such cases it may be possible to improve the design if the same samples of individuals can be used on two occasions, testing the control and the treatment on each individual. Thus we might be interested to discover whether a drug made patients sleep longer at night. For example, if the drug is given to ten patients and a placebo to another ten we might get results as shown in table 3.4a. The mean sleeping time for the treated individuals is 7.2 hr as compared with 6·7 hr for the controls. A t test between the means gives a value of only 0·75 which would be expected to occur by chance in almost half of all the cases where the two samples had been drawn from the same population. In other words there is no evidence that the drug has had any effect. In fact, however, the same ten individuals had been given the drug on one occasion and the placebo on another occasion, giving the data in table 3.4b. The actual sleeping times are the same as in table 3.4a, but they are in pairs, each pair applying to a single

TABLE 3.3.

Source of variation	Sum of squares	d.f.	V		F
Between samples	$\sum n(\bar{y} - \bar{\bar{y}})^2$	1	(B)	$\dfrac{\sum n(\bar{y} - \bar{\bar{y}})^2}{1}$	B/E
Within samples	$\sum (y_1 - \bar{y}_1)^2 + \sum (y_2 - \bar{y}_2)^2$	30	(E)	$\dfrac{\sum (y_1 - \bar{y}_1)^2 + \sum (y_2 - \bar{y}_2)^2}{30}$	
Total	$\sum (y - \bar{\bar{y}})^2$	31			

TABLE 3.4a. Results of experiments to determine the activity of a drug believed to induce sleep. First experiment.

Hours of sleep	
Untreated patients y_1	Treated patients y_2
7·2	5·3
4·8	4·6
6·7	7·7
8·9	9·4
4·1	7·2
6·8	7·9
7·4	8·9
5·7	7·3
8·4	7·5
7·0	6·2

Calculations

$\sum y$ = 67   = 72
$\sum y^2$ = 468·84   = 538·34
$(\sum y)^2/n$ = 448·9   = 518·4
$\sum (y - \bar{y})^2$ = 19·94   = 19·94
V = 2·216
$V\bar{y}$ = 0·2216   = 0·2216
$V(\bar{y}_1 - \bar{y}_2)$ = 0·4432
$s(\bar{y}_1 - \bar{y}_2)$ = 0·666
$\bar{y}_1 - \bar{y}_2$ = 0·5
t = 0·75 (18 degrees of freedom)

TABLE 3.4b. Second experiment.

Patient number	Sleeping time		Difference in sleeping time $y = y_2 - y_1$
	Control night y_1	Treatment night y_2	
1	7·2	7·7	+0·5
2	4·8	6·2	+1·4
3	6·7	7·3	+0·6
4	8·9	8·9	0
5	4·1	4·6	+0·5
6	6·8	7·5	+0·7
7	7·4	7·9	+0·5
8	5·7	5·3	−0·4
9	8·4	9·4	+1·0
10	7·0	7·2	+0·2

Calculations

$\sum y$ = 5·0 V = 0·2511
$\sum y^2$ = 4·76 $V\bar{y}$ = 0·0251
$(\sum y)^2/n$ = 2·5 $s\bar{y}$ = 0·159
$\sum (y - \bar{y})^2$ = 2·26 t = 3·15 (9 degrees of freedom)

person. If we disregard the pairing, a *t* test would yield the identical result to that obtained from the data of table 3.4a. We can, however, now consider the difference in sleeping time for each individual. On the basis of the null hypothesis, i.e. that the treatment has no effect, we would expect the mean difference to be zero. Thus we

know the population mean in this case and we can test the difference of the observed mean from the hypothetical directly. Thus, in this case;

$$t = \frac{\bar{y} - 0}{s_y}$$

and from this calculation we obtain a value of $t = 3·15$ which would occur by chance less than once in a hundred times if the drug had no effect. This example shows clearly the importance of using paired data whenever possible.

A word of warning is, however, necessary at this point. If all ten subjects were given the placebo on one night and the drug on the following night we would have to pause before jumping to the conclusion that the drug was effective. It might well be that some factor other than the drug had caused the change; thus the hospital ward might have been noisy on the first night and quiet on the second. We can protect ourselves against such extraneous factors by giving half the subjects the drug on the first occasion, the other half receiving the placebo; and then, on the second occasion reversing the situation. This type of design is often called a **cross-over experiment**.

Relationship between two variables

So far we have discussed the analysis of data where only one measurement is made on each individual studied. Frequently in biological observations or experiments, we

TABLE 3.5. Weights and systolic blood pressures of a group of ten men.

Man number	x Weight kg	y Systolic blood pressure mmHg
1	110·0	160
2	93·0	123
3	75·0	98
4	105·5	138
5	71·5	110
6	125·0	147
7	97·0	139
8	88·5	121
9	84·0	151
10	76·5	130

Calculations

$$r = \frac{\sum (x - \bar{x})(y - \bar{y})}{\sqrt{\sum (x - \bar{x})^2 \sum (y - \bar{y})^2}} = \frac{\sum xy - n\bar{x}\bar{y}}{\sqrt{(\sum x^2 - n\bar{x}^2)(\sum y^2 - n\bar{y}^2)}}$$

$\sum x$ = 926 $\sum y$ = 1317
$\bar{x}$ = 92·6 $\bar{y}$ = 131·7
$\sum x^2$ = 88 391 $\sum y^2$ = 176 749
$n\bar{x}^2$ = 85 747·6 $n\bar{y}^2$ = 173 448·9
$\sum x^2 - n\bar{x}^2$ = 2643·4 $\sum y^2 - n\bar{y}^2$ = 3300·1

$\sum xy$ = 124 008·5
$\bar{x}\bar{y}$ = 12 195·42
r = 0·696

are interested in the relationship that may exist between two measurements. Thus we may want to know the relationship, if any, between the blood pressure and the weight of a series of men or animals. This involves us in the further statistical technique of **correlation**.

If we made the two measurements on a sample of ten men we might get the data shown in table 3.5. The simplest way of illustrating any possible relationship between the two sets of measurements is to plot a **scatter diagram** as shown in fig. 3.3. Although the points are

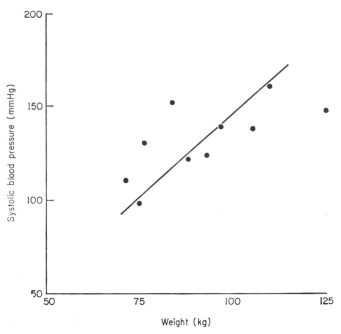

FIG. 3.3. Scatter diagram relating weight and systolic blood pressure of a group of men.

widely scattered a line can be drawn through the points indicating that as the weight increases so also does the blood pressure. When the scatter diagram shows this relationship the two measurements are said to be correlated. The **correlation coefficient** is a measure of this linear trend, and should not be used for relationships that follow patterns more complicated than a straight line. If the apparent relationship is obviously a curve there may, of course, be a linear relationship between some function of the data; e.g. the logarithm or square root of one measurement might be linearly related to the other measurement.

Correlation may be positive or negative. In the example in fig. 3.3 the blood pressure (BP) rises as the weight rises and the correlation is positive. If the BP fell as the weight rose the correlation would be negative. If there is a linear relation then it follows that, to some extent, the value of one measurement can be predicted if the other is known. If all the points lie on the line the prediction is without error; if there is no relationship we cannot predict at all. In the first instance the correlation co-

efficient is plus or minus one; in the second it is zero. Thus correlation coefficients must lie between plus and minus one.

Even when there is no relation between two sets of measurements, it is highly unlikely that a sample would give a correlation coefficient of exactly zero. A form of the *t* test is used to examine the significance of the sample value.

The coefficient, usually written as *r*, is calculated by the expression

$$r = \frac{\sum (x - \bar{x})\,(y - \bar{y})}{\sqrt{\sum (x - \bar{x})^2 \cdot \sum (y - \bar{y})^2}} \qquad (8)$$

With small samples, rather large numerical values of *r* (i.e. close to ± 1) are needed to provide convincing evidence for a relationship. For example, if we repeatedly took a sample of ten pairs of random numbers we should expect to obtain a value for *r* as high as 0·632 in one out of twenty samples.

If equation 8 is applied to the figures in table 3.4 we get *r* = +0·696 which is a value that would occur by chance, in the absence of any real correlation less than once in twenty times. We can therefore conclude that there is probably a real correlation. The value of *r* corresponding to various probabilities is provided in published tables for different values of *n*.

INTERPRETATION OF A CORRELATION

Even if a significant correlation between two variables is demonstrated, careful interpretation is necessary. It does not mean that a change in one variable causes a change in the other. Thus the fact that a correlation was established between the populations of storks in various provinces of Germany and the birth rates in these provinces did not mean that if more storks had been introduced the birth rate would inevitably have risen.

Secondly we must not extrapolate beyond the limits of the data. Thus if weight and blood pressure are shown to be correlated in men between the weights of 70 and 125 kg it does not follow that they are still correlated in lighter or heavier men.

REGRESSION

The correlation coefficient measures the degree to which two quantitites are associated where there is no special reason for regarding one of them as an independent variable. However, in experimental work one variable is usually fixed independently and changes that occur in the other variable which is dependent are observed. The amount of contraction of smooth muscle after various doses of a drug may be measured. Here we plot not a scatter diagram but a graph relating the contraction (the **response**) to the dose or the logarithm of the dose (log dose) of the drug given (fig. 3.4). There is usually a linear relationship with the log dose over a certain dose range; and this is a useful fact as will be seen below.

Any linear relation may be described by the equation:

$$y = a + bx \quad \text{(where } a \text{ and } b \text{ are constants)}$$

a being the intercept on the y axis and b the slope. The 'best' straight line is calculated by the method of least squares. This chooses the line in such a way as to minimize the sum of the squares of the deviations from it of the observed values of the response. The formulae for calculating b, usually referred to as the **regression coefficient**, and a are:

$$b = \frac{\sum (x - \bar{x})(y - \bar{y})}{\sum (x - \bar{x})^2}$$

$$a = \bar{y} - b\bar{x}$$

where $\bar{x}$ and $\bar{y}$ are the means of the values of x and y. In the case where y is the response and x the log dose, b is the slope of the log **dose response line**.

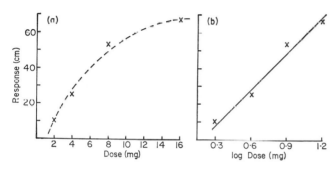

FIG. 3.4. Graphs relating (a) dose and (b) log dose of a drug to response, e.g. cm of contraction of smooth muscles.

USE OF DOSE RESPONSE LINES

The main use of dose response lines is in bioassay, where the strength of one sample of an active biological preparation, hormone or drug is measured in terms of the strength of another. Extracts of biological material are not pure chemicals and no two preparations can be relied on to be of equal strength. Hence bioassay is the normal method of controlling the strength of, for example, insulin preparations and most vaccines and antitoxins. Thus, to control the dose in experimental work or to protect the patient from fluctuations in strength when used clinically, each preparation must be tested against a standard preparation prepared and held for this purpose, and containing a definite number of units of activity per unit weight. This subject constitutes an important part of pharmacology and is discussed more fully in vol. 2, p. 3.3, but certain features are worthy of comment here.

Relative potency

If two preparations are compared by bioassay two dose-response lines can be plotted from the results. This usually

gives the sort of data illustrated in fig. 3.5. Here the mean response obtained with each preparation has been plotted against the log of the dose. It follows, if the lines are parallel, that for any level of response the horizontal distance between the lines (AB) is constant. This distance

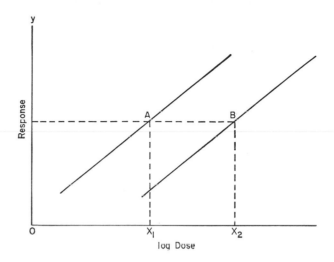

FIG. 3.5. Dose response lines in bioassay.

is the difference $(OX_2 - OX_1)$ between the logarithms of the two doses that produce the same response. Since the antilogarithm of the difference between two logarithms is the ratio of the two arithmetic values, we can therefore say that the ratio of equipotent doses is constant. This ratio is called the **potency ratio**. If the potency ratio of a preparation is 2·0 as compared with the standard, then all doses given must be halved to produce the same biological effect.

Limits of error

Since all measurements of response represent the means of varying responses in a number of animals, the dose response lines are not known without error. The potency ratio is thus only an estimate of the true value. It is thus customary to attach limits to the estimate beyond which it is improbable that the true value lies. The calculation of such limits is very complex.

It is important to remember that the best that can be done is to make a statement of probability. For example, after a particular test we can say that, unless a 1 in 20 chance has come off, the potency lies within two calculated limits. Nevertheless, if the 1 in 20 chance has come off, the real potency may lie well outside our limits.

This is one of the reasons why it is hard to control the potency of biological extracts of this kind. Thus a manufacturer may sell insulin labelled with a potency of 100 units/ml. This label is based on assays against the standard preparation of insulin tested by its potency to lower blood glucose and will, by law, have limits of error such that, unless a 1 in 20 chance has come off, the real potency will lie between 90 and 110 units/ml. But, occasionally, and despite the fact that most manufacturers work to even closer limits, the chance does come off, and the preparation is either stronger or weaker than is claimed. It is of the essence of statistics that this chance cannot be eliminated; it can only be quantified, thus allowing for reduction in the chance by proper experimental design.

ANALYSIS OF VARIANCE IN BIOASSAY

The power of the analysis of variance as a statistical tool is well illustrated by its application to bioassay. Suppose that a preparation of a biological preparation is given at two different dose levels and that the standard preparation is given at the same two dose levels, the responses of ten animals being measured for each dose. Thus forty animals in all are used in the test and four responses measured. An analysis of variance can be done in the following form:

Source of variation	d.f.	
Between doses	3	
Within doses	36	(9 within each of 4 doses)
Total	39	

But we can further partition the three degrees of freedom between doses as follows:

(1) between standard and test preparations   1
(2) between high and low doses   1
(3) interactions between preparations and doses   1
      —
      3

Here we are calculating the variance, about the overall mean, of the forty responses, attributable to:

(1) the means of the twenty responses to each preparation **independent of dose,**

(2) the means of the twenty responses to each dose **independent of preparation,**

(3) the mean of the ten responses to the high dose of the standard combined with the ten responses to the low dose of the test preparation, and of the ten responses to the low dose of the standard combined with the ten responses to the high dose of the test preparation.

These variances are compared with the error variance (the within doses variance) which is the irreducible measure of the biological variation of response in animals treated in exactly the same way.

If variance (1) is significantly larger than the error variance it means that the preparations vary significantly in strength. If variance (2) is significantly larger than the error variance it means that the slope of the dose response line is significantly greater than zero. If this is not true then there is no evidence that a larger dose will produce a larger response and the whole assay is worthless.

If variance (3) is significantly larger than the error variance it means that the two dose-response lines differ significantly from parallelism. This, in turn, means that the ratio of equipotent doses will vary depending on the level of the response; hence no valid potency ratio can be calculated and the assay is invalid. This may be the result of impurities in the test preparation modifying the responses.

Thus the analysis of variance can be used to test the validity of the assay in a number of ways. The more degrees of freedom that are available between doses, the more refined can the examination of the data become. Thus, when three doses of test and standard preparation are used, a further test is possible to see whether the dose response line is really linear or whether there is significant curvature. The concept is simple but the mathematics becomes increasingly complex.

Proportions

We have dealt so far with measurements made of various variables. In medicine there are many situations where the response that is observed is not continuously graded but is of the all-or-nothing variety. Thus a patient may live or die; a physiological event either does or does not take place. These responses are often called **quantal responses** to differentiate them from **graded responses**.

The logic of dealing with the statistics of quantal responses is the same as that used for graded responses, but the mathematics is different. One example must suffice for our argument.

Let us assume that we know that, of the population of patients who develop a given disease, the proportion, p, who die is 40 per cent. We draw a sample of 100 patients, and treat them by some new method. Suppose only 20 die. On the null hypothesis that the new treatment is without effect, in the long run we should expect that 40 per cent of the treated patients would also die. But, of course, in a particular sample of 100 patients it would be rather unlikely that exactly 40 would die. The real question of interest is: what are the chances that as many as 80 patients would survive if the treatment were ineffective? If the probability turns out to be sufficiently small, we shall be inclined to reject the null hypothesis. In principle we could calculate the exact probability by the binomial theorem, since the binomial distribution describes the situation exactly. Thus, for a sample of only 5 patients with, on the null hypothesis, a chance of survival of 0·6 and of death 0·4, the probability that:

5 survive	0 die	is $(0.6)^5 =$	7·8 per cent
4 survive	1 dies	is $5(0.6)^4 (0.4) =$	25·9 per cent
3 survive	2 die	is $10(0.6)^3 (0.4)^2 =$	34·6 per cent
2 survive	3 die	is $10(0.6)^2 (0.4)^3 =$	23·0 per cent
1 survives	4 die	is $5(0.6) (0.4)^4 =$	7·7 per cent
0 survive	5 die	is $(0.4)^5 =$	1·0 per cent

Thus, even if the null hypothesis is true, there is a 7·8 per cent probability that in our sample of 5 patients none will die and a 33·7 per cent (7·8+25·9%) chance that fewer than 2, the expected number, will die. Apart from showing the difficulty of drawing useful conclusions from small scale trials, the example demonstrates that the exact method is impractical for large samples. Fortunately, approximate methods are available. For large samples the binomial distribution approximates to a normal distribution. If the population probability is p, its standard error is given by the formula

$$s = \sqrt{\frac{p(1-p)}{n}}$$

and a test may be applied by calculating the deviation of our sample value from p in terms of its standard error. For a large enough sample, the quantity u, which is

$$\frac{\text{difference between population and sample proportions}}{s}$$

will be distributed in exactly the same way as shown in fig. 3.2b.

To return to our main example, working in percentages

$$s = \sqrt{\frac{40 \times 60}{100}} = 4·9$$

$$u = \frac{40-20}{4·9} = 4·1$$

There is less than one chance in 1000 of obtaining such a value for u on the null hypothesis. A reduction in mortality from 40 to 20 per cent in a sample of 100 is thus very much more convincing than an apparently greater improvement in a sample of 5.

Usually we do not know the value of the proportion in the population. This is the same problem as we discussed for graded responses. Here we rely on a comparison between a treated sample and a control sample.

DIFFERENCE BETWEEN PROPORTIONS

When we have two samples of sizes n_1 and n_2 with proportions p_1 and p_2, to test for a significant difference between the proportions we need a value for the standard error of their difference. An argument similar to the one on p. 3.7 shows that with the usual null hypothesis

$$s_{\text{diff}} = \sqrt{\frac{\bar{p}(1-\bar{p})}{n_1} + \frac{\bar{p}(1-\bar{p})}{n_2}}$$

where $\bar{p}$ is the proportion in the combined samples, used as the best estimate of the population probability.

Suppose we had two samples of 100 patients and one sample was treated and fifteen died, whereas in the other sample, used as controls, thirty died. The null hypothesis we test is that treatment has had no effect or in other words that both groups of patients are samples of the

same population. On this hypothesis the best estimate of $\bar{p}$, the proportion of the population who die, is made by combining the samples. We use this estimate to find the standard error of the proportion of both samples. Thus, of 200 patients, forty-five died, giving an estimate for $\bar{p}$ of 22·5. We thus have, working in percentages

$$s_{\text{diff}} = \sqrt{\frac{22·5 \times 77·5}{100} + \frac{22·5 \times 77·5}{100}}$$
$$= \sqrt{34·87}$$
$$= 5·9$$

and hence

$$u = \frac{p_1 - p_2}{s} = \frac{30-15}{5·9} = 2·54$$

In the long run such a value would be obtained in less than 1 in 100 samples, so that we conclude that the treatment was probably effective.

χ^2 test

When we wish to compare more than two proportions we must use another technique than that just described. This is comparable to the progression from the t test to the analysis of variance for graded responses. The χ^2 test, developed by Pearson, serves this purpose. χ^2 is a value computed from the difference between observed numbers and expected numbers. In a general form it can be calculated from

$$\chi^2 = \text{sum of } \frac{(\text{Observed number} - \text{Expected number})^2}{\text{Expected number}}$$

It is thus the sum of the squared deviations from expectation expressed as a ratio in relation to expectation. Tabulated values of χ^2 in relation to probability are available for any given number of summed differences. With two proportions only, the method gives identical results to the one already described.

Let us assume that the death rates from a disease of childhood are arranged in relation to the age. We might get figures such as those shown in table 3.6a. We might

TABLE 3.6a. Death rates for a disease of childhood arranged according to the age of the child.

Age in years	Number of cases of disease	Number dying	Per cent dying
<1	15	5	33·3
1	19	5	26·3
2	37	8	21·6
3	46	8	17·4
4	30	6	20·0
5	45	5	11·1
Total	192	37	19·3

TABLE 3.6b. Comparison of observed with expected deaths from diseases of childhood at different ages.

Age in years	Number of cases of disease	Number dying				Number recovering		
		Observed (O)	Expected (E)	$\frac{(O-E)^2}{E}$		Observed (O)	Expected (E)	$\frac{(O-E)^2}{E}$
<1	15	5	2·9	1·54		10	12·1	0·37
1	19	5	3·7	0·49		14	15·3	0·12
2	37	8	7·1	0·11		29	29·9	0·03
3	46	8	8·8	0·07		38	37·2	0·02
4	30	6	5·8	0·01		24	24·2	0·00
5	45	5	8·7	1·55		40	36·3	0·37
Total	192	37	37·0	3·77		155	155·0	0·91

$$\chi^2 = 3\cdot77 + 0\cdot91$$
$$= 4\cdot68$$
$$n = 5$$

suspect from the data that the chance of a child dying was greater the younger the age. How can this theory be tested? The null hypothesis is that age does not matter.

If it is assumed that there is no difference in the mortality at different ages, then we would expect that the overall mortality rate of 19·3 per cent would apply to all age groups. We can thus construct a new table giving the expected number of deaths at each age (table 3.6b). The total χ^2 as calculated is 4·68. It must always be remembered that the value of χ^2 is obtained both from the number dying and from the number recovering, although, since these are not independent figures, there are only six separate comparisons. Also one degree of freedom has been used up in determining the overall mortality rate, so finally $n = 5$. This value of χ^2, on consulting a table, would be expected to occur by chance in no less than 80 per cent of samples. There is thus no reason to reject the null hypothesis and no reason to think the disease more lethal in younger children.

FOURFOLD TABLE

When there is only one real comparison being made, there is a special quick way of calculating χ^2. This is a frequent situation in medicine. Thus, for example, we have thirty patients with coronary thrombosis treated with a new drug to prevent clotting of the blood and nineteen survive for 3 months; while of forty-one comparable cases not so treated only fifteen survive for 3 months. Is the treatment of any benefit as judged on this criterion of 3 months' survival? We can arrange the data as a fourfold table with marginal totals (table 3.7a). The general case is given in table 3.7b and the general equation for χ^2 is

$$\chi^2 = \frac{(ad-bc)^2(a+b+c+d)}{(a+b)(c+d)(a+c)(b+d)}$$

where $n = 1$

In principle this test is really the same as that for the difference between proportions described on p. 3.13.

Table 3.7. The fourfold table. Relationship between the number of patients, treated and untreated, who live or die.
(a) Figures for quoted example.

	Number living	Number dying	Total
Number treated	19	11	30
Number untreated	15	26	41
Total	34	37	71

(b) The general form of the fourfold table.

	Number living	Number dying	Total
Number treated	a	c	$a+c$
Number untreated	b	d	$b+d$
Total	$a+b$	$c+d$	$a+b+c+d$

In our example

$$\chi^2 = \frac{(26 \times 19 - 11 \times 15)^2 \times 71}{34 \times 37 \times 30 \times 41}$$
$$= 4\cdot97$$

This value will occur by chance in just over 1 in 100 samples. There is thus some reason for rejecting the null hypothesis and accepting that the treatment is of value.

It has been found that, when the numbers are small, the equation tends to overestimate χ^2. A correction is therefore used. Thus

$$\chi^2 = \frac{[ad-bc-\frac{1}{2}(a+b+c+d)]^2(a+b+c+d)}{(a+b)(c+d)(a+c)(b+d)}$$

Recalculating we get $\chi^2 = 3\cdot95$. This is a value which will occur by chance almost exactly once in twenty samples. Our conclusion is therefore still justified but not so firmly.

Quantal response assays

We may want to measure the regression line relating the proportion of individuals who recover when treated with varying doses of a drug. In this case we have to relate the percentage recovering to the dose, or preferably to the logarithm of the dose (p. 3.11). When such a log dose response line is plotted (fig. 3.6a) a **sigmoid** (S-shaped) curve is usually obtained. This created much statistical difficulty which was solved by Gaddum. His method, later modified by Bliss, depends on the transformation of the percentage response to a function called the **probit**. Probits are symmetrical about a central value 5·0 corresponding to a percentage response of 50 per cent; and the differences between probits get bigger the further away the response gets, in either direction, from 50 per cent. This has the effect of turning the sigmoid curve into a straight line (fig. 3.6b). When two preparations are being compared

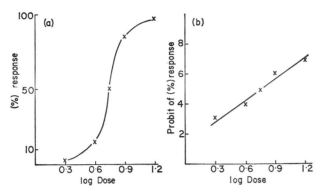

FIG. 3.6. Dose response relationships in a quantal response assay.

this linear relationship permits the calculation of a potency ratio and limits of error. The arithmetic is very complex, although the concept is simple. Values for probits are obtained in standard tables.

Errors of blood counting or radioactive counting

The distribution of the counts of cells or of disintegrating atoms follows a pattern called the **Poisson distribution.** It applies to random events which occur independently. Thus the chances of one particular atom disintegrating is not affected by the fact that some other atom has or has not disintegrated. The distribution can be described by a single number. If we know that a radioactive material is disintegrating at a rate of one per second we can calculate without any additional information the probabilities that exactly 0, 1, 2 and so on disintegrations will occur in any interval.

Another feature of a Poisson distribution is that its variance is equal to its mean. Thus if we count 100 cells, and regard this as the mean, the variance of the count is 100, and the standard deviation of the count is $\sqrt{100} = 10$ or 10 per cent. If we count 400 cells the standard deviation is 20 or 5 per cent; and if we count 10,000 cells it is 100 or 1 per cent. The same applies to radioactivity counts. The standard deviation is a measure of the error of the count. If the total number of cells actually counted is 100 or more, we can compare two separate counts by calculating the variance of the difference between them, using as before the theorem that the variance of a difference is the sum of the variances of the components.

Thus, if we have two counts of 180 and 220 respectively, we have a variance for the difference between them of $180 + 220 = 400$ and a standard error of this difference of 20. Since the difference (40) is twice its own standard error we might suspect that the two counts are not from the same population.

FURTHER READING

CAMPBELL R.C. (1967) *Statistics for Biologists.* London: Cambridge University Press.

COLQUHOUN D. (1971) *Lectures on Biostatistics: Introduction to Statistics with Applications in Biology and Medicine.* London: Oxford University Press.

HILL A. BRADFORD (1971) *Principles of Medical Statistics*, 9th Edition. London: The Lancet.

MORONEY M.J. (1969) *Facts from Figures.* Harmondsworth: Penguin.

Chapter 4
Supply and use of energy

Light, absorbed by plants for photosynthesis, is the initiator of all biological processes. Heat, given off by both animals and plants, is the final waste. Between light and heat, useful mechanical work is possible. Energy is a Greek word meaning work. In the nineteenth century, physicists made it a technical term, the capacity to do mechanical work. The interconversion of the various forms of energy such as light, heat, and the motions of wind, water or electricity and that stored in various fuels or reservoirs is possible but it is limited. The limits are set down and described by the science of energetics or thermodynamics.

Basic definitions

The definition of energy is the capacity to do work and is derived from mechanics. **Work** is defined as the overcoming of a force; for example, the lifting of a weight by a man is work done on the weight by some biological machinery against the force of gravity. The work done by the biological machinery must be at least equal to the obvious mechanical work done on the weight, i.e. work done = force × distance = mass × acceleration due to gravity × height. In the Système International d'Unités (SI) the unit of force is the **newton** (N) and is the force necessary to give a mass of 1 kg an acceleration of 1 metre per sec per sec (i.e. 1 kg m s^{-2}). If 1 newton moves 1 kg 1 metre, then 1 **joule** (J) of energy has been expended. Physiologists need a bigger unit. Most adult men and women when at rest expend energy at a rate between 3·5 and 5·0 kilojoules (kJ)/min. Physical activity raises the rate and daily energy expenditure usually lies between 8·0 and 15·0 megajoules (MJ).

The human body is a chemical engine. At rest it transduces the chemical energy present in food into mechanical work, as in the beating of the heart and the movements of the diaphragm in respiration. This accounts for less than 10 per cent of the resting energy, the remainder being utilized in the osmotic pumps which maintain the ionic gradients in the tissues and in the chemical syntheses needed to replace the molecules continually broken down in the turnover of the components of the cells. All of this energy is ultimately lost to the body in the form of heat.

The unit of heat formerly used in physiology was the **kilocalorie** (kcal) or the heat required to raise 1 kg of water from 14·5 to 15·5°C. For a long time it was also the accepted unit of energy. It is now replaced by the **kilojoule** (kJ). The conversion factor is 1 kcal = 4·184 kJ, but for most practical purposes the figure 4·2 suffices. The calorie is so deeply engrained in the minds of doctors and dietitians and also of all those who have to struggle to keep thin that it is unlikely that its use as a unit of energy will cease for a long time. Accordingly in many tables and in the text, energy values are expressed as both kJ and kcal.

Power is a measure of the rate of doing work. The electrical unit of power, the **watt** (W), is equivalent to 1 joule/sec. The domestic unit of electricity is the kilowatt-hour. Hence a one kilowatt domestic fire gives out about 60 kJ/min. This is about the same amount of heat as would be given out by twelve people sitting quietly in a room, as many hostesses know.

FUELS OF THE BODY

The fuels of the body are carbohydrate, fat, protein and ethyl alcohol, taken in the diet. Most of the energy bound in the carbon and hydrogen linkages of the molecules of these substances can be made available to the body, in the course of their breakdown by processes which are mostly oxidative. This energy is ultimately derived from the sun. The energy of solar radiation is fixed by the photosynthetic processes, when water and carbon dioxide are converted by green plants into carbohydrate. The energy so fixed can be utilized by plants for synthesis of other carbohydrates, fats, proteins and alcohols. Photosynthesis takes place only in the green leaves of plants, which are of limited use as human foods. Firstly, the cell walls of plants contain large amounts of fibre, which cannot be digested in the human alimentary canal. Secondly, the concentration of energy in green leaves is low. Animals, such as ruminants, whose diet is composed largely of green fodder, have to spend the greater part of their lives eating in order to obtain sufficient energy. Farmers aim to concentrate the energy originally present in green leaves either into the seeds of cereal grains and oil seeds or into the muscles, adipose tissue and milk and eggs of farm animals. Cereal grains, vegetable oils, meat and dairy products are the principal sources of energy in human diets. Farming can legitimately be considered a branch of chemical industry. Crops and farm animals are the 'plant' which the farmer uses to convert solar radiation into human food.

Energy content of foods

Since the gramme-molecular weight of glucose is 180 and by Avogadro's Law 1 gramme-molecule of a gas occupies 22·4 litres at STP, the combustion of 1 mole of glucose can be described thus:

$$C_6H_{12}O_6 + 6O_2 = 6CO_2 + 6H_2O + heat$$

$$180 \text{ g} \quad 6 \times 22 \cdot 4 \text{ l} \quad 6 \times 22 \cdot 4 \text{ l} \quad 6 \times 18 \text{ g} \quad 2.87 \text{ MJ}$$
$$(686 \text{ kcal})$$

The quantitative aspects of this equation are of great importance to physiologists. Glucose, of course, will not normally ignite until it has been raised to a high temperature and then the energy is liberated instantaneously. For glucose to serve as a fuel in the body, combustion must take place at a temperature around 37°C and it must be controlled so that the energy is liberated in small quantities, accurately graded to meet the local requirements of the tissues. Enzyme systems in the body effect the oxidation of glucose in a series of stages, of which at least six are associated with the liberation of energy. These reactions allow sufficient energy to become available to meet the needs of the tissues with a dissipation of heat so small that local temperature does not rise by more than 3 or 4°C at the most. How this is brought about will be described in chaps. 7, 8 & 9. The additive result of all these stages is the same as if the glucose had been ignited spontaneously and is given in the above equation. It also follows that the combustion of 1 g of glucose yields 15·9 kJ (3·81 kcal) (**heat of combustion**) and 0·6 g of H_2O (**metabolic water**). Further the volume of CO_2 produced is equal to the volume of O_2 utilized, so that the ratio,

$$\frac{CO_2 \text{ produced}}{O_2 \text{ used}} \text{ (respiratory quotient, RQ)} = 1$$

This ratio is nowadays often known as the **respiratory exchange**. Furthermore 1 litre of O_2, when used to oxidize glucose liberates 21·3 kJ (5·10 kcal) (**energy equivalent of oxygen**). Each of these values is of physiological importance, as will appear later.

These terms have been defined and explained with reference to glucose, because it is a foodstuff with a comparatively simple molecular structure. A similar procedure could have been employed, using a fat such as a triglyceride or a protein. As these molecules are larger and more complicated, equations are more cumbersome. Similar, but not identical, values for heat of combustion, metabolic water, respiratory quotient and energy equivalent of oxygen can be derived for these substances.

Heats of combustion

These are measured experimentally using a **bomb calorimeter** (fig. 4.1). This depends on the fact that foodstuffs can be readily ignited by a small electric current, when under high oxygen pressure. The bomb is a small steel cylinder, into which the food is placed in a platinum crucible. A small wire through which a current can be

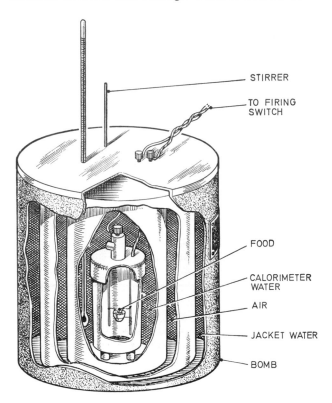

STIRRER

TO FIRING SWITCH

FOOD

CALORIMETER WATER

AIR

JACKET WATER

BOMB

FIG. 4.1. The bomb calorimeter.

passed is placed on the food. The bomb has a screw top, containing a valve through which oxygen can be passed to raise the pressure in the bomb. When the bomb is charged with food and the pressure raised, it is placed in a water calorimeter. The food is then ignited and the heat of combustion calculated from the rise in temperature in the calorimeter. Table 4.1 gives in the first column the heats of combustion of proteins, fats and carbohydrates derived from common foods and also of alcohol. These are precise physical measurements which represent the total energy available on oxidation. They do not represent the physiological values for the energy available to the tissues. Since the food is not completely digested and absorbed from the alimentary canal, and oxidation in the tissues is not always complete, some losses of energy are inevitable.

TABLE 4.1. Heats of combustion and availability of energy in the principal types of food.

	Heat of combustion kJ/g	kcal/g	Loss in urine kJ/g	kcal/g	Availability per cent	Atwater factors kJ/g	kcal/g
PROTEIN							
Meat	22·4	5·35 ⎫	5·23	1·25	92	17	4
Egg	23·4	5·58 ⎭					
FAT							
Butter	38·2	9·12 ⎫					
Animal fat	39·2	9·37 ⎬	—	—	95	37	9
Olive oil	39·3	9·38 ⎭					
CARBOHYDRATE							
Starch	17·2	4·12 ⎫	trace		99	16	4
Glucose	16·0	3·81 ⎭					
ETHYL ALCOHOL	29·7	7·10	trace		100	29	7

Losses in the faeces

The human alimentary tract is remarkably efficient. Many studies have shown that with a normal diet about 99 per cent of the carbohydrate, 95 per cent of the fat and 92 per cent of the protein is absorbed (table 4.1). The energy loss in the faeces is seldom more than 5 per cent of the intake. The figures above are not fixed values, but vary slightly from one individual to another and also according to the nature of the diet. With a diet based on undermilled cereals and coarse vegetables, the bulk of the faeces is large owing to the big intake of indigestible fibre and this is usually associated with a slight diminution in the absorption of the digestible components.

Losses in the urine

Proteins are not completely broken down in the tissues. The nitrogen is excreted in the urine largely in the form of urea, but also as uric acid, creatinine and other substances. Energy is lost in the urine, in amounts corresponding to about 5·23 kJ (1·25 kcal)/g of dietary protein. About one-quarter of the energy present in the dietary protein is thus not available to the tissues. In health, the breakdown of carbohydrates and fats is for practical purposes complete. A large number of organic acids and other substances derived from fat and carbohydrate appear in the urine but the daily output of each is measured in milligrams and the total output does not normally amount to 1 g. In disease, however, large amounts of energy may be lost in the urine. For example, in diabetes up to 25 per cent of the dietary intake of energy may be excreted in the urine in the form of glucose and acetoacetate.

Calculation of the energy value of human diets

Table 4.2 gives values for the protein, fat, carbohydrate and energy content of some common foods. The figures are taken from a report prepared by McCance and Widdowson, which gives analyses of 663 foods commonly eaten in Great Britain. Tables giving analyses of the principal foods consumed locally have been prepared in at least 35 countries. Any particular food gives approximately the same analysis in whatever part of the world the sample is taken, but it is best to use tables prepared from analyses of local foods. With the aid of such tables it is possible to prescribe a diet in which the energy content is known with an accuracy of ± 10 per cent. This degree of accuracy usually suffices in laying down ration scales (e.g. for boarding schools and other institutions and also for the armed services) and for clinical purposes (e.g. the treatment of obesity and diabetes). If in any investigation it is necessary to know more accurately the energy intake of a given person, it is essential to weigh out and homogenize a duplicate portion of everything that is eaten and then to analyse an aliquot.

In practical dietetics, physiological values for the energy content of the nutrients in a human diet, which take into account the losses of energy in the urine and faeces, must be used. Many years ago, the American physiologist Atwater rounded off the figures in the first three columns in table 4.1 to give the values 4, 9, 4 kcal/g for the energy available to the tissues from protein, fat and carbohydrate respectively. The **Atwater factors** (17, 37, 16 in kJ/g) are useful approximations widely used in making up dietary prescriptions. Physiological losses of alcohol in the urine and expired air are small, and a value of 29 kJ (7 kcal)/g may be taken as correct.

The detailed prescription of the items of food in a diet is properly the task of a dietitian, who is trained in the use of food tables.

Sources of energy in diets

Within fairly wide limits proteins, fats and carbohydrate are interchangeable as sources of energy. All diets

TABLE 4.2. Energy value and nutrient content of some common foods (values per 100 g). From McCance and Widdowson (1960).

	Energy kJ	kcal	Water g	Protein g	Fat g	Carbohydrate g	Alcohol g
Whole wheat flour	1420	339	15·0	13·6	2·5	69·1	—
White bread	1020	243	38·3	7·8	1·4	52·7	—
Rice, raw	1510	361	11·7	6·2	1·0	86·8	—
Milk, fresh, whole	276	66	87·0	3·4	3·7	4·8	—
Butter	3320	793	13·9	0·4	85·1	tr	—
Cheese, Cheddar	1780	425	37·0	25·4	34·5	tr	—
Beef steak, fried	1140	273	56·9	20·4	20·4	0	—
Haddock, fried	733	175	65·1	20·4	8·3	3·6	—
Potatoes	293	70	80·0	2·5	tr	15·9	—
Peas, canned	360	86	72·7	5·9	tr	16·5	—
Cabbage, boiled	38	9	95·7	1·3	tr	1·1	—
Orange, with peel	113	27	64·8	0·6	tr	6·4	—
Apple	197	47	84·1	0·3	tr	12·2	—
White sugar	1650	394	tr	tr	0	105·0	—
Beer,* bitter	130	31	96·7	0·2	tr	2·2	3·1
Spirits* (gin, whisky 70% proof)	929	222	63·5	tr	0	tr	31·5

* Values per 100 ml.

must contain some protein to provide nitrogen and essential amino acids (p. 11.12). Throughout the world most national diets provide between 10 per cent and 15 per cent of the energy as protein. Eskimos, South American gauchos and pastoral tribes such as the Masai in East Africa, who may live almost entirely on foods of animal origin, may take more protein, and there is no evidence that this does them any good or any harm. It is possible to live on diets containing very little of either fat or carbohydrate. Poor people whose diet is based largely on cereal grains have a predominantly carbohydrate diet. In many peasant communities energy may be provided by 12 per cent protein, 10 per cent fat and 78 per cent carbohydrate, although such a diet must be unappetizing and may well be lacking in vitamins. With increasing wealth a family always increases its fat intake. In prosperous western countries about 40 per cent of the energy is derived from fat. In the national diets of the United Kingdom, U.S.A. and other countries whose populations are well fed, the energy distribution is approximately 12 per cent protein, 40 per cent fat and 48 per cent carbohydrate. Increasing material prosperity, increasing dietary fat and increasing heart disease have been common features of many countries in the twentieth century and it has been held widely that these associations are causal (vol. 3, p. 17.13).

Table 4.3 sets out how the energy might be distributed in the diet of a healthy adult man and of a middle aged woman who wishes to reduce weight.

ENERGY EXPENDITURE AND HUMAN CALORIMETRY

The great French chemist Lavoisier, who first established the role of oxygen in the combustion of inorganic substances, defined clearly the problems associated with the use of energy in animals. He put a guinea-pig in a box surrounded by ice and measured the rate at which the ice melted and at which CO_2 was produced and showed that the two rates were related. He also measured the rate of oxygen consumption by a man at rest and showed that it was increased three or four times by light exercise. Lavoisier died on the guillotine during the Reign of Terror in 1794. After his death many chemists and physiologists in the nineteenth century developed methods to study the relationship between heat output, work done and the respiratory exchanges in man and animals.

TABLE 4.3. The provision of energy in two diets. (a) Diet suitable for an adult man. (b) Diet low in energy and in carbohydrate, suitable for a middle-aged woman who wishes to reduce her weight.

Nutrient	Daily intake g	Energy value kJ/g	kcal/g	Energy intake MJ	kcal
(a) Protein	100	17	4	1·7	400
Fat	100	37	9	3·7	900
Carbohydrate	400	16	4	6·7	1600
				12·1	2900
(b) Protein	60	17	4	1·0	240
Fat	40	37	9	1·5	360
Carbohydrate	100	16	4	1·7	400
				4·2	1000

By 1900, the American physiologist Atwater, assisted by an engineer Rosa, had developed a human calorimeter. This consisted of a chamber in which a man could live and work for several days, and at the same time the total output of heat could be measured (fig. 4.2). This could be related to the net energy intake, which is the energy in the food minus the energy lost in the urine and faeces. In experiments lasting 4 days he measured both the energy intake and the energy output of his subjects and was able to get agreement within ± 1 per cent. This demonstration, that the law of conservation of energy applies to man, was a great technical achievement. It was also important in killing the idea, common in the nineteenth century, that living creatures possessed 'a vital force' which in some way allowed them to operate outside of the laws of physics and chemistry. This idea is not yet quite dead and many obese people think that their fat accumulates in some mysterious way unrelated to the energy content of their diet. Unfortunately they are sometimes supported in this view by their doctors. 'Calories don't count' is a slogan of some advertised slimming regimes. Atwater counted them very accurately.

The measurement of the total heat output of a man (**direct calorimetry**) remains a very difficult procedure

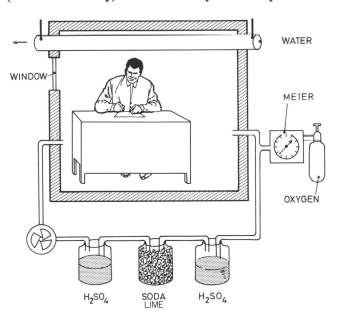

FIG. 4.2. The Atwater–Rosa human calorimeter.

and is seldom attempted nowadays. The heat output is, however, related quantitatively to the oxygen utilization. The measurement of oxygen consumption (**indirect calorimetry**) is a relatively easy technical procedure, which can be used to measure rates of energy expenditure in daily activities at work and during recreations, and any changes in the rates that may be brought about by disease.

Theoretical background of indirect calorimetry

If the reader turns back to p. 4.2, he will find the energy equivalent of oxygen, when glucose is being utilized. Values for each of the other nutrients can be calculated similarly and accepted values are set out in table 4.4, together with the respiratory quotients. It will be seen that the values of the energy equivalent do not differ greatly. In practice, the human body is nearly always running on a mixture of fuels. The usual assumption that the utilization of 1 litre of O_2 corresponds to the production of 20 kJ (4.8 kcal) of energy involves an error of at most ± 4 per cent.

As fats have a much lower proportion of oxygen in

TABLE 4.4. The energy equivalent of one litre of oxygen and the respiratory quotient associated with the combustion of the principal nutrients.

Nutrient	kJ	kcal	RQ
Protein	19·2	4·60	0·81
Fat	19·6	4·69	0·71
Carbohydrate (starch)	21·0	5·01	1·00
Ethyl alcohol	20·3	4·86	0·66

their molecules than carbohydrates, the RQ associated with their oxidation is lower than the value of 1·0 for carbohydrate. An observed value of the RQ of below 0·80 or over 0·90 indicates that the energy is being produced predominantly from fat or carbohydrate respectively.

The amount of protein broken down in the tissues can be determined from the amount of nitrogen excreted in the urine (p. 5.3) provided kidney function is normal. If over a given period of time the intake of O_2 and the output of CO_2 by the lungs and the urinary nitrogen are determined, then it is possible to calculate the amount of protein, fat and carbohydrate utilized by the tissues (**metabolic mixture**) and the relative proportion of the energy derived from each fuel. The arithmetic necessary for this calculation is essentially simple but is cumbersome. It can be found in the books recommended for further reading.

MEASUREMENT OF OXYGEN CONSUMPTION

There are three established methods in common use. The Benedict–Roth spirometer is the simplest when the subject is at rest and is employed for measuring metabolic rates in hospital patients. The Douglas bag method is the most accurate and reliable and is the method of choice in the physiology laboratory. The Max Planck respirometer is a convenient instrument to use in industry and in field conditions.

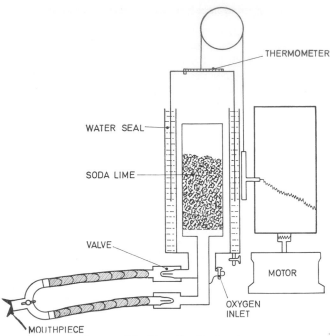

FIG. 4.3. The Benedict–Roth spirometer.

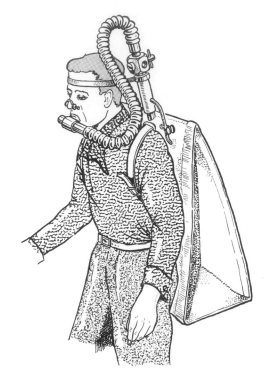

FIG. 4.4. The Douglas bag

The **Benedict–Roth spirometer** (fig. 4.3) is a closed-circuit breathing apparatus, which is filled with oxygen. It has a capacity of about 6 litres. The O_2 is contained in a metal drum which floats on a water seal. The subject breathes in from this drum through an inspiratory valve. His expired air passes back into the drum through an expiratory valve and a soda lime canister, in which the CO_2 produced is absorbed. As the O_2 is used up, the drum sinks and its movement is recorded on a paper chart; from this the rate of O_2 consumption can be read. The apparatus is simple to use and accurate. It has the disadvantage that it can be used only when the subject is at rest or doing very light exercise and that, as the CO_2 output is not measured, the RQ cannot be calculated.

The **Douglas bag** (fig. 4.4) is a canvas or plastic bag, normally of 100 litre capacity. The subject breathes through a metal or plastic mouthpiece which houses inspiratory and expiratory valves. Room air is breathed in and all the expired air is collected in the bag. The bag is then emptied through a gas meter and a sample of the expired air taken for analysis of the O_2 and CO_2 content. Rates of O_2 utilization and CO_2 production can then be calculated. The method is ideal for subjects either at rest or exercising on a treadmill or bicycle ergometer.

The **Max Planck respirometer** (fig. 4.5) was introduced in Germany for use in industry. The principle is the same as that in the Douglas bag method, but the volume of the expired air is measured directly in a dry gas meter. This is worn on the subject's back, like a haversack, and weighs 3–4 kg. The spirometer contains a sampling de-

vice, which diverts an adjustable portion of the expired air, less than 1 per cent, into a small rubber football bladder. This will not fill up for 5–10 min, even if the work is heavy. The sample of expired air in the bag is then analysed. This instrument is ideal for measuring O_2 consumption rates during light and moderate work. With very heavy work involving an expiratory output of more than 50 l/min, the meter tends to under-record and it imposes also a significant resistance on the subject's breathing at high rates.

Other apparatus is available for measuring very high

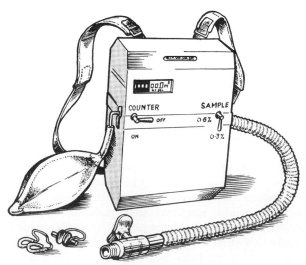

FIG. 4.5. The Max Planck respirometer.

rates of O_2 consumption, as in competitive athletics, and for the continuous recording for several hours of both O_2 intake and CO_2 output by hospital patients or subjects at rest. In both these circumstances, there are considerable technical difficulties and the methods are suitable only for use by experienced workers.

RATES OF ENERGY EXPENDITURE

The amount of energy which each of us requires to take in our food is determined by the amount of energy that we put out in the activities of everyday life. In many of the poor and underdeveloped countries the food supply is insufficient to meet the energy needs of a working population and of their growing children. In rich countries, where food is abundant, intake of energy frequently exceeds output. Inevitably then the excess is stored as fat, and obesity with its attendant disadvantages results. There is now much interest in determining rates of energy expenditure, and the findings are used for assessing dietary requirements, both at national and at individual level.

Energy expenditure lying at rest

An adult male lying at rest may use O_2 at the rate of some 250 ml/min corresponding to an energy output of about 5·0 kJ (1·20 kcal)/min. This figure may be modified according to his size, and for sex and age, by climate and diet and also by disease. As there are 1440 min in the day, 7·5 MJ (1800 kcal) is approximately the amount of energy which should be provided by the diet for a man confined to bed.

For over 70 years it has been customary to refer to the resting energy output as the **basal metabolic rate** (BMR). The BMR is described and discussed in many textbooks and has an immense literature. This is largely theoretical. The term implies that for each individual there is a fixed minimum level of metabolism on which life depends. However, the minimum level of metabolism of any individual is not always the same. It depends on the previous nutritional history, on the body temperature and may be affected by drugs and hormones. It is impossible to define a 'vital minimum' or basal metabolism. A more accurate and descriptive term is **resting metabolism**, which has no theoretical overtones.

EFFECT OF BODY SIZE

Table 4.5 illustrates a general biological law. The metabolic rate of a mouse is more than ten times that of an ox, expressed per unit of weight, but is of the same order for all mammals when expressed per unit of surface area. The small animal has a big surface, relative to weight, from which heat is lost. To maintain body temperature relatively more heat must be produced. Accordingly it became conventional to express values of resting metabolism in units of surface area. Standard values for a man and a woman aged 20 are 162 and 148 kJ (38·6 and

TABLE 4.5. Resting metabolism in various species related to size.

Species	Weight kg	Surface area m²	Resting metabolism/day kJ	kJ/kg	kJ/m²
Mouse	0·0285	0·007	22	754	3090
Rat	0·3	0·0384	110	377	2870
Monkey	3·22	0·257	653	209	2550
Dog	14·9	0·652	2270	151	3480
Sheep	29·5	0·805	2900	96	3600
Man	65·0	1·83	6980	113	3810
Pig	186·0	2·67	11 100	59	4160
Cattle	366·0	4·56	23 800	63	5210

35·3 kcal) $m^{-2} h^{-1}$. The surface area of human subjects is by tradition derived from a measurement of height and weight using a nomogram (fig. 4.6). This nomogram was constructed over 50 years ago and is based on measurements of the area of paper required to cover completely the nude bodies of less than twenty United States citizens.

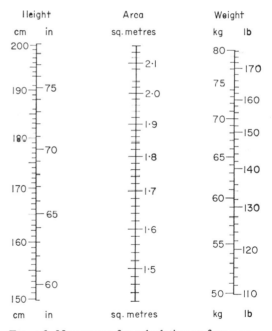

FIG. 4.6. Nomogram for calculating surface area.

It is generally agreed that women have a lower resting metabolic rate than men when the rates are expressed per unit of surface area. However, this does not mean, Mary, that the 'fire of life' burns less intensely in you than in Tom. It is only a reflection of the fact that you are fatter than he is. Table 4.6 presents data obtained by Edinburgh students in one of their physiological practical classes. The resting O_2 consumption was measured using the Benedict–Roth spirometer. The percentage of body fat was calculated from body density, determined by weighing each subject first in air and then

TABLE 4.6. Body fat, lean body mass and resting oxygen consumption of young men and women.

	Height cm	Weight kg	Surface area m²	Lean body mass kg	Body fat kg	Body fat %	Resting oxygen ml/min
24 young men							
Mean	176	68·5	1·83	61·1	7·5	10·7	258
Range	168–190	53·1–88·3	1·60–2·16	44·8–74·6	3·1–20·7	4·5–26·9	188–326
Standard deviation	5·9	8·2	0·13	6·93	4·3	5·6	30
25 young women							
Mean	165	58·2	1·62	43·1	15·1	25·6	186
Range	156–179	42·4–70·5	1·35–1·87	37·8–55·3	9·0–23·7	18·4–34·8	148–225
Standard deviation	4·2	7·1	0·10	4·1	4·0	4·57	22

TABLE 4.7. Normal values for the resting rate of energy expenditure of adults (kJ/min).

Men	Women	Fat %	45 kg	50 kg	55 kg	60 kg	65 kg	70 kg	75 kg	80 kg
Thin	—	5	—	4·1	4·4	4·7	5·0	5·3	5·5	5·8
Average	—	10	—	3·9	4·2	4·5	4·8	5·1	5·3	5·6
Plump	Thin	15	3·4	3·7	4·0	4·3	4·6	4·9	5·1	5·4
Fat	Average	20	3·3	3·5	3·8	4·1	4·4	4·7	4·9	5·2
—	Plump	25	—	3·3	3·6	3·9	4·2	4·5	4·7	5·0
—	Fat	30	—	—	3·4	3·7	4·0	4·3	4·5	4·8

under water. As the density of fat is about 0·9 and of the fat free tissues or lean body mass is about 1·1, the proportion of fat in the body can be calculated from a measurement of the density. The average O_2 consumption is higher for the men than for the women and this difference remains after correction for surface area (141 and 115 ml m^{-2} min^{-1} respectively). If the fat free body or lean body mass is used as the index of comparison, the sex difference disappears. The average O_2 consumptions are 4·2 and 4·3 ml min^{-1} kg^{-1} lean body for the men and women.

Several workers have now shown that the lean body mass predicts resting metabolic rates more accurately than does surface area and that there is no sex difference with the use of this variable. This is important theoretically. The surface area law implies that energy production is graded accurately to meet heat losses. This is not so, at least in civilized human communities. We adjust our body temperature so that we are comfortable by altering our clothing, going closer to or farther away from a fire, opening a window or putting on a fan. The rate of energy production is more probably determined by inherent properties within the cells. In 1902, the great German pioneer of human energy studies, Carl Voit, wrote: 'The unknown causes of metabolism are found in the cells of the organism. The mass of these cells and their power to decompose materials determines the metabolism. All kinds of influences may act upon the cells to modify their ability to metabolize, some increasing it or others decreasing it.'

Table 4.7 sets out standards for the normal resting metabolism related to body size. Figures are given for a range of body weight and fat content. The student is warned that this table differs from the conventional table found in textbooks for over 50 years and based on surface area. The table is simple to use. An estimate of body fat can be made from measurements of the thickness of subcutaneous folds of fat at various sites, using special calipers, and even the visual assessments given in the table may well be less inaccurate than calculation of surface area from the conventional nomogram.

Most people spend about 8 out of the 24 hours resting in bed. During this period the mean metabolic rate does not differ significantly from the value predicted in table 4.7. Measurements made throughout the night have shown that values are usually a little higher on first going to bed, probably due to the effect of the last meal (p. 4.9), but they generally fall a little below the standard between 2 and 4 in the morning when the body's temperature is at a minimum. A night's rest normally costs 1·7–2·1 MJ (400–500 kcal).

PARTITIONING OF RESTING O_2 UTILIZATION
AMONGST THE SEVERAL ORGANS
Table 4.8 shows how the resting metabolism may be divided among the principal organs of the body. To obtain this data it is necessary to measure the rate of blood flow in the organs (p. 30.49) and also the O_2 content of their arterial and venous blood and then apply the Fick principle (p. 30.36). The development in the last 20 years of small plastic catheters which enable samples of blood from deep veins to be taken in man has made this possible.

TABLE 4.8. The partition of the resting oxygen utilization among the principal organs of a healthy man weighing 65 kg.

Organ	Oxygen used ml/min	Resting metabolism %
Liver (including the splanchnic area)	67	27
Brain	47	19
Heart	17	7
Kidney	26	10
Skeletal muscle	45	18
Remainder (by difference)	48	19
Total	250	100

The brain, which makes up less than 2·5 per cent of the body weight, is responsible for about 20 per cent of the energy consumption at rest. Students and office workers may be disappointed to learn that their hard work at the books involves no appreciable extra energy. In many experiments it has been impossible to show any increase in O_2 uptake when a subject previously resting and dozing is suddenly set complicated problems in mental arithmetic. By contrast, the rate of O_2 consumption of a resting muscle may be increased a hundredfold on exercise. The reader may also be surprised to find that his kidneys do more work than his heart—at least when he is resting. After reading chap. 35, he will appreciate what a complex task is the manufacture of urine.

EFFECT OF AGE

A newborn baby has an O_2 consumption of about 7·0 ml kg^{-1} min^{-1}, twice the rate of an adult on a basis of weight. The high rate of metabolism is caused by the energy requirements for growth. As the growth rate declines, the metabolism approaches the adult level. Table 4.9 gives values for the resting metabolism

TABLE 4.9. Resting metabolism of infants and young children.

Weight kg	Resting metabolism MJ/24 h	Resting metabolism kcal/24 h	Weight kg	Resting metabolism MJ/24 h	Resting metabolism kcal/24 h
3	0·6	150	7	1·6	390
4	0·9	210	8	1·9	445
5	1·1	270	9	2·1	495
6	1·4	330	10	2·5	590

of infants and very young children. As is customary, the figures are given in MJ (kcal)/24 h, which are convenient for calculating dietary energy needs. Table 4.10 gives values for older children and adolescents, which may be compared with the adult values in table 4.7. It can be seen that adolescents have a slightly higher metabolic

TABLE 4.10. Resting metabolism of older children and adolescents.

Weight kg	Boys kJ/min	Girls kJ/min	Weight kg	Boys kJ/min	Girls kJ/min
15	2·1	2·1	40	3·9	3·6
20	2·5	2·5	45	4·1	3·8
25	3·0	2·8	50	4·3	4·1
30	3·3	3·1	55	4·6	4·3
35	3·6	3·4	60	4·8	4·5

rate than adults of the same weight. The sex difference in table 4.10 arises because little girls are fatter than little boys, a distinction that occurs long before puberty.

The resting metabolic rate continues to decline throughout adult life, but slowly at a rate of about 2 per cent per decade. Standard values for octogenarians are about 85 per cent of those for young adults (table 4.7).

EFFECT OF FOOD

The metabolic rate is raised soon after a meal has been eaten and may continue above the fasting level for 4–6 hr. This is known as the **specific dynamic action** (SDA) of food. This is a very variable phenomenon. After most meals, it usually amounts to an increase of about 10–15 per cent, but if the meal is rich in protein the SDA may be as much as 30 per cent. After a test meal consisting of fat or carbohydrate only, it is sometimes absent or less than 5 per cent. The SDA immediately after a meal rich in protein is probably due to work done by the stomach in secreting digestive juices; later the effect certainly arises from the liver, associated with the metabolism of amino acids. Even after a large meal the metabolic rate is back to the normal resting level in the small hours of the next morning. Man has no means of 'burning off' the effects of gluttony. A dietary energy excess must either be worked off by exercise or stored as fat.

Starvation, either partial or complete and due either to disease or famine, invariably causes a fall in the resting metabolic rate. This is certainly due to a shrinkage of the cell mass and possibly also to a reduction in the metabolism in the tissues. This is an adaptive mechanism which helps to protect the body in times of scarcity.

EFFECT OF CLIMATE

Standards for resting metabolic rates were first drawn up in North America and in Western Europe. It was shown later that these were about 10 per cent too high for Calcutta, Singapore and elsewhere in the tropics. A racial difference was first suggested, but this is almost certainly not a fact. Careful studies on European visitors to Asia have shown that a fall in resting metabolic rate usually occurs in them, but this is not invariable. The change takes place slowly over 3–6 months. Conversely many students from tropical countries who have measured their resting metabolism in our laboratory have usually found values similar to those obtained by natives of Edinburgh. How climatic changes bring about these alterations is not understood.

EFFECT OF THYROID ACTIVITY

The thyroid hormones stimulate oxidations and heat production within the cells. In experimental animals, removal of the gland causes a marked fall in resting O_2 consumption, which is increased by injections of extracts of the gland. The disease, myxoedema (hypothyroidism) due to atrophy of the thyroid gland, is associated with very low levels of resting metabolic rates, which can be raised by treatment with thyroid hormones. Overactivity of the gland (hyperthyroidism) raises the metabolic rates sometimes to as much as double the normal rate. How the thyroid hormones work is discussed in chap. 27.

With a careful technique, measurements for resting metabolism should usually fall within ± 15 per cent of the standard values, but a few individuals with normal thyroid gland activity may have higher or lower rates. For many years the measurement of the resting metabolic rate was the most reliable method of assessing thyroid function and of checking progress in thyroid disease. Nowadays it is seldom used for this purpose, as other tests of thyroid function which are more convenient for both patient and doctor are available (vol. 3, p. 23.17).

EFFECTS OF PREGNANCY AND LACTATION

These are discussed in chap. 38.

Energy expenditure in everyday life

MAXIMUM RATES OF WORK

A student who is physically fit should be able to undertake exercise which involves an O_2 consumption of 4 l/min. This means multiplying his resting rate by sixteen times. In a few exceptional athletes, a **maximum oxygen uptake** of 5 l/min or even higher has been recorded. Many students can do no better than 3 l/min. An ability to work at high rates is essential for those who undertake heavy manual labour or compete in strenuous sports and recreations. However, a middle-aged or elderly man or someone with a disability of the heart or lungs is able to move around comfortably, do light work and enjoy light exercise, provided he can increase his resting O_2 consumption rate four times, i.e. up to 1 l/min with an energy expenditure of 20 kJ (5 kcal)/min. The details of the respiratory and cardiovascular adjustments needed to increase the supply of O_2 to the tissues are a main theme of chaps. 30 and 31.

CLASSIFICATION OF PHYSICAL ACTIVITIES

Table 4.11 gives a classification based on rates of energy expenditure. This was first drawn up from the measurements of rates of O_2 consumption by men in the Swedish iron-industry. However, it is also applicable to other industries and to sports and games. With a suitable modification for body weight, it can be applied to women. By dividing by twenty, the figures can be

TABLE 4.11. The grading of industrial work and physical activity.

| | Energy expenditure | |
| | Men kJ min^{-1} 65 kg^{-1} | Women kJ min^{-1} 55 kg^{-1} |
Grade		
Light	10–19	6–14
Moderate	20–29	15–23
Heavy	30–39	24–32
Very heavy	40–49	33–41
Unduly heavy	50–	42–

transposed into rates of O_2 consumption in l/min. This is the more convenient unit for the physiologist or doctor concerned with studies on the heart and lungs. The table provides a numerical definition of **light, moderate** and **heavy work**.

Table 4.12 gives examples of the energy expenditure of various physical activities. It is based on many thousands of measurements by indirect calorimetry. Obviously the grading can be only approximate. Thus most jobs

TABLE 4.12. Examples of the energy expenditure of various physical activities.

Light work at 10–19 kJ/min		Moderate work at 20–29 kJ/min	Heavy work at 30–39 kJ/min	Very heavy work at over 40 kJ/min
Assemby work	Building industry	General labouring (pick and shovel)	Coal mining (hewing and loading)	Lumber work
Light industry	Bricklaying	Agricultural work (non-mechanized)	Football	Furnace men (steel industry)
Electrical industry	Plastering	Route march with rifle and pack	Country dancing	Swimming (crawl)
Carpentry	Painting	Ballroom dancing		Cross country running
Military drill	Agricultural work (mechanized)	Gardening		Hill climbing
Most domestic work with modern appliances	Driving a truck	Tennis		
Gymnastic exercises	Golf	Cycling (up to 10 miles/h)		
	Bowling			

on a farm involve **moderate** work, but some are **heavy** and a few **light**. Similarly for most of us tennis is a sport demanding **moderate** physical activity, but a Wimbledon champion must do **heavy** work and some performers on our public courts appear to be taking very **light** exercise.

Sitting and standing

Each of us spends a large part of the day sitting and standing, when energy is needed by the muscles responsible for maintaining the posture of the body. Work may also be done using the muscles of the arms. These factors do not greatly increase the metabolic rate. When we are mobile and active, the major part of the work done is usually expended in moving the weight of the body. The energy expenditure of some 160 Glasgow men and women has been measured when sitting and standing in their homes and engaged in reading, listening to radio and watching television, etc. The mean values were above the mean resting value by 20 per cent when sitting and 50 per cent when standing. The maximum increases were 70 per cent when sitting and 100 per cent when standing. Fidgeting and apparent 'tension' does not raise the energy expenditure greatly. It is impossible to increase your rate of energy expenditure significantly without getting up and moving about.

Walking

Walking at a moderate speed of three and a half miles an hour (5·6 km/h) involves increasing the energy expenditure fourfold, up to about 20 kJ/min for an average man. Most of the work involved in walking is utilized in raising the centre of gravity at each step. The energy cost of walking is directly proportional to body weight and also to the speed, except at very low and very fast speeds, when the movements become relatively less efficient. The cost of walking is the same in both sexes. Table 4.13 gives predicted values for the cost of walking by persons of varying weight at different speeds. These predictions are based on many hundreds of measurements and are unlikely to be out by more than ±15 per cent. Walking is the most common physical activity. It may be prescribed by a doctor who wishes to alter the energy balance of an obese patient.

TABLE 4.13. Energy expended (kJ) during 10 min walking related to speed of walking and gross body weight.

Speed		Weight (kg)					
km/h	miles/h	45	55	65	75	85	95
3	1·9	90	110	120	135	150	165
4	2·5	110	130	145	165	180	200
5	3·1	130	150	170	190	215	235
6	3·8	150	175	195	215	245	270
7	4·4	170	195	220	250	275	305

DAILY RATES OF ENERGY EXPENDITURE

If the time spent by an individual in each of his various activities throughout the 24 hours is recorded and also the metabolic cost of each activity determined, then the daily energy expenditure rate can be calculated.

Energy expenditure (kJ or kcal/day)=time spent in activity (min) × metabolic cost of activity (kJ or kcal/min).

Table 4.14 shows examples of how healthy men might each spend a day. There is, of course, a wide variation in the nature of work done by persons in the same nominal occupation. A rough guide applicable to Britain is as follows:

Sedentary occupations, for which on average 11·0 MJ or 2700 kcal/day are required include office workers (all clerical tasks), drivers, pilots, teachers, journalists, clergy, doctors, lawyers, architects and shop workers.

Moderately active occupations, for which 12·5 MJ or 3000 kcal/day are required include virtually all those engaged in light industry and assembly plants, railway workers, postmen, joiners, slaters, plumbers and bus conductors; most farm workers and builders' labourers fall in this group.

Very active occupations, for which 15·0 MJ or 3600 kcal/day are required include coal miners, steel workers, dockers, foresters and army recruits; some farm workers, builders' labourers and unskilled labourers fall in this group.

The energy requirements of workers in many occupations depend on the amount of mechanical power available. For instance many farmers and workers in the building industry do heavy work, but on a modern farm or building site their occupation could not be classified as more than moderately active.

Most groups of women require on average 9·0 MJ or about 2200 kcal/day. This may be subdivided into

TABLE 4.14. Energy expenditure and range of requirements of food for individuals and recommended intakes for groups of men in different occupational groups. Modified from *Recommended Intakes of Nutrients for the United Kingdom*.

	Sedentary	Moderately active	Very active
	MJ/8 h	MJ/8 h	MJ/8 h
Energy expenditure			
In bed	2·0	2·0	2·0
At work	3·5	5·0	7·5
Non-occupational	3·5–7·5	3·5–7·5	3·5–7·5
	MJ/24 h	MJ/24 h	MJ/24 h
Energy requirement from food	9·0–13·0	10·5–14·5	13·0–17·0
Recommended intake for a group	11·0	12·5	15·0

1·75 MJ or about 420 kcal/8 h in bed, 3·50 MJ or about 880 kcal/8 h for occupational activity in the home, an office or light industry and 3·75 MJ or about 900 kcal/8 h for non-occupational activity.

How far the requirement indicated above represents a true value for any population is uncertain. Table 4.15 sets out the results of surveys of the energy expenditure of various occupational groups amongst the people of

TABLE 4.15. Daily rates of energy expenditure by individuals with varying occupations.

Occupation	Energy expenditure MJ/day		
	Mean	Minimum	Maximum
MEN			
Elderly retired	9·6	7·2	11·6
Office workers	10·4	7·5	13·5
Colliery clerks	11·6	9·6	13·6
Laboratory technicians	11·7	9·3	15·8
Elderly industrial workers	11·7	9·0	15·3
University students	12·1	9·4	18·2
Building workers	12·4	10·1	15·5
Steel workers	13·6	10·8	16·4
Farmers	14·1	12·0	16·5
Coal miners	15·1	12·3	18·9
Forestry workers	15·2	11·8	19·0
WOMEN			
Elderly housewives	7·9	6·1	10·0
Middle-aged housewives	8·6	7·3	9·6
Laboratory technicians	8·8	5·5	10·5
Assistants in department stores	9·3	7·5	11·8
University students	9·5	5·7	10·8
Factory workers	9·6	8·1	12·3
Bakery workers	10·4	8·2	14·0

Scotland, carried out by Dr John Durnin of Glasgow University. Each survey covered a whole week. The reader will notice the enormous variations in each group; thus the most active university student, both male and female, expended almost twice as much energy as the most sedentary. This is due to the different uses of leisure time. In a modern industrial society very few people do much heavy work in the course of earning their living and this is usually achieved by a man with about 5·0 MJ (1200 kcal)/day or less. He may expend far more energy, over 8·3 MJ (2000 kcal)/day, if he pursues active recreations enthusiastically. On the other hand nowadays there is an increasing number of people who prefer to spend their leisure time sitting, perhaps watching television, or driving around in their car admiring what is left of the countryside. The new modern man, *homo sedentarius*, expends much less energy than his predecessor. So does the modern woman. Housework may appear tiring, but this is usually because many women

find it boring. Except in a large house, where there are several small children, it seldom involves heavy work.

The existence of *homo sedentarius* is well recognized in the United States. The Food and Nutrition Board of the United States Academy of Science in 1968 reduced the food allowances to 10·8 MJ (2600 kcal)/day for men aged 35–55 years and to 8·3 MJ (2000 kcal)/day for women. This certainly is in keeping with the modern American way of life, in which no one appears to walk if this can possibly be avoided. Yet this recommendation that Americans need less food may be unsound and perhaps the real need is for more exercise. *Homo sedentarius* may not be a healthy specimen. He is certainly prone to obesity, and obesity, as the figures of the American life insurance companies show, predisposes to heart disease and diabetes.

The regulation of food intake to meet requirements is dependent upon the central nervous system (chap. 25). The various factors that may disturb this regulation and lead to obesity are discussed in vol. 3, p. 24.37.

PEASANT AGRICULTURALISTS

The majority of the people of the world do not live in prosperous industrial urban societies. They are peasants, who get their living from their land. How hard do peasants work? Certainly the answer is very heavy at harvest and seed time, when 12 hours a day may be spent in the fields. Much agricultural work involves energy expenditure rates of 21 kJ (5 kcal)/min or over. However, all agricultural work is seasonal. Surveys in Africa and India have indicated that peasants spend from 855 to 1700 h a year at work in their fields. These figures correspond to 16–33 h/week. Thus the overall rate of energy expenditure may be no more than that of an industrial population.

THE FUTURE

Until 200 years ago, when the industrial revolution began, human muscles, supplemented by those of horses and oxen, provided the power that made civilization possible. Muscles did the work of the field, built the great temples and cathedrals, transported men and their armies about the world, spun and wove the fibres for clothing and tapestries, thrashed and ground the corn. Only in the last respect was a little power available from wind and water mills. In industrial societies all this has changed. Men and women have become creatures who flick switches that control large sources of power. In such societies, there is little necessity for them to use their muscles for anything but the lightest activity. At the same time working hours have been greatly reduced and the 35-hour week is now commonplace. With the better organization of industries, there is little doubt that a 20-hour week would suffice for doing the necessary work in a modern technical society. There is already much more time for leisure than formerly and this is likely to increase greatly.

NATIONAL FOOD NEEDS

The countries of the world can be divided roughly into two groups. In the rich countries in North America, Europe and in Oceania, agriculture and trade produce a plentiful supply of food. Indeed surplus crops have become an economic embarrassment. In these countries obesity is common, with all its consequent ill health. In the poor countries mostly in Asia, Africa and in Latin America, where the majority of the world's population live as peasant farmers, the food supply rarely measures up to the energy needs of the population. Hunger is commonplace, especially at the season before the harvest is due. The threat of famine and starvation is often not far away.

The transfer of the surplus crops and food products of the rich countries to the poor countries has been effectively carried out on occasions to meet special needs. Many millions of children have benefited from the dried milk supplied through the United Nations and national agencies. Surplus grains from the U.S.A. and other countries have averted serious famine in Asia and in Africa. However, the economic processes of normal trade have proved unable to distribute the world's food according to the physiological needs of the people and there is no sign that this will ever become possible. The poor countries have, for the most part, little to export which can balance their imports of foods. In most poor countries, agricultural production is increasing, but at a rate which is barely keeping up with the increase in population and in some countries it is falling behind. The only solution to the problem other than a catastrophic increase in the death rate due to war, famine or epidemic disease appears to be a rational and planned limitation of the birth rate. Fortunately, this is at last becoming generally realized and many poor countries have now commenced active family planning programmes (vol. 3,

p. 71.8). Whether these can be developed sufficiently rapidly to prevent the catastrophes which must arise when the people of a country outgrow their food supplies, only the future can tell.

It is probable that many, perhaps most, of the present generation of medical students will practise their profession in a country where there is either a superabundance of food or an inadequate supply. In either instance their clinical practice will include many difficult nutritional problems resulting from energy imbalance. They will also have the opportunity to use their influence to bring about administrative measures to alleviate or reduce such imbalances. In planning and carrying out a sound food policy for their country, all governments should depend upon the advice of their medical profession.

FURTHER READING

DAVIDSON SIR STANLEY, PASSMORE R., BROCK J.F. & TRUSWELL A.S. (1975) *Human Nutrition and Dietetics*, 6th Edition. Edinburgh: Churchill Livingstone.

DEPARTMENT OF HEALTH AND SOCIAL SECURITY (1969) Recommended Intakes of Nutrients for the United Kingdom. *Reports on Public Health and Medical Subjects* No. 120. London: H.M.S.O.

DURNIN J.V.G.A. & PASSMORE R. (1967) *Energy, Work and Leisure*. London: Heinemann.

FAO/WHO EXPERT COMMITTEE (1973) Energy and Protein Requirements. *Technical Reports of the World Health Organization* No. 522.

McCANCE R.A. & WIDDOWSON E.M. (1960) The Composition of Foods, 3rd Edition. *Medical Research Council Special Report Series* No. 297. London: H.M.S.O.

URBELOHDE A.R. (1963) *Man and Energy*. Harmondsworth: Penguin.

Chapter 5
Essential materials and waste

A policeman in the course of his duty may have to observe carefully everything and everybody who enters and leaves a house. His observations are likely to provide police headquarters with valuable clues, but not with sufficient evidence to charge anyone for criminal behaviour within the house. Before this can be done, it is usually necessary to get a warrant to enter and search.

It is comparatively easy for a physiologist to study both qualitatively and quantitatively the food and water consumed by a human body, and also the expired air, urine and faeces that leave it. Material is also lost in the sweat, in the menstrual fluid and milk, and in the form of a new-born baby. This chapter is concerned with the daily credits and debits of material, which are required to maintain the structures within the body and provide its energy. The cells and tissues of the body are not static structures. They are continually being turned over, and substances replaced at varying rates. Many of the chemical components set free by the breakdown of substances within the cells are utilized again to synthesize new tissues. Some, however, cannot be so used and are lost in the excreta, and these have to be made good from the diet. In a healthy adult, who is neither gaining nor losing weight, the dietary intake of each of the elements must exactly balance the excretory losses. It is a common practice both in clinical medicine and in research to draw up a balance for N, Ca, Na and K. It is also possible, but much more difficult, to determine the balance for C, H, Fe, S and indeed for any element which forms part of the structure of the body.

NUTRIENTS

The chemical components of a diet are referred to as nutrients. These may be classified as carbohydrates, fats, proteins and alcohol (the sources of energy), water and electrolytes, minerals and vitamins.

CARBOHYDRATES

These provide the chief source of energy in most diets. About 50 per cent of the total energy in the diet of a prosperous industrial community comes from carbohydrate. In a poor agricultural community, living largely on cereals, the proportion is higher and may be up to 85 per cent.

Masai warriors, Eskimos, South American gauchos and others who may live on foods entirely of animal origin have practically no carbohydrate in their diet. As these people are vigorous and healthy, carbohydrate is not a dietary essential. The explanation is that the body can form glucose from certain amino acids (p. 11.20) and from glycerol which is a component of fat (p. 10.2).

Starch

The chief dietary carbohydrate is starch, which is present in all cereal grains, roots and tubers. The starch molecule is a polysaccharide composed of several hundred glucose units linked together and forming two chains (p. 9.4). The small amount of glycogen (animal starch, p. 9.9) present in meat and other tissues makes only a trivial contribution to the diet.

Unavailable carbohydrate or dietary fibre

Plant cells have walls which are mainly composed of hemicellulose and cellulose. These, like starch, are polymers of smaller carbohydrate molecules. These chains cannot be broken down by the digestive juices of man and other mammals. However, protozoa and bacteria present in the alimentary canal of ruminants (cattle and sheep) and herbivores (rabbits and horses) contain cellulase and so can digest them and make the resultant material available as a source of energy for the animal host. The average British diet provides 4·2 g/day of fibre, of which 61, 26 and 13 per cent come from vegetables, fruit and nuts, and cereals respectively. Vegetarians may consume up to 20 g/day. Peasant communities living on coarse cereals, in Africa and elsewhere, may have fibre intakes as high as 25 g/day. A high fibre diet increases the bulk of the faeces and accelerates the passage of food through the intestines. This may be responsible for the much lower incidence of diverticular disease in many African countries than in Europe and North America (vol. 3, p. 19.108). The amount and nature of the dietary fibre affect the bacterial flora in the gut. Bacterial metabolism in the gut is partly responsible for the fate of the bile salts (p. 33.7) and so may modify concentrations of plasma cholesterol. These effects and their possible consequences to health are now the subject of much research.

Sugar

The familiar table sugar is **sucrose**, a disaccharide in which the constituent hexose units are glucose and fructose. Sucrose is manufactured from sugar-cane in the tropics and from sugar-beet in temperate regions. **Lactose** is the disaccharide present in the milk of all mammals and is made up of glucose and galactose units. **Maltose** is a disaccharide composed of two glucose units. It is formed from starch in the malting of barley and other cereals for brewing. The two monosaccharides **glucose** and **fructose** are made commercially by the hydrolysis of sucrose. They are present, in small quantities, in most fruits. Significant amounts of glucose may be present in grapes and of fructose in honey.

A normal diet may contain from 300 to 500 g of carbohydrate daily, providing 5·0–8·0 MJ (about 1200–2000 kcal). In traditional diets most of this is provided as starch in cereal grains, but in recent years in all prosperous countries an increasing proportion has come from sugar.

Nearly all the dietary carbohydrate is oxidized in the body to carbon dioxide and water, and the carbon is excreted as CO_2 in the expired air. The faeces contain all the fibre present in the diet, but negligible amounts of other carbohydrates. The urine contains citric acid, lactic acid and other intermediary products of carbohydrate metabolism and it may also contain traces of sugars. In health, the daily excretion of these substances is measured in milligrams. Less than 0·2 per cent of the carbon in the dietary intake of carbohydrate appears in the urine.

FATS

This is the second largest source of energy in most diets. In the United Kingdom fat supplies about 40 per cent of our energy. A normal diet for an active man may contain 140 g of fat, providing 5·2 MJ (1260 kcal)/day. In a modern diet about half the fat is eaten as table fat and about half is 'hidden fat', present in cakes, puddings, sauces, etc. Foods rich in fat are expensive and there is a close association between average national income and fat intake. Many people living in poverty get only 10–20 g of fat/day and such diets are almost always deficient in the fat-soluble vitamin A (p. 5.13). There are also certain fatty acids, the essential fatty acids (EFA), which animal tissues cannot synthesize and which must be supplied in the diet. These are polyunsaturated fatty acids (p. 10.1).

Animals fed on artificial diets devoid of these acids fail to thrive and develop a scaly dermatitis, but EFA deficiency has never been satisfactorily demonstrated in human beings on natural diets. Human requirements for EFA are certainly low, probably only 2–3 g/day, an amount which is provided by even the poorest natural diets. Diets rich in EFA lower the concentration of cholesterol and other lipids in the plasma and this may have a protective action against the development of atherosclerosis which is one form of arterial disease responsible for most cases of coronary thrombosis (vol. 3, p. 17.13).

Fat has an energy value more than twice that of carbohydrate and hence it provides a more concentrated form of energy. Polar explorers and others who may need 25 MJ (6000 kcal)/day may eat up to 300 g of fat daily, otherwise their diet would be impossibly bulky. Such large amounts of fat can be digested, absorbed and metabolized by very active men.

The diet contains many lipids, but the most important as a source of energy are the triglycerides, whose chemical structure is discussed in detail on p. 10.2. Here it is sufficient to state that a high proportion of saturated fatty acids in the triglyceride molecule gives fat which is solid at room temperature. This includes all animal and dairy fats, except marine fats. The triglycerides present in plants and in marine oils contain relatively more unsaturated fatty acids and are liquid at room temperature. The artificial hardening of these oils by hydrogenation of the double bonds in the unsaturated fatty acids is the basis of the margarine industry.

Fats play an important part in making foods palatable and a good cook needs a plentiful and varied supply. During World War II, the supply of oils and fats in the United Kingdom fell from the pre-war figures of 45·3 to 37·0 lb/head/year. This caused much discontent, although the supply remained far greater than was essential for physiological purposes.

The greater part of the dietary fat is oxidized in the body and the carbon is excreted as CO_2. The faeces always contain some fat, usually less than 5 per cent of the intake. The urine also contains traces of an intermediary product of fat metabolism, acetoacetic acid, and of its derivative β-hydroxybutyric acid. In health the amounts are so small that they can be neglected, but if the metabolism of carbohydrate is reduced greatly, as may happen in partial starvation or in diabetes mellitus, these acids are produced in large amounts and are then excreted in the urine. This condition is known as ketoacidosis and is discussed on p. 10.14.

PROTEINS

Protein in the diet is essential to replace the continuous breakdown of the body proteins. Each day in a normal man 200–400 g of protein, about 3·5 per cent of the total protein present in the body, may be destroyed and resynthesized. The amino acids formed by the breakdown may in part be used again, but an additional dietary source is also necessary. The national diet in the United Kingdom provides on average 93 g/day of protein, but this is certainly more than is necessary to maintain the tissues. This could be done by most adults with a daily dietary intake of 20–40 g. Many years ago it was recommended that the diet should contain 1 g protein/kg body weight and this is still sound advice. It provides a wide margin of safety and allows for the great variation in the minimal needs of individuals which is known to exist.

The protein needs of children are relatively greater than those of adults. A newborn baby requires about five times as much protein as an adult per unit of body weight. This requirement falls as the rate of growth declines, but toddlers need about two and a half times as much as adults and adolescents about one and a half times more. Unless these amounts are provided in the diet the child will not grow to its full potential. Poor children in all countries are liable to get an inadequate supply of protein. As a result they grow up small and stunted. In the poorer countries of the world, many children are weaned from the breast on to a diet containing little or no milk and in which the main constituent is carbohydrate of cereal origin. Amongst such children a severe and often fatal wasting disease with the West African name of kwashiorkor is common (vol. 3, p. 24.8). The production and distribution of protein foods suitable for very young children and the education of mothers in their use is perhaps the most important medical problem in many underdeveloped countries of the world.

Amino acids

Proteins are made up of amino acids, joined together by peptide bonds. The varying arrangements of the sequence of the amino acids in protein molecules give them different chemical properties and also their individuality. Each of us contains some proteins which are different from those of our neighbour (unless he is our identical twin). The number of amino acids commonly found in the proteins of the human body is approximately the same as the numbers of letters in the alphabet. The various combinations in which they can be arranged (p. 12.4) allow an infinite variety of proteins to be synthesized, in the same way as the letters of the alphabet allow an infinite number of sentences to be constructed. Some of the amino acids cannot be synthesized in the body and a dietary supply is necessary. These are known as essential amino acids and are discussed on p. 11.14.

Quality of proteins

Certain proteins, e.g. those in eggs and human milk, supply the amino acids in proportions well suited for the synthesis of human proteins. Other proteins are relatively deficient in one or more amino acids. These proteins are thus of relatively less value in the diet. Maize proteins are relatively lacking in tryptophan, wheat proteins in lysine, potato, cassava and many other vegetable proteins in the sulphur-containing amino acids. These amino acids are called the **limiting amino acids** of the particular proteins; the relative amount of this acid in a dietary protein determines its biological value (p. 11.16). Most dietary proteins have a biological value of 40–80 per cent of that of an ideal mixture of proteins such as is present in egg. Fortunately different vegetable proteins have different limiting amino acids and they are able to **supplement** each other. Thus it is possible, by blending suitable vegetable proteins, to produce a mixture which has almost the same biological value as casein in milk. In underdeveloped countries, where the milk supply is defective, artificial vegetable 'milks' can be manufactured and this is an important public health measure. For adults also, especially in underdeveloped countries, it is important that too large a proportion of the dietary protein should not come from one source. Traditional mixtures such as 'bread and cheese' and 'rice and dhal' are practical examples of the value of a mixture of proteins in a poor man's diet.

Nitrogen balance

As already mentioned the N present in the proteins is excreted in the urine mostly in the form of urea. By comparing the N in the diet with the total N excreted it is possible to tell whether a subject is gaining or losing protein from the tissues. A negative N balance (N excretion greater than the dietary N intake) occurs in starvation and in wasting diseases such as prolonged infections or fevers. A positive N balance occurs in a growing child or in a patient who is recovering from a wasting disease. Table 5.1 is an example of the effect of varying the dietary protein intake on the N balance. The subject was a young woman whose diet was restricted because of obesity and contained only 24 g of protein. The intake of N was 3·9 g/day and the total excretion estimated at 6·5 g/day. The N balance was therefore $3·9 - 6·5 = -2·6$ g/day. This is equivalent to a loss of tissue protein of $2·6 \times 6·25 = 16·25$ g/day. Her dietary protein was therefore insufficient and, as the object of the diet was to remove excess fat and not to cause wasting of muscle and other tissues, the diet was changed; part of the carbohydrate and fat was replaced by protein to make the total protein intake 80 g/day. Table 5.1 shows that on this diet she was in positive N balance, indicating that the dietary protein was now more than adequate for her needs.

It will be seen that most of the N output is in the urine and the amount in the faeces is small and in this instance not increased by the extra dietary protein. The faecal N comes in part from undigested food, but also from the

TABLE 5.1. Nitrogen balances of a young woman on two reducing diets: A containing 24, and B containing 80 g protein/day. All values expressed as g N/day.

	A	B
Intake		
Food	3·9	12·7
Output		
Urine	5·3	9·3
Faeces	0·7	0·6
Skin	(0·5)	(0·5)
	6·5	10·4
Balance	−2·6	+2·3

protein present in the digestive juices and in the epithelial lining of the gut, which is being continuously shed and renewed. There is also a continuous loss of N in the dead superficial cells, which are rubbed off the skin, in sweat and in the growth of nails and hair. These losses are small compared with those in the urine and are also extremely difficult to measure. In table 5.1 an arbitrary figure has been inserted, based on figures in the literature. It is much easier to collect and analyse urine than faeces. As the faecal losses are relatively small, in the absence of diarrhoea, faecal collection is often omitted. The subject can usually be assumed to be in positive balance if less than 90 per cent of the dietary intake of N appears in the urine.

Sulphur (S at.wt. 32)

The sulphur-containing amino acids, cysteine and methionine, provide from 20–50 mmol (0·6–1·6 g) of sulphur in the diet. The exact amount depends on both the quantity and quality of the dietary protein. In the metabolism of these amino acids H^+ and SO_4^{--} ions are formed. A high protein diet in this way contributes to the acidity of the urine (p. 5.29). The diet also contains a little sulphate and the total urinary sulphur may be up to 60 mmol (2 g)/day. Most of this is excreted as sulphate, but there is always a little organic sulphur present.

WATER

The body has three sources of water, (1) the water present in the food, (2) the water drunk and (3) the water formed by the oxidation in the tissues of the hydrogen present in the foodstuffs (metabolic water).

Water is lost in three ways, (1) in the urine, (2) in the alimentary canal and (3) by evaporation. There is an obligatory water loss by evaporation from the lungs and skin. The expired air is always saturated with water vapour at body temperature and water is evaporated from the skin, even when there is no sweating. Much of this is absorbed by underclothes, which are heavier and damper in the evening than when they were put on fresh in the morning.

Table 5.2 shows the measured intake and output of water by a young man leading a sedentary life in a temperate climate. These are normal values. The amount of water in the food depends on the nature of the diet and is normally about 1000 g but may be much less on a dry diet. The water drunk is also variable and usually amounts to between 1000 and 1500 g/day. However, several litres may be drunk in a hot climate or by someone who works in a hot environment. The metabolic water depends on how much carbohydrate, fat and protein is oxidized and amounts to between 200 and 400 g/day.

TABLE 5.2. The water balance in a young man leading a sedentary life (data are g/day and the mean of measurements over a 4 day period).

Intake		Output	
Water in food	800	Urinary water	1515
Water drunk	1300	Faecal water	25
Metabolic water	255	Evaporative water	810
	2355		2350

The urinary water is usually between 1000 and 1500 g/day. Normally very little water is lost from the alimentary canal and in formed faeces the output is up to 150 g/day. The evaporative water plays an important part in cooling the body. It is related to energy expenditure and usually accounts for about 25 per cent of total heat losses.

A negative water balance can arise in the following ways:

(1) if the water supply is curtailed or if, for any reason, a patient is unable to drink,

(2) if there are excessive losses from the alimentary tract, as occurs in diarrhoea and vomiting. Many litres of fluid may be lost in this way,

(3) if there is excessive sweating. Men working in hot climates may readily lose 6 kg/day of water in the sweat and losses as high as 12 kg/day have been reported,

(4) if there is excessive loss in the expired air. On high mountains the air is very cold and dry and so more water is required to humidify the expired air. Further, the volume of expired air is increased owing to the stimulus to respiration from the lowered oxygen pressure in the atmosphere (p. 46.2). It has been estimated that Everest climbers may lose water at the rate of 2–3 kg/day by this route and it is probable that members of several expeditions became dehydrated in this way,

(5) if the kidneys fail to retain water, as may occur in diabetes insipidus and in other uncommon diseases.

There is no true reserve of water in the human body. A normal adult male contains about 40 kg in his body. If he is 2 kg short, he is likely to be very thirsty; if he is 4 kg short he may well be very ill; and he will probably be dead before he has lost 8 kg. Even in a cold climate with no excessive sweating, a man will not survive more than about 4–6 days without water on account of the continuous obligatory water losses.

The full water balance that is set out in table 5.2 cannot easily be determined and a well equipped laboratory or metabolic ward is needed to do so. Fortunately it is seldom necessary for this to be done. It will be observed that in the table the water drunk approximately equals the urinary water. A fluid chart, on which all that a patient drinks and all the fluid that may be given intravenously and also the urinary output, are recorded, is frequently kept in hospitals. Clinical disturbances of water balance are described in vol. 3, p. 49.2.

ELECTROLYTES AND MINERALS

Sodium (Na$^+$ at.wt. 23)

The body of a healthy adult man contains just under 4 mol of sodium. The greater part of this is present in the extracellular fluids. This, together with the much smaller portion in the cells, can be measured by the dilution technique using ^{24}Na. The total exchangeable sodium amounts to about 40 mmol/kg of body weight. Up to 1·4 mol of sodium is present in bone, mostly in an unionized form which does not exchange rapidly with sodium in the extracellular fluid. Hence it does not provide a mobile reserve which can be drawn upon in acute sodium deficiency.

The dietary intake is very variable and in different individuals usually ranges from 70 to 350 mmol/day, corresponding to about 4–20 g of NaCl. The sodium content of the earth is not high and most natural foods contain little sodium. There are still a few primitive people in the world who are ignorant of the use of common salt and their daily intake may be only 30 mmol/day or less. Early in all civilizations common salt came into use as a food preservative and man rapidly developed a taste for it. Besides the table salt we each may add to our food, bakers and dairymen add salt to our bread and to our butter. All preserved and canned meats contain large amounts, as do most sauces, and cooks salt all vegetables. A diet low in salt is valuable in several types of diseases of the kidneys, the heart and the liver. All patients find even a minor restriction of their salt intake unpleasant and a severe restriction is almost intolerable and can seldom be borne for more than two or three weeks. Civilized man is certainly habituated to salt and perhaps can even be described as being dependent on it.

The output of salt by the kidneys closely parallels the dietary intake. However large the dietary intake, salt is not retained by a healthy individual and is promptly excreted in the urine. All land animals have evolved in an environment which is poor in sodium. The ability to conserve this element has been essential for survival. The human kidney is capable of protecting the salt content of the body and, if the need arises, can secrete a urine which is almost free of sodium and chloride (p. 35.17).

The faeces normally only contain about 5 mmol/day, but considerable loss may occur if there is diarrhoea. Visible sweat contains from 20–80 mmol/l. No salt is lost in the insensible evaporative water losses from the skin. Table 5.3 shows the balance in a young man leading a sedentary life in a temperate climate.

A negative sodium balance leading to sodium deficiency is common in hospital patients in the tropics. Their normal diet is often low in sodium and there is a continual loss in the sweat, which may easily amount to 200 mmol/day. A fever with the consequent increase in sweating, or a minor gastrointestinal disturbance with diarrhoea, each increases sodium losses and hence may precipitate sodium deficiency. Sodium depletion occurs less commonly in temperate climates, and arises from severe or prolonged vomiting or diarrhoea, and in some forms of kidney and endocrine disease.

Salt deficiency leads to a reduction in the volume of the extracellular fluid and of the blood. When it develops slowly and is of moderate severity, the symptoms are dizziness, fainting, weakness and mental confusion; there may be hypotension on standing. Acute severe

TABLE 5.3. The daily sodium and potassium balance of a young man leading a sedentary life on a normal diet. Mean of five daily measurements.

	Sodium mmol/day	Potassium mmol/day
Intake		
Food	135	60
Condiments	0	0
	135	60
Output		
Urine	130	55
Faeces	5	10
Skin	negligible	negligible
	135	65
Balance	0	−5

deficiency leads to shock with a marked fall in blood pressure (p. 30.51). It is also the cause of miner's cramp, well known to those who work underground in hot mines in any part of the world. A traditional remedy is for the miner to add salt to his beer. Clinical disturbances of sodium metabolism are described in vol. 3, p. 49.9.

Potassium (K+ at.wt. 39)

The body of a healthy adult male contains about 3·5 mol of potassium. Over 95 per cent of this is present as intracellular potassium and can be measured by the dilution technique using ^{42}K or by using a whole body counter to measure the natural isotope ^{40}K. Exchangeable potassium amounts to about 70 mmol/kg lean body mass and 55 mmol/kg total body weight.

All cells in both animals and plants are rich in potassium and in consequence most natural whole foods contain the element. Fruit juices are an especially rich source. Probably potassium deficiency never occurs as a result of a natural dietary deficiency. Intakes usually range between 40 and 90 mmol/day. The faeces contain a little more potassium than sodium, usually about 10 mmol/day. The sweat contains very little potassium. The urinary potassium normally approximates to the dietary intake. Table 5.3 shows the potassium balance in a young man.

Potassium depletion commonly arises from the increased losses associated with vomiting and diarrhoea. It may also follow from the continued use of purgatives. Excessive loss in the urine may occur in renal and endocrine disease and as a result of the use of certain drugs, notably diuretics (vol. 2, p. 11.6).

In all wasting diseases and following trauma where there is a breakdown in the cell structure, the intracellular potassium escapes into the extracellular fluid and blood and is in part excreted in the urine. All patients who are wasted, from whatever the cause, are liable to be deficient in potassium, which must be made good as part of their rehabilitation.

Deficiency of potassium causes muscle weakness, dizziness, thirst, polyuria, and mental confusion. It also interferes with the excitability of tissues, demonstrable in the heart by changes in the electrocardiogram (p. 30.13). Clinical disturbances of potassium metabolism are described in Vol. 3, p. 49.21.

Anions

The chief anions in the diet are chloride and phosphate. The chloride intake is similar to the sodium intake because of their association in dietary salt. The excretory losses of chloride usually run parallel to those of sodium, but the effect of Cl^- depletion as distinct from Na^+ is described on p. 35.35. Intake and output of phosphate are best discussed in relation to calcium, because of their close association in bone formation.

Calcium (Ca++ at.wt. 40)

Calcium is necessary for the formation and maintenance of bone, as is iron for the manufacture of the pigment haemoglobin, present in the red blood cells.

It has been mentioned already that very little sodium and potassium is present in the faeces. This is because the salts of these two elements are soluble in water and so are readily absorbed from the gut. In contrast, calcium, magnesium and iron form many salts which are either insoluble or only sparingly soluble. All diets contain calcium, magnesium and iron in quantities which easily meet the body's need, if they could be absorbed. However, the greater part of the dietary divalent ions and iron passes through the alimentary canal and is lost in the faeces. The problems of the supply of both calcium and iron are essentially the provision of a diet from which they can be absorbed in adequate amounts.

An adult human skeleton contains about 30 mol (1·2 kg) of calcium. This takes about 20 years to manufacture, so the growing child and adolescent must retain on average about 4 mmol or 160 mg/day of calcium. The skeleton is not a permanent structure, but is being continually renewed. Studies with isotopes indicate that in an adult about 17 mmol or 700 mg of calcium are reabsorbed from bone and replaced daily (p. 17.17). Some of this calcium can be utilized again, but there is always a loss in the urine which must be made good from the diet. Fig. 5.1 shows the calcium exchanges in a young European.

Typical European diets provide about 25 mmol (1 g)/day of calcium and about 20 mmol passes into the faeces. The only rich dietary source is milk. Cow's milk contains about 30 mmol/l (120 mg/100 ml), so 0·5 litre (just under 1 pint) goes a long way to meet the requirements of either

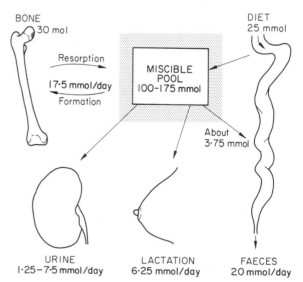

FIG. 5.1. Typical values for the calcium exchanges in the human body.

a child or adult. The calcium in milk is concentrated in cheese and most cheeses are very rich sources, providing about 600 mg/100 g. Human milk contains much less calcium than cow's milk, about 6 mmol/l (25 mg/100 ml). A mother who is nursing her baby will put out up to 6·5 mmol (250 mg)/day of calcium in her milk, and this must be replaced in her diet. Milk is a good source of protein as well as calcium and the protein probably facilitates the absorption of calcium, as the calcium salts of amino acids are relatively soluble.

Cereals, fruits and vegetables all contain calcium, but in very varying amounts. The calcium in cereals is made in part unavailable by the presence in the whole cereal grain of an organic acid, phytic acid, which forms an insoluble calcium salt. Phytic acid is not absorbed from the gut and calcium phytate is lost in the faeces. Most of the phytic acid is in the germ and outer pericarp of the grain, which is removed by milling. Thus calcium is much more readily absorbed from bread made from highly-milled white flour than from bread made from whole-meal flour. In the United Kingdom calcium lactate is artificially added to flour. The reason for this is as follows.

In making white bread about 70 per cent of the whole wheat grain is used. The remaining 30 per cent, which includes the indigestible fibre (p. 5.1) in the outer coats, is sold by the millers as cattle food. In 1940–1, many ships carrying grain from Canada and the USA to the UK were sunk by German submarines in the Battle of the Atlantic. In these circumstances, it seemed wasteful to use only 70 per cent of the cargo for human food, so it was decided to make all bread from a flour in which 85 per cent of the whole grain was extracted. This 'national flour' contained more phytic acid than white flour: experiments on man showed that its use increased the losses of calcium in the faeces. To make good these losses, the flour was 'enriched' by the addition of calcium lactate. This was sensible. However, when in peace time we reverted to bread made from white flour, the order to enrich the flour was not repealed. We continue to add calcium to our bread. Whether anyone now derives any benefit from this measure is uncertain.

Other substances that may make calcium unavailable include oxalic acid and free fatty acids. Rhubarb and certain other vegetables and fruits contain oxalates, but the amounts normally eaten are not sufficient to have any practical effect on calcium absorption. If fats are improperly absorbed as may happen in disease of the small intestine, there is an excess of unesterified fatty acids in the gut and these form insoluble calcium soaps, which are excreted in the faeces. Thinning and weakening of the bones, arising in this way, is a common consequence of long standing intestinal disease.

It was formerly thought that the intake of phosphates had an important effect on calcium absorption. However, it has been shown in adults that large intakes of phosphorus do not inhibit calcium absorption. Nevertheless, the phosphate intake may be more important for infants, and in artificial milk preparations for infant feeding it is probably wise to keep the phosphate and calcium proportions within the limits normally found in natural milk (table 5.6, p. 5.23).

TABLE 5.4. The principal sources of calcium in national diets (mg/head/day).

	Total calcium	Calcium from milk	Calcium from cereals	Calcium from vegetables
United Kingdom	1024	591	290*	46
USA	1116	856	29	135
India	347	147	165†	23

* Of this 243 mg was artificially added calcium.
† Of this 67 mg was provided by pulses.

So far this account of calcium has been an essentially European one. Table 5.4 sets out the national intake of calcium in the United Kingdom, the USA, where European diets are eaten, and in India. The figures for India are typical of many countries in Asia and Africa where the milk supply is small. Despite the low calcium intake there is no evidence that Asian and African bones are in any way inferior to European and American bones. They have the same calcium content and are no more liable to fractures. It is certain that on these low calcium diets, Asians and Africans absorb a higher proportion of the calcium than Europeans do on their diets. Those who live on diets rich in calcium are probably 'dis-adapted' to calcium absorption in some way. This may be due to the loss of an enzyme phytase in the alimentary canal, which can split the calcium phytate. When Europeans have been given low calcium diets experimentally, most of them have acquired the ability to absorb a greater proportion of the calcium than when on their usual diets. This change takes place gradually over many months.

Although the bones of people who are brought up in countries where there is little milk are of good quality, they are usually small. Milk provides protein and calcium necessary for bone formation, but the lack of dietary protein is probably the factor that most commonly limits growth. It has been shown that giving calcium lactate to children on diets which contain little milk does not accelerate growth. Giving extra protein does. It would be much easier and cheaper for a country such as India to enrich rice with calcium than to provide extra protein for the growing children. Unfortunately this measure would probably do no good.

The urinary output of calcium varies widely in individuals and 1–7 mmol (50–300 mg)/day is the normal adult range in health. This may be related to variations in intestinal absorption and in turnover rates in bone.

Calcium besides being necessary for bone development is also essential for the normal excitability of tissues. In severe calcium deficiency the motor nerves become readily excitable and twitching and spasm of the muscles, especially of the face, hands and feet occurs. This is known as tetany (p. 27.25). The roles of Ca^{++} in muscle contractility and blood coagulation are described on pp. 16.8 and 28.15 respectively.

Magnesium (Mg^{++} at.wt. 24)

The body of a healthy man contains about 1 mol (24 g) of magnesium. About two-thirds of this is present as bone mineral and most of the remainder is in the intracellular fluid where it is the most important cation after potassium. The ion plays an essential role in many enzymic reactions.

A typical diet contains 10–20 mmol (240–480 mg) most of which is not absorbed and appears in the faeces. Only about 4 mmol/day appears in the urine. Like potassium, magnesium is widely distributed in foods and a primary dietary deficiency probably never arises. Magnesium depletion, however, is often present in patients with prolonged diarrhoea whatever the cause. The chief features are depression, weakness and increased irritability. Clinical disturbances of magnesium metabolism are described in vol. 3, p. 49.31

Strontium (Sr at.wt. 88)

Interest in this metal arose when it was discovered that the radioactive isotope ^{90}Sr was present in the fall-out of atomic explosions. This contaminates crops and the isotope becomes incorporated into plants and animals, which are used as human food.

Strontium is a divalent metal in the same group in the periodic table as magnesium and calcium. It is treated biologically in a similar manner, being stored in bone. As ^{90}Sr has a half-life of 28 years, it is a potential danger to bone marrow and other tissues. The testing of nuclear weapons led to significant amounts of ^{90}Sr being found in milk and vegetables in many parts of the world. The amount of ^{90}Sr detectable in the bones of young children also rose, but not sufficiently to cause a level of radioactivity that is considered dangerous. Accidents at local atomic power stations are another potential danger. The Agricultural Research Council Radiobiological Laboratory in the U.K. and the Atomic Energy Commission in the USA each publish at regular intervals analyses of the radioactivity of samples of food.

Strontium derives its name from Strontian, a village in Argyllshire in the West of Scotland. It was first isolated at the end of the eighteenth century from mineral ore obtained from local lead mines.

Phosphorus (P at.wt. 31)

The human body contains from 20–30 mol (600–900 g) of phosphorus, of which over 80 per cent is present in bone and most of the remainder is within the cells. Phosphates are widely distributed in the earth's crust and are present in all plant and animal tissues. Phosphorus deficiency is known to veterinarians as occurring occasionally in cattle that graze on very poor land. A primary dietary deficiency of phosphorus probably never occurs in man. A diet that is adequate in calcium certainly contains sufficient phosphorus.

The roles of phosphates in the body are numerous and are discussed frequently in other chapters.

Iron (Fe at.wt. 56)

The body contains about 70 mmol (4 g) of iron, approximately the weight of a 2 inch nail. About 45 mmol are present in the pigment haemoglobin and about 18 mmol as ferritin and haemosiderin, the forms in which iron is stored in the cells. The remainder is present in myoglobin, the cytochromes and other cell constituents.

The life of a human red cell is about 120 days and just under 1 per cent of the total haemoglobin in the body must be resynthesized daily. For this purpose about 360 μmol (20 mg) of iron are needed. Most of this is obtained from the haemoglobin in the broken down red cells, but about 18 μmol (1 mg) is needed to make good body losses and this must be provided by the diet.

The body does not excrete iron. All the iron present in the plasma is bound to protein and this does not appear in the urine. A small iron loss occurs in the desquamation of cells from the skin and from the epithelium of urinary and respiratory tracts. More important is the iron loss in the menstrual blood. This normally amounts to about 500 μmol/menstrual period or the equivalent of 18 μmol/day but it may be much more. Furthermore if a woman becomes pregnant she needs additional iron to supply the needs of the fetus and later for her milk. During reproductive life a woman requires to absorb about 36 μmol/day of iron, about twice as much as a man.

All human diets contain more iron than the body needs; yet anaemia due to iron deficiency is extremely common. This is because most of the dietary iron is present in a form which cannot be absorbed. Good human diets provide 215–265 μmol (12–15 mg) iron daily and with this intake the 1 mg of iron needed by adult men is readily absorbed, but it is only marginally adequate for women and mild degrees of anaemia are likely to be found. When diets provide less than 160 μmol/day, anaemia is widespread and often severe in women, though it rarely occurs in men unless there is a chronic source of blood loss, e.g. bleeding piles or infection with the blood-sucking hookworm.

Some iron is present in all natural foods. Liver and other offal are rich sources; meat, fruit and vegetables are usually good sources. Whole cereal grains also contain much iron, but it is mostly made unavailable by the presence of phytic acid (p. 5.7), which forms insoluble iron phytate, similar to calcium phytate. Ferric iron is not absorbed and dietary iron must first be reduced to ferrous iron before it can pass across the gut wall and this reduction is probably assisted by ascorbic acid and the —SH groups in the sulphur-containing amino acids. A good mixed diet by providing plenty of ascorbic acid and protein facilitates iron absorption.

The role of the stomach and hydrochloric acid in iron

absorption has been much disputed. Atrophic gastric mucous membrane, producing little or no hydrochloric acid, and anaemia due to iron deficiency are frequently found together. Which of these is cause and which is effect has been disputed for 50 years and the problem is not yet solved.

Iron absorption is greatly increased if the body stores are reduced or the rate of formation of red blood cells is increased. For instance after a severe haemorrhage a man, instead of absorbing only 10 per cent of his dietary intake, may absorb 20–30 per cent. Clearly there is some control of the alimentary absorption of iron and this is related to iron needs. The nature of this control, which is situated in the walls of the small intestines, is discussed on p. 32.45.

In many parts of Africa iron cooking-vessels are used and extraneous iron gets into the diet so that intakes of iron may reach 2 mmol/day. Cheap wines and cider may be very rich in iron, possibly due to contamination from vessels in which they have been stored or prepared. In France and in the poorer sections of the USA many heavy wine-drinkers have a large dietary intake of iron. In these circumstances the control of absorption may break down and part of the dietary excess enters the body. As there is no means of excreting excess iron, it accumulates in the tissues and a condition known as siderosis arises (Greek *sideros*=iron). Siderosis may be found by chemical analysis in the organs at post mortem in a person who has died as a result of an accident, who was otherwise well. However, severe siderosis may contribute to the liver cirrhosis which is common in many parts of Africa and also in heavy wine-drinkers.

Acute iron poisoning may also occur and fatalities have been reported in children who have consumed a bottle of their mother's iron tablets, thinking them to be sweets.

Trace elements

The earth is composed of rocks made of mineral salts which are sparingly soluble in water. These enter the soil and are incorporated in plants and animals used for human foods. Man also digs mines and uses the minerals in industry. Many elements enter the body in the food, in the drinking water or in the inspired air and are present in the body in concentrations measured in μmol or nmol/kg. Some of the trace elements are components of enzyme systems and are therefore essential nutrients; others have a toxic action and are potentially lethal; some have no known biological action and their presence in tissues seems to be adventitious.

Accurate analysis of these elements in biological material was until recently either impossible or very difficult. The development of atomic absorption spectrometry and other methods is now providing precise information and there is an upsurge of interest in their

biological role. A few disorders, for the most part uncommon, are already known to be either associated with a deficiency of one of these elements or due to poisoning by excessive intake.

IODINE (I at.wt. 127)

Iodine is an essential component of thyroxine and other secretions of the thyroid gland. In the absence of an adequate supply the gland enlarges and a visible swelling appears in the neck, known as a goitre. Goitres may become very large and unsightly; they are associated with a varying degree of failure of thyroid function.

The body contains from 160 to 400 μmol (20–50 mg) of iodine and a daily intake of about 1·2 μmol (150 μg) is required. The iodine content of foods is very variable and depends on the iodine content of the soil on which they are grown. Iodine was first discovered in seaweed by Courtois in 1811, who was using it as a source of nitre for gunpowder for Napoleon's army. All sea foods are rich sources of iodine.

There are at least a million people in the world suffering from goitre. They are mostly found in isolated villages high up in the Himalayas and in the Andes and in many parts of Africa. Goitre can be prevented by adding potassium iodide to table salt. This is done in many countries, but not in the United Kingdom. Sporadic cases of goitre are still found in most countries and this is due to the fact that individual needs for iodine vary greatly. Goitres are most common in adolescent girls. Sea fish eaten at one or two meals a week provides more than the requirement of 1·2 μmol (150 μg)/day of iodine and goitre is prevented (vol. 3, p. 23.40).

FLUORINE (F at.wt. 19)

Most drinking waters contain from 50–150 μmol/l (1–3 parts per million). Epidemiological studies have shown that where the water contains less than 50 μmol/l dental caries is more common than elsewhere. In many districts of the world with water supplies low in fluoride it has been shown that the addition of fluoride to bring the concentration to one part per million reduces the incidence of dental decay in children.

If the fluoride content of the water is high (150–250 μmol/l) a brown mottling of the teeth occurs. This is unsightly, but the teeth are sound. Mottling of the teeth and fluoride intakes of this level are common in many countries and are not associated with any disease or signs of ill heath. However, there are a few isolated villages where wells provide water containing 500 μmol/l (10 parts per million) or even more of fluoride. This high intake causes an increased density of the bones and calcification of the ligaments. The spine is especially affected and the resulting poker back is a serious disability. Fluorosis is described in vol. 3, p. 55.6.

Medical and dental authorities are agreed that where the fluoride content of the drinking water is low, the addition of fluoride to bring the concentration up to 50 μmol/l is safe and reduces the incidence of dental decay in children. Water engineers are also agreed that this procedure is cheap and practical. However, the provision of adequate water supplies to a community is a responsibility of local governments. Although many local authorities in Europe and America have fluoridated their water with a consequent improvement in the teeth of their children, many others, including we regret to say Edinburgh, have not done so. Fluoridation has been bitterly opposed in local councils by those who state that it is an unnatural tampering with the water and that individuals have no choice to opt out of a scheme and drink, if they wish, unfluoridated water. Fluoridation is claimed to be a governmental interference with the rights of the individual. Most anti-fluoridators have an irrational fear of 'chemicals' without which a modern society could not exist. Undoubtedly they are responsible for our children continuing to have many bad teeth.

ZINC (Zn at.wt. 65)

Zinc is an essential nutrient and functions as a cofactor (p. 7.12) for many enzymes, including alcohol dehydrogenase, carbonic anhydrase and carboxypeptidase. The total amount in the body is 30–45 mmol (2–3 g), the bulk of which lies within the cells. Dietary intake is usually 150–230 μmol (10–15 mg)/day, but most of this is unabsorbed and appears in the faeces.

A clinical syndrome of stunted growth, delayed puberty and mild anaemia is common in some villages in Iran and other parts of the Middle East. Plasma zinc is low, and giving zinc supplements has been followed by accelerated growth and the development of puberty. The syndrome may well be due to zinc deficiency caused by the diet which consists mainly of unleavened wholemeal bread containing much phytic acid. This binds the zinc and prevents its absorption. Zinc is present in plasma bound to albumin, and plasma albumin concentrations are also low in these cases, perhaps due to an inadequate protein intake. Plasma zinc is also low in other diseases where the plasma albumin is reduced, e.g. in some liver and kidney diseases and in protein-energy malnutrition. It is possible that zinc deficiency may contribute to the clinical features in such cases.

COPPER (Cu at.wt. 64)

Copper is an essential nutrient and functions as a cofactor for tyrosinase and cytochrome oxidase. A copper-containing protein called haemocuprein, or erythrocuprein, is present in erythrocytes. A normal diet provides about 30 μmol (2 mg)/day, but a primary copper deficiency never arises in man, although it is well known as a cause of anaemia in cattle grazing on pastures which are copper-deficient. There is a rare genetically determined disorder due to a defect in copper absorption and known as Menkes' syndrome. Affected infants fail to thrive, show progressive mental deterioration, defective keratinization of hair and degenerative changes in the metaphyses and in aortic elastin. Previously all such children died before the age of 3 years. Now the nature of the disease is known, the outlook with copper therapy may be good. There is also a defect of copper metabolism in which there is a reduced concentration of the copper-binding protein caeruloplasmin. Affected individuals appear to absorb more copper from the diet than do normal subjects and they have a greater proportion of the copper in the plasma in a free state. Under these conditions excessive amounts of copper are deposited in certain tissues. The condition is called Wilson's disease (vol. 3, p. 47.25).

CHROMIUM (Cr at.wt. 52)

Chromium is present in all organic matter and appears to be an essential nutrient. Dietary intakes in the USA vary from 0·1–2 μmol (5–100 μg)/day.

In experimental animals chromium deficiency leads to a reduced rate of removal of a load of glucose from the blood, due to a low sensitivity of peripheral tissues to insulin. In some patients an impaired glucose tolerance has improved after giving chromium. Analytical methods for chromium are still difficult and its role in biology remains uncertain.

SELENIUM (Se at.wt. 79)

Soils and herbage growing on them vary greatly in their content of selenium. In some areas of the USA horses are liable to develop a chronic disease called the 'staggers' which is due to selenium intoxication. In parts of the USA and in New Zealand, lambs and calves may develop 'white muscle disease' which can be prevented by giving selenium supplements and is due to selenium deficiency. Although human plasma selenium in different parts of the world ranges from below 1·0 to over 10 μmol/l, no human counterparts of these diseases are known. Attempts to correlate the selenium content of the soil with the prevalence of dental caries, cancer and other diseases have been unsuccessful and selenium has as yet no known role in human nutrition.

Selenium can react with sulphydryl groups and replace sulphur in some amino acids and proteins. Such selenium compounds have an antioxidant action similar to that of vitamin E. In experimental animals the amount of selenium in the diet needed to prevent signs of deficiency depends on the intake of vitamin E.

COBALT (Co at.wt. 59)

Cobalt is a constituent of vitamin B_{12}, an essential nutrient (p. 5.17). Otherwise it has no known role in the body.

Most human diets contain 2·5–10 μmol (150–600 mg)/day. Cobalt salts used as a nonspecific remedy for anaemia have had serious adverse effects when given in doses of 500 μmol/day. An outbreak of severe cardiomyopathy affecting 48 beer drinkers in Quebec may have been due to cobalt deliberately added to the beer to improve its head. The beer contained 25 μmol/l and some of the men were said to be drinking 12 l/day.

MANGANESE (Mn at.wt. 55)

Manganese is a cofactor for arginase and phosphotransferase. Manganese deficiency can be produced in experimental animals and occurs in cattle grazing on peat pastures which are lacking in the element. The symptoms are poor growth, anaemia, bone changes and disturbances of the CNS. Human diets provide 35–160 μmol (2–9 mg)/day and human deficiency is not known. 'Manganese madness' is a well known disorder amongst workers in manganese mines in Chile.

VANADIUM (V at.wt. 51)

Vanadium deficiency has been produced in chicks and rats. High concentrations of vanadium in the liver decrease synthesis of cholesterol and in the aorta lead to mobilization of cholesterol. Reports of vanadium contents of foods vary greatly, in part due to analytical difficulties. There is no known role for vanadium in human nutrition, but the recent demonstration that it is an essential nutrient in other species makes it an element to watch.

TIN (Sn at.wt. 119)

There is some evidence that tin is an essential nutrient for rats. More interesting is its possible adverse effect, owing to the widespread use of tin and tinfoil in cans and in the packaging of foods. Human diets have been reported to contain from 30 to 170 μmol (3·5–20 mg)/day, more than would be present in natural foods. The toxic dose for man is about 40–60 μmol/kg, so there is a large safety margin.

MOLYBDENUM (Mo at.wt. 96)

Molybdenum has been shown to be an essential nutrient for small animals and it is a cofactor for a flavoprotein enzyme, xanthine oxidase. The amounts present in the soil and plants vary greatly. Most human diets provide between 0·5 and 2·0 μmol (50–200 μg)/day; in different geographical areas there is a wide variation in the concentration in human blood; there is a store in the liver which usually contains from 30 to 50 μmol/kg. Molybdenum deficiency is not known in man, but it might be a contributory factor in some disturbances of iron metabolism, since xanthine oxidase may influence the release of iron from ferritin.

NON-ESSENTIAL TRACE ELEMENTS

Cadmium, lead and mercury have as far as is known no biological role. However they are present in the tissues, occasionally in toxic amounts.

Cadmium (Cd at.wt. 112)

Cadmium is virtually absent from the body at birth, but accumulates in it slowly and by the age of 50 years there may be 200–300 μmol. It is concentrated in the renal cortex and if the amount present reaches 2 mmol/kg it causes renal damage. There appears to be a specific protein in the kidney which binds cadmium. This is known as metallothionein.

Cadmium is present in the geosphere, but increased exposure follows its various industrial uses. Superphosphates, used as fertilizers, may contain 130–180 μmol/kg and municipal drinking water usually contains 10 nmol/l. Rats given drinking water containing 50 μmol/l develop high blood pressure which can be lowered by giving zinc. Toxicity tests on animals show complex relations between cadmium and zinc, copper and selenium, perhaps due to competition for binding sites on protein. An industrial society should keep a watchful eye on its environmental cadmium.

Lead (Pb at.wt. 207)

Ever since lead was first mined and smelted, people have been at risk of absorbing toxic amounts in their drinking water, in their food and in the air. Lead poisoning may cause anaemia, a neuropathy or an encephalopathy. Lead is now mainly a hazard of industrial workers, but there are still homes with old lead water pipes, lead toys which children suck, and people who make home-made wines using old pewter vessels. Pewter is an alloy of lead and tin. The atmosphere may be a danger in the vicinity of an industrial plant or where there is much traffic giving out lead in exhaust fumes.

In an industrial society the intake of lead in food is about 2–4 μmol (400–800 μg)/day, 90 per cent of which is unabsorbed and is lost in the faeces. The amounts of lead of concern to biologists are measured in μmol and nmol and, by contrast, US industry processes over 1×10^6 tons/year. The fact that a doctor only occasionally sees a case of lead poisoning is due to the continuing supervision of industrial plant and workers by engineers and doctors (vol. 3, p. 73.8).

Mercury (Hg at.wt. 200)

Mercury has been used for centuries as a medicine and the effects of mercury poisoning from overdosage are well known. Organic mercurials are now increasingly used in industry, and industrial waste dumped into rivers or the sea has led to high concentrations of mercury in the fish in certain areas. Following a scare in the USA in 1969 the government chemist in Britain analysed 50 samples of canned tuna, and mercury was present in amounts from

0·5 to 4·0 μmol/kg. An FAO/WHO Committee has stated that the tolerable dietary intake of mercury is up to 1·5 μmol (300 μg)/week. That mercury in tuna fish is more than a potential hazard is shown by the case of a lady in New York who developed a neurological disorder which baffled her doctors for several months. The cause of the illness became clear when it was found that she was a dietary crank and in the habit of eating about 500 g of canned tuna daily; her blood mercury was high.

VITAMINS

Vitamins are organic compounds which the body is unable to synthesize and which must be supplied in the diet. Many of them have been shown to be components of enzyme systems (p. 7.13).

Five major diseases, scurvy, beriberi, pellagra, keratomalacia and rickets, arise as a result of a dietary lack of one of the vitamins. In the past these diseases have been responsible for much ill health and many deaths. As each can be prevented by appropriate dietary means, they should no longer occur. However, even in prosperous communities they are not extinct though nowadays rare and in many parts of the world they remain important medical problems. Only by the education of the public and the constant vigilance of individual doctors and the public health authorities is their prevention assured.

The discovery of vitamins is comparatively recent. The concept of dietary deficiencies was unknown to ancient and medieval physicians. In 1497 on Vasco da Gama's voyage from Portugal round the Cape of Good Hope to the Malabar coast in South India, one hundred out of his one hundred and sixty men died of scurvy. Thereafter scurvy was a common scourge of all those who went on long sea voyages. Some people, notably the great explorer Captain Cook and the Scottish naval surgeon James Lind, were well aware that the disease could be prevented by an adequate supply of fresh fruit or vegetables. In the late eighteenth century, Americans began to use the term 'limeys' for the British because lime juice was then a regular issue on ships of the British Navy. Yet the general concept of deficiency diseases was still not appreciated.

In the nineteenth century, nutritional research was directed primarily to elucidating the roles of protein, fat and carbohydrate of the diet in supplying the energy needs of the body. In the last third of the century, the discovery of bacteria and the realization of the enormous role which they and other parasites play in causing infectious diseases emphasized the importance of positive environmental factors in pathological processes. This led to a great search for infective agents and toxic factors to account for all diseases, which distracted the attention of most doctors and research workers from considering the possible role of dietary deficiencies as a cause of disease. Although a few far-sighted men realized that an inadequate diet might be a primary cause of disease, this was not generally appreciated, until the publication in 1912 of a famous experiment by Hopkins, the first Professor of Biochemistry in Cambridge. One group of rats were fed on a diet of pure protein, fat and carbohydrate together with minerals. Another group received the same diet but in addition each rat was given 3 ml of milk. Those rats on the pure diet failed to grow, but those receiving the milk developed normally. After 18 days the milk was taken away from the second group, which then ceased to grow, and given to the first group, which then grew normally. Clearly there was an 'accessory factor' in the milk.

It was soon shown that there were several accessory factors and as these were discovered they were called vitamin A, B, C, D etc. The word vitamine was introduced by the Polish biochemist, Funk, because he thought that all the factors were vital amines. It is now known that only a few of the vitamins are amines, but the name has stuck although the final 'e' was soon removed. In the last 40 years most of the vitamins have been isolated, synthesized and given new names, according to accepted chemical terminology. In general these new names will be used in this book. The old letters are, however, still in use and some of them are likely to remain. They are simpler, though less informative than the chemical names, and are preferable in popular expositions for the education of the general public.

The vitamins can be divided into two main classes: the fat-soluble and water-soluble vitamins. The body cannot maintain a large store of the water-soluble vitamins except for vitamin B_{12}, and so deficiency disease is likely to arise after only a few weeks on a diet deficient in these vitamins. By contrast there is a large store of most of the fat-soluble vitamins in the liver fats and in a previously well-fed adult these stores are sufficient to prevent the appearance of evidence of deficiency even after many months or perhaps years on an inadequate diet. Diseases due to deficiency of the fat-soluble vitamins usually occur in children who have been on a defective diet since weaning.

The water-soluble vitamins circulate freely in the blood and are excreted readily by the kidneys. If for therapeutic purposes a large excess is given, the excess is rapidly lost in the urine and so they are not toxic. By contrast the fat-soluble vitamins are not excreted. If an excess is given, it is stored in the liver and after a time toxic symptoms may arise. A popular and mistaken belief is that, if a little of something does one good, more of it will do you more good. It is very important to see that children are not overdosed with fat-soluble vitamins. An over-conscientious mother can be as great a danger to her child as a feckless one. This has practical aspects in the prevention of rickets.

Fat-soluble vitamins

VITAMIN A OR RETINOL (mol. wt. 286)

Retinol is a highly unsaturated aromatic hydrocarbon which is soluble in fats, but not in water. The structural formula is given on p. 10.25. It is present only in some foods of animal origin. Dairy products, butter, cheese and milk are rich sources as is margarine, to which the vitamin is now added artificially. Liver is also a rich source since it is the site where the vitamin is stored in the body. Fish-liver oils are exceptionally rich. Meats contain only traces of the vitamin as it is not stored or concentrated in any body fat outside the liver.

The body is not entirely dependent on a dietary source of vitamin A, as it can be formed in the body from carotene precursors, especially β-carotene. The carotenes are pigments which are widespread in fruits and vegetables. Dietary β-carotene can be converted into vitamin A in the wall of the small intestine. How much of the dietary carotene is converted is always uncertain; it is probably about one-third and may be less. In this country most of us get about half of our vitamin A direct from dairy products and about half from the precursors in fruits and vegetables. Vitamin A deficiency is now a rare condition in prosperous communities. It is still very common in many parts of the tropics, where there are few productive dairy cattle and where fruits and vegetables may be scarce and expensive.

The first sign of vitamin A deficiency is difficulty in vision when the light is dim (night blindness). The rods of the retina are stimulated when a retinal pigment, rhodopsin or visual purple, is bleached by light (p. 10.26). An aldehyde formed from retinol is an essential part of the visual purple. Vitamin A is also necessary for growth, normal bone formation and the normal process of shedding and repair of epithelial tissues. In the absence of an adequate supply, epithelial surfaces fail to shed their dead cells and become dry and thickened (keratinized). In particular this may affect the cornea of the eye, which becomes opaque and soft (keratomalacia). If not promptly treated, the cornea may collapse, disorganization and infection follow and lead to the loss of the eye. Every year, tens of thousands of young children in the poorer countries of the world go permanently blind for lack of a milligram or so of vitamin A. Did that last sentence make you feel uncomfortable? There is no cause in medicine that is more worth fighting than a campaign against keratomalacia.

As most diets contain both retinol and carotene it is convenient to express their vitamin A activity in terms of retinol equivalents. 1 retinol equivalent = 1 µg retinol or 6 µg of β-carotene or 12 µg of other carotenes. Recommended daily intakes for a young child and for an adult are 1·0 and 2·5 µmol (300 and 750 µg) of retinol equivalents respectively.

VITAMIN D OR CHOLECALCIFEROL (mol. wt. 385)

The word rickets comes from the Anglo-Saxon *wrikken* meaning to twist. It describes the twisting of the long bones, especially of the legs, and of the spine. The pelvis may also be twisted and contracted and this was formerly responsible for many difficult labours. The disease was first described by English physicians in the seventeenth century. At this time London began to take on the appearance of an industrial city and was often covered by a cloud of smoke. Rickets became a common disease amongst poor children in industrial cities throughout the world and was particularly severe amongst the families of Muslims living in purdah. The children of wealthy parents and country children, though not immune, were less often and less severely affected.

Soon after Hopkins had discovered vitamins, Mellanby and others were able to show that rickets was due to deficiency of a fat-soluble vitamin, vitamin D. The disease was produced experimentally by dietary means in dogs. Young puppies are very susceptible to rickets, and today medical students are perhaps more likely to see a case of rickets in a young puppy than in a child. It is easy to gain prestige by advising the owner to give her pup some cod liver oil. The bow legs will then soon straighten. Cod liver oil, like many other fish-liver oils, is a rich source of the vitamin. Vitamin D is found in dairy products, butter, milk and cheese, and also in eggs and liver. It is not naturally present in other foods, but is artificially added to margarines and to some infant foods.

Many adults live on diets providing little or no vitamin D and neither human nor cow's milk is a rich source. Vitamin D deficiency would be widespread if there were no alternative source. It can be synthesized from precursors in the skin by the action of ultraviolet light. Most people get the greater part of their supply in this way. Industrial smoke and the purdah system each reduce the exposure of children to sunlight and so contribute to rickets.

Cholecalciferol is hydroxylated in the liver and kidneys to more active compounds which promote bone formation by facilitating calcium absorption in the gut and also possibly by a direct effect on bone. These actions are discussed with those of other hormones affecting calcium metabolism on p. 27.24. The structural formula of cholecalciferol is given on p. 10.26.

Another form of the vitamin, calciferol, used in therapeutics is formed by irradiation of ergosterol, a sterol present in fungi and yeasts.

Overdosage with vitamin D leads to a high concentration of calcium in the blood, followed by pathological calcification of various organs of the body and is sometimes fatal.

It is difficult to estimate dietary needs for vitamin D because of the uncertainty of how much can be synthesized in the skin. An intake of 6·5 nmol (2·5 µg)/day is sufficient to prevent rickets, but few natural diets provide this amount.

VITAMIN E (mol. wt. about 430)

When rats are fed on certain artificial diets, they fail to reproduce. The females abort and the males become sterile. In addition degenerative processes occur in the muscle which becomes partially converted into fibrous tissue. All these changes can be prevented by adding vegetable oils to the diet. A concentrate obtained from wheat germ oil proved very effective and was named vitamin E. Vitamin E is now known to be a mixture of tocopherols (p. 10.25). These are oily liquids which have the property of protecting fatty acids against oxidation. There are a number of other antioxidants present in biological material.

There is no good evidence that vitamin E deficiency ever occurs in man, and probably all human diets contain a sufficiency of the necessary tocopherols. Vitamin E therapy has been tried for a wide variety of human ailments, including repeated abortions and various muscular dystrophies. Extravagant claims have been made which have not stood up to critical analysis. Vitamin E helps to correct anaemia that occurs in some infants born prematurely, but otherwise has no place in modern therapy.

A good mixed diet provides about 35 μmol (15 mg)/day of vitamin E.

VITAMIN K (mol. wt. 451)

The Danish biochemist, Dam, described how a bleeding disease of chicks could be prevented by feeding them with a number of foodstuffs, including lucerne and putrid fish-meal. From these he extracted a vitamin, which was called vitamin K (Koagulation Vitamin). There are several substances with vitamin K activity. All are fat-soluble and derivatives of naphthoquinone (p. 10.25).

Vitamin K is essential for the formation of prothrombin in the liver. Prothrombin is a necessary component of the complex mechanism for the clotting of blood (p. 28.14).

Vitamin K preparations are used in medicine in a variety of bleeding conditions. These may arise as a result of a failure to absorb vitamin K in disorders of the alimentary tract.

A primary dietary deficiency of vitamin K has not been produced in laboratory animals and probably never arises in man. It is readily synthesized by *Escherichia coli* and other bacteria that inhabit the intestines.

A good mixed diet provides daily from 650 to 1000 nmol (300–500 μg) of the vitamin.

Water-soluble vitamins

ASCORBIC ACID OR VITAMIN C (mol. wt. 176)

The widespread incidence of scurvy at one time in ships' crews and the fact that the disease could be prevented by fresh fruit and vegetables have already been described (p. 5.12). The essential feature of scurvy is haemorrhage, which may occur in the skin, giving the appearance of large bruises, or in the internal organs, where the consequences may be fatal. The disease is often most conspicuous in the gums, which appear swollen and bleeding.

The elucidation of the nature of the responsible vitamin had to await the discovery of a suitable experimental animal. In 1907, guinea-pigs were shown to be very susceptible to scurvy. Only guinea-pigs and primates develop the disease on experimental diets. Although all animals need a supply of this protective vitamin, other species are able to synthesize it in their own tissues. Man and other susceptible animals appear to have lost the mechanism for doing this.

Using the guinea-pig as an experimental animal, various extracts of citrus fruit juices were concentrated and tested. In 1928, the vitamin was obtained in a crystalline form and soon after synthesized. Previously referred to as vitamin C, it was renamed ascorbic acid and shown to be a simple sugar. The formula of ascorbic acid and its chief chemical properties are described on p. 9.4. Here it is sufficient to state that it is water-soluble and easily destroyed by oxidation at moderate temperatures. In consequence there may be large losses of the vitamin in washing, preparing, cooking and serving vegetables and fruit. These losses may be minimized by good techniques in the kitchen, but a serving of cooked vegetables or fruit is unlikely to contain more than half of the vitamin originally present. Often much less remains. The pleasant American custom of starting the day with a glass of fresh fruit juice at breakfast ensures an adequate intake of the vitamin.

Apart from fruit and vegetables there are no other important dietary sources. Milk, meat and eggs contain only traces. Of vegetable sources, green, leafy vegetables such as cabbage are the richest. The concentration of the vitamin in potatoes is not high, but as large amounts are eaten they are a useful source. In Scotland, much less fruit and vegetables are eaten than in the south of England, and potatoes provide the major portion of the supply of the vitamin. The amount present in potatoes falls off on storage and in the spring and early summer, before new potatoes become available, they contain very little. At this season of the year it is not unusual to find a case of scurvy in Edinburgh. The patient is usually an old man living alone, who either dislikes or cannot afford to buy fruit and fresh vegetables.

As already stated, milk contains very little ascorbic acid and what there is will be destroyed if the milk is boiled. In consequence young children are especially liable to scurvy and at one time infantile scurvy was very common. Nowadays, due to the better education of mothers in child feeding it has become rare. However, some 50 cases are diagnosed in young children in the United Kingdom each year.

Adult scurvy is specially likely to occur in dry and semi-desert countries, where vegetable gardens and orchards are difficult to maintain. In such countries scurvy is not uncommonly found when famine conditions arise. Less than 55 μmol (10 mg)/day of ascorbic acid is needed to prevent the onset of scurvy and many people appear to be perfectly healthy on such an intake. However, as an insurance 170 μmol (30 mg)/day is recommended by British authorities. In America the recommended intake is 340 μmol/day—a very liberal 'safety margin' which is generally considered in Britain to be unnecessary.

An ordinary helping of cabbage or other green vegetables (30–60 g or 1–2 oz) provides 110–140 μmol of ascorbic acid. A good helping of boiled potatoes (100 g or 3 oz) gives 30–85 μmol. An orange or other citrus fruit provides about 55–110 μmol in 30 g or 1 oz either of the fresh fruit or the juice.

THIAMIN OR VITAMIN B₁ (mol. wt. 301)

Beriberi is an ancient oriental disease, which affects chiefly rice eaters. There are two forms. In **dry beriberi** the patient is wasted and may be partially paralysed; he may be able to walk only with the aid of sticks; there may be a severe loss of function of the peripheral nerves. In **wet beriberi**, the heart is affected and the peripheral tissues become waterlogged, partly due to a loss of function of the capillary walls and partly due to heart failure. Large numbers of persons may be incapacitated by the disease and deaths are not infrequent.

Our understanding of the nature of beriberi began in 1890. A Dutch military physician, Eijkman, working in Indonesia, found that fowls fed on the food provided for his hospital patients developed weakness and paralysis similar in some ways to that present in his beriberi patients. It was found possible to produce a disease closely resembling human beriberi in a convenient laboratory animal, the pigeon, by feeding the birds on highly-milled, polished rice. This could be prevented if the birds were given a small portion of the outer pericarp or germ of the rice grain; this is normally removed in the milling process. Active extracts of rice germ were concentrated and finally a pure crystalline product was obtained. As little as 17 μmol (5 mg) of the crystals, if given to a patient with beriberi dying of heart failure can transform him in less than one hour. The laboured breathing is eased, the rapid pulse slows and the congestion relieved. There is perhaps no more dramatic spectacle in medicine than the relief of acute beriberi with a few crystals of the vitamin.

The responsible vitamin was first called vitamin B and subsequently vitamin B₁ to distinguish it from other water-soluble vitamins in the crude extract. The structure of the vitamin was soon elucidated and found to be an amine containing a sulphur atom. Thereupon it was renamed thiamin. The structure of thiamin is given on p. 7.13, together with its principal chemical functions.

The brain of a pigeon suffering from beriberi, if minced or sliced and suspended in 0·15 molar NaCl, takes up oxygen in the presence of carbohydrate more slowly than the brain of a normal pigeon. In 1931, the writer, then a medical student, was one of a group of assistants in the Biochemistry Department at Oxford who helped Professor Peters to show that if the vitamin was added to the brain suspension *in vitro* in catalytic amounts the defect in oxidation of carbohydrates was reversed. In beriberi the biochemical lesion, a term introduced by Peters, has been shown to be a specific defect in the complex mechanism for the breakdown of carbohydrate in the cells. The exact role of the vitamin is described on p. 9.12. This was the first demonstration that a vitamin was part of a specific enzyme system, essential for the metabolism of living cells. Subsequently many other vitamins have been shown to play an essential role in cell metabolism.

Thiamin is present in small amounts in all living cells. Consequently it is found in all whole natural foods. Not being soluble in fats, it is absent from butter, animal fats and vegetable oils. It is also absent in sugar and present in very small quantities in highly refined cereal flours. Thiamin can be stored in relatively large amounts in the seed grains of cereals and pulses. Consequently rich sources are whole cereal grains and pulses (peas and beans). Yeast is also rich and a well-known remedy for beriberi. Wholemeal wheat flour and hand-pounded rice provide ample thiamin. In the machine milling of both wheat and rice most of the thiamin is removed. Orientals are largely protected against beriberi by the thiamin in the pulses traditionally eaten with rice. In the past, outbreaks of beriberi have on occasions been reported in the West associated with excessive consumption of white bread. Synthetic thiamin is cheap and in many countries it must be added to white flour used for bread making. Thiamin tablets are widely available in most big Eastern towns, where beriberi is now a rare disease.

Thiamin circulates in the blood and is present in all the body fluids. If a mother is on a diet deficient in the vitamin, her milk will also be defective and her infant may suffer from beriberi.

Thiamin is not needed for the metabolism of fats and thiamin requirements are related to the carbohydrate content of the diet. A daily intake of 3·3 μmol (1 mg) provides good protection against beriberi.

NICOTINIC ACID (mol. wt. 123)

Maize or Indian corn is one of the gifts of the New World to the Old. Wherever it has been widely cultivated—in the southern states of the USA, in Central America, in Spain, Italy, the Balkans, Egypt, North Africa and many other countries—there have been widespread outbreaks of pellagra. It first occurred in Southern Europe in the eighteenth century. The word is of Italian origin and derived from *pelle* skin and *agra* rough. A characteristic feature is an eczematous condition of the skin, occurring over those parts of the body exposed to sunlight. There are also mental changes and diarrhoea which may lead to severe wasting. It may be remembered as the disease of the three D's—dermatitis, dementia and diarrhoea. It is a chronic disease recurring every spring with the increasing sunlight. Many thousands of people in any maize-eating area may be affected with a mild form, but there are also severe cases with some deaths.

At one time it was thought that maize contained some toxin or carried some infective agent, but the fact that it is a deficiency disease was proved by a series of classical epidemiological studies and human dietary studies carried out by an American doctor, Goldberger, in the Southern States between 1913 and 1928. He was able to show that pellagra could be prevented by the addition of milk and a variety of other foods to the diet and that it could be cured rapidly by yeast and yeast extracts. The accessory factor was shown to be heat stable and water soluble. It was first called vitamin B_2 or vitamin P-P (pellagra-preventing). At first the elucidation of its nature was held back by the lack of a suitable laboratory animal and all testing of extracts had to be carried out on human patients. When a condition known as black tongue in dogs was found to be in many ways analogous to pellagra, progress was rapid and in 1937 it was found that nicotinic acid or its derivative nicotinamide was the active substance. A dose of 800 μmol (100 mg) of either substance, or even less, will relieve the symptoms of a severe case of pellagra within a few hours.

The chemical structure and roles are given on p. 7.13.

Maize is a poor source of nicotinic acid, but highly milled rice usually contains even less. Although cases of pellagra may be found not infrequently amongst rice eaters they do not suffer from large epidemics of the disease. The explanation is that the body is not entirely dependent on a dietary source of nicotinic acid. It has a limited power of synthesis from the amino acid tryptophan. Maize protein contains little of this amino acid, but it is present in good amounts in rice and other cereals. About 300 μmol (60 mg) of tryptophan are equivalent to 8 μmol (1 mg) of nicotinic acid. Occasional cases of pellagra are still found in all countries, due usually to chronic intestinal disease interfering with absorption or to an inadequate diet associated with alcoholism. At one time it was not uncommon in the old lunatic asylums in Europe. Occasionally the characteristic and obvious skin condition is absent and the mental features predominate. Such a patient may receive psychotherapy for many months before it is realized that all he needs is a little nicotinic acid.

Like thiamin, nicotinic acid is present in the wholewheat grain in good quantities, but most is removed by the millers in preparing fine flours or polished rice. Butcher's meat, especially offal, and fish are good sources. Yeast and yeast extracts are very rich, but the vitamin does not pass in significant amounts into fermented liquors. Fruit and vegetables are poor sources, as are milk and dairy products. The pellagra-preventing action of milk, well known to Goldberger, is due largely to the rich content of tryptophan. The nicotine which smokers absorb cannot be converted into the vitamin.

A daily intake of 100 μmol (12 mg) of nicotinic acid provides an ample safety margin against pellagra.

RIBOFLAVIN (mol. wt. 376)

In the early days of accessory food factors, rats were found to need for normal growth a heat-stable water-soluble substance. This could be extracted from milk. In 1932, the German Nobel laureate, Warburg, described a yellow pigment, which acted as a respiratory catalyst in many tissue preparations. These were soon shown to be the same substance. The chemical structure and role are given on p. 7.13.

Riboflavin is certainly an essential dietary factor for man. In people subsisting on poor diets, a variety of degenerative conditions of the skin and mucous membranes is found. The junction of the skin with a mucous membrane is likely to be involved and particularly at the angle of the mouth, where the appearance of raw and often infected fissures radiating outwards is known as angular stomatitis. This condition, very common in many parts of the tropics, often responds promptly to treatment with riboflavin. Other causes, such as ill-fitting dentures and iron deficiency, are more likely to be responsible for angular stomatitis in Britain. The conditions which have been attributed to riboflavin deficiency are common in some parts of the world, where they serve as a useful index of unsatisfactory diet.

Lack of riboflavin, unlike ascorbic acid, thiamin and nicotinic acid, is not associated with the appearance of a major disease. The reason for this is not quite clear. Perhaps it is because the vitamin is widely distributed and almost all foods contain a little. Milk is a good source and whole cereals, pulses and offal are rich. It is the only vitamin present in significant amounts in British beer. A dietary intake of 2.5–5.0 μmol (about 1–2 mg)/day appears to be sufficient for human needs.

Anti-anaemic vitamins

The red blood cells have a life span of about 120 days. The continuous production of new blood cells is a major synthetic task for the body. If any one of three substances, iron and the two vitamins, cyanocobalamin and folic acid, is present in inadequate amounts, production is liable to be limited and anaemia may arise. As already stated, iron is an essential component of haemoglobin. Iron deficiency leads to a type of anaemia in which the haemoglobin level of the blood is reduced disproportionately to the number of red cells. By contrast when the supply of vitamins is defective, pigment production is not primarily affected, but the mature red cells do not develop normally from their large primitive precursors in the bone marrow (p. 28.9). There is a marked reduction in the number of cells, but these each contain a normal amount of haemoglobin.

CYANOCOBALAMIN OR VITAMIN B₁₂ (mol. wt. 1355)

The story of the discovery of this vitamin is one of the most exciting in medicine. A severe and invariably fatal form of anaemia was described first by Addison and known as pernicious anaemia. Thomas Addison (1793–1860) was a distinguished physician who, after graduating at Edinburgh, made his reputation at Guy's Hospital in London, where he was a contemporary of Bright and Hodgkin. His name is also associated with the disease that arises from destructive lesions of the adrenal glands. There was no hope for patients with pernicious or Addisonian anaemia. They invariably went downhill slowly and after many months or a few years died with the numbers of red blood cells in the blood reduced to only about one-fifth the normal level. This outlook was changed when Minot, Professor of Medicine in Harvard, showed in 1921 that the anaemia could be relieved if the patient consumed a pound of raw or lightly cooked liver each day. The writer well remembers when he was a schoolboy watching an uncle, who visited his home, struggling with this therapy. This desperate remedy at least provided hope.

Minot's pupil, Castle, made the next important discovery. He showed that if beef was digested by gastric juice obtained from a healthy person and then fed to a patient with Addisonian anaemia, a rapid improvement in the blood occurred. Beef previously digested by gastric juice from a patient with Addisonian anaemia had no such effect. He postulated that to cure the anaemia a dietary substance (the extrinsic factor) was necessary, but that this could only be effective in the presence of substance produced by normal gastric juice (the intrinsic factor). In patients with Addisonian anaemia, the defect was a failure to produce intrinsic factor, which was necessary either for the absorption or utilization of extrinsic factor. This has now been shown to be correct, but the discovery produced no immediate benefit to patients.

Throughout the 1930's, chemists prepared various extracts from liver containing the active blood forming principle. These extracts could be given by injection, a great advantage for the patients. Progress was slow, because each stage of the extractions could be tested only on a patient suffering from Addisonian anaemia, which fortunately was not a common disease. When it was discovered that the active factor was also a growth factor for the micro-organism *Lactobacillus lactis dorner* the pace quickened. Finally 20 mg of crystalline substance was extracted from 1 ton of fresh liver. A dose as small as 1 μg of this substance given to an anaemic patient stimulated red blood cell formation and produced remission in a few days. The substance was first known as vitamin B₁₂. When it was synthesized and shown to be a complex porphyrin derivative containing the element cobalt, it was renamed cyanocobalamin. The structure and role of the vitamin is given on p. 7.14.

The patient with pernicious anaemia formerly died, because he was unable to transport one-millionth of a gram of the vitamin daily across one or two millimetres of the gut wall. Nowadays he receives an injection of the vitamin at fortnightly or monthly intervals and has to continue these for life. In the great majority of cases there is no further sign of the disorder.

The nature of the intrinsic factor and of the defect in the gastric mucosa responsible for the failure of production are still not fully understood.

How the vitamin may act in the tissues is discussed on p. 28.9. It probably is essential for all growing tissue. Deficiency manifests itself first as a failure in blood formation because of the rapid turnover of blood in the body.

Cyanocobalamin is absent from all plant products. The dietary source is from foods of animal origin and may amount to around 10 nmol (15 μg)/day, but poor diets may contain as little as 2·5 nmol (3μg) or even less. The vitamin is formed by many moulds and fungi. Commercially it is made cheaply as a by-product in the manufacture of streptomycin.

Many animals grow more rapidly if they have a small addition of foods of animal origin to their diet. This is probably due to the action of vitamin B₁₂, which has been used for this purpose in animal husbandry. Antibiotics, such as penicillin and tetracycline, have been widely used by farmers to accelerate growth of chicks, pigs and young cattle. They probably act by so altering the intestinal flora as to favour the production or stabilization of vitamin B₁₂.

At one time it was thought that vitamin B₁₂ deficiency arose only as a result of a failure of the absorption mechanism and never as a primary dietary deficiency disease. There is now no doubt that a dietary lack of the vitamin is responsible for the anaemia that arises in some young Indian children, who have been suckled by mothers who are strict vegetarians or whose diet is otherwise unsatisfactory.

FOLIC ACID (mol. wt. 441)

At the time when only crude liver extracts were available for the treatment of pernicious anaemia, Dr Lucy Wills was studying in Bombay the severe anaemias that frequently occur in pregnant women in India. She found that some women had an anaemia with a blood picture identical with that in pernicious anaemia. Yet these patients did not respond to liver extracts known to be able to cure pernicious anaemia, but they did respond to dried yeast and yeast extracts. Here was another 'accessory factor'.

Later a substance obtained from spinach and called folic acid was shown to be an essential growth factor for certain micro-organisms. It was subsequently isolated and synthesized. The pure folic acid was found to be identical with the 'Wills factor'. Anaemia due directly to dietary deficiency of folic acid is common in many tropical countries, especially in pregnancy. Pregnancy appears to increase the requirements of this vitamin and folate deficiency is responsible for a proportion of the anaemias that occur in pregnancy in all countries. Anaemia due to a failure of absorption of the vitamin occurs in some patients with chronic disease of the alimentary canal. The structure of folic acid is given on p. 7.13 and its roles in tissue metabolism and in erythropoiesis are discussed on pp. 11.27 and 28.9 respectively.

Green vegetables and liver are rich sources of the vitamin. Cereals contain small quantities, but much may be lost in the milling process. Meat and fish contain the vitamin in variable amounts, but are not rich sources. Most fruits contain very little. Human diets in this country provide between 100 and 450 nmol (50–200 µg)/day of folic acid which seems to be an adequate amount.

OTHER WATER-SOLUBLE VITAMINS

Many other substances have been shown to be essential dietary factors for experimental animals or for micro-organisms. Some of them, such as pyridoxine and pantothenic acid, are almost certainly essential in the diet of man. However, they appear to be so widely distributed in human foods that it is doubtful if dietary deficiencies ever arise. Although pyridoxine and pantothenic acid are vitamins which appear to have little clinical importance, each is a component of an essential enzyme system. Their chemical structures and biochemical roles are given on p. 7.13. Very rarely an infant becomes increasingly irritable and develops convulsions, which can be immediately relieved by an injection of 10 mg of pyridoxine, far more than an ordinary infant receives in the diet. This is important as an example of a dietary idiosyncrasy. Human beings undoubtedly vary considerably in their requirements for vitamins. Occasionally a patient is found suffering from a deficiency disease, although his diet appears to be adequate in every respect. Such patients may respond well to large doses of a vitamin. The student must appreciate the variability of man. Inevitably his teachers and textbooks must concentrate on describing the properties of the average or normal individual.

FOODS

So far we have been considering the proteins, fats, carbohydrates, minerals and vitamins needed by the body. These are the essential nutrients. It is now time to desscribe the principal foods of man and how they can be mixed together to form suitable diets. Foods can be conveniently classified as follows: cereals and cereal products; starchy roots; pulses and legumes; vegetables and fruits; sugars, preserves and syrups; meat, fish and eggs; milk and milk products; fats and oils; beverages.

A good diet often contains foods from all nine classes, although no single one is essential.

CEREALS

Primitive man was a hunter who also collected wild fruits and berries. Civilization was not possible until the art of domesticating grasses was acquired. Grass seeds (cereals) could be harvested and stored for many months and so provided a source of food which was not dependent on the day-to-day activities of hunters. Cereals now form the principal food of the overwhelming majority of mankind. For many poor peasants in Asia and Africa they provide 80 per cent or more of the total energy in the diet. With increasing wealth, diets become more mixed but even in the richest countries cereals provide 25 per cent of total energy and are the largest single item of food.

The principal cereals of the world are rice, wheat, maize, the millets, barley, oats and rye. Corn is an old Saxon word which can properly be used to describe any cereal grain. In the USA its use has been restricted to maize, which is usually referred to as corn, but in other parts of the world corn may be used to describe the main cereal crop.

Botanically the cereals are closely allied. The seeds have the same general structure and chemical composition and so all whole cereals have similar nutritive properties; their value may be profoundly altered by the millers. Fig. 5.2 shows a diagram of a typical grain. The main bulk is the starchy inner endosperm to which at one end is attached the germ or embryo by a structure known as the scutellum. The outer endosperm and aleurone layer and pericarp surround the grain; the whole is encased in a woody husk.

The whole grain contains very little water and over 80 per cent is made up of starch. Contrary to a popular view, cereals contain a considerable amount of protein, which usually provides from 8 to 12 per cent of the energy present in the grain. However, as already described (p. 5.3), the quality of the protein in a single cereal is not ideally suited to human needs and a mixture of suitable sources of plant proteins is required. The whole grain contains about 3 per cent of fat.

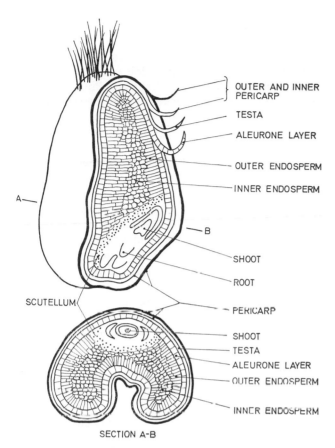

OUTER AND INNER PERICARP
TESTA
ALEURONE LAYER
OUTER ENDOSPERM
INNER ENDOSPERM
A —
— B
SHOOT
ROOT
SCUTELLUM
PERICARP
SHOOT
TESTA
ALEURONE LAYER
OUTER ENDOSPERM
INNER ENDOSPERM
SECTION A-B

FIG. 5.2. The structure of the wheat grain. From McCance R. A, (1946) *Lancet* i, 77.

Cereals provide significant amounts of the minerals calcium and iron, but owing to the presence of phytic acid, which forms insoluble phytates with these elements, they are poorly absorbed. Diets based largely on cereals are thus often barely adequate in these nutrients.

Whole cereal grains are rich sources of most of the B group of vitamins, especially thiamin. They contain no vitamin C. Of the fat-soluble vitamins, A and D are completely absent. Most cereals contain no significant amount of the vitamin A precursor, β-carotene, but several varieties of maize are comparatively rich. Vitamin E is present in the oil which can be extracted from cereals.

Wheat and rice

Wheat and rice are always eaten after part of the grain has been removed by milling. Milling removes the indigestible cellulose, which is present in the outer coats of the grain and adds bulk to the faeces. A sudden change to a diet based on whole or lightly-milled cereals may cause slight diarrhoea but this is only temporary. Milling also makes the resulting wheat flour or rice grain white. Whiteness has always been prized as a quality in flour and rice, per-

haps because of its association with purity. White flour and white rice were available to the ancient Greeks and Romans and to their contemporary Indians, but it was expensive. To grind and sieve a white flour by traditional methods with stone mills and to prepare a white rice by hand pounding were arduous tasks and such foods were only for the rich. With the advent of the industrial revolution, steel mills became available, which could readily produce fine white flour and rice. These then became the staple food of the poor. By tradition millers have always kept the millings, which they sell as cattle food. To make white flour or rice about 30 per cent of the whole grain must be removed. Mills have always spread rapidly with industrialization. They spare the peasant cultivators an arduous task and provide them with a white food, which gives social prestige. The millers appreciate the extra millings, which they can sell. The removal of the small amount of oil improves the keeping qualities of flour or rice and so makes a more suitable product for trade.

However, a high extraction wheat or rice containing only 70 per cent of the whole cereal has lost most of the B vitamins present and particularly nearly all the thiamin. This matters little in contemporary Western diets, where there are many other sources of the vitamins, but it is of paramount importance to poor rice eaters. Beri-beri, due to thiamin deficiency became common in rice-eating countries after the introduction of mills producing polished white rice. India and Pakistan are exceptions, and beriberi in epidemic proportions has been confined to a region on the east coast of India. This is because in these countries most paddy (rice in the husk) is parboiled or steamed before milling. Parboiling partially protects the grain against losses in milling, probably by making the germ more adherent.

Nowadays it is possible to replace some of the losses in milling by the addition of synthetic vitamins. White flour in Britain is enriched with thiamin and iron, but it is not possible to replace all the losses. It is much more difficult technically to enrich rice in this way.

Wheat or rice is the cereal of choice for most people. Improved varieties enable both crops to be cultivated on poor soils and under climatic conditions which were previously impossible.

Millets

The millets are the poor man's cereal. They grow well under conditions where the cultivation of rice or wheat is difficult or impossible. There are large numbers of millets, with an even greater number of names. The commonest are:

(1) *Sorghum vulgare* or the large millet, also known as dura in Africa and juar or cholam in India,

(2) *Eleusine coracanna* or finger millet, known as ragi in South India,

(3) *Pennisetum typhoideum*, known as bajra or cambu in India.

Millets are nutritious foods; like all cereals they have to be husked, but they are not highly milled. They are usually eaten after making into a porridge.

Maize

Maize is a cereal of American origin, but now grown widely in the Mediterranean region and in many parts of Africa and Asia. Although associated with pellagra (p. 5.16), it is an excellent food, provided it does not form too high a proportion of the diet. It is eaten by many of us as a breakfast cereal.

Barley, oats and rye

Barley and oats are good cereals formerly widely eaten in Europe. Barley is nowadays grown mostly for brewing, and oats as a cattle food. Even the Scots are eating less and less porridge. Rye is a hardy cereal formerly widely grown in north and east Europe. It is now being replaced by wheat, but rye is still grown in many parts of eastern Europe and rye bread is widely appreciated especially in Scandinavia and the United States.

Bread

Wheat flour can be made to rise and form a good loaf because it contains two proteins, gliadin and glutelin, which give wheat flour its characteristic stickiness. Wheat may be eaten unleavened as is traditional in the Middle East and in Pakistan and North India, and for this purpose wholemeal flour is used. Wheat flour may also be leavened by yeast; the dough so formed is then made into bread by baking. Wholemeal flour yields a dough which does not rise well and to get a good large loaf white flour is best. USA and Canadian wheats give a 'strong' flour which makes bread with a firm texture, so that the loaf stands up well. British wheats are 'weak' and are not good for breadmaking, but are ideal for biscuits. British biscuits are the best in the world.

Most bread contains about one-third of its weight as water. Bread is often made into toast; dry heat applied has little or no effect on the nutritive value, but a variable part of the moisture is driven off. An ounce of toast thus has a higher energy content than an ounce of bread, an important fact for those on a reducing diet. Italian wheats have a high content of gliadin and glutelin and are very hard. They are ideal for making 'pasta' which can then be moulded into macaroni and spaghetti.

In conclusion it may be said that the nutritive value of cereals is often underestimated in prosperous countries. Good bread and good rice are excellent foods. They are tasty and nutritious, provide energy, proteins and the B group of vitamins, and some calcium and iron. Only when an excessive proportion of the energy is derived from cereals does a diet become unbalanced.

Potatoes

This American plant was introduced into Europe early in the sixteenth century and by the middle of the seventeenth century its cultivation was widespread. Potatoes were more easily cultivated than cereals and they give a higher yield of energy per acre. This provision of an alternative crop serving as a second source of energy-rich food ended the history of famines in Western Europe, which had previously arisen from failure of the cereal harvests. However, in Ireland, potatoes completely replaced cereals in agriculture. When in 1845 and again in 1846 and 1847, the potato crops were almost entirely destroyed by blight, famine, perhaps the most disastrous in human history, occurred. Over a million people died and probably as many emigrated. Their descendants form an important part of the modern populations of such cities as Boston, Glasgow and Liverpool.

The potato is an excellent food. In 1910, a Danish 'keep fit' man lived for a year on a diet consisting solely of potatoes. He was investigated carefully by physiologists and shown to remain in good health. On no other single food could an adult man survive indefinitely. This is because, unlike cereals, potatoes contain a significant amount of vitamin C and small quantities of carotene. Potatoes contain a little less protein than cereals and are not so rich in the B group of vitamins, but the amounts present are at least adequate for an adult. Potatoes contain about 70 per cent of water. A given weight of potatoes thus provides about one-third of the starch and one-third of the energy present in the same weight of a cereal.

Potatoes have a reputation for being fattening. If you eat so many potatoes that the energy intake exceeds the expenditure, then inevitably excess fat is laid down. Potatoes have, however, no specific fattening properties and, eaten in moderation, are an excellent food.

The sweet potato is a traditional dish in the Southern States of the USA. It is grown extensively in many hot climates. The roots have the same general properties as other potatoes. Many varieties are coloured and the carotene present may be an important source of vitamin A activity.

Cassava and other tropical roots

Cassava shrubs, of which there are many varieties, come from South America, but are now widely grown in tropical Africa and in some parts of Asia. As they are easily cultivated and give a high yield, they are valuable as a source of energy. However, the roots contain little protein, which contributes only 3 per cent to the total energy. In any tropical area where cassava is a principal food, evidence of protein deficiency is usually widespread especially in the children. Many of the varieties are poisonous when freshly harvested owing to the presence of cyanides. These can be removed by washing and drying in the sun. Tapioca is prepared from cassava. The products available in Western shops are usually highly refined and nutritionally may be considered as pure starch.

Yams are climbing plants and **taro** a herbaceous perennial of the *colocasia* family, which are grown in many tropical areas. They are easily cultivated and the yield of tubers, which in the case of some yams may be as big as a football, is large. Hence, they are invaluable to many communities as a source of energy. Their protein content is not high; it may be sufficient to meet the needs of adults, but is inadequate for growing children.

Sago is another starchy food, but it is not a root, being derived from the pith of the sago palm.

Many invalid foods available in Western countries are based on tapioca, sago or ground rice. For practical purposes they are little more than pure starch, but as an easily digestible form of energy they have a place in the diets of convalescents. It is of course necessary to supplement them with a good source of protein and other nutrients, such as milk and eggs.

PULSES AND LEGUMES

Pulses, lentils or dhals are the dried seeds of various species of *leguminosae*. They have a traditional place in cereal diets in tropical and subtropical countries, where rice and dhal may be the equivalent of the poor man's bread and cheese in the west. Pulses are invaluable in supplementing the protein content of cereal diets. Their protein content is usually about double that of cereals. They also supplement the amino acid mixture, being especially rich in lysine, in which many cereals are poor. Pulses are not milled and all species are rich in the B group of vitamins in which cereal diets are often deficient. Greater cultivation and so more consumption of pulses would improve greatly many types of poor diet and reduce the incidence of protein deficiency in young children.

The soya bean is a pulse which forms the basis of much of the culinary art of the Chinese. It differs from other pulses in containing about 18 per cent of fat, but this gives it no nutritional advantages over the pulses more commonly used in other countries.

In Western diets there are a great variety of peas and beans. They are eaten in many different ways, but are far less important from the nutritional viewpoint than are the pulses in tropical diets. They are generally classified as 'vegetables' and their nutritive properties are discussed below under this general heading.

VEGETABLES AND FRUITS

A number of plant structures serve as vegetables in human diets. These are green leaves (cabbage and let-tuce), flowers (cauliflower and artichoke), seeds (peas and broad beans), gourds (egg plant, ladies' fingers and cucumber), stems (leeks and celery) and roots (beetroot, parsnip and onion). Broadly speaking, all have similar nutritive values and they can be discussed together as a class of food. First we eat vegetables because they are pleasant and their flavours add to the variety of our foods. Secondly, all vegetables contain 70 per cent or more of water. They contribute little energy and protein. Vegetables are recommended to those on reducing diets, because they may fill the stomach and give a sense of repletion without providing much energy. The fibre present in the plant structures adds bulk to the faeces and so prevents constipation. Most vegetables contain calcium and iron in amounts that could be useful, but they are often in a form that is poorly absorbed from the gut. The water-soluble B group of vitamins is present in all vegetables, but none is a particularly rich source. Vegetables also contain vitamin C, but the amounts are very variable and the vitamin is often lost during storage, preparation and cooking. Vegetables are chiefly valuable as a source of carotene, the precursor of vitamin A. The amount present is again extremely variable, but there is a rough relation between the colour of the vegetable and the carotene content. Carrots are exceptionally rich and are the chief source of vitamin A activity in the diet of many British people.

The minerals and vitamins present in vegetables can make a valuable contribution to the nutritive value of poor cereal diets. There is no doubt that in many village communities in the tropics, vitamin deficiencies could be abolished and general health improved if the people were persuaded to cultivate vegetable gardens. The importance of the nutritive value of vegetables in mixed Western diets has probably been exaggerated in popular teaching. The Scots don't like vegetables; at least they eat only about half as much as Londoners. There is no evidence that their health is any worse on this account.

Fruits in general contain more water and even less energy and protein than vegetables. Most contain small quantities of minerals and also vitamins of the B group and carotene. The main nutritional value of fruits lies in their vitamin C content; almost all fruits are good sources and some are very rich. A single helping of fresh fruit, canned fruit or fruit juice each day ensures that the vitamin C intake is adequate. Fruits and fruit juices are a pleasant and valuable source of potassium for many patients. Fruits contain a great number of organic acids. Citric acid derives its name from lemons, malic acid from apples and pyruvic acid from burnt grapes. These acids are all readily broken down and metabolized by enzyme systems within the body and so do not upset the acid–base balance.

Bananas require a special mention. They are a fruit which provides carbohydrate in quantities as much as

20 g/100 g. A great many varieties are grown and in some parts of the tropics they form a major food of the population. However, they contain little protein and children fed on diets in which bananas are the chief constituent are likely to suffer severely from protein deficiency. Of course in small quantities bananas are a pleasant food, easily digestible and especially appreciated by invalids and convalescents.

SUGAR, PRESERVES AND SYRUPS

In the United Kingdom we eat about 45 kg (100 lb)/head/year of sugar. Table 5.5 shows the great increase in sugar consumption in the last 80 years and a corresponding decline in cereal consumption. Similar figures are available from the USA. This is the largest change in our dietary habits that has taken place this century. Sugar consumption in Britain rose steadily for over 100 years, except when sugar was rationed in World Wars I and II, until 1960. Since then it has fallen very slightly. It appears that our appetite for sugar is at last satiated. The cane sugar or sucrose that the grocer sells is a pure chemical

TABLE 5.5. Changes in the amounts of sugar and cereal grains in the food supplies of the United Kingdom (lb/head/year).

	1880	1924–8	1953	1962	1971
Sugar	64	87	98	111	99
Wheat flour	280	198	193	161	146
Other cereals	?	16	16	16	13

almost up to the standard of an analytical reagent. It provides energy, but no other nutrients. The same is almost true of many fats and most alcoholic drinks, and these foods are said to provide 'empty calories'. This large sugar intake has to be complemented by foods rich in proteins, minerals and vitamins. It certainly contributes to the high incidence of dental caries, obesity, diabetes and possibly atherosclerosis in numerous countries. Many people said to have 'a sweet tooth' can be more accurately described as sugar addicts.

Sugar is a food preservative and it is used to make jams and preserves, which usually contain about 70 per cent of sucrose. Most jams retain only a small portion of the vitamin C originally present in the fruit.

Syrups such as molasses, treacles and Golden Syrup ® are concentrated sugar solutions. They contain 20–30 per cent of water, but negligible amounts of nutrients except sucrose. There are some natural syrups such as the famous maple syrup in North America, but these have no nutritive property other than their sugar content. Honey also contains about 75 per cent of sugars, mostly fructose; regrettably the bees neglect to add vitamins. It is a plea-

sant food, but the reputation for medicinal properties which it has acquired with some people is unmerited.

Sugar is the main ingredient in boiled sweets, which may contain 90 per cent. Toffees and candy are a mixture of sugar, syrup and fats. Most chocolates are a mixture of cane sugar and cocoa powder. These sweets contribute energy but little else to the diet.

MEAT, FISH AND EGGS

Muscle contains about 18 per cent of protein. Meat, as ordinarily eaten, always contains a large amount of fat and a composition of 20 per cent protein, 20 per cent fat and 60 per cent water is usual. There is, however, a wide range for all these values. The protein present in meat is of a high biological value. Meats contain little calcium, but are good sources of iron. They contain useful amounts of the B group of vitamins, especially nicotinic acid and riboflavin; pork muscle is rich in thiamin. There is a little vitamin C in fresh meat, but most of this is destroyed in cooking. Animal fats contain only very little vitamin A, except those from the liver.

All meats have approximately the same nutritive value, although they may differ markedly in their flavour and tenderness, which give them 'their quality'. At one time physicians taught that white meat (poultry and game) was more easily digested than red meat (beef and mutton) and so more suitable for invalids. This is a myth. All muscle is readily digested; however, the fibrous connective tissue, fascia and tendon, which may be present in a helping of any meat is less digestible. As animals age, their muscle develops more fibrous tissue and their meat becomes less tender.

Most people are very conservative in their taste for meats and normally eat the flesh of only a few species. Many Englishmen are revolted by the thought of eating frogs and snails, which a Frenchman considers a delicacy. A laboratory worker would be appalled if told to eat a guinea-pig, which may be much appreciated in many South American homes. Necessity may change established habits. Soldiers in beleaguered garrisons, after eating their horses, have turned to cats and dogs and even rats have been eaten. In many parts of Africa and in some areas in Asia a great variety of animal foods may be eaten, including locusts, lizards, snakes and monkeys. All these may be useful foods, especially as sources of protein, and so can contribute to health.

Liver, kidneys and other offal are of good nutritional value. In general they resemble butchers' meat, but liver is much richer in vitamins and in iron.

Beef teas, Oxo ®, Bovril ® and other meat extractives have a reputation as nourishing food. In fact they contain very little solid matter and so provide few nutrients. They do, however, contain the flavouring agents present in meat. These may well promote the appetite and so make a valuable contribution to the feeding of invalids.

Fish and other sea foods are a valuable source of protein. Many species have a high oil content, which may be rich in vitamins A and D. Small fish, if eaten whole, including the bones, provide calcium. This may be important in many tropical areas, especially in the deltas of great rivers, where the calcium intake is often low.

A hen's egg weighing 60 g contains about 6 g of first class protein, 6 g of fat and provides 330 kJ (80 kcal) and also some calcium and iron. The yolk is rich in vitamin A and also contains the water–soluble vitamins. Eggs have a deservedly high reputation as a human food.

MILK AND MILK PRODUCTS

Table 5.6 shows the composition of typical samples of human and cow's milk. Milk serves as a complete food for an infant during the early months, and although human milk is perhaps ideally suited to this purpose, cow's milk after some modification is also effective. There are many different reasons which may make a mother decide to breast feed or bottle feed her baby. She need have no fear that her baby will not receive adequate nourishment from a suitable preparation based on cow's milk made by reputable firms. The table shows that

TABLE 5·6 The composition of human and cow's milk.

	Human	Cow's
	values per 100 g	
Energy (kJ)	290	275
(kcal)	70	66
Carbohydrate (g)	7	5
Protein (g)	2	3·5
Fat (g)	4·0	3·5
Calcium (mg)	25	120
Phosphorus (mg)	16	95
Iron (mg)	0·1	0·1
Retinol equivalents (μg)	50	30–45
Cholecalciferol (ng)	25	10–40
Thiamin (μg)	17	40
Riboflavin (μg)	30	150
Nicotinic acid (μg)	170	80
Ascorbic acid (mg)	3·5	2·0
	values per litre	
Calcium (mmol)	6	30
Phosphorus (mmol)	5	31
Iron (μmol)	18	18
Retinol equivalents (nmol)	180	100–160
Cholecalciferol (pmol)	650	260–1020
Thiamin (μmol)	0·5	1·3
Riboflavin (μmol)	0·8	4·0
Nicotinic acid (μmol)	14	6·5
Ascorbic acid (μmol)	200	110

cow's milk is richer in protein and poorer in carbohydrate than human milk. An approximation to human milk can be made by diluting cow's milk with water and adding sugar.

All milks are rich in calcium, but poor in iron. An infant usually starts life with some reserves of iron laid down mostly in the liver in the later stages of uterine life. If mixed feeding with foods rich in iron is delayed for more than 6 months, anaemia due to iron deficiency is likely to occur. Indeed in all countries this type of anaemia is common in infants and young children. Milk contains all the vitamins that an infant requires. If, however, a mother receives a diet lacking in thiamin, her milk will be low in this vitamin and beriberi may develop in the infant. If a baby is being fed on a cow's milk preparation and this milk is boiled, all the vitamin C may be destroyed. In these circumstances infantile scurvy may arise. Many studies have shown that mothers on inadequate diets generally produce milk of good quality. The quantity of milk, however, may be insufficient to allow the baby to grow at the normal rate. Milk production appears to receive high priority in the metabolism of starving or undernourished women who are lactating.

It would be difficult, though not impossible, to feed young children or adolescents so that they could attain their normal growth potential without some milk in the diet. If milk is not available or available in only small amounts, then special care must be taken to see that both the quantity and quality of the protein intake is satisfactory and that there are good alternative sources of vitamin A and calcium.

Milk is a suitable food for those adults who like it, but it is not an essential constituent in adult diets. Milk fat is composed mainly of triglycerides containing saturated fatty acids. It is widely believed that a high intake of such acids predisposes to arterial disease, though the evidence is far from conclusive. Milk preparations are now available in the USA in which the butter fat has been removed and replaced by fats of vegetable origin containing a high proportion of unsaturated fatty acids. This is a good example of the foods which may be produced in a sophisticated society which possesses great technical ability.

Sour milks

In many countries it is the custom deliberately to sour milk by fermenting it with bacteria. *Lactobacillus bulgaricus* and *Streptococcus thermophilus* are the main micro-organisms used for this purpose. It breaks down the lactose in the milk, but the protein, calcium and vitamins remain. There are many local recipes for making sour milk or yogurt and all yield a product of high nutritive value. As the fermenting bacteria overgrow and destroy any pathogenic bacteria that may be present in the original milk, it is hygienic; it is also delicious.

Butter

It has long been the custom to separate the fats from surplus milk and make butter. The nutritive value of butter is discussed in the next section.

Skimmed milk

This is milk from which the butter fat has been removed. Traditionally in European farms it was given to young pigs, who thrived on it. Large quantities are now available from the big butter industries in the USA, New Zealand and elsewhere. It is easily dried and then forms a stable powder. As it contains all the protein and calcium present in the original milk, it forms, after reconstitution with water, a valuable food for growing children. With the aid of the United Nations, many thousands of tons of dried skim milk have been distributed in countries where the local milk supply is inadequate. There is much evidence that this has benefited the health of the children.

Cheese

Cheese making is an ancient art, used by farmers' wives to dispose of surplus milk. The basic process is to allow the milk to clot, usually under the action of the enzyme rennet. The clot is then separated and this contains most of the protein and a variable proportion of the fat present in the original milk. The clot is then dried and pressed. Cheeses are thus highly nutritious foods, rich in protein. There are many recipes which provide cheeses of different flavour and consistency. These are named after villages and small towns in the countries of Europe where they originated. Nowadays few farmers' wives find the time to make cheese, which is almost all produced commercially. You can no longer buy a Stilton cheese in Stilton.

FATS AND OILS

The chief fats of animal origin used in human diets are dairy fats (butter and ghee), suet from beef and lard from pork. Important vegetable oils include olive oil, groundnut oil, cotton seed oil, sesame or gingelli oil, mustard oil, coconut oil, red palm oil and corn oil from maize. Margarine is an artificial fat made largely from mixtures of vegetable oil and whale oil. It will be noticed that animal fats, except those of marine origin, are solid, whereas vegetable fats are liquid. The melting point of a fat is determined by the relative proportion of unsaturated to saturated fatty acids present. Margarine is made by reducing the proportion of unsaturated fats in natural oils by hydrogenation.

Fats are a concentrated source of energy. The diets of active men who do much work, such as lumber men and arctic explorers, would be very bulky if they did not contain a large amount of fat. Some fats are important because they carry the fat-soluble vitamins. However, fats are used in diets chiefly because we like them and they are essential for good cooking. In most prosperous countries, fats provide 35–40 per cent of the total calories, far more than is necessary to meet the physiological needs for essential fatty acids.

Butter fat contains vitamins A and D. The amounts of vitamin A depend on the quality of the pasture on which the cattle graze. Summer butter is usually very rich in this vitamin and there is appreciably less in winter butter. Vitamins A and D are artificially added to margarines to the levels present in summer butter. It is impossible to distinguish by feeding experiments between the nutritive values of margarine and butter and nowadays many people cannot distinguish their tastes. Margarine is perhaps the best example of the skill of food technologists in producing an artificial food.

Vegetable oils contain no vitamins, but are valuable as a source of energy and for their culinary properties. An exception to this is the red palm oil, which is rich in carotene. This palm, *Elaeis guineensis*, is a native of West Africa, but plantations are now present in other parts of Africa and also in Asia. In Nigeria it has been shown that children are healthier in areas where red palm oil is used than in areas where the diets are similar, except that they contain other vegetable oils. A great extension in the plantation of these palm trees would be of immense benefit to the health of many tropical communities.

BEVERAGES

Although a man drinks from 1 to 2 litres of water each day, he does not appear to like it very much, at least in its pure form. He prefers to drink one of a number of beverages. These are appreciated for their flavours and perhaps for the drugs which may be present; they may also contain nutrients. Flavours are provided by the essential oils of herbs, berries, fruits and grains. Their chemistry is little understood. Many traditional skills are employed to produce the aroma of a fine tea or the bouquet of a good whisky. Their manufacture is still a craft rather than a science.

Alcoholic beverages

A wit has said that *homo sapiens* can be distinguished from the other primates by the fact that, wherever two or three of them are gathered together, there you will find theological argument and fermented liquor. Ethanol is produced by the fermentation of carbohydrates present in grain or fruit by wild or cultivated yeasts. Ethanol is a remarkable substance. It is a nutrient which is easily absorbed, and so may be a valuable source of energy. On the other hand if taken regularly, it may contribute to the excess energy which causes obesity. As a drug, its sedative action gives it a place in medical practice. By inhibiting those centres in the brain on which the most developed mental faculties depend, it produces a sense of well-being and so promotes social intercourse. In many men and women the critical faculties are overdeveloped, so that it is difficult for them to appreciate the views of others. Alcohol may help to bring about the compromises which are essential in a good society. On the other hand excessive use of alcohol causes loss of judgement and, if continued, leads to addiction, which disrupts the person and may ruin his family. Alcohol is also a disinfectant and a preservative; these properties give it a useful, if small, place in medicine and in the food industry. Many people are so impressed by the evils which arise from the improper use of alcohol that they are total abstainers. Some of these try to enforce their views on others and sometimes succeed in bringing about a legal prohibition of alcohol in their country or community. Experience has shown that the law cannot prevent the abuses of alcohol. This is a matter of education.

Beers are made from cereal grains, chiefly barley. By keeping the grain in the warm, damp atmosphere of a malting house the starch in it is converted into maltose. The malt is steeped in water to form a wort which is then fermented by yeast. Beers contain from 2 to 6 per cent of alcohol according to their strength and similar amounts of carbohydrate. The energy value of beer ranges from 100–300 kJ (25–70 kcal)/100 ml. Although yeasts are very rich in the B group of vitamins, these do not come out of the cells. Beers are poor sources of these vitamins, except for riboflavin, significant amounts of which are found in most beers. These remarks do not always apply to home made and country beers, especially those in which wild yeasts are used. There have been reports of missionary teachers, ardent for total abstinence, causing the appearance in primitive rural people of multiple vitamin deficiencies by prohibiting the brewing of their country beer.

Wines are made by the fermentation of grapes and occasionally other fruits. Table wines contain from 8 to 10 per cent of alcohol and provide from 250–330 kJ (60–80 kcal)/100 ml. Port and sherry are strengthened by the addition of extra alcohol to bring the concentration up to 15 per cent. Wines are devoid of vitamins, but they sometimes contain large amounts of iron, parts of which may be absorbed and contribute to liver disease.

Spirits are made by the distillation of various fermented liquors. Brandy, whisky and rum contain just over 30 per cent of ethanol and provide 920 kJ (220 kcal)/100 ml. For practical purposes they are devoid of other nutrients. The distiller's art in forming the bouquet is most subtle and a fine brandy or a good whisky provides one of the elegant luxuries of European civilization. Illicit distillation by crooks or amateurs is a dangerous process; spirits so produced may contain methanol and other alcohols which are toxic. The drinking of such crude liquor may cause permanent blindness and death.

Coffee and tea

It is difficult to appreciate what European society was like less than 400 years ago when there was no tea or coffee. The coffee beans and tea leaves came from shrubs grown in tropical or subtropical gardens which are very beautiful. Much art is required in the preparation of the final products so as to preserve the aromas for which they are appreciated. The first infusions contain xanthine derivatives which have pharmacological properties. Caffeine, theophylline and theobromine are present, of which caffeine is the most important. It stimulates the nervous system and so often prevents fatigue; it also acts on the kidneys to increase the flow of urine. Tannins which are weak protein precipitants are present in both tea and coffee. There are no harmful effects from one or two cups of coffee or tea and probably no medical contra-indications to their use. The caffeine in excessive amounts of coffee may cause sleeplessness. Gastritis, which is sometimes found in those who drink many cups of strong tea, has been attributed, on no good grounds, to the tannin present. Tea and coffee by themselves are of no nutritive value. They are often drunk with added sugar and milk. In this way the tea and coffee drinking habit may contribute to the excess intakes of energy which cause obesity.

Soft drinks

Fruit juices, lemonades and squashes are pleasant drinks. If freshly prepared they are rich sources of vitamin C, as are many commercial preparations. The energy content is variable and depends on the amount of sugar added. This may be up to 15 per cent, or occasionally even more, giving a value of about 250 kJ (60 kcal)/100 ml. Fruit juices are all rich in potassium and so helpful in the diets of convalescents, who have to rebuild lost tissue.

'Colas' and many other synthetic soft drinks on the market are widely advertised. The exact composition of most of these is a trade secret. Many people find them pleasant drinks, but the advertisements, in so far as they claim any special nutritive or health promoting properties, may be misleading.

Mineral waters

Many natural waters contain inorganic salts to which medicinal properties have been attributed. The well at Epsom near London from which Epsom salts, magnesium sulphate, was first isolated, proved in the seventeenth century very profitable to its owner. Mineral waters contain carbonates, bicarbonates and sulphates and sometimes iron and hydrogen sulphide. For the most part these are present in such low concentrations that they have no medicinal or toxic properties. Mineral waters are pleasant drinks, but quite discredited as therapeutic agents. Nevertheless spa treatment remains popular. It is nowadays fashionable in Western Germany and the famous old Bohemian spas are well patronized by modern Czechoslovakians. For many successful and prosperous men and women, whose way of life may have led them to dietary excesses of energy and alcohol, a period on a disciplined regime is beneficial. Water, applied either internally or externally, does no harm; its use may serve as a ritual which can help to a more balanced way of life.

CHEMICALS ON THE FARM AND IN THE FOOD INDUSTRY

Farmers use artificial chemicals as fertilizers, to control weeds and to destroy insects and other pests. Food technologists use chemicals as preservatives, colouring agents, flavouring agents, anti-oxidants, flour improvers, fat extenders and emulsifiers. Some of these chemicals inevitably find their way in small quantities into the diet. It would be idle to pretend that they do not involve a hazard to health. However, in all advanced countries their use is controlled by legislation. For this purpose governments are advised by expert committees, who can draw on the findings of analytical and pharmacological laboratories. A doctor cannot be expected to appreciate the details of these problems, though some knowledge of their pharmacological testing is necessary. Suffice it to say that there is no evidence that any of the many permissible chemicals used in the concentrations and in the manner prescribed by law, represents a significant hazard to health.

There are people who think that the artificial use of chemicals in the preparation of food is wrong. These are the 'natural farmers' and 'health food' advocates. They are enthusiastic for the traditional way of life, which our ancestors found good. One may sympathize with their views, but in the modern world they are quite impractical. Farmers could not possibly produce the crops needed to feed the present population of the world without the use of chemicals. Nor could the shops provide the modern city dweller with the food to which he has become accustomed without the aid of chemicals used by the food industry. You may have had for breakfast fruit juice (from California), a cereal (from Iowa), some fish (caught off Iceland), bread (from Canadian flour), butter (from New Zealand), marmalade (from Seville oranges), coffee (from Brazil) with sugar (from Jamaica) and milk (from a dairy herd 200 miles from your home). It would be quite impossible to enjoy such a breakfast, unless there was an elaborate food industry able to use intelligently a variety of chemicals.

We cannot go back to the traditional way of life in which 80 per cent of the population lived in the country and grew food for themselves and also sufficient to sell in the markets of the nearby towns to meet the needs of the small numbers in the urban population. All the evidence, and there is much of it, indicates that the nutritive value of the diets of those who live in great cities like London and New York is as good as that of the diets eaten by their grandfathers and great grandfathers, who were mostly countrymen. The modern townsman is also immune from the effects of local failures of crops. He can enjoy any of the luxuries of the table all the year round, many of them at a low cost. All this is owed to an efficient food industry, which uses chemicals widely, but carefully. Whether modern foods taste better or worse than country fare can only be a matter of opinion.

Frozen and canned foods

No manufacturer can sell foods preserved by freezing or canning or indeed by any method, unless they taste good. In general, the chemical substances responsible for flavour are more unstable than vitamins and other nutrients. Any frozen or canned foods in which the original flavours are well preserved are therefore likely to contain most of their original nutrients. It would be foolish to claim that such foods are always as good as those fresh from one's garden or a nearby orchard or farm, but they may well be more nutritious than 'fresh' foods which have spent days in city markets and shops.

RECOMMENDED INTAKES

Ration scales have to be drawn up for the armed services and for those who live in institutions such as boarding schools, hospitals, prisons, etc. It is important that such scales provide nutrients in sufficient amounts to meet the physiological needs of the people for whom they are intended. Physiological standards of requirements are also needed to assess the significance of the findings in dietary surveys in which the food consumption of sections of a community may be measured. National governments nowadays direct agricultural and trade policies to try to ensure an adequate food supply for the people. Such policies are ultimately based on estimates of physiological needs.

Many countries and also the Food and Agricultural Organization of the United Nations have drawn up recommended dietary intakes. Table 5.7 is from the Department of Health and Social Security of the UK. The recommendations are for groups of people and not for individuals and provide a margin of safety to cover individual variations and common stresses. An individual whose dietary intake does not come up to these standards in all respects will not necessarily be malnourished. The US recommendations are similar to the British in most respects, but three differences merit brief mention. The intake of ascorbic acid recommended for an adult man is 340 µmol (60 mg), double the British figure. Few people in Britain take more than 30 mg/day, which is far more

TABLE 5·7 Recommended daily intakes of energy and nutrients for the UK.

Age range	Occupational category	Energy weight kg	Energy kcal	Energy MJ (a)	Protein (b) g	Thiamin (c) mg	Thiamin µmol	Riboflavin mg	Riboflavin µmol	Nicotinic acid equiv. (d) mg	Nicotinic µmol	Ascorbic acid mg	Ascorbic µmol	Vitamin A retinol equiv. (e) µg	Vit A µmol	Vitamin D cholecalciferol (f) µg	Vit D nmol	Calcium mg	Calcium mmol	Iron mg	Iron µmol
BOYS AND GIRLS																					
0 up to 1 year		7.3	800	3.3	20	0.3	1.0	0.4	1.1	5	40	15	85	450	1.6	10.0	26	600	15 (g)	6	110
1 up to 2 years		11.4	1200	5.0	30	0.5	1.7	0.6	1.6	7	55	20	110	300	1.0	10.0	26	500	13	7	125
2 up to 3 years		13.5	1400	5.9	35	0.6	2.0	0.7	1.9	8	65	20	110	300	1.0	10.0	26	500	13	7	125
3 up to 5 years		16.5	1600	6.7	40	0.6	2.0	0.8	2.1	9	75	20	110	300	1.0	10.0	26	500	13	8	140
5 up to 7 years		20.5	1800	7.5	45	0.7	2.3	0.9	2.3	10	80	20	110	300	1.0	2.5	6.5	500	13	8	140
7 up to 9 years		25.1	2100	8.8	53	0.8	2.7	1.0	2.6	11	90	20	110	400	1.4	2.5	6.5	500	13	10	180
BOYS																					
9 up to 12 years		31.9	2500	10.5	63	1.0	3.3	1.2	3.2	14	115	25	140	575	2.0	2.5	6.5	700	18	13	230
12 up to 15 years		45.5	2800	11.7	70	1.1	3.7	1.4	3.7	16	130	25	140	725	2.4	2.5	6.5	700	18	14	250
15 up to 18 years		61.0	3000	12.6	75	1.2	4.0	1.7	4.5	19	150	30	170	750	2.5	2.5	6.5	600	15	15	265
GIRLS																					
9 up to 12 years		33.0	2300	9.6	58	0.9	3.0	1.2	3.2	13	105	25	140	575	2.0	2.5	6.5	700	18	13	230
12 up to 15 years		48.6	2300	9.6	58	0.9	3.0	1.4	3.7	16	130	25	140	725	2.4	2.5	6.5	700	18	14	250
15 up to 18 years		56.1	2300	9.6	58	0.9	3.0	1.4	3.7	16	130	30	170	750	2.5	2.5	6.5	600	15	15	265
MEN																					
18 up to 35 years	Sedentary	65	2700	11.3	68	1.1	3.7	1.7	4.5	18	150	30	170	750	2.5	2.5	6.5	500	13	10	180
	Moderately active		3000	12.6	75	1.2	4.0	1.7	4.5	18	150	30	170	750	2.5	2.5	6.5	500	13	10	180
	Very active		3600	15.1	90	1.4	4.6	1.7	4.5	18	150	30	170	750	2.5	2.5	6.5	500	13	10	180
35 up to 65 years	Sedentary	65	2600	10.9	65	1.0	3.7	1.7	4.5	18	150	30	170	750	2.5	2.5	6.5	500	13	10	180
	Moderately active		2900	12.1	73	1.2	4.0	1.7	4.5	18	150	30	170	750	2.5	2.5	6.5	500	13	10	180
	Very active		3600	15.1	90	1.4	4.6	1.7	4.5	18	150	30	170	750	2.5	2.5	6.5	500	13	10	180
65 up to 75 years	} Assuming a sedentary life	63	2350	9.8	59	0.9	3.0	1.7	4.5	18	150	30	170	750	2.5	2.5	6.5	500	13	10	180
75 and over		63	2100	8.8	53	0.8	2.7	1.7	4.5	18	150	30	170	750	2.5	2.5	6.5	500	13	10	180
WOMEN																					
18 up to 55 years	Most occupations	55	2200	9.2	55	0.9	3.0	1.3	3.5	15	120	30	170	750	2.5	2.5	6.5	500	13	12	180
	Very active		2500	10.5	63	1.0	3.3	1.3	3.5	15	120	30	170	750	2.5	2.5	6.5	500	13	12	180
55 up to 75 years	} Assuming a sedentary life	53	2050	8.6	51	0.8	2.7	1.3	3.5	15	120	30	170	750	2.5	2.5	6.5	500	13	10	180
75 and over		53	1900	8.0	48	0.7	2.3	1.3	3.5	15	120	30	170	750	2.5	2.5	6.5	500	13	10	180
Pregnancy, 2nd and 3rd trimester			2400	10.0	60	1.0	3.3	1.6	4.2	18	150	60	340	750	2.5	10.0	26	1200	30	15	265
Lactation			2700	11.3	68	1.1	3.7	1.8	4.8	21	170	60	340	1200	3.5	10.0	26	1200	30	15	265

(a) Megajoules (10⁶ joules). Calculated from the relation 1 kilocalorie = 4·186 kilojoules.
(b) Recommended intakes calculated as providing 10 per cent of energy requirements.
(c) The figures, calculated from energy requirements and the recommended intake of thiamin of 0·4 mg/1000 kcal.
(d) 1 nicotinic acid equivalent = 1 mg available nicotinic acid or 60 mg tryptophan.
(e) 1 retinol equivalent = 1 µg retinol or 6 µg β-carotene or 12 µg other biologically active carotenoids.
(f) No dietary source may be necessary for those adequately exposed to sunlight, but the requirement for the housebound may be greater than that recommended.
(g) These figures apply to infants who are not breast fed. Infants who are entirely breast fed receive smaller quantities; these are adequate since absorption from breast milk is higher.

than is needed to prevent scurvy, and there is no evidence that we are any less healthy than Americans because we drink less fruit juice. The US figure for iron for women during their reproductive life is set at 320 μmol (18 mg)/day. This aims to cover the extra needs of women who have large menstrual losses. It is not easy to draw up a diet containing so much iron using only normal foods and this recommendation implies a policy of enriching some food, e.g. bread, with iron. It is not yet practical to add iron to bread in a form which is absorbable and yet does not impair the quality of the bread. Women with large menstrual losses need gynaecological treatment or medicinal iron or both. The energy allowances for adults are a little lower. The reason for this is that the majority of Americans appear to lead a more sedentary and less physically active life.

The recommendations in table 5.7 are liberal and provide a wide margin of safety. If surveys show that they are not met in any section of a community, it does not follow that malnutrition is present, but it is an indication for careful clinical examinations for evidence of deficiency states.

WASTE

Waste products leave the body by four routes, in the expired air, in the urine, in the faeces and in the sweat.

EXPIRED AIR

This usually contains from 3 to 5 per cent CO_2. The total amount of CO_2 expired daily normally ranges from 350–600 litres and contains about 17–25 mol (200–300 g) of carbon. Thus the lungs excrete a far greater bulk of waste matter than do the kidneys.

The expired air is always saturated with water vapour at approximately body temperature and from 250 to 500 g of water are lost from the body daily in this way. This is an obligatory water loss and not subject to physiological control.

The volatile substances ethanol and acetone can be detected in the expired air, if they are present in the blood in sufficient concentrations. These substances diffuse across the lung membranes and into the expired air in amounts directly proportional to concentration in the blood. Hence an analysis of the alcohol content of the expired air indicates to the police the concentration in blood. The total quantity of both alcohol and acetone that can be lost from the body in this way is small and the lungs play an insignificant role in the clearing of these substances from the blood.

Nitrogenous waste products are not excreted via the lungs.

URINE

Table 5.8 shows the composition of a 24-hour specimen of urine from a healthy young man.

TABLE 5.8. The usual range of the amounts of the main constituents in a 24-hr specimen of urine from a healthy young man.

WATER (ml)	1000–2500
ELECTROLYTES (mmol)	
Cations	
Sodium	100–250
Potassium	40–80
Magnesium	5–15
Calcium	1·2–8
Ammonia	30–60
Hydrogen	pH 5·0–7·0
Titratable acidity	20–40
Anions	
Chloride	100–250
Inorganic sulphate	50–120
Bicarbonate	0–20
Phosphate	20–50
NITROGEN CONTAINING SUBSTANCES (mmol)*	
Urea	300–650
Creatinine	5–15
Uric acid	1·2–8
Ammonia	30–60
Total amino acids	up to 150

* The urine also contains protein in amounts up to 50 mg/day. This is not detectable by the methods of analysis in common clinical use.

Water

The urinary output of water is regulated so that the concentration of the plasma is kept within the range of 275–295 mosmol/l. It is also the means by which the total water content of the body is controlled. This varies slightly from day to day and anyone who weighs himself regularly before breakfast frequently finds daily variations of 0·5 kg, and a gain or loss of 1 kg is not unusual. Most of this variation in body weight is due to changes in body water.

The water also acts as a vehicle for the other urinary constituents, which for a healthy man on a normal diet amount to about 50 g/day, most of which is urea and sodium chloride. Consider a subject eating 100 g of protein daily. There will be about 16 g of N to excrete. By far the greater part of this is excreted as urea and there will be about 500 mmol (30 g) of urea in the urine (60 g of urea contains 28 g of N). If the diet contains 170 mmol (10 g) NaCl, about the same amount will appear in the urine. The other urinary constituents may number over one hundred, but together they usually add up to about 160 mmol or 10 g. Theoretically these constitute an osmolal load of $500+(2\times170)+160=1000$ mosmol. In fact this slightly overestimates the osmolal load as determined by the degree of the depression of freezing point. This is because in a solution of electrolytes in water, interionic and electrostatic changes modify the osmotic effects of the ionized particles (osmotic coefficient).

The amount of water necessary for the excretion of these substances is determined by the ability of the kidney to concentrate urine. In health the kidney cannot produce a urine with a concentration greater than about 1200 mosmol/l, about four times the concentration of plasma. To excrete the osmolal load the kidneys must be provided with a minimum of $1000/1200=830$ ml of water. This is the **obligatory water** in the urine. Its volume depends on the nature of the diet. If this amount of water is not available from the normal intake, water is drawn from the tissues and the body becomes dehydrated, as may happen to the castaway in a lifeboat. Most of us drink more water than is necessary to excrete the urinary solids and it is unusual for urine to be excreted at its maximum concentration. With a urinary output of 1500 ml, the 1000 mosmol solute load will give a concentration of 660 mosmol/l.

The osmolal concentration of urine can be derived from a determination of its freezing point, which can be easily carried out in the laboratory on a small sample. A doctor can, however, get a good approximation in his consulting room or office by measuring its specific gravity using a simple hydrometer. The relation between sp gr and osmolality varies with the composition of the urine and the molecular weights of its constituents. Urine from a healthy subject on a normal diet shows the following general relationships:

sp gr	1·010	1·015	1·020	1·025	1·030	1·035
mosmol/l	400	600	800	1000	1200	1400

The 24-hour sample of urine from the subject on the diet described above thus has a specific gravity of approximately 1·017.

It is difficult to dry urine and so determine directly the urinary solids. However, it was pointed out in a German thesis over one hundred years ago that the last two figures in the specific gravity multiplied by two give the grammes of solids present in a litre of urine. For our subject 1 litre of urine will be calculated to contain $17\times2=34$ g of solids, and so his daily output of 1500 ml would contain 51 g of solids. This is approximately the figure suggested for the urinary solids based on a consideration of his diet.

Acid

Human urine is usually acid and the pH may range from 4·0 to 8·0. In health, the degree of acidity is determined by the amount of metabolic acid produced in the body and eliminated in the urine. Oxidation of sulphur-containing proteins is an important source of H^+, and 100 g protein produce the equivalent of about 30 mmol of sulphuric acid. This acid is of course buffered in the urine mainly by phosphate and NH_3 secreted into the urine by the kidney. In fruits and some vegetables, potassium and to a lesser extent sodium may be present as salts of organic acids, which are metabolized in the body and not excreted in significant amounts in the urine. Those who eat large quantities of fruits and vegetables may have alkaline urine. Alkaline urine is, of course, commonly found in patients who have been taking sodium bicarbonate. The kidney is able to manufacture ammonia and to excrete ammonium ions in the urine. In this way it can contribute to the maintenance acid–base balance of the body (p. 6.1). The role of the kidney in regulating the acid–base balance is very important in many pathological states. However the amount of acid that the kidney normally secretes is relatively small and amounts to between 50–100 mmol/day.

Nitrogenous substances

In the healthy adult the total amount of nitrogen in the urine is determined by the dietary intake and with typical European diets about 85 per cent is excreted as urea. By contrast in Asian diets the proportion of the urinary nitrogen excreted as urea is often less and may be as low as 60 per cent, but the reason for this is unknown.

The creatinine excretion in the urine is remarkably constant in any one individual and is independent of the diet. It is probably related to the muscle mass and, indeed, creatinine excretion is sometimes taken as a measure of the muscle mass in studies of body composition.

Uric acid is derived from purine metabolism. The urinary output comes mostly from the endogenous breakdown of the purines of the body and it is little affected, if at all, by the purine content of the diet.

The urinary ammonia is discussed on p. 35.32. The kidney normally conserves amino acids and only small amounts of these substances are found in the urine in health. There are a number of diseases, each fortunately rare, when, owing to a hereditary defect of kidney function, one or more of the amino acids may appear in the urine. A very small amount of protein is present in the urine, derived from the plasma and by exudation from the urinary tract.

Other urinary constituents

The urine contains small amounts of almost all other soluble body constituents. Its yellow colour is due to the presence of urochrome which is derived from one of the bile pigments. All the water-soluble vitamins and hormones and their metabolites can be detected in the urine. The amounts present are small and the losses are normally of no significance. However, the urinary output of a particular vitamin or hormone is often of interest both in physiological and pathological studies.

The kidney is readily conceived of as an organ for removing waste products from the body. It is much more than this, for it is the principal means of regulating the chemical composition of the internal environment of the body. This aspect is the main theme of chap. 35.

The composition of the urine and its volume are largely determined by the nature of the diet. In many renal diseases where the ability of the kidneys to carry out their functions is impaired, modification of the diet is an important aid in treatment. Recently we saw a patient receiving an elaborate and expensive treatment for assisting the removal of an excess of sodium from the body. This patient had been given a kipper for breakfast.

FAECES

Table 5.9 gives the composition of the normal faecal output over 24 hours of a young man on a European diet. Both the formation and output of faeces are irregular, so an analysis of a single sample cannot give an accurate picture of the daily output. Such an assessment is best made by collecting the faeces passed over at least 3 and preferably 5 days.

TABLE 5.9. The usual range of the amounts of main constituents in the faeces over a 24-h period in a healthy young man on a European diet.

Total weight (g)	75–200
Water (g)	50–175
Dry weight (g)	15–30
Protein* (g)	4–7
Fat (g)	3–5
Soluble carbohydrate	trace
Fibre	about 5
Sodium (mmol)	5–10
Potassium (mmol)	8–15
Calcium (mmol)	12·5–25
Iron (μmol)	180–270
Total ash (g)	3–6

* The figures for protein are analyses of $N \times 6\cdot25$. About half the N in the faeces is actually present as protein.

Faeces consist of dietary matter which the alimentary canal has been unable to absorb, together with the remnants of the mucous membranes of the alimentary tract, which are constantly being shed and renewed. Other substances are excreted into the gut lumen with the digestive juices. It is not easy to determine how much of any constituent of the faeces is dietary waste (exogenous) and how much is a true excretion (endogenous).

The bulk of faeces depends largely on the fibre content of the diet. Most European diets provide about 5 g of fibre daily, but 15 g would not be unusual in a vegetarian. All of this appears in the faeces as 'roughage'.

The intestinal contents are greatly modified by bacterial action in the large intestine. Bacteria form from 5 to 10 per cent of the dry weight of the faeces. They produce gas and most people pass up to 200 ml of flatus daily, part of which is probably derived from swallowed air. Flatus contains up to 30 per cent of methane, but the loss of energy in this way by man is very small. Cattle lose about 10 per cent of the gross energy content of the diets as methane.

SWEAT

The sweat is a means of getting rid of waste heat. The body is cooled by the evaporation of the sweat on the skin and sweat which simply drips off is ineffective in this regard. The evaporation of 1 litre of sweat removes 2·4 MJ (580 kcal) of heat from the body. The usual range for rates of sweating is from 0·1 to 1·0 l/h and this corresponds to heat losses of from 2·5–25 kJ (0·6–6·0 kcal)/min (figures which may be compared with rates of energy expenditure given in chap. 4). When the temperature of the environment is greater than the temperature of the surface of the skin, cooling by radiation and convection is impossible (p. 43.4). All heat loss can then take place only by evaporation of sweat. In very hot climates as much as 12–20 MJ (3000–5000 kcal)/day may be lost in the sweat.

Sweat varies greatly in chemical composition, but is essentially a hypotonic solution of sodium chloride. The osmolality lies between 100 and 200 mosmol/l. (plasma 285 mosmol/l). Table 5.10 gives some normal values for sweat. Losses of sodium can easily be as much as 250 mmol/day, which might require a doubling of the normal intake. In exceptional cases the losses can be greater.

Excretion of urea in the sweat is small and sweating is not of practical assistance to patients with kidney disease.

TABLE 5.10. The composition of normal sweat

Cations	
Sodium	20–70 mmol/l
Potassium	5–15 mmol/l
Anions	
Chloride	20–76 mmol/l
Lactate	10–30 mmol/l
Urea	4–20 mmol/l
pH	4–6·5
Freezing point	−0·18 to −0·37°C
Osmolality	100–200mosmol/l

FURTHER READING

DAVIDSON, SIR STANLEY, PASSMORE R., BROCK J.F. & TRUSWELL A.S. (1975) *Human Nutrition and Dietetics*, 6th Edition. Edinburgh: Churchill Livingstone.

GOODHART R.S. & SHILS M.E. (1973) *Modern Nutrition in Health and Disease*, 5th Revised Edition. Philadelphia: Lea & Febiger.

TABLES OF FOOD ANALYSES

McCANCE R.A. & WIDDOWSON E.M. (1960) The Composition of Foods, 3rd Edition. *Medical Research Council Special Report Series* No. 297. London: H.M.S.O.

WATT B.K. & MERRILL A.L. (1963) *Composition of Foods*. U.S. Dept. Agric. Handbook No. 8, Washington: Govt. Printing Office.

These tables give analyses of foods commonly consumed in the UK and the USA. Tables for other countries are available and Davidson *et al.* list 30 of these and give the addresses from which they may be obtained.

Chapter 6
Acids, bases and buffer mechanisms

This chapter is concerned with the physicochemical properties of biological fluids which are involved in the control of their 'reaction', i.e. their degree of acidity or alkalinity. Mammalian cells derive energy from oxidative processes which produce acidic waste products. These substances pass into the fluids of the body and are subsequently excreted (p. 35.29). A series of mechanisms stabilize the concentration of hydrogen ions in the body fluids within relatively narrow limits. This degree of control of hydrogen ion concentration is characteristic of mammals and greater variation in the reaction of body fluids occurs in fishes or insects. It is not known why the hydrogen concentration is so finely regulated because, although enzymes are sensitive to changes in acidity, they usually exhibit optimum activity (p. 7.6) over a much wider range of hydrogen ion concentration than is maintained in the plasma. However, cell membranes and subcellular particle membranes consist of specific proteins which are amphiprotic (p. 11.3) and are sensitive to small changes in the hydrogen ion concentration of their environment. It seems likely that the high degree of specificity shown by cell membranes may be attributed to highly organized lipoproteins arranged in a specific orientation (p. 13.6). It is possible that the tertiary and quaternary structure of the lipoprotein membranes, and hence the membrane characteristics, may be altered by the hydrogen ion concentration of the bathing fluid. Thus the normal metabolic activity of the cell and of the whole animal is adversely affected by wide changes in hydrogen ion concentration.

Acids

In 1923, Bronsted in Denmark and Lowry in England suggested that an acid be defined as a proton donor and a base be defined as a proton acceptor. Thus the relationship between acids and bases can be described as follows:

$$AH \rightleftharpoons A^- + H^+ \qquad (1)$$
Acid — Base — Hydrogen ion or proton

In aqueous solution hydrogen ions exist in hydrated form $[H_3O^+]$ and are termed **hydroxonium ions**. So when an acid ionizes in water this equation is more correctly written:

$$AH + H_2O \rightleftharpoons A^- + H_3O^+ \qquad (2)$$
Acid — Water — Base — Hydroxonium ion

By custom, however, the symbol for the concentration of hydrogen ions is usually represented as $[H^+]$ rather than in its hydrated form $[H_3O^+]$, the square brackets denoting concentration. An acid and its equivalent base are described as **conjugate** or a **conjugate pair**. Table 6.1

TABLE 6.1. The ionization of acids, the formation of the hydroxonium ions and the resultant conjugate bases.

	Acids	Conjugate bases
Water	$H_2O + H_2O$	$\leftrightharpoons H_3O^+ + OH^-$
Hydrochloric acid	$HCl + H_2O$	$\leftrightharpoons H_3O^+ + Cl^-$
Carbonic acid	$H_2CO_3 + H_2O$	$\leftrightharpoons H_3O^+ + HCO_0^-$
	$HCO_3^- + H_2O$	$\leftrightharpoons H_3O^+ + CO_0^{--}$
Phosphoric acid	$H_3PO_4 + H_2O$	$\leftrightharpoons H_3O^+ + H_2PO_4^-$
	$H_2PO_4^- + H_2O$	$\leftrightharpoons H_3O^+ + HPO_4^{--}$
	$HPO_4^{--} + H_2O$	$\leftrightharpoons H_3O^+ + PO_4^{---}$
Ammonia	$NH_4^+ + H_2O$	$\leftrightharpoons H_3O^+ + NH_3$
Protein	H. Protein $+ H_2O \leftrightharpoons H_3O^+ + $ Proteinate$^-$	

illustrates the ionization of acids, the formation of the hydroxonium ions and the resultant conjugate bases. The list also shows that acids may be neutral molecules, anions or cations. It will be noted that some acids ionize to give a single hydrogen ion or proton and the appropriate conjugate base, for example, water or HCl. These acids are monoprotic (monobasic) acids because each molecule of the acid produces one hydrogen ion. On the other hand, carbonic acid dissociates into two hydrogen ions and is a diprotic (dibasic) acid. The two ionizations of the acid are quite distinct and there is experimental evidence to support the concept of the reaction occurring in two separate steps.

(1) $\qquad H_2CO_3 + H_2O \rightleftharpoons HCO_3^- + H_3O^+$
Carbonic acid $\qquad$ Bicarbonate

(2) $\qquad HCO_3^- + H_2O \rightleftharpoons CO_3^{--} + H_3O^+$
Bicarbonate $\qquad$ Carbonate

According to the law of mass action the velocity of any chemical reaction is directly proportional to the product of the molal concentrations of the reactants and at equilibrium the dissociations are represented by two distinct dissociation constants. Thus for carbonic acid

$$K_1' = \frac{[HCO_3^-][H^+]}{[H_2CO_3][H_2O]}$$

and

$$K_2' = \frac{[CO_3^{--}][H^+]}{[HCO_3^-][H_2O]}$$

Because the concentration of water is very large compared with that of solute it is customary to regard it as being constant and to include it in the equilibrium constant, thus,

$$K_1'[H_2O] = K_1 \quad \text{and} \quad K_2'[H_2O] = K_2$$

The above equations are then more conveniently expressed

$$K_1 = \frac{[HCO_3^-][H^+]}{[H_2CO_3]} \tag{3}$$

and

$$K_2 = \frac{[CO_3^{--}][H^+]}{[HCO_3^-]} \tag{4}$$

Similarly there are polyprotic acids, such as phosphoric acid, which are capable of ionizing to yield three hydrogen ions. In these cases the conjugate base produced in the first ionization is the acid of the second ionization, and similarly the conjugate base produced in the second ionization is the acid involved in the third ionization.

Thus monoprotic acids have only a single K value and diprotic acids have K_1 and K_2 values; for triprotic acids there are K_1, K_2 and K_3 values. The strength of an acid depends upon the degree to which the acid is dissociated in solution and a strong acid is almost completely ionized. In other words a strong acid is one in which the tendency to release H^+ is much greater than for the conjugate base to accept them. A strong acid is therefore always associated with a weak base. For example, HCl is almost entirely ionized and yields the chloride ion, a very weak base. By contrast carbonic acid is a weak acid and is only slightly dissociated in aqueous solution to yield the strong base, HCO_3^-. The value of the dissociation constant of the acid K_a indicates the strength of the acid. It is normally given as the negative logarithm to the base 10 of the dissociation constant of the appropriate reaction (pK_a). A list of common acids of biological importance with values for K_a and pK_a is given in table 6.2.

Water can behave as an acid and a base because it dissociates into a $H^+ + OH^-$ and it can also accept an H^+ to give H_3O^+. A substance that behaves as an acid and a base is said to be amphiprotic (amphoteric). Many biological substances, notably proteins and amino acids, are amphiprotic (p. 11.3).

TABLE 6.2. K_a and pK_a values for acids of biological importance.

Acids		K_a	pK_a
Acetoacetic acid		2.6×10^{-4}	3.6
Benzoic acid		6.6×10^{-5}	4.2
Acetic acid		1.8×10^{-5}	4.7
β-Hydroxybutyric acid		1.6×10^{-5}	4.8
Carbonic acid	K_1	7.2×10^{-7}	6.1
	K_2	5.6×10^{-11}	10.3
Phosphoric acid	K_1	7.5×10^{-3}	2.1
	K_2	1.7×10^{-7}	6.8
	K_3	2.2×10^{-13}	12.7
Ammonium ion		1.8×10^{-5}	4.8
Lactic acid		1.4×10^{-4}	3.9

Ionization product of water and the pH scale

The ionization of water may be written:

$$H_2O \rightleftharpoons H^+ + OH^- \tag{5}$$

or

$$H_2O + H^+ \rightleftharpoons H_3O^+ \tag{6}$$

The equilibrium constant of the first reaction is given by:

$$K = \frac{[H^+][OH^-]}{[H_2O]} \tag{7}$$

The equilibrium point of this reaction falls very far to the left hand side of the ionization equation so that for all practical purposes the concentration of undissociated water remains constant and hence K is very small. This means that for a given temperature:

$$[H^+][OH^-] = K_w \tag{8}$$

At 24°C the ionic product of water is 10^{-14}; since $[H^+]$ must equal $[OH^-]$ at neutrality, $[H^+]$ of water under these conditions is 10^{-7} g ion/l. The constancy of the ionization constant for water at any given temperature means that if $[H^+]$ is increased, $[OH^-]$ must be decreased correspondingly. It follows that the reaction of an aqueous solution may be expressed either in terms of $[H^+]$ or $[OH^-]$. Conventionally $[H^+]$ is used for this purpose. Furthermore if $[H^+]$ of an aqueous solution is greater than it is in pure water, i.e. 10^{-7} g ion/l, the solution is said to be acid while if less than this it is said to be alkaline.

Following the studies of Sorensen in 1909 and others, the method of expressing hydrogen ion concentrations as g ion/l was changed to employ the common logarithmic expression of those values. In this nomenclature the hydrogen ion concentration is related to its $\log_{10}$ value (pH).

$$pH = \log_{10} \frac{1}{[H^+]} \tag{9}$$

Thus, water with $[H^+]$ of 10^{-7} g ion/l has a pH of 7.0. Acid solutions then have a pH less than 7.0 and alkaline solutions a pH greater than 7·0 and the pH scale representing $[H^+]$ ranges as a series of simple numbers from 0 to 14. Although the above equation relating pH and the logarithm of the reciprocal of $[H^+]$ is widely used in biology and medicine, it is more correctly expressed as the $\log_{10}$ of the reciprocal of the activity of the H^+, i.e.

$$pH = \log_{10} \frac{1}{a [H^+]} \qquad (10)$$

The concept of the activity of an ion in solution has been evolved to explain deviations from ideal thermodynamic behaviour of ions at certain concentrations.

Ideally when an electrolyte is dissolved in a liquid of high dielectric constant such as water, the resultant ions should, apart from hydration, be free from the influence of other substances in the solution. This ideal state is rarely achieved except at infinite dilution, because the electrostatic and other influences of other ions in the solution affect the behaviour of the ions under study. Thus an activity function has been evolved to designate the apparent concentration of an electrolyte in solution. In general the activity coefficient may be calculated from the following ratio:

$$\frac{\text{Activity}}{\text{Coefficient}} = \frac{\text{Observed activity of ionic species}}{\text{Molal concentration of ionic species}} \qquad (11)$$

The activity of an ionic species is dependent upon the concentration of charged particles of all species present in the solution. Thus, as the concentration of an electrolyte decreases so the activity coefficient tends towards unity. This coefficient is influenced by temperature, valence of the ions and by the concentration of ions or ionic strength.

On the Debye–Huckel treatment of activities, if Z is the valence of the ion and μ the ionic strength of the solution, then at a given temperature the activity coefficient in a dilute solution is given by:

$$-\log_{10} \text{ activity coefficient} = 0·5\,Z^2\,\sqrt{\mu} \qquad (12)$$

The activity coefficient for H^+ is not accurately known so that the pH measured electrometrically by a glass electrode and a pH meter is not in fact a precise measure of actual hydrogen ion concentration and bears a complex and indeterminate relation to it. For these reasons the pH of a solution is always determined by reference to pH of one or more standards whose assigned pH is given by the National Bureau of Standards in Washington.

These considerations do not reduce the meaning or importance of pH determinations in biological work. Absolute values for pH and changes which occur in pH of biological fluids closely reflect changes in the activity of hydrogen ions. Furthermore, the expression of the reaction of a complex biological solution in terms of $[H^+]$ is also often valuable and does not lead to misconceptions provided the above reservations are kept in mind.

Concept of buffers

Many intracellular metabolic processes, such as those which result in the decarboxylation of keto acids producing CO_2 (the anhydride of H_2CO_3) or the oxidation of S or P derived from dietary proteins and fats, and many others which yield hydrogen ions, could result in a marked change in the tissue fluid hydrogen ion concentration. As discussed previously, body fluids contain special physicochemical mechanisms which resist changes in hydrogen ion concentration.

A weak acid dissociates in aqueous solution to a limited extent so that at equilibrium most of the acid is undissociated. The equilibrium constant of this reaction is:

$$K = \frac{[A^-][H^+]}{[HA]} \qquad (13)$$

in which the value of K is small. By transposition:

$$[H^+] = K \frac{[HA]}{[A^-]} \qquad (14)$$

This indicates that the $[H^+]$ in a solution of a weak acid is a function of the ratio of the concentration of the undissociated acid and its conjugate base. If a solution of the salt of the acid is now added to the weak acid, the concentration of the conjugate base will be greatly increased since almost all the A^- ions will be derived from the salt.

Acid $HA \rightleftharpoons H^+ + A^-$ (weakly dissociated)

Salt $BA \rightarrow B^+ + A^-$ (completely dissociated)

From the mass action equation the increase in $[A^-]$ must reduce the degree of dissociation of HA and so the $[H^+]$ falls. Furthermore equation 14 becomes approximately equal to

$$[H^+] = K \frac{[\text{acid}]}{[\text{salt}]} \qquad (15)$$

This means that $[H^+]$ of a solution of a weak acid and its salt is proportional to the ratio of the concentration of the acid to the salt. Now if H^+ are added to such a solution the great bulk of them combine with the strong conjugate base (A^-) to form the weak largely undissociated acid (HA) and free H^+ are removed from the solution. The $[H^+]$ is therefore very much less than would have occurred if the same number had been added to water. Conversely if H^+ are removed from such a solution further ionization of the weak acid occurs so that the $[H^+]$ is maintained. In so far as such a solution tends to remove H^+ when these are added, and contribute H^+ when they are removed, this type of solution tends to stabilize the $[H^+]$ due to the presence of the conjugate pairs. For this reason the solution is said to be buffered and the conjugate pairs constitute a **buffer solution** or a **buffer system**.

The classic mass action equation 15 may be used to determine the hydrogen ion concentration if the dissociation constant K_a of the acid and the molar ratio of the acid to salt in the buffer solution are known. The equation is customarily expressed in logarithms and was converted to this form by a German physiologist, Hasselbalch, from the original devised in 1909 by Henderson in America. Consequently it is known as the Henderson–Hasselbalch equation:

$$pH = -\log [H^+]$$
$$= -\log K_a - \log \frac{[HA]}{[BA]} \qquad (16)$$

Since $-\log K_a$ is pK_a by definition

and $\quad -\log \dfrac{[HA]}{[BA]} = \log \dfrac{[BA]}{[HA]}$ we may write equation 16

$$pH = pK_a + \log \frac{[salt]}{[acid]} \qquad (17)$$

or

$$pH = pK_a + \log \frac{[proton\ acceptor]}{[proton\ donor]} \qquad (18)$$

$$= pK_a + \log \frac{[base]}{[acid]} \qquad (19)$$

The effectiveness of a buffer system can be illustrated by the so-called pH–titration curve. Such a curve for NaOH and H_3PO_4 is shown in fig. 6.1. In this diagram the

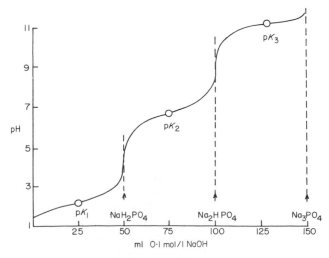

Fig. 6.1. Titration of H_3PO_4 with NaOH.

change in pH with respect to the volume of standard NaOH added $\left(\dfrac{dpH}{dA^-}\right)$ is minimal in the regions of pK_1, pK_2 and pK_3, i.e. the buffering capacity is greatest when

pH = pK. It is clear from equation 18 that at the values of pH which correspond to the values of pK, the ratios $\dfrac{[conjugate\ base]}{[conjugate\ acid]} = 1$.

Physiological buffer solutions

With the exception of H_2O and HCl, the acids and their conjugate bases, whose ionization is given in table 6.1, constitute the principal buffers in tissue and body fluids and help to maintain hydrogen ion concentration within limits compatible with life.

BICARBONATE BUFFER SYSTEM

The gas CO_2 is the anhydride of carbonic acid and the concentration of carbonic acid in an aqueous solution is related to the partial pressure of CO_2 in equilibrium with this solution (Henry's law)

$$[CO_2] = k_o \cdot P_{CO_2} \qquad (20)$$

where $[CO_2]$ is the concentration of CO_2 in liquid
$\qquad k_O$ is the solubility coefficient
$\qquad P_{CO_2}$ is the partial pressure of CO_2 in the gas phase in equilibrium with the liquid.

When CO_2 is dissolved in an aqueous solution such as plasma the dissolved gas slowly undergoes hydration with water to produce carbonic acid. This reaction is quite slow in plasma but in red blood cells there is an enzyme, carbonic anhydrase, which catalyses this hydration reaction (p. 31.21). As carbonic acid is a weak acid, it only weakly dissociates to H^+ and its conjugate base. The equilibrium falls very far to the left hand side of this equation. The bicarbonate buffer system consists of an aqueous solution containing a highly dissociated bicarbonate salt in equilibrium with a gas phase containing CO_2 at a fixed partial pressure.

$$CO_2 + H_2O \rightleftharpoons H_2CO_3 \rightleftharpoons H^+ + HCO_3^- \qquad (21)$$
$$BHCO_3 \rightleftharpoons B^+ + HCO_3^- \qquad (22)$$

Thus the P_{CO_2} dictates the concentration of H_2CO_3, and the concentration of the bicarbonate ions (base) depends upon the particular solution under study. Since the pK_1 of carbonic acid is a constant, at a given temperature, the pH of the buffer solution depends upon the P_{CO_2} and $[HCO_3^-]$, and is given by the Henderson–Hasselbalch equation:

$$pH = pK_1 + \log_{10} \frac{[HCO_3^-]}{[H_2CO_3] + [CO_2]} \qquad (23)$$

The apparent pK_1 of carbonic acid is 6·10. Thus the pH of a solution buffered by this system will be:

$$pH = 6·10 + \log_{10} \frac{[HCO_3^-]}{[H_2CO_3] + [CO_2]} \qquad (24)$$

The partial pressure of CO_2 in human arterial blood is 5·3 kPa or 40 mmHg (p. 31.23). At this pressure and 37°C the solubility of CO_2 in water is approximately 1·34 mmol/kg. Although only a small part of dissolved CO_2 is combined with water to form H_2CO_3 it is customary to regard the whole of the CO_2, dissolved and combined, as carbonic acid, i.e. 1·34 mmol/l. Each litre of human plasma also contains approximately 25 mmol HCO_3^-. The ratio of HCO_3^-/H_2CO_3 is therefore approximately 20, the log of which is 1·30. When this is added to the pK of carbonic acid, 6·10, the calculated value for pH is 7·37 which is the pH of the blood. The bicarbonate ion is the principal buffer base in extracellular fluids and the control of its concentration within narrow limits is one of the most important functions of the kidney (chap. 35). The concentration of the conjugate acid carbonic acid is also subject to accurate physiological control by the lungs (chap. 31). The system is of great importance in clinical medicine because $P\text{CO}_2$ and $[HCO_3^-]$ in blood may be relatively easily measured or calculated and estimates of the two are widely used to detect and assess abnormalities in acid-base balance which arise in the course of disease.

PHOSPHORIC ACID BUFFER SYSTEM

On purely chemical grounds the phosphate buffer system should provide a better buffering system than the carbonic acid–bicarbonate system over the physiological range of pH. This arises from the fact that its pK_2 is 6·8 and is near the pH of extracellular fluids. The total concentration of phosphate in the extracellular fluid is too low for the phosphate system to make a major contribution to buffering in this compartment. Phosphate, however, is present in urine in large amounts and it constitutes an important urinary buffer, the role of which is described on p. 35.31.

PROTEIN BUFFER SYSTEM

Plasma and tissue proteins are buffers because they possess a number of groups listed in table 6.3 which are capable of acting as proton acceptors or donors. These include the amino and carboxyl groups which occur at the ends of protein chains (p. 11.3). In addition, the dicarboxylic amino acids, aspartic and glutamic acids, provide free carboxyl groups. Tyrosine possesses a phenolic group, lysine contains a free amino group, while arginine and histidine provide guanidino and imidazole groups respectively. Since protein molecules composed of many amino acids contain large numbers of acidic and basic groups each with its own dissociation constant, they can act as buffers over a wide range of $[H^+]$.

Haemoglobin plays a specially important role in buffering carbonic acid; it is mainly due to the imidazole groups of histidine. This is described on p. 31.19.

TABLE 6.3. Titratable groups present in proteins.

Conjugate acid	Conjugate base	
(Pr)—COOH	(Pr)—COO⁻	Carboxyl
(Pr)—NH₃⁺	(Pr)—NH₂	Amino
(Pr)—OH	(Pr)—O⁻	Phenolic
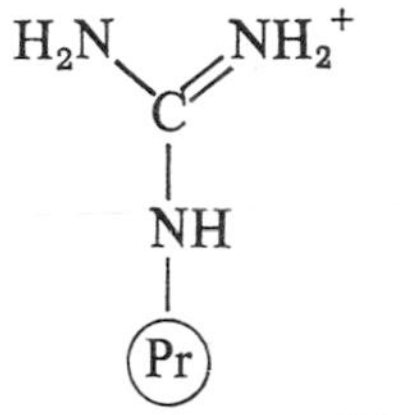	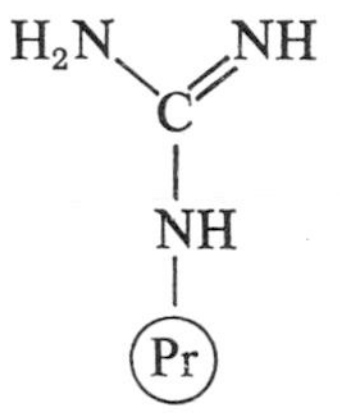	Guanidino
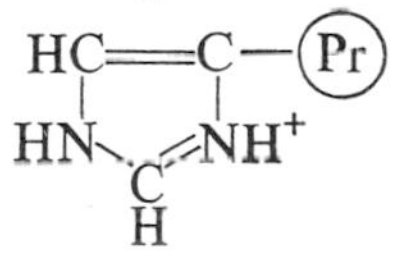	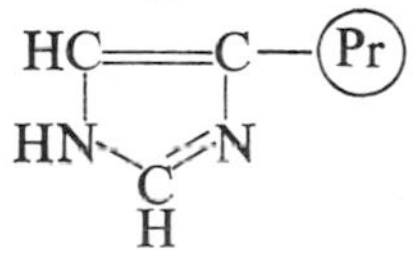	Imidazole

(Pr), protein molecule.

AMMONIUM BUFFER SYSTEM

The contribution of ammonia to the control of hydrogen ion concentration is confined to the urine and is described on p. 35.32.

Whole body as a buffer system

The body contains a complex system of buffers which are contained within the proteins of tissues and the cellular and extracellular fluids. In a solution containing a mixture of buffers the conjugate acid/base ratio is determined at any pH by its pK. Any change in pH is reflected in a change in the acid/base ratios of all the buffers accessible to the hydrogen ions. In experiments in which acids have been given to dogs it has been shown that the acids are largely buffered within cells but the bicarbonate system is the most important in the extracellular fluids.

Concentration of hydrogen ions in body fluids

Normal human plasma is usually described as being blandly alkaline with a pH of between 7·45–7·35 (mean 7·40). This corresponds to a mean $[H^+]$ of 40 nmol/l. It seems likely that pH of interstitial fluid is similar to that of the plasma after allowance has been made for the Donnan effect. Much less is known of the intracellular $[H^+]$ but both direct and indirect observations suggest that the majority of cells are appreciably more acid and possess an aggregate pH of about 6·8. The hydrogen ion concentration of some body fluids is given in table 6.4, where their values are expressed as nmol/l and in the pH notation.

TABLE 6.4. Hydrogen ion concentration of some body fluids

	pH units	[H⁺] nmol/l
Plasma	7·40 (7·35–7·45)	40
Urine	4·0–8·0	100,000–10
Gastric juice	1·0	100,000,000
Pancreatic juice	8·0	10
CSF	7·33	47
Bile	5·7–8·6	2000–2·5
Intracellular fluid		
muscle*	6·8	160
RBC	7·2	63

*Determined indirectly.

A word of warning is needed concerning the use of the pH notation. The hydrogen ion concentrations in most body fluids are very small fractions of a mole per litre. The pH notation was introduced to avoid the use of cumbersome small numbers and because electrodes used in the measurements of $[H^+]$ give readings logarithmically proportional to their activity. The relationship pH bears to $[H^+]$ is, however, complex as it is both curvi-

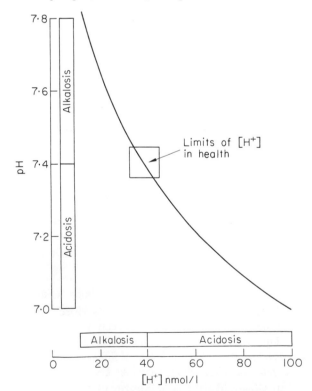

FIG. 6.2. Range of $[H^+]$ in blood compatible with life.

linear and inverse. Fig. 6.2 gives the range of $[H^+]$ in blood compatible with human life and the corresponding values for pH on the vertical axis, with the limits for $[H^+]$ and pH in health. Clearly the conversion from one nomenclature to the other cannot be done in the head.

The main danger of the use of the pH notation in medicine is that it obscures the fact that the difference in $[H^+]$ between two pH units low in the scale is greater than the difference between two pH units in the higher reaches of the scale. Thus a rise in the pH of from 7·20 to 7·40 represents a fall in $[H^+]$ of 23 nmol/l while a rise in pH from 7·40 to 7·60 represents a fall in $[H^+]$ of only 15 nmol/l.

The range from pH 7·0 to 7·8 compatible with life corresponds to $[H^+]$ of from 100 to 16 nmol/l. The extreme values are only found in serious disease. Since the mean normal $[H^+]$ in blood is about 40 nmol/l it will be seen that the body is better able to survive an increase in $[H^+]$ (**acidosis**) than to withstand an equal fall in its concentration (**alkalosis**). This may have an evolutionary origin and be due to the fact that mammalian tissues are obliged to dispose of acid produced by their metabolism.

Disturbances in acid–base balance

Fluctuations in plasma $[H^+]$ arise in many circumstances in health and disease, and their diagnosis and treatment constitute an important part of clinical practice. Four primary types are recognized and the simple examples below occur in circumstances that can be appreciated by those as yet unaware of the complexities of disease processes.

METABOLIC ACIDOSIS

During exercise and starvation, lactic acid and acetoacetic acid respectively accumulate in the tissues and tissue fluids. Lactic acid also accumulates in disorders that cause inadequate oxygenation of tissues. The $[H^+]$ in the blood rises but this is mitigated by the physiological buffers and equation 21 is moved from its point of equilibrium to the left. The production of CO_2 is increased as the acids are neutralized by the HCO_3^-/H_2CO_3 buffer system and arterial $[HCO_3^-]$ falls. The importance of this reaction arises from the fact that if the production of metabolic acid continued without further adjustment, $[HCO_3^-]$ would fall to vanishingly low values when the HCO_3^-/H_2CO_3 would cease to be an effective buffer; for this reason Van Slyke called the $[HCO_3^-]$ of the blood the **alkali reserve**.

However, the rise in arterial $[H^+]$ is sufficient to stimulate the rate and depth of ventilation (p. 31.27); CO_2 is eliminated by the lungs in increased amounts and in severe exercise (p. 45.8) P_{CO_2} falls below normal values. In metabolic acidosis the $[HCO_3^-]$ is always reduced and the pH of the blood is determined by this fall and by the extent to which P_{CO_2} is reduced by increased pulmonary ventilation, a physiological response termed **respiratory compensation**. During recovery, the depleted alkali reserve is restored by the regeneration of HCO_3^- by the renal tubular cells (p. 35.30).

RESPIRATORY ACIDOSIS

If the ability of the lungs to expel CO_2 is impaired, for example by depression of the respiratory region in the CNS such as occurs in barbiturate or morphine poisoning, or by paralysis of respiratory muscles, CO_2 is retained in the body and P_{CO_2} rises. Consequently, equation 21 is moved to the right and the $[H^+]$ in the tissues and blood rises; this again is mitigated by the acceptance of H^+ by non-bicarbonate buffer with the generation of HCO_3^-. The extent to which the pH changes is now influenced by the retention of HCO_3^- by the kidneys which increases blood $[HCO_3^-]$, a physiological response called **renal compensation** (p. 35.31).

METABOLIC ALKALOSIS

During digestion of a large meal the acid gastric secretion leads to withdrawal of H^+ from the blood (p. 32.17). If vomiting occurs, these ions with Cl^- are lost from the body and blood $[H^+]$ falls; equation 21 is therefore moved to the right and the $[HCO_3^-]$ rises. Thus metabolic alkalosis is necessarily accompanied by a rise in $[HCO_3^-]$. The fall in $[H^+]$ in turn reduces the stimulus to respiration, CO_2 elimination by the lungs is reduced and P_{CO_2} therefore rises, a compensatory respiratory response similar but in the opposite direction to that which occurs in metabolic acidosis.

RESPIRATORY ALKALOSIS

On climbing a mountain to about 12,000 feet, oxygen lack becomes a significant stimulus to respiration (p. 46.3); then CO_2 is eliminated in larger amounts than occurs at sea level. As P_{CO_2} falls, $[H^+]$ is inevitably reduced but the absolute change in arterial blood $[H^+]$ is again mitigated by the release of H^+ by non-bicarbonate buffers, a compensatory renal excretion of HCO_3^- occurs and the urine becomes alkaline (p. 35.35).

In clinical practice each of these four types of simple acid–base disturbance occurs commonly in the course of a large number of diseases. These include primary pulmonary or renal disease, diabetic ketoacidosis and disturbances in fluid and electrolyte balance in which there is excessive loss of acids or bases. Clearly the ability of the kidneys and lungs to effect adequate compensatory changes depends upon the extent to which these organs are also involved in the disorder of function. In all cases, successful treatment and sometimes the life of the patient depends upon an accurate interpretation of the variables of the Henderson–Hasselbalch equation, i.e. P_{CO_2}, pH and $[HCO_3^-]$. These three variables can either be measured directly in blood or, if values for two only are known, that of the third can be derived using the equation. Some of the problems of their measurement and their interpolation are considered in vol. 3, p. 49.54.

FURTHER READING

BELL R.P. (1971) *Acids and Bases: their Quantitative Behaviour.* London: Chapman & Hall.

DAVIS R.P. (1967) Logland: a Gibbsian view of acid–base balance. *American Journal of Medicine* **42**, 159–162.

EDSALL J.T. & WYMAN J. (1958) *Biophysical Chemistry.* New York: Academic Press.

GLASSTONE S. (1960) *Textbook of Physical Chemistry,* 2nd Edition, pp. 974–1009. London: Macmillan.

NAHAS G.G. (1966) Current concepts of acid–base measurement. *Annals of the New York Academy of Sciences* **133**, 3–4.

ROBINSON J.R. (1975) *Fundamentals of Acid–Base Regulation,* 5th Edition. Oxford: Blackwell Scientific Publications.

ROBSON J.S., BONE J.M. & LAMBIE A.T. (1968) Intracellular pH. *Advances in Clinical Chemistry* **11**, 213–275.

WADDELL W.J. & BATES R.G. (1969) Intracellular pH. *Physiological Reviews* **49**, 285–329.

Chapter 7
Enzymes

The vast majority of the metabolic reactions which occur in organisms, both inside and outside cells, proceed only extremely slowly, or not at all, in the absence of a catalyst. Enzymes are proteins, each of which catalyses one or a small group of these reactions. Many enzymes have been isolated in a pure state, and in the case of many more, in which this has not been done, their metabolic importance is well understood.

The rate of reaction catalysed by an enzyme is proportional to its concentration. The rate of reaction also depends on the concentration of the compound whose reaction is catalysed (the substrate), on pH and temperature as well as on the concentration of various types of activators, coenzymes and inhibitors. The study of the effects of these variables has led to important conclusions about the way in which enzymes act and to reliable methods for their estimation or assay.

In living tissues complex metabolic reactions must be co-ordinated, and this is achieved largely through regulation of the activity of particular enzymes by alteration of the concentrations of the enzyme, its substrates, inhibitors, activators or coenzymes. Many coenzymes are chemically related to and formed from vitamins so that it is not surprising that vitamin deficiencies lead to serious and widespread disturbances of metabolism. A full discussion of the regulation of metabolism appears in chap. 14.

Protein biosynthesis is catalysed by a complex of enzymes, and some structural proteins, e.g. the contractile protein of muscle, also have enzymic properties. Thus enzymes are not only important functional units but also act as units of structure. These generalizations are as true for disease-causing bacteria as they are for their human or animal hosts, and the successful use of antibiotics must ultimately be based on a sound understanding of the enzymology of both host and pathogen. It is possible now to describe a few comparatively uncommon diseases in terms of a failure of enzyme function, and this number is likely to increase. It is reasonable to think that in the not too distant future, practising doctors will need a much fuller understanding of the properties of enzymes than they do now.

Throughout this chapter the following symbols and abbreviations are used:

E	enzyme
S	substrate
ES	enzyme-substrate complex
P	products
I	inhibitor
[ ]	concentration of the substance in the brackets
T	temperature (°K)
t	time
K	a constant having the dimensions of an equilibrium constant
K_a	an acid dissociation constant
pK_a	$-\log K_a$
K_m	Michaelis constant
k	a velocity constant
v	initial velocity of a reaction
V	maximum initial velocity of a reaction

In chemical equations:

Ⓔ or ⒠H	an enzyme
P_i	inorganic orthophosphate
PP_i	inorganic pyrophosphate
Ⓟ	an organic phosphate radical

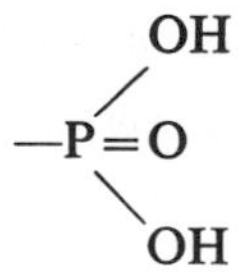

$$-\underset{\diagdown OH}{\overset{\diagup OH}{P}}=O$$ without reference to its state of ionization

ATP, ADP, AMP	adenosine triphosphate, adenosine diphosphate, adenosine monophosphate
NAD, NADH$_2$	oxidized and reduced forms of nicotinamide adenine dinucleotide
CoA, CoASH	coenzyme A
FAD	flavin-adenine-dinucleotide

BIOLOGICAL CATALYSIS

Within living organisms a host of organic compounds take part in degradative and synthetic reactions and undergo interconversion. A few of these metabolic reactions, like the reversible combination of water and carbon dioxide to form carbonic acid, occur at a measurable rate at physiological pH and temperature outside living systems but the majority proceed immeasurably slowly in the absence of a suitable catalyst.

Enzymes, like other catalysts, are active in small amounts and do not alter the equilibrium constant or the free energy change of the reaction catalysed (p. 8.2); they simply increase the rate of approach of the reaction to equilibrium. Like inorganic catalysts enzymes can be poisoned or inhibited and this is of great biological importance.

As they are proteins, enzymes are denatured by extremes of pH, by heat, and by high concentrations of organic solvents, the ions of heavy metals or bulky anions like trichloroacetate. All enzymes lose their catalytic activity on denaturation and, for an enzyme, the terms denaturation and inactivation merely reflect different ways of looking at the same phenomenon.

ENZYME SPECIFICITY

Inorganic catalysts like platinum black can catalyse a wide variety of reactions; enzymes differ markedly from such catalysts in that they show a high degree of specificity. With few exceptions each individual enzyme catalyses only one reaction or a group of closely related reactions. Since so many different metabolic reactions are known, it follows that there are very many enzymes and the list of the International Enzyme Commission includes almost 2000 well-defined enzymic activities from different animals, plants and micro-organisms. It seems likely that no two of these catalytic activities are due to the same protein.

Degrees of specificity

A great many enzymes show a specificity which is absolute, i.e. they are found to catalyse, in forward and reverse directions, only one reaction. Many others, especially hydrolysing enzymes, show a lower degree of specificity and are capable of catalysing the reactions of a group of related compounds. Thus a β-galactosidase catalyses the hydrolysis of a variety of β-D-galactosides at rates which vary somewhat with the nature of the aglycone R, but it does not catalyse the hydrolysis of α-galactosides or of glucosides.

Proteolytic enzymes also generally show a low degree of specificity and catalyse the hydrolysis of peptide bonds

linking many different types of amino acid residues, though they may show preferences for particular residues on one or other side of the bond. The pancreatic enzyme trypsin is more specific than most and it hydrolyses only those bonds in which the acyl group is a residue of one of the basic amino acids, lysine or arginine.

Sites of attack by trypsin

Chymotrypsin, also produced by the pancreas, rapidly hydrolyses bonds involving the carbonyl groups of amino acids with aromatic or bulky aliphatic side chains. Neither enzyme is entirely specific for peptides and they also catalyse the hydrolysis of unsubstituted amides and even of esters while showing the same specificity for the amino acid residue providing the carbonyl group. In fact, esters of arginine and of tyrosine are often used in the laboratory as substrates for assay of trypsin and chymotrypsin respectively.

The high specificity of most enzymes, together with much other evidence, some of which is discussed later, suggests that on the surface of the enzyme molecule there is one or perhaps a few sites specifically adapted for binding the correct substrate and bringing about the reaction. This region of the enzyme surface is called the **active centre** or **active site.**

Stereospecificity

The β-galactosidase quoted above attacks only derivatives of D-galactose, and trypsin and chymotrypsin catalyse only the hydrolysis of peptide or ester bonds of amino acids of the L-configuration. This enzymic requirement for only one optical isomer of a substrate is another general feature of enzymic catalysis. Also if an asymmetric product is formed from symmetric substrates, the reaction is found to proceed stereospecifically, and only one optical isomer is formed. Thus, the enzyme in the liver which converts glycerol to 1-glycerophosphate forms only the L-isomer. Using Fischer projection formulae:

$$
\begin{array}{ccc}
\text{CH}_2\text{OH} & & \text{CH}_2\text{OH} \\
| & & | \\
\text{HO—C—H} + \text{ATP} \longrightarrow & \text{HO—C—H} + \text{ADP} \\
| & & | \\
\text{CH}_2\text{OH} & & \text{CH}_2\text{O}\text{\textcircled{P}} \\
\text{Glycerol} & & \text{L-1-Glycerophosphate}
\end{array}
$$

Similarly citrate synthase which catalyses the formation of citrate in the citric acid cycle (p. 9.15) does so stereospecifically. The citrate is then dehydrated and rehydrated by aconitate hydratase. This occurs stereospecifically on the side of the molecule which originated from oxaloacetate to form D-(+)-isocitrate, possibly via the intermediate cis-aconitate. This was demonstrated by the use of isotopically labelled oxaloacetate:

(a, b and c in fig. 7.1). In the aconitate hydratase—citrate system, the groups on the substrate with which a, b and c respectively interact may be the 3-OH and 3-COOH and

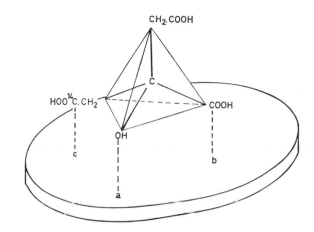

FIG. 7.1. Hypothetical interaction of citrate (formed enzymatically from ^{14}C-labelled oxaloacetate) with the surface of aconitate hydratase.

one of the terminal —CH_2COOH groups of the citrate. There is only one side of the tetrahedral arrangement of the groups around the symmetric C-3 atom that presents the three groups in the correct spatial arrangement for interaction with the three specific groups on the enzyme

$$
\begin{array}{ccccccc}
\text{COOH} & & & \text{COOH} & & \text{COOH} & & \text{COOH} \\
| & & & | & & | & & | \\
\text{CO} & +\text{CH}_3\text{CO.SCoA} & & \text{CH}_2 & & \text{CH}_2 & & \text{CH}_2 \\
| & & \xrightarrow[\text{synthase}]{\text{citrate}} & | & \xrightarrow[\text{hydratase}]{\text{aconitate}} & | & \xrightarrow[\text{hydratase}]{\text{aconitate}} & | \\
\text{CH}_2 & +\text{H}_2\text{O} & & \text{HO—C—COOH} & & \text{C—COOH} & +\text{H}_2\text{O} & \text{H—C—COOH} \\
| & & & | & & || & & | \\
^{14}\text{COOH} & & & \text{CH}_2 & & \text{CH} & & \text{HO—C—H} \\
& & & | & & | & & | \\
& & & ^{14}\text{COOH} & & ^{14}\text{COOH} & & ^{14}\text{COOH} \\
\text{Oxaloacetate} & & & \text{Citrate} & & \textit{Cis}\text{-aconitate} & & \text{D-}\textit{Iso}\text{-citrate}
\end{array}
$$

The ability of an enzyme to distinguish between the two chemically identical —CH_2COOH groups of the symmetric citrate molecule is at first sight surprising, but it stems from the fact that the enzyme, being made from asymmetric L-amino acid units, is itself asymmetric. Just as our own inherent asymmetry (right- or left-handedness) enables us to recognize the right side of another outwardly symmetric human being, without having to consider such minutiae as the side on which the hair is parted or the hand which wields a tennis racquet, so the enzyme is able to distinguish two like sides of a symmetric molecule, which a symmetric agent cannot do. More particularly it is only necessary that the enzyme showing such stereospecificity should interact with the substrate at three specific groups on its surface

surface. Thus, binding always takes place at the same face of the tetrahedron and the dehydration occurs stereospecifically. For a further explanation of stereoisomerism and other examples of stereospecificity, see p. 9.4.

Enzyme specificity and metabolic regulation

The high degree of specificity shown by enzymes is of great biological importance, since it allows the rate of individual enzymic reactions to be independently regulated by variation of either the concentration of the particular enzyme or its degree of activity. The whole pattern of enzymes in a cell thus becomes a very sensitive and flexible instrument for the regulation of the cellular metabolism.

CLASSIFICATION AND NOMENCLATURE

The specificity of the enzymes leads naturally to a system of classification based on the nature of the reaction catalysed. In the systematic nomenclature, the name of each enzyme denotes the substrate or substrates and the type of reaction catalysed, and all the systematic names have the suffix -ase. Trivial names of abbreviated form are more generally used but those based on the name of the substrate only are no longer recommended. Thus aconitate hydratase has the systematic name citrate (isocitrate) hydrolyase but the old trivial name aconitase is no longer used. Some of the best known enzymes (e.g., pepsin, trypsin) have names which do not end in -ase.

The Enzyme Commission has set out a system for classification of enzymes which also serves as a basis for assigning code numbers to them. These code numbers which contain four elements separated by points are given in the Recommendations (1972) of the Commission on Biochemical Nomenclature on the Nomenclature and Classification of Enzymes.

The enzymes fall into six main divisions; examples of each with trivial and systematic names appear below.

(1) **Oxidoreductases**: *lactate dehydrogenase* (L-lactate: NAD oxidoreductase)

$$CH_3CHOHCOOH + NAD \rightleftharpoons$$
$$CH_3COCOOH + NADH_2$$

cytochrome oxidase   (ferrocytochrome c: oxygen oxidoreductase)

$$4 \text{ ferrocytochrome } c + O_2 + 4H^+ \rightleftharpoons$$
$$4 \text{ ferricytochrome } c + 2H_2O$$

(2) **Transferases**: *aspartate aminotransferase* (L-aspartate: 2-oxoglutarate aminotransferase) (formerly glutamic-oxaloacetic transaminase).

COOH		COOH	
CH₂	COOH	CH₂	COOH
CH₂ + CH₂ ⇌ CH₂ + CH₂
CO	CHNH₂	CHNH₂	CO
COOH	COOH	COOH	COOH
2-Oxo-glutarate	L-Aspartate	L-Glutamate	Oxalo-acetate

Hexokinase   (ATP:D-hexose-6-phosphatephosphotransferase)

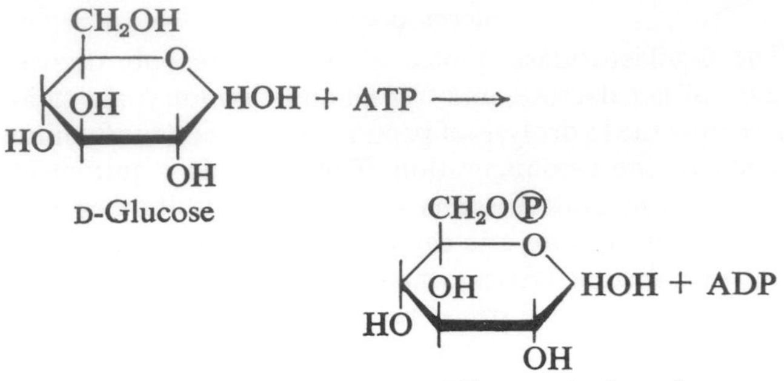

D-Glucose   HOH + ATP ⟶

D-Glucose-6-phosphate   HOH + ADP

Glycogen phosphorylase (α-1,4-glucan: orthophosphate glucosyl transferase)

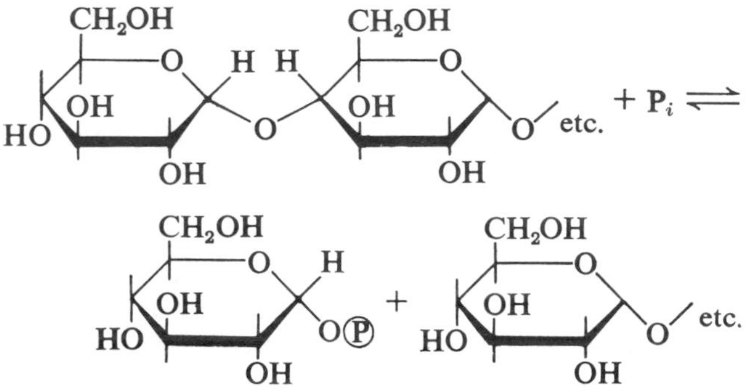

(3) **Hydrolases**: *alkaline phosphatase* (orthophosphoric monoester phosphohydrolase)

$$RO\textcircled{P} + H_2O \longrightarrow ROH + \textcircled{P}OH$$
Phosphoester   Alcohol   Orthophosphate

Lipase (glycerol ester hydrolase)

CH₂OCOR¹		CH₂OCOR¹	
CHOCOR² + H₂O ⟶ CHOCOR² + R³COOH
CH₂OCOR³		CH₂OH	
Triglyceride		Diglyceride	Fatty acid

(4) **Lyases** (**splitting enzymes**):   *fumarate hydratase* (L-malate hydrolyase)

COOH	COOH
CH₂	CH
H—C—OH ⇌ CH + H₂O
COOH	COOH
L-Malate	Fumarate

Oxaloacetate decarboxylase (oxaloacetate carboxylyase)

$$COOHCOCH_2COOH \longrightarrow COOHCOCH_3 + CO_2$$
Oxaloacetate   Pyruvate

Carbonic anhydrase (carbonate hydrolyase)

$$H_2CO_3 \rightleftharpoons H_2O + CO_2$$

(5) **Isomerases**: *triose phosphate isomerase* (D-glyceraldehyde-3-phosphate ketol-isomerase)

$$
\begin{array}{ccc}
\text{CHO} & & \text{CH}_2\text{OH} \\
| & & | \\
\text{HCOH} & \rightleftharpoons & \text{C}=\text{O} \\
| & & | \\
\text{CH}_2\text{O}\circledP & & \text{CH}_2\text{O}\circledP \\
\text{D-Glyceraldehyde-3-} & & \text{Dihydroxyacetone} \\
\text{phosphate} & & \text{phosphate}
\end{array}
$$

(6) **Ligases** (**joining enzymes**): *acetyl CoA synthase* (acetate: CoA ligase (AMP))

$$ATP + CH_3COOH + CoASH \longrightarrow$$
$$CH_3CO.SCoA + AMP + PP_i$$

A close examination of these divisions shows that some of them are rather arbitrary; hydrolases are just a special group of transferases as indeed are most enzymes.

PURIFICATION OF ENZYMES

Although some enzymic investigations can be successfully pursued with crude or only partially purified preparations, it is essential for many purposes, like the detailed investigation of the mode of action of an enzyme, to use a pure preparation. One of the first requirements when attempting to purify an enzyme is a suitable method of assay, or measurement of the amount of the enzyme, and a discussion of assay methods is given on p. 7.19.

Since enzymes are proteins, they are purified by the methods of protein fractionation (chap. 11), including isoelectric precipitation, salting-out, precipitation with organic solvents, ion exchange chromatography, exclusion chromatography, zone electrophoresis and isoelectric focusing. By a combination of these techniques many enzymes have been obtained in a pure, sometimes crystalline, state. In the development of a new purification scheme, each projected step is tested on a small sample of the material, and the total amount of protein and total amount of enzyme is determined before and after the treatment. If the step provides a good increase in the specific activity (units of enzyme/mg protein) and a good percentage recovery of the activity, the whole batch is treated in the same way and the next step is then investigated. There is no set recipe for the purification of an enzyme.

RATE OF ENZYME-CATALYSED REACTIONS

Measurement of the rate

In order to measure the rate or velocity of a reaction, it is necessary to measure, either continuously or at suitably chosen intervals of time, the concentration of products formed or the concentration of substrate remaining. It is usually better to measure the concentration of a product since estimation of quite small decreases in the initially high substrate concentration is likely to be less accurate. Colorimetric, spectrophotometric and fluorometric methods are most commonly used, because they are both sensitive and convenient for routine purposes, and may readily be used in continuous fashion with automatic recording of the absorbance of the reaction mixture so that a permanent record of the course of the reaction is obtained. When the reaction involves removal of hydrogen ions from the solution or their addition to the solution the technique of continuous titration at constant pH can be employed. Here an unbuffered solution is used and acid or alkali is added so as to keep the pH constant; the method can also be used with automatic recording. Reactions involving uptake or liberation of a gas can be followed by manometric methods.

Fig. 7.2 shows a typical progress curve for an enzymic

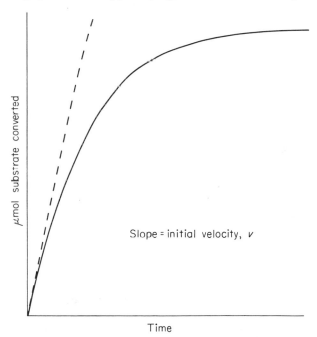

Slope = initial velocity, v

Time

FIG. 7.2. Typical progress curve of an enzyme-catalysed reaction. The initial velocity v is given by the slope of the dotted line. From Hendley D.D. & Beers R.F. (1961) *J. biol. Chem.* **236**, 2050.

reaction. In this, as in all reactions whether catalysed or not, the slope of the curve, i.e. the rate of the reaction, eventually falls to zero but in an enzyme-catalysed reaction the rate in the initial stages may be very nearly constant. The eventual decline in rate in both an enzymic and a non-enzymic reaction may be caused by the approach of the reaction to equilibrium, but in an enzymic reaction there are other possible causes. These include inhibition of the enzyme by one of the products of the reaction, fall of the concentration of substrate below levels which effectively saturate the enzyme (p. 7.8) and instability of the enzyme at the temperature and pH of the assay. The initial rate of the reaction, given by the slope of the progress curve at zero time, cannot be affected by any of these causes and it is therefore with this measure of the rate of the reaction that we shall be concerned. Valuable information can sometimes be obtained by analysis of the rest of the curve but such methods are beyond the scope of this book.

Effect of enzyme concentration on the rate

It is found empirically that at a fixed temperature, pH and initial concentration of substrate, the initial velocity of an enzymic reaction is directly proportional to the concentration of the enzyme, provided that the molar concentration of the enzyme is very much less than that of the substrate.

Effect of hydrogen ion concentration on the rate

Although enzymes *in vivo* act at a nearly constant pH, this effect is important in choosing a suitable pH for an enzymic assay and also because its study has helped the understanding of the way in which enzymes catalyse reactions.

If the initial rate of an enzymic reaction is determined at a number of different pH values (all other conditions being unchanged) it is usually found that there is one value (fig. 7.3a) or a range of values (fig. 7.3b) at which the rate is greatest. This optimal pH is usually not far from neutrality, in the range pH 5 to pH 9, but a few enzymes have optima outside this range; pepsin attacks some substrates optimally at pH 2 and arginase hydrolyses arginine optimally at about pH 10 at high and unphysiological concentrations of substrate.

It is noticeable that the ascending and descending limbs of a plot of activity against pH, at least where the two limbs are separated by a marked plateau as in fig. 7.3b, are sigmoid. That is to say, they have the same shape as the titration curve of an acid or base. This observation leads to an explanation of the pH optimum. Enzymes, being proteins, possess numerous ionizable groups on the surface of their molecules, largely those of the side chains of aspartic acid, glutamic acid, arginine, lysine and histidine and the phenolic hydroxyl of tyrosine and the thiol group of cysteine. There may also be free amino and carboxyl groups from the ends of the polypeptide chain or chains. Table 7.1 shows the pK_a values of these groups as they occur in proteins, but they may in particular cases be considerably altered by neighbouring charged groups. At the optimal pH of an enzyme, some of these groups are protonated and some unprotonated. Consider in an enzyme two such ionizable groups, —AH and —BH, which have well separated pK_a values, that of —AH being the lower. The

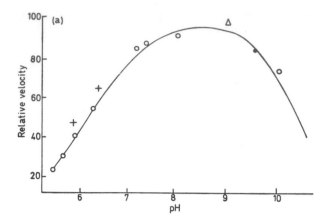

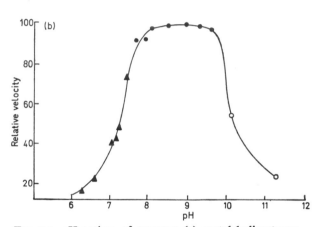

FIG. 7.3. pH-optima of enzymes (a) acetylcholinesterase (b) proline iminopeptidase. Symbols show experiments conducted in different buffer systems. From Wilson I.B. & Bergmann F. (1950) *J. biol. Chem.* **186**, 683, and Sarid S., Berger, A. & Katchalski E. (1959) *J. biol. Chem.* **234**, 1740.

TABLE 7.1. pK_a values of ionizable groups in proteins. (For labelling of C atoms in amino acids see p. 11.1.)

Group	pK_a
1- or α-Carboxyl	3·0–3·2
4- or β-Carboxyl (aspartic acid)	3·0–4·7
5- or γ-Carboxyl (glutamic acid)	3·0–4·7
Imidazolium (histidine)	5·6–7·0
2- or α-Amino	7·6–8·4
Sulphydryl (cysteine)	8·3–8·6
6- or ε-Amino (lysine)	9·4–10·6
Phenolic hydroxyl (tyrosine)	9·8–10·4
Guanidinium (arginine)	11·6–12·6

absence of a written positive charge does not mean that either may not be an imidazolium, guanidinium or substituted ammonium group. A plot, against pH, of the fraction of the enzyme molecules in which —AH is dissociated and —BH undissociated, without regard to the state of ionization of any other groups, would be like that of fig. 7.4. The points of inflection of the ascending and descending limbs are at the pK_a values of —AH and —BH respectively. This curve is clearly very similar to that of fig. 7.3.b, and it suggests that, for any enzyme showing a curve of this sort, there are two ionizable groups which must be in a particular state of ionization for the enzyme to be active, and that a pH-activity curve is simply a plot of the fraction of the enzyme present in this state against pH. There may be other ionizable groups essential for the activity, either for binding the substrate to the enzyme or

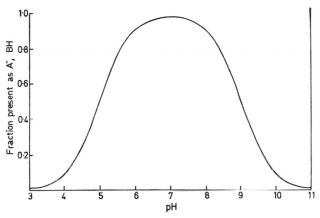

FIG. 7.4. Dissociation of molecule with two dissociable groups AH and BH whose pK_a values are 5·0 and 9·0 respectively.

bringing about its conversion, but if their pK_a values are further removed from the pH optimum of the enzyme they will have little effect on the shape of the curve. When the substrate is capable of ionization the curve may reflect the pK_a value of a substrate rather than an enzyme group.

It is possible from a detailed analysis of the effects of pH on activity to determine the pK_a values of essential groups and so to start to identify their nature.

Effect of temperature on the rate

The relationship between temperature and the rate of any chemical reaction is given by the Arrhenius equation:

$$\ln k = C - A/RT; \qquad 2.3 \log_{10}k = C - A/RT$$

or

$$\frac{d \ln k}{dT} = \frac{A}{RT^2}; \qquad \frac{d \log_{10} k}{dT} = \frac{A}{2 \cdot 3RT^2}$$

where k is the velocity constant of the reaction, R the gas constant (approx. $8 \cdot 3$ J mol^{-1} deg^{-1}), T the absolute temperature, A the energy of activation and C a constant. Enzyme-catalysed reactions show the same relationship so that a plot of initial velocity against temperature would look like that shown in fig. 7.5a, and a plot of log v against $1/T$ is a straight line whose slope is $-A/2 \cdot 3R$ as in fig. 7.5b. From such a plot, the value of A, the energy of activation of the reaction, can be obtained.

In the few cases where the spontaneous reaction is sufficiently fast to measure, it is found that the energy of activation for the catalysed reaction is lower than that for the spontaneous one; this is, of course, the expected result since catalysts lower the energy of activation of the reactions they catalyse (p. 8.2).

It is often difficult to measure the initial velocity of an enzymic reaction over a wide range of temperatures and one sometimes sees curves relating 'enzymic activity' to

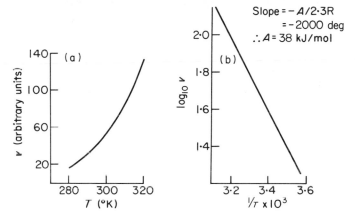

FIG. 7.5. Variation of rate of a reaction with temperature.

temperature with an optimum somewhere about 50°C. Such a curve appears in fig. 7.6. Here 'enzymic activity' is not the initial rate of the reaction, but is the amount of products formed in some fixed time and an 'optimum temperature' is found because two processes are involved i.e. the simple increase in the rate of the catalysed reaction and the increase in the rate of denaturation (inactivation) of the enzyme. Proteins generally have high energies of

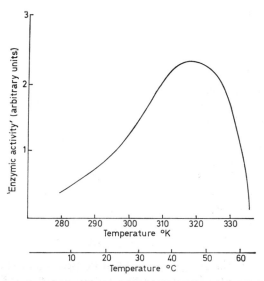

FIG. 7.6. Effect of temperature on amount of catalysed reaction occurring in a fixed time. 'Enzyme activity' is the amount of substrate converted in a fixed time.

activation of denaturation which means a marked temperature dependence of the rate of denaturation. This rate may increase several hundredfold over a 10°C rise in temperature in contrast to the approximate doubling of the rate for most reactions including those catalysed by enzymes. At temperatures over about 60°C, the enzyme is rapidly inactivated and has little opportunity to act at all. The rising part of the temperature activity curve reflects the increase in the rate of the catalysed reaction and the falling part reflects the inactivation of the enzyme.

This lability of enzymes to heat allows preparations which have been inactivated at 100°C for 5 min to serve as 'controls' in enzyme studies. However, not all enzymes are irreversibly and totally inactivated by such treatment.

Effect of concentration of substrate on the rate

Fig. 7.7 shows measurements of initial velocity plotted against initial substrate concentration for an enzyme in a series of experiments in which the pH, temperature and enzyme concentration are unchanged. At low substrate

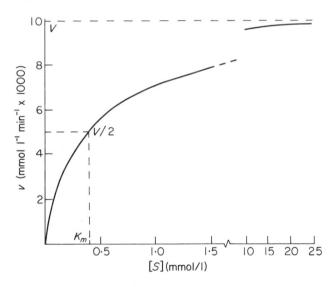

FIG. 7.7. Variation of velocity of a catalysed reaction with substrate concentration. $V = 0.01$ mmol l^{-1} min^{-1}, $K_m = 0.4$ mmol/l.

concentrations the velocity increases with substrate concentration but eventually a plateau of maximum velocity is reached. This behaviour was explained by Michaelis and Menten in 1913 on the assumption that enzyme and substrate combined together to form an enzyme-substrate complex with which they were in equilibrium:

$$E + S \rightleftharpoons ES$$

This explanation was modified by Briggs and Haldane who made the less demanding assumption that the complex is not in equilibrium with the enzyme and substrate but that a steady state is rapidly reached in which the concentration of the complex is constant. The reactions to be considered are:

$$E + S \underset{k_{-1}}{\overset{k_{+1}}{\rightleftharpoons}} ES \overset{k_{+2}}{\longrightarrow} E + P$$

to which we assign the velocity constants shown on the appropriate arrows. The reverse reaction:

$$ES \underset{k_{-2}}{\longleftarrow} E + P$$

is ignored because only the initial velocity of the reaction is being considered so that there are no products and hence no back reaction.

Usually the total concentration of enzyme $[E]$ is very much smaller than the concentration of substrate $[S]$; the substrate concentrations investigated may be in the range 10^{-5} to 10^{-3} mol/l, while the enzyme may well be as dilute as 1 mg/l which, assuming a molecular weight of 50,000, corresponds to 2×10^{-8} mol/l. When the steady state concentration of the enzyme-substrate complex has been attained, its rate of formation must be equal to its rate of breakdown in the forward and backward directions. Each of these rates is given by the product of the appropriate velocity constant and the concentrations of the interacting compounds. If $[E]$ is the total concentration of enzyme the concentration of free enzyme is $([E] - [ES])$. The concentration of free substrate will be very nearly equal to $[S]$ since $[ES] < [E] \ll [S]$.

Describing the steady state algebraically:

$$[S]([E] - [ES])k_{+1} = [ES]k_{-1} + [ES]k_{+2}$$

The velocity $v = k_{+2} [ES]$. We therefore extract $[ES]$, a variable often difficult to measure experimentally:

$$k_{+1}[E][S] - k_{+1}[ES][S] = (k_{-1} + k_{+2})[ES]$$

$$\therefore (k_{-1} + k_{+2})ES + k_{+1}[ES][S] = k_{+1}[E][S]$$

$$\therefore ES(k_{-1} + k_{+2} + k_{+1}[S]) = k_{+1}[E][S]$$

$$\therefore [ES] = \frac{k_{+1}[E][S]}{k_{-1} + k_{+2} + k_{+1}[S]}$$

$$\therefore [ES] = \frac{[E][S]}{\dfrac{k_{-1} + k_{+2}}{k_{+1}} + [S]}$$

and multiply both sides by k_{+2}:

$$k_{+2}[ES] = \frac{k_{+2}[E][S]}{\dfrac{k_{-1} + k_{+2}}{k_{+1}} + [S]} \tag{1}$$

The velocity $v = k_{+2}[ES]$ and at high substrate concentrations the maximum initial velocity, V, is reached when the enzyme is saturated with substrate, and is all present as enzyme-substrate complex whose maximal concentration is $[E]$, i.e.,

$$V = k_{+2}[E]$$

The expression $(k_{-1}+k_{+2})/k_{+1}$ is itself a constant, known as the **Michaelis constant**, K_m, and making the appropriate substitutions equation (1) becomes

$$v = V \frac{[S]}{K_m+[S]} \qquad (2)$$

This equation has the form of a rectangular hyperbola, as does a plot of initial velocity against substrate concentration (fig. 7.7). The equation simply states that the initial velocity at any given substrate concentration is the maximum initial velocity multiplied by the fractional saturation of the enzyme with substrate at the given substrate concentration.

In equation (2) v and V have the dimensions mol litre^{-1} sec^{-1}; K_m, being the ratio of the first order velocity constants k_{-1} and k_{+2} (sec^{-1}) and the second order constant k_{+1}(litre mol^{-1} sec^{-1}), has the dimensions of mol litre^{-1}, i.e., of concentration.

If the situation where the substrate concentration is such that the initial velocity is half the maximal initial velocity is considered:

$$\frac{V}{2} = \frac{V[S]}{K_m+[S]}$$

$$\therefore\ K_m+[S] = 2[S]$$

$$\therefore\ K_m = [S]$$

The value of K_m is therefore given by the substrate concentration which gives half the maximal initial velocity and this may, in some cases, be found from a curve like that in fig. 7.7. The Michaelis constant is a characteristic of the enzyme (for a given substrate and given reaction conditions) and can be determined even if the enzyme concentration is unknown, as is clear from equation (2) in which $[E]$ does not appear. V is dependent on the enzyme concentration, but if this is known in molar terms, k_{+2} may be found since $V=k_{+2}[E]$.

K_m is sometimes regarded as though it were the dissociation constant of the enzyme-substrate complex, k_{-1}/k_{+1}, but this is valid only when $k_{-1}\gg k_{+2}$ which is not always the case. When K_m does approximate to this dissociation constant it becomes analogous to the inverse of the binding constants of agonists and antagonists used in pharmacological studies (vol. 2, p. 3.9).

Determination of K_m and V

The determination of K_m and V from curves such as that of fig. 7.7 is not always possible or convenient; it may not be possible to reach the theoretical maximal velocity because the substrate is insufficiently soluble, or because high concentrations of substrate inhibit the enzyme (p. 7.10) or merely because the substrate can be obtained only in small amounts. It is in any case more convenient to use a linear expression and one is obtained in the following way.

Inverting equation (2) we get

$$\frac{1}{v} = \frac{K_m+[S]}{V[S]} \qquad (3)$$

and multiplying by $[S]$:

$$\frac{[S]}{v} = \frac{[S]}{V}+\frac{K_m}{V} \qquad (4)$$

If S/v is plotted against S, a straight line is obtained (fig. 7.8 plotted for the same data as fig. 7.7) having slope $1/V$ and intercepts on the ordinate and abscissa of K_m/V and $-K_m$. This method of plotting results has advantages over the plot of $1/v$ against $1/[S]$, based on equation (3), in that the points at higher substrate concentrations, which tend to be more accurate, are better

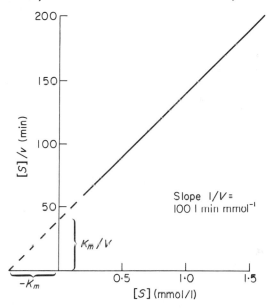

FIG. 7.8. Graphical determination of K_m and V.
$K_m = 0.4$ mmol/l,
$V = 0.01$ m moll^{-1} min^{-1}.
The figure shows a linear plot of the data of fig. 7.7.

spaced out, and thus have more weight in the fitting of the best straight line.

Determinations of K_m and k_{+2}, particularly under varying conditions of pH or solvent, or with different substrates, are valuable in investigations into the specific mode of action of individual enzymes. Such evidence has helped to identify groups in the active centres of many enzymes which are responsible for binding their substrates or for their catalytic activity; in several examples these identifications have been supported by studies involving chemical modification or by X-ray crystallographic determination of the three-dimensional structure of the enzyme-substrate complex. Values of K_m are important in assessing the physiological significance of enzymes especially when the regulation of alternative paths of reactions by changes in the concentrations of metabolites is involved. Values of k_{+2} have less importance in metabolic studies. If one is interested in deciding whether a tissue contains enough of a particular enzyme to account for the observed rate of metabolic conversion, it is sufficient to be able to measure the amount of the enzyme in terms of the rate of the catalysed reaction, and it is not necessary to know the molar concentrations of the enzyme or the value of k_{+2}.

INHIBITORS

Enzyme-catalysed reactions are affected also by agents which reduce their rates and investigation of how these effects are produced has been of great importance in inquiries into the mode of action of enzymes and more recently in understanding the ways in which the complex of metabolic reactions is regulated *in vivo*.

Many agents destroy the activity of enzymes unspecifically by denaturing the protein irreversibly. Such agents as strong acids or alkalis, trichloroacetic acid, detergents and high concentrations of heavy metal ions or organic solvents all act in this way and though they are useful experimentally when one wishes to stop an enzymic reaction, they are not of great theoretical interest and are not usually classed as inhibitors.

Competitive and non-competitive inhibition

The more interesting and informative inhibitors are those which show some degree of specificity, that is to say they lower the activity of only a few enzymes and do so at low concentrations. Such inhibition may be either reversible or irreversible; if the inhibitor can be removed and activity restored by dialysis or chromatography or precipitation of the enzyme, it is classed as reversible. Detailed analysis of specific, reversible inhibitors shows that they may be divided into two broad classes of competitive and non-competitive inhibitors, although examples with intermediate properties are known.

The difference between the two classes is illustrated in fig. 7.9 which shows data for the hypothetical enzyme of figs. 7.7 and 7.8. At a constant concentration of inhibitor, the initial velocity of reaction given by a constant concentration of enzyme at constant pH and temperature increases with substrate concentration, in a manner similar to that found in the absence of any inhibitor. If, at high substrate concentrations, the inhibition is eventually abolished so that V is the same as that found in the absence of inhibitor, the inhibitor is said to be competitive. It appears that the substrate and inhibitor, which often have similar chemical structures, compete with one another in binding at the active centre. Either one or the other can be bound but not both. Examples of such competition include the inhibition of succinate dehydrogenase by other dicarboxylic acids such as malate and

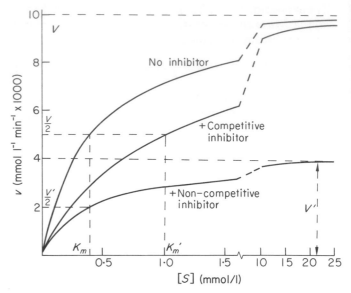

FIG. 7.9. Variation of velocity of a catalysed reaction with substrate concentration in the presence of a constant concentration of a competitive and of a non-competitive inhibitor.
$K_m = 0.4$ mmol/l, $V = 0.01$ mmol l^{-1} min^{-1},
$[I] = 3.0$ mmol/l, $K_i = 2.0$ mmol/l.

oxaloacetate, which like succinate are intermediates in the citric acid cycle (p. 9.15), and malonate which is not a metabolite. The fraction of enzyme molecules which bind substrate at any instant depends on the concentration of the substrate and of the inhibitor and on the dissociation constant of the enzyme-inhibitor complex K_i, and on the value of K_m. Only the enzyme-substrate complex can break down to give products. The reactions involved are:

$$E+S \rightleftharpoons ES \longrightarrow E+P$$
$$E+I \stackrel{K_i}{\rightleftharpoons} EI$$

At a sufficiently high substrate concentration the enzyme is almost entirely bound to substrate and the normal maximum velocity is found.

A non-competitive inhibitor at constant concentration produces the same fractional inhibition of the enzyme no matter what the concentration of the substrate, and such inhibitors show no chemical similarity to the substrate. Fumarate hydratase, for example, is non-competitively inhibited by thiocyanate ions. In a case of truly non-competitive inhibition, binding of inhibitor to the enzyme does not affect the binding of the substrate, nor does binding of the substrate affect the binding of the inhibitor, but binding of the inhibitor does prevent the breakdown of the enzyme-substrate complex in the forward direction to enzyme and products.

We must now introduce K_s, the true dissociation constant of the enzyme-substrate complex, which must also be the constant for dissociation of the substrate from the enzyme-inhibitor-substrate complex; the reactions involved are:

$$E+S \rightleftharpoons ES \longrightarrow E+P$$

$$E+I \overset{K_i}{\rightleftharpoons} EI$$

$$EI+S \overset{K_s}{\rightleftharpoons} EIS$$

$$ES+I \overset{K_i}{\rightleftharpoons} EIS$$

Analysis of the competitive and non-competitive situations by arguments similar to those used on p. 7.8 leads to the modified Michaelis equations shown below:

No inhibitor

$$v = \frac{V[S]}{K_m+[S]} \qquad \text{or} \qquad \frac{[S]}{v} = \frac{[S]}{V} + \frac{K_m}{V}$$

Competitive inhibition

$$v = \frac{V[S]}{K_m(1+[I]/K_i)+[S]} \quad \text{or} \quad \frac{[S]}{v} = \frac{[S]}{V} + \frac{K_m(1+[I]/K_i)}{V}$$

Non-competitive inhibition

$$v = \frac{V[S]}{(K_m+[S])(1+[I]/K_i)} \quad \text{or} \quad \frac{[S]}{v} = \left(\frac{[S]}{V} + \frac{K_m}{V}\right)(1+[I]/K_i)$$

These equations mean that in the case of competitive inhibition, an apparent value for K_m is found, higher than that found in the absence of inhibitor, being

$$K_m' = K_m(1+[I]/K_i)$$

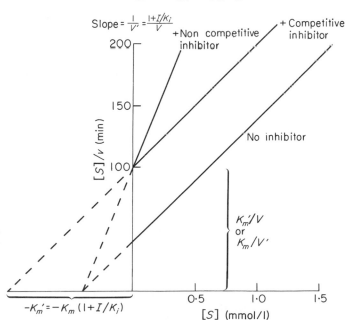

FIG. 7.10. Linear plots of competitive and non-competitive inhibition.
$K_m = 0.4$ mmol/l; $V = 0.01$ mmol l^{-1} min^{-1}. For both inhibitors,
$[I] = 3.0$ mmol/l, $K_i = 2.0$ mmol/l.

but the value of V is unchanged. With a non-competitive inhibitor K_m is unchanged, but a lower value is found for the maximal initial velocity, being

$$V' = V/(1+[I]/K_i)$$

The nature of an inhibition and the value of K_i may thus be found by plotting S/v against S for the reaction in the absence of inhibitor and in the presence of a constant known concentration of inhibitor. As shown in fig. 7.10 (the data of fig. 7.9. replotted) non-competitive inhibition gives a line of increased slope and unchanged intercept on the abscissa, while competitive inhibition gives a line with unchanged slope but increased intercepts on both axes.

Specific irreversible inhibitors

Some of the most potent enzyme inhibitors are those which react with the enzyme stoichiometrically and irreversibly with the formation of a new covalent bond. The inhibition of a number of esterases by organophosphorus compounds or of many thiol-enzymes by alkylating agents like iodoacetic acid are reactions of this type:

$$\text{(E)}H + F{-}P(OR)_2 \longrightarrow \text{(E)}{-}P(OR)_2 + HF$$
$$\underset{O}{\overset{\|}{}} \qquad\qquad \underset{O}{\overset{\|}{}}$$

$$\text{(E)}{-}SH + ICH_2COOH \longrightarrow \text{(E)}{-}S.CH_2COOH + HI$$

In many such cases as, for example, the inhibition of cholinesterase with di*iso*propylphosphorofluoridate (DFP) it has been shown that prior addition of substrate or a reversible competitive inhibitor at least partly protects the enzyme from the irreversible inhibition. This suggests that there is competition between the agents for the active site of the enzyme, so that it seems likely that the irreversible inhibitor reacts with a group in the active centre.

A new development has been the production of inhibitors designed specifically to inhibit one particular enzyme. Affinity labels are designed to contain a group which satisfies the specificity requirements of the enzyme and facilitates binding of the inhibitor to the active site, and a second, chemically reactive group which it is hoped will react irreversibly with some functional group in the active site. Tosyl phenylalanyl chloroketone,

$$CH_3C_6H_4SO_2.NH.CH(CH_2C_6H_5).COCH_2Cl$$

specifically inhibits chymotrypsin but not trypsin, while the analogous derivative of lysine shows the reverse specificity. In both enzymes a specific histidine residue is alkylated by the inhibitor. Bromoacetyl carnitine similarly alkylates and inactivates carnitine acetyl transferase (p. 10.8). Results like these suggest that if enough were known about the specificity and mode of action of enzymes important in the metabolism of pathogens but not in that of the host, the development of chemotherapeutic agents would become more rational and effective.

Metallic inhibitors

Many enzymes, especially those containing thiol groups essential for their activity, are inhibited by low concentrations of the ions of heavy metals or by metallo-organic compounds like *p*-chloromercuribenzoate,

$$Cl^- \dotsc Hg^+ \langle \bigcirc \rangle COO^-$$

This effect should be distinguished from the denaturation of proteins produced by high concentrations (of the order of 0·1 mol/l or more) of the salts of heavy metals. It is usually reversible, especially by the addition of metal-binding agents like cyanide, cysteine or ethylenediamine-tetra-acetate (EDTA, Versene). Sensitive enzymes are inhibited even by the concentrations of metal ions found in ordinary distilled water so that glass distilled or de-ionized water is necessary in work with enzymes, and addition of EDTA is often useful during their isolation.

Inhibition by excess of substrate

It was mentioned earlier (p. 7.9) that with some enzymes

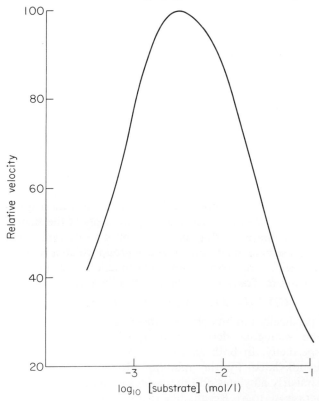

FIG. 7.11. Inhibition by excess of substrate. Erythrocyte acetylcholinesterase acting on acetylcholine. From Augustinsson K-B (1949) *Arch. Biochem. Biophys.* **23**, 111.

it is not possible in practice to attain the theoretical maximum velocity (determined from a plot of S/v against S), because at high substrate concentrations the substrate itself acts as an inhibitor (fig. 7.11). In some of these cases it has been shown that the substrate finally inhibits by removing from the enzyme an essential activating metal ion or by competing with a second substrate, often water, for its binding site. In others it appears that two substrate molecules are bound at one site on the enzyme surface, but neither is correctly bound and so no reaction takes place. Cholinesterase is inhibited by excess of acetylcholine in this way.

ACTIVATORS

The rates of some enzyme catalysed reactions are found to be increased by the presence of compounds or ions which do not themselves appear in the overall reaction and which are termed activators. Carbonic anhydrase requires Zn^{++} for its activity and phosphokinases are activated by Mg^{++}. Many other examples of activation by metal ions are known and for some there is evidence that the metal ion is involved in binding the substrate to the enzyme.

With other enzymes the activator may be an organic molecule, perhaps a metabolite in some chain of metabolic reactions, a hormone, or even the substrate itself. If the substrate acts as an activator, the relationship between the velocity and substrate concentration is not the normal one (p. 7.9); the rate of reaction increases faster than the substrate concentration at low substrate concentrations, so that the curve becomes S-shaped (fig. 7.12).

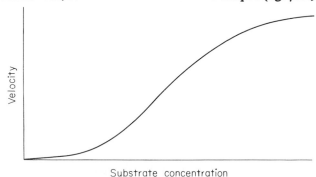

FIG. 7.12. Activation by substrate.

The activation and inhibition of enzymes by metabolites may play an important part in the regulation of the metabolism of both micro-organisms and mammals and these effects are discussed on p. 7.16.

PROSTHETIC GROUPS, COENZYMES AND VITAMINS

Although the majority of enzymes are proteins composed only of amino acids joined to one another by peptide

TABLE 7.2. Prosthetic groups, coenzymes and vitamins.

Growth factor or vitamin	Structure	Related prosthetic group or coenzyme	Function
Thiamin (B_1)	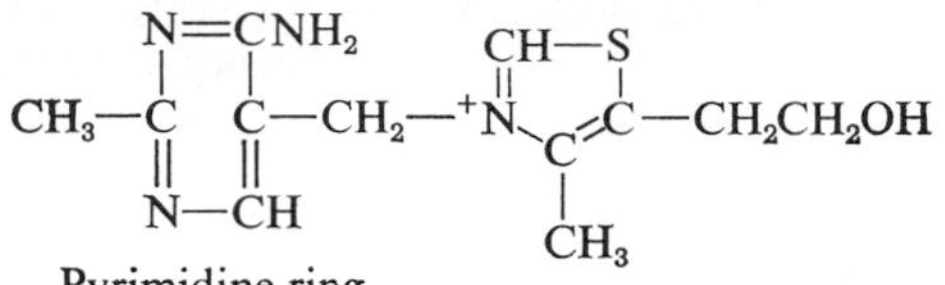 Pyrimidine ring Thiazole ring	Thiamin pyrophosphate	Transfer of some aldehyde groups e.g. pyruvate dehydrogenase system, transketolase.
Lipoic acid	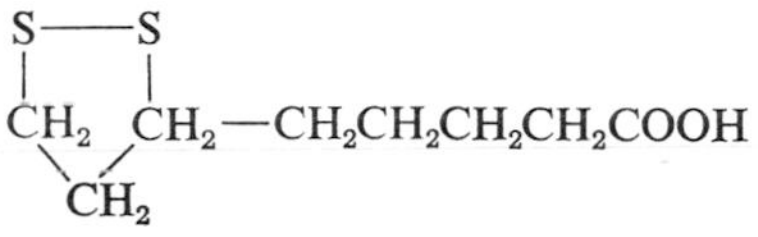	Enzyme-bound lipoic acid	Acceptance of some aldehyde groups and their oxidation to acyl complexes, e.g. pyruvate dehydrogenase complex.
Pantothenic acid	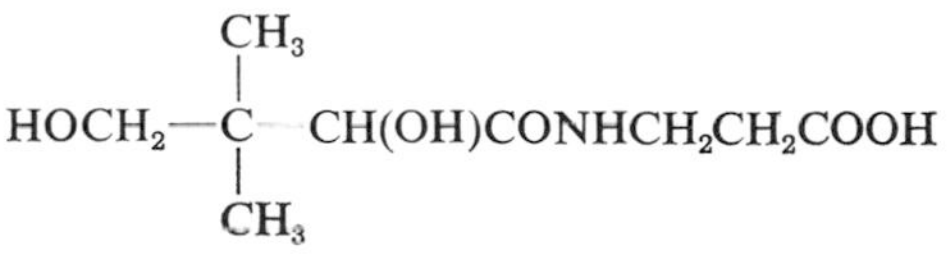	Coenzyme A	Acyl transfer and alteration, e.g. pyruvate dehydrogenase system, fatty acid oxidation.
Nicotinic acid (niacin)	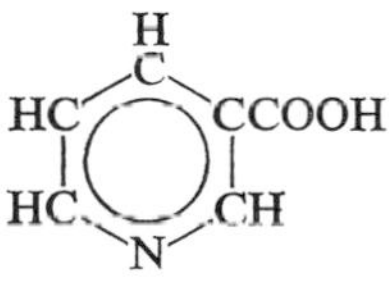 Nicotinic acid (niacin) 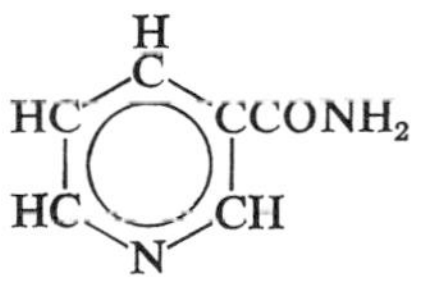 Nicotinamide	NAD, NADP	Transfer of H $\equiv$ e$^-$ + H$^+$
Riboflavin	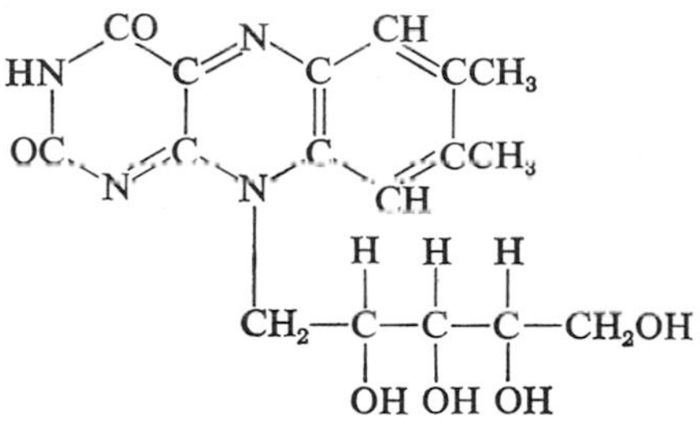	FMN, FAD	Transfer of H $\equiv$ e$^-$ + H$^+$
Pyridoxal and derivatives (B_6)	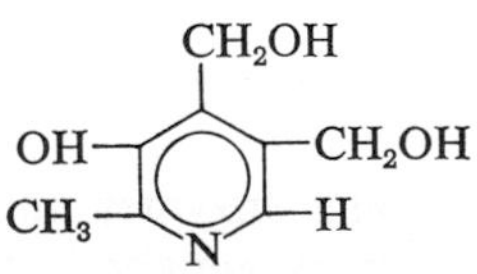 Pyridoxine 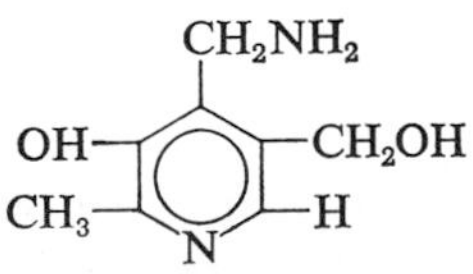 Pyridoxamine	Pyridoxal phosphate	Transfer of amino groups, generally by the formation of Schiff's bases, e.g. aminotransferases, serine hydroxymethyltransferase.
Folic acid	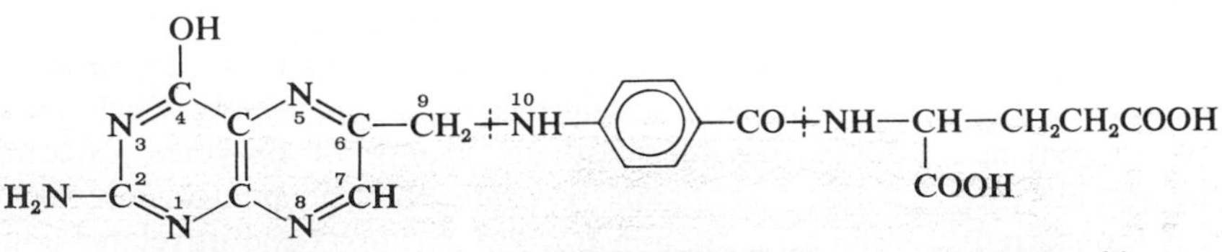 Pterin residue *p*-Amino-benzoic acid residue Glutamic acid residue	Tetrahydrofolic acid	Transfer and interconversion of C_1 units at level of oxidation of formate, formaldehyde and methanol, e.g. in purine synthesis, serine transhydroxymethylase, methionine synthesis.

TABLE 7.2—*continued*.

Growth factor or vitamin	Structure	Related prosthetic group or coenzyme	Function
Cyanocobalamin (B$_{12}$)	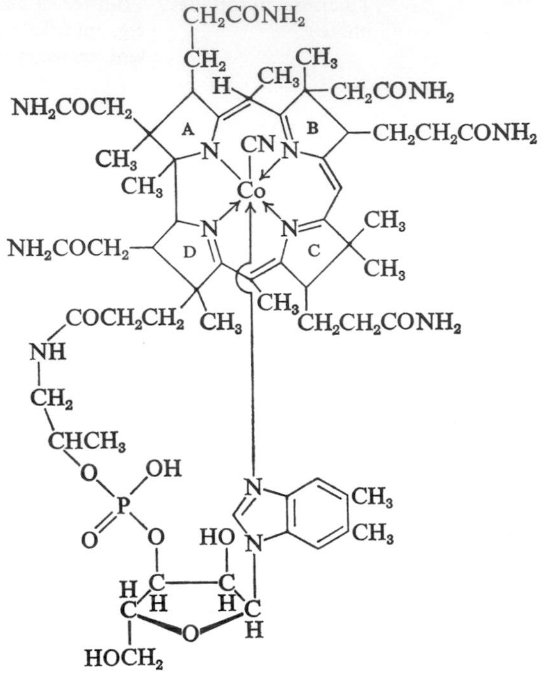	Cobamide coenzymes	Molecular rearrangements and formation of methyl groups.
Biotin	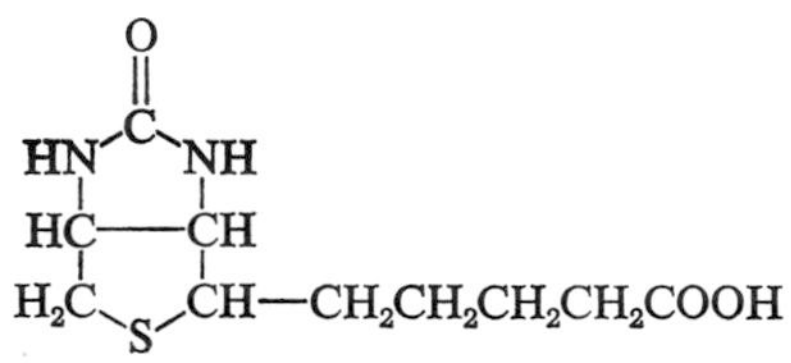	Enzyme-bound biotin	Carboxylations, e.g. acetyl CoA carboxylase.
—	—	Nucleoside diphosphates	
—	—	Haem	

bonds, some are conjugated proteins and contain in addition a relatively firmly, even covalently, bound organic compound which plays an important part in the catalytic activity. Such non-amino acid components are called prosthetic groups and the protein without its prosthetic group is called an apoenzyme. Each prosthetic group acts as a temporary acceptor of some metabolic fragment in its transfer from one compound to another. Since the prosthetic group remains attached to one apoenzyme molecule and since the enzymes are highly specific the fate of the fragment is determined when it is transferred to the prosthetic group.

The coenzymes are also organic compounds essential for the activity of some enzymes and they too act as intermediate acceptors of metabolic fragments. Unlike prosthetic groups they are not firmly bound to their enzymes but are freely dissociable.

Many of the substances which act as vitamins of the B group in the diet of man or animals, or which are essential growth factors for certain micro-organisms, are found to be chemically closely related to compounds which act as coenzymes or prosthetic groups of enzymes. Nicotinamide, riboflavin, thiamin, biotin, pantothenic acid. folic acid, vitamin B$_{12}$ and pyridoxal and its related compounds, all show this relationship. These substances cannot be synthesized either at all or at an adequate rate by the organisms requiring them, but if provided in the diet or growth medium they can be utilized for the synthesis of the essential coenzymes and prosthetic groups. Typical examples of prosthetic groups and coenzymes along with the growth factors or vitamins which are an essential part of their structure are shown in table 7.2.

ACTION OF COENZYMES

The first coenzyme (nicotinamide adenine dinucleotide, NAD) was discovered as a factor necessary for the fermentation of sugar by cell-free yeast extracts. It was diffusible and stable to heat and was clearly not itself an enzyme. The name coenzyme was given to indicate its role in co-operating with the enzymes to produce the fermentation reactions. Many other coenzymes have been discovered since.

The function of this coenzyme in yeast fermentation is to accept hydrogen from glyceraldehyde-3-phosphate in a reaction catalysed by a specific dehydrogenase (and involving phosphorylation of the substrate) and then to donate it in a reaction catalysed by alcohol dehydrogenase in which acetaldehyde is reduced to ethanol. In glycolysis in muscle the role is similar; the NAD is reduced in the same reaction but is reoxidized by transferring the hydrogen to pyruvate to form lactate in a reaction catalysed by lactate dehydrogenase.

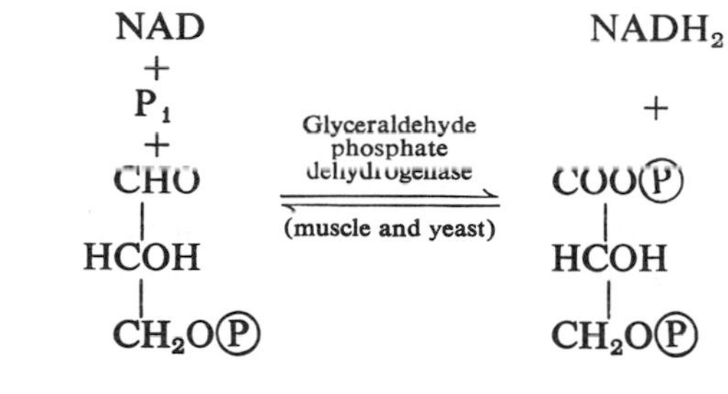

the $NADH_2$ may be oxidized by yet another series of reactions ultimately involving the oxidation of the hydrogen to water. Most of the $NADH_2$ is oxidized in one of these ways, but there are many other reactions in which it may be oxidized. There are also many ways in which NAD may be reduced to $NADH_2$. Thus neither the origin nor the fate of the hydrogen attached to NAD is in any way determined. The coenzyme can carry the hydrogen from any reaction in which it may become available to any reaction in which it can be utilized. Coenzyme A acts as a carrier of acyl groups and nucleoside diphosphates act as carriers of phosphate in an analogous way.

The manner in which the above reactions are written indicates that it would be legitimate to regard the coenzyme as a substrate in the reactions, and indeed the rate of the catalysed reaction depends on the coenzyme concentration in the same way as it depends on substrate concentration. The distinction between a coenzyme and a substrate lies more in the metabolic role of the compound than on the way in which it behaves in any enzymic reaction. A molecule of a coenzyme may be used over and over again in the same group of reactions, while in general a substrate molecule passes only once down one particular pathway.

Even the distinction based on metabolic role is not always clear. Phosphoglucomutase catalyses as an overall reaction the interconversion of glucose-1-phosphate and glucose-6-phosphate but does so only in the presence of small amounts of glucose-1,6-diphosphate. This has been shown by isotopic labelling studies to donate its phosphate to one reactant, converting it to the diphosphate, while it itself becomes the monophosphate product.

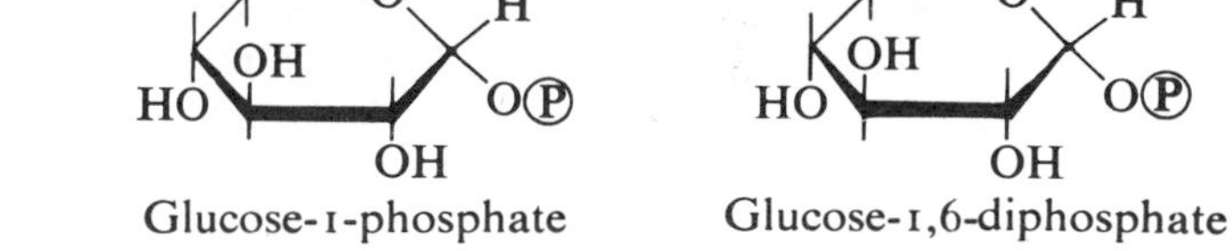

D-Glyceraldehyde-3-phosphate

1,3-Diphosphoglycerate

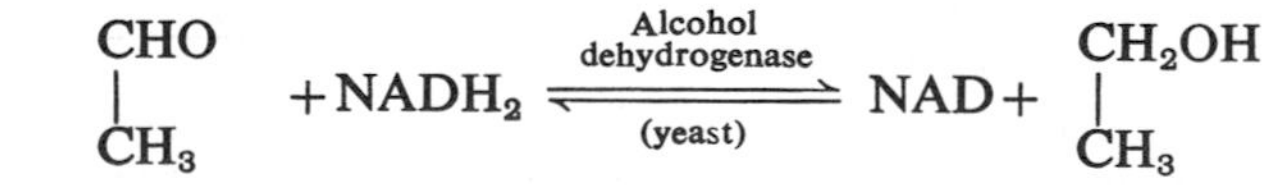

Acetaldehyde

Ethanol

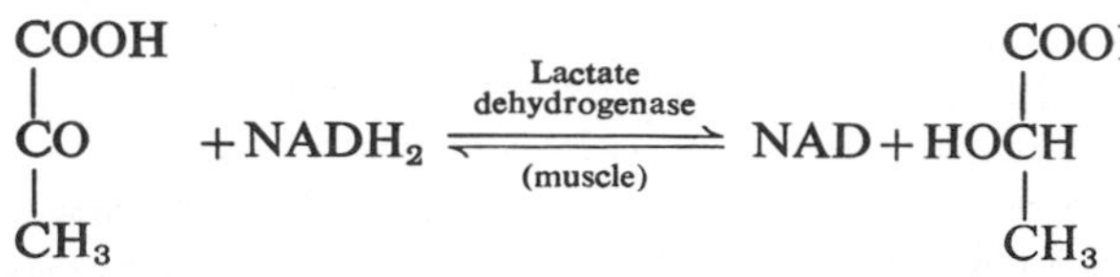

Pyruvate

L-Lactate

Under aerobic conditions in both yeast and muscle

Glucose-1,6-diphosphate

Glucose-6-phosphate

Glucose-1-phosphate

Glucose-1,6-diphosphate

Thus, although the concentration of the diphosphate remains constant the individual molecules are continually being changed. In fact, the reaction is more complex than that shown above; the enzyme itself acts as an intermediate acceptor of the phosphate between the glucose mono- and diphosphate.

ENZYME SUBSTRATE COMPLEXES AND ACTIVE CENTRES

The kinetic analysis, given on p. 7.8, of the effect of varying substrate concentration on the rate of enzymic reactions, was based on the assumption that the enzyme and substrate bind together to form a complex. In some cases the formation of such a complex has been shown more directly. Several metal containing or metal activated enzymes undergo a change of absorption spectrum on addition of substrate. Thus peroxidase which is a haem-enzyme catalysing reactions of the type

$$AH_2 + H_2O_2 \longrightarrow A + 2H_2O$$

shows a change in the absorption spectrum of the haem group when hydrogen peroxide is added to the solution, and this has been used for following the rate of formation of the peroxidase-hydrogen peroxide complex in detailed studies of the kinetics of the system.

Since enzymes usually attack substrates much smaller than themselves, and since, in those studied, only one or a few substrate molecules are bound to the enzyme at one time, it seems likely that the substrate is bound at one or a few special parts of the enzyme surface, i.e. the active site or centre. The nature of the groups involved in binding the substrate and of the groups with which it is thus brought into close proximity must be such that they induce changes in the electronic configuration of the substrate or substrates, so that their conversion into products occurs more easily (i.e. with a lower energy of activation) than is the case for substrate not bound to the active centre.

It is obviously of interest to obtain more detailed information on the nature of active centres and their mechanism of action and studies of this sort have been undertaken in many laboratories on a variety of different enzymes. The techniques used include studies of the changes in the kinetic parameters brought about by alterations in the substrate molecule or by changes of pH, dielectric constant or temperature, and chemical studies using specific irreversible inhibitors. Crystalline preparations of a complex of lysozyme with a trisaccharide competitive inhibitor and of carboxypeptidase with a dipeptide substrate have been obtained and examined by X-ray diffraction, and the precise locations of these ligands in the active centres of these enzymes have thus been identified.

The approach using specific reversible inhibitors can best be illustrated by the experiments performed with a group of esterases and peptidases which includes trypsin, the cholinesterase of the plasma and the acetyl-cholinesterase of the erythrocytes. These enzymes are all rapidly and irreversibly inhibited by a number of organo-phosphorus compounds including DFP and the inhibition is due to the attachment of one di-*iso*propylphosphoryl group to the active centre of each enzyme molecule:

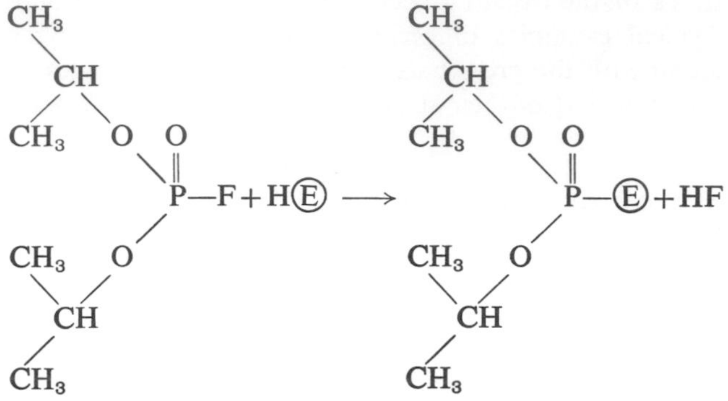

The amino acid residue at the active site to which the di-isopropylphosphoryl group is attached has been investigated in several of these enzymes by chemical or enzymic degradation. In every instance the reaction is found to have occurred by formation of a serine phosphoester derivative. The serine is always found in one of two sequences, either -Asp.Ser.Gly- or -Glu.Ser.Ala-, and with trypsin and chymotrypsin the similarity of the sequence extends even further. It thus seems likely that this serine sequence lies at or near the active centre of each enzyme.

There is also kinetic evidence for the involvement of histidine at the active site of these enzymes, but in chymotrypsin, for which the complete amino acid sequence is known, this residue has been identified at position 57 (numbering from the N-terminus) far from the serine residue at position 195. The two residues are brought close together by the secondary and tertiary folding of the polypeptide chain. We can now write plausible mechanisms for the action of these and two or three other enzymes.

ISOENZYMES

In the preceding discussion it has been tacitly assumed that in any one tissue only one protein is responsible for any one catalytic activity. The development of refined techniques of protein fractionation has shown that this is by no means always true. The important method of electrophoresis in starch or polyacrylamide gel allows one to separate proteins by small differences in their molecular charge and size and by this means many enzymes have been shown to exist in tissues in multiple molecular forms, which are known as isoenzymes or isozymes.

The best known example is lactate dehydrogenase. It exists in five forms which can be separated by electrophoresis in starch gel or starch grains at a mildly alkaline pH; they are detected in the gel by their specific enzymic activity, the reduction of NAD by lactate being coupled

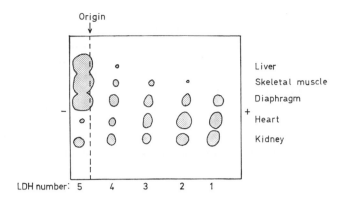

FIG. 7.13. Separation of the lactate dehydrogenases of tissues of the adult rat by electrophoresis in a bed of starch grains. Modified from Fine I.H., Kaplan N.O. & Kuftinec D. (1963) *Biochemistry* **2**, 116.

to the reduction of a colourless compound to an insoluble dye (fig. 7.13).

Analysis of tissue extracts by this method shows that tissues differ from one another in the proportions of the five isoenzymes they contain. Each isoenzyme of mammalian lactate dehydrogenase consists of four sub-units (polypeptide chains), each with an active centre for binding NAD and lactate, but there are only two types of sub-unit (H and M). The isoenzyme which migrates fastest towards the anode (LD1) is found in greatest abundance in heart muscle and consists of four H sub-units; the slowest migrating (LD5), is most abundant in skeletal muscle, and consists of four M sub-units; three intermediate forms have the compositions H_3M, H_2M_2, and HM_3. The physiological significance of this and other systems of isoenzymes is not certain.

Lactate dehydrogenases are also found in the plasma and the identification of the particular isoenzymes present is becoming of clinical importance as a diagnostic aid since damaged tissues release their enzymes into the blood; thus the pattern of isoenzymes in the serum may help to identify the tissue which has been damaged.

REGULATION OF METABOLISM AT THE ENZYME LEVEL

In a complex organism like a mammal the metabolic activity of the organs and tissues is regulated in a number of ways, usually involving the nervous and endocrine systems. At a lower level within the cell the properties of the enzymes suggest ways in which the flow of substrates along a metabolic pathway might be regulated. The rate of an enzyme-catalysed reaction is dependent on pH, temperature, and concentrations of the enzyme, substrates, coenzymes, activators and inhibitors. The activity of some enzymes is also sensitive to changes in the ionic strength of the medium, although these have not been

discussed. Three of these variables, pH, temperature and ionic strength, seem unlikely to play a role as part of a sensitive regulatory mechanism. Changes in any one of them would result in changes in the rates of a great number of metabolic reactions, and of course organisms regulate their internal pH and ionic strength, and warm blooded animals their temperature too, within narrow limits.

Examination of equation (2) shows that variation of the rate of reaction catalysed by a particular enzyme can be achieved by altering the substrate concentration or either of the 'constants' V and K_m. The maximum velocity, V, comprises two factors, the enzyme concentration and a rate constant, and of these the first can be varied by alteration of the rate of synthesis or degradation of the enzyme. The two kinetic parameters, K_m and the rate constant, are both susceptible to apparent variation by inhibitors or activators. All these methods of regulation occur.

Mass action effects

Variations of the concentrations of substrates or coenzymes affect the rate of catalysed reactions in which they play a part in a way which depends on the relationship between the K_m of the enzyme and the concentration of the substrate concerned. If the initial concentration of a substrate is of the same order as or lower than the K_m of the enzyme, so that the enzyme is not saturated and this concentration is then increased, for example by dietary intake, the rate of conversion of the substrate to products will automatically increase so that the concentration of the substrate tends to return to its original lower level. The reverse effect would operate if the initial substrate concentration should fall by a reduction in its rate of supply or by increase in the rate of some competing pathway. If, however, the concentration of the substrate is already much higher than the K_m of the enzyme, so that the enzyme is effectively saturated, changes in the concentration of the substrate do not produce changes in its rate of conversion to products. An interesting situation arises when a metabolite is a substrate for two different enzymes, each catalysing the initial reaction of a different chain as in the scheme below:

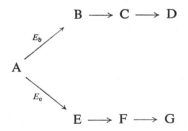

If we assume that in this scheme the enzyme E_b has a low K_m so that it is always saturated with the substrate

A, the rate of conversion of A to B will not depend on the concentration of A. If the enzyme E_e has a higher K_m so that it is only one-third saturated at the initial concentration of A, the rate of conversion of A to E will be only one-third of the maximum. If now the concentration of A is raised tenfold, the enzyme E_e will become five-sixths saturated (you should check this figure for yourself), and the rate of conversion of A to E will be 2·5 times what it was before. The important result is that a change occurs in the ratio in which A is divided between the two pathways. Such a situation is found in yeast where pyruvate is oxidized by an enzyme with a K_m of about 10^{-4} mol/l and decarboxylated to aldehyde by an enzyme with a K_m of about 10^{-3} mol/l. When the supply of pyruvate increases a greater fraction of it is used for acetaldehyde formation (fermentation) while the rate of oxidation remains relatively unchanged. Changes in the concentration of coenzymes produce similar effects, and since the same coenzymes are used by many different enzyme systems these effects provide a means of co-ordinating the rates of different metabolic pathways, e.g. the Pasteur effect, p. 9.14.

Changes of enzymic activity

Another possible means of metabolic regulation depends on alteration of the activity of an enzyme by changes in the concentrations of activators or inhibitors which may be hormones or metabolites or coenzymes involved in other metabolic pathways or may even be the substrate or the product of the reaction. An important example of such a regulator enzyme is phosphofructo-kinase which catalyses an irreversible reaction at the beginning of the glycolytic pathway (p. 9.6). The enzyme is inhibited by high concentrations of ATP and also by citrate. ATP is not only a substrate for the enzyme but also a distant end product of its activity, as is citrate. The enzyme is inhibited by ADP and inorganic orthophosphate. These effects occur at physiological concentrations of the effectors and account for a large part of the regulation of glycolysis and the Pasteur effect (p. 9.14). They are probably examples of allosteric effects, caused by binding of the effectors to the enzyme at sites different from that at which the substrate is bound and mediated by consequent changes in the conformation of the protein. There are many other examples of such activation and inhibition, but it is as well to bear in mind that it is much easier to demonstrate the effect on the enzyme than to show that the effect is in fact important in the regulation of the metabolism of the organism.

The inhibition of phosphofructokinase by ATP and by citrate is an example of the general phenomenon of end product inhibition. The end product of a pathway inhibits the enzyme catalysing the first step which leads exclusively to its formation. Since the pathway involved may be long,

the end product often has little structural similarity to the substrate of the enzyme catalysing the first step and in such cases the inhibition is likely to be allosteric, at least if it shows competitive kinetics. Other allosteric inhibitors however need not be direct or indirect products of the enzymes they inhibit.

It seems likely that the importance of isoenzymes may lie in the possibility they provide for the catalytic activity of different tissues to show different degrees of sensitivity to metabolites which act as activators or inhibitors.

Covalent modification of enzymes

Some systems of enzymes are regulated by their phosphorylation by specific protein kinases and dephosphorylation by specific phosphatases. One such system is the glycogen phosphorylase and glycogen synthase of muscle (p. 9.9). The kinases and phosphatases are themselves subject to regulation, ultimately by glucagon, adrenaline and insulin via the intracellular concentration of cyclic AMP. Analogous systems are thought to operate in the mobilization of triglyceride in adipose tissue.

Changes in the concentration of enzyme; induction and repression

The control of the rate of an enzymic reaction by inhibition or activation produces a rapid, fine control but the rate may also be altered more coarsely, and more slowly, by changes in the concentration of the enzyme itself.

Induction is a process in which the substrate of a reaction or a closely related compound specifically provokes an increase in the rate of synthesis of the enzyme. Repression is the converse process in which an intermediate or final product of an enzyme reaction reduces the rate of synthesis of the enzyme. The effect is to increase the rate of removal of the inducing substrate or to reduce the rate of formation of a product which is already present. In *Esch. coli* the formation of threonine dehydratase is repressed by the presence of isoleucine in the growth medium. In a growing culture of cells the pre-existing enzyme is continuously diluted by division of the cells so that isoleucine not only inhibits the enzyme already present but also allows its concentration in the cells to fall. The bacterium thus not only stops synthesizing an amino acid it can obtain from the growth medium but also stops synthesizing an enzyme for which it has no current need. The likely mechanism is discussed on p. 12.16.

Induction and repression have been studied most in bacterial systems but there are some examples in mammalian metabolism in which changes in the concentration of an enzyme are important (p. 33.10).

Zymogens

Some of the proteolytic enzymes of the digestive tract are secreted into the tract not as the active enzyme but in the form of an inactive precursor or zymogen. Thus pepsinogen is secreted into the stomach by the gastric mucosa and is activated by the acid of the stomach as well as by pepsin itself. The pancreas also secretes its major proteases or peptidases as the zymogens trypsinogen, chymotrypsinogen and procarboxypeptidase. Trypsinogen is activated by the enterokinase of the small intestine and by trypsin which also acts as the activator for chymotrypsinogen and procarboxypeptidase. All these activation reactions start when the pancreatic juice is mixed with enterokinase in the small intestine and involve selective hydrolysis of a few of the peptide bonds of the zymogens. It seems likely that the proteolytic enzymes of the pancreas are produced in an inactive form because the active enzymes would hydrolyse the proteins of the cells which form them. This would be biologically disadvantageous and does occur in acute pancreatitis. It is significant that the pancreas also contains and secretes a protein, trypsin inhibitor, whose function is presumably to prevent activation of the zymogens in the gland by any small quantity of trypsin which may be formed. In the small intestine, large amounts of trypsin formed by the action of enterokinase swamp the inhibitor. Pepsin is rapidly inactivated at pH values above 6 so that it would be rapidly destroyed at the intracellular pH and here the zymogen mechanism may be a protection for the enzyme rather than the cell.

ASSAY OF ENZYMES

The assay or measurement of the amount of an enzyme is important in experimental biochemistry. A suitable assay system is essential in any attempt at purification of an enzyme and is also important in metabolic studies where it is necessary to show that the amounts of all the enzymes involved in a proposed metabolic pathway in a tissue are sufficient to account for the observed rate of metabolic conversion. The proper assay of enzymes is also of great and growing importance in clinical practice where measurement of the amounts of particular enzymes in tissues or fluids is used as an aid in diagnosis, prognosis and control of treatment.

The isolation of an enzyme in pure state is usually a tedious process involving many different treatments in succession and the final recovery may often be less than 10 per cent of the enzyme in the starting material. Isolation and weighing of the purified enzyme would be a hopelessly impractical way of determining the amount of the enzyme in a tissue. The obvious practical way is to make use of the fact that the initial rate of the catalysed reaction is proportional to the concentration of the enzyme, other conditions being constant, and to measure initial velocities under suitably chosen conditions.

Assay conditions

The conditions to be considered are those whose effects have been discussed in the previous sections. The pH must be kept constant either by using a buffer or by continuous titration. The pH chosen is usually the optimum pH of the enzyme not only because the assay is most sensitive at this pH but also because the rate of reaction varies only slightly with small variations in pH in this region and errors are minimized.

The temperature must be kept constant with a thermostatically controlled water bath. The assay is more sensitive at higher temperatures because the reaction is faster, but a limit is set by the instability of the enzyme. Temperatures of 25°, 30° or 37°C are often employed. If the enzyme is found to be unstable at the pH and temperature first chosen it may be necessary to work at a lower temperature or even at a pH other than the optimum.

The substrate concentration should be high enough to keep the enzyme saturated during the reaction so that the rate does not decline because of removal of the substrate, but it may not be possible to achieve this condition if the substrate has a very low solubility or is merely very expensive. In such cases a declining rate of reaction is to be expected.

If the enzyme requires activators or coenzymes these should also be present in saturating concentrations, and ideally the incubation mixture should contain no inhibitors of the enzyme. This last condition may not be easily achieved in assays of enzymes in tissue extracts, and one may not even know whether inhibitors are present or not; it must be borne in mind that the activity found may be less than the maximum activity of the uninhibited enzyme.

In every enzyme assay it is necessary to carry out a suitable blank reaction using boiled or otherwise inactivated enzyme in order to be able to correct the rate found for any spontaneous or non-enzymic reaction or for any apparent reaction due only to the reagents used for analysis. The intensity of the reagent blank reaction varies from one method of following the reaction to another; methods of following the course of the reactions have already been discussed in general terms.

Units of enzymic activity

The International Commission on Enzymes recommended in 1964 that one unit of enzyme be defined as that amount of enzyme which causes the conversion of one micromole of substrate per minute under standard conditions, usually optimum pH, 30°C and saturating concentrations of substrate, etc. From 1972 this unit was superseded by the **katal**, the quantity of enzyme activity that causes the conversion of one mole of substrate per second under the same conditions. With either of these units one can express the specific activity of an enzyme preparation as units of activity per milligram of protein or per milligram of protein nitrogen. The latter measure of the amount of protein is often used since dry protein preparations may contain high and variable proportions of water or of the salts used in their precipitation or crystallization and the nitrogen content of a dialysed protein preparation is easily determined.

If the enzyme preparation is pure and the molecular weight is determined, one can calculate the molecular activity. This is the number of moles of substrate converted per mole of enzyme per minute at optimal substrate concentration, and is related to the older, less well-defined term, turnover number, which is no longer in use. The catalytic activity of an enzyme is defined as the number of moles of substrate converted per active centre per minute at optimal substrate concentration and is thus identical with the molecular activity for enzymes having only one active centre per molecule.

For some enzymes it is not possible to express the activity in micromoles of a substrate converted because the substrate or the reaction is ill defined. This is especially so with enzymes like proteases and nucleases which attack substrates of high molecular weight and catalyse the hydrolysis of several bonds in each substrate molecule. In such cases the units of activity have to be arbitrarily defined as for example the amount of enzyme giving a specified increase in the optical absorption of the products of the reaction soluble in a suitable precipitating reagent.

SUBCELLULAR LOCATION OF ENZYMES

Study of the metabolic pathways described later in this volume will show that biopolymers (proteins, nucleic acids and polysaccharides) and also simpler compounds like fatty acids or glucose are synthesized by routes which are not the reverse of their routes of degradation. Clearly if the enzymes involved in both the synthetic and the degradative routes were present and active simultaneously nothing would be achieved apart from the expenditure of the free energy of hydrolysis of ATP and its conversion to heat. This wasteful process is prevented in two ways. Some enzymes are subject to specific inhibition under metabolic conditions when their action is not required; examples of this are seen in phosphofructokinase, involved in the degradation of glucose, and fructose diphosphatase, involved in its synthesis (see chap. 9). Further control is achieved by spatial separation of enzymes or enzyme systems among the subcellular organelles and the cytosol. The latter is the supernatant aqueous phase produced when a cell is disrupted and centrifuged to sediment all the subcellular organelles. The locations of some enzymes are shown in table 7.3 which contains examples of the separation of synthetic and degradative systems.

TABLE 7.3. Subcellular localization of enzymes in mammalian systems.

Subcellular particles (p. 13.5)	Enzyme or enzyme complex
NUCLEUS	DNA replicase
	DNA-dependent RNA polymerase
	NAD and NADP synthesizing enzymes
	Histone synthesizing enzymes
MITOCHONDRIA	Tricarboxylic acid cycle enzymes
	Fatty acid oxidizing enzymes
	Respiratory chain and oxidative phosphorylation enzymes
	Haem synthesizing enzymes
LYSOSOMES	Deoxyribonuclease
	Ribonuclease
	Cathepsins
	Lipases
	Phosphatases
	Glucosidases
	β-Glucuronidase
	Sulphatase
	Esterases
ROUGH ENDOPLASMIC RETICULUM (microsomes)	Protein synthesizing enzymes
SMOOTH ENDOPLASMIC RETICULUM	Phospholipid synthesizing enzymes
	Cholesterol synthesizing enzymes
	Glucuronide synthesizing enzymes
	Hydroxylases or mixed function oxidases
	Lipid peroxidizing systems
CYTOSOL (cell sap)	Glycolytic enzyme system
	Fatty acid synthesizing system
	Pentose cycle enzymes
	Amino acid 'activating' enzymes
CELL BOUNDARY AND LIMITING MEMBRANES WITHIN THE CELL	Adenosinetriphosphatase
	Adenyl cyclase

CLINICAL APPLICATIONS OF ENZYMOLOGY

Assay of metabolites

The specificity of enzymic assays gives them a great advantage over chemical methods in estimating the concentrations of some metabolites in blood and urine. Thus the use of glucose oxidase in a system in which the by-product hydrogen peroxide is allowed to oxidize a suitable colourless compound to a coloured product makes the estimation completely specific for glucose and unaffected by other reducing compounds which may interfere in chemical estimations. Uric acid may be estimated specifically with uricase.

The drawback of such enzyme-based assays is the high cost of the enzymes. For this reason there is great interest in the development of enzymes covalently bound to an insoluble powdered support or the interior of a tube, so that the enzyme may be used over and over again.

Assay of enzymes

Enzymes may be released from cells into the bloodstream in two ways in different kinds of disorders. The soluble enzymes of a tissue appear in the blood in any condition which involves extensive cell damage or death. Lactate dehydrogenase is liberated from the heart in myocardial infarction and estimates of its activity in the blood are useful in the clinical assessment of the patient. Since different tissues contain different lactate dehydrogenase isoenzymes (p. 7.16) those from different tissues may be distinguished by assay under appropriate conditions. Thus, LD1, found predominantly in heart, is stable to mild heating or to urea (2 mol/l) and can still be estimated after such treatment, while LD5 (characteristic of liver) is destroyed and cannot be detected.

Insoluble enzymes are released into the blood only in certain specific conditions. Biliary obstruction apparently induces formation of alkaline phosphatase by the liver, and some of the enzyme appears in the blood. The tissue of origin of this enzyme detected by assay in the blood can be identified by the isoenzyme pattern found on gel electrophoresis.

Hereditary disorders

Some inborn errors of metabolism (vol. 3, chap. 47) are due to a biochemical lesion resulting from absence or diminished activity of a single enzyme system. Their accurate diagnosis may depend on an enzyme assay in a sample of tissue obtained by biopsy. There are ten different glycogen storage diseases affecting either liver or muscle which can be identified in this way (vol. 3, p. 47.12).

There is at present considerable interest in replacing the missing enzyme in patients with a hereditary lack. Experiments are still at an early stage but some success has been found in model experiments, in introducing a β-fructofuranosidase into rats, which do not possess such an enzyme. The enzyme was injected entrapped in particles prepared by emulsification of a solution of the enzyme with phosphatidyl choline, cholesterol and phosphatidic acid and these particles were shown to be taken up by the lysosomes of the liver and spleen. These results are promising, though there are many problems, not least of immunological reaction to a foreign protein, to be overcome.

FURTHER READING

BENDER M.L. & BRUBACHER L.J. (1973) *Catalysis and Enzyme Action.* New York: McGraw-Hill.

DE DUVE C. (1975) Exploring cells with a centrifuge. *Science* 189, 186–194.

DESNICK R.J., THORPE S.R. & FIDDLER M.B. (1976) Towards enzyme therapy for lysosomal storage diseases. *Physiological Reviews* 56, 57–99.

DICKERSON R.E. & GEIS I. (1969) *The Structure and Action of Proteins.* New York: Harper & Row.

DIXON M. & WEBB E.C. (1964) *Enzymes*, 2nd Edition. London: Longman.

GUTFREUND H. & KNOWLES J.R. (1967) The foundations of enzyme action. In *Essays in Biochemistry*, Vol. 3, ed. Campbell P.N. & Greville G.D. New York: Academic Press.

MOSS D.W. & BUTTERWORTH P.J. (1974) *Enzymology and Medicine.* London: Pitman Medical.

WILKINSON J.H. (1970) *Isoenzymes*, 2nd Revised Edition. London: Chapman & Hall.

Chapter 8
Energetics of living cells

Energy is the capacity to perform work. It may be stored as within molecules (chemical energy) or appear in different forms such as kinetic, electrical, thermal and radiant energy, the basic units of which are discussed on p. 4.1.

The continued viability of living matter depends on controlled energy transformations. As described on p. 4.1, solar energy is harnessed by the photosynthetic apparatus of the green plants in which it is converted into chemical energy, first in the form of a simple carbohydrate. Plants then convert this into other molecules such as complex sugars, proteins and lipids which may then be consumed by an animal. Subsequently the energy may be utilized for mechanical, osmotic, electrical or other work in the animal organism. The animal tissues may in turn be consumed as a source of chemical energy and essential nutrients by another animal or by man. The energy cycle is then completed by the oxidative sequences of reactions occurring in animal tissues in which dietary and tissue metabolites are converted by chemical transformations to substances of lower potential energy. These are carbon dioxide, water, urea, etc. and are excreted as waste products to serve in turn other living systems such as plants and bacteria. Much of the science of biochemistry is concerned with studies of the specific processes whereby animal tissues transfer energy between different molecules and store and utilize it to perform work.

The combustion of glucose in a bomb calorimeter where it is converted almost instantaneously into carbon dioxide and water with the liberation of energy as heat is described on p. 4.2. In the body at 37°C glucose is broken down slowly to the same products and some of the energy liberated can be used to do work, the remainder being dissipated as heat. On the other hand, glucose remains unchanged almost indefinitely if kept in a bottle on the laboratory bench or in the larder. Further, in green plants carbon dioxide and water can be converted into glucose by solar radiation and at the same time oxygen is given off.

Dynamic equilibrium

Consider a general reaction in which an equilibrium is reached:

$$A + B \rightleftharpoons C + D$$

According to the Law of Mass Action the rate (v) of the forward reaction is proportional to the concentrations of A and B

$$v_1 \text{ (forward)} = k_{+1}[A] \times [B]$$

similarly for the backward reaction

$$v_2 \text{ (backward)} = k_{-1}[C] \times [D]$$

k_{+1} and k_{-1} are the appropriate velocity constants. At equilibrium the two rates must be the same and so,

$$K = \frac{k_{+1}}{k_{-1}} = \frac{[C] \times [D]}{[A] \times [B]}$$

K is defined as the **equilibrium constant**.

The correct expression for true or thermodynamic equilibrium involves activities rather than molar concentrations, as the velocity of a chemical reaction depends upon activities rather than the concentration of the reacting substances. In biological work it is usual to assume that solutes and solutions behave in an ideal thermodynamic fashion in which case the activities and concentrations may be taken as identical.

For reactions which proceed forwards and far to the right K is large and for reactions which do not proceed far to the right K is small. The equilibrium constant is dependent upon temperature and many reactions can be forced in the desired direction by raising or lowering the temperature. Unfortunately this device is not available to mammals who are obliged to operate at a constant temperature. The equilibrium constant K is therefore a useful measure of the degree of spontaneity of a given chemical reaction. However, a favourable equilibrium constant implies only that the reaction may proceed and is theoretically possible. There may be impediments to its progress.

Thermodynamic considerations

All energy transformations that take place in living systems obey fundamental laws of thermodynamics which is a branch of science devoted to the study of energy exchanges. Thermodynamics is concerned with the conditions under which a reaction will proceed and with the overall energy transformations, not with the route through which this transformation occurs or the rate at which the reaction occurs.

The **first law of thermodynamics** states that the total energy within a closed system, such as the universe, remains constant. Thus, energy cannot be created or destroyed. As indicated on p. 4.1 this law implies an exact equivalence between different forms of energy such as chemical energy, kinetic energy, electrical energy and heat.

The **second law of thermodynamics** sets the limits which restrict the transformation of one type of energy into another which then may become available for useful work. This energy (G) is called free energy. The relation it bears to the total energy of a system (enthalpy H) and the energy not available for work (entropy TS) is concisely stated in the form of the equation.

$$H = G + TS$$

These terms must now be defined.

Enthalpy (H) is the sum of the total energy initially present in a system. In a biological system this is usually equivalent to the heats of combustion of the reactants. Thus it can be readily measured.

Free energy (G) of a system is that fraction of the total energy which is available for useful work. When a chemical reaction occurs the reaction proceeds with a decrease in free energy until an equilibrium point is reached. The symbol G is taken from the name of the American physical chemist Willard Gibbs.

Entropy is a measure of that part of the total energy of the system that is not available for work. Entropy is a function of the temperature (T) of the molecules involved in a particular system. The symbol S is a capacity factor expressed as joules/degree. The total entropy is obtained by multiplying it by the intensity factor T.

Entropy is related to the degree of disorder or randomness in a system. At the molecular level it reflects the probability that a particular reaction will occur. Thus in a freely reversible reaction the change in entropy is zero while in an irreversible process the entropy steadily increases. In a closed system entropy can only increase and is reduced only if a source of energy is introduced from outside.

CALCULATION OF FREE ENERGY CHANGES

Biochemists are concerned with the problem of whether reactions can proceed by themselves in the presence of suitable catalysts, or whether an extraneous source of energy is needed to drive them. This involves consideration of the changes in free energy involved in reactions. The changes that can occur in a system are more important than the absolute amounts of energy present. In consequence the second law is more useful if written in the following form:

$$\Delta G = \Delta H - T \Delta S$$

ΔG cannot be determined directly by experiment, but can be derived in the following manner. It can be shown on theoretical grounds that:

$$\Delta G^0 = -RT \log_e K$$

G^0 is the **standard free energy** when the concentrations of all the components of a reaction are molal. R is the gas constant and equals $8\cdot314 \, J \, mol^{-1} \, deg^{-1}$. T is the absolute temperature and K the equilibrium constant of a reversible reaction. Hence, for reactions taking place at 37°C

$$\Delta G^0 = -8\cdot314 \times 310 \times 2\cdot3 \log_{10} K.$$

Thus for a reaction with an equilibrium constant of 1000

$$\Delta G^0 = -8\cdot314 \times 310 \times 2\cdot3 \times 3$$
$$= -17\cdot78 \, kJ$$

Provided the value of ΔG^0 is negative (at a fixed temperature and pressure), then the reaction theoretically can proceed of its own accord and will be energy yielding or **exergonic**. On the other hand if a reaction has a positive ΔG^0, it cannot proceed unless it is coupled to another process which provides energy. Such reactions are said to be **endergonic**. There are many examples of exergonic reactions being coupled to endergonic processes. If ΔG^0 is zero the reaction is in chemical equilibrium.

Because a reaction is capable of proceeding, it does not follow that it will necessarily take place. Petrol can be combusted and the energy used to drive a car. Yet it can remain stable indefinitely in the tank. Before combustion can begin, it has to be ignited by a spark. This provides **activation energy** which raises the total energy level sufficiently to allow combustion to take place. In the case of a

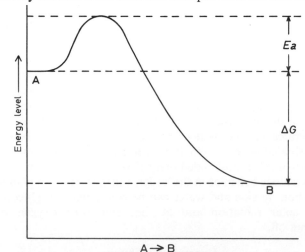

FIG. 8.1. For the conversion of A to B, energy of activation *Ea* is required. This energy is recovered and made available together with the change of free energy ΔG of the reaction.

petrol engine the activation energy is provided by the heat from the spark. In general, cells do not influence the rate of metabolic reactions by changes in temperature. Enzymes and other catalysts are able in some ways to decrease the activation energy of biological reactions sufficiently to allow them to proceed. No enzyme or catalyst, however, can cause a reaction to proceed that is not capable of taking place on energetic grounds. Fig. 8.1 illustrates diagrammatically the changes in energy level in the course of a reaction.

Immediate source of energy in cells

One of the problems is to unravel the precise mechanisms by which living tissues control the release of energy with only very small changes in temperature. In all cells there is a continuous process of repair and maintenance in which the chemical components are disassembled and resynthesized. This cellular activity requires energy and is expensive from the short term energetic standpoint. However, on a long term view it is efficient because these processes allow the entire cellular architecture to be replaced without disturbing the normal activity of the cell. The value of this system will become apparent when problems arising from cell injury are encountered.

Many cells vary their rates of metabolic activity greatly. They must be geared to the demands made upon them by other cells and tissues and this necessitates the use of energy which must be immediately available. In the case of a resting muscle called upon to contract and so do work, the energy must be available in a matter of milliseconds. The cells of the kidneys and cardiac muscle, for instance, adjust their metabolic rates to provide the energy necessary for the concentration of ions or for the work of the heart.

Nutrients derived from the diet provide the energy necessary for all these processes. Supplied at irregular intervals, they must be stored in suitable compounds which act as energy reserves. The main store, of course, is in the form of fat in the adipose tissue, but it takes time for this to be mobilized and transported to cells which require it. Certain organic phosphorylated compounds play a key role in this capacity and their contribution to the energetics of living tissues is now described.

'HIGH ENERGY PHOSPHATE' COMPOUNDS

Phosphoric acid is a weak inorganic tribasic acid whose function in bodily buffer systems is discussed on p. 6.5. This acid has the structure

$$\text{HO}-\overset{\displaystyle \overset{O}{\|}}{\underset{\displaystyle \underset{OH}{|}}{P}}-\text{OH} \quad \text{or} \quad H_3PO_4$$

Phosphoric acid can react with alcohols to form esters, e.g.

$$H_3PO_4 + ROH \rightleftharpoons RO\overset{\displaystyle \overset{}{}}{\underset{\displaystyle \underset{O}{\|}}{P}}(OH)_2 + H_2O$$

The acid can also react with amines,

$$H_3PO_4 + RNH_2 \rightleftharpoons RNH\overset{}{\underset{\underset{O}{\|}}{P}}(OH)_2 + H_2O$$

or combine with organic acids to form mixed anhydrides, e.g.

$$H_3PO_4 + RCOOH \rightleftharpoons RCOO\overset{}{\underset{\underset{O}{\|}}{P}}(OH)_2 + H_2O$$

In living tissues there is a wide range of phosphorylated compounds, including phosphorylated derivatives of carbohydrates, proteins and lipids (phospholipids), many of which have complex structures. Some of the phosphorylated derivatives are phosphate esters or phosphate anhydrides, and fig. 8.2 shows the specific groupings between the phosphate moiety and the rest of the molecule. The **free energy of hydrolysis** of most phosphate esters is low and for these ΔG^0 lies between -4 and -17 kJ/mol; α-glycerophosphate and glucose-6-phosphate are examples of this group. In a much smaller group, of which the other substances in fig. 8.2 are examples, the free energy of hydrolysis is high and ΔG^0 lies between -21 and -46 kJ/mol. These two groups, first distinguished by Lipmann, are now called 'low energy phosphate' compounds and 'high energy phosphate' compounds respectively. This is a loose, albeit convenient, terminology and refers to the actual free energy of hydrolysis of the bonds and not to a specific energy state of the compound as a whole. One example helps to illustrate this point.

Adenosine triphosphate $\xrightarrow{\text{H}_2\text{O}}$
(ATP)

adenosine diphosphate $+ H_3PO_4 +$ energy
(ADP)

Here ATP is hydrolysed in the presence of water and perhaps by an enzyme such as an ATPase to give rise to ADP with the release of the free energy of hydrolysis of the terminal phosphate bond. For this reaction ΔG^0 is about -33 kJ/mol. Consider a second reaction in which ADP is hydrolysed in the presence of water to yield adenosine monophosphate (AMP) + inorganic phosphate + energy.

$$\text{ADP} \xrightarrow{\text{H}_2\text{O}} \text{AMP} + H_3PO_4 + \text{energy}$$

Again ΔG^0 for the hydrolysis of the terminal phosphate bond of ADP is comparable to that of the terminal phosphate bond of ATP and about -33 kJ/mol. Consider now the third hydrolysis of AMP to yield adenosine + inorganic phosphate. This reaction results in a lower release of free energy of hydrolysis and consequently the

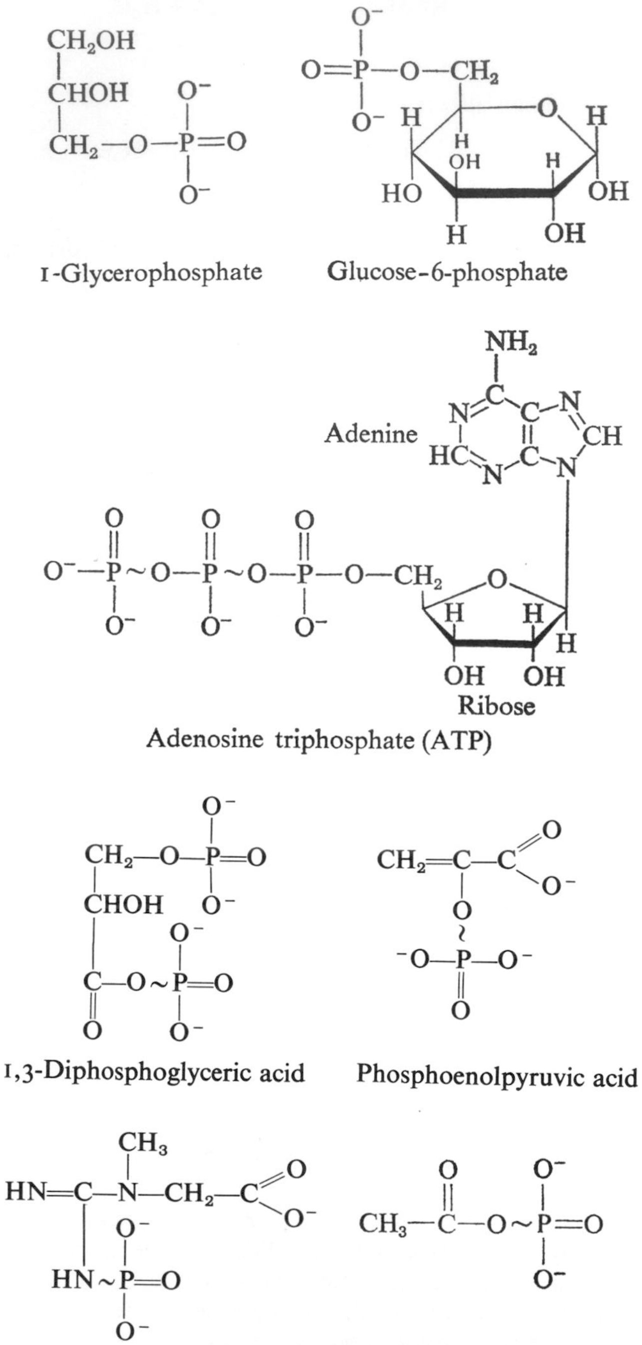

1-Glycerophosphate   Glucose-6-phosphate

Adenosine triphosphate (ATP)

1,3-Diphosphoglyceric acid   Phosphoenolpyruvic acid

Creatine phosphate   Acetyl phosphate

FIG. 8.2. Phosphorylated derivatives which are phosphate esters or phosphate anhydrides.

bond which links the sugar moiety of adenosine to the phosphoric acid moiety is a 'low energy phosphate bond' whereas, more correctly, the observation is that the bond had a low free energy of hydrolysis. The overall energy changes in the controlled hydrolysis of the phosphate moieties of ATP are as follows:

ATP $\longrightarrow$ ADP + inorganic phosphate + 33 kJ

ADP $\longrightarrow$ AMP + inorganic phosphate + 33 kJ

AMP $\longrightarrow$ adenosine + inorganic phosphate + about 13 kJ

It is customary to represent the high energy phosphate groups as $\sim \circledP$. Thus the structure of ATP may be expressed as $A—P \sim \circledP \sim \circledP$. The reasons for high levels of energy of the phosphate bonds are complex and there is no simple satisfactory explanation. The high free energy of hydrolysis of the terminal phosphate group of ATP is in part due to the stabilization by resonance of one of the products of the reaction, ADP. Similar considerations apply to the conversion of ADP to AMP. In the breakdown of carbohydrates, phosphorylated derivatives are first formed at the expense of ATP. A typical example is the phosphorylation of glucose by the enzyme hexokinase to form glucose-6-phosphate (G-6-P).

It is possible to predict the direction in which such a reaction is likely to proceed by breaking it down to its component parts. As stated previously ATP is hydrolysed as follows:

$$ATP + H_2O \longrightarrow ADP + H_3PO_4 + 33 \text{ kJ}$$

G-6-P has a low free energy of hydrolysis and the reaction is:

$$G\text{-}6\text{-}P + H_2O \longrightarrow \text{glucose} + H_3PO_4 + 13 \text{ kJ}$$

Hence when glucose is phosphorylated at the expense of ATP there is a decrease in free energy so that this is a spontaneous reaction:

$$\text{Glucose} + ATP \longrightarrow G\text{-}6\text{-}P + ADP + 21 \text{ kJ}$$

Here we have an example of a low energy phosphate compound being synthesized at the expense of a high energy compound.

The above values are for the standard free energy changes (ΔG^0) and so are obtainable only under standard conditions where the concentrations of the reactants are expressed in mol/kg. As a rule reactants are not at this concentration and hence changes are usually expressed as ΔG values and related to ΔG^0 by the equation:

$$\Delta G = \Delta G^0 + RT \log_e \frac{\text{(products)}}{\text{(reactants)}}$$

It is important to note this effect of concentration on ΔG because where the ΔG in a reaction is small, the direction of the reaction can be affected by the change in the concentration of one or other of the reactants. This is demonstrated by the reactions which lead to the storage of high energy phosphate bonds in compounds like creatine phosphate as follows:

$$ATP + \text{creatine} \rightleftharpoons ADP + \text{creatine phosphate}$$

This reaction has a ΔG^0 which is positive, although small and about 8·5 kJ. However, it is possible for the reaction to proceed in the direction of creatine phosphate in spite of this by increasing the concentration of ATP. This is the situation in the living cell where for reasons not understood the intracellular concentrations of ATP and ADP are kept low, about 10^{-2} mol/kg to 10^{-3} mol/kg. As ATP is essential to the economy of the cell, a ready source must be available. When reactions in the cell generate ATP and other high energy phosphate compounds, any excess of high energy phosphates is thus stored as creatine phosphate. If a demand for ATP arises, the creatine phosphate reacts with the ADP to give ATP and creatine. Thus, although ΔG^0 of the above reaction is small and positive, the manipulation of the concentrations of the ADP and ATP in the cell makes it possible to drive the reaction in the forward or backward direction depending upon whether there is a need to restore the ATP levels or to increase the energy reserve of creatine phosphate.

In certain instances phosphorylated intermediate products of metabolism may be modified by further enzymic action which changes the structure of the bond linking the organic moiety to the phosphate group. For example, in the oxidation of an alcoholic phospho-ester to a carboxylic acid phosphate anhydride, a phosphate ester bond with a low free energy of hydrolysis is transformed into a phospho-anhydride bond with a high free energy of hydrolysis. This is a reaction in which electrons are withdrawn from the molecule.

$$RCH_2CH_2O\textcircled{P} \longrightarrow RCH_2COO \sim \textcircled{P} + 4e$$

In the chemical laboratory, an alcohol is converted into a carboxylic acid by heating with acidified dichromate:

$$CH_3CH_2OH \longrightarrow CH_3CHO \longrightarrow CH_3COOH$$

This is a spontaneous reaction and the free energy associated with the conversion is dissipated as heat. However, in the animal organism the oxidation of such an alcohol into a carboxylic acid results in much of the energy of the reaction being trapped in high energy phosphate compounds. Subsequently this energy may either be utilized or transferred to a store by a suitable controlled exchange reaction.

Many of the key mechanisms which link oxidative reactions with the regeneration of ATP from ADP + inorganic phosphate occur in subcellular particles called mitochondria. The resultant oxidation reactions are the principal energy yielding reactions in the cell, and much effort has been exerted towards elucidating the links between oxidation and high energy phosphate bond formation.

Mitochondria and cellular energetics

In many mammalian cells there are about 1000 of these organelles. They contain two discrete membrane systems; the external membrane is smooth and continuous while the internal membrane is gathered together in a series of folds or cristae. Fig. 13.6 shows that the surface area of the cristae is much greater than the surface area of the smooth external membrane.

Fractionation procedures which disrupt cellular architecture can be used to disperse the subcellular organelles throughout a tissue homogenate. Then by differential centrifugation, the cellular components can be separated into nuclei, mitochondria, lysosomes, endoplasmic reticulum and the cell sap. Of these subcellular particles, the mitochondria have by far the highest rate of oxygen uptake *in vitro*. They can be disrupted by ultrasound or detergents, and it is then possible to make separate preparations of external membrane, of cristae and of the fluid matrix which fills the centre of the mitochondrion. Most of the enzymes of the citric acid cycle are located in the matrix and those associated with electron transfer reactions in the cristae.

The cristae are complex lipoprotein structures and physical, chemical and biological approaches indicate that within them there reside a great number of respiratory enzymes and coenzymes.

Oxidation

Oxidation is defined as a reaction involving loss of electrons and conversely reduction is a reaction in which electrons are gained. The oxidation of a substance may therefore be written:

$$A \longrightarrow A^+ + 1e^-$$

Clearly there must be provision for some suitable electron acceptor. In general, oxidation reactions are coupled to reduction reactions and electrons flow from the substance which is undergoing oxidation to the substance which is undergoing reduction.

$$A + B \rightleftharpoons A^+ + B^-$$

It is also characteristic of biological oxidations that they are often linked together to form a chain along which the electrons flow. Further stages in the above reaction might be:

$$B^- + C \rightleftharpoons B + C^-$$
$$C^- + D \rightleftharpoons C + D^-$$

The net result of such a chain of reactions would be:

$$A + D \longrightarrow A^+ + D^-$$

In biological systems a common oxidizing agent is molecular oxygen which accepts electrons as follows:

$$O_2 \xrightarrow{+1e^-} O_2^-$$
$$O_2^- \xrightarrow{+1e^-} O_2^=$$
$$O_2^= \xrightarrow{+1e^-} O_2^{\equiv}$$
$$O_2^{\equiv} \xrightarrow{+1e^-} O_2^{\equiv}$$

These reactions ultimately lead to the conversion of molecular oxygen into metabolic water since

$$2O^= + 4H^+ \longrightarrow 2H_2O$$

It is a simple matter to calculate the volume of water produced per day (metabolic water) by an individual at rest, given that the oxygen consumption is about 250 ml/min and about one-half of the oxygen is used as an electron acceptor.

As a consequence of studies on the enzymes and coenzymes located in the inner cristae of the mitochondrion, a number of enzyme redox systems have been isolated from the complex lipoprotein cristae. The structures of many of these enzymes have been deduced and attempts made to predict the function of these redox systems to establish how the participation of these compounds in electron transfer reactions results in the trapping of energy in a utilizable form.

RESPIRATORY COENZYMES

An important group of substances, respiratory coenzymes, serve as intermediates in the chain of events between the initial stage of the oxidation of a substrate in a cell and the final stage of oxidation which is the formation of water by molecular oxidation. A brief account of their role as coenzymes or prosthetic groups is given on p. 7.13. Before describing in more detail their modes of action in the cell, their chemical structures are discussed.

Pyridine nucleotides

Two electron acceptors widely distributed in the cells are **nicotinamide-adenine dinucleotide (NAD)** and **nicotinamide-adenine dinucleotide phosphate (NADP)**. The structure of NAD is:

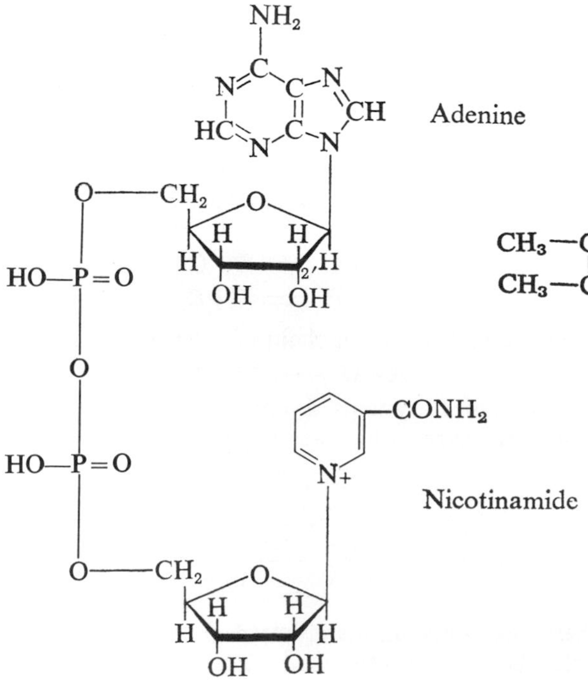

NADP has the same structure as NAD with the addition of a phosphate on position 2' of the ribose molecule attached to adenine.

The business part of the molecule is the pyridine ring of nicotinamide. A substrate, XH_2, provides the oxidized form of the coenzyme with two electrons, in this instance accompanied by $2H^+$, i.e. $2H^+ + 2e^- = 2H$. The pyridine ring takes up two electrons and one proton and the other proton is set free in the medium.

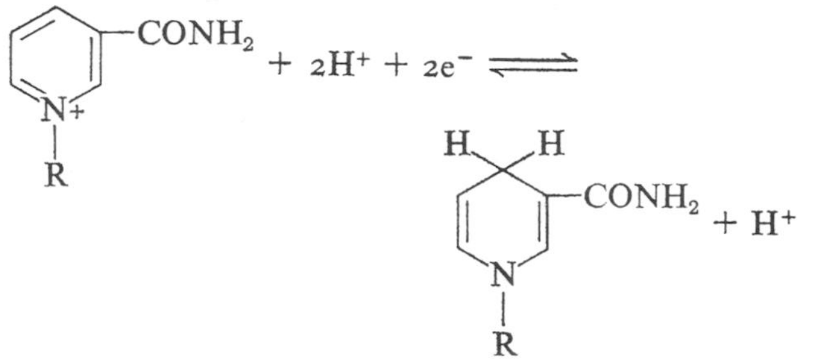

In the reverse direction $NADH_2$ gives up two electrons and one H^+.

$$NAD + 2e^- + H^+ \rightleftharpoons NADH_2$$

This type of reaction can be followed easily because there are big differences between the ultra-violet absorption spectra of NAD and $NADH_2$. Changes in the concentrations of the two forms are measured by determining the absorbance of the solution at 340 nm.

Flavoproteins

The flavoproteins are enzymes involved in oxidation-reduction reactions and contain **flavin-adenine dinucleotide (FAD)** or **flavin mononucleotide (FMN)** as prosthetic groups. FAD is a derivative of adenosine and the vitamin riboflavin with the following structure:

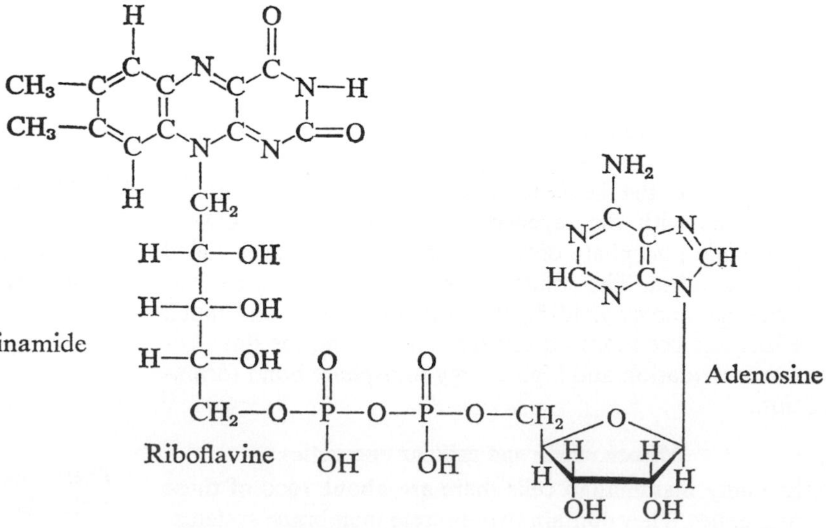

Nicotinamide-adenine dinucleotide (NAD)

Flavine-adenine dinucleotide (FAD)

FAD can take up to two electrons and two H^+ (two hydrogen atoms) on two nitrogen atoms in the *iso*alloxazine ring of riboflavin to form $FADH_2$ as follows:

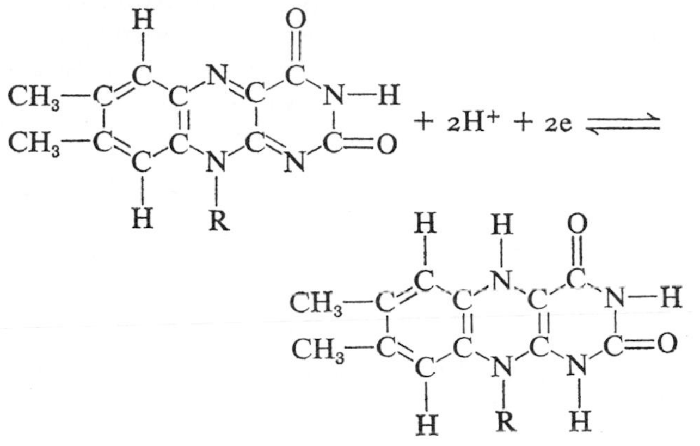

FMN, which is the 5' phosphate of riroflavin, also takes up to two electrons and two H^+ in a similar manner, to form $FMNH_2$.

Thus in the flavoprotein groups of oxidation-reduction enzymes the prosthetic groups FAD or FMN act as acceptors of electrons or hydrogen atoms from suitable substrates. In mitochondria $NADH_2$ dehydrogenase-catalyses the reduction of the flavin coenzyme at the expense of hydrogen atoms (or electrons) derived from $NADH_2$. Thus, a substrate XH_2 undergoes dehydrogenation at the expense of a dehydrogenase enzyme with NAD as a prosthetic group. The reaction is therefore

$$XH_2 + NAD = X + NADH_2$$

The two additional electrons on the pyridine nucleotide molecule are then transferred to the prosthetic group of the flavoprotein as follows:

$$NADH_2 + FAD = NAD + FADH_2$$

In certain circumstances, the substrate oxidized XH_2 may bypass the first step in this sequence. For example, the oxidation of succinate in mitochondria is as follows:

Succinate + succinic dehydrogenase flavoprotein (SDFp)
$$= fumarate + SDFpH_2$$

Electron-transporting quinones
Several electron-transporting quinones are present in mitochondria; one example is **ubiquinone** whose general formula is shown below; n may vary from 6 to 10 in different species, but is usually 10 in mammals.

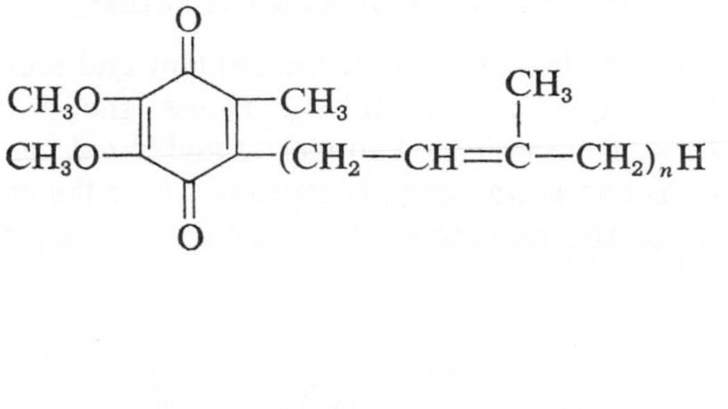

Ubiquinones are capable of accepting one or two electrons to form stable semiquinones or quinones on reduction, and are usually referred to as **coenzyme Q (CoQ)**. Vitamin K may also act as an electron carrier but it is uncertain if it acts in this way in mitochondria. The reduced form of the $NADH_2$ dehydrogenase flavoprotein and the reduced form of succinic dehydrogenase flavoprotein can both be reoxidized by CoQ under certain circumstances. This reaction would therefore be

$$FpH_2 + CoQ = Fp + CoQH_2$$
or $$SDFpH_2 + CoQ = SDFp + CoQH_2$$

Cytochromes
These are haemoproteins found in the cristae of mitochondria. Each cytochrome contains one atom of iron in a porphyrin structure and forms a prosthetic group which is bound to a specific protein.

Cytochrome b has the same iron porphyrin as haemoglobin. As in the case of haemoglobin, this haem prosthetic group is dissociable, that is it can be removed from cytochrome b and reinserted into the molecule to reconstitute the active 'cytochrome b'. The iron ion liganded to the porphyrin and the protein undergoes a reversible redox reaction

$$Fe^{++} \rightleftharpoons Fe^{+++} + e^-$$

Cytochrome c is a haemoprotein with a molecular weight of about 12 500. The vinyl groups ($-CH=CH_2$) in the porphyrin component are reduced and linked to cysteine residues of the protein by thiol ether bonds.

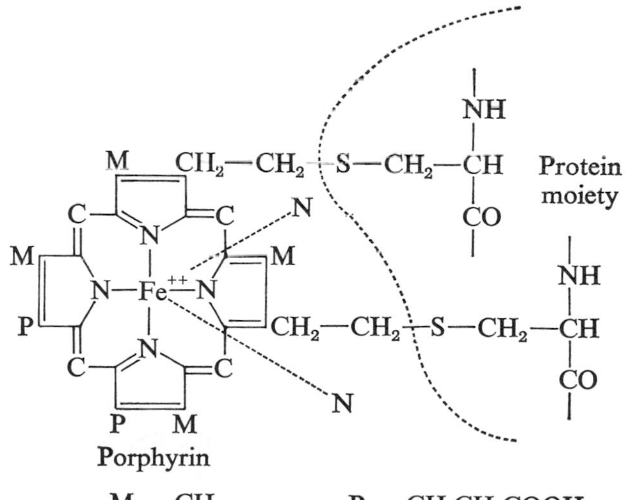

$$M = CH_3 \qquad P = CH_2CH_2COOH$$

Cytochrome c

The iron ion is associated with both the resonating porphyrin structure and amino acids in the protein moiety and again the iron ion, Fe^{++}/Fe^{+++} participates in a redox reaction.

Cytochrome a is also found in the cristae but has not been as well characterized as cytochromes b and c. It and the related cytochrome a_3 are collectively known as cytochrome oxidase; Cu^{++} ions play a key role in its function.

Thus the enzymes present in mitochondrial cristae include at least two flavoproteins, CoQ and cytochromes b, c and $a+a_3$. How these operate within mitochondria to form a redox chain has been elucidated by separating, using physical methods, the cristae into four small partially functional units or complexes.

Complex I is a combination of a flavoprotein with an iron sulphur protein and is capable of accepting electrons from $NADH_2$; it cannot be reoxidized by oxygen but can be by CoQ.

Complex II contains the flavoprotein of the succin-oxidase system together with an iron sulphur protein; it cannot be reoxidized by oxygen but can be by CoQ.

Complex III contains cytochrome b and also a derivative of cytochrome c termed cytochrome c_1; it cannot accept electrons directly from $NADH_2$ or from succinate but it can do so from $CoQH_2$; it cannot be re-oxidized by oxygen but it can donate electrons to cytochrome c.

Complex IV contains cytochrome $a+a_3$ in association with Cu^{++} ions. It appears to accept electrons from reduced cytochrome c and can be reoxidized by molecular oxygen.

The separation of these four complexes and their association with different respiratory coenzymes suggests that the order in which they are rearranged in the lipo-protein of the cristae may be as shown in fig. 8.3.

These observations on the possible order in which events in the electron transport chain occur are supported by studies using specific inhibitors of different parts of the redox chain. Thus some barbiturates, e.g. amylobarbitone, block the chain between $NADH_2$ and the flavoprotein acceptor; the insecticide, rotenone, blocks it between flavoprotein and CoQ and the antibiotic, antimycin a, blocks it between cytochrome b and cytochrome c. Finally, the well-known poison, cyanide, blocks the chain at the level of cytochrome a_3. It is possible to apply spectral methods to measure the ratio of oxidized: reduced flavoprotein, or oxidized:reduced cytochrome b, or oxidized:reduced cytochrome c. The action of specific inhibitors together with the isolation of complexes I–IV and the application of spectral studies justifies the concept that the flavoproteins, ubiquinones and the cytochromes function in electron transfer reactions from the oxidizable substrate to the ultimate electron acceptor, oxygen.

OXIDATION-REDUCTION POTENTIALS

In oxidation-reduction studies the hydrogen electrode is used as the reference system. It consists of a cell in which hydrogen gas at I atmosphere pressure is bubbled over a platinum black electrode which is partly immersed in a solution of hydrogen ions whose activity is unity. In actual practice this corresponds to an aqueous solution of hydrochloric acid containing about 1·18 mol/l. The overall reaction is therefore

$$2H^+ + 2e^- = H_2$$

Oxidation-reduction (redox) systems can be directly or indirectly compared with this reference electrode. Since the ease with which an electron leaves one molecular species differs from the ease with which an electron leaves another, it is possible to compare the redox potential of pairs of molecules or ions, provided they can undergo an electron transfer reaction. Thus the oxidized over the reduced forms of a number of inorganic or organic molecules can be compared, e.g. Fe^{+++}/Fe^{++}, $NAD/NADH_2$, pyruvate/lactate and $2H^+/H_2$. In each case the oxidized form can be transformed into the reduced form by the addition of one or two electrons. While in some cases H^+ are also involved, their role is passive and they interfere little with the overall energetics. The oxidation–reduction equations involving the trans-ference of electrons can be treated as normal chemical reactions:

$$\underset{\text{(reductant)}}{X} + \underset{\text{(oxidant)}}{Y} \rightleftharpoons \underset{\text{(oxidant)}}{X^+} + \underset{\text{(reductant)}}{Y^-}$$

The equilibrium constant (K) will be derived in the usual way.

$$K = \frac{[X^+][Y^-]}{[X]\,[Y]}$$

It is possible to treat this reaction as two dependent functions, namely the loss of an electron by X to yield X^+ and the gain of this electron by Y to yield Y^-. The actual value of K is then dependent on the relative affinities of X and Y for the electron. By means of the hydrogen electrode and suitable equipment it is possible to set up 'half cells' to establish the relative affinities of different systems for electrons.

In this way the $2H^+/H_2$ system can be connected to the Fe^{+++}/Fe^{++} system or to the $NAD/NADH_2$ system or to any other redox couple. Such observations make it possible to arrange redox systems in an electrochemical order and those with a more positive electrode potential value are capable of oxidizing a less positive system. Thus the flavoproteins (Fp) can oxidize $NADH_2$ since they have a more positive electrode potential value than the $NAD/NADH_2$ system. Naturally in order to standardize the electrode potentials it is necessary to specify the concentration of the reactants in the general equation:

$$\text{Oxidant} \rightleftharpoons \text{reductant} + \text{electron(s)}$$

The usual conditions are that the oxidant and reductant are both expressed in mol/kg. Hence the electrode potentials are compared under standarized physical conditions and in an aqueous solution where the concen-trations of the reductants and oxidants are equal. As most biological redox systems are measured at pH 7·0, standard potentials (E'_0) are quoted in comparison with the hydrogen reference electrode at this pH. This has a value E'_0 of -0.42 of a volt with reference to the hydrogen electrode at pH 0. Consequently by means of tables of standard redox potentials it is possible to predict the tendency for electrons to pass from one system to another. Table 8.1 sets out a selection of redox

TABLE 8.1. Redox potentials E'_0 in aqueous solution at pH 7·0

Respiratory coenzymes	E'_0
O_2/H_2O	$+0.82$
Cytochrome a	$+0.29$
Cytochrome c	$+0.23$
Ubiquinone (CoQ)	$+0.10$
Cytochrome b	-0.04
Flavoproteins (Fp)	-0.06
FAD	-0.20
NAD (or NADP)	-0.32
H^+/H	-0.42
Other redox systems	
Ascorbic/Dehydroascorbic acid	$+0.08$
Fumarate/Succinate	0.00
Pyruvate/Lactate	-0.18
Pyruvate/Malate	-0.33
GSSG/GSH (Glutathione)	-0.34
2-Oxoglutarate/Succinate	-0.67

potentials of biological interest. The upper part shows the values for the important respiratory coenzymes and these lie between $+0.82$ volts for molecular oxygen and -0.42 volts for the hydrogen electrode. The lower part contains E_0 values for four important biochemical reactions and also for ascorbic acid and glutathione. These two substances which are readily oxidized are both widespread in the tissues, but their functional role is still largely unknown. From table 8.1 it would therefore be predicted that a redox coupled system such as $NAD/NADH_2$ ($E'_0 -0.32$ volts) would be capable of reducing a flavoprotein to the corresponding reduced flavoprotein. Similarly one might predict that flavoproteins could in turn reduce the succinate-fumarate system. However, because a system has a redox potential which is more negative than some other system, this does not imply that the reduction reaction necessarily occurs. It only indicates that, other considerations being favourable, the system moves in the direction of the more positive E'_0.

Energetics of redox reactions

Redox potentials are valuable physical constants because they are precisely related to free energy changes. It will be apparent that the energy available as a consequence of the electron moving from a more negative system to a more positive system and ultimately to oxygen can be made available for useful work.

Redox potentials allow us to calculate the free energy change, since when one or more electrons move from a donor redox system to an acceptor redox system ΔG is directly related to (E) the difference in redox potential.

If E_1 is the standard redox potential of system A the donor and E_2 is the standard redox potential of system B the acceptor then

$$E_1 - E_2 = \Delta E$$

It can be shown that $\Delta G^0 = -nF\,\Delta E_0$ where n is the number of electrons transferred and F is the charge/mol $= 96{,}500$ coulombs $= 96$ kJ.

In redox systems it is desirable to separate the donor and acceptor systems and consider the overall reaction as being composed of two 'half cells'.
Thus if

$$K = \frac{\text{oxidized}}{\text{reduced}}$$

then

$$\Delta G^0 = -RT\log_e K = -RT\log_e \frac{\text{oxidized}}{\text{reduced}}$$

$$\Delta G^0 = -nF\Delta E = -RT\log_e \frac{\text{oxidized}}{\text{reduced}}$$

$$\Delta E = \frac{RT}{nF}\log_e \frac{\text{oxidized}}{\text{reduced}}$$

For example in the oxidation of lactic acid to pyruvic acid we have the following reaction:

$$\text{lactic acid} + NAD \rightleftharpoons \text{pyruvic acid} + NADH_2$$

The free energy of a redox system in terms of the electrical energy available for useful work can be measured in terms of the number of electrons involved in the movement and the relative electrode potentials of the two systems involved, that is the electrode potential of the donor system and the electrode potential of the acceptor system. Thus in the former reaction the equilibrium constant K for the reaction is given as follows:

$$K = \frac{[\text{pyruvate}][NADH_2]}{[\text{lactate}]\ \ [NAD]}$$

The actual value of the change in free energy in this reaction is given by the equation which was derived previously:

$$n\Delta G^0 = -RT\log_e K$$

It is therefore easy to deduce that the change in free energy in a redox system is related to the change in the standard potential of the oxidized system compared to the standard potential of the reduced system. Thus the general equation for the change in free energy in a redox system is given by

$$\Delta G^0 = -nF\Delta E$$

Synthesis of ATP in mitochondria

If mitochondria are suspended in the appropriate buffer solution of the correct ionic strength and oxidizable substrates such as pyruvate and oxaloacetate are added to the medium in the presence of ADP and inorganic phosphate under aerobic conditions, there is a decrease in the concentration of ADP and inorganic phosphate together with uptake of oxygen and the appearance of ATP. The overall equation can be represented as

$$O_2 + 2XH_2 + 4P_i + 4ADP \rightarrow 4ATP + 2H_2O + 2X$$

This process is often referred to as **oxidative phosphorylation**. The number of ATP molecules generated per atom of oxygen varies depending upon the substrate oxidized, i.e. depending upon the electron donor; thus the above equation with a different substrate YH_2 might give a result as follows

$$O_2 + 2YH_2 + 6P_i + 6ADP \rightarrow 6ATP + 2H_2O + 2Y$$

It will be noted that in the first equation, 2 molecules of XH_2 have generated 4 ATP molecules as a result of the oxidation by 1 molecule of oxygen. This is equivalent to 2 ATPs generated per atom of oxygen, or, as usually stated, a P/O ratio of 2. In the second instance oxidation of substrate YH_2 has achieved a P/O ratio of 3. Thus different oxidation processes in mitochondria may give different amounts of ATP and if, as stated previously, ATP is the principal chemical transducer in the cell, the efficiency of the chemical reaction within the mitochondria can govern the available cellular ATP. Since energy can neither be created nor destroyed, if the efficiency is low, a greater amount of energy is not trapped as ATP, but dissipated in some other form such as heat.

Mitochondria also contain enzymes with ATPase activity. Hence experiments designed to measure P/O ratios in mitochondria are fraught with difficulties and rely upon the use of specific ATPase inhibitors. If mitochondria are properly prepared in a medium of the correct ionic strength and if they are supplied with inorganic phosphate and an oxidizable substrate such as XH_2, they have a small oxygen uptake. When ADP is supplied, respiration rate rises markedly. Such reactions are said to be tightly coupled, implying that the equations described above are in fact operative in the mitochondria and that the uptake of oxygen by the organelles is dependent upon a supply of exogenous ADP. It has been deduced that under certain circumstances, transit of two electrons through the respiratory chain generates three high-energy phosphate bonds. The two electrons eventually move to oxygen which acts as an electron sink where, together with two protons, they produce metabolic water. Under other circumstances some substrates only generate 2 ATPs per atom of oxygen giving a P/O ratio of 2. This is important in establishing the mechanism and the sites of synthesis of high-energy phosphate bonds in the respiratory chain. Substances such as succinate, which

by-pass the initial NAD coenzyme and donate electrons directly to succinate dehydrogenase flavoprotein, give a P/O ratio of 2. By inference this suggests that one possible site for the generation of a high-energy phosphate bond may lie between the reduced NAD ($NADH_2$) and the flavoprotein. The application of standard biochemical methods to intact mitochondria and to the various mitochondrial complexes has produced evidence that there are three possible sites in the redox chain for the generation of ATP from ADP. The first is between $NADH_2$ and the flavoprotein, as already discussed. The second is between the flavoproteins and the first of the cytochromes, while the third is between the cytochromes and oxygen (fig. 8.3).

Applying the concepts of energetics, the electrode potential of the $NADH_2/NAD$ system is -0.32 V and that of the oxygen is $+0.82$ V. The change in electrode potential (ΔE) is therefore 1.14 V. This electrode PD is equivalent to a ΔG of over 200 kJ. This is the maximum energy available to the system and as the mitochondrial particles appear capable of producing three phosphate bonds, of high free energy of hydrolysis, each with a ΔG of over 30 kJ, the efficiency of the process is probably of the order of $3 \times 30/200 \approx 50$ per cent.

The mechanism by which these phosphorylations are coupled to the oxidation of coenzymes and prosthetic groups is still subject to debate. There are at least three theories which attempt to account for the process of oxidative phosphorylation.

CHEMICAL COUPLING HYPOTHESIS

An anhydride-phosphate with a high free energy of hydrolysis is generated when glyceraldehyde-3-phosphate is oxidized to glyceric acid 1,3-diphosphate outside the mitochondria. This observation stimulated a search for phosphorylated forms of the electron (hydrogen) carriers in mitochondria. The concept is advanced that as a substrate AH_2 is oxidized at the expense of an oxidant B, a transient intermediate may be formed of the type $A \sim I$. This intermediate might then react with other intermediates eventually to form an $X \sim D$ intermediate complex which could react with ADP to form ATP. One possible theoretical sequence of events is shown on the following four equations

$$AH_2 + B + I \rightleftharpoons A \sim I + BH_2$$
$$A \sim I + X \rightleftharpoons A + X \sim I$$
$$X \sim I + P_i \rightleftharpoons X \sim P + I$$
$$X \sim P + ADP \rightleftharpoons X + ATP$$

While any of the redox couples in mitochondria can be substituted for AH_2 or B, so far none of the hypothetical intermediates $A \sim I$ or $X \sim P$ has been isolated or characterized. Thus although the chemical coupling hypothesis is based upon known examples of the generation of a high energy phosphate compound during oxidations in

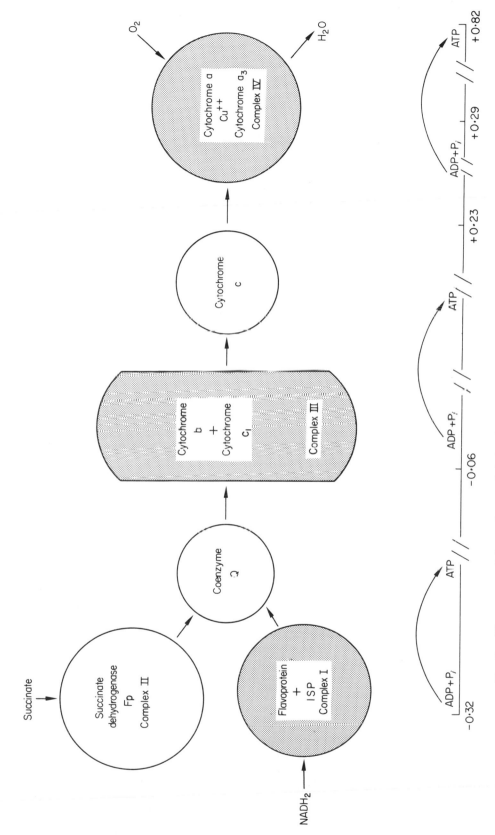

FIG. 8.3. The enzymes of the respiratory chain in mitochondria positioned according to their redox potentials.

other systems, it has not been possible to justify this theory by isolating the postulated intermediates from mitochondria. Despite this failure the concept is retained because it does explain the tight coupling between phosphorylation and electron transport in so far as the oxygen consumption is dependent on the supply of ADP. Furthermore, physiological and pharmacological agents which interfere *in vitro* with the efficiency of oxidative phosphorylation, e.g. thyroxine, free fatty acids, dinitrophenol and a variety of antibiotics, all decrease the P/O ratio in mitochondrial preparations. The uncoupling action of these compounds in mitochondria can be explained by the chemical coupling hypothesis, as due to interference with either the generation of one of the postulated intermediates or the hydrolysis of one of the intermediates prior to ATP formation.

CHEMI-OSMOTIC HYPOTHESIS

This hypothesis arose from the observation that oxidative phosphorylation occurs in intact cristae of mitochondria but not in fragmented particles of it unless the fragments are allowed to coalesce into closed vesicles. The hypothesis suggests first that as electrons are transported through the various components of the electron transport chain, protons (H^+) are lost from the outer surface of the membrane, and secondly that the components of the electron transport chain are orientated in a specific fashion so that they can translocate protons from the inside of the membrane and extrude them to the outside of the membrane. It will be seen that on this theory $[H^+]$ within the matrix of the mitochondrion tends to fall whereas $[H^+]$ in the intermembrane space of the mitochondrion tends to rise. Therefore there should be a marked change in $[H^+]$ across the narrow cristae which should result in the production of an electrical potential gradient across the cristae. The proponents of this theory suggest that within the lipoprotein environment of the cristae such a $[H^+]$ gradient could in fact be employed to drive the reaction as follows

$$ADP + Pi \longrightarrow ATP$$

If the pH in the matrix of the mitochondrion was about pH 9 and if the pH in the intermembrane space was about pH 5, then this electrochemical gradient would be sufficient to drive the reaction in favour of ATP synthesis.

CHEMICAL CONFORMATION HYPOTHESIS

The hypothesis suggests that during the transit of electrons throughout the respiratory chain, events may occur at specific sites which change the conformation (shape) of specific proteins and so force some of them into a high energy state. Thus, instead of the specific high energy intermediary $A \sim I$ of the chemical coupling hypothesis, a protein might assume a specific conformation at a higher energy level. By appropriate interaction with ADP and P_i this high energy state could be channelled

into ATP. While there is evidence for the existence of proteins in different energy states in other systems, these have not been shown to occur in mitochondria.

It has proved unexpectedly difficult to elucidate the mechanism of oxidative phosphorylation, possibly because the system is effective only when the proteins catalysing the reactions are integral parts of the mitochondrial membrane structure and thus cannot easily be investigated chemically. A large number of physiological and pharmacological agents can influence the delicate architecture of mitochondria and so influence the efficiency of the chemical events. The interlocked chain of electron carriers in the inner cristae is essential for the successful trapping of the free energy generated by the transit of electrons from the substrates to molecular oxygen.

Mitochondrial respiratory states

When the concentration and availability of ADP, substrates and oxygen in a preparation of mitochondria are controlled *in vitro*, five states of mitochondrial respiration can be described (fig. 8.4).

(1) In the absence of ADP and substrate, oxygen uptake is minimal;

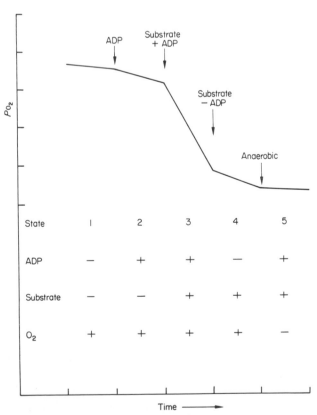

FIG. 8.4. The rate of uptake of oxygen by a mitochondrial preparation *in vitro*. Oxygen uptake is expressed as P_{O_2}/dt so that the greater the fall in P_{O_2} in the system, the greater is the uptake of oxygen.

(2) when ADP is supplied but there is no substrate, oxygen uptake changes very little;

(3) when ADP, substrate and oxygen are freely available oxygen uptake is maximal;

(4) when ADP is limited but substrate and oxygen are freely available, respiration is tightly coupled, oxygen uptake is low and geared to the available ADP; and

(5) when ADP and substrate are present but there is no oxygen, there is of course no oxygen uptake.

Mitochondria tend to swell in state 1 but they shrink in states 2 and 3; they swell again in state 4 and shrink in state 5.

The role of the ratio ATP/ADP and of $NADH_2$/NAD in the control of mitochondrial respiration is further considered in chap. 14 along with the contribution of the mitochondria to the supply of ATP and the utilization of ADP in mammalian cells.

Agents affecting mitochondria

A number of antibiotics, drugs and other agents block the mitochondrial respiratory chain. The sites of inhibition vary with different agents and it is possible to identify their point of action by observing the changes in the redox state of the several redox couples in the mitochondrial cristae.

In the presence of oxidizable substrates, oxygen, ADP and inorganic phosphate, mitochondria are inhibited by cyanide or carbon monoxide. Under these conditions all the components of the respiratory chain are pushed into a fully reduced state with the exception of cytochrome oxidase. It is possible to deduce that cyanide and carbon monoxide block Complex IV, i.e. cytochrome oxidase, and this can be confirmed by independent enzyme inhibitor studies.

Similarly, the insecticide rotenone can be shown to inhibit the electron transport chain between the flavoprotein in Complex I and CoQ. The antibiotic antimycin a blocks the respiratory chain between Complex III–cytochrome b and cytochrome c, while the barbiturates block the respiratory chain between $NADH_2$ and the flavoprotein of Complex I.

These drugs and many others have proved useful tools in exploring mitochondrial structure and function. It is doubtful whether any drugs do in fact exert their metabolic or therapeutic effects by interfering with the mitochondrial electron transport chain. However certain toxic agents such as dinitrophenol, dinitro-orthocresol and some other compounds are capable of reducing the efficiency of mitochondrial function, so causing a decrease in the tight coupling of respiration to oxidative phosphorylation. Under these circumstances the failure to generate ATP is associated with the dissipation of the electrical energy as heat, and in consequence the temperature of the organism rises. It is thought that certain agents which induce hyperpyrexia do so by interfering with the mitochondrial efficiency in this way. The rapid and often lethal rise in body temperature referred to as malignant hyperpyrexia, that occurs in some patients exposed to anaesthetics, may be due to the anaesthetic uncoupling oxidative phosphorylation either directly or indirectly.

The interscapular depots of fat cells in some species are brown in colour (p. 34.2). This brown tissue contains a high proportion of mitochondria, often located close to fat droplets. When examined *in vitro*, these mitochondria appear to be substantially uncoupled. It seems that in brown adipose tissue, fatty acids can be oxidized under conditions where there is little, if any, ATP net production and consequently most of the energy of this process is dissipated as heat (p. 34.8). In some species, brown adipose tissue plays an important part in maintaining body temperature in the newborn but its role in man is disputed.

Biogenesis of mitochondria

There is evidence that mitochondria contain a circular DNA and the enzymes necessary to utilize this DNA in a replicative function. The mitochondria contain enzymes for RNA synthesis and mitochondrial ribosomes. Mitochondria have the ability to synthesize certain specific proteins. The protein synthesis occurring in mitochondria can be differentiated from that in extramitochondrial sites by the fact that the synthesis of protein in mitochondria is inhibited by chloramphenicol. Although some of the mitochondrial proteins are made within the mitochondria, many of the enzymes involved in mitochondrial activities have an extramitochondrial origin, are synthesized on ribosomes and transported into mitochondria. It is possible that mitochondria synthesize essentially structural proteins, and provide a skeleton or framework on which certain of the respiratory enzymes and other catalysts associated with mitochondrial function can subsequently be assembled and stored.

FURTHER READING

BORST P. (1972) Mitochondrial nucleic acids. *Annual Review of Biochemistry* 41, 333–376.

DAM K. VAN & MEYER A.J. Oxidation and energy conservation by mitochondria. *Annual Review of Biochemistry* 40, 115–160.

KING T.E., MASON H.S. & MORRISON M. (1973). *Oxidases and Related Redox Systems*, vols. 1 & 2. Baltimore: University Park Press.

KLINGENBERG M. (1970) Metabolite transport in mitochondria. *Essays in Biochemistry* 6, 119–159.

LEHNINGER A.L. (1971) *Bioenergetics*, 2nd Edition. New York: Benjamin.

RACKER E. (1970) The two faces of the inner mitochondrial membrane. *Essays in Biochemistry* 6, 1–22.

SCHATZ G. & MASON T.L. (1974). The biosynthesis of mitochondrial proteins. *Annual Review of Biochemistry*, 43, 51–87.

Chapter 9
Carbohydrate metabolism

D-Glucose is probably the most abundant organic chemical on earth, surpassing in quantity even the vast masses of paraffin hydrocarbons which are known to be hidden beneath the earth's crust. Glucose can be made from the simplest chemicals, water and carbon dioxide, using only the energy of sunlight, and it can act as the sole source of carbon for a vast number of living organisms. Even in man glucose need be supplemented by only a very few chemicals, including, of course, amino acids as a source of nitrogen, for it to be able to support life indefinitely. It is clear, therefore, that knowledge of the pathways of metabolism open to glucose and its derivatives is important in the study of human biology.

When the word 'glucose' is used it must be remembered that free glucose occurs only rarely and it is polymers of glucose, mostly of high molecular weight, which are so abundant. For better or worse, the most abundant of all these polymers, cellulose, cannot be utilized directly by vertebrates, which can metabolize only the partial breakdown products provided by symbiotic bacteria (p. 5.2). This symbiosis is most highly developed in ruminants, e.g. cattle or sheep, and hardly exists at all in man. Empirical exploitation of these facts by our forefathers led first to organized herding of ruminants and later to the intensive production of the glucose polymer which can be digested by man, i.e. starch, in cereal agriculture.

CHEMISTRY OF CARBOHYDRATES

Narrowly defined, carbohydrates are chemicals of the composition $(CH_2O)_n$, where n is usually greater than 3. The presence of so many oxygen atoms in the molecule, together with the strict tetravalency of carbon, imposes stringent limitations on the structural possibilities. The word carbohydrate is now taken to mean not only organic compounds of this precise composition, but also carbohydrate derivatives, and di- and polysaccharides, whose empirical formulae depart somewhat from the basic pattern.

The formula $(CH_2O)_n$ implies a linear array of carbon atoms, one of which must carry a carbonyl group (aldehyde or ketone), and all the rest must carry an alcohol (−OH) group. The simplest such compound is glyoxal, but **glyceraldehyde**

$$
\begin{array}{ll}
1 & CHO \\
  & | \\
2 & CHOH \\
  & | \\
3 & CH_2OH
\end{array}
$$

is usually taken to be the parent compound, because it is the simplest carbohydrate to show stereoisomerism which is explained on p. 9.4; all optically active carbohydrates are named with reference to L- or D-glyceraldehyde. The most common carbohydrates, the **monosaccharides**, have five or six carbon atoms and are called pentoses and hexoses, and their carbon atoms are numbered from the aldehyde or ketone end.

The presence of so many hydroxyl groups makes the molecule **polar**, which means in effect that carbohydrates are chemically reactive, soluble in water and insoluble in non-polar or fat solvents. This is not true, however, of cellulose. Carbohydrates and related sugar alcohols are also, as a class, sweet to the taste; this is even true of glycerol.

The main chemical reactions of carbohydrates which occur in the body depend on the carbonyl and the alcohol groups. These reactions are acetal formation, oxidation-reduction and esterification.

ACETAL AND HEMI-ACETAL FORMATION

Many of the properties of aldehydes and ketones are better understood if the carbonyl form is written in the hydrated form as it largely exists in aqueous solution:

$$
\begin{array}{ccc}
R & & R\quad\;\; OH \\
\diagdown & & \diagdown\;\diagup \\
CO+H_2O & \rightleftharpoons & C \\
\diagup & & \diagup\;\diagdown \\
R_1 & & R_1\quad\;\; OH \\
I & & II
\end{array}
$$

Acetal formation can then be regarded as a reaction of

molecule II with one or more alcohols with the elimination of water:

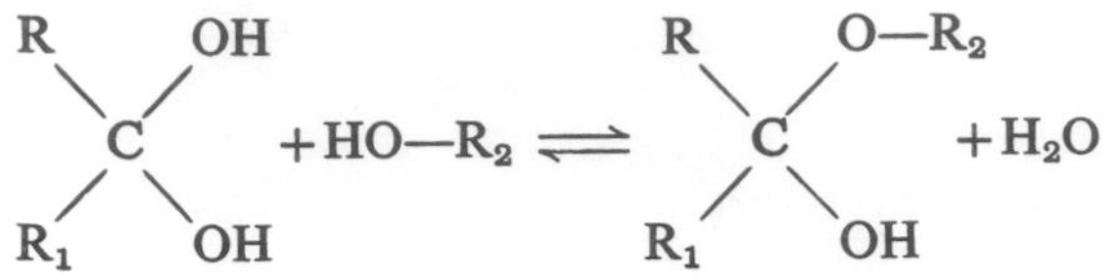

Hemi-acetal

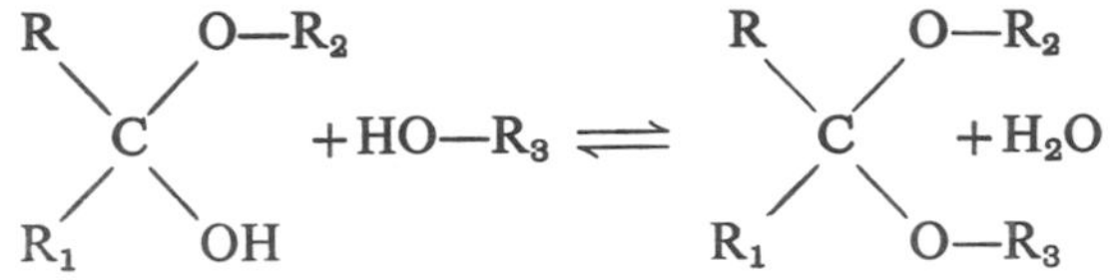

Acetal

Hemi-acetals are sufficiently unstable to form and break up spontaneously, especially in aqueous solution; acetals are more stable, although easily hydrolysed by acid.

The importance of this in sugar chemistry is that the alcohols R_2—OH and R_3—OH can be hydroxyl groups in the same molecule, or in similar molecules. Thus the aldehyde group of D-glucose can form a hemi-acetal with the —OH on either C-4 or C-5 of its own chain:

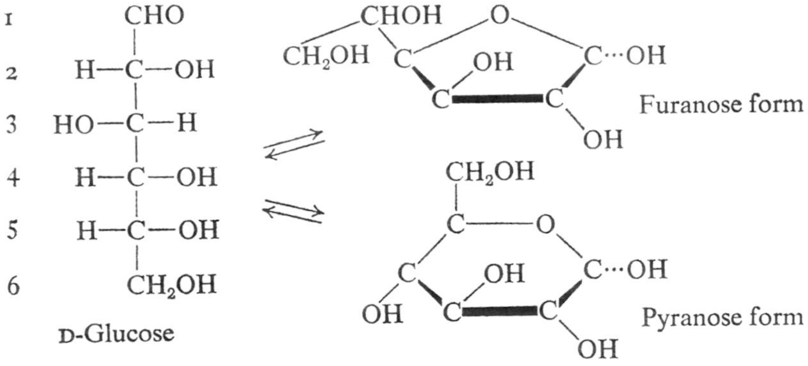

Since the second sugar molecule in this example still has a free carbonyl group, it can also form an acetal, and so long chains or **polysaccharides** can be built up. The —OH-donating monosaccharide used need not be identical with the hemi-acetal, so that non-symmetrical disaccharides, such as lactose, or polysaccharides with repeating patterns, such as in the **proteoglycans** may be built up. The structure and function of proteoglycans is given on p. 17.7.

The acetals, whether polysaccharide or not, are called **glycosides,** and energy is necessary for their formation; an interesting point in carbohydrate metabolism is the method by which the reactants are activated in nature. They are stable once formed, unless attacked by acids or enzymes. In particular, both the pyranose or furanose configuration of the hemi-acetal ring, and the α- or β-configuration of the hydroxyl, are stable until the glycoside bond is destroyed.

OXIDATION AND REDUCTION

In sugars containing an aldehyde group (aldoses), the aldehyde can easily be oxidized to the corresponding carboxylic acid and somewhat less readily reduced to the

Furanose form

Pyranose form

D-Glucose

The dotted lines joining C-1 with the new —OH indicate the existence of two stereoisomers, denoted as α- and β-D-glucose. The three compounds in the diagram form and reform spontaneously in a solution of glucose, a phenomenon known as **mutarotation.**

The hemi-acetal ring forms of the sugars can clearly react with a second alcohol. While this can be of almost any type, the most interesting acetals are those in which the second hydroxyl belongs to another monosaccharide giving, for example, the **disaccharide** maltose:

alcohol. In ketoses, the ketone cannot be oxidized without breaking the carbon chain, but it can be reduced just like an aldose. The **sugar alcohols** do not occur widely in nature, and are not readily metabolized in man. For this reason they can be used as sweetening agents for diabetic patients, who should not eat sugar in excess. Fructose and glucose both give the same alcohol, **sorbitol**.

Aldoses can also be oxidized at the primary alcohol group to the corresponding **uronic acids** by gentle

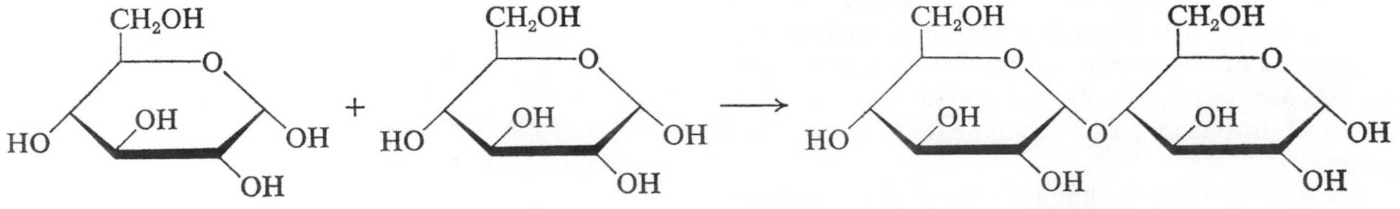

D-Glucose   +   D-Glucose   →   Maltose

oxidizing agents, e.g. hypoiodite. This test distinguishes between aldoses and ketoses. The biological synthesis of uronic acids is important and **glucuronic acid** $COOH-(CHOH)_4CHO$ is widely distributed in the body (p. 16.7).

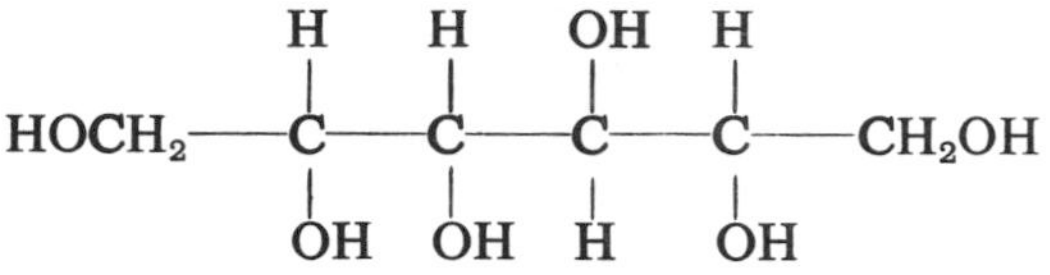

D-Sorbitol

The usual oxidizing agents used in the laboratory, e.g. hot alkaline copper solutions, oxidize both aldoses and ketoses with break-up of the molecule.

ESTER FORMATION

Any of the primary or secondary alcohol groups of a monosaccharide or polysaccharide can be esterified by reaction with an acid. The most common biological esters are those of phosphoric and sulphuric acids.

Both sulphuric and phosphoric acids are polyprotic. It follows that the mono-esters are acids, and also that the possibility of di-ester formation exists. The phosphoric acid di-esters are widely distributed in nature and are important, e.g. cyclic adenosine monophosphate, the dinucleotides, and the polynucleotides or nucleic acids.

Sulphate di-esters are not known, but the acidity of the sulphate-containing proteoglycans gives them considerable solubility in water, while on the other hand their calcium salts have a rigid structure which may be important in explaining the physical properties of bone.

Some important mono- and polysaccharides

As already explained, there are two trioses; D- and L-glyceraldehyde. The occurrence of stereoisomerism means that there are four tetroses, eight pentoses and sixteen hexoses in the aldose series and eight ketohexoses. Most of these occur in traces in nature. Three hexoses, two pentoses and three disaccharides of importance are:

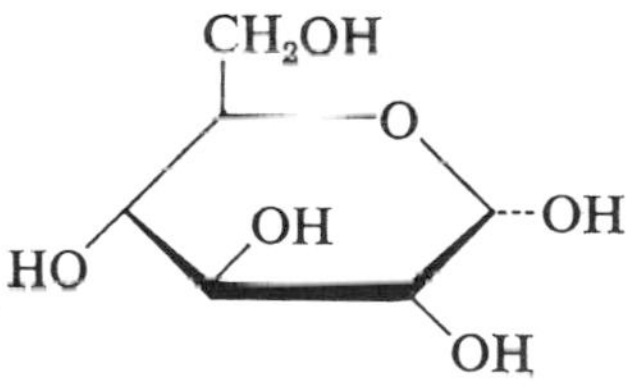

D-Glucose

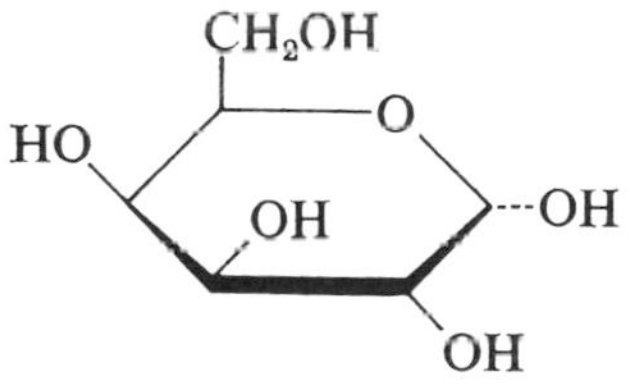

D-Galactose

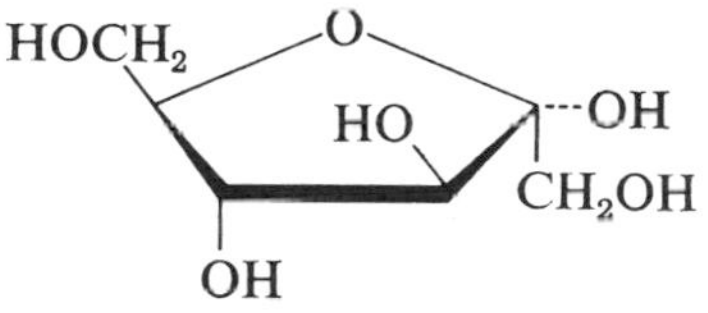

D-Fructose

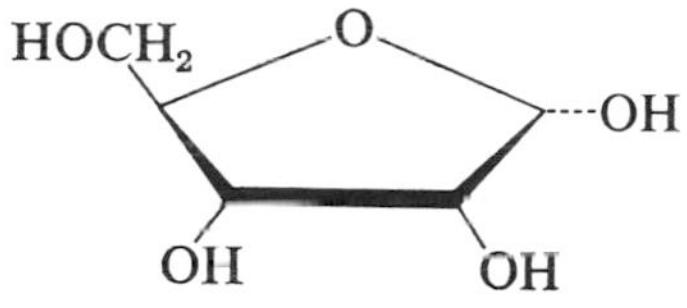

D-Ribose

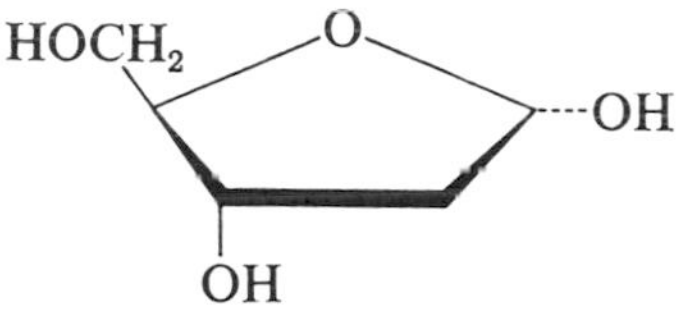

D-2-Deoxyribose

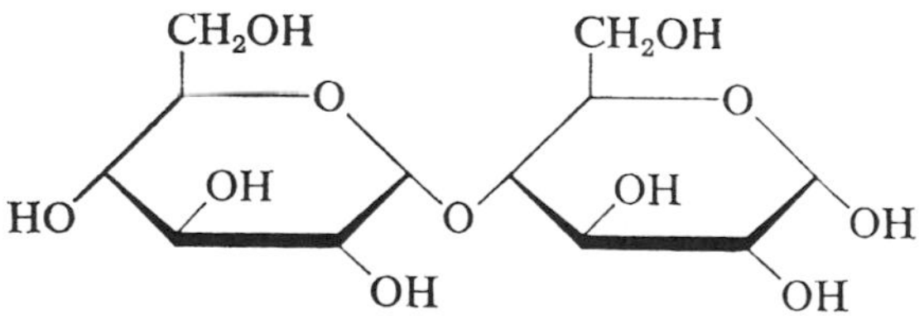

α-Maltose
(α-D-glucosyl-1,4-D-glucose)

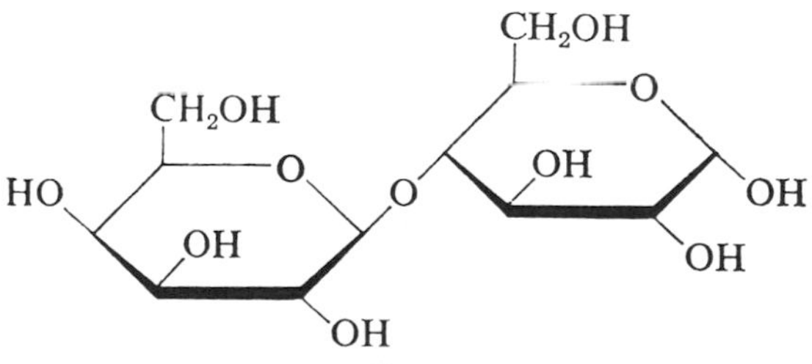

α-Lactose
(β-D-galactosyl-1,4-D-glucose)

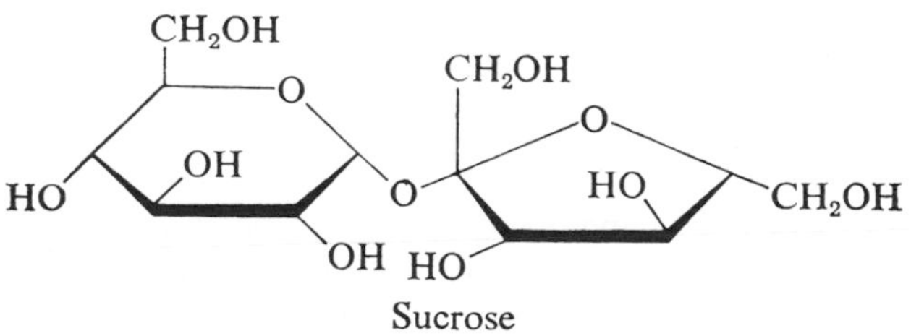

Sucrose
(α-D-glucosyl-β-D-fructoside)

Starch has two components, amylopectin, whose structure is like that of glycogen but is less highly branched, and amylose, which is a straight-chain polymer of α-1,4-glucosyl residues. **Cellulose** is a straight-chain polymer of β-1,4-glucosyl residues. **Acid polysaccharides** containing either sulphate esters or uronic acids are discussed on p. 17.7 and **glycogen** on p. 9.9.

Ascorbic acid, the antiscorbutic vitamin is a hexose derivative:

$$
\begin{array}{l}
\text{CO} \\
\text{HO—C} \\
\text{HO—C} \quad \text{O} \\
\text{HC} \\
\text{HO—CH} \\
\text{CH}_2\text{OH}
\end{array}
$$

It is the lactone of a uronic acid, and is strongly acidic, because the proton of the —OH on C-2 dissociates readily. The **enediol** grouping can be oxidized by very mild oxidizing agents:

$$
\begin{array}{ccc}
\text{HO—C} & & \text{O=C} \\
\text{HO—C} & \rightleftharpoons & \text{O=C}
\end{array}
$$

and the product, **dehydroascorbic acid**, retains antiscorbutic activity. With more vigorous oxidation, however, the molecule splits up into oxalic acid and other products. Even dissolved O_2 in aqueous solution does this, and the process is greatly accelerated by traces of copper ions, alkaline pH, sunlight and heat. Solutions of ascorbic acid can to some extent be stabilized by strong acids, but the crystalline solid is stable indefinitely in the dark. It is very soluble in water. Although ascorbic acid is made biologically from D-glucose, the active form is the L-isomer.

Stereoisomerism

The electron orbitals (valency bonds) of individual atoms are orientated in three-dimensional space. The four single bonds of carbon are directed towards the apices of a regular tetrahedron, if the nucleus is imagined to be at the centre of the polygon. It follows that if the four bonds of a single carbon atom are united with four different atoms or groups, two arrangements are possible which are not identical, and therefore two different isomers of the compound exist.

The situation is sometimes described by saying that the mirror image of one isomer is not identical with the isomer itself. What this means can be seen in fig. 9.1.

If the forms in the diagram are regarded as tetrahedra

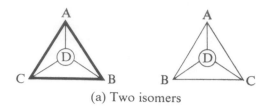

(a) Two isomers

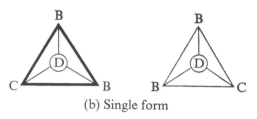

(b) Single form

FIG. 9.1. Stereoisomers.

with their bases resting on the paper, and their apices projecting upwards, so that the radical 'D' is in each case pointing towards the reader's face, it will be appreciated that the right hand tetrahedron in both instances is the mirror image of the left. In the upper part of the figure the right hand tetrahedron cannot be superimposed on the left, e.g. by twisting it round; the only way in which A can be superimposed on A, B on B, and C on C, is by inverting one tetrahedron, and then, of course, it is impossible to superimpose D on D. In the lower part of the figure, the right-hand tetrahedron can be imposed on the left by rotating it 120° clockwise. This is to say that there are two isomers of the compound (ABCD) but only one of the compound (BBCD).

In a molecule containing more than one carbon atom, each may be asymmetric, and the number of possible isomers is then 2^n. There are 2^4, or 16, isomers of a hexose and 2^5 or 32 if it is in the hemi-acetal form. The physical differences between the isomers are very small if there is only one asymmetric atom, but with several, real differences begin to appear. For example, there are noticeable differences between the hexoses in chemical reactivity, solubility and sweetness.

The most remarkable differences between stereoisomers are, however, in their biological activity and in optical properties. All stereoisomers, unless they are internally compensated, rotate the plane of polarized light. There is no satisfactory simple explanation of this phenomenon. However a ray of light may be thought of as a bundle of wave forms, each vibrating in a different fixed plane stretching between the light source and the receptor. If the ray passes through certain crystals which have non-symmetrical lattices, only wave forms vibrating in certain preferred planes may be let through, the rest of the beam being absorbed. The emergent light beam is said to be **plane polarized**. If it passes through a second similar crystal, all the remaining light is absorbed unless the orientation of the lattice of the second crystal in space is identical with that of the first. This is the principle of the polarimeter.

Optically active substances, i.e. those containing an asymmetric carbon atom, rotate the plane of polarized light to an extent dependent on the substance, its concentration in solution, and the length of the light path. The rotation may be to the right (dextrorotatory) or to the left (laevorotatory) when viewed along the light path. The extent of the rotation may be measured by observing how much the second of a pair of polarizing crystals must be rotated to let the beam of light through again, after the stereoisomer has been introduced into the light path.

Stereoisomerism would be of academic interest were it not that the great majority of biological processes make use of only one of a pair of stereoisomers. All but one of the amino acids are optically active and naturally occurring proteins are constructed only from L-amino acids. Moreover the great majority of enzymes accept only one of the possible stereoisomers of a compound as a substrate (p. 7.3).

Furthermore even certain coenzymes exhibit stereo-isomerism. C-4 of NAD or NADP accepts 1 e and 1 H$^+$ and then contains 2 H atoms which project on opposite sides of the pyridine ring, but these 2 H atoms at C-4 are not equivalent. Certain enzymes selectively remove an H$^+$ + e from one face of the reduced coenzyme. When the reduced coenzyme structure is written with the —CONH$_2$ to the right hand side of the formula the plane facing the reader is termed A and the hydrogen atom sticking out of this plane towards the reader at C-4 is termed H$_A$. The other hydrogen atom is then H$_B$. Certain dehydrogenases are A or B specific with respect to the donor NADH$_2$ or NADPH$_2$ systems.

Thus cells and tissues not only contain, in general, a large number of optically active compounds, but the 'unnatural' isomers are either biologically inactive or have biological properties differing from the natural ones. For example, D-ascorbic acid is not an antiscorbutic substance. D-thyroxine has no more than one third of the effect of L-thyroxine on the basal metabolism. The unnatural isomer of acyl carnitine is a competitive inhibitor of the natural isomer, and so may block transfer of fatty acid metabolites in and out of mitochondria. These examples show that at least an awareness of the need to specify a stereoisomer in considering biological phenomena is essential in medical science and especially in pharmacology (vol. 2, p. 3.16).

RACEMIZATION

A mixture containing equal proportions of both isomers of an optically active compound shows no optical activity because the effects of the two isomers cancel each other out. The biological activity is usually only 50 per cent of

that of the pure natural isomer. Such a mixture is called a **racemic mixture**, and is the usual product when a compound is made chemically.

Racemization also occurs when a compound with an asymmetric carbon atom acquires a double bond and loses it in a subsequent reaction, unless the process is under stereospecific control. For example, L-lactic acid can be oxidized to pyruvic acid, where C-2 is no longer a centre of asymmetry. If pyruvic acid is reduced artificially, the product is DL-lactic acid, unless a specific L- or D-lactate dehydrogenase is used.

NOMENCLATURE

Originally, optically active compounds were called **dextrorotatory** or **laevorotatory** on the basis of their rotation of polarized light, hence dextrose (glucose) and laevulose (fructose). The prefixes D- or L- were also used. The system fell into confusion when it was found that closely related compounds could have opposite rotations. For example, we know that lactic acid is made in nature from dextrorotatory glyceraldehyde (phosphate) but in animals the lactic acid is laevorotatory, although its salts are dextrorotatory. The difficulty has been avoided by establishing chemically the relationship of each natural isomer to a reference compound. All carbohydrates are classified by reference to D-glyceraldehyde (with a capital letter); amino acids with reference to L-serine. The actual rotation is then indicated by a sign (+) or (−); thus lactic acid produced in animals is L(+) lactic acid; bacteria may produce the D(−) compound.

CARBOHYDRATE METABOLISM
Catabolism of glucose

Only one reaction directly involving glucose is of importance in animals. This consists of a transfer of a phosphate radical from adenosine triphosphate (ATP) to the OH group on carbon atom 6 of glucose. The other product is adenosine diphosphate (ADP). This reaction is catalysed by the enzyme **hexokinase** and is in practice irreversible for thermodynamic reasons.

Glucose-6-phosphate (G-6-P) is a substrate for several enzymes; one catalyses isomerization to glucose-1-phosphate (G-1-P), one to fructose-6-phosphate (F-6-P), and one the oxidation to 6-phosphogluconic acid (6-P-G). A fourth enzyme, found only in certain tissues, is a specific **glucose-6-phosphatase** which converts the ester back to free glucose and inorganic phosphate (P$_i$). Thus the multiplicity of pathways of the carbon atoms of glucose really begins with G-6-P and not with glucose (fig. 9.2).

Each of these pathways is considered in turn, beginning with that initiated by the conversion to F-6-P. The final product of this pathway is the C-3 compound pyruvate, each molecule of glucose being split into two. In most cells pyruvate can be readily oxidized to CO$_2$ and water, and in animal tissues this route to the complete oxidation of glucose is the most important. The sequence of reactions leading to pyruvate is usually known as the **Embden–Meyerhof pathway** (fig. 9.4).

While the interconversion of G-6-P and F-6-P is freely reversible, the next step, involving the transfer of another phosphate radical from ATP to form F-1,6-di-P (FDP),

is almost irreversible. The enzyme responsible, **phosphofructokinase**, has several interesting properties. It is inhibited by ATP, its own substrate, at concentrations of about 4 mmol/l which is towards the upper end of the concentrations found in tissues, by phosphocreatine and by citrate. A number of substances prevent the inhibition of phosphofructokinase; they include AMP, cyclic AMP

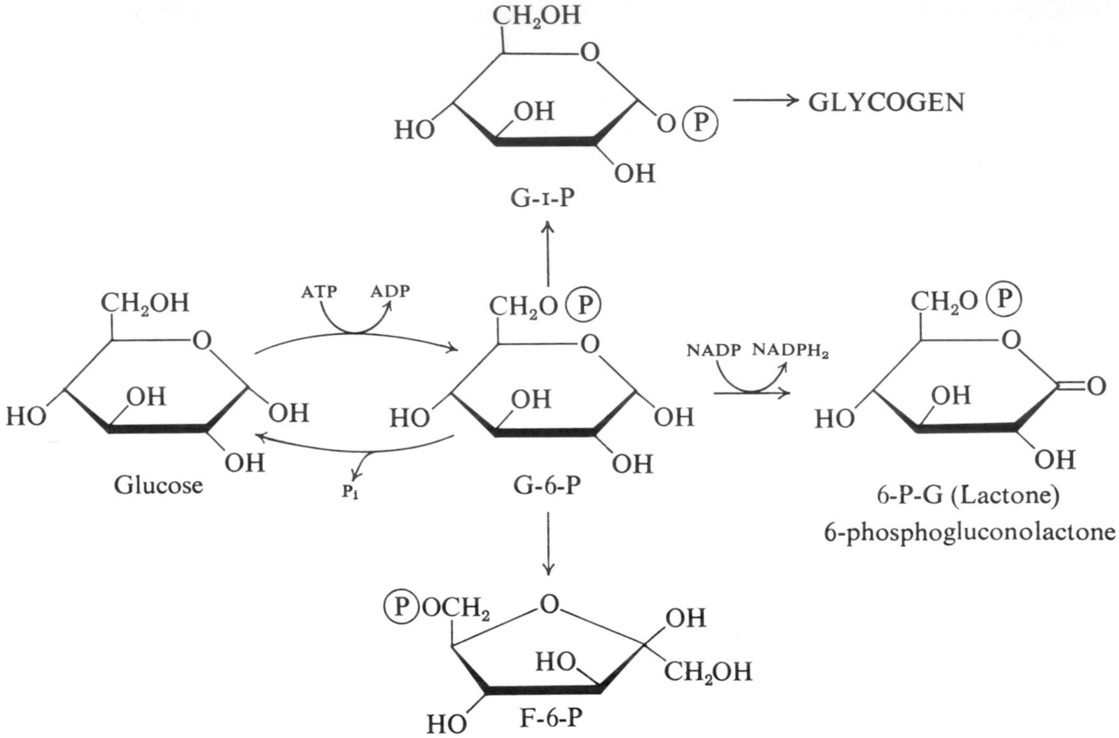

FIG. 9.2. Interrelationships of glucose-6-phosphate.

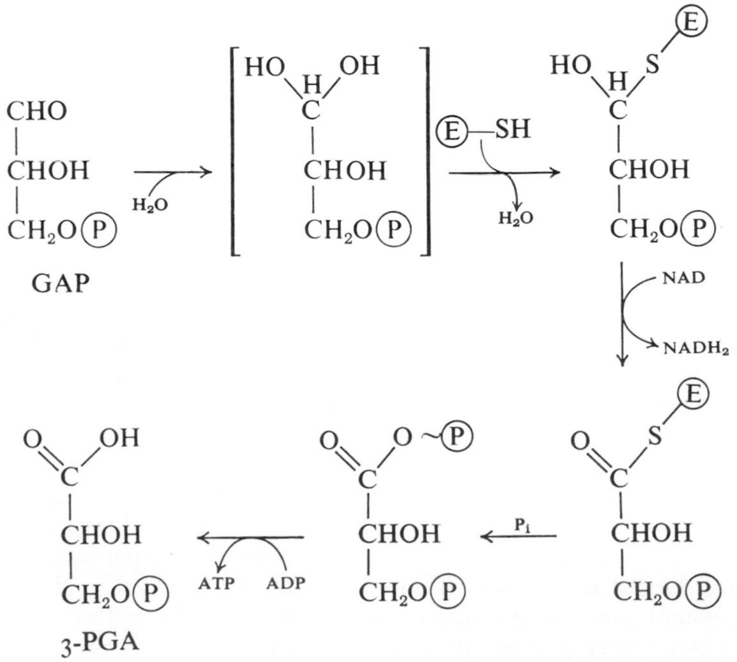

FIG. 9.3. The conversion of glyceraldehyde-3-phosphate (GAP) to 3-phosphoglycerate (3-PGA).

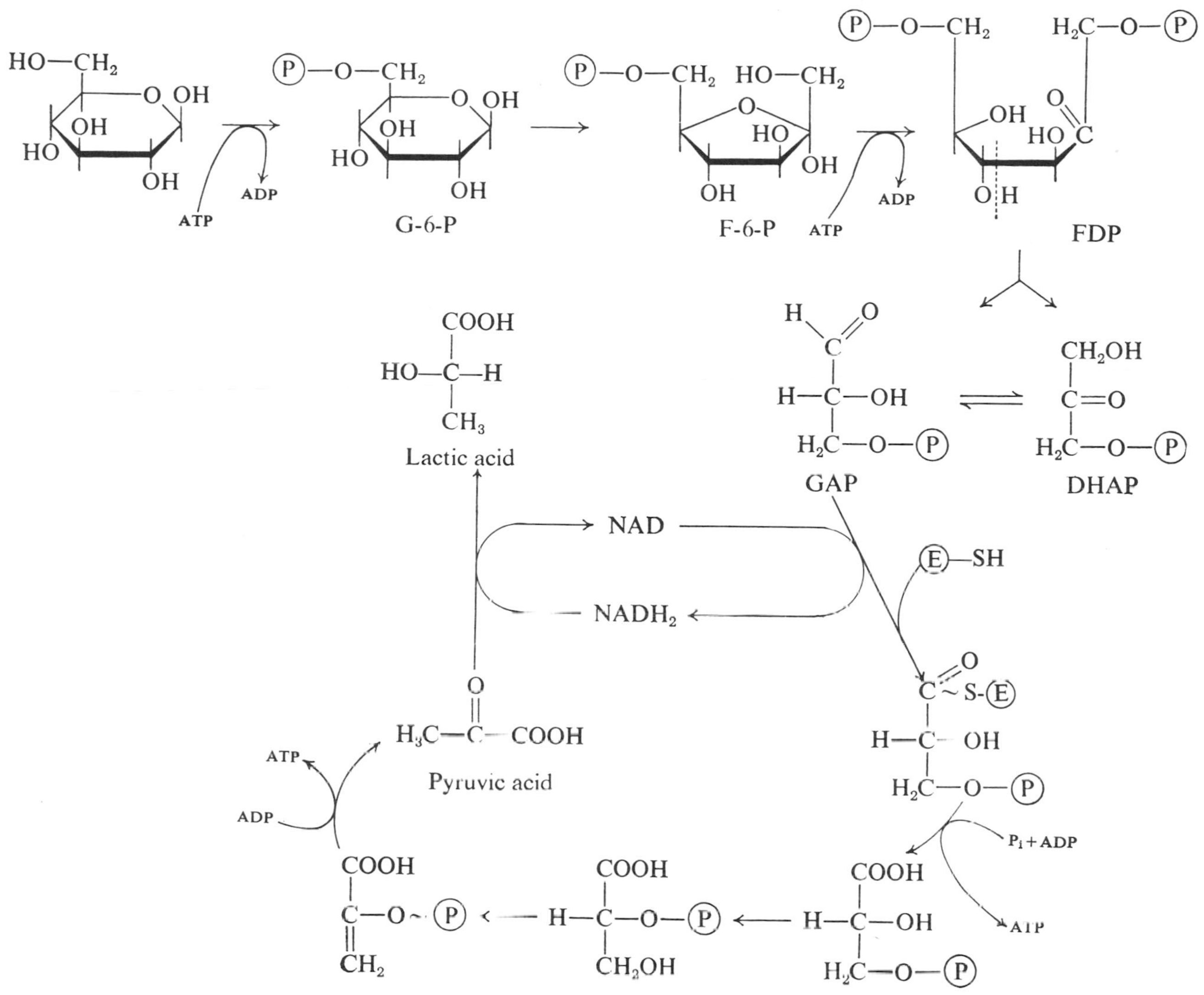

FIG. 9.4. The Embden–Meyerhof pathway.

(p. 9.9), ADP, inorganic phosphate, FDP and F-6-P. All except the last can also enhance the activity of the enzyme in the absence of inhibitors. It will be noted that many of the **effectors** are neither substrates nor products of the reaction catalysed by phosphofructokinase, but are chemicals important in other reactions of intermediary metabolism. As explained in chap. 14, there is good reason to believe that these unusual kinetic properties help in the control of the flux rate through the complete pathway.

In the next reaction FDP splits between C-3 and C-4 to yield the trioses, glyceraldehyde-3-phosphate (GAP) and dihydroxyacetone phosphate (DHAP). Because there are two products and only one reactant, the position of equilibrium is very dependent on the absolute concentrations of all three. At the concentrations obtaining in tissues, either breakdown or synthesis (p. 9.10) of hexoses

may be favoured by slight changes in conditions. DHAP is metabolized only by a side reaction and so might be expected to accumulate. It does not do so, because an **isomerase** catalyses the interconversion of DHAP and GAP, and the latter compound is continuously removed.

The reaction which follows is an oxidation, accompanied by a considerable decrease in the free energy of the system. In this case, however, a new phosphate compound is synthesized, a mixed anhydride, and the phosphate radical is then transferred to ADP, forming ATP. This was the first example of 'energy-trapping' to be discovered. The details of the overall reaction are given in fig. 9.3. The active site of the responsible enzyme (E) contains an SH group, probably firmly bound as glutathione.

A reactive thio-ester is formed as an intermediate, and this is phosphorylated to yield 1:3 diphosphoglycerate and the free enzyme once again. Thus the net result is:

$$GAP + P_i + NAD + ADP \longrightarrow 3\text{-}PGA + ATP + NADH_2$$

This is an example of 'substrate level phosphorylation' (see also fig. 9.10 and p. 9.7). 3-Phosphoglycerate is isomerized to 2-phosphoglycerate and the latter readily loses a molecule of water, with the formation of phosphoenolpyruvate. This enol ester grouping is again very reactive and the transfer of the phosphate radical to ADP occurs readily, catalysed by **pyruvate kinase.** This enzyme is allosterically inhibited (p. 14.6) by its own substrate, and the inhibition is relieved by FDP. This feed-forward control is important in the control of flux through the Embden–Meyerhof pathway.

The pathway can be summarized as follows:

$$Glucose + 2ATP \longrightarrow FDP + 2ADP$$
$$FDP + 4ADP + 2P_i + 2NAD \longrightarrow$$
$$2Pyruvate + 4ATP + 2NADH_2$$

Thus there is a net gain of 2ATP for each molecule of glucose catabolized.

Pyruvate is an important intermediate compound, but before describing its metabolism, the other three possible reactions of glucose-6-phosphate are considered.

HEXOSE MONOPHOSPHATE (PENTOSE) PATHWAY (fig. 9.5)

In many tissues, but not in muscle, there exists a pattern of enzymes in addition to those already described, which is capable of directly oxidizing G-6-P to pentose phosphates, and which together with the enzymes of the Embden–Meyerhof pathway, can oxidize G-6-P completely to CO_2 and H_2O (or $NADPH_2$). The enzymes are first **glucose-6-phosphate dehydrogenase,** which oxidizes the ring form of G-6-P to the acid lactone; a **lactonase** catalyses the production of the straight-chain form of the acid. The dehydrogenase requires NADP specifically as hydrogen acceptor, as does the associated enzyme, **phosphogluconic acid dehydrogenase.** Although the product of this latter reaction should be a 3-oxo acid, it must spontaneously decarboxylate at the enzyme site, as it has never been isolated, and the observed products are ribulose-5-phosphate and CO_2.

Ribulose-5-phosphate can be isomerized to ribose-5-phosphate, the starting material for purine nucleotide synthesis (p. 12.26). It may be that in some tissues this is the main function of this enzyme sequence; in other tissues, however, e.g. liver, the rate at which G-6-P is metabolized by this alternative pathway can be shown to be much faster than the rate of nucleic acid synthesis and the pentose phosphates must therefore be metabolized in some other way. With the help of two enzymes, **transketolase** and **transaldolase,** which have been found to occur together with G-6-P dehydrogenase, it is possible to rearrange the thirty carbon atoms present in six molecules of the pentose ribulose-5-phosphate into five molecules of the

hexose glucose-6-phosphate, as shown in fig. 9.5. In summary, the sequence gives

$$6G\text{-}6\text{-}P + 12NADP \longrightarrow 5G\text{-}6\text{-}P + 12NADPH_2 + 6CO_2.$$

In effect, one molecule of glucose has been completely oxidized. Since no energy has been directly trapped as in the Embden–Meyerhof scheme, the value of this oxidation may be questioned. Its importance may well be the production of twelve molecules of $NADPH_2$ per molecule of glucose oxidized; this is required for fatty acid synthesis, since this and most synthetic reactions in cells which involve reduction are catalysed by enzymes specific for $NADPH_2$, whereas most cell dehydrogenases are specific for NAD. The point of the alternative pathway may therefore be in providing

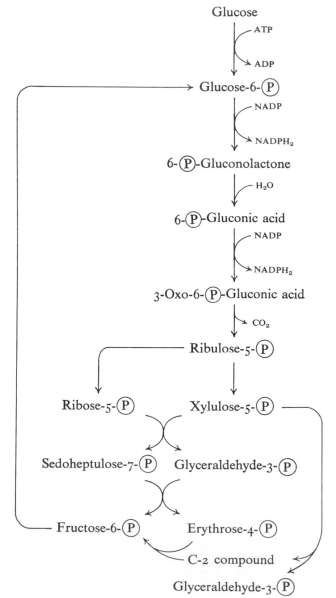

FIG. 9.5. The hexose monophosphate pathway.

the appropriate reduced coenzyme, rather than in producing ATP directly.

Glycogen metabolism

Glycogen is found in most animal cells, but more particularly in muscle and liver. The concentration in muscle is about 10 g/kg of the wet weight, and may vary from 0 to 50 g/kg; in the liver the concentration is usually about 50 g/kg, but may be as high as 100 g/kg; it falls in starvation and other circumstances practically to zero, for reasons which will become apparent later.

Glycogen is a large polymer of glucose, mol. wt. 1–5 million; it contains only α-glucose residues. These are connected to each other mostly by 1:4 linkages thus:

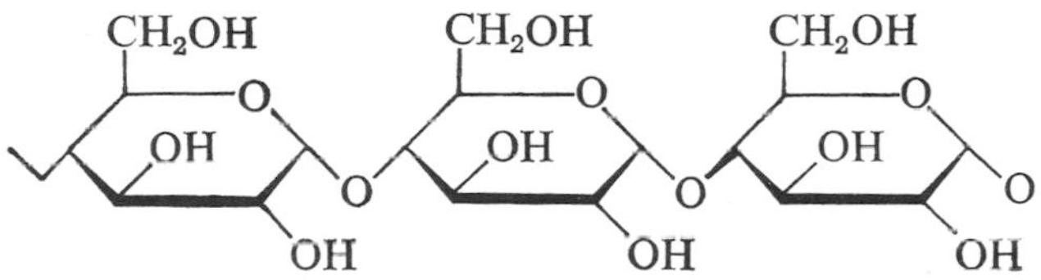

but there also occur 1:6 linkages at so-called branch points. In the inner part of the molecule there is a branch point every three to four residues and the outer branches are six to eight residues long.

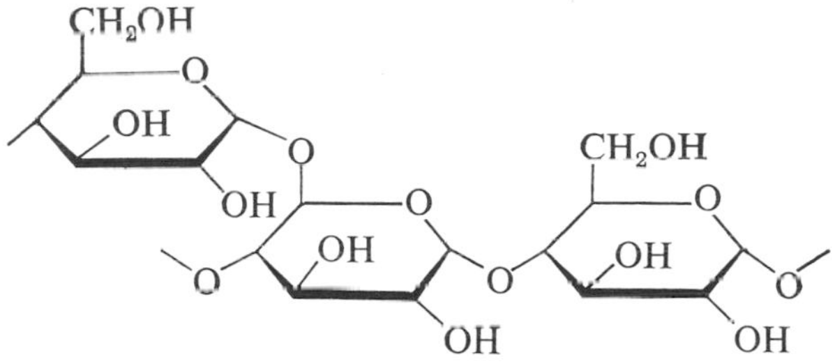

The whole structure has a tree-like appearance, as shown

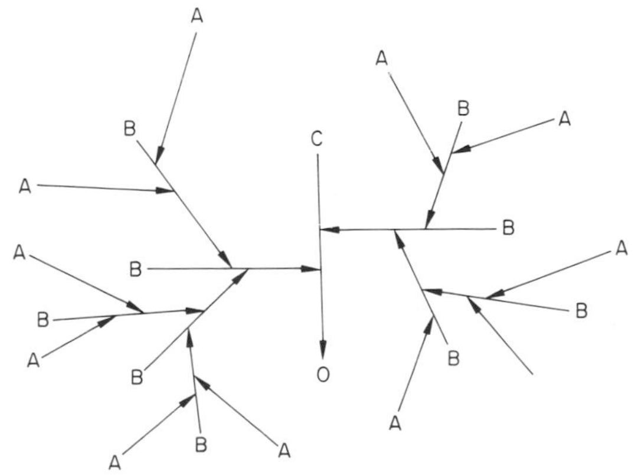

FIG. 9.6. Structure of glycogen. An **A** chain is defined as a chain connected to the remainder of the molecule through its reducing end. A **B** chain is also joined through its reducing end, but in addition carries other **A** and/or **B** chains at one or more of its primary hydroxyls. Each molecule has a single **C** chain which is unsubstituted at its reducing end, marked with an **O** in this diagram. Adapted from Whelan W.J. (1970) *FEBS Letters* **12**, 103.

in fig. 9.6. This highly branched structure of the molecule is very significant for the metabolism of glycogen.

BREAKDOWN OF GLYCOGEN

Residues which are attached at the outermost end of the terminal branches by a 1:4 link can be transferred to inorganic phosphate and so form α-glucose-1-phosphate (G-1-P). This reaction is catalysed by an enzyme called **phosphorylase**, which has complicated properties. It exists in tissues in two forms, one active (phosphorylase *a*) and one inactive (phosphorylase *b*). Muscle phosphorylase *b* has half the molecular weight of the muscle *a* enzyme. The conversion of *a* to *b* is accompanied by the release of inorganic phosphate, and conversely the reactivation process requires phosphorylation by ATP. Thus we have:

$$
\left.
\begin{array}{l}
\text{Phosphorylase } a \longrightarrow \\
\quad \text{phosphorylase } b + 2P_i \\
\text{Phosphorylase } b + 2ATP \longrightarrow \\
\quad \text{phosphorylase } a + 2ADP
\end{array}
\right\} \text{Liver}
$$

$$
\left.
\begin{array}{l}
\text{Phosphorylase } a \longrightarrow \\
\quad 2 \text{ phosphorylase } b + 4P_i \\
2 \text{ phosphorylase } b + 4ATP \longrightarrow \\
\quad \text{phosphorylase } a + 4ADP
\end{array}
\right\} \text{Muscle}
$$

The dephosphorylating and rephosphorylating processes are each catalysed by a specific enzyme.

In normal aerobic tissues it is found that most of the phosphorylase and most of the rephosphorylating enzyme are inactive. The latter can be reactivated by yet a third enzyme which requires **cyclic AMP** (3′: 5′-cyclic AMP). This nucleotide which has a key role in the control of metabolism is a cyclic compound with the phosphoric acid moiety double esterified between the alcoholic hydroxyls on carbon atoms 3 and 5 of the ribose portion of the nucleotide as follows:

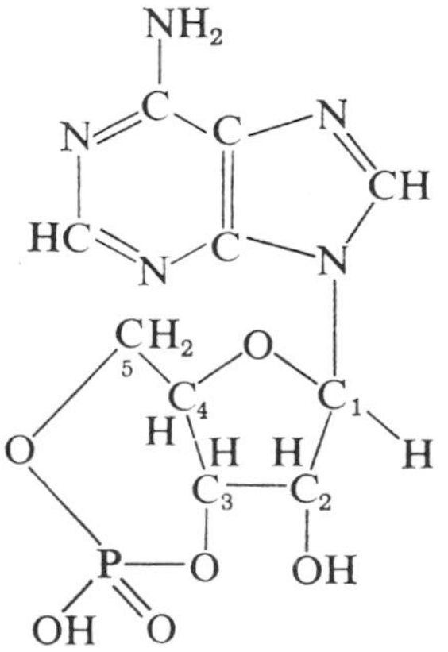

It is formed from ATP by the action of an enzyme, **adenylate cyclase**

$$
\text{ATP} \longrightarrow \text{cyclic AMP} + PP_i \text{ (pyrophosphate)}
$$

The cyclic AMP is also attacked by an enzyme or

enzymes present in most tissues termed **phosphodiesterases** which hydrolytically split the cyclic phosphate structure between the C-3 of the ribose and the phosphate as follows

$$\text{cyclic AMP} \longrightarrow 5'\text{AMP}$$

The concentration of cyclic AMP in a given tissue is accordingly dependent upon the supply of ATP and the relative activities of the adenyl cyclase and the phosphodiesterases. It is never present in a concentration more than a few per cent of the concentration of either ATP or 5'AMP.

Cyclic AMP is a chemical mediator in the mechanism of action of various hormones (p. 14.13). Thus glucagon, parathyroid hormone and adrenaline activate the adenyl cyclase system and quickly increase the tissue concentration of cyclic AMP. In liver an increased cyclic AMP level facilitates the conversion of inactive phosphorylase (phosphorylase *b*) into active phosphorylase (phosphorylase *a*). This is quite distinct from the activation of phosphorylase *b* itself by 5'AMP.

Thus the explanation of the glycogenolytic effect of adrenaline is that it facilitates the conversion of ATP to cyclic AMP. This latter substance in turn enhances the formation of phosphorylase *a* which then attacks the glycogen molecule to give G-1-P and so triggers off glycogenolysis (p. 14.8). Cyclic AMP takes part in several other control systems by activating a protein kinase, but this is not its only mode of action. The direct action on phosphofructokinase has already been mentioned (p. 9.6) and in certain tissues it may have an effect upon nucleic acid synthesis.

G-1-P and G-6-P are kept in equilibrium by a reaction catalysed by **phosphohexoisomerase.** This reaction is shown in fig. 9.2. Thus the glucose residues liberated from glycogen by phosphorylase can enter either the Embden–Meyerhof or hexose monophosphate pathways of glucose metabolism.

It is only the α-1:4 linked glucose residues of glycogen which can be broken off by phosphorylase and the enzyme is unable to attack 1:4 bonds interior to a 1:6 branch point. For the complete breakdown of glycogen, another system is required, which can attack the 1:6 bonds. This enzyme, the debranching enzyme or **amylo-6-glucosidase,** simply hydrolyses the glucose residue attached by a 1:6 bond to produce free glucose.

To produce the branched structure of glycogen a **branching enzyme** (transglycosylase) is necessary. This is in fact a transferase, acting as shown in the diagram below:

(○ represents a glucose residue)

The reaction catalysed by phosphorylase is essentially reversible and *in vitro* glycogen can be synthesized in a system consisting of a primer (a fragment of polysaccharide), a suitably high concentration of G-1-P, a low concentration of inorganic phosphate and branching enzyme. The concentrations of G-1-P and P_i found *in vivo* do not favour the synthetic reaction; furthermore patients have been found whose liver or muscle cells contain no phosphorylase, but yet are loaded with glycogen. An independent mechanism of glycogen synthesis explains these awkward facts.

GLYCOGEN SYNTHESIS

This mechanism of glycogen synthesis depends on glycosyl transfer from a coenzyme called uridine diphosphate glucose (UDPG). The following sequence of reactions occurs:

$$\text{UTP} + \text{G-1-P} \longrightarrow \text{UDPG} + \text{PP}_i$$
$$\text{UDPG} + (\text{glucose})_n \rightleftarrows \text{UDP} + (\text{glucose})_{n+1}$$
$$\text{UDP} + \text{ATP} \longrightarrow \text{UTP} + \text{ADP}$$

This reaction sequence is energetically less economical for the cell, since two molecules of ATP are required for each glucose residue added. On the other hand, the large drop in free energy on the fission of the UDP–G bond means that the transfer reaction is essentially irreversible and synthesis is therefore always favoured. All the evidence suggests that glycogen synthesis and breakdown proceeds by the action of the two enzyme systems **UDP glucosyl transferase** and **phosphorylase** respectively. UDP glucosyltransferase (glycogen synthase) exists in two forms. One of these (D) depends on the presence of G-6-P for activity, and is effectively not active in conditions *in vivo*. The other form (I) is independent of the presence of G-6-P. The conversion from the active (I) to the inactive (D) form is catalysed by a specific kinase which transfers a phosphoryl group from ATP. This kinase is different from the more general protein kinase and is not sensitive to cyclic AMP. The reverse process, activation of the synthase by dephosphorylation, is stimulated by insulin in a way still unknown.

INBORN ERRORS OF GLYCOGEN METABOLISM

A number of uncommon disorders are associated with increased storage of glycogen in the various tissues (vol. 3, p. 47.12). These do not arise from increased formation of glycogen but are due to a lack of one of several enzymes involved in its handling. The defects usually become obvious in infancy and often lead to death before adult life.

Table 9.1 gives a summary of the various types of glycogen storage disease with the enzymes whose absence leads to glycogenosis. In some patients more than one enzyme may be absent or have a very low activity.

TABLE 9.1. Enzyme defects in glycogen storage diseases.

Type	Enzyme defect	Tissues Affected
I	Glucose-6-phosphatase	Liver, kidney, gut
II	Lysosomal α–1,4–glucosidase	Generalized, particularly heart, tongue, brain
III	Amylo-1,6-glucosidase (Debranching enzyme)	Liver, heart, muscle, RBC, WBC
IV	Branching enzyme (amylo 1,4–1,6 transglycosylase)	Liver, spleen, heart, muscle, RBC, CNS
V	Muscle phosphorylase	Skeletal muscle
VI	Liver phosphorylase	Liver, WBC

Other carbohydrate pathways

UDPG is a component of a number of other important pathways in carbohydrate metabolism:

LACTOSE SYNTHESIS

Lactose is the disaccharide found in milk and formed from glucose and galactose (Gal). It is synthesized only in mammary tissue.

$$UDPG \longrightarrow UDP \; Gal$$

$$UDPGal + G\text{-}1\text{-}P \longrightarrow UDP + Lactose\text{-}1\text{-}P$$

$$Lactose\text{-}1\text{-}P \longrightarrow Lactose + P_1$$

GALACTOSE METABOLISM

Lactose in the diet is hydrolysed in the gut wall to glucose and galactose. The latter sugar is transformed to glucose.

$$Gal + ATP \longrightarrow Gal\text{-}1\text{-}P + ADP$$

$$Gal\text{-}1\text{-}P + UDPG \longrightarrow UDPGal + G\text{-}1\text{-}P$$

$$UDPGal \longrightarrow UDPG$$

The enzyme which catalyses the first reaction is an epimerase. It inverts the configuration of —H and —OH at C-4, thus converting the galactose residue into a glucose residue.

The epimerase is found in liver and curiously also in erythrocytes. Clearly the immediate formation of UDPG favours direct synthesis of glycogen from galactose in liver.

Due to a lack of one or other of the enzymes in the above sequence a child may be unable to convert galactose to glucose. Galactose accumulates in the blood and tissues. These infants do not thrive, and develop cataracts and mental defects, unless on an artificial diet without galactose (vol. 3, p. 47.10).

GLUCURONIC ACID METABOLISM

The oxidation of glucose residues is shown in fig. 9.7. Glucuronic acid occurs combined in two types of compound. Firstly it is present in many of the mucopolysaccharides which act as lubricants and are also important

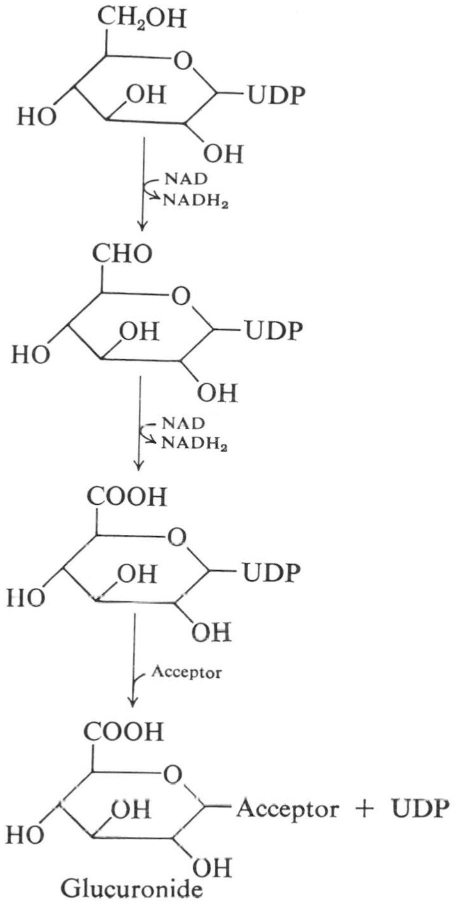

FIG. 9.7. The formation of glucuronides.

constituents of connective tissue (p. 17.7). Secondly, in the liver it can combine with many toxic or potentially toxic substances to form water soluble glucuronides, which may then be excreted in the bile. The bile pigment, bilirubin diglucuronide, a product of haemoglobin catabolism, is an important example. The mechanism by which this is formed is described on p. 33.13. Free glucuronic acid is seldom found in the body.

FRUCTOSE METABOLISM

Fructose is not normally a constituent of the diet but the disaccharide sucrose is consumed in large quantities. It is hydrolysed in the gut wall to equimolar amounts of fructose and glucose. Fructose can be phosphorylated to F-6-P by hexokinase, but this reaction is inhibited in the presence of glucose and it seems likely that fructose is metabolized by means of a special fructokinase.

$$Fructose + ATP \longrightarrow F\text{-}1\text{-}P + ADP$$

F-1-P can be split by an aldolase to form dihydroxyacetone phosphate and glyceraldehyde. The latter is phosphorylated either directly or after oxidation to glyceric acid. In either case the two trioses join the Embden–Meyerhof pathway.

Pyruvic acid metabolism

Pyruvate has a central position in carbohydrate metabolism (fig. 9.8). There are at least seven reactions involving pyruvate or the close relative, phosphoenolpyruvate. These are numbered in the figure and discussed in turn.

(1) The reaction catalysed by **pyruvate kinase** has already been mentioned as converting phosphoenolpyruvate to pyruvate at the end of the Embden–Meyerhof pathway. For all practical purposes it is irreversible, so that phosphoenolpyruvate and thus other triose phosphates cannot be made directly from pyruvate.

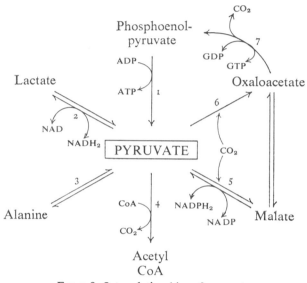

FIG. 9.8. Interrelationships of pyruvate.

(2) Most animal cells contain in their cytoplasm large quantities of **lactate dehydrogenase**, which requires NAD and catalyses the reversible oxidation of lactate. Lactate undergoes no other known reaction in animals. Its formation is important under anaerobic circumstances since it allows the reoxidation of $NADH_2$ formed in the oxidation of glyceraldehyde phosphate. The $NADH_2$ is normally oxidized by the aerobic pathway described later in the chapter. If for any reason the cells have an inadequate supply of oxygen, this reoxidation does not occur fast enough for their energy needs; glucose can still be catabolized and ATP consequently produced by the coupling of the two reactions and the whole of the Embden–Meyerhof pathway then becomes self-contained. Anaerobiosis is thus usually accompanied by increased lactate formation (see opposite).

The activity of the lactate dehydrogenase is so great that the redox couples pyruvate/lactate and NAD/$NADH_2$ are nearly always in equilibrium within the cytoplasm (p. 8.9). The pyruvate/lactate ratio in blood is quite frequently used as an indicator of the NAD/$NADH_2$ ratio or redox state of cells. This is, however, unwise as muscle cells contain a lactate permease and possibly also a pyruvate permease, so that the extra-cellular concentrations of these two substances may be widely different from the cytoplasmic concentrations. It is also certain that the NAD/$NADH_2$ ratio is different in the mitochondria and in the cytoplasm.

(3) An aminotransferase, widely distributed in cells, can convert alanine (ala) to pyruvate (pyr):

$$ala + \text{2-oxoglutaric acid} \xrightleftharpoons{} pyr + \text{glutamic acid}$$

Formation of alanine by transamination, followed by leakage of the amino acid into the blood, and uptake by the liver, is the major route by which $-NH_2$ groups, released by amino acid catabolism in muscle, are transferred to liver, a so-called 'alanine cycle'.

(4) The oxidative decarboxylation of pyruvate (fig. 9.9) is the main pathway of metabolism for this compound and thus for carbohydrate. Essentially, pyruvate is split into CO_2 and acetaldehyde. In animal tissues the latter is not set free but combines first with the prosthetic group thiamine pyrophosphate, from which it is transferred to a second prosthetic group, lipoic acid. This can exist in two forms called lipoic acid I and lipoic acid II.

The acetaldehyde is transferred to form I, which becomes reduced, while the acetaldehyde group is oxidized to an acetyl residue.

This acetyl residue is then transferred to coenzyme A, and the reduced lipoic acid is re-oxidized to form I by NAD. The overall reaction is:

$$CH_3COCOOH + CoASH$$
$$\downarrow {\small\begin{array}{l} NAD \\ \rightsquigarrow NADH_2 \end{array}}$$
$$CH_3CO.SCoA + CO_2$$

The acetyl group can be oxidized to CO_2 and H_2O as described on p. 9.15, or it can be used to synthesize fatty acids or other lipids. The decarboxylation reaction is almost irreversible, so that the acetyl group cannot be used to synthesize pyruvate.

The enzymes which catalyse the oxidative decarboxylation of pyruvate are organized in a **multi-enzyme complex**, of mol. wt. about 10^6 daltons. They are not present in equimolar quantities, there being most of the transacetylase, but they are packed in an ordered, quasi-crystalline fashion. It is of great interest that the activity of the first enzyme, pyruvate dehydrogenase, is completely inhibited by phosphorylation of a specific site on the enzyme protein, catalysed by a specific kinase (cf. glycogen synthase, p. 9.10). Activity is restored by dephosphorylation, catalysed by a phosphatase. Much effort has gone into attempts to identify the method by which this cycle of events is controlled, but at present it seems that the rate of pyruvate oxidation is largely controlled by the activity of the permease which translocates pyruvate into mitochondria, and which is strongly inhibited by palmityl-carnitine (p. 10.8).

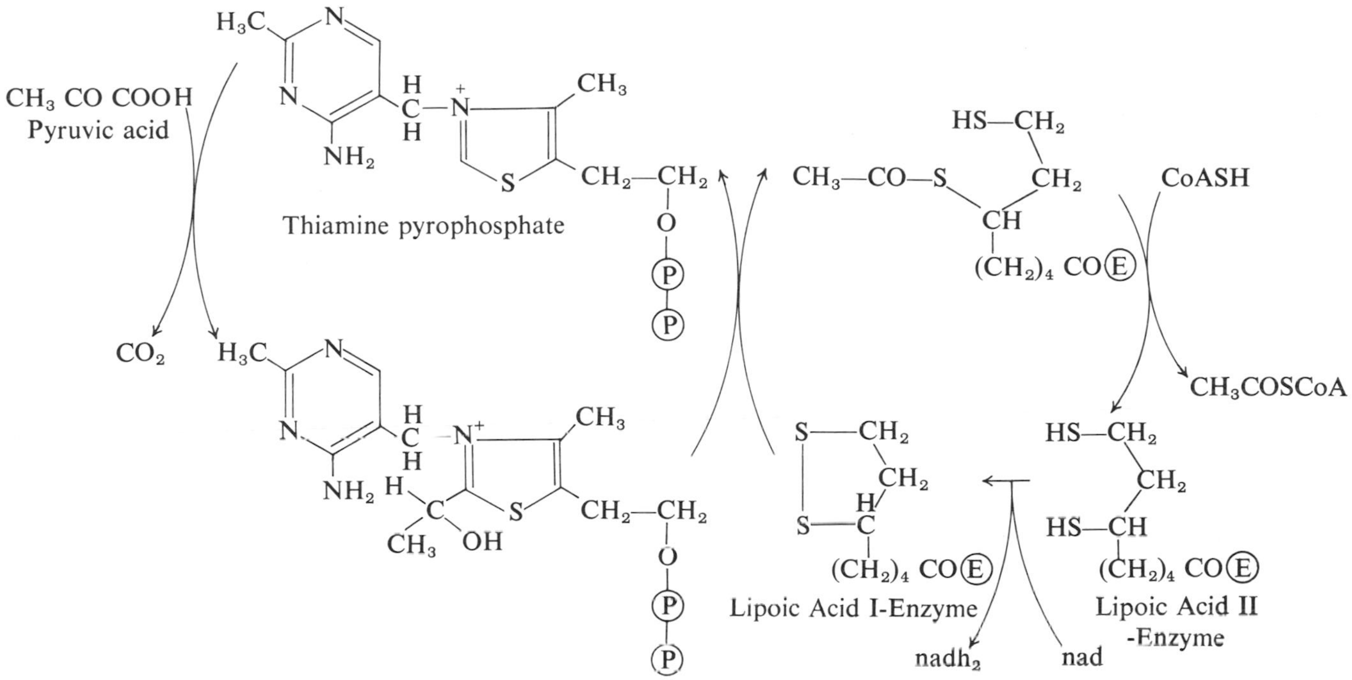

FIG. 9.9. The formation of acetyl CoA.

2-Oxoglutarate oxidation (p. 9.15) is catalysed by a very similar multi-enzyme complex, but its activity is not regulated by a protein kinase.

Reactions 5, 6 and 7 in fig. 9.8 represent various ways in which a connection can be made between pyruvate and the 4 carbon acids of the citric acid cycle (fig. 9.10).

(5) The **malic enzyme** catalyses the reversible reaction to malic acid.

$$CH_3COCOOH + CO_2$$

$$\downarrow \begin{array}{l} \text{NADPH}_2 \\ \text{NADP} \end{array}$$

$$HOOCCH_2CHOHCOOH$$

(6) **Pyruvate carboxylase** is an enzyme found in mitochondria which catalyses the reaction to oxaloacetic acid.

$$CH_3COCOOH + CO_2$$

$$\downarrow$$

$$HOOCCH_2COCOOH$$

It contains biotin as prosthetic group and, as with acetyl-CoA carboxylase, ATP has to be used to activate the CO_2 before it can be used. The reaction, therefore, goes only from left to right, as written, and not in the reverse direction, as might be expected.

Pyruvate carboxylase is active only in the presence of acetyl CoA although this compound is not used in the reaction. It appears that this requirement for activity could be a very important control mechanism regulating the oxaloacetate concentration in the mitochondria, and hence their ability to oxidize acetyl groups.

(7) **Phosphoenolpyruvic acid carboxylase,** the last enzyme of this group, does not involve pyruvate directly but converts oxaloacetate to phosphoenolpyruvate. Guanosine triphosphate (GTP), an energy rich compound, is involved.

$$HOOCCH_2COCOOH$$

$$\downarrow \begin{array}{l} \text{GTP} \\ \text{GDP} \end{array}$$

$$CH_2CO\textcircled{P}COOH + CO_2$$

The enzyme is found in the cytoplasm and is thought to be very important in enabling hexoses to be formed from non-carbohydrate precursors. It permits the pyruvate kinase reaction to be by-passed and hence carbohydrate to be formed from amino acids and lactate.

Although we are concerned here with the metabolism of carbohydrates, it is worth pointing out that the citric acid cycle alone will not catalyse the complete oxidation of the carbon skeleton of amino acids, because it contains no mechanism for converting the 4-carbon acids to acetyl groups. It is the latter which are actually completely oxidized in the cycle. The citric acid cycle (fig. 9.10) provides a mechanism, when taken together with reactions 5 or 6, and 7 of fig. 9.8, for the complete oxidation of amino acids as well as for their partial conversion to carbohydrate, since the carbon skeletons of the glucogenic amino acids can be converted either to pyruvate, or to a member of the citric acid cycle, and hence to oxaloacetate or malate.

This fact is important in **gluconeogenesis,** since carbon

skeletons of many amino acids are the most important non-carbohydrate precursors of glucose molecules. If the pyruvate kinase barrier is passed, fructose diphosphate can relatively easily be formed from phosphoenol pyruvate, provided the ATP and $NADH_2$ levels in the cytoplasm are sufficiently high to force the reversal of the triose phosphate dehydrogenase step. The phosphorylations which produce FDP (and G-6-P) are on energetic grounds not reversible, however, and fructose-6-phosphate (and free glucose) can be formed only by 'by-pass' reactions. In some tissues there exists **fructose diphosphatase** which can catalyse the reaction:

$$FDP \longrightarrow F\text{-}6\text{-}P + P$$

Fructose diphosphatase is allosterically inhibited by AMP, thus it is only active when the ATP concentration in the cell is high (p. 14.18). In these conditions phosphofructokinase is inhibited and thus, in liver, either glycolysis or gluconeogenesis is favoured, but not both together.

In liver, and also to a small extent in kidney, there exists a specific **glucose-6-phosphatase**.

The liver is thus, in effect, the only organ which can form free glucose, either from glycogen or from small molecule precursors. This is a very important function of this organ, since there is a continual uptake of glucose from the blood by many organs, notably the brain, which cannot readily utilize other sources of energy. In man, if the blood glucose level falls below a certain limit, whether or not carbohydrate is being taken in from the gut, dysfunction of the central nervous system, which can be fatal, ensues.

Pasteur effect

A phenomenon which is very widely observed in both animal tissues and micro-organisms was first pointed out by Pasteur. If the conditions are made wholly or partially anaerobic, as by restricting the O_2 supply, there is not only an increase in the rate of production of lactic acid (or of ethanol, by yeasts) but also an increase in the rate of utilization of glucose or of glycogen. The rates fall to their normal level again on the re-admission of air.

The value of this phenomenon is quite clear. The major part of the ATP synthesis in most cells is a product of the oxidative reactions going on in mitochondria. If these stop because of lack of oxygen, the corresponding ATP output ceases too. Nevertheless, the cell's demand for ATP may be unchanged or even increased. Glycolysis does produce some ATP, as already described, and it is the only kind of metabolism which can continue in the absence of an adequate supply of oxygen, because of the self-contained reduction of pyruvate to lactate (or acetaldehyde to ethanol in yeast). One might therefore expect, in theory, the aerobic rate of utilization of glucose to be increased nineteenfold when the oxygen source is removed, since this is the ratio of ATP produced

aerobically to anaerobically per mole of glucose. In practice, the ratio does not increase beyond five, so some cell functions must be starved of energy.

The anaerobic breakdown of glucose is not in itself inefficient, since most of the free energy of the glucose is still present in the lactic acid. The latter must, however, be disposed of; in animals it is usually reoxidized to pyruvate in the liver when aerobic conditions return.

It is of considerable interest to find out the mechanism of the Pasteur effect, in terms of enzymology, since this would provide insight into the control of cell metabolism in general. In a linear sequence of enzyme reactions which are more or less reversible, the rate of each is controlled by the rate of substrate supply from its predecessors and the rate of product removal by its successor. There needs to be only one rate-limiting or pace-making reaction, not necessarily the first. Application of this idea to the Embden–Meyerhof pathway is complicated by the fact that there are three reactions generally thought of as irreversible, those catalysed by hexokinase, phosphofructokinase and pyruvate kinase, and one which is reversible only with difficulty, the oxidation of glyceraldehyde phosphate. It is difficult to see how the rate of earlier reactions can be controlled by later ones in the sequence.

The breakdown of glycogen in anaerobic conditions can readily be explained in terms of the known properties of enzymes. Phosphorylase *b* is rapidly reactivated to phosphorylase *a*, and muscle phosphorylase b is in any case active in the presence of AMP (see below). This leads to a greater rate of formation of hexose phosphates. Phosphofructokinase will be activated by a slight fall in the concentration of ATP, a rise in the concentration of AMP, and an increase in concentration of F-6-P. It is at this point appropriate to explain why a rise in concentration of AMP is to be expected. An enzyme known originally as Lohmann's enzyme, or myokinase, and now known as **adenylate kinase**, is present in most tissues and is very active. It catalyses the reaction:

$$ATP + AMP \underset{\longleftarrow}{\overset{\longrightarrow}{\rightleftharpoons}} 2\ ADP$$

In anaerobic circumstances, when the concentration of ADP might originally start to rise and of ATP to fall, because of the cessation of oxidative phosphorylation, adenylate kinase, working from right to left of the equation given above, rapidly reforms ATP, and the net result is an increase in AMP concentration in the tissue, and, for a short time at least, little change in ATP or ADP levels. Changes of this kind have been observed to occur within a few seconds of stopping the blood flow to the liver.

The rate of the triose phosphate dehydrogenase reaction increases largely because of increased concentrations of the substrate, rather than of the co-factors ADP and P_i. The over-riding requirement is that NAD should continuously be supplied, and this can happen because the $NADH_2$ produced in the oxidation of glyceraldehyde phosphate is re-oxidized by the reduction of pyruvate to lactate. All the other enzymes in the pathway respond to increased rates of production of their substrates, and the overall effect is an increase in the rate of production of lactate at the expense of glycogen.

It is more difficult to explain an increase in the rate of consumption of glucose by cells and tissues in anaerobic conditions, because there is no universal way in which hexokinase can be activated. We are forced to conclude that the rate of utilization of glucose is controlled by the rate at which it permeates the cell membrane, without being able at present to specify how the latter might be affected by changes in Po_2 or demands for ATP.

Glycerol phosphate

Glycerol phosphate is necessary for the formation of tri-glycerides and phospholipids, and it can be made from carbohydrate by a dehydrogenase which catalyses the reaction:

$$
\begin{array}{ccc}
CH_2OH & & CH_2OH \\
| & & | \\
CO & +NADH_2 \rightleftharpoons & HOCH \quad +NAD \\
| & & | \\
CH_2O\textcircled{P} & & CH_2O\textcircled{P} \\
DHAP & & \text{3-}sn\text{-glycerol phosphate}
\end{array}
$$

Glycerol phosphate unlike DHAP is optically active and *sn* is an abbreviation for stereospecific numbering. By convention when the molecule is displayed with the —OH to the left, as above, the backbone is numbered from 1 to 3 starting at the top. Only 3-*sn*-glycerol phosphate is metabolically active.

The system GAP/DHAP is also a possible candidate for the transfer of reducing equivalents to or from mitochondria and cytoplasm, but in general the levels of the two enzymes are too low in animal tissues for this to be very effective.

Citric acid cycle

The complete oxidation of carbohydrate and indeed also of fats and amino acids is accomplished by means of a cyclic sequence of enzymic reactions, whose substrates and products are present only in catalytic quantities within the cell. This sequence is commonly known as the citric acid cycle, but sometimes as the tricarboxylic acid or Krebs cycle.

We have already seen that pyruvate, the sole end product of the catabolism of glucose, can be oxidized to acetyl CoA ($CH_3CO.SCoA$), and CO_2. In chap. 10, it is also shown that the long-chain fatty acids, the most important constituents of fats, are oxidized to

acetyl CoA by means of the β-oxidation cycle. Since these two nutrients, glucose and fatty acids, provide between them over 85 per cent of the energy intake in almost all diets, the further fate of acetyl CoA is clearly of considerable interest. Although the acetyl residue can be used for a number of syntheses, it is mostly oxidized by way of the citric acid cycle to provide energy for tissue functions.

Acetyl CoA reacts with oxaloacetic acid to produce citric acid; free CoA is also released.

$$
\begin{array}{ccc}
CH_3CO.SCoA & & CH_2COOH + HSCoA \\
+ & & | \\
COCOOH & \longrightarrow & HOCCOOH \\
| & & | \\
CH_2COOH & & CH_2COOH \\
\text{Oxaloacetic acid} & & \text{Citric acid}
\end{array}
$$

The enzyme which catalyses this reaction is **citrate synthase**. It is inhibited by ATP.

Citric acid is converted into *iso*-citric acid by the action of the enzyme **aconitase**:

$$
\begin{array}{ccc}
CH_2COOH & & CH_2COOH \\
| & & | \\
HOCCOOH & \longrightarrow & CCOOH \\
| & & \| \\
CH_2COOH & & CHCOOH \\
\text{Citric acid} & & \textit{Cis}\text{-aconitic acid}
\end{array}
$$

$$
\begin{array}{c}
\downarrow \\
CH_2COOH \\
| \\
HCCOOH \\
| \\
HOCHCOOH \\
\textit{Iso}\text{-citric acid}
\end{array}
$$

Iso-citric acid is oxidized by two enzymes, one specific for NAD and occurring in mitochondria, and the other specific for NADP and found in cytoplasm. The product is extremely unstable and decomposes spontaneously, especially in the presence of *iso*-citric dehydrogenase, to give 2-oxoglutaric acid and CO_2. The reaction catalysed by the NAD-linked enzyme is not reversible.

$$
\begin{array}{ccc}
CH_2COOH & \quad NAD \quad\quad NADH_2 \quad & CH_2COOH \\
| & & | \\
HCCOOH & \longrightarrow & CH_2 \\
| & \quad CO_2 \quad & | \\
HOCHCOOH & & COCOOH \\
\textit{Iso}\text{-citric acid} & & \text{2-Oxoglutaric acid}
\end{array}
$$

The oxidation of 2-oxoglutaric acid which follows proceeds by a mechanism similar to that by which pyruvic acid is oxidized (p. 9.12). The enzyme contains thiamine pyrophosphate as a prosthetic group and a CoA derivative, succinyl CoA, is the product. The latter is

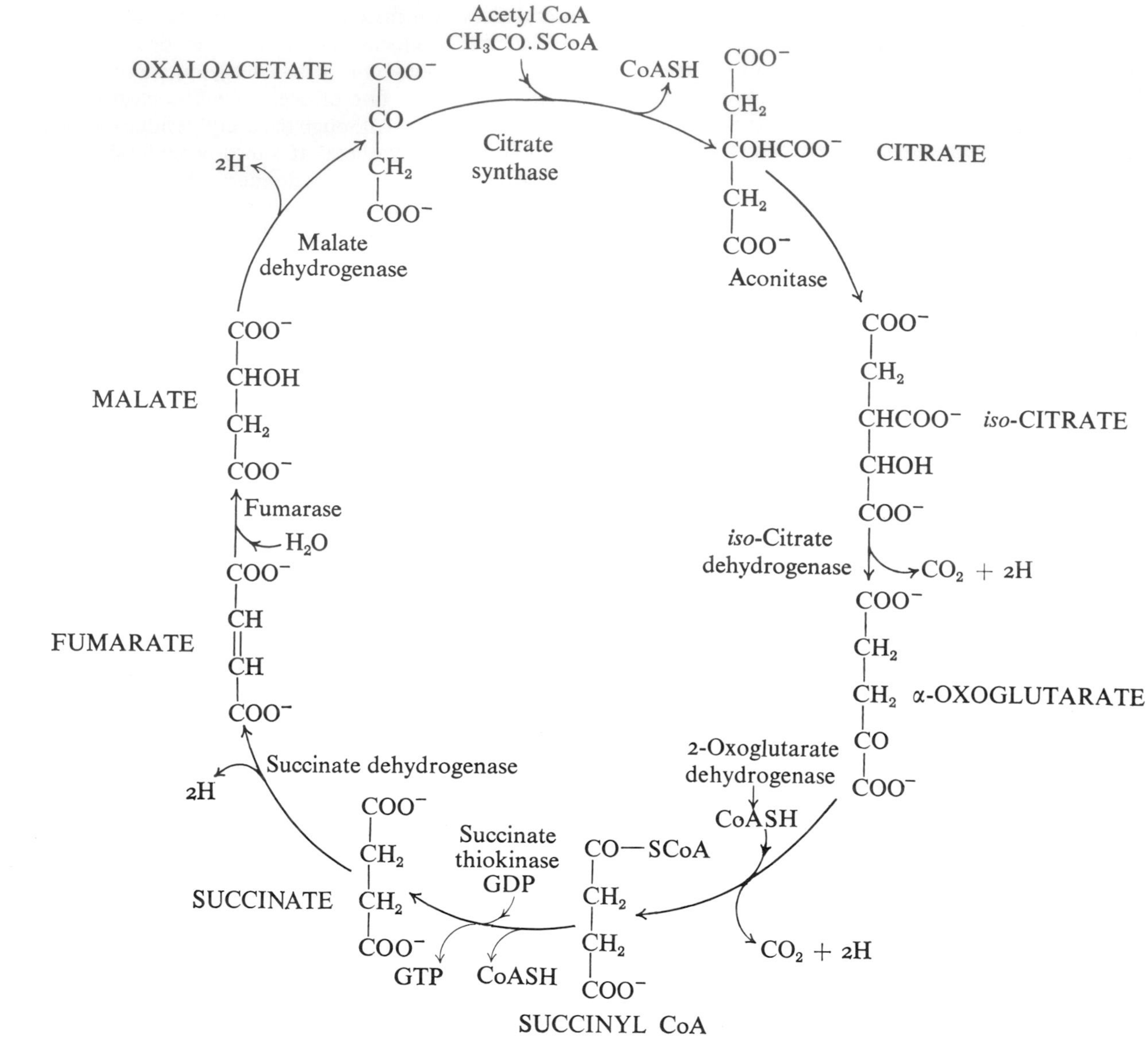

Fig. 9.10. The citric acid cycle.

immediately converted to free succinic acid by the following reaction:

$$
\begin{array}{ll}
\text{CO.SCoA} & \text{COOH} \\
| & | \\
\text{CH}_2 \quad +\text{GDP}+\text{P}_i \rightleftharpoons \text{CH}_2 \quad +\text{GTP}+\text{CoASH} \\
| & | \\
\text{CH}_2 & \text{CH} \\
| & | \\
\text{COOH} & \text{COOH} \\
\text{Succinyl CoA} & \text{Succinic acid}
\end{array}
$$

Notice that the free energy of the succinyl CoA thio-ester link is preserved by the formation of a high-energy bond in guanosine triphosphate (GTP).

Succinic acid is oxidized to fumaric acid by **succinic dehydrogenase**, which contains an atypical flavin as a prosthetic group.

$$HOOCCH_2\,CH_2\,COOH$$
$$\downarrow$$
$$HOOCCH{=}CHCOOH + 2H$$

Fumaric acid is converted to malic acid by the addition of a molecule of water, catalysed by **fumarase.**

$$HOOCCH{=}CHCOOH + H_2O$$
$$\downarrow$$
$$HOOCCH_2\,CHOHCOOH$$

Finally, malic acid is oxidized to oxaloacetic acid to complete the cycle:

$$HOOCCH\,CH_2\,CHOHCOOH + NAD$$
$$\downarrow$$
$$HOOCCH_2\,COCOOH + NADH_2$$

The net result of this cyclic process, set out in schematic form in fig. 9.10, is the oxidation of the acetyl group $CH_3CO—$, to two molecules of CO_2 and four sets each of two electrons and two H^+ (2H). In the cycle three $NADH_2$ and one FpH_2 are formed. More hydrogen appears here than in the original $CH_3CO—$ radical because two molecules of H_2O are consumed, one in the formation of citrate and one in the formation of malate.

ELECTRON TRANSPORT REACTIONS

The oxidation of these reduced co-factors is carried out by a complex sequence of enzymes. The enzymes of the citric acid cycle, with the exception of special forms of *iso*citric and malic dehydrogenases, are in mitochondria to which the electron transport chain is confined. The substrate oxidizing and co-factor oxidizing enzymes are co-ordinated in a way that allows the efficient trapping of the energy yielded by the oxidations.

The probable sequence of reactions in the oxidation of mitochondrial $NADH_2$ is shown in fig. 9.11. The precise nature of the flavoprotein coupling $NADH_2$ to the cytochromes has not been elucidated, and there is some disagreement about the relative positions of cytochrome b and ubiquinone (p. 8.7). Cytochromes a and a_3 have been distinguished spectrophotometrically, but as cytochrome oxidase is a complex enzyme it is quite possible that the two different haem groups are attached to the same lipoprotein.

The linkage between Fp redox steps and the cytochromes, each prosthetic group of which can accept only one electron, is by means of the —SH and Fe groups shown in fig. 9.11. These are probably not separate prosthetic groups; the —SH groups at least are part of the appropriate flavoproteins, and it has long been known that these enzymes are accompanied by non-haem iron.

Succinate is oxidized directly by a flavoprotein, and the electrons from this arrive in the main chain at the level of cytochrome b–ubiquinone. This can be shown by the use of poisons, e.g. certain barbiturates, which block the oxidation of $NADH_2$, but not of succinate. Antimycin A, on the other hand, blocks the oxidation of cytochrome b, and inhibits the oxidation of both $NADH_2$ and succinate.

The oxidation of fatty acids also takes place in mitochondria, and the flavoprotein acyl CoA dehydrogenases are said to be re-oxidized by an electron-transferring factor which links to the main chain at the level of cytochrome c.

Mitochondria freshly prepared from tissues do not oxidize added $NADH_2$, and it is not known how cytoplasmic $NADH_2$ is re-oxidized. A 'shuttle', i.e. the reduction in the cytoplasm by $NADH_2$ of a compound, the reduced form of which can enter the mitochondria and there be re-oxidized, is one possible solution of this difficulty. A number of possible shuttle redox pairs of this type have been proposed.

Energetics of intermediary metabolism

As discussed in chap. 8 the oxidation of one mole of $NADH_2$ by molecular oxygen leads to a decrease in free energy of about 210 kJ. This energy does not all appear as heat, but the oxidation is accompanied by the synthesis of 3 moles of ATP per mole of $NADH_2$. If succinate is used as a substrate, rather than a compound which produces $NADH_2$, the ratio of ATP formed to each pair of electrons transferred (the P/O ratio) approaches 2 rather than 3. From this it is clear that one ATP is synthesized during the transfer of two electrons from $NADH_2$ to cytochrome b, and two ATP are synthesized during the transfer of two electrons from cytochrome b to oxygen.

The complete oxidation of one mole of glucose to CO_2 and H_2O yields 2870 kJ. The oxidation of glycogen yields a little more energy from the splitting of the glycosidic bond. Table 9.2 shows the free energy still available at various stages of the process, and makes it clear how much of the total energy is released during the oxidation of acetyl CoA (about 60 per cent of the total). For lactate $\triangle G^0$ is 2720 for complete oxidation to CO_2 and H_2O. For the conversion of glucose to lactate $\triangle G^0 = -150$ which is only about 5 per cent of the total energy which can be made available by the complete oxidation of

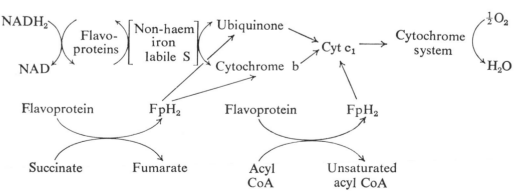

FIG. 9.11. Sequence of reaction in the oxidation of mitochondrial $NADH_2$.

glucose. There is a close correlation between the amount of $NADH_2$ formed and the free energy released. In the oxidation of carbohydrate almost all the energy is transferred to NAD, producing $NADH_2$. Subsequently this energy is released in the re-oxidation to NAD.

Since the amount of ATP formed during intramito-chondrial oxidation of $NADH_2$ is known from direct measurement, and the stages at which substrate level phosphorylation occur are also known, it is possible to estimate both the moles of ATP formed per mole of carbo-

TABLE 9.2. Free energy available during intermediary metabolism.

	Free energy of oxidation to CO_2 and H_2O (kJ/mol)		NAD reduced (mol)
	$-\triangle G^0$ to CO_2	Partial $-\triangle G^0$	
Glucose	2870		
		150	0
2 Lactate	2720		
		360	2
2 Pyruvate	2360		
		553	2
2 Acetyl CoA	1807		
		1807	6 (and 2 flavoprotein directly)
$4CO_2 + 4H_2O$	0		

hydrate oxidized, and the efficiency with which energy is 'trapped' as chemical energy useful to the cell during the oxidation (fig. 9.12).

Since the free energy of hydrolysis of ATP is about 33 kJ, the breakdown of one mole of glucose with the formation of 38 moles of ATP has an efficiency of $33 \times 38/2870$ or just over 40 per cent. However efficiencies may be very different because the net ATP yield is:

from glucose to 2 pyruvate	+ 8 ATP
from glucose to 2 lactate	+ 2 ATP
from glycogen to 2 lactate	+ 3 ATP
from 2 pyruvate to CO_2 and H_2O	+30 ATP
from glucose to CO_2 and H_2O	+38 ATP

The figures indicate the order of magnitude of energy trapping through ATP and stress the dominant role of mitochondrial oxidations in the provision of energy for cellular functions.

FURTHER READING

DICKENS F., RANDLE P.J. & WHELAN W.J. eds. (1968) *Carbohydrate Metabolism and its Disorders*, vols. I & II. New York: Academic Press.

LEHNINGER A.L. (1971) *Bioenergetics*, 2nd Edition. New York: Benjamin.

PIGMAN W. & HORTON D. eds. (1970–72) *The Carbohydrates*, vols. I & II. New York: Academic Press.

RACKER E. (1965) *Mechanisms in Bioenergetics*. New York: Academic Press.

Scientific American Offprints No. 36, 41, 69 & 91. San Francisco: W.H. Freeman.

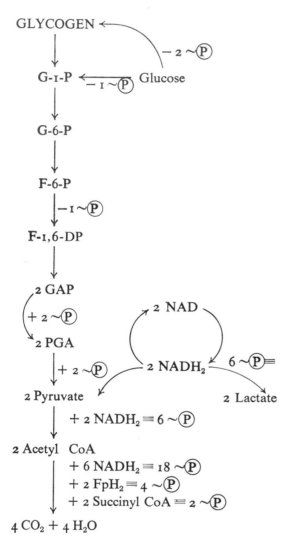

FIG. 9.12. Formation of ATP.

Chapter 10
Lipid metabolism

Some account of the importance of fat in the diet has already been given (p. 5.2). This chapter is concerned with the metabolism of fats in the body, where they are of the utmost importance in providing a compact store of fuel, which can be rapidly mobilized when needed. The housewife knows well what she means when she uses the word fat, but she includes a number of different types of chemical substances which collectively biochemists call **lipids**. They are all characterized by being soluble in fat solvents such as chloroform or ether, but almost insoluble in water. Although all lipids share this property, they possess a wide variety of chemical structures, physicochemical properties and metabolic characteristics. Lipids may be divided into five classes:

(1) fatty acids,
(2) triglycerides,
(3) phospholipids and glycolipids,
(4) cholesterol and its derivatives,
(5) complex lipids, such as sphingolipids and vitamins A, D, E and K.

CHEMISTRY OF SIMPLE LIPIDS

Fatty acids

These are monocarboxylic acids, homologues of acetic acid with longer, almost invariably unbranched chains. Only about eighteen are found in significant amounts in mammalian tissues and these are shown in table 10.1. All the important acids have an even number of carbon atoms which are referred to by numbers or by Greek letters, as follows:

$$\underset{\omega}{\overset{16}{CH_3}}(CH_2)_{11}\underset{\gamma}{\overset{4}{CH_2}}\underset{\beta}{\overset{3}{CH_2}}\underset{\alpha}{\overset{2}{CH_2}}\overset{1}{COOH}$$

The carbon atom furthest from the carboxyl group is called the ω carbon atom, regardless of the length of the fatty acid chain. In addition an acid is described as mono-, di-, tri or polyenoic depending on whether it has one, two, three or more double bonds. The shorthand designation for linolenic acid with eighteen carbon atoms and three double bonds is $C_{18:3}$, or in more detail $C_{18:3}\triangle^{9,12,15}$ which indicates the positions of the double bonds in the chain. There are two geometrically isomeric configurations

at each double bond. The naturally occurring unsaturated fatty acids are all *cis* form with the molecules bent back at the double bond. Thus they cannot pack as closely together as saturated chains or those in the *trans* form:

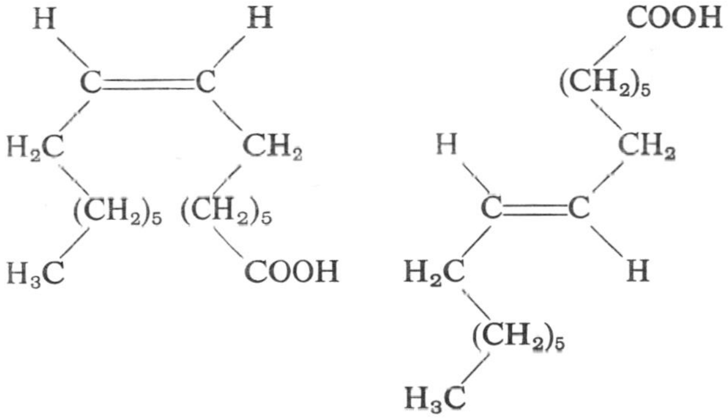

Cis: natural form   *Trans:* not found in nature

TABLE 10.1. Structure of fatty acids of biological importance.

Molecular formula	Common name	Systematic name
Saturated acids		
$C_4H_8O_2$	Butyric	n-Butanoic
$C_6H_{12}O_2$	Caproic	n-Hexanoic
$C_{10}H_{20}O_2$	Capric	Decanoic
$C_{12}H_{24}O_2$	Lauric	Dodecanoic
$C_{14}H_{28}O_2$	Myristic	Tetradecanoic
$C_{16}H_{32}O_2$	Palmitic	Hexadecanoic
$C_{18}H_{36}O_2$	Stearic	Octadecanoic
$C_{20}H_{40}O_2$	Arachidic	Eicosadecanoic
$C_{24}H_{48}O_2$	Lignoceric	Tetracosanoic
Unsaturated acids		
$C_{16}H_{30}O_2$	Palmitoleic	Hexadec-9-enoic
$C_{18}H_{34}O_2$	Oleic	Octadec-9-enoic
$C_{22}H_{42}O_2$	Erucic	Docos-13-enoic
$C_{24}H_{46}O_2$	Nervonic	Tetracos-15-enoic
$C_{18}H_{32}O_2$	Linoleic	Octadeca-9,12-dienoic
$C_{18}H_{30}O_2$	Linolenic	Octadeca-9,12,15-trienoic
$C_{20}H_{32}O_2$	Arachidonic	Eicosa-5,8,11,14-tetraenoic
Hydroxy acids		
$C_{24}H_{48}O_3$	Cerebronic	α-HO-Tetracosanoic
$C_{24}H_{46}O_3$	α-HO-Nervonic	α-HO-Tetracos-15-enoic

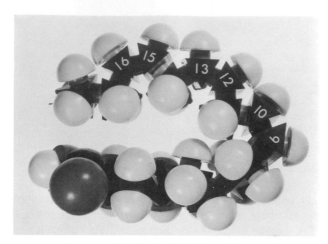

FIG. 10.1. Model of a linolenic acid molecule.

When multiple double bonds are present in natural fatty acids, the double and single bonds do not alternate and are therefore not conjugated. A model of the linolenic acid molecule is illustrated in fig. 10.1.

Because butyric acid has a short chain, it is slightly soluble in water (pK 4·76). Acids with longer chains are almost insoluble in water and have much higher pK values. All fatty acids form esters with alcohols:

$$RCOOH + R'OH \rightleftharpoons RCOOR' + H_2O$$

They also form salts with alkalis; these are the familiar soaps of commerce. The detergent properties of soaps are due to their ability to form a stable emulsion in water and the emulsion dissolves oily material in its fatty chains.

The melting point of a fatty acid of a given chain length decreases with the increase in the number of double bonds. Thus oleic, linoleic and linolenic acids are oils, liquid at room temperature, unlike stearic and palmitic acids. The degree of unsaturation of a sample of fatty acids may be defined by the iodine number. This is the amount of iodine taken up by unit weight of the material:

$$\underset{\substack{| \quad | \\ H \quad H}}{R-C=C-COOH} \xrightarrow{I_2} \underset{\substack{| \quad | \\ I \quad I}}{\overset{\substack{H \quad H \\ | \quad |}}{R-C-C-COOH}}$$

Saturated acids are formed commercially in some margarines by hydrogenating unsaturated fatty acids using metallic catalysts. In this way the more unsaturated vegetable oils are altered to resemble animal fats. Unsaturated fatty acid chains tend to become oxidized in air, yielding unstable products, probably peroxides, which decompose to keto and hydroxy acids; these have a characteristic rancid smell.

The nature and proportion of each fatty acid in a mixture can be determined by gas liquid chromatography. In this method the acids are converted to their more volatile methyl esters and a sample (a few μg only) of

the mixture is swept by a stream of inert gas at elevated temperature over a liquid such as a silicone oil spread on an inert solid. The components of the vapour partition between the gas and liquid phases as they pass along the tube, the more volatile and shorter chain esters emerging before the longer chain esters. By recording the presence of an ester in the effluent gas and the retention time, the relative amounts of each component may be compared with those of standard fatty acid esters (fig. 10.2). Since for each series of saturated, mono-, di- and

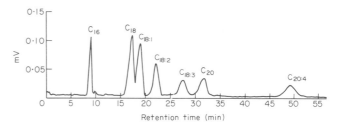

FIG. 10.2. Separation of a mixture of fatty and methyl esters on a column of silicone oil.

trienoic acids, the log of the retention time is proportional to the chain length, it is possible to determine the identity of an unknown fatty acid.

Triglycerides

Most of the dietary fat is composed of a mixture of triglycerides (TG). The three carbon atoms in the glycerol molecule are designated by numbers:

$$
\begin{array}{ll}
1 & CH_2OH \\
 & | \\
2 & CHOH \\
 & | \\
3 & CH_2OH
\end{array}
$$

These numbers replace α, β and α', formerly used and so familiar in some glycerol esters that their use may persist. In most natural TG molecules glycerol is esterified with 2 or 3 different fatty acids. A typical example is:

$$
\begin{array}{c}
\overset{O}{\overset{\|}{}} \\
H_2COC(CH_2)_{14}CH_3 \\
\overset{O}{\overset{\|}{}} \quad | \\
CH_3(CH_2)_7CH=CH(CH_2)_7COCH \\
| \quad \overset{O}{\overset{\|}{}} \\
H_2COC(CH_2)_{16}CH_3
\end{array}
$$

1-palmityl-2 oleyl-3-stearyl-*sn* glycerol

Fats used in the food industry may be of animal origin, e.g. lard, butter and fish liver oil, or of vegetable origin, e.g. soya, groundnut, maize (corn), cotton seed, sesame, coconut and olive oils. Since they are all triglycerides, the difference between them lies in the nature and

TABLE 10.2. Pattern of fatty acids in fats and oils (approximate percentage of total fatty acids).

	C_{4-12} saturated	$C_{14:0}$	$C_{16:0}$	$C_{18:0}$	$C_{16:1}$ + $C_{18:1}$	$C_{18:2}$	Other PUFA	Other FA
Butter, cream and milk	11	10	26	11	36	4	1†	—
Beef	—	3	29	21	44	2	—	—
Bacon and pork	—	1	26	12	50	10	—	—
Chicken	—	1	26	7	44	21	—	—
Fish oil	—	5	15	3	27	7	43*	—
Coconut oil	58	18	10	3	8	2	—	—
Palm oil	—	1	40	4	45	9	—	—
Cocoa butter	—	—	24	35	38	2	—	—
Rapeseed oil	—	—	3	1	16	14	9†	50‡
Olive oil	—	—	13	3	71	10	—	—
Groundnut oil	—	—	12	3	55	30	—	—
Sesame oil	—	—	9	5	40	43	—	—
Cottonseed oil	—	1	25	3	19	51	—	—
Corn (maize) oil	—	—	12	3	31	53	1	—
Soya bean oil	—	—	10	4	24	53	7†	—
Sunflower seed oil	—	—	7	4	25	63	—	—
Safflower seed oil	—	—	7	2	15	72	—	—
Margarine	3	10	23	9	31	7	1	5‡
Polyunsaturated margarine	2	1	12	8	22	52	1	—

* Long chain polyunsaturated fatty acids (C_{20} and C_{22}). † $C_{18:3}$ (linolenic). ‡ $C_{22:1}$ (erucic).

Note: The composition of all these fats and oils varies depending on methods of animal husbandry and crop production. In margarines the proportion of fats and oils for the blend depends on world market prices.

proportions of the particular fatty acids esterified to the glycerol moieties (table 10.2). Milk fats are exceptional in that 10 per cent of the fatty acids have short chains of four to twelve carbon atoms. Mammalian tissues, including human fat, contain predominantly C_{16} and C_{18} acids, some saturated and others unsaturated. Olive oil has $C_{18:1}$ as a major component and corn oil $C_{18:2}$. The high proportion of polyunsaturated fatty acids or PUFA, as they are called by nutritionists, in fish oils keeps them liquid at the temperature of sea water, whereas the solid fat, lard, has about 50 per cent of fatty acids $C_{16:0}$ and $C_{18:0}$. It must be emphasized that a fat such as butter is not a chemically pure substance consisting of millions of identical molecules, as is the case with a spoonful of cane sugar. It is a mixture of different triglyceride molecules. Thus a sample of human fat, in which the fatty acids are oleic acid (R_1) 50 per cent, palmitic acid (R_2) 23 per cent, linoleic acid (R_3) 10 per cent, stearic acid (R_4) 6 per cent and palmitoleic acid (R_5) 5 per cent, consists of many different molecules such as:

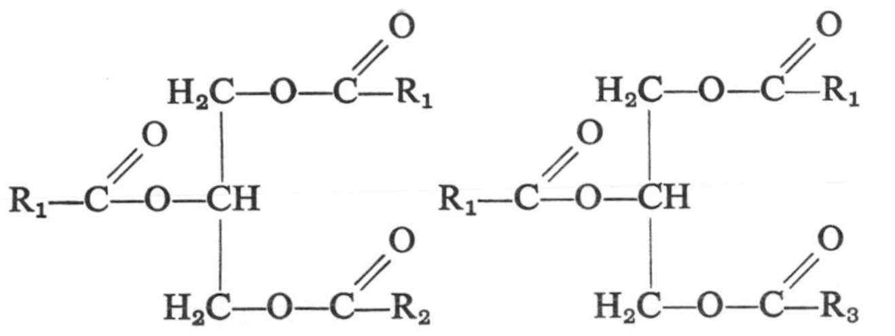

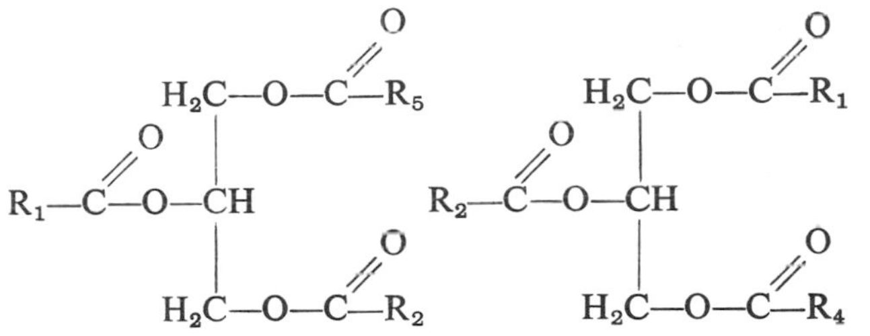

The glycerol portion may be esterified with any three of these five acids in any one of the three positions on the molecule.

The triglycerides can be separated by gas liquid chromatography without prior hydrolysis. Obviously saponification and subsequent analysis of the liberated fatty acids by gas liquid chromatography, which is easier to perform, gives an overall picture rather than information about the individual triglyceride molecules which are present. A molecule in which all three fatty acids are the same is very seldom encountered in nature and each usually contains at least one saturated and one unsaturated fatty acid.

Phospholipids

There are two main groups of phospholipids, the phosphatides and the sphingolipids. They all contain phosphorus and frequently nitrogen as well as carbon, hydrogen and oxygen. They are important constituents of biological membranes and are present in blood plasma.

Egg yolk is a rich source. The chemistry of the phosphatides is discussed here and that of the sphingolipids, which are more complex phospholipids, on p. 10.16.

PHOSPHATIDES

These are derived from L-**phosphatidic acid** and have the general formula:

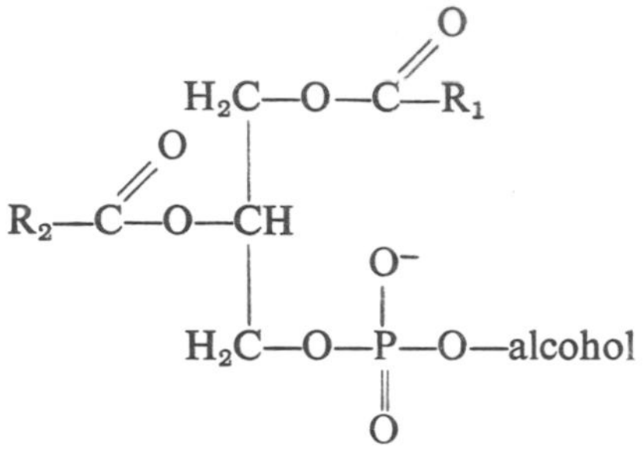

$$H_2C-O-\overset{\displaystyle O}{\overset{\|}{C}}-R_1$$
$$R_2-\overset{\displaystyle O}{\overset{\|}{C}}-O-CH$$
$$H_2C-O-\overset{O^-}{\underset{\|}{\overset{|}{P}}}-O-alcohol$$

Position 3 on the glycerol molecule is esterified by phosphoric acid and the other two by fatty acids. The hydroxyl group on the phosphate is also esterified by one of the following alcohols:

Choline $\quad HO-CH_2CH_2\overset{+}{N}(CH_3)_3$
Ethanolamine $\quad HO-CH_2CH_2NH_2$
Serine $\quad HO-CH_2CHNH_2COOH$

Inositol

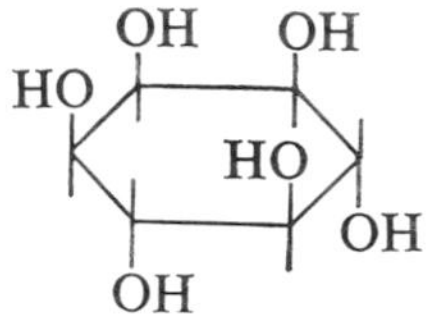

Glycerol $\quad HOCH_2CHOHCH_2OH$
Phosphorylated inositol $\quad C_6H_6(OH)_4[OPO(OH)_2]_2$

There are thus a series of phosphatidyl esters, of which the best known, phosphatidyl choline or **lecithin,** is readily isolated from egg yolk.

The mitochondrial lipid in heart muscle contains **cardiolipin.** Unlike the other phospholipids it is not found in brain. The structure is given below; the esterified fatty acids are mainly polyenoic.

It can be seen that phospholipids, unlike triglycerides, are charged polar compounds. Since lecithin is neutral and the others show varying acidity, it is possible to separate the classes by adsorption chromatography on silicic acid columns. In general the fatty acids on the 2 position are unsaturated, while those on the 1 position are saturated. One or other of these may be absent, for example in the 1-acyl and 2-acylglyceryl phosphoryl cholines. These substances are called **lysolecithins** as they have the ability to lyse or break cell membranes. These lysophosphatides are not normally found in tissues in significant amounts and their physiological role is uncertain.

The **plasmalogens** have an unsaturated ether group, rather than an ester group, on position 1. Those of ethanolamine and choline form a big proportion of the phospholipids of brain and heart.

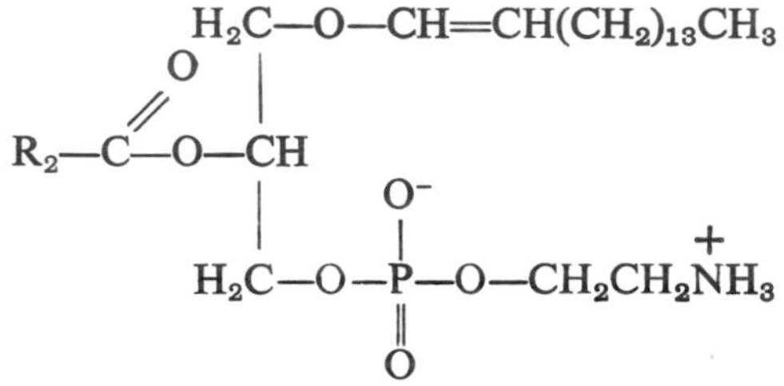

$$H_2C-O-CH{=}CH(CH_2)_{13}CH_3$$
$$R_2-\overset{\displaystyle O}{\overset{\|}{C}}-O-CH$$
$$H_2C-O-\overset{O^-}{\underset{\|}{\overset{|}{P}}}-O-CH_2CH_2\overset{+}{N}H_3$$

An ethanolamine plasmalogen

The suffix 'alogen' in their name is used since, on mild hydrolysis, they yield an aldehyde. In the compound shown, this would be $CH_3(CH_2)_{13}CHO$.

Cholesterol

The steroids form a large class of lipids, which includes the hormones of the adrenal cortex and sex glands, vitamin D and the bile acids. These substances are produced in the body from cholesterol which is widespread in nature and present in all normal diets in amounts up to 1 g daily. About 2 g more are synthesized daily in various

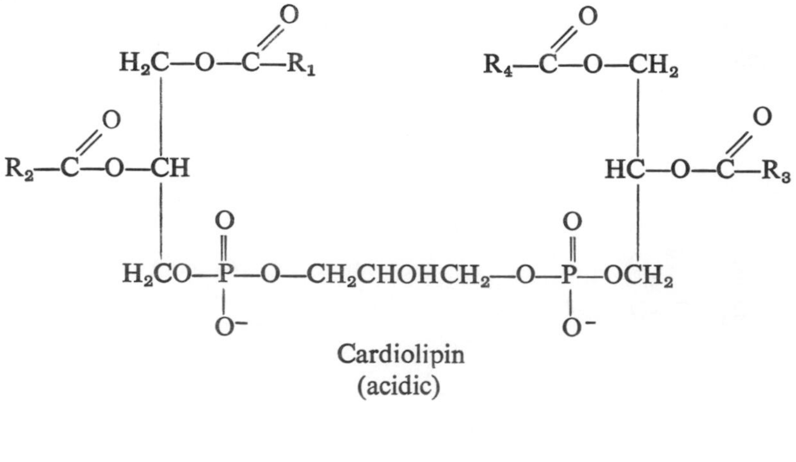

Cardiolipin
(acidic)

tissues, mainly in the liver. Cholesterol has the structural formula:

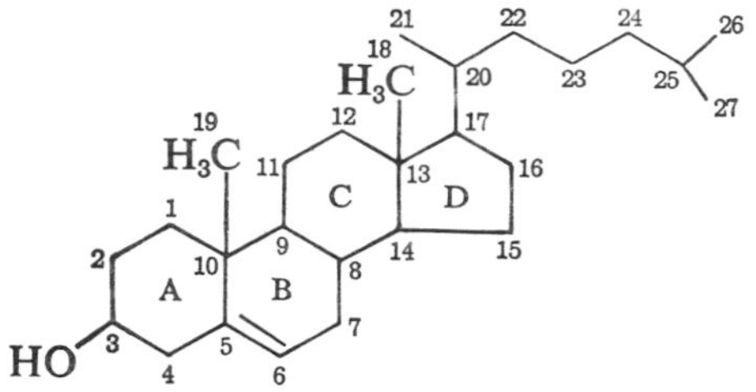

Many biological compounds have the same ring structure but with different substituents, especially at positions 3, 11 and 17.

The essential functions of cholesterol and related compounds at the molecular level are not precisely known. These are undoubtedly related to the shape and general configuration of the basic steroid structure, discussed on p. 10.21.

METABOLISM OF LIPIDS

Alimentary absorption

Adults on a normal Western diet absorb 100–120 g of lipid per day; most of this is triglyceride but there is also cholesterol and phospholipid. The ingested material enters the duodenum as a coarse emulsion. Here some of the fatty acids are split off the TG molecules by pancreatic lipase, and 2-monoglycerides and a little glycerol are liberated (p. 32.43).

Since the fatty acids and monoglycerides are not water-soluble, one might foresee difficulties in transporting them into the intestinal mucosal cells. This is overcome by the action of bile salts which combine with them to form aggregates or micelles. These particles are less than 0·5 μm in diameter, about one-hundredth the size of those in the original TG emulsion. They form a clear solution in water from which the fatty acids and glycerides can enter the villi of the mucosal cells, along with the glycerol and other water-soluble compounds. Within the cells the monoglycerides are then re-esterified by activated fatty acids. The resulting TG droplets are not identical with those ingested, since the dietary fatty acids change position on the glycerol molecule, and are mixed with those entering the mucosal cells from the blood. Some short chain acids with fewer than fourteen carbon atoms pass directly into the portal blood along with any free glycerol, due probably to their greater water solubility and rejection by the esterifying enzymes. The bile salts do not appear to enter the intestinal cells but pass into the ileum where they diffuse into the blood and recirculate to the liver. The cholesterol and phosphatidyl choline excreted in bile are also largely reabsorbed.

Dietary cholesterol esters are hydrolysed in the gut along with TG. The products pass into the intestinal epithelial cells where they mix with cholesterol formed endogenously and are almost all esterified. The acids used are mainly unsaturated, presumably selected from the fatty acid pool by the enzymes involved. Phospholipids are also formed within the intestinal cells.

The lipids accumulating in the cells pass out into the lymph in the form of **chylomicrons**. These are particles consisting mostly of TG with some cholesterol, phospholipid and protein in proportions which vary slightly and are indicated in table 10.3. Being 0·1–1 μm in diameter, they scatter light and so a suspension of chylomicrons appears milky. This is readily observed in lymph or plasma sampled 3 or 4 hours after a meal rich in fat.

Transport of lipids in the blood

The chylomicrons pass into the lymph, through the thoracic duct and into the blood in the great veins of the neck. Lipoproteins formed by the liver from endogenous TG are also transported in the plasma. Lipoproteins are macromolecules with a central core of TG surrounded by cholesterol and its esters, phospholipid, mainly phosphatidyl choline and sphingomyelin, and a little protein, the apoproteins. The phosphate groups of phospholipids are in contact with the aqueous phase and their charge may stabilize the colloid. Phospholipid in lipoproteins turns over more rapidly than the triglyceride portion. Lipoproteins may be looked upon as transporters which carry TG and cholesterol. In the tissues TG is unloaded for use and the transporter is returned for reloading, usually in the liver.

The three types of lipoprotein formed in the Golgi apparatus of the liver are designated α, pre-β and β from their mobility relative to the globulins during the electrophoresis of serum (p. 11.7). Each has its own structure and chemical composition, although in fact each consists of many lipid components. The apoprotein of α-lipoproteins appears to differ from that of the β-lipoproteins, judging from their amino acid content and their antigenicity. The structure of some of these apoproteins has been established. The β-apoprotein of low density lipoproteins (LDL) is a polymer of several units. It is also found in pre-β or very low density lipoproteins (VLDL) along with at least four other distinct peptides. The α- or high density lipoprotein (HDL) apoprotein may be two proteins each with constituent subunits. Some confirmation for this is obtained by studying patients with the rare disease abetalipoproteinaemia. They cannot synthesize the apoprotein for both β- and pre-β (LDL VLDL) and so cannot make chylomicrons. In another hereditary condition normal α- or HDL apoprotein is not formed (vol. 3, p. 47.15).

The apoproteins contain 3–4 per cent carbohydrate. They are formed in the liver and have a half-life (3–4 days) shorter than that of other plasma proteins.

TABLE 10.3. Lipoproteins in plasma.

Lipoprotein	Electrophoretic mobility	Density kg/l	Approximate normal concentrations g/l	Percentage composition (dry weight)			
				Protein and carbohydrate	TG	Total cholesterol	Phospholipid
Chylomicrons	None	<0·96	0–0·5	2	83	9	7
Very low density (VLDL)	pre-β	0·96–1·006	1·5	9	50	22	18
Low density (LDL)	β	1·006–1·063	4·0	21	10	47	22
High density (HDL)	α	>1·063	3·5	50	8	19	22

When the lipoproteins are considered in order of increasing density (table 10.3), it will be seen that the TG content falls, while that of the phospholipid and protein rises. It is possible to achieve a large scale separation of the different plasma lipoproteins by making stepwise additions of sodium bromide in order to raise the specific gravity to fixed values. The lipoproteins lighter than the density of the solution can then be centrifuged at high speeds to the top of the tube. In this way successive lipoprotein fractions of defined density can be obtained. It has not been common practice to determine plasma concentrations of lipoproteins. More convenient is the measurement of cholesterol and TG which, if the sample is taken in the fasting state, reflect concentrations of LDL and VLDL respectively (table 10.3). Table 10.4 shows the normal ranges for these and also for phospholipids, though the latter are seldom measured. Normally about 70 per cent of the cholesterol is esterified. When, in a fasting man, the TG level in the plasma falls to about 0.6 mmol/l (50 mg/100 ml), only about 30 per cent of the fatty acid present is in TG molecules. After a meal containing at least 30 g of fat, however, the quantity of TG rises and chylomicrons appear. The cholesterol and phospholipid concentrations remain virtually unchanged.

The lipoprotein content of the blood depends on the quantities of the different types of lipids to be transported, the availability of amino acids and phospholipids and on a normally functioning liver.

TABLE 10.4. The normal range of values of plasma lipids in healthy young fasting adults.

	mmol/l	mg/100 ml
Cholesterol	3·6–6·7	140–260
Triglyceride	0·6–1·8	50–150
Phospholipids	0·7–4·2	50–300

There are familial (hereditary) conditions in which plasma lipids are abnormally high These can be divided into five types (vol. 3, p. 47.15) on the basis of which plasma lipoproteins are raised, either singly or in combination. Types IIa, IIb and IV are important, the others being rare.

Type IIa hyperlipoproteinaemia is inherited as an autosomal dominant and presents in childhood or early adult life. Plasma concentrations of cholesterol and β-lipoproteins (LDL) are high. Deposits of lipids, xanthomata, occur in tendons, particularly the tendo calcaneus, in the skin mainly on extensor surfaces and in the eyelids. The lipid is mainly cholesterol taken up from plasma into cells of the mononuclear phagocytic system. From this it can be deduced that LDL is involved in cholesterol transport. It has also been observed that in the normal individual the rate of turnover of ^{14}C-cholesterol carried on HDL is greater than for cholesterol carried on LDL. Possibly HDL is required to carry cholesterol from the peripheral sites to the liver for conversion to bile salts and excretion. Those of lower density are necessary for the transport of triglycerides from the liver and intestinal mucosal cells. Tissues other than the liver remove ^{14}C-cholesterol from the plasma, though to a much smaller extent. The cholesterol esters of the HDL contain a larger proportion of arachidonic acid and other polyunsaturated essential fatty acids than do those in the low density fraction which resemble the liver cholesterol esters. High concentrations of plasma cholesterol fall if unsaturated vegetable oils are substituted in the diet for saturated fats. It seems probable that this effect is produced by changing the distribution of cholesterol between the plasma and cellular compartments of the body rather than by decreasing its rate of synthesis or increasing its rate of degradation.

Type IV hyperlipoproteinaemia is common and usually only detected in adult life. It is of great importance because it predisposes to atherosclerosis and ischaemic heart disease. In atherosclerosis there is deposition of lipid in the intima of arteries, but the mechanism by which this is brought about is uncertain (vol. 3, p. 17.7). Plasma TG and cholesterol concentrations are both raised. The rise in plasma TG is probably greater and perhaps more important, but the condition was first identified by the rise in plasma cholesterol about which far more is known. In prosperous communities, the mean value for plasma cholesterol increases with age. Values above 6.7 mmol/l (260 mg/100 ml) carry an increased risk of ischaemic heart disease. The increase begins in the third decade, but is not marked in the female population until after the menopause due to the protective action of female sex hormones. Other factors predisposing to a high plasma cholesterol are lack of exercise and the diet, which in prosperous countries is high in saturated fatty acid and sucrose. These may exaggerate the genetic tendency of some individuals to maintain a high plasma cholesterol level. It should be emphasized however that a direct cause and effect relationship between hypercholesterolaemia and atherosclerosis has not been proved (vol. 3, p. 17.14).

Plasma concentrations of TG are frequently high in patients with obesity and diabetes, and many such patients may have an abnormal metabolism of VLDL associated with impaired tolerance of dietary carbohydrate.

Breakdown of lipoprotein

Chylomicrons and VLDL are removed from the blood by adipose tissue and muscle (including heart muscle) through the action of an enzyme, **liprotein lipase** (LPL). In this way the plasma is 'cleared' of its milky appearance. The fatty acids which are split off the TG core by the enzyme enter the tissues. In adipose cells they are reformed into TG with 1-glycerophosphate derived from blood glucose. In muscle they are used directly for oxidation. The liberated glycerol and other components remain in the blood and return to the liver. The activity of plasma LPL is increased after a meal. It is decreased in fasting, but on the other hand the **TG lipase** present in adipose tissue has its activity increased by fasting and decreased by feeding. The function of the two enzymes is different. LPL is used to put triglycerides into the stores and is required only when there is already sufficient metabolic fuel (carbohydrate). The other lipase breaks down stored TG. The liberated free fatty acids then pass out of the adipose tissue, enter the circulation and are used by the tissues as a source of energy.

Electron microscopy shows chylomicrons to be sequestered on the walls of blood capillaries, possibly attached to LPL by HDL-apoprotein. The complex sulphated polysaccharide heparin also seems to be associated with the enzyme, perhaps by an allosteric effect promoting its binding with the substrate. During fasting the tissues show little LPL activity, and the enzyme appears to be within the adipose cell. However, feeding carbohydrate releases it to the capillary endothelium and the activity rises. An injection of heparin is able to discharge the enzyme into the blood, but normally the blood activity is very low. After an injection of heparin the activity of the enzyme in the plasma is increased. This is possibly due to activation of the enzyme but may also result from increased release from a storage site.

LPL activity may be controlled by the level of cyclic AMP within the tissues. Thus noradrenaline, adrenaline and growth hormone secreted during fasting increase cyclic AMP and decrease LPL, while the converse is true of insulin secreted when food has been taken. The decrease in plasma TG observed during exercise or when food is taken after fasting may be caused both by decreased release of lipoproteins from the liver and by enhanced uptake within the peripheral tissues.

The liver differs from other tissues in that lipoproteins are taken up directly without prior breakdown by lipase. Within the parenchymal cells they are disrupted, yielding oily drops of TG which may be subsequently hydrolysed. As labelled plasma free fatty acids (FFA) are not incorporated into plasma lipoproteins in hepatectomized animals, the probable site of lipoprotein formation is the liver. The fatty acid pattern of the lipoprotein-TG resembles less closely that of the recently ingested triglycerides than does that of the chylomicrons. This is because the liver fatty acids from which they are built up include those brought in as FFA from the adipose stores (laid down over a considerable period) and those formed endogenously by the liver. In the liver, FFA molecules are incorporated into TG molecules and also tailored by the lengthening and desaturation of their chains.

Drugs and plasma lipids

Extensive search has been made for drugs which reduce elevated plasma lipid concentrations. The most commonly used is clofibrate which lowers VLDL and to some extent LDL in hyperlipoprotinaemia. The active agent, chlorophenoxy*iso*butyrate, competes with other acids for binding sites on the plasma albumin. This may diminish the transport of FFA from adipose tissue (p. 34.5) and may possibly release bound thyroid hormone which would enhance the breakdown of lipids. It may also interfere with early steps in cholesterol synthesis and in the secretion of lipoproteins by the liver (vol. 2, p. 8.11).

Cholestyramine, a basic ion-exchange resin, increases the excretion of bile salts, leading to a decrease in LDL and plasma cholesterol (vol. 2, p. 10.12). However it is unable to affect Type IIb hyperlipoproteinaemia, characterized by high levels of TG (vol. 3 p. 47. 14).

Oxidation of fatty acids

Fatty acids on oxidation yield a large quantity of energy and in the form of TG function principally as an energy store. When they are required by the body, TG are broken down by lipases to yield glycerol and free fatty acids (FFA). Both products pass out of the fat storage cells into the blood stream, where the FFA are transported bound to plasma albumin, being thereby made soluble in water.

Isotopically labelled fatty acids injected into the blood are taken up by the liver, heart, kidney, muscle and other organs. There they may be reformed into TG and other lipids or oxidized within the mitochondria of the cells. To cross from the cytoplasm through the outer mitochondrial membranes for oxidation, the fatty acids must probably first be esterified with coenzyme A and then with carnitine; once inside, the carnitine is split off.

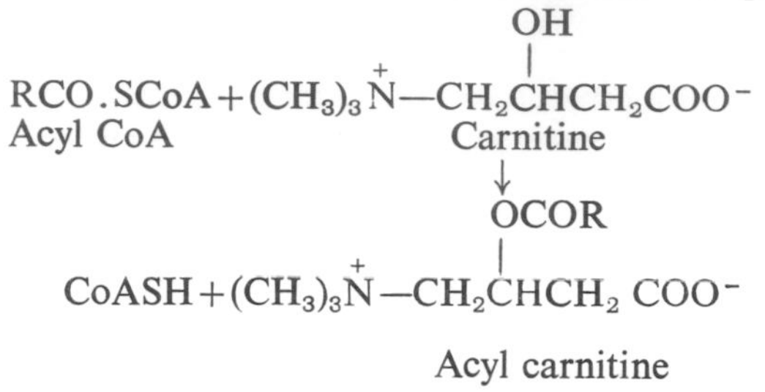

$$RCO . SCoA + (CH_3)_3 \overset{+}{N} \underset{\text{Carnitine}}{-CH_2 \overset{\overset{\displaystyle OH}{|}}{C} HCH_2 COO^-}$$
Acyl CoA

$$\downarrow$$

$$CoASH + (CH_3)_3 \overset{+}{N} \underset{\text{Acyl carnitine}}{-CH_2 \overset{\overset{\displaystyle OCOR}{|}}{C} HCH_2 \ COO^-}$$

The necessary transferase enzyme is more active when cytoplasmic FFA concentration is rising, as in starvation. At the same time glycolysis is inhibited and so entry of pyruvate into the mitochondria is reduced.

Four classes of enzymes, found in the mitochondria of liver and other tissues, break down fatty acid chains by stepwise removal of two carbon fragments. The removal of a fragment involves:

(1) activation by esterification with coenzyme A,
(2) oxidation at the 3 (or β) position,
(3) hydration,
(4) reoxidation, followed by
(5) liberation of acetyl CoA.

The chain is then shorter by two carbon atoms (fig. 10.3).

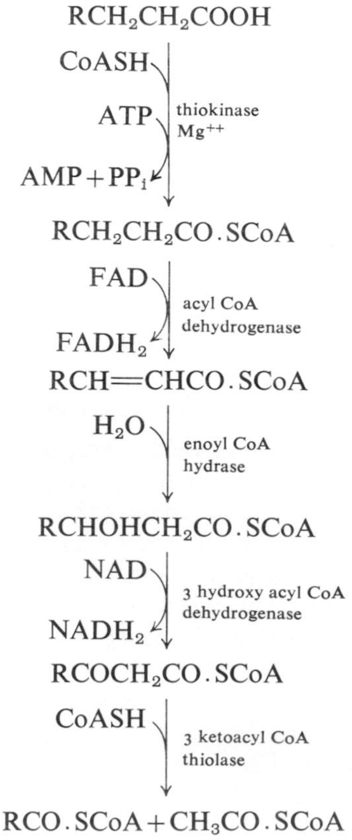

$$RCH_2CH_2COOH$$

CoASH

ATP ⎱ thiokinase
⎰ Mg^{++}

AMP + PP_i

$$RCH_2CH_2CO . SCoA$$

FAD ⎱ acyl CoA
⎰ dehydrogenase

$FADH_2$

$$RCH = CHCO . SCoA$$

H_2O ⎱ enoyl CoA
⎰ hydrase

$$RCHOHCH_2CO . SCoA$$

NAD ⎱ 3 hydroxy acyl CoA
⎰ dehydrogenase

$NADH_2$

$$RCOCH_2CO . SCoA$$

CoASH ⎱ 3 ketoacyl CoA
⎰ thiolase

$$RCO . SCoA + CH_3CO . SCoA$$

FIG. 10.3. β-oxidation of fatty acids.

Thus in a series of steps a C_{18} chain is broken down to nine acetyl CoA units. This is the β-oxidation pathway. When all the necessary enzymes are present, no fatty acids with C_4 to C_{14} chains or other intermediates can be isolated. Each step is apparently co-ordinated with the following one in such a way that the products do not accumulate but pass straight down through the reaction sequence to acetyl CoA. The polyunsaturated fatty acids, linoleic and arachidonic, are as rapidly oxidized as the saturated ones. The same route is used, but an isomerase is necessary to allow oxidation to pass beyond the original double bond.

For every two carbon atoms split off, one molecule of FAD and one of NAD is reduced (steps 2 and 4). These enter the respiratory chain for oxidation by the cytochromes and generate five ATP molecules. The liberated acetyl CoA molecules join the common pool, mixing with those formed by oxidation of pyruvate derived from glucose or amino acids. They may also be used to form fatty acids or cholesterol (p. 10.22). However, in the tissues of a fasted individual who has little carbohydrate available, most of the acetyl CoA present has been derived from fat and is used for energy production rather than for synthetic purposes.

The energy which may be obtained by the oxidation of one molecule of stearic acid ($C_{18:0}$) may be calculated as follows: (1) for each of the eight stages where an acetyl CoA molecule is formed five molecules of ATP are produced as described above; (2) each of the nine acetyl CoA units may enter the citric acid cycle and generate twelve ATP molecules on one revolution. Thus C_{18} acid forms $(8 \times 5) + (9 \times 12) = 148$ ATP molecules. This may be compared with three molecules of glucose (also eighteen carbon atoms) which can form $3 \times 39 = 117$ ATP molecules. As the heats of combustion of stearic acid and glucose are 39 and 15.5 kJ/g respectively, fat is a more concentrated store of chemical energy than carbohydrate. Taking the free energy of hydrolysis of ATP as 30 kJ/mol, the efficiency of conversion of energy from stearic acid to ATP is approximately $\dfrac{148 \times 30}{284 \times 39} = 40$ per cent. The corresponding figure for glucose is 42 per cent.

It has been observed that in brain tissue palmitic acid is oxidized *in vitro* more rapidly than palmityl CoA. This is contrary to the findings for other tissues and suggests that a different oxidative pathway is followed. A hint is given by the presence of odd numbered and 2-hydroxy fatty acids in the cerebrosides of the white matter. It appears that fatty acids in the brain are oxidized primarily to 2-hydroxy acids which are then decarboxylated to acids with one less carbon atom. This probably occurs through a series of oxidative steps including an enzyme-bound oxo-compound.

Liver microsomes and also certain bacteria can oxidize fatty acids of intermediate chain length at the final or ω

(or $\omega-1$) position. The process seems to involve oxygen, a haem-containing protein (cytochrome P_{450}), a flavoprotein and $NADPH_2$. The resulting ω-hydroxy compounds are further oxidized to the dicarboxylic acids which may be excreted or split by the β-oxidative pathway. The physiological importance of the ω-oxidation of fatty acids is not yet clear, but the mechanism is used in the hydroxylation of drugs.

Fatty acid synthesis

It is a common observation that the body appears to lay down fat when the diet is rich in carbohydrate. The conversion of carbohydrate into fat was demonstrated in 1853 by Lawes and Gilbert, the pioneers of agricultural chemistry. They showed that the carcasses of young pigs contained more than four times as much fat as had been present in their previous diet. In recent experiments performed *in vivo* and *in vitro* the labelled carbon atoms of ^{14}C-glucose have been traced to both the fatty acid and glycerol parts of the tissue TG molecules. Not unexpectedly, ^{14}C-acetate is also converted to fatty acids, suggesting that glucose may first be broken down to this two-carbon fragment before the long chains are built up. The action of the mitochondrial enzymes which oxidize fatty acids is not reversible and so these enzymes cannot form long chain fatty acids from acetate. As this synthesis occurs in the cell cytosol from which all the subcellular particles have been removed, a different system containing only soluble enzymes must be involved. A cytoplasmic enzyme preparation can synthesize fatty acids from acetyl CoA, if $NADPH_2$ and manganese are added. Much of the $NADPH_2$ is formed by the oxidation of glucose-6-phosphate in the hexose monophosphate pathway, which is normally active in tissues which are sites of fatty acid synthesis. When acetate is used as substrate, then ATP and CoA must also be supplied. When the unfractionated enzyme system is used palmitic acid is the only product which can be isolated. However, by using $^{14}CO_2$ and only one fraction of the enzyme mixture, the formation of malonyl CoA by the carboxylation of acetyl CoA can be demonstrated.

Fig. 10.4 shows how an isotopically labelled carbon atom can be followed through a series of reactions. The single enzyme involved is acetyl CoA carboxylase. The step which it catalyses appears to be the slowest or limiting one in the whole pathway from acetyl CoA to long chain fatty acid. As a consequence, it is a probable site for the operation of physiological controls. Biotin binds to the protein portion of acetyl CoA carboxylase to form the active enzyme, shown as biotin Ⓔ in fig. 10.4, which acts as a carrier of carbon dioxide.

When 1-[^{14}C]malonyl CoA is provided as substrate along with acetyl CoA, the resulting palmitic acid contains no ^{14}C. On the other hand, if 2-[^{14}C]malonyl CoA is used, the even carbon atoms 2–14 in the palmitic acid

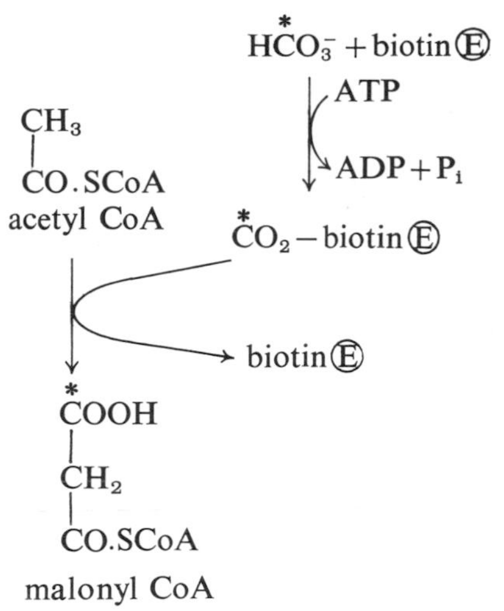

FIG. 10.4. The function of biotin in acetyl CoA carboxylase in the synthesis of malonyl CoA.

are labelled. This allows the system to be visualized overall as:

$$\text{Acetyl SCoA} + 7\ 1\text{-}[^{14}\text{C}]\text{malonyl SCoA} + 14\text{NADPH}_2$$
$$\longrightarrow CH_3(CH_2)_{14}COOH + 7^{14}CO_2 + 14NADP +$$
$$6H_2O + 8CoASH$$

Experimentally the quantity of $NADPH_2$ oxidized per mole of palmitic acid formed was found to be almost fourteen moles, or two for each two carbon residue added to the original acetyl group.

The multi-enzyme group, fatty acid synthase, which links on the malonyl groups and performs the remainder of the synthesis, has a molecular weight of many hundreds of thousands when isolated from mammalian tissue. It has still to be resolved into its constituent enzymes. However, when the bacterium, *Esch. coli*, was used rather than mammalian cells as source of the synthase, the various enzymes could be separated out, along with an 'acylcarrier' protein (ACP) of molecular weight about 10,000. The latter contained one —SH group as a 4-phosphopantotheine residue (p. 7.13). Its role may be as a carrier of the substrate molecules to the condensing enzyme. The activated malonyl group may then condense with the acetyl group on the carrier, yielding acetoacetyl-S-ACP, with release of a carbon atom as carbon dioxide:

$$\left. \begin{array}{l} \text{Acetyl SCoA} + \text{ACP-SH} \xrightarrow{\text{CoASH}} \text{acetyl S-ACP} \\ \text{Malonyl SCoA} + \text{ACP-SH} \xrightarrow{\text{CoASH}} \text{malonyl S-ACP} \end{array} \right\} \longrightarrow$$
$$CH_3COCH_2CO.S\text{-ACP} + CO_2 + \text{ACP-SH}$$

Subsequently the acetoacetyl S-ACP is reduced, using $NADPH_2$ as hydrogen donor, to D(-)3-hydroxybutyryl S-ACP, which has the configuration at the 3 carbon atom opposite to that of the corresponding intermediate in fatty acid oxidation. The product is then dehydrated and again reduced, to butyryl S-ACP, by a process involving $NADPH_2$ (fig. 10.5).

$$CH_3COCH_2CO.S\text{-}ACP$$

$$\downarrow \overset{NADPH_2}{\underset{NADP}{}}$$

$$D(-)CH_3CHOHCH_2CO.S\text{-}ACP$$

$$\downarrow H_2O$$

$$CH_3CH\!=\!CHCO.S\text{-}ACP$$

$$\downarrow \overset{NADPH_2}{\underset{NADP}{}}$$

$$CH_3CH_2CH_2CO.S\text{-}ACP$$

FIG. 10.5. Reduction of acetoacetyl-ACP in the synthesis of fatty acids.

The product is a saturated chain bound to the 'acyl carrier' protein and able to pick up another molecule of malonyl S-ACP. This leads to the formation of hexanoyl S-ACP with a 6C chain. The process can be continued until the 16C acyl S-ACP is reached. At this point, the palmitic acid is freed from the carrier protein.

A carrier protein of mammalian origin has not yet been isolated but the fatty acid synthase in mammals appears to resemble that in yeast, which has been extensively investigated. In this organism the various enzyme components required to perform the different steps of the synthesis have not yet been separated in an active state as they have been in *Esch. coli*, but evidence has been obtained for the presence in the multi-enzyme complex of two functional thiol groups. One, designated S′ below, binds the acyl group and the other, S″, part of 4-phosphopantotheine, binds the incoming malonyl group. The elongation and reduction steps are represented in fig 10.6.

$$R(CH_2CH_2)_nCO.S'\text{Ⓔ}S''COCH_2COOH$$

$$\downarrow CO_2$$

$$R(CH_2CH_2)_nCOCH_2CO.S''\text{Ⓔ}S'H$$

$$\downarrow \text{reductive steps}$$

$$R(CH_2CH_2)_{n+1}CO.S''\text{Ⓔ}S'H$$

FIG. 10.6. The role of thiol groups on a multi-enzyme complex in lengthening fatty acid chains.

The thiolase which finally removes the acyl chain from the enzyme complex has low activity when chains are less than C_{12} and is most active for C_{16}. This may be why the *de novo* synthesis of fatty acids stops with palmitic acid. The major difference between the bacterial enzyme system and that of the higher organisms appears to lie in the strength of the forces binding these catalytic proteins to the structural components of the cell. However, a mixture of acetyl S-ACP and malonyl S-ACP derived from *Esch. coli* can be converted to a long chain fatty acid by the fatty acid synthase system of adipose tissue. This and the fact that liver adipose tissue and lactating mammary gland require carbon dioxide and biotin for fatty acid synthesis lead to the conclusion that this cytoplasmic system is operative in these tissues as well as in the cells of micro-organisms. The natural primer may however be butyryl rather than acetyl CoA.

Control of fatty acid synthesis in animals

At least three enzymes in the complicated chain of events leading to the synthesis of fatty acids have been considered as sites of control, responding to physiological changes in the state of the animal:

(1) the state of aggregation of acetyl CoA carboxylase,
(2) the supply of cytoplasmic acetyl CoA through the activity of citrate cleavage enzyme, and
(3) the quantity of fatty acid synthase present.

In chicken liver preparation citrate reacts with the biotin prosthetic group of acetyl CoA carboxylase causing aggregation to a much more active form 10 to 20 times the size:

$$\underset{\text{(inactive)}}{\text{protomer}} \overset{\text{citrate}}{\underset{}{\rightleftharpoons}} \underset{\text{(active)}}{\text{polymer}}$$

The relevance of this physiological condition is uncertain since the level of available citrate in the cytoplasm is not known and likely to be low. Most of the citrate which passes out of the mitochondrion is split by the citrate cleavage enzyme to yield acetyl CoA for building the fatty acid chains and oxaloacetate (p.14.6).

There is little fatty acid synthesis in the fasting animal but it becomes more rapid when the animal is refed or if, as on weaning, it changes to a diet lower in fat. Accordingly attempts have been made to relate the activity of citrate cleavage enzyme and hence provision of cytoplasmic acetyl CoA to the nutritional state. These have not shown that the fall in enzyme activity on fasting and the rise on refeeding always closely parallel the changes in the rate of fatty acid synthesis. Another control system had to be sought.

Immunological assay has shown that the amount of the fatty acid synthase complex in liver falls on fasting and rises again on refeeding. It also falls when a high fat diet is given and rises on changing to one low in fat. The chemical signal for this enzyme induction is not known but the amount of available enzyme parallels the rate of formation of fatty acid as nutritional conditions are changed. The synthase in brain is independently controlled and varies with age.

Another factor is likely to be the rate at which the newly synthesized fatty acid is removed into TG and lipoprotein. Any negative feedback that exists would thus be released. In the same way it is possible that the high level of FFA present in the tissues of a fasting animal (p. 10.13) has an inhibitory effect on acetyl CoA carboxylase and other enzymes of fatty acid synthesis.

Formation of unsaturated fatty acids

These arise from the corresponding saturated acids. The process requires $NADPH_2$ and molecular oxygen. For this reason yeasts grown anaerobically need a supply of oleic acid, but not when in air. In yeasts and rat liver microsomes, there are particulate enzyme systems including a flavoprotein $NADPH_2$ reductase, cytochrome b_5 and a cyanide-sensitive factor apparently able to activate the oxygen. They can convert stearic acid to oleic acid, $C_{18:1}\Delta^9$, and also $C_{20:3}\Delta^{8,11,14}$ to arachidonic acid, $C_{20:4}\Delta^{5,8,11,14}$.

In experimental diabetic animals there is poor conversion of saturated to unsaturated fatty acids. Injection of insulin allows recovery of this process to take place, but only after a delay of about 24 hours. Actinomycin, an inhibitor of protein synthesis, also inhibits this response to insulin. Perhaps insulin promotes the synthesis of the desaturation enzymes by lifting the repression of the appropriate genes. In the normal rat, the $C_{18}\Delta^9$ desaturase activity is low in fasting and restored on refeeding.

An alternative route for the synthesis of unsaturated acids must exist in anaerobic organisms. Here the cytoplasmic synthesis proceeds as already described. When 3-hydroxydecanoyl-ACP is formed, it can be dehydrated in the 2-3 position and then reduced to the saturated acyl-ACP (path A, fig. 10.7); alternatively dehydration can occur in the 3-4 position. The resulting double bond is not reduced, but persists throughout the subsequent chain-lengthening steps (path B, fig. 10.7).

Ingested or synthesized fatty acids may be transformed, mainly in the liver, into fatty acids particular to the specific lipids of the body. The unsaturated fatty acids and intermediate length saturated acids are elongated in the microsomes by addition of 2C units reacting as malonyl CoA. In contrast, chain lengthening in the mitochondrial fraction of liver occurs also by a second route, which is independent of biotin, apparently by reversal of β-oxidation. Evidence for this was provided by incubating mitochondria with 2-[^{14}C]acetyl CoA and a number of cofactors. Most of the incorporated ^{14}C became located in

Path A

$$CH_3(CH_2)_6CHOHCH_2\,CO.S\text{-}ACP$$

$$CH_3(CH_2)_6\overset{3}{C}H=\overset{2}{C}H\,CO.S\text{-}ACP$$

$$CH_3(CH_2)_8CO.S\text{-}ACP$$

$$\downarrow \text{3 Malonyl S CoA}$$

$$CH_3(CH_2)_{14}\,COOH + 3CO_2$$
Palmitic acid $C_{16:0}$

Path B

$$CH_3(CH_2)_6CHOHCH_2\,CO.S\text{-}ACP$$

$$CH_3(CH_2)_5\overset{4}{C}H=\overset{3}{C}H\,\overset{2}{C}H_2CO.S\text{-}ACP$$

$$\downarrow \text{Malonyl S CoA}$$

$$CH_3(CH_2)_5CH=CH\,CH_2CO\,CH_2CO.S\text{-}ACP$$

$$CH_3(CH_2)_5CH=CH\,(CH_2)_3\,CO.S\text{-}ACP$$

$$\downarrow \text{3 Malonyl S-ACP}$$

$$CH_3(CH_2)_5CH=CH\,(CH_2)_9\,COOH$$
cis-Vaccenic acid $C_{18:1}\Delta^{11}$

FIG. 10.7. Pathways of fatty acid formation.

the second carbon atom of the chain rather than on alternate atoms right along the chain. Existing or added fatty acids were being lengthened in the mitochondria rather than *de novo* synthesis taking place.

The fatty acid composition of lipids in the tissues differs in different species, but may be modified by environmental factors. Fats from animals raised by intensive feeding on farms have a lower ratio of polyunsaturated to saturated fatty acids (P/S ratio) than free-living animals. Some success has been achieved in producing meat and milk with higher proportions of polyunsaturated fatty acids by dietary measures. The linoleic acid content of adipose tissue fat in human subjects has been raised from 11 to 32 per cent by feeding corn oil, but the change takes many months. It has been known for a long time that exposure of animals to cold lowers the melting point and raises the iodine value of their fat.

Essential fatty acids

The chain lengthening and desaturation processes are

important for the provision of adequate supplies of the essential fatty acids. Dietary linoleic acid is converted by the microsomes to arachidonic acid (fig. 10.8).

Linoleic acid

Desaturase | O_2 / $NADPH_2$

γ-Linolenic acid

Malonyl CoA / Desaturase | O_2 / $NADPH_2$

Arachidonic acid

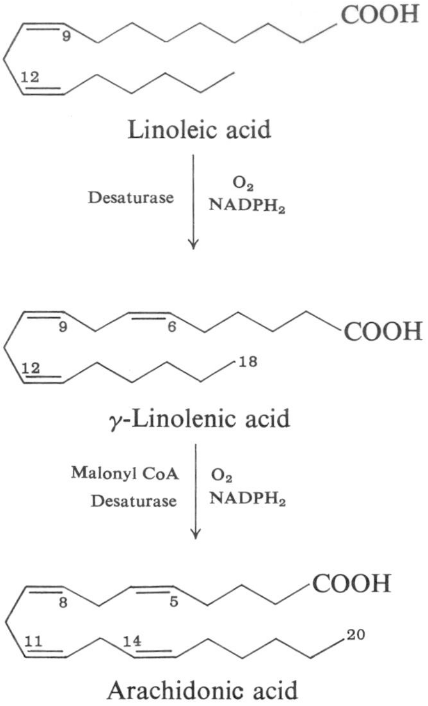

FIG. 10.8. The conversion of linoleic to arachidonic acid.

Note that these essential acids have their last double bond six places away from the methyl end. An isomer of γ-linolenic acid, $C_{18:3}\Delta^{9,12,15}$, is transformed into $C_{20:3}\Delta^{11,14,17}$. This substance is present in the tissues but is not an essential fatty acid. Oleic acid is also useless in preventing the symptoms of essential fatty acid deficiency, for desaturation can occur only at a site on the carboxyl side of the existing double bond, i.e. $C_{18:1}\Delta^9$ cannot be converted to $C_{18:2}\Delta^{9,12}$ with the necessary double bond six places away from the methyl group.

Arachidonic acid is found in highest concentration in the lipids of the endocrine organs, adrenal cortex, ovary, testis and pituitary, and in the brain.

To be effective, polyunsaturated acids must be in the all-*cis* form. Thus arachidonic acid all-*cis* $C_{20:4}\Delta^{5,8,11,14}$ is curved. The all-*trans* form would be linear, similar to a saturated chain. A phospholipid or cholesterol ester containing an all-*cis* polyunsaturated acid is therefore of a very different shape from one with a saturated or *trans* unsaturated acid.

Apart from the special role of arachidonic acid as a precursor of the prostaglandins (see below), provision of phospholipids containing the essential fatty acids appears to be necessary for the integrity of membranes and for the electron transport system of mitochondria (p. 8.5). Why linolenic acid should be less effective in this regard is not

known since it differs only in having its double bonds lying nearer the methyl end of the chain.

SYNTHESIS OF PROSTAGLANDINS

The prostaglandins or prostanoids discovered by von Euler are local hormones (p. 27.50) present in all tissues, with the highest concentrations in the seminal vesicles. They are synthesized from C_{20} unsaturated fatty acids. Several forms are known. PGE_1 is derived from eicosa-8,11,14-trienoic acid (a derivative of γ-linolenic acid) and PGE_2 from eicosa-5,8,11,14-tetraenoic acid (arachidonic acid). Fig 10.9 shows their structure:

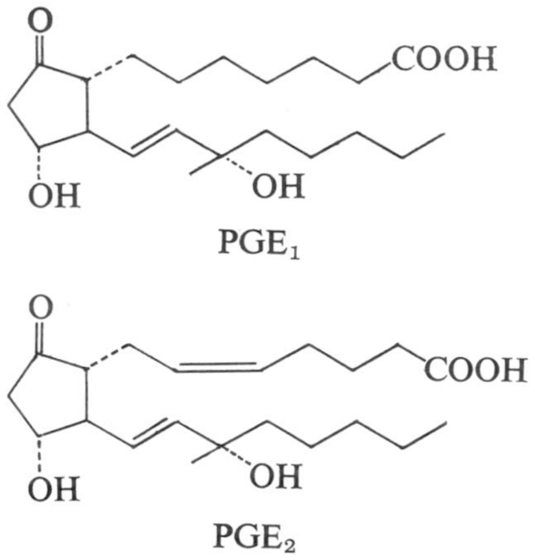

PGE_1

PGE_2

FIG. 10.9. Structure of two of the prostaglandins.

A microsomal preparation of the prostate gland of sheep can convert labelled arachidonic acid into PGE_2, in the presence of oxygen and a reducing agent, glutathione. The oxygen introduced into the fatty acid at specific points in the molecule is derived from the gas phase and hence the reaction is typical of oxygenases. The reaction is in fact a di-oxygenase because the molecule of oxygen introduced into the molecule at one site provides two of the hydroxyls in the molecule.

Triglyceride synthesis and breakdown

The microsomes of liver and adipose tissue cells appear to be the principal sites of TG synthesis. The glyceride portion of the molecule is provided by 1-glycerophosphate formed by phosphorylation of glycerol, except in the adipose tissue which has little of the necessary enzyme, glycerokinase. In the fat cell of adipose tissue the compound is derived by reduction of the triose phosphate, dihydroxyacetone phosphate, formed in glycolysis. Fat synthesis in adipose tissue is therefore dependent on carbohydrate metabolism and does not take place or is greatly reduced in starvation when carbohydrate is not readily available.

The condensing fatty acids are first activated by CoA and then possibly transferred to an acyl carrier protein. Two of them esterify the free hydroxyl groups of

1-glycerophosphate to give a phosphatidic acid. Usually an unsaturated fatty acid condenses at the 3 position, while either a saturated or an unsaturated acid may go on the other hydroxyl. The phosphate group is finally split off by a phosphatase, and a third fatty acid substituted to give a molecule of TG (see fig. 10.13). In intestinal mucosal cells 2-acylglycerols may be acylated directly to diglycerides and triglycerides.

The TG are stacks of energy-yielding fatty acid chains. Since the tissues in which they are synthesized also contain lipases which break them down again to free glycerol and FFA, the laying down and removal occurs freely, providing a flexible system. The control by means of hormones as well as by the availability of substrates is considered on p. 34.6. Pancreatic lipase differs from the other lipases so far studied in that it splits off only the 1 and 3 fatty acids from TG. The bulk of the dietary TG is therefore broken down in the duodenum and first part of the jejunum only as far as the 2-monoglyceride.

Role of free fatty acids (FFA) in metabolism

FFA is the form in which lipid is transported in the blood from adipose tissue depots to the tissues where it is used as a source of energy. The concentration of FFA in plasma is low but very variable. Whereas after an overnight fast the level of blood glucose usually lies between 4 and 5 mmol/l, the level of plasma FFA is usually between 400 and 600 μmol/l. The level is sensitive to the nutritional state of the subject. If he continues to fast but takes exercise, the level rises rapidly and in one to two hours may reach as high as 2000 μmol/l. On the other hand if a normal breakfast or 50 g of glucose is taken, it falls in about 30 min to 200 μmol/l or sometimes less.

The level in the plasma differs in different blood vessels. In one fasting subject after a short period of light exercise blood was drawn from an artery and two veins in the leg, a superficial vein draining mostly adipose tissue and a deep vein draining muscle. The levels of plasma FFA were 820 (artery), 1390 (superficial vein) and 540 (deep vein) μmol/l. These figures indicate an entry of FFA into the circulation from adipose tissue and an uptake by muscle. After giving glucose and an injection of insulin, the plasma FFA level fell to 190 μmol/l in the superficial vein. The utilization of glucose shuts off the outflow of FFA from adipose tissue and prevents its uptake by muscle. Using the same technique in animals it has been shown that the brain does not remove FFA from the blood even in the fasting state.

By injecting palmitic acid labelled with ^{14}C into the circulation, it is possible to calculate the turnover rate of FFA in the blood. Surprisingly it has been found that each molecule of FFA exists on average in the plasma for only a few minutes. In one experiment the value was 2·7 minutes. Now if 750 μmol, the amount normally present in the plasma, is replaced every 2·7 min, then

about 100 g of lipid is carried into and out of the blood as FFA in 24 hours. This is equivalent to just under 4·2 MJ (1000 kcal)/day which is sufficient to meet about two-thirds of the energy needs at rest. Obviously this FFA component of the blood is of the utmost importance in the metabolic economy of the body.

Dynamic aspects of lipid metabolism

The classical methods of analysis of plasma and tissue lipids give limited information as to where the constituents have come from, how they are transformed and to what extent this occurs. By injecting ^{14}C-fatty acids into animals it has been found that 30 per cent is taken up by the liver. Within 5 min this is practically all esterified, being found mainly in the neutral lipid rather than in the phospholipids which have a slower turnover rate. The ^{14}C leaves the liver first in the VLDL and later appears in the LDL.

The slower turnover of ^{14}C-labelled chylomicrons in fasted dogs after hepatectomy indicates that the liver is the major site of removal of lipoprotein from the blood–liver pool. TG is hydrolysed there and the fatty acids oxidized or converted to ketone bodies. In contrast, in the fed animal, removal from the plasma by other tissues becomes more important and about one-third is removed by the liver, and one-fifth by the adipose tissues. The triglyceride fatty acid of lipoprotein enters adipose and muscle cells in the fed animal through activation or formation of lipoprotein lipase. It is not necessary for the triglyceride fatty acids present in the chylomicrons to pass first through the liver for transformation to LDL before being taken up by the peripheral tissues.

Isotope studies also show that the exchange of cholesterol phospholipid or fatty acid molecules from one component (plasma lipoprotein, cell membrane or storage depot) to another takes place without necessarily involving a net change of that component. Lipid molecules, except those in the nervous system, are being continuously transformed and transported about the body. Thus, the apparent constancy of the body fat has been shown to be illusory.

Ketosis

In fasting or during prolonged exercise, energy is obtained by mobilization of the fat stores and there is a tendency towards overproduction of acetyl CoA in the liver. More is formed than can enter the citric acid cycle. Instead it is converted to acetoacetyl CoA and thence to acetoacetate, which enters the blood stream (fig. 10.10).

The metabolism of acetoacetate is described on p. 33.6. Tissues other than liver, such as muscle and kidney, can reactivate the ketone bodies by the following reactions:

(1) β-hydroxybutyrate $\longrightarrow$ acetoacetate

(2) acetoacetate + HSCoA + ATP

     thiokinase

     $\longrightarrow$ acetoacetyl CoA + AMP + PP$_i$

(3) acetoacetate + succinyl CoA

     thiophorase

     $\longrightarrow$ acetoacetyl CoA + succinate

The resulting compounds are utilized as metabolic fuel along with the lipid stored in these tissues. However, the rate of utilization of these ketone bodies is limited. When the rate of production by the liver exceeds that of removal by the peripheral tissues, then the blood level rises. As the pK values of β-hydroxybutyric acid and acetoacetic acid are 4·8 and 3·8 respectively, the ketone bodies circulate in the blood plasma in ionized form. Consequently the dissociation of the carbonic acid (pK 6·1) is affected, and the ratio $[HCO_3{}^-]/[H_2CO_3]$ falls (keto-acidosis).

The only means of controlling acetoacetate formation in the body appears to be by the secretion of insulin. This tapers off as the blood glucose falls and allows FFA mobilization to occur by suppressing re-esterification. This results in increased FFA oxidation (fig. 10.10). As a result more acetyl CoA is formed and more NAD is reduced. Most of the additional acetyl CoA is converted to acetoacetyl CoA, but they also inhibit oxidation of pyruvate and promote its conversion instead to phosphoenol pyruvate (PEP) and ultimately to glucose (gluconeogenesis). At the same time the high $NADH_2/NAD$ ratio within the mitochondria reduces much of the oxaloacetate to malate. The quantity of oxaloacetate

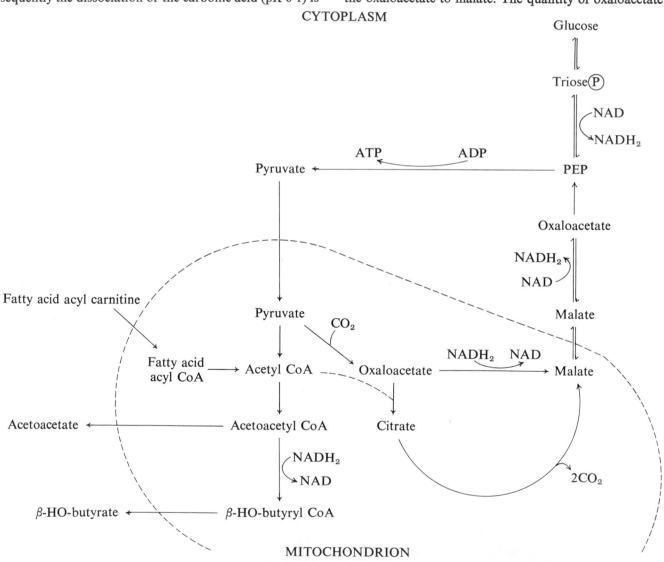

Fig. 10.10. Reactions occurring in the liver during ketosis. Ketone body formation is increased from the enlarged pool of acetyl CoA. Gluconeogenesis is increased by inhibition of pyruvate oxidation and increased conversion of pyruvate to oxaloacetate in the mitochondria. This oxaloacetate is reduced to malate which passes out into the cytoplasm.

available for condensation with acetyl CoA in the citric acid cycle is therefore diminished. Malate passes out, providing reducing capacity necessary for the synthesis of glucose. Even in prolonged fasting, gluconeogenesis seems to be sufficient to maintain some insulin secretion. Insulin depresses activity of the lipase present in the adipose tissue which is particularly active in this situation (p. 34.5). As a consequence, the flow of FFA into the blood and thence to the liver is controlled. Without insulin, the acetoacetate derived from the flood of FFA entering the liver would be poured out unchecked. This may lead to a grave condition and occurs in some patients with diabetes mellitus in whom the supply of endogenous insulin is inadequate.

Interrelations between lipid and carbohydrate metabolism

Since fatty acids and carbohydrate are broken down to acetyl CoA, both can supply energy to the body through the citric acid cycle and the respiratory chain. Table 10.5 is an estimate of the sources of energy used by the tissues

TABLE 10.5. An estimate of the fuels used by a normal man at rest in the postabsorptive state, modified from Fritz I.B. (1961) *Physiol. Rev.* **41**, 52.

Fuel	Site of oxidation	mmol/min oxidized	O_2 used mmol/min
Glucose	Chiefly brain	0·33	2·0
FFA—Ketones	Liver	0·04	
FFA—CO_2	Liver	0·10 ⎫ 0·32	6·0
FFA—CO_2	Extrahepatic tissues	0·18 ⎭	
Ketones	All tissues, except liver	0·16	0·6
Glycerol	All tissues	0·09	0·3
Amino acids	Chiefly liver	35 mg	1·1
			10·0

of a man at rest in the postabsorptive state. Great accuracy cannot be claimed for any individual figure. However, there is little doubt that FFA provides the major part of the energy under these conditions, glucose provides about one-fifth, nearly all used by the brain, amino acids about one-tenth and ketones and glycerol significant but smaller amounts. The proportions utilized may be altered greatly by a meal and by exercise. After giving glucose or taking a meal containing carbohydrate, the RQ rises to close to unity suggesting that, during carbohydrate absorption, glucose rather than fat is used to provide energy. More direct evidence for this may be obtained by injecting ^{14}C–palmitic acid. Then $^{14}CO_2$ appears in the expired air, but

the amount can be reduced by taking glucose. This indicates that glucose diminishes the rate of oxidation of fatty acids. The mechanism for the switch over of fuels is probably as follows; glucose entering the blood from the intestines causes a rise in the amount of circulating insulin (p. 27.46), which facilitates the passage of glucose into the cells and so allows it to be metabolized. Part of this glucose is converted in the liver and adipose tissue to glycogen, and the remainder is broken down to triose

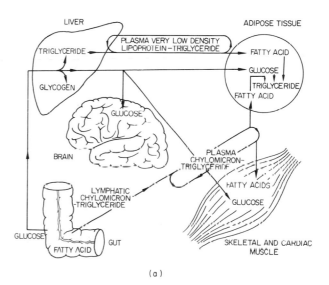

(a)

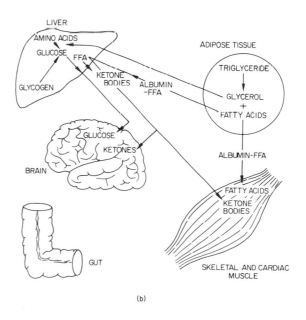

(b)

FIG. 10.11. Transport, storage and utilization of fat in the tissues related to carbohydrate metabolism; (a) after a meal, (b) when fasting. Modified from Galton D.J. (1975) in *Obesity: Pathogenesis and Management*, ed. Silverstone J.T. London: M.T.P.

phosphate by the glycolytic pathway and the hexose monophosphate pathway. In this way, 1-glycerophosphate becomes available, particularly in the adipose cells, to lock up most of the liberated FFA by re-esterifying them to TG. As a consequence the FFA leave the adipose cells at a reduced rate and the lowered plasma level no longer allows the tissues to use FFA as a fuel. Instead, glucose is readily available for oxidation, by breaking down to pyruvate and on to acetyl CoA, finally yielding carbon dioxide and $NADH_2$. Acetyl CoA produced in excess of energy requirements is transformed within the liver and adipose cells to fatty acid. The hexose monophosphate pathway can provide much of the $NADPH_2$ necessary for this synthesis. Thus excess of dietary carbohydrate may be stored as glycogen or converted to fat. The amount converted into fat may depend upon how full the glycogen store is.

During sharp bursts of exercise, carbohydrate (glycogen) is the immediate source of the extra fuel and energy is provided by glycolysis within the muscle cells. Within a few minutes of the start of exercise muscles begin to withdraw large amounts of FFA from the blood. The factors responsible for the mobilization of fat during muscular exercise are discussed on p. 34.6.

In fasting when glucose is no longer being absorbed, depletion of the liver glycogen occurs and the blood glucose falls to about 3 mmol/l (54 mg/100 ml). Glucose utilization is reduced in the tissues, other than in the nervous system, and this keeps the blood level from falling further, a situation which would soon cause damage to the brain.

The major change is that less glucose enters the adipose cell to act as a brake on the output of FFA. As a result, the concentration of plasma FFA may be doubled or more by an 18 hour fast in spite of the FFA being removed by the tissues in increasing amounts. The FFA are oxidized in place of glucose and become the major source of energy for the tissues.

Fig. 10.11 summarizes the sites of the main reactions in the transport, storage and utilization of fat in the tissues and its relation to carbohydrate metabolism.

CHEMISTRY OF SPHINGOLIPIDS

The sphingolipids are a relatively complex group of lipids containing the base sphingosine.

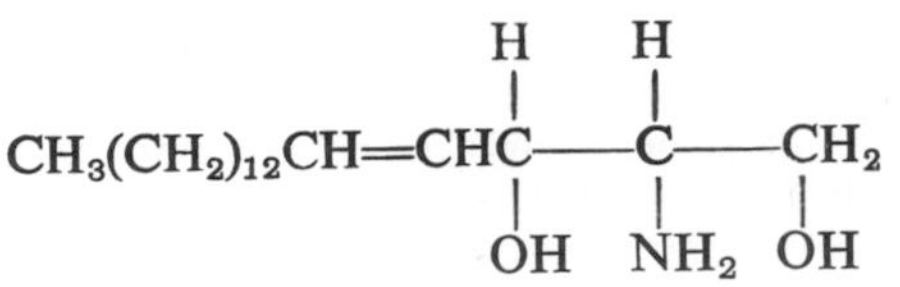

Sphingosine

Sphingomyelins found in nervous tissue, particularly myelin sheath, and in blood contain sphingosine, phosphoryl choline and a molecule of fatty acid. The phosphoryl choline is esterified to the primary alcohol group and an amide link joins the fatty acid to the amino group. Sphingomyelins are thus phospholipids.

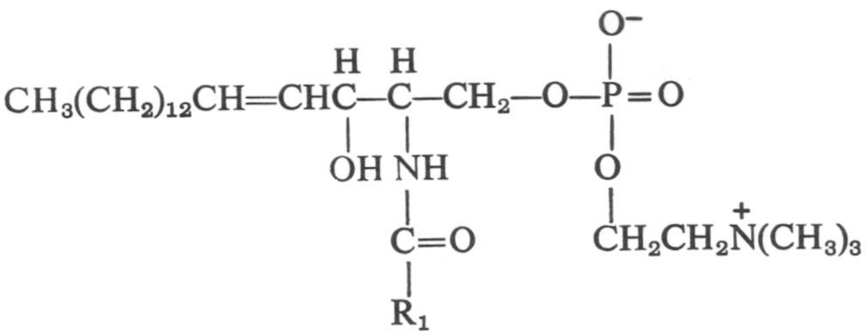

N-acylsphingosine　　　　Phosphoryl choline

Cerebrosides are similar compounds with a hexose, usually galactose, joined to sphingosine in place of the phosphoryl choline, i.e. they contain no phosphorus and so are not phospholipids. The fatty acid mixture obtained after hydrolysing brain cerebrosides contains $C_{24:0}$ fatty acids and C_{24}-2-hydroxyacids as major components.

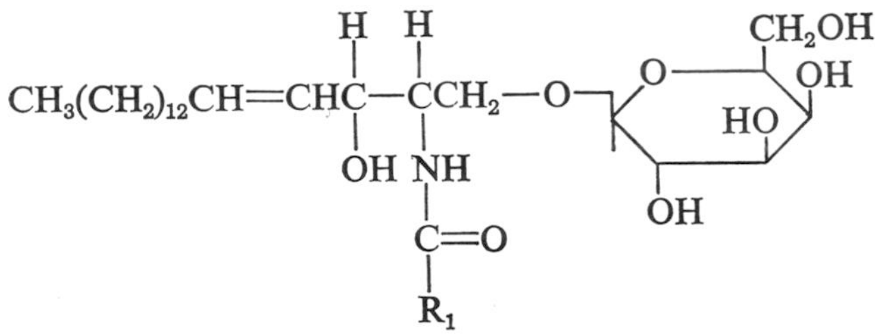

N-acylsphingosine　　　　Galactose

A cerebroside (glycolipid)

Gangliosides are found in erythrocytes, spleen and nervous tissue, and resemble cerebrosides but are more complex. They have the following structure:

N-acylsphingosine
|
glucose-galactose-*N*-acetylglucosamine
|
N-acetylneuraminic acid

Brain ganglioside

The carbohydrate side chain is longer and contains one molecule of *N*-acetylglucosamine and at least one of *N*-acetylneuraminic acid.

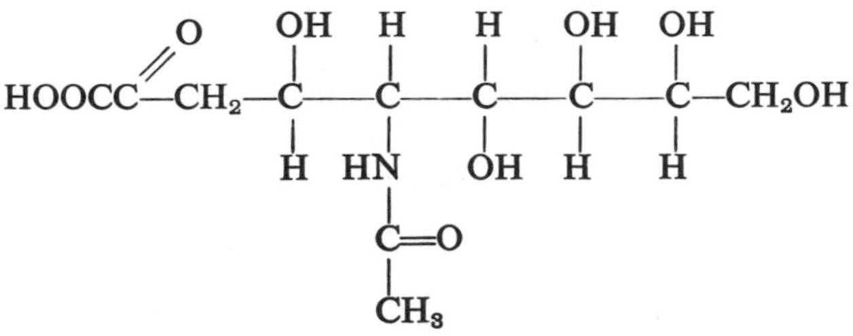

$$\text{HOOCC}\overset{\displaystyle\parallel}{}\!\!-\!\text{CH}_2\!-\!\underset{\text{H}}{\overset{\text{OH}}{\text{C}}}\!-\!\underset{\text{HN}}{\overset{\text{H}}{\text{C}}}\!-\!\underset{\text{OH}}{\overset{\text{H}}{\text{C}}}\!-\!\underset{\text{H}}{\overset{\text{OH}}{\text{C}}}\!-\!\underset{\text{H}}{\overset{\text{OH}}{\text{C}}}\!-\!\text{CH}_2\text{OH}$$

N-acetylneuraminic acid

The distribution of lipids in the nervous system is shown in table 25.5. Defects in the enzyme systems which degrade sphingolipids are responsible for a group of rare disorders, the lipidoses (vol. 3, p. 47.18).

METABOLISM OF PHOSPHOLIPIDS

The metabolism of phosphatides and of sphingolipids are discussed together although, in the latter group, neither the cerebrosides nor the gangliosides contain phosphorus. This is justified by their similarity of function.

Synthesis of phospholipids

The use of isotopically labelled precursors, such as [^{32}P] phosphate, [^{14}C] choline and [^{14}C] fatty acids, shows that phospholipids are formed in all tissues. The pathways involved have been deduced by adding possible coenzymes and intermediates and observing the effect on the incorporation of the isotope into the product.

Thus when phosphatidic acid is mixed with [^{14}C] [^{32}P] phosphoryl choline and a preparation from rat brain, the ^{32}P is found to be incorporated into the newly formed phosphatidyl choline and is not split out during condensation, i.e. no labelled inorganic P is produced. As the

incorporation is stimulated by the addition of cytidine triphosphate (CTP), CDP-choline is probably an intermediary stage, as shown in fig. 10.12.

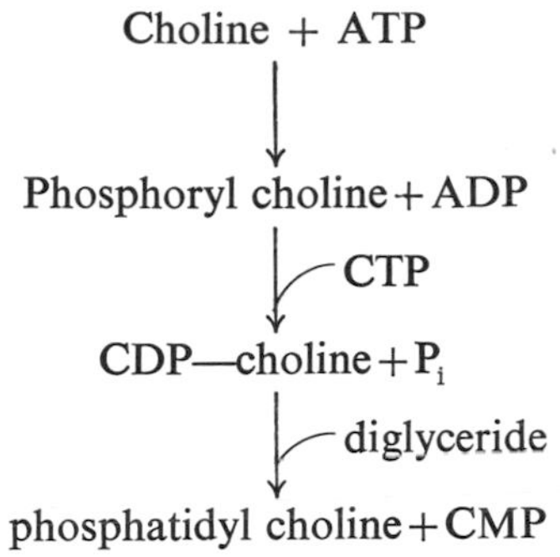

$$\text{Choline} + \text{ATP}$$
$$\downarrow$$
$$\text{Phosphoryl choline} + \text{ADP}$$
$$\downarrow\!\!\diagup\!\text{CTP}$$
$$\text{CDP}\!-\!\text{choline} + \text{P}_i$$
$$\downarrow\!\!\diagup\!\text{diglyceride}$$
$$\text{phosphatidyl choline} + \text{CMP}$$

Fig. 10.12. Synthesis of phosphatidyl choline.

The same argument applies to the formation of phosphatidyl ethanolamine from ethanolamine and probably also for the plasmalogens. Fig. 10.13 shows the pathway for the formation of phosphatidyl ethanolamine and also of phosphatidyl serine and phosphatidyl inositol which follow a different route.

Although phosphatidic acid is on the pathway to triglycerides as well as to phospholipids, these may not be formed within the cell from the same precursor pools. There is some evidence that high concentrations of palmityl CoA inhibit phosphatidic acid phosphatase. This might be expected to divert phosphatidic acids to phospholipids by the route shown on the left of fig. 10.13 rather than to di- and triglyceride formation.

Synthesis of sphingolipids

Experiments with labelled serine and palmityl CoA show these to be precursors of sphingosine. Palmityl aldehyde is first formed and then condenses with serine, the product

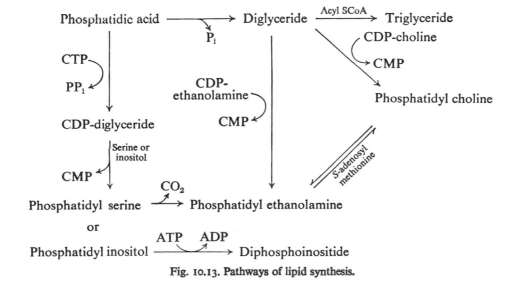

Fig. 10.13. Pathways of lipid synthesis.

being subsequently oxidized by a flavoprotein yielding sphingosine (fig. 10.14).

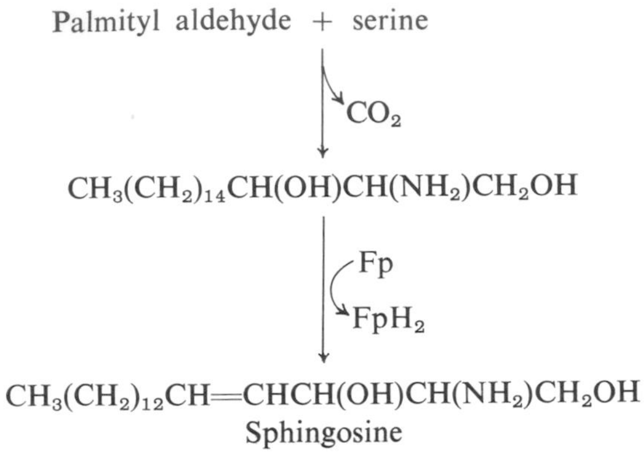

$$\text{Palmityl aldehyde} + \text{serine}$$

$$\downarrow CO_2$$

$$CH_3(CH_2)_{14}CH(OH)CH(NH_2)CH_2OH$$

$$\downarrow \begin{array}{c} Fp \\ FpH_2 \end{array}$$

$$CH_3(CH_2)_{12}CH{=}CHCH(OH)CH(NH_2)CH_2OH$$
Sphingosine

FIG. 10.14. Formation of sphingosine.

This is acylated by an activated fatty acid and may further react with CDP-choline to give sphingomyelin or these reactions may occur in the reverse order. The synthetic routes to the cerebrosides and gangliosides are shown in fig. 10.15.

Degradation of phospholipids

Mammalian tissues contain active enzymes which degrade glycerophosphatides. Two groups, phospholipases A1 and A2 and lysophospholipases, both remove the acyl groups (fig. 10.16) while acyl transferases can rebuild them, selecting appropriate acyl groups from the available pool.

The product of the attack by phospholipase A2 on phosphatidyl choline (lecithin) is A2-lysolecithin (1-acyl, 3-phosphoryl choline glyceride). Two molecules of this can dissimulate yielding phosphatidyl choline and glycerylphosphoryl choline. There is another class of enzyme in many tissues called phospholipase C, which splits the phosphoryl ester, leaving a diglyceride.

The plasmalogens, glycolipids and sphingolipids also turn over during the life of the cell. Thus enzymes are present to break them down, by hydrolysing off their ether or acyl groups, sugar residues or phosphoryl choline.

Rarely in individuals these enzymes are absent. Then undegraded phospholipids accumulate, especially in nervous tissues. Mental retardation and other defects develop (vol. 3, p. 47.18).

The liberated acyl groups are probably used to acylate other compounds such as cholesterol. The specificity of these lipases and the enzymes involved in reacylating to phosphatidyl choline, etc., is such that compounds are formed of the required structure, i.e. those with a particular saturated fatty acid at the 1-position and an unsaturated one at position 2.

LECITHIN-CHOLESTEROL ACYLTRANSFERASE (LCAT)

A lecithin acyltransferase is present in plasma. Its substrate is HDL to which phosphatidyl choline and cholesterol pass from VLDL. The lecithin donates its 2-acyl group to cholesterol (fig. 10.17) and, if the cholesterol is previously isotopically labelled, the new cholesterol

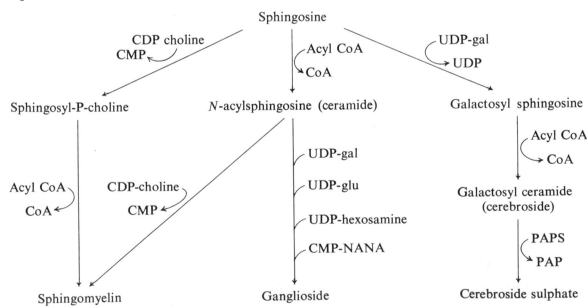

PAPS = 3'-phosphoadenosine-5'phosphosulphate
NANA = *N*-acetylneuraminic acid

FIG. 10.15. Formation of complex sphingolipids.

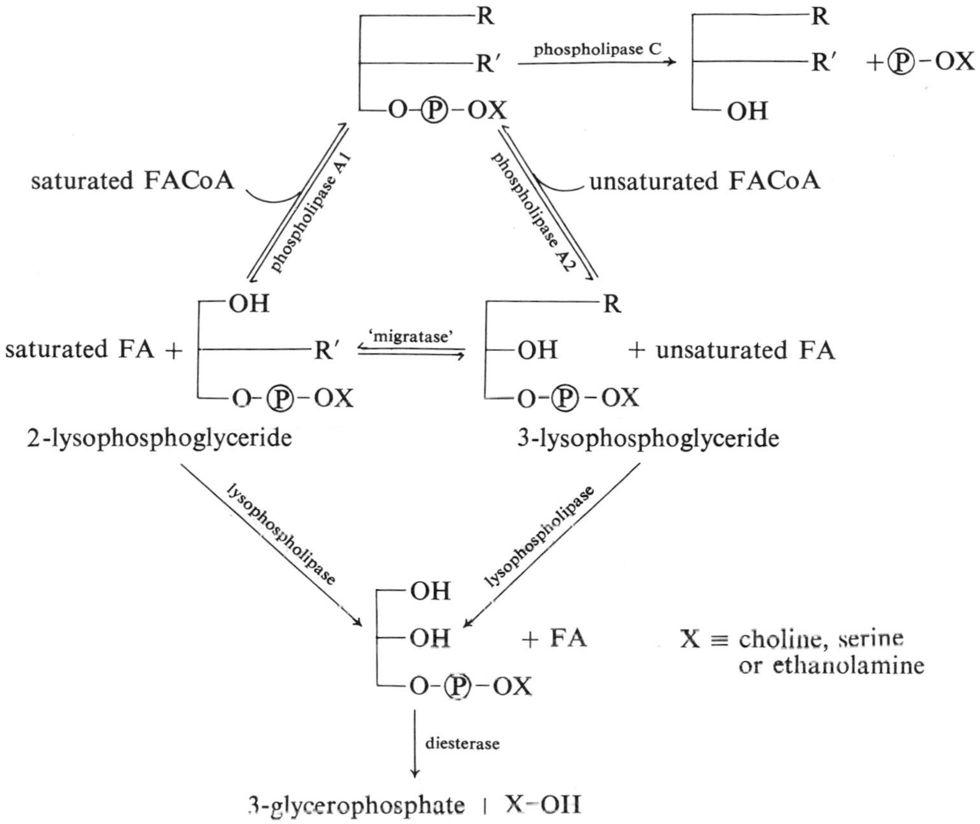

FIG. 10.16. Action of phospholipases.

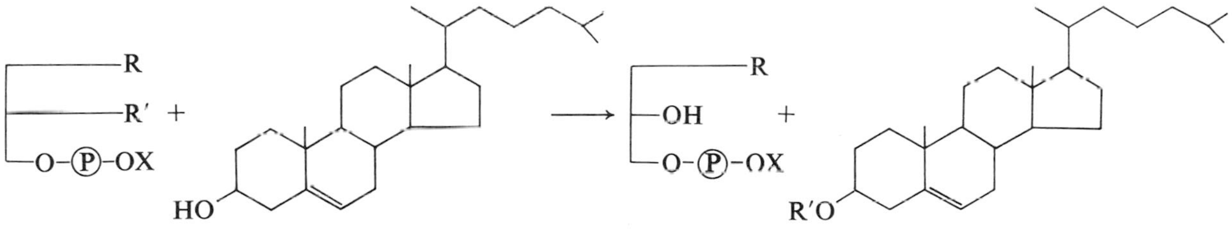

Fig. 10.17.   Acylation of cholesterol.

can be seen to travel back to less dense lipoproteins while the lysolecithin becomes bound to albumin.

A few individuals have been found who have insufficient of the enzyme (vol. 3, p. 47.15). Their blood plasma has the low ratio of esterified to free cholesterol and the high phosphatidyl choline concentrations expected if this was normally a major pathway in the body. Its function may be to turn over the unsaturated fatty acids present in phosphatidyl choline rather than to esterify cholesterol for which there is another efficient enzyme system in the liver, the site where the lipoproteins are assembled (p. 10.24). It may also be involved in the transport of cholesterol from the cell membranes for excretion by the liver.

Functions of phospholipids

The phospholipids are found in the cellular and sub-cellular membranes of all organisms to the extent of 20–30 per cent of the dry weight. An obvious molecular property is their dual nature, for like bile salts they consist of hydrophilic and hydrophobic portions.

COMPONENTS OF MEMBRANES

Membranes are thought to behave as two-dimensional oriented viscous solutions of globular proteins in a phospholipid bilayer, which also contains a small quantity of cholesterol. The integral proteins protrude partially or completely into the lipid matrix to which they are strongly held by hydrophobic association. This leaves the ionic or hydrophilic portions of the protein on the outside free to bind other hydrophilic molecules, such as the peripheral proteins, and to react with water molecules and ions. Short sugar chains are attached covalently to many of the proteins at the outer surface. Membranes are therefore asymmetrical with regard to the position of carbohydrate and also to the structure and position of the protein components. The non-polar regions of the folded polypeptide chains are embedded among particular fatty acid chains in a manner depending on the chemistry of the protein. A diagram of a fragment of membrane is shown in fig. 10.18.

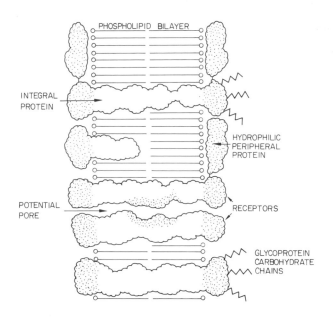

FIG. 10.18. Model of a membrane.

In the plasma membrane electron microscopy reveals a flat vesicular closed structure whereas in the inner mitochondrial membrane, containing the enzymes involved in electron transport, the sheets may be rolled into tubes capable of being flattened out, e.g. by the presence of calcium or sodium ions. Most membrane-bound enzymes are integral proteins but peripheral proteins which have been identified include cytochrome c on the mitochondrial membrane and the ribosomal proteins of the endoplasmic reticulum.

The plasma membrane separates the extracellular fluid from the cytoplasm of the cell. In addition it allows the controlled entry and exit of small molecules, nutrients and waste products and the free passage of water. Studies on the rate of entry of glucose and cations into cells have led to the hypothesis that this is limited by the availability of carriers existing in the cell membrane. Transport systems for the passage of such small molecules may consist of specific peripheral receptor lipoproteins attached to pairs of adjacent proteins spanning the inside of the membrane. If a quaternary change in these proteins widened the gap between them, this would correspond to the pore through which molecules

have been imagined to pass. We can visualize the acidic phosphatides, phosphatidyl serine and phosphatidyl inositol, on the outside of the lipoprotein receptor binding calcium ions and also perhaps being a component of the lipoprotein ATPase, the basis of movement of sodium and potassium ions in and out of cells (p. 15.7). Thus the ability of calcium to increase the permeability of the cell membrane to other small molecules may lie in its ability to alter the spatial structure of the constituent proteins. Such a transformation can be used to describe the process whereby the plasma membrane of an isolated fat cell becomes more permeable to glucose after controlled treatment with phospholipase C. Presumably the phospholipids are digested away, changing the characteristics of the membrane, while the carrier mechanism, common also to the insulin-facilitated transport of glucose, is unaffected (p. 18.8).

The phospholipids of membranes are not chemically inert building blocks but are dynamic components continually broken down by phospholipases and replaced. The mean half-life of the lipids in mitochondrial membranes is about 10 days in liver and 30 days in brain. However, in each tissue there is a structural fraction turning over more slowly than the rest. The enzymes involved in the breakdown have greater affinity for fatty acid chains of a particular length or degree of unsaturation, thus allowing the structural pattern to be retained.

SUBCELLULAR PARTICLES

It is probable that the phospholipids present in the endoplasmic reticulum are involved in protein synthesis through their capacity to orientate the messenger-RNA molecules (p. 12.5). Within the cell nucleus the small amount of phospholipid rapidly incorporates ^{32}P in periods of great mitotic activity. More conclusive information is available from studies of mitochondria.

In mitochondria the oxidation of $NADH_2$ and its coupling to the synthesis of ATP depends on the lipid components of the inner membrane. In subcellular particles respiration stops after they have been subjected to the action of phospholipases or lipid solvents. Moreover the activity of the oxidizing enzymes, e.g. cytochrome oxidase, is restored by adding phospholipid extracts. Thus removal of the lipid results in destruction of the organized systems, as shown by loss of activity, which is restored by returning the phospholipid. The mitochondrial enzymes appear to be located together in groups according to their function, e.g. those for electron transport (p. 8.5) and those for fatty acid oxidation. The functional constituents, flavin, haem and nonhaem iron, are all hydrophobic, and the lipoprotein may provide a medium necessary for the electron flow and for the correct conformation of the enzymic proteins.

An additional role has been allocated to mitochondrial phospholipids. They are known to promote the activities of certain enzymes. Thus cytochrome c oxidase requires an acidic lipid, its substrate apparently being a phospholipid complex of cytochrome c. Perhaps this is to bind NAD and provide a hydrophobic environment for the enzymic reaction. In a similar way, β-hydroxybutyrate dehydrogenase requires phosphatidyl choline. As the mechanism of the active transport processes becomes known, so the role of the phospholipids in the plasma membrane may be shown to be more than structural.

PHOSPHOLIPIDS IN BLOOD PLASMA

These are known to have two important functions in the blood, one as constituents of the plasma lipoproteins (p. 10.5) and the other in blood coagulation (p. 28.14). A phospholipoprotein is contributed by the platelets to the mechanism involved in prothrombin activation; it perhaps provides a catalytic surface on the platelet.

STRUCTURE OF STEROIDS

Steroids may be regarded as derivatives of a parent substance, perhydro*cyclo*pentenophenanthrene.

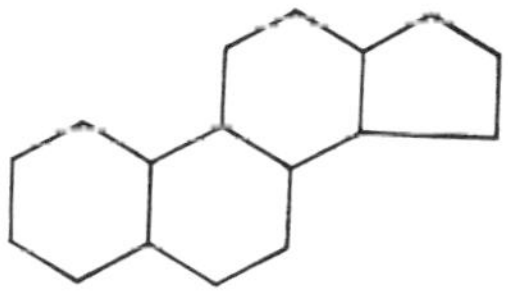

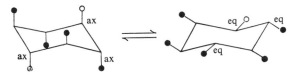

As the rings, unlike those of aromatic compounds such as benzene, are fully saturated, the bond angle of the six membered rings is 120°. Now the tetrahedral angles of the bonds about an isolated carbon atom are about 109°. Consequently in these rings the carbon–carbon bonds would be strained from this optimum angle, if the rings did not buckle.

Consider first the single ring compound, *cyclo*hexane, C_6H_{12}, which can exist in two non-planar forms, the chair and the boat (fig. 10.19). The chair form has carbon

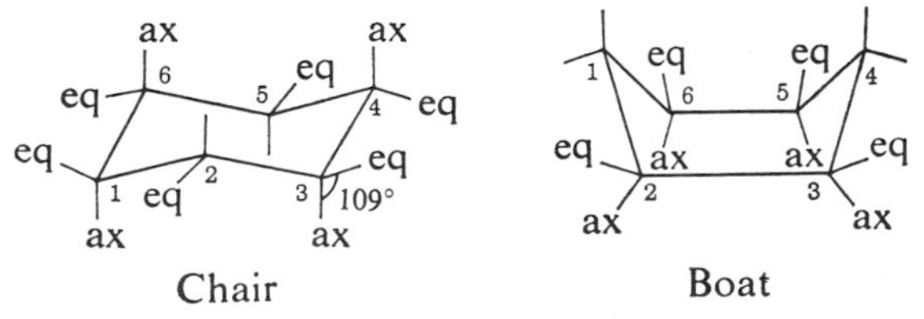

Chair   Boat

FIG. 10.19. The *cyclo*hexane ring in two non-planar forms.

atoms 1, 3 and 5 in one plane and the rest in a parallel plane a little above. It is the form in which most of the molecules exist. In it there are two kinds of bonds, those parallel to the threefold axis of symmetry of the molecule (axial) and those which make an angle of 109° with the axis of the ring (equatorial). By rotating the ring

FIG. 10.20. Two chair forms of *cyclo*hexane.

valence bonds, two chair forms can be visualized (fig. 10.20). They are equivalent, unless the groups represented in the open and closed circles are different, as in the mono-substituted compound, *cyclo*hexanol. Then the two forms exist in equilibrium with one another. The one with the hydroxyl group in the less crowded equatorial position is more stable and present in greater amount.

Turning now to the situation in which two rings are fused together, as in the steroids, we can visualize two ways in which this could be done. One is the *trans* form in which the bonds to hydrogen at the ends of the ring junction are both axial (fig. 10.21). In the *cis* form they lie in the equatorial and axial positions. If a group is substituted for hydrogen, to regain stability, i.e. with minimum interference from other groups, this larger group should be in the equatorial position (fig. 10.22.). By convention a

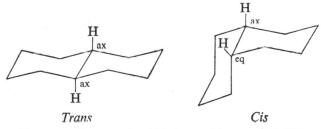

Trans   *Cis*

FIG. 10.21. Two ways in which two *cyclo*hexane rings may be fused together.

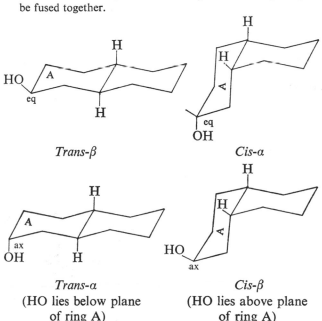

Trans-β   *Cis-α*

Trans-α
(HO lies below plane of ring A)

Cis-β
(HO lies above plane of ring A)

FIG. 10.22. Four forms of 3-HO-*cyclo*decalin.

group which sticks down below the junction of the rings is described as α to the junction, while the other possibility is described as β to the junction. Consequently, for stability the 3-hydroxyl should be α in a *cis* form and β in the *trans* form. This is the situation in the common sterols. Cholestanol, derived from cholesterol, a compound with the *trans* configuration, is a 3-β-ol while the bile acids are *cis* 3-α-ols. Using the easier flat diagrams it is customary to indicate that a group is α or below the plane of the ring junction by using a dotted bond. In this way the formulae below show part of the molecules of the bile acids and of cholestanol:

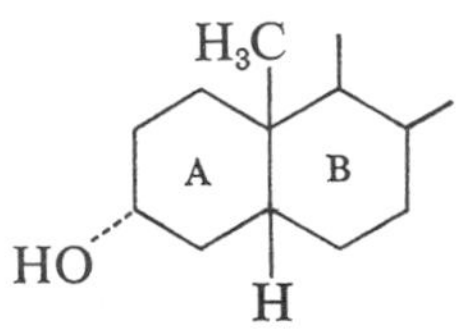

Cis-3-α-ol
Bile acid

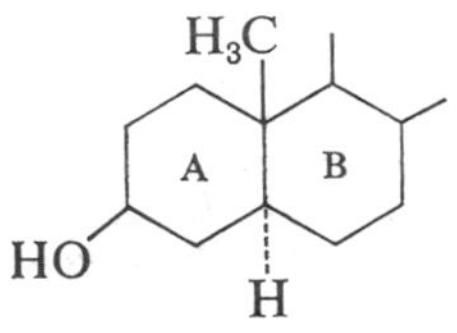

Trans-3-β-ol
Cholestanol

Cholesterol is generally written as on p. 10.5. Notice that the double bond is adjacent to the junction between rings A and B. Cholestanol is shown in fig. 10.23, in which the spatial relationships between the atoms are indicated.

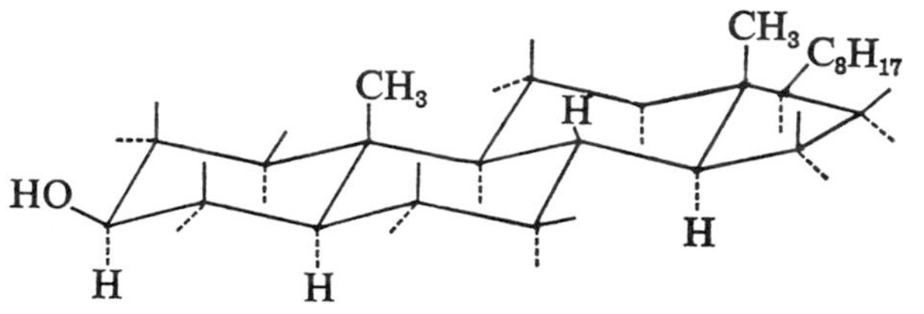

FIG. 10.23   Cholestanol.

The rings are locked together between 5, 10 and 8, 9 C atoms, resulting in the occurrence of asymmetric centres at carbon atoms 3, 5, 8, 9, 10, 13, 14, 17 and 20. The groups pointing below the molecule (downwards on the paper) are α orientated. They are written joined to the

nucleus by broken lines, while those above (β groups) are joined by continuous lines. The 3-hydroxy and angular methyl groups at 18 and 19 and the side chain are all β orientated. Fig. 10.24 shows a model of the cholesterol molecule.

Since cholesterol with its hydroxyl group is an alcohol, it is capable of forming esters with acids. Those of biological importance are with long chain fatty acids or with sulphate. On reduction of the double bond at position 5, two arrangements at C_5 are possible. Some products of microbial reduction in the gut are in the *trans* form while the *cis* form is found in the bile acids.

METABOLISM OF CHOLESTEROL

Synthesis of cholesterol

The basic building block of cholesterol, like that of fatty acids, is acetate of which three molecules after activation unite to form hydroxymethylglutaryl CoA (fig. 10.25).

Next the product is reduced to mevalonate, a process requiring $NADPH_2$ (fig. 10.26). Successive phosphorylations with ATP yield a triphospho-compound which then splits off P_i and CO_2. In this way mevalonate is converted to isopentenyl pyrophosphate which is a

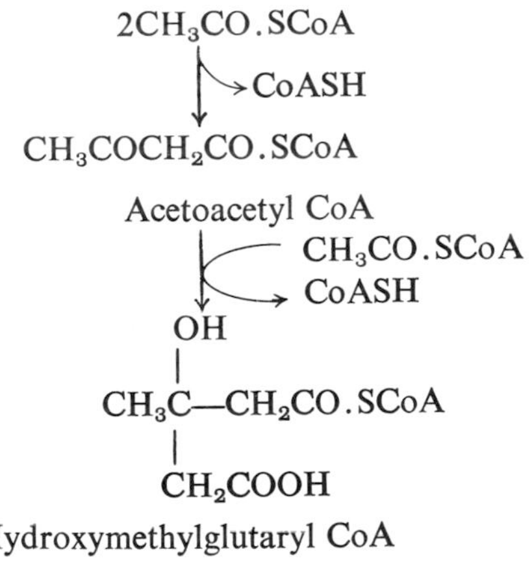

$$2CH_3CO.SCoA$$

$$\searrow CoASH$$

$$CH_3COCH_2CO.SCoA$$

Acetoacetyl CoA

$$CH_3CO.SCoA$$

$$\searrow CoASH$$

OH
|
$$CH_3C-CH_2CO.SCoA$$
|
$$CH_2COOH$$

Hydroxymethylglutaryl CoA

FIG. 10.25. Formation of hydroxymethylglutaryl CoA.

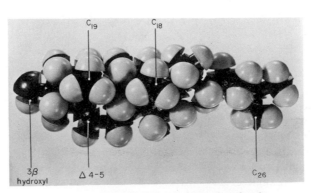

FIG. 10.24. Model of the cholesterol molecule.

derivative of the isoprene unit, a building block of long chain naturally occurring compounds, for example rubber and the carotenoid pigments (p. 10.25).

Three of these C_5 units join to form the C_{15} farnesyl pyrophosphate (fig. 10.27), two molecules of which condense to the C_{30} squalene by a reductive step utilizing $NADPH_2$. The whole process from acetate to squalene goes on in an anaerobic environment.

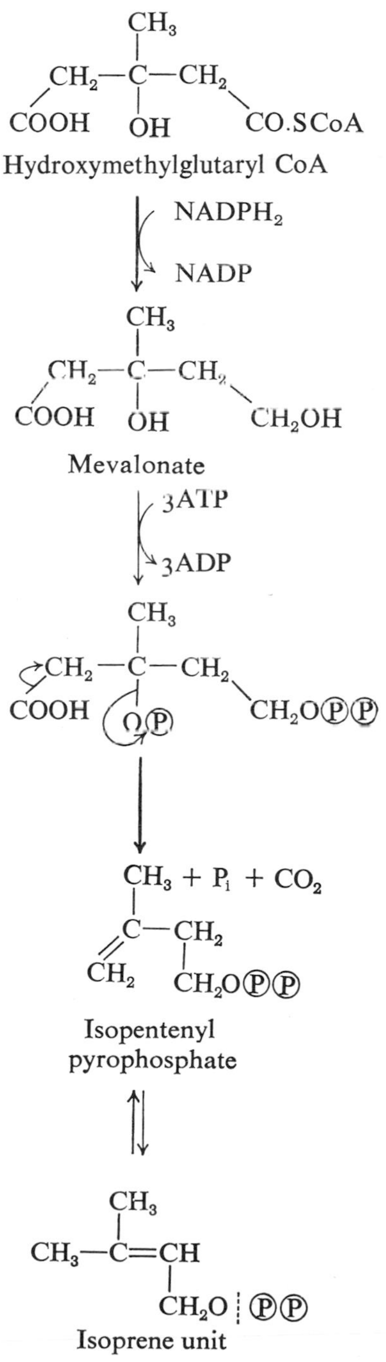

FIG. 10.26. Formation of an isoprene unit from hydroxymethylglutaryl CoA.

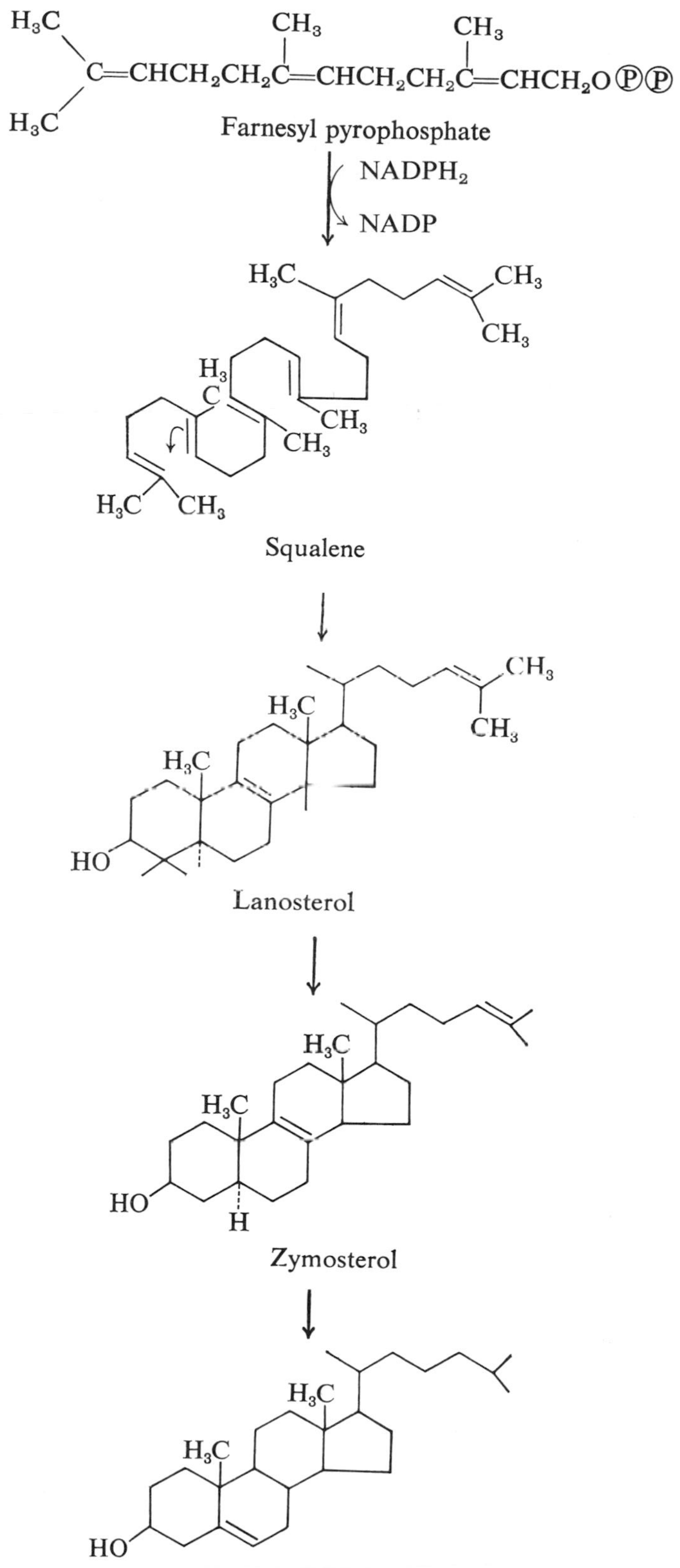

FIG. 10.27. Formation of cholesterol from farnesyl pyrophosphate.

The subsequent steps are oxidative. The C_{30} chain is folded and tailored to the 3-β-hydroxy steroid molecule, cholesterol (fig. 10.27). The sequence of steps involves oxidation by oxygen and migration of CH_3 groups from the positions held in squalene. Three other CH_3 groups are lost as CO_2. This biosynthesis is stereospecific with regard to each of the sixteen asymmetric centres of the steroid molecule. It is presumably achieved by rigid fixing of the molecule to the enzymes performing the cyclization steps.

Cholesterol is synthesized in all the tissues of the body. The slowest step which therefore determines the rate is the reduction to mevalonate. At this point a negative feedback mechanism operates in the liver, when as is usual the diet contains significant amounts of cholesterol. The responsible agent could be bile acids derived in part from the dietary cholesterol. Starvation also depresses the formation of cholesterol by the liver, hydroxymethylglutaryl CoA being degraded instead to ketone bodies (p. 10.13). In contrast, the synthesis in the extrahepatic tissues, the source of 70 per cent of the plasma cholesterol, is less sensitive to starvation.

Cholesterol esters

Cholesterol may be esterified at its free hydroxyl group by fatty acids, which are first activated to fatty acyl CoA, but in the intestinal mucosal cell esterification of the entering cholesterol is obligatory for its release into the lymph. A variety of fatty acids is found in the cholesterol esters in man, the composition depending on the tissue examined. Little of the cholesterol in the liver is esterified compared with 70 per cent in plasma or the adrenal gland.

Plasma cholesterol esters may be formed in the liver where they enter the lipoprotein fraction and subsequently appear in the blood. However, most of the newly synthesized cholesterol is secreted into plasma as free cholesterol. The free cholesterol in the plasma lipoproteins may be transesterified from the 2-fatty acyl groups of the plasma phosphatidyl choline by the LCAT enzyme (p. 10.18). The importance of the two sources of plasma cholesterol esters is not clear but after injecting ^{14}C-mevalonate into an animal there is a delay between the label appearing in the free cholesterol and in the cholesterol esters of the plasma. This suggests that the free cholesterol of liver and plasma is a precursor of plasma cholesterol esters.

Since in man all the cholesterol esters of a given plasma lipoprotein fraction turn over at the same rate, they are probably formed by the same mechanism, regardless of the fatty acid residue present. These may be saturated, mono-, di- or polyunsaturated C_{16} to C_{20} acids. The biggest proportion of plasma cholesterol esters is found in the HDL (p. 10.5) which turn over more rapidly than the LDL. Cholesterol esters may stabilize the lipoproteins in some way through their hydrophobic long fatty acid chains. They do not appear to be involved in transport of cholesterol from one tissue to another.

The cholesterol esters of the tissues are probably formed by esterification of cholesterol synthesized within the tissues themselves. They predominate over free cholesterol in those tissues in which cholesterol is a metabolic intermediate, as in the adrenal gland where steroid hormones are formed. Thus the cholesterol esters may be a reservoir of cholesterol 'nuclei' and of fatty acids available on hydrolysis for synthetic purposes. The control of cholesterol ester hydrolase, like glycogen phosphorylase, is through the phosphorylation of an enzyme under the influence of cyclic AMP.

Cholesterol is present in the free rather than the esterified form in subcellular or plasma membranes.

Bile acids

These are oxidation products of cholesterol in which one, two or three α-hydroxy groups have been introduced by a process within the microsomes involving $NADPH_2$ and oxygen. Mitochondrial oxidation partially removes the side chain with formation of a carboxyl group, and the double bond at C_{5-6} is reduced. The *cis* configuration is found at the junction of rings A and B.

Cholic acid and chenodeoxycholic acid are the primary bile acids. Fig. 10.28 indicates their structure. They are formed in the liver; two other bile acids, deoxycholic acid and lithocholic acid, are formed from them by intestinal bacterial action (p. 33.7).

Compounds with a free 3β-hydroxy group, e.g. cholesterol, are precipitated by digitonin which is itself a steroid glycoside. This provides a method of separating cholesterol from other steroids and 3α-hydroxy acids. A quantitative method of assaying cholesterol is the Liebermann–Burchardt reaction. It is based on the blue–green colour formed when cholesterol is mixed with

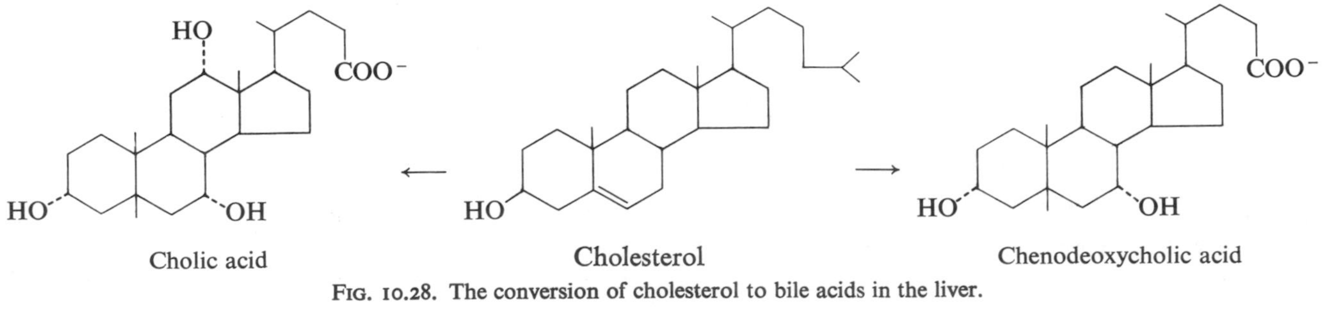

Cholic acid   Cholesterol   Chenodeoxycholic acid

FIG. 10.28. The conversion of cholesterol to bile acids in the liver.

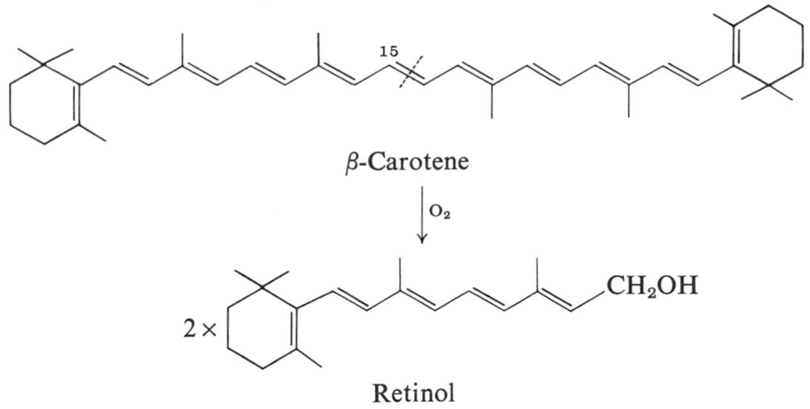

FIG. 10.29. The conversion of β-carotene to retinol.

concentrated sulphuric acid and acetic anhydride. The bile acids with three α hydroxy groups at 3, 7 and 12, or two hydroxy groups at 3 and 7 or 3 and 12, give a pink colour with furfural under acid conditions. This is the Pettenkofer reaction.

FAT-SOLUBLE VITAMINS

An account of the nutritional aspects of these substances is given on p. 5.13.

VITAMIN A
Vitamin A or retinol is a pale yellow substance quite insoluble in water. As already described, part is supplied preformed in the diet and part is derived by oxidation in the body of carotenes, which are water-insoluble, coloured pigments present in plants. β-Carotene, which is orange in colour, is the main source of retinol and the conversion is shown in fig. 10.29.

Retinol and carotene are stable to heat and temperatures normally used in cooking but are readily oxidized. With the high temperatures used in frying, losses are small if exposure to air is limited as in deep frying, but with shallow frying pans all vitamin activity may be lost.

Retinol reacts with antimony trichloride to form a bright blue compound with an absorption maximum at 620 nm and this property is used for assay purposes both in foods and in tissues.

VITAMIN D
Vitamin D exists in several forms. The natural form, cholecalciferol or vitamin D_3, is formed by the action of sunlight on 7-dehydrocholesterol, a sterol widely distributed in the skin and all animal fats. Vitamin D_2 (calciferol), used in therapeutics, is formed from the irradiation of ergosterol, a sterol found in fungi and yeast. This compound differs from 7-dehydrocholesterol in having, as a side chain, C_9H_{17}. In the body it is the 1,25 dihydroxy derivatives of cholecalciferol and calciferol that are active. In the body, the liver first inserts the C_{25} hydroxyl group and then the kidneys insert the C_1 hydroxyl group (fig. 10.30). This reaction is diminished

in certain kidney diseases in which evidence of vitamin D deficiency persists, in spite of administration of calciferol (vol. 3, p. 22.10).

VITAMIN E
Vitamin E is a mixture of tocopherols, which are yellow oily liquids remarkably stable to heat. α-Tocopherol has the following structure:

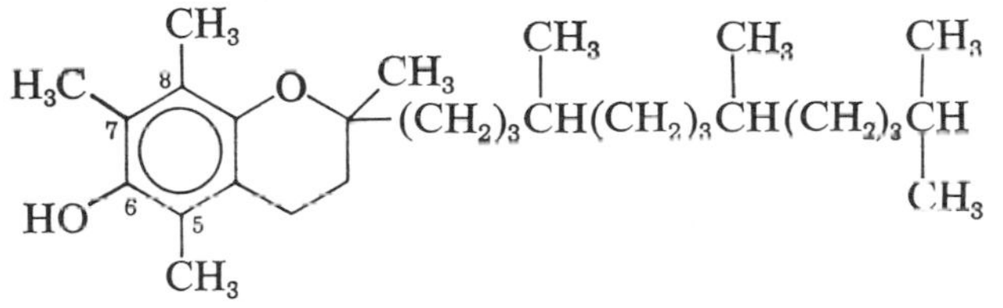

Vitamin E; α-(or trimethyl)-tocopherol

Five other tocopherols have vitamin E activity; they differ structurally in having only one or two methyl groups in the 5, 7 or 8 positions.

VITAMIN K
Vitamin K exists in nature in two forms and several synthetic analogues are used clinically. Vitamins K_1 and K_2 are both derivatives of the cyclic structure naphthoquinone and each has a long side chain designated R in the formula:

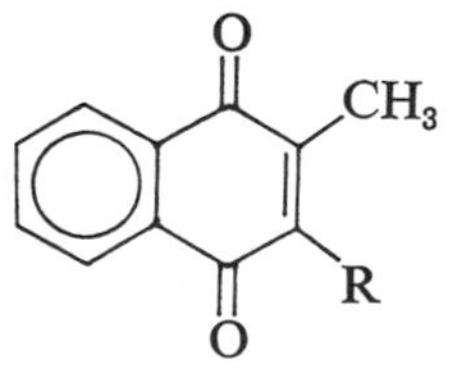

In K_1, 2-methyl-3-phytyl-1,4-naphthoquinone, R is

$$-CH_2-CH=\overset{\overset{\displaystyle CH_3}{|}}{C}-(CH_2-CH_2-CH_2-\overset{\overset{\displaystyle CH_3}{|}}{CH}-)_3CH_3$$

In K_2, 2-methyl-3-difarnesyl-1, 4-naphthoquinone, R is

$$-CH_2-(CH=\overset{\overset{\displaystyle CH_3}{|}}{C}-CH_2-CH_2-)_5CH=\overset{\overset{\displaystyle CH_3}{|}}{C}-CH_3$$

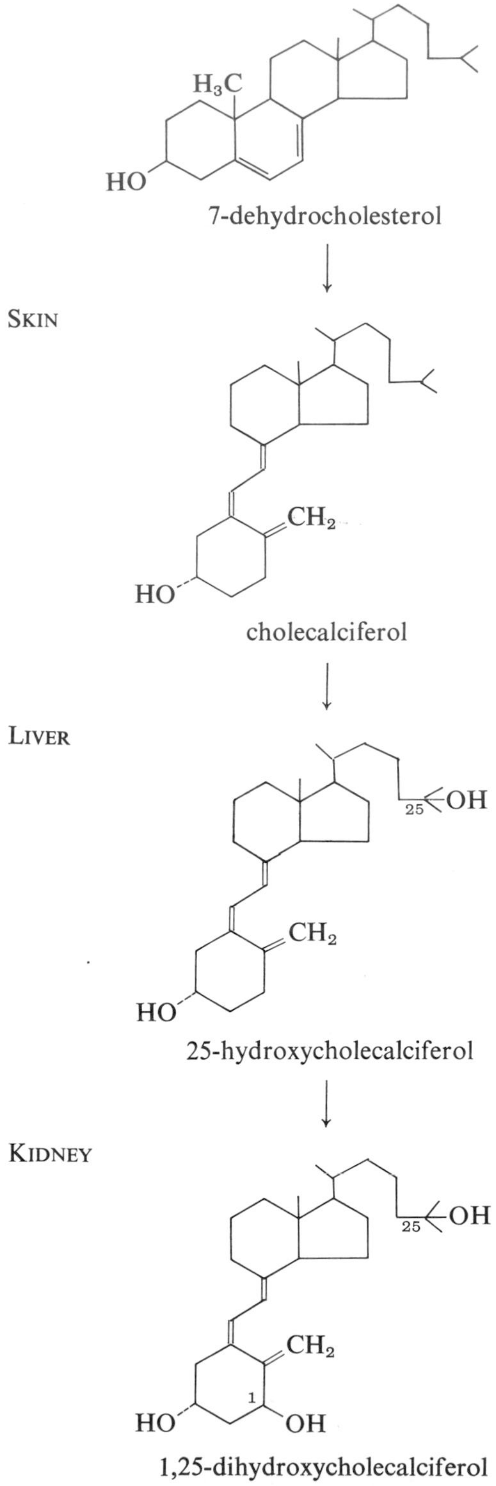

7-dehydrocholesterol

SKIN

cholecalciferol

LIVER

25-hydroxycholecalciferol

KIDNEY

1,25-dihydroxycholecalciferol

METABOLIC ROLES OF THE FAT-SOLUBLE VITAMINS

The precise role of vitamin A is established only in respect of its action in night vision. The *cis* form of the aldehyde retinal, which is derived from the vitamin, combines with a protein (opsin) to form the visual pigment, rhodopsin. When this is bleached by light, it breaks down into opsin and retinal, this time in the *trans* form. This is converted back into the vitamin which then undergoes conversion to the *cis* form, which is ready for reoxidation to retinal (*cis*). The conversions are summarized in fig. 10.31:

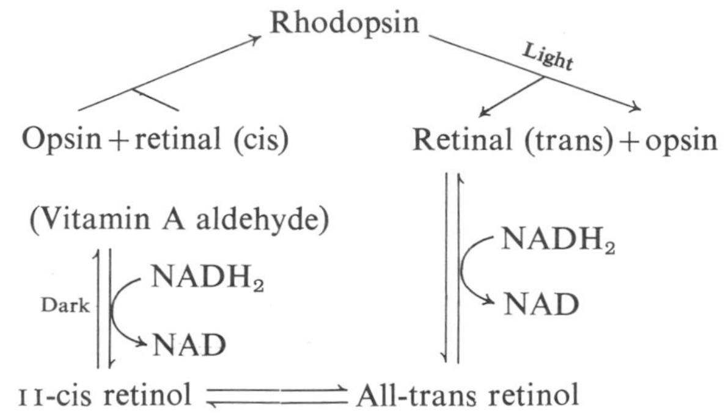

FIG. 10.31. Relation of rhodopsin to retinol.

Other aspects of night vision are discussed on pp. 5.13 and 26.14. As the regeneration process is slow, a sufficient quantity of vitamin A aldehyde must be present if vision in poor light is to be maintained.

The part retinol plays in the metabolism of epithelial cells, bone and other tissues is far from certain. In rats deficient in vitamin A there is a decrease in synthesis in the goblet cells of the small intestine of a fucose-containing glycopeptide and also in synthesis in the liver of a glycolipid containing mannose. It is possible that retinol acts as a carrier for carbohydrates necessary for the manufacture of components of intracellular membranes.

Vitamin D is essential for the normal absorption of calcium from the small intestine and for its deposition in growing bone; these effects are probably brought about by inducing a specific RNA required in the synthesis of a protein carrier for Ca^{++}.

The polyunsaturated fatty acids such as linoleic acid are sensitive to autoxidation in the presence of oxygen. This is a free radical attack.

$$R_1CH_2CH=CHCH_2CH=CHCH_2R_2$$
$$\downarrow O_2$$
$$R_1CH_2CH=CHCH=CHCHCH_2R_2$$
$$|$$
$$OO\cdot$$

It can be suppressed by anti-oxidants such as the tocopherols. This autoxidation is most readily demonstrated in chicks fed a diet rich in polyunsaturated fatty acids and low in vitamin E. In the absence of vitamin E peroxidation reactions in membranes seem to be accelerated. Whether vitamin E has a significant action in these respects in health is uncertain.

Vitamin K is necessary for the formation of prothrombin and other clotting factors in the liver, but how it affects the synthesis of these proteins is not known. Uncoupling of oxidative phosphorylation in mitochondria obtained from vitamin K-deficient chicks has been observed.

FURTHER READING

DEUEL H.J. (1951–57). *The Lipids; their Chemistry and Biochemistry*, vols. I–III. New York: Interscience.

GUNSTONE F.D. (1968) *An Introduction to the Chemistry and Biochemistry of Fatty Acids and their Glycerides*, 2nd Edition. London: Chapman & Hall.

GURR M.I. & JAMES A.T. (1975) *Lipid Biochemistry; an Introduction*, 2nd Edition. London: Chapman & Hall.

MASORO E.J. (1968) *Physiological Chemistry of Lipids in Mammals*. Philadelphia: Saunders.

PAOLETTI R. & KRITCHEVSKY D. eds. (1963–75) *Advances in Lipid Research*, vols. 1–13. New York: Academic Press.

Chapter 11
Protein metabolism

The proteins form a group of macromolecular nitrogenous substances with such a wide range of physical and chemical properties that they serve diverse physiological functions. Some highly insoluble proteins, such as the keratins of skin, hair and nails are comparatively inert, but are indispensable structural components; others, including the proteins of muscle and connective tissue, are concerned with mechanical function as well as structure. Some more soluble proteins are used for transporting oxygen, iron, copper, lipids and a variety of hormones about the body. Perhaps the most striking fact is that all enzymes are proteins.

Living organisms must therefore obtain compounds containing nitrogen as well as carbon, hydrogen and oxygen for the synthesis of proteins. Higher animals, including man, are unable to utilize inorganic nitrogenous compounds to a significant extent, and are therefore dependent on other forms of life for a suitable dietary supply of nitrogen. For them protein is an important and indispensable constituent of the diet. More than 90 per cent of the nitrogen of all living cells is present in the form of protein, which is the ultimate product of a complex system of intracellular synthetic machinery. The nitrogen content of nearly all proteins is close to 16 per cent. It is therefore common practice to determine protein approximately in crude biological materials by measuring the nitrogen content and applying the simple equation: protein $= N \times 6 \cdot 25$.

In spite of the great diversity of their properties, all proteins can be hydrolysed, either by treatment with a series of enzymes or by boiling for some hours with moderately concentrated acid (5–6 mol/l HCl) to give a mixture of amino acids. **Simple proteins** give only amino acids on hydrolysis. **Conjugated proteins** give, in addition, other substances. A molecule, other than an amino acid, obtained by the hydrolysis of a conjugated protein is called a **prosthetic group** (p. 7.13). These vary greatly in the nature and strength of the bonds which link them to the main part of the protein molecule, and many of them are liberated by treatment which is too mild to hydrolyse the protein into its constituent amino acids. Conjugated proteins are classified according to the nature of the prosthetic group. Thus, haemoproteins contain haem,

phosphoproteins phosphate and glycoproteins carbohydrate. Many enzymes are conjugated proteins.

AMINO ACIDS

As their name indicates, amino acids are substances which contain both amino and acidic groups. Very large numbers of such compounds are known to organic chemistry but only about twenty are found as products of the hydrolysis of proteins. All but two of these are 2-amino acids, i.e. the amino group is linked to the carbon atom adjacent to the carboxyl group:

$$R-\overset{\displaystyle COOH}{\underset{\displaystyle NH_2}{CH}}$$

Formerly, carbon atoms in amino acids were labelled α, β, γ, etc., the α carbon atom being adjacent to the carboxyl group, i.e. in the two position. This system is still much used.

In the simplest amino acid, aminoacetic acid or glycine, $R = H$. In other amino acids, R may be a straight chain or branched aliphatic radical; it may contain a hydroxyl group, a thiol or a thioether group; it may possess additional basic or acidic groups or a cyclic radical. The important amino acids are given, with their formulae and commonly used abbreviations, in table 11.1.

The formulae show that all the amino acids except glycine ought to be optically active and this has been found to be so. However, only the L-form of each acid, i.e. the isomer which is theoretically derived from L(—)serine, is found as a product of protein hydrolysis, although there are rare instances of the biological occurrence of D-amino acids, particularly D-glutamic acid.

General chemical properties
The individual amino acids possess specific properties which depend on the nature of R and general properties

TABLE 11.1. Some biologically important aminoacids. Those marked E cannot be synthesized by adult men and are essential constituents of the diet. (p. 11.14.)

Name		Standard abbreviation	R
Glycine		Gly	$H-$
Alanine		Ala	CH_3-
Valine	E	Val	$(CH_3)_2CH-$
Leucine	E	Leu	$(CH_3)_2CH-CH_2-$
Isoleucine	E	Ile	$C_2H_5-CH(CH_3)-$
Serine		Ser	CH_2OH-
Threonine	E	Thr	$CH_3-CHOH-$
Aspartic acid		Asp	$HOOC-CH_2-$
Asparagine		Asn	$H_2NOC-CH_2-$
Glutamic acid		Glu	$HOOC-CH_2-CH_2-$
Glutamine		Gln	$H_2NOC-CH_2-CH_2-$
Lysine	E	Lys	$H_2N(CH_2)_4-$
Ornithine*		Orn	$H_2N(CH_2)_3-$
Arginine		Arg	(guanidino structure) $\begin{array}{c}H_2N \\ HN\end{array}\!\!\!>\!\!C-NH-(CH_2)_3-$
Histidine		His	(imidazole) CH_2- ring
Phenylalanine	E	Phe	(phenyl) $-CH_2-$
Tyrosine		Tyr	$HO-$(phenyl)$-CH_2-$
Tryptophan	E	Trp	(indole) CH_2-
Cysteine		Cys	$HSCH_2-$
Cystine		CySSCy	Formed from 2Cys
Methionine	E	Met	$CH_3-S-(CH_2)_2-$

FORMULA

Name	Standard abbreviation	
Proline	Pro	(pyrrolidine ring) $\overset{N}{\underset{H}{}}\!\!-COOH$
Hydroxyproline	Hyp	HO-(pyrrolidine ring) $\overset{N}{\underset{H}{}}\!\!-COOH$

3-Alanine*			$H_2N-CH_2-CH_2-COOH$
γ-Aminobutyric acid*			$H_2N-CH_2-CH_2-CH_2-COOH$

* These amino acids are not found in proteins, although of biological importance.

which are determined largely by the 2-amino-carboxyl group. The latter vary slightly on account of the influence of R. The amino group itself is responsible for a purple colour produced when amino acids are warmed with ninhydrin, a complex triketone. This reaction is useful for the detection of amino acids on paper chromatograms or electrophoresis strips. Proteins give a similar but much weaker reaction.

The amino group reacts readily with 1-fluoro-2-4-dinitrobenzene to give a dinitrophenyl derivative of the amino acid:

$$R-\underset{\underset{NH_2}{|}}{\overset{\overset{COOH}{|}}{CH}} + \text{(F, NO}_2\text{, NO}_2\text{ ring)} \longrightarrow R-\underset{\underset{NH}{|}}{\overset{\overset{COOH}{|}}{CH}} \text{(NO}_2\text{, NO}_2\text{ ring)} + HF$$

The compounds produced are bright yellow and easily identified on chromatograms. The reaction is useful for identifying free amino groups in protein molecules.

When an amino acid is dissolved in water, the carboxyl group tends to lose a proton while the amino group becomes protonated:

$$R-\underset{\underset{NH_2}{|}}{\overset{\overset{COOH}{|}}{CH}} \rightleftharpoons R-\underset{\underset{NH_3^+}{|}}{\overset{\overset{COO^-}{|}}{CH}}$$

The resulting structure has both a positive and a negative charge, but the net charge is zero unless there are other ionizable groups in the molecule. Such a structure is called a **zwitterion**. In an electric field it migrates neither to the cathode nor the anode (fig. 11.2).

The addition of acid to a solution containing the zwitterion form of an amino acid causes the carboxyl group to become protonated:

$$R-\underset{\underset{NH_3^+}{|}}{\overset{\overset{COO^-}{|}}{CH}} + H^+ \rightleftharpoons R-\underset{\underset{NH_3^+}{|}}{\overset{\overset{COOH}{|}}{CH}}$$

This equilibrium depends to some extent on the influence of R, but for most amino acids pK_{a_1} is around 2·6.

Conversely, the addition of base to a zwitterion solution detaches the proton from the amino group, leaving the carboxyl fully dissociated:

$$R-\underset{\underset{NH_3^+}{|}}{\overset{\overset{COO^-}{|}}{CH}} + OH^- \rightleftharpoons H_2O + R-\underset{\underset{NH_2}{|}}{\overset{\overset{COO^-}{|}}{CH}}$$

This dissociation again depends slightly on R, but for most amino acids pK_{a_2} is about 9·6.

The pH range over which an amino acid assumes the zwitterion structure is called the isoelectric region and the arithmetic midpoint of this is the **isoelectric point**. Both above and below the isoelectric region the solution acts as a buffer. These important physiochemical points are summarized in fig. 11.1, which shows graphically the

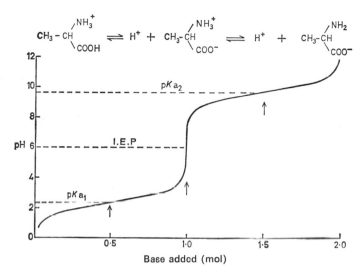

FIG. 11·1. Titration curve of alanine, showing pK values, isoelectric point, and the structural formulae corresponding to the stages of the titration.

pH changes which follow the addition of base to the acid form of the amino acid alanine.

Separation of amino acid mixtures

Electrophoresis is the migration of a charged solute, e.g. an amino acid in an electric field. Unless the pH is near the isoelectric point, the amino acid migrates towards one of the electrodes. In a buffer of suitably chosen pH the properties of a wide range of amino acids are sufficiently different for effective separations to be made by electrophoresis on supporting media like paper, cellulose acetate or polyacrylamide gel. Fig. 11.2 shows a paper electropherogram of the amino acids found in the urine of a healthy subject and one with cystinuria, a hereditary condition in which the patient's urine contains excessive quantities of cystine and basic amino acids (vol. 3, p. 47.3).

Ion exchange is a more effective technique of separation for larger quantities of amino acids when quantitative analysis is required. A buffered amino acid solution is allowed to percolate slowly through a long narrow column packed with a highly polymerized insoluble substance containing free acidic or basic groups. If the pH is suitable, the amino acid ions are electrostatically

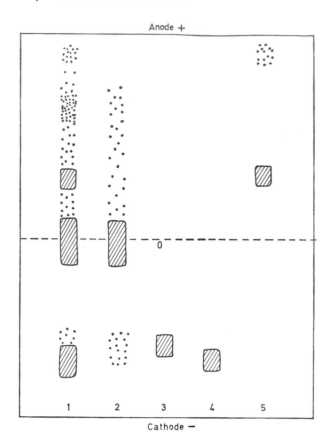

FIG. 11.2. Amino acid patterns of urines after paper electrophoresis at pH 8·6. 0, line on which the spots of urine or amino acid solution were applied. 1, Cystinuric urine; 2, Normal urine; 3, 4, 5, standards of lysine, arginine and cystine, respectively. The monobasic, monoacidic amino acids migrate very little at pH 8·6 and are clustered round the point of application of the urine. From Goulden B.E. & Leaver J.L. (1967) *Vet. Rec.*, **80**, 244.

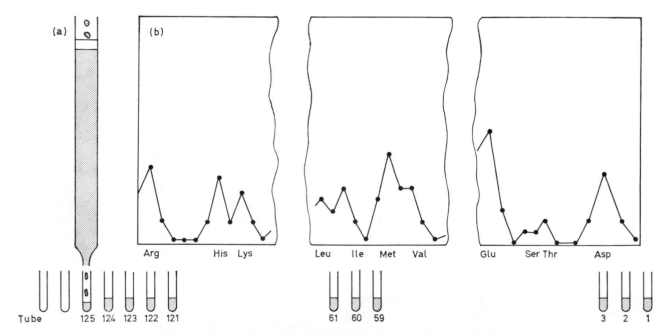

FIG. 11.3. Separation of amino acids by ion exchange chromatography. (a) Column packed with ion exchange resin and loaded with amino acid mixture through which is dripped a series of buffer solutions. The eluate is collected in constant volume fractions which are analysed quantitatively by the ninhydrin reaction. The points on the chart (b) represent intensities of colour given with ninhydrin in individual tubes.

bonded to the ion exchanger and may be liberated serially, according to their properties, by altering the composition of the buffer which drips through the column. The process, which is illustrated in fig. 11.3, is widely used in studying the amino acid mixtures obtained by hydrolysis of purified proteins.

Paper chromatography is an ingenious and popular separation technique which uses the differences both in distribution coefficients of amino acids between various pairs of solvent mixtures and in the extent to which different amino acids are adsorbed to paper. The diversity in the structure of R (table 11.1) causes distinct changes in the solubilities of the amino acids in different solvents. In an atmosphere containing solvent vapours, the fibres of a piece of filter paper become saturated with the solvent. Even in the absence of other solvents, paper contains a good deal of water. If a small spot of a solution of amino acids is placed near one end of a piece of filter paper and a suitable mixture of solvents, e.g. *n*-butanol, water and acetic acid, is allowed to flow across the paper, the amino acids migrate across the paper at different rates, determined partly by differential adsorption but chiefly by differences between their relative solubilities in the mobile solvent mixture and the solvent (water) in the paper fibres. When the paper has been almost completely covered by the moving solvent it is dried, sprayed with ninhydrin and warmed to colour the amino acid spots. Individual compounds can be identified by comparing the rate of flow (R_f = distance travelled by substance/distance travelled by solvent front) with that of known amino acids applied to the paper as separate spots. Separations by paper chromatography can often be improved by turning the dried paper (without staining it) through 90° and making a second run with a different solvent mixture. Fig. 11.4 illustrates such a two-dimensional paper chromatogram given by an amino acid mixture.

Thin layer chromatography (TLC) is a chromatographic process in which a thin layer of cellulose powder, silica gel or other suitable material is spread on a glass plate for use in much the same way as paper chromatography. One of its advantages is that excellent separations can often be obtained on small plates in an hour or two whereas the paper technique may need a whole day. Both techniques are also useful for the separation, purification and identification of drugs and other substances of medical interest.

Properties of individual amino acids

The radical R confers on the individual amino acids many specific chemical properties. Thus glutamic and aspartic acids have each an additional carboxyl group, the properties of which are superimposed on those of the amino-carboxyl group. Sometimes the additional carboxyl groups are found as amides, e.g. in glutamine and asparagine, which are no longer markedly acidic. Other 2-amino acids have additional amino groups (lysine, ornithine) or other basic groups (histidine, arginine).

Several of the more complex radicals found in the amino acids, e.g. the phenolic ring in tyrosine, the indole ring in tryptophan and the guanidinyl group in arginine, give characteristic colour reactions which are useful for either identifying the compounds or their quantitative determination. Usually the reaction is given not only by the free amino acid but also, perhaps in a modified form, by proteins which contain it.

Although all the amino acids are colourless, some, notably tyrosine and tryptophan, have striking absorption bands in the ultraviolet, with maxima close to 275 and 280 nm respectively. The intensity of absorption in this region of the spectrum is often used for the quantitative estimation of these amino acids or of proteins which contain them, in the same way as absorption at 260 nm is used as a measure of nucleic acid concentration.

The sulphydryl group of cysteine is readily split off by warming with dilute alkali and, in the presence of lead acetate, a black precipitate or dark brown coloration of lead sulphide is produced. The sulphydryl group is also very susceptible to oxidation, when two of the groups react together to give a disulphide:

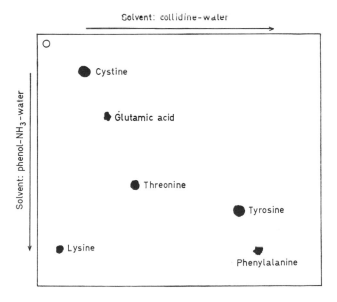

FIG. 11.4. Two-dimensional paper chromatography of amino acids. ○, point of application of mixture. From McElroy W.D. (1964) *Cell Physiology and Biochemistry*, 2nd Edition. New Jersey: Prentice-Hall.

$$\begin{matrix} COOH \\ | \\ CHNH_2 \\ | \\ CH_2SH \end{matrix} + \begin{matrix} COOH \\ | \\ CHNH_2 \\ | \\ HSCH_2 \end{matrix} \underset{+2H}{\overset{-2H}{\rightleftharpoons}} \begin{matrix} COOH \\ | \\ CHNH_2 \\ | \\ CH_2-S \end{matrix} \begin{matrix} COOH \\ | \\ CHNH_2 \\ | \\ -S-CH_2 \end{matrix}$$

The double molecule of the free amino acid is called cystine. This redox reaction is freely reversible.

PEPTIDES

When a protein free extract of yeast is treated with cuprous oxide, the insoluble cuprous salt of an amino acid derivative called **glutathione** is precipitated. Although first isolated in this way from yeast, glutathione is present in most, perhaps in all living cells. It has a molecular weight of 307 and belongs to the class of substances known as peptides. When boiled with acid it gives equimolar proportions of glutamic acid, glycine and cysteine. The last named is usually obtained in the oxidized form, cystine. On treatment with dilute NaOH and a trace of copper sulphate, glutathione gives a purple colour. This test is positive with biuret (NH_2—CO—NH—CO—NH_2) and with all substances containing more than one peptide link or bond (—CO—NH—). In glutathione the three amino acids are linked together by two peptide bonds:

$$
\begin{array}{l}
\text{COOH} \\
|\\
\text{CHNH}_2 \qquad\qquad \text{Peptide bonds}\\
|\\
\text{CH}_2 \qquad\qquad\quad \text{CH}_2\text{SH}\\
|\\
\text{CH}_2\text{—CO—NH—CH—CO—NH—CH}_2\text{—COOH}
\end{array}
$$

4-Glutamyl   Cysteinyl   Glycine

One unusual feature of the structure is the linking of the glutamic acid to the rest of the molecule by a peptide bond involving the 4-carboxyl group. Even in the case of the dicarboxylic acids, almost all peptide bonds involve the carboxyl group next to the —NH_2.

A characteristic property of glutathione is its reversible oxidation to the disulphide form:

$$ 2GSH \underset{+2H}{\overset{-2H}{\rightleftharpoons}} G\text{—S—S—G} $$

This type of reaction takes place with all peptide structures, including proteins, which contain cysteine.

Glutathione, which contains three amino acid residues, is a tripeptide, as is TRH the thyrotrophin releasing hormone secreted by the hypothalamus. The molecules of oxytocin and vasopressin, the neurohypophyseal hormones (p. 27.16) each contain nine amino acid residues while those of the hormones glucagon and ACTH contain twenty-nine and thirty-nine respectively. Such compounds are called polypeptides. Peptides of varying molecular weights are widespread in low concentrations and fulfil an assortment of functions. They are also formed in the gut by the action of digestive enzymes on proteins in food.

PROTEINS

Proteins, like peptides, give a positive biuret test and can be hydrolysed to give a mixture of amino acids. Protein solutions give many of the amino acid tests which do not depend on the 2-aminocarboxyl radical. Analysis shows that —COOH and —NH_2 are produced in equivalent amounts during the hydrolysis of a protein. It therefore appears that protein molecules consist of amino acids linked together by peptide bonds:

$$
\begin{array}{ccc}
R_1 & R_2 & R_3 \\
| & | & | \\
\end{array}
$$
$$ \text{—NH—CH—CO—NH—CH—CO—NH—CH—CO—} $$

Such a statement, however, only begins to describe the structure of a protein molecule. How large is the molecule? How many molecules of each amino acid are present in a protein molecule? In what order are the amino acids arranged? Does the molecule consist of one large polypeptide chain, or of two or more linked together? Is the molecule freely flexible or does it assume some definite shape? What forces or bonds maintain the shape of a protein? In the case of a conjugated protein, it is also necessary to consider the location of the prosthetic group and the way in which it is bound to the polypeptide chain.

The answers to these questions are of two kinds: those which deal with such purely chemical matters as amino acid numbers and sequence, and those which deal with physical matters like the actual shape of the molecules. The first group is said to deal with the primary structure of proteins, the second with secondary and tertiary structure.

Purification of proteins

No solution can be found to these problems until a protein has been isolated in a pure state, free from other proteins. Protein molecules with rare exceptions are insoluble in organic solvents. These often also damage their delicate structure and consequently interfere with their properties. Even moderate heat is often harmful. Hence the common techniques for the purification of organic compounds are usually not applicable to proteins. Special techniques have been developed, many of which have found applications in clinical biochemistry and other fields of medical interest.

DIALYSIS

Early in the history of proteins it was observed that they are not dialysable; if a protein solution containing also substances of low molecular weight (salts, sugars, urea or amino acids) is placed in a cellophane sac, permeable only to substances of low molecular weight, and the sac is suspended in a vessel of water, then the protein remains in the sac while the other substances diffuse out. If the external liquid contains salts or a buffer or some other dialysable substance, then this passes into the sac, so that by using repeated changes of the external liquid, or a continuous flow, the other constituents of a protein solution can be changed in any desired way. Dialysis is widely used in the isolation and purification of proteins in the automated clinical chemical analysis of blood plasma or serum, and in procedures where the separation of proteins from small molecules is required. The discovery that proteins are not dialysable gave an early indication that they are substances of high molecular weight.

GEL FILTRATION

This is a modern development of dialysis in which a small volume of protein solution, followed by a continuous flow of water or a salt solution or a buffer, is passed down a vertical glass column packed with fine particles of gel (dextran or polyacrylamide). The gel particles function as tiny dialysis sacs into which substances of low molecular weight diffuse freely, while the protein molecules are excluded by their large size, being restricted to the space between the gel particles. Hence, as the constituents of the original protein solution flow down the column, solutes of low molecular weight pass more or less freely in and out of the gel particles, while the proteins, not being delayed in this way, flow more rapidly and therefore emerge from the foot of the column first. The procedure is illustrated in fig. 11.5. Gel filtration can

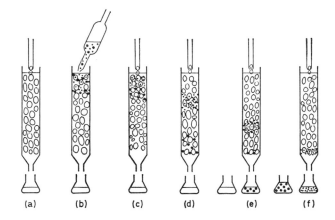

FIG. 11.5. Gel filtration: (a) prepared column; ○, gel particles, magnified several thousand times. (b) Application of sample; ●, large protein molecules, ⫶⫶⫶ solutes of low-molecular weight. (c, d); Separation commences; low molecular weight solutes travel more slowly because the molecules permeate the gel particles. (e, f) Collection of the separated materials in different flasks.

be adapted to the separation of proteins of different molecular weight by the use of gel particles specially made to have exclusion limits well into the range of molecular weights of proteins.

ELECTROPHORESIS

In the molecule of a protein there are very many ionizable groups and, as the properties of these are modified by neighbouring groups, the pattern of change in ionization with change in pH is very much more complex than in the case of any of the amino acids. As the pH moves from the acid side, where the positive charges of protonated amino groups predominate, to the alkaline side, where the negative charges of ionized carboxyls are more numerous, a definite point is passed where the sums of the charges of opposite sign are equal. This is the isoelectric point, and at this pH the protein does not migrate in an electric field. Strictly speaking, the above definition refers to the theoretical **isoionic point,** and the experimentally observed isoelectric point is slightly different because of the effects of ions adsorbed from the chosen buffer. However, in general there will be an excess of positively or negatively charged groups, and it is possible to separate proteins in a mixture into groups which have similar ratios of net charge to mass. Electrophoresis is commonly carried out on a strip of filter paper or cellulose acetate, or in a small glass tube containing clear polyacrylamide gel. It is used to check the homogeneity of a purified protein preparation or to ascertain the relative proportions of different groups of proteins in plasma or other body fluids. Most proteins are colourless but they can be located by staining with the dark blue dye naphthalene black. The intensity of the stain corresponds approximately to the amount of each protein present. A diagram showing the separation by electrophoresis of the major groups of proteins in normal serum is given on p. 33.17. This technique can be made more sensitive and more informative if the protein fractions are identified by reaction with specific immunological antibodies. It is then called **immuno-electrophoresis.**

Proteins can also be separated by ion exchange (p. 11.3). With such complex mixtures of proteins as are found in plasma, this is too tedious for routine analysis, but the technique is invaluable for the purification of many individual proteins.

SALT PRECIPITATION

An older but still useful technique makes use of the fact that many proteins are precipitated from solution by high concentrations of inorganic salts, e.g. ammonium sulphate. A once popular classification of the proteins was based on differences in solubility in water and salt solutions of different concentration. By definition, albumins are proteins which are soluble in water and dilute salt solutions and are only precipitated by complete saturation of the solution with ammonium sulphate. Globulins are insoluble in water, soluble in dilute salt and precipitated by lower concentrations of ammonium sulphate; the original standard was half the concentration required to saturate the solution, but many globulins are more easily precipitated. An interesting clinical application of the salting out technique is the distinction of haemoglobin from the closely related pigment myoglobin; this distinction may be important, because both pigments may be present in the urine after crush injuries. Haemoglobin is precipitated in ammonium sulphate solution, 2·8 mol/l, but myoglobin remains soluble until the concentration reaches 3·4 mol/l.

AFFINITY CHROMATOGRAPHY

This technique may effect a high degree of purification in a single step. The procedure depends on the use of an inert material, often a polysaccharide, which is suitable both for use in a column and for chemical combination with some reagent having a specific affinity for the substance to be isolated. After the reagent has been attached to its inert support, the column is packed, and when a solution containing the desired substance (perhaps after only a moderate degree of preliminary purification) is passed through, the substance is retained by means of its affinity for the previously bound specific reagent. Unwanted material can be washed out before elution of the desired substance by an appropriate procedure. The technique is used widely in the field of immunochemistry both for the isolation of proteins after the attachment of specific antibodies to the column material and for the isolation of antibodies by the converse procedure. It is also used in the technically difficult separation of functionally related types of RNA, e.g. fractionation of m-RNA.

Molecular weights of proteins

Although protein molecules are too large to pass through a dialysis membrane, those of the common soluble proteins are much too small to settle out of solution under the simple force of gravity. Modern centrifugal methods, however, can easily give gravitational fields of the order of 10^5–10^6 g, and under these conditions the molecules of proteins can be sedimented and to some extent separated according to their size and weight.

Most of the recorded molecular weights of proteins have been determined by centrifugal methods. The rate at which the molecules of a protein sediment in the gravitational field of a high-speed centrifuge depends on several factors:

(1) the molecular weight of the protein,

(2) the partial specific volume, which is a measure of the contribution of the protein to the total volume of the solution,

(3) the gravitational force, which is related to the angular velocity (a function of the speed of revolution) and the effective radius of the centrifuge rotor,

(4) the diffusion coefficient, which is a measure of the effect of the solvent (usually water) and the salts, buffer components or other solutes of low mol. wt. on the movement of the protein molecules.

Since there are independent methods for the evaluation of both diffusion coefficients and partial specific volumes, and the gravitational force is easily calculated for the particular centrifuge used, it is possible to estimate the mol. wt. of any protein by measuring, usually by an optical method, its rate of sedimentation.

Physical techniques such as gel filtration and electrophoresis can be adapted to the estimation of the molecular weights of proteins, and these methods are often less laborious than those which use the analytical ultracentrifuge.

Sometimes the molecule, usually of a conjugated protein, contains such a small proportion of some element or chemical grouping that this gives a minimum value for the mol. wt. For example, both haemoglobin and myoglobin contain about 0·34 per cent Fe. If it is assumed that each protein molecule contains one atom of iron, the mol. wt. in both cases works out at about 16 400. Osmotic and centrifugal methods show that in fact the mol. wt. of myoglobin is close to this figure, but that of haemoglobin is about four times as high, 65 000. The original assumption is therefore correct for myoglobin, but not for haemoglobin. The exercise thus discloses that the molecule of haemoglobin must contain four atoms of iron.

Table 11.2 gives examples of the mol. wt. of proteins.

TABLE 11.2. The molecular weights of some proteins.

Protein	Molecular weight (daltons)
Insulin	5 700
Cytochrome c	12 500
Pepsin	35 000
Haemoglobin (human)	65 000
Catalase	250 000
Apoferritin	440 000

Primary structure of proteins

The proportions of the different amino acids which make up a protein molecule can be ascertained by quantitative hydrolysis, ion-exchange separation and estimation of the amounts of the individual amino acids. Representative figures are given in table 11.3. For the complete elucidation of structure the next task is the immense one of determining the order in which the various amino acid residues are linked together. A useful starting point is the amino acid bearing a free amino group at one end of the polypeptide chain. This can be identified by application of the fluorodinitrobenzene reaction (p. 11.3). The pure protein is allowed to react with the reagent, when only free amino groups, present at the end of the chain and in any lysine residues form the yellow dinitrophenyl derivatives. Subsequent hydrolysis, paper chromatography and identification of the yellow spot or spots should disclose the number and nature of the end groups. Each polypeptide chain present in the original material should yield one α-2,4-dinitro-phenyl derivative, so that the finding of two or more indicates a complex molecule with more than one polypeptide chain. The presence of a single N-terminal amino acid does not, of course, exclude the possibility of the existence of multiple chains in the molecule. For example, the molecule of normal adult human haemoglobin contains a pair of α- and a pair of β-chains. Although these differ in amino acid make-up, the N-terminal amino acid in both cases is valine. Where a molecule proves to have more than one chain, the links between the chains may be stable covalent disulphide bonds between cysteine residues or weaker bonds of the type of hydrogen bonds.

Identification of the carboxyl terminal amino acid is more difficult, because no reagent has yet come into use which reacts specifically with the terminal —COOH quite as effectively and simply as fluorodinitrobenzene reacts with the —NH$_2$. Useful information can sometimes be obtained by brief treatment of the protein in solution with carboxypeptidase, an enzyme which specifically catalyses the hydrolysis of the peptide bond nearest to the free —COOH. The results of such experiments need critical study, because the removal of the terminal amino acid automatically exposes a new one, also capable of removal by the enzyme.

Determination of the complete sequence of the amino acid residues in a polypeptide chain involves a rigorous and painstaking analysis. In one method the protein (or, if the molecule contains multiple chains, a preparation containing only one kind of chain) is subjected to partial hydrolysis by a range of different techniques, e.g. varying concentrations of acid, allowed to act for different times at different temperatures or a variety of specific enzymes, used singly or in sequence. The peptides obtained in each case must be separated, hydrolysed and identified. Application of the fluoro-dinitrobenzene reaction either to the original material or to the mixture of peptides may assist in the identification. The use of hydrolytic reagents of different specificities and different rates of reaction gives a series of peptides which overlap when placed in correct sequence along the chain, and in favourable cases it may be possible to build up gradually a picture of the complete structure. Alternatively, the amino acids may be identified chromatographically after being lopped off one by one from the N-terminal end of the peptide with the Edman reagent, phenyl isothiocyanate. The amino acid sequences of several hundred proteins and polypeptides have now been established. Insulin (p. 27.41) is a good example.

A simple variant of this technique has proved of great value in the study of differences between the structures of closely related polypeptides and proteins. The hydrolysis of a pure protein with a pure peptidase of high specificity should always give the same mixture of peptides. If these are separated by a standard procedure involving electrophoresis followed by chromatography the same final pattern (**finger print**) should always be observed. If the same procedure is applied to a protein which differs only slightly from the first, perhaps in the identity of only a single amino acid, the peptide pattern or finger print should also show a slight, but clearly defined difference. This technique was first used for the study of species differences in the structure of insulin, but is best known for its application to the study of abnormal genetic variants of human haemoglobin. Over 150 of these variants have now been recognized. In many of these, the abnormality consists only of a difference in a single amino acid in the β-chain. For example, in sickle-cell haemoglobin, commonly called haemoglobin S, a single glutamic acid in the normal β-chain is replaced by valine. Such a difference would be almost impossible to detect by

TABLE 11.3. The amino acid composition of some proteins (molecules amino acid/molecule of protein). Hydroxyproline is not listed because it is found only in connective tissue proteins like collagen.

	Haemoglobin (Human A) mol. wt. 65 000	Albumin (Human serum) mol. wt. 70 000	Cytochrome c (Human heart) mol. wt. 12 500
Gly	40	15	13
Ala	72	60	6
Ser	32	25	2
Thr	32	29	7
Pro	28	31	4
Val	62	46	3
Ile	0	9	8
Leu	72	64	5
Phe	30	33	3
Tyr	12	18	5
Trp	6	1	1
Cys*	6	36	2
Met	6	6	3
Asp	30	55	3
Asn	20	—†	5
Glu	22	83	8
Gln	10	—†	2
Arg	12	25	2
His	38	16	3
Lys	44	59	18
Total	574	611	103

* Cysteine + cystine. † Amides not separately determined.
Haemoglobin figures compiled from complete amino acid sequence by Perutz M.F. (1962) *Proteins and Nucleic Acids*. Amsterdam: Elsevier; cytochrome c recalculated from data of Tristram G.R. & Smith R.H. (1963) *Adv. Prot. Chem.* **18**, 227; albumin from Neurath H. (1970) *The Proteins*, 2nd Edition, vol. IV, New York: Academic Press.

any conventional method of analysis, but, as may be seen from fig. 11.6, it is easily disclosed by finger printing.

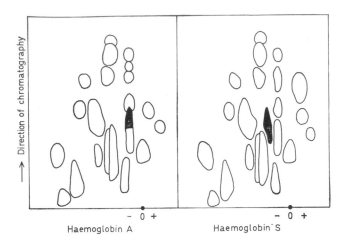

FIG. 11.6. Fingerprints of tryptic hydrolysates of haemoglobins A and S. ○, point of application of hydrolysate; + −, direction of electric field. The peptides which differ in behaviour and composition are marked black, the one containing valine (in HbS) has moved slightly further towards the cathode. Modified from Ingram V. (1958) *Biochim. Biophys. Acta*, **28**, 539.

Secondary and tertiary structure of proteins

The backbone of the polypeptide chain contains the repeating unit —N—C—C— of which the atoms are linked by single covalent bonds. If there were free rotation about these bonds, the chain would twist and coil at random, without assuming any definite and reproducible structure or shape. Measurements of the rates of diffusion and sedimentation of protein molecules in solution show that the facts are not consistent with such an hypothesis. Haemoglobin, serum albumin, many enzymes and a host of other proteins behave as if the molecules were uniform, relatively compact particles (**globular proteins**). The molecules of other proteins, e.g. collagen, fibrin, silk fibroin, appear to exist in a more or less rigid, greatly elongated form (**fibrous proteins**). Many fibrous proteins are insoluble and information about their shape has been obtained by the use of the EM and other techniques, such as X-ray crystallography, which are also applicable to crystals prepared from soluble proteins.

When a beam of X-rays traverses a molecule, the rays are diffracted by the component atoms to an extent which depends on the number of electrons in each atom. In a crystal, where the molecules are orientated in a regular manner, and to some extent in other organized molecular structures, the diffraction effects accumulate to give a well-defined pattern. The patterns given by complete crystals can be photographed, and the analysis of many photographs taken from different angles enables a picture to be built up of the location and spacing of the

atoms in the repeating unit of the crystal. The interpretation of the diffraction patterns given by the crystals of substances composed of atoms of elements of low atomic number is much easier if crystals can be made which incorporate occasional atoms of heavy metals such as mercury, and where possible this device is utilized in the X-ray crystallography of proteins. The natural occurrence of iron in myoglobin and haemoglobin makes these ideal proteins for investigation by this technique, especially because they can be made to crystallize well.

The X-ray diffraction patterns given by many proteins give prominence to a frequently repeated interatomic spacing of such a magnitude that it could not occur in extended polypeptide chains. This indicates some permanent folding or twisting in a way which must be conditioned and maintained by the groups of atoms (—NH——CH—CO—) of which the backbone of the polypeptide is constructed. The kind of twist which best fits some of the experimental results is illustrated in fig. 11.7. Each turn of the α-helix contains 3·6 amino acid residues. The figure shows how each —NH— or —CO— is in close proximity to a —CO— or —NH— in the neighbouring turn, so that the structure is maintained by —CO... HN— hydrogen bonds. In another type of structure similar hydrogen bonds are formed between peptide linkages in different peptide chains or different parts of the same chain. This gives the β-structure. If the β-structure extends over many polypeptide chains, as in silk fibroin, a pleated sheet is formed. Protein structure at this level is called **secondary structure**, while the final shape of the complete polypeptide molecule is described as **tertiary structure**. Where the complete molecule is comprised of a number of subunits each of which is itself a polypeptide, their spatial relationship is called **quaternary structure**.

Since many proteins are found in solution in the living body, it is important to know whether the secondary structure is characteristic only of the crystalline state, or whether it persists when the molecule is dissolved. The optical rotatory properties of protein solutions suggest that in most proteins there is a marked tendency for the α-helix to persist in solution. The extent to which this occurs depends partly on pH, so that electrostatic bonds between side chain groups must play a part in the maintenance of the helix. Among the few proteins which show little or no evidence of α-helical structure in solution are the milk phosphoprotein casein and the immunologically important γ-globulins of plasma.

Wherever the amino acids proline or hydroxyproline occur in a polypeptide chain, the common α-helical secondary structure cannot be formed. This situation, which is found in collagen and other connective tissue proteins, as well as sporadically elsewhere, develops partly because the nitrogen atom forms part of a rigid heterocyclic ring which does not fit perfectly into the shape of the α-helix, and partly because the nitrogen carries no hydrogen to form a hydrogen bond. The difficulty is surmounted in different ways. In most proteins, where there is only an occasional proline molecule, the α-helix is temporarily interrupted and the chain as a whole takes an angle determined by the other forces

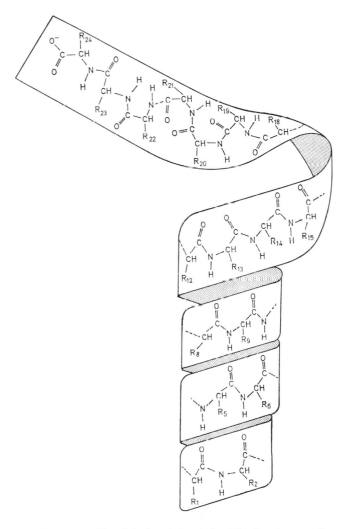

FIG. 11.7. The right-handed α-helix. The lower part of the ribbon, with the polypeptide structure drawn upon it, shows the helical structure. Note that the relative positions of —NH— and —CO— in successive coils are favourable for hydrogen bond formation. Further up the ribbon there is random folding, with full extension of the chain at the upper end. From Haggis G. *et al.* (1964) *Introduction to Molecular Biology*. London : Longman.

involved. In collagen about a quarter of the molecules are either proline or hydroxyproline, spread evenly along the chain, so that the common α-helix cannot be stabilized at all. A different type of helix develops, in which three similar polypeptide chains are twisted together. The formation of the structure is facilitated by the fact that every third position in the collagen polypeptide chains is occupied by glycine, which has only a hydrogen atom for side chain and therefore occupies little space.

The formation of the α-helix cannot itself account for the observed fact that the molecules of many proteins adopt a globular shape, both in solution and in the crystalline state. The stability of the α-helix depends to some extent on bonds between side-chain groups in neighbouring parts of the chain. There seems no *a priori* reason why the formation of hydrogen bonds or electrostatic interaction should not take place between side chain groups in different parts of the molecule thrown sufficiently close together. Such bonds would then hold together different parts of the polypeptide chain in much the same way as —S—S— bonds between remotely separated cysteine residues, and a sufficient number of these points of interaction might well produce an approximately globular structure.

Another factor arises from the presence in several amino acids of R-groups which contain only carbon and hydrogen atoms, and thus have no tendency to form charged or polarized areas. The molecule tends to arrange itself in such a way that these non-polar groups come together, often in the interior of a more or less globular structure. Such a 'hydrophobic pocket' in haemoglobin is partly responsible for holding in position the prosthetic group, haem. The quaternary structure of haemoglobin, in which the two α- and two β-chains are knit together in a roughly spherical shape, involves the interaction of side-chain groups in different polypeptide chains. A model of the haemoglobin molecule is shown in fig. 11.8. Careful inspection indicates that the α-helix, indicated by flat discs piled on top of one another, breaks down at various points and at many of these there is a definite inflexion of the axis of the chain. This happens because here and there the forces tending to draw the amino acids away from their neighbours are stronger than those which tend to knit the α-helix together. Some, but by no means all, of the corners occur, as would be expected, at points where the chain contains proline.

The secondary, tertiary and quaternary structures of proteins are a matter of highly complex physical chemistry with, however, an increasing number of repercussions in physiology and medicine. X-ray crystallography has disclosed changes in the quaternary structure of haemoglobin which are associated both with the equilibrium between haemoglobin and oxygen and with the physiologically important differences between the acid-base properties of haemoglobin and oxyhaemoglobin (p. 31.19). The difference in the primary structures of haemoglobin A and haemoglobin S, to which reference has already been made, is associated with differences in shape and solubility. The changes in the structure of γ-globulins which confer on them a wide range of specific immunochemical properties are of immense importance, although the changes themselves are not yet fully understood (vol. 2, p. 22.11).

Denaturation

The bonds which maintain the spatial configuration of protein molecules are weak and easily broken, with consequent loss of structural integrity, by heat or sometimes even by alteration of the physicochemical conditions, such as by the addition of acid or alkali. The loss of structure caused by any such method is called denaturation, provided that the treatment is not vigorous enough to alter the primary structure; the reductive fission of disulphide bonds is, however, sometimes regarded as denaturation. Denaturation is associated with the loss of

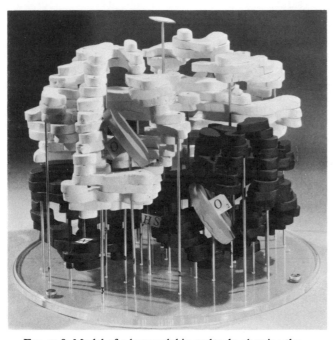

FIG. 11.8. Model of a haemoglobin molecule, showing the α chains in white and the β chains in black. The large diagonally sloping discs are haem molecules in their respective pockets in one α and one β chain. The oxygen molecules are shown correctly located.

such biochemical properties as enzymic activity and with marked alterations in physicochemical properties. For example solubility, more especially near the isoelectric point, is often greatly diminished by denaturation.

Detergents are powerful denaturing agents. Heating a protein in a solution of the detergent sodium dodecyl sulphate (SDS), especially in the presence of a thiol to reduce —S—S bonds, destroys secondary, tertiary and quaternary structure. All proteins are thus converted to polypeptide chains having only primary structure. These take up SDS by a physical process which depends on the length of the chain. The material is then suitable for molecular weight determinations by electrophoresis on polyacrylamide gel.

AMINO ACIDS AND PROTEINS IN NUTRITION

Broadly speaking, nutrition serves two purposes which are inextricably woven together; these are the building and maintenance of the essential constituents of the living body, and the provision of energy for all the physical and chemical activities of life (chap. 4). Fats, carbohydrates and proteins all serve as sources of energy, but only proteins can supply the nitrogen and the sulphur for the synthesis of proteins and other compounds containing these elements.

The quantitative study of human protein needs and how to meet them is of practical importance in several circumstances. It is necessary to know the protein requirements of an individual when planning a therapeutic diet in which certain foods are restricted, e.g. for a patient with obesity or chronic nephritis (vol. 3, chap. 50). The protein needs of a community should be considered by those responsible for agricultural policies. All who advise on the feeding of infants and young children and manufacturers of infants' food should be aware of the special needs of the very young. As more land is required to produce protein than carbohydrate, foods rich in protein are relatively expensive. The protein requirements of individuals, from which those of a community can be computed, may be evaluated by experimental methods.

Nitrogen requirements

One useful approach is to determine the amount of nitrogen which dietary protein has to supply to meet daily losses of N. Even on a protein-free diet there is a continuing loss of N from the body by several routes and the sum of the amounts going by each route is termed the **obligatory nitrogen loss.** The replacement of this is clearly a mandatory call on the metabolism of protein. Additional N is needed to allow for all kinds of stress, even minor infections and injuries, which stimulate protein catabolism (vol. 3, p. 3.16). Additional N is also required for growth in childhood, during pregnancy and lactation, and to make good tissue losses during convalescence from wasting illnesses, e.g. a prolonged fever or a severe accident or surgical operation.

Nitrogen is lost from the body surface (in sweat, hair and nails and by loss of the superficial layers of the skin), in the faeces and in the urine. Surface N losses do not normally amount to more than 5 mg/kg body weight/day, and may be less.

Faecal N is derived partly from digestive secretions and intestinal cell debris, and partly from undigested dietary protein. There is more undigested protein when the diet is bulky and when the protein is of vegetable origin, two factors which often go together. Faecal N ranges from 10 to 20 mg/kg body weight/day; measurement is tedious

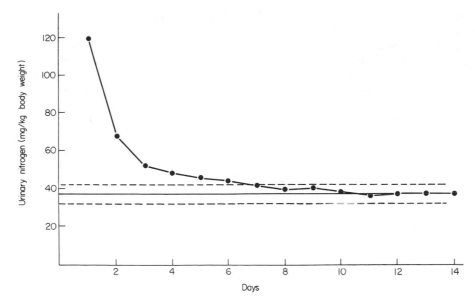

FIG. II.9. Urinary nitrogen (mg/kg body weight/day) in men on a protein-free diet. Recalculated from Scrimshaw N.S. *et al.* (1972) *J. Nutr.* **102**, 1595. Horizontal straight lines indicate mean ± S.D. for all subjects (83) between 10 and 14 days.

and unpleasant, and with most diets it is reasonable to assume a figure of 12 mg/kg/day.

Urinary N varies greatly and depends on the N content of the diet. When young men are given a protein-free diet adequate in other respects, the urinary N falls in a few days from around 120 to 37 mg/kg body weight/day (fig. II.9). This low value stays remarkably constant during the second week of such a diet, and thereafter falls very slowly. Figures obtained in this way are taken to represent obligatory urinary N loss. Values for women are slightly lower, since the body weight includes a greater proportion of adipose tissue, comparatively inert in nitrogen metabolism.

Miscellaneous additional minor obligatory N losses may include menstrual blood, accidental minor blood losses, exhaled ammonia and possibly gaseous nitrogen. In neither sex does the total exceed 2 mg/kg body weight/day.

The experimental determination of obligatory nitrogen losses is tedious and difficult. Since most of the losses are in the form of normal metabolic products, it is not surprising that the sum is closely related to the basal metabolic rate, which is much more easily measured. The accepted value for adult men, 0·48 mg N/kJ basal metabolism, is probably equally applicable to women and older children. It is in error for infants, but on the 'safe' side, since it overestimates their obligatory N losses, perhaps by 25–30 per cent.

All the above figures are mean values and if the distribution in a population is symmetrical, an allowance to cover only the mean requirement is insufficient for nearly half the total numbers, depending on how many

are clustered round the mean. An addition of 30 per cent or 2 s.d. to the mean value adequately covers random variations of biological and technical origin.

Requirement for growth is calculated from the known rate of growth of well-nourished children and the experimental observation that N (mainly in protein) accounts for 2·9 per cent of the weight gain during growth. The figures obtained require a statistical correction similar to that used for obligatory N losses. Table II.4 gives mean values for the calculated N requirements of both sexes at selected ages.

TABLE II.4. Nitrogen requirements (mg/kg body weight/day); obligatory losses with growth supplement where appropriate. From FAO/WHO (1973).

Age (yr)	Obligatory N loss		Growth supplement		Total	
	M	F	M	F	M	F
6/12–8/12	112		42		154	
9/12–11/12	110		26		136	
2	100		12		112	
5	86		9·5		96	
8	76		7		83	
12	66	60	8	10	74	70
16	57	54	4	1	61	55
Adult	54	49	0	0	54	49

The additional N requirement imposed by pregnancy amounts to an average 80 mg/day during the first trimester and rises more than tenfold to 860 mg/day during the last trimester. The extra N required for lactation is about 1·6 g/day, with much individual variation. The N requirements for convalescence from acute or chronic wasting diseases and for the rehabilitation of mal-nourished children need individual consideration. The principles of refeeding an undernourished or marasmic child are now well established (vol. 3, chap. 24).

Experimental figures for N requirements provide a base from which to work, but cannot be translated directly into dietary protein needs by simple arithmetic. Difficulty arises because individual proteins or mixtures of proteins are used with varying efficiency. Also the rates of many of the enzymic reactions involved in amino acid metabolism are directly and indirectly affected by the concentrations of their substrates. The inescapable N losses of a person on an ordinary diet, no matter what the source of protein, are therefore somewhat greater than those on a protein-free diet.

Utilization of dietary protein

Most methods of investigating the utilization of dietary protein involve the measurement of nitrogen intake (I) and output. The latter is usually experimentally confined to urinary (U) and faecal (F) nitrogen. When $I > U + F$, as for example in normal growth, the subject is said to be in positive N balance. If he is starved, febrile or beginning to recover after breaking his femur, $I < U + F$ and he is in negative N balance. In a normal adult on a normal diet, $I = U + F$, and he is said to be in N equilibrium or simply N balance. All studies of N balance should cover at least four days to allow for chance variations.

Studies of N balance in adult subjects on diets containing known amounts of specified sources of protein are used to find the minimum quantity of such protein which maintains N equilibrium. Such studies are simple in theory, although the actual experiments are expensive, tedious and difficult to organize. Careful work has shown that adult men are, on average, maintained in N balance on a diet containing 77 mg N/kg body weight/day as whole egg or milk protein; this figure is higher than the requirement of 54 mg N/kg body weight/day, calculated from the obligatory N loss. When plant proteins are fed, 85–120 mg N/kg body weight/day is needed to maintain N balance, and so these are less efficiently utilized.

In a similar way the relative dietary qualities of individual proteins or sources of protein can be evaluated. The most effective comparisons are obtained by feeding the test proteins to growing animals in suboptimal amounts, when the maximum proportionate retention of nitrogen is observed. Opportunities for conducting human experiments along these lines have been rare, but fortunately results agree well with those obtained on rats. The best index of quality is **net protein utilization (NPU)**, calculated as the percentage of the N intake which is retained in the body:

$$NPU = \frac{I - U - F}{I} \times 100$$

Whole egg protein has been much used as a reference protein because in young rats it gives an NPU of 95, close to the theoretical ideal of 100. Human milk proteins give a similar value. Tests on human subjects under dietary conditions involving normal protein intake give somewhat lower results, although these proteins still come out at the

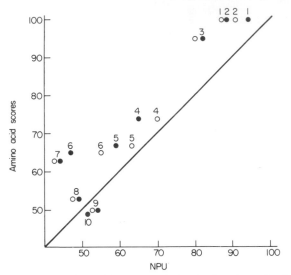

FIG. 11.10. Amino acid scores and NPU values determined in rats (●) and children (o). Numbers on the figures refer to sources of protein: 1, whole egg; 2, human milk; 3, cow's milk; 4, soya bean; 5, polished rice; 6, groundnut; 7, millet; 8, whole wheat; 9, sesame; 10, maize. Complete agreement between the two systems would give the straight line. (FAO/WHO 1973.)

top of the list. Some examples of experimental NPU values, related to chemical score (p. 11.16), are given in fig. 11.10.

Essential amino acids

The differences in quality of dietary proteins which are now being quantified were first defined some sixty years ago. Osborne and Mendel found that ovovitellin from egg yolk and lactalbumin from milk promoted the growth of young rats extremely well, but casein, also from milk, was less satisfactory (fig. 11.11). The wheat protein gliadin just maintained the weight of the animals, while on zein from maize they lost weight steadily. Increasing the proportion in the diet improved the growth-promoting properties of casein, and gave a slight benefit with gliadin but had no effect with zein. That these findings were attributable to differences in amino acid composition was shown by the sequel; gliadin contains all the amino acids but only very little lysine, and the addition of lysine to the gliadin diet conferred on it good growth-promoting properties. Zein contains little lysine and no tryptophan, and in that case supplements of both amino acids were required.

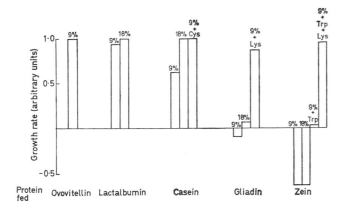

FIG. 11.11. Comparison of the growth promoting properties of different proteins. The proteins were fed to young rats at a level of 9 per cent and 18 per cent of the weight of an otherwise adequate diet with and without supplements of amino acids as indicated. Data from Osborne T.B. & Mendel L.B. (1914) *J. biol. Chem.* **17**, 325.

It can be concluded that neither lysine nor tryptophan can be synthesized in the animal body, even when there is an ample supply of nitrogen. They were the first of the essential or indispensable amino acids to be discovered. An essential amino acid is one which cannot be synthesized in the body from readily available precursors at a rate sufficient to meet metabolic needs. The division between essential and non-essential is not absolute. Tyrosine, for example, can be synthesized in the body, but only from the essential amino acid phenylalanine. Hence in the absence of dietary tyrosine, a deficiency of phenylalanine leads to a deficiency of tyrosine. Conversely, an ample supply of tyrosine may diminish, although it cannot abolish, the need for phenylalanine. In practice the two aromatic amino acids are bracketed together when the essential amino acid content of dietary proteins is considered. The sulphur-containing amino acids are related in a somewhat similar way. Cystine can be synthesized, but only by a process (p. 11.21) in which the sulphur is provided by the essential amino acid methionine. In nutritional work these two amino acids are also considered together. Casein contains methionine in a proportion similar to that in many other proteins, but is rather low in cystine. The supply of cystine can be augmented in three ways, two of which are illustrated in fig. 11.11: by increasing the casein intake or by supplementing the diet with cystine. The third method, supplementation with methionine, could not be tested by Osborne and Mendel because that amino acid was not discovered until some years after their work was done. The classification of an amino acid as essential depends only on the need to supply it in the diet, and not at all on its metabolic significance. No one amino acid could be singled out as having a peculiar essentiality in protein

structure and several of the non-essential amino acids fulfil specific and important metabolic functions.

There are age and species differences in essential amino acid requirements. Chicks, for example, require a dietary supply of glycine but mature fowls do not. Young rats cannot synthesize arginine sufficiently rapidly to permit full growth on an arginine deficient diet. In the same way histidine is an essential amino acid for human infants but not for older children or adults, although the age of transition has not been determined exactly. The other amino acids essential in human nutrition are isoleucine, leucine, lysine, methionine+cystine, phenylalanine+tyrosine, threonine, tryptophan and valine.

Much of the variation in the nutritional quality of proteins depends on their amino acid composition, and animal proteins are usually richer than plant proteins in essential amino acids. It can now be seen that from the point of view of protein nutrition the advice that the diet should consist of a range of different foods is sound, for proteins of different amino acid composition are likely to complement one another.

A necessary step towards the exact description of protein quality in terms of amino acid composition is the quantitative measurement of human requirements for essential amino acids. Elaborate feeding experiments in subjects of different age groups have given estimates which are summarized in table 11.5. In relation to the

TABLE 11.5. Estimated essential amino acid requirements of adults, children (10–12 yr) and infants. From FAO/WHO (1973).

Amino acid	Amino acid requirements mg/kg/day		
	Adult	Child	Infant
Histidine	—	—	28
Isoleucine	10	30	70
Leucine	14	45	161
Lysine	12	60	103
Methionine+cystine	13	27	58
Phenylalanine+tyrosine	14	27	125
Threonine	7	35	87
Tryptophan	3·5	4	17
Valine	10	33	93
Total EAA	83·5	261	742
Total EAA nitrogen	10	34	93

weights of the subjects, the requirements of infants are much the highest. When the N content of the estimated essential amino acid requirement is compared with the total N requirement given in table 11.4 it is seen that the adult may need about 20 per cent of his dietary N requirement in essential amino acids, a child about 40 per cent and an infant 50–60 per cent. Later work may modify the figures, but there can be no doubt about the trend. A

TABLE 11.6. Provisional reference pattern for dietary protein and essential amino acid composition of whole egg protein. From FAO/WHO (1973).

Amino acid	Provisional reference pattern mg/g protein	Whole egg protein mg/g protein
Histidine	—	22
Isoleucine	40	54
Leucine	70	86
Lysine	55	70
Methionine + cystine	35	57
Phenylalanine + tyrosine	60	93
Threonine	40	47
Tryptophan	10	17
Valine	50	66
Total EAA	360	512
Total EAA nitrogen	43*	64*

* Calculated on the assumption that equimolar amounts of the pairs cys and met, phe and tyr are present.

provisional amino acid reference pattern is given in table 11.6 with, for comparison, the reported essential amino acid content of the common reference mixture of whole egg proteins.

The next step is calculating the nutritional quality of a protein by comparing its content of the essential amino acid in which it is poorest with a chosen standard. This chemical approach shares with the biological method the difficulty of finding a suitable standard. Either whole egg protein or a reference amino acid pattern, based on knowledge of human amino acid requirements, may be used (table 11.6). The calculation is made as follows:

Amino acid score

$$= \frac{\text{mg amino acid/g test protein}}{\text{mg amino acid/g reference standard}} \times 100$$

It is repeated for each of the essential amino acids in turn, and the lowest figure obtained is the one used. The amino acid concerned is called the **limiting amino acid.** The limiting amino acids most frequently encountered are lysine and the sulphur-containing amino acids, and occasionally tryptophan.

Ideally the chemical and biological methods should give identical results, and as fig. 11.10 shows, some progress has been made in this direction. It appears that in comparison with NPU amino acid scores currently used overestimate the value of many proteins, perhaps because the score takes account of only the most limiting amino acid, whereas the biological method estimates the effect of a lack of more than one. Present advice is that both amino acid scores and NPU are useful for initial prediction, but that the quantitative efficiency of planned diets should be checked by actual nitrogen balance or growth promotion experiments. When well known sources of protein are being considered, an abundance of sufficiently useful if not absolutely precise information is available.

Recommended protein intake

Calculations are at present based on whole egg protein, which is assumed to have NPU or amino acid score not significantly different from 100. The empirical procedure used is as follows:

(1) determine total N requirements (mg/kg/day) as for table 11.4,

(2) add 30 per cent to allow for the differences between obligatory loss measurements and balance studies,

(3) add a further 30 per cent as a statistical compensation for individual variability,

TABLE 11.7. Calculation of the safe level of protein intake in terms of diets containing whole egg protein and other protein of NPU or amino acid score 70%. Numbers at the heads of columns in the table refer to steps in the calculation as given above.

Age yr	Body wt. kg	N requirement mg/kg/day basal 1	N requirement mg/kg/day adjusted 2, 3	Whole egg protein requirement g/kg/day 4	Whole egg protein requirement g/day	Mixed protein (score 70%) requirement g/day 5
Infants 6/12–11/12	9	150	254	1.53	14	20
Children 5–6	21	94	159	0.99	21	30
Adolescents						
Male 15	52	63	106	0.66	34	50
Female 15	50	56	95	0.60	30	43
Adult						
Male	65	54	91	0.57	37	53
Female	55	49	83	0.52	29	41

(4) convert to safe protein intake (whole egg protein), using the relation: $N \times 6 \cdot 25 =$ protein and

(5) convert to safe levels of other proteins by using the formula $S_x = S \, 100/x$ where $S =$ safe level of intake of whole egg protein and $S_x =$ safe level of intake of protein of NPU or amino acid score x. The examples given in table 11.7 include the supplement for growth where applicable. Supplements for pregnancy, lactation and clinical purposes must be added separately, and also require correction for the quality of the actual dietary protein. It is probable that this method of calculating the desired protein intake allows sufficient margin to cover the variable errors in NPU and amino acid score. The NPU of the mixed proteins in diets commonly consumed in prosperous countries is around 75, and average protein intake usually exceeds the recommended safe level.

Protein nutrition and energy supply

There are important relations between protein intake and energy supply. At one end of the scale, the utilization of protein is more effective when energy needs are met largely by other foodstuffs. When the diet lacks carbohydrate, as in some much-advertised reducing regimes, gluconeogenesis is stimulated and amino acids are thereby used extensively to supply energy; in this way protein deficiency may develop. On the other hand, if the bulk or energy content of a diet is high relative to the protein content, the food eaten may be insufficient to supply protein needs. This may happen in infants on a diet of a cereal mash or cassava after premature weaning (p. 5.20). Clearly, also, the poorer the quality of the protein, the higher the amount needed in the diet. When protein accounts for less than 8–10 per cent of the dietary energy, some individuals, e.g. the very young and the very old, are likely to be unable to eat enough to obtain sufficient protein. Eight per cent may be a satisfactory threshold where the quality of protein is high, but 10 per cent may be required if the protein in the staple food is of poor quality as in diets based on cassava and maize, eaten by millions of people in tropical Africa and America.

Where the diet suffers from this type of shortcoming, it can be improved by the addition of foods in which protein provides a high proportion of the energy. The amount required may be quite small, especially if the added protein is of high NPU and rich in the limiting amino acid of the original diet. Skimmed milk, whether dried or fresh, is better for this purpose than whole milk because the fat in the latter more than doubles the energy from non-protein sources. More than 30 per cent of the energy of skimmed milk is derived from protein. Very effective mixtures of vegetable proteins prepared in accordance with the principles discussed can be used in countries where it is difficult to obtain sufficient milk.

INTERMEDIATE METABOLISM OF AMINO ACIDS

The intermediate metabolism of amino acids embraces a wider range of biochemical reactions than that of either carbohydrates or fats. There are several reasons for this; firstly, proteins always contain nitrogen and almost always sulphur as well as carbon, hydrogen and oxygen, so that the metabolism of amino acids includes the elaboration of nitrogenous and sulphur-containing end products (mainly urea and sulphate); secondly, many different types of structure are found among the carbon skeletons of amino acids, and each is metabolized in its own more or less specific way. While the ultimate end products are carbon dioxide and water, produced in the citric acid cycle and by the re-oxidation of dehydrogenase coenzymes, the various amino acids enter the cycle only after conversion to intermediate products, most of which also arise in carbohydrate and fat metabolism. Again, since proteins are, apart from traces of some of the vitamins and other highly specialized compounds, the only source of nitrogen available to the animal body, amino acid metabolism includes the biosynthesis not only of proteins (chap. 12) but also of almost all other nitrogenous compounds, including nonessential amino acids. The carbon skeletons of these are synthesized mainly but not exclusively from precursors which are not amino acids, although the nitrogen is provided by other amino acids. Many other nitrogenous compounds, including purine and pyrimidine bases, porphyrins and creatine are synthesized in specific reactions from particular amino acids. Fig. 11.12 summarizes the main pathways.

Such a wide variety of biochemical processes necessarily involves a large number of enzymes. Many of these require the presence of coenzymes. As there are so many possibilities for the development of a nutritional or metabolic defect leading to error in, or failure of, the synthesis of a coenzyme or enzyme, it is not surprising to find a large variety of pathological conditions, fortunately many of them exceedingly rare, associated with specific failures of reactions in the metabolism of one or more of the amino acids. When the basic defect is an inherited failure to synthesize a specific enzyme, the condition is known as a hereditary or **inborn error of metabolism**. Where a reaction fails because of some other cause, such as deficiency of a vitamin, leading to lack of a particular coenzyme, the condition is an **acquired error of metabolism**. The study of metabolic errors is important in specific cases for clinical reasons and has also been of great value in the elucidation of metabolic processes. Failure of one link in a chain of reactions may lead either to accumulation of an intermediate, as in alkaptonuria (an inborn error of tyrosine metabolism) or to diversion into an abnormal metabolic pathway, as in phenylketonuria (an inborn error of the

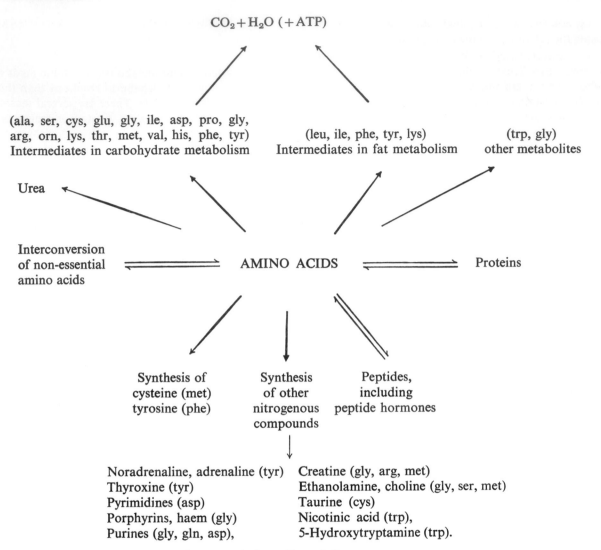

$$CO_2 + H_2O \ (+ATP)$$

(ala, ser, cys, glu, gly, ile, asp, pro, gly,
arg, orn, lys, thr, met, val, his, phe, tyr)
Intermediates in carbohydrate metabolism

(leu, ile, phe, tyr, lys)
Intermediates in fat metabolism

(trp, gly)
other metabolites

Urea

Interconversion
of non-essential
amino acids

AMINO ACIDS

Proteins

Synthesis of
cysteine (met)
tyrosine (phe)

Synthesis
of other
nitrogenous
compounds

Peptides,
including
peptide hormones

Noradrenaline, adrenaline (tyr)
Thyroxine (tyr)
Pyrimidines (asp)
Porphyrins, haem (gly)
Purines (gly, gln, asp),

Creatine (gly, arg, met)
Ethanolamine, choline (gly, ser, met)
Taurine (cys)
Nicotinic acid (trp),
5-Hydroxytryptamine (trp).

FIG. 11.12. Amino acid metabolism.

metabolism of phenylalanine). Inborn errors were first recognized in the field of amino acid metabolism, where more than fifty have now been identified (vol. 3, chap. 47).

Amino acids in body fluids

In comparison with the amounts present in chemical combination as protein, concentrations of free amino acids in body fluids are low. Plasma contains a total concentration of 2–4 mmol/l, to which the individual amino acids make very different contributions. Glutamine, alanine and lysine are among the most plentiful, methionine and aspartic acid the least so.

The amino acids in all the body fluids are of mixed origin, and, while there is free diffusion between plasma and interstitial fluid, there is no simple relation between extracellular and intracellular amino acids. The plasma amino acids are derived from the products of protein digestion, which are actively absorbed across the wall of the small intestine (p. 32.43) and from the products of hydrolysis of extracellular proteins, those of dead or decaying cells (e.g. aged erythrocytes) or, in the case of the non-essential acids, new synthesis. It has been known for half a century that all cells take up amino acids avidly from the interstitial fluid and may accumulate some of them against the concentration gradient. Inside the cell molecules mingle with those of newly synthesized amino acids and perhaps those of amino acids liberated from proteins in the course of the life of the cell. The intracellular concentration of amino acids varies greatly, but may be five to ten times greater than that outside the cells.

The composition of the mixture of amino acids available to the enzyme systems of any cell depends not only on the mixture in the extracellular fluid bathing that cell (and this may vary from one part of the body to another) but also on the extent to which metabolism in that cell contributes to the mixture.

Urinary losses normally amount to no more than about 5 mmol per day of free amino acids, with about as much again in the form of some easily hydrolysed substances of unknown nature. Losses are small because amino acids are actively reabsorbed in the renal tubules by mechanisms which resemble those involved in intestinal absorption. In cystinuria, an inborn error, there is a failure of the active absorption of cystine as well as of the di-amino acids, lysine and arginine, in both the kidney and the intestine. As might be expected, the pattern of renal excretion of amino acids is altered both qualitatively and quantitatively in a number of pathological conditions, including nutritional disorders, some diseases of the liver and many inborn errors of metabolism.

Fate of the nitrogen of amino acids

Many of the biochemical processes which effect the removal of the 2-amino group and its subsequent metabolism are common to all the amino acids and are conveniently treated before discussion of the metabolism of the individual amino acids.

One method by which the amino group can be removed from an amino acid molecule is **oxidative deamination**, in which the amino acid is converted to a 2-keto acid and the amino group to ammonia.

The first enzyme found to catalyse oxidative deamination in animal tissues, mainly kidney, was a flavoprotein named D-amino acid oxidase because of its surprising specificity for the D-amino acids. Its natural function remains obscure but it appears to be identical with glycine oxidase or glycine dehydrogenase, which catalyses the same type of reaction with glycine as substrate. The more recently discovered L-amino acid oxidase, another flavoprotein, is only weakly active with most amino acids.

Another specific oxidative deamination is that catalysed by L-glutamate dehydrogenase which utilizes NAD or NADP as coenzyme.

$$COOHCH_2CH_2CHNH_2COOH + NAD$$
Glutamic acid

$$H_2O \quad \updownarrow \quad H_2O$$

$$COOHCH_2CH_2COCOOH + NH_3 + NADH_2$$
2-Oxoglutaric acid

This reaction is important partly because in conjunction with a series of transaminations it serves as a general method of deamination and also because it is readily reversible and is believed to play an important part in the transfer of energy across the membranes of mitochondria. The thermodynamic equilibrium point lies far in favour of glutamate synthesis, and the reaction is also of importance in connection with amino acid synthesis. It is one of the fundamental reactions of nitrogen fixation in plants.

In 1937 the Russian biochemist Braunstein discovered a process of very wide significance, **transamination**. This is the reaction in which an amino acid reacts with a 2-keto acid. The 2-keto acid is converted to the amino acid with the same carbon skeleton, while the original amino acid is deaminated with the production of the corresponding oxo acid. These reactions are reversible and are catalysed by a series of enzymes called aminotransferases. Two of these widespread enzymes, aspartate aminotransferase and alanine aminotransferase, commonly called GOT and GPT (abbreviations of the former names glutamic oxaloacetic transaminase and glutamic pyruvic transaminase), have a special clinical interest because they escape into the plasma when there is damage to various tissues, notably the myocardium and the liver (p. 33.18). Aminotransferases require a phosphorylated derivative of pyridoxine, vitamin B_6, as coenzyme. The active compound is an aldehyde, pyridoxal 5-phosphate, which is reversibly converted in the course of its action to the corresponding amine, pyridoxamine 5-phosphate:

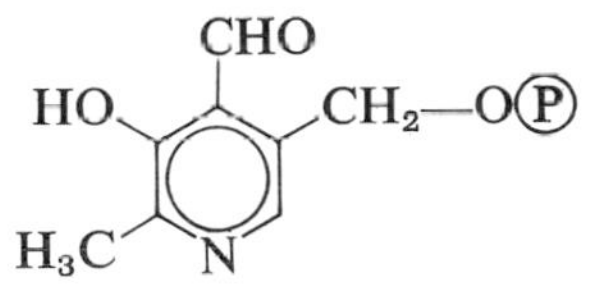

Pyridoxal 5-phosphate 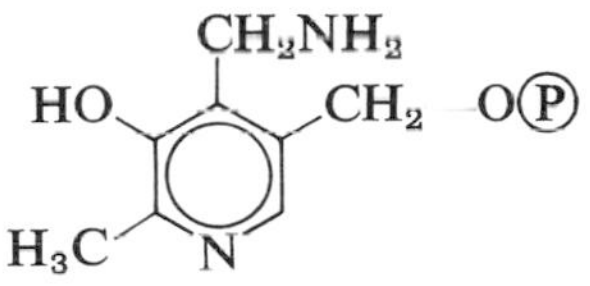   Pyridoxamine 5-phosphate

The course of the reaction can be represented in fig. 11.13. For simplicity, one-way arrows have been used, but all the reactions are reversible.

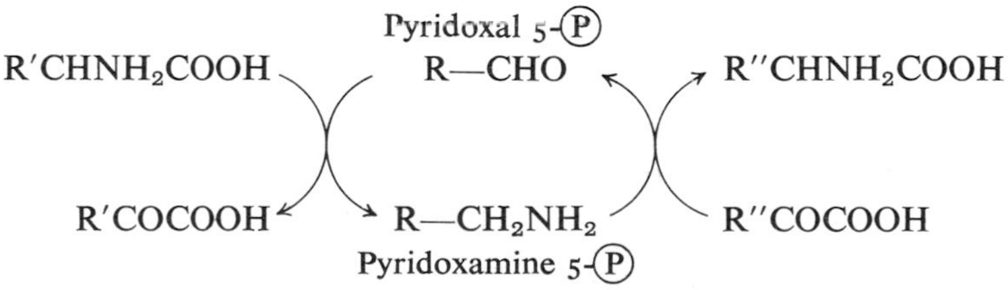

Fig. 11.13. Action of aminotransferase.

All the amino acids, except threonine and lysine, can undergo transamination and glutamate, aspartate and alanine or one of the corresponding keto compounds appear to participate in every reaction. Furthermore, the wide distribution of aminotransferases linking glutamate with aspartate or alanine means that the nitrogen of any other amino acid can very easily appear in one of these three acids. If it should appear in glutamate, this may then be oxidatively deaminated by the action of glutamic dehydrogenase to give ammonia and 2-oxoglutarate. The latter substance can then serve as the acceptor for another amino group, so that we have here the machinery for the continuous deamination of a wide range of amino acids:

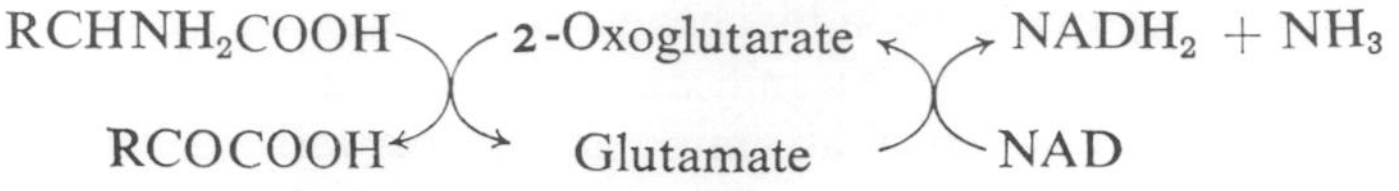

$$\text{RCHNH}_2\text{COOH} \rightleftharpoons \text{2-Oxoglutarate} \rightleftharpoons \text{NADH}_2 + \text{NH}_3$$
$$\text{RCOCOOH} \rightleftharpoons \text{Glutamate} \rightleftharpoons \text{NAD}$$

Ammonia is highly toxic, and either free or protonated is present only in minute concentration in normal body fluids, with the exception of urine. In the bodies of mammals, ammonia is ultimately converted to **urea** by a cyclic process which takes place in the liver (p. 33.3). The first intermediate in that process and some others (p. 12.27) is **carbamyl phosphate**, an amide of the mixed anhydride of carbonic and phosphoric acids $\text{NH}_2\text{COO}\textcircled{P}$. It is very unstable and present in tissues in only very low concentration.

Glutamine, another metabolic derivative of ammonia, is much more stable and is found in greater quantities all over the body. Like carbamyl phosphate it is synthesized only with the aid of ATP.

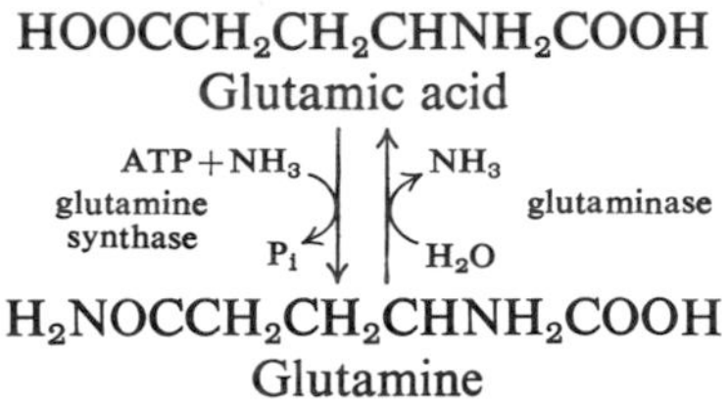

$$\text{HOOCCH}_2\text{CH}_2\text{CHNH}_2\text{COOH}$$
Glutamic acid

ATP+NH$_3$ → NH$_3$
glutamine synthase   glutaminase
P$_i$ H$_2$O

$$\text{H}_2\text{NOCCH}_2\text{CH}_2\text{CHNH}_2\text{COOH}$$
Glutamine

The formation of glutamine may be regarded as a temporary store and the ammonia can be liberated through the action of a specific hydrolase, glutaminase (p. 35.32).

Fate of the carbon of amino acids

Most of the carbon in amino acids is finally oxidized to carbon dioxide. The use of alanine as the donor of an amino group in a transamination leaves pyruvate which may then undergo oxidative decarboxylation to acetyl coenzyme A. The oxo acids formed from glutamic and aspartic acids are themselves intermediates in the citric acid cycle, so that their oxidation presents no new problem. The question also arises, however, whether these intermediates may be converted to glucose or other carbohydrate derivatives, rather than to carbon dioxide. Evidence of this has been available for 60 years from experiments in which lean meat, proteins or amino acids were fed to phlorizinized dogs. Phlorizin poisons the renal tubules, inhibits the reabsorption of glucose and leads to large losses of sugar in the urine. Lean meat and purified proteins caused the excretion of glucose corresponding, on the average, to 58 per cent of the

protein fed and also to the excretion of a little aceto-acetate and β-hydroxybutyrate. After amino acids were given the products varied; most of the amino acids were converted largely to glucose, but leucine, isoleucine, phenylalanine and tyrosine gave rise to acetoacetate. Thus, in this experiment many amino acids were glucogenic and a few ketogenic. Modern evidence confirms that gluconeogenesis from amino acids is a process of normal metabolic significance which may be quantitatively affected in a number of disease conditions. Its rate is subject to control by such hormones as insulin (p. 27.44), glucagon and corticosteroids (p. 27.35). The glucogenic pathways for individual amino acids are described below.

Metabolism of individual amino acids

ASPARTIC ACID AND ASPARAGINE

The fate of the carbon and the general importance of this amino acid in transamination have already been noted, as well as the part it plays in donating the nitrogen for the final stages of the synthesis of arginine and adenylic acid (p. 33.3 and 12.24). A carbamyl derivative of aspartic acid is the starting point for the synthesis of pyrimidine bases (p. 12.26). The amide asparagine is also found in proteins, and in many glycoproteins the carbohydrate (moiety) is bound to the protein through the amide group of asparagine. Normal tissues synthesize asparagine readily, but some malignant cells do not. Tumours of this type depend on an external source of asparagine, and treatment with the hydrolytic enzyme asparaginase may hinder the supply sufficiently to cause some regression (vol. 2, pp. 28.13 and 29.13).

GLUTAMIC ACID AND GLUTAMINE

The general importance of glutamic acid should be already obvious. It has a few highly specialized functions, e.g. in brain where it is decarboxylated to give γ-amino-butyric acid This neurotransmitter is subsequently inactivated by oxidation to succinic semialdehyde, which may be converted to succinyl-SCoA and used in the tricarboxylic acid cycle.

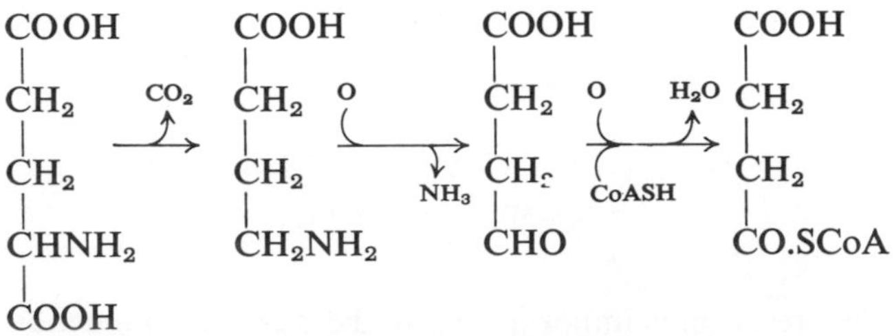

COOH   COOH   COOH   COOH
| | | |
CH$_2$ CO$_2$ CH$_2$ O CH$_2$ O H$_2$O CH$_2$
| → | | |
CH$_2$ CH$_2$ CH$_2$ CH$_2$
| | NH$_3$ CH$_2$ CoASH |
CHNH$_2$ CH$_2$NH$_2$ CHO   CO.SCoA
|
COOH

FIG. 11.14. γ-Aminobutyric acid formation and metabolism

Glutamine serves as the donor of an amino group in the synthesis of many important compounds, including aminosugars and purine bases (p. 12.24).

METHIONINE

This is an essential amino acid which in the normal course of its metabolism provides the sulphur for the synthesis of cysteine and cystine. The carbon atoms for these amino acids are provided by serine. Methionine also has a key role in transmethylation (p. 11.27), the process by which methyl groups are transferred to appropriate acceptors to give physiologically important compounds such as creatine and adrenaline. The loss of the methyl group from methionine in this way leaves homocysteine which condenses with serine to give a thioether cystathionine. Under the influence of the enzyme cystathionine 3-lyase, cystathionine is split to give cysteine, 2-oxobutyric acid and ammonia, a reaction which requires the coenzyme pyridoxal phosphate. Oxidative decarboxylation of the 2-oxobutyric acid (in the same way as occurs in the metabolism of the oxo acids pyruvic acid and 2-oxoglutaric acid) then yields propionyl coenzyme A. Succinyl coenzyme A, formed by an intramolecular rearrangement, is an intermediate in the tricarboxylic acid cycle and may be either oxidized or converted to carbohydrate. This accounts for the glucogenic properties of methionine.

$$CH_3SCH_2CH_2CHNH_2COOH$$
Methionine

$$HSCH_2CH_2CHNH_2COOH$$
Homocysteine

Serine $\longrightarrow$ H$_2$O

$$HOOCCHNH_2CH_2SCH_2CH_2CHNH_2COOH$$
Cystathionine

Cysteine $\longleftarrow$ Cystathionine 3-lyase

$$CH_3CH_2COCOOH$$
2-Oxobutyric acid

CoASH

CO$_2$

$$CH_3CH_2CO \cdot SCoA$$
Propionyl coenzyme A

CO$_2$

$$CH_3CHCOOHCO.SCoA$$
Methylmalonyl coenzyme A

B_{12} coenzyme

$$HOOCCH_2CH_2CO.SCoA$$
Succinyl coenzyme A

The oxidative decarboxylation of 2-oxobutyrate takes place in the same way as that of pyruvate.

CYSTINE AND CYSTEINE

Before further metabolism cystine is reduced to cysteine which is metabolized through one or other of three pathways, each of which involves deamination, formation of pyruvate and ultimate oxidation of the thiol sulphur to inorganic sulphate. Many inborn errors affecting the metabolism of the sulphur-containing amino acids are known (vol. 3, pp. 47.3 and 4). As cystine is sparingly soluble, patients with cysteinuria, due to a defect in renal reabsorption of cystine, form urinary calculi consisting almost entirely of cystine. Homocysteinuria occurs when cystathionine synthase is defective (vol. 2, p. 31.9). Cystathionine is found in the urine when cystathionine β-lyase is defective; in this very rare condition some patients respond to large doses of pyridoxine.

SULPHUR METABOLISM

In addition to the sulphur-containing amino acids and derivatives of those which have been mentioned, a wide variety of sulphur compounds is found in the body. Blood group polysaccharides, heparin and several connective tissue polysaccharides are sulphate esters, and some hydroxy compounds are excreted in the urine as sulphate esters formed with the aid of the coenzyme 3'-phosphoadenosine 5'-phosphosulphate. Some halogenated hydrocarbons are detoxicated by conjugation with cysteine to give mercapturic acids. Coenzyme A is a thiol incorporating a derivative of the cysteine molecule. Taurine, a sulphonic acid conjugated with bile acids, is derived from cysteine. Saliva contains thiocyanate, which is non-toxic in contrast to cyanide from which it is derived. Certain animal tissues contain proteins rich in sulphur and non-haem iron which are present in a polymeric structure associated with the protein. These proteins are related to the photosynthetic plant protein ferredoxin and have functions in specific oxidations, such as the introduction of a hydroxyl group into the molecule of a steroid hormone or a drug (p. 33.11).

The excretion of sulphur in the urine varies mainly with the intake of the amino acids containing sulphur and hence with the intake of protein, although there is a little preformed sulphate in most foods. With most satisfactory diets the total daily output is of the order of 1g sulphur. About three-quarters of this is inorganic sulphate formed from cysteine and methionine in the way outlined above. Most of the remainder consists of sulphate esters of organic hydroxy compounds.

VALINE

This glucogenic essential amino acid is catabolized in a long series of reactions involving transamination, oxidative deamination and oxidation of one of the methyl groups to methylmalonyl coenzyme A and hence to succinyl coenzyme A.

CH$_3$—CHCHNH$_2$COOH (CH$_3$ branch)
Valine

↓

CH$_3$—CHCOCOOH
2-Oxoisovaleric acid

↓

CH$_3$—CHCO.SCoA
Isobutyryl coenzyme A

↓

CH$_3$—CHCO.SCoA
|
COOH
Methylmalonyl coenzyme A

LEUCINE

Transamination to a 2-keto acid is again followed by oxidative decarboxylation. After further metabolic changes the products are equimolar amounts of acetoacetate (which accounts for the ketogenic properties of leucine) and acetyl coenzyme A.

CH$_3$—CHCH$_2$CHNH$_2$COOH
Leucine

↓

CH$_3$COCH$_2$COOH + CH$_3$CO.SCoA
Acetoacetic acid   Acetyl coenzyme A

ISOLEUCINE

The third branched-chain essential amino acid is also transaminated to a 2-keto acid, oxidatively decarboxylated and subjected to several further reactions, with the formation in the end of equimolar proportions of acetyl coenzyme A and propionyl coenzyme A.

The branched-chain 2-keto acids which are produced from valine, leucine and isoleucine are probably all oxidatively decarboxylated by the same enzyme. Maple syrup urine disease, so rare as to be a clinical curiosity, is an inborn error of metabolism in which there is a deficiency of this enzyme. The 2-keto acids are excreted in the urine to which they impart a characteristic odour. The intracellular transport and metabolism of pyruvate is inhibited by this group of 2-keto acids as well as by phenyl pyruvate (p. 11.23). Since the brain normally relies almost entirely on carbohydrate metabolism for its energy, inborn errors which cause the accumulation of these 2-keto acids lead to mental incapacity.

The metabolism of valine leads directly, and that of methionine and isoleucine indirectly, after carboxylation of propionyl coenzyme A, to the formation of methylmalonyl coenzyme A. The intramolecular rearrangement by which this is transformed to succinyl coenzyme A requires a coenzyme derived from vitamin B$_{12}$. In pernicious anaemia deficiency of the vitamin leads to a deficiency of the coenzyme and the methylmalonyl coenzyme A is hydrolyzed to the free acid, which is excreted in the urine. This acquired metabolic error forms the basis of a chemical test for vitamin B$_{12}$ deficiency.

THREONINE

This is metabolized in two different ways. The more important is by way of a reaction catalyzed by an enzyme requiring pyridoxal phosphate, threonine dehydratase. Its action gives ammonia and 2-oxobutyric acid, which is also an intermediate in methionine metabolism. Threonine can also be metabolized after being split by threonine aldolase to acetaldehyde and glycine.

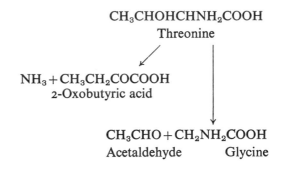

CH$_3$CHOHCHNH$_2$COOH
Threonine

NH$_3$ + CH$_3$CH$_2$COCOOH
2-Oxobutyric acid

CH$_3$CHO + CH$_2$NH$_2$COOH
Acetaldehyde   Glycine

PROLINE AND HYDROXYPROLINE

These non-essential amino acids are synthesized from glutamic acid. The 4-carboxyl group is reduced to —CHO and the five-membered ring is then formed by condensation. Reduction gives proline. Hydroxyproline is formed only by hydroxylation of proline in the course of the synthesis of collagen. The catabolism of proline apparently follows the reverse pathway to glutamic acid. The urinary excretion of hydroxyproline is used as an index of collagen metabolism in malnutrition and in diseases of supporting tissues.

LYSINE

Lysine is an essential amino acid. Although no evidence has been found that it can be transaminated, it is undoubtedly metabolized, presumably after oxidative deamination by L-amino acid oxidase. The subsequent reactions are complex and lead to one molecule of acetoacetyl coenzyme A for each molecule of lysine catabolized. As in the case of proline, some of the lysine molecules present are hydroxylated during collagen synthesis.

HISTIDINE

This can be transaminated, but is chiefly catabolized through a long series of reactions which starts with a specific deamination of an unusual kind and leads to the formation of formiminoglutamic acid (FIGLU). In the presence of a coenzyme derived from the vitamin folic acid, FIGLU is converted to glutamic acid. In folic acid deficiency, FIGLU is excreted in the urine, where it can be estimated readily (p. 28.9).

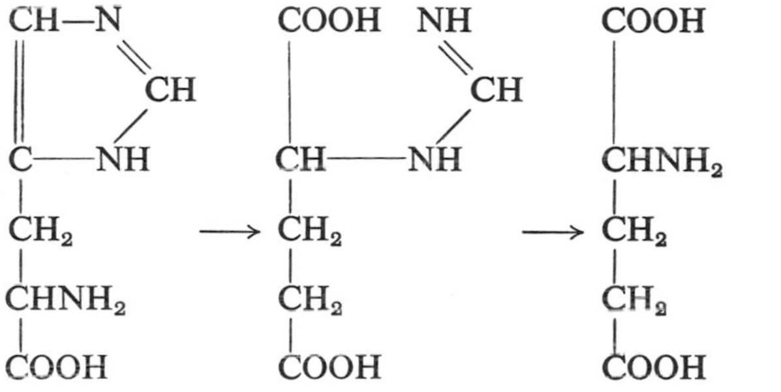

Histidine   FIGLU   Glutamic acid

The biosynthesis of histidine is not sufficiently rapid in infants to meet all their needs. For them histidine is an essential amino acid.

The pharmacologically important substance histamine is formed from histidine by decarboxylation. It is metabolized in several ways, of which the most important is by methylation and subsequent oxidation to methylimidazole acetaldehyde and methylimidazole acetic acid (vol. 2, p. 14.9).

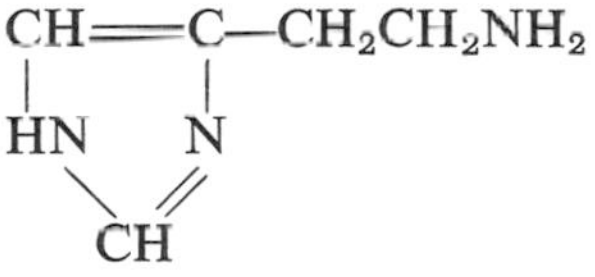

Histamine

ARGININE

This is of immense importance in urea synthesis (p. 33.3), and since the raw material of arginine, ornithine, is readily synthesized from glutamic acid, arginine itself is non-essential. The catabolism of arginine again takes place through ornithine to glutamic acid. Arginine serves as a source of the guanidinyl group for the synthesis of other compounds containing this group, notably creatine.

Creatine is synthesized from arginine, glycine and methionine. The first two are condensed together in the kidney in the presence of the enzyme glycine transamidinase with the formation of guanidinoacetic acid, which is subsequently methylated in the liver to give creatine.

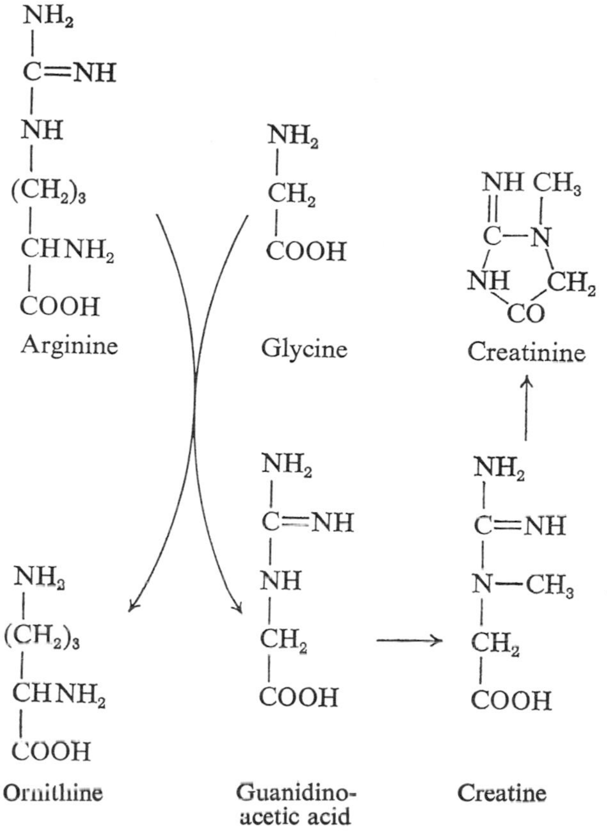

Ornithine   Guanidino-acetic acid   Creatine

Creatine is transported to the muscles where it is converted to phosphoryl creatine (p. 16.13). Creatine is excreted in varying amounts by women and children, but only traces are present in the urine of men. A cyclic anhydride, **creatinine**, is excreted by both sexes. The daily excretion of creatinine is remarkably constant and has been used as an index of muscle mass.

PHENYLALANINE AND TYROSINE (fig. 11.15)

Phenylalanine is an essential amino acid, but tyrosine is not, since it can be synthesized from phenylalanine. Indeed, the normal catabolism of phenylalanine proceeds by hydroxylation to tyrosine. Hereditary lack of the necessary enzyme, phenylalanine 4-monooxygenase leads to an inborn error of metabolism, phenylketonuria, in which phenylalanine, instead, is transaminated extensively to phenylpyruvic acid. This is excreted to the extent of 1–2 g/day and is also metabolized further to phenyllactic acid and related compounds. When the hydroxylase system is present, these other pathways are not followed to any extent. Presence of phenylpyruvic acid in the blood and central nervous system leads to mental retardation. Arrangements to test the blood of every child soon after birth for phenylpyruvic acid have been made in many places. Restriction of the intake of phenylalanine at a sufficiently early age has enabled many infants with this defect to develop normally. Such a treatment is expensive

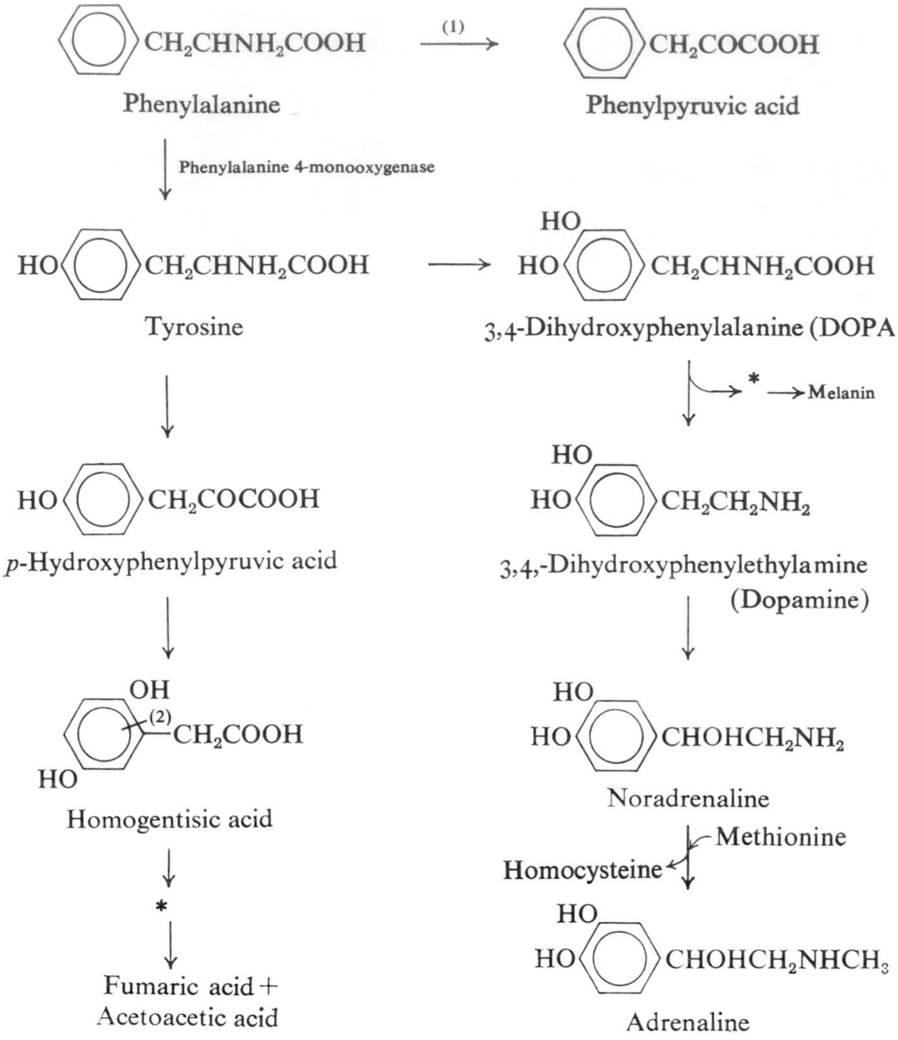

Phenylalanine → Phenylpyruvic acid (1)

Phenylalanine 4-monooxygenase

Tyrosine → 3,4-Dihydroxyphenylalanine (DOPA)

DOPA → * → Melanin

p-Hydroxyphenylpyruvic acid

3,4,-Dihydroxyphenylethylamine (Dopamine)

Homogentisic acid (2)

Noradrenaline

Methionine / Homocysteine

*

Fumaric acid + Acetoacetic acid

Adrenaline

FIG. 11.15. Phenylalanine and tyrosine metabolism. (1) Abnormal pathway followed in subjects with phenylketonuria. (2) Site of cleavage of the aromatic ring; in alkaptonuria the enzyme required is absent. *Successive arrows indicate multiple reactions.

for the community, but the cost is less than that of keeping a mental defective for life (vol. 3, p. 47.6).

After transamination to *p*-hydroxyphenylpyruvic acid the catabolism of the aromatic amino acids proceeds by the formation of homogentisic acid, 2, 5-dihydroxyphenylacetic acid. Compounds like this are readily oxidized; the ring is split open and the resulting dicarboxylic acid, 4-maleylacetoacetic acid, is converted to a mixture of equimolar amounts of fumaric acid and acetoacetic acid. Alkaptonuria is an inborn error of metabolism in which there is a lack of homogentisic acid oxidase. The free acid is excreted in the urine, which darkens greatly as a result of atmospheric oxidation. The connective tissue of people with this inborn error may become pigmented and they are prone to arthritis.

A small amount of tyrosine is metabolized by further

hydroxylation to 3,4-dihydroxyphenylalanine (DOPA), a reaction catalysed by the liver enzyme tyrosinase. DOPA serves as a precursor of the skin pigment melanin (p. 37.10). In the adrenal medulla and the nervous system DOPA is decarboxylated to give the corresponding amine dopamine, which is then used for the synthesis of noradrenaline and of adrenaline in the adrenal medulla.

The iodine-containing thyroid hormones are also derivatives of tyrosine.

TRYPTOPHAN

The bulk of the tryptophan which is metabolized passes under the influence of the hepatic enzyme tryptophan 2,3-dioxygenase, which opens the five membered ring to give *N*-formyl kynurenine (fig. 11.16). Removal of the formyl group leaves kynurenine, which is metabolized

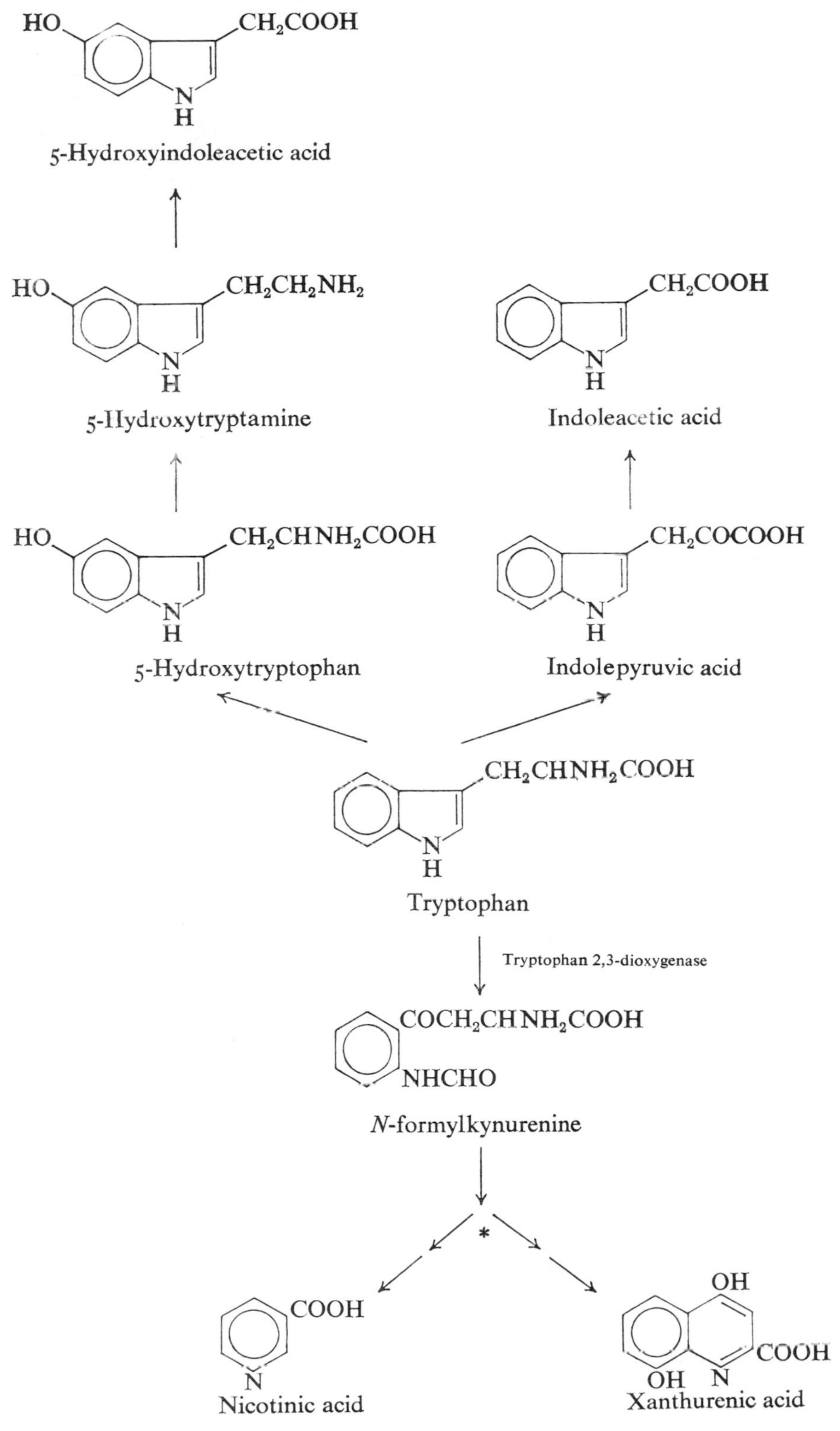

HO — [indole ring] — CH₂COOH
5-Hydroxyindoleacetic acid

HO — [indole ring] — CH₂CH₂NH₂
5-Hydroxytryptamine

[indole ring] — CH₂COOH
Indoleacetic acid

HO — [indole ring] — CH₂CHNH₂COOH
5-Hydroxytryptophan

[indole ring] — CH₂COCOOH
Indolepyruvic acid

[indole ring] — CH₂CHNH₂COOH
Tryptophan

Tryptophan 2,3-dioxygenase

[benzene ring] — COCH₂CHNH₂COOH, NHCHO
N-formylkynurenine

[pyridine ring] — COOH
Nicotinic acid

[quinoline ring] — OH, COOH, OH
Xanthurenic acid

Fɪɢ. 11.16. Some aspects of tryptophan metabolism. *Multiple reactions in both pathways.

through complex pathways to give nicotinic acid as a major normal end-product. Tryptophan is thus to be regarded as a provitamin for nicotinamide. Several of the intermediate reactions require the coenzyme pyridoxal phosphate, and in pyridoxine-deficient conditions the normal pathway may be more or less blocked. The urinary excretion of by-products such as xanthurenic acid is greatly increased, particularly after the patient is given a test dose of tryptophan. Such tests sometimes give abnormal results in pregnancy and in women on oral contraceptives, but the significance of these findings is not clear.

Tryptophan can also be hydroxylated to 5-hydroxytryptophan, which undergoes decarboxylation to 5-hydroxytryptamine (5-HT), an important neurophysiological agent (p. 27.51; vol. 2, p. 16.1). Its formation accounts for little of the daily utilization of tryptophan. 5-HT is deaminated to 5-hydroxyindoleacetic acid before excretion, but a very small amount appears as the alcohol 5-hydroxytryptophol (5-hydroxyindolylethanol). Administration of ethanol makes this a major pathway of 5-HT metabolism.

Melatonin is a derivative of 5-HT which has been isolated from the pineal gland, hypothalamic tissue and peripheral nerve. It promotes the aggregation of melanin granules in melanocytes (p. 37.9) and has indirect functions in the control of reproductive processes in species where these are photosensitive.

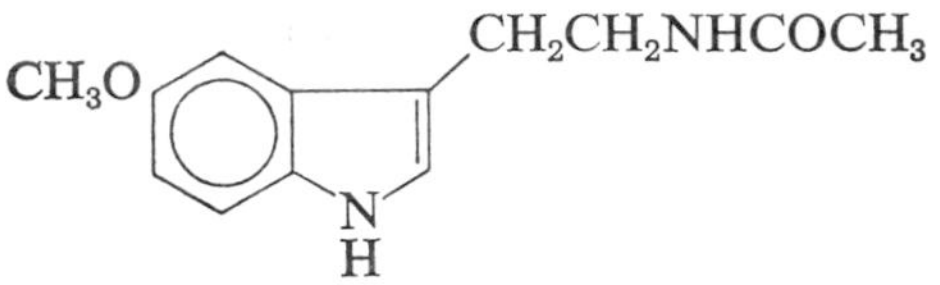

$$CH_3O \quad \underset{H}{\overset{CH_2CH_2NHCOCH_3}{\text{indole}}}$$

Melatonin (*N*-acetyl-5-methoxytryptamine)

Another pathway of tryptophan metabolism involves transamination to indolepyruvi cacid and oxidative decarboxylation to indoleacetic acid, also known as a plant hormone. Several inborn errors of tryptophan metabolism are known (vol. 3, p. 47.4).

Intestinal micro-organisms convert tryptophan to indole and derivatives such as skatole and indoxyl. These may be absorbed and re-excreted. Indoxyl is conjugated in the liver with sulphate to give an ester of which the K salt, indican, is excreted in the urine.

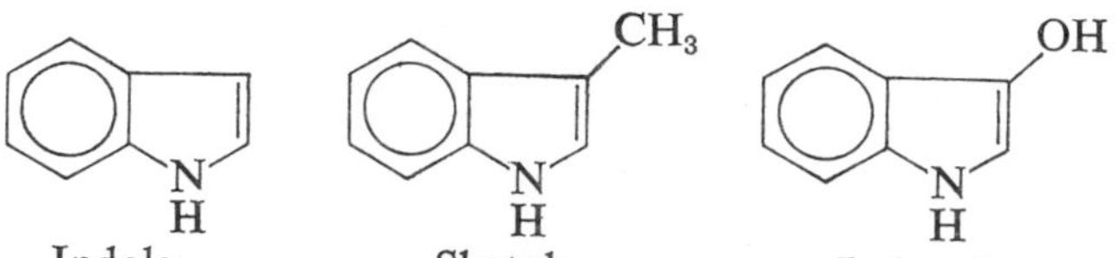

Indole   Skatole   Indoxyl

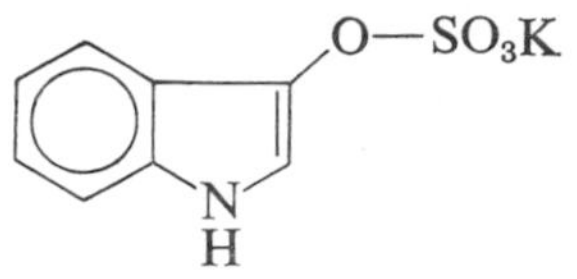

Indican

SERINE

Serine is found in high proportion in the phosphoproteins of milk and eggs, where the hydroxyl groups of serine residues are esterified with phosphate. It is synthesized in the body from either glycine or 3-phosphoglyceric acid, an intermediate in glycolysis. Both pathways are reversible.

GLYCINE

Glycine is the simplest amino acid and is readily formed from carbohydrate, e.g. via 3-phosphoglyceric acid and serine. It is important because it takes part in several biosynthetic processes. These include the synthesis of creatine (p. 11.23) and the synthesis of purine nucleotides (p. 12.24). It reacts with succinyl coenzyme A to give δ-aminolaevulinic acid, an intermediate in the synthesis of porphyrins and haem (p. 28.7).

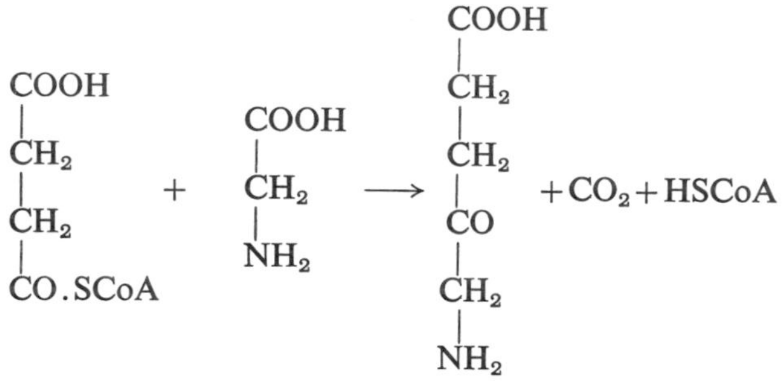

$$\begin{array}{c} COOH \\ | \\ CH_2 \\ | \\ CH_2 \\ | \\ CO.SCoA \end{array} + \begin{array}{c} COOH \\ | \\ CH_2 \\ | \\ NH_2 \end{array} \longrightarrow \begin{array}{c} COOH \\ | \\ CH_2 \\ | \\ CH_2 \\ | \\ CO \\ | \\ CH_2 \\ | \\ NH_2 \end{array} + CO_2 + HSCoA$$

Succinyl coenzyme A   Glycine   δ-Aminolaevulinic acid

Since the reaction which gives glycine from serine is reversible, it is possible for the catabolism of glycine to take place in the same way as that of serine. There are, however, other pathways, notably that in which the amino acid is deaminated by glycine oxidase with the formation of glyoxylic acid and ammonia. The glyoxylic acid may either be oxidized to oxalic acid and excreted in the urine or oxidatively split to formic acid and carbon dioxide. The formic acid may then enter the pathways of 'one-carbon' metabolism.

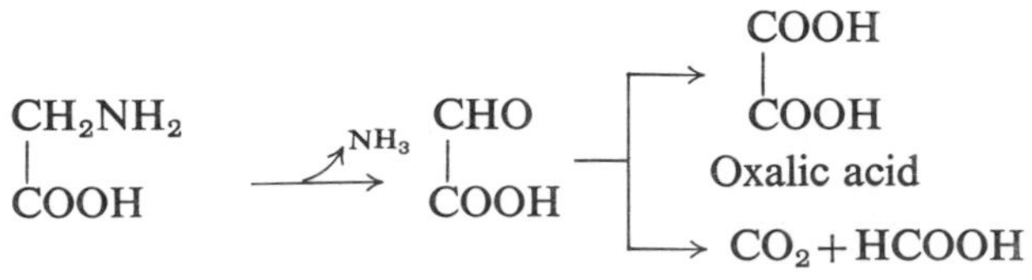

$$\begin{array}{c} CH_2NH_2 \\ | \\ COOH \end{array} \xrightarrow{-NH_3} \begin{array}{c} CHO \\ | \\ COOH \end{array} \begin{array}{c} \nearrow \begin{array}{c} COOH \\ | \\ COOH \end{array} \text{Oxalic acid} \\ \searrow CO_2 + HCOOH \end{array}$$

Glycine   Glyoxylic acid   Formic acid

One-carbon metabolism

In the course of this outline of amino acid metabolism, at least three radicals containing only one carbon atom have been encountered: $-CH_3$, $-CH_2OH$ and $-CHO$. The last of these is familiar as an aldehyde group, but it is also a formyl radical and is usually known by this name in relation to one-carbon metabolism. These radicals appear in the course of the metabolism of methionine, glycine, serine, histidine and tryptophan and may be used in the synthesis of methylated compounds like creatine or choline, or in processes where single carbon atoms have to be inserted into complex structures, as in the synthesis of purine nucleotides (p. 12.26). Isotopic studies show that these radicals, no matter what their origin, pass through a common metabolic pathway. Their metabolism involves the participation of a coenzyme, tetrahydrofolic acid (THF), derived from the water-soluble vitamin folic acid. THF (p. 7.13) binds one-carbon radicals at each of two nitrogen atoms, N^5 and N^{10}. When serine is converted to glycine, the hydroxymethyl group is transferred to the coenzyme to give N^{10}-hydroxymethyl THF. Dehydration gives N^5, N^{10}-methylene THF which can also be formed reversibly from methionine via the intermediate N^5-methyl THF. The N^5, N^{10}-methylene compound can be reversibly oxidized to N^5, N^{10}-anhydroformyl THF which is also produced by the deamination of N^5-formimino THF. The anhydroformyl compound is derived from N^{10}-formyl THF which is itself formed from formate and THF with the help of ATP. Both N^5, N^{10}-anhydroformyl THF and N^{10}-formyl THF are used in the synthesis of purine nucleotides and hence

nucleic acids. Moreover, the other one-carbon derivatives can all be transformed to N^5-methyl THF, an intermediate source of methyl groups for transmethylation. The interrelations of these various substances are summarized in fig. 11.17.

Certain drugs which cause remissions in leukaemia owe their activity to chemical similarity to folic acid (vol. 2, p. 29.7 and vol. 3, p. 21.75). In appropriate cases the effects of overdosage with these powerful drugs can be treated with tetrahydrofolic acid.

Transmethylation

Methionine loses its methyl group to form homocysteine by the process of transmethylation, through which many biologically important methyl compounds are synthesized (table 11.8). Reaction with ATP gives an intermediate high energy compound, *S*-adenosylmethionine, which serves as the methyl donor. The synthesis of creatine from guanidinoacetic acid is given as an example (fig. 11.18).

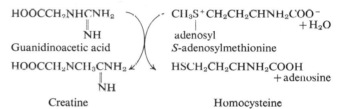

FIG. 11.18. Transmethylation in the synthesis of creatine.

Although methionine is an essential amino acid, it can be synthesized to a limited extent from homocysteine and N^5-methyltetrahydrofolic acid. A methyl group for this purpose can also be derived from betaine, a metabolic oxidation product from choline.

TABLE 11.8. Transmethylation reactions in which *S*-adenosylmethionine is involved.

Methyl acceptor	Product
Guanidinoacetic acid	Creatine
Noradrenaline	Adrenaline
Catecholamines	4,*O*-methylcatecholamines
Nicotinamide	*N*-methylnicotinamide
Phosphatidyl ethanolamine	Phosphatidyl choline

Polyamine synthesis

Aliphatic polyamines derived from the basic amino acids are of widespread biological occurrence. They are strong bases and interact readily with nucleic acids. Under experimental conditions they can affect the rate of DNA replication and the synthesis of aminoacyl t-RNA compounds. Polyamine concentrations rise in transforming lymphocytes and rat liver undergoing regeneration after partial hepatectomy or poisoning with carbon

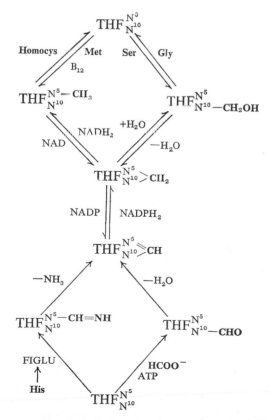

Fig. 11.17. Tetrahydrofolic acid and one-carbon metabolism.

tetrachloride, but the full physiological significance of these observations is unknown. The simplest member of the group, putrescine or 1,4-diaminobutane, is formed by the decarboxylation of ornithine and is used for the synthesis of the more complex compounds spermidine and spermine. Spermidine is formed when *S*-adenosylmethionine donates the nitrogen and three carbon atoms between the sulphur and the methionine carboxyl to putrescine. A repetition of the process at the opposite end of the diaminobutane residue gives spermine, which seems to be the most active of these compounds in biological systems (fig. 11.19).

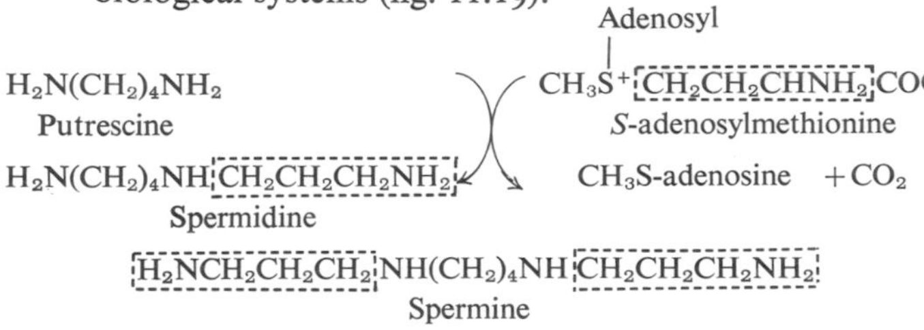

$$H_2N(CH_2)_4NH_2$$
Putrescine

Adenosyl
$$CH_3S^+ \overline{CH_2CH_2CHNH_2}COO^-$$
S-adenosylmethionine

$$H_2N(CH_2)_4NH\overline{CH_2CH_2CH_2NH_2}$$
Spermidine

$$CH_3S\text{-adenosine} + CO_2$$

$$\overline{H_2NCH_2CH_2CH_2}NH(CH_2)_4NH\overline{CH_2CH_2CH_2NH_2}$$
Spermine

FIG. 11.19. Synthesis of spermidine and spermine. The broken lines indicate the portion of the *S*-adenosylmethionine molecule transferred in the synthetic reactions.

TURNOVER OF PROTEINS

The picture of amino acid and protein metabolism is incomplete without some knowledge of the ways in which body proteins are destroyed and the rate at which they are replaced. Apart from the specialized case of the proteins of skin, hair and nails, which are lost altogether, the body proteins are believed to be destroyed by hydrolysis. Isotopic labelling experiments show that there is some re-utilization of the amino acids during the replacement of intracellular proteins, which indicates that the destructive process must be one in which amino acids are liberated. Proteolytic enzymes, the cathepsins, are widely distributed in tissues. They are found especially in lysosomes (p. 13.8), but the extent to which they are active during life is unknown.

How long the molecules of any given protein persist before replacement is a complex problem. Experiment shows that many extracellular proteins are destroyed at random, but at very different rates. At one extreme, measurement of the rate of disappearance of the label after an initial brief period of synthesis from isotopically labelled amino acids has shown that, in the rat, bone collagen synthesized in infancy persists with little destruction for at least 300 days (half the life span). Collagen from other sources is less persistent. On the other hand, the use of purified proteins labelled with ^{131}I has shown that human serum albumin may be replaced at a rate of about 3 per cent/day and fibrinogen at 25 per cent/day.

The position with intracellular proteins is more complicated, because the pattern of cell life, with the synthesis of protein during cell division balanced by protein destruction on the death of the cell, is superimposed on possible metabolic patterns during the life of the cell. The study of individual proteins, e.g. liver aldolase and muscle myosin, indicates that some turnover takes place during the life of the cell. This varies greatly from tissue to tissue and from protein to protein, e.g. liver proteins are more labile than those of muscle, but is small compared with the initial rate of synthesis or the final rate of degradation when the cell is destroyed. In the case of erythrocytes, no metabolism of haemoglobin takes place while the mature cell is circulating and the daily renewal of 0·8 per cent of the cells accounts for a turnover of about 90 mg protein/kg/day. At the other extreme the cells of the jejunal mucosa undergo renewal every 1–2 days and even although the rate of protein replacement might in other circumstances appear quite substantial, it is negligible in comparison with the high turnover of protein associated with the rapid replacement of the cells themselves. When these cells are exfoliated, their protein is added to the dietary protein in the alimentary tract, which is also augmented by the proteins of the digestive juices themselves and a small but significant portion of escaped plasma proteins, particularly albumin. In protein-deficient rats regeneration of jejunal mucosal cells takes place at less than half the normal rate.

It is difficult to arrive at a sound overall value for the rate of replacement of protein in the entire body, largely because the extent to which the re-utilization of amino acids takes place cannot yet be fully evaluated. One careful study suggests that the daily rates of protein synthesis in newborn babies, young adults and elderly persons are about 17, 3 and 2 g/kg respectively, values which become similar when seen as proportions of the resting metabolic rate for the age groups studied. These and other figures agree in showing that protein turnover is several times greater than the normal daily dietary intake, so that the latter clearly performs an indispensable topping-up function. Nevertheless, the daily absorption of amino acids is many times greater than the sum of the pools of free amino acids within the body, but although fluctuations in plasma amino acid concentrations do occur they are transient and smaller than might be expected. Increase in dietary protein raises the amino acid concentration in the portal blood, from which the liver removes much of the excess, so that the rise in the systemic circulation is less. The rate of synthesis of secreted proteins like albumin rises, and an increased synthesis of urea cycle enzymes accounts for the increase in synthesis and excretion of urea.

When a subject consumes a protein free diet the output of nitrogen in the urine takes several days to fall to the value which reflects inevitable wastage of tissue proteins (fig. 11.9). Negative nitrogen balance is thus most marked in the early stages of such an experiment.

The weight and protein content of certain organs, notably the liver, spleen and other visceral structures, follow a similar downward curve. Some of the plasma proteins, in particular albumin and transferrin, behave similarly. There is a fall in haemoglobin which is secondary to a diminution in the numbers of erythrocytes. If the diet is low in protein, the changes are qualitatively similar but quantitatively less, although different organs and proteins are affected to different extents. The protein content and weight of the liver, for example, fall even when the change in protein intake is not sufficient to cause overt signs of protein deficiency. When normal protein intake is resumed, all these changes are reversed. The subject goes into positive nitrogen balance which only reverts to equilibrium after several days. The nitrogen retained appears as an increase in the total protein of the body, distributed appropriately over those organs which lose protein on a protein deficient diet. That part of the body protein which fluctuates according to the dietary intake is called **labile body protein**. Even under the most favourable conditions, the labile body protein is not more than 5 per cent of the total body protein or 600 g in an adult male. It is usually much less. It is generally assumed that modest diminution in the various components of labile body protein does no harm, so that at times this fraction has been regarded as a short term store. Even if this view is correct the effect does not seem to be important. There is also no evidence that those of us in prosperous countries, who are accustomed to eat much more protein than the amounts necessary to ensure that physiological needs are met, derive any benefit thereby.

CONTROL MECHANISMS

Like other metabolic processes, those of amino acid and protein metabolism are controlled at the molecular level by the rates of enzymically catalysed reactions, which may be altered in three ways: directly through the mass action effect of substrate concentration, by allosteric effects on enzyme activity and by changes in enzyme concentration.

Since they are themselves the constituents of enzyme molecules, amino acids may be regulatory vehicles in a way which is without parallel in carbohydrate or fat metabolism. Tryptophan is found in low concentration in most proteins and plays a part as a metabolic limiting factor which is analogous to its role under some conditions as a limiting amino acid in the dietary protein. The synthesis of liver proteins, including enzymes concerned both in protein synthesis and in amino acid metabolism, depends on the supply of tryptophan. Such effects may be mediated by setting a limit to the rate of translation of messenger RNA. The same amino acid provides a different example of control. The first reaction in the major pathway of tryptophan metabolism is catalysed by tryptophan 2,3-dioxygenase, an enzyme which is sta-

bilized in the presence of its substrate. This ensures an adequate supply of the enzyme when there is ample tryptophan and, perhaps more important, ensures the conservation of the amino acid when it is not freely available. Tryptophan affords the best known example of this type of control, but in other circumstances another amino acid, e.g. methionine, may limit the rate of protein synthesis, and many enzymes are stabilized by their substrates.

ACTIONS OF HORMONES

A rise in plasma amino acids, e.g. from dietary causes, stimulates the secretion of insulin (p. 27.46), corticosteroids and hypophyseal growth hormone. All these hormones, as well as thyroxine and the sex hormones, affect the metabolism of amino acids and proteins. In muscle and adipose tissue insulin promotes the uptake of amino acids and stimulates the synthesis of protein, perhaps because it also stimulates the synthesis of some kinds of RNA. In liver the effects of insulin develop more slowly and appear to depend very much on the individual proteins considered. The suppression of hepatic gluconeogenesis is one of the best known of the effects of insulin, and this may be caused by a diminution in the activity or quantity of the key enzyme phosphoenolpyruvate carboxykinase.

Cortisol, on the other hand, stimulates gluconeogenesis. This may be caused by a stimulation of RNA synthesis, leading to increased synthesis of liver proteins, including enzymes (pp. 14.15 & 27.35). Since cortisol inhibits protein synthesis and amino acid uptake by muscle, the general result is a diversion of amino acids to the liver and its metabolic processes. Cortisol in this way stimulates the catabolism of protein, with increase in plasma amino acids and urea excretion. This is an early consequence of stress, e.g. accidental or surgical trauma, and it is attractive to speculate that the transient increased availability of amino acids facilitates the anabolic stage of recovery. Gluconeogenesis is also stimulated by glucagon (p. 27.48).

Growth hormone appears to stimulate the uptake of amino acids and protein synthesis by all cells. Thyroxine causes an indirect RNA-mediated stimulation of protein synthesis, and also promotes protein breakdown in all cells, an effect which predominates whenever the hormone is above the physiological level.

Several androgenic steroids including testosterone stimulate the synthesis of protein in muscle, possibly because of the increase in activity of the nuclear enzyme RNA polymerase. This so-called anabolic effect is easily demonstrable in rats. Numerous analogues of testosterone have been used by athletes in the hope of increasing muscle mass, although this is forbidden by athletic codes, and in the treatment of patients with various wasting diseases. The effect, if present, is usually slight and of doubtful value in adults. However the sudden increase of muscle mass in boys at puberty is probably attributable to the increased secretion of testosterone at that period.

The extent to which any metabolic pathway is used depends on the amounts of enzymes or polypeptide hormones made available by synthesis and, as their specific biological properties are determined by the amino acid sequence, all the processes of protein synthesis (chap. 12) are an important part of the mechanism for the regulation of metabolism (chap. 14).

FURTHER READING

FAO/WHO EXPERT COMMITTEE (1973) Energy and Protein Requirements. *Technical Reports of the World Health Organization* No. 522.

FLORKIN M. & STOTZ E.H. eds. (1975) *Comprehensive Biochemistry*, vol. 25. Regulatory Functions—Mechanisms of Hormone Action. Amsterdam: Elsevier.

FLORKIN M. & STOTZ E.H. eds. (1975) *Comprehensive Biochemistry*, vol. 31. A History of Biochemistry, part III, chap. 35. From amino acids to the tricarboxylic acid cycle. Amsterdam: Elsevier.

LEHMANN H. & HUNTSMAN R.G. (1974) *Man's Haemoglobins*, 2nd Edition. Amsterdam: North Holland.

MUNRO H.N. & ALLISON J.B. eds. (1964–70) *Mammalian Protein Metabolism*, vols. I–IV, New York: Academic Press.

NEURATH H. (1963–70) *The Proteins*, 2nd Edition, vols. I–V. New York: Academic Press.

ROSE W.C. (1957) The amino acid requirements of adult man. *Nutrition Abstracts & Reviews* 27, 631–647.

ROSENBERG L.E. & SCRIVER C.R. (1974) Disorders of amino acid metabolism. In *Diseases of Metabolism*, 7th Edition, vol. I, chap. 10, pp. 465–654, ed. Bondy P.K. & Rosenberg L.E. Philadelphia: Saunders.

WATERLOW J.C. (1975) Protein turnover in the whole body. *Nature* 253, 157.

YOUNG V.R., J, STEFFEE W.P. *et al.* (1975) Total human body protein synthesis. *Nature* 253, 192–193.

Chapter 12
Cell growth and division

The growth and division of a unicellular organism, such as a **bacterial** (prokaryotic) or a **protozoal** (eukaryotic) cell, leads ultimately to the formation of two copies of a structure of which there was originally only one. If, as is usually the case, the two daughter cells are identical, every molecule and atom of the parent cell is duplicated in the daughter. With **metazoan cells** the duplication is frequently less clear cut since differentiation of the daughter cells is more likely to occur in the course of growth. However, in general, the growth and division of a metazoan cell requires the duplication of the great majority of the molecules and structures in the parent.

The distribution of newly-synthesized cell material between the daughter cells broadly follows one of two patterns; it is either shared between the daughters, or it all finds its way to one of them. Most mammalian cells share their cell compounds more or less equally between their daughters, but the second type of division, usually called **budding**, is encountered in some plants and primitive animals. Among the yeasts, for example, both types of division are found and this leads to the description of a yeast as a 'budding' or a 'fission' yeast.

The duplication of cell material involves the synthesis of many types of macromolecules, apart from the provision of sufficient compounds of low molecular weight to allow macromolecular synthesis to occur. The biosynthesis of most types of macromolecules is described in chaps. 9 & 10. This chapter is concerned primarily with two processes:

(1) the method by which inherited information is interpreted and used to make the protein part of the new cell material, i.e. the mechanism of protein synthesis and the role of the gene,

(2) the method by which the information necessary to synthesize a cell or indeed a whole new organism is transferred from cell to cell and from organism to organism.

The key molecule in both these processes is deoxyribonucleic acid (DNA), since the information needed to allow the synthesis of all the proteins and enzymes of the cell, bacterial or mammalian, lies in the nucleotide base sequence of the DNA (p. 12.2). It is the same base sequence that provides the information which allows a duplicate copy of the DNA to be made for the daughter cell. In this section therefore, the structure of DNA is first discussed in some detail since the informational role of this molecule is implicit in its structure. Then the way in which the information in the DNA is used to make proteins is considered. Finally the method whereby the information is passed to daughter cells and organisms is described.

STRUCTURE OF DNA

The DNA molecule is an extremely long chemical thread made up of two strands. Unlike most threads, however, the strands are not wound round one another but are held as a pair which are wound round an imaginary central core to form a spiral or 'double helix' (fig. 12.1). This arrangement means that the gross structure of the helix looks like a long screw from the side; but if it is examined from one end, a hole can be seen passing from one end to the other up the centre of the helix.

Each strand of the double helix consists of a long chain of the sugar deoxyribose and phosphate residues arranged as shown in fig. 12.2. These chains are formed by the loss of two water molecules to condense a phosphoric acid residue with two deoxyribose molecules, one being attached through its 5'-hydroxyl and the other through its 3'-hydroxyl. Each of these deoxyribose molecules is, in turn, connected to further phosphate residues, and so the chain is built up. Every sugar molecule in the chain is substituted through its 3'- and 5'-hydroxyl groups and all the phosphates are doubly substituted except the residues at the ends of the chain. One end is a singly-substituted phosphate on a 3'-hydroxyl of a deoxyribose, and the other is a similar phosphate on a deoxyribose 5'-hydroxyl. This difference allows the chemical identification of the two ends of a DNA strand; and any process, such as a stepwise enzyme action (p. 12.16), which moves along the strand, can be considered to move in a definite direction, either $5' \rightarrow 3'$ or $3' \rightarrow 5'$. This concept of 'direction' along a DNA deoxyribose-phosphate backbone is important since the two strands that go to make up the double helical thread are arranged to lie in

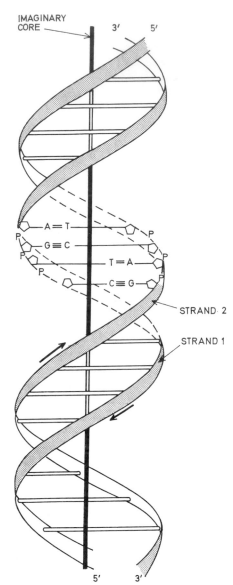

FIG. 12.1. DNA thread of two strands round an imaginary core in an anti-parallel manner. A, T, G and C represent the complementary base pairs adenine, thymine, guanine and cytosine (p. 12.2).

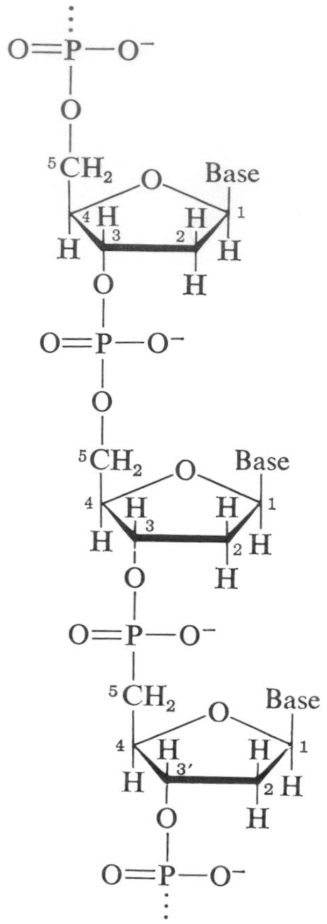

opposite directions: reading along the strands from one end of the double helix to the other, one strand runs in the direction $3' \rightarrow 5'$ and the other $5' \rightarrow 3'$. For this reason, the DNA thread is said to consist of an anti-parallel double helix.

In addition to the phosphate residues at the $3'$ and $5'$ positions, each of the deoxyribose residues in the strands is further substituted at the C-1 position with a purine or pyrimidine base (fig. 12.2). Two purines, adenine and guanine, and two pyrimidines, thymine and cytosine, are commonly found in DNA (fig. 12.3). Although no intrinsic pattern seems to emerge when the order of the

FIG. 12.2. Three residues from the middle of the polydeoxyribosephosphate backbone of DNA.

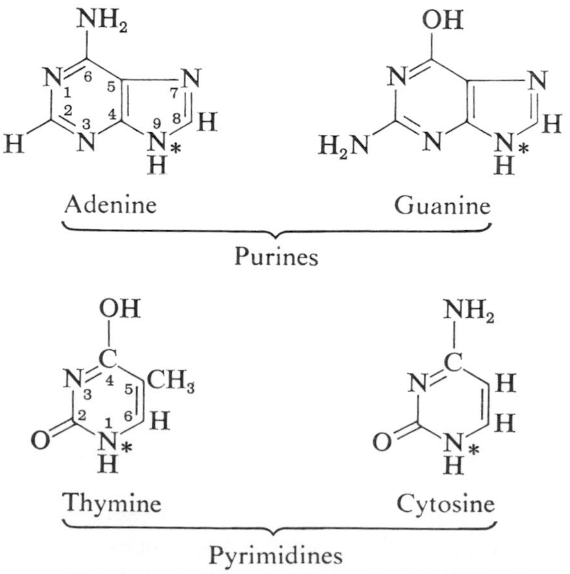

FIG. 12.3. Structure of the purine and pyrimidine bases found in DNA. The asterisk marks the atom involved in bonding to the C-1 of deoxyribose.

bases along the strand is examined, the bases on one strand are clearly related to the bases on the strand opposite. In the DNA double-helical thread the purine and pyrimidine bases of the two strands lie opposite one another in the structure (fig. 12.4) and the pattern is always one in which

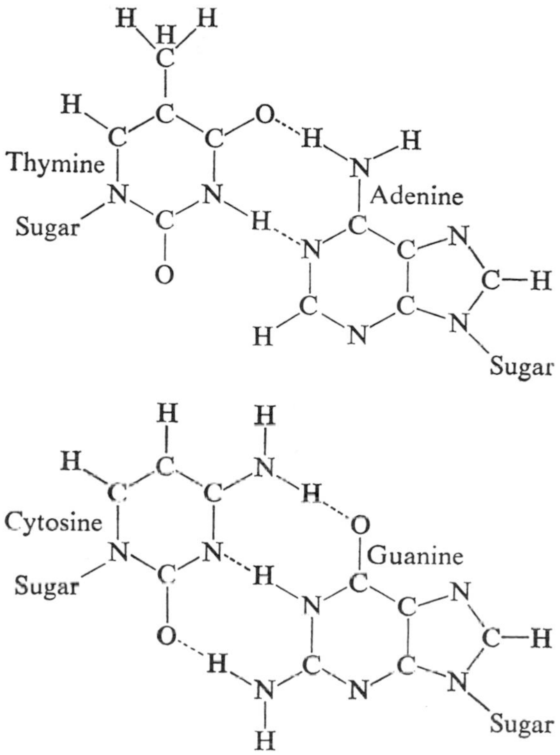

FIG. 12.4. Complementary base pairs drawn to show intermolecular hydrogen bonds (dotted lines).

a thymine on one strand is faced by an adenine and a guanine by a cytosine. Thus thymine and adenine are said to be a complementary base pair and so are guanine and cytosine. This arrangement is largely responsible for holding the two strands in their correct juxtaposition in the double-helical thread; adenine–thymine and guanine–cytosine base pairs are particularly effective in doing this because they form closely-fitting intermolecular links through hydrogen bonds, two in the case of the adenine–thymine pair and three with guanine–cytosine (fig. 12.4). The presence of an adenine opposite a thymine and a guanine opposite a cytosine means that there is always one molecule of adenine to every molecule of thymine and one guanine for every cytosine in DNA; chemical analysis shows this to be so.

Although the ratio of each base in a pair is 1 : 1, the ratio of the two types of base pairs, (adenine + thymine) to (guanine + cytosine), varies widely in DNA from different species. Examination of the (adenine + thymine) to (guanine + cytosine) ratios for various organisms shows that the more extreme ratios are carried by bac-

teria, whereas the mammalia form a closer group around an (adenine + thymine)/(guanine + cytosine) ratio of 60 : 40 (table 12.1). The similar base ratio of all mammalia is usually taken to indicate a relatively close evolutionary relationship when compared with different species of bacteria.

TABLE 12.1. Guanine + cytosine per cent of base pairs in DNA of some bacteria, invertebrates and vertebrates.

Bacteria and rickettsiae	Invertebrates	Vertebrates
30 *Clostridium welchii*		
32 *Rickettsia prowazeki*		
34 *Staphylococcus aureus*	34 Sea urchin sp.	
36 *Proteus vulgaris*	36 Sea urchin sp.	
38 *Pneumococcus*	38 Clam	
40		40 MAN
42 *Bacillus subtilis*	42 Earthworm, locust	42 Ox, sheep, pig, mouse, rat, salmon, trout, herring, frog.
44 *Rickettsia burneti*		44 Horse, hen, turtle
46		
48 *Corynebacterium acne*		
50 *Neisseria gonorrhoeae*		
52 *Escherichia coli*		
54 *Salmonella typhi*		
56 *Aerobacter aerogenes*		
58 *Brucella abortus*		
60		
64 *Pseudomonas fluorescens*		
66 *Pseudomonas aeruginosa*		
68 *Mycobacterium tuberculosis*		
70		
72 *Micrococcus lysodeikticus*		
74 *Actinomyces bovis*		

The very precise alignment of base pairs in the double-stranded molecule of DNA leads to a structure of great regularity, whatever the ratio of (A + T) / (G + C). The overall diameter of the helical thread is about 1·8 nm and there are about ten base pairs per turn. The base pairs, being virtually planar structures, are stacked on top of one another like a pile of coins and their interaction with the other atoms of the helix ensures that they are spaced regularly about 0·34 nm apart. The intramolecular hydrogen bonding also holds the —C-3′—O—P—O—C-5′— polydeoxyribosephosphate strands in a fixed position at an angle of about 70° to the longitudinal axis of the DNA.

When the double helix is looked at from the side, the polydeoxyribosephosphate chains, which contribute most to the screw-like appearance of the structure, are seen to be unequally spaced to give a major and a minor groove. This arrangement is also a direct consequence of the interatomic hydrogen bonds and the precise geometry of the grooves may be very important in the action of certain antibiotics used in clinical medicine.

It must be stressed that all the dimensions given so far refer to double-stranded DNA when examined in the crystalline state by X-ray crystallography. In this state the structure is very compressed and the extent of inter-atomic bonding within the molecule at its greatest. In solution, or in the cell, there is little doubt that base pairing exists, but it is clear that the rigidly crystalline structure cannot occur. The molecular weight of DNA isolated from cells is usually between 5×10^8 and 1.5×10^9 (average about 8×10^8) and such DNA is usually some-what degraded. A molecular weight of 8×10^8 corresponds to a helical length of about 5 μm and clearly therefore some super-coiling of the helix is essential if it is to be accommodated in the chromosome. A well-documented case of the impossibility of accommodating helical DNA in a cell concerns the DNA from bacteriophage (bacterial viruses). In this case the DNA from the phage is about 3 μm long, if stretched out in the helical state, yet the phage head is only about 0.08 μm in diameter.

Single-stranded DNA

Although virtually all the DNA in cell nuclei is double-stranded, some bacterial viruses have single-stranded DNA. The molecular weight of the DNA in these viruses is about 1.7×10^6, and they are organisms with probably the smallest quantity of genetic information. These viruses are probably single-stranded only when outside the host cell; once within the cell they immediately set about synthesizing the strand complementary to the one carried by the free virus.

Determination of DNA structure

The structure of DNA outlined above has been deduced from extensive study of the products of chemical and en-zymic hydrolysis together with the X-ray crystallographic examination of crystalline DNA. The polydeoxyribo-nucleotide nature of the molecule was deduced by chemical means and careful analysis gave the following molecular characteristics:

(1) The sum of the purine nucleotides in hydrolysates equals the sum of pyrimidine nucleotides, i.e. $(A+G) = (T+C)$.

(2) Adenine and thymine are present in equal amounts, and so are guanine and cytosine, i.e. $(A=T)$ and $(G=C)$.

(3) The number of 6-amino groups on the purine and pyrimidine bases equals the number of 6-keto or hydroxyl groups. In this respect, $(A+C) = (G+T)$. The underlying structural reason for these constants, however, was not apparent until the actual position of the atoms in a crystal of DNA was visualized by X-ray crystallographic analysis. When this was done, Watson and Crick were able to suggest their complementary anti-parallel base pairing model to rationalize all the analytical and crystallographic evidence on DNA structure.

Although the overall structural features of the DNA molecule are now clear, the actual base sequence of any gene is still not known completely. Some considerable lengths of some genes have been elucidated, and this has thrown interesting light on how genes comes to be trans-cribed but in no case is the sequence anything like com-plete.

Genetic code

As mentioned previously, the order of the base pairs in the DNA double helix appears to be completely random apart from the specific pairing across from strand to strand, but actually it contains very precise information. In the process of protein synthesis (p. 12.4) the order of the amino acids in the strand-like polypeptide chains of a protein is determined by the order of purine and pyrimi-dine bases on one of the strands of the DNA double helix. Thus the essentially linear molecule of DNA determines the structure of the essentially linear polypeptide chain, and the apparently random order of bases on the DNA reflects the apparently random order of amino acids in a polypeptide chain. In practice it is found that only one strand of the DNA is used in protein synthesis and that sets of three adjacent bases on this strand provide the information that leads ultimately to the insertion of one amino acid into the growing polypeptide chain. For this reason the DNA is said to carry a code constructed out of 'base triplets'.

Since four different purine and pyrimidine bases are found in DNA, sixty-four different base triplets are possible, if it is assumed that the base order can only be read in one direction along the DNA strand and that the triplets do not overlap (see p. 12.1 for a discussion of 'direction' in DNA). Since only twenty different amino acids are found in proteins under natural conditions (p. 11.1) more than one 'triplet' is available for each type of amino acid. Identification of the triplets that correspond to each amino acid, the problem of 'cracking the genetic code', has shown that certain amino acids can be coded by up to six different base triplets whereas others only have one (see p. 12.12). The reason for this variation is not yet understood.

PROTEIN SYNTHESIS: THE COMPONENTS OF THE SYSTEM

It has already been stated that one of the central roles of DNA in the cell is to provide information to enable amino acids to be inserted into their correct places in a growing polypeptide chain during protein synthesis.

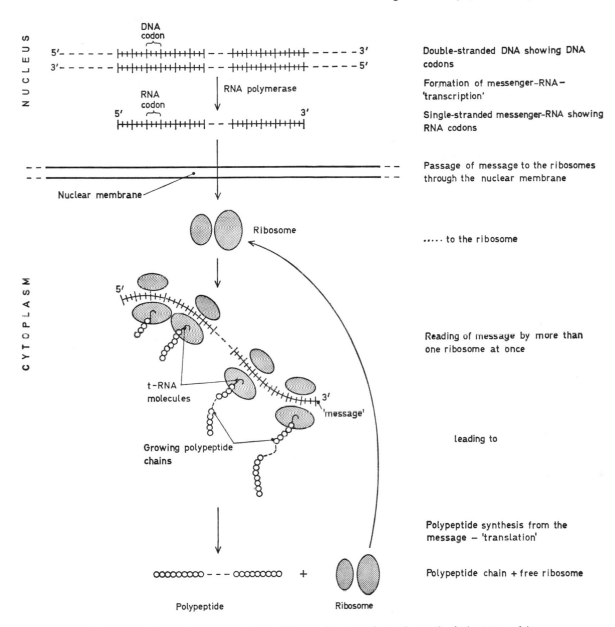

NUCLEUS

5′ – – – – – |+|+|+|+|+|+|+|+|+|+| – – – |+|+|+|+|+|+|+|+|+| – – – – – 3′   Double-stranded DNA showing DNA
3′ – – – – – |+|+|+|+|+|+|+|+|+|+| – – – |+|+|+|+|+|+|+|+|+| – – – – – 5′   codons

DNA codon

RNA polymerase

Formation of messenger-RNA –
'transcription'

RNA codon

5′ |+|+|+|+|+|+|+|+|+| – – – |+|+|+|+|+|+|+|+|+| 3′   Single-stranded messenger-RNA showing
RNA codons

Passage of message to the ribosomes
through the nuclear membrane

Nuclear membrane

CYTOPLASM

Ribosome   ..... to the ribosome

5′

Reading of message by more than
one ribosome at once

t-RNA
molecules

3′
'message'

Growing polypeptide
chains

leading to

Polypeptide synthesis from the
message – 'translation'

Polypeptide chain + free ribosome

Polypeptide   Ribosome

FIG. 12.5. Schematic representation of the mechanism of protein synthesis (not to scale).

Proteins are synthesized on ribosomes by the stepwise addition of amino acids to a growing polypeptide chain (p. 12.10); one problem in protein synthesis can therefore be stated precisely. How can the information contained in the DNA as a succession of base triplets be translated to ensure the correct order of insertion of amino acids in a growing protein? This problem is exacerbated in eukaryotic cells by the fact that the DNA lies in a nucleus whereas most of the ribosomal sites of protein synthesis are outside the nuclear membrane.

The problem is solved in the cell by the use of a second type of informational macromolecule, once again a strand-like nucleic acid with repeating structure (fig. 12.5).

The information is transcribed from the purine–pyrimidine 'language' of the DNA to the similar language of ribonucleic acid (RNA) and then translated to the amino acid language of protein at the ribosome. The intermediary nucleic acid molecule is a special type of RNA, often called **messenger RNA** in recognition of its role. Once at the ribosome the information in the messenger RNA is translated into a polypeptide chain by the use of a number of further RNA molecules which are adapted to recognize both specific purine–pyrimidine triplets of the message and also amino acids. These **translating RNAs** are often called the **transfer** or **t-RNAs**. They are not bound permanently to the message on the ribosome, but are free in solution in the neighbourhood of the protein-synthesizing sites and appear to be drawn into the system when required to insert a given amino acid. After carrying out this process they are then liberated until required again.

In the succeeding sections, therefore, the chemical structure of the messenger RNA, transfer RNAs and ribosomes are examined to see how their structure is adapted to their role in protein synthesis before proceeding to discuss the mechanism of protein synthesis itself in detail.

Structure of messenger RNA (m-RNA)

Superficially, messenger RNA has considerable structural similarities to DNA. Once again there is the long chain of alternating sugar–phosphate residues; although in RNA the sugar is ribose not deoxyribose. As in DNA, the phosphates are doubly substituted, one bond being to the 3'-hydroxyl of the sugar and the other to the 5'. Once again the ends of the strand can be distinguished, one by having a free 5'-phosphate and the other by a 3'-phosphate. Unlike DNA, however, there is no evidence that messenger RNA contains base pairs and therefore the molecule is single stranded. Furthermore, since there are no base pairs there is no mechanism for forming a stable helical structure and a length of messenger RNA is probably a great deal more flexible than an equivalent length of DNA.

DNA chains are extremely long, and they are not transcribed into messenger RNA in one piece. Rather, the DNA is transcribed section by section, as a series of messages, so the RNA transcripts are much shorter than the DNA. At the lower limit, messenger RNAs may be as little as 150 bases long, and it seems unlikely that they can ever contain more than 7000–10,000 bases. The means whereby the DNA is transcribed section by section, rather than as a continuous messenger-RNA molecule, is discussed later.

As with DNA, the information necessary to ensure the insertion of an amino acid in the correct position in a growing polypeptide chain is carried in the sequence of purines and pyrimidines substituted at the C-1 position of the ribose residues of messenger RNA. However, the bases found in RNA are not all the same as in DNA. The purines adenine and guanine and the pyrimidine cytosine are present in both DNA and RNA, but thymine does not occur in RNA whereas another related pyrimidine, uracil (fig. 12.6), does. So the sixty-four base triplets of DNA, which are constructed from the four bases adenine, guanine, cytosine and thymine, are transcribed into sixty-four RNA triplets compiled from adenine, guanine, cytosine and uracil. These RNA base triplets are frequently called **RNA codons**, since they are the code units carrying the essential information to ensure the unambiguous insertion of a single amino acid when

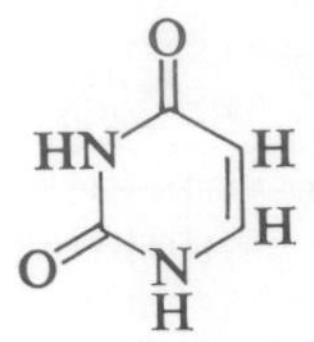

FIG. 12.6. Structure of the pyrimidine uracil.

the message comes to be translated into protein. Because of the method of synthesis, however, the base sequence of a given piece of DNA is not transcribed into a piece of messenger RNA having an identical base sequence, even excepting the replacement of thymine by uracil. Rather the messenger RNA base sequence is complementary to the DNA sequence, as if a base-paired double strand had formed between the informational strand of the DNA and a strand of messenger RNA during synthesis (see p. 12.2). Thus the messenger carries a complementary cytosine when DNA carries guanine (or vice versa) and uracil where DNA has adenine (or vice versa).

Structure of transfer RNA (t-RNA)

Since the messenger RNAs are transcripts of portions of the DNA and are capable of leaving the nucleus to reach the ribosomal sites of protein synthesis (p. 12.5), their use solves the first problem of the transfer of information from the DNA to the ribosome, the problem of translocation. However, the messenger RNA molecules, as in DNA, carry their information in terms of their purine and pyrimidine base sequence and there remains the problem of 'translating' the language of purine–pyrimidine triplets into amino acid sequence. This step is achieved by the transfer RNAs with the help of the ribosomes.

The structure of the transfer RNAs, of which there are certainly large numbers of different types in a cell, is based in each case on the polyribosephosphate backbone characteristic of the nucleic acid molecules examined so far. Once more the molecule has 'ends' consisting of free 3'- and 5'-phosphates, and the ribose molecules are substituted at C-1 with purine and pyrimidine bases. As with the messenger RNAs, the bases adenine, guanine, cytosine and uracil are common, but the transfer RNAs often contain an additional sprinkling of other purines and pyrimidines, often called the 'unnatural' or 'abnormal' bases (fig. 12.7). Transfer RNAs are considerably smaller than most RNAs, and the complete structure of a number has now been worked out.

So far, two parts of the alanine t-RNA structure have been clearly identified in its activity, and similar regions occur in all transfer RNAs:

(1) the final base at the 3' end of the molecule. In practice the final three bases at the $P^{3'}$ end (CCA) are common to all t-RNAs that have yet been examined. These are numbered 75–77 in fig. 12.8;

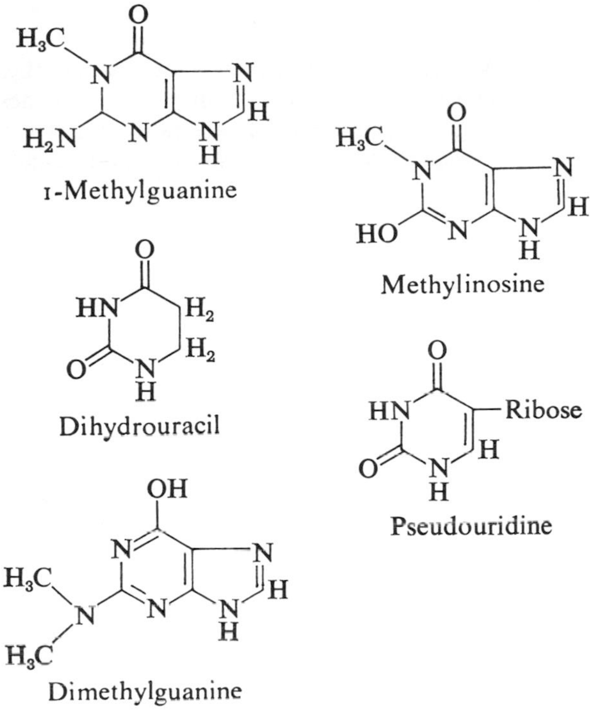

1-Methylguanine

Methylinosine

Dihydrouracil

Pseudouridine

Dimethylguanine

FIG. 12.7. The 'unnatural' purines and pyrimidines found in alanine transfer-RNA from yeast. In addition to these compounds, thymine (normally considered to be a pyrimidine characteristic of DNA) is found in alanine transfer-RNA.

$$\overset{1\,2\,3}{\overbrace{}}\qquad\overset{Me}{|}$$
HO.P$^{5'}$.G.G.G.C.G.U.G.U.G.G.C.G.C.G.U··

$$\overset{DiH}{|}\qquad\overset{DiH}{|}\qquad\overset{DiMe}{|}$$
···A.G.U.C.G.G.U.A.G.C.G.C.G.C.U.C.C.C.U···

$$\overset{36\,37\,38}{\overbrace{}}\overset{Me}{|}$$
···U.I.G.C.I.ψ.G.G.G.A.G.A.G.U.C.U.C.C···

···G.G.T.ψ.C.G.A.U.U.C.C.G.G.A.C.U.C.G···

$$\overset{75\,76\,77}{\overbrace{}}$$
···U.C.C.A.C.C.A.P$^{3'}$.OH

FIG. 12.8. Structure of alanine transfer-RNA from yeast.

A=adenine, G=guanine, C=cytosine, U=uracil

'Abnormal' bases
I: hypoxanthine (base-pairs as guanine)
T: thymine (normally a DNA component)
DiH.U: 5, 6 dihydrouracil
DiMe.G: N, N dimethylguanine
Me.G: 1-methylguanine
Me.I: methylhypoxanthine
ψ: pseudouridine

(2) a group of bases near the middle of the molecule, numbered 36–38 in fig. 12.8.

The first of these two regions is responsible for binding the alanine. Since this region of the molecule is the same in all t-RNAs it confers no specificity to the molecule. The terminal A residue merely accepts the activated amino acid to form the transfer RNA-amino acid complex.

The second region is the one responsible for recognizing the relevant base triplet on the messenger RNA. As we have seen, the sequence of base triplets, each of which specifies an amino acid, is transcribed from DNA into the complementary base sequence of messenger RNA and it is these RNA triplets, or **RNA codons**, that have each to be identified by part of the transfer RNA structure. The part of the transfer RNA which recognizes the codon is called the **anticodon** and consists of residues 36–38 in the structure shown in fig. 12.8. Recognition is by base-pairing between the codon and the anticodon in an antiparallel manner, as though that section of the RNA was double-stranded. This interaction is shown in fig. 12.9.

$$3' \longrightarrow 5'$$
Anticodon   ...C G I...   (in transfer RNA)
Codon   ...G C C...   (in messenger RNA)
$$5' \longleftarrow 3'$$

FIG. 12.9. Codon-anticodon pairing between alanine transfer RNA (anticodon: CGI) and one of the alanine RNA codons (CCG).

The remainder of the t-RNA structure is concerned with recognition of the enzyme responsible for loading the relevant amino acid (*via* the amino acid adenylate, see p. 12.9) onto the carrier adenine residue at the 3' end of the molecule.

Examination of the base sequence of the various transfer RNAs, whose structure is now known in detail, shows that certain regions are diverse in base sequence while others are relatively conservative, and this is thought to be connected with the way in which these small RNA molecules fold. In practice they seem to have regions of internal base-pairing to give a clover-leaf structure (fig. 12.10), and all transfer RNAs can be drawn in a similar form. It will be noted that the two regions set aside for specific comment above do not contribute to the base-paired regions. With the anticodon, at least, the reason is clear enough; it must be able to participate in base-pairing with the codon.

Although it is possible to draw the structure of all t-RNAs in the clover-leaf form, it would be misleading to think of them having this conformation in the cell. There is almost certainly additional superfolding, and indeed the clover-leaf pattern takes no account of possible further base-pairing between the regions of the molecule that remain single stranded in the conformation shown in fig. 12.10.

Before leaving the topic of t-RNAs, it is important to mention that each RNA codon in the message may well have more than one t-RNA carrying the appropriate anticodon. The reason for this multiplicity of t-RNAs is

Ribosomes

The ribosomes are the site of protein synthesis and their microscopic structure and location in the cell are described on p. 13.8. Chemically they are fairly uniform in composition regardless of their source, and usually

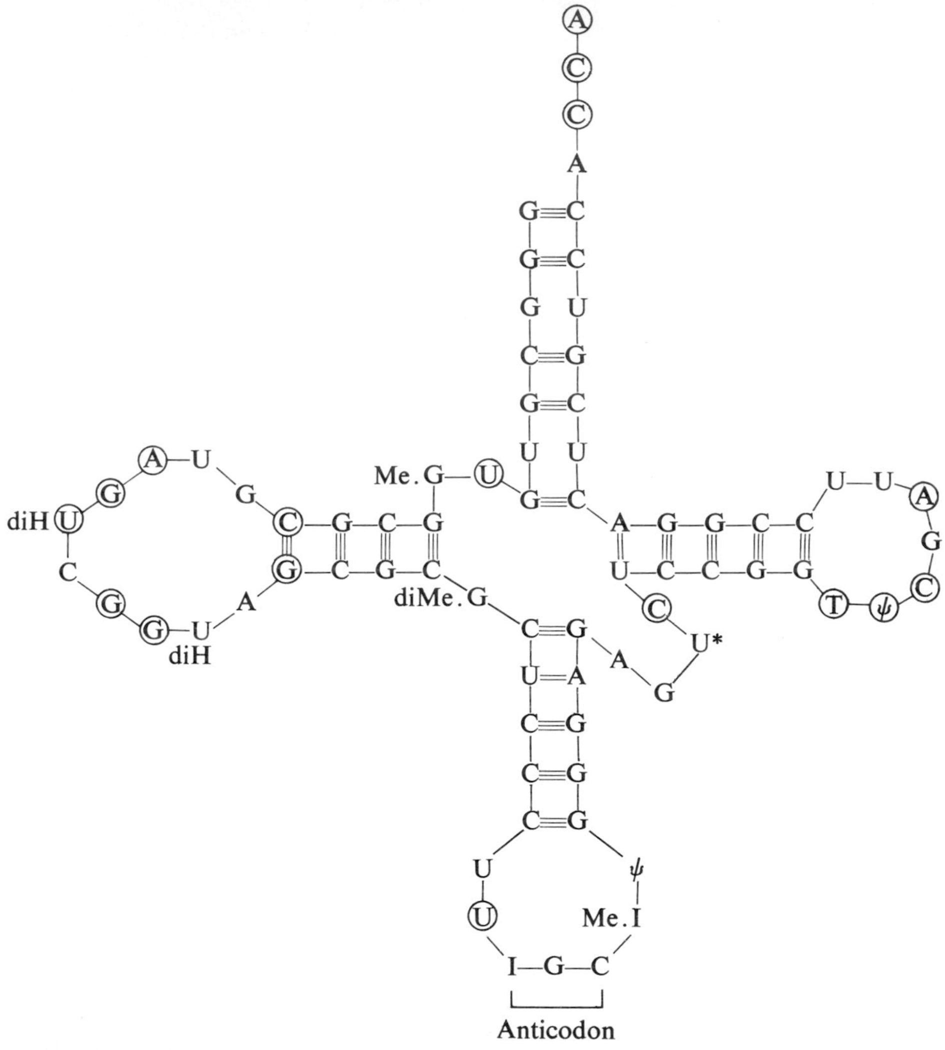

FIG. 12.10. Alanine transfer RNA from yeast, drawn in the 'clover-leaf' form. See also figs. 12.8 & 9.

not yet known. However, one possibility is that it is a means of protecting the protein-synthesizing system of the cell from the effects of mutation. Since the bases of the anticodon reflect the DNA base sequence of the gene that specifies the t-RNA directly, mutation in the appropriate part of that gene could lead to alteration of the anticodon without modifying any other parts of the t-RNA. This, in turn, could lead to the widespread insertion of the 'wrong' amino acid in many cell proteins. In this case, therefore, duplication of t-RNAs may be solely protective.

contain about 60 per cent protein and 40 per cent RNA (r-RNA). The protein component is not a single protein but a relatively large number of different proteins, the majority of which appear to be basic, and the r-RNAs have the polyribosephosphate structure, substituted with purine and pyrimidine bases, which has become familiar from the discussion of messenger and transfer RNA. In the laboratory, ribosomes can be made to fall into two unequal pieces, one about 65 per cent of the total and the other about 35 per cent, although whether this occurs in the cell is very doubtful. The relative proportion of protein to nucleic acid in these fragments seems to be about the same as in the parent structure, but it is likely that the larger fragment carries two RNA chains whereas the smaller has only one. Each RNA chain contains about 1500–2000 bases but the extent of inter-base pairing and helical structure is much disputed. The function of ribosomal RNA is not yet clear.

PROTEIN SYNTHESIS: THE MECHANISM

The process of protein synthesis involves two separate series of biochemical reactions:

(1) the reactions that each amino acid has to undergo to achieve an activated chemical state from which it can form a peptide bond and thus extend the growing peptide chain by one unit,

(2) the reactions by which the information in the DNA is transferred via the messenger RNA to the site of protein synthesis on the ribosome.

These two biochemical processes impinge at the site of protein synthesis on the ribosome and are co-ordinated there by the transfer RNAs. The process is shown diagrammatically in fig. 12.5.

AMINO ACID ACTIVATION

This process occurs in two stages and is carried out by enzymes called **aminoacyl-RNA synthetases.** The first reaction consists of the coupling of an amino acid with adenosine triphosphate (ATP) to form an aminoacyl-adenylate, with the liberation of pyrophosphate. The amino acid adenylate is not liberated from the enzyme surface during this reaction but the pyrophosphate is, and the course of amino acid activation may be followed experimentally by measuring the liberation of this compound:

$$\text{ATP} + \text{\textcircled{E}} + \text{HOOCCHNH}_2 \overset{R}{|}$$

$$(1) \downarrow \text{PP}_i$$

$$\text{\textcircled{E}} . \text{AMP} . \text{OCCHNH}_2 \overset{R}{|}$$

t-RNA—C—3'—$\text{\textcircled{P}}$—5'—C—3'—$\text{\textcircled{P}}$—5'—A—3'—$\text{\textcircled{P}}$

$$\text{\textcircled{E}} + \text{AMP} + \text{P}_i \xleftarrow{(2)}$$

t-RNA—C—3'—$\text{\textcircled{P}}$—5'—C—3'—$\text{\textcircled{P}}$—5'—A—COCHNH$_2$ $\overset{R}{|}$

The second stage of the reaction involves transfer of the amino acid residue from adenosine monophosphate (AMP), still on the surface of the enzyme, to the terminal adenine residue of the *adenyl.cytidyl.cytidyl*··· portion of the relevant transfer RNA (p. 12.7). Once formed, the cleavage of the bond joining the amino acid to the t-RNA

can provide the free energy for the formation of a peptide bond.

There is probably a synthetase enzyme for each type of transfer RNA found in the cell and the specificity of interaction between these molecules lies in the structure of the enzyme and the RNA sequence of those parts of the t-RNA not involved in accepting the amino acid or binding to the RNA codon in the message.

PEPTIDE BOND SYNTHESIS

Once activated in this way and carried on a specific transfer RNA, the amino acid is capable of reacting with the carboxyl end of a growing polypeptide chain according to reaction 3a (p. 12.10). During synthesis of the protein chain, the end of the growing peptide chain is occupied by an amino acid (R_1, reaction 3a) still attached through its carboxyl group to the terminal adenine of its own transfer RNA (t-RNA$_1$); thus its terminal amino acid is still in the activated state. The incoming activated amino acid (R_2, coupled to t-RNA$_2$) reacts through its free amino group to form a peptide bond with the activated terminal carboxyl of the peptide chain (reaction 3a). The energy necessary for this chemical reaction comes from the splitting of the bond between the terminal carboxyl group and the adenine of t-RNA$_1$. At the end of this reaction, therefore, the amino acid chain has been lengthened by an amino acid which is still activated with t-RNA$_2$ on its carboxyl group, and t-RNA$_1$ is liberated. The next amino acid (R_3, carried by t-RNA$_3$) is then added to the growing chain by an identical series of reactions (reaction 3b), and in this way the polypeptide chain grows to the full length determined by the number of triplets in the message. Which of the twenty amino acids is inserted at each position in the peptide chain seems to be determined solely by the coding triplet in the message attracting an anticodon grouping on a t-RNA which is already loaded with an amino acid.

POLYRIBOSOMES

Since the ribosome is intimately involved in the processes described above, the point of contact between the message and the ribosome must move along the messenger RNA as the polypeptide chain grows. Electron microscope (EM) studies of ribosomes photographed in the act of synthesizing proteins suggest that more than one ribosome can pass along a messenger RNA molecule at one time; that is, synthesis of a second polypeptide chain may start before the previous one is complete. The structures in which the ribosomes are found at intervals along the length of a messenger RNA molecule are often called polyribosomes.

FORMATION OF MESSENGER RNA

We have seen how the amino acids are activated and are inserted one at a time into the growing polypeptide

$$
\begin{array}{c}
\overset{\text{t-RNA}_1}{\underset{}{|}} \\
\overset{R}{\underset{|}{}}\ \overset{R}{\underset{|}{}}\ \overset{R}{\underset{|}{}}\ \overset{R_1\ 3'}{\underset{|}{}} \\
\text{NH}_2\text{CHCONHCHCONHCHCONHCHCO}
\end{array}
\quad + \quad
\begin{array}{c}
\overset{\text{t-RNA}_2}{\underset{}{|}} \\
\overset{R_2\ 3'}{\underset{|}{}} \\
\text{NH}_2\text{CHCO}
\end{array}
\tag{3a}
$$

$$\downarrow$$

$$
\begin{array}{c}
\overset{\text{t-RNA}_2}{\underset{}{|}} \\
\overset{R}{\underset{|}{}}\ \overset{R}{\underset{|}{}}\ \overset{R}{\underset{|}{}}\ \overset{R_1}{\underset{|}{}}\ \overset{R_2\ 3'}{\underset{|}{}} \\
\text{NH}_2\text{CHCONHCHCONHCHCONHCHCONHCHCO}
\end{array}
\quad + \quad
\begin{array}{c}
\overset{\text{t-RNA}_1}{\underset{}{|}} \\
3' \\
\text{OH} \\
\text{(released)}
\end{array}
$$

$$
\begin{array}{c}
\overset{\text{t-RNA}_2}{\underset{}{|}} \\
\overset{R}{\underset{|}{}}\ \overset{R}{\underset{|}{}}\ \overset{R}{\underset{|}{}}\ \overset{R_1}{\underset{|}{}}\ \overset{R_2\ 3'}{\underset{|}{}} \\
\text{NH}_2\text{CHCONHCHCONHCHCONHCHCONHCHCO}
\end{array}
\quad + \quad
\begin{array}{c}
\overset{\text{t-RNA}_3}{\underset{}{|}} \\
\overset{R_3\ 3'}{\underset{|}{}} \\
\text{NH}_2\text{CHCO}
\end{array}
\tag{3b}
$$

$$\downarrow$$

$$
\begin{array}{c}
\overset{\text{t-RNA}_3}{\underset{}{|}} \\
\overset{R}{\underset{|}{}}\ \overset{R}{\underset{|}{}}\ \overset{R}{\underset{|}{}}\ \overset{R_1}{\underset{|}{}}\ \overset{R_2}{\underset{|}{}}\ \overset{R_3\ 3'}{\underset{|}{}} \\
\text{NH}_2\text{CHCONHCHCONHCHCONHCHCONHCHCONHCHCO}
\end{array}
\quad + \quad
\begin{array}{c}
\overset{\text{t-RNA}_2}{\underset{}{|}} \\
3' \\
\text{OH} \\
\text{(released)}
\end{array}
$$

chain at the behest of the triplet codons on the messenger RNA. The only biochemical process that remains to be described is the formation of messenger RNA. The exact biochemical reactions involved in messenger RNA synthesis are unknown although *in vitro* studies have given an indication of what must be involved. The synthesis of RNA in normal cells appears to be brought about by an enzyme known as **DNA-dependent RNA polymerase**. This enzyme is capable of synthesizing RNA by the stepwise addition of nucleotides according to the following general reaction, where XTP represents the nucleotide triphosphates of adenine, guanine, cytosine or uracil.

$$
\begin{array}{c}
\overset{\text{RNA}}{\underset{|}{}} \\
\overset{5'}{\underset{|}{}} \\
\circledP
\end{array}
\ + \text{XTP} \rightarrow\
\begin{array}{c}
\overset{\text{RNA}}{\underset{|}{}} \\
5' \\
\circledP \\
| \\
3' \\
| \\
X \\
| \\
5' \\
| \\
\circledP
\end{array}
\ + \text{PP}_i
$$

The enzyme requires a 'primer' of double-stranded DNA and the order in which the nucleotides are inserted into the growing nucleotide chains is determined by the nucleotide order of the primer DNA. When studied in the test tube, using double-stranded DNA, two types of RNA chain are synthesized, each complementary in structure to one of the DNA strands of the double helix. Thus the action of the enzyme on a piece of DNA having the following composition,

$$3'-\text{A}-\text{G}-\text{C}-\text{T}-\text{T}-\text{C}-\text{G}-\text{A}\cdots 5' \quad (1)$$
$$5'-\text{T}-\text{C}-\text{G}-\text{A}-\text{A}-\text{G}-\text{C}-\text{T}\cdots 3' \quad (2)$$

would be to yield two single-stranded RNA chains, one having the sequence

$$5'-\text{U}-\text{C}-\text{G}-\text{A}-\text{A}-\text{G}-\text{C}-\text{U}-3'$$

(i.e. complementary to strand 1) and the other having the sequence

$$3'-\text{A}-\text{G}-\text{C}-\text{U}-\text{U}-\text{C}-\text{G}-\text{A}-5'$$

(complementary to strand 2). In the living cell, however, only one of the DNA strands is transcribed into an RNA chain.

Actinomycin D inhibits DNA replication by binding to DNA and thus blocking DNA-primed RNA polymerase (vol. 2, p. 20.14). Rifampicin acts by binding directly to DNA-primed RNA polymerase.

'CRACKING THE GENETIC CODE'

Before leaving the topic of protein synthesis and the involvement of DNA in the process, it is valuable to examine briefly the experimental approaches that were used to elucidate the genetic code, that is, to decide which of the sixty-four possible DNA and RNA base triplets can lead to the insertion of given amino acids in the growing peptide chain.

The main experimental routes which have been used are:

(1) determination of the amino acid sequence of pure proteins,

(2) examination of the effect of mutagens on amino acid sequence, and

(3) synthesis of model polynucleotide 'messengers' and their use for protein synthesis *in vitro*.

The first step was the discovery that minor differences in amino acid sequence existed in the structure of proteins and enzymes obtained from various species. Even within a species, genetically-determined variations in protein structure can be found. In man the haemoglobins provide an example (p. 28.5). The amino acid sequence of haemoglobin from most individuals conforms to a structure now accepted as 'normal' haemoglobin but, rarely, molecular variants of the 'normal' structure are found (p. 11.9). One of these is the haemoglobin associated with sickle-cell anaemia, a very common disorder in negro races. This haemoglobin differs from 'normal' in the substitution of a single amino acid in the structure (valine) for another (glutamic acid). Since the sickle-cell trait is heritable it was assumed that the change of amino acids in the haemoglobin was genetically determined and due to a one-step mutation. Other 'variant' haemoglobins have been detected in the human population and these can be be shown to be due to a single, or at the most two, amino acid transpositions. Examination of all the alternative amino acids which are found at a single point in these variants of the haemoglobin molecule has shown that certain amino acid transpositions are common while others have never yet appeared. These results suggest, therefore, that amino acids that can be exchanged are separated by a single mutational step, whereas those which cannot are separated more widely. Since one mutation will change the nature of one of the bases in a coding triplet in the DNA, it follows that amino acids which can be exchanged at a single point in the structure in haemoglobin, or any other protein for that matter, will have DNA codons which differ in the nature of only one of the three bases. Although this approach gives some idea of the relationships between the amino acids and their codons it gives no idea of the nature of the bases involved.

In view of these results the next stage was clearly to try to induce mutations with mutagens known to have specific chemical effects, in an attempt to link certain types of chemical change in the DNA to certain types of amino acid transposition in the proteins. By and large this approach has been bedevilled by the broad specificity

of most mutagens and it is never possible to be absolutely sure that a given chemical change has actually occurred in the DNA.

Despite these difficulties, however, two mutagens yielded useful results. The first was nitrous acid, which was known from previous chemical work to change an $-NH_2$ group to an $-OH$ group; for example, adenine to hypoxanthine and cytosine to uracil. Although neither of these products are normal components of DNA, it became clear that they could act, at least in the coding role, and by the careful study of HNO_2 mutations certain amino acid transpositions could be identified as associated with changes in either guanine or cytosine.

The other mutagens that yielded valuable results were members of the acridine series of dyes. Their action was either to add or subtract a base from DNA by insertion or excision during synthesis. Although the line of argument is involved it became clear that insertion or excision of one base leads to disappearance of the product protein in recognizable form and that the insertion or excision of two additional bases was necessary for the reappearance of recognizable protein. These arguments were the first to hint at the presence of a **triplet code**, a solution that had been anticipated on theoretical grounds.

The final proof of the triplet nature of the code came from experiments in which the composition of the protein synthesized was examined after certain model messenger-RNA molecules had been added to an *in vitro* protein-synthesizing system. In the first experiments of this kind a 'message' of polyuridylic acid led to the synthesis of polyphenylalanine, suggesting that the RNA triplet UUU coded for phenylalanine. More complex messages, such as poly UC, caused the synthesis of polypeptides consisting of two alternating amino acids, thus:

$$UCU, \ CUC, \ UCU, \ CUC, \ UCU, \ \cdots$$
$$\downarrow$$
$$Ser, \quad Leu, \quad Ser, \quad Leu, \quad Ser, \quad \cdots$$

These results suggested that the 'code' was probably triplet but could theoretically involve any odd number of bases. The clinching experiment was one in which the primers were poly AAG, poly AGA, and poly GAA. These three polymers led to the synthesis of three different polypeptides each containing one amino acid, thus:

$$AAG, \ AAG, \ AAG, \ AAG, \ AAG, \ \cdots$$
$$\downarrow$$
$$Lys, \ Lys, \ Lys, \ Lys, \ Lys, \ \cdots$$

and
$$AGA, \ AGA, \ AGA, \ AGA, \ AGA, \ \cdots$$
$$\downarrow$$
$$Arg, \ Arg, \ Arg, \ Arg, \ Arg, \ \cdots$$

and　　GAA, GAA, GAA, GAA, GAA, ⋯

$$\downarrow$$

Glu,　Glu,　Glu,　Glu,　Glu,　⋯

Thus the code must be 'triplet' and AAG, AGA and GAA are RNA codons for Lys, Arg and Glu respectively. The complete list of RNA codons is shown in table 12.2.

TABLE 12.2. The RNA version of the genetic code.

First base	Second base				Third base
	U	C	A	G	
U	Phe	Ser	Tyr	Cys	U
	Phe	Ser	Tyr	Cys	C
	Leu	Ser	C.T.	C.T.	A
	Leu	Ser	C.T.	Trp	G
C	Leu	Pro	His	Arg	U
	Leu	Pro	His	Arg	C
	Leu	Pro	GluNH$_2$	Arg	A
	Leu	Pro	GluNH$_2$	Arg	G
A	Ile	Thr	AspNH$_2$	Ser	U
	Ile	Thr	AspNH$_2$	Ser	C
	Ile	Thr	Lys	Arg	A
	Met*	Thr	Lys	Arg	G
G	Val	Ala	Asp	Gly	U
	Val	Ala	Asp	Gly	C
	Val	Ala	Glu	Gly	A
	Val	Ala	Glu	Gly	G

C.T., chain termination triplets. *AUG is the initiator codon in bacterial and mammalian cells. In bacteria it leads to the insertion of *N*-formyl-methionine.

The DNA version consists of the complementary sequences of deoxyribonucleotides. It is interesting that this list now contains three codons which can lead to chain termination in the polypeptide. UGA is the most likely to act extensively *in vivo*.

Punctuation

The RNA version of the genetic code (table 12.2) contains two types of so-called **punctuation triplets** which influence the translation of messenger RNA. The first type is the single **initiator triplet**, AUG, which is involved in the onset of message translation. The other type, comprising the three **terminator triplets**, UAA, UAG and UGA, do not code for the insertion of an amino acid, but rather lead to chain termination and the release of the newly completed polypeptide from the ribosome. The genetic code is therefore responsible for providing the information to start and stop translation as well as for deciding the order of amino acid insertion during polypeptide synthesis.

INITIATION

In both bacterial and mammalian cells a single triplet (AUG) is responsible for initiation although the exact process is slightly different in the two types of cell. In both cases the triplet used is one which, were it not the first in the message to recognize the t-RNA, would lead to the insertion of methionine. Unlike termination (see below) initiation involves an amino acid insertion and the difference between the mammalian and bacterial processes lies in the chemical nature of the amino acid used. In mammalian cells it seems to be methionine itself, while in bacteria *N*-formyl-methionine (fig. 12.11) is involved. In both cases this initiating residue is removed immediately after the completion of the polypeptide chain, so in practice the first residue in the mature polypeptide chain is coded for by the triplet in the message immediately succeeding AUG.

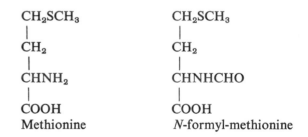

FIG. 12.11. Structure of methionine and *N*-formyl-methionine.

In both mammalian and bacterial cells a number of proteins, probably three, are concerned in initiation and the process involves some conformational changes in the ribosome. Initially the ribosome dissociates into its 30S and 50S components and messenger RNA is bound to the 30S subunit, using the first initiator protein as a catalyst. Then the t-RNA corresponding to AUG binds by codon/anticodon interaction, a process catalysed by the second initiator protein. In both bacterial and mammalian cells a special t-RNA (known as t-RNA$_f$) is used for this purpose. In both cases it has the anticodon needed to recognize AUG but in mammalian cells it is loaded with a methionine residue, while in bacteria the *N*-formylated derivative of this amino acid is used. Once the complex consisting of 30S subunit/message/loaded t-RNA$_f$ (the so-called initiation complex) has formed, the 50S subunit is attached, and the process of polypeptide synthesis proper begins. This sequence is summarized in fig. 12.12. The precise role of the third initiator protein is still unclear.

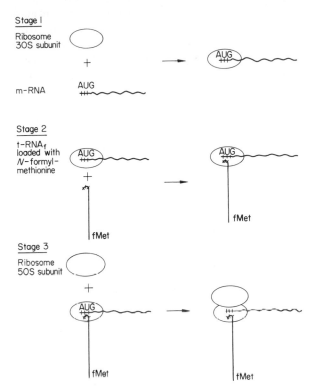

Stage 1
Ribosome
30S subunit

+

m-RNA   AUG

Stage 2
t-RNA$_f$
loaded with
N-formyl-
methionine

+

fMet

fMet

Stage 3
Ribosome
50S subunit

+

AUG

fMet

fMet

Fig. 12.12. Diagrammatic representation of the initiation of translation.

It is important to stress at this stage that the initiator triplet may not be the first in the message. Messenger RNA molecules vary greatly in their size and constitution depending on the job they have to do. In some cases they may be responsible for the synthesis of a single polypeptide chain in a relatively unregulated manner, and in this case the initiator triplet may indeed lie near the beginning of the message. But even in such a simple case, regions responsible for binding to the ribosome will be needed and these will have to lie between the start of the messenger RNA molecule itself and that part of it which leads to the synthesis of polypeptide chains.

In many living systems much more complex messenger RNA molecules exist. Commonly the message is responsible for the synthesis of a number of polypeptide chains which go to form a series of proteins, often of metabolically related function. Such polycistronic messages, as they are known, will clearly have some regions related to polypeptide chain synthesis, while other parts are concerned with ribosome binding and with the beginning and end of translation. Polycistronic messages therefore have a number of initiator codons corresponding to the sites for starting the synthesis of each polypeptide chain; and since many proteins have more than one polypeptide chain per molecule, each mature protein may need more than one initiator.

TERMINATION

Unlike initiation, where one triplet is involved, termination may use one of three (UAA, UAG and UGA, see table 12.2), although it is still not certain that all these are used in all types of cell. Probably most species use one of the three predominantly. Another dissimilarity from initiation is that the termination triplets do not lead to the insertion of an amino acid. Rather, with the help of terminator proteins, they lead to the release of the polypeptide chain from the ribosome. This release, in both bacterial and mammalian cells, is controlled by two proteins R1 and R2, and both recognize the termination triplets directly. R1 recognizes UAA or UAG while R2 binds to UAA or UGA.

As with initiation triplets, there will be one termination triplet in a message for each polypeptide chain that is specified. Whether the last triplet of a message is a termination triplet is still uncertain. Certain very simple RNA viruses, which may themselves be regarded as RNA messages in some respects, end in the sequence UAAUGA, i.e. with two termination codons one after the other, but whether this arrangement is to be found in all messages is not known as yet.

REGULATION OF PROTEIN SYNTHESIS

Although most cells carry a single copy of a given gene as part of their DNA it is obvious that living cells have widely varying needs for individual proteins. For example, the number of molecules of pantothenic acid needed by a cell as a metabolic cofactor is much smaller than its requirement for leucine as a protein constituent, and accordingly it is important for the cell to be able to balance its biosynthetic activities against its requirements. Similar adjustments are needed for the various catabolic reactions of the cell and, in general, all the metabolic activities of living organisms need to be regulated precisely to the needs of the moment. One way of doing this is to modify the activity of enzymes, and this is a commonly used method of regulation in both bacterial and mammalian cells. But in many circumstances it is more economical to regulate the amount of enzyme protein available to do a job; this type of regulation is the primary concern here since it involves a perturbation of the rate of synthesis of individual proteins.

The earlier parts of this chapter have described how the base sequence of the DNA is transcribed into the RNA of the message, and then how this message is translated, with the aid of ribosomes, into the polypeptide chains that go to make up the mature proteins (fig. 12.5). This system means that the rate of synthesis of a given protein could be regulated at two main points; either the formation of message can be influenced or its translation into protein adjusted. In practice both occur and are known as transcriptional and translational control, respectively.

Transcriptional control

Transcriptional control is exercised ultimately by regulation of the activity of RNA polymerase, the enzyme that catalyses the synthesis of messenger RNA from the relevant stretch of DNA (fig. 12.5). This type of control takes two forms; either the binding of the RNA polymerase enzyme to its attachment site on the DNA is regulated, or its ability to start its journey along the DNA and synthesize the messenger as it goes is controlled. Bacterial cells undergo interference at both points and both result in a regulation of the amount of protein synthesized. These two mechanisms tend to produce different effects. The first tends to set the rate of transcription of the particular piece of DNA in question, and is a type of control where the level of expression is not easily altered without mutational change. The second is much more flexible and allows the intervention of specific molecules so that the extent of transcription, and therefore the synthesis of individual proteins, may be specifically controlled by small inducer or repressor molecules.

Laboratory studies have shown that RNA polymerase binds specifically to certain regions of the DNA known as **polymerase binding sites.** These sites probably consist of a number of consecutive bases on one or both of the DNA strands. Not only do the sequences in these regions control the recognition of the polymerase molecule, they also affect the strength, or affinity, of binding to the site. In this way the detailed sequence of the site may influence the effectiveness of the polymerase to achieve transcription.

Genetic studies suggest strongly that an alteration in the affinity between the RNA polymerase and the DNA in the binding sites affects the rate of protein synthesis, since mutations within the binding site significantly affect the rate of transcription. Originally these mutations, which were sometimes known as 'pace-setter mutations' in view of their consequences, were shown to map in a region named the **promoter**, but this region is now thought to be precisely equivalent to the polymerase binding site. Certainly mutants mapping in this region can influence the rate of synthesis of certain bacterial proteins by a factor of several hundred-fold, but each promoter binding site is specific for a given message and single mutational alteration therefore only affects the rate of synthesis of that particular message.

In regions of the DNA where there are no other regulatory sites, the binding of the RNA polymerase to the binding site seems to be solely responsible for setting the rate of message transcription, and the polymerase transcribes an RNA molecule from the DNA template until instructed to stop by a transcription termination region (see below). However, with other genes or groups of genes, the passage of the polymerase from the binding site to those regions of the DNA eligible for transcription

into message may be subject to a further control, and it is at this point of the process that many specific **regulator molecules** exert their effect on those parts of the whole protein synthetic effort under their control. For example, it is here that β-galactosides ultimately act to allow β-galactosidase, and the other proteins associated with it, to be synthesized (p. 14.14).

The specific effects which hinder the access of the polymerase molecule to those parts of the DNA sequence which are to be expressed as messenger RNA are also achieved by the binding of specific effector proteins to the DNA. This **repressor binding site, o (operator)**, lies between the **polymerase binding site** p and the start of the section of the DNA to be transcribed (structural gene) (fig. 12.13). In practice this type of interaction leads

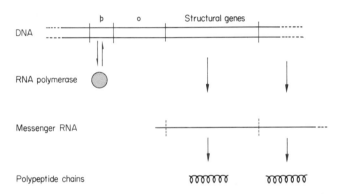

FIG. 12.13. Transcriptional regulation of messenger synthesis at the RNA polymerase binding site, p. The amount of messenger RNA, and consequently the amount of polypeptide synthesized, depend primarily on the affinity of the RNA polymerase molecule for the polymerase binding site.

to a great variety of regulatory possibilities even though the actual effect may be simple; the binding of the effector to the DNA impairs the passage of the RNA polymerase along the DNA, perhaps even mechanically just by getting in the way. The potential variety in such a process arises from the fact that this effector is a protein and, like many such molecules, is capable of a range of modified behaviour in the presence of small molecules. In practice each effector seems to have two basic properties. On the one hand it recognizes the repressor binding region on the DNA, and on the other it recognizes those small molecules whose regulatory effect it has to mediate. Thus, with this protein, interaction with the small molecules may alter its conformation and this, in turn, may influence its binding to the DNA. If the small molecule acts to make the effector protein lose its power of binding to the DNA, the block to the passage of RNA polymerase will be removed and transcription will take place (fig. 12.14). Such a process is a classical enzyme induction where the small molecule is the **enzyme inducer.**

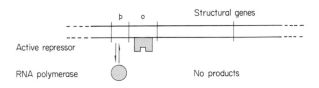

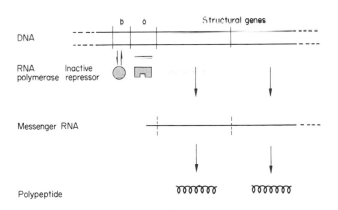

FIG. 12.14. Inducible protein synthesis. Polymerase binding site, p; repressor binding site, o. *Only inactive when complexed with small molecule inducer.

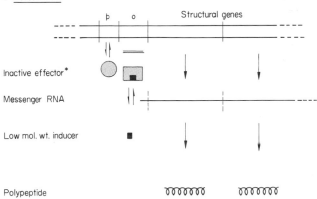

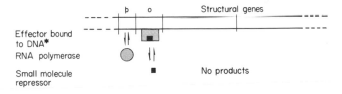

FIG. 12.15. Repressible protein synthesis. *Only occurs when effector is complexed with small molecule repressor.

Interaction of an effector molecule with small molecules does not always lead to the breakdown of the complex between effector and DNA. Indeed in some cases such an interaction may be essential for binding to the DNA to occur at all. In this case, then, the passage of the RNA polymerase along the DNA is only impaired in the presence of the small molecule, that is the effect is one of repression of enzyme synthesis (fig. 12.15).

Any type of regulation where there is a combination of a protein with DNA, itself requires the presence of additional genes which code for the effector proteins. Such genes are one of the types of **regulatory genes** found in many types of living cell.

Both the inducible and repressible systems described up to this point are examples of negative control systems, since they only allow transcription to occur when an effector molecule fails to block the passage of RNA polymerase. However certain systems of positive control are known, even if their precise molecular properties are not so well understood. In such systems combination between a protein and a small molecule is essential for transcription to occur. One possible mechanism for this type of control is for a small molecule to be necessary for RNA polymerase to bind to the polymerase binding site or, alternatively, that some complex with the polymerase molecule is needed to make the enzyme active. Although there is some suggestion that such a mechanism of regulation may exist in bacteria, little is known about the precise details at the molecular level. Indeed, up to this point the presence of most positive control systems has been inferred solely from the genetic properties of the regulatory mutants concerned.

Once the transcription of the message has commenced, RNA polymerase will read the DNA template until instructed to stop. Little is yet known of the mechanisms involved in this step and what is known has come from laboratory studies on the transcription of bacterial viruses. Certainly a protein, known as *rho*, seems to cause the RNA polymerase to drop off the DNA template; but what it is that determines the site of function of *rho* is unknown. It may be a particular base sequence in the DNA template, but if so its identity has not yet been decided.

Translational control

Messenger RNA in living cells frequently leads to the synthesis of more than one polypeptide chain. However the amounts of each polypeptide made from such a polycistronic message may not be equal. Indeed the translation of many such messages exhibits 'polarity', that is, more copies of the genes represented at the beginning of the message are expressed as protein than of those at the end. For example, the lactose operon in *Escherichia coli* consists of three genes, for β-galactosidase, β-galactoside permease and β-galactoside transacetylase synthesis, as well as the regulatory genes that control the expression of the whole group, or **operon**. This operon is transcribed as a polycistronic message, which in turn is translated into those polypeptide chains that go to make up the individual enzyme proteins. However, the polarity of translation ensures that more β-galactosidase is made than permease, and that this protein in turn is more abundant that the transacetylase.

Such gradients in translation efficiency seem to be caused by the behaviour of the ribosomes as they pass from the region on the message responsible for coding for one polypeptide chain to the part responsible for the next. When the ribosome reaches the termination triplet in the message (p. 12.13) some of the ribosomes seem to drop off and a smaller number then continue to translate the next section of the message. At present it is unclear whether this reduction is because all ribosomes drop off the message on reaching a termination triplet, with a smaller number reattaching at the next initiation signal, or whether only a small proportion actually drop off at termination to leave the remaining ribosomes to continue their journey. Even so, the overall result is the same; the later genes of an operon are expressed at a lower level than the early ones.

How widespread such polarity in the expression of polycistronic messages may be is uncertain, but it occurs in many metabolic pathways of naturally occurring bacterial species.

As far as we know at present no specific regulatory effects are mediated at the translation level. All small molecule inductions and repressions seem to be implemented at the level of transcription, a situation which is certainly more economical as far as the cell is concerned, since no message need be synthesized in the uninduced or the repressed state.

In summary, the regulation of protein synthesis occurs at both the level of transcription and the level of translation. However the former is probably the more widespread and certainly allows specific influences of small molecules, such as are found in enzyme induction and repression. Much of what has been discovered so far about these systems has been achieved by examining bacteria, where the combined use of genetic and biochemical techniques has proved particularly fruitful. Attention is now turning to similar processes in mammalian systems, and perhaps the most interesting aspect of this work is that it is beginning to give us clues as to how some hormones, agents impossible to study in bacterial populations, may exert their effects in mammals. This aspect of the problem is discussed more fully on p. 14.12. Knowledge of regulatory processes is also being extended to other eukaryotic systems where processes of development are being investigated. Much remains to be known about the mechanisms and role of regulating

processes in biology, and it is certain that the occurrence of such systems is widespread in all types of cell.

NUCLEAR DIVISION

Up to this point we have been concerned with the biochemical reactions by which the information carried in the genetic material of the cell is used in the synthesis of the protein components of new cell material. The primary concern from now on will be with the replication of genetic material and its distribution into the daughter cells. This process may be considered in two separate parts:

(1) the biochemical reactions whereby a second copy of the parental DNA is prepared for distribution to the daughter cell, and

(2) the processes whereby the two copies of the genetic material are separated and one copy passed to each daughter cell.

The second of these processes probably always involves the use of specialized cell structures which are strictly nothing to do with the replication of the DNA molecule itself; and in diploid cells, where there are many chromosomes to distribute equally to the daughter cells, these structures can be seen with a microscope in appropriately stained preparations.

The overall process of duplication of chromosomes and their distribution to the daughter cells in diploid organisms is called **mitosis,** and nuclei undergoing this process have a very characteristic appearance when stained by methods which distinguish the chromosomes. In diploid organisms, the formation of gametes is accompanied by a halving of the total number of chromosomes in the nucleus and this process of reduction division or **meiosis,** involves further variations in the pattern of DNA replication and chromosomal transfer. The succeeding section deals with the chemical process of DNA replication and the movements of chromosomes during mitosis and meiosis.

Replication of DNA

For the genetic information in a cell to be transferred to its progeny on division, replication of parental DNA must precede cell separation. At the present time enzymes from bacterial and mammalian sources which fulfil most of the biochemical requirements for replication of DNA have been studied *in vitro*; but it is not yet known whether these are the enzymes which carry out the duplication in the living cell. The DNA synthesizing enzymes which are active in the test tube are known as the DNA polymerases and they catalyse the formation of DNA from the 5′-triphosphates of deoxyadenine, deoxyguanosine, deoxycytidine and deoxythymidine.

The actual chemical reactions involved are shown in fig. 12.16. As with the DNA-primed RNA polymerase (p. 12.10) the overall reaction involves the transfer of a

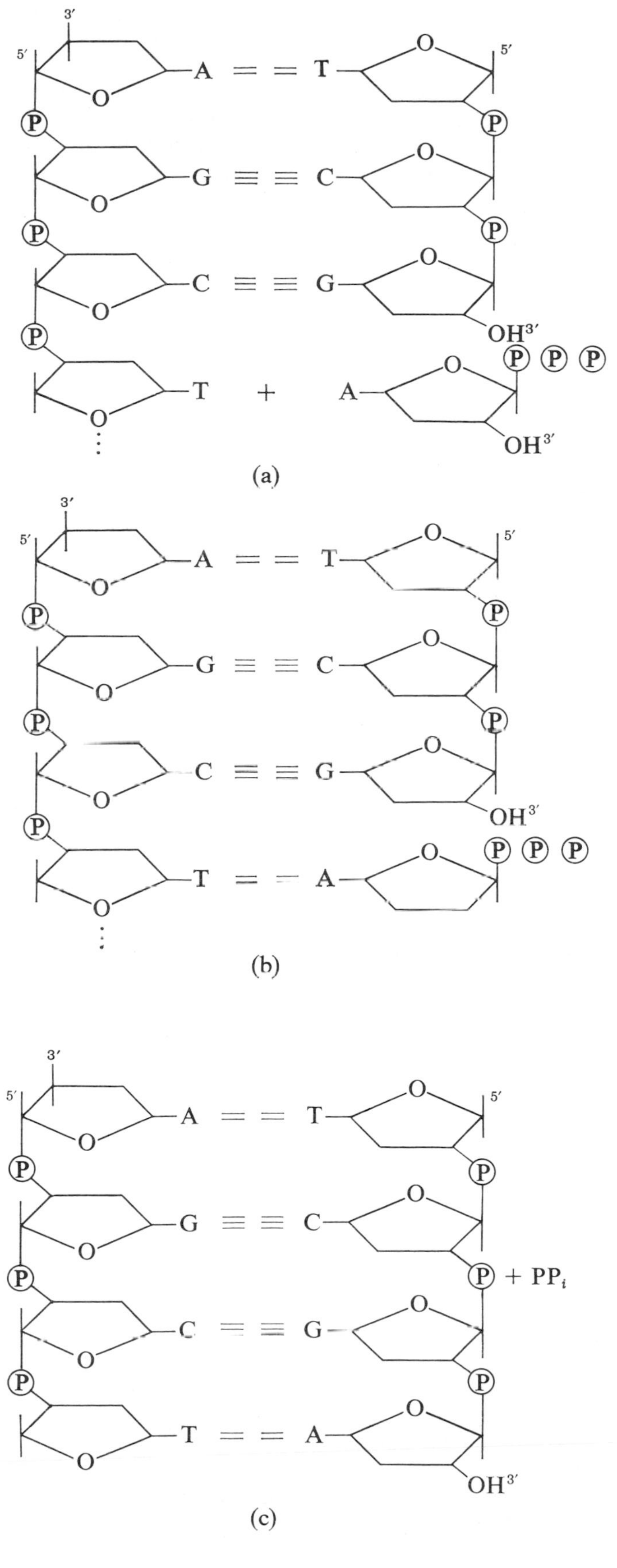

(a)

(b)

(c)

nucleotide to the 5′ end of a DNA chain with the concomitant liberation of pyrophosphate. Also, as with that enzyme, these enzymes will not act without the presence of some 'primer' DNA and, as with the RNA enzyme, the product of polymerase action has the same overall base composition as the primer. The way in which the primer may be involved in this process is shown in fig. 12.16. Moreover, with the DNA polymerases, the product has the base-paired double helical form of native DNA and it seems extremely likely that two DNA strands which are synthesized by the enzyme, and which form the base-paired double helix of the product, are complementary in structure to the two strands of the 'primer' DNA.

One difficulty that is not yet resolved concerns the direction of synthesis of the DNA polymerase. Since DNA consists of an anti-parallel double helix (p. 12.2), the 3′-phosphate on one strand of the helix will lie opposite a 5′-phosphate on the complementary strand. Yet autoradiograph studies in bacteria show that DNA replication passes in one direction only along a DNA helix; that is, one strand would seem to be synthesized in the 3′→5′ direction and the other in the direction 5′→3′. The isolated DNA polymerases are all most active *in vitro* in the 3′→5′ direction, and the means by which the synthesis of both complementary strands is achieved *in vivo* is not understood. Furthermore, there is some doubt as to whether the DNA polymerases that have been isolated so far are sufficiently active to achieve the amount of DNA synthesis needed to duplicate all the DNA of a cell within one cycle. Despite all these difficulties, however, there is little doubt that the replication of DNA in the living cell involves an enzyme (or enzymes) which form a replica molecule by synthesizing two DNA strands complementary in structure to the two strands of the parental helix. Fig. 12.17 shows that such a product is indistinguishable from the parent structure.

In organisms such as bacteria, which have a single chromosome, DNA replication is continuous throughout the division cycle, but in nucleated cells the replication of DNA is completed before the distribution of the chromosomes to the daughter cells commences. Thus autoradiograph studies show that the maximum rate of DNA synthesis occurs in nucleated cells during interphase and little during mitosis or meiosis.

Arrangement of DNA into chromosomes

In bacteriophages, which are viruses that live within

Fig. 12.16. The possible chemical reactions involved in DNA replication. (a) The existing double-stranded DNA molecule has opened to give a free thymidine residue. To retain the base-paired structure of the original DNA, this thymidine must be faced by deoxyadenosine triphosphate (dATP). (b) The incoming dATP residue is aligned opposite the thymidine residue. (c) A chemical reaction occurs between the dATP molecule and the 3′-OH group of the preceding residue of the same strand, with the concomitant liberation of the pyrophosphate (PP$_i$) residue.

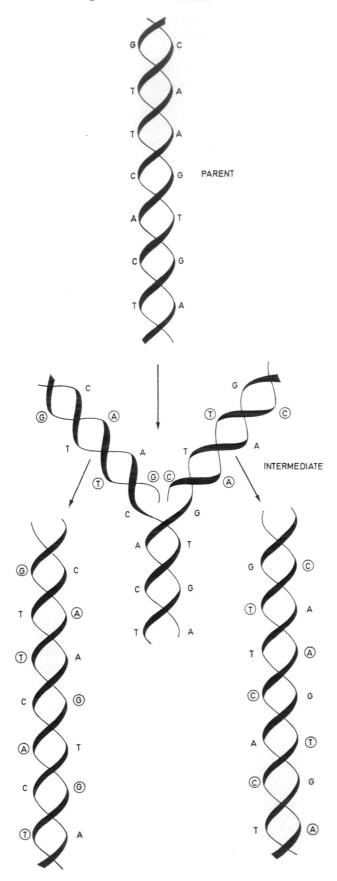

bacteria, the genetic material consists of a single molecule of DNA which in a number of instances has been shown to be circular. The replication of the DNA molecule is therefore the same thing as the replication of the genetic material of the organism. In bacteria also, genetic and cytological evidence indicates that the genetic material is composed of one large DNA molecule. In higher organisms, however, the situation is much more complicated. Firstly, there is a great increase in the total amount of DNA. The length of DNA molecules is usually measured in terms of the number of 'base pairs' and the length found in various species increases in step with the complexity of the organism and its position in the evolutionary tree. Virus particles have between 10^4 and 10^5 base pairs, bacteria have between 10^6 and 10^7 and higher organisms have anything up to 10^9. Secondly, in mammalian cells the DNA is closely associated with protein. This nucleoprotein complex is termed **chromatin** and confers on nuclear material special staining properties. Feulgen stain is highly specific for chromatin but is difficult to apply in practice. Other stains which are easier to use though less specific, for example orcein or Giemsa, are often used to stain chromosomes. Acridine orange is also used and has the useful property of giving a yellow fluorescence with DNA-containing structures and a red fluorescence with RNA-containing structures. Thus in the nucleus the red fluorescence of the nucleoli can be clearly seen against the yellow chromatin. More recently it has been shown that different regions of the chromosomes stain differentially under certain conditions with dyes such as Giemsa, Leishman, quinacrine hydrochloride and quinacrine mustard. The precise chemical basis of these staining differences, which give the chromosomes a banded appearance, is not known but it seems probable that they reflect differences in the configuration of the nucleoprotein in different regions of the chromosome.

The proteins which are found complexed with DNA in nucleated cells are mostly basic proteins, often containing large amounts of the amino acids lysine and arginine. In general these basic proteins are called histones but in certain specific locations they may have special names; for example, the protamines that are found with the DNA of spermatozoa. There has been much speculation over the years about the role of the histones in the mammalian cell and this has been sharpened by the realization that they are absent in bacteria and viruses. One hypothesis is that they 'blank off' portions of the DNA of the chromosomes to limit expression of some of the genetic material in differentiated cells. Smaller amounts of acidic proteins are also found associated with the DNA and these may play a vital role in controlling gene expression.

The DNA of the mammalian cell along with its associated protein is divided into a number of separate blocks,

FIG. 12.17. Biosynthesis of DNA. Ringed bases are components of the newly-synthesized strand.

the **chromosomes**, so called because of the staining properties already described. The single DNA thread of bacteria and viruses is often loosely called a 'chromosome' but it differs considerably in structure from those of mammals and other nucleated cells. The number of chromosomes in a cell is characteristic of the species (table 12.3). All the cells of the body with the exception of the gametes and a few cells in the liver and bone marrow have the same number of chromosomes. The precise

arrangement of the DNA and histone in the chromosome is not known. There are several hypotheses. There may be a number of DNA molecules lying parallel to each other along the length of the chromosome or lying end to end and joined by protein bridges. Autoradiographic examination of loosely coiled chromosomes suggests that they are multi-stranded. Another suggestion is that the entire chromosome is a single DNA molecule of enormous size. If the DNA is in the form of a single long thread its packing into a chromosome is bound to be complex. EM has so far shed little light on this problem. The light microscope shows that the chromosome is a coiled structure with, sometimes, a suggestion of secondary coiling. This coiling should not, however, be confused with the helical structure of the DNA molecule because there is a difference of several orders of magnitude in the scale. The staining procedures which demonstrate banding patterns have given much new information, since a combination of the different methods reveals marked differences in the staining characteristics of particular regions. However, how this relates to the configuration of the DNA in the chromosome, except for a small number of regions which have been shown to contain highly repetitive DNA, is unknown. In short, the detailed

TABLE 12.3. Diploid chromosome numbers.

Moulds		*Mollusc*	
Neurospora sp.	14	Snail	54
Plants		*Vertebrates*	
Cucumber	14	Cat	38
Pea	14	Mouse, pig	40
Onion	16	Monkey	42
Cabbage	18	Rabbit	44
Bean	22	MAN	46
Water melon	22	Sheep	54
Tomato	24	Cattle	60
Pine tree	24	Guinea-pig	64
Insects		Horse	66
Drosophila	8	Dog	78
House fly	12	Hen	78
Bee	32	Pigeon	80

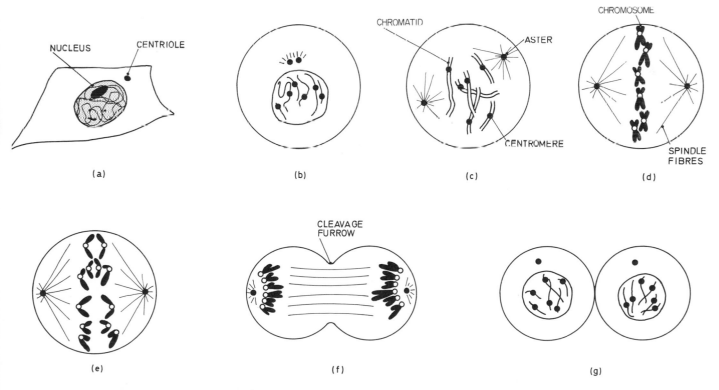

FIG. 12.18. Mitosis. (a) Interphase (46 chromosomes). (b) Early prophase. Centriole divides, chromosomes appear as threads. (c) Late prophase. Centrioles separate. Aster and spindles form, chromosomes seen to be double, nuclear membrane disappears. (d) Metaphase. Chromosomes line up in equatorial plane. (e) Early anaphase. Centromeres divide, chromatids begin to separate. (f) Late anaphase. Separation of chromatids continues, cleavage furrow forms. (g) Telophase. Two daughter cells each with 46 chromosomes.

structure of the chomosomes of higher organisms is not known in spite of intense study.

Mitosis

In order to conserve the specific number of chromosomes (the diploid or 2n number) the division of the genetic material of the cell occurs by the precisely controlled process of mitosis (fig. 12.18). Mitotic division is the type of cell division which occurs in somatic cells during periods of growth when the total number of cells is increasing, or during repair processes when lost or damaged cells are being replaced. In the resting cell (interphase) the chromosomes cannot be detected inside the nucleus as discrete structures. There are sometimes a few condensations of DNA (chromocenters) which can be recognized in the interphase nucleus. One of these, the sex chromatin body or Barr body, occurs only in female cells and is discussed in more detail on p. 12.21. The interphase part of the cell cycle is normally split into three periods. During the G1 phase RNA synthesis, protein synthesis and cell growth proceed, but there is no DNA synthesis. In the second stage (the S phase) the DNA of the chromosomes is replicated. The replication is not exactly synchronous, some chromosomes completing their synthesis before others. Between the end of DNA synthesis and the next cell division there is a second growth period (G2).

As a cell approaches mitosis, the chromosomes become visible as threads within the nucleus (prophase). At the same time cytoplasmic bodies, the centrioles, divide and the two new centrioles move to opposite poles of the cell. It is from these bodies that the protein fibres (the spindle) which control the mechanical separation of the chromosomes radiate. At the end of prophase the nuclear membrane disappears and the chromosomes which are now obviously double structures continue to contract. Each half of these double structures is known as a chromatid (fig. 12.19). They are held together at one point, the centromere, which is the point of attachment of the chromosome to the spindle. The chromosomes line up in the equatorial plane of the cell (metaphase)

and it is at this stage that the chromosomes are normally examined. The two chromatids separate following a longitudinal division of the centromere. The spindle fibres now appear to contract, pulling the chromatids which become the chromosomes of the two daughter nuclei towards opposite poles of the cell (anaphase). A cleavage furrow begins to divide the cytoplasm of the cell, the chromosomes elongate and a nuclear membrane reforms around them. This stage is termed telophase and it results in the reconstitution of two daughter nuclei which are genetically identical with the parent nucleus.

Normal human chromosomes

The chromosomes of man can be examined directly using the light microscope. Some tissues, for example bone marrow, are dividing sufficiently rapidly for preparations to be made directly from the body, while other tissues such as peripheral blood cells or skin fibroblasts can be made to divide out of the body by growing in tissue culture for a short period. A large number of dividing cells is accumulated in the culture with the use of the drug colchicine which inhibits the formation of the spindle so that cells enter mitosis but are arrested at the metaphase stage. The cells are now treated with a hypotonic solution which helps to improve the spreading of the chromosomes at a later stage. They are fixed to preserve their morphology and then flattened by drying the cells out onto a glass microscope slide. The chromosomes may be stained using either a conventional procedure which stains the chromosomes uniformly or one which reveals the banding pattern. These latter are of several types. Most commonly used are the G-banding technique using a Giemsa stain, or the Q-banding technique using quinacrine derivatives. These chromosomes which are forty-six in number can be arranged as twenty-three pairs, one member of each pair being derived from the mother and one member from the father (homologous chromosomes). Such an array is termed a **karyotype** (fig. 12.20). There is one pair of chromosomes, the sex chromosomes, which is involved in the determination of sex. The other twenty-two pairs, which are not involved in sex determination, are termed **autosomes**. For the description of chromosomes, the length, the position of the centromere and the banding pattern are taken into account. A chromosome with the centromere near the middle is said to be metacentric, while a chromosome with the centromere near one end is said to be acrocentric. If the centromere occupies an intermediate position it is said to be submetacentric (fig. 12.19). The presence of satellites or secondary constrictions, and the use of autoradiography can also help in identification. The chromosomes are normally numbered according to an international convention (Paris nomenture) the largest chromosome being number 1 and the smallest number 22. By conventional staining techniques only a few of the chromosomes can be recognized indivi-

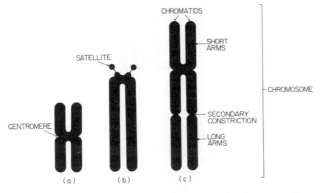

FIG. 12.19. Metaphase chromosomes. (a) Metacentric, (b) acrocentric, (c) submetacentric.

dually, e.g. nos. 1, 2, 3 and 16, but all can be placed in a chromosome group. It is usual to assign letters to these

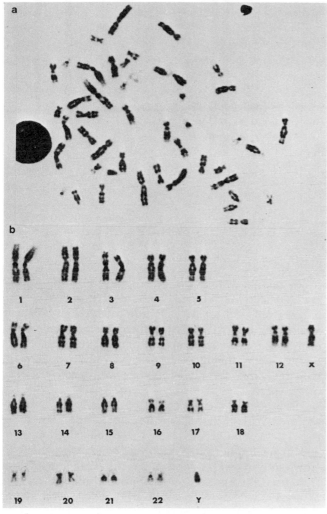

FIG. 12.20. Human chromosomes. Chromosomes of a normal male cell from a culture of peripheral blood; (a) Giemsa stain showing G-banding (× 1600); (b) chromosomes of the same cell arranged in pairs according to the Paris (1971) nomenclature.

groups as follows: chromosomes 1–3 group A, chromosomes 4 and 5 group B, chromosomes 6–12 group C chromosomes 13–15 group D, chromosomes 16–18 group E, chromosomes 19–20 group F, chromosomes 21–22 group G. The use of banding techniques however allows each chromosome to be identified and assists in the detection of chromosome abnormalities.

The sex chromosomes are not assigned numbers. In the female the two sex chromosomes are alike and are called X chromosomes which belong to the C group. In the male, however, there is one X chromosome like those of the female and one Y chromosome which is quite different in appearance. It resembles chromosomes 21–22 and is therefore a G group chromosome, but it can normally

be distinguished from 21–22 in good conventional preparations. Since the long arm of the Y chromosome shows a very bright fluorescence when stained with quinacrine, the Y chromosome can now be identified easily. Even in interphase cells the fluorescent Y chromosome can be recognized as a characteristic fluorescent Y body. In future this may prove of value, for example in recognizing Y-bearing spermatozoa, in checking the sex of amniotic fluid and in recognizing certain chromosome abnormalities.

The Y chromosome in man is strongly male determining and in certain abnormal situations can ensure masculinization in the presence of as many as four X chromosomes. Two X chromosomes are necessary for normal female sexual development. However, there is evidence to suggest that all or part of one X chromosome is inactive after a certain stage in development. Autoradiographic evidence shows that this X chromosome synthesizes DNA much later in the S period than do the other chromosomes. This late-labelling X can be seen in a proportion of female interphase nuclei as the X-chromatin body (Barr body). This body stains deeply with DNA-specific stains but it can also be recognized with less specific stains such as cresyl violet. It is normally seen applied to the inside of the nuclear membrane (fig. 12.21).

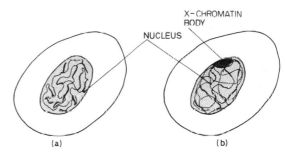

FIG. 12.21. X-chromatin. (a) Male cell, chromatin negative. (b) Female cell, chromatin positive.

Normal females have 40–70 per cent of cells with a single X-chromatin body (chromatin positive) while male cells have no X-chromatin body (chromatin negative). This is of great practical importance since the number of X chromosomes carried by an individual can be determined very simply by examining cells from the oral mucosa in a buccal smear. Certain abnormalities of sexual development can be detected in this way. The number of sex chromatin bodies is always one less than the number of X chromosomes in the cell. Morphological abnormalities of the X chromosome may be reflected in the altered size of the sex chromatin body, while chromosome mosaic individuals may have an unusually low percentage of cells with a sex chromatin body.

Meiosis

As we have seen, mitosis is the mechanism for maintaining

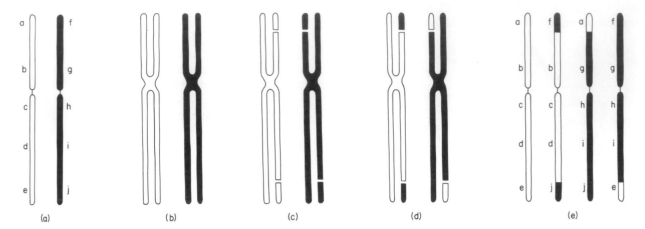

FIG. 12.22. Crossing over. (a) Pairing of homologous chromosomes; a–f, b–g, c–h, d–i, e–j are pairs of allelic genes. (b) Each chromosome replicates and is now composed of two chromatids. (c) Breakage occurs in some of the chromatids. (d) Crossing over occurs as a result of incorrect joining. (e) Four new chromosomes; in each, crossing over has resulted in the recombination of the genetic material.

the constancy of the genetic material from cell to cell, but as the chromosome number is characteristic of the species there must also be a mechanism for maintaining the constancy of the chromosome number from generation to generation. The cells in all tissues of the body have forty-six chromosomes, with the exception of some cells in the bone marrow and in the liver which have 2, 4 or 8 times the normal number of chromosomes (polyploid cells). If, however, the gametes also contained forty-six chromosomes the fusion of an egg and a sperm would result in the production of an individual with ninety-two chromosomes. During the formation of the gametes, therefore, a special type of cell division, meiosis, reduces the number of chromosomes in the gametes to half the number found in the somatic cells, in this case twenty-three chromosomes, the haploid or n number of chromosomes. It is important to note, however, that meiosis is not merely a reduction division, since during this process a mixing of genetic material takes place between homologous chromosomes. In simple organisms reproduction can occur by simple fission of the genetic material and the cell into two identical daughter cells. However, in many instances even in lower organisms reproduction cannot be continued indefinitely in this way, e.g. if a stock of Paramecium is kept under conditions which permit only asexual reproduction it quite rapidly becomes degenerate. The stock can be rejuvenated by permitting sexual reproduction which involves the mixing of genetic material from two separate individuals to occur. Similarly mammalian cells in tissue culture, which of course divide by mitosis, have a finite lifetime after which they cease to divide and they eventually degenerate. During meiosis breaks occur when the two homologous chromosomes are lying close together, and in the rejoining process 'crossing over' occurs so that each individual chromosome

in the mature gamete will have a portion of its genetic material derived from a maternal chromosome and part derived from a paternal chromosome. This breakage and rejoining is an essential feature of the normal process of meiosis (fig. 12.22), and is responsible for maintaining the genetic variability which ensures the uniqueness of each individual, and probably the continued existence of the species.

The process of meiosis consists essentially of two separate divisions which follow one closely upon the other (fig. 12.23). The first division is the reduction division, and it has an elongated prophase which can be subdivided into several different stages. In the first stage (**leptotene**) the chromosomes appear within the nucleus as unpaired thread-like structures, but very soon homologous chromosomes come to lie closely together (**zygotene**). Each of these paired structures is termed a bivalent. In the next stage (**pachytene**), each chromosome reduplicates itself so that each bivalent is composed of four threads lying closely parallel to each other. As the shortening of the chromosome progresses it becomes apparent that the homologous chromosomes are not held together along their entire length, but only at particular points (**diplotene**). These points, termed **chiasmata,** are the points where crossing over occurs. Meiosis in the female is normally arrested at this point for a prolonged period (the dictyate phase) which lasts from the late intra-uterine period of development until just prior to the shedding of the ovum from the ovary several decades later. During spermatogenesis there is no such delay. In either case meiosis proceeds by further contraction of the chromosomes (**diakinesis**) and the chiasmata begin to move towards the ends of the chromosome (terminalization). Shortly after this process is complete the nuclear membrane disappears marking the end of prophase. The chromosomes, still in homologous pairs, line up in the equatorial plane of the cell (first meiotic metaphase). One member of each homologous pair then moves to opposite poles of the cell without any division of the centromeres (first meiotic anaphase). The mechanical processes involved appear to be the same as those underlying mitosis, but the result is quite different in that the two daughter nuclei which reconstitute at the first telo-

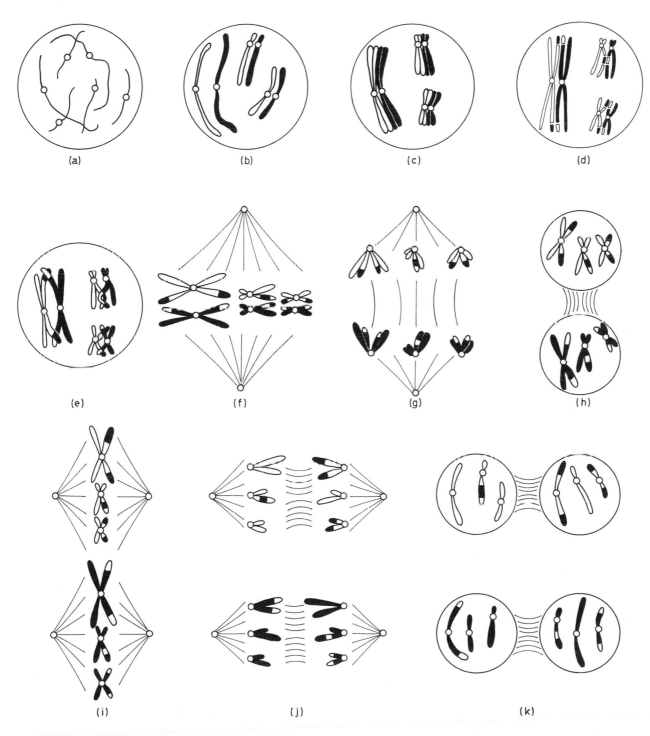

FIG. 12.23. Meiosis. (a) Leptotene, 46 chromosomes; (b) zygotene; (c) pachytene; (d) diplotene; (e) diakinesis; (f) first metaphase; (g) first anaphase; (h) first telophase, 23 pairs of chromatids; (i) second metaphase; (j) second anaphase; (k) second telophase. 23 chromosomes in each of four cells.

TABLE 12.4 Names and abbreviations of purine and pyrimidine nucleotides and related compounds

Base	Nucleoside	Nucleotide (nucleotide monophosphate)	Nucleotide diphosphate	Nucleotide triphosphate
Adenine	Adenosine Adenine riboside	Adenine ribotide Adenosine monophosphate (adenylic acid) AMP A-5'-P	Adenosine diphosphate ADP	Adenosine triphosphate ATP
Guanine	Guanosine Guanine riboside	Guanine ribotide Guanosine monophosphate (guanylic acid) GMP G-5'-P	Guanosine diphosphate GDP	Guanosine triphosphate GTP
Cytosine	Cytidine Cytosine riboside	Cytosine ribotide Cytidine monophosphate (cytidylic acid) CMP C-5'-P	Cytidine diphosphate CDP	Cytidine triphosphate CTP
Uracil	Uridine Uracil riboside	Uracil ribotide Uridine monophosphate (uridylic acid) UMP U-5'-P	Uridine diphosphate UDP	Uridine triphosphate UTP
Thymine	Thymidine Thymine deoxyriboside	Thymine deoxyribotide Thymidine monophosphate (thymidylic acid) d-TMP* d-T-5'-P*	Thymidine diphosphate d-TDP*	Thymidine triphosphate d-TTP*
Orotic acid	Orotidine Orotic acid riboside	Orotic acid ribotide Orotidine monophosphate (orotidylic acid) OMP O-5'-P	—	—
Hypoxanthine	Inosine Hypoxanthine riboside	Hypoxanthine ribotide Inosine monophosphate (inosinic acid) IMP I-5'-P	—	—

Where *deoxy*ribosides and *deoxy*ribotides are involved, the abbreviations are prefixed with d-, e.g. *deoxy*guanosine diphosphate is d-GDP.

* Thymine derivatives, although containing *deoxy*ribose, are frequently abbreviated without the d-: thymine deoxyriboside diphosphate = thymidine diphosphate = TDP.

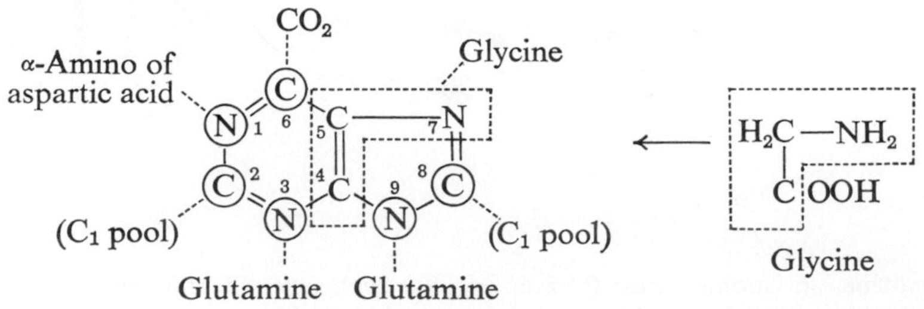

FIG. 12.24. Basic purine structure showing the metabolic origin of the C, O and N atoms that go to make up the ring structure.

phase each have only twenty-three chromosomes, each of which is composed of two chromatids. The second meiotic division usually follows closely after the first, and resembles an ordinary mitotic division. The overall result of meiosis, therefore, is the production of four cells each with twenty-three chromosomes from a single primary germ cell with forty-six chromosomes. In the male each of these four cells undergoes differentiation to form a spermatozoon, but in the female unequal division of cytoplasm between the divisions results in the production of one very large cell which matures to form the ovum and three small cells termed polar bodies which degenerate. At fertilization the diploid number is reconstituted by the union of two nuclei each containing twenty-three chromosomes. A female has two X chromosomes and therefore all the ova will have a single X chromosome (**homogametic**), but in the male half of the spermatozoa will contain an X chromosome and half will contain a Y chromosome (**heterogametic**). Fertilization of an ovum by a Y–bearing sperm results in a male fertilized egg or zygote, and fertilization by an X–bearing

sperm results in a female zygote. Thus sex determination occurs at the instant of conception. Abnormalities of cell division are discussed on p. 39.10.

SYNTHESIS OF NUCLEIC ACID PRE-CURSORS AND THE BREAKDOWN OF MACROMOLECULAR RNA AND DNA

For nucleic acid synthesis to occur the cell must have a ready supply of the precursor nucleotides, which in turn, require adenine, guanine, cytosine, uracil, thymine, ribose and deoxyribose in suitable molecular combination. It is the biosynthesis of these compounds which is first described here.

Nucleic acid components are liberated from macromolecular RNA and DNA by the concerted action of nucleases and phosphatases, and the purines and pyrimidines liberated are further degraded by pathways completely unrelated to their synthesis. The specificity of nuclcolytic enzymes and the subsequent degradation of purines and pyrimidines is dealt with in the second part

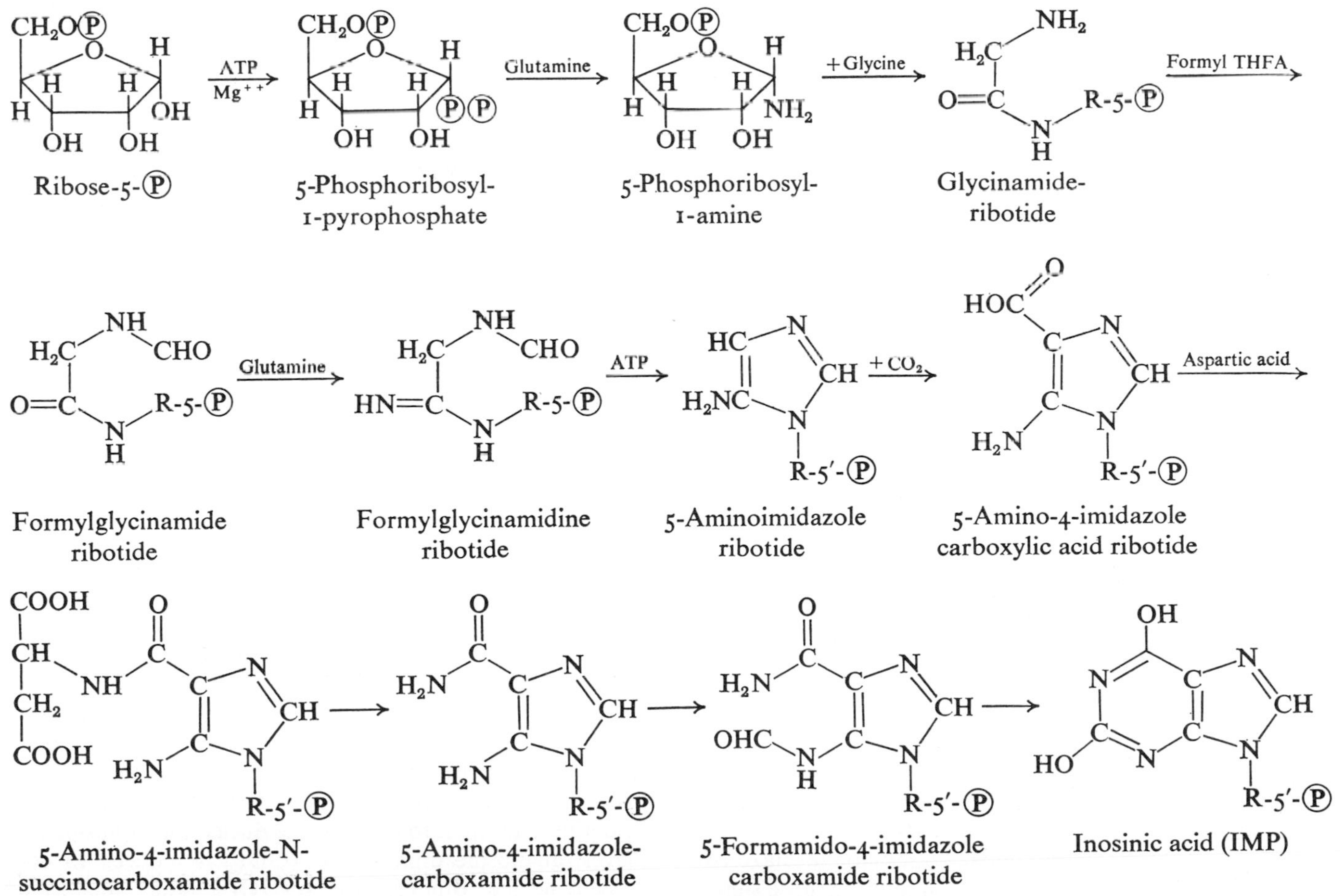

FIG. 12.25. Purine nucleotide biosynthetic pathway. Formyltetrahydrofolic acid (Formyl THFA).

of this section. The names, structures and abbreviations of the various (chiefly) nucleotide derivatives of the purine and pyrimidine bases are set out in table 12.4.

Purine and pyrimidine biosynthesis

SYNTHESIS OF PURINE RIBONUCLEOTIDE MONO-PHOSPHATES

The basic molecular structure of all purines is shown in fig. 12.24; while adenine has an amino group at position 6, guanine has an —OH at that position and —NH_2 at position 2. Both adenine and guanine are synthesized via inosinic acid, IMP, by the same biosynthetic pathway. In the course of this process the purine nucleus is built up stepwise from glycine, NH_3 and a source of C-1 units. Fig. 12.24 shows also how the various nitrogen and carbon atoms of the purine ring are derived from their precursors; thus C-4, C-5 and N-7 come from glycine; C-6 comes from CO_2; N-1 from NH_3 via the α-amino of aspartic acid; N-3 and N-9 come from NH_3 via the amino group of glutamine; and C-2 and C-8 come from the C-1 pool with the intervention of formyltetrahydrofolic acid. The exact sequence of biosynthetic reactions is shown in fig. 12.25. Since the immediate precursors of the nucleic acids are the

these enzymes by their structural resemblance to glutamine. Once at the active centre, they inactivate the enzymes by blocking an essential —SH group.

PURINE NUCLEOTIDES, NUCLEOSIDES AND FREE BASES

Once in the form of the ribonucleotide monophosphates, the nucleotides can be converted freely, if a sufficient supply of energy is available, to the related nucleotide di- and triphosphates, and it is as the triphosphates that they are used in the biosynthesis of RNA (fig. 12.26). Alterna-

$$\text{XMP} \underset{\substack{\downarrow \\ \text{ATP} \quad \text{ADP}}}{\overset{\substack{\text{ATP} \quad \text{ADP} \\ \downarrow}}{\rightleftharpoons}} \text{XDP} \underset{\substack{\downarrow \\ \text{ATP} \quad \text{ADP}}}{\overset{\substack{\text{ATP} \quad \text{ADP} \\ \downarrow}}{\rightleftharpoons}} \text{XTP}$$

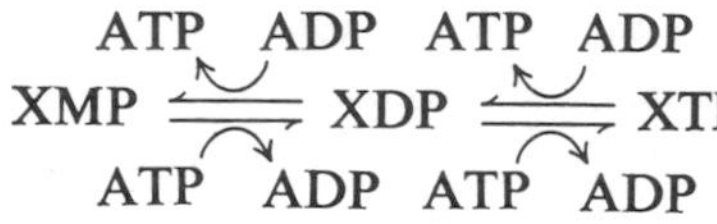

FIG. 12.26. Interconversion of nucleotide mono-, di- and triphosphates. X, any purine or pyrimidine base; XMP, nucleotide monophosphate; XDP, nucleotide diphosphate; XTP, nucleotide triphosphate.

tively the terminal phosphate may be removed by phosphomonoesterase to form purine ribosides and thence, by removal of the ribose, to form the free bases. It is this last reaction that liberates free adenine and guanine from

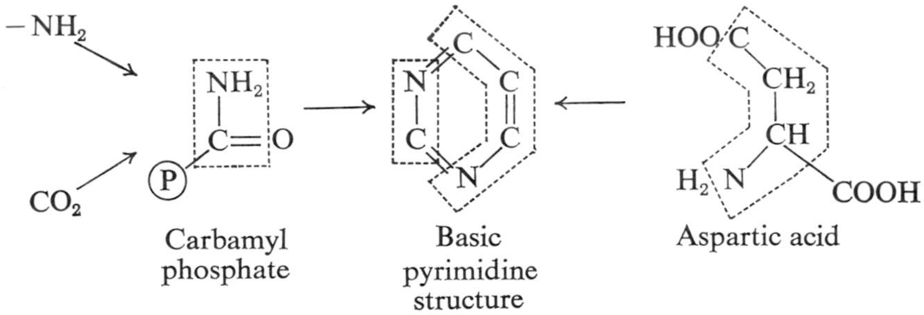

FIG. 12.27. Basic pyrimidine structure showing the metabolic origin of the C, O and N atoms that go to make up the ring structure.

purine and pyrimidine nucleotide triphosphates, it is these compounds rather than the free bases, that are the end-products of the biosynthetic pathways. Free bases, if found at all, occur transiently as intermediates in the breakdown of nucleic acids and possibly in the formation of deoxyribonucleotides. The biosynthetic pathways proper end at the nucleotide monophosphates, and since the pathway starts with ribose 5-phosphate every molecule up to the final adenine and guanine ribonucleotide is already in the nucleotide monophosphate state.

Two antibiotic compounds, azaserine and diazo-oxonorleucine, exert their action by inhibiting those steps of the purine biosynthetic pathway which involve the use of glutamine. The antibiotics are drawn to the active sites of

RNA and DNA during hydrolysis by a combination of nucleases and phosphatases (p. 12.29).

CONVERSION OF PURINE RIBONUCLEOTIDES TO DEOXYRIBONUCLEOTIDES

Just as adenine and guanine *ribo*nucleotide triphosphates are the precursors of RNA, so the *deoxyribo*nucleotide triphosphates are the precursors of DNA (p. 12.10). The conversion from the ribonucleotide to the deoxyribonucleotide is thought to occur at the nucleotide diphosphate level; guanosine diphosphate (GDP) is reduced to deoxyguanosine diphosphate (d-GDP), and adenosine diphosphate (ADP) to deoxyadenosine diphosphate (d-ADP). These deoxyribonucleotide diphosphates are

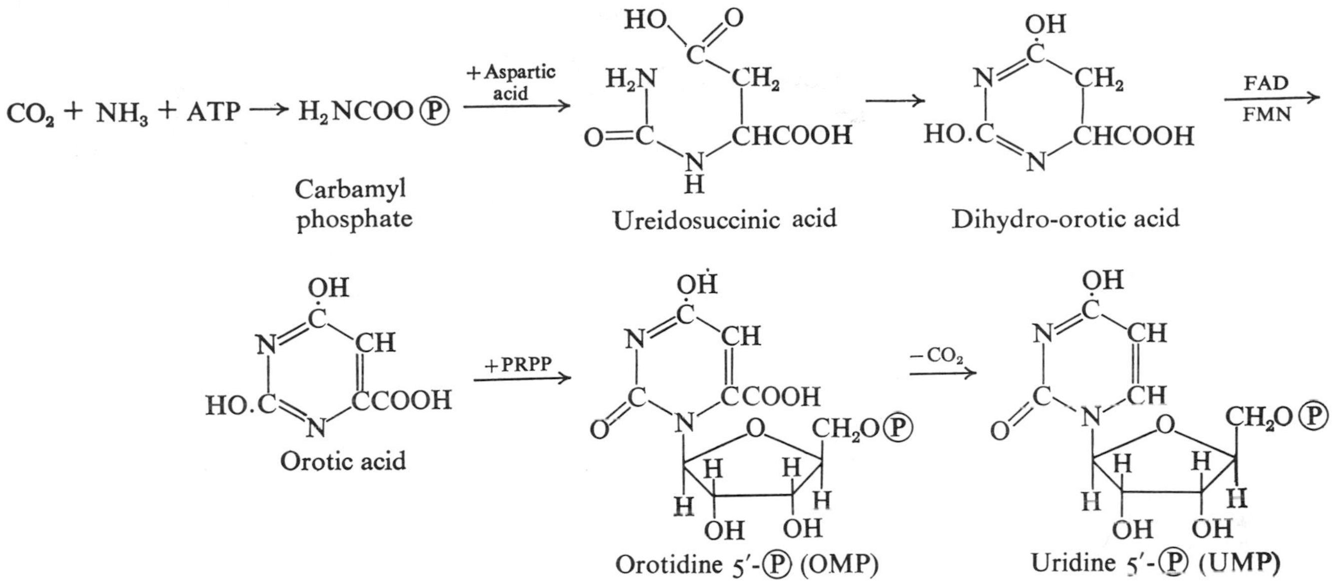

FIG. 12.28. Pyrimidine biosynthetic pathway. PRPP, phosphoribosylpyrophosphate.

then converted, exactly as with the ribonucleotide di-phosphates, to the triphosphates before being used for DNA synthesis.

PYRIMIDINE RIBONUCLEOTIDES AND DEOXYRIBO-NUCLEOTIDES

The basic structure of all pyrimidines is shown in fig. 12.27, the actual structures of uracil, cytosine and thy-mine being shown in figs. 12.3 & 6. All pyrimidines are synthesized by the same pathway, the ring structure being built up from CO_2, NH_3 and aspartic acid. Fig. 12.27 also shows how the various atoms of the pyrimidine ring are derived from its precursors: N-1 from NH_3 and C-2 from CO_2 via carbamyl phosphate; N-3, C-4, C-5 and C-6 from the α-amino group and C-2, C-3 and C-4 of aspartic acid, respectively. The α-carboxyl group of aspartic acid is lost as CO_2 during this synthesis. The exact sequence of reactions is shown in fig. 12.28.

As in the case of purines, the end-product of the path-way is in the ribonucleotide. Uridine ribonucleotide (UMP) is derived from orotidine 5'-phosphate by decar-boxylation, and cytidine ribonucleotide (CMP) from UMP by replacement of an —OH group by —NH_2. The amino group for this conversion is supplied by the amide residue glutamine (fig. 12.29).

As with the purine ribonucleotides, conversion of the pyrimidine ribonucleotides to the di- and triphosphates occurs readily in the presence of a suitable energy source, and the triphosphates are used for RNA synthesis (p. 12.5). Hydrolysis by the appropriate monoesterases yield uridine and cytidine from which uracil and cytosine are formed, in turn, by nucleosidase action (p. 12.30). As in the case of purines, these routes are normally only degradative.

The origin of the pyrimidine deoxyribonucleotides is unclear. Probably, as with the purines, the conversion occurs at the diphosphate level, i.e. uridine ribonucleotide

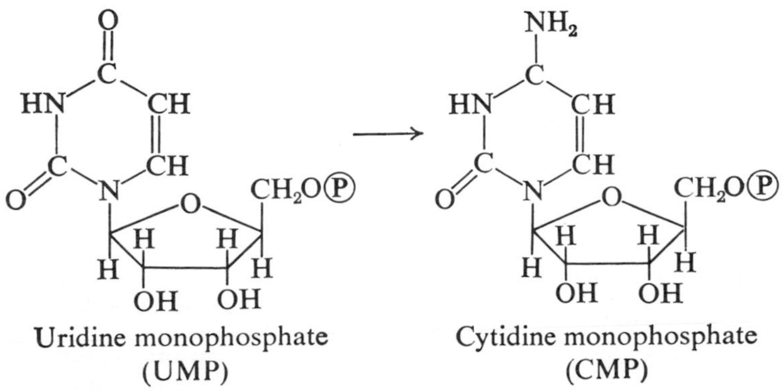

FIG. 12.29 Conversion of uridine monophosphate to cytidine monophosphate.

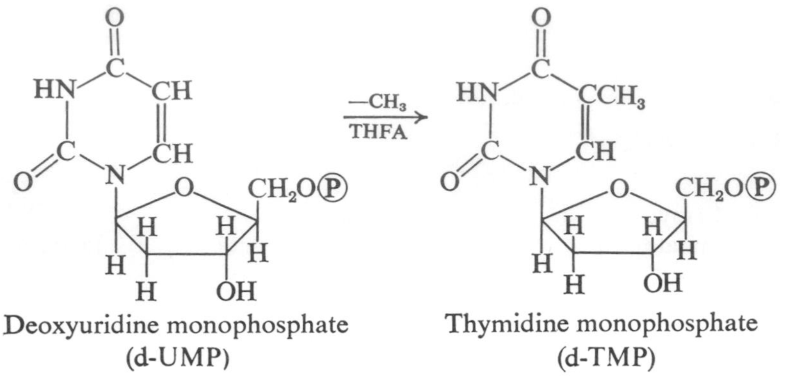

FIG. 12.30. Conversion of deoxyuridine monophosphate to thymidine monophosphate.

diphosphate (UDP) is reduced to uridine deoxyribonucleotide diphosphate (d-UDP) and cytidine ribonucleotide diphosphate (CDP) is reduced to cytidine deoxyribonucleotide diphosphate (d-CDP).

The thymine derivatives necessary for DNA synthesis probably arise from d-UMP by methylation at the C-5 position using formyltetrahydrofolic acid as the C-1 source (fig. 12.30). The involvement of folic acid at this stage is shown by the extreme sensitivity of this reaction to inhibition by antifolic drugs such as aminopterin and amethopterin. Once thymine deoxyribonucleotide (d-TMP) is formed, interconversion to d-TDP and d-TTP occurs in the same way as is found with d-CMP.

'ABNORMAL' PURINES AND PYRIMIDINES
Certain RNA fractions, notably transfer RNA (p. 12.6), contain about 10 per cent of their purine and pyrimidine residues in the form of bases other than those commonly associated with DNA and RNA. Little is known about their synthesis except that 2,6-diaminopurine, 6-methyl purine and N,N-dimethylaminopurine are almost certainly synthesized as the ribonucleotide monophosphates from AMP. Among the pyrimidines, dihydrouracil is on the degradative pathway from uracil, and thymine *ribo*nucleotide is probably synthesized via the nucleoside from free thymine. Pseudouridine (p. 12.7) is derived from uracil, possibly with the intervention of phosphoribosyl pyrophosphate.

Biosynthesis of ribose and deoxyribose
D-ribose is used for the biosynthesis of purine and pyrimidine ribonucleosides and ribonucleotides as 5-phosphoribosyl-1-pyrophosphate (fig. 12.25), and this compound is synthesized in the cell from ribose 5-phosphate and ATP, according to the reaction:

$$\text{ribose 5- P} + \text{ATP} \longrightarrow \text{5-phosphoribosyl-1-} \atop \text{pyrophosphate} + \text{AMP}$$

In some organisms, the ribose 5-phosphate used for RNA synthesis is a by-product of the hexose monophosphate pathway of glucose metabolism (p. 9.8). In this

series of reactions, glucose is converted to ribulose 5-phosphate via 6-phosphogluconic acid and 6-phospho-3-ketogluconic acid. The ribulose 5-phosphate is then isomerised to ribose 5-phosphate by the widely distributed ribulose 5-phosphate isomerase enzyme. Although this reaction sequence occurs widely, it may not be used to make the majority of ribose in the cell. An alternative pathway to ribose 5-phosphate has been postulated in which there is a transketolase-catalysed transfer of a $CH_2(OH)C=O$... residue from fructose to glyceraldehyde-3-phosphate.

Deoxyribose, as stated above, can certainly be formed by reduction of a ribose residue which is already part of a nucleotide (p. 12.24). However, there is a possibility that a condensation of glyceraldehyde 3-phosphate with acetaldehyde to form deoxyribose 5-phosphate can be catalysed by an enzyme present in many types of cell. How this compound is used for deoxyribonucleotide synthesis is not yet clear.

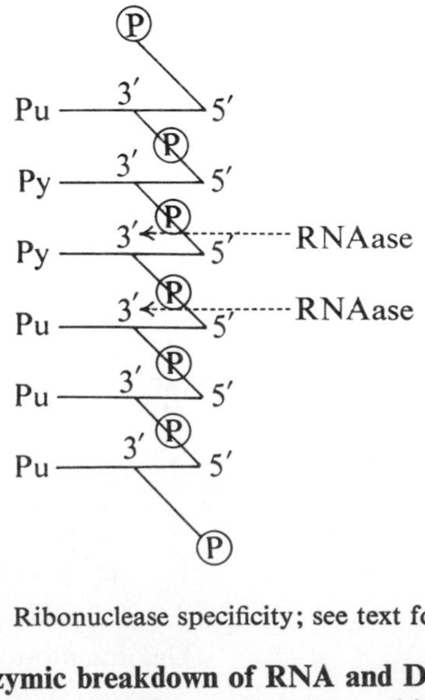

FIG. 12.31. Ribonuclease specificity; see text for details.

Enzymic breakdown of RNA and DNA
A large number of different enzymes which hydrolyse macromolecular RNA and DNA have been classified

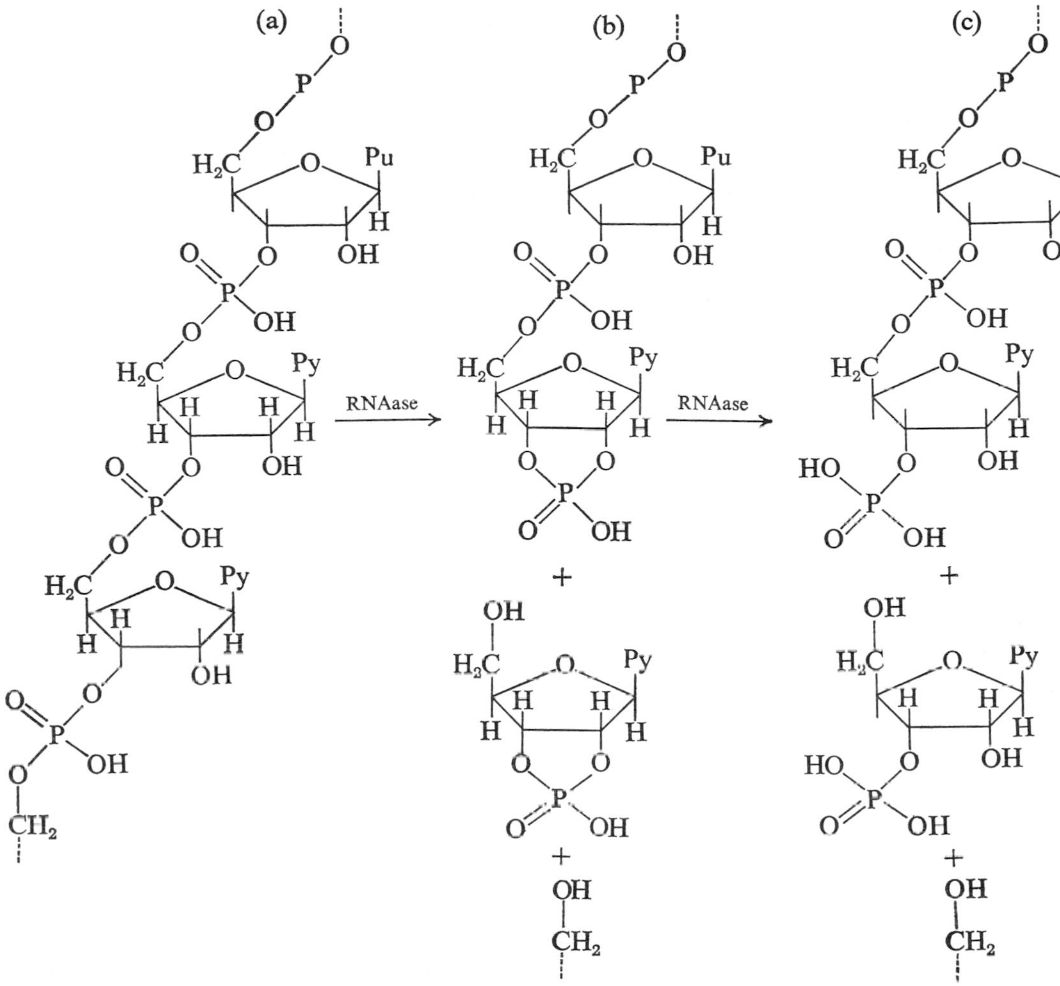

FIG. 12.32. Intermediate structures formed during ribonuclease action. (a) Intact RNA structure. (b) Intermediate cyclic 2'-, 3'-diphosphate. (c) Final product. Pu, purine; Py, pyrimidine.

among the broad group of nucleases, but only in relatively few cases has the exact specificity of the enzyme been worked out. The enzymes, which act on nucleic acids and their breakdown products, may be classified as follows:

(1) depolymerases: ribonucleases and deoxyribonucleases. In general, enzymes in this group which are active on RNA are inactive on DNA and vice versa;

(2) phosphodiesterases and phosphomonoesterases. These enzymes act on the oligonucleotide breakdown products of both RNA and DNA;

(3) nucleosidases.

DEPOLYMERASES

In man, the large molecular weight nucleic acids, which enter the alimentary tract as part of the food, are degraded in the duodenum by ribonuclease and deoxyribonuclease which are part of the pancreatic secretion. Both enzymes have been purified and a considerable amount is known about their properties.

Ribonuclease

Pancreatic ribonuclease is specifically adapted to split the bond linking the phosphoryl group of pyrimidine nucleoside 3'-phosphate to the 5-hydroxyl of the adjacent purine or pyrimidine nucleoside (fig. 12.31, see p. 12.6 for the details of RNA structures). With model compounds as substrates, the enzyme can be shown to produce a 2',3'-cyclic phosphate as an intermediate in the hydrolytic process (fig. 12.32). When the enzyme acts on intact RNA the macromolecule is degraded to free cytidine 3'-phosphate and uridine 3'-phosphate together with some larger oligonucleotides which, as a consequence of the enzyme specificity, are rich in purines.

Deoxyribonuclease

Pancreatic deoxyribonuclease hydrolyses DNA with the formation of 5'-nucleotides, dinucleotides and relatively large amounts of material that are partly degraded but which can be hydrolysed no further (fig. 12.33a). The

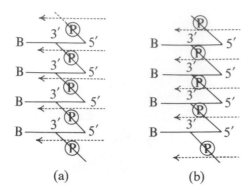

(a)   (b)

FIG. 12.33. Specificity of different types of deoxyribonuclease. (a) Pancreatic DNAase. (b) Spleen DNAase. The horizontal broken arrows indicate the sites of hydrolytic cleavage.

exact specificity of the enzyme is not known. Spleen tissue contains a second type of deoxyribonuclease which degrades DNA to oligonucleotides having a free 3′-phosphate group (fig. 12.33b). Streptococci produce an enzyme similiar in action to pancreatic deoxyribonuclease except that little free mononucleotide is produced.

PHOSPHODIESTERASES

These enzymes hydrolyse the phosphodiester bonds which link ribose and deoxyribose moieties to phosphate in the polynucleotide chain. Two types of diesterase are known; one hydrolyses the polynucleotide chain to 3′-monophosphates (spleen diesterase is commonly used for this purpose) and the other yields 5′-monophosphates (fig. 12.34). The latter type of enzyme is found in the venom of several species of snakes. Both these enzymes have been used extensively for the preparation of specific nucleotides from nucleic acids and also in structure determination on oligonucleotides from RNA and DNA.

PHOSPHOMONOESTERASE

These enzymes remove orthophosphate from the terminal esterified phosphate group in mono- or oligonucleotides (fig. 12.35). A 5′-nucleotidase is present with the di-

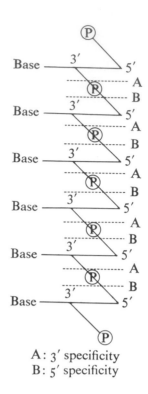

A: 3′ specificity
B: 5′ specificity

FIG. 12.34. Specificity of 3′- and 5′-phosphodiesterase.

esterase in snake venom and rye-grass is a source of 3′-monoesterase.

NUCLEOSIDASES

The combined action of the depolymerases, phosphodiesterases and phosphomonoesterases is to degrade RNA and DNA to the state of nucleosides. The nucleosidases then split the sugar-base bond in these compounds to liberate the free purine or pyrimidine and ribose or deoxyribose (fig. 12.36).

Breakdown of free purines and pyrimidines

BREAKDOWN OF PURINES

Once adenine and guanine have been liberated from the nucleic acids by the appropriate degradative enzymes,

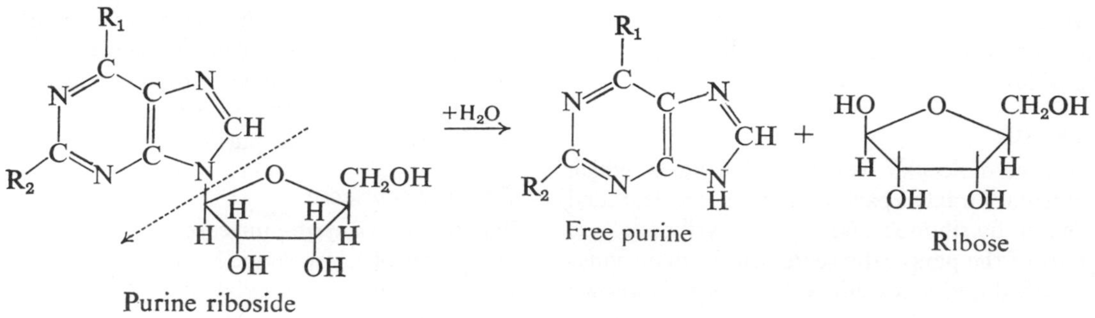

Purine riboside   +H_2O →   Free purine   +   Ribose

FIG. 12.36 Nucleosidase action.

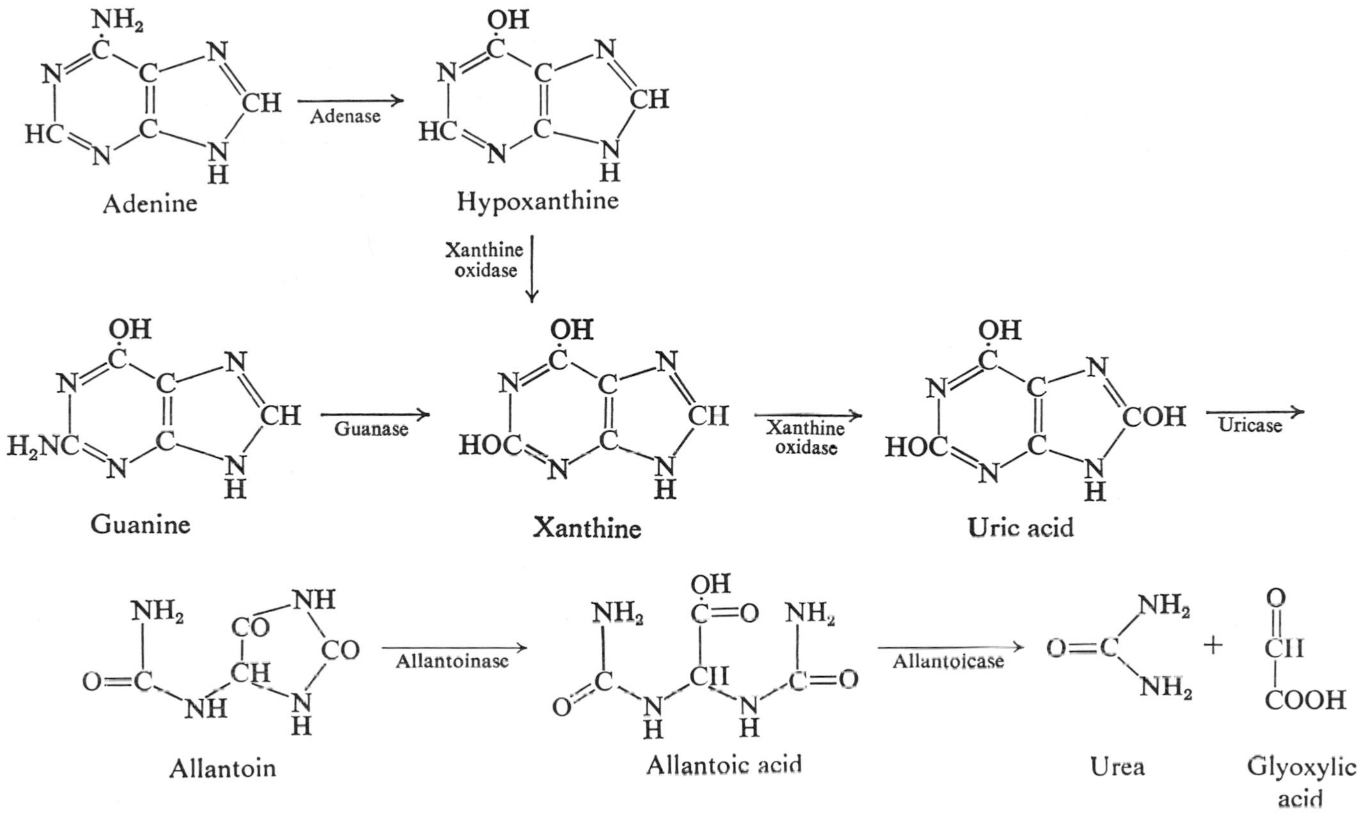

FIG. 12.37. Purine degradative pathways.

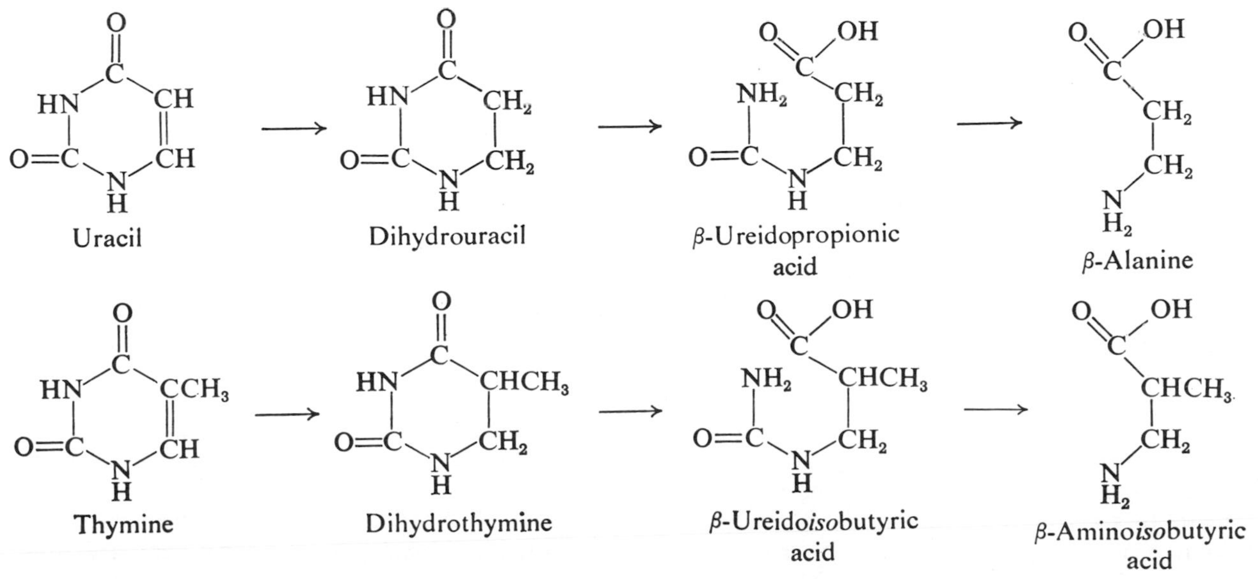

FIG. 12.38. Pyrimidine degradative pathways.

they may be degraded further by a series of reactions which in certain organisms ultimately yield urea (fig. 12.37). The first step in this pathway is the conversion of both adenine and guanine to xanthine (via hypoxanthine in the case of adenine) and this compound is then converted to uric acid by the action of xanthine oxidase. In some species, uric acid can then be further degraded to urea via allantoin and allantoic acid.

Although not all the enzymes necessary to achieve these reactions are found in all species, they seem to form the main route of degradation of the purines, at least in metazoa. Man and the apes are unusual since they have

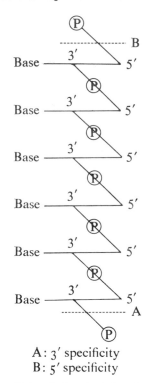

A: 3′ specificity
B: 5′ specificity

FIG. 12.35. Specificity of 3′- and 5′-phosphomonoesterase.

no uricase and therefore uric acid is excreted as the end-product of the purine breakdown. In most mammals, however, uric acid is degraded to allantoin, which is excreted, whereas many fish excrete allantoic acid. Further pathways exist in micro-organisms; thus some *Pseudomonas* species degrade purines to urea and glyoxylic acid, while the anaerobic *Clostridia* yield glycine via 5-aminoimidazole.

Purine catabolism is directly implicated in at least one disease since an increased urate body pool is a feature of gout (vol. 3, p. 25.40). In many such patients there is an acceleration of the first rate-limiting step of purine synthesis in the conversion of 5-phosphoribosyl-1-pyrophosphate to 5-phosphoribosyl-1-amine (p. 12.25). This condition occurs in primates and some birds and is characterized by the deposition of crystals of urates in the joints.

BREAKDOWN OF PYRIMIDINES

The free pyrimidines liberated from RNA and DNA by the concerted action of nucleases and phosphatases may be further degraded to one of three β-substituted amino acids, depending whether uracil, cytosine or thymine is involved (fig. 12.38). These β-amino acids are the main nitrogenous excretory products derived from pyrimidines in mammals.

An alternative degradative pathway to urea and malonic acid exists in some bacteria. In this case the first step of the pathway is the conversion of pyrimidines to the corresponding substituted barbituric acids.

FURTHER READING

ALLFREY V.G. & MIRSKY A.E. (1961) How cells make molecules. *Scientific American* **205**, September, 74–82.

BERGSMA D., HAMERTON J.L. *et al.* eds. (1972) *Paris Conference (1971)*. Standardisation in Human Cytogenetics. Birth Defects; Original Article Series, 8, No. 7.

BOSCH L. ed. (1972) *The Mechanism of Protein Synthesis and its Regulation*. Amsterdam: North Holland Publishing Co.

DAVIDSON J.N. (1972) *The Biochemistry of the Nucleic Acids*, 7th Edition. New York: Academic Press.

HAMERTON J.L. (1971) *Human Cytogenetics*, vol. 1. New York: Academic Press.

HAYES W. ed. (1973) Advances in molecular genetics. *British Medical Bulletin* **29**, 185–271.

HANAWALT P.C. & HAYNES R.H. eds. (1973) *The Chemical Basis of Life: An Introduction to Molecular and Cell Biology*. Readings from *Scientific American* San Francisco: Freeman.

LAST J.A. & LASKIN A.I. (1972) *Protein Biosynthesis in Non-Bacterial Systems*. New York: Dekker.

LEWIN B.M. (1970) *The Molecular Basis of Gene Expression*. Chichester: Wiley.

MANDELSTAM J. & McQUILLEN K. (1973) *Biochemistry of Bacterial Growth*, 2nd Edition. Oxford: Blackwell Scientific Publications.

NIRENBERG M. (1963) The genetic code. *Scientific American* **208**, March, 80–94.

OCHOA S. (1963) Synthetic polynucleotides and the genetic code. In *Informational Macromolecules*, ed. Vogel H., Bryson V. & Lampen J.O., New York: Academic Press.

SILVESTRI L.G. ed. (1970) *Ribonucleic Acid-Polymerase and Transcription*. 1st Lepetit Colloquium on Biology and Medicine. Amsterdam: North Holland Publishing Co.

STEIN W.H. & MOORE S. (1961) The chemical structure of proteins. *Scientific American* **204**, February, 81–92.

STENT G.S. (1971) *Molecular Genetics: An Introductory Narrative*. San Francisco: Freeman.

THOMPSON J.S. & THOMPSON M.W. (1973) *Genetics in Medicine*, 2nd Edition. Philadelphia: Saunders.

WATSON J.D. (1970) *Molecular Biology of the Gene*, 2nd Edition. New York: Benjamin.

WELLS R.D. & INMAN R.B. (1973) *DNA Synthesis in vitro*. Lancaster: Medical & Technical Publishing Co.

WHITE M.J.D. (1973) *The Chromosomes*, 6th Edition. London: Chapman & Hall.

WOESE C.R. (1967) *The Genetic Code*. New York: Harper & Row.

YUDKIN M. & OFFORD R. (1974). *Comprehensible Biochemistry*. London: Longman.

Chapter 13
Cell structure

This chapter is concerned with the structural organization of cells, with particular emphasis on mammalian cells. Living cells vary greatly in their size and complexity. **Prokaryotic cells** are very small and are surrounded by a single cell membrane and have no other intracellular membrane or nucleus; the eubacteria and spirochaetes and rickettsiae are examples. They are considered in vol. 2. **Eukaryotic cells** are found in mammals and in all higher organisms including protozoa and fungi. They are very much larger than prokaryotic cells and contain a nucleus surrounded by a membrane which contains their genetic material in the form of chromosomes.

The fertilized ovum is one of the largest human cells; against a dark background, it can just be seen by the naked eye. By repeated mitotic division, this cell produces the co-ordinated population of cells and their products which we recognize as an adult human being. The number of generations of cells between the adult and its ovum is surprisingly small; a series of 50 divisions produces over 10^{15} cells. The processes of intermediary metabolism occur within each of these cells, but during this period of cellular multiplication differentiation is taking place so that groups of cells become specialized for their particular role in the body.

Differentiation

The earliest changes in differentiation affect the nucleic acids and thus the types of proteins produced in any cell; these changes cannot be seen in microscopic preparations as alterations in cell structure. When chemical differentiation is accompanied by cellular differentiation, the shape or contents of the cell can be seen to be different from those of its unspecialized neighbours. Tissue differentiation, **histogenesis**, occurs when differentiated cells aggregate to form tissues, and organ differentiation, **organogenesis**, follows as groups of tissues combine to form functioning organs. The division of the ovum and its subsequent differentiation produce all the cells of the body, but as this differentiation proceeds cells become restricted in the range of cell types which they can produce. As they specialize, they lose the capacity for cell division. A complex organism contains highly specialized cells which cannot divide, and it also produces dividing cells for repair and replacement. So the cells of the body can be graded according to their mitotic capabilities; it is a continuous gradation which can be roughly separated into three groups.

Cells which cannot divide in the adult: a full complement of these cells is obtained during development and their life may be as long as that of the individual. Any damage or loss is irrevocable as they cannot be replaced from less specialized cells. Nerve cells, which establish complex connections during their differentiation, and muscle cells which combine to form a skeletal muscle fibre are examples of this group of mitotically inactive cells. Satellite muscle cells can undergo mitotic division (p. 16.9). *Cells which divide infrequently and irregularly in health:* these can be stimulated to rapid division. The connective tissue cells belong to this group, and after injury a burst of mitotic activity will produce the cells necessary for repair. Similarly, the cells of adipose tissue and of glands proliferate in response to a demand for increased function.

Cells which reproduce rapidly and regularly in the healthy adult: in these populations, the offspring of the rapidly dividing cells differentiate into specialized cells which have a short life span. The epithelia of the skin and alimentary tract and the precursors of erythrocytes are good examples of this type, for an adult produces and destroys about a million erythrocytes every second and replaces the lining of the intestine every few days.

Size and shape of differentiated cells

The large independent protozoon cell performs all the functions of living matter and is directly exposed to the external environment. The small size and varied shapes of higher animal cells are incompatible with an exposed independent existence. Human specialized cells can live only in an environment whose limits of temperature, osmolality and ionic balance are controlled by the activities of other specialized cells. Most of the cells of the body are between 10 and 40 μm in diameter, the lymphocyte (7–8 μm) being the smallest and the ovum (about 100 μm) and some nerve cells by far the largest. Consider a nerve cell which supplies the skin of the big toe. The cell body and nucleus are in the 5th lumbar intervertebral space, just above the sacrum; a process from the cell body branches, one part going down to the toe, and the other up to the spinal cord to reach the medulla in the skull. The cell body has a diameter of about 50 μm and the cylindrical processes are only about 5 μm in diameter, but they extend almost 2 m (2 000 000 μm). At the magnification of fig. 13.1 these processes would run for almost half a mile. Similarly, skeletal muscle is formed of multinucleated cylindrical fibres which run the whole length of most of our muscles. To facilitate diffusion through the walls of blood vessels the lining endothelial cells are flattened so that they are less than 1 μm thick. The erythrocyte provides another example of modification of external shape (fig.

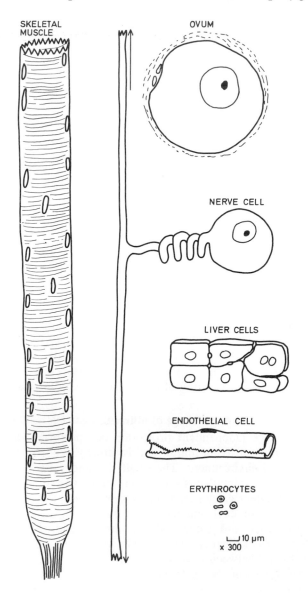

FIG. 13.1. Variations in the size and shape of cells.

13.2). This non-nucleated disc is packed with haemoglobin and as oxygen combines with and is released from the haemoglobin it must diffuse into and out of the cell. Near the periphery of a disc (X), the contents are exposed to a greater surface area of membrane than at the centre (Y). Hence it is possible to contain at the periphery more haemoglobin which is effective, so that the biconcave disc is the most efficient shape.

Internal structure is modified so that each type of cell becomes adapted for its particular role. Thus it is difficult to describe a 'typical cell'. It is best to consider first those features which are common to all cells and necessary

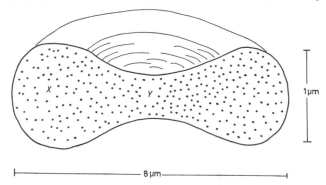

FIG. 13.2. An erythrocyte.

for the maintenance of each cell's life; later the components which are found only in specialized cells are discussed.

No single technique can show all the features of cell structure; the concept of a cell to be described is a synthesis of the information provided by several methods. It is unnecessary for students to know the details of these techniques, but it is worthwhile understanding the particular contributions and limitations of each method.

Investigative techniques

LIGHT MICROSCOPY

With an ordinary **light microscope** little can be seen in a living cell. Almost all its constituents are colourless so that it appears as a drop of clear jelly. Although the absorption of light by cell constituents is similar, some of these possess different refractive indices. This property is used in the **phase contrast microscope**, where the combination of two beams of light, one of which has been retarded by a quarter of its wavelength, succeeds in converting slight differences in refractive index into different intensities.

If the cell contains closely packed orientated material, this can be demonstrated by its effect on polarized light, so that when viewed through a **polarizing microscope** with a polarizer and analyser at right angles, oriented fibrils and membranes appear bright against a black background. These structures are then said to be **birefringent** or **anisotropic**. The detection and even measurement of certain constituents of living cells, of which nucleic acids and haemoglobins are examples, can be accomplished by illuminating them with monochromatic light of appropriate wavelength and measuring its absorption in a **microspectrophotometer**.

All these microscopes can be used on single free cells, like blood cells and spermatozoa, and can also be applied to intact cells dispersed from complex organs. They are useful for examining cells growing outside the body in organ, tissue and cell culture. Cell movements, growth and multiplication can be directly observed in cultured cells and the changes in structure produced by irradiation, toxic agents and deprivation of essential nutrients can be seen. As a tissue cell growing in culture has lost the environment and intercellular contacts of the intact tissue, changes in the cell shape are inevitable and obvious, but other changes may be undetected. The value of cell culture as employed in the study of human chromosomes is described on p. 12.20.

FIXATION AND EMBEDDING

Attainment of satisfactory resolution with the light microscope depends on the specimen being thin; to separate objects which are less than 1 μm apart the whole thickness should not be more than 10 μm. Small free cells satisfy this criterion, but many cells are larger than 10 μm and in the tissues they are so tightly packed that adequate resolution can be achieved only by cutting the tissue into very thin slices. As it is difficult to cut fresh tissues, it is usual first to **fix** the tissues, to retain their contents more or less as at the moment of death. This process of fixation denatures the cell proteins, and so prevents the autolysis which would otherwise follow cell death; it can be achieved by chemicals such as alcohol, formaldehyde and osmium tetroxide. After the tissue is fixed it must be supported in a medium such as paraffin wax which allows it to be cut into thin slices. The fixed tissue must first be dehydrated with alcohol and other chemicals and then infiltrated with molten paraffin wax before it is cast into a block and cooled. The paraffin block can then be cut on a microtome and a series of thin sections produced.

STAINING

If the sections are examined immediately, after the wax has been removed with a solvent such as xylol, no more can be seen than in the direct examination of a living cell. It is therefore necessary to stain selectively certain cell components. A multitude of staining methods are used; many of the best, like the dyer's old art, are empirical. Nowadays new methods are often based on known chemical reactions and these are termed **histochemical** methods. **Haematoxylin and eosin** is the best known empirical method; it stains the nuclei blue-black, and the cytoplasm and extracellular fibres pink. Certain basic dyes, like toluidine blue, stain the nucleic acids in both nucleus and cytoplasm. Metallic impregnation methods

demonstrate fine nerve processes, delicate reticulin fibres and even intracellular organelles. Collagen can be specifically stained with aniline dyes and if these are combined with cytoplasmic and nuclear stains, the triple staining method will distinguish extracellular connective tissues from the cells themselves. Elastin protein can be stained by an empirical method in elastic connective tissues.

Typical examples of histochemical methods are provided by the prussian blue reaction (PBR), which stains iron and the periodic acid-Schiff (PAS) method for polysaccharides. In this method, the periodic acid first oxidizes the glycol groups which will then react with the Schiff's reagent and produce a red colour. If the section is first treated with salivary amylase the glycogen present will be hydrolysed; this procedure makes it possible to distinguish this polysaccharide from the glycoproteins of connective tissues and mucin which are not affected by the enzyme.

All information obtained from fixed, embedded and sectioned cells is static, and any dynamic changes can be inferred only by examining cells at different periods in their life span or secretory cycle. Dynamic interpretations from static material can be assisted by studying the sites of incorporation of radioactive materials. The cells or animals are first exposed to a radioactive substance for a certain time; the tissue is then fixed and sections cut and covered with a photographic emulsion. The emissions from the radioactive elements incorporated into the tissue components affect the overlying emulsion and silver grains are produced at these sites. After subsequent staining of this section, the position of the radio-activity can be related to the structure of the tissues. This method of **autoradiography** can demonstrate, for example, cell production and cell secretion by identifying those cells which have incorporated radioactive thymidine into their DNA. It is thus largely responsible for the present knowledge of the dynamics of cell populations (p. 13.1).

It should be appreciated that in sections of chemically fixed tissues which have been cut in paraffin wax, all the water and those components which are soluble in water, alcohol, benzene or molten wax have been removed. The residue of insoluble material is merely a scaffolding composed of precipitated, denatured proteins, effete enzymes and highly polymerized insoluble molecules such as nucleic acids and polysaccharides. Some lipoprotein complexes remain, but all other lipids have been dissolved. Conceding that only a travesty of the original cell remains, it must be recognized that the technique of chemical fixation and wax embedding has provided most of our present knowledge of the arrangement and shape of tissue cells, and of the pathological changes in diseased tissues. It is probable that almost all the slides in a student's collection will be specimens of this nature and it is essential that the drastic treatment given to the material should be remembered during their examination.

FROZEN SECTIONS

Many methods attempt to preserve more of the cell's structure. The removal of lipid can be avoided by freezing fresh or fixed tissue; the ice block provides sufficient support to produce **frozen sections**, in which the lipid can be stained with a dye like Sudan III. These frozen sections are useful also as a method of rapid diagnosis on tissues removed at a surgical operation, and can be prepared while the operation is still in progress. Some enzymes retain part of their activity after the use of certain fixatives, but, apart from the phosphatases, practically no enzymes survive paraffin embedding. For **enzyme histochemistry** therefore, fixed or fresh **frozen** sections are used; autolysis is prevented by rapid freezing and the resulting ice block is cut on a cold microtome. Rapidly frozen tissue can also be dehydrated for embedding in paraffin wax by sublimation of the ice in a vacuum. This **freeze-dried** tissue preserves some enzyme activity and retains small soluble molecules which are washed away in any form of aqueous chemical fixation. The enzymes are located in the cells by incubating the section with an appropriate substrate in a medium which precipitates one of the end products at the site of enzyme activity.

IMMUNOFLUORESCENCE

The highly selective nature of immunological reactions can be used to identify and localize particular proteins in cells and tissues. This complicated technique is easily explained by taking a specific example. To locate the protein heavy meromyosin (HMM), a pure preparation of HMM is injected into a rabbit and, after a suitable period, the animal produces an antibody to this protein (anti-HMM). This antibody is a protein present in the plasma of the rabbit. Blood can then be removed and the purified antibody chemically combined with a fluorescent dye to form anti-HMM-F. If frozen sections or fragments of muscle are now treated with anti-HMM-F, the strong bonds between HMM and anti-HMM-F hold the fluorescent dye at the sites where HMM is distributed in the muscle. The uncombined anti-HMM-F is then washed away and the fluorescence revealed by illumination in ultraviolet light. This ingenious technique of **immunofluorescence** has proved valuable in many investigations of normal structure and of human immunological diseases in which, for example, the presence of specific immunoglobulins may be detected (p. 29.8).

ELECTRON MICROSCOPY AND ALLIED TECHNIQUES

All the methods mentioned so far are ultimately limited by the resolving power of the light microscope ($0.3\ \mu\text{m}$) which is about three orders of magnitude greater than the size of the smaller molecular components of the

cells. It follows that much of the organization of the cell would forever remain unknown if investigations were limited by this resolution. Employment of the transmission **electron microscope** (EM) for greater resolution (1.0 nm) increases the technical difficulties, since the specimen must be in a vacuum and less than 50 nm thick. These conditions virtually exclude the examination of living cells, which cannot therefore be used as a criterion for the faithfulness of preservation of the fine structure revealed by the EM. The most successful method of examining tissues in the EM has been a copy of the chemical fixation paraffin embedding method of light microscopy. The most common fixative is osmium tetroxide but glutaraldehyde is now frequently used in combination with it or alone; potassium permanganate gives comparable results and frozen dried specimens may be used. Cutting sections thin enough for the EM is accomplished by replacing paraffin wax by plastic embedding media. Finely engineered ultramicrotomes using broken glass or diamond knives cut the tissues in these plastics into sections less than 60 nm thick. These sections are supported on copper mesh grids for examination and photography in the EM. The autoradiographic, histochemical and immunological methods of light microscopy have all been adapted so that they can be employed in electron microscopy.

Much useful information about intracellular structures has come from a combination of electron microscopy and **differential centrifugation**. Small portions of a tissue are fixed, embedded and sectioned for electron microscopy to determine the form of its intracellular structures. If a large portion of the same tissue is homogenized, various constituents can be separated by centrifuging at different speeds. These pellets of segregated constituents can then be prepared for EM examination. Similar pellets can be analysed for their chemical constitution and enzymic activity. In this way, chemical structure and function can be assigned to the particular components of the original intact cell. As an example, mitochondria can be isolated by centrifugation and shown to possess oxidoreductases (p. 7.4). A more recent development is the application of the **scanning electron microscope** to biological tissues. Electrons instead of being transmitted through the specimen are focussed on its surface where they stimulate emission of secondary electrons. In this way, the surface topography of tissues or of individual cells may be seen (fig. 34.1 & vol. 3, fig. 21.8).

The resolving power of the EM and especially the inadequacies of methods of fixation and sectioning prevent these techniques revealing actual atomic structure. The general form of macromolecules can be seen, but the atomic structure of a collagen fibre or myosin filament cannot be revealed by EM. **X-ray diffraction** patterns from pure crystalline biological materials will indicate their atomic architecture. The necessary purity can be achieved only by chemical isolation of the material, but if the location of a macromolecule can be determined by EM it is justifiable to interpolate the known atomic structure to this site.

Hence by combining the information produced by all the techniques of structural examination it is possible to create a mental image of the architecture of all parts of the body at all levels of organization. This goal has already been achieved in some tissues (fig. 13.3) where it is possible to draw the plan for the whole range.

FUNDAMENTAL CELL STRUCTURE

There are certain features of cell structure which are present in all cells capable of continued life. These features are described before considering more specialized cellular

Cell Boundary
Cytoplasm
    Cytoplasmic matrix
    Endoplasmic reticulum
    Golgi apparatus
    Mitochondria
    Ribosomes
    Lysosomes
    Microbodies
    Centrioles

Nucleus
    Nuclear envelope
    Nucleoplasm
    Sex chromatin
    Nucleolus

structures which are found only in cells adapted for particular functions. Mature erythrocytes and blood

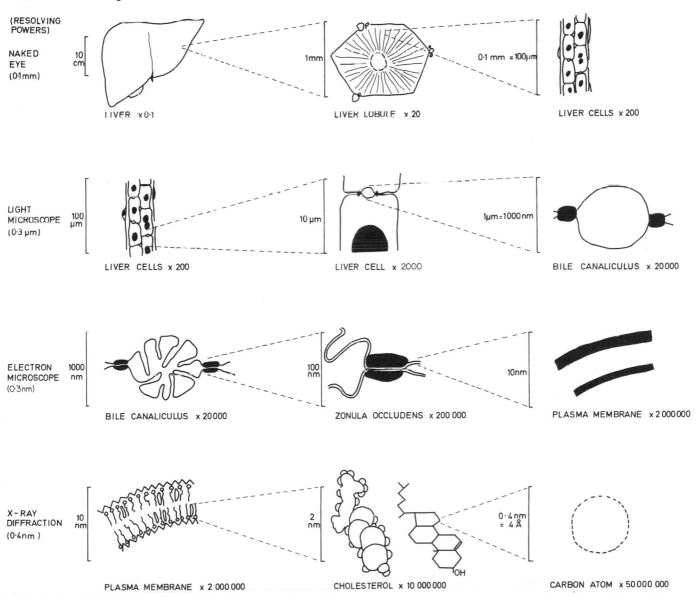

Fig. 13.3. Naked eye examination, light microscopy, electron microscopy and X-ray diffraction each give different views of the body. These sketches of the liver show the contribution of each method. If they are combined, an understanding of the molecular architecture of the organ is obtained.

platelets are non-nucleated; they have a brief life and cannot reproduce, so they must be regarded as exceptions to the scheme.

Cell boundary

When a living cell moves in its supporting medium, its edge can be detected in the phase contrast microscope as a sudden change in refractive index. Even after staining the cytoplasm, little can be seen at the boundary of most cells by light microscopy. With the EM however, a clearly defined membrane separates the contained cytoplasm from the surrounding medium. In a thin section of osmium-fixed material, the membrane appears as shown in fig. 13.4; this structure is a feature of all animal and plant cells. It had been predicted from studies of cell permeability that the cell surface would include a membrane composed of a bimolecular leaflet of phospholi-

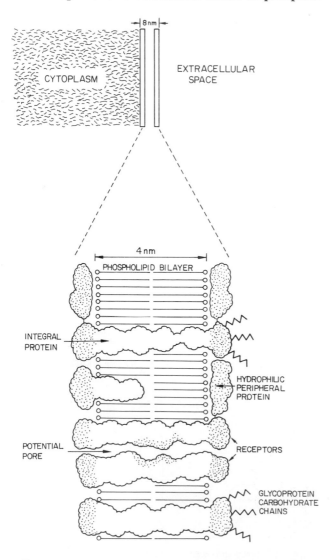

FIG. 13.4. The plasma membrane as it appears in an electron micrograph, showing its molecular architecture.

pids. The dimensions of the membrane now observed with the EM fit such a structure; for this and other reasons, it is now believed that the tripartite membrane illustrated in the upper part of fig. 13.4 has the general chemical architecture shown in the lower part. This limiting membrane is known as the **plasma membrane** and is, by definition, the layer which provides the main control of the exit and entry of ions and small molecules. Changes in the plasma membrane's permeability to ions affect the normal negative electrical potential of the cytoplasm, and the consequent electrical events can be recorded as the action potential (p. 15.16).

The plasma membrane is not static or rigid; it is in active motion, extending pseudopodia and contributing to the movement of the whole cell. These activities are probably caused by forces developed in the underlying cytoplasmic proteins.

The structure with two rows of packed lipids seen in fig. 13.4 is analogous to the micellar arrangement assumed by phospholipids in the absence of protein. Nevertheless one cannot be certain that this is the arrangement of phospholipid and protein in membranes in the living cell. The complex permeability properties of membranes indicate that the structure is less simple; protein-lined pores penetrate the phospholipid portion and proteins extend throughout the central portion (p. 10.20).

The surface of the cell also carries identification marks which are characteristic of the cell, the species and even the individual. Our capacity to reject tissues grafted from other people is effected by the reactions which follow the recognition of a foreign cell surface. The proteins and possibly carbohydrates in the outer lamella of the plasma membrane must therefore incorporate specific antigenic patterns which are determined by the genetic machinery of the cell.

Cytoplasm

The term cytoplasm refers to all the material within the cell, except that contained in the nucleus. As more and more cytoplasmic structures have been discovered and named, the definition of cytoplasm has become confused. If it refers to all the extranuclear material, the term **cytosol** can be used for the portion which is not contained in any recognizable organelle.

The cytosol of a living cell appears homogeneous in the phase contrast microscope. This amorphous mass of colloidal proteins, carbohydrates and simple solutions of all the small molecules and ions involved in metabolism is maintained in an internal cellular environment. The internal medium is partially insulated from changes in the extracellular fluid by the plasma membrane. This is necessary, as precise physicochemical conditions must prevail within the cell to maintain the colloidal dispersion and intrinsic shape of the protein molecules. The cytoplasm has a uniform affinity for stains like eosin, although chemical fixation can cause artefactual clumping. Rapid freezing avoids this coalescence and by preserving enzyme activity allows subsequent histochemical incubation to show the presence of cytoplasmic enzymes.

The EM shows that, beyond the resolution of the light microscope, internal cell membranes produce an elaborate division of the cytoplasm into compartments with different chemical constitutions. These internal membranes have structures similar to those of the plasma membrane and are made of phospholipid. The EM allows their description and classification. A satisfactory nomenclature is not available and with the variations which accompany any cell specialization it is difficult to describe a general arrangement. However, in all cells membranous sacs, tubes and vesicles are present; their lumina usually appear empty in contrast to the surrounding cytoplasmic matrix with its denatured proteins, polymerized carbohydrates and nucleic acids. Originally this internal organization was thought to be a network confined to the centre of the cell, and it was thus named **endoplasmic reticulum**. Although this form and distribution is not constant, the name has been preserved.

The **Golgi apparatus** is one portion of the endoplasmic reticulum which forms an organelle present near the nucleus of all cells. It consists of a stack of flattened sacs surrounded by a cloud of microvesicles and a few larger vacuoles (fig. 13.5). This complex can be impregnated

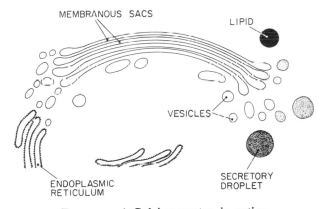

FIG. 13.5a. A Golgi apparatus, in section.

with silver and gold salts for light microscopic examination, where it appears as a network around the nucleus. It is a prominent feature of secreting cells where it lies on the side of the nucleus nearest to the secreting surface. It provides the membrane to package the secretion and is also closely associated with polysaccharide synthesis and lysosome formation.

Mitochondria are also membranous organelles; since they have a unique structure and are not known to be continuous with or formed from the endoplasmic reticulum, they are considered as separate bodies. Mitochondria can be seen by phase contrast microscopy,

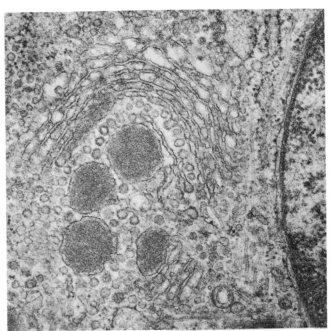

FIG. 13.5b. Golgi region of a secreting cell showing presence of partially formed secreting granules within Golgi zone ($\times 50\ 050$).

often as long thread-like bodies about 1 μm wide, and this is the origin of their name (Gr. *mitos* = thread, *chondros* = granule). They may number thousands in a single cell, and are in continuous motion, segmenting and rejoining and they can be seen to grow in length. If cells are exposed to the dye Janus green during life (intravital staining) the mitochondria are specifically stained. The ultrastructure of mitochondria is very characteristic (fig. 13.6); they are surrounded by two membranes and the internal membrane is invaginated to form cristae. Between the cristae the dense matrix contains some dark granules. Differential centrifugation, EM and histochemical methods show that mitochondria contain the enzymes for the citric acid cycle and the cytochromes of the electron transfer system (p. 8.7). Thus mitochondria should be regarded as the furnaces where the cell's fuel is burned and the released energy harnessed.

Many enzymes and cytochromes are integral parts of the phospholipid mitochondrial membranes, and the matrix contains the nicotinamide nucleotides and certain enzymes. At very high resolution, electron micrographs show bead-like projections on the cristae which are probably the individual molecules of the enzymes. The cristae appear to act as a scaffolding which holds the enzymes in relation to each other, very probably in the order in which they operate. Mitochondria contain a very small amount of DNA, enough to provide the genetic information necessary for the synthesis of their own structural proteins.

Most of the RNA of the cell is found in the cytoplasm; it can be demonstrated by its absorption of ultraviolet

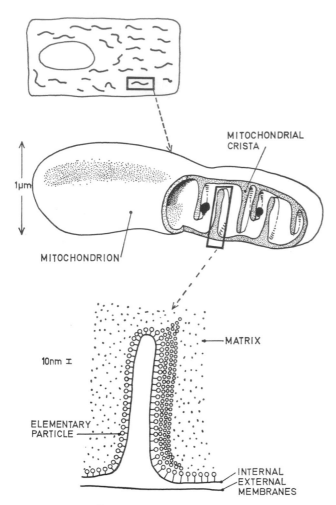

FIG. 13.6a. A mitochondrion.

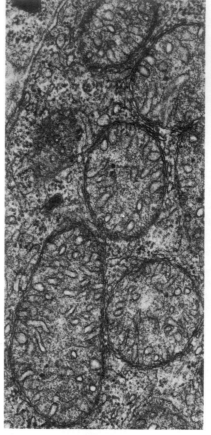
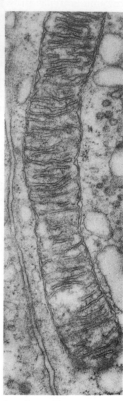

FIG. 13.6. (b) Part of an adrenal cell showing cell components notably mitochondria with 'tubular' cristae (×46 000); (c) mitochondria with 'shelf' type cristae (×35 900).

light, even in a living cell. Although fixation and embedding removes the lower molecular weight transfer RNA, cytoplasmic nucleic acids can be shown in these specimens as cytoplasmic basophilia after staining with basic dyes like toluidine blue. Since the DNA is virtually restricted to the nucleus, this staining demonstrates the presence of RNA in the cytoplasm and the previous treatment indicates that this RNA is in an insoluble form. Dense particles, 15 nm in diameter, are seen by EM in the cytoplasmic matrix of all cells; after isolation by centrifugation, these particles are shown to be a RNA-protein complex and they are known as **ribosomes.** A string of ribosomes is attached to a strand of messenger RNA to produce a polyribosome in the synthesis of a protein (fig. 13.20). Hence a ribosome particle in an EM indicates the point where a protein molecule can be produced. If a cell is not growing or secreting protein there are few ribosomes, but some are always present to replace the proteins lost in normal turnover.

Most cells contain organelles which are smaller and denser than mitochondria, and these are called **primary lysosomes.** They have a single limiting membrane and contain hydrolytic and proteolytic enzymes; one of the former, acid phosphatase, can be recognized histochemically and this reaction is used to identify lysosomes.

A primary lysosome fuses with a **phagosome,** containing ingested material, or with an **autophagic vacuole,** which, being a zone of internal scavenging, is surrounded by two layers of membrane (fig. 13.21). After fusion, a **secondary lysosome** is formed and the released enzymes begin to digest the contents prior to absorption into the cytoplasm (fig. 13.7).

Peroxisomes and microbodies (fig. 13.21) are also membranous vesicles which store enzymes, sometimes in crystalline form. One variety is known to contain uricase but there are probably many types as yet undifferentiated.

Apart from the group of cells (p. 13.1) which have relinquished the power to divide, all other cells contain bodies which lie close to the nucleus, near the Golgi apparatus; these are the **centrioles.** Each is an open ended barrel-shaped body, less than 0·5 μm long and 0·2 μm in diameter; the wall is made of nine sets of three longitudinal tubules arranged in an overlapping fashion (figs. 13.8 and 13.9). Throughout the interphase period,

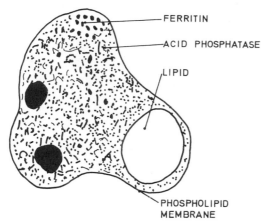

FIG. 13.7. A secondary lysosome.

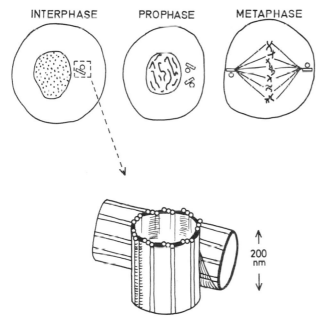

FIG. 13.8. The centrioles in an interphase cell.

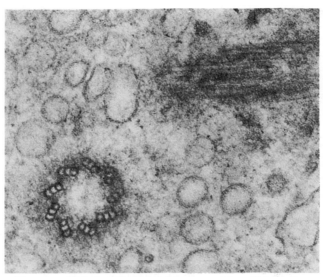

FIG. 13.9. EM of a pair of centrioles in a rat thyroid follicular cell (×91 900).

macromolecules. Thus there is a **nuclear envelope** which can constrain the DNA and histones of the nucleus without interfering with the passage of metabolites. The nuclear envelope consists of two lipoprotein membranes which form a flattened sac, the perinuclear cisterna, surrounding the **nucleoplasm**. The inner membrane is applied to the nucleoplasm and the outer to the cytoplasm. The perinuclear cisterna is a part of the lumen of the endoplasmic reticulum, since in places the outer nuclear membrane is continuous with the endoplasmic reticulum in the cytoplasm (fig. 13.10). Circular pores between the nucleoplasm and cytoplasm are formed by the fusion of the outer and inner membranes of the nuclear envelope; these pores are about 50 nm in diameter and they are probably partially occluded. When the prophase stage of cell division is completed the nuclear envelope breaks up into a series of vesicles which reaggregate around the nuclei of the two daughter cells at telophase.

the cell contains a pair of centrioles often orientated at right angles to each other. Immediately before prophase, both centrioles divide to produce two pairs, which move to the opposite sides of the nucleus. Only one member of each pair seems to be involved in mitosis, and from this one, a leash of **microtubules** (fig. 13.21) extends into the nucleus to form the spindle (p. 12.20). Microtubules are a normal constituent of the cytoplasm of interphase cells, about 25 nm in diameter, but only in mitosis are they seen to connect with the centriole to form the spindle.

Nucleus

The margins of the nucleus are sharply defined in living and stained cells. Intact nuclei can be isolated from cells. Water and small molecules penetrate the nucleus rapidly but there is a barrier to the passage of

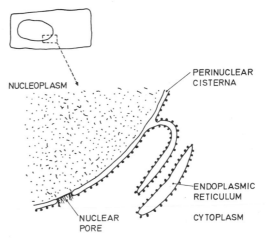

FIG. 13.10a. A nuclear envelope.

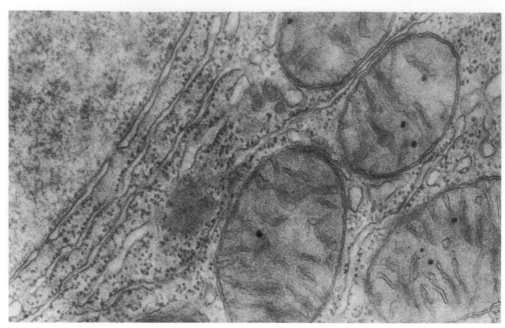

FIG. 13.10b. EM showing pores in the nuclear envelope, abundant rough-surfaced endoplasmic reticulum and several mitochondria containing dense granules (× 60 000).

The changes in the nucleus which are associated with the appearance of chromosomes and their movements during cell division are described on p. 12.20, so we are concerned now with the 'resting nucleus'. This structure is badly named because it is during this interphase period that the DNA controls the production of RNA and at the appropriate time the DNA replicates, ready for the next division. As these events are invisible and follow the dramatic microscopic events of mitosis, a false impression of inactivity is given.

In the living cell under phase contrast, the nucleus appears homogeneous, with a slightly higher refractive index than the cytoplasm, in which it moves and gently rotates. In the interphase nucleus, the DNA is uncoiled and extended to its full length, making the actual length of the DNA molecules in each nucleus about a metre. Even remembering that each double helix is only 1·8 nm wide, it is hard to visualize so much being packed into a sphere perhaps 5 μm in diameter; the nucleus also contains the special nuclear proteins, the histones. The packing is random, so the nucleus can be likened to a ball of very fine thread; EM confirms this arrangement as the nucleoplasm appears as a uniform mass of dots and short lengths of fine fibres.

The nucleic acid attracts stains such as haematoxylin, and the DNA can be specifically stained with Schiff's reagent after partial hydrolysis, the **Feulgen reaction**. Most fixatives for light microscopy cause some clumping of the nuclear contents, so that the nucleus appears to contain darkly staining masses which may be condensed near the nuclear membrane or form a network throughout the nucleus. This artefact is called **chromatin** and

since there is some constancy in its arrangement in particular cells treated in standard fashion, its distribution can be useful in identification.

The sex chromatin or Barr body, which is present in the nuclei of normal interphase female cells, represents a mass of unextended DNA. It is not an artefact and as the number and distribution of these bodies indicate the fate of the sex chromosome during division and fertilization they are clinically important.

Apart from the chromatin produced from the DNA content, the nuclei usually contain aggregations of RNA which are called **nucleoli**. Nucleoli are dark spheres about 1 μm in diameter; they are known to contain RNA because they disappear after ribonuclease digestion, they do not stain with the Feulgen reaction and yet they attract the nucleic acid stains. Nucleoli are especially prominent in protein-secreting cells and they always disappear before mitosis.

Nuclei vary in size and shape, their size increasing with that of the cell. Very large cells such as osteoclasts and skeletal muscle fibres are multinucleated. The shape of the nucleus conforms to the shape of the cell, thin flat discs in endothelial cells, long ovoids in smooth muscle cells and spheres in cubical epithelial cells. Some nuclei acquire bizarre shapes, being multilobulated in the polymorphonuclear leucocyte and kidney-shaped in monocytes.

If all the cellular constituents so far described were assembled in their simplest form, the cell produced would appear as in fig. 13.11. This cell would be capable of movement, maintenance and cell division. It could absorb from the surrounding medium the nutrients and oxygen necessary to produce energy. It could discharge its waste

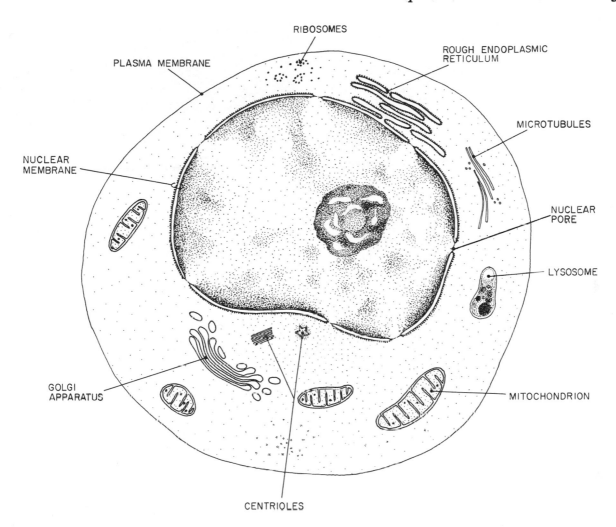

FIG. 13.11. A section of a cell containing the structures which are essential for its survival.

products and could synthesize its own constituents. This theoretical cell is strikingly similar to an actual cell, the lymphocyte. The immunological functions which are currently assigned to this important white blood cell do not make any functional demands which could not be accomplished by this fundamental cell structure.

SPECIALIZED CELL STRUCTURES

In differentiated cells, certain features of the fundamental structure just described become exaggerated and other cellular structures appear. It is these specialized features which, by increasing the mobility, absorptive capacity, synthetic ability etc., determine the role of any particular cell, and it is the recognition of these features which makes it possible to identify a cell in the tissues. No cell possesses more than a few of these special features and they are conveniently described as modifications of the fundamental structure under these headings.

The cell boundary
  Extracellular constituents
  Intercellular adhesion
  Pinocytosis, phagocytosis and secretion
  Increase in surface area
  Cilia and flagella
Cytoplasmic membranous organelles
  Rough-surfaced endoplasmic reticulum
  Smooth-surfaced endoplasmic reticulum
  Mitochondria
Cytoplasmic proteins, lipids and carbohydrates
Pigments

Cell boundary

EXTRACELLULAR CONSTITUENTS

When two tissue cells are in apposition, their plasma membranes do not usually come into direct contact, there being an extracellular gap about 15 nm wide. This gap is permeable to water and ions and probably serves to expose a large area of the plasma membranes of closely packed cells to the interstitial fluid. This space between cells exists because each membrane has an outer coating of glycoprotein, the carbohydrate-protein complexes, which in the extracellular spaces of the body form a part of the connective tissue ground substance. The bonds between these opposed cells are not strong, since the gap can be enlarged by osmotic changes, and other cells, e.g. lymphocytes, can migrate into the gap (fig. 13.12).

The strength of the surface can be increased by formation of a **basement membrane**; this is probably produced by incorporating collagenous protein in the surrounding glycoprotein coat. The basement membrane can be shown by light microscopy either by impregnating with silver salts or by staining by the PAS reaction. Different surfaces of a single cell can have varying amounts of extracellular covering. Thus an epithelial cell (fig. 13.12) has a naked plasma membrane facing the lumen, a polysaccharide-containing extra-cellular space along its sides and a well developed basement membrane at the base of the cell.

About one third of the body is extracellular (p. 1.3) and the physical characteristics of this part can vary from a watery interstitial fluid to the calcified collagenous matrix of bone. The form of the extracellular materials determines the properties of the connective tissues (chap. 17). Here it is only necessary to recognize that these tissues are extensions of the extracellular coats around

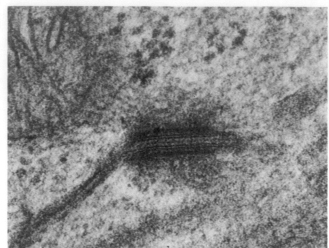

FIG. 13.13a. Desmosome (macula adhaerens) (× 142 000).

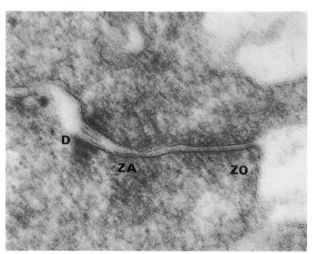

FIG. 13.13b. EM of intercellular adhesions between adjacent absorptive cells of rat small intestine (× 117 500). D = desmosome; ZA = zonula adhaerens; ZO = zonula occludens.

cells. Cellular activity is responsible for the synthesis of the connective tissue proteins (collagen, reticulin, elastin, plasma proteins, etc.) and carbohydrates, e.g. sulphated glycosaminoglycans in cartilage; it also maintains them during life and controls the deposition of minerals in these tissues.

INTERCELLULAR ADHESION
If body cells did not stick together, we would collapse into a slimy mass of assorted cells around our skeletal remains. The attachments of cells to each other create organs and provide barriers to enclose such fluids as bile, blood and urine (chap. 18). The specific adherence of cells is an important factor in controlling differentiation, and the loss of this property, which is one of the features of malignant change, releases the neoplastic cell to roam the body.

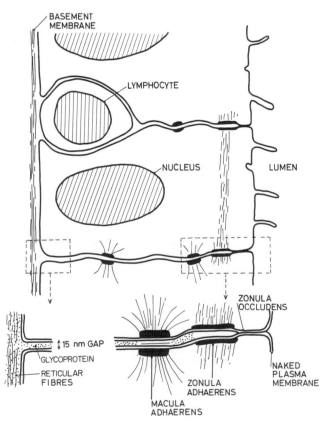

FIG. 13.12. Intercellular adhesions.

Where cells adhere strongly to their neighbours, special structures are seen at the surface. These structures are found only between cells of a similar type, muscle to muscle and epithelial cell to epithelial cell, and although their distribution varies in different tissues they are constant in structure. A useful nomenclature for these specialized regions of adhesion is as follows.

Macula adhaerens or desmosome (figs. 13.12 and 13.13) is a 'spot-weld' between adjacent cells, where the cytoplasmic sides of the plasma membranes are thickened to receive the attachment of intracellular filaments. In the gap between these thickenings, an organization of the intercellular materials reveals itself as a bisecting line. Structures like half desmosomes attach cells to the surrounding connective tissue. This is well seen at the end of a muscle cell where the contractile force of a myofibril is transmitted through the plasma membrane to the collagen fibres of the tendon.

Zonula adhaerens (figs. 13.12 and 13.13) is similar to a desmosome but more extensive; in epithelia it forms a continuous girdle around the cell, formerly known as the terminal bar. A zonula adhaerens does not have such a prominent bisecting line and may not have intracellular filaments radiating out into the cytoplasm.

Zonula occludens (figs. 13.12 and 13.13) is the junction where intercellular space is obliterated by the cohesion of the outer layers of the apposed plasma membranes. An obvious function of this **tight junction** is to eliminate intercellular diffusion and thus it is an essential feature of epithelial organization. In certain locations, e.g. between cardiac and smooth muscle cells, the adhering membranes permit the passage between them of small particles, about 3 nm in diameter, while still resembling structurally the 'tight' junction of the zonula occludens. In these circumstances, they are known as 'gap' junctions and probably facilitate electrical contact between the cells.

Some cells fuse even closer to each other, so that the intervening plasma membranes disappear, forming a **syncytium.** This is seen in the syncytial structure of the skeletal muscle fibre, the syncytiotrophoblast of the placenta and the large osteoclast.

PINOCYTOSIS, PHAGOCYTOSIS AND SECRETION

While the passage of water, gases, ions and small molecules through the plasma membrane occurs passively or by active transport mechanisms (p. 18.8) built into the plasma membrane itself, a special method is employed for the entry and exit of larger soluble molecules and of particles. Fig. 13.14a shows how the formation of a small vesicle can carry a macromolecule into the cell without disrupting the ionic permeability characteristics of the surface. These minute vesicles, 20–40 nm in diameter, are present at the surface of most cells and the name of the process is **pinocytosis** or 'cell drinking' (fig.

13.15). The production of the vesicle and its movement depends on energy, and ATPase can be demonstrated in the walls of pinocytotic vesicles. As the first step in the process is adhesion of the particle to the surface, pinocytosis can select molecules from the surrounding medium.

Phagocytosis or 'cell-eating' is a similar process, but here the ingested material is particulate; and adheres to the surface of the cell before being engulfed. Bacteria, effete erythrocytes and dead cells are ingested by phagocytosis (p. 29.3). Pinocytosis is seen in almost all cells; by contrast, the capacity for phagocytosis is virtually

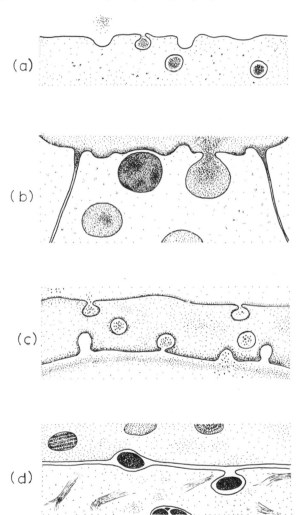

FIG. 13.14. Various forms of membrane transport. (a) pinocytosis: a macromolecular particle is indicated as a black dot; its entrance into the cytoplasm through a small vesicle is shown. (b) The discharge of a secretory droplet. (c) The passage of a particle through a cell as seen in capillary endothelia; note that the particle remains enclosed in a membranous vesicle. (d) The transfer of material from one cell to its neighbour: this could indicate the passage of a melanin granule from a melanocyte on the left to an epithelial cell on the right.

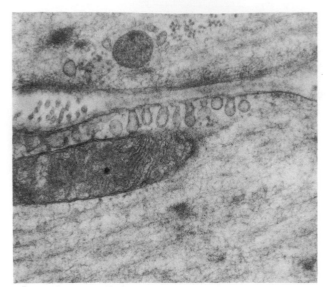

FIG. 13.15. EM of pinocytic vesicles beneath the plasma membrane of smooth muscle cells (× 46 270).

restricted to macrophages and polymorphonuclear leucocytes (chap. 29). Although the differentiation made between pinocytosis and phagocytosis is as described here, the words are sometimes used almost interchangeably, and the term **endocytosis** may be used to cover both situations.

Just as these contortions of the cell surface take substances into the cell, so the reverse process, emiocytosis, is used for the discharge of macromolecular material into the surrounding medium. At the apex of an enzyme-secreting cell, the stored protein enzymes approach the surface as secretory granules; their membranous envelopes join the plasma membrane and the contents are liberated (fig. 13.14b). Many thousands of small vesicles are held at nerve terminals, to release their contained transmitter material on stimulation of the nerve (p. 15.25).

A combination of these input and output mechanisms allows material to be transferred directly from one cell to another. For instance the melanocytes in the skin which manufacture the pigment melanin pass it directly to the ordinary epithelial cells where it is stored (fig. 13.14d). Pinocytosis is also a means of transfer straight through a cell without the material coming into direct contact with the other cell contents; the permeability of capillary walls probably depends in small part on this process (fig. 13.14c).

INCREASE IN SURFACE AREA

The area of exposed plasma membrane can be increased by various geometric patterns. Finger-like projections are common and if packed close together they form a refractile luminal surface to the cell known as a brush border (fig. 13.16). Similarly, infoldings of the membrane

which accommodate the processes of adjacent cells increase the surface area (fig. 13.17). These adaptations are probably more complex than a simple increase in the surface area, for the membranes of the brush border and basal infoldings carry specific enzymes; they should therefore be regarded also as supports for enzymes concerned with ion pumping and active transport. They thus have

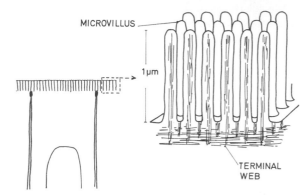

FIG. 13.16a. Microvilli forming a brush border.

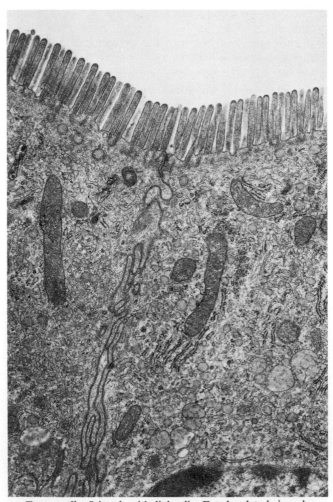

FIG. 13.16b. Jejunal epithelial cells. Fat droplets being absorbed (× 13 500).

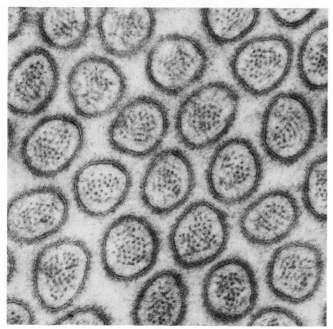

FIG. 13.16c. Microvilli in transverse section (× 13 500).

(p. 32.15) and the very fine T-tubules of striated muscle carry the surface action potential deep into the fibre (p. 16.8).

The myelin sheath of a nerve fibre is also an extension and modification of the surface plasma membrane (p. 15.4).

CILIA AND FLAGELLA

Cilia are cell projections which are actively motile; they are like oars which can move a protozoan cell. In tissues composed of stationary cells the cilia move the fluid bathing the surface. Ciliary movement has a sense of direction, all the cilia on one cell or on an epithelial sheet of cells beating the same way. During the forceful stroke the cilium is a rigid rod, about 4 μm long, which recoils in a bent flaccid state ready for the next cycle (fig. 13.18). The ultrastructure of a cilium is intriguing and complicated; it is attached to a root body which resembles a centriole (p. 13.9). Fine tubules extend from the root

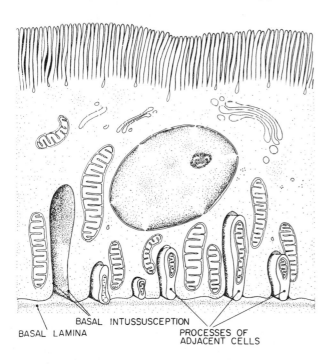

FIG. 13.17. Increase in the surface area by basal intussusceptions, as found in the renal tubules.

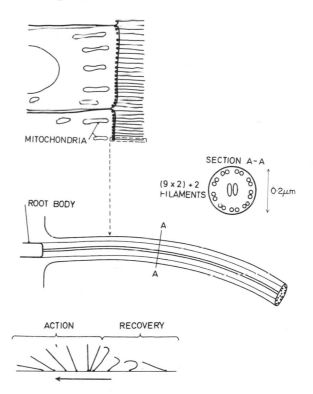

FIG. 13.18. Cilia, movements and ultrastructure.

a supporting role similar to that of the cristae in mitochondria. A further example of membranes playing a supportive role is provided by the retinal rods and cones, where invaginations of the plasma membranes carry the photosensitive pigments.

The surface area can be increased also by tubular invaginations. Intracellular canaliculi provide a passage for acid secretion by the oxyntic cells of the stomach

body up the axis of the cilium, nine pairs of tubules being arranged peripherally around a central thicker pair (fig. 13.19).

Flagella are much longer than cilia, the human sperm tail reaching 50 μm, but the basic structure of a flagellum is the same as that of cilium with some extrafibrillar material symmetrically arranged around the ring of

$(9\times2)+2$ tubules (fig. 13.18). Many other types of cell carry a single cilium which resembles normal cilia in all cytoplasmic basophilia; the deep blue-staining cytoplasm of the immature red cell which is synthesizing haemoglobin provides a good example.

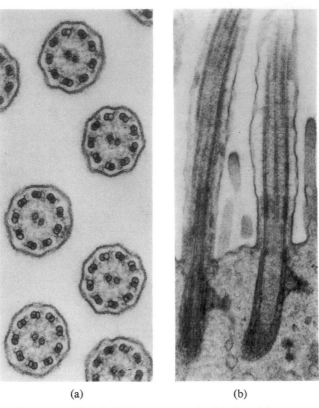

(a)   (b)

FIG. 13.19. EM of cilia in rat tracheal epithelium (a) transverse section ($\times$ 79 920); (b) longitudinal section ($\times$ 36 000).

respects except that it lacks the central thicker pair of tubules. Such single cilia may be akin to the retinal rod in their structure but their function is as yet unknown; they are thought to be non-motile.

On some secreting cells, very long tapered processes provide sites for the discharge of secretion; these are called stereocilia. They are easily seen by light microscopy, being 10–20 µm long, and their resemblance to cilia is only superficial as they are non-motile and do not have an organized internal structure.

Cytoplasmic membranous organelles

As described on p. 13.8, some **ribosomes** are always present in cells for the natural turnover of the cell's own proteins. A high concentration of ribosomes in the cytoplasm indicates more active protein synthesis. If the proteins produced are for the growth of the cell, as in embryonic development, or if they are retained in the cell, the polyribosomes are found floating freely in the cytoplasm. This concentration of RNA causes an intense

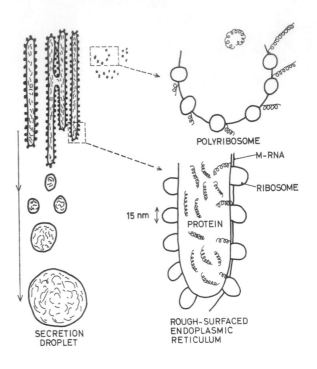

FIG. 13.20a. Protein synthesis at polyribosomes. At the top right this is shown as it would occur free in the cytoplasm. On the left the ribosomes are attached to membranes of the endoplasmic reticulum and the synthesized proteins pass into the lumen of the reticulum.

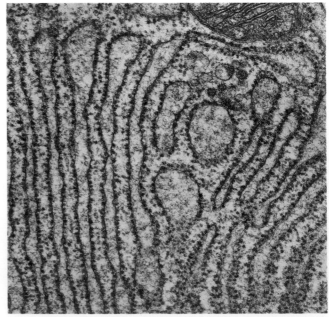

FIG. 13.20b. 'Granular' endoplasmic reticulum ($\times$ 5400).

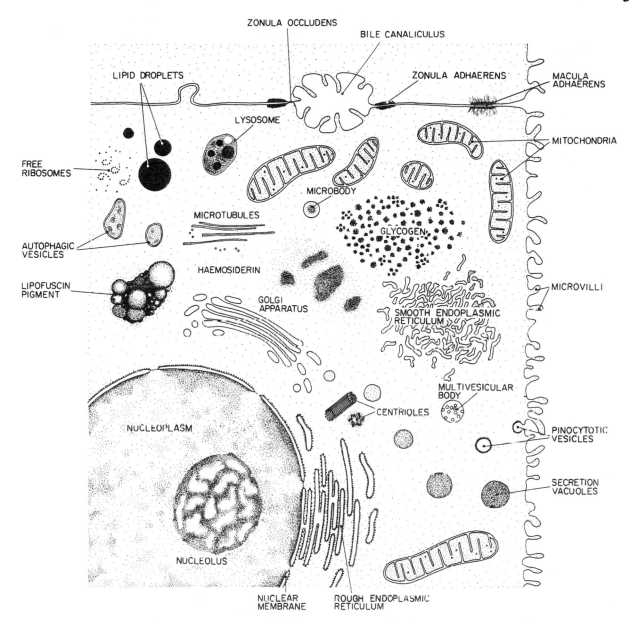

FIG. 13.21. A composite diagram showing the structures which can be seen in a parenchymal cell in the liver (hepatocyte).

ENDOPLASMIC RETICULUM(ER)

When a large number of ribosomes is attached to the membranes of the endoplasmic reticulum, this is described as **rough-surfaced ER** (fig. 13.20). This combination also indicates protein synthesis, but here the newly formed protein molecules in the lumen of the endoplasmic reticulum move into the Golgi region of the cell transported by microvesicles. Here they aggregate into secretory granules before passing to the surface for discharge. Thus the endoplasmic reticulum and the Golgi region can be regarded as a packaging and delivery apparatus. Note that these cells will also be basophilic in the light microscope; the EM, by showing the relationship between the ribosomes and the internal membranes, can show whether the products are mainly exported or stored. Hence the protein-secreting cells of the pancreas and the plasma cells secreting antibodies contain large amounts of rough-surfaced ER. Elaborate proliferations of membranous tubules and sacs without attached ribosomes are known as **smooth-surfaced ER** (fig. 13.21). This is found in cells which are synthesizing carbohydrates, like glycogen, and steroids. In striated muscle, smooth-surfaced endoplasmic reticulum is called the sarcoplasmic reticulum. It is concerned with calcium ion binding and constitutes a support for the enzymes of anaerobic glycolysis.

Microsomes are an artefact of homogenization. When

the endoplasmic reticulum is disrupted, it forms vesicles which can be separated by ultracentrifugation. These may be derived from rough- or smooth-surfaced reticulum; microsomes from the former contain ribosomes.

MITOCHONDRIA

As the main site for energy conversion in cells, a complement of these organelles is almost always present. An obvious specialization is the provision of large numbers of large mitochondria with an increased area of closely packed cristae in those cells which need a great deal of energy. The continually beating heart muscle, the cells of the kidney tubules pumping ions back into the plasma and the parietal cells of the stomach secreting hydrochloric acid are all packed with large complex mitochondria.

Cytoplasmic proteins, lipids and carbohydrates

PROTEINS

Many of the enzymatic and structural proteins form an integral part of the organelles already described, but some are in colloidal solution in the cytoplasmic matrix. Cellular differentiation can be shown by locating an enzyme system associated with a particular function; for instance, the epithelial cells of the prostate have a high acid phosphatase activity. In the EM, a diffuse density in the cytoplasmic matrix is all that remains of this colloidal solution. However, one particular globular protein (ferritin) is made obvious by its extraordinary capacity to store iron. Ferritin has an iron-containing core which by scattering electrons appears as a dense particle 5 nm in diameter.

Fibrous proteins fulfil diverse roles in the cytoplasm of many cells. They are responsible for the movement of cilia and flagella and for the contraction of muscle (p. 16.4). They confer strength and turgidity on the cytoplasm as tonofibrils in the epithelial layers of the skin. Similarly, in a cell with a brush border an underlying feltwork of fibrils extends into each microvillus, and this is known as the terminal web (fig. 13.16). The outermost layers of the epidermis contain the fibrous protein keratin, the substance which forms nails and hair.

LIPIDS

Phospholipid protein complexes are the basis of the plasma and internal membranes; as such they are present in the organelles and structures like the myelin sheath. Whorled electron-dense structures, myelin figures, are occasionally found, as a result of fixation of phospholipid, in cells. The simpler lipids, the triglycerides, are present in varying quantities and, as they are immiscible with water, even a small amount will aggregate to form a lipid droplet. Large amounts form a single spherical droplet around which the cell is reduced to a thin cyto-

plasmic film, as in an adipose tissue cell (p. 34.1). Numerous smaller lipid droplets are seen in the cells of brown adipose tissue and in cells which secrete and store steroid hormones or the fat-soluble vitamins A and D.

Embedding in paraffin wax removes all the simple lipids, so a lipid-containing cytoplasm can appear either frothy or show a single large spherical space. Frozen sections retain the lipid which can then be stained. In EM, osmium fixation, by combining with the lipids, makes them less soluble, so they can be recognized as homogeneous inclusions in the cytoplasm.

CARBOHYDRATES

Monosaccharides and disaccharides, being soluble, are removed by all preparative procedures except freeze drying. Histochemical staining with the PAS type of reaction can show only the highly polymerized and relatively insoluble polysaccharides, like starch and glycogen. Digestion with salivary amylase provides a useful control, since this treatment hydrolyses glycogen. Glycogen is present in most cells, but is stored mainly in muscle and liver. In EM, glycogen particles can be recognized as clumps of dense granules each larger than a ribosome.

Mucous secretions contain large amounts of mucoprotein and glycoprotein which are polysaccharide-protein combinations. These substances are also PAS positive but they resist digestion with amylase. If they are stained with certain dyes, they take on a colour different from that of the original dye, that is, they exhibit **metachromasia**. Metachromasia is shown also by the sulphated glycosaminoglycans of cartilage and by another similar substance, heparin.

Pigments

Compared with the vivid colours of plants, insects and birds, mammals are drab creatures and man is one of the least colourful. Much of our colour we receive fortuitously from the iron-containing haemoglobin and its iron-free but coloured derivatives, bilirubin, urobilinogen and stercobilin. Likewise our muscles are reddish because the iron-containing myoglobin is present in them. Even the subtle and seductive natural colours of the eyes and hair are merely interference patterns formed by a black pigment, melanin, which appears as black spherical granules in which the actual melanin is combined with protein (chap. 37).

In pathological conditions, many pigments may be present, but in normal unstained cells, apart from melanin, only visual purple, lipofuscin, haemosiderin and ingested foreign matter can be seen. Visual purple is a photosensitive pigment, present in the rods and cones of the retina where it is presented to the light, in monomolecular layers, by being attached to flat sheets of lipoprotein membrane. Carotene and other carotenoid substances can also colour cells if they are present in sufficient amounts.

Lipofuscin, one of the commonest cellular pigments, is known by a variety of names (wear and tear pigment, haemofuscin, lipochrome, brown atrophy and age pigment), a selection which demonstrates its complexity as well as ignorance of its function, and indicates that it contains some lipid and some iron. The lipofuscin content increases with the age of a cell. In nerve cells of old people large masses of this yellow pigment may surround the nucleus. There are structural resemblances and so possibly a relationship between secondary lysosomes (p. 13.8) and lipofuscin granules, although the latter do not have the acid phosphatase activity of the former. Haemosiderin, which consists of large aggregations of ferritin molecules, also appears as yellowish-brown granules, but its intense prussian blue staining distinguishes it from lipofuscin.

Exogenous substances, such as dust, carbon particles or tattooed dyes, remain obvious in the cells which have phagocytosed these particles.

COMMENT

This survey of the types of organelles and structures found in cells is not comprehensive. Additional features are still being discovered and biochemical and functional information is being allotted to known structures. Continued research, even with existing techniques, should clarify many points in the immediate future. It is bound to be difficult to determine precisely the relation between structure and function in the cell; the size of the structures, their interdependence and the disturbance which any method of examination produces, all make the task formidable. This is not surprising since a complete understanding of the machinery of the cell would mean an explanation of life itself. It is encouraging to compare a modern description of the cell with an account written before the application of electron microscopy, X-ray diffraction and refined biochemical techniques.

As illustrative of the present position, the parenchymal cell of the liver may be used as an example. The liver functions as an exocrine gland, as the main site for a multitude of reactions in intermediary metabolism and as a store of materials (chap. 33); it is therefore not surprising that this cell contains a larger collection of organelles than most of our more limited cells. In fig.

13.21, all the structures mentioned in the preceding pages are illustrated as they appear in the liver cell.

Finally, although the general pattern of cell structure has been summarized, descriptions of the infinite variety of different cells have not been attempted. Many of these differences, in secreting cells, are due to the nature of the secretion product. Even when this product cannot be chemically defined, empirical staining methods can distinguish these cells from their neighbours. Consideration of all these cells is best deferred until the structure and function of the systems is discussed (chaps. 25–38).

FURTHER READING

Practical details of various techniques:

Hayat M.A. ed. (1973) *Principles and Techniques of Electron Microscopy.* Vol. 3. Biological applications. London: Van Nostrand Reinhold.

Kay D. (1965) *Techniques for Electron Microscopy,* 2nd Edition. Oxford: Blackwell Scientific Publications.

Pearse A.G.E. (1968) *Histochemistry, Theoretical and Applied,* 3rd Edition. London: Churchill.

Well-illustrated histology textbooks:

Bloom W. & Fawcett D.W. (1968) *A Textbook of Histology,* 9th Edition. Philadelphia: Saunders.

Fawcett D.W. (1966) *The Cell: Its Organelles and Inclusions.* Philadelphia: Saunders.

Ham A.W. (1974) *Histology,* 7th Edition. Philadelphia: Lippincott.

Accounts of cell structure which emphasize dynamic aspects:

De Robertis E.D.P., Nowinski W.W. & Saez F.A. (1960) *General Cytology,* 3rd Edition. Philadelphia: Saunders.

Loewy A.G. & Siekevitz P. (1970) *Cell Structure and Function,* 2nd Revised Edition. New York: Holt, Rinehart & Winston.

Toner P.G. & Carr K.E. (1971) *Cell Structure,* 2nd Revised Edition. Edinburgh: Churchill Livingstone.

Comprehensive reviews:

Brachet J. & Mirsky A.E. eds. (1959–64) *The Cell,* vols. 1–6. New York: Academic Press.

Lima-de-Faria A. ed. (1969) *Handbook of Molecular Cytology.* Amsterdam: Elsevier.

Chapter 14
Control of metabolism

With modern chemical and physical techniques reliable information has been obtained about the chemical composition of living cells, and it may soon be possible to locate exactly all their molecules and ions. Even this will not explain the nature of life in chemical terms, since it will only identify the position of the constituents at a particular moment of time. Attempts to convert such a static picture into a dynamic one by repeating analyses on identical cells at intervals have met with only limited success. A more promising approach became possible with the development of spectroscopic methods for continuous monitoring in life of concentrations of specific intracellular substances. These methods, to be useful, must be specific and sensitive and be harmless to the living system. They are difficult to apply to the mixed cell population of mammalian tissues. Yet they have already given information on some of the controls that determine rates of chemical reactions within isolated cells and thereby regulate metabolism.

VARIATIONS OBSERVABLE IN MAN

A fundamental feature, observed by all who study living systems, is that no system is ever steady, but all are continuously oscillating, apparently spontaneously.

One of the simplest examples in a human subject is his weight. This can be measured using a clinical balance to an accuracy of 10 g. If the subject weighs 70 kg the precision of the observation is nearly 0·01 per cent. Let us assume that his energy requirement is known and that food commensurate with his needs is fed at three intervals throughout the day. If the subject is weighed hourly, his weight will be seen to fluctuate depending on the time of food intake, urinary excretion, defaecation, sweat loss, etc. However, it is possible to calculate an average weight over a period of observation. In this case the factors which contribute to the variability about the mean are easy to evaluate. Similar observations can be made on height, rectal temperature, blood pressure, oxygen consumption, etc. The gross fluctuations measured in each case are the sum of minute changes occurring within single cells.

A large number of observations have been made on the changes in concentration of metabolites in mammalian plasma. Plasma glucose, free fatty acids, potassium,

calcium, sodium and bicarbonate concentrations all fluctuate about a mean value. Changes in the concentration of glucose and free fatty acids in plasma are shown in fig. 14.1. The plasma glucose rises a short time after

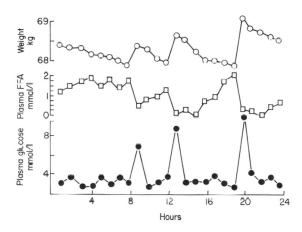

FIG. 14.1. Variations in weight and in the plasma concentrations of glucose and FFA in a normal healthy subject during a 24-h period.

the consumption of food; the plasma free fatty acid concentration falls as plasma glucose rises. These changes are not due to primary events occurring in plasma, but reflect alterations in the rates of entry and exit of metabolites in or out of the plasma. Thus the changes are explicable on the basis of many events occurring in the gut and tissues. The task which confronts anyone attempting to understand how molecular processes are controlled is to make serial, accurate observations under standardized conditions on, say, a component in plasma, and develop a hypothesis to explain the observed fluctuations. If the hypothesis is sound, it should be possible to use it to predict the concentration of the specific compound under different conditions. If anomalies emerge, the hypothesis has to be modified to accommodate the new data.

Although it is possible to obtain by biopsy, samples of many human tissues, for technical and ethical reasons measurements of the concentration of metabolites are usually made only on plasma. Most studies on tissues

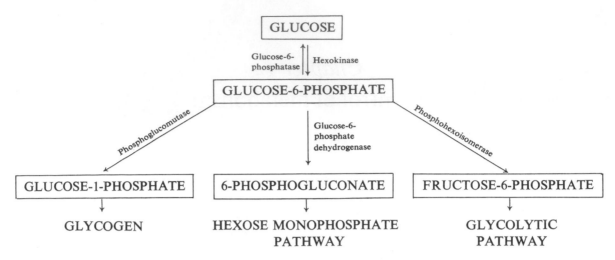

FIG. 14.2. The central position of glucose-6-phosphate in the intermediary metabolism of carbohydrate.

have to be made on other species and their relevance to man has to be assessed.

REGULATION OF METABOLISM

Metabolism describes the transformation and translocation of molecules in living systems. Thus the control of metabolism embraces the chemical regulatory systems which operate in living cells. These permit the living cell to keep the concentrations of many intracellular and extracellular metabolites close to set values.

In mammalian tissues the problem is to discover how cells adjust their energy expenditure and internal composition in the face of relatively large changes in the composition of the extracellular environment. Eating habits vary and, as most nutrients are readily absorbed, dietary components rapidly find their way into the extracellular fluid. Thus the concentrations of glucose, triglycerides, free fatty acids, amino acids and other nutrients in plasma vary substantially with dietary intake, and these variations influence the intracellular concentration of metabolites.

Most people vary their food intake from time to time throughout the day and also from day to day. During the week there are periods of greater or lesser activity and of increased or diminished food intake. The control of metabolism must cope with these fluctuations in food intake and energy expenditure and also with other factors.

The control of metabolism is discussed under the following topics:

(1) Regulation of enzymic activity.
(2) Mitochondria.
(3) Regulation of glycolysis.
(4) Generation and use of NADPH$_2$.
(5) Control of amino acid metabolism.
(6) Membranes and control of metabolism.
(7) Action of hormones.
(8) Metabolic adaptations to environmental stress.

Regulation of enzymic activity

Nutrients enter mammalian cells from the ECF through the plasma membranes, and then take part in reactions, most of which are controlled enzymically. The catalytic activity of an enzyme depends on the number of enzyme molecules per unit volume (p. 7.6). The control of metabolism is closely associated with modifications of enzyme activity. For example, when a metabolite such as glucose enters the cytosol, the molecule may be utilized as a substrate in a reaction activated by hexokinase.

$$\text{Glucose} + \text{ATP} \longrightarrow \text{Glucose-6-phosphate} + \text{ADP}$$

If ATP is present in excess and if the hexokinase is not saturated with substrate, additional glucose entering the cell is phosphorylated to G-6-P. This can then be transformed enzymically into fructose-6-phosphate or glucose-1-phosphate (p. 9.5 and fig. 14.2). Furthermore in liver, G-6-P may be acted on by glucose-6-phosphatase to yield glucose and inorganic phosphate inside the cell. At this metabolic branchpoint G-6-P may be diverted to the glycolytic pathway, to glycogen, to glucose or to 6-phosphogluconolactone and the hexose monophosphate pathway (fig. 9.2, p. 9.6). Thus the absolute amount and the K_m of hexokinase, phosphohexoisomerase, phosphoglucomutase and phosphatase are important factors which dictate the fate of glucose.

Some enzymes are stored in cells as larger proteins or enzymes, which are inactive. To generate the catalytically active enzyme, the proenzyme is acted on by a peptidase.

$$\text{Proenzyme} \xrightarrow{\text{peptidase}} \text{Enzyme} + \text{peptide}$$

Storage as a proenzyme is a form of control of enzyme activity and is seen mainly in extracellular enzymes associated with the function of the alimentary tract, e.g.

pepsinogen/pepsin, trypsinogen/trypsin and chymotrypsinogen/chymotrypsin. Another protein, the hormone insulin, is stored as a prohormone and activated in a similar way (p. 27.41). In these instances, the proenzyme or prohormone has no known biological activity until it is cleaved by a specific peptidase which generates the potent enzyme or hormone.

One of the simplest controls of metabolic events in living cells is that of **end-product inhibition** (fig. 14.3a). This type of feedback control is illustrated in the metabolic sequence in the synthesis of long chain fatty acids.

$$\text{Acetyl CoA} \xrightarrow[\text{ATP}]{\text{CO}_2} \text{Malonyl CoA} \dashrightarrow$$

$$\text{Butyryl CoA} \dashrightarrow \text{Palmityl CoA}$$

The end-product, palmityl CoA, inhibits the acetyl CoA carboxylase pacemaker, while citrate activates this enzyme. Acetyl CoA carboxylase exists as monomeric units which are inactive until they aggregate into protomeric forms.

$$\underset{\substack{\text{carboxylase}\\\text{monomeric form}\\\text{(inactive)}}}{\text{Acetyl CoA}} \underset{\substack{\text{fatty acyl}\\\text{CoA}}}{\overset{\text{citrate}}{\rightleftharpoons}} \underset{\substack{\text{carboxylase}\\\text{protomeric form}\\\text{(active)}}}{\text{Acetyl CoA}}$$

A number of other feedback control systems are more elaborate and involve the control of branched metabolic pathways. Where the pathway is as shown in fig. 14.3b,

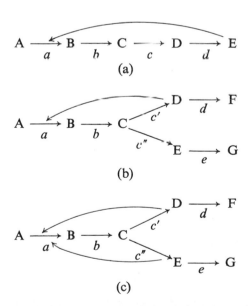

FIG. 14.3. Examples of enzymic feedback control. (a) Feedback control of the end-product E on the enzyme *a* responsible for the conversion of A to B where this first reaction is the rate-controlling step; (b) single path feedback control of intermediate product D on the rate-controlling step catalysed by enzyme *a*; (c) cumulative feedback control of products D and E on enzyme *a*.

the feedback to the enzyme *a* responsible for the conversion of A to B could be exerted by metabolites B, C, D or E. If enzyme *a* was sensitive to metabolite D, then the rate of production of D and E is modulated by metabolite D. This may or may not be an advantage. In some instances enzymes are known in which control at enzyme *a* is mediated by a combination of substrate D plus substrate E. This is sometimes termed **concerted feedback inhibition** and another variant is termed **cumulative feedback inhibition** (fig. 14.3c).

The rate of a reaction in cells may also be influenced by other factors involved in the reaction. Thus lactate dehydrogenase which converts pyruvate to lactate is influenced by the concentrations of both pyruvate and $NADH_2$, the electron donor. Similarly the rate of phosphorylation of glucose by ATP under the influence of hexokinase in hepatocytes depends on the concentrations of both glucose and ATP. The glucose may have come from the diet, while the ATP may be supplied to the enzyme in the cytosol by activities in the mitochondria. Thus mitochondrial respiratory processes influence and control the utilization of glucose by phosphorylation. Similarly some reactions requiring ATP are inhibited by high concentrations of ATP. For example, the phosphorylation of fructose-6-P by ATP in the presence of phosphofructokinase is inhibited by high concentrations of ATP, an effect potentiated by citrate, and this is discussed on p. 14.5.

COVALENT MODIFICATION OF ENZYMES

There are many situations in which covalent modification of an enzyme by phosphorylation results in either activation or deactivation of its catalytic function (p. 7.18). Phosphorylation of the enzyme is effected by a protein kinase and ATP; dephosphorylation by a phosphoprotein phosphatase. The phosphorylation occurs in some instances at one or more of the serine or threonine residues. In some cases the active form of the enzyme is the phosphorylated protein; in others it is the dephosphorylated form which is active. The general reaction is as follows:

$$\text{Dephosphoprotein} \underset{\substack{\text{Phosphoprotein}\\\text{phosphatase}}}{\overset{\substack{\text{Protein kinase}\\+\text{ATP}}}{\rightleftharpoons}} \text{Phosphorylated protein}$$

Glycogen breakdown is effected in part by a phosphorylase. This enzyme exists as a protein monomer, phosphorylase *b*, which is inactive. Two monomers are converted into the active form, phosphorylase *a*, by phosphorylase kinase and ATP (p. 9.9). Inactivation is catalysed by phosphorylase phosphatase. Generation of the active phosphorylase depends on the activity of the kinase and inactivity of the phosphatase. Phosphorylase kinase itself may exist in an inactive form and be activated by phosphorylation. This requires a phospho-

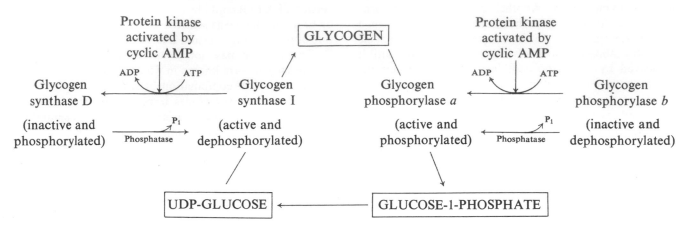

FIG. 14.4. Two amplifying reactions involved in the control of glycogen metabolism.

rylase kinase kinase and also ATP. There are differences between the phosphorylase *a* in skeletal muscle and in liver. In liver it is activated by a kinase dependent on cyclic AMP, whereas in skeletal muscle the kinase is dependent on Ca^{++}. These reactions illustrate the general rule that the route by which a substance B is formed from a precursor A is different from the route used to regenerate A from B, and the mechanism of activation of a mammalian enzyme may depend on the tissue source of the enzyme. An example is the breakdown of glycogen to glucose-1-phosphate and the reverse reaction in which glycogen is synthesized (fig. 14.4).

Glycogen synthesis occurs after glucose-1-phosphate has reacted with uridine triphosphate (UTP) to form UDPG and PP_i. The UDPG then reacts with α-1,4-glucan, $(glucose)_n$, to form a glucosyl glycan, $(glucose)_{n+1}$, and UDP (p. 9.10). This reaction is catalysed by glycogen synthase which exists in active and inactive forms, known as I and D. The I form is converted to the inactive phosphorylated D form by a kinase and ATP. Dephosphorylation of the enzyme is catalysed by a phosphatase and this regenerates the active form.

Thus the key enzyme for glycogen breakdown is active in its phosphorylated form and the key enzyme for glycogen synthesis is active when dephosphorylated. In the liver the phosphorylase kinase is activated by cyclic AMP. Hence conditions which increase intracellular cyclic AMP concentrations, e.g. circulating catecholamines, favour the breakdown of glycogen.

BIOLOGICAL AMPLIFIERS

The control of glycogen metabolism through a series of enzymic reactions is an example of a biological amplifier system. Here the change in the concentration of a coenzyme or cofactor, in this case cyclic AMP, activates an enzyme which in turn activates another enzyme system and the sequence may be repeated several times so that a cascade of reactions results. In the control of glycogen metabolism in liver there are in fact two cascades operating in opposition in such a way that glycogen synthesis and breakdown are finely controlled. As the phosphorylase kinases in different tissues are sensitive to different activators, the control of glycogen metabolism in liver is different from that in muscle, kidney, brain or other tissues. The concentration of cyclic AMP is therefore critical to this control. Another enzyme in carbohydrate metabolism whose activity is controlled by phosphorylation is the pyruvate dehydrogenase complex which is discussed later (p. 14.13).

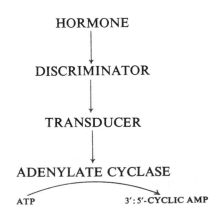

FIG. 14.5. Components of the adenylate cyclase system.

There are many other examples of the control of biochemical events by biological amplifiers. Among the best known is the sequence of events in blood coagulation, where the conversion of soluble plasma fibrinogen to insoluble fibrin involves a long series of enzymic reactions (p. 28.14).

The controls of lipid metabolism through lipolysis, and

of carbohydrate metabolism through glycogenolysis have much in common. In lipolysis the rate-limiting step is the mobilization of free fatty acids by hormone-sensitive lipase (p. 34.5). This enzyme is activated through phosphorylation by a protein kinase which is dependent on cyclic AMP. The cyclic AMP is generated from ATP by adenylate cyclase, which may be activated in adipocyte plasma membrane by the hormones adrenaline, noradrenaline, glucagon and ACTH. This is another example of a cascade reaction.

In muscle, troponin associated with actomyosin (p. 16.4) is essential for the sensitivity of actomyosin ATPase to Ca^{++}. This protein is also made active by phosphorylation by ATP and a protein kinase.

In the adrenal cortex of most species, cholesterol is stored as cholesterol esters in lipid droplets. The steroid hormones are synthesized from non-esterified cholesterol, and the rate-limiting event in steroidogenesis is the cleavage of the cholesterol side chain which converts free cholesterol to pregnenolone (p. 27.34). The rate of release of free cholesterol from esterified cholesterol is influenced by cholesterol ester hydrolase. The active form of this enzyme is phosphorylated and is produced by a protein kinase and ATP. The protein kinase itself appears to be activated by cyclic AMP whose concentration is controlled by ACTH. In a similar fashion the luteinizing hormone (LH) may activate a hormone-sensitive cholesterol ester hydrolase in corpora lutea (p. 38.16). This action again results in an intracellular release of free cholesterol which becomes available to mitochondria for pregnenolone and, subsequently, progesterone production.

The adenylate cyclase system is apparently composed of three parts, a discriminator site to which a hormone binds, a transducer component which may contain GTP, and adenylate cyclase itself (fig. 14.5).

ALLOSTERIC EFFECTS

Another method of control involves the interaction of an enzyme with an effector molecule, i.e. a substance that is not a substrate or cofactor for the reaction, but a ligand which alters the catalytic characteristics of the enzyme. This type of ligand is referred to as an **allosteric effector molecule.** The term allosteric means 'other site' and implies that the effector molecule binds to the enzyme at a site other than the active one. Allosteric enzymes exhibit a sigmoidal relationship between the substrate concentration and the velocity of the reaction (p. 7.8, and so the Michaelis–Menten kinetics must be modified. A positive allosteric effector molecule decreases the initial velocity of the reaction at low substrate concentrations. Then, over a small range of substrate concentration there is a dramatic increase in initial velocity for a small change in substrate concentration. A number of enzymes exhibit

allosterism and some of these effects may represent complex control systems.

A typical example is phosphofructokinase which exhibits allosteric modification in the presence of ATP, ADP, AMP and many other effectors (fig. 14.6). The

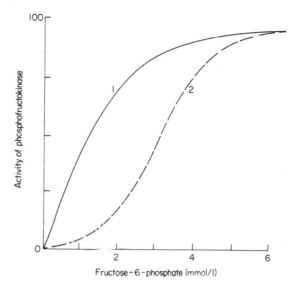

FIG. 14.6. Allosteric modification of phosphofructokinase by nucleotides.

conversion of fructose-6-phosphate to fructose-1,6-diphosphate is under the control of phosphofructokinase and ATP. This is a key enzyme in the glycolytic pathway and it can be deduced that when ATP is required in the cell, glycolysis ought to be activated. As the concentration of ATP in the cytosol falls, the ADP and AMP concentrations tend to rise because the sum of the nucleotides ATP + ADP + AMP is roughly constant. AMP and ADP act as positive allosteric effectors of the phosphofructokinase reaction, while ATP exerts a negative effect. As discussed later, citrate is also a negative allosteric effector of phosphofructokinase.

There are two main situations. In one, the allosteric effector alters the kinetics so that the K_m of the enzyme is altered while the V_{max} remains unchanged. In the other, the K_m is unchanged but the V_{max} is altered. There are many situations in metabolism where allosteric effectors appear to influence enzymic reactions by altering either the K_m or V_{max} of potentially important enzymes. The control of intracellular events by allosteric effectors has been much studied because it could play an important role as a primitive or self-regulating intracellular mechanism.

In some cases, as the substrate concentration rises, the presence of substrate molecules on sites adjacent to or remote from the active centre of the enzyme alters the structure of the active centre. This phenomenon is known as **positive** or **negative cooperativity,** according to whether activity is increased or decreased. Likewise, the extent of complex formation between haemoglobin (Hb) and oxygen to give HbO_2 responds to the concentration of oxygen (Po_2), as discussed on p. 31.19. For this reason Hb has been called an honorary enzyme.

Thus the substrate or another small molecule is involved in activating or deactivating the active centre of the enzyme; it is significant that all the allosteric enzymes studied are composed of several subunits, the structural arrangements of which are the basis of the Koshland theory of induced fit, as shown in fig. 14.7.

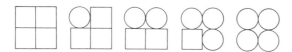

FIG. 14.7. In allosteric enzymes the enzyme exists in oligomeric forms. The less active monomer is shown by a square and the more active monomer by a circle. Thus, the relatively inactive tetramer is converted to an active tetramer. In the case of pyruvate kinase □ has a low affinity for PEP and a high affinity for ATP and ○ has a high affinity for PEP and FDP.

An example of an allosteric enzyme is acetyl CoA carboxylase involved in fatty acid synthesis. This key enzymic step converts acetyl CoA into malonyl CoA (p. 10.9 and fig. 14.8). Under conditions of active

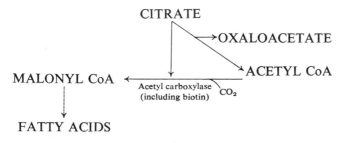

FIG. 14.8. Allosteric effect of citrate on the enzyme acetyl CoA carboxylase, a key enzyme in lipogenesis. This enzyme is sensitive to a number of other allosteric effectors such as fatty acid acyl CoAs.

lipogenesis in adipose tissue, the acetyl CoA is supplied from citrate generated in mitochondria, whence it is exported to the cytosol and there split by citrate lyase.

$$\text{CoASH} + \text{Citrate} \xrightarrow{\text{citrate lyase}} \text{Oxaloacetate} + \text{acetyl CoA}$$

The acetyl CoA carboxylase reaction exhibits a positive allosteric response to citrate. Hence, when too much citrate is produced in the cell, the excess provides acetyl CoA on the one hand and also activates allosterically the carboxylase enzyme responsible for converting the acetyl CoA to malonyl CoA, and hence to long chain fatty acids.

Another example of a key enzyme which may be modified allosterically by the substrate and by ATP is pyruvate kinase, which converts phosphoenolpyruvate to pyruvate and ATP.

$$\text{Phosphoenolpyruvate} + \text{ADP} \longrightarrow \text{Pyruvate} + \text{ATP}$$

This important reaction in glycolysis occurs in the cytosol and is virtually irreversible; hence in gluconeogenesis, where glucose has to be produced from precursors such as alanine or pyruvate, an alternative route from pyruvate to phosphoenolpyruvate must be found. Such a route occurs when pyruvate moves into the mitochondrion where it undergoes a carboxylation.

$$\text{Pyruvate} + \text{ATP} + CO_2 \longrightarrow \text{Oxaloacetate} + \text{ADP} + P_i$$

The pyruvate carboxylase enzyme exhibits allosteric characteristics and acetyl CoA is a positive effector of this enzyme, as shown in fig. 14.9.

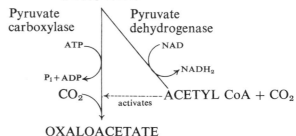

FIG. 14.9. Acetyl CoA as a positive allosteric effector of pyruvate carboxylase.

The reaction, like the acetyl CoA carboxylation reaction, is dependent on biotin as a cofactor. Pyruvate can also be converted by a complex series of reactions in the mitochondrion to acetyl CoA and CO_2.

$$\text{CoASH} + \text{Pyruvate} + \text{NAD} \longrightarrow \text{Acetyl CoA} + \text{NADH}_2 + CO_2$$

In most mammalian cells the distribution of metabolites between the cytosol and the mitochondria is an important factor in the regulation of metabolism, and their flow in and out of the mitochondria is under delicate control. Although the enzymes of the citric acid cycle are localized in mitochondria, metabolites of the cycle may be present in the cytosol. Oxaloacetate does not permeate out of the mitochondria but its reduction product, malic acid, does. Malate may be reoxidized in the cytosol to oxaloacetate. This is converted by phosphoenolpyruvic carboxykinase and GTP to phosphoenolpyruvate (fig. 14.10). This reaction bypasses the pyruvate kinase reaction and permits gluconeogenesis from amino acids and lactate in the liver (p. 9.13).

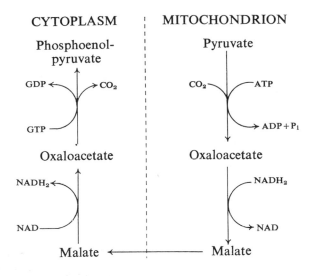

FIG. 14.10. The malate shuttle between mitochondria and cytosol as a means of transferring electrons or reducing equivalents from inside mitochondria to cytosol.

Mitochondria

Oxidative phosphorylation in mitochondria requires not only a supply of electrons from suitable donors but also ADP and P_i. As ADP is converted into ATP, respiration in the mitochondrion is reduced so that, within limits, oxygen consumption is related to the availability of ADP. As the ratio of ATP/ADP falls, respiration is switched on, while, as the ratio of ATP/ADP rises, respiration is switched off (p. 8.10).

It is also possible to monitor metabolism from the $NAD/NADH_2$ ratio in mitochondria. The NAD concentration exceeds that of $NADH_2$ when the Po_2 is high, and as the Po_2 falls to low values, the concentration of $NADH_2$ rises. The presence of $NADH_2$ ensures the availability of reducing power (or electrons) for other reduction reactions, such as the conversion of pyruvate to lactate in the cytosol, which is a method of oxidation of $NADH_2$ without the intervention of oxygen; for this reason it may be said to spare oxygen, and is partly responsible for the lactic acid component of the oxygen debt discussed on p. 45.6.

Intact mitochondria appear to be impermeable to $NADH_2$, so that $NADH_2$ generated in the cytosol cannot enter them to be reoxidized. However dihydroxy-acetonephosphate (DHAP) produced in glycolysis can be reduced by $NADH_2$ in the cytosol to 1-glycerophosphate by a cytosol 1-glycerophosphate dehydrogenase. Mitochondria are permeable to 1-glycerophosphate which is then reoxidized in the mitochondria by a different 1-glycerophosphate dehydrogenase which utilizes FAD as the electron acceptor. The product of this reaction, i.e. dihydroxyacetonephosphate, diffuses out of the mitochondrion to be a substrate in the cytosol. Thus this mechanism serves as an electron shuttle allowing the $NADH_2$ in the cytosol to be reoxidized without generating lactate from pyruvate. The control of the mitochondrial 1-glycerophosphate dehydrogenase appears to be influenced by thyroxine. This is referred to on p. 14.16

Mitochondria have the ability to catabolize oxidatively long chain fatty acyl carnitine derivatives to acetyl CoA (p. 10.7) and can then metabolize the latter to CO_2 and H_2O with the production of ATP. The entry of a typical fatty acid such as palmityl carnitine into mitochondria stimulates the processes of fatty acid oxidation, with the generation of $NADH_2$ and hence ATP, as well as the production of large amounts of acetyl CoA. The acetyl CoA can enter the citric acid cycle through the activity of citrate synthase. This enzyme is sensitive to the concentration of ATP in the mitochondria; high concentrations of ATP inhibit the enzyme allosterically, while low concentrations of ATP or high concentrations of ADP activate citrate synthase. Under some conditions in the mitochondrion, the concentration of the key metabolite, oxaloacetate, falls below the K_m for citrate synthase.

When fatty acid oxidation is increased, as in starvation, diabetes and when a diet high in fat and low in carbohydrate is taken, the production of ketone bodies is increased. The ketone bodies originate from the condensation of acetyl CoA molecules as discussed on p. 33.6. The evidence suggests that when the rate of production of acetyl CoA from acyl carnitine is markedly increased, the citrate synthase system is saturated and hence alternative metabolic channels are used to dispose of acetyl CoA; one such route is the condensation of two of these molecules to give acetoacetyl CoA.

When palmityl carnitine is oxidized by coupled mitochondria (p. 8.12) under conditions where the supply of ADP is not limiting, the mitochondria produce citrate and acetoacetate; where the supply of ADP is limiting, they produce citrate and β-hydroxybutyrate, the reduction product of acetoacetate. When palmityl carnitine is oxidized by uncoupled mitochondria, the principal product is citrate. This important control point in mitochondrial metabolism is shown in fig. 14.11.

In mammals the liver is the principal site for the production of the ketone bodies, acetoacetate, β-hydroxybutyrate and acetone. These metabolites pass into the ECF and are taken up by tissues such as cardiac and skeletal muscle, kidney, and in certain circumstances brain, where, except acetone, they are metabolized to provide energy.

Under normal circumstances the mitochondrial source of acetyl CoA is fatty acids and pyruvic acid. As discussed previously, acetyl CoA acts as a positive effector on pyruvate carboxylase so that, as long as there is a generous supply of pyruvic acid available in the mitochondrion,

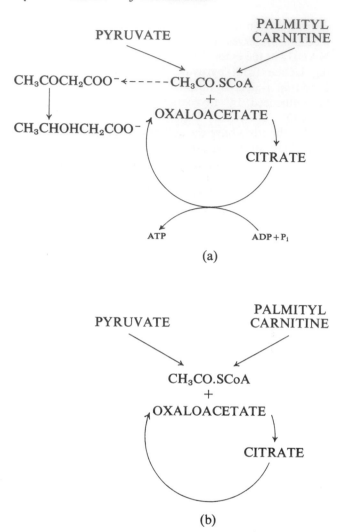

(a)

(b)

FIG. 14.11. Conditions for the generation of ketone bodies in liver; (a) in coupled mitochondria where both citrate and ketone bodies are generated, (b) in uncoupled mitochondria where the main product is citrate.

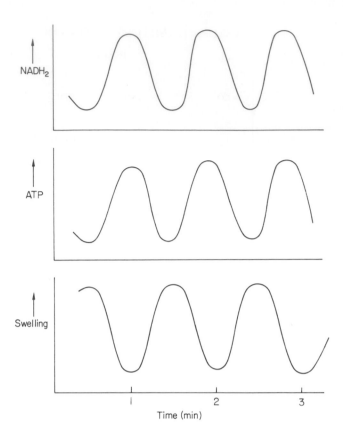

FIG. 14.12. Oscillations in the concentrations of ATP and NADH$_2$ associated with different states of the mitochondrion. Concentrations of ATP when high tend to shrink the mitochondria and when low to swell them. Modified from Boiteux A. and Hess B. (1974).

there is the potential to generate the key intermediate oxaloacetate, needed in the citrate synthase system (fig. 14.8). One unanswered question is whether in ketosis the intramitochondrial oxaloacetate concentration is decreased, causing acetyl CoA to be channelled to acetoacetate production, or whether citrate synthase is inhibited by elevated levels of ATP producing the same effect.

The ratio of ATP/ADP exerts an important control on many intramitochondrial events in a manner similar to that in which it tends to dominate the control of glycolysis in the cytosol. The intramitochondrial concentrations of NADH$_2$ and ATP fluctuate in phase together in a regular manner, with a periodicity of about one minute. When the concentration of ATP falls the mitochondria swell, and when the concentration rises the mitochondria shrink (fig. 14.12).

Regulation of glycolysis

Glycolysis is the conversion of glucose or glycogen to pyruvate and is effected by a network of enzymic reactions occurring in the cytosol of most cells. Glycolytic enzymes form a concentrated viscous solution with their substrates and cofactors in a single homogeneous phase. Studies on yeast cells suggest that glycolysis is controlled through metabolic intermediates, such as organic and inorganic phosphates, ammonium ions and others which act as effector ligands on the enzyme systems.

The control of glycolysis in yeast is not identical with that in mammalian cells. Indeed, the control differs in different mammalian cells. Some cells such as those of the liver synthesize and export glucose as well as oxidizing it. However, the intermediates in glycolysis in different cell types and the enzymes and coenzymes involved are almost identical. As yeast cells are easier to study than mammalian cells, much of the study of glycolysis has been carried out on them.

The coenzymes and substrates involved have been studied both in intact yeast cells and in cell-free extracts, and some components show marked regular fluctuations. Concentrations of intermediates in the cytoplasm may oscillate within the range of 10^{-5} to 10^{-3} mol/l. Plotting concentrations of some of these substances against time shows that the oscillations have a periodicity of several minutes. Fig. 14.13 shows that the concentrations of G-6-P and F-6-P change together, suggesting that hexose isomerase is not an important control point. On the other hand, when the F-6-P concentration is high, the fructose-1,6-diphosphate (FDP) concentration is low. This suggests that phosphofructokinase (PFK) could be an important controlling enzyme, a fact substantiated from other studies.

Fig. 14.13 also shows that concentrations of pyruvate (Pyr), ADP and $NADH_2$ oscillate reciprocally with those

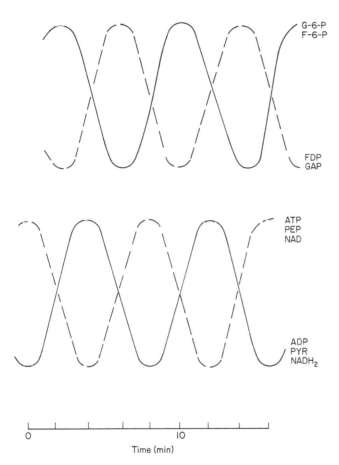

FIG. 14.13. Oscillations of glucose-6-phosphate and fructose-6-phosphate compared to fructose-1,6-diphosphate and glyceraldehyde phosphate in the cytosol of cells. Similar oscillations in ATP, phosphoenolpyruvate and NAD versus ADP, pyruvate and $NADH_2$ are out of phase with the former oscillating couples. Modified from Boiteux A. & Hess B. (1974).

of phosphoenolpyruvate (PEP), ATP and NAD. This implies that pyruvate kinase (PK) as the link between PEP and Pyr could be a rate-limiting controller enzyme. It is also seen that the oscillating couple F-6-P/FDP are out of phase with the oscillating couple PEP/Pyr. This

phase shift results in important changes in the concentration of specific nucleotides and factors which influence the two key enzymes PFK and PK.

$$F\text{-}6\text{-}P + ATP \longrightarrow FDP + ADP$$
$$PEP + ADP \longrightarrow Pyr + ATP$$

The product of each enzymic reaction, i.e. ADP and ATP is the substrate of the other reaction, and thus the reactions are coupled.

PFK is an allosteric enzyme sensitive to ATP and ADP while PK, also an allosteric enzyme, is sensitive to ADP alone. Since F-6-P exhibits the largest swing in concentration it is assumed to be an important if not the primary oscillator in the glycolytic system.

The enzymes which control glycolysis have multiple feedback controls exerted through specific nucleotides and substrates.

As the glycolytic chain is never in a steady state, all the reactions are operating far from their equilibrium points and the system is said to be 'open'. In these oscillating systems the rates of the reactions and the concentration changes of the reactants appear to arise as a result of allosteric modifications of key enzymes. As far as can be established, these changes are not due to alterations in the absolute amounts of the enzymes involved through enzyme induction, as discussed on pp. 14.14 and 33.10.

Generation and utilization of $NADPH_2$

Although the coenzymes NAD and NADP are closely related structurally, they are differently distributed in the cell and have quite different roles in metabolism. NAD and NADP are synthesized as follows:

Nicotinamide + phosphoribosylpyrophosphate $\longrightarrow$
Nicotinamide mononucleotide + PP_1,
Nicotinamide mononucleotide + ATP $\longrightarrow$
$NAD + PP_1$,
and
$$NAD + ATP \longrightarrow NADP + ADP$$

In most cells there is markedly less NADP than NAD. The redox potential of the $NAD/NADH_2$ couple is almost identical with that of the $NADP/NADPH_2$ couple. In mammalian cells most of the latter couple is present in the reduced form as $NADPH_2$, whilst most of the former couple is present in the oxidized state as NAD.

One of the reasons for this difference is that NAD is largely confined to the mitochondria while the NADP is mainly in the cytosol. There is a little NADP in the mitochondria and some of the $NADH_2$ in the mitochondria can be reoxidized by an energy-linked reaction as follows:

$$NADH_2 + NADP + ATP \longrightarrow$$
$$NAD + NADPH_2 + ADP + P_1$$

This reaction is catalysed by a transhydrogenase enzyme present in the mitochondria.

A few dehydrogenases can utilize either NAD or NADP as electron acceptors or donors. In this case it is possible to achieve a transhydrogenation as follows:

$$XH_2 + NAD \rightleftharpoons X + NADH_2$$
$$X + NADPH_2 \rightleftharpoons XH_2 + NADP$$

the overall reaction being

$$NAD + NADPH_2 \rightleftharpoons NADH_2 + NADP$$

A similar effect can be obtained in the cell by the shuttling of metabolites between mitochondria and cytosol. Thus oxaloacetate is generated in the mitochondrion where it can be reduced by $NADH_2$ to give malate. This may pass through the mitochondrial membrane into the cytosol, where it can be converted into pyruvate plus CO_2 and $NADPH_2$. The pyruvate may then pass back into the mitochondria and be converted into oxaloacetate (p. 14.7).

$$Oxaloacetate + NADH_2 \rightleftharpoons$$
$$Malate + NAD \text{ (mitochondria)}$$
$$Malate + NADP \rightleftharpoons$$
$$Pyruvate + CO_2 + NADPH_2 \text{ (cytosol)}$$
$$Pyruvate + CO_2 + ATP =$$
$$Oxaloacetate + ADP + P_1 \text{ (mitochondria)}$$

the net effect being

$$NADH_2 + NADP + ATP =$$
$$NAD + NADPH_2 + ADP + P_1$$

Possibly the most important route for the production of $NADPH_2$ is via the hexose monophosphate pathway in which two dehydrogenases generate two molecules of $NADPH_2$ from each molecule of glucose-6-phosphate (fig. 9.5, p. 9.8). This pathway is a significant source of $NADPH_2$ which is an important commodity in the economy of the cell.

$NADPH_2$ is an obligatory cofactor in a number of cellular reactions and its supply could regulate some of the following processes.

The synthesis of long chain fatty acids in the cytoplasm has an absolute requirement for $NADPH_2$. In the formation of one molecule of palmitic acid from 8 molecules of acetyl CoA, 14 molecules of $NADPH_2$ are required (p. 10.10).

The synthesis of cholesterol has a requirement for $NADPH_2$ at various stages, such as the reduction of β-hydroxy-β-methylglutaryl CoA to mevalonic acid, the condensation of two molecules of farnesyl pyrophosphate to squalene, the oxidative cyclization of squalene to lanosterol and the oxidative demethylation of lanosterol to cholesterol (pp. 10.22–24).

$NADPH_2$ is an obligatory cofactor in the mixed function oxidases which are involved in the hydroxylation of physiological substrates and foreign substances by the smooth endoplasmic reticulum of organs such as the liver. The general equation for the reaction is

$$NADPH_2 + XH + O_2 \longrightarrow NADP + XOH + H_2O$$

Oxidations effected in this manner include those of phenylalanine to tyrosine, fatty acids to ω-hydroxy fatty acids, cholesterol to 7α-hydroxycholesterol, aromatic hydro-carbon to phenol, and barbiturates to hydroxylated barbiturates.

$NADPH_2$ is also an obligatory cofactor in a complex reaction, apparently a dehydroxylation, in which the deoxyribonucleotides required in the synthesis of DNA are synthesized from the corresponding ribonucleotides. At least four enzymes are involved. The overall reaction when applied to ADP is

$$ADP + NADPH_2 \longrightarrow dADP + H_2O + NADP$$

Similar reactions occur with the other nucleotides. A balanced supply of the deoxyribonucleotides is required for the effective production of DNA.

$NADPH_2$ is also required in the oxidative desaturation of long chain fatty acyl CoA derivatives such as stearyl CoA to oleyl CoA (p. 10.11), in the reduction of the oxidized form of glutathione and in a variety of amino acid transformations, e.g. glutamate dehydrogenase.

Control of amino acid metabolism

Since mammals are able to synthesize some of the amino acids required in the structure of cellular proteins, the supply of these represents one possible control point in the regulation of their metabolism. The general rule, that the route by which a substance is synthesized is different from that by which it is degraded, applies also to the metabolism of the amino acids. The amino groups of amino acids can be formed by transamination from the non-essential amino acid, glutamic acid (p. 11.19), and this acid plays an important role in the control of amino acid metabolism in mammalian systems. It is formed from 2-oxoglutarate, an intermediate occurring in carbohydrate metabolism, in the presence of ammonia and $NADPH_2$ by the enzyme glutamate dehydrogenase. It can then be used as a donor of amino groups to suitable acceptors in aminotransferase reactions.

There appears to be a specific aminotransferase enzyme for each amino acid. The equilibrium constant of the reaction is close to unity, so that the direction of the reaction is largely influenced by the concentration of the reactants and the amount of the aminotransferase. Some aminotransferases in liver, such as tyrosine aminotransferase, are induced by adrenocorticosteroids and by high dietary intakes of protein.

Glutamic acid and other amino acids, when acted on by D-amino acid oxidase present in the liver and kidneys, yield ammonia which is then removed and converted into carbamyl phosphate, an intermediate in the synthesis of urea (pp. 11.20 and 33.3).

$$NH_4^+ + HCO_3^- + 2ATP \longrightarrow$$
$$NH_2COO\textcircled{P} + 2ADP + P_i$$

The removal of ammonium influences the equilibria of the reactions. Hence the amount and the activity of the enzymes in the urea cycle affect amino acid metabolism in general.

Glutamic acid is also an important substance in the sequestration of toxic ammonia into the relatively innocuous glutamine (p. 11.20). Glutamine synthase is extremely sensitive to a range of nucleotides and other

the metabolism of amino acids, comparable to the position of glucose-6-phosphate in carbohydrate metabolism. Its metabolic fate in common with that of many key substrates depends upon the availability and the activity of the various enzymes which utilize it. In turn, the activity of these enzymes may be altered by various metabolic intermediates, allosteric effectors or hormones, so that the channelling of glutamine in specific directions is dictated by a variety of intracellular signals (fig. 14.14).

Apart from the reactions already discussed, aminotransferase reactions convert aspartic acid into oxaloacetate and alanine into pyruvic acid. The amino acids histidine, arginine and proline are relatively easily transformed into 2-oxoglutarate, while valine and isoleucine can be converted into succinate. Other conversions of

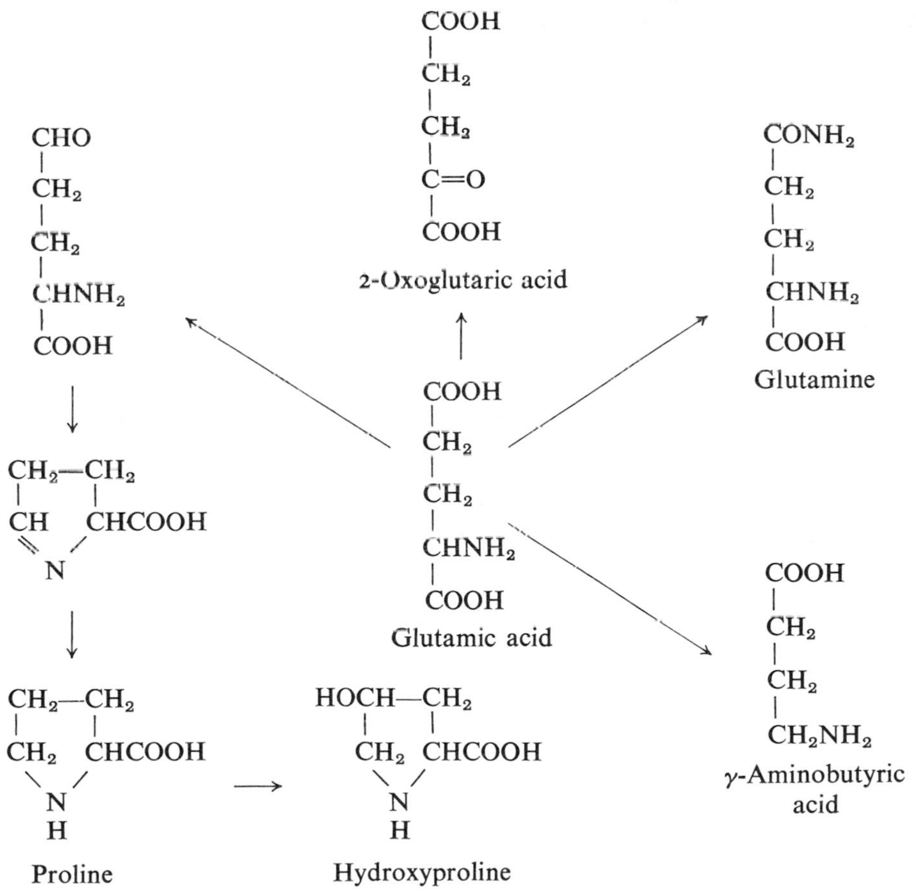

FIG. 14.14. The central position of glutamic acid in the metabolism of amino acids.

molecules which exert allosteric controls over its activity. Glutamine, apart from its role as 'inactivator' of ammonia, serves as a donor of amino groups in the synthesis of a number of amino acids, purine and pyrimidine bases (pp. 11.20 and 12.24).

Glutamic acid therefore occupies a central position in

amino acids are described on pp. 11.21–27.

The delicate balance which exists between liver and muscle with respect to amino acid metabolism is important. The turnover of protein in muscle is considerable, and some of the amino acids released in this way pass to the liver where, together with lactate and glycerol, they provide essential building units for gluconeogenesis. Raised plasma concentration of these precursors promotes gluconeogenesis. Production of glucose in the liver and kidneys plays a key role in the adjustment of the whole organism to fasting and in the metabolic response to injury (vol. 3, p. 3.14).

Membranes and the control of metabolism

The regulation of metabolism depends upon the compartmental nature of the eukaryotic cell. The enzymes and metabolites involved in a specific reaction sequence do not float freely in the cytosol, but are contained in specific organelles or membranes. For example, the enzymes of the citric acid cycle are in the matrix of the mitochondria. Operation of the cycle depends on the integrity and efficiency of the respiratory chain. These enzymes and cofactors are grouped together in the mitochondrial cristae in an essentially non-aqueous environment, a situation which improves the efficiency of electron transport.

Grouping of multi-enzyme sequences together in subcellular organelles and locking the enzymes to lipoproteins in membranes allows a much greater overall effectiveness than would be possible if the events took place in free solution.

The organization of cellular events on a topographical basis is illustrated by the biochemical description of the structure of membranes. The apparent flimsy ultrastructure of plasma membranes and subcellular particle membranes seen with the electron microscope is essentially a lipoprotein matrix to which are attached various specific proteins whose function is to act as carriers, enzymes, receptors and other highly specific centres of activity. These membranes appear to consist of repeating units of structural and active proteins. The structure can be deduced to exhibit a definite 'sidedness' in that there is an 'inside' and an 'outside' of the plasma membrane, the mitochondrial cristae and the endoplasmic reticulum (pp. 10.20 and 13.6).

These characteristics give a vectorial component to metabolic processes and set the stage for the maintenance of electrochemical gradients involving Na^+, K^+, H^+ and other cations; similarly the membranes treat fatty acids, oxo acids, amino acids, Cl^- and other anions in a highly selective fashion. The 'sidedness' of the mitochondrial cristae is an essential factor in the chemiosmotic explanation of oxidative phosphorylation.

It is possible to demonstrate the existence of highly specific carriers in cell membranes for many amino acids and carbohydrates. The uptake of these molecules therefore depends in part on the saturation kinetics of these carrier functions. Similarly the uptake of free fatty acids by certain cells or the uptake of free fatty acids by mitochondria depend on the selective characteristics of specific

acyl translocating systems, e.g. the carnitine acyltransferase system in mitochondria (p. 10.8).

Action of hormones

One of the principal ways in which metabolism is controlled is by the action of hormones secreted by the endocrine glands. These not only induce metabolic effects within the cell but they exert their action exclusively or mainly on specific or target organs, and their nature and individual effects are described in chaps. 27 and 38.

There are three main ways by which hormones appear to affect metabolic processes in mammalian cells: (1) some hormones by their effects on adenylate cyclase alter the intracellular concentration of cyclic AMP and this secondary messenger in turn influences intracellular metabolism, (2) some hormones operate at the cell surface by some as yet unknown carrier mechanism and (3) other hormones interact with a receptor in the cytoplasm of the cell, enter the nucleus and ultimately alter protein synthesis in that cell.

HORMONES OPERATING THROUGH CYCLIC AMP

Some of the protein hormones of the anterior pituitary exert their effect by first becoming attached to specific receptors or discriminators in the plasma membrane of the responsive cells. This produces a change in the plasma membrane, perhaps involving a chemical transducer molecule and GTP. As shown in fig. 14.5, this conformational change in the cell membrane affects adenylate cyclase, perhaps by an allosteric modification of the enzyme. The change is virtually instantaneous and, as a result, production of cyclic AMP from ATP inside the cells is increased within a few seconds. Since adenylate cyclase appears to be located on the inner surface of the specific cells, all that is required is the external contact of the protein hormone which need not penetrate the cell.

In some cells several different discriminators respond to different hormones, but these all produce an identical effect inside the cell, i.e. an increase in concentration of cyclic AMP. Thus, adipose tissue cells respond to catecholamines, ACTH and other hormone signals in this way. A discriminator usually responds to a particular polypeptide sequence, but some appear to respond to peptides other than the appropriate hormone. An example occurs in the thyroid gland which is normally activated by TSH, but can also be activated by the immunoglobulin, LATS (p. 27.24).

In some cells there are proteins which appear to play a dual role; on the one hand they bind to some protein kinases and inactivate them, while on the other hand they bind to cyclic AMP. As the cyclic AMP concentration rises in such a cell, the protein kinase is activated either directly or because of the removal of the inhibitor or binding protein. In other cases the rise in cyclic AMP activates a protein kinase kinase. The net result in all cases is that the rise in the intracellular cyclic AMP concentration in the presence of ATP results in phosphorylation of certain proteins. One of the problems in endocrinology is to identify which proteins have been phosphorylated and to determine whether these phosphorylated proteins have an increased or decreased enzymic activity.

$$\text{Protein} \xrightarrow[\text{ATP} \quad \text{ADP}]{\text{cAMP + protein kinase}} \text{Phosphorylated protein}$$

This reaction, influenced by the elevated cyclic AMP concentration, is offset by at least two mechanisms. On the one hand, cyclic AMP phosphodiesterase inside the cells is capable of splitting the cyclic ester to 5′-AMP (p. 9.10). Secondly, a phosphoprotein phosphatase is present in cells capable of hydrolysing the phosphoprotein to the protein and inorganic phosphate, as discussed previously.

Examples of liver and muscle phosphorylase, glycogen synthase, adipose tissue hormone-sensitive lipase and other enzymes modified by phosphorylation have been cited earlier. The hormones which are known to change the intracellular cyclic AMP concentration of specific cells include glucagon, catecholamines, hypothalamic releasing hormones, trophic hormones of the anterior pituitary such as ACTH, TSH, FSH and LH, as well as vasopressin, calcitonin and the parathyroid hormone. The specificity of action is often marked. Thus, while ACTH activates adenylate cyclase of the adrenal cortex, it does not affect liver or heart cells. Similarly, parathyroid hormone and vasopressin affect only the renal cortex and the renal medulla respectively. In adipose tissue, adenylate cyclase activity is altered by ACTH, TSH, catecholamines and glucagon, each hormone influencing a single adenylate cyclase system. Glucagon and the catecholamines also affect the liver cell but, unlike the catecholamines, glucagon does not affect skeletal muscle.

HORMONES OPERATING AT CELL SURFACES BY UNKNOWN MECHANISMS

Other hormones operate on the cell surface by some as yet obscure membrane carrier mechanism. Thus, insulin acts on the plasma membrane of skeletal and cardiac muscle and on adipose tissue to increase the rate of uptake of glucose. By contrast, the uptake of glucose into the cells of the brain, the liver and the intestinal mucosa is not much affected by this hormone. By increasing its rate of entry into certain cells its flux through glycolysis, glycogen synthesis and the hexose

monophosphate pathway is increased. In this way insulin promotes utilization of glucose by muscle, and lipogenesis in adipose tissue. Elevated blood glucose results in increased uptake of glucose by the pancreatic β-cells. It seems likely that the elevated intracellular glucose in these specialized cells activates the release and later the production of a specific m-RNA involved in proinsulin synthesis and this, in turn, results in an increased secretion of insulin by the β-cells. Insulin also promotes the uptake of amino acids by muscle and increases protein synthesis in that tissue.

Apart from the effect of insulin on adipose tissue which promotes lipogenesis, insulin may decrease the adipose tissue cyclic AMP concentration and thereby lower the activity of the hormone-sensitive lipase. Alternatively, through a receptor in the membrane it may block the production of cyclic AMP and therefore interfere with the formation of an active protein kinase, and hence prevent the lipolytic response to hormones such as the catecholamines. Fig 14.15 summarizes some of these effects.

Insulin, therefore, is a hormone which in part through a reduction in cyclic AMP increases the activity of glycogen synthase, and decreases the activity of glycogen phosphorylase and triglyceride lipase enzyme systems. Since these enzymes are regulated by phosphorylation-dephosphorylation cycles, the hormone in this case may produce its effect through action on protein kinase or protein phosphatase.

Pyruvic dehydrogenase is an intramitochondrial pacemaker enzyme which appears to be markedly affected by insulin. By contrast, this multi-enzyme complex which converts pyruvate into acetyl CoA is affected by insulin but not by cyclic AMP. The enzyme is inactivated by phosphorylation and reactivated by dephosphorylation. The phosphorylation is effected by an ATP-dependent protein kinase, while the dephosphorylation is effected by a protein phosphatase.

$$\text{Phosphatase} \underset{H_2O}{\overset{P_i}{\rightleftharpoons}} \left(\begin{array}{c} \text{Pyruvate dehydrogenase} \\ \text{(active)} \\ \text{Pyruvate dehydrogenase} \\ \text{(inactive)} \end{array} \right) \underset{ADP}{\overset{ATP}{\rightleftharpoons}} \text{Protein kinase}$$

It is possible that the activity of the enzyme is controlled by the ATP concentration. At high ATP concentrations intracellular Mg^{++} is bound and the phosphatase which would dephosphorylate and activate the enzyme is inhibited by the lack of magnesium. This enzyme is inhibited by ATP and activated by glucose, fructose and pyruvate.

Acetyl CoA carboxylase is also markedly stimulated by insulin and, as this is a pacemaker enzyme in fatty acid synthesis, insulin increases lipogenesis (fig. 14.8). The metabolic disorder which develops in insulin deficiency, namely diabetes mellitus, is of great clinical

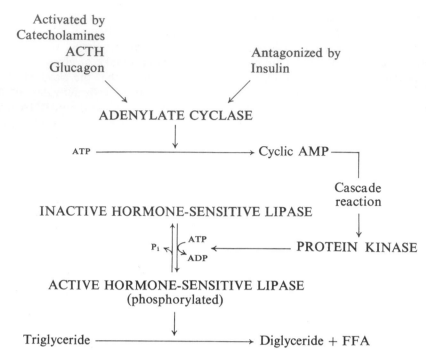

FIG. 14.15. Metabolic processes affected by insulin.

importance. Failure of the pancreas to produce insulin in sufficient amounts results in a failure to utilize glucose by muscle and adipose tissue. This leads to hyperglycaemia and glycosuria. The decreased uptake of glucose by adipose tissue is associated with an increased lipolysis; as a result, the concentration of plasma FFA rises and the additional load of free fatty acids to the liver increases ketone body formation (p. 10.14). These changes are similar but more severe than those which occur in healthy subjects during a mild fast.

HORMONES OPERATING THROUGH NUCLEAR EVENTS

Much effort has been spent on attempts to understand the nature of the control of enzyme production and regulation in biological systems. Some simple organisms such as *Escherichia coli*, when grown in a medium containing lactose, adapt to their environment by producing enzymes capable of utilizing this substrate. This discovery has led to the concept that the DNA of the organism has specific segments which can be transcribed into complementary RNA molecules, such as m-RNA, t-RNA and r-RNA. The m-RNAs can be translated into specific polypeptides (enzymes) on the ribosomes. An account of the control of protein synthesis is given on p. 12.14 where it is suggested that a section of the DNA called the regulator gene codes for a specific m-RNA. This latter molecule is concerned with the production of a specific repressor protein. Other sections in the DNA code for other m-RNAs and hence for specific

proteins such as enzymes, and are termed the structural parts of the gene. Between the regulator gene and the structural gene, there may be two other sites, (1) an operator to which the repressor protein is able to bind and block effective transcription of the adjacent portions of the genome which contains the structural genes, and (2) an RNA polymerase binding site (promoter) between the regulator and the operator (p. 12.14).

If another molecule such as a metabolite capable of binding to the repressor protein is present, a conformational change may be produced in the repressor protein so that it no longer represses the operator. As a consequence of this phenomenon of **derepression**, the exposed operator allows the RNA polymerase to bind to the promoter region of the genome and permit transcription of the structural genes for their specific m-RNAs. This in turn results in the translation of the m-RNAs and the production of the appropriate proteins or enzymes in the ribosomes (fig. 12.15).

In the case of *Esch. coli*, lactose binds to the repressor protein which then fails to bind to the operator, and as a result the structural enzymes, galactose permease, β-galactosidase and thiogalactosidase acetylase are produced. How far can these observations on prokaryotic systems be applied to the mammalian situation? While in *Esch. coli* the quantity of enzyme under different situations may vary one thousandfold, man is never exposed to environmental changes which would induce comparable changes in enzyme concentration. Nevertheless, the principles of enzyme repression, derepression and induction discovered in these simple organisms appear to have counterparts in mammalian systems.

One obvious link is the fact that some micro-organisms, like mammals, use cyclic AMP as a secondary messenger in certain control situations. The nucleotide plays a part as a chemical transducer in the bacterial phenomenon known as catabolite repression, and the cyclic AMP concentration is regulated by metabolites in bacteria in much the same way as certain hormones influence intracellular cyclic AMP concentration in mammalian systems. Through the intervention of a regulator gene, repressor proteins and the operator genes, it is possible to evolve a plausible explanation for the participation of cyclic AMP in the increased production of selected enzymes from specific tissues.

There is now much evidence that control of metabolism in mammalian systems exercised by some hormones is mediated through control of transcription or translation of the mammalian genome. The hormones which are believed to act in this way include the steroid hormones cortisol, aldosterone, oestrogens, androgens and progesterone, and the thyroid hormones thyroxine and triiodothyronine.

Steroid hormones

The steroid hormones do not appear to influence tissue cyclic AMP concentration or to have receptors on the external surface of the cell. They penetrate the plasma membrane and enter the cytosol where they bind to receptor proteins. There is then a lag period of from 20–500 min before specific physiological or biochemical effects can be observed in the target tissue. The protein-hormone complex appears to aggregate and change shape before being translocated into the nucleus. The complex interacts with the chromatin or genetic apparatus in the nucleus and increases or decreases the rate of formation of some specific m-RNAs or related macromolecules, and hence ultimately increases production of specific proteins. Although these hormones exert effects on carbohydrate, protein, lipid and electrolyte metabolism, special attention has been paid to specific enzymes considered important in metabolic control (fig. 14.16).

The effect of a hormone such as cortisol on liver is very different from its effect on lymphoid tissue or muscle. In liver, cortisol exerts an anabolic effect, while in muscle the same hormone is catabolic. The net effect of increased secretion of cortisol in a mammal is to raise the plasma amino acids, largely derived from muscle, and increase the utilization of amino acids by the liver. Several studies have shown that certain hepatic enzyme activities which may reflect concentrations are affected by cortisol. These enzymes include tyrosine aminotransferase, tryptophan-2,3-dioxygenase and some related enzymes. These enzymes are readily inducible by adrenocorticosteroids, have short biological half-lives, and have

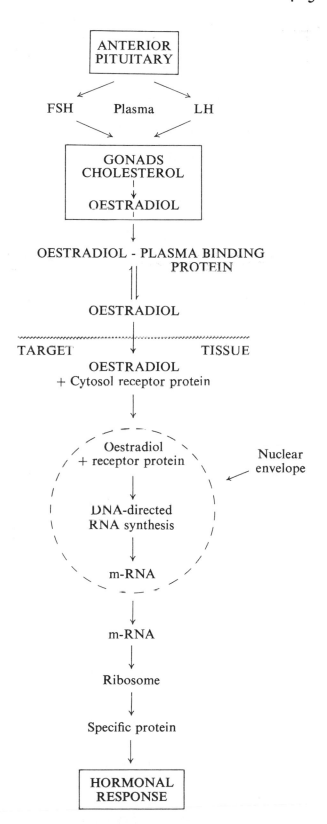

FIG. 14.16. The possible mode of action of some steroid hormones.

cofactors which are easily dissociable. Their induction could explain some of the metabolic effects of adrenocorticosteroids in protein metabolism and the negative nitrogen balance associated with increased adrenocorticosteroid secretion. The elevated plasma concentration of amino acids could be a factor in the elevated hepatic gluconeogenesis. It is also possible that the increased deposition of glycogen in liver known to occur with adrenocorticosteroids could be mediated through activation of glycogen synthase.

Some of the steroid hormones such as progesterone, androgens and oestrogens, appear to have highly specific target tissues. Thus, unlike the adrenocorticosteroids which affect a great many cells, these sex steroids have a highly selective effect on certain specific tissues such as the uterine endometrium, prostate, epididymis and seminal vesicles. The mode of action of oestrogens is comparable to that of corticosteroids. Oestrogenic hormones penetrate the plasma membrane of tissues such as the uterus and bind to certain specific protein receptors in the cytosol. The hormone-protein complex aggregates, changes size and moves into the nucleus. Again, as a result of an interaction with the genetic apparatus in the nucleus, there is evidence for increased synthesis of certain specific m-RNAs which in turn leads to the increased synthesis of certain specific proteins. For example, in the chick oviduct it has been possible to show that the synthesis of the protein, ovalbumin, is specifically under the control of oestrogenic hormones.

In much the same way progesterone has specific receptors in the cytosol of the uterus, and the protein receptor complex is translocated into the nucleus. The production of a specific m-RNA is increased and studies in the chick show that a specific protein, avidin, is produced. This protein is produced only when the tissue is specifically activated by the progestational hormone.

Similar studies show that androgens find specific receptors in the cytosol of tissues such as the prostate and epididymis, and that there is subsequent production of specific m-RNAs with presumably the production of certain specific proteins.

Aldosterone probably acts by first finding specific protein receptors in the cytosol of the renal tubule cells. A steroid-protein complex is then formed and migrates into the nucleus where it increases production of certain m-RNAs and later of specific proteins as yet unidentified. Since the main action of the hormone is to alter the rate of Na^+ transport, it may be assumed that the protein is either involved in the sodium pump or acts as a permease, so influencing the transport of Na^+.

Thyroid hormones

Thyroxine administration to animals results in a variety of metabolic responses which include effects on carbohydrate, lipid, protein and electrolyte metabolism. The hormone raises the metabolic rate (the rate of consumption of oxygen) and as the site of oxygen consumption in the cell is known to be in the mitochondria, attention was turned to these organelles for an explanation of how this iodinated amino acid altered the oxygen consumption rate. Thyroxine, at non-physiological doses, 'uncoupled' mitochondria *in vitro* but it is unlikely that this is the mode of action. When thyroxine is given to a euthyroid or to a hypothyroid individual, there is a lag of from 12 to 36 h before metabolic rate increases. One of the earliest effects of the hormone is to elevate the activity of a DNA-directed RNA polymerase and this is followed by an increase in m-RNA. There follows an increase in the production of certain specific proteins. One of the most intensively studied of these proteins is 1-glycerophosphate dehydrogenase. The activity of this enzyme in mitochondria is greatly elevated in the hyperthyroid state. The increase in its activity in mitochondria allows a greater use of the 1-glycerophosphate shuttle which leads to an increased oxidation of the extramitochondrial $NADH_2$ via the mitochondrial pathway. This and related observations emphasize that the mode of action of thyroxine is exerted at the nuclear level in the first instance and the ultimate effects of the hormone are due to elevations of certain specific proteins or enzymes such as the case cited above. It must be borne in mind that thyroxine affects almost all cells in the body and it may have effects on a number of enzymes (p. 27.23).

$$\begin{array}{cc} \text{Cytosol} & \text{Mitochondria} \end{array}$$

$$\text{G-6-P} \diagdown \quad \text{NAD} \diagdown \quad \text{1-GP} \longrightarrow \text{1-GP} \diagdown \text{FAD}$$

$$\text{PEP} \diagup \diagdown \text{NADH}_2 \diagup \diagdown \text{DHAP} \longleftarrow \text{DHAP} \diagup \diagdown \text{FADH}_2$$

Metabolic adaptations to environmental stress in man

Some metabolic adaptations in man which illustrate possible biochemical control processes activated in response to selected constraints are now considered. These are adaptations to fasting, to overfeeding to an extent which may induce obesity with diets containing excess carbohydrate, fat or protein, and to temporary and long term oxygen deficit.

FASTING

After food has been withheld from a man for 4–6 h the small intestine is empty; with no alimentary absorption the plasma concentration of glucose falls before becoming stabilized at a slightly lower level.

The liver has a role as a glucostat; when plasma glucose falls a little, the pancreas responds by lowering the secretion of insulin and increasing the secretion of glucagon. The latter has two main target tissues, muscle and adipose tissue, where it increases cyclic AMP concentration. In the liver, cyclic AMP has a negative allosteric effect on the glycogen synthase system which is accordingly diminished. On the other hand the same signal has a positive allosteric effect on the phosphorylase enzyme complex resulting in increased breakdown of glycogen to glucose-1-phosphate. This is converted to glucose-6-phosphate (p. 9.6) which is subsequently hydrolysed to glucose and enters the blood and replaces glucose used by the brain and other tissues.

In adipose tissue, the action of glucagon and perhaps catecholamines raises cyclic AMP concentration which activates the hormone-sensitive lipase, leading to an efflux of free fatty acids into the plasma for utilization by peripheral tissues. The carnitine acyl transferase enzyme system needed for the metabolism of fatty acyl CoA derivatives by liver mitochondria is markedly raised in fasting. During this phase the RQ falls to about 0·75.

During a fast, synthesis of long chain fatty acids from glucose in adipose tissue and liver virtually stops as the activity of the key enzyme in lipogenesis, acetyl CoA carboxylase, drops to a very low value. Activity of the citrate cleavage enzyme system also falls during fasting, as does the lipoprotein lipase or clearing factor lipase of adipose tissue. When hepatic glycogen reservoirs diminish, the control systems which permit the utilization of the carbon skeletons of amino acids for conversion into carbohydrates (gluconeogenesis) begin to operate. The enzymes whose activities have to be moderated include those responsible for the reversal of glycolysis. Starvation activates the pituitary-adrenal axis with increased secretion of adrenocorticosteroids. These steroids decrease peripheral utilization of glucose so that cardiac and skeletal muscle use free fatty acids for fuel in place of glucose. They also increase breakdown of protein to amino acids in peripheral tissue (p. 27.35). This effect,

together with diminished protein synthesis from amino acids, leads to a rise in the concentration of amino acids in plasma. Hence, during a fast, more amino acids are made available to the liver. Some of these are glucogenic and others ketogenic (p. 11.20). Many of the aminotransferases are markedly increased in activity during periods of starvation. This results in the increased availability of several oxo acids and the production of ammonia which is rapidly converted to urea and excreted. Some steps in the glycolytic sequence are not easily reversible and hence collateral routes may be needed.

The substantial flow of metabolites to the liver during fasting produces intracellular pyruvate, lactate, oxaloacetate and acetyl CoA. The liver uses these substances for gluconeogenesis to maintain the blood glucose. All the stages of the breakdown of glucose in the Embden–Meyerhof pathway are readily reversible, except the final conversion of phosphoenolpyruvate to pyruvate by pyruvate kinase (p. 9.7). During fasting phosphoenolpyruvate may be formed by the route described on p. 14.7. An increase in activity of pyruvate carboxylase in mitochondria converts pyruvate into oxaloacetate which is then reduced to malate. The malate diffuses into the cytosol where it is reoxidized to oxaloacetate which phosphoenolpyruvate carboxylase converts into phosphoenolpyruvate, using GTP as the source of phosphate.

Another possible block in the reversal of glycolysis is overcome by fructose-1, 6-diphosphate-1-phosphohydrolase which converts fructose-1,6-diphosphate into fructose-6-phosphate (p. 9.6). This enzyme is activated by ATP and inhibited by AMP, while the forward phosphofructokinase enzyme is allosterically negatively affected by ATP. Fasting also increases the activity of

TABLE 14.1. Location and control of rate-limiting enzymes.

	Rate-limiting or controlling enzyme	Intracellular location	Activator (A) or inhibitor (I)
Glycogenesis	Hexokinase	Cytosol	3':5'-cyclic AMP (I)
	Glycogen synthase	Cytosol	3':5'-cyclic AMP (I)
Glycogenolysis	Phosphorylase	Cytosol	3':5'-cyclic AMP (A)
Glycolysis	Phosphofructokinase	Cytosol	ADP (A), AMP (A), FADP (A)
			3':5'-cyclic AMP (A)
			ATP (I)
Gluconeogenesis	Glucose-6-phosphatase	Cytosol	
	Fructose-1,6-diphosphate-1-phosphohydrolase	Cytosol	ATP (A)
			AMP (I), FDP (I)
	Pyruvate carboxykinase	Cytosol	
	Pyruvate carboxylase	Mitochondria	Acetyl CoA (A)
Citric acid cycle	Pyruvate dehydrogenase	Mitochondria	ATP (I), Acetyl CoA (I)
	Isocitrate dehydrogenase	Mitochondria	ADP (A)
			ATP (I)
Lipogenesis	Acetyl CoA carboxylase	Cytosol	Citrate (A)
			Palmityl CoA (I)
Lipolysis	Hormone-sensitive lipase	Cytosol	3':5'-cyclic AMP (A)

glucose-6-phosphatase, which releases glucose from glucose-6-phosphate, generated by gluconeogenesis in the liver. The key metabolic processes and some of the controller enzymes involved are set out in table 14.1.

One important aspect of the adjustments to metabolism which occur during a fast is regeneration of key intermediates. This process, sometimes termed **anaplerosis,** includes several reactions some of which have been discussed previously. The withdrawal of key intermediates in the citric acid cycle for anabolic reactions, such as the utilization of oxaloacetate for the generation of aspartate, blocks the operation of the cycle. Then oxaloacetate can be regenerated in the liver from pyruvate and CO_2 by pyruvate carboxylase (fig. 14.8 and p. 9.13). Similarly, malate can be formed from pyruvate and CO_2 by the malic enzyme. Thus anaplerotic reactions regenerate oxaloacetate or malate from glycolytic intermediates such as pyruvate. The activity of these enzymes is increased during fasting.

As a consequence of increased mobilization of fatty acids from adipose tissue and their increased oxidative catabolism by liver mitochondria, there is increased production of acetyl CoA. This can be converted into acetoacetyl CoA in liver, and the latter molecule can condense with another molecule of acetyl CoA to produce β-hydroxy-β-methylglutaryl CoA or HMG CoA (p. 10.22). This branched chain thioester is an important intermediate in the generation of sterols and free acetoacetic acid. The first stage in the conversion of HMG CoA to sterols is its reduction to mevalonate by HMG CoA reductase (p. 10.23). This reductase reaction is possibly the most important rate-determining step in sterol synthesis. The liver is a main site of cholesterol synthesis in man and, in fasting, hepatic HMG CoA reductase activity virtually disappears and cholesterol synthesis from acetate stops. On the other hand HMG CoA production proceeds at an increased rate in the liver. This activates HMG CoA lyase which splits HMG CoA into acetyl CoA and free acetoacetic acid (p. 33.6). The free acetoacetic acid diffuses out of the liver cells into plasma and is utilized by tissues such as cardiac and skeletal muscle, kidney and also, in prolonged fasts, brain. When the plasma insulin level is low, ketone body production is increased; as the plasma insulin level rises, ketone body production falls.

PROLONGED UNDERNUTRITION

In prolonged undernutrition reserve stores of fat and glycogen are utilized and tissue protein is also broken down to provide energy. Over 2 kg of tissue protein in man (about 20 per cent of the total) can be lost before the subject is in danger of death from starvation. As a result of this loss the resting metabolic rate is reduced and so the energy requirement falls. This, together with curtailment of all unnecessary physical activity, allows some degree of adaptation to starvation and enables many of the victims of famine to survive until relief is brought.

The effect of chronic undernutrition easiest to observe in children is diminution or cessation of growth. Amino acids from the inadequate supply of dietary protein are used as a source of energy in preference to synthesis of tissue protein. This diversion is brought about by changes in activity of liver enzymes. Table 14.2 records data from biopsy samples of liver from undernourished Jamaican children on admission to hospital and after dietary rehabilitation. On admission, activity of amino acid-activating enzymes was high and it fell on rehabilitation. Argininosuccinase activity responsible for the formation of urea was low on admission, but rose when adequate dietary protein was provided.

In prolonged undernutrition, essential amino acids are conserved for protein turnover, and their plasma concentration falls (vol. 3, p. 24.11). Non-essential amino acids continue to be used for gluconeogenesis and their plasma concentration may be normal or raised. The ratio of plasma concentrations of essential to non-essential amino acids has been used as an index of severity of malnutrition.

TABLE 14.2. Enzymic activity of the livers of children with malnutrition. The figures for the amino acid-activating enzymes are the mean of 18 measurements and expressed in μmol P exchanged/mg protein h^{-1}; for argininosuccinase the figures are the mean of 11 measurements and expressed in μmol urea/mg protein h^{-1}. The changes on recovery are statistically significant. From data of Stephen Joan L.M. & Waterlow J.C. (1968) *Lancet* i, 118.

	Amino acid-activating enzymes	Arginino-succinase
Soon after admission	1·44	1·06
1–2 months later	0·91	1·46

OVERNUTRITION

A high intake of carbohydrate elicits a response from the pancreas to produce more insulin, which promotes the uptake of glucose by liver, muscle and adipose tissue. There is an increase in glucokinase in the liver which promotes the formation of glycogen. There is also a rapid increase in the activity of acetyl CoA carboxylase, a rate-limiting enzyme in lipogenesis. This, together with an increase in the fatty acid synthase complex, and an increase in glucose-6-phosphate dehydrogenase which generates $NADPH_2$, sets the stage for lipogenesis in adipose tissue and liver. The conversion of carbohydrate to fat raises the RQ, but in man it goes above unity only after repeated intakes of excess carbohydrate.

A different situation prevails if the subject eats a high energy diet with excess triglyceride. For effective absorption of the triglyceride pancreatic lipase activity is increased. The hepatic carnitine acyl transferase activity is elevated, allowing increased oxidation of fatty acids in the mitochondria. This also occurs in the fasting state where the liver has to deal with an increased load of fatty acids from adipose tissue. Many of the enzymes involved in gluconeogenesis are stimulated by a high energy, high fat diet. Thus in the liver various amino-transferases, glucose-6-phosphatase and fructose-1,6-diphosphate-1-phosphohydrolase increase in activity. Lipoprotein lipase (clearing factor lipase) activity is also raised.

If the diet is high in protein and low in carbohydrate and fat, there is a need for additional pancreatic peptidases, and there is increased activity of all the enzymes involved in the operation of the urea cycle. The activity of many aminotransferases is increased by such a diet, as is the activity of the key enzymes involved in gluconeogenesis.

It is a common observation that some people who have good appetites and are hearty eaters remain thin, whilst others who appear to eat very little readily become obese. This has led to the view that there is a control mechanism for disposing of excess dietary carbohydrate and fat which may be lacking in those with a tendency to obesity. However, there is no biochemical evidence that the tissues dispose of excess energy other than by storage as glycogen and triglyceride. In man it is very difficult to measure accurately over prolonged periods both energy intake in the diet and energy output in physical activities It is also impossible to determine accurately to what extent a small change in body weight is due to changes in the fat content or in total body water. How body weight is controlled in the long term and why control is no problem for some and a continuing struggle for others is unknown.

There is evidence that obese people channel more carbohydrate through the hexose monophosphate pathway than those of normal weight. Hence they have more $NADPH_2$ available for lipogenesis. However, whether this is a result or a contributory cause of their obesity is unknown.

TISSUE HYPOXIA

When the rate of utilization of oxygen by a tissue exceeds the rate of delivery by the circulation, tissue hypoxia results. This occurs during anaerobic work (p. 45.4), when the partial pressure of oxygen in the inspired air is reduced (p. 46.2) and in many diseases (vol. 3, p. 18.22). In cardiac and skeletal muscle the work load, and hence energy requirements, vary enormously throughout the day. The metabolic processes in resting muscle are adjusted so that the ratio of ATP/ADP is high, and the rate of production of ATP in the mitochondria is low because lack of ADP limits the respiratory rate. The high concentration of ATP inhibits phosphofructokinase, the key enzyme in the glycolytic pathway, and tends to decrease the activity of isocitrate dehydrogenase, so that the citric acid cycle is depressed.

As a muscle springs into action and performs work, ATP is utilized and after the reserve high energy phosphate (creatine phosphate) is used up, the ratio of ATP/ADP falls. This tends to drive the phosphofructokinase and isocitrate dehydrogenase reactions, so that glycolysis and the citric acid cycle reactions are stimulated. This is an example of the Pasteur effect (p. 9.14). Under physiological conditions when the oxygen supply to the tissues can be increased, increased oxygen consumption readjusts the ATP/ADP ratio. Should there be a deficit of oxygen for any reason, such as a diminished blood supply or inability of the respiratory apparatus to supply the extra oxygen, then the tissues are confronted with a challenge to their control systems.

During periods of physiological or pathological hypoxia, the intracellular ATP concentration is diminished because the rate of utilization exceeds the rate of supply. Some of the ADP in mitochondria can then yield ATP by the reaction

$$2\,ADP \longrightarrow ATP + AMP$$

This dismutation generates AMP and, since this is a potent positive allosteric effector of the phosphofructokinase reaction, gives a surge to glycolysis. In this way, when aerobic production of ATP cannot sustain cell activities, the less efficient glycolytic pathway acts as an emergency producer of ATP. This reserve route produces pyruvate and $NADH_2$. As tissue Po_2 is too low to allow the mitochondrial respiratory chain to transfer electrons to oxygen, the $NADH_2$ is reoxidized at the expense of pyruvate with formation of lactate.

Unfortunately there are limitations to the extent to which this scheme can operate in cells, because both pyruvic and lactic acids are strong acids and affect the internal pH of the cell with repercussions on the activities of other enzymes and on the characteristics of the cell and the subcellular membranes. Under physiological circumstances when the blood supply is intact, the lactate generated diffuses out of the cells and is transported to the liver for conversion to glycogen. If the period of hypoxia is short, these intracellular changes in the ATP, ADP, pyruvate and lactate concentrations are rapidly returned to normal values as the Po_2 in the tissues returns to its usual level. If the period of hypoxia is prolonged or severe as in very heavy physical exercise, oxygen consumption continues to be raised after the work has stopped and in this way the metabolites such as lactate are oxidized. This is responsible for the lactic acid part of the oxygen debt (p. 45.6).

In prolonged and repeated muscular exercise and in exposure to high altitudes, hypoxia leads to adaptive changes, for example muscles hypertrophy and the red cell mass increases. This cell hypertrophy and hyperplasia resulting from environmental changes may be due to the effect of a local ATP deficit activating the genetic apparatus of the cells, so that they increase in size or number. Fig. 14.17 shows an increase in RNA synthesis and in DNA concentration in the rat ventricle during adaptation to altitude hypoxia.

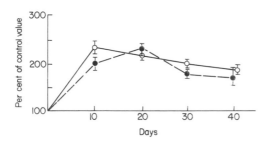

FIG. 14.17. DNA concentration (—) and incorporation of [14]C- orotic acid into m-RNA (---) of right ventricle of rat heart during altitude hypoxia. Per cent of control values is plotted vertically and time from beginning of adaptation horizontally. From Meerson F. Z. (1975) *Physiol Rev.* **55**, 79

Summary

One definition of life is the continuous ability to adjust to the external environment, and clearly the adjustments to metabolism employed by living systems are diverse.

This discussion presents some of the molecular mechanisms used by living systems for the control of molecular processes. The concentration of any metabolite in a cell or body fluid fluctuates about a mean or average value. The concentrations of certain key metabolites such as glucose and oxygen vary substantially but the concentrations of many other metabolites are restrained within narrow limits.

Regulation of metabolism is achieved by several complex controls exerted upon enzyme systems so that the activity and the absolute amounts of these catalysts are influenced by many factors operating in concert. This results in the concentrations of many metabolites in cells being controlled within prescribed limits. The metabolic pathways in a cell are organized in specific organelles and the end- and by-products of one set of reactions are the substrates and allosteric effectors of other reactions. Despite the complexity of cellular metabolic events it is possible to explore and identify rate-limiting foci or bottle-necks in these pathways. Attention has centred on the key reactions which might be exploited in the control of metabolism in cells and which might be influenced by chemotherapeutic substances in the correction of metabolic defects in disease.

By understanding the metabolic events in different living systems it is possible to attack bacteria in mammalian tissues by chemotherapeutic agents in the knowledge that they do not affect the metabolism of the host. Similarly, knowledge of the mode of action of hormones in mammalian systems has led to the discovery of other synthetic compounds which are more effective than the naturally occurring hormone. A fuller understanding of the controls in normal mammalian cells will increase understanding of the unusual metabolic features of tumour cells so that the differences in the metabolism of these cell types may be amenable to chemotherapy and lead to the control of neoplasia.

FURTHER READING

BOITEUX A. & HESS B. (1974) Oscillations in glycolysis, cellular respiration and communication. *Faraday Symposia of the Chemical Society*, No. 9, pp. 202–214.

LEVINE R. & LUFT R. eds. (1964–75) *Advances in Metabolic Disorders*, vols. 1–8. New York: Academic Press.

NEWSHOLME E.A. & START C. (1974) *Regulation in metabolism*. New York: Wiley.

WEBER G. ed. (1963–75) *Advances in Enzyme Regulation*, vols. 1–13. Oxford: Pergamon.

Chapter 15
Conducting tissues

Excitability is a characteristic of all living tissues and is present in both unicellular and multicellular organisms. A stimulus such as that applied by an electric current at one site may be transmitted to another part where it excites movement or other activity. A stimulus may also be inhibitory when it diminishes activity or movement. Although a general property of all cells, excitability and its spread or transmission are especially developed in nerve and muscle cells. Conduction occurs not only from one part of a cell to another but also from one nerve cell to another, from nerve to muscle cells, from muscle cell to muscle cell, in the case of some smooth muscle, and from nerve to secretory cell.

STRUCTURE OF NERVOUS TISSUE

In higher animals the nervous system is divided into two main parts, the central nervous system (brain and spinal cord) and the peripheral nervous system. The peripheral system consists of long nerve cables or fibres attached centrally to a nerve cell. It transmits information from peripheral sensory receptors by **afferent impulses** to the brain or spinal cord, where they are appreciated and co-ordinated. Cells within the central nervous system then transmit outgoing or **efferent impulses** to effector organs such as muscles or glands. In addition, there is a peripheral autonomic system of neurones, whose activity is less dependent on central nervous control and mainly concerned with the control of the internal organs such as the heart, intestine and glands. The nervous system is composed of the following structural units.

The nerve cells or neurones are the conducting units and although a great number of morphological variations exist, they are all able to receive impulses and transmit them to other cells.

The supporting cells of the central nervous system are called the **neuroglial cells. Schwann cells** play a similar role in the peripheral nervous system. The neuroglial cells are intimately related to the neurones and play an important part in the metabolism of the nervous system. In addition, they form the myelin sheaths which surround the larger nerve axons and act as insulating covers.

Connective tissue composes the fibrous tissue sheaths which surround the nerve fibres and ganglia of the peripheral nervous system. It is not normally present within the central nervous system, but connective tissue forms the protective meningeal membranes that cover the outsides of the brain and spinal cord. In addition many sensory nerve endings have elaborate connective tissue capsules.

The neurone

A neurone is a cell and consists of a cell body or perikaryon (*peri*, around, *karyon*, kernel or nucleus) and its associated processes. There are many varieties of neurones, differing in shape, size and in the number, length and form of their processes. The processes are of two basic types, **axons** and **dendrites**. A neurone may have many dendrites and these, together with the perikaryon which usually has the same cytological features, generally form the main receptive portion of the neurone. A mammalian neurone has only one axon and this process, which may be myelinated and lacks ribosomes in its cytoplasm, most frequently conducts nerve impulses away from the perikaryon in a non-decremental manner. These are only generalizations since, as more neurones have been examined both electrophysiologically and with the electron microscope, absolute definitions of axons and dendrites have become more difficult to make. Some of the problems are considered below.

One classification of neurones may be made on the basis of the length of the axon. **Golgi type I neurones** have long axons which leave their place of origin in the grey matter and either extend out of the central nervous system to enter peripheral nerves, or extend to another part of the central nervous system in the white matter. **Golgi type II neurones** have relatively short axons which end in the grey matter close to the parent perikaryon. Such neurones are very abundant in the cerebellar and cerebral cortices.

The term **nerve fibre** is sometimes used as synonymous with axon, but is more correctly applied to the axon with its investing sheath. A collection of nerve fibres lying outside the boundaries of the central nervous system forms a **peripheral nerve.**

Neurones may also be classified on the basis of the number of processes arising from the perikaryon.

Multipolar neurones are the most common type within the central nervous system; they have a single axon and many dendrites. The shapes of the neurones vary greatly; sometimes the dendrites arise in an apparently random fashion as in the anterior horn cells of the spinal cord (figs. 15.1 and 15.2). In other neurones such as the large

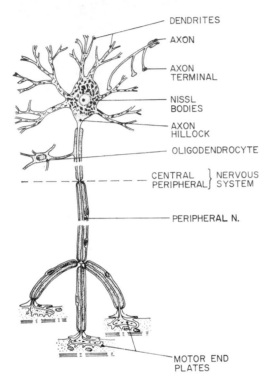

FIG. 15.1. Diagram of a ventral horn cell from the spinal cord. The broken line represents the limits of the central and peripheral nervous systems.

Purkinje cells of the cerebellum (fig. 15.3) the dendrites arise from only one pole of a pear-shaped perikaryon and although there may be only one main stem dendrite, this branches profusely to produce an extensive dendritic tree (fig. 15.3b). The pyramidal neurones of the cerebral cortex on the other hand have a single large apical dendrite, arising from the apex of a cone-shaped perikaryon, and a number of small dendrites which arise from the base of the perikaryon (fig. 15.3a). In all of these multipolar cells, the axon is a smooth and thin process of generally uniform diameter which conducts impulses away from the perikaryon. In contrast, the dendrites are irregularly contoured processes which taper rapidly. Dendrites receive most of the synapses formed with other neurones and for some neurones, such as the Purkinje cells (fig. 15.3b) and pyramidal cells

(fig. 15.3a), the main receptor sites are dendritic spines that protrude as short extensions of the dendrites.

Some multipolar neurones possess processes which are all identical to each other in terms of both their morphology and conduction properties. Such neurones lacking an axon are the amacrine and horizontal cells of the retina (p. 26.12) and the granule cells of the olfactory bulb (fig. 25.80).

Bipolar neurones have only two processes. The receptive process is considered to be a dendrite while the process that transmits impulses to other neurones is regarded as the axon. Such neurones are present in the bipolar layer of the retina; somewhat modified bipolar neurones are the rods and cones of the retina (fig. 26.17) and the receptor cells of the olfactory epithelium (fig. 15.3c). The neurones of the vestibular and cochlear ganglia of the eighth nerve are also bipolar (fig. 26.37). In these the receptor portion of the peripherally directed process may be considered as the dendrite and the part of the neurone beyond the commencement of the myelin sheath as the axon. Hence the perikaryon, which itself may be covered by a myelin sheath, may be regarded as interposed along the axon.

Unipolar neurones occur within the mesencephalic nucleus of the trigeminal nerve (fig. 25.54) and most of the neurones in the spinal and cranial nerve ganglia have this form (fig. 15.3d). These first order sensory neurones possess a single process which arises from the perikaryon and divides into a **peripheral process**, which carries impulses towards the cell body, and a **central process** which enters the brain or spinal cord (fig. 15.3d). When first formed, neurones of the spinal ganglia are bipolar, with a process extending from each end of the perikaryon. During development these two processes come together on one side of the cell body and their bases fuse into a single, short stem. Thus the neurone becomes unipolar; it is sometimes termed **pseudo-unipolar** because of its mode of development. There is no structural difference between the peripherally and centrally directed processes of the neurone; each has the cytological features of an axon in that it lacks ribosomes in its cytoplasm and may possess a myelin sheath. The perikaryon may therefore be regarded as lying along the length of the axon and the nerve impulses may bypass the perikaryon. As with vestibular and cochlear ganglia cells, the dendritic portion of the neurone can be considered to be the end of the peripheral process which receives sensory stimuli.

CYTOLOGY OF THE NEURONE

The form of the neurone so far described is that revealed by the Golgi silver impregnation technique which was used to great effect by the Spanish neuroanatomist, Ramon y Cajal. It is the best method for visualizing the full extent of a neurone and all its processes in three dimensions (fig. 15.3); the neurone appears brown or

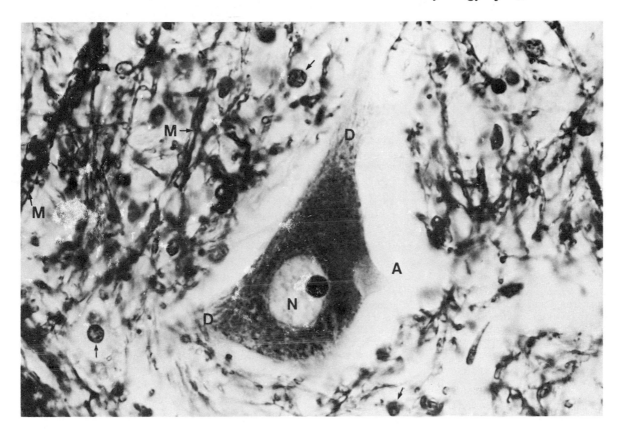

FIG. 15.2. Photomicrograph of a part of the anterior horn of the spinal cord stained with cresyl violet and luxol fast blue. The cresyl violet shows the large nucleolus in the pale nucleus (N) of the anterior horn cell, and the Nissl bodies of the perikaryon. Extending from the perikaryon are two dendrites (D) and the pale axon (A) which has a distinct axon hillock at its base. Surrounding the neurone is the neuropil in which the nuclei of neuroglial cells (arrows) appear, as well as parts of myelinated nerve fibres (M). (× 900).

black and none of its internal cytology can be seen. A similar result can be obtained by a method in which a micropipette is inserted into a neurone. The activity of the neurone can be recorded and then a dye, such as Procion yellow, injected into the cytoplasm spreads through the cytoplasm and shows the shape of the cell.

Other stains show the internal structure of neurones. Thus, basic dyes show the perikarya and bases of dendrites of neurones (fig. 15.2). Such dyes stain the **Nissl granules** of the cytoplasm by binding with the concentrations of ribosomes that are both attached to the surfaces of groups of cisternae or granular endoplasmic reticulum and lie free in the intervening cytoplasm. Nissl granules are present in the perikarya of almost all neurones and vary from the rather large and coarse granules of the motor cells (fig. 15.1) to the small dust-like particles of the sensory neurones. The granules also extend into the dendrites but are only sufficiently prominent in their bases to produce effective staining. In contrast, ribosomes are absent from axons and also from the axon hillock, where the axon arises from the perikaryon.

Dissolution of the Nissl granules, **chromatolysis**, is usually associated with injury to the body of the neurone (vol. 2, p. 25.9). Cutting the axon causes chromatolysis and this procedure is used experimentally to determine the position of its perikaryon.

Basic dyes also stain the nucleus of a neurone. This is usually spherical and situated in the centre of the perikaryon, although in chromatolysis it may assume a more eccentric position. In normal nuclei there are one or two prominent nucleoli, and the nuclear envelope is quite distinct (fig. 15.2).

Since dendrites contain only a few Nissl granules and axons contain none, basic dyes cannot stain these processes effectively. The neuronal processes are displayed by a variety of silver staining methods which deposit silver particles and reveal the **neurofibrils**. These run nearly parallel to each other in the processes and are particularly prominent in the axon. In the perikaryon they run in bundles between the Nissl granules. In EM studies, structures with the sizes and characteristics of neurofibrils have not been observed, but neurones and their processes contain two types of thinner and long organelles whose clumping together is probably respon-

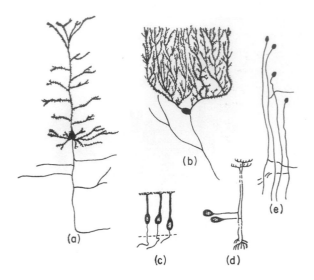

FIG. 15.3. Various types of neurones. Golgi preparations, redrawn from Cajal. (a) Pyramidal neurone from cerebral cortex, (b) Purkinje cell from cerebellum, (c) bipolar cells from olfactory mucosa, (d) dorsal root ganglion cells, (e) unipolar neurones from the mesencephalic nucleus of the trigeminal nerve.

sible for the formation of neurofibrils. These long organelles are the **neurofilaments**, each about 10 nm in diameter, and the 24 nm thick **microtubules** (fig. 15.4). Both are common in the perikaryon. In dendrites microtubules predominate, while neurofilaments are most common in larger axons. At the axon hillock some microtubules form compact bundles which extend into the **initial segment of the axon**. This also has a dense layer of material coating the cytoplasmic side of the plasma membrane, an undercoating which is thought to be involved in the generation of the axonal action potential, since it also occurs at the nodes of Ranvier (fig. 15.9).

In addition to the neurofilaments, microtubules and ribosomes, the cytoplasm of neurones contains mitochondria; those within the dendrites and axons are long and thin. The Golgi apparatus is well developed; indeed, it was in the perikarya of neurones that this organelle was first described by Golgi. Vacuoles, vesicles, glycogen and pigment, including lipofuscin, may occur as cytoplasmic inclusions. The pigment may be brown or black, as in cells of the substantia nigra.

DENDRITES

Dendrites do not extend far from the perikaryon and are characterized by their repeated branching and irregular outlines. Along with the perikaryon, dendrites are the main receptor portions of neurones, for the majority of synapses are formed on their surfaces. On some dendrites the synapses are borne on spines or thorns (fig. 15.1).

AXONS

The axon of a multipolar neurone arises from the axon hillock, and its first portion is the initial segment. Axons differ structurally from dendrites in that ribosomes do not occur beyond the initial segment and axons may be myelinated. Larger axons have more neurofilaments than microtubules in their cytoplasm (fig. 15.4). Axons branch at varying distances from the perikaryon, but they do not ramify like a dendrite; instead their branches come off the main stem at right angles and within the central nervous system the terminal branches always form bulbous expansions called **boutons** (fig. 25.1). If the boutons are at the ends of these terminal branches they are **terminal boutons** and when they occur along the length of an axon they are known as **boutons en passant.** These boutons or axon terminals are applied to the surfaces of dendrites, the perikaryon and axons or other neurones (fig. 15.1).

Axons that leave the central nervous system to run in peripheral nerves also end in expansions that may be applied to the surface of another neurone (as in the case of those axons of the sympathetic nervous system which form synapses upon the neurones of the autonomic ganglia). Axons may also end on the surface of a striated muscle fibre to form a motor end plate (fig. 15.45), or within the interstices of glandular and smooth muscle tissues.

The various sheaths of an axon are now described, as these affect the mode of conduction. Axon terminals or boutons are considered in chap. 25.

SHEATHS OF PERIPHERAL NERVE FIBRES

The sheath-forming cells of the peripheral nervous system are the Schwann cells. These are elongated cells with spindle-shaped nuclei which lie parallel to the length of the axons which they ensheath both completely and separately. It is on the basis of the form of the sheath that peripheral nerves are said to be either **myelinated** or **unmyelinated.**

In the following account, the term 'nerve fibre' refers to an ensheathed axon and so embraces all neuronal processes which may be carrying impulses towards the central nervous system (afferent fibres) or away from it (efferent fibres). Such nerve fibres may be myelinated or unmyelinated and, as pointed out above, both the centrally and peripherally directed processes of the sensory ganglion cells have the same structure.

Most peripheral nerves contain a mixture of myelinated and unmyelinated nerve fibres, but it is common for one type to predominate. In the living body, nerves that contain many unmyelinated nerve fibres appear dull and grey, while those that contain mostly myelinated nerve fibres are white and glistening. This white appearance is due to

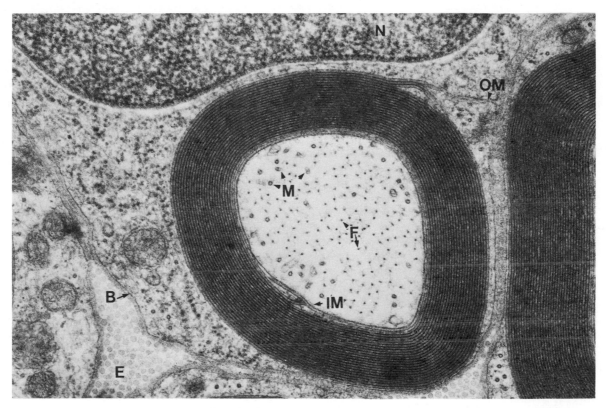

Fig. 15.4. Electronmicrograph of a transverse section of a myelinated peripheral axon. The axon has both neurofilaments (F) and microtubules (M) in its cytoplasm. Surrounding the axon is the myelin sheath which is a spiralled sheet of Schwann cell plasma membrane. The spiral begins at the internal mesaxon (IM) and ends at the outer mesaxon (OM). The myelinated axon is embedded in a Schwann cell, the nucleus (N) of which is partially visible. Surrounding the Schwann cell is a basal lamina (B) and the fibres of the endoneurium (E). ($\times$ 35 000).

the presence of myelin, a complex lipoprotein which blackens with osmic acid (fig. 15.5).

Unmyelinated nerve fibres

These are between 0·1 and 1·0 μm in diameter. EM studies show that many axons are invested by the same Schwann cell (fig. 15.6). The separation between axons is achieved by each being invaginated at a different site on the Schwann cell surface, so that in effect each lies in its own groove. Some axons are only partially enclosed by the Schwann cell but others are completely enfolded in such a way that the edges of the groove come together to form a mesaxon (fig. 15.6). A mesaxon is formed by the close apposition of the surfaces of two different areas of the plasma membrane of the same Schwann cell.

Since each Schwann cell extends for only a short distance along a group of axons, the total ensheathing of a peripheral unmyelinated nerve fibre is achieved by a series of Schwann cells lying end to end.

Myelinated nerve fibres

These include practically all those with a diameter of more than 2 μm. When myelin is blackened with osmic acid it is found that the myelin sheath is interrupted at regular intervals along its length by indentations. These interruptions are the **nodes of Ranvier** (fig. 15.5) and the length of myelin between two adjacent nodes is referred to as an **internode**. Generally, the greater the diameter of the fibre the less frequent are the nodes of Ranvier, so that the internodal length of a nerve fibre 5 μm in diameter is about 0·5 mm while that of a 10 μm fibre is about 2 mm (fig. 15.7). Another observation made with the light microscope is that only one Schwann cell nucleus is associated with one internodal length of myelin (fig. 15.5), since this length represents the extent of that Schwann cell.

Polarized light and X-ray diffraction techniques show that myelin is composed of lipid and protein laid down in a series of concentric layers or lamellae, each of which has a thickness of about 18 nm. EM observations confirm this finding and show that the lamellae are formed from the plasma membrane of the Schwann cell; it is for this reason, of course, that myelin has a high lipoprotein content. To understand the structure of the myelin sheath, it is necessary to refer to its development. In the first stage of myelin formation, a single axon is enclosed by a

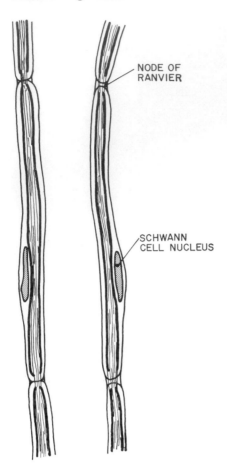

FIG. 15.5. Internodal segments of two nerves from a young animal. Stained with osmic acid.

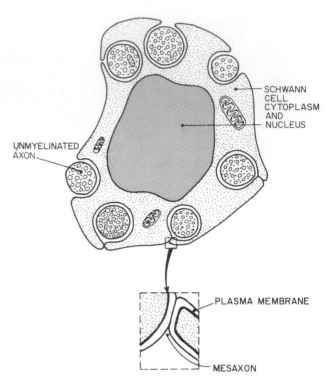

FIG. 15.6. Diagram to show the arrangement of unmyelinated axons within a Schwann cell; details of how plasma membrane surfaces come together to form a mesaxon are also given.

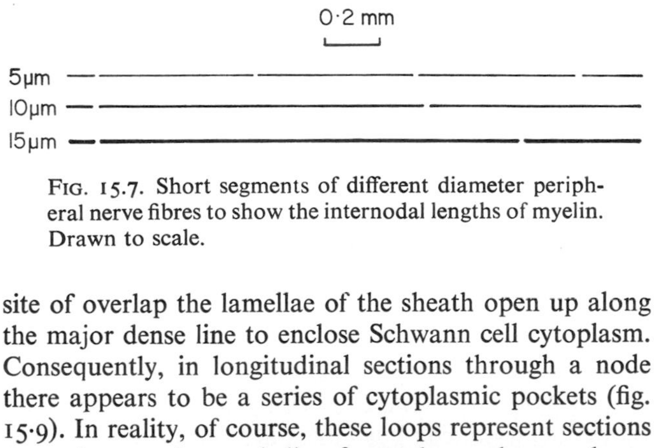

FIG. 15.7. Short segments of different diameter peripheral nerve fibres to show the internodal lengths of myelin. Drawn to scale.

Schwann cell (fig. 15.8a), in such a way that it indents the surface of that cell to lie within a groove. Next, the free edges of the Schwann cell come together to form a mesaxon (fig. 15.6), so that the two opposed plasma membranes form a gap junction between their outer surfaces (fig. 15.8b). The mesaxon then elongates in a spiral manner around the enclosed axon (fig. 15.8c). Initially the spiral is loose, but later the cytoplasm is lost from between the successive turns. At the site of fusion of the cytoplasmic surfaces of the plasma membrane forming the myelin sheath, a dense line is formed. This **major dense line** within the sheath alternates with the thinner, **intraperiod line** (fig. 15.8d), formed by the apposition of the outer surfaces of the same membrane. Thus compact myelin is formed, and each turn of the spiral is termed a lamella. Cytoplasm remains on the inside of the sheath, between the myelin and the axon as well as on the outside where the nucleus of the Schwann cell is seen (fig. 15.4).

At a node of Ranvier (fig. 15.5 and 15.9) the successive layers of the spirally arranged lamellae of myelin end. Each layer overlaps the one lying internal to it and at the site of overlap the lamellae of the sheath open up along the major dense line to enclose Schwann cell cytoplasm. Consequently, in longitudinal sections through a node there appears to be a series of cytoplasmic pockets (fig. 15.9). In reality, of course, these loops represent sections through a continuous helix of cytoplasm whose ends are in direct continuity with the cytoplasm on the inside and outside of the myelin sheath.

In the region of these loops the gap between the plasma membrane of the Schwann cell and that of the axon is very small, being only about 5 nm. It is thought that this is to limit the passage of ions into the extracellular space between the sheath and the axon. At a node, the myelin is interrupted, the interdigitating processes of the adjacent Schwann cells do not fuse together and the continuous basement membrane and endoneurium are permeable to ions (fig. 15.9). So here the plasma membrane of the axon

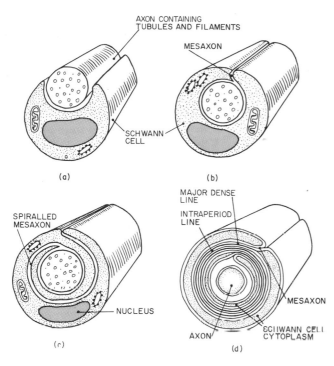

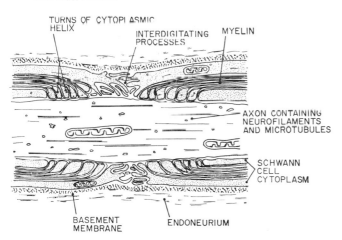

FIG. 15.8. The myelin sheath of peripheral nerve fibres. a–c, the development of the sheath; d, the structure of the adult sheath.

FIG. 15.9. Diagram of a longitudinal section through a node of Ranvier of a peripheral myelinated nerve fibre.

is bathed with extracellular ions. Ionic insulation of the internodal segment and exposure at the nodes are necessary for saltatory conduction (p. 15.22).

PERIPHERAL NERVE STRUCTURE

Nerve bundles, which make up a peripheral nerve, contain both myelinated and unmyelinated fibres. On the outside of each Schwann cell there is a basement membrane which forms a tube around each nerve fibre (fig. 15.9). Between the nerve fibres delicate connective tissue, **endoneurium**, fills the interior of nerve bundles. This is hardly visible with the light microscope. Around each

bundle of nerve fibres there is a sheath of connective tissue, the **perineurium**, which consists of layers of connective tissue fibres between which are fibroblasts (fig. 15.10). Binding these bundles together and forming the outer connective tissue sheath of the whole nerve is the **epineurium** (fig. 15.10).

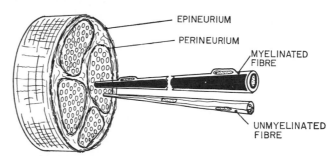

FIG. 15.10. Structure of a peripheral nerve containing myelinated and unmyelinated nerve fibres, showing the neural sheaths.

SHEATHS OF AXONS IN THE CENTRAL NERVOUS SYSTEM

Most axons within the central nervous system do not have sheaths and are separated from their neighbours by spaces only 20 nm wide. The sheaths of the myelinated axons, which are of course few in grey matter and predominate in white matter, are similar to those of peripheral nerves in that the myelin is formed by the spiral wrapping of the plasma membrane of the myelin-forming cell, in this case the oligodendrocyte (fig. 15.1 and 15.11).

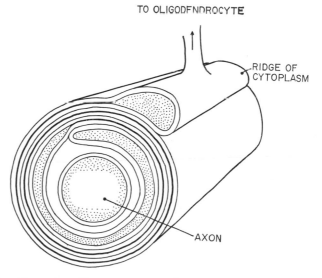

FIG. 15.11. The structure of the myelin sheath of the central nervous system. While the nucleus of the Schwann cell of the peripheral nervous system is contained within the cytoplasm on the outside of the sheath, the nucleus of the oligodendrocyte is within the cell body situated some distance away from the site of myelin formation. Also see fig. 15.8.

The main differences between the myelin sheaths in the peripheral and central nervous systems are as follows:

(1) An oligodendrocyte is responsible for the formation of a number of internodal lengths of myelin, not upon the same axon, but upon different axons. For this reason the oligodendrocyte nucleus is not found in intimate association with the outside of the sheath, as is the Schwann cell nucleus. Instead it is some distance away, the myelin sheath being formed at the end of an oligodendrocyte process.

(2) There is an incomplete layer of cytoplasm on the outside of a myelin sheath in the central nervous system, so that the outsides of adjacent myelin sheaths can come into direct contact with each other.

(3) At a node of Ranvier in the central nervous system the axon is bare and not covered by cytoplasmic processes of the myelin-forming cell as in peripheral nerves.

Thus a nerve fibre within the central nervous system has a myelin sheath formed by oligodendrocytes, but once that nerve fibre leaves the central nervous system its myelin is formed by Schwann cells (fig. 15.1).

Neuroglia

The neuroglia (*neuron*, nerve, *glia*, glue) are the supporting cells of the central nervous system and outnumber the neurones by at least 10 to 1. They are of four different types, the astrocytes, the oligodendrocytes, ependymal cells and microglia. The structural features of these cells are not apparent in preparations normally used for the histological study of the nervous system, since only their nuclei are visible. Consequently, special stains and EM methods have to be used for their study.

Astrocytes have numerous processes arising from the perikaryon and this star shape accounts for their name. They are of two types, fibrous astrocytes, which predominate in white matter, and protoplasmic astrocytes, which are found mainly in grey matter. The difference between the two types lies in the number of intracellular fibrils which they contain. Astrocytes occur throughout the central nervous system and their processes course between those of neurones. Single processes in grey matter may isolate certain neuronal components such as synapses from the surrounding structures, while in white matter groups of processes of fibrous astrocytes surround bundles of nerve fibres.

Some processes of astrocytes extend to the outside of the nervous tissue and expand into end feet which separate neurones and their processes from both the fluid and meninges on the outside of the central nervous system, as well as from the blood vessels that penetrate into it. Thus, end feet of astrocytes separate the nerve cells from all other tissues. Although substances entering or leaving the central nervous system have to pass through or between these end feet, the endothelial cells of the capillaries, which have tight junctions (p. 13.13) between them, form the blood–brain barrier. Nevertheless it is likely that astrocytes influence the composition of extracellular fluid close to excitable membranes and they probably take up neurotransmitters and other substances which might otherwise interfere with neuronal activity. Astrocytes react to pathological conditions by producing extensive scars that are thought to prevent the breakdown of remaining nervous tissue.

Oligodendrocytes are smaller and have fewer processes than astrocytes. They are found throughout the central nervous system and in white matter lie in rows between the myelinated nerve fibres, where one of their functions is the formation and maintenance of central myelin sheaths. In grey matter, oligodendrocytes are often found close to neurones, where they are referred to as perineuronal satellite cells. The role of these satellite cells is not certain.

Ependymal cells line the entire ventricular system of the brain and the central canal of the spinal cord. They retain their epithelial character, being low columnar in shape, ciliated and arranged in a single layer over the ventricular surface. Modified ependymal cells form the choroid plexuses from which the cerebrospinal fluid is produced.

Microglial cells are characterized by nuclei which stain deeply and have either an elongated or a rounded shape. Long branching processes arise from the cell bodies. Under normal conditions microglia appear to play no part in the maintenance of the central nervous system, but in pathological conditions they migrate towards the site of inflammation or degeneration and carry out phagocytosis and their cytoplasm becomes filled with lipid substances and cell debris (p. 29.5).

NERVE CONDUCTION

Much of the knowledge of the physiology of nerve and muscle cells is based on studies of the giant axon of the squid and of the frog sartorius muscle. Both preparations are sufficiently large for chemical analysis and remain excitable for several hours after excision. Excitability depends on the differences in ionic concentrations, especially of Na^+ and K^+, between extracellular and intracellular fluid, and also on the properties of the cell membrane. Table 15.1 gives the ionic composition for squid axon and frog muscle; these differ quantitatively but not qualitatively from nerve and muscle cells in man.

Physical systems in which two phases are separated by a membrane with one phase having a large impermeable ion were originally described by Nernst and by Donnan. Their work was based on that of a modest but outstanding member of Yale University, Professor Josiah Willard Gibbs, who by 1875 had described the general theoretical conditions for ionic equilibrium in such systems. By 1902

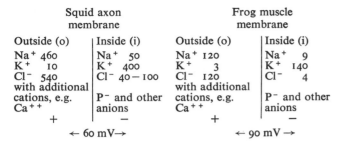

Squid axon membrane		Frog muscle membrane	
Outside (o)	Inside (i)	Outside (o)	Inside (i)
Na^+ 460	Na^+ 50	Na^+ 120	Na^+ 9
K^+ 10	K^+ 400	K^+ 3	K^+ 140
Cl^- 540	Cl^- 40 — 100	Cl^- 120	Cl^- 4
with additional cations, e.g. Ca^{++}	P^- and other anions	with additional cations, e.g. Ca^{++}	P^- and other anions
+	−	+	−
← 60 mV →		← 90 mV →	

TABLE 15.1. Concentrations of ions in mmol/l and electrical potential differences in millivolts across the cell membranes of the squid axon and frog muscle. P^- represents a negatively charged protein group, for which the membrane is impermeable.

an equilibrium system had been described for phases separated by a membrane with ionic distributions comparable to those in biological cells. In its simplest form this considers two solutions separated by a membrane freely permeable to the small ions present in the solution, e.g. Na^+, K^+ and Cl^-, but impermeable to others, e.g. protein ions, P^- (fig. 15.12). Then if (i) represents the

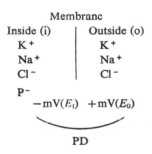

$$\text{Membrane}$$

Inside (i)	Outside (o)
K^+	K^+
Na^+	Na^+
Cl^-	Cl^-
P^-	
$-mV(E_i)$	$+mV(E_o)$

PD

FIG. 15.12. The effect of a semipermeable membrane on ionic potential distribution. The membrane is permeable to Na^+ and Cl^- but not to P^-. PD, potential difference.

inner compartment containing P^-, (o) the outer compartment, and the square brackets concentration, there are two conditions for equilibrium:

(1) the hydrostatic pressure in the compartment (i) must be greater than that in the compartment (o); this difference in pressure is called the osmotic pressure;

(2) there must be an electrical potential difference (PD or $E_i - E_o$) between the two phases related to the concentrations of the permeable ions.

For Na^+ and K^+ this relationship is given by the Nernst equation:

$$E_i - E_o = \frac{RT}{F} \ln \frac{[K^+]_o}{[K^+]_i} = \frac{RT}{F} \ln \frac{[Na^+]_o}{[Na^+]_i}$$

For the negative ion Cl^- it becomes:

$$E_i - E_o = \frac{RT}{F} \ln \frac{[Cl^-]_i}{[Cl^-]_o}$$

where R is the gas constant, T the absolute temperature, F the faraday and ln logarithms to the base e.

About this time, such a PD was demonstrated across biological cell membranes and is now called the **resting potential** or the **transmembrane potential.** Using the string galvanometer, it was shown that during nervous and muscular activity a zone of altered transmembrane potential, the **action potential**, moved along the axis of the cell and could be detected as it passed recording electrodes on the surface of the cell. The speed with which this zone of depolarization (fig. 15.13) moves along the axon or muscle cell is called the **conduction velocity** (p. 15.21). This had been measured in 1850 by Helmholtz who found values up to 30 m/sec in frog sciatic nerve muscle preparations.

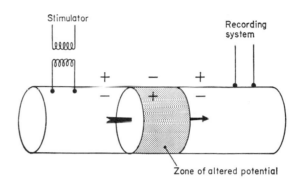

FIG. 15.13. Depolarization in a conducting nerve.

HISTORICAL NOTE AND THE BERNSTEIN THEORY

In 1902 Bernstein applied these new electrochemical theories to biological cells and suggested the following.

(1) In the resting state, only K^+ could pass through the membrane, which was impermeable to all other ions.

(2) As a result there was an equilibrium system similar to that demonstrated by Donnan with an electrical PD across the membrane (fig. 15.12). The value of this potential would be decided by K^+, the only permeable ion, and would have the value:

$$E_i - E_o = \frac{RT}{F} \ln \frac{[K^+]_o}{[K^+]_i}$$

(3) Bernstein postulated that on excitation the permeability of the cell membrane changed especially to anions, so that the cell was no longer in equilibrium with the extracellular fluid, but became a diffusion system of the kind described by Gibbs. Under these circumstances there would be diffusion of ions between the compartments. Gibbs had also demonstrated that such a system would give a potential difference between phases, and that this diffusion potential would be different in value and sign from the resting potential.

(4) Transmission of the action potential resulted because this region of altered permeability moved along the axon.

(5) Following the passage of the zone of altered permeability, the membrane reverted to its original state. The axon was then capable of further excitation.

Bernstein's view prevailed for over forty years and apparently explained the ionic composition of cell and extracellular fluid and the magnitude and direction of the resting potential. However, a critical test of the theory needed:

(1) accurate measurements of the resting potentials of individual cells in solutions identical with their normal extracellular fluid,

(2) better knowledge of the ions permeable to the cell membrane,

(3) accurate chemical analysis of intracellular and extracellular ionic content, and

(4) detailed analysis of the transmembrane voltage change and its time course when an action potential passes along the cell.

These measurements were not technically possible during the years when Bernstein's theory held and the factors which led to its modification illustrate the close interplay between new experimental techniques and theoretical ideas.

In early apparatus for measuring resting potentials (fig. 15.14) one silver electrode was in contact with the cell contents through a damaged area of the membrane and the other with the bathing solution, which represented the extracellular fluid. Short circuiting was prevented as far as possible by a barrier dividing the bath into two parts, in which the uninjured and damaged portion of the nerve or muscle lay. Precision depended largely on the effectiveness of this barrier. Values of up to -30 mV were obtained from frog muscle, whereas the value accepted today is -90 mV. Before 1940, chemical estimation of Na^+, K^+ and Ca^{++} was always difficult and often impossible in small samples; a single sodium estimation could take up to two days of tedious work and it was difficult to be certain whether these ions were permeable or impermeable. Chloride analysis was easier and Conway in Dublin had deduced that Cl^- was permeable.

In the late 1930s accurate extracellular recording of action potentials was advanced by the improved design of amplifiers and oscilloscopes, and the second World War indirectly contributed much to our present biological knowledge. In 1939, Hodgkin and Huxley in Cambridge developed the experimental approach which led to the revision of ideas about ionic distributions and their relation to excitability in the cell. The contribution of these two workers was recognized by the award of the Nobel prize.

Experimental considerations

Modern research depends on the following techniques:

(1) A micropipette is made by drawing fine glass tubing to a diameter of about 1 μm. It is filled with 3 mol/l KCl and, using a micromanipulator, is inserted through the membrane into a larger nerve or muscle cell. A silver-silver chloride wire in the 3 mol/l KCl solution enables it to serve as a microelectrode and a similar electrode in the extracellular fluid allows the electrical potential difference between the inside and outside of the cell to be measured (fig. 15.14).

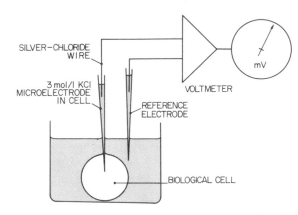

FIG. 15.14. Arrangements for measuring the electrical potential difference between the inside and outside of a cell.

(2) Voltage measuring devices which require virtually no current to be drawn from the system are used.

(3) Modern photometers enable accurate and rapid measurements to be made of the concentrations of K^+, Na^+ and other ions in very small samples of fluids.

(4) The use of radioactive isotopes makes possible the study of membrane permeability to all important ions.

A study of the squid axon with reference to Na^+ and K^+ is illustrated in table 15.2. A value of transmembrane

TABLE 15.2. Calculated values for $E_i - E_o$, if K^+ and Na^+ are to be in equilibrium across the squid axon membrane. Experimental value for $E_i - E_o = -60$ mV.

	Concentration (mmol/l)		$E_i - E_o$ (mV) required for equilibrium
	Inside cell	Outside cell	
Na^+	50	460	$+58$
K^+	400	10	-89

potential ($E_i - E_o$) for ionic equilibrium, calculated from the Nernst equation, is given for Na^+ and K^+. Using radioactive isotopes the membrane has been shown to be permeable to both ions. The measured value of ($E_i - E_o$) for squid axon is -60 mV. Since neither Na^+ nor K^+ is in equilibrium across the squid axon membrane, the resting potential is not a Nernst equilibrium potential and it will be shown that it is in fact a **diffusion potential**, i.e. an electrical potential between two phases caused by the interdiffusion of ions. Omitting theoretical considerations, discussed below, it can be stated that a value for the diffusion potential $(E_i - E_o)$ is given by the Goldman equation:

$$(E_i - E_o) = \frac{RT}{F} \ln \frac{P_{K^+}[K^+]_o + P_{Na^+}[Na^+]_o + P_{Cl^-}[Cl^-]_i}{P_{K^+}[K^+]_i + P_{Na^+}[Na^+]_i + P_{Cl^-}[Cl^-]_o}$$

In this expression P is the membrane permeability coefficient for any ion, e.g. P_{K^+} is a measure of the ease with which K^+ passes through a membrane.

At 20°C (293°A), and when the potential is in mV, the term RT/F ln is 58 millivolts $\log_{10}$ and the equation becomes

$$\begin{aligned}(E_i - E_o) \\ = 58 \log_{10} \frac{P_{K^+}[K^+]_o + P_{Na^+}[Na^+]_o + P_{Cl^-}[Cl^-]_i}{P_{K^+}[K^+]_i + P_{Na^+}[Na^+]_i + P_{Cl^-}[Cl^-]_o}.\text{mV}\end{aligned}$$

The importance of the Goldman equation is that it draws attention to the significance of membrane permeability in determining the transmembrane potential. A change in membrane permeability to any ion alters the transmembrane potential even if the gross concentrations of that ion inside or outside the cell do not change within chemically detectable levels. This is in marked contrast to the Nernst equation, where only large changes in internal or external concentrations produce a transmembrane potential change.

Theoretical considerations

Basic to the study of both equilibrium and diffusion systems is the concept of **chemical potential** introduced by Gibbs and for which the symbol μ is used; its units are Joules/mole. Gibbs showed that any species in equilibrium between phases had the same value for its chemical potential in those phases. In the case of a two-phase system with phases (i) and (o), at equilibrium for each permeable substance $\mu_i = \mu_o$.

For substances not in equilibrium Gibbs suggested that the flux at any point x in the diffusion system would be proportional to both the concentration of the substance and the gradient of its chemical potential at that point. Flux is defined as that number of moles or ions passing in one second through an area 1 cm² at right angles to the direction of diffusion of that substance. For diffusion systems we write:

$$J = -UC\frac{d\mu}{dx} \tag{1}$$

where J is the flux, U the thermodynamic mobility and C the concentration, in moles. The negative sign is necessary because the flux is always down the chemical potential gradient.

Theoretical studies suggest that the relationship between μ and C of a non-ionic substance is

$$\mu = {}^*\mu + RT \ln C \tag{2}$$

${}^*\mu$ is the standard reference chemical potential; as with

all potential functions, values of μ must be related to some arbitrary reference state. The value of ${}^*\mu$ depends upon the solvent and it is important to stress that this relation applies to solute species only.

The flux of any non-ionic species diffusing in a single solvent is obtained by combining equations (1) and (2)

$$J = -UC\frac{d}{dx}({}^*\mu + RT \ln C) \tag{3}$$

and since ${}^*\mu$ is constant

$$J = -UC\frac{d}{dx}(RT \ln C) \tag{4}$$

this reduces to

$$J = -URT\frac{dC}{dx} \tag{5}$$

This is a theoretical derivation of Fick's experimental law for non-ionic solutes under similar conditions

$$J = -D\frac{dC}{dx} \tag{6}$$

where D is the diffusion coefficient. Hence for non-ionic solutes flux depends only on their concentration gradient.

For ionic solute species in a phase at a voltage E there is an additional energy of ZFE Joules/mole because of ionic charge, where Z is the valency number and F the faraday (coulomb/mole of charge). The chemical potential for ions is written formally:

$$\bar{\mu} = {}^*\mu + RT \ln C + ZFE \tag{7}$$

It is divided into a chemical and an electrical component and is commonly referred to as the **electrochemical potential** and given the symbol $\bar{\mu}$. In equation (7) the standard state ${}^*\mu$ depends on the solvent of the phase but not on the electrical state.

As with non-ionic substances, the condition for equilibrium with permeable ions is that the electrochemical potential of any ion is the same in all phases. In the case of two phases i and o separated by a membrane, for any permeable ions $\bar{\mu}_i = \bar{\mu}_o$. Hence

$${}^*\mu_i + RT \ln C_i + ZFE_i = {}^*\mu_o + RT \ln C_o + ZFE_o \tag{8}$$

If the solvent is the same for each phase, then ${}^*\mu_i = {}^*\mu_o$ and rearrangement gives

$$E_i - E_o = \frac{RT}{ZF} \ln \frac{C_o}{C_i} \tag{9}$$

This is, of course, the Nernst equation for equilibrium given on p. 15.9. As set out there Z is omitted, because its value is 1 for Na^+ and K^+ but -1 for Cl^-.

For ionic diffusion systems the flux of any ion is

$$J = -UC\frac{d\bar{\mu}}{dx} \tag{10}$$

It is the simplicity of this expression which makes the concept of electrochemical potential so important. An ion always diffuses down its electrochemical potential gradient. However combining equations (7) and (10) gives the following expression for flux:

$$J = -UC\frac{d}{dx}(*\mu + RT\ln C + ZFE)$$

$$= -URT\frac{dC}{dx} - UCZF\frac{dE}{dx} \qquad (11)$$

Hence the flux of any ion is not only a function of its concentration gradient but also of the electrical potential gradient; these two gradients may act in opposition.

In these equations the ionic thermodynamic mobility U is not identical with the conventional ionic mobility U', as measured in solutions without concentration gradients. The relationship between U and U' is however linear and is $U = U'/F$. If the mobility factor is not clearly defined, apparent contradictions may arise in the details of equations used in electrophysiology.

Origin of the electrical potential in diffusion systems
Consider the ionic system in fig. 15.15 with 1 mol/l KCl and 1 mol/l NaCl in compartment (i) but 0·1 mol/l KCl

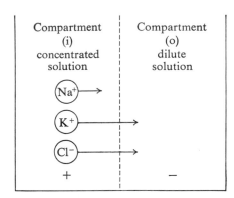

FIG. 15.15. Movements of ions in a diffusion zone.

and 0·1 mol/l NaCl in compartment (o). The barrier prevents mixing due to density differences and allows the formation of a diffusion zone without turbulence. For the moment any suggestion that it behaves as a selective membrane is not considered. When the cell is filled, Na$^+$ (mobility of 5·2 μsec volts^{-1} cm^{-1}) diffuses less rapidly from (i) to (o) than K$^+$ (mobility 7·6) or Cl$^-$ (mobility 7·9); for an instant, too short for practical measurement, there is an excess of Na$^+$ in compartment (i) and an excess of Cl$^-$ in compartment (o) giving rise to an electrical potential difference with a finite value across the interface between phases. The potential thus created opposes the movement of negative ions from (i) to (o) and aids the movement of positive ions. The excess of unmatched charge is very small, perhaps of the order of 10^{-12} mol in each compartment, and so cannot be detected by chemical means; only the electrical

effect is observable. At any given concentration of ions in each compartment and allowing free ionic diffusion in water from one compartment to the other, a unique diffusion potential $E_i - E_o$ is set up and at any region in the barrier the flux of any diffusing ion is given by equation 11. There is a diffusion rate for each ion from (i) to (o), which is for any ion at any instant a compromise between dC/dx and dE/dx. Such a system runs down in time. Ions diffuse from one compartment to the other until the composition of each is identical and $E_i - E_o$ is zero.

Once the idea of electrochemical potential and its relationship to chemical composition and electrical potential had been realized, it was an elementary step to devise the conditions for ionic equilibrium between phases and so to arrive at the Nernst equation. But is it equally possible using the flux equations to formulate a relationship between the diffusion potential ($E_i - E_o$) and the concentration of ions in compartments (i) and (o)? This intriguing problem roused the interest of many of the great men of science at the beginning of the twentieth century. Gibbs, Nernst, Planck and Einstein are all associated with attempted solutions, but the fact remains that without some simplifying assumption, either about concentration gradients or electrical potential gradient, no answer can be reached.

For electrophysiologists the most useful attempt is the Goldman equation (p. 15.11) published in 1943. This treatment assumes a layer between phases (o) and (i) where diffusion takes place, of width a (fig. 15.16). The

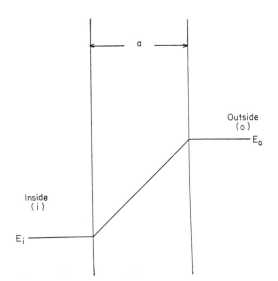

FIG. 15.16. The electrical gradient through a cell membrane.

simplifying assumption is that the gradient of electrical potential in this zone is linear, and that

$$\frac{dE}{dx} = \frac{E_i - E_o}{a} \qquad (12)$$

With this assumption it becomes possible to integrate the individual ionic flux equations. For example, for Na^+ the equation

$$J_{Na^+} = -U_{Na^+}RT\frac{d[Na^+]}{dx} - U_{Na^+}CF\frac{E_i - E_o}{a} \quad (13)$$

can now be integrated. If, as is usual, only the ions K^+, Na^+ and Cl^- are considered, the Goldman equation is obtained. It is now possible to define P, the permeability coefficient, precisely. For any ion P has the value URT/a, but as each ion species has a different U value, so it also has a different P value. P is not a permeability constant since in a biological membrane its value may change depending on the value of $E_i - E_o$. The Goldman equation was originally developed for a free diffusion zone. If a system is now considered where the barrier, like the biological membrane, has ion-selective properties, the value of U for any ion may be different depending upon whether the ion is in free solution outside the membrane or in a less well defined solution inside the membrane. But the Goldman integration still applies, although only from one inner surface of the membrane to the other inner surface, and values of $[K^+]$, $[Na^+]$ and $[Cl^-]$ must be those existing just on the insides of the membrane surface (fig. 15.17). These concentrations are not readily available, and the Goldman treatment has been modified by Hodgkin and Huxley using the membrane/solvent partition coefficient β for any ion. This is incorporated

Inside (i)	Membrane		Outside (o)
$[K^+]_i$ ⇌ $[K^+_{membrane}]_i$		$[K^+_{membrane}]_o$ ⇌ $[K^+]_o$	
$[Na^+]_i$ ⇌ $[Na^+_{membrane}]_i$		$[Na^+_{membrane}]_o$ ⇌ $[Na^+]_o$	
$[Cl^-]_i$ ⇌ $[Cl^-_{membrane}]_i$		$[Cl^-_{membrane}]_o$ ⇌ $[Cl^-]_o$	

FIG. 15.17. Ionic concentrations within and without the cell membrane $[K^+_{membrane}]_o = \beta[K^+]_o$, etc, see text.

into the permeability coefficient term. For example, if $[K^+_{membrane}]_o$ is the concentration of K^+ in the membrane at the interface membrane/outside solution, then $[K^+_{membrane}]_o = \beta [K^+]_o$. The permeability coefficient is then modified to $RTU_{K^+}\beta/a$. With this new value for P the Goldman equation retains its original form for membrane systems, and ionic concentrations are still those inside and outside the cell. This newly defined P may be measured experimentally for some ions, using the measured values for the resting potential and the flux of the radioactive ion across the membrane.

It has been shown by Hogg that the Goldman equation applies to PD gradients across the membrane which are antisymmetrical (fig. 15.18) about a plane at the midpoint of the membrane. This is theoretically more satisfying

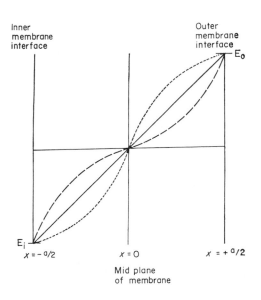

FIG. 15.18. Antisymmetric potential changes about membrane midplane.

than the narrow restriction of a linear potential change across the membrane.

Any change in the values of P for a membrane, for any ion, gives a different value of $E_i - E_o$ even without gross changes in the concentrations of ions in either phase.

Summary

In the previous section it was shown that:

(1) any ion in equilibrium across a membrane obeys the Nernst equation (p. 15.9);

(2) if the system is not in equilibrium but is a diffusion system, the value of the electrical potential across the membrane $(E_i - E_o)$ for any set of conditions is given by the Goldman equation (p. 15.11). It was stressed that the permeability coefficient of the membrane (P) to any ion is not constant, but may vary with the value of $E_i - E_o$, e.g. changes in the ionic concentration outside the cell may produce changes in the value of P for any ion. This makes interpretation of experimental data difficult;

(3) changes in the permeability coefficient of any one ion produce changes in the value of $E_i - E_o$ without changes which are detectable by chemical methods in either the internal or external concentrations of that ion. Fig. 15.19 may help in understanding how an increase in the value of P for each of the ions Na^+, K^+ and Cl^- affects the value of the transmembrane potential.

The resting potential in the diagram is that for frog sartorius muscle, although the changes are true for other systems. With the normal concentrations of ions outside and inside the cell, an increase in P_{Na^+} makes the resting potential more positive, i.e. it moves its value towards zero and may even put it into the positive region. Increases

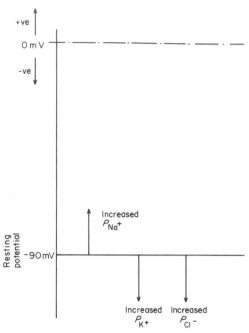

FIG. 15.19. The effect of changes in permeability coefficient on resting potential.

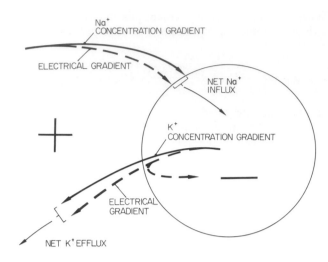

FIG. 15.20. Effect of concentration and electrical gradients on the diffusion of Na^+ and K^+.

in P_{K^+} and P_{Cl^-} make the resting potential more negative. The changes may be calculated from the Goldman equation. In the case of a general increase in P_{Na^+}, P_{K^+} and P_{Cl^-}, the trend is to make the transmembrane potential less negative (more positive). This is not immediately obvious from the Goldman equation but is an experimental fact. One must assume that the effect of an increase in P_{Na^+} is greater than the combined effects of increasing P_{K^+} and P_{Cl^-}. The summary of information about changes in permeability coefficients in fig. 15.19 is needed to understand the electrophysiology of the action potential, pre- and post-synaptic potentials and the neuromuscular junction.

Active transport

So far the biological cell has been examined only in terms of established physicochemical theories and the transmembrane potential explained as a diffusion potential. Equation (11) shows that in passive diffusion an ion has a flux down its concentration gradient and this flux may be increased or decreased by the electrical potential gradient. In nerve and muscle cells the flux direction for Na^+ is obvious. Both concentration and electrical gradient drive Na^+ into the cell. The case for K^+ is more complex. Here the concentration gradient helps to drive K^+ out of the cell, but the positively charged K^+ is attracted towards the negative charge inside the cell. However to compensate completely for the driving force due to the concentration gradient the transmembrane potential would have to be -89 mV (table 15.2) and not

the observed -60 mV. Potassium ions therefore diffuse out of the cell (fig. 15.20). Obviously such a system would run down, internal and external ionic concentrations becoming identical when the potential would fall to zero. As the internal ionic composition of the cell remains constant, we must postulate that in the framework of the membrane there is an active transport system which pumps out Na^+ and pumps in K^+, and so compensates for losses by passive diffusion. Fig. 15.21 represents such

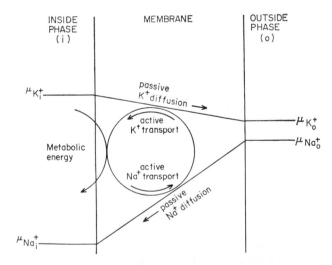

FIG. 15.21. Model of a membrane ionic pump.

a system, in which a pump compensates for the influx of Na^+ and the efflux of K^+. Such a mechanism working against chemical and electrical gradients, i.e. the electrochemical potential gradients, requires energy. Experimentally it has been established that this energy is supplied by the metabolic processes of the cell.

If a cell is poisoned with dinitrophenol (DNP), the formation of ATP is blocked and this decreases the rate at which Na^+ is extruded from the interior of the squid axon. An axon can be loaded with ^{24}Na by stimulating it in the radioactive solution; if it is then placed in an extracellular fluid containing no ^{24}Na, the rate at which the ^{24}Na leaves the axon is easily measured by counting the radioactivity in the extracellular fluid. The addition of DNP markedly decreases the rate at which ^{24}Na is extruded from the axon (fig. 15.22). When the DNP

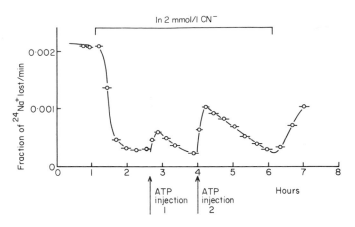

FIG. 15.23. The effect of injecting two different amounts of ATP into an axon poisoned with cyanide; injection 1 raised the ATP concentration in the axon by 1·2 mmol/l and injection 2 by 6·2 mmol/l. From Hodgkin (1964).

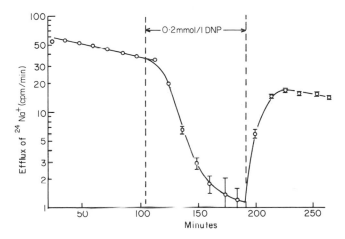

FIG. 15.22. Sodium efflux from a Sepia axon during treatment with dinitrophenol. At the beginning and end of the experiment the axon was in artificial sea water. Abscissa: time after end of stimulation in ^{24}Na sea water. Ordinate: rate at which ^{24}Na leaves axon. Unbroken vertical lines are $\pm 2 \times$ S.E. Temperature 18°C. From Hodgkin (1964).

is removed from the medium, Na^+ is extruded at the original rate, when allowance has been made for the decreasing concentration of ^{24}Na inside the axon. That the reaction $ATP \longrightarrow ADP + \Delta G$ is an essential step in the active extrusion of Na^+ is shown by poisoning an axon with cyanide. Cyanide blocks the oxidative processes necessary for the formation of ATP and the rate of extrusion of Na^+ from the cell drops, but rises again when ATP is injected into the axon (fig. 15.23).

Experiments with ^{42}K have shown that when the cell is poisoned, the influx of K^+ also decreases and this led to the concept of a Na^+/K^+ linked pump. More exact measurements, however, show that in some cells the 1:1 ratio between these ions does not hold. The attractive theory that for each Na^+ actively transported out of the cell a K^+ is transported in is an oversimplification. A detailed study of the contribution to the system by Cl^- is needed, but the half life of ^{35}Cl is so short (37 min) that experimental studies are difficult to carry out.

An enzyme which hydrolyses ATP to ADP was first identified in the membranes of red blood corpuscles and is known as **adenosine triphosphatase** or **ATPase**. It is

probably present in all cell membranes and is activated by a rise in either $[Na^+]_i$ or $[K^+]_o$, and by Mg^{++} in the presence of Na^+. It is inhibited by digoxin and other cardiac glycosides which inhibit the transport of Na^+ against a gradient. An $(Na^+ + K^+)$ activated ATPase has now been isolated from all tissues in which an active transport of Na^+ and K^+ is known to occur and it is probably responsible for the directional pumping of Na^+ and K^+ in all cells.

While this concept of the ionic state of the cell may be modified in the future, the idea of a diffusion system generating a transmembrane potential, and an active transport maintaining a constant ionic cell composition, is likely to persist.

The energy required is provided by metabolic processes that go to make up the resting metabolism. What proportion of the energy utilization by resting man goes to maintain ionic concentrations cannot be calculated.

Nerve impulse

Information is transmitted along nerves by means of a voltage change, which is of uniform shape in unmyelinated nerves. Because the frequency and the velocity at which nervous impulses are transmitted are both limited, the biological method differs in several respects from the methods used in telecommunication. Nevertheless, electrical engineering techniques and theory illustrate some points in the relation between structure and function in the nerve axons. Since the axon consists of an inner conducting medium separated from an outer extracellular conducting medium, it may be compared with the co-axial cable (fig. 15.24) used to join a television aerial to the set. Much time and thought has gone into the designing of cables which transmit complex voltage wave forms with a minimum voltage loss or distortion.

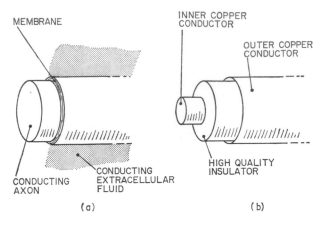

FIG. 15.24. Comparison of the structure of an axon (a) and a cable (b).

CABLE THEORY

A theoretical model of a co-axial cable is shown in fig. 15.25. Each unit of length (i) of the inner conductor has a resistance r_i. The inner conductor is separated from the outer one by an insulator. No insulator has infinite resistance and the leakage resistance across a unit length is r_m. The two conductors separated by an insulator form a condenser with capacity (C_m). If a square current pulse

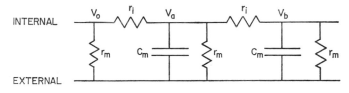

FIG. 15.25. The electrical properties of a cable.

(I_0) is injected into the cable at o, the recorded voltage pulse decreases the further along the cable it goes and at points $a, b, \ldots, n$ $V_a, V_b, \ldots, V_n$ become progressively less. The pulse wave also changes its shape and is no longer square, but the rising edge is curved in an exponential manner, as is the falling edge (fig. 15.26). Using the ratio V_0/V_n and the distance required for V_0 to reach V_n, it is possible to calculate values for r_i, r_m and C_m. V_0 decreases exponentially and the distance required for it to fall to $1/e$ ($e = 2\cdot73$) is known as the characteristic length λ and equals $\sqrt{r_m/r_i}$. In the squid axon λ is about 3 mm and so all voltage and current would have disappeared long before the end of the axon, if it behaved as a co-axial cable. Obviously transmission in nerves cannot be explained solely in terms of electrical engineering. For a motor neurone in the spinal cord of an adult man which gives off an axon which reaches the big toe, about one metre away, a different conducting process is necessary.

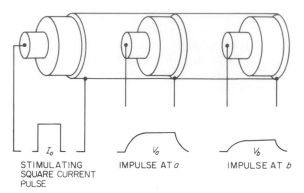

FIG. 15.26. The change in form of recorded voltage pulse during transmission in a cable.

ACTION POTENTIAL

On applying an increasing electrical stimulus to a nerve fibre, at first only the local changes to be expected in a co-axial cable (electronic effects) are recorded. Then a new mechanism, unknown to electrical engineers, is observed. If a voltage pulse (fig. 15.27) is applied to an axon,

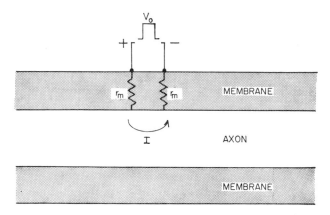

FIG. 15.27. Diagram showing the current (I) from an external stimulus flowing through the membrane and inside the axon.

current flows from the positive to the negative electrode. Some of this current (I) flowing through the membrane resistance decreases the transmembrane potential, i.e. it depolarizes the membrane. When this current is sufficiently great to change the potential from about -60 mV to -40 mV, a change takes place in the physical properties of the membrane. In the region of stimulation the permeability to sodium (P_{Na^+}) suddenly increases, and Na^+, with their positive charge, cross the membrane into the cell. The number of ions involved is minute and may be as small as 10^{-16} mol/cm length. This has very little effect on the $[Na^+]$ of the interior of the axon and cannot be detected chemically, but the electrical effect is easily observed. The movement of Na^+ further changes the transmembrane potential until it is reversed, the inside

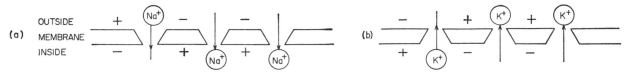

FIG. 15.28. (a) Na$^+$ entering the axon during the initial rising phase of the action potential, (b) K$^+$ leaving the axon during the final falling phase.

becoming positive relative to the outside (fig. 15.28a). A feedback now operates at the level of the single cell membrane which serves to limit this potential change. Hodgkin and Huxley showed that the voltage change across the membrane caused by the increase in P_{Na}^+ induces an increase in P_K^+ and that an outflow of K$^+$ restores the transmembrane potential to its pre-excitation value (fig. 15.28b). The movements of ions resulting from these changes in P_K^+ and P_{Na}^+ account for the changes in transmembrane potential across an axon when it is stimulated locally. The local electrical potential rises from -60 mV to about $+20$ mV and back again to -60 mV. This change is called an **action potential** or **spike potential** (fig. 15.29). This transmembrane voltage change is transmitted along the axon in an undistorted form and at a velocity much less than that at which any physical voltage impulse would be passed in a co-axial cable.

Although the experimental technique for depolarizing the membrane may seem artificial, in fact the physiological initiation of a nerve impulse is brought about by such a depolarization. In afferent nerve fibres this arises from sensory receptor cells, as a result of specific responses to changes in the body's internal or external environments; in efferent fibres the voltage is generated within the motor neurone by the action of the afferent nerves at the synapse. How this biological voltage change is transmitted must now be considered.

Once a local depolarization of the membrane has taken place, the situation arises where in effect two batteries are joined in series. Local currents flow in the directions shown by the arrows (fig. 15.30a). These local currents passing through the membrane depolarize it in the same manner as does an artificial stimulus. So a region of reversed polarity passes down the axon (fig. 15.30b). The velocity is slow, in terms of physical conduction, being about 15 m/sec; in the squid giant axon in general in unmyelinated axons the velocity of transmission is roughly proportional to the axon diameter. When two pairs of glass microelectrodes are used to measure the transmembrane potential, the action potential can be detected on an oscilloscope as it passes each point (fig. 15.31). The stimulus artefact is a voltage change induced physically in the recording system at the instant of stimulation. On the oscilloscope screen the distance between this artefact and the action potential is a measure of the time it takes for the action potential to reach the recording electrodes. This time, **the latent period** is illustrated for the two sets of

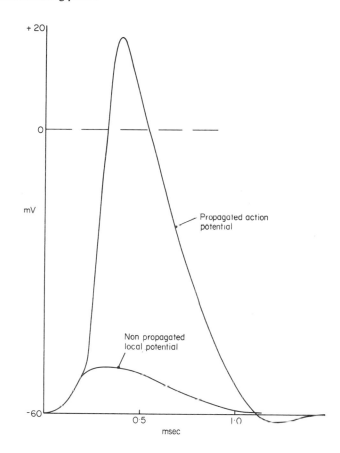

FIG. 15.29. Transmembrane voltage changes measured near the point of stimulation. A subthreshold stimulus produces local changes which are not propagated. A threshold stimulus produces a propagated action potential.

electrodes A and B in fig. 15.31. The latent period increases with the distance from the point of stimulation; such observations are used to calculate the velocity of conduction in nerves.

After the passage of the action potential there is a brief period of time, of the order 0·5 msec, during which it is impossible to stimulate the axon. This period is known as the **absolute refractory period**.

THEORY OF THE ACTION POTENTIAL

Confirmation for the theory that the origin of the action potential is a function solely of the interplay between sodium and potassium permeability has been given by

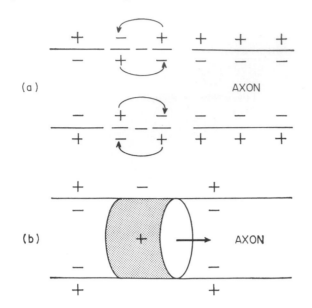

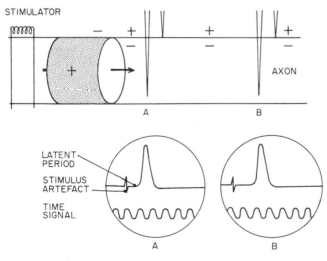

FIG. 15.30. (a) Local currents inside and outside the axon, (b) passage of reversed polarity down the axon.

FIG. 15.31. The action potential recorded at two different sites, A and B, on a nerve.

Hodgkin and Huxley. Direct measurement of P_{Na^+} and P_{K^+} is not possible in the millisecond taken for the nerve impulse. Instead, a new quantity, the **membrane conductance** (g) to these ions, which is more readily measured, has been defined on the basis of an empirical model of the membrane. However, Gibbs had already laid the theoretical foundations for such a model.

Equation (11) (p. 15.12) gives the flux for any ion and multiplying by ZF gives the current I carried by that ion

$$I = ZFJ = -URTZF\frac{dC}{dx} - UCZ^2F^2\frac{dE}{dx}$$

and rearranging

$$I \cdot \frac{1}{UCZ^2F^2} = -\frac{RT}{ZF}\frac{1}{C}\frac{dC}{dx} - \frac{dE}{dx} \qquad (14)$$

Integrating from the outside to the inside of the membrane and multiplying by dx, the equation becomes

$$I\int_0^1 \frac{dx}{UCZ^2F^2} = -\frac{RT}{ZF}\int_0^1 \frac{1}{C}.dC - \int_0^1 dE$$

On the right hand side both integrals are readily solved and this gives

$$I\int_0^1 \frac{dx}{UCZ^2F^2} = -\frac{RT}{ZF}\log_e\frac{C_i}{C_o} - (E_i - E_o)$$

or

$$I\int_0^1 \frac{dx}{UCZ^2F^2} = E_{\text{Nernst}} - E_{\text{membrane}} \qquad (15)$$

where E_{Nernst} is the equilibrium potential for the ion (p. 15.9), and E_{membrane} the cell transmembrane potential. On the right side the expressions are in terms of electrical voltage only, while on the left current is multiplied by an integral, which cannot be immediately evaluated, but by Ohm's Law it must have the dimensions of resistance and $\int_0^1 \frac{dx}{UCZ^2F^2}$ becomes the transmembrane resistance for any ion being considered. Taking Na^+ as an example we may write

$$I_{Na^+}(R_{Na^+}) = E_{\substack{Na^+ \\ \text{Nernst}}} - E_{\text{membrane}} \qquad (16)$$

Fig. 15.32 gives the electrical analogue to this equation.

The Hodgkin model is based on a number of ionic units of this type (fig. 15.33). For Na^+ the positive pole of the Nernst potential is directed towards the inside of the cell and for K^+ to the outside of the cell. Hodgkin also added another system (L, fig. 15.33) for the flux of ions other than

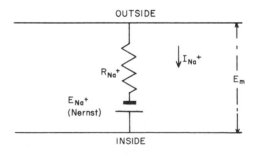

FIG. 15.32. Electrical analogue for the current flow by Na^+ through the membrane. $E_m = E_{\text{membrane}}$.

Na^+ and K^+. At the moment little is known about the contribution of these other ions; the most important are Ca^{++} and Cl^-, but neither of these alter the conclusions about the interplay between the permeability of Na^+ and K^+.

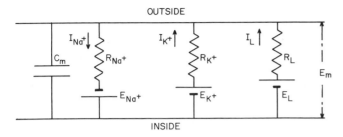

FIG. 15.33. The Hodgkin model for membrane ionic currents.

For squid axon in the resting state there can be no net flow of current across the cell membrane, i.e. any current carried into the cell by an ion must be equal and opposite to that carried out of the cell by other ions. It is now necessary to look more closely at the concept of membrane conductance. Equation (16) may be rewritten as

$$I_{Na^+} = \frac{1}{R_{Na^+}} \left(E_{\substack{Na^+ \\ Nernst}} - E_{membrane} \right) \quad (17)$$

and the quantity $1/R_{Na^+}$ is called the **conductance,** which is the inverse of resistance, and given the symbol g_{Na^+} expressed as mho. Any permeable ion has its own membrane conductance. We have already seen (p. 15.13) that the greater the value of the thermodynamic mobility for any ion the greater the permeability to that ion. Equations (15) and (16) relate g to the thermodynamic mobility as

$$g = \frac{UZ^2F^2}{\int_0^1 dx/C} \quad (18)$$

During the passage of an action potential the ionic concentration in the membrane does not change appreciably. Therefore any change in ionic mobility (U) is directly proportional to conductance; but permeability is also directly proportional to U (p. 15.13). Therefore during the action potential the behaviour of g reflects changes in P, and hence $P \propto g$. Experimental studies of the quantity g use the technique known as the **voltage clamp.**

The voltage clamp experiment changes the transmembrane potential along the entire axon to some predetermined value and maintains the axon at that value. In theory this can be done as shown in fig. 15.34. A

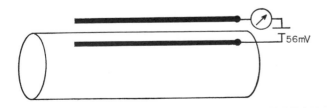

FIG. 15.34. Arrangement for a voltage clamp experiment.

battery of negligible internal resistance and of electrical potential 56 mV is connected suddenly to two lengths of silver wire, extending the full length of the axon internally and externally. In practice, because of electrode resistance and resistance of the extracellular and intracellular phases a more elaborate electronic feedback circuit is required for studies on animal cells, but a simple battery and very low resistance electrode system has been used with large cylindrical plant cells. Effectively the transmembrane potential has now been set at -56 mV. The value -56 mV is taken to illustrate one experiment; a series of experiments entails clamping the membrane to a range of such voltages. Fig. 15.35 shows that the problem at

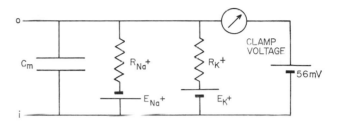

FIG. 15.35. Electrical circuit with a voltage clamp.

a physical level should be a simple demonstration of Kirchoff's Laws. The addition of the extra 56 mV battery gives a new current distribution in the circuit. If the values of R_{Na^+} and R_{K^+} remain constant, current flows in only one direction and there is no possibility in such a physical analogue of a reversal, at any time, of current flow. However, when an experiment of this kind is applied to a length of squid axon immersed in artificial extracellular fluid the results, as shown in fig. 15.36, suggest

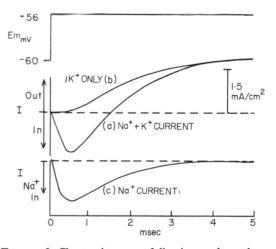

FIG. 15.36. Changes in current following a voltage clamp.

that once more physics or physical chemistry cannot be applied in their most elementary form to the biological membrane. Clamping the transmembrane potential to

−56 mV shows (fig. 15.36a) that for the first 1·5 msec current (*I*) flows into the cell, reaching a maximal influx at about 0·5 msec, returning to zero, and after 1·5 msec current flows out of the cell, the value increasing to a steady 1·5 mA/cm² for as long as this particular clamping voltage is applied. Hence the membrane system cannot be a simple physical arrangement as in fig. 15.35. The only possible interpretation is that the values of R_{Na^+} and R_{K^+} are changing during the time course of the experiment. That this is so has been demonstrated by Hodgkin and Huxley. They repeated the experiment using an extracellular fluid with the sodium replaced by choline, an ion which cannot traverse the membrane but does maintain osmolality. Fig. 15.36b shows that on applying the clamping voltage there is no inward flow of current, but a slow increase of outflowing current to a similar maximal value after about 3 msec. It was suggested from this experiment that the inward flow of current was caused by Na^+ and the outward flow by K^+, and that subtracting curve (b) from (a) would give the sodium current (c). Experiments of this type allow calculations from I_{Na^+} and I_{K^+} of how the conductance (*g*) of each ion varies with time. These show that g_{Na^+} increases to reach a maximum at about 0·5 msec and then returns to its original value within 3 msec and that g_{K^+} increases more slowly, reaching a maximum and keeping that value at about 5 msec (fig. 15.37). Thus g_{Na^+} and g_{K^+}

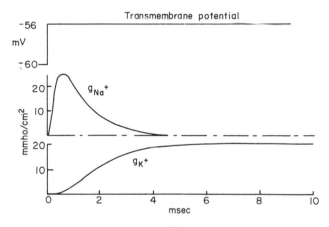

FIG. 15.37. Changes in conductance following a voltage clamp; mmho/cm² is the unit of conductance.

are not only functions of transmembrane potential, but also of the time during which such a potential is applied. Hodgkin and Huxley have studied the relationships of g_{Na^+} and g_{K^+} with time for a number of clamped transmembrane potentials in the squid axon, and derived a complex equation which describes changes in g_{Na^+} and g_{K^+} once the squid axon is depolarized. An equation has also been derived relating the theoretical change in *V* against time for the transmembrane potential, if

the squid axon is depolarized sufficiently to initiate an action potential. From this the shape and size of the action potential can be calculated, and the velocity of propagation worked out. There is little doubt that the transmission of an action potential involves changes in g_{Na^+} followed by changes in g_{K^+}. The calculated changes of these, and the calculated shape and duration of the transmitted action potential are given in fig. 15.38. The

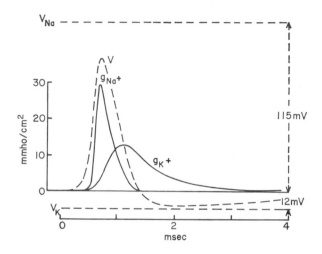

FIG. 15.38. Theoretical solution for propagated action potential and conductances at 18·5°C. Total entry of sodium = 4·33 pmol/cm²; total exit of potassium = 42·26 pmol/cm². From Hodgkin A.L. & Huxley A.F. (1952). *J. Physiol.* **117**, 500.

correlation between the calculated properties of the action potential and the observed experimental values is perhaps one of the most outstanding examples of the application of chemistry and physics to biology. The Na^+/K^+ permeability theory can account for both the origin and transmission of the voltage change, known as the action potential.

The all or none rule

Provided that the duration of the stimulating pulse is sufficiently long, the propagation of an action potential begins at a critical value of stimulating voltage, below which there is no propagation. Further increase of voltage does not change the shape of the propagated action potential, not does it alter the conduction velocity or the refractory period. The action potential follows an all or none rule, i.e. if the voltage is just sufficient to generate it, the response is maximal and in no way changed by a further increase of the stimulus.

Duration of the action potential

It is of interest to calculate the length of the squid axon occupied by the passage of a single action potential. If the velocity is 15 m/sec and the duration of the impulse is

1 msec, the length of the axon occupied, like that of a train running past the platform of a station, will be

$$\text{velocity} \times \text{duration}$$

which in this case is 1·5 cm. This may seem a surprising length of nerve to be occupied by the action potential, but in human motor nerve axons up to 10 cm may be taken up by the passage of a single action potential.

MEMBRANE STRUCTURE

An interpretation of membrane structure based on the Hodgkin and Huxley analysis has been described as electromechanical. Such an interpretation is both correct and unfair, ignoring as it does the many clues implied or stated in the model which have helped to interpret later work, using biochemical analysis, X-ray diffraction, electron microscopy and nuclear magnetic techniques.

Fig. 15.33 is relevant to an understanding of membrane structure. It suggests the membrane as a capacitance (which can be measured experimentally) short-circuited by pathways selectively conducting Na$^+$ and K$^+$. This selectivity is experimentally verified by the voltage clamp experiment, and by experiments using specific poisons. Thus tetrodotoxin, a poison isolated from the puffer fish, stops Na$^+$ currents in the membrane, but is effective only if applied to the outside of the squid axon membrane; and tetraethylammonium ions block K$^+$ currents, but are effective only inside the squid axon membrane.

The Hodgkin and Huxley analysis of Na$^+$ and K$^+$ conductance during the action potential used rate constants to describe an opening and closing of the Na$^+$ conducting pathway and an opening of the K$^+$ conducting pathway. This is consistent with the idea that the conducting channels may be controlled by gates, possibly formed by protein molecules, which control the entry of Na$^+$ and exit of K$^+$, and which change their configuration with electric field strength across the membrane.

A compromise diagram of the cell membrane is shown in fig. 10.18. Here a phospholipid bimolecular layer acts as an insulator and is responsible for the membrane capacitance. The protein phases outside and inside the membrane have complex functions. Some give the membrane structural stability, while others penetrate the membrane and may form the channels, which allow ionic diffusion, and also the specialized gates. Protein molecules which partly penetrate the membrane form part of active transport systems for either ionic or non-ionic substances. Nuclear magnetic resonance studies have shown that the membrane is not a static system; its structure changes continually and the system is in fact fluid.

MEMBRANE PUMPS

In fig. 15.21 the fact that Na$^+$ are pumped out of the cell and K$^+$ pumped in is represented in very schematic form. In fact such active transport, driven by metabolic energy, is a more complex problem and presents another membrane challenge. It appears to contradict a basic law of physics (Curie's Law) which states that in a homogeneous system, chemical energy cannot impart directional (vectorial) transport to any of the reactants. A qualitative solution to the problem would seem to lie in the fact that we now assume the membrane to be very inhomogeneous.

As an example it is suggested that one of the penetrating lipoproteins is part of an ATPase enzyme system, and that part of the energy-bonding process for ATP requires Na$^+$ from the inside of the cell, but hydrolysis needs K$^+$ from the outside. The fixed orientation of the ATPase within the membrane imparts the required vectorial (directional) properties needed for ionic transport.

CONDUCTION IN MYELINATED FIBRES

In these myelin is present in regions round the axon, but the nodes of Ranvier are left unmyelinated (p. 15.5). The result is an interesting compromise between the biological mechanism of transmission and that of the co-axial cable. The thick myelin sheath increases the transmembrane resistance and decreases the transmembrane capacitance so that the myelinated regions of an axon behave as a co-axial cable (fig. 15.39). At a node transmission takes

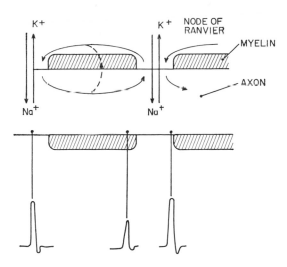

FIG. 15.39. Saltatory conduction. An action potential at a node causes a local current to flow down the interior of the axon. A small part of this current leaks through the myelin and the potential is attenuated. Sufficient current reaches the next node to depolarize it and so regenerate the full action potential.

place as already described in the unmyelinated squid axon. When an action potential is generated at one node, then local currents tend to flow at the next node and depolarize it. The action potentials thus jump from one node to the next, i.e. **saltatory conduction**. However, between nodes the nerve behaves as a co-axial conductor and the velocity of conduction approximates to that in engineered cable, i.e. 0·7 to 0·9 × speed of light.

The shape and size of the action potential between the nodes follows physical laws and is attenuated, i.e. the height decreases and the shape is distorted, but the voltage change at each node remains sufficient to bring about the same change in membrane ionic permeability to regenerate the action potential. Conduction in myelinated nerves is not unlike transmission in a transatlantic cable, containing amplifiers sunk at intervals so that they can restore the shape and form of the impulses before there is serious attenuation. Up to three nodes can be blocked before conduction ceases. There is an inbuilt safety factor.

EXTERNAL RECORDING OF THE ACTION POTENTIAL

It is possible to use intracellular microelectrodes to study transmission only in large nerve axons. In most nerves the action potential can be recorded only by placing silver electrodes on the surface of the axon. Fig. 15.40 shows the electrical events, recorded at external electrodes, as the action potential passes down an axon. Such a record is a diphasic action potential. In practice it is difficult to obtain the symmetry suggested in the figure because the zone of altered polarity may overlap both recording electrodes. A better record is obtained if the axon membrane is crushed between the electrodes, thereby destroying the membrane, but keeping the electrical continuity of the axoplasm (fig. 15.40f). Then only the first phase of the action potential is recorded, because the zone of altered polarity cannot reach the second electrode. Conventionally the direction in which the oscilloscope beam is displaced is reversed when recording the external monophasic action potential. This record must not be confused with that recorded from internal electrodes. In these, as we have seen, the potential changes from about -60 mV to about $+20$ mV and returns to the original value, i.e. it is positive going. With external recording the potential changes from 0 mV to a negative value, the size of which depends on the geometry of the axon, and back to 0 mV, i.e. it is negative going.

The technique of recording externally from single axons has been widely used with fibres carefully dissected from mixed nerves.

EXTERNALLY RECORDED ACTION POTENTIALS FROM MIXED NERVES

Fig. 15.41 shows a record obtained by stimulating a frog sciatic nerve with a gradually increasing stimulus. The record is a summation of a number of responses from different axons. With a small stimulus only a few of the large axons respond. With increasing stimulus more and more of the large fibres respond until a maximum is

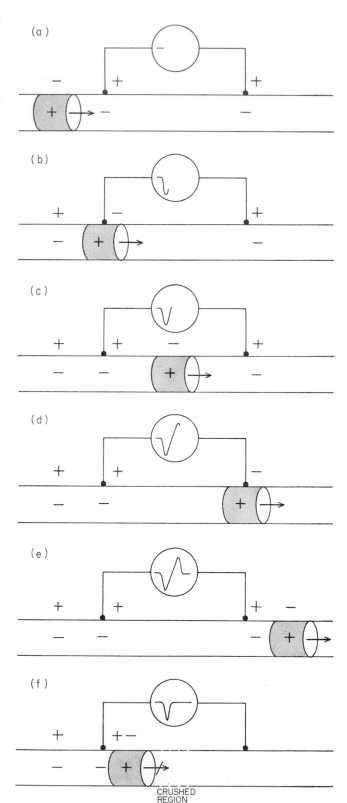

FIG. 15.40 (a–e). Electrical events recorded by surface electrodes as an impulse passes down an axon; (*f*) the effect of crushing the axon.

reached (e) and further small increases (f and g) produce no change in the size or shape of the response. This is because more and more of the large fibres conduct until all become active. Only a much larger increase in stimulus excites the smaller fibres.

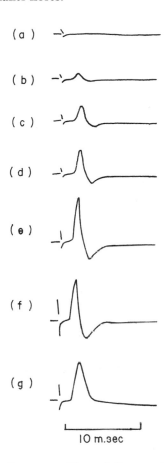

(a)

(b)

(c)

(d)

(e)

(f)

(g)

10 m.sec

FIG. 15.41. Response of frog sciatic nerve to gradually increasing strength of stimulus. From Bures J., Petran M. & Zachar J. (1967) *Electrophysiological Methods in Biological Research*, 3rd Revised Edition. New York: Academic Press.

The speed of conduction of the impulse depends on the diameter of the fibre, being slowest in the small ones (fig. 15.42). Hence the electrical changes produced in the small fibres reach the recording electrodes after those produced in the large fibres. The result is a **compound action potential** (fig. 15.43) in which three distinct peaks may be seen.

Fibre size and speed of conduction

A large nerve bundle contains fibres which vary in diameter from < 1 to 22 μm. For mammalian medullated fibres at 37°C the speed of conduction in m/sec is approximately 6 times the diameter measured in μm. Both fibre size and speed of conduction are used to classify nerve fibres.

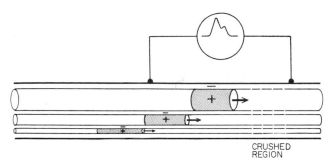

FIG. 15.42. The separation of the action potential of fibres of different size.

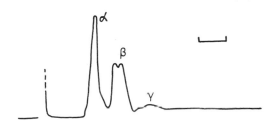

FIG. 15.43. A compound action potential recorded from frog sciatic nerve, showing the α, β and γ components of the A wave. Time scale 5 msec. From Bures J., Petran M. & Zachar J. (1967).

The compound action potential shows three waves A, B, C. The major A wave is the contribution of the large rapidly-conducting fibres and these include the ordinary motor neurone fibres running to muscle. Conduction rates range from 15 to 120 m/sec in this group, which is further subdivided into α, β and γ fibres. The γ fibres are the smallest and slowest conducting fibres running to striated muscle (fig. 15.43).

The B wave arises from fibres with a speed of 3–15 m/sec and are efferent preganglionic sympathetic fibres. C fibres are unmyelinated and conduct slowly at 0·5–1 m/sec.

Experimentally it is difficult to demonstrate the existence of the B and C waves in student practical classes. Large stimulating voltages are required because of their

TABLE 15.3. Classification of sensory fibres.

Group	Diameter (μm)	From
I	12–20	Muscle spindles and Golgi tendon organs
II	8–9	Skin; some fibres from muscle spindles
III	3–4	Various sources
IV	1·5	Various sources

small size and a logarithmic time base display is needed because of their slow conduction.

A different classification, which depends on fibre diameter and not on conduction velocity, is generally used for sensory fibres. Fibres of different size usually carry information from different sources (table 15.3).

RELATIVE AND ABSOLUTE REFRACTORY PERIOD

If a frog sciatic nerve preparation is stimulated twice then, provided the time interval between stimuli is sufficiently great, two identical action potentials are recorded (fig. 15.44a). If the time interval is then decreased in stages, the stimulus strength being kept constant, the height of the second action potential starts to fall (b). The

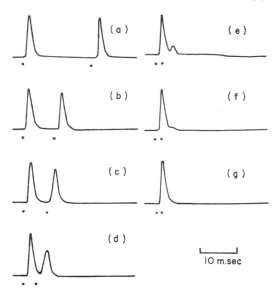

FIG. 15.44. The responses of a frog sciatic nerve to two identical stimuli separated by a decreasing interval of time (a–g). The spike amplitude from the second stimulus declines as the interval between the two stimuli is reduced. A measure of the absolute refractory period is provided by (g). From Bures J., Petran M. & Zachar J. (1967).

time between the stimuli at this point is the **relative refractory period**, and as the time interval is further decreased, the height continues to fall (c–f) and eventually disappears (g). At this point the second stimulus is said to fall within the **absolute refractory period**. During the absolute refractory period no increase in stimulus can produce a second action potential, but during the relative refractory period the size of the second action potential may be restored by increasing the strength of the second stimulus.

TRANSMISSION OF EXCITATION FROM CELL TO CELL

The electron microscope has shown that in vertebrates there appears to be no direct continuity between the end

of an axon and another nerve cell or cell of an effector organ such as muscle. The cytoplasm of the axon and of the excitable tissue to which the impulse is transmitted are each enclosed within their own membranes and these are separated by a gap. The nerve impulse has to cross this gap, and if, as seems likely, the electrical resistance and capacities of the junctional membrane and intercellular space possess the same properties as the nerve fibres, the action potential cannot cross it directly, the discontinuity of the junction is overcome by the liberation of a chemical substance which crosses the gap between the cells and stimulates or inhibits the next cell. This it does by altering the membrane permeability of the cell so as to set up or inhibit another potential, which in turn is transmitted onwards. The first example of chemical transmission was provided by the experiments of Otto Loewi in 1920. The heart is slowed by stimulating the vagus nerve and Loewi showed that if this is done with the heart of a frog, perfusion of the blood from this heart through the heart of a second frog causes it also to be slowed. He concluded that vagal stimulation liberated a substance, 'Vagusstoffe', which affected the excitability of cardiac muscle. It is now known that this substance is **acetylcholine.** The drug atropine causes the heart to beat faster by interfering with the action of acetylcholine at the nerve-muscle junction.

The heart is innervated by a second group of nerves which accelerate it, the sympathetic nerves. Loewi also showed that a similar 'accelerator substance' was liberated by sympathetic nerve stimulation. The similarity between the effect of sympathetic nerve stimulation and the actions of adrenaline, called by Cannon sympathin, had already been pointed out by Langley and Elliott at the turn of the century, and it is now clear that the accelerator substance is **noradrenaline**, a close derivative of adrenaline. The role of noradrenaline in neurotransmission is discussed in vol. 2, p. 15.16.

Neuromuscular transmission

NEUROMUSCULAR JUNCTION

Somatic efferent axons end upon the surfaces of skeletal muscle cells to form **end plates**. The neurones giving rise to these axons are the motor cells of the ventral horn of the spinal cord and of the cranial nerve nuclei. A nerve fibre after reaching a muscle enters the perimysium of the muscle before it terminates by bifurcating several times, each bifurcation occurring at a node of Ranvier. By this means, each motor neurone may innervate a number of muscle fibres which collectively form a motor unit (p. 16.10).

When the terminal branch of a motor nerve fibre reaches the muscle cell, it loses its myelin sheath and the axon expands on to the surface of the muscle in the form of a number of terminal arborizations to form the **motor end**

plate (figs. 15.45–15.47). At the end plate these short terminal branches lie in finger-like **synaptic gutters,** and there they are covered by thin extensions of the last

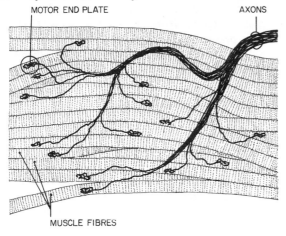

FIG. 15.45a. Skeletal muscle fibres, each showing a single motor end plate (neuromuscular junction). Low power.

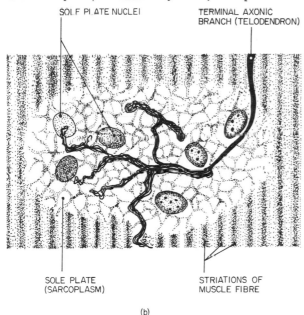

FIG. 15.45b. High power view (en face) of motor end plate indicated in fig. 15.45a. Redrawn after Cajal.

Schwann cell. At the bottoms of these synaptic gutters, the sarcolemma or plasma membrane of the muscle cell is thrown into a series of folds, the junctional folds, which run at right angles to the terminal branch of the nerve; these branch in such a way that when viewed from above they appear as a finger print. The sarcolemma at the tops of these folds is separated from the plasma membrane of the axon terminal by a distance of about 50 nm, and in the interval between the two plasma membranes there is an ill-defined layer, about 20 nm thick, that represents

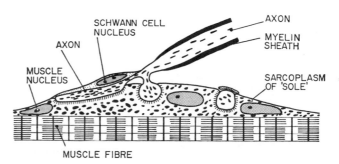

FIG. 15.46. Representation of a motor end plate as seen in longitudinal section. The terminal nerve branches lie in synaptic gutters in which the plasma membrane of the sarcolemma is thrown into folds. In the muscle fibre there is an accumulation of sarcoplasm, the sole, that contains many mitochondria and muscle cell nuclei. Modified from Couteaux R. (1959) *C. R. Acad. Sci.* **249**, 964.

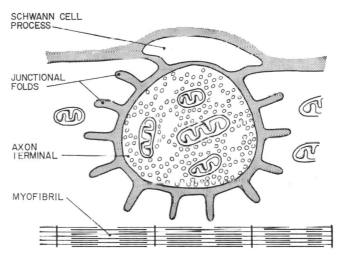

FIG. 15.47. Diagram of portion of a motor end plate to show the axon terminal lying within the synaptic gutter. The sarcolemma, which forms the junctional folds, is separated from the axon terminal by a distance of 50 nm.

the fused basal laminae of the muscle cell and axon (fig. 15.47).

The region of a muscle cell which receives the end of a nerve is called the sole. This is an elevation of muscle fibre characterized by an accumulation of sarcoplasm containing numerous mitochondria and nuclei. The junctional folds at the sole contain acetylcholinesterase (p. 15.26).

TRANSMISSION AT THE NEUROMUSCULAR JUNCTION

In those regions of the axon which lie in close proximity to the skeletal muscle cell there are many vesicles. These contain acetylcholine and it is thought that an action potential transmitted down each of the branches of the axon produces depolarization of the nerve ending and causes the vesicles to burst with an increased frequency at the surface of the axon terminal and so release their acetylcholine. This transmitter substance then diffuses across the gap between the axon terminal and the muscle fibre to react with specific receptor sites in the muscle membrane at the end plate, causing an increase in permeability to Na^+ and K^+ simultaneously and to other cations. This effect is only transient, for **acetylcholinesterase** located at the muscle cell surface quickly destroys the acetylcholine. The ionic movements resulting from the permeability increase cause the membrane potential in the end plate to become more positive (depolarized). An end plate potential (EPP) is set up and local currents flow, which are sufficient to depolarize the nearby muscle cell membrane to a point where the membrane permeability to Na^+ increases markedly; and at this region an action potential originates in the muscle cell and is generated by the processes previously described for the nerve axon. The duration of the action potential is longer and in skeletal muscle may be as much as 5 msec.

Experimental evidence

The classical preparation is the frog sartorius muscle with its attached nerve, but mammalian tissues have also been used. The transmission of the impulse across the neuro-muscular junction can be shown by placing a microelectrode between the nerve and the muscle at the point of junction. The potential generated in the nerve as the impulse arrives at the junction is distinct from the action potential in the post-junctional tissue which occurs 0·8 msec later. This delay indicates electrical discontinuity and strongly favours the idea of non-electrical transmission.

That the acetylcholine comes from the nerve and not as a result of the muscle contraction can be shown by adding eserine and curare to a nerve muscle preparation. Eserine, the active principle of the Calabar bean and used as an ordeal poison in West Africa, competitively inhibits the enzyme responsible for the destruction of acetylcholine. When the nerve is stimulated increasing quantities of acetylcholine can be detected in the perfusate. Curare is used as an arrow poison by Peruvian Indians and has the effect of paralysing the man or animal injured by the arrow. If the nerve of a curarized muscle-nerve preparation is stimulated, the muscle does not contract, but acetylcholine appears in the perfusate in amounts similar to those when contraction occurs.

That acetylcholine acts only on the end plate can be shown by applying it by a micropipette to the postsynaptic junction of a neuromuscular junction. Very small amounts (10^{-15} mol) of acetylcholine are able to excite a muscle fibre if applied directly on an end plate. Movement of the pipette a fraction of a millimetre or so to the surface of the muscle results in failure to induce a response.

There is no histochemical test for acetylcholine, but acetylcholinesterase can be detected histochemically and the brown reaction product formed is located at the end plates.

Acetylcholine is synthesized by choline acetyl transferase (acetylase) from choline and acetyl CoA. The enzyme is present in neurones whose axons liberate acetylcholine. It is manufactured in the cell bodies and is carried down the axon. When a cholinergic nerve fibre is

$$\text{Acetate} \rightleftharpoons \overset{\text{CoA}}{\underset{\text{Acetyl CoA}}{}} \rightleftharpoons \overset{\text{Acetylcholine}}{\underset{\text{Choline}}{}}$$

cut the enzyme is detectable at the cut end while the cell body becomes depleted. Acetylcholine is manufactured throughout the neurone but especially at terminal boutons and is rapidly replaced as it is secreted. The choline is continuously absorbed from the extracellular fluid by nerve endings and when sympathetic ganglia are suspended in a medium free of choline they soon become depleted of acetylcholine. The vesicles in the presynaptic nerve endings visible under the EM contain physiologically inactive acetylcholine.

Small amounts of acetylcholine are released from nerve endings even at rest. This is shown by the existence in resting muscle of spontaneous miniature EPPs which occur about once a second and do not fully depolarize the post-junctional membrane. When a nerve impulse reaches the prejunctional nerve terminal a large increase in the secretory rate occurs. By comparing the responses of acetylcholine applied to an end plate by ionophoresis it can be calculated that acetylcholine is released in quanta or packets containing thousands of molecules at a time.

Acetylcholine release is associated with the migration of Ca^{++} into the cytoplasm of the nerve terminal and the amount released is proportional to the concentration of Ca^{++} in the ECF. Magnesium ions have an effect opposite to Ca^{++}; increasing the Mg^{++} in the ECF depresses acetylcholine secretion.

Acetylcholine must be rapidly removed from the myoneural or synaptic junction if repolarization is to take place and an enzymatic mechanism to carry this out was postulated by Dale in 1914. Acetylcholine is hydrolysed extremely quickly by one of a series of enzymes called cholinesterases. Cholinesterases are found in red cells, nervous tissue and striated muscle and are responsible for the destruction of acetylcholine.

SPREAD OF THE IMPULSE IN MUSCLE

When an end plate potential reaches a sufficient level, it generates an action potential which spreads through the muscle fibre in a manner similar to the spread in a nerve fibre. There is a resting potential with the inside of the cell negative compared to the surface and the potential is due to the passage of Na$^+$ into the cell from the extracellular fluid. The shape of the action potential depends on the nature and position of the recording electrodes. In muscle it travels at a rate of several m/sec and is able to activate the contractile apparatus within the cell. In animals it is possible to record from intracellular electrodes as with the squid axon. It is also possible to record the electrical activity of human muscles.

The **electromyogram** can be obtained using an electrode about the size of a hypodermic needle which is inserted through the skin into the belly of the muscle; the electrode is insulated except at the tip. Recordings can also be made using surface electrodes on the skin. The activity so recorded comes in each case from many fibres, often composing several motor units (p. 16.11) whose nerve fibres may not be firing synchronously; hence it is not a precise record of the activity in any one fibre. There is little electrical activity from a resting muscle, although spontaneous random discharges may occur, but a burst of discharges arises whenever a muscle contracts voluntarily. Electromyography has a limited clinical application in the investigation of certain diseases of muscle and motor neurones. If simultaneous records can be made from several groups of muscles, these can be used to analyse the muscles employed and their timing in a complex movement. Golfers have had their swings studied in this way.

SMOOTH MUSCLE AND OTHER TISSUES
Their nerve fibres form plexuses within the viscera and there are dilations of the nerve fibres that contain vesicles but do not form synaptic junctions with the surrounding cells; the chemical transmitter is discharged into the surrounding extracellular space.

The electrical activity of smooth muscle varies greatly from time to time and from tissue to tissue. Spikes of potential can be recorded from the gut, but here and in other sites the potential changes are small and represent only partial depolarization. Stretching a smooth muscle depolarizes the membrane and may cause firing and subsequent contraction.

Smooth muscle may continue to function after it has been separated from its nerve supply. After the nerves to a skeletal muscle have been cut, the muscle is completely paralysed and is flaccid. Smooth muscle after section of the nerves may still contract and show electrical activity. The nerves regulate rather than initiate activity. Many smooth muscles have a double nerve supply, receiving one set of fibres which release acetylcholine and another set which release noradrenaline. These oppose each other, one being excitatory and the other inhibitory, but their roles in this respect differ in different parts of the body. Both the spontaneous activity of smooth muscle and the responses to nervous stimulation may be modified greatly by hormones and this is most marked in the case of uterine muscle. Activity of smooth muscle is also modified by local hormones, notably the prostaglandins.

FURTHER READING

BOURNE G.H. (1968–70) *The Structure and Function of Nervous Tissue*, vols. 1–6. New York: Academic Press.

COUTEAUX R. (1973) The motor end plate structure. In *The Structure and Function of Muscle*, 2nd Edition, vol. 2, pp. 483–530, ed. Bourne G.H. New York: Academic Press.

HODGKIN A.L. (1964) *The Conduction of the Nervous Impulse*. Liverpool: Liverpool University Press.

HOLMES R. ed. (1974) *Cells and their Ultrastructure*. S321, 1. *Membranes and Transport*. S321, 3 and 4. Milton Keynes: Open University.

KATZ B. (1966) *Nerve, Muscle and Synapse*. New York: McGraw-Hill.

NAUTA W.J.H. & EBBESSON S.O.E. eds. (1970) *Contemporary Research Methods in Neuroanatomy*. New York: Springer.

PAPPAS G.D. & PURPURA D.P. eds. (1972) *Structure and Function of Synapses*. New York: Raven Press.

PETERS A., PALAY S.L. & WEBSTER H. de F. (1976) *The Fine Structure of the Nervous System: the Neurons and Supporting Cells*. Philadelphia: Saunders.

Chapter 16
Contracting tissues

Apart from slow movements due to cilia and other cell processes, all motion in and of the body is the result of contraction in muscle cells. The finger movements of a violinist, the punch of a boxer, the beat of the heart, the expulsion of a fetus and the constriction and dilatation of the pupil of the eye illustrate the variety of these movements. Muscular tissues must be capable of contractions which are variable in speed, power and extent. Some of these tissues are under somatic nervous control and others are controlled by the autonomic nervous system or circulating hormones. Some normally contract only when stimulated by their nerve, while others have an inherent rhythmic contraction but this can be modified by external influences. These different contractile functions and methods of control are associated with differences in the structure of muscular tissues. The main differences lie in the shape, size and content of the muscle cells themselves. For reasons explained later, some muscle cells appear **striated** in the light microscope and others are **non-striated** or **smooth.**

It is useful to classify muscle into three types:

(1) **skeletal muscle** which appears striated and is under voluntary control,

(2) **cardiac muscle** which appears striated but is not under voluntary control, and

(3) **smooth muscle** which is not striated, is found in the viscera and is not under voluntary control.

In most mammals, including man, skeletal muscle makes up about half the body weight, contains more than half the body water and has an extracellular fluid content which is about one and a half times the volume of the blood plasma. When mild exercise is taken, such as walking at three and a half miles an hour (5·6 km/h), the oxygen consumption can increase to between five and six times the basal level. Thus the pattern of energy metabolism in the body is determined almost entirely by skeletal muscle.

STRUCTURE OF MUSCLE

SKELETAL MUSCLE (fig. 16.1a)

The cross-striated cells are very long, up to 10 cm. Some run from the origin of a muscle to its insertion. The diameter of these cylindrical cells is from 30–60 μm, and each contains thousands of nuclei, which usually lie near the surface of the cell. Each cell receives, near its centre, the termination of a spinal or cranial nerve fibre. At the site of the nerve ending, the muscle cell and the nerve combine to produce a complex structure, the myoneural junction or motor end plate (p. 15.24).

CARDIAC MUSCLE (fig. 16.1b)

These cells are much shorter than in skeletal muscle. They do not exceed 150 μm in length. They have an irregular shape and are often branched. Individual cells stick to their neighbours and so the whole muscle consists of a network. The points of adhesion between adjacent cells are called intercalated discs (p. 16.8). The cross striations are similar to those in skeletal muscle, but there are only one or two nuclei in each cell and these are near the centre.

Each of these cells has its own inherent rhythm but, since they are all joined together, the cell with the most rapid rhythm drives all the others. After an impulse has been produced, it spreads over the intercalated discs to affect the whole muscle. The fastest cells are usually located in the sinuatrial node (p. 30.13), but all the other cells are capable of driving the heart at slower rates, if the nodal cells are ineffective.

SMOOTH MUSCLE (fig. 16.1c)

These non-striated spindle-shaped cells are narrower than either of the other types. Usually they are about 200 μm long and less than 10 μm in diameter; in the pregnant uterus (p. 38.51) they increase to at least twice the normal size. One long ovoid nucleus occupies the middle of each cell.

All the smooth muscles are under the control of the autonomic nervous system, but the degree of control varies greatly. Some smooth muscle, like that in the pupil or the wall of the ductus deferens, is richly supplied with sympathetic and parasympathetic nerves, while other smooth muscle, e.g. in the intestinal wall, resembles cardiac muscle in having an inherent rhythm which is only modulated by its motor nerve supply. Smooth

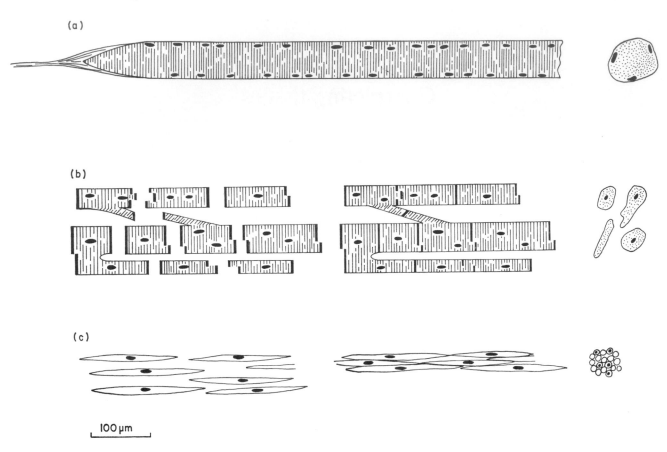

FIG. 16.1. Three types of muscle (a) part of a skeletal muscle in longitudinal (left) and transverse (right) section; (b) cardiac muscle cells artificially dissociated (left), normally linked (centre) and in tranverse section (right); (c) smooth muscle cells dissociated (left), normally linked (centre) and in cross section (right).

muscle is stimulated to contract by being stretched and this property accounts for much of its activity.

Muscular tissue also includes the connective tissues, lymphatic and blood vessels, motor nerves to the muscle and to the vessels, and sensory nerves from muscle spindles and Golgi tendon organs. The macroscopic arrangement of muscular tissues is described on p. 20.11. As the cells are always elongated, they are often called muscle fibres, but this term is confusing as it may be applied not to a single cell or line of cells, but also to the bundles of cells which can be seen with the naked eye. Also, in muscle the word fibre refers to a living cell while, in the connective tissues, it means the extracellular components which give the connective tissues their properties.

Muscle cell

It is convenient to consider the general design of a muscle cell, which includes the features found in all types of muscle. It has many of the features of the typical cell (chap. 13) but it has been adapted for the conversion of chemical energy into a contractile force. The cell is always elongated in the line of contraction and it is surrounded by an excitable membrane known as the **sarcolemma**

(fig. 16.2). The cytoplasm has the special name of **sarcoplasm**; it possesses all the normal elements of cytoplasm (p. 13.6) and also the contractile protein filaments, **myofilaments**, which run along the long axis of the cell. When these filaments group together and become visible in the light microscope, they are called **myofibrils**. The mitochondria are usually large and numerous. The smooth endoplasmic reticulum is disposed around the myofibrils and is known as the **sarcoplasmic reticulum.**

The special cytology of muscle cells is described under the following headings:

(1) myofilaments,
(2) sarcolemma and sarcoplasmic reticulum,
(3) development, growth and regeneration.

MYOFILAMENTS

All myofilaments contain at least three proteins, actin, myosin and 'native' tropomyosin and are of two types, thick and thin.

Tropomyosin

'Native' tropomyosin consists of two components, tropomyosin (mol. wt. 70 000) and troponin (mol. wt.

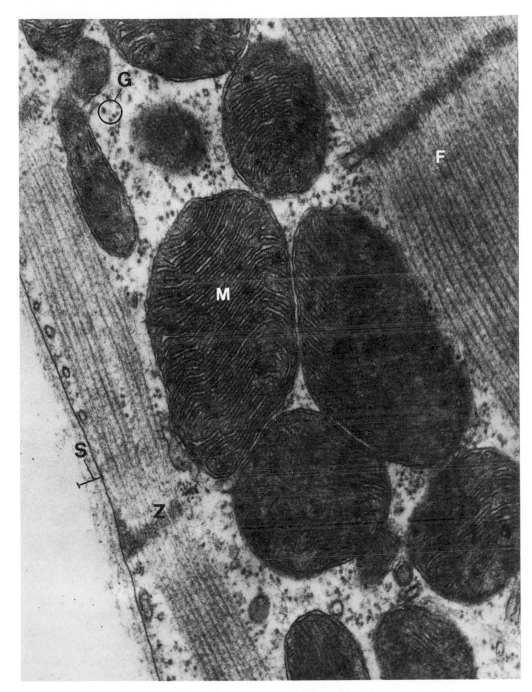

FIG.16.2. A cardiac muscle cell.

An electron micrograph of a rat cardiac muscle cell showing the sarcolemma (S), myofilaments (F), mito-chondria (M), Z-discs (Z, p. 16.5) and glycogen granules (G); osmium fixation, araldite embedding (× 63 000).

50 000). Troponin binds Ca^{++} ions very tightly and in this way may make actin and myosin react together sensitively in response to the [Ca^{++}] of the system, as described later.

Actin
Actin can exist in a globular form **G–actin** (mol. wt.

42 000) with a diameter of 5·5 nm. It contains bound ATP. G–actin readily aggregates in moderately concentrated salt solutions to form long filaments, each filament containing two strands of spherical actin molecules, twisted on each other (fig. 16.3). This fibrillar form is called **F–actin**. The thin filaments in muscle consist of F–actin, probably combined with tropomyosin. Each

G–actin unit in F–actin contains a group capable of combining with myosin.

Myosin

Myosin is a much larger protein (mol. wt. 500 000) and it has a more complex shape. One portion contains extended α-helices and resembles tropomyosin. This light meromyosin (LMM) portion is 93 nm long and joins the heavy

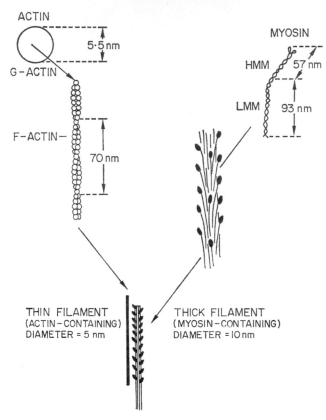

FIG. 16.3 The molecular structure of myofilaments.

meromyosin (HMM) portion, which is double headed, at a flexible joint (figs. 16.3 & 4). It is this heavy portion which contains the two heads, ATPase activity, and can combine with actin and split ATP. When the molecules aggregate to form filaments, their LMM portions fit in parallel to form the core of the thick filaments. The heads of the myosin molecules project, in a radial fashion, from the sides of the thick filaments. As the heads all point in the same direction, the intrinsic structure of the myosin-containing filaments is polarized in one direction (fig. 16.3). Although the actin filaments are apparently unpolarized (fig. 16.3), it can be shown that, on each globular molecule, the myosin-combining site points to the same end of the filament (fig. 16.4).

In the sarcoplasm these myosin- and actin-containing filaments lie side by side and the contractile force is produced at the points of apposition between the projecting

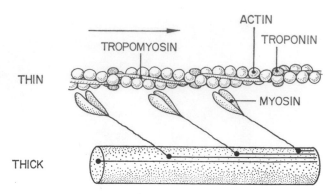

FIG. 16.4. The double headed myosin molecules react with the actin to split ATP and produce a contractile force in the direction of the arrow.

heads of the myosin molecules and the globular actin molecules. These points of apposition are often called cross bridges. Since both filaments are polarized, the force can be exerted in only one direction. A muscle can contract actively but it cannot lengthen actively. If shortening occurs, successive G–actin molecules come into contact with myosin heads. When shortening is not allowed, as in isometric contraction (p. 16.10), the same pairs of G–actin molecules and myosin molecule heads are interacting throughout the attempted contraction (fig. 16.4).

In smooth muscle, the filaments run along the long axis of the cell, but do not group together to form myofibrils. There is no regular pattern of particular lengths of each type of filament, so cross striations are not evident by light microscopy. This arrangement of filaments imposes no limit to the range of shortening as one filament can continue sliding past its counterpart. The power of the movement is directly related to the number of filaments and hence to the number of contact points between actin and myosin molecules. The expulsive force exerted by the uterus at parturition demonstrates the power of smooth muscle. Smooth muscles contract relatively slowly but are capable of maintaining the same tension for long periods. This **tonic activity** of smooth muscles in the visceral and vascular walls, which is controlled by the autonomic nervous system and by circulating hormones, plays an important part in regulating the function of the cardiovascular, gastrointestinal, urogenital and respiratory systems.

Rapid contraction in mammalian skeletal muscles is associated with a regular arrangement of the two types of filaments. This results in a cross-striated pattern being seen in the light microscope. It is associated with clear grouping of the filaments to form definite myofibrils. The dimensions and disposition of the filaments in a myofibril from striated muscle are shown in figs. 16.5 and 6. The thick myosin-containing filaments are 1·6 μm long and they are held in a regular hexagonal packing by cross connections situated halfway along their length. At

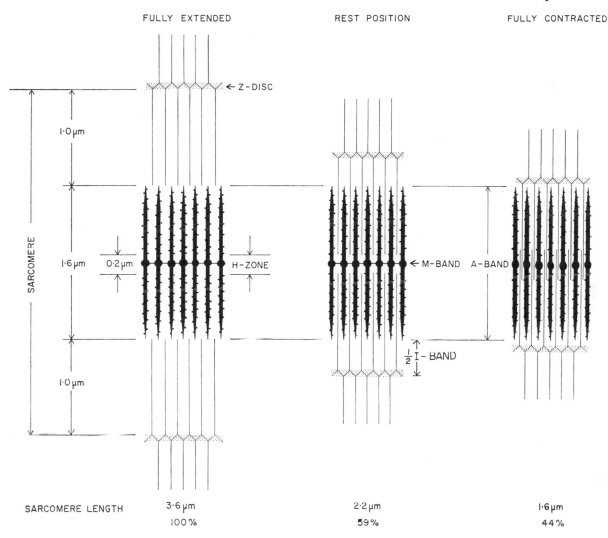

FULLY EXTENDED   REST POSITION   FULLY CONTRACTED

FIG. 16.5a. The arrangement of myofilaments in a myofibril. From Muir A. R. (1967). *Vet. Rec.* **80,** 456

this point the polarity of the myosin molecules changes so that all the heads point away from the centre. Thus the contractile force is directed towards the centre. Where the polarity changes, the tails of the myosin molecules overlap so there are no projecting heads for a distance of 200 nm in the centre. The thin actin-containing filaments are 1μm long and they are anchored at one end to a meshwork of tropomyosin known as the **Z-disc**. These two arrays of filaments fit into each other, so that each thin filament is surrounded by three thick ones and each thick filament is directly related to six thin filaments (fig. 16.6).

In this manner a composite contractile unit, the **sarcomere**, is formed. Its various parts are known by the letters shown in figs. 16.5 & 7. A myofibril from the biceps muscle runs perhaps 6 cm from origin to insertion and contains about 30 000 sarcomeres. The thick filaments produce birefringence in polarized light (anisotropy) and so are called the A-band. The width of the A-band does not change, but a paler, isotropic I-band con-

tains only thin filaments and this band narrows during contraction. The architecture of the sarcomere imposes precise limits on the amount of shortening which can occur. It is obvious from fig. 16.5 that the total range of movement of one sarcomere is 2μm, that is from 3.6μm to 1.6μm. Thus a muscle fibre can shorten by more than 50 per cent. In fact, our skeletal muscles need to shorten to 43 per cent of their fully extended length to produce the full movement at the single joint where they act. This shortening is almost exactly the same, proportionately, as the shortening which can occur at each of its sarcomeres.

A myofibril is about 1μm thick and the regular series of A- and I-bands is due to its constituent sarcomeres. All the myofibrils in a cell are placed and kept in register with each other; this remarkable fact is still unexplained. Thus the whole cell shows the cross-striated pattern which is truly the property of single myofibrils. Fig. 16.7 shows how myofilaments are assembled and organized in a whole skeletal muscle fibre.

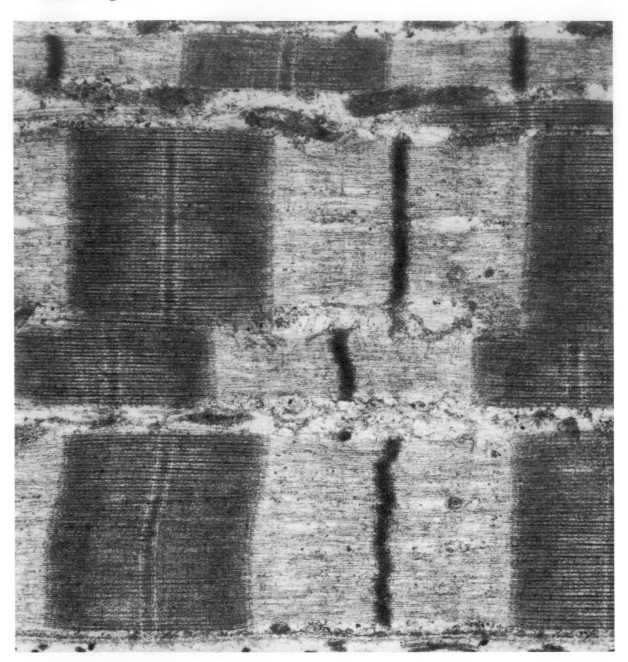

FIG. 16.5b. EM of skeletal muscle in relaxed position showing arrangement of myofilaments in myofibrils (× 37 500).

Fig. 16.8 indicates the isometric tension exerted at different degrees of overlap between thick and thin filaments. Zero overlap gives zero tension. Extreme overlap causes the thin filaments themselves to overlap each other, and tension falls off. In between is the optimal overlap of thick and thin filaments, where the available tension is maximal.

Connective tissue, largely composed of collagen, surrounds all the cells and limits extension of the cells beyond the physiological range which is dictated by the sarcomere design. The connective tissue is organized in three ways:

(1) the sheath around the whole muscle is called the **epimysium**.

(2) the sheath around the bundles of cells producing the 'muscle fibres' visible to the naked eye is the **perimysium**.

(3) each cell has a connective tissue tube called the **endomysium**.

All these sheaths are continuous with and form a large part of the tendon or bony attachment. The contractile force produced in the myofibrils is transmitted to the tendon at the end of the cell. Here the myofibrils are

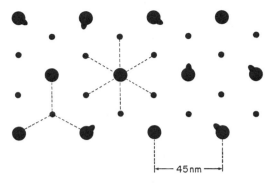

FIG. 16.6. A transverse section through an A-band.

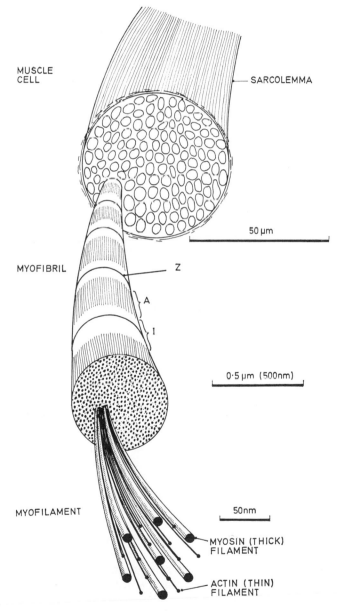

Fig. 16.7. The arrangement of myofilaments and myofibrils in a skeletal muscle fibre.

attached to the inside of the plasma membrane, from the outside of which reticular and collagen fibres run to the ultimate attachment.

SARCOLEMMA AND SARCOPLASMIC RETICULUM

The sarcolemma forms the boundary of individual muscle cells (fig. 16.2). It has a structure similar to the boundary of all other cells (p. 13.6) consisting of a plasma membrane with an outer condensation of connective tissue forming a basement membrane. Changes in the permeability of this membrane allow the ionic movements which create an action potential (p. 15.18).

The basement membrane is well developed around a multinucleated skeletal muscle cell and it blends with the collagenous endomysial tube. So the plasma membrane of a skeletal muscle fibre is always separated from the plasma membrane of neighbouring cells. Each skeletal muscle cell receives a nerve ending, and depolarization of its plasma membrane is normally due to nerve impulses causing discharge of transmitter substance at this motor end plate. Smooth-muscle cells which receive a rich autonomic nerve supply are similarly isolated from each other, although the basement membrane sheath is thinner. This fact explains the older view that smooth muscle did not possess a sarcolemma.

In cardiac muscle, the basement membrane covers only the sides of the fibres, so at the intercalated discs the

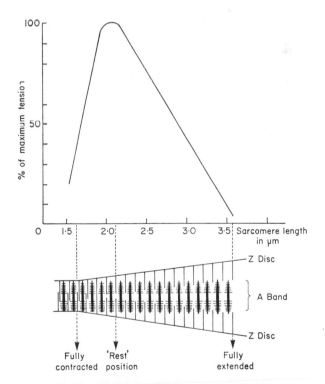

FIG. 16.8. The relationship between the length of a sarcomere and the isometric tension which its muscle cell can produce. From data of Gordon A.M., Huxley A.F. & Julian F.J. (1966) *J. Physiol.* **184**, 143.

plasma membranes of the two cells fuse to become an undulating double membrane between two adjacent cells (fig. 16.9), a structure similar to a zonula occludens. Because of the fusion, depolarization of one cell spreads to its neighbours and so through the whole heart. Smooth muscle which has a meagre nerve supply also has groups of cells joined together by plasma cell fusions with the same spread of depolarization.

The ionic changes in the sarcoplasm due to depolarization lead to contraction of the myofibrils. This process is

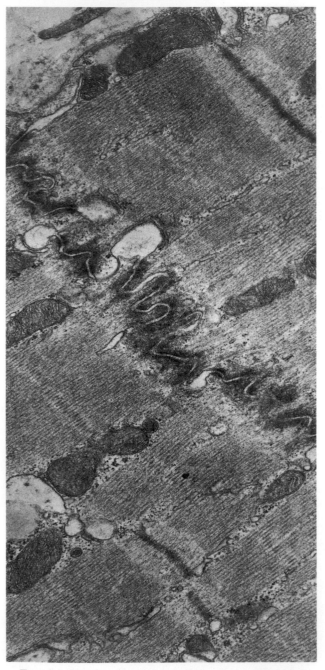

FIG. 16.9. EM of cardiac muscle showing also an intercalated disc (× 27 000).

called excitation–contraction coupling and recently two aspects of the process have been clarified.

Firstly, it has been shown that the sarcolemma is not confined to the surface of striated muscle cells. Tubules of plasma membrane leave the sarcolemma and penetrate the cell, passing close to all the contained myofibrils. These are the **T-tubules** and they are spatially related to the

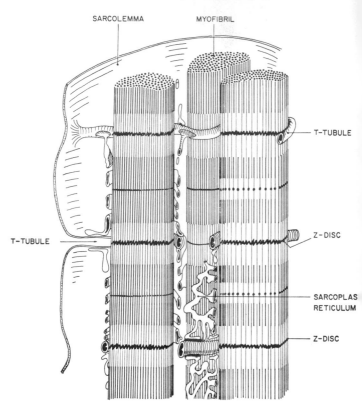

FIG. 16.10. The internal cellular membranes of cardiac muscle.

cross striations, being at the level of the Z-disc in cardiac muscle (fig. 16.10) and at the junction of the A and I bands in skeletal muscle. Thus the impulse to contract spreads along these tubules to permeate the whole cell as well as spreading along the surface.

Secondly, the myofibrils are embraced by a system of fine intracellular tubules called the **sarcoplasmic reticulum**. The membranes of this reticulum have peculiar Ca^{++} binding properties and it is thought that they initiate contraction by liberating Ca^{++} into the sarcoplasm. It is also established that Ca^{++} are necessary for the ATPase activity of the myosin. The sarcoplasmic reticulum comes into contact with the sarcolemma and the T-tubule and it may be here that the signal passes from the surface membrane to the sarcoplasmic reticulum.

Thus the sequence of events which initiates a contraction is as follows:

(1) A propagated action potential passes along the sarcolemma and spreads inward along the T-tubules,

depolarizing their membranes; this is the electrical signal.

(2) Ca^{++} are consequently released from the sarcoplasmic reticulum adjoining the T-tubules. A rise in [Ca^{++}] from 10^{-7} mol/l to 10^{-5} mol/l is sufficient for maximal effect and is the ionic signal.

(3) At this new higher concentration Ca^{++} bind to troponin; this causes a configurational change in the molecule and in tropomyosin which causes myosin and actin to interact to release the activity of ATPase and so contraction.

(4) During relaxation, the released Ca^{++} are recovered by the sarcoplasmic reticulum and the changes in (3) are reversed.

DEVELOPMENT, GROWTH AND REGENERATION OF MUSCLE

All striated muscle and practically all smooth muscle develops from mesoderm. The smooth muscles of the iris, the arrector pili muscles (fig. 37.9) and the contractile cells in secreting epithelia, myoepithelial cells (p. 18.10), are exceptions in that they may arise from ectoderm. The cells which are to become striated muscle are seen first in the segmentally arranged somites. Clusters of spindle-shaped cells, **myoblasts**, form discrete lateral masses in the somites known as **myotomes**. Some of the muscles remain segmentally arranged, e.g. the intercostal muscles, but most of the myoblasts migrate and rearrange to form the non-segmented muscles. In the limbs there is probably also some differentiation of myoblasts, but the early migration of myoblasts does seem to be followed by the outgrowth from the central nervous system of the motor nerve supply. In this manner the pattern of muscle innervation is determined even if there is differentiation of myoblasts at the site of the final muscle. The migration of the myoblasts from the myotomes in the occipital region into the tongue is established in evolution even though it cannot be observed in human embryos; it explains the course and distribution of the hypoglossal nerve.

Prior to the differentiation of a muscle, the myoblasts proliferate and then stick together to form long columns of cells. Suddenly, the intercellular barriers disappear and a multinucleated tube is formed. Myofibrils with cross striations first appear just inside the sarcolemma of this multinucleated cell and the content of myofibrils gradually increases. At a later stage, the nuclei move from the centre of the cell to take up their mature position under the sarcolemma. When the sarcomeres are seen first in the early embryo, they have the same dimensions as in the adult, so growth in length of the muscle is associated with the addition of new sarcomeres. Not quite all the myoblasts fuse together; a small proportion, perhaps 5–10 per cent of the nuclei in a skeletal muscle, remain as undifferentiated cells sandwiched between the basement membrane and the sarcolemma of the adult muscle cell. These are the **satellite cells** and they play an important part in

muscle regeneration. For regeneration of skeletal muscle to occur the damage must not be severe enough to impair the blood or nerve supply or to destroy completely the endomysial tubes. Under these conditions proliferation of myoblasts, probably derived from satellite cells, is followed by a recapitulation of the process of embryonic development.

The myoblasts which are to form cardiac muscle appear in the cephalic part of the lateral plate mesoderm (fig. 19.6). As in skeletal muscle they adhere to each other, but in this tissue the intervening cell membranes do not disintegrate since the adhesions form the intercalated discs. Myofibrils appear in the same position as in skeletal muscle but the nuclei do not move out to the periphery of the cell. There are no satellite cells in cardiac muscle and there is no regeneration of myocardium.

The differentiation of smooth muscle is much simpler as the mesodermal cells need only to elongate and to synthesize the contractile proteins. In contrast to the striated varieties, the body remains capable of developing smooth muscle throughout adult life. In the uterine wall during pregnancy, for instance, there is an actual increase in the number of smooth muscle cells (hyperplasia) as well as an increase in the size of individual cells (hypertrophy).

Hyperplasia does not occur in skeletal or cardiac muscle after birth, so all the growth is due to increase in size of the cells. This hypertrophy is augmented by exercise and by sex hormones, particularly testosterone, at puberty. Disuse leads rapidly to atrophy of skeletal muscle, for it can be detected within a few hours of the immobilization of a limb in plaster. Loss of the motor nerve supply produces severe wasting of muscles, but central nervous system lesions do not have the same effect.

Whole skeletal muscle

There are numerous patterns for the arrangement of the muscle cells (p. 20.11), which are determined by the available sites for skeletal attachment and the need to ensure that the cells are just long enough to produce the movements at the joints affected by the muscle. A fusiform muscle belly with a tendinous insertion is the simplest arrangement. The muscle cells are bound together, fasciculated and supported by the epi-, peri- and endomysium mentioned above. The collagen of the tendon is derived partly from these sheaths and partly from fibres arising from the ends of the muscle cells themselves. The muscle cells may either run the whole length of the belly or end at intermediate points by being attached to other muscle cells. In the former case all the motor end plates are in a band at the centre of the belly; in the latter they are scattered through the whole substance of the muscle.

Each cell has only one motor end plate (p. 15.25), which includes the end of a spinal or cranial nerve fibre.

Each ventral horn nerve cell, or its cranial equivalent, sends one axon which branches in the muscle to supply a number of muscle cells. Since the nerve cell exhibits an 'all or none' property and as the arrival of an impulse at its motor end plates causes a similar 'all or none' depolarization of the muscle cells it supplies, this combination of muscle cells and their innervating neurone forms a structural and functional unit. It is known as the **motor unit** and the number of muscle cells in such a unit varies with the delicacy of the movement which that muscle produces. In the small muscles moving the eyes and fingers one nerve cell supplies only 10–12 muscle cells; in the coarse muscles of the limbs and back a motor unit may have as many as 300 muscle cells. The individual muscle cells in a motor unit are scattered throughout the substance of the muscle; they do not correspond to the bundles of cells enclosed by perimysium. As well as these motor axons, every skeletal muscle contains sensory axons attached to receptors such as muscle spindles and tendon organs.

An electrode placed over a muscle, or inserted into the extracellular tissue in the muscle, can detect the electrical activities of adjacent motor units. When these are amplified and recorded they produce an electromyograph which demonstrates the activity of that muscle in a particular action (vol. 3, p. 34.17).

FUNCTION OF SKELETAL MUSCLE

Excitability

All skeletal muscles have motor nerve supplies, which are the normal channels of excitation, and all can be excited by stimulation of their motor nerves. But the region of the muscle fibre which does not have a motor end plate is also electrically excitable. Like peripheral nerve, it exhibits a threshold to electrical stimulation, a latent period between stimulation and response and absolute and relative refractory periods, i.e. a period of unresponsiveness to any stimulus, which is followed by a period in which there is an increase in the magnitude of the threshold stimulus. Thus it can be taken that the muscle cell itself belongs to the same class of irritable tissue as the nerve fibre.

Characteristics of muscular contraction

If a muscle is excited by applying a single shock to its motor nerve it responds by exhibiting:

(1) an action potential which appears after a short latency,

(2) a contraction which occurs after a further latent period.

If the nerve is stimulated repetitively at a sufficiently low frequency there is a series of discrete action potentials but the contractile activity is of a continuous nature.

The form taken by the contractile activity depends on circumstances. If the attachments of the muscle are fixed, the activity takes the form of development of tension in the muscle, and the contraction is called **isometric**. If one or both of the attachments can move, then the muscle may be able to shorten without the development of any increase in tension, and this sort of contraction is called **isotonic**. If one sets out to draw a cork from a bottle, the arm muscles used initially contract isometrically until the tension developed is sufficient to put the cork into motion. They contract isotonically during withdrawal until the cork is practically free and thereafter contraction is neither purely isotonic nor purely isometric. Thus when we speak of muscular contraction we use 'contraction' in a technical sense. In common speech, contraction means shortening. In muscle physiology it means that physiological activity which can lead to shortening if the circumstances allow. One should always be on guard in medical science to keep general and technical meanings separate.

TWITCH AND TETANUS

A single shock to a motor nerve produces a contraction which is called a **twitch**. Depending on the species and on the anatomical site and the temperature of the muscle, the time before return to resting tension in an isometric twitch may be 100–600 msec.

If a second stimulus is applied after an interval exceeding the refractory period, which is usually of the order of a millisecond, the tension rises further than in a twitch, even if the peak of twitch tension has been passed before the second stimulus is applied. If a series of stimuli at regular intervals is applied, the tension continues to rise more and more slowly until it becomes constant or oscillates at the frequency of stimulation around a constant mean which can be several times as great as maximum twitch tension. Tension declines to zero 100–600 msec after the last stimulus, as in a twitch. This kind of contraction is called a **tetanus**. This word must be distinguished from tetany, a state of increased excitability of motor nerves. Tetanus is also the name of a disease in which tetanic contractions of muscle arise as a result of poisoning by a bacterial toxin.

During a tetanus (or tetanic contraction) action potentials can be observed in the muscle. There is one action potential of a normal kind for every stimulus applied. Thus action potentials remain discrete, whilst contractions fuse, but fusion takes place only if the interval between stimuli is much shorter than twitch time. A frequency of 10/sec may give fused contraction, but a smooth tetanic contraction needs a frequency of 100/sec or more. It should be noted that this high frequency is not required for a natural smooth movement, in which motor units are not stimulated synchronously as they are during an experiment. When units are naturally stimulated, as during a voluntary movement, any slight jerkiness in the action of one unit is entirely smoothed by the asynchronous contributions of other units (see below).

ACTIVE STATE

It is difficult to devise apparatus for recording muscular contractions in which there is no lag in response and no distortion. The isometric contraction should be the easier to record faithfully, but the maximum isometric twitch tension of the medial head of the cat gastrocnemius can exceed 6 kg and even the gastrocnemius of the small English frog (*Rana temporaria*) gives a tension of 2 kg, so fairly substantial devices are needed.

Further difficulties arise within the muscle itself. What one is trying to record is the tension that the muscle fibres themselves would develop if they were directly attached to undistortable and immediately responsive detectors. But the muscle cells are attached to each other and to the attachments of the muscle by the connective tissue elements already described which are being stretched in some measure all the time that the tension in the muscle cells is rising. These elements will therefore not have achieved full stretch at the moment at which tension in the muscle cells begins to fall, and the tension transmitted by them to their attachments will not be, at its maximum, the maximum tension which the muscle cells can develop.

This same argument can be applied to the relation between the muscle as a whole and the recording apparatus, in which a tension must be developed if a tension is to be recorded. So we expect the recorded twitch tension to be lower than the tension that the muscle is capable of developing in a twitch. The tension that we ought to be able to record if there were none of these obstacles has been called the **active state tension**.

The technique of determining the time course of the active state is too complex to be described here, but the outcome is important: active state tension rises almost instantaneously to its maximal value which is equal to maximal tetanic tension (fig. 16.11). The active state tension is maintained for a little shorter time than that taken for a twitch to reach peak tension and then declines. Since this has been established, several other pieces of evidence have been shown to fit in. For instance, the effects of a number of drugs which change the form of the normally recorded isometric twitch have been shown to be explicable by their effect on the length of the plateau of active state tension.

Thus the picture of a contracting muscle is very different from what we should expect from personal experience of the fineness with which it can be adapted to our needs. The individual elements have to be thought of as contracting maximally or not at all, with no gradations possible except those inherent in the transition between fully isometric and fully isotonic. The picture that emerges from the work on active state reinforces the notion of the individual muscle cell as something that acts in an all or none fashion, and this is of importance in theories of muscular contraction.

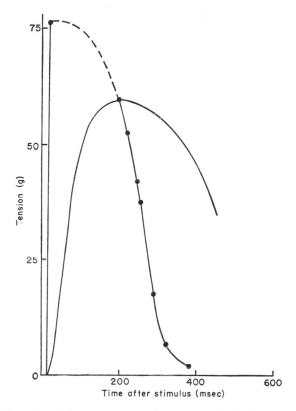

FIG. 16.11. Time-course of active state tension in frog sartorius at 0°C. The interrupted part of the line was drawn by extrapolation. An ordinary muscle twitch is also shown. From Ritchie J.M. (1954) *J. Physiol.* **126**, 155.

Gradation of muscular activity

So far we have considered the properties of muscle maximally stimulated either directly or through its motor nerve so that all the muscle cells act together. The muscles, however, consist of numerous motor units, normally acting independently, each consisting of the muscle cells which are innervated by the terminal branches of the axon of the single motor neurone. Since motor neurones in the ventral horn of the spinal cord are stimulated individually, it is very unlikely that the twitches of different motor units will be synchronous. In any sustained muscular activity a set of motor units contracts asynchronously in such a way that some are fully active, some are relaxing and some are quiescent at any given instant. If there is a rotation of states of activity among a constant number of such units, the muscle will be in a more or less steady state of activity, although no single unit will be in a steady state of tetanic contraction. The all-or-none responses of the individual contractile units are masked by the asynchronous nature of the activity and by the non-rigid nature of the connective structure of the muscle through which the contractile activity has to be transmitted to origins and insertions.

Fatigue

When an isolated frog gastrocnemius muscle is made to twitch repetitively by electrical stimulation of its nerve, the contraction steadily becomes smaller, even if the muscle is kept in oxygen. A sufficiently long period of rest restores the ability to contract.

This effect is usually due to the circumstances of the experiment. Every contraction causes an efflux of potassium from the excited cells, as with nerve. The potassium added to the extracellular water cannot be removed by the circulation, as would happen *in vivo*, and accumulates. Increase in extracellular potassium renders the muscle cells inexcitable. If such muscles are soaked in fresh physiological saline they regain excitability. If a small volume of saline is used for a series of such muscles it ultimately loses its ability to restore excitability and is then found to contain three to four times the normal potassium concentration.

Isolated muscles can become exhausted as well as inexcitable. They require energy for contraction, even if they are not doing external work. Muscle cells store carbohydrate in the form of glycogen and lipid in the form of triglyceride, but these stores are limited and in isolated muscle failure to respond may be due to exhaustion of reserves of nutrients.

Rigor

When muscles become irreversibly exhausted they fail to relax, i.e., they go into rigor, rather than fail to contract. Although there are complicating factors, the onset of rigor is determined chiefly by failure of energy supply. As soon as oxygen is no longer supplied by the circulation the sole available energy source is glycogen, which can be converted anaerobically to lactic acid. When glycogen is exhausted rigor follows. The onset of rigor is accelerated in an animal which has been violently exercised immediately before death, and rigor is instantaneous in an animal which has been poisoned with iodoacetic acid, which prevents the formation of lactic acid. It is important to keep in mind that lack of energy seems to destroy the capacity to relax, not the capacity to contract.

Rigor mortis, the rigor that occurs after death, passes off with time. This probably has no significance for an understanding of muscle function. Autolytic processes occur in cells after death and their internal structure gradually disintegrates; this disintegration involves the contractile elements.

Relation between muscle length and contraction

If the ability of a muscle to contract is due to interaction between the myosin and actin filaments in its sarcomeres,

it is to be expected that passive stretching to the point where there is no overlap of these filaments would make it incapable of contraction. When muscles are stretched in this way and then stimulated it can be seen under the light microscope that sarcomeres do not in fact contract.

The amount of work which a muscle can perform when it is maximally stimulated depends on its initial length. If it is initially not under tension, the contractile elements must shorten and the connective tissue must be stretched before tension can be developed at the attachments of the muscle, and the development of such tension is a prerequisite of the performance of external work. During these preliminaries work is done in overcoming internal friction and in deforming the connective tissue elements. Only a fraction of the energy liberated in each twitch can be used for external work in such circumstances. With increase in initial extension of the muscle less energy is needed for these unproductive activities so that more external work can be done; when the degree of initial extension is reached at which some of the sarcomeres have attained such lengths that they can no longer contract, the ability to perform work begins to fall. Thus there is an optimal extension, at which the muscle can perform maximal work in a single twitch.

This relation is not directly applicable to normal muscular activity *in vivo*. In these circumstances some of the muscle fibres undergo passive stretching every time a twitch takes place in adjacent motor units, so that the passive viscous and elastic properties of muscle fibres enter more into this situation than into the experimental one. But as the pattern of excitation of motor units in any voluntary contraction *in vivo* is at present impossible to determine, it is not possible to analyse profitably the performance of muscle *in situ*.

Heat production in muscle

Metabolic energy which cannot be used to perform mechanical, electrical or chemical work must be dissipated as heat. Frog sartorius muscle at rest, metabolizing nutrients at the rest rate, dissipates about $8 \cdot 4$ J/kg^{-1} min^{-1} at 20°C. The only way of measuring such small heat production is by means of a sensitive thermopile. Accurate measurements on active muscle can be made only with muscles that can be brought into close contact with a suitable thermopile and kept in contact. In the frog sartorius the heat production during a single maximal isometric twitch is about $12 \cdot 6$ J/kg the exact value depending on the amount of work done. Energy is liberated in a twitch in three forms:

(1) initial heat, which starts before a mechanical response is seen; this is sometimes called the heat of activation,

(2) heat of shortening which is directly proportional to the extent of shortening,

(3) mechanical work.

It has been pointed out that the magnitudes of these components are quite independent of one another; there is never any question of reducing the amount of activation or shortening heat by making the muscle do more work. No heat is liberated during relaxation. These changes occur equally well in the presence or absence of oxygen. If oxygen is available, there is a subsequent slow production of additional heat which is about equal in magnitude to the sum total of activation heat, shortening heat and external work. Comparable data are not available for the muscles of warm-blooded animals. The general similarity in structure of amphibian and mammalian muscle, however, makes it unlikely that there are fundamental differences between their basic modes of action, so we may take it that a similar pattern of energy liberation would occur in mammalian muscle, and that any effective theory of muscular contraction should take into account this pattern of heat production.

The sarcoplasm contains all the enzymes of the Embden–Meyerhof pathway, which was indeed first studied in muscle, and all the enzymes of β-oxidation of fatty acids, together with all the enzymes of the citric acid cycle and of the terminal respiratory pathway. It can therefore generate ATP at the expense of energy derived from carbohydrate or fat.

Energy source for contraction

ATP is generally held to be the specific means by which the energy produced in the oxidation of nutrients can be utilized for the performance of work by muscles. If this is true, the theory of muscular contraction must find a central place for ATP, although it is generated outside the contractile myofibrils.

There is nothing specialized in the processes of ATP generation in muscle cells. It arises in the ways described on p. 8.10. But there is something specialized about the pattern of needs for it. As we have seen, individual muscle cells go into activity in all or none fashion and they do this repetitively in any overt muscular activity. In addition, the increased energy requirement of the muscles in mild activity is large, judging from the increase in oxygen requirement of the whole animal, so individual muscle cells need a great deal of ATP frequently at very short notice.

On the other hand, we shall see that muscular contraction would be difficult or impossible if the ATP concentration was very high, so that it is not feasible to store a large reserve of ATP in the cell.

The difficulty is overcome by storing the reserve of high energy phosphate in another form, phosphocreatine:

$$\text{Phosphocreatine} + \text{ADP} \xrightleftharpoons[\text{kinase}]{\text{creatine}} \text{Creatine} + \text{ATP}$$

This tends to go to the left, so that the equilibrium concentration of ATP is low. In resting mammalian muscle the ATP concentration is about 5 μmoles/g and the phosphocreatine concentration about 20–30 μmoles/g.

The creatine kinase activity in muscle is sufficiently high to make re-equilibration almost instantaneous; if oxidative phosphorylation cannot generate ATP from ADP as rapidly as necessary, the creatine kinase automatically makes up the deficit to a limited extent. The total store of energy as ATP and phosphocreatine in human muscle is sufficient to keep a man running for less than 5 sec.

Muscle logistics

Muscle is ultimately dependent for its supply of ATP on the nutrients and oxygen brought to it in the bloodstream. (p. 30.1). But the circulation cannot supply these needs just at the time when they are most wanted. It has been shown that in vigorous contraction the pressure set up within the muscle is enough to arrest blood flow. It may be expected that in parts of a muscle where units are contracting the capillaries will be squeezed and supplies will often be temporarily cut off. Thus, there is a tendency for the muscle to be deprived at its time of greatest need.

There is another supply difficulty; at rest, muscle blood flow is about 20–50 ml kg^{-1} min^{-1}. If all the oxygen were abstracted from this it would supply 120–300 ml O_2/min to all the muscles of the body. This compares with a resting oxygen requirement of the whole body of 250 ml/min. The oxygen requirement for walking at 5·6 km/h is more than four times the resting requirement, and almost all this extra oxygen is used by the muscles. Thus, even in mild exercise there has to be a considerable adaptation of the circulation, involving increased cardiac output and redistribution of the output between destinations to give a larger share to the muscles. This adaptation is rapid, but not instantaneous. During it the muscles have to get energy from somewhere, and it cannot be obtained on credit. Muscle glycogen can be broken down by the normal pathways to pyruvate. In the absence of adequate oxygen, the pyruvate can act as hydrogen acceptor from NADH generated in the oxidation of triose phosphate to phosphoglyceric acid. The pyruvate is reduced to lactate. The overall effect of this transformation is to liberate about one-fifth of the energy of the glycogen for use by the muscle. If oxygen is available, the pyruvate can be completely oxidized by way of the citric acid cycle. It is in this stage that the remaining four-fifths of the energy of the glycogen is liberated.

Muscle normally contains 5–10 g of glycogen/kg but the lipid content is appreciably higher and can be oxidized to provide energy. However when muscles most urgently need a store of utilizable energy they are also most deficient in oxygen, and therefore tend to be restricted to the partial use of their glycogen by converting it to lactate.

This ability of muscle to obtain energy anaerobically was responsible for the early belief that carbohydrate was the fuel of muscle. In fact, it appears that carbohydrate is important because of its availability as a short term anaerobic source of energy at the beginning of exercise, but in sustained activity the major source of energy supply is the free fatty acids of the blood. However, quite a lot can be done without external supplies. The athlete who runs 100 metres is unlikely to obtain more than a tiny fraction of the energy he dissipates from anything other than glycolysis of muscle glycogen. A fuller discussion of the effects of muscular exercise is given in chap. 45.

Oxygen supply to muscle

For the same reasons that make it difficult to supply nutrients to muscle there is a problem in maintaining oxygen supply. Muscles used rhythmically as in rowing or running may have a highly intermittent blood supply and may be forced to depend on glycolysis of a diminishing glycogen supply if they lack adequate continuous oxygen supply. However, they can make their glycogen last five times as long if they can oxidize it.

Some muscles of birds and mammals are equipped with a means of diminishing the effects of oxygen deprivation. These are the red muscles. They owe their darker colour to their content of myoglobin, which is a haem protein of the same general character as haemoglobin, and has the property of combining with oxygen in the same way. The haemoglobin molecule is made up of four sub-units whose molecular weight is about 16 000 (p. 11.12). The myoglobin molecule consists of one such unit, but this unit is not identical in amino acid composition with any of the subunits in the haemoglobin of the same species.

Myoglobin differs from haemoglobin also in its oxygen dissociation curve. As described on p. 31.20, myoglobin can pick up and store in the cells the oxygen brought by the blood even when the circulation is too inadequate to maintain a high oxygen tension in the tissue fluid interposed between capillaries and muscle cells.

Red muscles and white muscles

In the blood-free state, all organs have some colour due to the natural intracellular pigments such as the yellow flavins, the orange carotenoids and the red cytochromes. But these are pale shades usually, compared with the colour of myoglobin, so that muscles containing much of this pigment are strikingly red, The difference in colour between pectoral muscle of the domestic fowl and that of the pigeon, partridge or grouse shows that corresponding muscles in different species can contain a lot of myoglobin or a little. Muscles which have to maintain activity for long periods, such as the pectoral muscles of flying birds and the extensors of the limbs used in walking, are more likely to contain red muscle.

In some species it has been found that the time course of the maximal twitch of a red muscle is much more prolonged than that of a white muscle. This is true in the cat. If the motor nerves of a pair of muscles in the hind limb of a kitten are cut, one muscle being red and one white, and if the distal end of each cut nerve is sutured to the proximal end of the other nerve, so that, after regeneration, each nerve comes to innervate the wrong muscle, then the twitch of the red muscle becomes brisker and that of the white muscle less brisk. However, it is doubtful if this association between whiteness and speed of contraction is a general one. Furthermore, recent work suggests that the classification into white and red fibres is an oversimplification, confused by the sometimes inadequate criteria adopted by some research workers. More work on more muscles, including analyses of contraction in terms of active state, is desirable before too much is built on this evidence.

Limiting oxygen pressure in muscle

As the oxygen pressure in arterial blood is of the order of 13 kPa, we tend to think that muscles need to be supplied with oxygen at quite high oxygen pressure. Since the advent of oxygen electrodes it has become clear that the oxygen pressure needed at the surface of a cell in order to provide a high enough concentration to meet the needs of the cell can be very low indeed. A diagram which gives oxygen pressures at various sites in the human body is on p. 46.2. No figures are available for human muscle, but in general the critical concentration is less than 0·1 kPa. Since intracellular concentrations must be lower than extracellular ones in order that there shall be diffusion of oxygen into and across the cells, the ability of myoglobin to hold on to oxygen until the oxygen tension is less than 1 kPa is of no disadvantage.

The need for relatively high oxygen pressures in blood arises because the oxygen has to diffuse across the capillary wall and through the extracellular fluid to reach the cell. There must therefore be a concentration gradient from capillary lumen to cell surface and this must be capable of being made large enough to meet the needs for rapid transport in conditions of vigorous activity. Since one cannot raise the arterial tension appreciably, the cells need to be able to operate energetically when the oxygen tension at their surfaces is low.

The gradient of concentration of oxygen, and incidentally of any other metabolite, between capillary and muscle cell is affected not only by the concentration difference between these structures but also by their mean distance apart. This distance is dependent on the mean number of patent capillaries per unit cross-sectional area of the muscle. This number rises markedly during muscular activity (p. 30.30).

FURTHER READING

BOURNE G.H. ed. (1972–73) *The Structure and Function of Muscle*, 2nd Edition, vols. I–IV. New York: Academic Press.

BÜLBRING E., BRADING A., JONES A. & TOMITA T. eds. (1970) *Smooth Muscle*. London: Arnold.

CARLSON F.D. & WILKIE D.R. (1974) *Muscle Physiology*. Englewood Cliffs, N.J.: Prentice-Hall.

COHEN CAROLYN (1975) The protein switch of muscle contraction. *Scientific American* **233**, November, 36–45.

PORTER R.L. FITZSIMONS D.W. eds. (1974) *The Physiological Basis of Starling's Law of the Heart*. Ciba Foundation Symposium No. 24, N.S. Amsterdam: Associated Scientific Publishers

WILKIE D.R. (1968) *Muscle*. London: Arnold.

Chapter 17
Supporting tissues

Since the middle of the last century, when the cell theory became widely accepted, medicine has been primarily concerned with cellular functions in organs. This is understandable because breakdown in a cellular system such as the heart, the liver or the kidney often produces dramatic effects within a few hours. However, as knowledge of organ functions has increased and therapeutic procedures have become more effective, attention has been directed increasingly to a group of diseases whose progress is usually measured in years or decades. Examples of these are the hardening of the walls of the arteries, some rheumatic diseases and the slow atrophy of bones with age. These diseases arise because of a metabolic failure in tissues which are rich in extracellular fibrous proteins but poor in cells. In consequence the metabolism of such tissue is slow compared with that of the cellular tissues of such organs as the liver, kidney or heart, but the tissue is far from inert as was once believed.

CONNECTIVE TISSUE

Connective tissues are derived from mesoderm and they make up a large part of the body, including all tissues which are not epithelial, or nervous or muscle. This covers such widely varying tissues as bone, cartilage, fibrous tissue, elastic tissue, blood and lymph. In spite of their variety, these tissues share the common property that their function is dependent on the quality of their extracellular component. Undifferentiated mesoderm, which can become any of the above tissues, is widespread in embryos and persists even in an adult. It is called **mesenchyme.**

Supporting tissue consists of extracellular fluid, proteins and minerals which support the cells in their various organs and by means of the bony skeleton support the whole body. Connective tissue contains cells which are responsible for manufacturing and maintaining the extracellular material but they themselves play only a small part in its actual function.

The properties of most connective tissues are due to their content and arrangement of **fibrous proteins.** They also contain an interfibrillar substance commonly known as connective tissue **ground substance,** the properties of which depend upon complex protein-polysaccharide macromolecules. These compounds constitute an important and ubiquitous system present in all extracellular fluid and tend to make the aqueous phase more like a jelly. Its consistency depends upon the amount and nature of the protein polysaccharides; this can vary from the rigidity of hyaline cartilage through the jelly-like content of the umbilical cord to the watery extracellular fluid found in skeletal muscle, which is the extracellular fluid of the physiologists.

Fat cells are widely distributed throughout connective tissue and in places such as the skin they have the important physical functions of insulation and padding. In view of the metabolic importance of adipose tissue in health and disease, it is considered separately (chap. 34).

Quantitative aspects of connective tissues

The significance of connective tissue is better appreciated if the components of the body are considered in terms of their functional contribution. Thus there are tissues which are predominantly cellular, though they include a little fibrous tissue in their stroma; typical examples are the liver, skeletal muscle and brain, and in these organs the major part of the metabolism takes place. Then there are those tissues which are predominantly fibrous, but which include a few cells. The function of these tissues is mostly mechanical; the rigidity and strength of bone is produced by a highly organized mineralization of the fibrous protein collagen which is found in bone, as well as in tendons and fasciae. A third group of tissues, not often regarded as connective tissue, is the blood and extracellular fluids whose functions are nutritive.

Table 17.1 sets out the composition of a 65 kg man in terms of tissues and organs. If the predominantly cellular organs, such as the muscles, liver, brain and endocrine organs, are added together they come to about 38 kg. This cell or organ mass includes some connective tissue in the form of stromal collagen, the collagen of the arteries and some extracellular fluid. Making allowance for these, the true cell mass is about 34 kg or just over half the total weight of the standard man (65 kg). Thus the cells of the

TABLE 17.1. The tissues of a 65 kg man (kg fresh tissue).

Skeletal muscle	30·0
Internal organs	7·3
Bone	9·0
Skin and subcutaneous tissue	7·8
Adipose tissue	4·0
Blood	5·5
Structural connective tissue (tendons, fasciae, etc.)	1·0
Loculated fluids (joints, eye balls, etc.) and miscellaneous connective tissue fluids	0·4
Total	65·0

body which are most concerned with the processes of metabolism and movement are supported structurally and nutritionally by about their own weight of connective tissue. Tissues such as skin and bone contain relatively few cells, and so cytoplasm makes up a smaller proportion of their total volume. It can be seen that skin and bone together make up a large part of the body (16·8 kg) and that the contribution of all the other structural components such as tendons is relatively small (1 kg). The remaining mass of the body is largely accounted for by two tissues of great nutritional importance; these are blood and fat (9·5 kg).

TABLE 17.2. A normal chemical composition of a man weighing 65 kg and the distribution of substances in supporting tissue.

Component	Mass (kg)	Amount in supporting tissue (kg)
Protein	11·0	3·0 Connective tissue including bone
Fat	9·0	6·2 Adipose tissue and skin
Water	40·0	12·0 Interstitial fluid
		3·0 Loosely bound in bones, joint capsules, eyes, etc.
		3·0 Plasma
Minerals	4·0	3·8 Bone
Carbohydrate	1·0	0.5 Connective tissue polysaccharides
Totals	65·0	31·5 (48·5 per cent of body weight)

Table 17.2 sets out the chemical composition of the normal body in terms of protein, fat, carbohydrate, minerals and water, and gives an estimated partition of these constituents between the cells and supporting tissue. Inspection shows, not unexpectedly, that the bulk of the protein and water of the body is found in association with cells, whereas 95 per cent of all the minerals in the body is in the connective tissue, principally in the skeleton. Cells and connective tissue have a small quantity of carbohydrate attached to them. The polysaccharide of the cell (glycogen) can be easily broken down to glucose and so made available as a source of energy. However, the complex polysaccharides of the connective tissue are relatively inert as befits their structural and polyanionic function which is discussed on p. 17.7.

Chemical composition of individual tissues

Table 17.3 gives the chemical constituents of some typical tissues. Here skin is considered as a connective tissue organ because the ectodermal contribution of cells and keratin is relatively small. About 95 per cent of all protein in the skin is collagen and is thus of mesenchymal origin. It can be seen that protein is an important component of all structural tissues and tendon has the highest concentration of protein of any tissue, although as mentioned previously, the total mass of all tendons is small. In contrast, the protein content of plasma and adipose tissue is low. It is perhaps surprising that the protein content of tissues as widely different as bone and muscle is virtually the same although it is, of course, extracellular in bone and intracellular in muscle.

Each of the tissues listed in table 17.3 has an extracellular fluid (ECF) compartment, the composition of which corresponds closely to that of plasma as far as the minerals listed are concerned. Since ECF occupies only a small part of the volume of the tissue, the content of each mineral should be less than that found in a kg of plasma provided it is largely extracellular in distribution. If this is not so then the mineral must be present attached to a special compartment in the tissue. As table 17.3 shows, connective tissues have a mineral composition very

TABLE 17.3. Composition of 1 kg of various fresh tissues.

Constituent	Tendons	Cartilage	Bone	Skin	Adipose tissue	Skeletal muscle	Plasma
Protein (g)	360	170	200	270	20	210	66
Fat (g)	—	—	50	100	850	75	7
Water (g)	600	740	250	620	130	700	913
K (mmol)	12	12	40	22	5	105	5
Na (mmol)	90	170	230	70	22	25	144
Ca (mmol)	3·5	24	4500	4	—	1	2·5
Mg (mmol)	7	5	100	1·5	—	10	0·9
Cl (mmol)	90	40	30	80	—	16	104
Polysaccharide (g)	30	80	30	10	—	10	1

different from a typical cellular tissue such as muscle. A further discrepancy is that each connective tissue shows a characteristic difference from the expected content of sodium and to a lesser extent of calcium and magnesium judged by comparison with plasma. In bone this is at first sight not surprising, particularly for calcium, but the actual site of the large amount of magnesium and sodium present is unknown. Similarly in tendon there is slight excess of sodium and chloride, and surprisingly a large excess of magnesium which is essentially an intracellular mineral. In bone, sodium is held mainly in a water free state in association with the mineral crystals of the matrix. Studies with ^{24}Na have shown that part of bone sodium is readily exchangeable with plasma sodium. The calcium and phosphate of bone play an important role in maintaining the concentrations of these substances in the blood, and in some diseases demineralization of the skeleton can proceed to such an extent that the bones become very weak and may break after trivial injuries.

Structure of connective tissues

The basic ingredients of connective tissues remain similar in different parts of the body but the relative proportions of the constituents vary widely. There are two main systems of fibres, each composed of a characteristic protein, **collagen** and **elastin**, associated with which there are numbers of proteoglycan macromolecules. These substances are characteristic of the ground substance of connective tissue, i.e. the watery phase bathing the fibres and cells. Three types of cell are found:

(1) **fibroblasts** which manufacture the collagen fibre systems and proteoglycans. (p. 17.8)

(2) **mast cells** which are specifically concerned with the proteoglycan, heparin, and

(3) **macrophages** which may be fixed or free to move about and scavenge for cellular and other debris.

A more detailed consideration of the various cells and fibres found in connective tissue is given in vol. 2, table 30.1.

The fibrous proteins of connective tissue are different from any intracellular substances and can be stained characteristically by simple histological procedures. Elastin, the chief protein of elastic tissue, is stained by the dyes orcein and resorcin-fuchsin, brown and dark blue respectively, but is not stained selectively by acidic dyes like eosin. Whether or not collagen stains with aniline dyes seems to depend on the size of the strands, which are made up of small subunit fibrils of collagen associated with proteoglycans. Thus, in loose connective tissue, the EM reveals many small strands of collagen less than 0·5 μm in diameter; these do not stain with dyes such as aniline blue, which stain the larger strands (1–5 μm). In addition, some delicate fibres commonly found in the connective tissue of glandular organs do not stain easily,

although the EM shows that fine collagen fibrils are their principal components; they are known as **reticulin fibres**. Impregnation with silver under special conditions is the best way to demonstrate them. Finally, mention should be made of a structure called the **basement membrane** or more accurately the basal lamina (p. 18.1). This contains very fine elements of specialized collagen, particularly rich in carbohydrate, which can be stained with the PAS method (plate 18.1b, facing p. 18.2).

In growing tissues, where cells and fibrous proteins are being manufactured, the nucleic acids of the nucleus and cytoplasm stain with a basic dye such as haematoxylin, and the cell population stands out clearly against the background of extracellular components which take up acidic counterstains such as eosin or aniline blue. In mature non-proliferating tissues the cell nuclei still stain prominently a deep purple with haematoxylin but the cytoplasm now stains only with the counterstain, if at all, and thus a superficial examination can give the impression that some cells are virtually all nucleus.

One further staining phenomenon is of importance, i.e. metachromasia or metachromatic staining. This means that certain stains of a single colour stain some elements of tissues a different colour. An example of this is the staining red of the cytoplasmic granules of mast cells by toluidine blue. This is because of the granule's content of the sulphated proteoglycan heparin. The explanation of the important phenomenon of metachromatic staining is thought to be that groups of molecules of the dye are coupled to macromolecules in such a way that the absorptive behaviour of the molecular complex is altered, and thus the colour of the transmitted light observed down the microscope is changed.

LOOSE CONNECTIVE TISSUE

This is also known as areolar connective tissue because the early histologists thought that it contained empty spaces, like a sponge (areola = a small space). There are, however, no spaces and normally no fluid. The extracellular, or interstitial space is permeated by gel-like ground substance which is microscopically structureless. This tissue can serve as a model for the structure of all connective tissue. It is found typically beneath the skin, around viscera, in serous membranes, around organs and muscles and in the nooks and crannies of the body such as occur between the tendons and around joints. Fig. 17.1 is a drawing of a section of typical areolar tissue stained with haematoxylin and eosin. Large numbers of strands, 2–10 μm in diameter, are each made up of fibres smaller than 1 μm, which in turn are formed of bundles of microfibrils. The fibres branch by splitting and can be fanned out like the cords making up a rope. These are collagen fibres. Another and different kind of fibrous material can also be seen. These are the elastic fibres, which occur less frequently than the collagen fibres in most connective

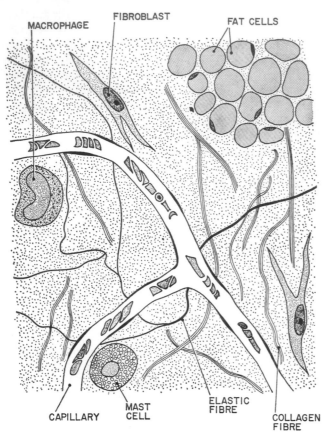

FIG. 17.1. Diagram of the structure of loose connective tissue (× 500).

tissues; they characteristically branch and link up with each other.

The fibrous structure of loose connective tissue resembles a sponge which gives easily when it is pulled and has sufficient elasticity to return to its original shape when released. The loose mesh is ideal for holding the water. Because of the content of proteoglycans and the mesh of fibres, water is not free to move about easily, and yet like water in a filter-paper there is no barrier to diffusion of small molecules or ions.

The cells of loose connective tissue are few in number but characteristic. Fibroblasts, macrophages, mast cells and fat cells are found scattered through the meshwork of fibrils. Loose connective tissue is a living tissue and it contains a blood supply. Furthermore, because the slow movement of water is an important part of its function some lymphatic capillaries are also present in association with the blood capillaries.

FIBROBLASTS

The fibroblast is the cell type most commonly seen in connective tissue (fig. 17.1). It has a prominent round or slightly elongated vesiculate nucleus with a prominent nucleolus and the cell body tends to be drawn out into a number of projections. In the EM abundant rough sur-

faced endoplasmic reticulum, pinocytotic vesicles, lysosomes, modest numbers of mitochondria and granules of varying size are seen (fig. 17.2). In tissues that are actively growing, e.g. in young animals or around a healing wound, the cytoplasm of the fibroblast is basophilic and easily seen in light microscopy. In old tissues such as a contracted scar the fibroblasts become less active and protein synthesis diminishes. The nucleus elongates and there is only a thin layer of cytoplasm, hard to demonstrate in conventional histological preparations. These changes are reflected in fine structure; rough surfaced endoplasmic reticulum decreases and the Golgi zone is less prominent.

MACROPHAGES

Macrophages are known also by other names such as fixed and wandering histiocytes, phagocytic cells, or as littoral cells, in those situations where they provide a flattened lining for sinusoidal channels. They probably all originate from blood monocytes and so are known as the mononuclear phagocytes (chap. 29). Macrophages are present in most connective tissue and are approximately as numerous as the fibroblasts from which they are distinguished by having an indented bean-shaped nucleus. If a dye such as colloidal trypan blue is injected into connective tissue a day or two before the tissue is taken for histological examination, the difference between a macrophage and a fibroblast is apparent, for only the cytoplasm of the macrophage contains appreciable numbers of granules of dye. This experiment demonstrates that one of the important functions of the macrophage is to scavenge for foreign particles, fragments of cells or extracellular material.

Another distinction between macrophages and fibroblasts is found in their general disposition. Fibroblasts tend to occur in relation to collagen fibres, whereas macrophages congregate, sometimes in clusters, in the region of blood vessels. Some tissues such as tendons or ligaments may be practically free of macrophages, while other tissues such as the omentum have many.

MAST CELLS

Mast cells are relatively common in connective tissue, particularly in association with the blood vessels in adipose tissue. The name comes from the German word *masten*, to feed, and they were so named by Paul Ehrlich, who when a medical student discovered them in 1877, because they are full of granules and were thought to be phagocytic. We now know that they manufacture macromolecules of carbohydrate and are producers of granules and not overfed cells. The granules are not seen well in sections stained with haematoxylin and eosin, but in squashed preparations of connective tissue, methylene blue stains the mast cells and their masses of granules

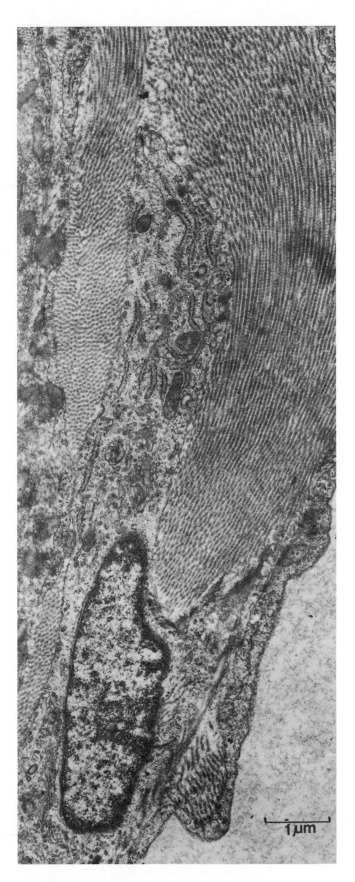

clearly. Mast cells are about the same size as fibroblasts and are more spherical with round nuclei, when this is visible through the granules (fig. 17.1).

Mast cells are known to produce a number of substances, including heparin, which is used to prevent clotting of blood and has other possibly important roles. These granules of complex macromolecules are responsible for the characteristic metachromasia of mast cells. Thus the dye, toluidine blue, stains them red instead of the expected blue. Histamine and 5-hydroxytryptamine are also made by mast cells although the latter is produced in very low concentrations, if at all, in human mast cells. The biological role of histamine is discussed in vol. 2, chap. 14.

FAT CELLS

Fat cells are highly specialized and play a big role in metabolism; they occur in most loose connective tissues in small clumps or even singly and in some situations they form large aggregates organized into lobules by strands of connective tissue (chap. 34).

The four types of cell described are not the only cells that can be found in connective tissue, but they are the most common. White cells from the blood, polymorphs, lymphocytes and monocytes are occasionally found in loose connective tissue particularly, and these cells appear in large numbers when there is inflammation. A specialized cell known as a **plasma cell** is frequently found. This cell has a basophilic cytoplasm and an eccentrically placed nucleus with a prominent Golgi region which usually shows up as a pale area, centrally placed, near the nucleus. Plasma cells have an important function in the manufacture of antibodies (chap. 29). As might be expected, plasma cells are found where foreign proteins are likely to gain entrance to the body, e.g. beneath the epithelial membranes lining the respiratory and alimentary tracts.

DENSE CONNECTIVE TISSUE

This tissue is found in tendons and fasciae where strength and flexibility are needed and in such structures as the ligamentum nuchae or the aortic wall where distensibility as well as strength is required. The strength is achieved by a great increase of fibrous material which in tendons consists almost entirely of collagen fibrils arranged in parallel bundles. Although collagen has little elasticity in comparison with elastin, it has high tensile strength. The tension sustained by the Achilles tendon during games such as tennis is a measure of its strength; it has been estimated that the tensile strength of a tendon is about four times the maximum isometric tension generated by its muscle, and is of the order of 150–300 N/mm². In

FIG. 17.2. EM of fibroblast, in active synthetic phase, lying between two bundles of collagen fibrils ($\times 17\ 700$).

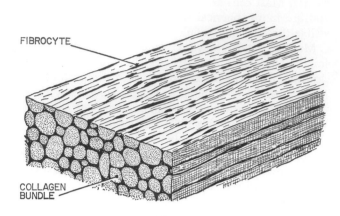

FIBROCYTE

COLLAGEN
BUNDLE

FIG. 17.3. Dense connective tissue. A section cut from a large mature tendon. This shows the flattened fibrocytes sparsely distributed among the collagen fibres (× 200).

terms of loading, the ability of the fibrocartilaginous intervertebral discs, largely collagen, to withstand pressures of up to 250 kg/cm² is an index of the resistance of collagen to distortion. In big tendons groups of collagen bundles are organized into fascicles by loose connective tissue in which the blood vessels run, but both the blood supply and cell population are relatively small. The only cells seen in sections of tendons are strings of flattened fibrocytes running between groups of fibres (fig. 17.3). In structures where distensibility as well as strength is important, such as the aortic wall, elastic tissue is prominent. Fresh elastic tissue is yellow and tissues with a predominance of elastic tissue have a distinct yellow tint. In sections the elastic tissue is characteristically coiled and branched in configurations which are quite distinct from the regular arrangement found in collagen fibre bundles.

Fascial sheets of tissue as in the fascia lata need strength and flexibility in many directions and so the collagen fibres are randomly arranged in thick bundles somewhat similar to the cellulose fibres in a sheet of paper.

Serous membranes

These tissues line the pleural, pericardial and peritoneal cavities, and consist of thin layers of loose connective tissue, covered by a layer of simple squamous epithelium called **mesothelium.** Folds of serous membrane, called 'ligaments', mesenteries or omenta, are associated with various viscera and may contain large amounts of adipose tissue in well nourished subjects. In health they are covered by thin films of fluid which make them slippery. This is a most important property of the membranes which allows, for example, the coils of the gut to glide over each other without difficulty. The lubricant is a proteoglycan complex, chiefly hyaluronic acid, which is discussed more fully on p. 17.8. In some diseases large volumes of fluid may accumulate in the peritoneal, pericardial or pleural cavities.

Proteins and proteoglycans of connective tissue

COLLAGEN

Collagen is remarkable both because of its amino acid composition and because of the amazingly regular way in which the molecules of protein are put together to make

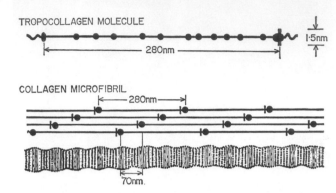

TROPOCOLLAGEN MOLECULE

1·5nm

280nm

COLLAGEN MICROFIBRIL

280nm

70nm.

FIG. 17.4. Diagrammatic view of the way tropocollagen molecules are arranged in the formation of collagen microfibrils.

the basic fibre unit. Individual protein chains of the microfibril are in register with neighbouring chains so that a characteristic banded appearance is seen under the EM. This is diagnostic of collagen as no other fibrous protein possesses this particular periodicity. Fig. 17.4 shows a diagrammatic EM view of a collagen microfibril. The major periodicity of about 70 nm is illustrated. In tissues the microfibrils line up when running parallel, so that the corresponding part of each band matches. Thus characteristic dark and light bands run across bundles of microfibrils. (fig. 17.5)

At higher magnifications and with different preparative techniques, the basic 2 band 70 nm periodicity can be seen to be itself made up of some 10 or 11 sub-bands (fig. 17.4). In the actual formation of a microfibril the basic molecular units must aggregate in an overlapping ordered fashion. The ordering of the tens of thousands of molecules so precisely in a microfibril is a most remarkable phenomenon.

The basic molecule is **tropocollagen.** These molecules are synthesized inside the fibroblast cell, but the microfibrils are assembled outside the cell (fig. 17.6). It is possible to disintegrate collagen into tropocollagen and to demonstrate the ability of these molecules to aggregate side by side in suitable environments, and so build the microfibril complete with periodicity in a test tube. Thus the fibroblasts secrete tropocollagen into the regions about the cells where the molecules line up end to end and side by side to form long microfibrils which can be seen to grow thicker as they are pushed away from the cell of origin by more secretion. The fibrils near a cell are thin and gradually become thicker at a distance from the cell. The long fibrils found in connective tissue imply a remarkable degree of co-ordination between neighbouring fibroblasts.

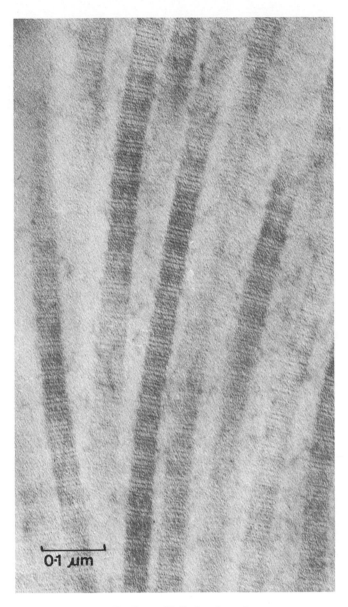

FIG. 17.5. EM of collagen fibrils (× 165 000).

The secreted tropocollagen molecules have a length of about 280 nm and a diameter of some 1·5 nm with a molecular weight of about 350 000. Each molecule consists of a helical arrangement of three separate polypeptide chains, each made of about a thousand amino acids. In the chain of amino acids, nearly every fourth one is glycine, followed by either a hydroxyproline or a proline molecule. Collagen is unique in containing about 13 per cent of hydroxyproline. This can be estimated chemically and thus the amount of collagen in a tissue can be calculated from the amount of hydroxyproline present. Hydroxyproline excretion in urine is also used to study collagen metabolism. Normally it is about 0·5 mmol or 60 mg/24 hr in growing children, falling to half

this value in healthy adults. In some diseases, such as hyperthyroidism or Paget's disease of bone, hydroxyproline excretion is increased. An interesting feature concerning the hydroxyproline and hydroxylysine of collagen is that they are formed by hydroxylation of proline and lysine in the formation of tropocollagen molecules. This is unusual because most other amino acids in proteins are supplied from the pool of amino acids. This means that they are not coded for genetically. Collagen contains only small amounts of methionine, cysteine, phenylalanine and tyrosine.

ELASTIN

Elastin is, like collagen, a fibrous protein, but its rod-like molecules are packed in a random fashion and so the EM reveals no ordered ultrastructure. Elastin occurs in tissues either as interconnected threads, as in the skin, or as more massive fibres, as in the ligamentum nuchae, or as fenestrated plates, as in the wall of the aorta, where as many as fifty plates may make up the thickness of the elastic tissue in the wall. Elastin is resistant to drying and survives in good condition in Egyptian mummies.

The amino acid composition of elastin differs from that of collagen most notably in that its content of hydroxyproline is low, as is its content of dicarboxylic amino acids. Apart from these differences the proteins have a similar composition. Both have important associated carbohydrate complexes and are therefore glycoproteins. These giant molecules may lace the protein molecules together to give the highly ordered collagen structure. Elastin is associated with lipid material and sphingolipid and galactosides have been extracted from it.

PROTEOGLYCANS

The proteoglycans are complexes of specific proteins and repeating monosaccharide residues, i.e. A B A B etc., forming acidic polysaccharide chains. Each molecule of proteoglycan (PG) contains many such polysaccharide chains which, when free of protein, are called **glycosaminoglycans** (GAG). The glycosaminoglycans are only synthesized when the appropriate protein is available for linkage. Historically the obsolete term mucopolysaccharide was used to mean either the proteoglycan complex or the free polysaccharides. Table 17.4 gives some of the properties of six well characterized proteoglycans associated with connective tissue.

Although the proteoglycans of connective tissue account for only 1–5 g/kg of fresh tissue their relationship to water and hormone metabolism is important. Thus in severe hypothyroidism the skin is characteristically thickened (myxoedema) and this is associated with increased hydration and an accumulation of proteoglycans. The dramatic water-holding capacity of some of

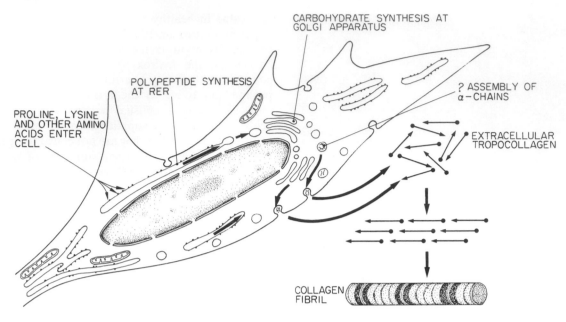

FIG. 17.6. Diagrammatic summary of the sequence of events in collagen synthesis. Redrawn from Bloom and Fawcett, after Gross.

the molecules is apparent in the tissues of the cock's comb. In the mature bird this is a massive headpiece of firm consistency yet it is over 90 per cent water. It contains some 2 per cent of collagen and about 7 per cent of hyaluronic acid. The mass of the comb is dependent upon the levels of androgen in the blood, so much so that the weight of the castrated cock's comb was formerly used to assay quantities of androgens. The size of the tissue and its turgidity are due to the quantity of hyaluronic acid present and this in turn is dependent on the quantity of androgen present. Wharton's jelly of the umbilical cord and the vitreous humour of the eye are

other examples of protein-glycosaminoglycan gels.

Another example of the hydration of proteoglycans is the massive increase in size of the sexual skin in certain species of monkey that is dependent on blood levels of oestrogen. This can be abolished by the administration of progesterone or the local injection of hyaluronidase.

Fig. 17.7 shows that the essential difference is the position of the OH or CHOH groups above or below the plane of the pyranose ring of the molecule. In the common hexuronic acids the CH_2OH group at position 6 is replaced by COOH to give D-glucuronic acid or L-iduronic acid. The hexosamines have NH_2 at C-2 instead of OH;

TABLE 17.4. Properties of some common proteoglycans.

Proteoglycan	Component monosaccharides of glycosaminoglycan	Occurrence
Hyaluronic acid	D-Glucuronic acid, 2-acetamido-2-deoxy-D-glucose	Vitreous humour, ground substance of connective tissues, umbilical cord, plasma, synovial fluids, cardiac valves
Chondroitin-4-sulphate (chondroitin sulphate A)	D-Glucuronic acid, 2-acetamido-2-deoxy-4-O-sulpho-D-galactose	Aortic tissue, cartilage, adult bone, ligamentum nuchae, cornea
Dermatan sulphate (chondroitin sulphate B)	L-Iduronic acid, 2-acetamido-2-deoxy-4-O-sulpho-D-galactose	Cardiac valves, skin, bovine lung tissue, bovine sclera
Chondroitin-6-sulphate (chondroitin sulphate C)	D-Glucuronic acid, 2-acetamido-2-deoxy-6-O-sulpho-D-galactose	Aortic tissue, cartilage, adult bone, cardiac valves, umbilical cord
Keratan sulphate (keratosulphate)	D-Galactose, 2-acetamido-2-deoxy-6-O-sulpho-D-glucose	Nucleus pulposus, costal cartilage, corneal tissue, aortic tissue
Heparin	D-Glucuronic acid, 2-deoxy-2-sulphoamino-D-glucose with additional O-sulphate groups	Liver, mast cells, spleen, muscle, lung, thymus, blood, heart

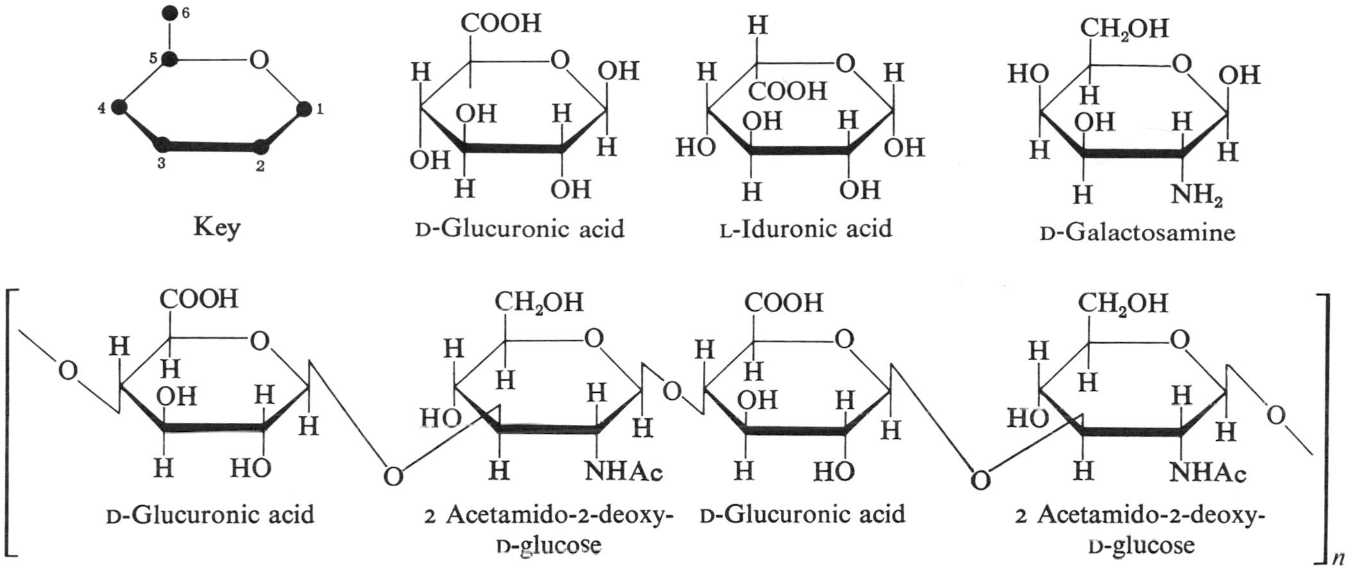

Segment of carbohydrate chain of hyaluronic acid

Fig. 17.7. Basic structural elements of glycosaminoglycans

glucosamine and galactosamine are the usual hexosamines found in glycosaminoglycans. The repetitive unit is usually a disaccharide hexuronic acid-acetylated hexosamine combination. This is shown in fig. 17.7 where the basic structure of hyaluronic acid is depicted. In the chondroitin sulphates, sulphate groups are found on the C-4 or C-6 positions of the hexosamine. Heparin is more complex in that it is based on a tetrasaccharide unit with five or six sulphate groups, one of which is found attached to the nitrogen group at C-2 of the hexosamine and another at the C-2 carbon position of the hexuronic acid.

In the same way as proteins are composed of twenty or so amino acids, glycosaminoglycans are built up from a few basic molecules. The shape of the monomer appears to be of importance to carbohydrate polymers because small changes in the configuration make a difference in the properties of the glycosaminoglycans which are formed from them. For example, the basic unit of chondroitin-4-sulphate and dermatan sulphate (table 17.4) differs only in the orientation of the carboxyl groups on C-5 of the hexuronic acid. Such small changes in orientation are not easy to identify, and this is one reason why knowledge of these important molecules has lagged behind that of proteins and lipids. Another factor is that the proteoglycans are intimately associated with other proteins and sometimes with lipids to form macromolecular complexes.

HYALURONIC ACID

Hyaluronic acid is the best known of the proteoglycans and it has the widest distribution in connective tissue. In tissues it is closely associated with water and has a molecular weight of about 10^7 daltons. The different properties of hyaluronic acid extracted from tissue ground substance and from synovial fluid may be due to the nature of the associated proteins.

Apart from its water holding capacity hyaluronic acid has the property of increasing the slipperiness of fluids and of lubricating the joints. However, this property is shared with other glycoprotein components which are present in the synovial fluid. In rheumatic diseases of joints, disturbances in hyaluronic acid metabolism occur.

CHONDROITIN SULPHATES

Chondroitin sulphates have a wide distribution in tissues but as their name suggests they are particularly important in the structure of cartilage. The intercellular elements of hyaline cartilage consist of a network of fine collagen fibrils, visible only with the EM, supported by a chondroitin–sulphate–protein complex which varies in different parts, as is shown by staining with toluidine blue which reacts metachromatically with chondroitin sulphates. Radioactive sulphur has been used to study the sulphate metabolism of cartilage.

Table 17.4 shows that proteoglycans such as dermatan sulphate and keratan sulphate have a wide distribution. Dermatan sulphate is particularly associated with tissues such as skin in which coarse collagen strands are prominent. As a person ages, the proportion of keratan sulphate increases relative to the chondroitin sulphates and is, in fact, linked to the same protein to make mixed glycosaminoglycan-protein complexes. The list of tissues in table 17.4 reflects merely those tissues which have been studied.

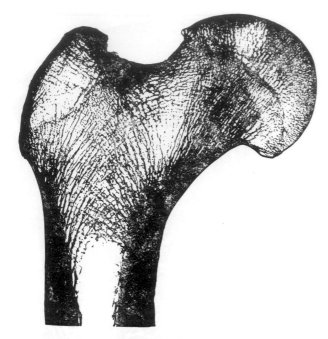

FIG. 17.17. The arrangement of trabeculae shown in this X-ray of a femoral head is as characteristic of the femur as its external form. Like cancellous bone elsewhere in the body its structure is so organized as to provide great strength with economy of material.

between osteoblastic and osteoclastic activity. During the growing period both processes are highly active although bone formation clearly exceeds destruction. In adult life until middle age the amount of bone remains constant, but during this time there is a continuous process of repair and replacement of the skeleton so that there is a complete turnover of bone approximately every 20 years.

In old age resorption exceeds formation leading to an atrophy of the skeleton which is called osteoporosis. If this atrophic process is severe the safety margin of skeletal strength is reduced and fractures may result from slight trauma (vol. 3, p. 26.9).

Periosteum

The periosteum is the ensheathing membrane which covers bone, except where it is covered by articular cartilage. It consists of an inner layer composed of osteoblasts which is conspicuous during the growing period and contributes largely to the increase in diameter of the bone, and an outer fibrous layer which carries part of the blood supply to the bone and provides attachment for muscles and ligaments. During the growing period the periosteum is firmly attached only at the circumference of the epiphyseal cartilage plate. Elsewhere it can be peeled off the bone as easily as a banana skin. Because of this loose attachment the muscles and ligaments which are attached to the periosteum may move their attachments over the under-

lying bone, during the growth of the bone. If this were not so, the fact that bone growth in length takes place only at the epiphyseal cartilage plates would result in a bizarre situation where many muscle origins and insertions were restricted to a narrow zone somewhere near the centre of each long bone.

It is only after growth ceases and the periosteum no longer slides like an elastic sheet over the underlying bone that firmer attachments develop and muscles acquire an anchorage through collagen fibres which pass directly into the bone tissue itself.

For powerful muscles such as the biceps, quadriceps and gastrocnemius, the periosteal attachment described above would not be strong enough and in these instances the muscles acquire a direct attachment to bone during the growth period through the medium of secondary centres of ossification.

Blood supply of bone

As with many other features of the anatomy of bone the blood supply has a different arrangement before and after growth has ceased (p. 19.38). A typical long bone has four principal groups of vessels (fig. 17.18).

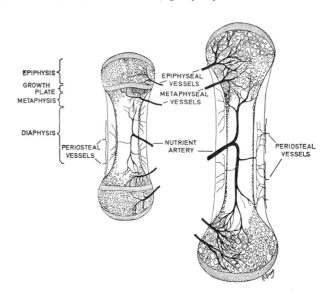

FIG. 17.18. Diagram showing the arrangement of blood vessels in bone before and after the growth period. Note that the growth plate isolates the epiphyseal from the metaphyseal circulation during the growing period, but that they anastomose freely after growth has ceased. The periosteal vessels supply the osteogenic layer on the bone surface during the growth period, but penetrate the cortex and supplement the nutrient artery in adult life.

The **epiphyseal** vessels supply the epiphyseal centres of ossification and are concerned also with the nutrition of growth cartilage. These vessels do not anastomose with the **metaphyseal** vessels since the cartilage acts as an avascular septum. The metaphyseal vessels sustain the vigorous new bone formation and remodelling which takes place on the metaphyseal side of the growth cartilage. The diaphysis is supplied mainly by one or more large **nutrient arteries** which penetrate the cortex to branch within the medullary cavity supplying the marrow and the greater part of the bone shaft.

The **periosteal** contribution to the blood supply of bone is slight during the growing period but increases when growth ceases and the periosteum acquires a firm and stable relationship to the underlying bone. As the growth plate disappears a free anastomosis develops between the epiphyseal and metaphyseal circulations.

The separate sources of blood supply in the growth period leads to a risk of avascular necrosis of bone. Thus infection of bone which may thrombose the nutrient artery can lead to death and sequestration of an entire diaphysis in childhood, whereas this complication is less common in adult life when loss of the nutrient artery can be replaced by the periosteal blood supply.

Relationship of bone and marrow

At first sight the association of bone and haemopoietic marrow appears to be a marriage of convenience; bone in order to combine strength with lightness is arranged in a tubular form which affords ideal protection for the delicate marrow tissue. However, the relationship is more profound than this for frequently haemopoietic marrow tends to develop in association with bone which forms outside the skeleton, e.g. in damaged muscle or tendon. When this happens, the bone becomes organized into a capsular form with a thin cortex containing the marrow. From evidence such as this it has been suggested that the marrow may be one of the several factors which help to determine the structure of bone. The common origin of bone and marrow cells is referred to on p. 17.12.

CARTILAGE

Structure and function of cartilage

Cartilage is the other major component of the skeleton and like bone has several roles to perform. The greater part of the skeleton is first represented by cartilage, which in due course is replaced by bone through the process of endochondral ossification considered in chap. 19. The cartilage model is responsible for both the shape and ultimate size of the individual bones. During fetal life or soon after birth the cartilage in each bone becomes restricted to two regions, the **epiphyseal cartilage plate** or plates which are responsible for the continued growth in length of the long bones and which disappear in adolescence, and the articular surface of bone.

The **articular cartilage** contributes to the growth of the epiphyses, or the whole bone in the case of the carpal and tarsal bones which lack separate cartilage plates. The superficial layers form a highly efficient joint surface which possesses enduring low friction properties which are the envy of engineers. The coefficient of friction of articular cartilage is approximately 0·013 which is almost three times more slippery than ice articulating with ice. Finally articular cartilage serves as a cushion which helps to protect the underlying bone from the effects of sudden loading. Cartilage also persists into adult life as an integral part of the skeleton notably in the rib cartilages.

Other types of cartilage tissues exist outside the skeleton in the framework of the ear and respiratory system.

Structure of cartilage

Cartilage is a firm gel bound together by the fibrous proteins collagen and elastin in varying proportions. The descriptive terms hyaline, fibrous or elastic are applied to it according to the relative amount of collagen or elastin. Hyaline cartilage is clear homogeneous tissue (Greek *hyalos*: glass) from which articular and rib cartilage is formed. Fibrocartilage is a firmer opaque material found in the menisci of the knee joint. Elastic cartilage, which is yellow in colour, is found in the structure of the ear and epiglottis.

Hyaline cartilage contains 75 per cent water, the remaining 25 per cent consisting of collagen and proteoglycan in approximately equal proportions. In ordinary preparations, studied by optical microscopy, the collagen fibres are invisible, since they have the same refractive index as the ground substance (proteoglycans). The proteoglycans of articular cartilage are chondroitin sulphates and keratan sulphate. The hydrophilic properties of the proteoglycans are responsible for maintaining the high water content of cartilage. The collagen network binds the cartilage to the adjacent bone, supports and contains the proteoglycans and provides the tensile strength of the cartilage. These two components acting as a functional unit are responsible for the mechanical properties of cartilage, which in articular cartilage include the capacity to be deformed and to recover its shape, compensating for irregularities in the shape of the bone ends, so that load is distributed more widely and evenly during movement. Articular cartilage also acts as a damper or shock absorber to reduce the damaging effect of sudden load on the bone ends. To achieve this mechanical purpose the components of cartilage show a high degree of organization. In articular cartilage four zones can be identified:

(1) a narrow superficial zone in which collagen fibres are closely packed and arranged parallel to the surface. The chondrocytes here are discoid with their long axes parallel to the surface;

(2) a thicker intermediate zone in which the collagen fibres form an irregular interlacing mesh. The chondrocytes here are larger, rounder and more evenly spaced;

(3) a deeper zone in which the collagen fibres are arranged perpendicularly to the underlying bone and the chondrocytes likewise are disposed in columns parallel to the fibres, and

(4) a very narrow calcified border adjacent to the underlying bone.

The growth cartilage of the epiphyseal plate likewise shows zonal differences of arrangement which are described in chap. 19.

Chondroblast and chondrocyte

The chondrocyte is the cell responsible for production and maintenance of the cartilage matrix. Its size, shape and structure vary according to its situation. At sites of rapid cartilage growth such as the proliferative zone of the epiphyseal cartilage (fig. 17.19b and fig. 19.67) the cells are small, flattened and may show mitotic activity. These cells are referred to as **chondroblasts.** Chondroblasts and chondrocytes can continue to elaborate more matrix, i.e. collagen fibres and ground substance, even when completely surrounded by matrix. This means that cartilage can grow by interstitial growth (p. 19.38). By contrast, osteoblasts can elaborate more matrix only when they lie on a surface; bone grows by appositional growth only, this difference being determined by the comparative softness of cartilage on the one hand and the unyielding rigidity of bone on the other. The mature chondrocyte may be flattened, as in the superficial zone of articular cartilage, but more usually is a plump, circular cell with large rounded nucleus filling the lacuna within the cartilage matrix. The histological appearance

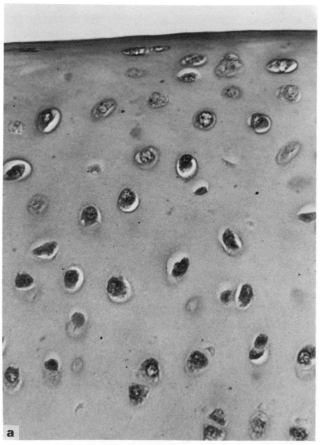

FIG. 17.19. Cartilage structure.

(a) Articular cartilage, in which the chondrocytes are large circular cells, fairly uniformly distributed throughout the matrix. Near the surface they are flattened (× 375).

(b) Epiphyseal cartilage plate, in which the cartilage cells are organized into columns in the axis of growth. Towards the epiphyseal side (top) the cells are actively proliferating and appear small and flattened. Further down the column the cells enlarge and eventually degenerate. They are then invaded by the metaphyseal blood vessels and new bone is laid down on the persisting scaffold of cartilage matrix. Note that the nutrition of the cartilage plate is derived from the vessels on the epiphyseal side (× 90).

of the chondrocyte however varies with its site in the different zones of articular and epiphyseal cartilage as shown in fig. 17.18. Chondrocytes are separated from each other by matrix and, although processes extend from the cells into the surrounding matrix, they do not appear to link up with other cells as is the case with osteocytes. EM studies show that rough endoplasmic reticulum is seen in most chondrocytes and is probably the site of collagen synthesis. The Golgi complex is well developed and contains large smooth-walled vacuoles. Radioactive tracer studies using ^{35}S indicate that the Golgi complex is concerned with the synthesis or storage of chondroitin sulphate and keratan sulphate, which are transported to the cell surface within the vacuoles. Degenerating chondrocytes have shrunken crenated nuclei, swollen disorganized mitochondria and dilated cisternae of endoplasmic reticulum. Mitotic activity is rarely observed in mature chondrocytes and the turnover of these cells therefore must be very slow; yet these cells are not inactive, for even after the cartilage matrix is fully elaborated chondrocytes continue to show considerable metabolic activity associated with a continual turnover of the cartilage matrix throughout life. Chondrocytes have a very limited capacity to repair large defects such as may arise as a result of injury or disease, and although such defects may fill with a fibrocartilaginous tissue derived from fibrous ingrowth, this material provides a poor substitute for articular cartilage and degenerative change may subsequently develop.

Calcification

Cartilage, like bone, may become calcified (mineralized). This is most evident in the deepest zone of articular cartilage and in the hypertrophic zone of the epiphyseal cartilage plate where it is an essential precursor of the subsequent endochondral ossification. If mineralization is prevented, as in rickets, the invasion of vascular tissue and bone is inhibited and the hypertrophic zone becomes greatly widened. Alkaline phosphatase can be demonstrated at sites of cartilage mineralization and presumably acts in the same way as it does at sites of bone mineralization (p. 17.11). The mineral is a calcium apatite crystal similar to that of bone.

Nutrition

Cartilage is largely avascular and acquires its nutrition by diffusion of nutrients from the surrounding tissue fluids. In the epiphyseal cartilage plate the major source of nutrition is the vascular plexus on the epiphyseal side of the plate next to the proliferating zone, the rich metaphyseal blood supply being concerned mainly with endochondral ossification. This observation has clinical importance, for fractures commonly take place in childhood through the hypertrophied zone of cartilage, a site of considerable structural weakness. These fractures never disturb the nutrition and growth of the cartilage plate, whereas the more unusual epiphyseal fracture which may damage the epiphyseal vessels frequently disturbs cartilage growth, with subsequent shortening or deformity of the affected bone. Articular cartilage derives its nutrition largely by diffusion from the joint synovial fluid, except during the growth period when the deeper layers receive a supply from the epiphyseal vessels. Mechanical activity acts as a pump which aids diffusion of nutrients through cartilage. If for any reason a joint or limb is disused, nutrition is impaired and both articular and growth cartilage may degenerate and may even become wholly destroyed; a limb severely paralyzed by poliomyelitis in childhood is frequently shorter than the unaffected limb for this reason.

Synovial tissue

The lining membrane of joints and tendon sheaths is referred to as the synovial membrane. It presents a smooth glistening surface with occasional villi and covers all intra-articular surfaces except the articular cartilage and menisci. Its purpose is to secrete synovial fluid which acts as a lubricant for joint movement and a source of nutrition for articular cartilage, and as a scavenging membrane it clears the joints of unwanted fluid, metabolites and particulate matter. Synovial cells are derived from embryonic mesenchyme of the skeletal blastema and are, therefore, similar in origin to other connective tissue cells. They form a discontinuous layer from one to four cells deep and are linked to each other by interlacing cytoplasmic processes. On light microscopy synovial cells are variable in shape, some flattened polygonal and others spindle-shaped. EM reveals two types of synovial cell, types A and B. A cells which are the more numerous are characterized by prominent Golgi complexes and many smooth walled vacuoles, but have little rough endoplasmic reticulum, while B cells contain much rough endoplasmic reticulum and have less developed Golgi complexes and fewer vacuoles. The synovial membrane is supported by a fibrocellular subsynovial tissue richly supplied with blood vessels and lymphatics containing many mast cells and macrophages.

SYNOVIAL FLUID

This is a clear viscous fluid consisting of a protein rich dialysate of blood plasma with added mucin composed mainly of hyaluronic acid. The proteoglycan confers visco-elastic properties on the fluid and the viscous component is of the non-Newtonian type, i.e. the viscosity falls with increasing shear rate. When the hyaluronic acid molecules are randomly cross-linked, the fluid has a high resistance to compression characteristic of an immobile joint. When the joint is moved the hyaluronic acid molecules line up in parallel and this greatly reduces viscous drag.

Synovial fluid is secreted by the A type synovial cells. Its protein content is largely derived from the plasma but some is probably secreted by the B cells. The scavenging role of synovial membrane is remarkably efficient. Crystalloid and similar very small particles are absorbed by the venous circulation, larger particles by the lymphatics, and very large particles are phagocytosed by the synovial lining cells which can remove whole erythrocytes and cell fragments. Multicellular loose fragments which may be shed by the articular cartilage in such diseases as osteoarthrosis or following trauma may become embedded in the synovial membrane where they are walled off by fibrous tissue. They are then anchored and so cannot cause symptoms by moving about the joint cavity.

FURTHER READING

BLOOM W. & FAWCETT D.W. (1968) *A Textbook of Histology*, 9th Edition. Philadelphia: Saunders.

BOURNE G.H. ed. (1971–72) *The Biochemistry and Physiology of Bone*, 2nd Edition, vols. I & II. New York: Academic Press.

BRIMACOMBE J.S. & WEBBER J.M. (1964) *Mucopolysaccharides. Chemical Structure, Distribution and Isolation.* BBA Library, vol. 6. Amsterdam: Elsevier.

EVANS F.G. (1957) *Stress and Strain in Bones*. American Lecture Series No. 296. Springfield, Ill.: Thomas.

FREEMAN M.A.R. (1973) *Adult Articular Cartilage*. London: Pitman Medical.

GHADIALLY F.N. & ROY S. (1969) *Ultrastructure of Synovial Joints in Health and Disease*. London: Butterworth.

GROSS J. (1961) Collagen *Scientific American* **204**, 121–130.

HAM A.W. (1974) *Histology*, 7th Edition. Philadelphia: Lippincott.

HANCOX N.M. (1972) *Biology of Bone*. London: Cambridge University Press.

HARKNESS R.D. (1961) Biological functions of collagen. *Biological Reviews* **36**, 399–463.

LACROIX P. (1951) *Organization of Bones*. London: Churchill.

RASMUSSEN H. & BORDIER P. (1974) *The Physiological and Cellular Basis of Metabolic Bone Disease*. Baltimore: Williams & Wilkins.

SMILEY J.D. & ZIFF M. (1964) Urinary hydroxyproline excretion and growth. *Physiological Reviews* **44**, 30–44.

SMITH J.W. & SERAFINI-FRACASSINI A. (1974) *The Structure and Biochemistry of Cartilage*. Edinburgh: Churchill Livingstone.

THOMPSON SIR D'ARCY W. (1961) *On Growth and Form*, abridged edition. London: Cambridge University Press.

VAUGHAN JANET M. (1975) *The Physiology of Bone*. Oxford: Clarendon Press.

WIDDOWSON E.M. & DICKERSON J.W.T. (1964) Chemical composition of the body. In *Mineral Metabolism*, ed. Comar C.L. & Bronner F., vol. II, part A. New York: Academic Press.

Chapter 18
Lining and secreting tissues

Bile, urine and intestinal contents are examples of fluids which are produced in the body, and life demands that they be kept separate from each other and from the rest of the tissues. Cells which serve these functions of secretion and lining are collectively called **epithelium**. An epithelium controls the passage of materials which cross the cells, and often a chemical or electrical gradient is established and maintained across it. Large molecular complexes may be absorbed or secreted and, in a gland, the epithelium becomes specialized for a secretory rather than a lining purpose. Epithelia do not have a single embryological origin and may arise from ectoderm, mesoderm or endoderm.

The epithelia form both the internal and external surfaces of the body and they possess two characteristic features. Firstly, they consist almost entirely of cells with little intervening extracellular space and no blood vessels. The uninterrupted layer of cells is needed to control the passage of material across their surface. The details of the close adhesions between adjacent epithelial cells are described on p. 13.12. Secondly, they are separated from the underlying tissue by a layer called the **basement membrane**, which is composed mainly of glycoproteins and collagen, rich in carbohydrate; this can be demonstrated on light microscopy by the PAS reaction (plate 18.1b, facing p. 18.2). With the electron microscope the basement membrane appears as an electron-lucent lamina and an electron-dense **basal lamina**, each usually about 30 nm thick. The clear lamina is nearest to the plasma membrane of the epithelial cell and the basal lamina lies next to the connective tissue underlying the epithelium. The basal lamina is composed of amorphous material consisting of proteoglycan, but it tends to be filamentous in character, with reticular fibres on its deep aspect where it merges with the connective tissue. However, much of the basal lamina material is produced by the epithelial cells and does not represent condensed connective tissue. It promotes cell adhesion but also exerts a regulatory function on materials passing to or from the basal aspect of the epithelial cells. This 'barrier' function is developed to a high degree in the case of the renal glomerulus (p. 35.7).

After fulfilling these two general requirements, there is variation in the arrangement, shape and number of cells which make up the various types of lining epithelia. This variety arises from different functional requirements and the wide range of physical, chemical and osmotic forces to which the surfaces are exposed. The external surface of the body is probably that most at risk; it is a dry surface lined by a strong epidermis. Many of the wet internal surfaces of the body lined by epithelia, for example that of the gastrointestinal tract (p. 32.1), are lined by **mucous membranes** which consist of an epithelium lying upon a basement membrane, supported by a connective tissue layer called **lamina propria**, and usually containing glands of various kinds; the surface of the mucous membrane, sometimes called a **mucosa**, is kept moist by the glandular secretions, which are often mucinous and slimy. The body cavities, pleural, pericardial and peritoneal, are lined by **serous membranes.** These consist of a lining of mesothelium (p. 18.2) supported by loose connective tissue and kept moist by a thin film of non-mucinous fluid.

Classification of epithelia

The first character used to classify an epithelium is that of the number of layers of cells separating the basement membrane from the external surface or lumen. When there is only one layer and all the cells have a luminal and basement membrane surface, it is called a **simple epithelium**. When it is more than one cell thick and no single cell extends through the whole depth of the layer, it is a **stratified epithelium**. A less common form, **pseudostratified epithelium**, contains some cells which extend from the basement membrane to the lumen and some which are in contact only with the basement membrane.

The next characteristic which is used is the shape of the cell which abuts on the lumen; this can be **squamous, cubical** or **columnar**. Various other features such as the possession of cilia or of a brush border characterize some epithelial cells.

SIMPLE SQUAMOUS EPITHELIUM (fig. 18.1 and plate 18.1a.)
The single layer of cells is very thin, often less than 2 μm

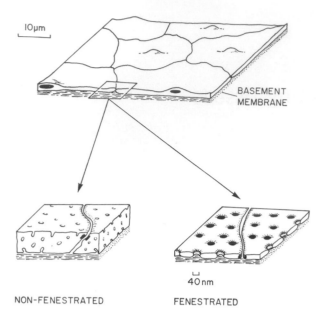

FIG. 18.1. Simple squamous epithelium.

thick and the cells are like scales, hence the term squamous. Each cell extends over a large surface area, perhaps 1000 μm², and its edges are stuck to those of its neighbours. From the surface this epithelium resembles crazy paving. The EM shows that there are two types of simple squamous epithelium, **non-fenestrated** and **fenestrated**. In the latter the thin cells are perforated by numerous circular pores each about 40 nm in diameter. In the cytoplasm of the non-fenestrated type many small pinocytotic vesicles are present and, since some of these fuse with the inner and outer plasma membranes, they are probably involved in transporting macromolecules.

These cells form the lining of blood vessels and heart, and are then referred to as **endothelium**; the serous sacs are also lined by these cells, and here they are known as **mesothelium**.

SIMPLE CUBICAL EPITHELIUM (fig. 18.2)

This consists of a regular palisade of cubical cells, each one having a centrally placed nucleus.

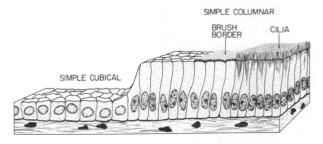

FIG. 18.2. Simple cubical and columnar epithelium.

SIMPLE COLUMNAR EPITHELIUM (fig. 18.2 and plate 18.1c)

Columnar cells are taller than they are broad, and their nucleus is nearer to the basal end of the cell. Such cells line many glands and mucosal surfaces. Simple columnar epithelium sometimes possesses a brush border or cilia on its luminal side, e.g. in the bronchi, where it is referred to as **ciliated columnar epithelium.**

STRATIFIED SQUAMOUS EPITHELIUM (fig. 18.3)

Many layers of polygonal cells underlie the flattened cells of the surface. The squamous cells on the surface may retain their nuclei or they may become non-nucleated squames, full of the protein keratin. Thus there are two varieties of stratified squamous epithelium **keratinized** (cornified) and **non-keratinized** (non-cornified).

Keratinized squamous epithelium forms the epidermis of the skin, and the non-keratinized type is found in the oesophagus.

STRATIFIED COLUMNAR EPITHELIUM (fig. 18.3 and plate 18.1d)

The adherent columnar cells on the surface are separated from the basement membrane by at least one layer of smaller cells as in the larger ducts of glands.

PSEUDOSTRATIFIED COLUMNAR EPITHELIUM

This appears to contain more than one layer of columnar cells, but close inspection shows that all cells abut on the basement membrane. However, the apices of some cells do not reach the luminal surface of the epithelium and hence the distribution of cell nuclei gives the observer the impression of a stratified epithelium. The columnar cells of this type of epithelium often bear cilia, and the upper respiratory tract is lined in this manner.

TRANSITIONAL EPITHELIUM (fig. 18.3 and plate 35.1b, facing p. 35.12)

Epithelium of this type presents a line of swollen cells to the lumen and has a number of layers of smaller cells below the surface. This name is confusing and inappropriate but there does not appear to be an acceptable alternative. The lower urinary tract, i.e. pelvis of the kidney, ureter and bladder, is lined by transitional epithelium.

Functions and distribution of epithelia

LINING EPITHELIUM

The thinness of a simple squamous epithelial layer facilitates passive diffusion, but as it has such a small cytoplasmic volume in relation to surface area it cannot perform active transport of material or secretion. Its flat moist surface provides a frictionless boundary. Since the cells allow diffusion, they provide a suitable lining for the blood and lymph vessels; the fenestrated type is present where the material transferred is greater than average, for example in the capillaries of the endocrine glands,

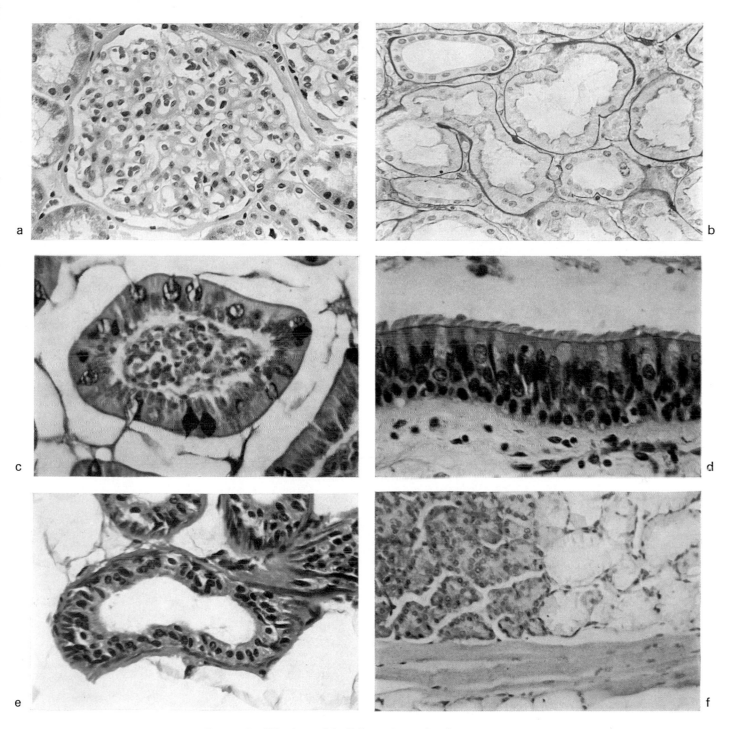

PLATE 18.1. Histology of the lining and secreting tissues.

(a) Simple squamous epithelium lines the capsule of the renal glomerulus (Bowman's capsule), and appears as a line of flattened nuclei. Simple cubical epithelium lines the distal convoluted tubules seen around the glomerulus. Human renal cortex, haem. & eosin (×400).

(c) Simple columnar epithelium with mucus-secreting goblet cells from a small intestinal villus. The brush border and the mucus is stained red by the PAS stain. Human jejunum, PAS (×400).

(e) Myoepithelial cells in the walls of sweat gland acini. These elongated, red-staining cells are seen cut in various planes of section. Human skin, Masson (×450).

(b) The basement membranes of the proximal and distal convoluted tubules and the collecting tubule appear as fine red lines. The brush border of the proximal tubules stains pink; their lumina are abnormally dilated. Human renal cortex, PAS & tartrazine (×375).

(d) Stratified, ciliated, columnar epithelium. Human trachea, haem. & eosin (×500).

(f) Serous and mucous acini with striated muscle fibres from the tongue. The pale cells with small basal nuclei in the mucous acini, on the right, are easily distinguished from the darker serous cells. Rabbit tongue, Van Gieson (×250).

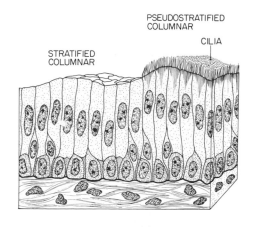

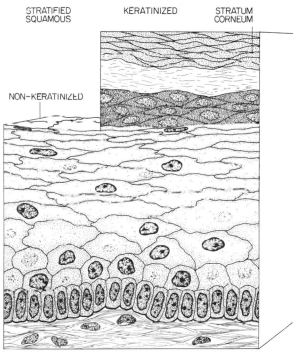

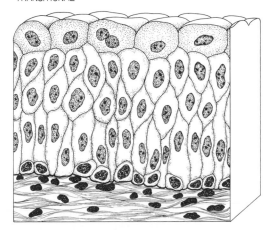

FIG. 18.3. Stratified epithelia.

renal glomerulus and mucosa of the small intestine. The alveolar epithelium in the lung is simple squamous, which allows the passage of gases. The serous cavities, such as the pleura and peritoneum, have a simple squamous lining which allows the contained organs to slide over each other.

There is some justification for considering endothelia and mesothelia as types of lining different from other epithelia. They always develop from mesoderm and retain, in the adult, the capacity of regeneration from primitive mesenchymal cells. Pathological conditions, such as tumours, arising in the endothelia and mesothelia differ in many respects from those arising in epithelia, so pathologists usually consider them as separate categories and apply the term 'epithelium' only to the other lining tissues.

Active absorption requires the use of energy and the volume of cytoplasm necessary to contain the mitochondria is provided by cubical or columnar epithelium. The luminal surface of the cells is often increased by the formation of a brush border (p. 13.14). Absorption would be hindered by a stratified type of epithelium and absorptive surfaces are of the simple cubical or columnar type. Examples are the lining of the small intestine and the proximal convoluted tubules in the kidney, which also have brush borders. Less active absorption occurs in the large intestine, gall bladder, stomach and the larger ducts of glands, where the epithelium is simple cubical or columnar and does not have a true brush border, although there are a few microvilli on each cell. The simple cubical epithelium forming the distal convoluted renal tubules absorbs actively but here it is the basal surface of the cell which is increased (p. 35.4).

Ciliary activity also consumes energy and so cilia are always associated with a columnar type of cell. Ciliated columnar epithelium may be simple, stratified or pseudostratified. It is present in the respiratory passages and the uterine tubes.

Resistance to surface friction is the characteristic feature of stratified squamous epithelium. It also provides a relatively impervious layer, and so it forms the epithelium of the skin, and the lining of the mouth, pharynx, oesophagus and vagina. When it lines a moist surface such as the mouth or conjunctival sac, it is non-keratinized with nuclei in the surface layer of cells. On the dry surfaces there is always a layer of cells, without nuclei but loaded with keratin, which form a stratum corneum, and the thickness of this layer is directly related to the amount of surface friction. A series of elaborate modifications allows this type of epithelium to withstand friction; (1) the basement membrane is indented by the underlying connective tissue so that it forms an irregular plane which helps to prevent the whole epithelium from shearing away from its support; (2) the epithelial cells are

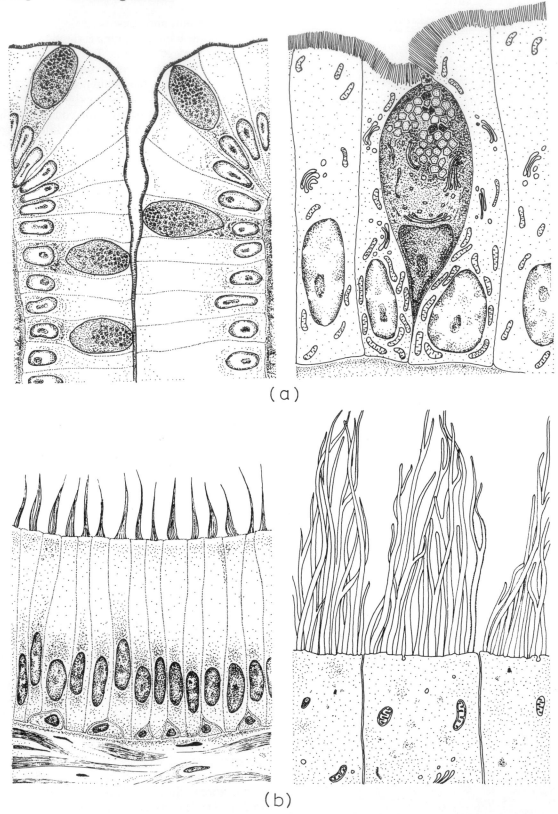

(a)

(b)

FIG. 18.4. (a) Goblet cells in simple columnar epithelium; left, light microscopy; right, electron microscopy; (b) non-motile stereocilia on simple columnar cells of ductus epididymidis; left, light microscopy; right, electron microscopy.

toughened by a fibrous protein forming tonofibrils within the cells, and (3) at the adhesion points between adjacent cells, desmosomes, the tonofibrils are attached to the adhesion plaques. Thus a stratified squamous epithelium provides a thin, tough, almost watertight surface layer which is firmly tacked down to the tissue beneath.

Transitional epithelium seems to be the only variety which can withstand the hypertonicity and special composition of urine. It is therefore always and only found on surfaces like those of the ureter and bladder which are constantly in contact with urine. These organs vary their contained volume and transitional epithelium allows for stretching.

SECRETORY EPITHELIUM

Secretion is another important epithelial function and the height of the epithelial cells can indicate their secretory activity. This is seen in the thyroid gland where the lining of a follicle is simple squamous in a quiescent follicle but becomes cubical or columnar with increasing activity. The secretory products are usually stored in the cytoplasm of the epithelial cell; mucus, for instance, can be stained in the inner half of the cells which line the surface of the gastric mucosa. Goblet cells in a columnar epithelium are specialized mucus-secreting cells which have this shape because of their large store of mucus (fig. 18.4 and plate 18.1c, facing p. 18.2). Some secreting epithelial cells have long non-motile processes which project into the lumen; these stereocilia (fig. 18.4) are best seen on the columnar cells of the duct of the epididymis.

ORIGIN OF EPITHELIA

Since epithelial structure has to conform to the function of a surface, it is not influenced by its embryological origin. Non-keratinized stratified squamous epithelium, for instance, is derived from all three germ layers from ectoderm in the conjunctiva, from entoderm in the oesophagus and from mesoderm in the upper part of the vagina. Endothelia and mesothelia arise only from mesoderm.

Regeneration of epithelia

The relatively undifferentiated type of cells lining blood vessels (endothelium) and serous cavities (mesothelium) seems to be able to recruit cells from the surrounding mesenchyme. In the healing of a wound, some of the new capillaries differentiate *in situ* and they are not all produced by outgrowths from neighbouring vessels. Most epithelia, after the earliest embryonic stages, can grow only from themselves. The basement membrane does not always prevent the migration of cells into an epithelium, and lymphocytes are regular visitors, but none of these migratory cells are capable of differentiating into

epithelial cells. Conversely, epithelial cell proliferation is confined by the basement membrane which epithelial cells do not normally penetrate. A carcinoma is a malignant neoplasm in which epithelial cells lose their mutual adhesion and penetrate into the underlying tissue.

The loss of a cell in the single layer of a simple epithelium is replaced by cell division and lateral movement to fill the gap. If large numbers of undifferentiated epithelial cells are interposed in a simple epithelium, the pseudostratified variety is produced. When the number of regenerating cells is sufficient to separate all the surface cells from the basement membrane, a true stratified epithelium is present. The exposed epithelia which are liable to suffer damage are of the stratified type. A journey down the air passages of the respiratory system shows epithelium changing from pseudostratified to simple as more protected cavities are reached. In the stratified squamous epithelia there is a constant replacement of the surface cells as they die; the basal cells of this epithelium tend to divide at night when the body is at rest, although diurnal periodicity is more conspicuous in mice than in men.

It is initially surprising that the intestinal epithelium, which is so exposed to dietary indiscretions, should be of a simple type. Its absorptive function is assisted by its being only one cell thick and its replacement is now known to be effected by a rapid migration from regenerating cells which enjoy the seclusion of the tubular crypts. So each intestinal epithelial cell has a short active life.

If an area of epithelium is destroyed, an ulcer is produced. The ulcerated region is repaired by migration and proliferation of cells in the intact epithelium around the edges of the ulcer. Another example of the independent property of epithelia is given by skin grafting, for a superficial slice of skin, including epidermis, can be cut off and transplanted to carry epithelial cells to a completely denuded area. The epidermis at the site of removal is renewed by epithelial cells which grow out of the truncated sweat glands and hair follicles to populate the surface.

EPITHELIAL DERIVATIVES

The epithelia are modified to produce a variety of structures. The origin of hairs and nails from the epidermis is described with the skin (p. 37.7). The manner in which the enamel of the teeth develops on the basal surface of the epithelium forming an enamel organ is mentioned elsewhere (p. 22.50). Glands are also derived from epithelia and, as described below, some lose their connection with the surface.

Secretory tissue

All cells, of course, must be able to transport substances across their membranes; they must be able to take up nutrients and extrude waste matter. Some cells, however, extrude substances which are useful to the body, and these are called **secretory cells**. These cells may be part of the structure of an organ, as in the pancreas, or they may be grouped together and organized as glands which are developed as epithelial outgrowths.

Glands which retain a connection with the surface from which they are developed and discharge their secretion on to it, such as the sweat glands and those which produce digestive juices, are called **exocrine** glands. Those which lose their connection with the surface, and secrete **hormones** directly into the blood stream, are called **endocrine** glands. These hormones are carried in the blood stream to act on target organs at a distant site. In all cases nutrients must be transferred from the blood of the surrounding capillaries to the cells, and products elaborated in the secretory cells must be passed into the **ducts** or blood stream.

EXOCRINE GLANDS

In order to increase the volume of secretory epithelial

cytoplasm which discharges on to a surface, the glandular outgrowths assume different shapes (fig. 18.5). Tubular outgrowths can be simple, branched or coiled, while saccular outgrowths are, in man, only branched. A compound gland is one in which the original outgrowth forms a complex branching duct system before becoming the secretory portion; the secretory portion can be tubular or saccular or, as in the liver, exhibit a laminar arrangement of its secretory cells. The saccules of a compound gland are called **acini**, because each one resembles a berry (Latin: *acinus*) on the end of the branching stalk or duct.

The type of secretory product affects the structure of a gland. If it is synthesizing enzymes, it has **serous (zymogenic) acini** whose cells have basophilic cytoplasm due to their high RNA content. A large oval nucleus with prominent nucleoli lies near the centre of the serous cell and its apical cytoplasm contains stores of its protein secretion as zymogen granules (p. 18.7). Glycoproteins forming the basis of mucous secretion appear clear after routine staining methods, so that **mucous acini** have an

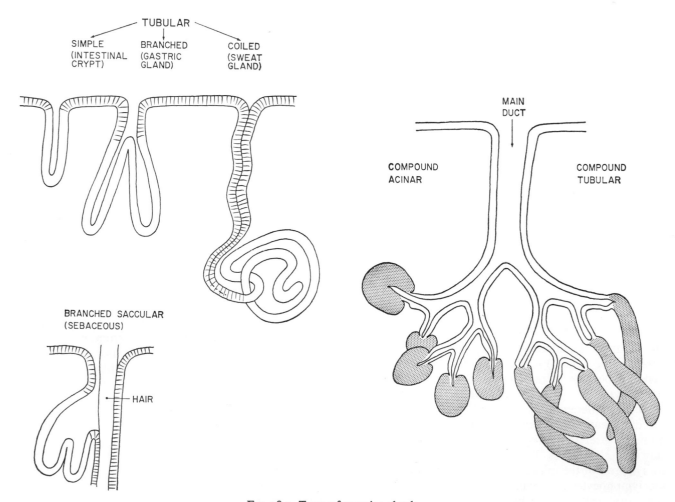

FIG. 18.5. Types of exocrine glands.

empty appearance with compressed nuclei near the base of each cell (fig. 18.6 & plate 18.1f, facing p. 18.2). The mucus can be stained by the PAS reaction (p. 13.3). The goblet cells mentioned above are isolated mucus-secreting cells.

Most exocrine glands are either mucus-secreting, e.g. sublingual, or serous in type, e.g. pancreas. In a mixed gland, such as the submandibular, the acini are usually of one or other type with the mixing occurring in the duct. There are, however, some mucous acini in which a segment of the secretory unit is composed of serous cells. In some planes of section, the serous cells as a group form a crescentic shape apparently at the periphery of the mucous acinus; such crescents are known as serous demilunes (fig. 18.6b). In the parotid gland, even the individual secretory granule may contain both serous and mucous (seromucous) components.

Apart from proteins and glycoproteins, some gland cells secrete electrolytes and water. The secretory cells of the sweat glands expel a hypotonic NaCl solution but the outstanding example of this type of secretion is the parietal cell of the stomach which produces a hydrochloric acid solution. Lipoid materials are also secreted by certain glands, notably the cutaneous sebaceous and apocrine sweat glands.

The range of secretory products mentioned above demands different methods of discharge. Electrolytes and water can be pumped through the cell membrane without any structural change being observed in that membrane; this is **eccrine** secretion. In **apocrine** secretion the materials accumulate in the luminal part of the cell, which then breaks off into the lumen. Stereocilia represent a form of apocrine secretion as these long cytoplasmic processes project into the lumen and accumulate blebs of secretion which are pinched off. A third method of secretion is **holocrine**, where the whole cell accumulates the product; the sebaceous glands of the skin are a characteristic example of this type of discharge.

The fourth and most common method of secretion is **merocrine**. In many of the enzyme-producing exocrine

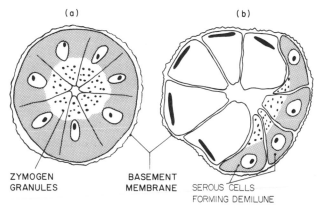

FIG. 18.6. Serous (a) and mucous (b) acini.

glands such as those of the pancreas, microscopic examination shows the presence of granules, which are the precursors or storage forms of the active enzymes secreted by the cells. By time–lapse cinephotography of living tissues, it can be shown that these **zymogen granules** are in constant motion in the cells, and that their numbers are depleted when the gland is active. They build up again in the resting cells. They appear to be semi-fluid in nature, and dissolve when they are liberated into the ducts of the glands. EM studies show that the granules are first formed in the rough endoplasmic reticulum. Later they aggregate in the Golgi region where they are surrounded by smooth endoplasmic reticulum, which becomes continuous with the membrane of the free surface of the cell during secretion. The granule then breaks through this membrane, while the cell membrane remains intact (fig. 13.14b).

ENDOCRINE GLANDS

Secretory granules may be seen also in the cells of endocrine glands. The secretory granules demonstrated in the anterior pituitary gland appear to be similar to those seen in the exocrine pancreas. EM also emphasizes their similarity, since here too the granules are surrounded by a smooth membrane, and are formed near the Golgi apparatus. The mechanism of release of the hormone is similar to the release of enzyme from exocrine glands.

Hormones may be stored in one of two ways; (1) within the cell, e.g. as granules of insulin in the β-cells of the pancreatic islets, and (2) as a spheroidal mass of secretory product enclosed by a single layer of secretory cells, as in the thyroid follicle. The endocrine glands are described in greater detail in chap. 27.

Secretory processes and transport across membranes

As already indicated cell and cytoplasmic membranes exist in order to keep certain molecular species apart either qualitatively or quantitatively. In some cases transport across the boundary membrane of cells and cytoplasmic membranes can be explained in terms of either bulk flow or diffusion. Bulk flow results from differences in hydrostatic pressure and the transmembrane pressure difference determines the direction and magnitude of flow. Examples are the formation of glomerular filtrate (p. 35.7) and intercellular transport in the wall of the gall bladder (p. 32.38). Diffusion consists of the random movement of molecules, the velocity of which at constant temperature depends upon molecular size. The number of molecules which cross a unit area of a membrane in a given time is termed the **flux** or **exchange** and directional movement is determined by their relative transmembranous concentrations. Thus

$$f = K(C_1 - C_2)$$

where f = flux, K is a constant which depends upon the chemical nature of the molecule and the permeability coefficient of the membrane, and C_1 and C_1 the concentrations on each side of the boundary membrane. Many nutrients such as O_2 pass through cell membranes by diffusion (p. 31.25) and exchange between intravascular and extracellular fluids is mediated by this process. Such processes are called **passive** or **non-mediated transport.**

Cell membranes which consist of a phospholipid bilayer (p. 13.6) constitute a barrier to diffusion, and large molecules such as proteins, most polar molecules and smaller highly charged molecules diffuse across very slowly or not at all. However, molecules which are lipid-soluble diffuse through membranes more readily. These considerations are of importance in relation to the flux of physiological materials and drugs (vol. 2, p. 2.1).

At many sites in the body, net flux of a substance across a cell membrane occurs more rapidly or more completely than can be accounted for by their chemical or electrochemical gradients. By this means the intracellular composition of many tissues becomes very different from that of the surrounding extracellular fluid. For example, the secretory cells of the salivary glands take up iodide ions from the blood, where they are in low concentration, and achieve a high intracellular concentration. If a solute moves across a membrane at a rate or in a direction which cannot be predicted on the basis of molecular size, solubility or electrochemical gradient, or if this flux can be shown to occur only when energy is provided by metabolism, the process is either one of **mediated** or **active transport.**

MEDIATED TRANSPORT

The common characteristic of this form of transport is that the substance transported is bound to a component of the cell membrane. The simplest situation is one in which a solute is carried across a cell membrane from a concentrated to a dilute solution more rapidly than would be expected by diffusion. This may be explained by assuming that the solute becomes chemically bound to a carrier molecule at the surface of the membrane. If there are identical carrier molecules throughout the thickness of the membrane, the solute can rapidly move from one side to another. The carrier molecules themselves need not move. This is called **facilitated diffusion.**

Another form of mediated transport involves a carrier molecule which picks up at one surface of a membrane

Membrane

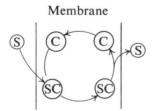

FIG. 18.7. Carrier-mediated transport. S, substrate; C, carrier molecule.

molecules of a particular species. The carrier-solute complex then moves rapidly through the membrane and the solute is released at the other side (fig. 18.7). If the carrier travels in both directions equally readily, net flux of the solute occurs down the concentration gradient, but at an increased rate. If, however, the carrier molecule is generated at one side of a membrane and inactivated when it releases solute at the other side, a one-way system is created, capable of transferring a substance from a dilute to a more concentrated solution.

In such mediated systems, the flux of the solute depends on the availability of the specific carrier molecules at the membrane surface and does not vary linearly with the concentration gradient across the membrane. Instead, the kinetics of the system are similar to those of an enzyme-catalysed reaction (p. 7.8). Thus when all the specific sites of the membrane are occupied, the carrier system is saturated and flux reaches a maximum. An example is the renal tubular reabsorption of glucose (p. 35.12).

Such systems are usually highly discriminating for different types of solute molecules but may be specifically inhibited by compounds with closely similar chemical groups. It is for this reason that phlorizin, which occurs in the bark of apple and contains glucose in its structure, blocks the renal tubular reabsorption of glucose without itself being reabsorbed. However, competition between similar molecules may occur for the available carrier molecules; this is seen, for example, in the small intestine where one monosaccharide can competitively inhibit the active absorption of another, or in renal tubular absorption of amino acids (p. 35.13). Again the characteristics of the flux are similar to ES and EI effects on the velocities of enzyme-catabolized reactions, where the carrier molecule can be substituted for the enzyme (E) and the flux of substance S is being investigated in the presence of an inhibitory substance (I) (p. 7.10).

While the carrier-mediated transport theory offers an explanation of the specific ability to transport physiological materials into or out of cells, the nature of the carriers is unknown, though they are probably specific proteins which require to be continuously regenerated.

ACTIVE TRANSPORT

Several transport processes of vital importance to cellular function are more directly linked to metabolic energy than are those of mediated transport and so are able to work against chemical or electrical gradients. This is especially the case for the creation and maintenance of concentration differences of ions inside and outside excitable cells, such as those of muscle and nerve. One of the most important active transport systems in the body involves the movement of Na^+ across cell membranes and depends for its energy upon the hydrolysis of ATP by ATPase within the cell membrane. This is carried out by one of two mechanisms. In one, extrusion of Na^+ from cells is linked with the transport of K^+ into cells. This is called a **coupled pump** and is electrically neutral. Activated by ATPase, it is described on pp. 15.14 and 32.44. In the other, directional Na^+ transport is not compensated for by corresponding K^+ transport and so an electrochemical gradient is created. This type of active transport is called **electrogenic**. A good example is the secretion of HCl by the parietal cells of the gastric mucosa (p. 32.15). Another example is the Ca^{++} transporting ATPase in the intracellular sarcoplasm membrane involved in muscular contraction (p. 16.9).

Active transport depends on the integrity of the cell membrane. It involves large amounts of energy and an increased blood supply is needed to support the metabolic requirements of actively secreting tissue. Thus, for example, about 70 per cent of O_2 used by the kidney is utilized for active transport.

Pinocytosis is another form of active transport visible histologically and described on p. 13.13; it is employed to a very limited extent and rates of transport are relatively slow.

Work of secretion

If the standard free energy changes in the chemical reactions involved in secretion are known, together with the activities of the secreted substances, the minimum work done in secretion can be calculated. However, these values are extremely difficult, if not impossible, to determine for complex molecules such as enzymes and hormones. Estimates, based on many unsupported assumptions, suggest that 1·7 kJ energy are required to produce the protein present in the gastric juice secreted by a dog after a meal of 200 g meat.

For the energy requirements for the secretion of ions, the calculation is simpler at least to the extent that their concentrations can be determined accurately. If we consider the transport of H^+ from the blood (pH 7·4) to gastric juice (pH 1·0), we use the formula:

$$\triangle G = RT \ln \frac{C_1}{C_2}$$

where $\triangle G$ is the work done (i.e. the free energy change) per mole HCl transported, R is the gas constant, T the absolute temperature, and C_1 and C_2 the pH values (negative logarithms of the H^+ concentration). Rewriting, and using $\log_{10}$, we have at 37°C

$$\triangle G = RT \times 2·303 \, (\log_{10} C_1 - \log_{10} C_2) \text{ Joules}$$
$$= RT \times 2·303 \times 26·8 \text{ Joules}$$
$$= 38 \text{ kJ}$$

This calculation is obviously an approximation, in that no account has been taken of the free energy change that may have arisen as a result of changes in electrical potential.

Control of secretion

Some glands secrete continuously, while others are activated only by specific stimuli. This applies to both exocrine and endocrine glands. The type of control is intimately related to the resting rate of secretion, the duration of secretion in response to the stimulus, and the feedback systems inhibiting the process. The following factors influence the rate of secretion.

BLOOD FLOW

During secretory activity the blood supply of a gland is greatly increased, thereby ensuring a plentiful supply of nutrients and oxygen to produce the energy required and of water and electrolytes necessary for elaboration into the secretion.

In three situations a specific mechanism to achieve this vasodilation has been described. These are in salivary secretion, sweat production, and the exocrine secretion of the pancreas. Here it is believed that when activity of the glands begins, a proteolytic enzyme is released which reacts with tissue fluid protein to form the polypeptide **bradykinin**. This potent vasodilator substance probably has a local effect in increasing blood flow. This increase has, of course, no necessary influence on the rate of secretion from the gland, but may aid it by supplying increased amounts of oxygen and nutrients. Bradykinin is likely to be active in other secretory tissues (vol. 2, p. 17.1).

NERVOUS FACTORS

Nervous control mechanisms occur when a rapid onset of secretion is required from an otherwise inactive gland or a rapid increase above a low resting rate of secretion. The adrenal medulla and salivary glands are examples of secretory tissues under nervous control.

CHEMICAL FACTORS

Chemical control of secretion occurs in glands such as the parathyroids, where the level of plasma calcium determines the rate of secretion of parathyroid hormone which in turn regulates the plasma calcium concentration.

HORMONAL FACTORS

Hormonal control mechanisms exist where a less rapid, less finely graded but prolonged secretion is required, such as the production of hormones by the adrenal cortex and of bile by the liver.

Some glands require both a rapid onset of secretion and a prolonged response, and in these cases a combination of nervous and hormonal control is found. For example, the secretion of gastric juice is rapidly raised above the resting level by nerve impulses and its secretion is maintained by a hormone, gastrin.

PHYSICAL FACTORS

Physical factors are involved in sweat secretion, which

depends ultimately on deep body temperature, though this information is transmitted by nerve impulses.

MECHANICAL FACTORS

Mechanical stimuli are probably involved in the secretion of mucus. Its secretion in the gastrointestinal tract is thought to be caused by mechanical stimulation of the mucosa.

These and other examples of simple and mixed control of secretory processes are described more fully in other chapters, where the mechanisms are dealt with in greater detail.

Myoepithelium

Around the cells of some glands (sweat, salivary, mammary and lacrimal), there are specialized cells of ectodermal origin, which resemble smooth muscle in appearance (plate 18.1e, facing p. 18.2). The cytoplasmic processes of these **myoepithelial** cells surround the secretory units, and have been shown by EM studies to contain myofilaments. The contraction of these is thought to assist in expelling the secretion of the glands. This may be brought about by either nervous or hormonal mechanisms.

Other secretory processes

By our original definition that secretory cells are those which extrude substances useful to the body, we should include also nerve synapses, nerve endings, and the neurosecretory cells of the hypothalamus. The synapses and nerve endings produce the chemical mediators necessary for the transmission of the nerve impulse. The hypothalamus produces releasing hormones and the posterior pituitary hormones. These forms of neurosecretion are, however, outside the usual concept of secretory tissue, and are dealt with in chaps 15 and 27.

FURTHER READING

BLOOM W. and FAWCETT D.W. (1968). In *A Textbook of Histology*, 9th Edition, Chapter 3. Philadelphia: Saunders.

DAVSON H. (1970) *A Textbook of General Physiology* 4th Edition, vols. I & II. London: Churchill.

FINEAN J.B., COLEMAN R. & MICHELL R.H. (1974) *Membranes and their Cellular Functions*. Oxford: Blackwell Scientific Publications.

HARRIS E.J. (1972) *Transport and Accumulation in Biological Systems*, 3rd Edition. London: Butterworth.

LIN E.C.C. (1972) The molecular basis of membrane transport systems. In *Structure and Function of Biological Membranes*, ed. Rothfield L.I., pp. 285–341. New York: Academic Press.

NEAME K.D. & RICHARDS T.G. (1972) *Elementary Kinetics of Membrane Carrier Transport*. Oxford: Blackwell Scientific Publications.

ROBINSON J.R. (1975) *A Prelude to Physiology*. Oxford: Blackwell Scientific Publications.

Chapter 19
Early development

For the new individual, life begins in the ampulla of the uterine tube with the act of fertilization, when the nuclei of the ovum and sperm fuse (p. 38.38). At fertilization the diploid number of chromosomes is restored, the chromosomal sex of the new individual is determined and the ovum is activated to proceed to the first **cleavage division** (fig. 19.1).

EMBRYOGENESIS

After fertilization a series of divisions known as **cleavage** converts the single fertilized ovum, **zygote**, into a large number of cells or **blastomeres**. The first few cleavage divisions take place in fixed symmetrical planes, but subsequent divisions appear to be irregular. Since the human zygote, as that of other mammals, contains little yolk in the cytoplasm, cleavage involves the whole zygote and all the blastomeres are of about equal size. Cleavage divisions occur within an intact zona pellucida, which limits the size of the **conceptus**. The blastomeres are arranged as a solid ball of cells called the **morula**. With continuing cell division, the cells form a hollow ball, the blastula or **blastocyst** (fig. 19.1b), whose wall is closely applied to the inner surface of the intact zona pellucida. The cavity of the blastocyst is the **blastocoele**; its outer wall is a single layer of cells called the **trophoblast**. Attached to the inner surface of the trophoblast is a small cluster of cells, the **inner cell mass**. The trophoblast makes no direct contribution to the embryo but is concerned with its nutrition. It is the part of the conceptus which will make intimate contact with the maternal tissues. The inner cell mass, on the other hand, is the source of cells of the embryo itself and of two of its membranes, the **amnion** and the **yolk sac**. At this stage the blastocyst is distended with fluid (fig. 19.1c).

The conceptus is now nearing the end of its first week of life. Three or four days are spent in passage down the uterine tube and two or three days lying free within the narrow uterine lumen. The investing cells of the corona radiata have been shed and the zona pellucida becomes thin and shortly disappears. The conceptus is still only a little larger than the fertilized ovum. Cleavage produces a large number of small cells, with a normal ratio of nuclear to cytoplasmic mass, from a single large ovum which had a disproportionately large amount of cytoplasm.

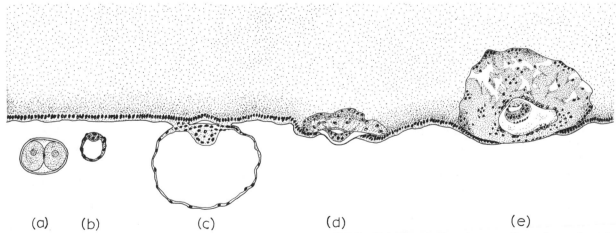

(a)   (b)   (c)   (d)   (e)

FIG. 19.1 The development of the conceptus during the first 9 days after fertilization. (a) First cleavage (from the uterine tube); (b) early blastocyst, 107 cells (from uterus); (c) blastocyst at stage of attachment; (d) 7 day embryo; (e) 9 day embryo. After O'Rahilly.

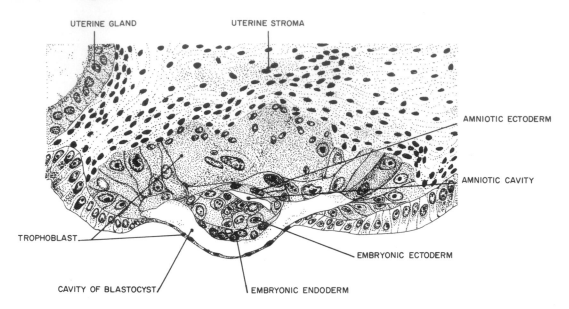

UTERINE GLAND

UTERINE STROMA

AMNIOTIC ECTODERM

AMNIOTIC CAVITY

EMBRYONIC ECTODERM

TROPHOBLAST

CAVITY OF BLASTOCYST

EMBRYONIC ENDODERM

FIG. 19.2 Human conceptus, aged about 7 days after fertilization. After Hertig & Rock (1945) *Contr. Embryol.* **31.**

The conceptus is now ready to implant in the endometrium and this phenomenon is described on p. 38.39.

CONCEPTUS AT 7 DAYS

Fig. 19.2 shows a section through the youngest known implanted human embryo. It is not yet completely buried in the endometrium, but its point of penetration has still to be repaired by regeneration of uterine epithelium. The primitive blastocyst cavity has temporarily collapsed. Where the trophoblastic wall of the blastocyst is not in direct contact with maternal tissue it remains a simple squamous epithelium. Elsewhere it has grown rapidly by ingesting and digesting cells of the endometrium.

The embryo itself is forming from the inner cell mass (fig. 19.2). A slit-like **amniotic cavity** has just appeared. Its roof is a thin layer of **amniotic ectoderm**, probably formed by splitting off from the trophoblast; its floor is a thicker layer, the **primitive embryonic ectoderm**. The **endoderm** is a thin layer of cells, which has split off from and remains closely applied to the lower surface of the primitive ectoderm.

CONCEPTUS IN THE SECOND WEEK (fig. 19.3)

At fourteen days, the conceptus is completely implanted within the endometrium. It consists of a roughly spherical sac, whose thick wall is the trophoblast, and whose cavity may now be called the **extraembryonic coelom**, since it surrounds the embryo. Two epithelial sacs, the amniotic cavity and the yolk sac, are suspended within this coelom. They are roughly spherical and are flattened where they lie in contact with one another, like two hollow rubber balls pressed together. The embryo itself consists of two flat sheets of epithelial cells at

this area of contact. One layer, which is continuous at its margins with the epithelium of the amnion, is the **embryonic ectoderm,** the other, continuous at its margins with the epithelium of the yolk sac, is the **embryonic endoderm.**

The inner surface of the trophoblast and the outer surface of the amniotic and yolk sacs, in fact all surfaces facing into the extraembryonic coelom, are covered by a layer of a loose, primitive mesenchymal tissue, the **extraembryonic mesoderm.** This is thought to have developed initially from the trophoblast and forms, with it, the outermost layer of the conceptus, the **chorion.** Strands of extraembryonic mesoderm suspend the amniotic and yolk sacs from the inner surface of the chorion, and form the **connecting stalk** which provides the main mesodermal basis of the umbilical cord.

It is important to appreciate that the whole conceptus is still minute at this stage, the external diameter being about 1–2 mm. It is superficially embedded in an endometrium which is about 8 mm thick. Small though it is, however, the conceptus has grown rapidly during the week since implantation began; its diameter has increased about five times. Some of this increase is due to distension of the extraembryonic coelom by fluid derived from the endometrium, but comparison of figs. 19.2 & 3 shows that the trophoblast in particular has grown rapidly. The outer shell shows no cellular boundaries and is therefore called **syncytiotrophoblast**; the inner layer remains cellular and is called **cytotrophoblast.**

Nutrients required for this rapid trophoblastic growth are obtained from maternal tissues. The syncytiotrophoblast is spongy and is penetrated by irregular, intercommunicating spaces, or lacunae. The invading trophoblast necessarily erodes maternal vessels, mostly enlarged capil-

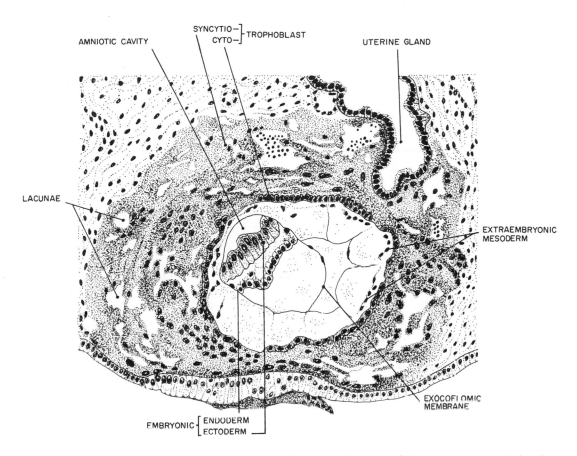

AMNIOTIC CAVITY

SYNCYTIO—
CYTO— ⌐TROPHOBLAST

UTERINE GLAND

LACUNAE

EXTRAEMBRYONIC
MESODERM

EXOCOELOMIC
MEMBRANE

EMBRYONIC ⌐ENDODERM
└ECTODERM

FIG. 19.3. Human conceptus aged about 12 days after fertilization. After Hertig & Rock (1941) *Contr. Embryol.* **29.**

laries and venules, and these discharge blood into the lacunae. The trophoblast is nourished by the fluid element of this extravasated blood, by interstitial fluid of the succulent endometrial stroma and by maternal blood and connective tissue cells which it ingests by phagocytosis. Nutritive material for the growing embryo itself can be derived only from the same sources. This primitive nutritive material is called **histotrophe**. It provides for the survival and growth of the conceptus during these early stages before circulation of maternal blood through the trophoblastic lacunae is fully active and before any embryonic vessels have developed in the chorion.

CONCEPTUS IN THE THIRD WEEK

The third week is a period of rapid development. The **chorionic sac** increases in diameter from about 2 mm to between 5 and 15 mm. It is covered externally by well-developed **chorionic villi**. These are bathed in maternal blood which now circulates through **intervillous spaces**, and, within their mesodermal cores, chorionic blood vessels develop (p. 38.41).

The most important change in the embryo itself is the establishment of the third of the germ layers, the **intraembryonic mesoderm**. It is best appreciated by imagining the chorionic sac to be opened and the amnion cut away close to the margin of the bilaminar germ disc where it becomes continuous with the embryonic ectoderm. The dorsal surface of the embryonic disc may now be inspected (fig. 19.4a). A linear thickening of the ectoderm appears in the midline of the disc and establishes both the polarity of the disc, since it lies at what will be the caudal end, and its bilateral symmetry. If one could study fresh human embryos at this stage, this **primitive streak** would appear opaque as compared with the rest of the ectoderm which would be almost translucent. A transverse section through the primitive streak (fig. 19.4f) shows that it lies at the bottom of a shallow **primitive groove**. Streams of mesodermal cells arise from it and spread laterally and forwards towards the head end of the disc. These form the intraembryonic mesoderm which occupies the interval between ectoderm dorsally and endoderm ventrally.

At the cranial end of the streak there is a slight thickening, the **primitive node**, from which a rod of cells, the **notochordal** or **head process**, extends forwards in a plane between ectoderm and endoderm (fig. 19.4d and e). In its forward growth, the cranial end of the notochordal process soon meets the **buccopharyngeal membrane**, which is a small circular mid-line area where ectoderm and endo-

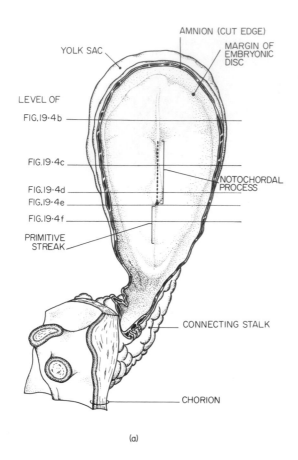

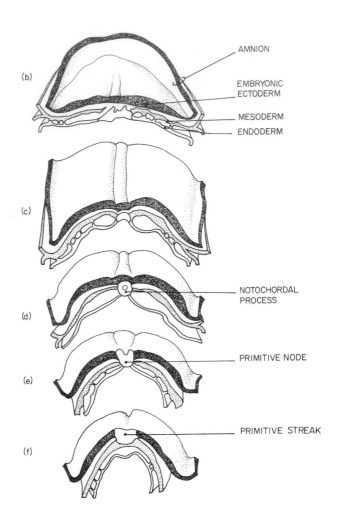

FIG. 19.4. Embryonic disc of estimated age 20 days after fertilization. (a) Dorsal view exposed by removal of the amnion to show the primitive streak and the notochordal process; (b–f) transerverse sections through the embryonic disc at levels indicated in (a). After Heuser (1932) *Contr. Embryol.* **23**.

derm remain in contact, not having been separated from one another by the spreading intraembryonic mesoderm. The notochordal process extends to the hinder edge of the buccopharyngeal membrane and no further (fig. 19.12).

A similar area of immediate contact between ectoderm and endoderm is found at the caudal end of the primitive streak. This is the **cloacal membrane**.

With the development of the intraembryonic mesoderm, the germ disc is now three-layered. The notochordal process, and with it the disc as a whole, elongates rapidly, and the primitive streak comes to lie more and more caudally. The primitive streak plays the dominant role in these changes (fig. 19.5)

Quite apart from forming a primitive, temporary, midline skeletal axis, the notochordal process plays an important part in the next major event in embryonic development, the formation of the **neural plate**, the forerunner of the **neural tube.** The **neural plate** arises as a

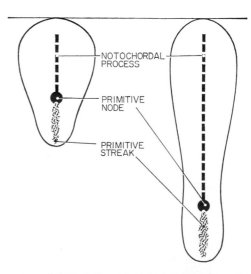

FIG. 19.5. Dorsal views of the germ disc to show how the disc grows in length by the proliferation of new cells from the primitive node and primitive streak. Based on Streeter.

thickened area of embryonic ectoderm overlying the notochordal process and its associated (paraxial) mesoderm. This relationship is not simply topographical; the ectoderm is induced to form the neural plate by the underlying tissue which acts as a **primary inductor.**

CONCEPTUS IN THE FOURTH WEEK

Changes in the intraembryonic mesoderm

These are most easily understood in a transverse section through the middle of the germ disc (fig. 19.6).

(1) The **paraxial mesoderm** which lies on either side of the axially placed notochord divides into a series of segmental blocks, the **mesodermal somites.** These develop in craniocaudal sequence; the caudally retreating primitive node and streak add new somites to the caudal end of the series, until the total of about forty-two pairs is completed. The number of somites present in a particular embryo is a better guide to its general developmental state than is its length.

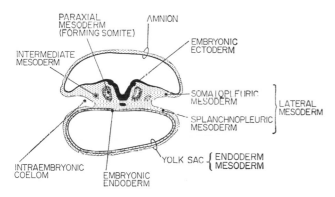

FIG. 19.6. Transverse section through the three-layered germ disc, showing subdivisions of the intraembryonic mesoderm.

(2) The **lateral mesoderm** lies towards the lateral edge of the flat, trilaminar embryonic disc. It is not segmented. A cavity, **the intraembryonic coelom** appears within it, dividing the mesoderm into two layers. The upper of these two layers, together with the embryonic ectoderm, forms the **somatopleure,** so called because it is the forerunner of the body wall. The lower layer, together with the embryonic endoderm, forms the **splanchnopleure** as the forerunner of the wall of the gut.

The intra- and extraembryonic coeloms soon communicate with one another. This provides a route of entry into the embryo of fluid from the maternal tissues, via the chorion and extraembryonic coelom. It should be noted that the embryonic somatopleure may be traced without interruption into the amniotic somatopleure, and the embryonic splanchnopleure into the yolk sac splanchnopleure.

(3) The **intermediate mesoderm** lies between paraxial and lateral mesoderm. It is neither segmented into somites nor divided into two layers. Most of the genito-urinary system develops in this mesoderm.

Development of the yolk sac (fig. 19.7.)

The early development of the yolk sac is illustrated in figs. 19.4 and 6. While the extraembryonic coelom is developing, endoderm originating from the embryonic disc grows round the inner aspect of the mesothelial membrane of the primary yolk sac to form a **secondary yolk sac.**

As the result of the formation of the head and tail folds in the embryonic disc, parts of the secondary yolk sac become enclosed within the embryo as the foregut and hindgut respectively. The intervening part now forming the roof of the yolk sac is the midgut.

With the development of the lateral body folds in relation to the sides of the midgut the communication between the midgut and the yolk sac becomes constricted, and the latter is excluded from the inside of the embryo proper. The yolk sac, which now communicates with the midgut by means of a **vitello-intestinal duct,** is known as the **definitive yolk sac.** This structure reaches a size of about 5 mm diameter and persists until term as a small vesicle applied to the inner surface of the chorion. The vitello-intestinal duct normally disappears after the loop of midgut has returned to the developing abdominal cavity.

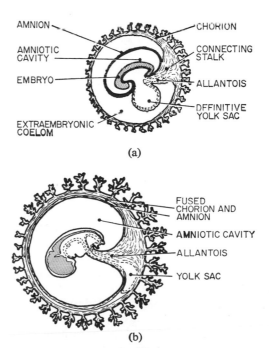

(a)

(b)

FIG. 19.7. Formation of the amnion and yolk sac; (a) and (b) represent successive stages of development.

Pericardial coelom and pericardioperitoneal canals

The intraembryonic coelom forms a continuous, horse-shoe-shaped cavity (fig. 19.8). The **pericardial coelom** lies towards the cranial end of the germ disc. The mesoderm in front of it remains intact, separating the pericardial and extraembryonic coeloms. It is called the **septum transversum**. The **pericardioperitoneal canals** are paired tubes which link the pericardial and peritoneal coeloms. It is important to realize that so long as the embryo remains a flat, trilaminar disc, the various parts of the coelom all lie in the same flat plane, and that only the peritoneal part of the coelom communicates with the extraembryonic coelom.

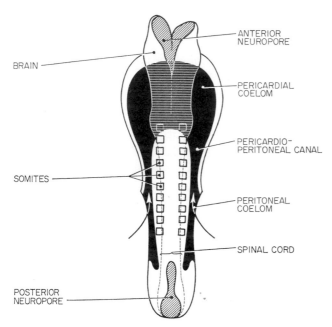

FIG. 19.8. Dorsal view of the embryo at the beginning of the fourth week showing the outline of intraembryonic coelom, a continuous series of spaces within the intraembryonic mesoderm. The amnion has been removed and the coelom is shown as if seen through a translucent ectoderm. The peritoneal part of the coelom communicates with the extraembryonic coelom (arrows).

Formation of the neural tube (figs. 19.9 & 19.10)

The thickened ectoderm of the neural plate forms a pair of longitudinal neural folds, one on each side of the midline neural groove. The **neural folds** fuse with one another dorsally to form a closed **neural tube**, forerunner of the brain and spinal cord. Fusion begins in the centre of the tube in embryos with seven paired somites and extends cranially and caudally. As the embryo grows in length, the neural tube is progressively added to at its caudal end. New neural plate ectoderm arises by cellular proliferation from the primitive streak, and this in turn thickens, folds, and closes. The importance of the primitive streak as a growth centre is again apparent.

For a time, the neural tube remains open both cranially and caudally. The cranial opening or **anterior neuropore** closes at the end of the 4th week. Because the neural tube grows by additions to its caudal end, closure of the caudal or **posterior neuropore** is delayed until the 6th week, when new somite formation from the primitive streak ceases.

When the neural folds fuse, some neural ectoderm at the lateral edges of the neural plate is not included within

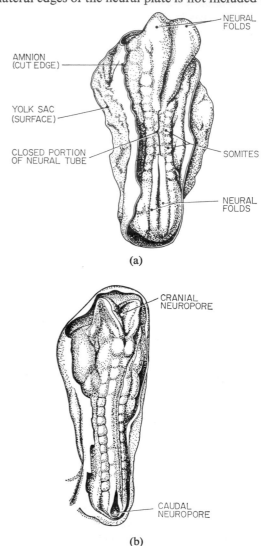

FIG. 19.9. Dorsal views of embryos of 7 somites (a) and 10 somites (b) showing the formation of the neural tube by fusion of the neural folds. After Payne (a) and Corner (b).

the neural tube. This is the **neural crest** (fig. 19.10). In the spinal region of the neural tube, this forms a series of segmental masses, corresponding to the mesodermal somites. In the cranial region, the neural crest forms irregular non-segmental masses. From both the cranial and the spinal neural crest a wide variety of cells arise:

(1) **primitive neuroblasts**, from which develop the first order sensory neurones, whose cell bodies are found in the cranial and spinal sensory ganglia,

(2) **lemnoblasts**, the forerunners of Schwann cells of peripheral nerve fibres,

(3) **sympathoblasts**, which give rise to the postganglionic effector neurones of the autonomic nervous system,

(4) **phaeochromoblasts**, which migrate to form the adrenal medulla and other chromaffin tissue,

(5) **melanoblasts**, which migrate to the epidermis where they form the pigmented melanocytes.

Folding of the body (fig. 19.11)

The trilaminar germ disc lies upon the yolk sac. This flat plate is converted into a cylindrical embryo by bending or folding in both transverse and longitudinal planes. Transverse folding produces the **lateral body folds** (fig. 19.11). A number of important changes should be noted.

(1) After folding is complete, the embryo lies almost entirely within the amniotic cavity.

(2) The lateral and ventral abdominal wall has been formed from the somatopleure.

(3) The continuity between intra- and extraembryonic coeloms has been restricted.

(4) The gut tube has been pinched off from the yolk sac, but the two still communicate by a **vitello-intestinal duct.**

(5) As the gut tube separates from the yolk sac, it draws away from the dorsal abdominal wall, and the initially broad mesodermal attachment becomes thinned to form a **dorsal mesentery.**

(6) The intermediate mesoderm comes to lie ventral to the somites and as it thickens, it bulges into the coelom as the **urogenital ridge.**

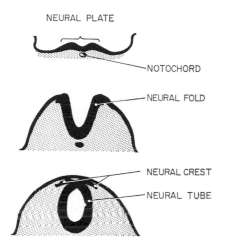

FIG. 19.10. Cross-sections to show successive stages in the formation of the neural folds, their fusion to form the neural tube, and the origin of the neural crest.

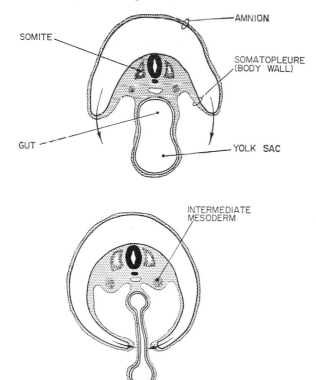

FIG. 19.11. Transverse sections showing development of the lateral body folds which convert the flat germ disc into a cylindrical embryo.

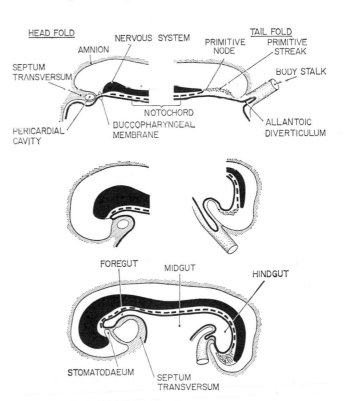

FIG. 19.12. Sagittal sections showing the formation of head and tail folds.

Similarly longitudinal folding forms the head and tail folds (fig. 19.12). This folding occurs because dorsal structures, particularly the neural tube, grow more rapidly than ventral structures. Several changes should be noted.

(1) As the septum transversum and the pericardial cavity have swung into a ventral position, a diverticulum of the gut has been pinched off from the yolk sac. This diverticulum is the **foregut**; it lies between the pericardial coelom and the neural tube and ends blindly in front at the **buccopharyngeal membrane**.

(2) The brain is now the most cranial part of the embryo. The ectoderm-lined diverticulum which lies between neural tube dorsally and pericardium ventrally is the **stomatodaeum**; it is separated from the foregut by the buccopharyngeal membrane.

(3) The septum transversum, originally the most cranial structure in the embryo, now forms the caudal wall of the pericardial coelom. It lies beneath the endoderm of the ventral wall of the caudal part of the foregut. When the liver develops as a ventral outgrowth from this part of the gut wall it grows immediately into the septum transversum.

The effect of the formation of the head fold on the pericardioperitoneal canals obviously cannot be seen in a midsagittal section. Fig. 19.13 shows the canal leading

dorsally from the pericardial coelom to lie at the side of the caudal end of the foregut, and passing dorsal to the septum transversum before opening into the peritoneal coelom.

The **tail fold** appears somewhat later than the head fold, and again a blind-ending diverticulum, the **hindgut**, is pinched off from the yolk sac. It is separated from the amniotic cavity by the cloacal membrane. Note, too, the changed relations of the primitive node, primitive streak, cloacal membrane, **body (connecting) stalk** and its contained endodermal **allantois** (allantoic diverticulum). In the formation of the tail fold the craniocaudal sequence of these structures is reversed, and the formation of the head fold has a similar effect on the craniocaudal sequence of septum transversum, pericardial cavity and buccopharyngeal membrane. For this reason, this sequence of changes is sometimes called **reversal** of the embryo.

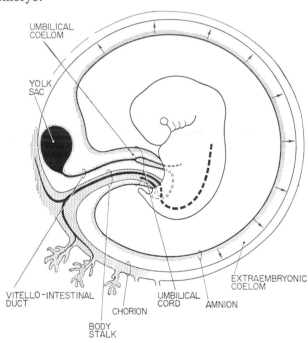

FIG. 19.14. The mode of formation of the umbilical cord. As the amnion expands, it obliterates the extraembryonic coelom by fusing with the chorion, and provides an investment for the umbilical cord. Part of the extraembryonic coelom persists for a time within the umbilical cord as the umbilical coelom. The body (connecting) stalk contains the allantoic diverticulum and umbilical vessels, only one of the two umbilical arteries is shown.

The formation of the lateral body, head and tail folds is not a sequence of separate events, but part of a general process of constriction at the junction between embryo and yolk sac. As the amnion expands to obliterate the extraembryonic coelom, it forms an external investment for the **umbilical cord**. The body stalk provides the meso-derm for the umbilical cord and it also contains the um-

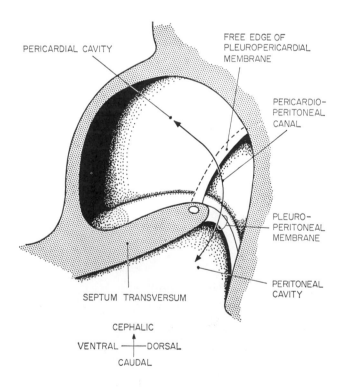

FIG. 19.13. The pericardioperitoneal canal. The embryo has been sectioned in a parasagittal plane, to the right of the midline, and the heart removed. The diagram shows the inner cut surface of the right hand portion of the sectioned embryo.

bilical vessels, the endodermal allantoic diverticulum, the vitello-intestinal duct, and the remains of the extra-embryonic coelom (fig. 19.14).

Development of the allantois

The allantois develops as a diverticulum from the caudal wall of the yolk sac and its site of origin comes to lie at the junction between the hindgut and the definitive yolk sac. The allantois grows into the mesoderm of the connecting stalk in which blood vessels develop which finally become the paired umbilical arteries and the single umbilical vein. In man the allantois remains small, but as the vascularization of the placenta is effected through the blood vessels which differentiate in the mesoderm around the allantois, it is of great functional significance and the human placenta is described as being **chorioallantoic**.

Development of the amnion and umbilical cord

The amniotic cavity appears as a split in the inner cell mass. The size of the cavity rapidly increases and becomes lined by cells delaminated from the inner aspect of the related trophoblast and by ectodermal cells growing up from the margins of the embryonic disc.

The amnion is initially attached to the chorion by a very broad connecting stalk of extraembryonic mesoderm. With extension of the extraembryonic coelom into the mesoderm of the connecting stalk, the amnion becomes separated from the inner aspect of the chorion by the extraembryonic coelom except in relation to the caudal end of the embryo. Here the attachment of the embryonic disc and the amnion to the chorion persists as the definitive connecting stalk.

The separation of the amnion from the chorion allows the amnion to expand in the enlarging extraembryonic coelom. Growth of the amnion brings its superficial aspect into contact with the inner aspect of the chorion so that the extraembryonic coelom is progressively obliterated until only a cleft remains, separating the amnion and chorion.

With the development of head, tail and lateral body folds, and with the growth and differentiation of embryonic form, the junction between the amnion and the ectoderm of the embryo comes to be situated progressively on its ventral aspect. Thus a large **umbilicus** is established. In the early stages of its development the umbilicus transmits the vitelline duct, coils of intestine and possibly the allantois, all flanked by the communication between the intraembryonic and the extra-embryonic coeloms. As the amnion expands it comes to ensheath the connecting stalk, the vitello-intestinal duct and extraembryonic coelom, and the region contained within the resulting tubular sheath of amnion is the **umbilical cord.**

The mesodermal cells forming the core of the umbilical cord become converted into loose mesenchyme embedded in a jelly-like intercellular matrix. This is Wharton's jelly, through which the umbilical vessels and the allantois pass. At first the umbilical cord is short but it lengthens rapidly.

As pregnancy advances, the outer surface of the amnion fuses with varying degrees of intimacy with the inner aspect of the chorion so that at term the two membranes may be partially fused. From the foregoing description it will be realized that the amnion forms a closed bag which, because it is filled with a watery fluid, **amniotic fluid**, provides a supporting aquatic environment in which the embryo is free to move as it develops.

MAIN FEATURES OF THE EMBRYO

The following account presents a composite picture of embryos of about one month of age. The somites are almost completely formed. The embryonic length ranges from 4–7 mm, and the diameter of the chorionic sac from 20–38 mm. Most of the organ systems are now present in rudimentary form, and the student should find this a useful general baseline from which he can proceed to their more detailed study.

The outer surface of the **chorionic sac** is thickly clothed by villi which have an outer covering of trophoblast and a central core of extraembryonic mesoderm, containing blood vessels through which circulates embryonic blood. The chorionic villi are bathed in circulating extravasated maternal blood and exchange of nutritive and waste material and of respiratory gases takes place between the two blood streams. This type of nutrition is called haemotrophic, in contradistinction to the histotrophic nutrition of the early conceptus.

The embryo is suspended from the inner surface of the chorion by the body stalk, through which run two umbilical arteries carrying blood to the chorionic circulation and two umbilical veins returning blood to the embryo. The amnion invests the embryo and contains the amniotic fluid. The watery environment of the amniotic fluid is particularly important in providing physical support in these early stages, when the embryo has the consistency of a soft jelly. A narrow tubular stalk (the yolk stalk or vitello-intestinal duct) connects the embryonic gut with the yolk sac, which lies within the extraembryonic coelom. The yolk sac is bathed in coelomic fluid, and its wall is richly supplied with embryonic blood by the vitelline artery.

MAIN EXTERNAL FEATURES (fig. 19.15)

The C-shaped curvature is characteristic; this is a further effect of the growth of the nervous system which has already helped to form the head and tail folds.

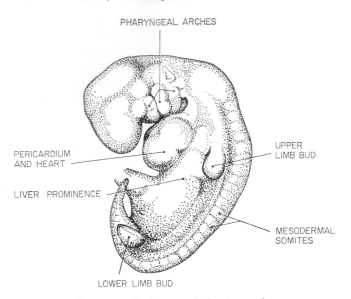

PHARYNGEAL ARCHES

PERICARDIUM
AND HEART

LIVER PROMINENCE

UPPER
LIMB BUD

MESODERMAL
SOMITES

LOWER LIMB BUD

FIG. 19.15. Embryo aged about 4 weeks.

The head is disproportionately large, mainly because of the precocious development and growth of the brain. The **pharyngeal** or **branchial arches**, from whose mesoderm develop, among other things, the skeleton and musculature of the jaws, are conspicuous. In the absence of a neck the developing face and jaws rest directly on the primitive

pericardium through whose translucent wall the heart can be seen.

On each side of the dorsal part of the trunk, flanking the spinal cord, is a series of segmental mesodermal blocks, the somites. Ventral to these are the **limb buds**, simple stubby outgrowths from the trunk. The upper limb is more advanced in development than the lower, in keeping with the general precocity of the front end of the embryo. The surface bulge between the heart and the upper limb bud is produced by the liver. The ventral abdominal wall, between the pericardium and the root of the tail, is occupied entirely by the umbilical ring, the line of continuity between amniotic ectoderm and the embryonic epidermis.

NERVOUS SYSTEM (fig. 19.16)

The **neural tube** extends throughout the length of the embryo and possesses a large **neural canal** and a wall which is still essentially epithelial. Brain and spinal cord are not sharply demarcated but the divisions into fore-, mid- and hindbrain are recognizable.

The ganglia of cranial and spinal nerves develop from the **neural crest** which, in the spinal region, forms a series of cell clumps lying beside the neural tube, in segmental arrangement corresponding to the mesodermal somites. The cranial neural crest, on the other hand, is not

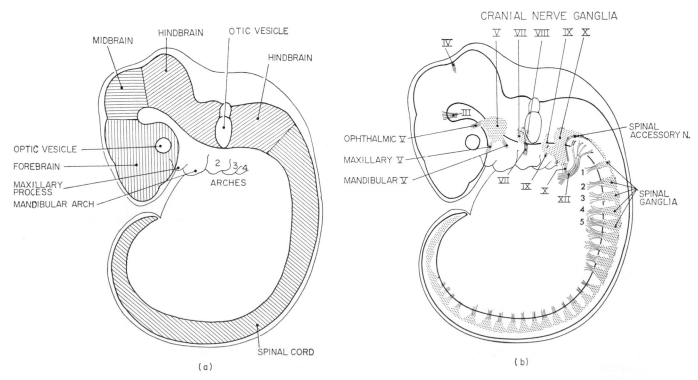

FIG. 19.16. The nervous system in an embryo of about 4 weeks; (a) subdivisions, (b) cranial and spinal ganglia. After Streeter.

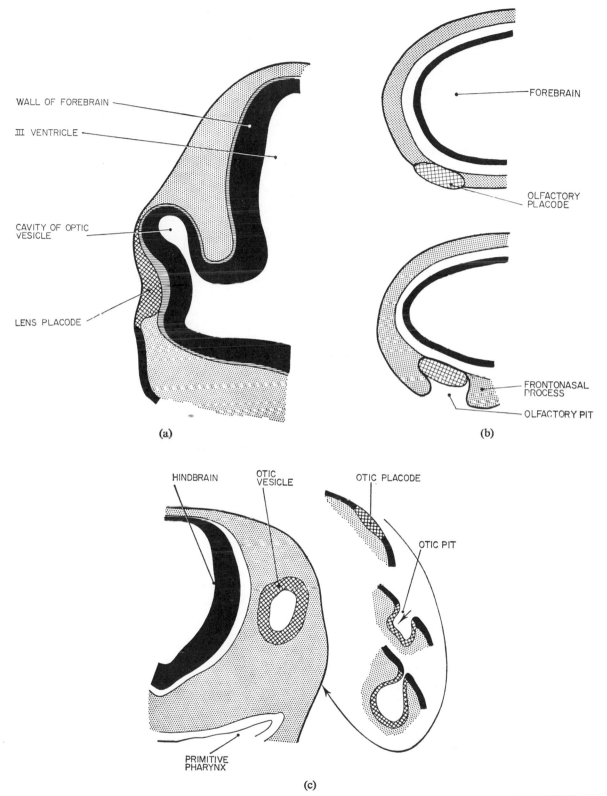

WALL OF FOREBRAIN

III VENTRICLE

CAVITY OF OPTIC
VESICLE

LENS PLACODE

(a)

FOREBRAIN

OLFACTORY
PLACODE

FRONTONASAL
PROCESS

OLFACTORY PIT

(b)

HINDBRAIN

OTIC
VESICLE

OTIC PLACODE

OTIC PIT

PRIMITIVE
PHARYNX

(c)

FIG. 19.17. The forerunners of the special sense organs in embryos of about 4 weeks. (a) The optic vesicle, a hollow outgrowth from the forebrain will form, among other things, the future retina. The lens develops from the surface ectoderm, under the inductive influence of the optic vesicle; (b) olfactory epithelium develops from areas of surface ectoderm, the olfactory placodes; (c) the lining epithelium of the inner ear develops from the otic vesicle, a derivative of the otic placode.

arranged segmentally, but in clusters from which develop the ganglia of V, VII, VIII, IX and X cranial nerves. The young nerve cells, **neuroblasts**, of the craniospinal neural crest develop in a basically similar fashion. Each sends an axonic outgrowth into the neural tube, the **central process**, and an axonic outgrowth to a peripheral sensory terminal, the **peripheral process**. It is worth noting that these precursors of first order afferent neurones are initially isolated structures and establish secondarily their connections both with the central nervous system (the neural tube) and with peripheral sensory receptors.

The precocious appearance of the eye is matched by that of the **olfactory placodes**, thickened areas of surface ectoderm which sink beneath the surface as the olfactory pits. From the placodal epithelium will develop the smell receptors. The epithelial lining of the internal ear is already present as the **otic vesicle**, which lies beside the hind brain, close to the VII and VIII ganglia, an early association which persists into the adult. The otic vesicle develops as a localized ectodermal thickening, the **otic placode**, which sinks beneath the surface to form a pit and then becomes pinched off from the surface as a closed ectodermal vesicle (fig. 19.17).

NOTOCHORD AND MESODERMAL SOMITES

The pairs of segmentally arranged somites, derived from the paraxial mesoderm, are described in regional groupings; four occipital, eight cervical, twelve thoracic, five lumbar, five sacral and eight or nine coccygeal. A small, short lived cavity appears within each somite, dividing it into an outer sheet of cells, which constitutes the **myotome** and the so-called **dermatome**, and an inner, more loosely-arranged collection of cells, the **sclerotome** (fig. 19.18).

The myotome gives rise to much of the skeletal muscle whose histological development is described on p. 16.9. The more general features of rearrangement of the myotomal contributions may be summarized as follows.

(1) The early muscle fibres are arranged in a craniocaudal orientation, which is commonly lost later.

(2) Muscle primordia commonly undergo extensive migration, e.g. the latissimus dorsi which develops from cervical myotomes has attachments in the adult as far caudally as the iliac crest. Similarly the muscle of the diaphragm arises from cervical myotomes and undergoes an extensive shift caudally. These migrating muscle primordia draw after them their nerves of supply and the course followed by these nerves gives an indication of the direction and extent of migration.

(3) Few muscles arise from single myotomes; most are formed by fusion of parts of adjacent somites.

(4) Two muscles may arise by longitudinal splitting of a single primordium.

(5) Layers of muscles, such as those of the abdominal wall, may be formed by tangential splitting of primordia.

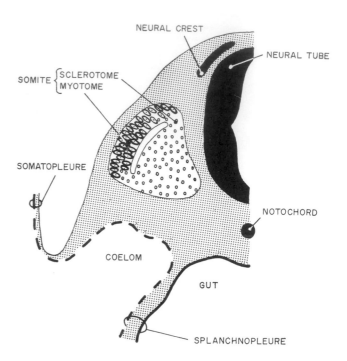

FIG. 19.18. The mesodermal somites are wedge-shaped blocks of paraxial mesoderm. Each shows an outer myotome and an inner sclerotome.

(6) Part, or all, of a myotomal primordium may degenerate, leaving, as a connective tissue remnant, an aponeurotic sheet or a ligament.

These various morphogenetic mechanisms lead to the laying down of the musculature of the trunk. Although the details are complex, the general pattern is simple and of some importance (fig. 19.19).

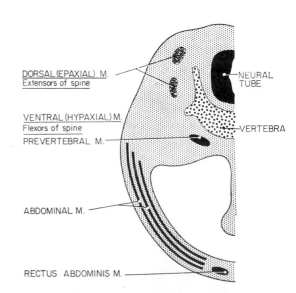

FIG. 19.19. The basic pattern of the body musculature derived by migration from the myotomes.

A **dorsal column** develops on a plane dorsal to the vertebral transverse processes and forms the postvertebral extensor muscles of the spine, which are innervated by the dorsal primary rami of the spinal nerves.

A **ventral column** forms the prevertebral musculature and, by migrating into the somatopleuric mesoderm, the lateral and ventral muscles of the thoracic and abdominal walls. These are innervated by the ventral primary rami of spinal nerves.

Branchial muscles, which arise from the branchial arch mesoderm (p. 19.33), are not of somite origin.

The dermatome was so named because its cells were believed to migrate to a position beneath the ectoderm, there to form the dermis, the connective tissue layer of the skin. At best, such a contribution is small, and the only justification for retaining the name is the segmental distribution of nerve fibres to the skin.

The sclerotome contributes, by proliferation and migration, to the general body mesenchyme. It also provides cellular streams, originally segmental like the somite, which flow medially to surround the notochord and the neural tube (fig. 19.20). These segmental masses become rearranged to form intersegmental blocks from which develop

subsequently replaced by bone by the process of endochondral ossification (p. 19.38).

The notochord disappears where it is surrounded by the developing centra; between them it expands to form the gelatinous centre of the intervertebral disc, the **nucleus pulposus**.

GUT TUBE AND ITS DERIVATIVES (fig. 19.21).

The gut tube, lined throughout by endodermal epithelium, extends from the buccopharyngeal membrane, now ruptured, to the cloacal membrane, by which it is closed off from the amniotic cavity. It is relatively simple at this stage, following the general C-curvature of the neural tube and the notochord. From it will develop a great variety of structures. The cranial end of the tube is the **primitive pharynx**. It is the broadest part of the gut, flattened between the pericardium which lies below its floor and the nervous system and notochord which lie above its roof. From each lateral wall there project four pouch-like extensions or bays, the **pharyngeal pouches**.

Behind the primitive pharynx the gut tube narrows into the oesophagus. The ventral wall of the foregut develops a blind-ending tube which provides the epithelial lining of the **trachea**, **bronchial tree** and **respiratory portion of the**

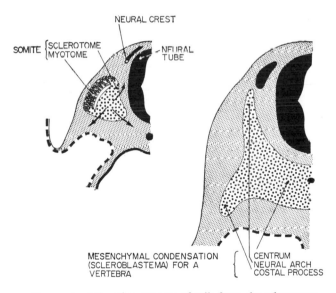

FIG. 19.20. Migrating streams of cells from the sclerotome form, among other things, the vertebrae and ribs.

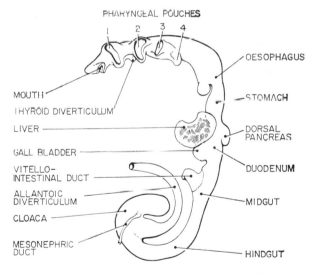

FIG. 19.21. Outline drawing, from the left side, of the gut tube and its derivatives, in an embryo of about 4 weeks. After Streeter.

the **centra of the vertebrae**. From sclerotomic material surrounding the neural tube arise the **neural arches** of the vertebrae, and ventrolateral extensions into the body wall form the **costal processes**. The three constituent elements of each vertebra, centrum, neural arch and costal process, are thus established in an intersegmental position and alternate therefore with the segmental spinal nerves and with the myotomic muscles. Each vertebra is laid down as a densely cellular mesenchymal precursor, the **scleroblastema**; this transforms into a cartilage model which is

lungs (p. 31.5). The respiratory function of the branchial region has been lost, to be replaced in air-breathing animals by the lungs which still arise, however, from the gut endoderm.

The **stomach** is already recognizable as a spindle-shaped dilation, which leads in turn into the **duodenum**. Two outgrowths of endodermal epithelium arise from the duodenum; a dorsal one that forms the major part of the **pancreas**, and a ventral one, from which develop the epithelial components of the **liver, gall bladder, bile ducts** and a minor part of the **pancreas**. The site of outgrowth of the liver bud is a valuable landmark as it defines the junction between the **foregut** and the **midgut**.

From the embryonic midgut there will develop part of the duodenum, distal to the entry of the common bile duct, the rest of the **small intestine**, in the **caecum, appendix** and **ascending colon**, and the greater part of the **transverse colon**. It is that part of the gut which in younger embryos was widely continuous with the yolk sac, and which is still connected with it by the vitello-intestinal duct. The midgut is that part of the gut which is supplied, in the adult, by the superior mesenteric artery, bordering cranially on the vascular territory of the coeliac artery, and caudally on that of the inferior mesenteric artery.

The midgut continues without demarcation into the **hindgut**; this in turn opens into the **cloaca** (Latin, a sewer) which receives the **mesonephric ducts** and the **allantois** (allantoic diverticulum).

When the general form of the endodermal gut tube has been appreciated we can look at its surroundings. It is immediately invested throughout its length by a loose cellular mesenchyme of the splanchnopleure from which will develop the connective tissue and muscle layers of the gut (figs. 19.6 & 11). The gut is also related to a series of spaces which form the **coelomic cavity** of the embryo.

COELOMIC TRACT

The three portions of the intraembryonic coelom: the pericardial cavity, pericardioperitoneal canals and peritoneal cavity, are continuous with one another. The peritoneal part of the coelom communicates with the extraembryonic coelom. This communication may be important for the survival of the embryo, since it provides a route for circulation of fluid and dissolved nutrients from the extraembryonic coelom into the intraembryonic coelomic tract. This may serve as an accessory route of supply for the early embryo.

The gut is closely related to the coelom. The primitive pharynx lies dorsally to the pericardial cavity (fig. 19.22a). The oesophagus and the tracheal outgrowth are flanked on either side by the pericardioperitoneal canals, forerunners of the pleural cavities (fig. 19.22b). The remainder of the foregut and the midgut lie within the peritoneal cavity, suspended from the dorsal abdominal wall by the dorsal mesentery (fig. 19.22c and d).

The **diaphragm**, which later separates the pleural and pericardial cavities from the peritoneal cavity, is represented at this stage by the septum transversum. As its name implies this is a mesodermal sheet lying transversely across the body. Ventrally it is continuous with the ventral abdominal wall; dorsally it is incomplete where it is traversed on either side of the midline by the pericardioperitoneal canals. Its cranial surface faces into the peri-

cardium, its caudal surface is being invaded by cords of liver cells derived from the hepatic bud (fig. 19.23). The **pleural cavity** develops as an extension of the pericardioperitoneal canal. The forerunner of the lung is called the **lung bud**, consisting of one of the primary divisions of the epithelial tracheal tube, with a covering layer of splanchnopleuric mesoderm.

To understand later changes in the coelomic cavities it is important to appreciate that, at this stage, the lung buds are very small relative to the heart and pericardial cavity. The primitive pleural cavities into which the lung buds grow are also relatively small, and they lie entirely dorsal to the pericardial cavity and open freely into its dorsal wall. The lung bud grows into a pleural cavity which expands before it. The cavity grows ventrally around the heart. It expands into the thick layer of loose mesenchyme which forms the wall of the pericardial cavity (fig. 19.24). Extension of the pleural cavity into this mesenchyme splits it into an outer layer which will form the **chest wall** and an inner layer, the **pleuropericardial membrane**, which will form the definitive **fibrous pericardium**. Hence this is clothed internally with serous pericardium and externally by parietal pleura. Each pleuropericardial membrane has a free edge dorsally; fusion of the two free edges in the midline with one another and with the mesoderm ventral to the oesophagus will later close off the pericardial from the two pleural cavities.

Expansion of the pleural cavities into the thick mesodermal bed of the primitive pericardial wall brings into existence a second membrane lying between the pleural cavity and the peritoneal cavity and called, therefore, the **pleuroperitoneal membrane** (fig. 19.25). Like the pleuropericardial membrane this too has a free edge dorsally and medially. Fusion between the mesoderm which surrounds the oesophagus in the midline and the free edge of the pleuroperitoneal membrane on each side will at about the 6th week separate each pleural cavity above from the peritoneal cavity below.

HEART AND CIRCULATION

The heart in an embryo of about 4 weeks is already an active pump, with rhythmical co-ordinated contractions passing from the venous (input) end of the heart to its arterial (output) end, which projects through the roof of the pericardium and, therefore, comes to lie below the floor of the primitive pharynx. The arterial and venous ends are relatively fixed points of anchorage; between them the heart is a free tubular loop lying within the pericardial coelom. It is essentially uniform in structure throughout its length (fig. 19.26).

(1) An inner lining of simple squamous epithelium, similar to the endothelial lining of the entire vascular tree, is called **endocardium**.

(2) An outer layer of developing muscle forms the

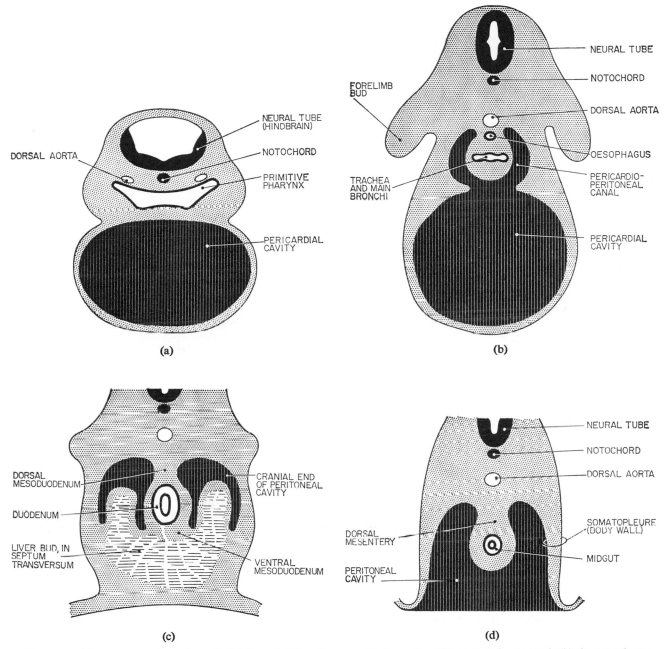

FIG. 19.22. Transverse sections through (a) the primitive pharynx with the pericardial cavity lying ventral; (b) the oesophagus and trachea, flanked by the pericardioperitoneal canals, which open from the dorsal wall of the pericardial cavity; (c) the septum transversum; (d) the midgut level.

myocardium. The outermost cells of this layer develop into connective tissue and form the **epicardium.**

(3) The **cardiac jelly** is a layer of connective tissue between the endocardium and the myocardium. It is sparsely cellular and rich in gelatinous intercellular matrix.

Regional variations in shape and thickness of myocardium and cardiac jelly distinguish the various chambers. Starting at the venous end these are: **sinus venosus,**

primitive atrium, primitive ventricle, bulbus cordis and **truncus arteriosus.**

The arteries are little more than endothelial tubes, relatively larger than they are in the adult and lacking the connective tissue and muscle elements which develop later from the surrounding mesenchyme. Their basic pattern is shown in fig. 19.27. The truncus arteriosus pierces the dorsal wall of the pericardium and opens into a dilated **aortic sac** which lies below (ventral to) the pharyngeal floor. From it arise on each side a series of **aortic arch arteries**. These run round the primitive pharynx to open into the paired dorsal aortae which lie dorsal to the pharynx. Each aortic arch artery lies within the mesoderm of a pharyngeal arch between two adjacent pharyngeal pouches.

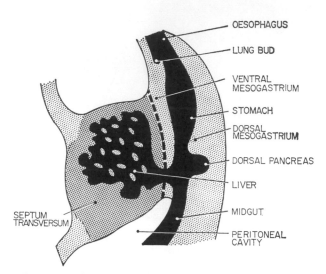

FIG. 19.23. Sagittal section to show the relationships of the septum transversum to the coelomic cavities, the gut and the liver.

The **paired dorsal aortae** extend caudally to the tail of the embryo, lying dorsally to the gut, ventrally to the neural tube, and following the C-curve of each. Their branches are distributed to a surface network of capillaries investing the neural tube, to arterial plexuses in the visceral mesoderm surrounding the gut tube, trachea and lung buds, to the intermediate mesoderm from which will develop, among other things, the kidneys and gonads, and to the somatopleure.

The largest branches of the dorsal aortae are their terminal ones, the **umbilical arteries**, which arise from plexuses lying beside the cloaca, and run in the body stalk on either side of the allantoic diverticulum, to the chorionic circulation. It is, of course, not surprising that the chorionic circulation should take the major share of the blood; by allowing exchange between embryonic and maternal circulations the chorion provides for the nutritive, respiratory and excretory needs of the embryo, quite apart from the endocrine function of its trophoblastic component.

The veins are distributed on a simple basic plan (fig. 19.28).

(1) From the head, and particularly the brain, blood is drained by the paired **anterior cardinal veins**; from the body caudal to the heart run the paired **posterior cardinal veins**. These join the anterior veins to form the **common cardinal veins**.

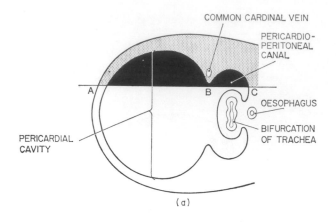

(a)

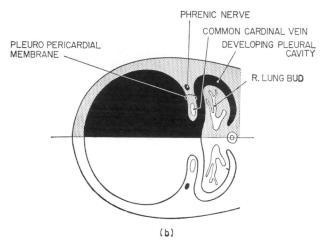

(b)

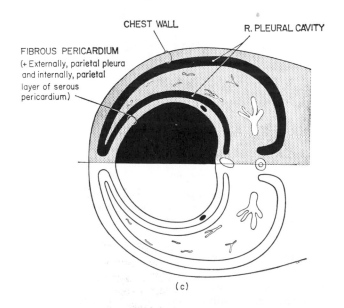

(c)

FIG. 19.24. Transverse sections to show (a) how the pleural cavity develops as an extension of the pericardioperitoneal canal, by splitting of the mesoderm of the primitive pericardial wall, (b) how the lung grows into the enlarging cavity prepared for it, (c) the adult relationships.

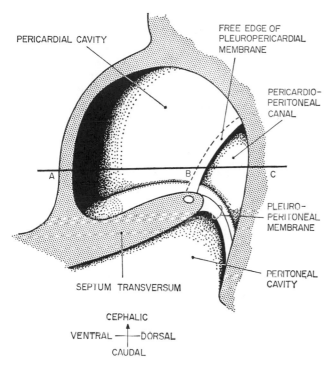

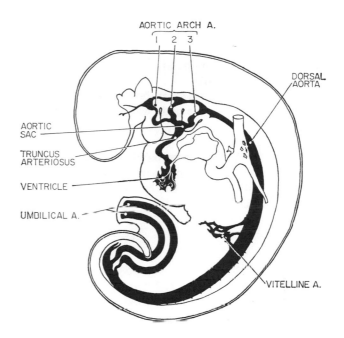

FIG. 19.27. The main arteries in an embryo of about 4 weeks. After Streeter.

FIG. 19.25. Drawing to show the development of the pleural cavity from the pericardioperitoneal canal. As in fig. 19.13, the embryo has been sectioned in a parasagittal plane, to the right of the midline, and the diagram shows the medial cut surface of the right hand part of the sectioned embryo. Cf. fig. 19.24a which shows the upper surface of a section cut in plane ABC. Based on Frazer, *Manual of Human Embryology*.

(2) Blood returns from the chorionic circulation by the paired **umbilical veins**.

(3) From the vascular yolk sac, blood returns by paired **vitelline veins**.

These three pairs of veins converge on the **sinus venosus**, a common venous reservoir embedded within the mesoderm of the septum transversum. The routes by which they reach the septum transversum are worthy of attention.

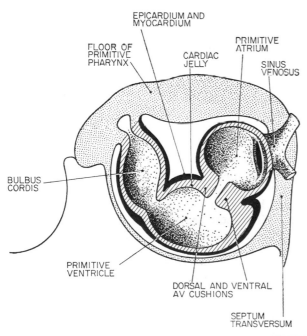

FIG. 19.26. Diagrammatic longitudinal section of primitive heart tube showing the basic structure of its wall and its fundamental subdivisions.

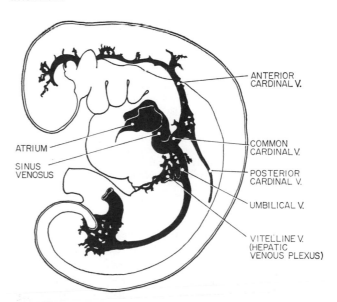

FIG. 19.28. The main veins in an embryo of about 4 weeks. After Streeter.

(1) The common cardinal veins which run caudally to enter the septum transversum lie in the pleuropericardial membrane close to its free border. The lung bud grows laterally into the expanding pleural cavity behind (dorsal to) this vein (fig. 19.29).

(2) The umbilical veins enter the embryo by way of the body stalk and run in the body wall mesoderm (somatopleure) to enter the septum transversum at its lateral edges. The umbilical veins do not, therefore, at this stage become involved with the cords of liver cells which are beginning to invade the septum transversum.

(3) The vitelline veins enter the embryo in the visceral mesoderm which surrounds the yolk sac stalk and turn

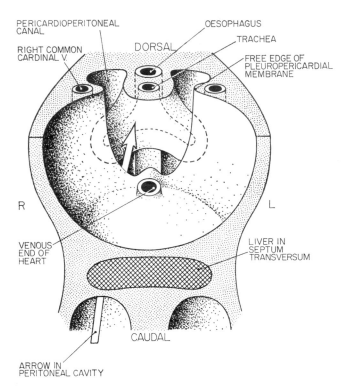

FIG. 19.29. The front wall of the pericardial cavity has been cut away, and the heart removed. The openings into the pericardioperitoneal canals lie on each side of the splanchnopleuric mesoderm which surrounds the oesophagus and trachea. The common cardinal veins run in the free edges of the pleuropericardial membranes. As the lung bud grows laterally into the primitive pleural cavity it passes dorsal to the vein. Modified from Frazer, *Manual of Human Embryology*.

cranially to enter the septum transversum where they are broken up into a complicated plexus of thin-walled vessels. This **hepatic venous plexus** becomes intimately intermingled with growing liver cords. Having circulated through the liver, this vitelline vein blood is collected into a symmetrical pair of **right** and **left hepatocardiac veins**.

These important relationships may be best illustrated by a semi-schematic ventral view (fig. 19.30). This shows

that (1) the sinus venosus occupies the full width of the septum transversum, extending laterally as **right** and **left horns**, (2) the common cardinal and umbilical veins enter the sinus laterally at the extremity of each horn, (3) the hepatocardiac veins enter the sinus nearer to the midline and (4) the opening of the sinus venosus into the primitive atrium, the sinuatrial orifice, is no longer in the midline but has moved to the right. This is one of the earliest indications of a developing asymmetry in the pattern of the major veins as they enter the heart.

The right hepatocardiac vein enlarges and forms the terminal segment of the inferior vena cava (fig. 19.31); the left closes off. The right umbilical vein becomes closed. The left umbilical vein establishes an anastomosis with the left vitelline vein as they enter the septum transversum.

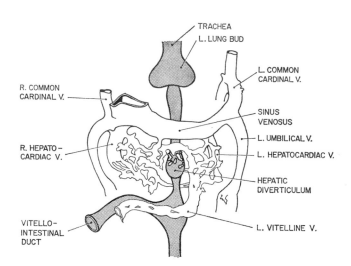

FIG. 19.30. Ventral view of the arrangement of veins entering the sinus venosus in an embryo of about 4 weeks. After Streeter.

This anastomosis diverts umbilical vein blood into the hepatic venous plexus. We have already seen that the chorionic circulation is the largest recipient of blood; a major part of the venous return is, therefore, through the left umbilical vein into the hepatic venous plexus. Because the left hepatocardiac vein is closing, umbilical vein blood runs obliquely through the hepatic plexus towards the right hepatocardiac vein near its entrance to the sinus venosus. The increased venous flow, obliquely from left to right, through the hepatic plexus, brings about the formation of a large venous channel, the **ductus venosus**, which provides a direct route of flow for oxygenated blood from the left umbilical vein to the inferior vena cava.

URINARY SYSTEM

The intermediate mesoderm which lies between the paraxial and lateral mesoderms forms an extended cellular mass, the **nephrogenic** (kidney forming) **cord**, which is found between lower cervical and sacral levels.

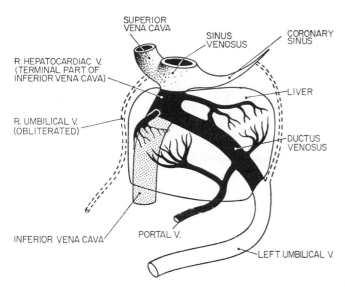

FIG. 19.31. Ventral view of the arrangement of veins entering the sinus venosus, at a later stage than fig. 19.30. The portal vein is derived from the vitelline veins.

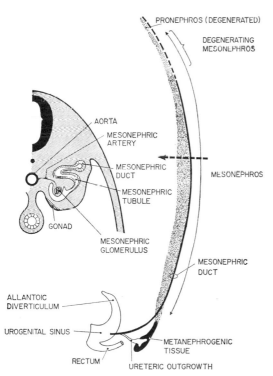

FIG. 19.32. The nephrogenic cord, showing the relative positions of pro-, meso- and metanephros. A transverse section of the mesonephros is shown on the left.

Kidney tubules develop directly from the cellular mesoderm of the nephrogenic cord; this development begins at the upper end of the cord and extends progressively towards its caudal end. As new tubules are added caudally, those at the head end of the cord regress. In essence,

therefore, a wave of kidney tubule formation spreads caudally through the nephrogenic cord.

The tubules which thus arise in succession are not identical and may be grouped into three sets (fig. 19.32).

(1) The **pronephros** (the head kidney) is confined to the extreme upper end of the cord, and is vestigial and functionless in the human embryo.

(2) The **mesonephros** (the middle kidney) extends from upper thoracic to lower lumbar segments, although it is not fully developed throughout its length at any one time. Its tubules are probably functional in the human embryo and open into a duct, the **mesonephric duct**, which began its development in connection with the pronephros, and which grows caudally to open into the **cloaca**.

(3) The **metanephros** forms the permanent, definitive kidney of man and other mammals, birds and reptiles. Its development is described with the urinary tract (p. 36.1).

GENITAL SYSTEM

The development of the genital system is described in detail on p. 38.57. Here we need say only that the **gonads** develop as paired swellings on the inner side of the mesonephros. They bulge into the peritoneal coelom and form the **urogenital ridge**.

SUMMARY

This account has sketched the outline of early embryogenesis and the further development of most of the systems is considered in the appropriate chapters. However, the cardiovascular system and the branchial arches form

TABLE 19.1. Timetable of human development

Age after fertilization (weeks)	Crown-rump length (mm)	
0–1		Fertilization and cleavage
1–2		Implantation
2–3		Embryo two layered
3–4		Embryo three layered, first somites formed, neural folds appear, intraembryonic coelom develops
4–5	4–7	35–38 pairs of somites, leg buds appear, lens placode develops, division of atrium in progress, one way circulation through heart
5–6	11–14	Limb bones, skull base and vertebrae are precartilaginous, closure of IV foramen, division of truncus arteriosus complete, palate development begins (completed at 12 weeks)
6–7	22	First bone formed, sex recognizable externally

such integral parts of the embryo that their whole development is described here.

Embryologists usually define the stage of development of an embryo by reference to its length or number of paired somites, but in this chapter the timing of events is related to postconceptional age. Interest in the timing of embryogenesis has increased greatly in recent years because of the recognition that various environmental influences may distort development. Severe damage occurs when dramatic changes are taking place in the development of an organ, and so the timing of exposure to the hazards determines the nature of the lesion. It must not be assumed that all developmental anomalies are the result of external influences. There is evidence that many defects are genetic in origin. Table 19.1 relates age and length with some important developmental events.

DEVELOPMENT OF THE HEART

The circulation of blood is well established in embryos at the end of the 4th week of development. The heart at this stage is a simple tubular structure which forms a U loop within the pericardial cavity. Blood returns to the heart at its venous end, the sinus venosus, which is embedded in the septum transversum. The sinus venosus opens into the single primitive atrium by way of the sinuatrial orifice which lies in the midline, is elongated dorsoventrally and is guarded by two flaps of endocardium, the right and left venous valves, which prevent reflux of blood from atrium to sinus. The primitive atrium, in its turn, leads into the primitive ventricle. The atrioventricular (AV) orifice is soon encroached upon by two local thickenings of the cardiac jelly (fig. 19.33a). Imagine yourself within the cavity of the primitive ventricle, looking towards the AV orifice and the primitive atrium (fig. 19.33b). As the dorsal and ventral cushions thicken and grow towards one another, the orifice becomes H shaped; later, when the cushions meet and fuse, the AV orifice is divided into right and left channels, separated by the **septum intermedium**, so called because of its position intermediate between atrium and ventricle.

From the primitive ventricle the blood flows into the bulbus cordis which gradually narrows and passes without a sharp line of demarcation into the truncus arteriosus. This is the arterial end of the heart; it pierces the pericardial roof to open into a thin-walled midline structure, the **aortic sac**, from which arise the aortic arteries.

In understanding the complex changes which follow, it is important to keep in mind several features of the primitive heart tube.

(1) It is attached to the pericardial wall only at its venous and arterial ends. Between these two fixed points it loops freely into the pericardial cavity. The dorsal mesocardium, a 'mesentery' which at an earlier stage

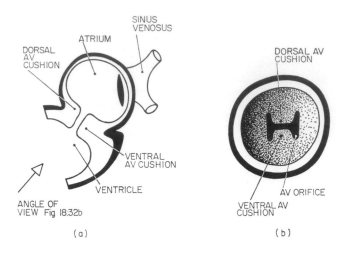

FIG. 19.33. Atrioventricular (AV) junction and the AV cushions. (a) Schematic longitudinal section; (b) diagrammatic view of the AV orifice and the AV cushions which encroach upon it, as seen from within the cavity of the ventricle.

suspended it within the pericardium, has disappeared.

(2) It lies in the midsagittal plane.

(3) It shows little regional specialization and the layers which constitute its wall are continuous without interruption from one chamber to the next. In particular, there is no interruption of the musculature at the junction between atrium and ventricle and the impulse for contraction spreads directly from the venous end, where it is initiated, to the arterial end. The venous end of the heart is already established as the **pacemaker**; a unidirectional flow of blood from venous to arterial end is maintained by the peristaltic wave of contraction. This is aided by the

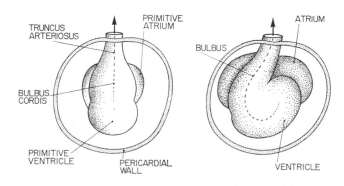

FIG. 19.34. Ventral views of the heart tube, showing the displacement of the bulbus cordis to the right and the ventricle to the left; changes brought about by the rapid elongation of the heart. Based on Frazer, *Manual of Human Embryology*.

peculiar inelastic property of the cardiac jelly which is thickened to form the endocardial cushions at the AV orifice. As the wave of contraction passes over the AV junction, the AV cushions are pressed together, effectively preventing reflux of blood and anticipating the effect, but not the mechanism, of the AV valves which develop later.

The heart tube now enters a period of rapid growth and becomes bent in the transverse as well as in the sagittal plane. The result of this can be seen by looking at the heart from the front (fig. 19.34); the bulbus cordis is now displaced towards the right and the ventricle towards the left. The primitive atrium lies dorsal and caudal to the ventricle and may be seen bulging forward on either side of the bulbus cordis.

The various chambers of the simple heart tube now become divided by septal partitions. To simplify understanding, these changes are dealt with chamber by chamber, although they occur more or less simultaneously.

PARTITIONING OF THE ATRIUM

The sinu-atrial opening moves from its original midline position on the dorso-caudal wall of the atrium to a position to the right of the midline. Division of the atrium into right and left sides by a flimsy **septum primum** now begins (fig. 19.35). This develops from the dorso-caudal wall of the atrium and extends in the midsagittal plane as a crescentic sheet of tissue which approaches and fuses with the septum intermedium. The hole which is bounded by its free edge is the **foramen primum**. This becomes progressively smaller as the septum primum grows to meet the septum intermedium and, before communication between the right and left sides of the

atrium is cut off, a new opening, the **foramen secundum**, appears, high up in the septum primum. This communication allows blood to flow into the left side of the atrium because the only venous return to the heart at this stage is via the sinus venosus which now opens into the right side of the atrium.

A second septum, **septum secundum**, later develops on the right side of septum primum. It differs from septum primum in certain important respects. Although it grows towards septum intermedium, it does not reach it; its growing margin remains as a free edge to form a conspicuous landmark on the right side of the atrial septum, the **limbus fossae ovalis** of the adult heart (fig. 30.5). It is also a thicker and more substantial structure than septum primum. Its growth normally continues until it overlaps foramen secundum completely. It does not, however, prevent the flow of blood from right to left atrium because the diaphanous septum primum is easily displaced to the left by the stream of blood which flows through the oblique passage between the two septa (fig. 19.36). So long as pressure in the right atrium is higher than that in the left, this flow of blood through the septum will continue. This is the state of affairs until pulmonary respiration begins at birth; then the venous return from the greatly increased pulmonary circulation brings the pressure in the left atrium to a level equal to, or slightly greater than, that in the right, and septum primum is pressed up against septum secundum. Thus it acts as a valve which closes off the passage through the septum. The oblique passage is the **foramen ovale**; the entrance to it is in the right atrium, bounded by the limbus fossae ovalis, the free margin of septum secundum; the exit from it is foramen secundum, opening into the left atrium (fig. 42.3).

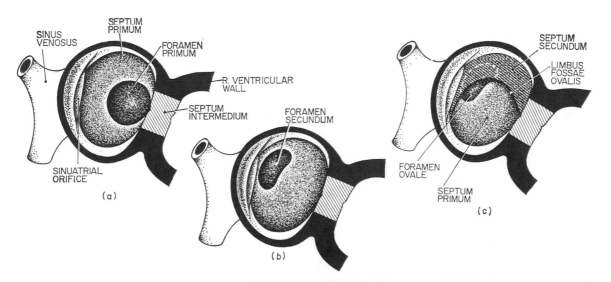

FIG. 19.35. The development of the interatrial septa. The right wall of the primitive atrium and of the ventricle have been removed and the developing septa are viewed from the right. (a) Septum primum and foramen primum, (b) septum primum and foramen secundum, (c) septum secundum.

PARTITIONING OF THE VENTRICLE

This is brought about by a very different mechanism. The greater parts of both the right and left ventricles develop from the single ventricle by expansion of its wall externally and hollowing out of its wall internally (fig. 19.37c). The interventricular septum is, as it were, left behind as a crescentic sheet of cardiac muscle, lying more or less in the sagittal plane, between the expanding right and left ventricles. We can only guess at the factors which bring about this expansion of right and left ventricles; perhaps the two streams of blood which enter the ventricle through the right and left AV orifices have a sculpturing action on the thick trabeculated ventricular muscle. Be

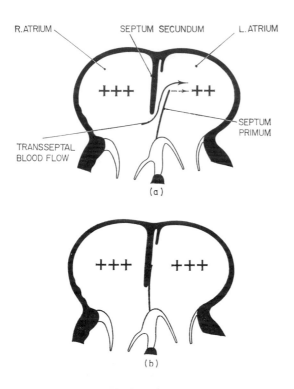

FIG. 19.36. Section of the heart to show the mechanism of the foramen ovale; (a) prenatal, (b) postnatal.

this as it may, the muscular part of the interventricular septum does not grow upwards into the ventricle; the ventricles expand on either side of it. The free edge of the **muscular septum** which is produced in this fashion obviously does not meet the septum intermedium; between the two is an **interventricular foramen** allowing communication between right and left ventricles. This is closed later by cardiac jelly from a variety of sources; the closing tissue is fibrous rather than muscular and forms the **membranous portion** of the interventricular septum (fig. 19.43). The mechanism of its formation is inseparable from the method of division of the bulbus cordis and truncus arteriosus.

PARTITIONING OF THE BULBUS CORDIS AND TRUNCUS ARTERIOSUS

The bulbus cordis and the truncus arteriosus together constitute the outflow tract of the developing heart which eventually delivers blood into a **systemic** circuit (derived from the fourth aortic arch) and a **pulmonary** circuit (derived from the sixth aortic arch). The bulbus cordis and truncus arteriosus must be divided in such a way that the right ventricle discharges into the pulmonary circuit, and the left into the systemic circuit.

Fig. 19.38 illustrates the interior of the ventricles and of the bulbus at the beginning of development of the continuous spiralling septum which will divide the bulbus and truncus throughout their length. It is important to appreciate the relationships of the ventricles to one another and to the bulbus at this stage. The ventricles lie side by side, the right lying slightly ventral to the left; each receives its own stream of blood through its own AV orifice. The bulbus lies in such a position that it can re-

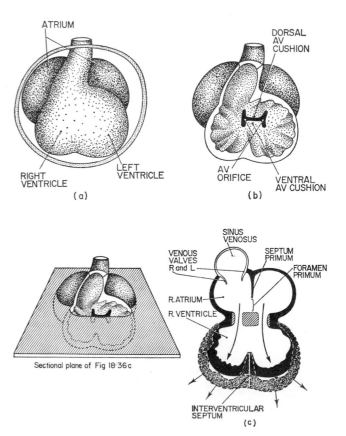

FIG. 19.37. The origin of the right and left ventricles from the primitive ventricle. (a) Ventral view of the unopened heart, (b) ventral view of the heart after removal of its ventral wall, (c) diagrammatic section of the heart cut in the plane shown. (a) and (b) based on Frazer, *Manual of Human Embryology*.

ceive two streams of blood, one from the right ventricle and one from the left.

Because the right ventricle lies slightly ventral to the left, the right ventricular stream is ejected into the front or ventral half of the bulbus, the left ventricular stream into the back or dorsal half. It is known from the study of hydrodynamic models that two fluid streams, ejected in parallel into a single tube, spiral around one another, the spiral turning clockwise as the two streams travel through the tube. There are good grounds for believing that the same sort of thing happens in the outflow tract of the heart at this stage and that the two spiralling streams exert a moulding effect on the thick layer of cardiac jelly which lies beneath the endocardium of the bulbus and truncus.

The effect of this moulding can be illustrated most simply by a transverse section through the bulbus cordis at the level indicated in fig. 19.38. Ridges of thickened cardiac jelly project into the bulbus from its right and left sides;

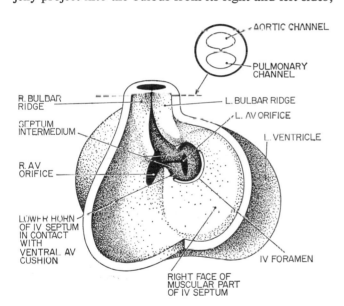

FIG. 19.38. The front wall of the bulbus cordis and of the right ventricle has been removed and the heart is viewed obliquely from the front and the right. This view allows the right face of the interventricular (IV) septum to be seen. Note (1) the relation of the two 'horns' of the interventricular septum to the septum intermedium, (2) the right and left bulbar ridges, thickenings of the cardiac jelly of the bulbus cordis shown also in a transverse section. After Frazer, *Manual of Human Embryology.*

these are the **right** and **left bulbar ridges**. Soon they meet and fuse, to form the **bulbar septum** which divides the bulbus into **anterior** and **posterior** channels. This septum is not confined to the bulbus but continues upwards into the truncus, spiralling as it goes. In the truncus it is called the **aorticopulmonary septum** because it divides the truncus into aortic and pulmonary channels. At the upper end of the truncus the **aortic channel** lies in front and ejects its

blood into the 4th aortic arches (systemic circuit), while the **pulmonary channel** lies behind and ejects its blood into the 6th aortic arches (pulmonary circuit) (fig. 19.39).

The bulbar ridges also extend downwards towards the ventricles; as they do so they spiral in such a way that the **right bulbar ridge** comes to lie on the caudal wall of the ventricle, where it grows across the dorsal end of the right AV orifice, before meeting and fusing with the free edge of the muscular part of the interventricular septum. The **left bulbar ridge** similarly spirals on to the cranial wall of the ventricle to meet and fuse with the free edge of the muscular part of the interventricular septum. The right and left bulbar ridges form a coronally disposed septum at level A (fig. 19.40), dividing the bulbus at this level into an anterior (pulmonary) channel and a posterior (aortic)

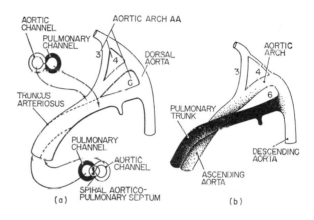

Fig. 19.39. (a) View of truncus arteriosus, aortic arch arteries 3, 4 and 6, and dorsal aorta from left side. The dotted lines trace the course of the attachment of the spiral aortico-pulmonary septum to the wall of the truncus. (b) Similar to (a), after splitting of the truncus into two separate channels, one of which, the aortic, leads into the 4th aortic arch, the other, the pulmonary, into the 6th arch.

channel. This septum spirals as it descends through the bulbus so that when it meets and fuses with the free edge of the muscular portion of the interventricular septum, it lies in the sagittal plane. The septum has divided the bulbus into two channels, one communicating with the right ventricle and forming the **infundibulum** of the adult right ventricle, the other communicating with the left ventricle and forming the **aortic vestibule** of the adult left ventricle. The bulbar septum has not only divided the bulbus, however; it has also sealed off the interventricular foramen, being the main contributor to the **membranous portion** of the interventricular septum (fig. 19.40).

ABSORPTION OF SINUS VENOSUS INTO RIGHT ATRIUM

Originally the sinus venosus is embedded within the septum transversum and is an independent chamber, opening in the midline into the caudal wall of the primitive atrium. It is symmetrical, receiving on each side the common cardinal, umbilical and vitelline veins (fig. 19.30). This pattern is soon replaced by a less complicated but asymmetrical one as the result of the following changes.

(1) The right anterior cardinal vein, the right common cardinal vein and the right horn of the sinus venosus form the **superior vena cava**. The right posterior cardinal vein remains as the arch of the vena azygos.

(2) The left common cardinal vein and the left horn of the sinus venosus cease to receive blood from the body wall. Their territory becomes restricted, at a later stage, to the wall of the heart itself, when they form the **coronary sinus**.

(3) The vitelline and umbilical veins undergo great modification, largely because of the invasion of the septum transversum by the developing liver.

In summary, the sinus venosus now receives three veins, the superior vena cava, inferior vena cava and coronary sinus, and opens into the back wall of the right atrium through an elongated sinu-atrial orifice, guarded by right and left venous valves.

The sinus venosus now becomes freed from the septum transversum and is absorbed or 'taken up' into the back wall of the right atrium. Thus, each of the three tributaries of the sinus venosus develops an independent opening (fig. 19.41). The part of the definitive atrial wall derived from sinus venosus is smooth internally, as befits its venous origin, while the remainder of the definitive

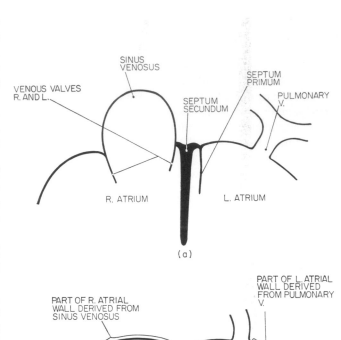

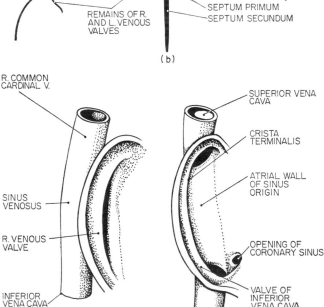

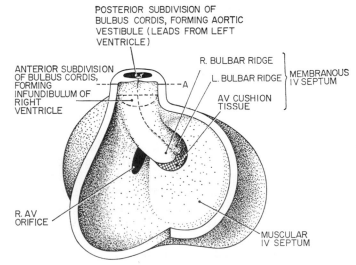

Fig. 19.40. A view of the opened heart, similar to that shown in fig. 19.38, at a later stage of development. The right and left bulbar ridges, which lie in the coronal plane at level A, spiral as they descend so that, when they reach the ventricles, they lie in the sagittal plane and can therefore fuse with the free edge of the muscular interventricular (IV) septum and seal off the interventricular foramen. After Frazer, *Manual of Human Embryology*.

FIG. 19.41. The absorption of the sinus venosus in the back wall of the right atrium. Transverse sections (a) before and (b) after absorption of sinus venosus into back of right atrium and of pulmonary veins into body of left atrium. Right lateral views (c) before and (d) after absorption.

atrium has a rough trabeculated interior, being derived from the primitive atrium. The venous valves lose their original significance with the disappearance of the single sinu-atrial orifice. The left venous valve fuses with the atrial septum; the right forms, dorsally, the **crista terminalis** and, ventrally, the valve of the inferior vena cava and the valve of the coronary sinus. Of these three structures, only the valve of the inferior vena cava has any functional importance. During fetal life it may help to direct the inferior caval blood stream across the right atrium towards the foramen ovale (fig. 42.2).

DEVELOPMENT OF PULMONARY VEINS

From the back wall of the left atrium a single pulmonary vein develops and divides; each branch in turn divides, so that two pulmonary veins from each lung return blood by a single common trunk to the left atrium. In much the same way that the sinus venosus was absorbed into the back of the right atrium, so the **common pulmonary vein** and its two primary divisions are absorbed into the back of the left atrium. Each of the four pulmonary veins now opens independently into the left atrium and the rectangular area bounded by their four orifices is smooth, being of venous origin, while the remainder of the interior of the definitive atrium is trabeculated, being derived from the primitive atrium (fig. 19.41).

DEVELOPMENT OF THE ATRIOVENTRICULAR VALVES

The right and left AV openings derive from the originally single AV opening which is divided by the septum intermedium. Each opening is surrounded by cardiac jelly from which the AV valves develop by growth, excavation and thinning.

The **left AV orifice** is the simpler. One valve cusp develops on each side of the slit, giving rise to the (bicuspid) **mitral valve**.

The **right AV orifice** is originally like the left, but the right bulbar ridge, as it grows down the back wall of the ventricle towards the free edge of the interventricular septum, cuts across the dorsal end of the opening, converting it from a slit into a triangular opening. Each boundary of the triangle is composed of cardiac jelly from which the three cusps of the **tricuspid valve** are sculptured.

DEVELOPMENT OF THE AORTIC AND PULMONARY VALVES

These develop from cardiac jelly. At the upper end of the bulbus cordis, the right and left bulbar ridges form a coronally disposed bulbar septum (fig. 19.38). Additional dorsal and ventral intercalated cushions of cardiac jelly develop at this level. When the upper bulbus divides to form aortic and pulmonary channels it does so in the plane of the bulbar septum. The anterior (pulmonary) channel and the posterior (aortic) channel each has

three masses of cardiac jelly from which the three cusps of its valve will be fashioned (fig. 19.42). In later development the entire heart rotates about its long axis, so that the right atrium and ventricle come to lie anteriorly and the left chambers posteriorly. This rotation alters the relative positions of the great vessels as they leave the heart; in the adult the pulmonary trunk, at the level of the valve, lies mainly to the left of the aorta.

DEVELOPMENT OF THE CONDUCTING SYSTEM

Peristaltic contraction of the primitive heart tube occurs in the absence both of a conducting system and of autonomic innervation, the sinus venosus acting as pacemaker. Initial continuity of atrial and ventricular muscle allows the spread of the impulse for contraction. This continuity is progressively interrupted in embryos of

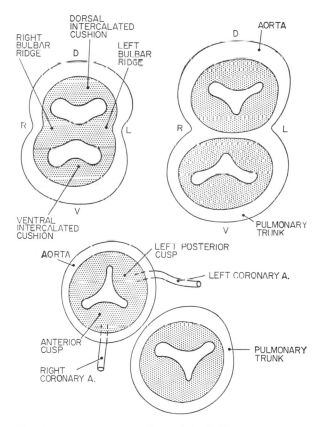

FIG. 19.42. Transverse sections of the bulbus cordis, seen from above, to show the mode of origin of the pulmonary and aortic valves.

30 days and older and the development of specialized conducting tissue becomes necessary. The **SA** and **AV nodes** appear as specializations of the myocardium and the **AV bundle**, continuous with the AV node, differentiates in the interventricular septum where it divides into **right** and **left bundle branches** (p. 30.13).

So far the development of the heart has been described

in a piecemeal fashion, chamber by chamber. Fig. 19.43 brings together, in a simple diagram, most of the important and clinically useful information about the septa of the heart. It shows schematically the appearance of a sectional plane passing through the atria and ventricles.

Interest in cardiac development has increased greatly in recent years, partly because of the development of surgical correction of several different kinds of cardiac malformation and partly because of the demonstration that some virus infections, notably rubella, of the mother at certain stages of pregnancy may cause cardiac defects. Congenital malformations of the heart are described in vol. 3, pp. 16.62 and 46.9.

Development of the aortic arch arteries

The aortic arch arteries are simple endothelial tubes which arise from the aortic sac; this lies in the midline, below the floor of the primitive pharynx and above the roof of the

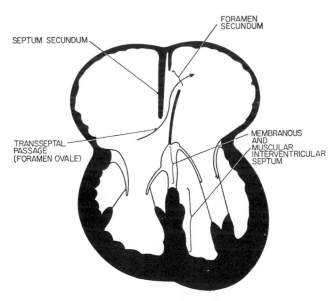

FIG. 19.43. Section through atria and ventricles, to show the developmental origin of the septa of the heart.

pericardium. These arteries run dorsally around the primitive pharynx within mesoderm of the pharyngeal (branchial) arches, and open dorsally into the dorsal aorta.

Initially, the aortic arch arteries form a bilaterally symmetrical pattern, but symmetry is lost as development proceeds. There are six pairs of them, numbered from 1–6, in order of their sequence of development. As more caudal members of the series appear, arteries 1 and 2 dwindle and largely disappear. Artery 5, while of some interest to the comparative embryologist, is ephemeral and can be disregarded.

Because later development is asymmetrical, it is convenient to study the changes which occur on each side in turn, as seen in lateral views of the embryo.

Fig. 19.44a shows the aortic arch arteries in an embryo of about 4 weeks. The 1st and 2nd arteries have disappeared, the 3rd and 4th are large and arise in common from the aortic sac ventrally. It is worth noting that there is no ventral aorta in the human embryo. The 6th or **pulmonary arch** is still small; it lies close to the site of origin of the lung buds, and the future left pulmonary artery arises from the middle of its caudal wall by sprouting of endothelial cells. The relation of the arteries to the pharyngeal pouches is also of importance. The 3rd pouch lies between the 3rd and 4th arteries; the caudal pharyngeal complex (p. 19.31) lies between the 4th and 6th arteries.

At 5 weeks (fig. 19.44b) division of the truncus arteriosus by the spiral aorticopulmonary septum is nearly complete. The upper end of the truncus and the aortic sac are divided into an anterior portion, from which arise the 3rd and 4th arteries, and a posterior portion, from which arises the 6th artery. In this way the outflow of the right

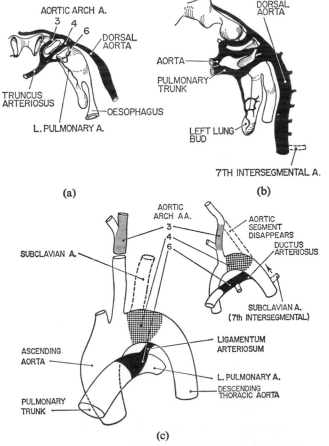

FIG. 19.44. (a) Aortic arch arteries of the left side in an embryo of about 4 weeks (5 mm). After Congdon. (b) Aortic arch arteries of the left side in an embryo of about 5 weeks (11 mm). (c) Scheme of the great vessels of the adult, seen from the left side, for comparison.

ventricle is directed to the pulmonary arteries and ductus arteriosus. The basic pattern of transformation on the left side is completed with the disappearance of the short segment of dorsal aorta between the points of entrance into it of 3rd and 4th arteries.

The left external carotid artery arises as a new outgrowth from the proximal end of the left 3rd aortic arch. The left subclavian artery is formed from the left 7th cervical intersegmental artery, which at this stage arises from the dorsal aorta below the opening into it of the 6th aortic arch. The left subclavian artery subsequently migrates headwards up the aorta to its definitive position.

Fig. 19.44c shows schematically the appearance of the great vessels as seen from the left side in the adult, and should make clear the developmental origin of the various vessels.

RIGHT SIDE

Fig. 19.45a shows the situation on the right, when the pattern is essentially the same as that on the left; fig. 19.45b shows the later changes and fig. 19.45c presents schematically the situation in the adult.

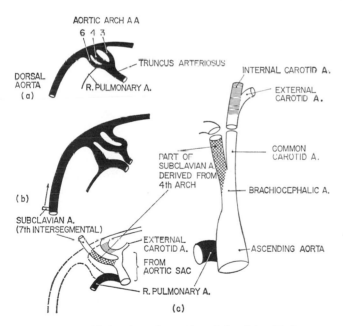

FIG. 19.45. (a) Aortic arch arteries of the right side in an embryo of about 4 weeks (5 mm). (b) Aortic arch arteries of the right side in an embryo of about 5 weeks (11 mm). (c) Scheme of the great vessels of the adult seen from the right side, for comparison.

Once the pattern of development of the aortic arches as seen separately on right and left sides is understood, fig. 19.46, which summarizes the entire story, may be appreciated. In studying this diagram the distortions necessary to depict the aortic sac and the dorsal aortae in the same plane should be remembered.

CAUSATIVE FACTORS IN AORTIC ARCH DEVELOPMENT

It would be unfortunate if preoccupation with the complex changes in the aortic arch system prevented brief comment on some of the factors thought to be responsible for the changing pattern.

(1) Embryonic vessels first appear as capillary-like tubes lined by a simple squamous epithelium, the endothelium, which arises from the flattening of aggregates of **angioblasts** of mesenchymal origin.

(2) Reduction of blood flow through one of these primitive endothelial tubes usually leads to a reduction in its size and eventual disappearance. This fate overtakes the 1st and 2nd aortic arches, e.g., when the 3rd and 4th vessels take over the output from the aortic sac.

(3) Contrariwise, increased blood flow through a primitive endothelial channel leads to its enlargement and subsequently to the differentiation of the various supporting layers which make up the definitive artery or vein.

(4) Genetic factors play an important part in shaping the pattern of development of the aortic arches and of other parts of the vascular system. For example, in mammals it is the left 4th aortic arch which persists as the main systemic vessel, in birds the right. It is not clear to what extent the genes operate indirectly through haemodynamic mechanisms. It is known, however, that experimental ligation of the right 4th arch in the chick embryo results in the left 4th arch taking over the blood flow from the aorta and persisting as the systemic trunk. Altered haemodynamic factors can, then, override genetic control.

(5) New vessels may arise from existing endothelial tubes as sprouts of solid endothelial cords which subsequently acquire a lumen. The distal portions of the pulmonary arteries arise in this way from the 6th aortic arches. In normal development actively growing parts seem to attract invasion by capillaries. In the adult, defects resulting from loss of tissue may be made good by granulation tissue, a mass of young connective tissue, richly vascularized by new capillary sprouts.

FUNCTIONAL IMPORTANCE OF THE DUCTUS ARTERIOSUS

The ductus arteriosus is a wide channel linking the left pulmonary artery with the aorta, and, in fetal life, carries a large part of the output of the right ventricle into the systemic circulation. Its fate at and after birth is discussed on p. 42.4. The lung, functionless throughout fetal life, must be prepared for function at birth. This involves the development of a pulmonary circulation, of no functional value to the fetus but vital to the establishment of pulmonary respiration. The capillaries in the unexpanded lung of the fetus offer high resistance to pulmonary circulation and there are two mechanisms by

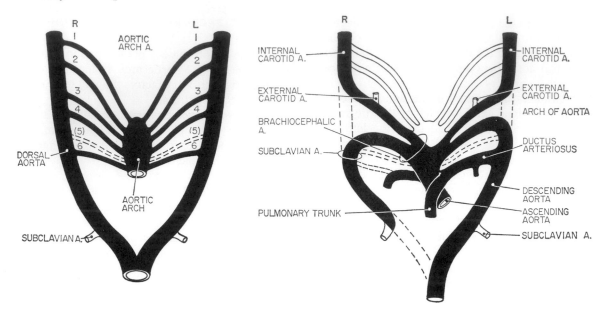

FIG. 19.46. Schematic drawing showing, in ventral view, the fate of the aortic arches.

which blood may be short-circuited away from the pulmonary circulation. First, the foramen ovale provides a route by which some of the blood returning to the right atrium is shunted to the left atrium and thence to the

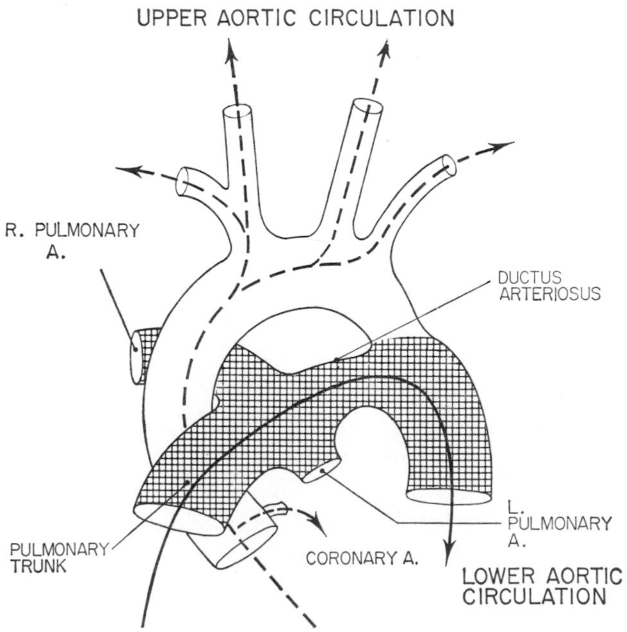

UPPER AORTIC CIRCULATION

FIG. 19.47. To show the two aortic circulations, an upper, to the head and neck, brain, upper limbs and the heart itself and a lower, distributed to the remainder of the body.

systemic circulation, by-passing the lungs. Secondly, much of the blood leaving the right ventricle via the pulmonary trunk follows the low pressure route into the

aorta via the ductus arteriosus, rather than the high pressure route through the pulmonary circulation.

These two bypasses of the pulmonary circulation may be thought of as providing two aortic circulations (fig. 19.47). (1) An **upper aortic circulation**, derives its blood from the placenta, via inferior vena cava, foramen ovale, left atrium, left ventricle and upper aorta, i.e. that part proximal to a conical narrowing on the proximal side of the opening of the ductus arteriosus. Blood to the upper aortic circulation is distributed to the head and neck brain, upper limbs and to the heart itself. (2) A **lower aortic circulation** derives its blood from the superior vena cava, via the right atrium, right ventricle, pulmonary trunk, left pulmonary artery and ductus arteriosus and distributes it to the rest of the body.

This concept is based essentially on two facts. First, the oxygen saturation in the upper circulation, e.g. in carotid blood, is consistently higher than that in the lower e.g. in femoral artery blood. Secondly, ligation of the aorta proximal to the ductus in the sheep fetus scarcely reduces blood flow in the lower aortic circulation. The two aortic circulations are of importance to the fetus in that blood of higher oxygen saturation is directed to the brain and the heart itself, while blood of lower oxygen saturation goes to the placenta.

At birth the ductus closes, and the events leading to its closure are discussed on p. 42.4. Here it need only be emphasized that the late fetal ductus has a structure different from the vessels which it connects; its wall contains substantial amounts of smooth muscle, arranged in interlacing spirals. Contraction of this muscle at birth brings about closure of the ductus by a combination of kinking, shortening and narrowing of the channel.

DEVELOPMENT OF PRIMITIVE PHARYNX AND OF THE PHARYNGEAL DERIVATIVES

GENERAL FEATURES

The **primitive pharynx** is the front end of the foregut. It is the widest part of the endodermal gut tube, is rather flattened between the pericardium ventrally and the neural tube dorsally and is at first closed anteriorly, and separated from the stomatodaeum, by the bucco-pharyngeal membrane.

The **pharyngeal (branchial) pouches** grow outwards as hollow balloon-like extensions of the pharynx. They develop in sequence, pouch 1, the first to appear, being most cranial. In the human embryo there are four true pouches on each side; they meet the surface ectoderm to form a two layered epithelial **closing membrane**. As the pouches develop and extend outwards, they divide the mesoderm which lies between the pharynx and the surface ectoderm into a series of bars, the **pharyngeal or branchial arches**. Each pouch lies between two arches, the first pouch, for example, lying between the 1st and 2nd arches. In the earlier stages of pharyngeal development, the mesoderm of the arches is readily distinguished from neighbouring paraxial mesoderm by being much more densely cellular.

From the mesoderm of each arch there develop

(1) an aortic arch **artery** running round the pharynx from aortic sac to dorsal aorta,

(2) a cartilaginous **skeletal** element and

(3) a branchial **muscle** element.

Within the mesoderm of each arch there also runs a **nervous** element, consisting of branchial (special visceral) motor fibres, which supplies the branchial muscle arising from that arch.

The whole complex of pouches and arches makes sense only in an evolutionary context. In aquatic vertebrates, the pouches and arches of the embryo form the gill pouches and bars of the adult; the aortic arch arteries carry blood to and from the gills (afferent and efferent branchial vessels); the branchial cartilages provide the supporting skeleton of the gill arch and are moved by the muscle element. All these structures have persisted in the earlier stages of avian and mammalian embryos. The development of pulmonary respiration makes them redundant as respiratory organs, but they have been retained and made use of in other ways.

The general form of the pouches and their immediate surroundings are illustrated in fig. 19.48 which shows the pharyngeal region from the exterior, and in two different sectional planes. Each pouch is, at first, widely continuous with the pharynx. It is flattened between two adjacent arches and has a cranial and a caudal wall, a dorsal and a ventral end and laterally it makes contact with the surface ectoderm at an elongated closing membrane. As seen from the outside of the embryo, the closing membrane lies in the depths of a furrow between two arches, an **external pharyngeal groove**.

The relations of a typical pouch to the aortic arch arteries and to the pericardium are particularly important.

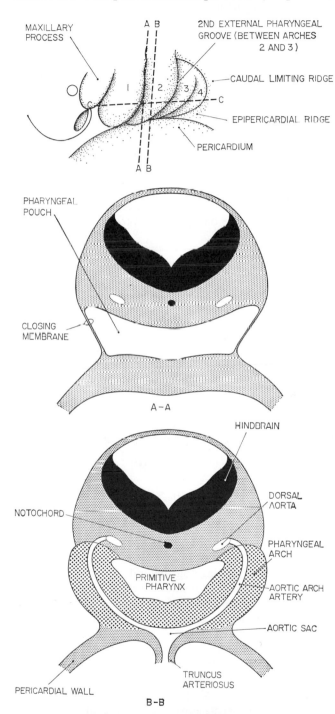

FIG. 19.48. External view of the pharyngeal region of an embryo aged about 4 weeks (5 mm). Schematic coronal sections in planes A–A and B–B are shown below. The floor of the pharynx after cutting in plane C–C is shown as fig. 19.56.

The 3rd pouch, for example, lies between the 3rd and 4th arteries and its ventral end lies close to the roof of the pericardium. At this early stage, the embryo has no neck; the floor of the primitive pharynx, from which the tongue and the floor of the mouth develop, is immediately above the pericardium.

MORPHOGENETIC FACTORS

A major morphogenetic factor in subsequent development of the region is the so-called descent of the heart. While it is not a strictly accurate description of what happens, it is a useful phrase. The extent of descent of the heart is made clear in fig. 19.49 which shows the level of the septum transversum relative to the somites in two embryos. In the younger, about 24 days, the dorsal edge of the septum transversum lies opposite the upper cervical somites; by the 7th week it has 'descended' to the level of the first lumbar somite. The change in position is, of course, a relative one and is due to the dorsal part of

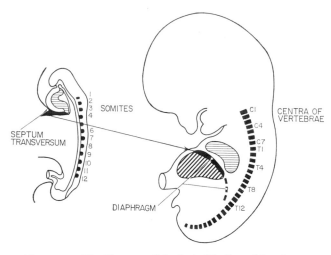

FIG. 19.49. The 'descent of the heart' indicated by the relation of the septum transversum (future diaphragm) to the somites. Based on Patten, *Human Embryology*.

the body, including the somites, growing faster than the ventral, which, in lagging behind, suffers a relative 'descent.' An important result of these changes is that the head, and with it the floor of the mouth, is lifted off the pericardium, as a neck comes into existence. Which of the various structures of the neck is the pace setter is unknown but the developing vertebral column is probably responsible. Several structures in the neck keep pace with this growth; the 3rd aortic arch (common and internal carotid arteries) is a simple example. It is, in a sense, drawn out between its lower end in the thorax and its upper end in the head. The process is not, of course, simply one of passive elongation; if it were, the vessel would narrow and break; growth of the vessel wall must also occur. In similar fashion the oesophagus, the larynx

and trachea and the vagus nerves grow with the growing neck.

This concept is useful in following the development of the pouches. Consider the 3rd pouch; at an early stage it lies between the 3rd and 4th aortic arches, with its dorsal end close to the dorsal aorta and its ventral end close to the pericardium. Its subsequent growth does not fully keep pace with that of the neck as a whole. Its ventral end maintains its primitive relationship to the pericardium; its dorsal end, however, does not maintain its position in the head but is left behind in the lower neck (fig. 19.51).

The fundamental developmental changes in the form and position of the 3rd and 4th pouches are largely determined by traction in the growing neck; they are made possible by the severance of the connection between the pouches and the primitive pharynx and between the pouches and the surface ectoderm. In other words, the 3rd and 4th pouches become free epithelial structures, subject to relative displacements among the tissues of the neck.

FATE OF THE POUCHES (fig. 19.51)

Pouch 1 lies between the 1st (mandibular) and 2nd (hyoid) arches. It incorporates part of the 2nd pouch and retains both its original continuity with the pharynx and its original contact with the ectoderm at the 1st closing membrane. Because it gives rise to the epithelial lining of the auditory tube and the tympanic cavity it is called the **tubotympanic recess**. The 1st closing membrane contributes to the formation of the **tympanic membrane**.

Pouch 2 in the main loses its identity in the tubotympanic recess. Part of it remains independent, however, and is said to be represented in the adult by the **intratonsillar fossa**. The development of the palatine tonsil in relation to this part of the 2nd pouch is one of a number of interesting lymphoepithelial associations, discussed more fully later in connection with the thymus.

Pouch 3 is the most typical of the series. In embryos of about 5 weeks, while the pouch is still a hollow structure attached to the pharyngeal wall, a **parathyroid gland (parathyroid III)** begins to differentiate from the endodermal epithelium of the wall of the dorsal end of the pouch. It lies close to the 3rd aortic arch artery from which it is precociously vascularized. There is experimental evidence of the very early onset of function in the mammalian parathyroid. The remainder of the pouch forms a solid cord of compactly arranged epithelial cells, the forerunner of the **thymus (thymus III)**. The pouch loses its connection with the pharynx and with the surface ectoderm. Its ventral end remains in contact with the pericardium and the thymic cord of cells becomes drawn out away from it, retaining for a time its connection with parathyroid III. The final positioning of parathyroid III and thymus III, and the histogenesis of the thymus are discussed on p. 19.32.

Pouch 4 appears later than pouch 3, is smaller and

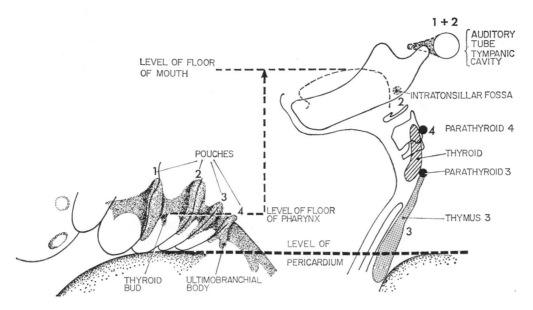

FIG. 19.50. The pharyngeal pouches, as seen from the left side. The overlying pharyngeal arches are imagined as transparent. Note particularly the position of the ventral ends of the pouches, immediately above the pericardium.

FIG. 19.51. The derivatives of the pharyngeal pouches. With the development and growth of the neck, the head has been lifted off the pericardium. The floor of the mouth has moved upwards, leaving the thyroid and the derivatives of pouches 3 and 4 behind, at various levels, in the neck. Note particularly that the ventral (lower) end of pouch 3 retains its primitive relation to the pericardium.

makes less contact with the surface ectoderm. In general, its behaviour follows that of pouch 3. However, from its caudal wall there arises a hollow outgrowth, the so-called **ultimobranchial body**. This grows rapidly and soon the boundaries between the pouch itself and the ultimobranchial body become obscure; the whole structure is now called the **caudal pharyngeal complex**. The other **parathyroid gland (parathyroid IV)** arises from the dorsal end of pouch 4; it is clearly serially homologous with parathyroid III. The connection between the caudal complex and the pharynx becomes attenuated and ruptures and the entire complex follows the 'descending' heart as the neck elongates. Just as pouch 3 lay between the 3rd and 4th aortic arches so the caudal pharyngeal complex lies between the 4th and 6th arteries. The final positioning of the complex and the fate of that part of it which does not give rise to parathyroid are considered later.

DEVELOPMENT OF THE THYROID GLAND

This is derived not from a pouch, but from the endodermal epithelium in the midline of the pharyngeal floor, between the 1st and 2nd arches. The aggregation of epithelial cells forms a **thyroid bud** which grows ventrally, away from the pharyngeal floor and towards the aortic sac, with which it soon comes into intimate contact (fig. 19.52). It follows the 'descending' heart and the growth of the slender solid cord of cells which links it to the parent pharyngeal endoderm fails to keep pace with that of the

surrounding tissues and normally it soon ruptures. As the neck elongates the thyroid leaves the 'descending' heart, losing its earlier contact with the aortic sac, and

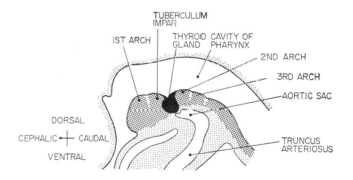

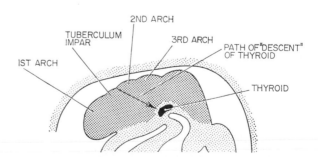

FIG. 19.52. Sagittal sections, to show the development of the thyroid gland from the endodermal epithelium of the floor of the pharynx.

becoming stranded in the lower part of the neck. Its cells proliferate actively, producing bilaminar cords of cells which spread out on either side of the midline, giving the gland a U-shaped appearance. The caudal pharyngeal complex becomes attached to the posterior aspect of the lateral lobe of the thyroid near its upper pole. Parathyroid III similarly is related to the back of the lateral lobe near the lower pole. Here it remains as the inferior parathyroid of the adult, severing its connection with the anlage of thymus III. Parathyroid IV forms the superior parathyroid, after severing its connection with the rest of the caudal pharyngeal complex. The fate of that part of the complex which does not form parathyroid IV is no longer in doubt. It becomes completely embedded in the substance of the lateral lobe and its very intimate association with the thyroid was taken by some to indicate that it made a contribution to the follicular epithelium of the gland. Recent work however shows that the ultimobranchial body forms epithelial cells scattered between the thyroid follicles, the so-called **parafollicular** or **C cells**, which are the source of calcitonin, a hormone involved, with parathyroid hormone, in calcium homeostasis (p. 27.18).

Between the bilaminar cords of thyroid epithelium is vascular connective tissue derived from surrounding mesenchyme. Precursors of secretion may be detected within thyroid cells of experimental animals by the use of ^{131}I, shortly before colloid-containing follicles are found. In man, follicles containing stainable colloid are first seen in embryos of 10 to 11 weeks.

Developmental anomalies

The thyroid may fail to follow the descending heart and then develops at the site of its formation in the developing tongue. Such a **lingual thyroid** is usually the patient's only thyroid tissue. The thyroid bud, in whole or in part, may follow the heart all the way in its descent, giving rise to thoracic ectopic thyroid tissue.

The slender cellular cord which links the thyroid bud and the pharyngeal floor until $5\frac{1}{2}$ weeks may persist as a tubular **thyroglossal duct**, lined by epithelium and reinforced externally by connective tissue. Its persistence, in whole or in part, may lead to the formation of cysts, sinuses or fistulae anywhere in the midline of the neck from the base of the tongue to the thyroid gland. Because of their origin, these remnants may be lined by a variety of epithelia and they may form ectopic thyroid tissue (fig. 19.58).

DEVELOPMENT OF THE THYMUS

The human thymus is a thymus III, derived from the ventral part of the 3rd pouch. Initially it is obviously epithelial, forming an elongated densely cellular cord on either side of the lower neck and extending into the thorax. At about 10 weeks the epithelium forms a looser cytoreticulum and lymphocytes begin to appear. Blood vessels and connective tissue invade the thymus from the surrounding mesenchyme, dividing it into the characteristic lobules. The epithelial cytoreticulum becomes obscured in the **cortex** because of the dense accumulation of lymphocytes, but it remains more obvious in the **medulla**, where lymphocytes are less abundant. **Hassall's corpuscles** are specialized differentiations of the epithelial cytoreticulum (p. 29.39).

The origin of the thymic lymphocytes is an embryological problem of long standing, whose solution has acquired a new urgency in recent years with the recognition of the great importance of the thymus in immune reactions. The problem is discussed in chap. 29.

DEVELOPMENT OF THE PHARYNGEAL ARCHES

Only four of the six arches can be seen externally; the 5th is small and short lived, while the 6th is deeply placed and lies in the parasagittal plane flanking the entrance to the respiratory tract in the floor of the caudal end of the pharynx.

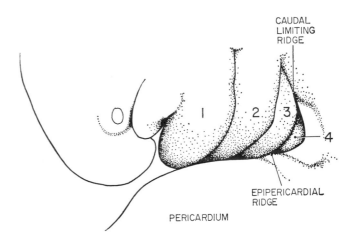

FIG. 19.53. External view of pharyngeal arches, showing the 3rd and 4th arches in the depths of the cervical sinus.

Arches 1 and 2 are the most prominent externally; 3 and 4 soon sink beneath the surface in the so-called **cervical sinus**, a depression in the side of the developing neck, bounded by the 2nd arch and by two low mesodermal ridges, the **caudal limiting** and **epipericardial ridges** (fig. 19.53).

Skeletal elements

Within each arch a skeletal element develops by condensation and chondrification of mesoderm. In the 1st and 2nd arches these **cartilage bars** extend throughout the length of the arch, but in the 3rd, 4th and 6th caudal arches they are present only at the ventral end of the arch. The fates of arch cartilages are varied; they may disappear, they may be replaced by bone, or they may be represented in the adult by 'ligaments' which are the remains of the perichondrium. Fig. 19.54 summarizes the fate of the cartilage bars.

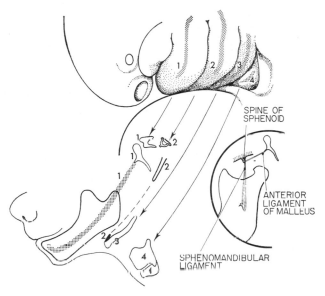

Fig. 19.54. Scheme of the fate of the pharyngeal arch cartilages.

The **first arch cartilage (Meckel's cartilage)** is closely related, at its dorsal end, to the tubotympanic recess, forerunner of the tympanic cavity, and from it develop two of the auditory ossicles, the **malleus** and the **incus**. The intermediate portion regresses, leaving its perichondrial sheath to form the **anterior 'ligament' of the malleus** and the **sphenomandibular 'ligament'**. The major ventral portion of Meckel's cartilage extends ventrally to the midline where it meets its fellow. The **mandible** develops in relation to Meckel's cartilage, but almost exclusively as a membrane bone, to which the cartilage makes essentially no contribution.

The **second arch cartilage**, like Meckel's cartilage, is related at its dorsal end to the developing middle ear, to which it contributes the **stapes**. From the rest of the cartilage, or its perichondrium, there develop the **styloid process** of the temporal bone, the **stylohyoid ligament** and the lesser cornu and upper part of the body of the **hyoid bone**.

The **third arch cartilage** is deficient dorsally; its ventral end forms the lower part of the body of the hyoid bone and its greater cornu.

The cartilages of the 4th and 6th arches are restricted to the ventral region; their fate is less precisely known than that of the 1st and 2nd arches but in general they form the **laryngeal cartilages.**

Muscular and branchial motor nervous elements. These may be considered together. The muscles derived from pharyngeal arch mesoderm consist of skeletal striated

muscle but, because of their origin, they are called branchial. The nerves which supply them are classified as branchial efferent. The fate of the muscle elements and the innervation of the muscle groups derived from them are summarized in table 19.2.

Sensory nervous elements

Some of the mesoderm of each arch contributes to the development of a particular area of skin, or mucous membrane, or both; this area, in a general way, receives its sensory innervation from the sensory component of the nerve appropriate to that arch.

Fig. 19.55 shows the pattern of sensory nerves in the arches. The sensory fibres have their cell bodies in ganglia of nerves V, VII, IX and X, which are derived mainly from the cranial neural crest. The ganglia of VII, IX and X receive additional contributions from the **epibranchial placodes**, which are localized thickenings of the ectoderm overlying the dorsal ends of the 2nd, 3rd and 4th arches. *The Vth cranial (trigeminal) nerve* is the nerve of the 1st arch. Its extensive distribution to skin and mucous membranes in the head reflects the widespread contributions of mesoderm of the 1st arch to skin and mucous membrane. The **ophthalmic division** of V is a nerve of the paraxial mesoderm, which forms the frontonasal process, and is not considered further here. The **maxillary division** of V is the nerve of the **maxillary process**, whose mesoderm contributes to the skin of the face, and to the mucous membrane of the nasal cavity and of the palate. These areas accordingly are innervated by the maxillary nerve.

TABLE 19.2

Arch	Muscles derived	Motor innervation
1 (Mandibular)	Muscles of mastication Anterior belly of digastric Mylohyoid Tensor veli palatini Tensor tympani	Mandibular division of trigeminal nerve (V)
2 (Hyoid)	Muscles of facial expression (including platysma) Stylohyoid Posterior belly of digastric Stapedius	Facial nerve (VII)
3	Stylopharyngeus	Glossopharyngeal nerve (IX)
4	Cricothyroid muscle	External laryngeal branch of superior laryngeal nerve (branch of vagus, X)
6	Constrictors of pharynx Intrinsic muscles of larynx Striated muscle of upper oesophagus	Vagus nerve (X) (principally fibres of the cranial accessory nerve, XI)

The **mandibular division** of V is the nerve of the mandibular arch itself, which contributes mesoderm to the skin of the face and the mucous membrane of the mouth and tongue, again determining the general pattern of sensory innervation.

The VII, IX and X nerves have little cutaneous sensory distribution, but they supply sensory fibres to the mucous membrane of the tongue, pharynx and larynx, whose distribution is related to developmental migrations of the appropriate arch mesoderm.

Relations of arteries and nerves of the arches

Relations in the neck can be understood only in terms of its development; the course of the recurrent laryngeal nerves serves as an example. These nerves are branches of the vagi and enter the 6th arch caudal to the 6th arch artery. Descent of the heart carries the 6th arch artery caudally and, on the left side, the recurrent laryngeal nerve must follow a looped course below the ductus arteriosus. On the right side, disappearance of the distal end of the 6th artery, and of the 5th artery, allows the recurrent nerve to loop below the 4th aortic arch, which forms the subclavian artery.

There is also an important functional relation between the nerves and arteries of the arches. Baroreceptor areas develop on the 3rd aortic arch (carotid sinus) in-

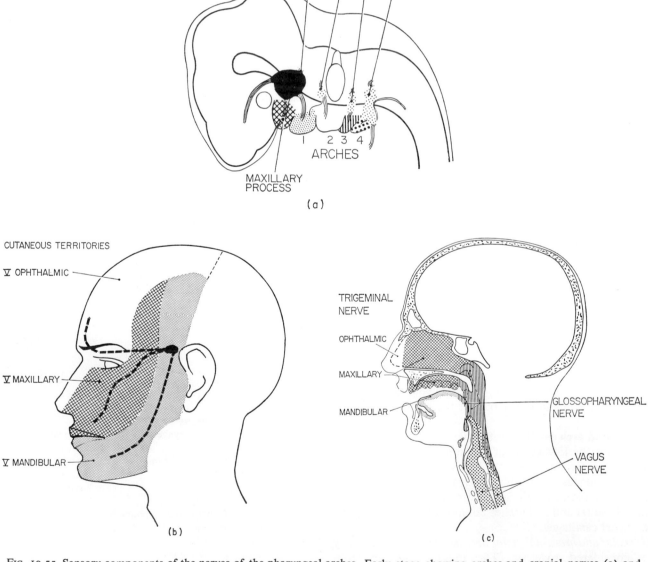

FIG. 19.55. Sensory components of the nerves of the pharyngeal arches. Early stage showing arches and cranial nerves (a) and superficial (b) and deep (c) distribution in the adult.

nervated by the IX nerve, and on the 4th aortic arch (aorta and right subclavian) innervated by the X nerve.

DEVELOPMENT OF THE TONGUE

The tongue develops from the pharyngeal arches in the floor of the primitive pharynx (fig. 19.56). The first pair

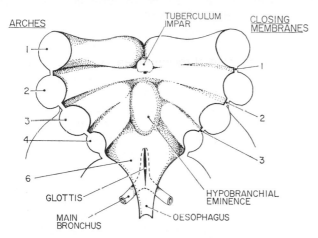

FIG. 19.56. The floor of the pharynx viewed from above. See plane C–C on fig. 19.48a.

of arches meet in the midline and contribute to the formation of a small unpaired midline elevation, the **tuberculum impar**. The second pair of arches also meet in the midline, but the third and fourth pairs fall short of the midline, their inner ends running into a low ridge on the pharyngeal floor, the **hypobranchial eminence**. Behind this and also in the midline is the **glottis**, flanked by the 6th pair of arches. This view of the pharynx makes clear why the sixth arches do not appear on the external surface.

The surface is covered by a mucous membrane, an epithelium and its supporting connective tissue. The epithelium covering the pharyngeal surface of the first arch is ectodermal; that of the remainder is endodermal.

Principal contributions to the tongue are made by paired **lingual swellings**, derived from the inner ends of the 1st pair of arches, and by mesoderm of the 3rd pair of arches which is said to migrate forwards beneath the epithelium and, in so doing, excludes the second pair of arches from the tongue (fig. 19.57). The sulcus terminalis, or rather the line of circumvallate papillae immediately in front of it, marks the junction of the body (anterior two-thirds) and the root (posterior third) of the tongue. These are derived respectively from first and third arches, and are innervated by the nerves of those arches, V and IX. The **foramen caecum** marks the site of origin of the thyroid diverticulum, which grew downwards from the pharyngeal floor between the tuberculum impar in front and the 2nd arches behind. This relationship is shown in fig. 19.58 which shows why a persistent thyroglossal duct lies in front of the body of the hyoid which develops, as we have seen, from the cartilage bars of the 2nd and 3rd arches.

The innervation of the taste buds of the body of the tongue by the **chorda tympani** (VII) is, at first sight, embryologically unsatisfactory, until it is recalled that chorda tympani may represent the **pretrematic branch** (pre —in front; trema—a hole) of VII, i.e. the branch which, in ancestral forms, came from the facial (VII), the nerve of the second arch, and ran in the first arch, in front of the **gill cleft** (fig. 19.55a).

The origin of the musculature of the tongue presents some interesting problems. The motor nerve is the hypoglossal (XII) which arises by a series of rootlets from the medulla, in line with the ventral roots of spinal nerves, and which is associated, in phylogeny, with the occipital

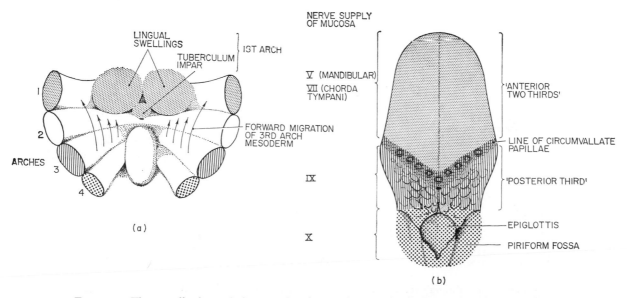

FIG. 19.57. The contributions of pharyngeal arch mesoderm to the development of the tongue.

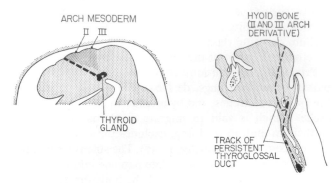

FIG. 19.58. Sagittal section showing the relationship of a thyroglossal duct to the 2nd and 3rd pharyngeal arches.

somites. In forms below the mammals, there seems no doubt that the tongue musculature arises by migration of occipital somite material which invades the developing tongue, accompanied by the XII nerve. In mammals, on the other hand, although premuscle tissue can be traced into the tongue from the caudal limiting ridge by way of the epipericardial ridge, the evidence for the origin of this material from occipital somites is very slender.

Formation and closure of the cervical sinus

The cervical sinus, as we have already seen, is a depression on the exterior of the pharyngeal region, bounded by the 2nd arch and the caudal limiting and epipericardial ridges. In its floor lie the 3rd and 4th arches and the 2nd, 3rd and 4th external grooves. These relationships are best seen in a section cutting horizontally through the sinus (fig. 19.59). The placode which contributes to the IX ganglion is an area of thickened ectoderm overlying the dorsal end of the 2nd external groove, while the placode of X covers the dorsal end of the 4th arch (fig. 19.55).

Growth of the boundaries of the sinus results in their gradual approximation to one another and in the closure of the sinus. The placodal ectoderm is buried beneath the surface as two vesicles (vesicle II = placode of IX, vesicle IV = placode of X) which normally disappear. The two **cervical vesicles** are of importance clinically because occasionally they may persist to form **branchial cysts** in the neck. **Branchial fistula** may also result from developmental aberrations during closure of the sinus. This is an epithelial tract running from an internal opening, in the pharyngeal region, to an external opening on the skin of the neck. The formation of such a fistula implies a combination of abnormal events (fig. 19.60) which includes (1) the persistence of a pharyngobranchial duct, the tubular connection between a pouch and the pharynx, (2) the establishment and persistence of a connection between one or other of the cervical vesicles and its associated pouch, (3) the persistence of a cord or tube of ectodermal epithelium between the vesicle and the surface ectoderm, and (4) the opening from the pouch to the cervical vesicle may develop later or be produced during surgical exploration. Branchial cyst and fistula are more fully described in vol. 3, p. 32.25.

GROWTH OF THE BODY

Growth is a complex process and it is not made easier to understand by the numerous definitions proposed for it. These range from the forthright and oversimplified, 'growth is increase in size' (T.H.Huxley) to the over-elaborate and almost meaningless 'growth is the co-ordinated expression of incremental and developmental factors and functions.'

We begin by looking at growth in length, or stature, before and after birth. Fig. 19.61 shows two kinds of

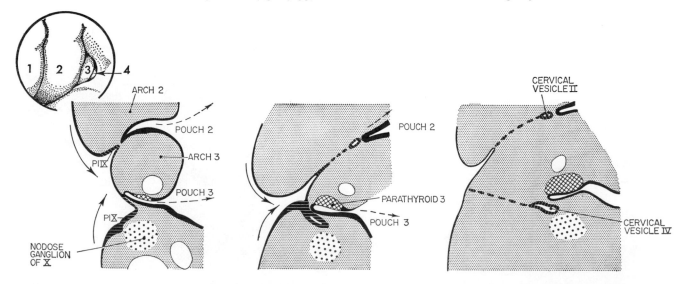

FIG. 19.59. Horizontal section through the cervical sinus before and after closure of the sinus. Two ectodermal vesicles are buried beneath the surface; they normally disappear.

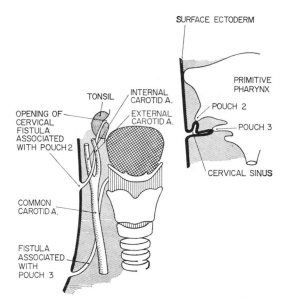

FIG. 19.60. Scheme to show the developmental origin of a fistulous connection between the pharynx and the skin of the neck.

growth curve: (a) a 'distance travelled' curve, giving **height achieved** at a particular age and (b) a 'velocity curve,' which gives the **rate of growth** during the journey. These curves show several features of interest.

(1) The rate of fetal growth is considerable. After a slow start during the first two months, which is the main period of embryogenesis and organogenesis, growth accelerates to a maximum at about four and a half months when it slows again. The newborn baby measures about 50 cm, representing an average increment in length of about 1·5 mm/day. If this rate of growth continued after birth, a 10-year-old child would stand 7 metres tall.

(2) Growth slows in late pregnancy and accelerates temporarily after birth.

(3) The rate of growth declines rapidly in the first four years after birth and more slowly until puberty, when a rapid acceleration occurs, the **adolescent growth spurt.**

(4) Growth in stature virtually ceases at about 18 years in boys, and 16 years in girls. This marks the end of the period of growth of long bones; the vertebral column continues to grow by a small amount, 3–5 mm in all, up to the age of about 30 years.

Height remains stationary until about 50 years when it begins to decline: 'In extreme old age the old man's frame is shrunken and it is but a memory that "he once was tall".' (D'Arcy Thompson).

In analysing growth in stature, we have examined what is really the simplest measure of growth, essentially the growth in one dimension, length, of a single tissue, bone. On closer examination, even this apparently simple measurement is found to be more complex. A man's height is the sum of the lengths of head, trunk and lower limbs and these make widely differing proportionate contributions to total height at different ages. This point is clearly seen in fig. 19.62; at the 4th month of fetal life, the head is a major contributor to body height, reflecting the precocious development of the brain, while the lower limbs make the smallest contribution. At maturity, on the contrary, the lower limbs make a larger contribution than the trunk, and the head is a poor third.

The child is father to the man, but the transformation of one to the other is not simply a matter of proportionate increase in stature. Before puberty, the legs grow faster than the trunk; boys are on average taller than girls after adolescence and this seems to be due to the longer period of prepubertal lower limb growth in boys. Most of the adolescent growth spurt in stature occurs in the trunk rather than in the limbs.

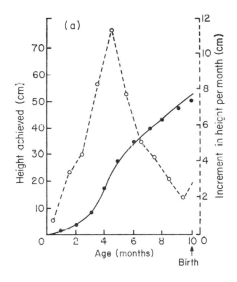

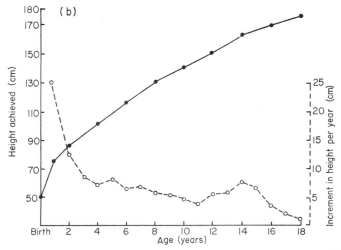

FIG. 19.61. Graphs of growth in length showing the height achieved (solid line) and the rate of growth (broken line), (a) prenatal, (b) postnatal at various ages. Based on Tanner (1964).

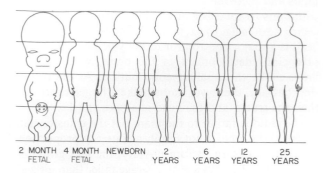

FIG. 19.62. To show the changing proportions of the body during growth and development.

Before the factors which control growth in stature are analysed, the way in which long bones develop and grow must be examined and this is most easily done in a developing limb.

Development of limbs and growth of long bones

The **limb buds** first appear as simple paddle-like outgrowths from the trunk. The forelimb buds appear first and are always in advance of the hindlimb buds in their development. The limb bud is essentially a mass of primitive mesenchyme, a loose gelatinous embryonic connective tissue, surrounded by a layer of ectodermal epithelium, the forerunner of the epidermis (fig. 19.63a). From the mesenchymal core of the limb bud there develop: (1) the skeletal axis of the limb, bones and periosteum, cartilage, joints and their capsules and ligaments, (2) the muscles, tendons and fasciae, (3) the dermis, the connective tissue layer of the skin, and the subcutaneous connective tissue and (4) the blood vessels and lymphatics.

The nerves of the limb do not develop in situ, but by the invasion of the limb bud at an early stage by axonic sprouts from cell bodies in the ventral grey horn, dorsal root ganglia and sympathetic ganglia.

DEVELOPMENT OF LONG BONE

The **scleroblastema** (fig. 19.63b) is formed by the aggregation and proliferation of mesenchymal cells to form a compact cellular mass which roughly anticipates the form of the future bone. Its cells differentiate into chondroblasts, which actively elaborate the matrix of cartilage. In short, the mesenchymal scleroblastema is transformed into embryonic hyaline cartilage which forms a rough but recognizable model of the future bone and is therefore called the **cartilage model**.

The cartilage model (fig. 19.63c) is everywhere surrounded by the primitive mesenchyme from which it developed. Where the cartilage models of adjacent bones meet, a joint space develops, lined by a connective tissue membrane, the synovial membrane, reinforced externally

by the joint capsule. Over all the remaining surface of the cartilage model the surrounding mesenchyme forms an investing membrane, the perichondrium, within which two rather poorly demarcated layers may be recognized, an inner, which is looser and more cellular, and an outer, which is more fibrous.

Growth of the cartilage model occurs by two mechanisms (figs. 19.64): (1) **interstitial growth** in which chondroblasts within the model divide and the daughter cells elaborate more matrix about themselves, and (2) **appositional growth** in which new chondroblasts are formed by differentiation of primitive mesenchymal cells of the inner, cellular, layer of the perichondrium. These newly formed chondroblasts produce matrix and the cartilage model increases in girth by the successive addition of cartilage to the external surface.

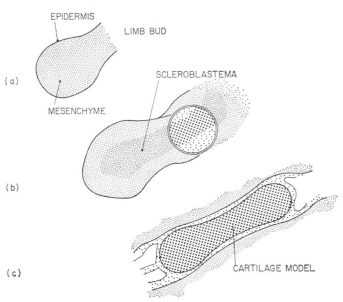

FIG. 19.63. Successive stages in the development of a long bone; (a) the limb bud, (b) the scleroblastema, (c) the cartilage model.

It is important to distinguish between these two methods of growth of cartilage because, as we shall see, the capacity of cartilage to grow interstitially is fundamental to the continued growth in length of long bones.

Division of cartilage cells is more active in two disc-shaped areas, each lying in a plane at right angles to the long axis of the cartilage model and at some distance from each end. The plane of division of each dividing cartilage cell is also in a plane at right angles to the long axis of the model. As the result of repeated cell divisions and the accompanying production of cartilage matrix, the cells of the model assume a characteristic pattern (fig. 19.65). While those at either end of the model, in the future epiphyses, divide in more random fashion and therefore retain a uniform pattern, cartilage cells of the future shaft or diaphysis are arranged in lines or rows along the long axis of the model. These lines or rows of cartilage cells are usually called cartilage columns.

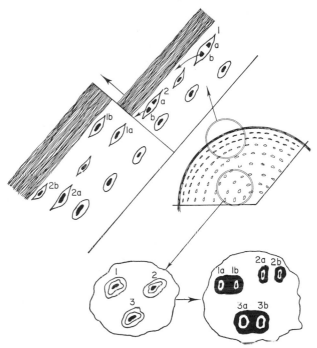

FIG. 19.64. Two mechanisms of growth of cartilage; above, appositional or growth by surface accretion; below, interstitial or growth from within.

Primary ossification centre

Two important events now occur at about the same time, but for convenience are described separately. The first consists of **degeneration of cartilage** in the centre of the cartilage model (fig. 19.66a). Cartilage cells at the centre of the future shaft enlarge greatly. This hypertrophy is associated with a corresponding enlargement of the spaces in the matrix, the **lacunae**, within which the cells lie, and with the deposition of calcium salts in the matrix which lies between the enlarged lacunae. Calcified cartilage matrix is apparently poorly permeable to tissue fluid and the hypertrophied cartilage cells die and shrivel. The centre of the shaft of the cartilage model now presents the appearance of a honeycomb; the spaces are empty lacunae, and the walls are calcified cartilage matrix. The second event is the **formation of the periosteal collar of bone** (fig. 19.66b). While these degenerative changes are going on, cells in the inner cellular layer of the perichondrium differentiate into bone forming cells or **osteoblasts**. These lay down a thin layer of **membrane bone**, so-called because it is developing within a connective tissue membrane. The essential stages in the formation of this periosteal collar are those involved in bone formation whenever or wherever it occurs in the body (p. 17.12).

The perichondrium within which the periosteal collar of bone has developed is now called **periosteum**. The change is one of name only, and neither of appearance nor developmental potentiality.

From the inner layer of the periosteum one or more **periosteal buds** now pass through spaces in the periosteal collar and invade the honeycomb of calcified cartilage matrix at the centre of the shaft (fig. 19.66c). The periosteal bud is essentially a loose vascular cellular connective tissue. It extends into the empty cartilage lacunae by breaking down the thin partitions of calcified cartilage matrix which lie between them. Its cells have a wide range of developmental potentiality and give rise to:

(1) **Osteoblasts** which align themselves on the surface of the bars, or trabeculae, of calcified cartilage matrix, and produce bone. This is called **endochondral bone** because it has developed within the cartilage model; it is distinguished from membrane bone by the fact that each trabecula contains a central core of calcified cartilage matrix. It must be stressed that, in endochondral ossification, cartilage is not transformed into bone; it is replaced by bone, the calcified cartilage matrix merely serving as an inert scaffolding upon which bone is deposited.

(2) **Osteoclasts** which play an important part in the removal or resorption of bone (p. 17.15).

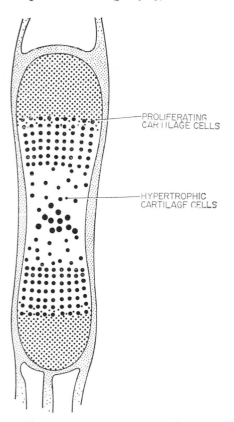

FIG. 19.65. To show the orientation of cartilage cells within the cartilage model; the pattern is determined by the plane of cell division in two disc shaped areas, the future epiphyseal plates.

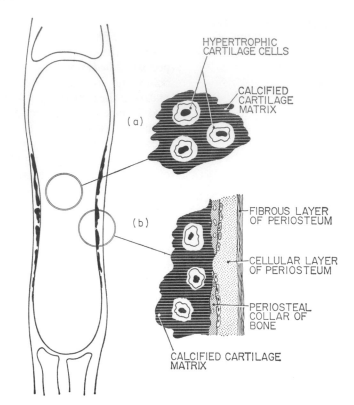

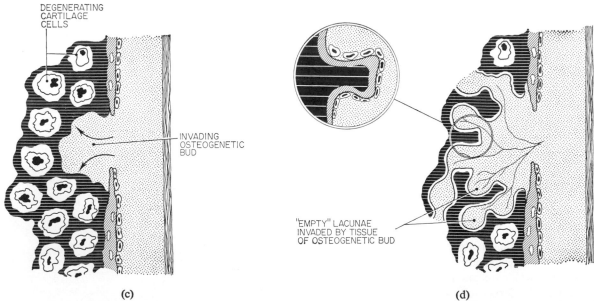

FIG. 19.66. Four stages in the establishment of the primary ossification centre in the middle of the shaft. (a) Enlargement and degeneration of cartilage cells and calcification of the cartilage matrix, (b) the formation of the periosteal collar of bone, (c) and (d) the invasion of the empty lacunae by the periosteal (osteogenetic) bud, consisting of bone-forming and bone-destroying cells, and developing blood vessels and bone marrow elements.

(3) Bone marrow precursors (p. 28.4).

(4) Blood vessels which are initially large thin walled sinusoids. These extend into the medullary cavity by sprouting of solid endothelial buds, which subsequently acquire a lumen.

The region of bone formation at the centre of the shaft

which has now been established is called the **primary centre of ossification**. It appears in most long bones in the 7th–8th week of intrauterine life and consists of the membrane bone of the periosteal collar and the endochondral bone within the cartilage model.

Having begun at the centre of the shaft, the process of

ossification extends towards each end. It is preceded by the same sequence of events that has already been described at the primary centre; hypertrophy of cartilage cells, enlargement of lacunae, calcification of cartilage matrix, degeneration of cartilage cells, invasion of empty lacunae by vascular loose connective tissue of the osteogenetic bud and the deposition of bone on the surface of calcified cartilage trabeculae.

The pattern in which this bone is produced is determined by the orientation of the columns of cartilage cells already referred to. In each column, the youngest cartilage cell, that most recently produced by cell division, lies furthest from the centre of the shaft; the oldest cell lies nearest to the centre of the shaft. Each column of cartilage cells is steadily encroached upon by degenerative change.

The osteogenetic tissue extends in succession into each new, empty, enlarged lacuna (fig. 19.67). Between the columns of empty lacunae the calcified cartilage matrix forms scalloped bars or trabeculae on the surface of which new bone is deposited. Although cartilage cells at the inner (central) end of each column are continually degenerating and disappearing, the length of the column is not thereby reduced, because there occurs continued cartilage cell division at the outer end of the column. The processes of new cartilage cell production at one end of the column, and cartilage cell degeneration at the other are nicely balanced; new endochondral bone is continually laid down on trabeculae of calcified cartilage matrix and the bone as a whole steadily increases in length. It cannot be emphasized too strongly that the continued growth of the bone in length is dependent on the continued multiplication of cartilage cells at the outer end of each cartilage cell column. Hence, the growth in length of a long bone depends upon the interstitial growth of cartilage.

That part of the bone which is ossified from the primary ossification centre is the **diaphysis**; usually a cartilaginous **epiphysis** remains at each end of the bone. Hence the plate or disc of proliferating, hypertrophying and degenerating cartilage cells is called the **epiphyseal plate.** The area of most recently formed endochondral bone, on the diaphyseal side of the epiphyseal plate, is the **metaphysis**.

Ossification of the epiphyses

At birth, the ends of most long bones still consist of cartilage; **secondary centres of ossification** appear within them in the first few years after birth. The sequence of changes is similar to that at the primary centre, with the important exception that no periosteal collar is formed at the surface. Cartilage cells at the centre of the epiphysis enlarge and die, leaving enlarged lacunae with walls of calcified cartilage matrix. In human epiphyses a periosteal bud is not the usual source of osteogenic and haemopoietic cells. These arise instead from the **cartilage canals**, irregular branching channels which carry vascular

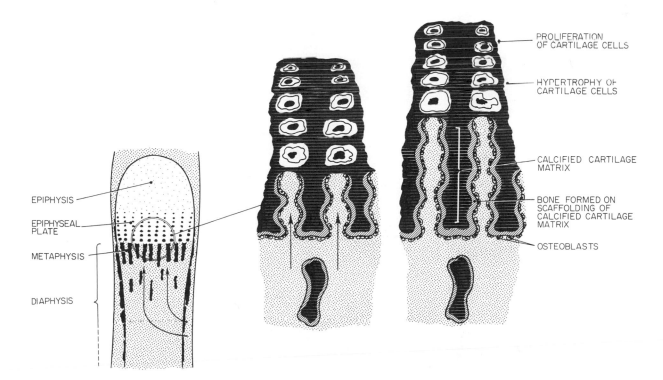

PROLIFERATION OF CARTILAGE CELLS

HYPERTROPHY OF CARTILAGE CELLS

CALCIFIED CARTILAGE MATRIX

BONE FORMED ON SCAFFOLDING OF CALCIFIED CARTILAGE MATRIX

OSTEOBLASTS

EPIPHYSIS

EPIPHYSEAL PLATE

METAPHYSIS

DIAPHYSIS

FIG. 19.67. Scheme to show the extension of the ossification process towards the end of the shaft.

mesenchyme from the surface deep into the centre of the epiphysis. Endochondral bone is now formed by the usual mechanism (fig. 19.68).

It is worth emphasizing that the epiphyses of a long bone are ossified later than and independently of the diaphysis. In fact, the epiphyses and diaphysis are three separate bones, united by the cartilaginous epiphyseal plates. These plates are the representatives, in postnatal life, of the original cartilage model, not yet replaced by bone. The continuing interstitial growth of the epiphyseal plate provides for continuing growth in length of a long bone; bone itself cannot grow interstitially.

Epiphyseal union
At the end of the growing period, division of cartilage cells in the epiphyseal plate ceases and the continuing invasion of the plate, from the diaphyseal side, by bone-forming tissue results in the complete replacement of the cartilaginous plate by bone. Epiphysis and diaphysis are now one, united by a thin disc of bone, somewhat denser than the remainder and, therefore, recognizable in a radiograph as the epiphyseal 'scar.' The process of bony union of epiphyses and diaphysis is called **synostosis**. In a typical long bone, with an epiphyseal plate at either end, one plate may make a larger contribution than the other to the total growth in length of the bone, either because its cartilage cells proliferate more rapidly, or because they proliferate for a longer period, or by a combination of the two reasons. This end of the bone is often referred to as 'the growing end'; clinically important examples are the lower end of the femur and the upper end of the tibia, the upper end of the humerus and the lower ends of radius and ulna. Premature arrest of growth may result from accidental damage to the epiphyseal plate. Occasionally the surgeon may use this as a therapeutic device.

Final shaping of the bone
The articular cartilage, which clothes the articulating surface of the epiphysis, persists throughout life. It represents part of the original cartilage model which has not been replaced by bone of the secondary ossification centre.

Growth in girth of the bone occurs by the continuing production of new bone within the cellular layer of the periosteum. This is appositional growth of bone and is intramembranous. As bone is added externally, it is removed internally (fig. 19.69); the shaft, therefore, retains a tubular form, which not only gives strength without excessive weight, but also provides space for the bone marrow. This combination of external deposition and internal resorption is the simplest example of a process of shaping of growing bone called **remodelling**.

Remodelling occurs also in the metaphyses, the two regions most recently formed by endochondral ossification on the diaphyseal side of the epiphyseal plate. Because the plate is a circular disc, the new bone formed at the metaphysis is a cylinder whose diameter is the same as that of the disc. The shaft retains its graceful form, widening slightly from its centre to its extremities, because, in the region of the metaphyses, bone is removed externally and added internally. Note that this is the

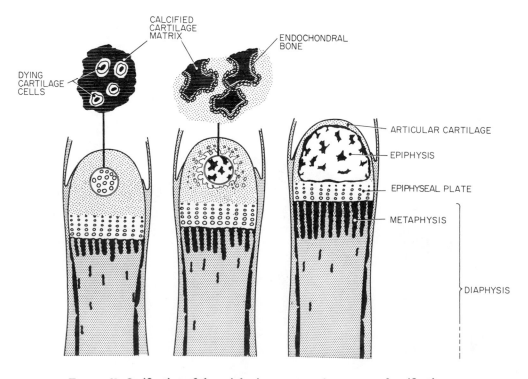

FIG. 19.68. Ossification of the epiphysis, at a secondary centre of ossification.

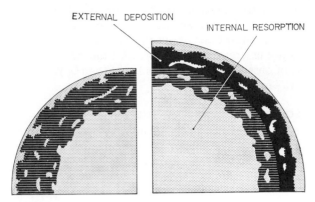

FIG. 19.69. Transverse sections of a growing bone to show increase in girth by external deposition and internal resorption.

reverse of what happens at the centre of the shaft (see fig. 19.70).

Control of growth in stature

Growth in stature of the whole body is largely determined by the growth in length of the long bones which, in turn, is finally dependent upon interstitial growth of the epiphyseal plates of cartilage. The rate of linear growth and the final stature attained are, therefore, essentially determined by the rate of proliferation of cartilage cells in the epiphyseal plate and the duration of the proliferative period.

Many factors affect the rate and duration of this proliferation.

Genetic

Studies on identical twins make it clear that genetic factors are of paramount importance in determining the final adult height. Even when reared apart, adult identical twins differ in height much less than do fraternal twins brought up together.

There is a popularly held view that there has been a secular increase in average adult height, but the evidence suggests that men of the Old Stone Age were no shorter than the average 167–170 cm today. However, when undernutrition is widespread and prolonged, the average height of adults falls.

The final expression of genetic constitution as adult height has become stable. It also appears that the genetic constitution manifests itself in early childhood; a child taller than average tends to remain taller and achieves a greater than average adult height. A reasonably accurate prediction of final height can be made by doubling the height of the child on its second birthday. It must be stressed, however, that there are greater differences in height between identical twins during the growing period than at the end of it. Further, there is no doubt that adult stature is achieved earlier, i.e. growth in childhood is accelerated, in children today.

Hormonal

(1) **Anterior pituitary somatotrophic hormone** or **growth hormone** is of major importance in controlling growth from birth to adolescence, exerting its main effect on cartilage cell proliferation and, therefore, on the growth in length of long bones. This is made clear by the dwarfism which results from deficient secretion of the hormone and gigantism when secretion is excessive (vol. 3, pp. 23.5 and 7).

(2) **Thyroid hormones** affect both the rate and the duration of cartilage cell proliferation in the epiphyseal plate; if secretion is deficient in the postnatal growing period, growth in stature, and particularly in length of long bones, is stunted.

(3) **Adrenal androgens**, which are first secreted in quantity at adolescence, are responsible for the adolescent growth spurt.

(4) **Testicular androgens** in boys are also involved. These hormones act upon the vertebral column rather than upon the long bones. Castration during the growth period leads to a failure of synostosis between epiphysis and diaphysis and, as a result, the period of growth in length of the limbs is prolonged.

Nutritional

Growth in stature is slowed by malnutrition but may accelerate, to return the individual almost to his genetically appropriate stature, when normal nutrition is restored.

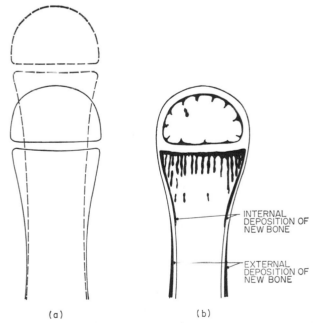

FIG. 19.70. Longitudinal sections of a growing bone to show remodelling of bone at the metaphysis. (a) Shows the change in shape and (b) shows the sites of new bone deposition.

Growth may also be retarded by non-specific factors such as severe illness. While cartilage proliferation and therefore growth in length are retarded, ossification in the metaphysis may proceed with little disturbance; a rather denser, thin plate of bone may be laid down during this period of growth retardation and may persist as a **line of arrested growth**, easily visible in a radiograph.

ADOLESCENT GROWTH SPURT

Although the rate of growth is greater in early embryonic life and in infancy than it is at puberty, the period of the adolescent growth spurt is more dramatic, not only be-

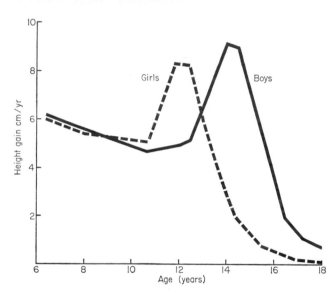

FIG. 19.71 Graphs to show the 'adolescent growth spurt'. Based on Tanner (1964).

cause it is a period of accelerated growth rate and follows a period of slowly declining rate but because of its associated changes and the onset of sexual maturity.

Fig. 19.71 gives velocity curves for growth in boys and girls and shows several important features.

(1) The growth spurt is of sudden onset. It is, in fact, the only substantial, sudden change of rate in the whole growth curve; apart from the adolescent spurt, children do not usually grow, as is sometimes popularly believed, by 'fits and starts.'

(2) The rate of growth accelerates from about 6 cm to about 10 cm/year (the fetus grows to a birth length of 50 cm in 10 months).

(3) Girls enter the growth spurt on average at age $11-13\frac{1}{2}$ years, earlier than boys by some two years. The intensity of the spurt is, however, greater in boys than in girls. These two facts help to explain the greater average height of men; boys continue their prepubertal growth in stature, mainly growth of the limbs, for a longer period than girls; growth in stature in the adolescent period in-

volves the trunk rather than the limbs, and the boys now benefit from the greater velocity of the spurt.

One important fact about the adolescent growth spurt does not emerge from fig. 19.71; it is the variability of its time of onset. The range is from $10\frac{1}{2}-16$ in boys and from $9\frac{1}{2}-14\frac{1}{2}$ in girls.

ASSOCIATED EVENTS AT PUBERTY

The changes which occur at puberty are probably triggered by the hypothalamus, bringing about release of

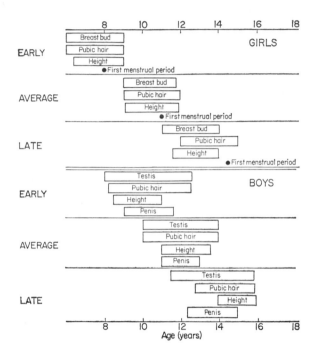

FIG. 19.72. The chronology of events at puberty. The chart shows the period of accelerated growth of organs, e.g. 'testis', and of the body as a whole, 'height'. Based on data of Tanner (1962) *Growth at Adolescence*, 2nd Edition. Oxford: Blackwell Scientific Publications.

pituitary gonadotrophins, which stimulate growth of the gonads and later the secretion of sex hormones, which evoke the secondary sex characters.

Fig. 19.72 summarizes the chronology of the major events in boys and girls. Again, the variability of their time of onset must be stressed. This means, of course, that chronological age, i.e. age by the calendar, is a poor index of physiological maturity; as Tanner points out, 'the statement that a boy is 14 is . . . hopelessly vague'; he may still be a boy, or almost a man. It is obviously important, therefore, for the doctor to be aware of the normal range of variation of onset of, for example, menstruation. Neither onset at age 10 nor delay until age 17 need necessarily, in the absence of other findings, be a matter for concern.

The doctor obviously needs a better yardstick than chronological age to measure the progress of the child and adolescent along the route to physiological maturity. Of various measures of **developmental age**, the developmental status of the skeleton is one of the most conveniently and objectively assessed. The times of appearance of ossification centres in short bones, e.g. of the carpus, and in the epiphyses of long bones, and their union with the diaphysis correlate well with the time of appearance of secondary sex characters. Thus skeletal maturity is a better index of physiological maturity than chronological age. Skeletal maturity is most conveniently assessed from radiographs of the wrist; appearances are compared with standards derived from similar radiographs of large numbers of 'normal' children. Menstruation begins in girls of 'bone age' of $12-14\frac{1}{2}$, although their chronological ages range from $10-17$.

Using skeletal age as an index, it appears that the girl who begins to menstruate early was already more mature physiologically at age 7, and probably earlier, than her more tardy classmates. The tempo of development of physiological maturity, i.e. the skeletal age, and the age of onset of puberty and of the growth spurt, is, in part at least, under genetic control; there is, for example, less difference between the time of onset of menstruation in identical than in non-identical twins.

CHRONOLOGICAL AND DEVELOPMENTAL AGE IN FETAL LIFE

In the first two-thirds of intrauterine life, chronological age correlates well with the developmental state of various organs and with the size, both weight and length, of the body as a whole. Towards the end of pregnancy, however, the weight of a particular fetus is no longer entirely reliable as a guide to its chronological, i.e. gestational, age or to its developmental status. An inadequate uterine environment may inhibit fetal growth. So it is important to distinguish between babies who are of low birth weight because of fetal growth retardation and those who are light because of shortened gestation (vol. 3, p. 45.31). The former show a characteristic lack of subcutaneous fat and the skin is loose and wrinkled, suggesting that fat has actually been lost. Brown fat which plays an important part in temperature regulation in the newborn is also reduced or absent (p. 42.6). Skeletal and brain size, and the maturity of the brain, as indicated by the complexity of the cerebral gyral pattern, are, however, little affected. Similarly, the developmental maturity of the lung is normal, as judged by histological appearances. In short, the baby who has suffered fetal growth retardation, shows signs of malnutrition rather than of a curtailed period of gestation.

While genetic factors are paramount in determining final adult stature this is not true of birth weight. Here maternal environment is more important; a small mother tends to produce a small baby because uterus and placenta are small and cannot provide for a large baby.

Tissue growth

SKELETAL MUSCLE

The development of the skeletal muscle fibres is described on p. 16.9. The formation of new fibres ceases about the fourth month of fetal life. Further growth of the muscle as a whole, therefore, depends upon (1) increase in length and diameter of existing fibres and (2) increase in the amount of noncontractile interstitial connective tissue. The growth in length of individual fibres commonly does not keep pace with the elongation of the whole muscle; the constituent fibres slide over one another, so that few of them eventually run the whole length of the muscle from tendon to tendon. Increase in diameter results from synthesis of new cytoplasm, both sarcoplasm and myofibrils; in the rat gastrocnemius muscle the weight of cytoplasm per nucleus increases more than five times between 17 and 95 days of age.

Several factors affect the final diameter of the muscle fibre; it varies from muscle to muscle in the same individual and in the same muscle in different species. Thus, fibres of the diaphragm of the shrew are several times smaller than those of the cow, but the difference is much less than that in the total bulk of the two animals. It seems that there are upper size limits for muscle fibres, beyond which they cannot grow without sacrificing efficiency. Androgenic hormones play an important part in development of the greater muscular bulk and strength in boys than in girls after puberty, the differences before puberty being small. The enlargement of muscle in response to increased work is a matter of common knowledge; it results from the enlargement (hypertrophy) of individual fibres, in which additional myofibrils appear. Since a muscle contains a substantial population of connective tissue cells, the total bulk of the muscle may not alter much in the earlier stages of work hypertrophy because the muscle fibres enlarge at the expense of the interstitial connective tissue.

The atrophy of muscle which occurs with disuse is no less familiar than work hypertrophy but is equally complex; its mechanisms involve such factors as increased interstitial connective tissue, reduced blood supply and, possibly, the purely 'trophic' effects of neuromuscular contact.

SKIN

As the body grows, the skin grows with it, maintaining itself as a well fitting tight covering. How is its growth so nicely adjusted to that of the underlying tissues? Experimental evidence suggests that skin grows interstitially in response to tension generated by growth of deeper structures. In the epidermis, interstitial growth involves proliferation of cells in the basal, germinative layer. In the dermis, proliferation of connective tissue cells is predominant in the earlier stages of growth; later, the production of fibrous intercellular material is of major importance. There are occasions when tensions arise so rapidly in the skin that it cannot grow pari passu with the deeper tissues; it becomes thinned and shiny, and tearing of the dermal connective tissue may occur.

FAT

The cells of adipose tissue arise from a cell resembling a fibroblast. Many small discrete droplets of fat appear within the cytoplasm, and eventually coalesce in a single large droplet, which displaces the flattened nucleus into the thin peripheral rim of cytoplasm. Adipose tissue grows by recruitment of new fat cells and by marked cell enlargement from the continued accumulation of fat. Deposition of subcutaneous fat in the human fetus does not begin until about 34 weeks. It increases in thickness until about 9 months postnatally, then decreases until 7 or 8 years, when it increases again.

The familiar sex differences become marked at adolescence. In boys, subcutaneous fat in the limbs is reduced, but changes little in the trunk; in girls, limb fat continues to increase and trunk fat even more so. These differences provide an obvious illustration of the importance of differential rates of growth in shaping body form.

NERVOUS TISSUE

Growth in the nervous system is complex, but involves, at least, the following:

(1) formation and proliferation of young nerve cells, neuroblasts, in the neural tube and in peripheral ganglia, somatic and autonomic;

(2) formation and proliferation of precursors of the special supporting tissue of the nervous system, the glia and sheath cells;

(3) growth of cell processes, axons and dendrites from the neuroblasts, i.e. the differentiation of the neurones;

(4) formation of investing sheaths, particularly myelin, round the nerve cell processes.

It is a commonplace of adult human anatomy that the spinal cord is larger where the nerves of the limb plexuses arise from it. Experiments on lower animals have shown that the size of central nuclear aggregates of nerve cells is largely determined by the size of the peripheral field innervated. Thus unilateral limb amputation in the chick embryo results in reduced growth of the appropriate part of the spinal cord. This is caused by the degeneration of large numbers of nerve cells. On the other hand increasing the peripheral field, as by transplanting supernumerary limbs in larval amphibians, leads to enlargement of those parts of the nervous system which supply the additional tissue. This response seems to be due to an increased differentiation of cells to form neurones, rather than to increased proliferation.

Axons and dendrites arise as protoplasmic sprouts from the cell body or perikaryon; the new cytoplasm is synthesized in the cell body and flows along the processes, whose tips make their way to peripheral connections by pseudopodial extensions, spinning out the fibre behind them as they advance. The factors which determine the direction followed by growing processes remain obscure, but the ultrastructural orientation of the region through which they are advancing seems to be of greatest significance. The diameter of the developing processes is determined by the size of neuroblast from which they arise.

Once an axon has established a peripheral connection it is, in a sense, anchored at each end; further growth occurs interstitially, the stimulus for growth probably being provided by the traction of, for example, the growing limb in which it lies.

In man proliferation of neurones occurs in fetal life, mainly during the second trimester of pregnancy, and ceases altogether by the end of the first year after birth. Thereafter their number declines; a reduction of cell counts with age has been found in both cerebral and cerebellar cortices.

Reference has been made to the precocious development and growth of the neural tube in the embryo, and this precocity continues to be evident after birth.

Myelin is formed round processes of nerve cells by the supporting cells (p. 15.4). Myelin formation begins in the spinal cord at about mid-fetal life and the process is not completed for several years. At birth, fibres of the brain are still largely unmyelinated, and continuing myelination accounts largely for the continuing increase of weight of the brain until adolescence.

Maintenance, regeneration and repair

So far, growth processes have been considered largely in relation to those changes which constitute the development of the individual; the same processes are no less important in maintenance, repair and regeneration of body tissues.

MAINTENANCE

The life span of the individual may differ greatly from that of his constituent cells. Thus dead cornified cells are constantly rubbed away from the surface of the epidermal layer of the skin and, since the epidermis maintains a relatively constant thickness, this loss must as constantly be made good by new cell production. This occurs by cell division in the deepest layer of the epidermis, the basal or germinative layer. Daughter cells move towards the surface, driven by the pressure of new cell production behind them, and undergo the series of structural changes, **cytomorphosis**, which in turn leads to their death and shedding in the cornified layer. Thus, the epidermis is maintained, although its constituent cells are constantly changing. This continual replacement of cells is called **cell turnover**, and its rate may be measured either by determining the proportion of cells which divide in unit time, or by autoradiography after labelling of dividing cells by tritiated thymidine. Cell populations have been classified, according to their rates of turnover, as renewing, expanding and static (p. 13.1).

REGENERATION AND REPAIR

In many tissues, growth by cell division virtually ceases in the adult, but may be resumed to make good losses due to disease or accident. The liver provides a model example; its cells constitute an expanding population during the growth period, but cell division declines to a normal rate of about 0·01 per cent in the adult. After partial excision of the liver, the remaining portion shows a great increase in mitotic activity, with rates estimated at more than 3·5 per cent. In a few days it declines to about 1 per cent and then more gradually to normal levels.

Damage to nerve cells, on the other hand, does not elicit a return of mitotic activity; if the axon is cut, regeneration may occur by outflow of cytoplasm from the cut end of the proximal stump, essentially an increase in the rate of the normal proximodistal flow.

In mammals, unlike some lower vertebrates, regeneration of parts such as a limb, or organs such as the eye, does not occur: regeneration is restricted to the cellular and tissue level. Regeneration in mammals is not, however, an unorganized process. In the repair of fractures of bones, essentially a process of regeneration of lost tissue, osteogenic cells inside and outside the shaft at the fracture site produce new bone, both directly by intramembranous ossification and by replacement of cartilaginous callus, endochondral ossification. Initially, an excess of bone is formed at the fracture site, but a remodelling process similar to that described in long bone development restores the normal contours of the bone, often so effectively that the original fracture site is scarcely evident. Not only has bone tissue been regenerated, but a bone organ has been repaired.

In liver regeneration, too, an essentially normal histological structural pattern may be restored.

GENERAL ASPECTS OF DEVELOPMENT

Morphogenesis

Although each system of the body presents its own complexities of developmental pattern, the processes of morphogenesis are few and relatively simple. They may involve increase in size of the constituent cells or, more commonly, in their number, through local proliferation or by migration of cells from surrounding areas. The production of intercellular material may make an important contribution. These processes are not, of course, in themselves responsible for the appearance of characteristic patterns of shape in the developing embryo. These patterns arise rather from **differential growth rates** of various parts of the embryo.

The formation of sheets or layers of cells is one of the basic developmental manoeuvres, and particularly the establishment of the three germ layers. The formation of the endoderm by delamination from the inner cell mass, and of the mesoderm by migrations of cells from the primitive streak is described on p. 19.3.

The formation of tubular structures may occur in a variety of ways, by the fusion of folds, e.g. neural tube, by the appearance of a lumen in a solid rod of cells, e.g. the duct of many glands, or even by the adhesion and subsequent disappearance of the epithelial walls at the centre of a hollow disc, e.g. semicircular canals. Undoubtedly, however, the most important event in development is cell differentiation.

Cell differentiation

The fertilized ovum, the embryo, the fetus and the adult are simply stages in the life of the individual. The developmental changes through which the individual passes involve great increases in size and in complexity. The single, large and apparently simple fertilized ovum gives way to the much larger and more complex embryo and adult, in whom there have appeared different regions (head, trunk, limbs) different organ systems and organs, different tissues, different cells, and different cell constituents. The term differentiation is used to describe the complex processes involved in the establishment of all these differences. On closer analysis the problem of differentiation is basically one of cell differentiation, whose nature and control are the fundamental problems of modern biology.

The differences between fully differentiated cells, e.g. an erythrocyte, a neurone and a skeletal muscle fibre, are obvious; each shows structural specializations which reflect specialized functions. Each is a discrete cell type; as Weiss pointed out long ago, there are no cells intermediate between any of them, and the transformation of one into either of the others is impossible. They are the stable end stages of differentiation; the erythrocyte is a dying cell, whereas the neurone and the skeletal muscle fibre are long lived but, under most conditions, are incapable of division.

The differences are less obvious between cells which are more closely related, e.g. cells of the epithelial layer of the cornea and cells of the epidermis. Both develop from the ectoderm and each forms part of a surface layer. One cell type, however, is transparent and non-cornified, while the other becomes fully cornified and is soon shed as a dead squame. These structural differences reflect functional differences and are appropriate to the different environments in which the cells occur naturally. Would a corneal epithelial cell retain its 'corneal' characters if it were transplanted to a skin site? In fact, it does; slivers of cornea transplanted to a defect in the skin of the chest in rabbits continue to behave like cornea, retaining their transparency.

Now let us look at two cell types even more closely related to one another; epidermal cells from body skin and from skin of the sole of the foot in the guinea-pig. Sole of foot epidermis is thick, with a prominent cornified layer, while body epidermis is thin and its cornified layer is poorly developed. Stimuli of various kinds, mechanical, chemical or thermal, may produce thickening of body skin epidermis, so that it comes to resemble epidermis on the sole of the foot, but the change is not permanent and is reversed when the stimulus is removed. Moreover, if skin from the sole of the foot is transplanted to an area of body skin, it continues to behave indefinitely as if it were still on the sole of the foot, exposed to mechanical trauma. There are, then, inherent differences between the cells of the two types of epidermis. These differences spring from a higher innate rate of cell proliferation in epidermis of the sole of the foot; they are evident in the foetus, before mechanical stimuli can act and they are altered only temporarily or not at all by environmental change.

Each of these three examples of the permanent character of cellular differentiation has been drawn from the adult organism. That presumptive epidermal cells can be permanently diverted into a different developmental pattern may be shown by growing skin from a 5-day chick embryo in a tissue culture medium containing an excess of vitamin A. Cells which normally would become epidermal cells synthesizing keratin, become mucus secreting and sometimes produce cilia. This experiment indicates that in the earlier stages of development, cells are more plastic and their developmental course is more easily altered by changes in their environment.

At still earlier stages of development, even more striking redirection of development may be shown to occur experimentally. If a patch of cells which would have formed the neural plate of an early amphibian embryo is transplanted to an area of potential epidermis, the potential nerve cells develop into epidermal cells. Contrariwise, potential epidermis transplanted to the future neural plate area develops into neural tissue. It appears from this that, in the earlier stages of development, prospective potency is much wider than presumptive fate, i.e. the direction in which a cell normally develops if left undisturbed is only one of several possibilities; it is, in fact, pluripotent and the full range of its developmental potentiality can be revealed only by experimental alterations in its environment.

EMBRYONIC INDUCTION

What factors determine the direction in which a particular cell or group of cells develop? In all vertebrates, the so-called **chorda mesoderm** plays a prime role in determining the basic structural plan of the embryo. Its mode of formation varies in different species; in mammals it is represented by the notochordal process and the paraxial mesoderm which flanks it. Experimental evidence indicates that the chorda mesoderm induces the ectodermal tissue, which overlies it, to form the neural plate. The evidence for this is threefold.

(1) If contact between the ectoderm and the chorda mesoderm is prevented, the neural tube fails to develop.

(2) Ectoderm normally destined to form epidermis, i.e. presumptive epidermis, forms neural plate if transplanted to a position overlying the chorda mesoderm.

(3) Chorda mesoderm transplanted to a new site beneath presumptive epidermis induces ectopic neural plate formation.

In amphibians the chorda mesoderm arises by the rolling in of cells into the blastocoele cavity, the invagination taking place at the blastopore. If tissue of the dorsal lip of the blastopore is transplanted beneath ectoderm of another amphibian embryo at the same stage, not only is a neural tube induced, but also most of the essential organs of a second embryo. It was for this reason that Spemann called the dorsal lip of the blastopore the **organizer** or **primary organizer**. There is no reason to doubt that the primitive streak and the cells which migrate from it, notochordal process and intra-embryonic mesoderm, serve a similar function in mammals.

Once the direction of development of the main axial organs has been induced by the primary organizer, a series of **secondary inductions** is set in train. This can best be illustrated by the example of the eye. The formation of the optic vesicle is the result of an inductive action on the neural plate. The optic vesicle in turn induces the formation of a lens placode, and subsequently of a lens, from the surface ectoderm with which it lies in contact. The evidence for the inductive action of the optic outgrowth is the same as that already given for the primary inductive action of the chorda mesoderm.

The chain reaction of induction does not end here. In amphibians the characteristic transparency of the cornea is due to the disappearance of pigment from its epithelial layer, and to the failure of pigment cells to appear in its stromal layer. These important events are induced by the lens and the optic cup.

Although the initial development of the optic vesicle is an induction, dependent upon another tissue, once the eye rudiment is established its development continues more or less normally when it is transplanted to a site removed from its inducer. This capacity for autonomous development is called **self differentiation**.

SELF REGULATION

That the development of an organ rudiment is already determined in a particular direction does not imply that each cell within it is irrevocably committed to a particular fate. The broad plan of future development may be laid down within the rudiment, but the individual cells can still follow a number of different developmental paths. This is illustrated very clearly in the development of a limb. The limb bud is already determined; if explanted to another site it continues its development normally. However, if it is split, it forms two limbs, each smaller than normal; if a second limb bud is transplanted alongside it, a single limb is formed, larger than normal; if it is excised, a new limb bud arises from the general area of the limb field. This ability of an experimentally altered rudiment to redirect its constituent cells so that they form a harmonious whole is called **self regulation**.

COMPETENCE

Induction involves two parties; the inducing tissue or inductor and the tissue which is induced. Competence is the ability of a particular tissue, at a particular time, to respond to a particular inductor.

Let us use the presumptive ectoderm of a young amphibian blastula as an example. As already described, when left undisturbed it will normally develop into epidermis; but if transplanted to the presumptive neural plate area it forms neural plate. Under a variety of normal or experimental circumstances it may develop into structures as diverse as pigment cells in the skin, cartilage cells in a branchial arch, craniospinal or autonomic ganglion cells, Schwann cells, the lens, the otic vesicle, or the anterior lobe of the pituitary. Under certain conditions it may form mesodermal or even endodermal structures.

As development proceeds, the wide range of competence of the presumptive ectoderm becomes restricted. Restriction of developmental potential, i.e. differentiation, is not, at first, expressed as structural change within the cell. That development is now determined in a particular direction is made clear by transferring the cells to the neutral environment of tissue culture when they self differentiate. The state of determination which precedes the histological signs of differentiation is sometimes called **chemodifferentiation**, a useful term in which to cloak our ignorance.

ROLE OF THE NUCLEUS IN DIFFERENTIATION

Differentiation is seen, then, as the result of the interaction of inducing agents, which are external and environmental, and the inherited potentialities of the tissue, transmitted by the genes. Does nuclear differentiation occur, or is the genetic complement of all the cells of an individual embryo the same? When the nucleus from one of the presumptive ectodermal cells of a frog blastula is transplanted to an enucleated activated frog ovum, normal development sometimes follows, indicating that, at this stage, the nuclei of the presumptive ectoderm, at least, are genetically equivalent. A similar conclusion may be drawn from the fact that small fragments of early chick blastoderm, which contains up to 60 000 cells or more, may, on rich culture medium, produce a small but complete embryo. In some of these fragments, none of the cells would normally have contributed to the embryo itself but would have formed extraembryonic membranes.

It must be said, however, that the nucleus from an endodermal cell of a frog blastula, when transplanted to an enucleated frog ovum, is less capable of directing normal development; it seems already to have undergone some differentiation. Moreover, in later stages of development there is clear evidence that nuclear differentiation has occurred. Indeed, some cells, such as lens epithelium or erythrocytes, lose their nuclei altogether, and the nuclei from postgastrulation stages of frog are not capable of directing normal development when transplanted to an enucleated frog egg.

These evidences of nuclear differentiation do not, however, establish that cell differentiation results from nuclear differentiation as a primary event. Rather are the nuclear changes to be regarded as the result of suppression or activation of gene loci by the local micro-environment, cytoplasmic or extracellular.

CHROMOSOMAL DIFFERENTIATION

There is direct evidence that environmental factors can affect the structure of chromosomes and, presumably, the activity of their genes. In certain flies, the giant chromosomes show, at various sites, cloud-like thickenings called puffs. At the site of puffing, there is evidence of RNA synthesis, and there are sound reasons for believing that puffing is the morphological expression of gene activation (p. 39.2). The time and site of appearance of puffs correlates with particular stages of differentiation. Most significantly it has been shown that the time of appearance of certain puffs is altered when premature moulting of the larva is induced by injections of the moulting hormone.

REVERSAL OF DIFFERENTIATION

The possibility of reversal depends largely on what is meant by differentiation.

Cells in tissue culture appear to lose some of their specific structural attributes, and tend to form sheet-like epithelial aggregates or more loosely associated cells like fibroblasts or isolated cells of macrophage type. This 'dedifferentiation' is often only apparent, however, and the cells may resume their former differential characters when restored to a more normal environment.

In a similar way, some cells look strikingly different under different conditions of hormonal stimulation. The epithelial cells of the prostate and seminal vesicle, for example, are shrunken and non-secreting in castrated animals, and resume their normal structure and functional activity under the influence of testosterone. The uterine epithelium responds similarly to oestrogens. There is good reason to believe that these hormones exert their effects by gene activation. It is doubtful, however, if these changes should be regarded as differentiation; the term **modulation**, with its implication that the changes are reversible and do not involve any fundamental change in the cell, is to be preferred.

Evidence is accumulating, however, that true dedifferentiation may occur. Cartilage cells, freed from their matrix and grown in tissue culture, may lose the capacity to synthesize matrix and may, apparently, differentiate again into other cells of the connective tissue lineage.

It is clear that purely cytological criteria are not sufficiently refined to allow the earlier stages of cell differentiation to be recognized. If differentiation is fundamentally the development of a specific pattern of protein synthesis, then studies of isoenzyme content and of tissue specific antigens will enable us to describe more precisely the sequence of differentiation.

SELECTIVE CELL ASSOCIATIONS

There are other, even more subtle, differences between cells, which are revealed by their interactions with one another. If the cells of a developing organ, such as the kidney, are dissociated by trypsin, and the resulting cell suspension is sown on the chorioallantoic membrane of the chick, they reorganize themselves into a mass which is recognizable as kidney. Moreover, kidney and liver cells, mixed together, sort themselves out into histologically organized fragments of liver and of kidney; no mixtures of the two cell types are found.

This preferential attachment of cells of like origin is believed to depend upon their surface properties. Its basis is probably the same as that of **contact inhibition**. Isolated cells, grown in culture on a glass surface, move about on the surface, and divide. When they make contact with other cells, movement and frequently division are inhibited. If the same phenomenon occurs in vivo, it is clearly important in the regulation of cell movement and cell division, both in normal tissues and at sites of repair of lost tissue. The spread of epithelial cells over a denuded surface, and the cessation of movement when the defect is covered may be described, although not explained, in terms of the removal and then the return of contact inhibition.

FURTHER READING

BELL E. ed. (1965) *Molecular and Cellular Aspects of Development*. (A collection of important original papers on modern developmental biology.) New York: Harper and Row.

DAVIES J. (1963) *Human Developmental Anatomy*. New York: The Ronald Press Co.

O'RAHILLY R. (1973) Developmental stages in human embryos. *Contributions to Embryology*, Carnegie Institution of Washington, Publication 631.

SINCLAIR D.C. (1973) *Human Growth after Birth*, 2nd Edition. London: Oxford University Press.

SPRATT N.T. (1964) *An Introduction to Cell Differentiation*. London: Chapman and Hall.

STREETER G.L. Developmental horizons in human embryos. *Contributions to Embryology*, Carnegie Institution of Washington, **30**, 1942; **31**, 1945; **32**, 1945; **34**, 1951.

TANNER J.M. (1964) Human growth and constitution. In *Human Biology*, ed. Harrison G.A., Weiner J.S., Tanner J.M. and Barnicot N.A. London: Oxford University Press.

WIDDOWSON ELSIE M. (1970) Harmony of growth. *Lancet* i, 901.

Chapter 20
Introduction to topographical anatomy

Topographical anatomy deals with the form, relationships and mechanical functioning of the component parts of the body. It is commonly studied by examining the arrangement of the organs and tissues in a given region and determining their function by appropriate methods.

The traditional method of obtaining topographical information is to dissect a dead body, and much present knowledge was originally obtained in this way. The advantages are that a leisurely investigation can be made, and that deep structures may be examined as easily as superficial ones. But most of the bodies used for this purpose are those of elderly people; their muscles are feeble and small, and many of their organs may be diseased or wasted. The embalming process shrinks and hardens the soft tissues, and may distort their relationships. It is therefore necessary to check the information provided by the dead body against the living subject before it can be accepted. New methods of study of the living body have led to a considerable revision of anatomical ideas, and this revision is by no means complete, especially as regards function.

Inspection of the living body reveals the swelling of muscles and their behaviour when a movement is made, the pulsation of arteries, and the position of superficial bones, tendons and veins. Examination by touch (**palpation**) gives more detail, and detects the resistance of bone, the contraction of buried muscles and the position of nerve trunks, dense connective tissue and solid viscera. Manipulation of joints demonstrates their construction and the types and ranges of movement of which they are capable. **Percussion**, in which a finger of one hand is laid flat on the body and struck firmly with a finger of the other hand, can map the boundaries of air-containing organs such as the lungs and stomach by the 'feel' of the vibrations set up and the dullness or resonance of the note produced.

With instruments, more is possible. The stethoscope can give an idea of the position and size of the heart and lungs, for their normal functioning creates noises which can be heard through it (**auscultation**). Recording electrodes can illustrate the part played by muscles in various movements. Instruments can be introduced through the orifices of the body to inspect such viscera as the urinary bladder, the stomach, the nose and the larynx, the rectum and the uterus. The eardrum and the retina can also be examined, using special equipment.

Surgical exploration of the living body is a fruitful source of information, and so is radiology. A plain radiograph can show not only the bones but also the shape, position and size of the heart and lungs in different phases of activity and in different postures. The hollow organs can be made visible if radio-opaque substances are swallowed or injected into them; air may be introduced to outline body cavities. Cineradiography demonstrates the mechanical functioning of the joints, the heart, lungs, and alimentary canal.

Surface anatomy

This is the name given to the rules describing the projection of deep structures on to the surface of the body; the importance of being able to locate and identify a given structure through the intact skin needs no emphasis.

Wherever possible bony prominences are used as reference points from which to take bearings, and measurements are often expressed in units derived from the patient's own body rather than in centimetres. If we say that in the average adult a given artery lies six centimetres away from a bony projection, we are faced with a complicated calculation when we try to work out how far away it would be in a 3-year-old child. But if it is described as lying three fingers' breadths away from the bone, we are expressing a general rule which does not vary with age or body size, since the patient's fingers grow with him, and large people have larger fingers than small ones. Other units used in this way are thumbs' breadths and hands' breadths.

It is often possible to avoid even this kind of measurement if two bony points are available. It may be, for example, that a nerve can be found two-thirds of the way along a line joining one bony point to the other, and proportional measurements of this kind are also general. In the abdomen, where easily identified bony landmarks are scanty, a grid of artificial lines can be superimposed as a substitute, and this grid will be used in the description of the abdominal viscera (fig. 21.54).

The mobility of the internal organs was not appreciated until quite recently, and the 'surface markings' of viscera were given in terms of the dead and embalmed body; acts such as breathing, sitting, or bending down alter the relationships of the internal organs to each other and to the surface of the body.

Language of anatomy

The language of anatomy is the basis of the language of medicine. It must therefore be clear, precise and unequivocal. In the early days of anatomy the same structure received different names in different countries. In 1895, an international conference at Basle adopted an agreed terminology based upon Latin, a language admirably suited for the purpose, since it was understood the world over, was sufficiently adaptable to accommodate new ideas and discoveries, and was not tainted with ideas of national prestige. The Basle Nomina Anatomica (BNA) represented a considerable advance from chaos, but several countries subsequently found some of the terms in it unsuitable and proceeded to make unilateral revisions: the Birmingham Revised terminology (BR) of 1933 and the Jena Nomina Anatomica (JNA) of 1936 are examples.

In 1955, another international Latin terminology was accepted; this Paris Nomina Anatomica (PNA) allows each country to make translations but not alterations of the basic terms.

Complete adoption of a new terminology cannot be achieved by a stroke of the pen. Clinicians and anatomists still tend to refer to structures by the names which they learned as students. Some of these eponymous terms perpetuate (often with little justification) the name of the supposed discoverer of the structure and this practice has some historical interest. But the Latin terms are more useful because they usually give some idea of the position, function, shape or construction of the structures to which they are applied. Those who have no Latin should use a medical dictionary to find out their meaning; it is much easier to do this than to try to remember the 5500 terms in the PNA parrot-wise.

Descriptive terms

Anatomical descriptions are based on the **anatomical position**, in which the body stands erect with the feet together and parallel; the arms are by the side, and the palms of the hands, the head, and the eyes all face directly forwards. Relationships described in this position retain their validity no matter what position the body subsequently takes up. For example, structures further away from the ground in the anatomical position are said to be **superior** to structures which are closer to the ground; the converse of superior is **inferior**. Thus the head is superior to the heart, and the heart is inferior to the head. This relationship is still expressed in the same way even if the patient stands on his head. A similar convention is used in map reading, where one place remains north of another on the map, even though the map may be twisted round or picked up and held in a different plane. In descriptive embryology the word **caudal** may be substituted for inferior, and the words **cranial** or **rostral** for superior; rostral means nearer the beak, caudal, nearer the tail.

Structures near the front of the body are **anterior** to those near the back; conversely, structures near the back are **posterior** to those near the front. The spine is always posterior to the heart, even though the patient may be lying down. Here again there are alternatives; **ventral** is a synonym for anterior and **dorsal** for posterior. The words **lateral** and **medial** refer to structures respectively further away from and nearer to the mid-line of the body; something exactly in the midline is said to be **median**.

In the limbs, other words may be used. In the forearm **ulnar** is equivalent to medial, and **radial** means lateral (the ulna is the medial bone of the forearm, and the radius the lateral bone). Similarly in the leg, **tibial** is the same as medial, and **fibular** the same as lateral. The words **palmar** and **plantar** describe respectively the anterior surface of the hand and the inferior surface of the foot (the palm and the sole), while the posterior surface of the hand and the superior surface of the foot are both usually called the **dorsum**. The pair of words **proximal** and **distal** substitute for superior and inferior.

Other pairs of more ordinary words are often employed. **Superficial** and **deep** refer to relative distance from the surface of the body, and the use of **external** and **internal** is usually restricted to the description of hollow viscera or the walls of cavities such as that of the chest. The words **central** and **peripheral** refer to relative distance from the centre of the body. Several ordinary words take on a more precise meaning. Thus **arm**, which in everyday speech may mean the whole upper limb, in anatomical description refers only to the territory between the shoulder and the elbow, and **leg** means only the part of the lower limb between knee and ankle.

Description of movements is often difficult, and the movements permitted at individual joints are explained when these joints are considered. The word **abduction** refers to movement away from the mid-line of the body, and its converse is **adduction**. In the hand, however, abduction and adduction are considered to occur away from and towards an arbitrary line through the middle digit, since this simplifies the description of the small muscles of the hand. In the foot a similar convention holds, but the arbitrary line is through the second digit, not the third. **Flexion** is defined as a movement of a joint in which the two movable parts are brought towards apposition, and its converse is **extension**. **Medial rotation** (pronation) turns the anterior surface of the limb to face medially; **lateral rotation** (supination) turns the anterior surface to face laterally.

Lastly, it is necessary to know the terms used to describe sections made through the body in various planes. An anteroposterior section exactly in the mid-line, dividing the body into two equal halves, is said to be in the **median sagittal plane**, and any other section parallel to this is known as a **sagittal** or **parasagittal section**. The reason for this is that one of the joints of the skull, known as the sagittal suture because of its resemblance to an arrow, lies in the median plane. A section at right angles to the median plane, dividing the body into anterior and posterior portions, is known as a **coronal section**, from the name of another skull suture. The terms **horizontal**, **transverse** and **oblique** as applied to sections of the body are self-explanatory, but it must be remembered that all such terms refer to the anatomical position.

Variation

In topographical anatomy quantitative variation is of considerable importance. The figures given in this book for the weights of different organs and the dimensions of cavities represent arithmetic means, and theoretically standard deviations or ranges should also be given. These are usually omitted for reasons of space and clarity but it should be remembered that the mean figure gives only limited information about the values likely to be obtained in individual patients.

Topographical anatomy also deals with qualitative variation. Such matters as the shape of a tooth, the position of an organ, the path of a blood vessel, or the pattern of cutaneous innervation, are important even though it is difficult to define them in mathematical terms. This book contains descriptions of the commonest anatomical arrangements, which may occur in only a minority of the population (chap. 3).

ORGANIZATION OF TISSUES

FASCIA

Superficial fascia

The connective tissue which surrounds and permeates the more highly differentiated tissues is itself organized, in certain situations, into specialized structures. The superficial fascia (panniculus adiposus) is a layer of loose areolar tissue deep to, and merging with, the dermis of the skin. Where it is plentiful, as in the forearm, it allows the skin to move freely over the underlying structures, but where it is virtually absent, as in the nose and the ear, the skin is firmly bound down. In the loose meshes of the superficial fascia the vessels and nerves running to the skin are protected by their mobility from injuries they might suffer if they were rigidly fixed in position.

In certain places the superficial fascia contains muscle fibres. These may be voluntary muscle, as in the muscles of facial expression and the platysma (p. 22.16), or involuntary, as in the nipple or the scrotum. In the region of the lower abdomen and groin the superficial fascia contains elastic and collagen fibres in sufficient numbers to make a recognizable membranous layer which helps the muscles of the abdominal wall to resist the intra-abdominal pressure (p. 21.30).

The main constituent of the superficial fascia is fat, which forms an insulating layer protecting the body against loss of heat; people with a heavy deposit of subcutaneous fat survive immersion in cold water longer than those not so well favoured. Whales and walruses have an immensely thick layer of blubber under their skins; hairy animals have little fat in the superficial fascia, the hair providing a sufficient insulation.

The fat in the superficial fascia also acts as a storage depot to be called upon in starvation, and it protects the underlying structures from rough usage by the environment. The rounded contours of the female body are due to the fact that females have relatively more subcutaneous fat than males. The distribution of this fat is a secondary sexual characteristic. For example, the female breast develops in the superficial fascia, and at puberty the glandular tissue of the breast is embedded in fat. Fat is also laid down at this time in the buttocks and thighs, and on the posterior aspect of the arms. Later in life fat is often deposited between the scapulae and at the back of the neck, forming the dowager's hump, and also in the subcutaneous tissue of the lower part of the abdomen. In the male abdominal wall fat tends to accumulate in the upper rather than the lower part of the region; the sexual difference has not been explained.

In certain places there is overgrowth and specialization of the superficial fascia. In the pads of the fingers it consists of dense fibrous strands which form a kind of honeycomb structure enclosing small collections of fat. A similar arrangement is found in the toes, and in the pad of the heel; the fatty tissue of the lower part of the buttock is honeycombed in much the same way. It is thought that this is a protective device developed in areas subjected to pressure by standing, sitting, handling tools, etc., in order to minimize damage to the underlying structures.

Deep fascia

Immediately deep to the superficial fascia lies a layer of dense connective tissue (p. 17.5), which is known as the deep fascia. Its thickness and strength vary considerably from one part of the body to another. It is thin and filmy over the small muscles of the thumb, and in the face it is so tenuous as to be considered absent. In contrast, it is immensely thick and strong in the lower part of the back and on the outer side of the thigh.

In the limbs, the deep fascia forms a sleeve which surrounds the muscles and dips between them to become attached to the periosteum of the bones. This arrangement divides the limb into osteofascial compartments, and many muscles attach themselves to the fascial walls of the compartment in which they lie. The fixation of the fascia to the bone stabilizes and supports these muscles, and also has an important influence on the circulation. When a muscle contracts within its tight tube of bone and fascia, the swelling of its belly compresses the deep veins and lymphatics which lie with it inside the tube. Since both veins and lymphatics are provided with non-return valves (p. 30.27), the compression always forces the venous blood and lymph towards the thorax. If this action is prevented through paralysis of the muscles or because the limb is enclosed in plaster of Paris, tissue fluid tends to accumulate in the periphery, particularly if the limb is dependent.

In the front of the leg there is no separate layer of deep fascia over the subcutaneous surface of the tibia, and similar fusions of fascia and periosteum occur over the mandible and the crest of the ilium. Sometimes the fascia is thickened to form specialized fibrous structures. In the front of the fingers it is represented by the fibrous sheath of the flexor tendons, and it is replaced on the back by the fibrous extensor hood (p. 23.26).

At the wrist and ankle the investing deep fascia is thickened and strengthened to strap the tendons down and prevent them from bow-stringing away from the bones when they are pulled on by their muscle bellies. Elsewhere special pulleys or slings may be formed to alter the direction of pull of tendons or to check their action. A good example is found in the orbit, where the tendon of the superior oblique muscle passes through such a pulley and turns back on itself to be attached to the eyeball (p. 26.4).

The deep fascia is not easily penetrated by fluid, and collections of fluid such as blood or pus tend to take the line of least resistance and spread along the 'fascial planes' Thus the various layers of deep fascia in the neck determine the direction in which infection may spread from the throat or mouth, and are therefore of clinical importance. Some glands have a dense layer of fascia immediately surrounding them, restricting them from expansion. If the gland becomes inflamed and swollen, the fibrous capsule is stretched, and since it is usually well supplied with sensory nerves, the process is very painful. This is part of the explanation of the pain in mumps, an infection involving particularly the parotid salivary gland.

LIGAMENTS

A ligament is a well-defined band or cord of white fibrous tissue, usually connecting two bones. Most ligaments are developed to resist movement of a joint in a particular direction; some of them are local thickenings of the fibrous joint capsule, and are called **intrinsic ligaments**. Others are completely isolated from the joint capsule, and are known as **extrinsic ligaments**. An example is the sacrotuberous ligament (p. 21.15), which helps to prevent the sacrum tilting on the ilium, but is some distance away from the sacroiliac joint. It is possible that such ligaments may be laid down by fibroblasts in response to unidirectional stresses tending to pull the bones apart, but the existence of other ligaments is more difficult to explain; thus, the coraco-acromial ligament and the ligament which bridges across the suprascapular notch of the scapula merely connect two different parts of the same bone, though the coraco-acromial ligament may play a protective role in the mechanism of the shoulder joint (p. 23.4).

Some structures which receive the name of ligaments are not strictly ligaments at all; the inguinal ligament and its extensions (p. 21.24) are simply the tendinous attachments of the external oblique muscle of the abdomen.

CARTILAGE

Cartilage is a light, strong, resilient material, which can survive prolonged pressure or friction without damage. It is classified according to the number and type of the fibres which occur in the matrix surrounding the cells (p. 17.19). If only fine fibres of collagen are present, it is called **hyaline cartilage**; if collagen fibres form dense coarse bundles, the name is **fibrocartilage**, and if elastic fibres predominate, the tissue is called **elastic cartilage**.

Hyaline cartilage is found in the adult in the respiratory tract (p. 31.4) where it stiffens and holds open the trachea and bronchi, in the costal cartilages which join the ribs to the sternum and to each other (p. 21.8), and as the articular cartilage of synovial joints (p. 17.19). In the infant and child it is more widespread, since it forms the precursor of the whole bony skeleton except the clavicle and the bones of the vault of the skull and of the face. The cartilaginous model is gradually invaded by bone-forming cells in the process of ossification (p. 19.39) and ultimately replaced by bone except at the joints. This replacement is complete in most bones by the age of 21, but a certain amount of replacement of hyaline cartilage by fibrocartilage and ultimately by bone or bone-like tissue continues in restricted situations until old age. This calcification or ossification of the costal cartilages is of importance as it may impede the free movements of the chest in respiration.

The thin cap of hyaline **articular cartilage** left at the ends of the bones to take part in the synovial joints is smooth and allows movement with a minimum of friction. Thin layers of hyaline cartilage receive an adequate nutrition by diffusion and thus require no blood vessels.

This is true for many of the smaller joints, where the cartilage is no more than 1 or 2 mm thick. In the larger joints, where the cartilage may reach a thickness of about 0·5 cm in a young person, it may be partly tunnelled through by cartilage canals, which contain blood vessels derived from the adjacent bone. The bearing surface, however, is always free from blood vessels. Articular cartilage is devoid of nerve fibres.

Fibrocartilage is found in symphyseal joints, such as those between the bodies of adjacent vertebrae (p. 21.3) and it also forms the intra-articular discs (menisci) which are found in many joints (p. 20.8), and which differ from most cartilage in having a considerable nerve supply. It is found in tendons where they are exposed to pressure, and sometimes where they are attached to bone. It is often difficult to distinguish between fibrocartilage and fibrous tissue, since the collagen fibres may be so numerous as to obscure the scanty cartilage cells.

Elastic cartilage occurs only in the mobile parts of the external ear and the nose, in the epiglottis, in parts of the arytenoid cartilages of the larynx (p. 22.52), and in the pharyngotympanic tube; its elastic qualities are shown by the springy return of these structures to their original shape if they are pulled or distorted. It has little tendency to ossify in old age.

If cartilage is injured or partly destroyed, a certain amount of regeneration can take place, through the activity of the cells of the thin covering membrane which is called the **perichondrium**, though cartilage may also be formed in ordinary connective tissue in response to friction, possibly through the conversion of fibroblasts to chondroblasts (p. 17.20). The surface of articular cartilage is continually being worn away because of the movements of the joint, and continuous growth is necessary to maintain its normal thickness. In this case the perichondrium can play no part, since the free surface has no covering of perichondrium.

BONE

The human skeleton has two embryological sources. The **visceral bones** are derived from the branchial arches, and comprise the facial skeleton, the hyoid bone, the auditory ossicles, and such bone as may replace the cartilaginous elements of the larynx in old age. The **somatic bones** of the rest of the body originate in the body wall, and belong to the axial skeleton, formed by the skull and vertebral column, or to the appendicular skeleton of the limbs. Some somatic bones occur in tendons or muscles, and are known as **sesamoids**. Most are small, and many are inconstant, but the patella (p. 24.9) is both large and important.

The bones form a supporting scaffolding and protection for the soft tissues, and enable the body to resist the action of gravity and other external forces. They act as a system of levers allowing one part of the body to move relative to another; this permits the body to move about in space, propelled along by the thrust of the lower limbs, or pulled about by the grasping hands. Some sesamoids apparently act as roller-bearings, such as those in the ball of the great toe (p. 24.23). Other bones have a protective function. The skull consists of several bones fixed together to form a box for the vulnerable brain; the ribs protect the thoracic and upper abdominal viscera. The skeleton is a store of calcium salts which can be called on when required; about 99 per cent of the calcium of the body is found in the bones. Lastly, the bones contain marrow which produces the myeloid elements of the blood; in the embryo most of the skeleton is used in this way, but after birth haemopoiesis becomes restricted to such places as the proximal ends of the limb bones, the bodies of the vertebrae, the sternum and the skull.

Bones vary greatly in shape and to a lesser extent in structure. The **long bones** of the limbs consist essentially of a shaft and two ends, which are expanded to provide stable surfaces for the adjacent joints. The shaft is a tube of dense (compact) bone (p. 17.16) and the medullary cavity in the centre is filled with marrow (p. 28.4). In the adult this is fatty and yellow, though in response to a need for extra blood formation it can revert to haemopoietic function and become red marrow again. The ends of long bones consist of spongy (cancellous) bone (p. 17.16) covered over by a thin rind of compact bone; the meshes of the spongy bone are filled by red marrow.

The same basic construction is found in the metacarpals, metatarsals and phalanges, which are classed as **miniature long bones** since they are much smaller than the humerus or the femur.

The **short bones** of the carpus and tarsus are roughly cubical; they are made of spongy bone surrounded by a thin layer of compact bone, like the ends of the long bones.

Flat bones consist of a sandwich of spongy bone between two layers of compact bone. Their surfaces are usually curved, as in the 'flat' bones of the vault of the skull. In this situation the layers of compact bone are known as **inner and outer tables**, and the spongy bone in the middle is called the **diploë**.

Any bones which cannot conveniently be included in the foregoing categories are classed as **irregular bones;** the vertebrae and the bones of the face are irregular. The central portion of some of the skull bones is absorbed and replaced, not by marrow, but by air sinuses extending from the nasal cavity. Such bones are sometimes included in a separate class of **pneumatic bones**.

The surface of a bone is roughened where ligaments or tendons are attached. Fleshy muscle attachments leave the surface relatively smooth. Vessels, nerves or tendons may make grooves or actually pierce the bone. These features on the surface of a bone are readily identified and given special names.

For example, any localized elevation or projection is called a **process**; sharp pointed processes may be called **spines**, and large round ones are **tuberosities** or **tubercles**. A hooked process may be called a **hamulus**, and a horn-shaped one a **cornu**. A sharply defined ridge is known as a **crest**, and a low one is called a **line**. Grooves are known as **sulci**, and tunnels as **canals**; a hole in a bone is a **foramen**, and a depression is called a **fossa**. An **articular surface** is a smooth area participating in a joint; it is covered in the living state by cartilage (p. 20.8). A **facet** is a small articular surface, a **condyle** a rounded one, and a **trochlea** is one shaped like a pulley. An **epicondyle** is a small process closely related to a condyle.

The internal construction of bones also varies according to local stresses and strains. If the bones were solid masses of compact bone, they would be very heavy, and enormous muscles would be needed to move them. On the other hand, cancellous bone is not so strong as compact bone, and a compromise is necessary. Every bone has an outer crust of compact bone, which varies in thickness according to the strains it must resist. In the short and irregular bones it is thin, but in the middle of the shafts of the long bones it is relatively thick and strong. Spongy bone is a meshwork of thin irregular plates or bars of bone called trabeculae, which are so disposed as to resist the stresses normally applied to the bone. In this way a characteristic pattern is formed for each bone of the skeleton (fig. 17.17).

Very little strength is lost by the shafts of the long bones being tubular instead of solid, since bending stresses are taken by the surfaces of the cylindrical shaft, and there is little need for a solid core. In the same way, bones such as the maxilla can be hollowed out with impunity; its surface must be large in order to make room for the teeth and the facial muscles, but a solid maxilla would impose a strain on the muscles at the back of the neck which hold the head upright.

Bone must also be strong where other tissues are attached to it. At such points the outer, fibrous layer of the periosteum (p. 17.18) becomes modified. The collagenous perforating fibres which fix it to the surface layers of the compact bone become more numerous and crowded together, forming a strong attachment continuous with the collagen of the tendon, muscle, or ligament and binding together the compact bone which it perforates. In the adult, a tendon may gradually become transformed into bone; as it approaches the bony surface, it develops a zone of fibrocartilage (p. 17.19), which is succeeded by a zone of calcified cartilage, and this in turn merges into the true compact bone.

The process of ossification and growth is described in chap. 19. Most of the primary centres of ossification appear before birth, as do some of the secondary centres.

Since closure of the epiphyseal plates does not begin to occur until late adolescence, the skeleton in childhood consists of a growing framework of cartilage and membrane, in which growing islands of bone are separated from each other by progressively diminishing intervals. The epiphyseal lines, which mark the site of the epiphyseal cartilages, are visible not only on the bone itself, but on its radiographic shadows, where they must be distinguished from the appearances caused by fractures. It is for this reason that the position of all epiphyseal lines has to be learned, though it is not necessary to commit to memory the exact times of appearance and closure of the individual centres of ossification. Such times vary within wide limits, and the average figure may be misleading when applied to an individual patient. Detailed information is of course needed when attempting to assess the age of an unidentified body, or the stage of growth reached by a patient whose development does not appear to be proceeding satisfactorily. It is usual for more growth to occur at one end of a long bone than the other, and the end at which most activity takes place is often called the **growing end**. This is a misleading term, for both ends grow, but it calls attention to the fact that an injury to this end will produce a more serious impairment of growth than damage to the other.

Secondary centres of ossification also play a part in the growth of some of the prominences and processes of individual bones, not only those which are found at the ends of the bone. For example, there are secondary centres for the medial border of the scapula and for its coracoid process (p. 23.42), but not, as a rule, for its lateral or superior border, which manage to grow satisfactorily without such an apparatus. This underlines the fact that very little is known about the reasons for the appearance of epiphyses. It was formerly customary to account for them as due to pressure, traction, or evolutionary fusion of bones which are separate in other animals. Such explanations leave many facts unaccounted for. Pressure-bearing points on bone frequently fail to develop epiphyses, and so do localized muscular or ligamentous attachments.

The region of the shaft of a long bone which immediately adjoins the epiphyseal plate is known as the **metaphysis**, and is important because it is here that infection tends to lodge. There is a very rich supply of blood to this area from **metaphyseal** vessels which encircle the bone and enter it through numerous small foramina. If the epiphyseal plate, or part of it, with the corresponding portion of metaphysis, is included within the line of attachment of the adjacent joint capsule, an abscess at the end of the bone may burst into the joint cavity; if the epiphyseal line is outside the joint capsule, this cannot occur. The relationship of the epiphyseal lines to the corresponding joint capsules is thus important clinically.

The metaphysis is the most vascular portion of the

bone, but the most obvious of the vessels supplying a long bone is the **nutrient artery**, which enters the shaft through the **nutrient foramen** at a position which is characteristic for the particular bone. Branches of the nutrient artery supply the bone marrow and the compact and spongy bone of the shaft. The compact bone of the shaft also receives some supply from the periosteal vessels. The ends of the long bones are supplied by **epiphyseal arteries**; in growing bones these seldom anastomose with terminal branches of the metaphyseal and nutrient arteries. The terminal branches of the blood vessels supplying compact bone lie in the Haversian canals (p. 17.16), which also convey fine sensory nerve fibres derived from the deeper layer of the periosteum covering the bone.

The blood and nerve supply of short and irregular bones is less stereotyped, but is often sufficiently constant to be of clinical importance; in the scaphoid bone, the pattern of the blood vessels and scanty blood supply slow the healing of a fracture in this bone (p. 23.15).

Normal healthy bone resists bending and twisting nearly as well as cast iron and there is a considerable safety factor protecting it against overloading. Nevertheless it is not proof against leverage, and violence applied to a part of the body some distance away may succeed in breaking a bone at its weakest point. It is even possible to snap a bone by a violent contraction of the patient's own muscles, if this happens to catch the protective mechanisms unawares.

In young people bones may crack in a spiral fashion, part of the bone remaining intact. This is called a **greenstick** fracture, from the resemblance to the way in which a green twig breaks incompletely. It is relatively easy to repair, since the ends of the bone remain closely apposed. In older people the bones are more brittle, and the break is often complete, with the result that the direction of the force applied and the contraction of the muscles attached to the fragments may produce a considerable deformity by twisting or pulling them apart.

The process of repair of a fracture is essentially similar to the process of ossification, and the bone-forming cells are derived from the periosteum. A large unwieldy lump of bony tissue called provisional callus is formed round the site of the fracture, and this has then to be remodelled to form a more streamlined structure known as the definitive callus. Sometimes bone formed by displaced periosteum may constitute a danger to the adjacent blood vessels; this is particularly liable to occur in the region of the elbow.

JOINTS

Joints occur where one component of the skeleton meets another; like a carpenter's or engineer's joints, they are not necessarily associated with movement. Nor are they

necessarily permanent. For example, the epiphysis and metaphysis of a long bone are united by hyaline cartilage in a **primary cartilaginous joint**, which allows no movement, and disappears when growth of the bone ceases.

There are three main classes of permanent joints. In **fibrous joints** the bones are united by fibrous tissue. In the variety known as a **suture**, the attachment is tight enough to prevent all movement, and such joints are found only in the skull, where they allow the bones to grow. Many of them are not strictly permanent, since after growth is finished they too tend to be invaded by bone and may eventually disappear in old age. A **syndesmosis** is a fibrous joint in which some stretching or twisting movement is possible, such as the distal tibiofibular joint (p. 24.15).

In the second kind of permanent joint the ends of the bones are covered by hyaline cartilage, and the two cartilaginous surfaces are then united by a plate of fibrocartilage to form a **secondary cartilaginous joint**, or **symphysis**. The middle of the plate of fibrocartilage may become softened, as in the intervertebral discs (p. 21.3), or it may develop a small cavity, as in the pubic symphysis (p. 21.14). Movement at such joints is naturally limited,

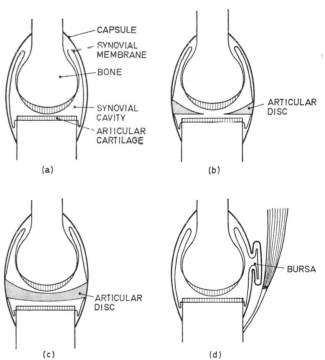

FIG. 20.1. Synovial joints (highly schematic). The synovial cavity is greatly exaggerated; in reality the cartilaginous surfaces are in contact, separated only by a thin film of synovial fluid. (a) Essential features. (b) Joint containing an incomplete disc of fibrocartilage. (c) Joint containing a complete disc. The joint cavity is divided into two, and the synovial membrane is attached to the margins of the disc. (d) Formation of a bursa. Its walls consist of synovial membrane plus a thin layer derived from the capsule; these are fused together in the living joint.

but the sum total of the individual movements between adjacent vertebrae can be considerable.

The third type of permanent joint is the **synovial joint**, which usually permits free movement (fig. 20.1). The moving surfaces are as a rule covered by a layer of hyaline cartilage, but in a few joints, such as the temporomandibular joint (p. 22.18), this may be replaced by fibrocartilage or even fibrous tissue. Stretching from one bone to another, and continuous with the fibrous periosteum on each, is the joint capsule, forming a sleeve of collagen fibres encircling the joint. Many of these fibres run randomly, but here and there they form definite bands of parallel fibres known as intrinsic ligaments. These may be connected to such structures as the cartilaginous discs or menisci which are found in certain joints, and most of them afford attachments for muscles and tendons. Some ligaments extend a considerable distance beyond the joint which they protect, as, for example, the tibial collateral ligament of the knee joint (p. 24.10), and others may pass over two or more joints, being functionally concerned with several movements.

The joint capsule is lined by a thin, smooth, vascular **synovial membrane**, which covers all surfaces within the capsule except those covered by articular cartilage. It also excludes from the joint cavity any tendons or ligaments which may lie within the capsule, and is attached to the margins of the articular cartilage and to any disc or meniscus which may be present.

In certain parts of the joint, where the bones do not fit each other well and the capsule might tend to slacken in certain phases of movement, there may be pads of fat between the fibrous capsule and the synovial membrane; these pads, which bulge into the dead space during movement, may help in the lubrication of the joint.

The synovial membrane usually develops folds and fringes in places well clear of the articular surfaces; occasionally some of them may be nipped by an unexpected movement, thereby causing one variety of internal injury of the joint. The fringes are highly vascular, and are the main source of synovial fluid. This clear or slightly yellow viscid fluid is a dialysate of blood plasma, with the addition of hyaluronic acid secreted by the connective tissue cells of the synovial membrane; it lubricates the joint, nourishes the articular cartilage, and provides macrophages to scavenge the debris from the working surfaces. Synovial fluid is present in very small quantities; even the knee joint normally contains less than 0·5 ml. But if the joint is injured, as by a sprain, fluid may accumulate in the joint cavity, separating the working surfaces and stretching the already damaged capsule. If this fluid becomes infected, locally produced toxins may enter the abundant blood and lymphatic capillaries of the synovial membrane. The synovial cavity can be regarded as a specialized connective tissue space.

In the ball and socket joints at the shoulder and hip a thin ring or labrum of fibrocartilage, triangular in cross-section, is attached round the margin of the socket, so deepening it to enclose more of the ball. In the knee joint (p. 24.10) the flat surfaces of the condyles of the tibia are deepened in a very similar way by two crescentic pieces of fibrocartilage called semilunar cartilages or menisci. Other joints, such as the sternoclavicular joint (p. 23.3) have a complete fibrocartilaginous disc dividing the joint into two separate compartments (fig. 20.1c). Such discs may be perforated (fig. 20.1b), and need not be round; for example, the 'disc' in the distal radioulnar joint (p. 23.13) is triangular in shape.

Several functions have been suggested for these **articular discs**. They may increase the stability of the joint by adapting to the different profiles of the articular surfaces during movement; they may act as shock absorbers, protecting the margins of the articular surfaces. It is probable that they help to distribute the synovial fluid more evenly through the joint cavity and so act as 'oilers' reducing friction. Finally, discs and menisci may allow different movements to take place in the two compartments into which the joint is divided; in the temporomandibular joint (p. 22.18) gliding movement occurs in the upper compartment and hinge movement in the lower.

In many joints the fibrous capsule has weaknesses or gaps through which the synovial membrane may protrude to form pockets lying on the surface of the joint (fig. 20.1d). Such **bursae** help to reduce friction, for instead of muscle rubbing against the capsule, one smooth surface of the bursa slips over the other, lubricated by synovial fluid. Bursae are not necessarily connected with the synovial cavity of a joint, and can develop in the connective tissue round muscles or tendons as smooth-walled cavities containing a viscid lubricant closely resembling synovial fluid. Sometimes a bursa may be wrapped round a tendon so as to enclose it almost completely (fig. 20.2) for much of its length; such elongated bursae are known as **synovial sheaths**.

Voluntary movements at synovial joints are naturally determined by the shape of the articular surfaces. **Hinge joints** permit flexion and extension (p. 20.2). **Pivot joints** resemble the hinges of a gate, and, like them, allow a movement of rotation; the superior radioulnar joint allows the radius to rotate around its axis in the movements of pronation and supination of the forearm (p. 23.14).

Plane joints, such as those between the bones of the carpus and tarsus (pp. 23.16 and 24.19) have surfaces which are more or less flat, and consequently permit gliding movements in several directions in the plane of the surface.

In a **condylar joint** one bone articulates with the other by two distinct and often completely separate articular condyles. Such joints in general behave like hinge joints, but if one condyle is made to rotate on its own axis the

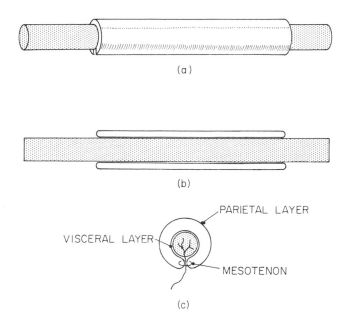

VISCERAL LAYER

PARIETAL LAYER

MESOTENON

(a)

(b)

(c)

FIG. 20.2. Construction of synovial tendon sheath. (a) Surface view. (b) Longitudinal section. (c) Cross section. Note how the blood supply enters the tendon.

other describes an arc centred on the point round which rotation takes place. In the knee joint (p. 24.10) the two condyles share a common synovial cavity, but in the atlanto-occipital joint (p. 22.23) there is a separate cavity for each condyle. Other joints, not normally described as condylar joints, have similar capacities for movement; the two temporomandibular joints (p. 22.18) together form a condylar joint in which the two condyles are separated by the width of the skull.

Saddle-shaped joints have surfaces shaped like two saddles, one placed cross-wise and upside-down on top of the other. Such joints allow rocking movements in two main planes at right angles to each other, and slight movements in other intermediate planes; a little rotation can also occur. The type specimen of such joints is the carpometacarpal joint of the thumb (p. 23.16), but this kind of surface can be detected in many other joints, though the curvatures of the saddles are not so marked.

Ball and socket joints allow movement round any axis drawn through the middle of the ball; thus flexion and extension, abduction and adduction, rotation, and any combination of these movements are all possible. If they occur sequentially, as when the toe is used to trace out a circle on the ground, the combination of movements is known as circumduction.

Ellipsoid joints, such as the radiocarpal joint, are ball and socket joints in which both ball and socket are ellipsoidal rather than spheroidal. They permit flexion and extension, abduction and adduction, and circumduction. Rotation is impossible.

This classification of synovial joints by the movements they permit is an oversimplification. The articular surfaces of any joint are not such as would be obtained by sectioning any regular geometric solid, and all voluntary movements are necessarily compound rather than simple. For example, the profiles of the trochlear surfaces of the humerus and talus have a screw-like spiral twist, so that flexion and extension at the elbow and ankle, which are both classed as hinge joints, are always accompanied by some axial rotation. In a similar manner most other movements, of whatever basic kind, are transformed into circumductions. Nor are voluntary movements the only movements which can occur at a joint. When a ball is gripped by the hand there is an easily observable rotation of the proximal phalanges of the fingers on the heads of the metacarpals. This movement results largely from the fingers meeting the resistance of the curved surface of the ball. It is of great functional importance. Movements of this kind are sometimes known as accessory movements.

Very few movements in the intact body involve only one joint. Certain joints are coupled together, such as those between the radius and ulna; rotation of the radius round the ulna must take place at both joints or it cannot take place at all. Again, many muscles and ligaments take part in the working of two or more joints, and a movement in one automatically produces a movement in the other; a good example is afforded by the movements of the shoulder girdle (p. 23.8), which necessarily involve several joints. Finally, the postures of the body, such as standing, are dependent on many joints, and an injury to one of them can lead to far-reaching alterations in the behaviour of the others.

Many factors limit the movements permitted at a joint, and some may be more important than others. For example, flexion of the elbow is limited by the development of the muscles on the front of the arm, for the soft parts are brought into apposition with each other. The bigger the biceps, the more it restricts the range of flexion. In most joints the first line of defence is the tension of the antagonist muscles. In cases where the muscles are paralysed, a greatly increased range of passive movement becomes possible, leading to stretching of the joint capsule and the formation of what is called a flail joint. On the other hand, if the tone of the muscles is increased, as in spastic paralysis, movements will be reduced in range. Should the muscles be inadequate, the duty of restricting movement falls to the ligaments, either intrinsic or extrinsic (p. 20.4). Ligaments are inextensible, and are therefore ill-adapted to withstand a suddenly imposed maximal strain, which might rupture their fibres. Sudden movements are therefore probably always restricted by muscles. On the other hand it appears that the continued stresses imposed on the hip joint and the arches of the foot by the maintenance of the upright posture (p. 24.26) must be taken mainly by the ligaments.

The stability of a joint is determined largely by the

muscles which surround it and hold the articular surfaces together. These have the advantage over the inelastic ligaments in that they can remain tense throughout the movement they resist, and pay out gradually as their opponents contract. Muscles such as those comprising the rotator cuff of the shoulder joint (p. 23.10) are sometimes referred to as **extensile ligaments**.

The action of muscles in maintaining stability may be assisted, in certain instances, by the tension of ligaments. For example, in hinge joints it is theoretically possible for the ligaments at either side of the joint to remain tense throughout the whole range of flexion and extension. The ligaments in the plane of movement can become tense only in extreme flexion or extreme extension, and are therefore of no use in holding the bones together during the movement.

A third factor in joint stability is the degree of congruence of the articular surfaces. In the sacroiliac joint (p. 21.15) many protuberances on one bone fit into depressions on the other, giving a mechanically strong joint. Such an arrangement naturally interferes with movement, and indeed one must think of strength and mobility as being to a certain extent incompatible. The factors which make for strength are good fit of bones, strong tight capsule and closely applied strong muscles; these necessarily interfere with freedom of movement. In contrast, joints with weak, lax capsules, marked incongruity of the articular surfaces, and controlling muscles situated some distance away from the capsule, have lost strength but gained mobility.

The congruence of the articular surfaces is usually minimal during the movement, and maximal at both extremes, when the joint is described as reaching a 'close-packed' position. Not only do the bones achieve the best fit in this position, but the ligaments are wound up and tensed by the rotation which is inherent in all simple movements. In contrast to the close-packed position, in which the joint is well adapted to resist stresses, is the **position of rest** taken up by the joint when it is not in use and when all the muscles acting on it are relaxed. The position of rest is naturally about the mid-point of the various movements undertaken by the joint.

The blood supply of joints is derived from a plexus of vessels lying outside the joint capsule, and its nerve supply comes from the adjacent nerve trunks. The fibrous capsule is freely supplied by sensory fibres, and so are any inclusions of fibrocartilage in the joint. The synovial membrane has a few sensory fibres, and the articular cartilage has none. The rich supply of the joint capsule is associated with receptors which feed information from the joint to the central nervous system. Since the capsule is supplied by nerves which also supply the muscles acting on the joint there is a possibility of establishing local reflex arcs which may play a part in maintaining stability.

MUSCLE

Smooth muscle (p. 16.1)
(Involuntary or visceral)

Smooth muscle tends to be arranged in sheets rather than in discrete bundles. It occurs in the walls of blood-vessels, where it regulates the blood supply to the tissues and helps to control the blood pressure. In the walls of the alimentary canal it mixes food and digestive secretions, propels them onwards, and expels their residues. Smooth muscle is concerned with the propulsion and ejection of urine, the passage of the ovum along the uterine tube to the uterus, and the movement of spermatozoa during ejaculation. It provides the motive force which empties the uterus at childbirth, and it may assist in supporting certain parts of the gut. Smooth and skeletal muscle fibres may be mixed together, as in the middle third of the oesophagus (p. 32.6) or the levator palpebrae superioris muscle (p. 26.2).

When simple constriction of a tube is required, as in the anal canal (p. 32.30) and urethra (p. 36.5), the smooth muscle fibres are arranged circularly to form a **sphincter**. When propulsion is called for, they tend to form two layers, which are usually termed **longitudinal and circular**, but which are in reality both spirals, one being loose and the other tight. The mechanics of this arrangement cause waves of contraction and relaxation to pass along the tube as the muscle is excited by its nerve supply.

Cardiac muscle
(Involuntary striated)

Cardiac muscle is restricted to the heart and the roots of the great vessels which enter and leave it. Like smooth muscle, it is arranged in sheets, whose characteristic spiral twist is important in the emptying of the heart (pp. 16.1 & 30.11).

Skeletal muscle (p. 16.1)
(Voluntary, striated or somatic)

Skeletal muscle fibres occur in bundles called fasciculi. Each fibre ends in a collagenous tip, which may be very short, or may form part of a recognizable tendon or aponeurosis.

Many muscles have attachments to several different structures, and are described as having two or more **heads**: this is often reflected in their name: biceps, triceps, quadriceps. Some of the attachments move relatively little when the muscle contracts: these are known as the **origin** of the muscle, while the more movable ones are called its **insertion**. These are only relative terms, and if the insertion of the muscle can be fixed the origin will then move towards it. For example, the pectoralis major muscle (p. 23.6) is described as taking origin from the chest wall and being inserted into the arm. But in climbing the upper limb is fixed by the grip of the hand, and the pectoralis major then acts from its fixed insertion to pull the chest towards the arm. Similarly, many muscles in the lower limb act from their insertions on their origins during walking, when the foot is fixed to the ground by friction.

The arrangement of the fasciculi within a muscle determines its external form and its range of movement. The fibres may run parallel to each other throughout the whole length of the muscle (fig. 20.3). Since a muscle fibre can only shorten by about one third of its extended length, the arrangement of the fibres in a **strap muscle** allows the maximum range of contraction. In the rectus abdominis muscles (p. 21.23) the strap arrangement is broken up into several segments by tendinous intersections which cross the muscle at intervals (fig. 20.3b). In the hand, where bulky muscles would get in the way of movement, the fleshy parts of the muscles are located in the forearm, and attached to their insertions by long thin **tendons**. Muscles of this kind are called **fusiform**, from the shape of their fleshy bellies (fig. 20.3), and the gain in the mobility of the part involves a sacrifice of range of movement, since the tendon is inert, and the contracting fibres are shorter than in a strap muscle of similar length. Occasionally a muscle has a belly at either end, with a connecting tendon in the middle (fig. 20.3); it is then said to be **digastric**. Finally, the muscle fibres may not form a straight line with the tendon, as in the fusiform muscle, but may run into it at an angle. In this way are formed the unipennate and bipennate muscles (fig. 20.3e, f), named because of the resemblance of the arrangement to a feather.

A fixed volume of muscle tissue can accommodate either a few long fibres or many short fibres. The range of movement depends on the average length of the fibres, but the strength of the muscle is a function of the number of fibres contracting. A pennate muscle therefore gains in strength what it loses in range, though some of the advantage is lost because of the angulated pull, which has a component at right angles to the tendon as well as one in line with it.

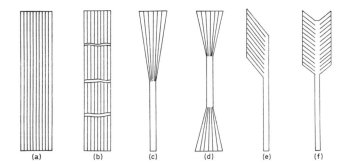

FIG. 20.3. Arrangement of fibres in somatic muscle (schematic). (a) Strap muscle. (b) Intersected muscle. (c) Fusiform muscle. (d) Digastric muscle. (e) Unipennate muscle. (f) Bipennate muscle.

The actions of a muscle depend on its attachments, and there are very few muscles in the body with only one action. Again, no muscle acts alone; it is always set into play together with several others as an integrated group. It is therefore misleading to think of one muscle in isolation, and better to consider the group as a whole. A muscle which crosses a joint in such a way that its contraction produces abduction and lateral rotation (p. 20.2) cannot be made to produce either of these movements separately. But when it acts as a member of a group, some of the other members can be employed to cancel out the unwanted action. Thus, if pure abduction is required, the lateral rotation can be nullified by combining its action with one or more medial rotators. Similarly if lateral rotation is desired, the muscle can be combined with a group of adductors which cancel the unwanted abduction.

A muscle is said to act as a **prime mover** in a given movement when it contracts primarily for the purpose of producing the movement. When it acts in a subsidiary capacity it is called a **synergist**. Synergists prevent the unwanted movements inherent in the contraction of the prime movers, and may also help them by fixing other joints to provide a stable base from which the prime movers can act. Muscles which oppose the prime movers are called their **antagonists**, and play a very important part in the movement because they pay out gradually as the prime movers contract, so providing a steady control.

Not all skeletal muscles act on joints, and some produce movement of soft tissues only; as examples may be cited the muscles which move the eyeball and the soft palate. It is also necessary to distinguish between the actions of which a muscle is capable, and the functions which it normally performs. Thus a number of the muscles which closely invest the shoulder joint and form the rotator cuff (p. 23.10) are capable of rotating the humerus in its socket, but their chief task is to act as extensile ligaments which prevent the bones from being separated during movement.

Fine movements, such as writing, are performed with the prime movers and antagonists contracting throughout, the necessary motions resulting from variations in the opposing forces. On the other hand, in movements such as kicking a football or serving at tennis, the prime movers and antagonists relax once the stroke has been made, the continuation of the movement being due to momentum. Such movements are terminated by contraction of the antagonists in order to prevent damage to inextensible structures.

NERVE

The basic unit of the nervous system is the neurone (p. 15.1), and the central nervous system, comprising the brain and spinal cord, consists of large numbers of neurones supported in a framework of cells known as neuroglia (p. 15.8). Sections through the central nervous system exhibit grey and white areas; the white matter is white because light is reflected from the myelin sheaths of the nerve fibres which preponderate in it; the grey matter is largely made up of cell bodies.

Masses of grey matter are called **nuclei**, some of which, e.g. the basal nuclei, are large and embedded in the depths of the brain. Other collections of neurones, forming grey matter, are outside the central nervous system and are known as **ganglia**. In the spinal cord the grey matter lies in a column surrounded by white matter, like the pattern in a stick of rock. In the cerebral hemispheres a thin cortex of grey matter on the surface is separated from the basal nuclei by white matter.

The peripheral nervous system is the name given to the nerves which bring information to the central nervous system and carry instructions from it to the periphery. Those which spring from the spinal cord are called the **spinal nerves**, while those attached to the brain are known as **cranial nerves**. The cell bodies of the motor neurones in the peripheral nerves lie in the grey matter of the central nervous system, while those of the sensory neurones lie in ganglia just outside it. The **autonomic nervous system** is the collective name for the neurones concerned in the supply of smooth muscle, cardiac muscle, and the cells of certain glands; the **cerebrospinal system** supplies the whole of the rest of the body. The autonomic system is purely motor, while the cerebrospinal system contains both motor and sensory neurones.

The spinal nerves are segmental structures, and are attached to the spinal cord in an orderly series. There are eight cervical nerves, twelve thoracic, five lumbar, five sacral and one coccygeal nerve. The first cervical nerve emerges from the spinal canal between the occipital bone and the first cervical vertebra (fig. 22.25) and the first seven cervical nerves therefore lie superior to the correspondingly numbered cervical vertebrae. Because there are only seven cervical vertebrae, the eighth cervical nerve emerges inferior to the seventh cervical vertebra, and from this point downwards the nerves emerge inferior to the correspondingly numbered vertebrae.

Each spinal nerve is attached to the spinal cord by two roots, ventral and dorsal. The dorsal root is almost entirely composed of sensory fibres, and their cell bodies lie in the dorsal root ganglion, which is situated in the intervertebral foramen (fig. 20.4). Their central processes enter the spinal cord along a vertical posterolateral furrow. The ventral roots leave the cord from its anterolateral aspect in a series of more compact bunches; they are exclusively composed of motor fibres whose cell bodies lie in the spinal grey matter.

The roots of the cervical nerves run more or less hori-

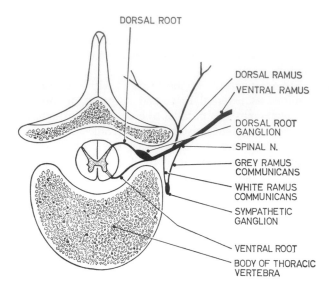

DORSAL ROOT

DORSAL RAMUS
VENTRAL RAMUS

DORSAL ROOT GANGLION
SPINAL N.
GREY RAMUS COMMUNICANS
WHITE RAMUS COMMUNICANS
SYMPATHETIC GANGLION

VENTRAL ROOT
BODY OF THORACIC VERTEBRA

FIG. 20.4. Formation and branching of a thoracic spinal nerve. The coverings of the spinal cord and nerve roots have been omitted for the sake of clarity.

zontally from the cord to emerge through the appropriate intervertebral foramen. But because the cord is shorter than the vertebral column, successive pairs of roots have to run more and more obliquely in order to escape. In consequence the length of the nerve roots increases from above downwards, and the lower part of the spinal canal, below the termination of the spinal cord, is occupied by a leash of nerve roots known as the cauda equina.

Just peripheral to the spinal ganglion, the dorsal and ventral nerve roots unite to form the spinal nerve, which therefore contains both motor and sensory fibres. After a very short course, the spinal nerve divides into two main branches, a **dorsal primary ramus** destined for structures on the posterior aspect of the trunk, and a larger **ventral primary ramus**, which is distributed to the ventral part of the body and to the limbs. Each ramus, like the parent trunk, contains both motor and sensory fibres.

Immediately after they are formed, the ventral rami of the thoracic and first two lumbar nerves give branches to a chain of ganglia lying alongside the bodies of the vertebrae and extending from the skull down to the coccyx. These **white rami communicantes** contain preganglionic fibres which constitute the thoracolumbar sympathetic outflow of the autonomic nervous system. The ganglia and the vertical communications between them are known as the **sympathetic trunk**. The fibres of the white ramus communicans may end locally in the corresponding ganglion, or they may turn upwards or downwards in the sympathetic trunk to reach another ganglion. In either case they synapse with a postganglionic sympathetic neurone, which then sends its axon either directly back into the corresponding spinal nerve, or

muscle only, and are referred to as **motor nerves**. Nevertheless, the sensory branches contain sympathetic motor fibres for the smooth muscles of the blood vessels and hairs of the skin, and the motor branches contain sensory fibres coming from the sense organs in the muscle.

The general redistribution of fibres in a plexus (fig. 20.6) means that a given branch of the plexus may contain fibres originating in several different nerve roots. Thus, the musculocutaneous nerve (p. 23.31), a mixed branch of the brachial plexus, contains fibres derived from the fifth, sixth and seventh cervical nerve roots. Conversely, the fibres leaving or entering the spinal cord in any one nerve root may be distributed along several different pathways to the periphery. For example, the fifth cervical nerve contributes fibres to seven other named branches of the brachial plexus, as well as giving off several branches before taking part in the plexus at all. The group of muscles to which fibres from a given ventral root are ultimately conveyed, possibly by many different peripheral pathways, develops originally from a segmental cluster of cells or **myotome**, part of a mesodermal somite (p. 19.5). The motor nerve which eventually enters a given muscle often contains fibres derived from two or

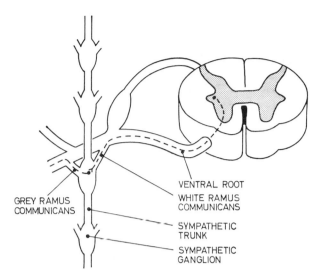

FIG. 20.5. White and grey rami communicantes. The dotted line shows the path of a sympathetic fibre originating in the thoracic part of the spinal cord. It runs through the ventral root of the spinal nerve and the white ramus communicans into the sympathetic ganglion, where it relays. The second order neurone runs in the grey ramus communicans to the ventral ramus of the nerve and will be distributed in one or more of its branches.

through the sympathetic trunk to enter another spinal nerve. The bundles of such secondary sympathetic neurones look grey because they have a negligible coating of myelin, and are therefore known as **grey rami communicantes**. In contrast to the white rami communicantes, which are restricted to the thoracic and first two lumbar nerves, the grey rami communicantes can and do reach every spinal nerve (fig. 20.5). Some of the fibres of the grey ramus communicans are distributed with the ventral ramus, while others find their way into the dorsal ramus of the nerve.

Each dorsal ramus is connected to the one above and the one below by bundles of nerve fibres passing from one to the other and so forming what is called a **simple loop plexus**. The arrangement allows a nerve fibre emerging in one spinal nerve either to continue to the periphery in a branch of that nerve, or, by passing along the connecting loops, to enter another nerve at a different level.

The plexuses connecting the ventral rami are more complicated because of the difficulties introduced by the limbs, but the principle is similar. The rami which feed the plexus communicate or combine, and from the peripheral side of the resulting plexus there spring branches, which may or may not receive special names. All these branches, like the rami from which they are derived, contain both motor and sensory fibres, and many of them supply both muscle and skin; these are known as mixed nerves. Others may be solely destined for skin, and are commonly called **sensory nerves**; others again supply

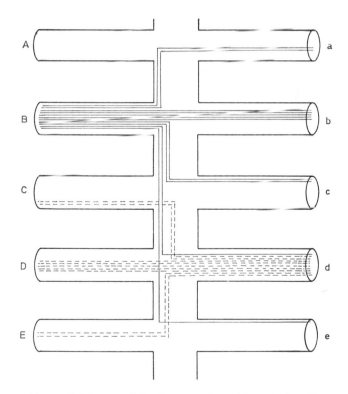

FIG. 20.6. Diagram of simple nerve plexus. The spinal rami running into the plexus are labelled A to E, and the nerves running away from it are labelled a to e. The fibres in B are mainly distributed through its direct continuation b, but some find their way into a, c, d and e. Conversely, the fibres in d can be traced back, not only to D, but also to B, C and E.

more central roots, so there is a degree of overlap between adjacent myotomes.

The skin supplied by a given dorsal nerve root is called its **dermatome**. Adjacent dermatomes overlap each other very extensively, and because of this it is difficult to map accurately the territory supplied by one spinal nerve root.

The cranial nerves differ from the spinal nerves in several ways. They do not form plexuses, though they may communicate with their neighbours on leaving the skull. Not all of them are mixed nerves, and there is no regular arrangement of motor and sensory roots. Some have a specialized role in connection with the organs of special sense, and one, the optic nerve, is really part of the brain and not a peripheral nerve at all. Several contain autonomic fibres derived from the cranial parasympathetic component of the autonomic nervous system, but others contain no autonomic fibres at all.

In summary, a peripheral nerve may contain both motor and sensory fibres of the cerebrospinal system. If it is a branch of a spinal nerve or plexus it will also contain sympathetic motor fibres; if it is a branch of a cranial nerve it may or may not contain parasympathetic fibres. The largest fibres in a peripheral nerve are those derived from the sensory endings in a skeletal muscle, which reach a diameter of about twenty μm, and the smallest are the axons of the secondary sympathetic neurones, which may be less than one μm in thickness.

FURTHER READING

BARNETT C.H., DAVIES D.V., & MACCONAILL M.A. (1961) *Synovial Joints; their structure and mechanics.* London: Longman.

CLARK W.E. LE GROS (1971) *The Tissues of the Body,* 6th Revised Edition. Oxford: Clarendon.

SINCLAIR D. (1975) *An Introduction to Functional Anatomy* 5th Edition. Oxford: Blackwell Scientific Publications.

TABER C.W. (1973) *Cyclopedic Medical Dictionary,* 12th Revised Edition. Philadelphia: Davis.

Chapter 21
Trunk

My book is wrote . . . in order, by a more frequent and a more convulsive elevation and depression of the diaphragm, and the succussations of the intercostal and abdominal muscles in laughter, to drive the *gall* and *bitter juices* from the gall-bladder, liver, and sweet-bread of his majesty's subjects with all the inimicitious passions which belong to them, down into their duodenums.

TRISTRAM SHANDY

The trunk is the central part of the body and is continuous, above with the neck, on either side with the upper limbs and below with the lower limbs. The outer tissues of the trunk constitute the **body wall**. This encloses two regions (fig. 21.1) which are described as cavities, al-

though in the natural state they are completely occupied by organs and their associated vessels, nerves and connective tissues. They are cavities only in the sense that the inside of a box is a cavity when it is filled with china and sawdust. The two cavities are separated by the **diaphragm**, a dome-shaped sheet of skeletal muscle whose fibres arise from the body wall and are inserted into a central tendon. The **thoracic cavity** lies above the diaphragm and the corresponding part of the trunk is described as the **thorax**. The **abdominal cavity** lies below the diaphragm and consists of two parts in wide communication. The larger upper part is the **abdominal cavity** proper. The smaller lower part is called the **pelvic cavity**; it lies within the lower part of the bony pelvis (the **lesser pelvis**), and is limited below by an inverted dome-shaped muscle sheet, the **pelvic diaphragm**. Below the pelvic cavity and between the thighs there is a region of the body wall which is traversed by the terminal parts of the gastrointestinal and genitourinary tracts; this is the **perineum**.

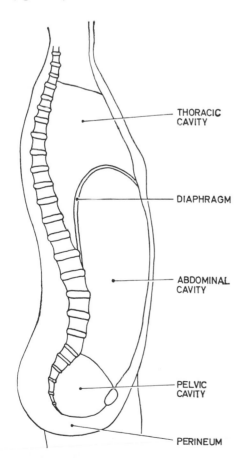

FIG. 21.1. Median section of trunk showing compartments.

THORACIC CAVITY

DIAPHRAGM

ABDOMINAL CAVITY

PELVIC CAVITY

PERINEUM

RELATIONSHIP OF STRUCTURE TO FUNCTION IN THE BODY WALL

The body wall, as well as providing protection to the internal organs, has other functions which vary in different parts and the structure is correspondingly modified. The common **posterior wall** of the thoracic, abdominal and pelvic cavities is formed by the relevant parts of the vertebral column and the related muscles. The vertebral column has three functions, namely, to surround and protect the spinal cord, to transmit body weight and to allow movement between one part of the trunk and another. Consequently it consists of a large number of vertebrae, bony rings of rather elaborate form, which articulate in series by intervertebral joints. The **wall of the pelvic cavity** is continuous laterally with the tissues of the lower limb and must consequently transmit much of the weight of the body from the vertebral column to the lower limb skeleton. For this reason it consists largely of bones, the joints between which allow little movement. The **lateral** and **anterior walls of the abdominal cavity** are largely formed by three layers of flat muscles, which run concentrically around it. On contraction, these muscles not only move the thorax in relation to the pelvis, but raise the intra-abdominal pressure, an essential step in defaecation and parturition.

In the **thoracic cavity**, on the other hand, a negative, or more accurately subatmospheric, pressure is necessary for respiration (chap. 31). Consequently the lateral and anterior walls of the thoracic cavity consist, not of muscle alone as in the abdominal wall, but of muscles and bones together. The bones are the sternum, anteriorly, and the ribs which extend round the chest wall between the sternum and the vertebral column. Three layers of intercostal muscles occupy each intercostal space and attach adjacent ribs to one another, while other larger muscles pass to the ribs from surrounding parts such as the neck, upper limbs and pelvis. Contraction of these muscles moves the ribs in relation to the vertebral column and sternum so that the volume of the thoracic cavity is increased, and the pressure within the cavity is diminished.

The **diaphragm** is concave towards the abdominal cavity and convex towards the thoracic cavity. Thus when this muscle contracts it reduces intrathoracic pressure and increases intra-abdominal pressure. Intrathoracic pressure can be raised only indirectly, by contracting the abdominal muscles and relaxing the diaphragm. The raised intra-abdominal pressure then displaces the diaphragm upwards and, by reducing the volume of the thoracic cavity, increases the pressure within it.

GENERAL ORGANIZATION OF THE BODY WALL

Developmentally the organization of the body wall is essentially segmental and, although in the adult this early pattern is partially obscured, much of the region still consists of a series of segments or zones, each of which contains similar structures. Thus each successive segment contains a vertebra, a costal or rib element in one form or another, a spinal nerve and a sympathetic ganglion, a somatic or body wall artery and a somatic vein.

Vertebral column

The vertebral column, which consists of the vertebrae and the joints and ligaments uniting these bones to one another, contains the spinal cord and its meninges within the vertebral canal. Each vertebra is thus a ring of bone surrounding a vertebral foramen which may be regarded as one segment of the vertebral canal (figs. 21.2 and 21.3).

The anterior part of the ring, the **body,** is roughly cylindrical, with more or less flat upper and lower surfaces. The posterior part of the ring, the **vertebral arch,** consists of paired **pedicles** and **laminae.** The pedicles are

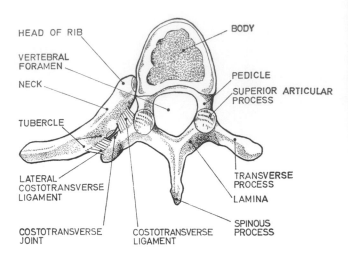

FIG. 21.2. Thoracic vertebra and rib seen from above.

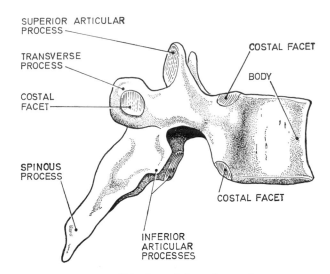

FIG. 21.3. Side view of thoracic vertebra.

continuous in front with the upper part of the posterior surface of the body. Behind they are continuous with the laminae which extend backwards and medially to fuse posteriorly. The **spinous process** projects backwards in the median plane from the junction of the laminae. Three additional processes project from the junction between each pedicle and lamina. The **transverse process** extends laterally; the **superior articular process** extends upwards and carries an articular facet on its posterior surface, and the **inferior articular process** extends downwards and has an articular facet on its anterior surface.

The vertebral column may be divided conveniently into five zones in which the individual vertebrae exhibit characteristic features. The seven cervical, the twelve thoracic and the five lumbar vertebrae are associated with the neck, the thorax and the abdomen proper, respectively. In the pelvic cavity and perineum, five sacral vertebrae are fused to form the single **sacrum** and three or four small and incomplete vertebrae are described collectively as the **coccyx.**

INTERVERTEBRAL JOINTS

The **intervertebral disc** (figs. 21.4 and 21.5) is a unique type of secondary cartilaginous joint which lies between

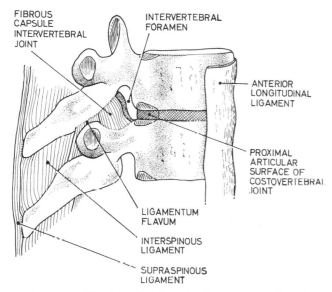

FIG. 21.4. Side view of articulation between two thoracic vertebrae.

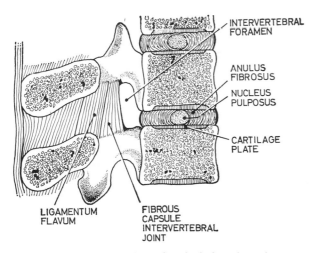

FIG. 21.5. Median section of articulating thoracic vertebrae.

adjacent vertebral bodies. The adjacent bony surfaces each present a central plate of avascular hyaline cartilage surrounded by a raised rim of bone. The peripheral parts of these surfaces are united by the **anulus fibrosus,** which consists of concentric layers of dense collagenous connective tissue in which the fibres follow oblique circular

courses from one bone to another. The region within the anulus fibrosus and between the cartilage plates is occupied by the **nucleus pulposus.** In the newborn this is a gelatinous material containing a high concentration of mucopolysaccharides; it is traversed by fine collagen fibres and contains groups of very large vesiculated cells which are derived from the notochord. In infancy and childhood the cells disappear, and throughout life the rigidity of the tissue progressively increases owing to an increase in its collagen.

This joint permits small degrees of angulation and rotation between adjacent vertebral bodies. At the same time the anulus fibrosus elastically resists these movements, so that, when the moving force ceases, the bones tend to recoil to a neutral position. The elasticity of the anulus and nucleus pulposus also absorbs a large part of the strain energy created by sudden stresses acting along the vertebral column. If these stresses are greater than the elastic limit of either the anulus or the cartilage plates, these tissues may rupture and allow herniation of the nucleus pulposus either backwards, where it may encroach upon the intervertebral foramen (figs. 21.4 and 21.5) or into the spongy bone of the vertebral body above or below.

The common accessory ligaments of all the intervertebral discs are the **anterior** and **posterior longitudinal ligaments.** The anterior ligament (fig. 21.4) is a broad band which covers, and is attached to, the anterior aspects of the vertebrae and intervertebral discs. The posterior ligament (fig. 21.6) lies on the anterior wall of the verte-

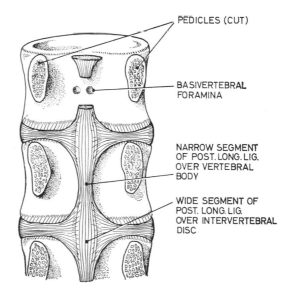

FIG. 21.6. The anterior wall of the vertebral canal.

bral canal. It is broad over the posterior aspects of the intervertebral discs to which it is very firmly attached; between the discs it is a narrow band which is quite separate from the posterior surfaces of the vertebral bodies. Both ligaments end at the upper border of the sacrum because below this level the sacral vertebrae are fused.

The **intervertebral joints** (figs. 21.4 and 21.5) are small paired synovial joints between the apposed articular facets on the superior and inferior articular processes of adjacent vertebrae; each is lined by synovial membrane and surrounded by a simple fibrous capsule. The shape and orientation of these joints dictate the kind and range of movement which can occur between vertebrae. The accessory ligaments of the intervertebral joints are the **ligamenta flava**, and the **interspinous** and **supraspinous ligaments** (figs. 21.4 and 21.5). The ligamenta flava are paired ligaments containing a high proportion of elastic fibres. Each pair joins the adjacent laminae of the articulating vertebrae. Behind they fuse and become continuous with the interspinous ligament, while in front each fuses with the fibrous capsule of the corresponding intervertebral joint. Adjacent spinous processes are joined by a mass of collagenous tissue; between these processes this forms the interspinous ligaments, whereas the tissue surmounting the tips of the processes is called the supraspinous ligament.

The **intervertebral foramina** (figs. 21.4 and 21.5) are paired gaps in the wall of the vertebral canal between each adjacent pair of vertebrae. They allow spinal nerves

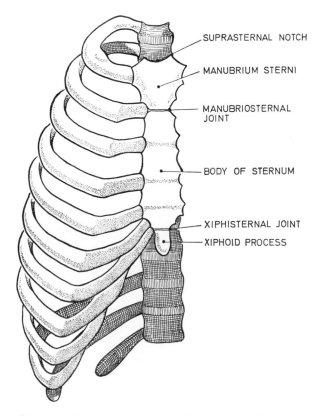

SUPRASTERNAL NOTCH

MANUBRIUM STERNI

MANUBRIOSTERNAL JOINT

BODY OF STERNUM

XIPHISTERNAL JOINT
XIPHOID PROCESS

FIG 21.7. The thoracic skeleton. The costal cartilages are stippled.

and veins to leave the canal and spinal arteries to enter it. In the sacral region their form is modified by the fusion of the vertebra to one another, but in the thoracic and lumbar regions all have the same general form. Here each foramen is bounded above and below by a pedicle, behind by an intervertebral joint, and in front by the upper vertebral body and an intervertebral disc. The foramina are only slightly larger than the structures which traverse them, so any narrowing of the foramina causes compression of these structures.

Ribs

A costal element is associated developmentally with each vertebra but the extent to which this element develops and its eventual fate vary greatly in different regions.

In the cervical region, the costal element is incorporated in the 'transverse process' (fig. 21.25c) and is usually small. When abnormally long it forms a cervical rib.

In the thoracic region, because of the need to produce negative intrathoracic pressures, the costal elements develop as twelve separate ribs each of which is continued anteriorly as a costal cartilage (fig. 21.7). Posteriorly each articulates with one or two adjacent vertebral bodies at the **costovertebral joints**, and the upper ten articulate with the corresponding transverse processes at the **costotransverse joints** (figs. 21.2 and 21.8). The upper seven ribs extend round the body wall and their costal cartilages articulate anteriorly with the sternum at the **sternocostal joints**. The lower five, sometimes known as false ribs, become progressively shorter and their costal cartilages end either as free extremities or by articulation with the costal cartilages immediately above at the **interchondral joints** (fig. 21.7). Because of the presence of the ribs, the segmental nature of the body wall is very evident in the thorax, and each **intercostal space** contains three intercostal muscles, an intercostal nerve, intercostal arteries and intercostal veins.

In the lumbar region the costal elements remain small and do not survive as separate bones. They become fused with the developing transverse processes so that an adult lumbar transverse process consists of a true transverse element and a costal element. As a result the segmentation of the body wall is less obvious in the lumbar than in the thoracic region.

Similarly in the sacral region the transverse and costal elements fuse to form the lateral part of the sacrum (fig. 21.25d).

Spinal nerves

The spinal nerves emerge from the vertebral canal into the tissues of the body wall through intervertebral foramina. The relationships they bear to their corresponding vertebrae are described on p. 20.12.

Immediately beyond the intervertebral foramen each

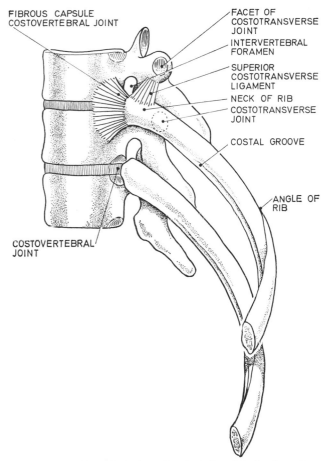

FIG. 21.8. The articulation of typical ribs with the thoracic vertebral column. Refer to figs. 21.3 and 21.4.

spinal nerve divides into **ventral** and **dorsal primary rami**, of which the dorsal is usually the smaller (fig. 21.9). The

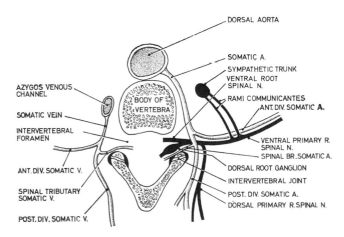

FIG. 21.9. Schematic diagram of the relationship of the main vessels and nerves of the trunk to the vertebral column.

dorsal primary rami turn backwards around the corresponding intervertebral joints, and, dividing into medial

and lateral branches, supply the postvertebral group of muscles and segmental strips of skin on the posterior aspect of the trunk. Each ventral primary ramus (VPR) passes laterally and its subsequent distribution depends on the extent of its association with the limbs. The VPR of T3–T12, which have no association with the limbs, extend round the body wall lying in the corresponding intercostal spaces (fig. 21.29). The other thoracic, lumbar and sacral VPR contribute in varying measure to the innervation of the body wall. Additionally, and in some cases predominantly, they contribute to the nerve plexuses which lie lateral to the cervical, lumbar, sacral and coccygeal parts of the vertebral column; from these plexuses, nerves carrying fibres from more than one spinal segment are distributed to the tissues of the upper and lower limbs.

Sympathetic trunk

Although its position varies in different regions of the body, in general the sympathetic trunk lies anterolateral to the vertebral bodies along the whole length of the vertebral column, and consequently anterior to the spinal nerves as they emerge from the intervertebral foramina (figs. 21.9, 21.27 and p. 20.12).

The VPR of T1–L2 or 3 are connected to the corresponding sympathetic ganglia by white rami communicantes (figs. 20.5 and 21.9). These are composed predominantly of the axons of the preganglionic cells in the lateral horn of the spinal grey matter and represent the entire outflow of sympathetic fibres from the central nervous system. Many of these fibres synapse with cells in the sympathetic ganglion which they reach first; others pass upwards or downwards along the trunk to synapse in the cervical, lower lumbar or sacral ganglia which have no white rami and therefore no direct supply of preganglionic fibres; some pass directly into the visceral branches of the sympathetic trunk to synapse in one of the prevertebral autonomic plexuses (fig. 21.50).

In contrast to the narrow inflow of fibres to the sympathetic trunk through the T1–L3 segments, postganglionic fibres leave all the ganglia of the trunk and pass through grey rami communicantes to the VPR of all the spinal nerves (figs. 20.5 and 21.9). Thereafter they are distributed through both the ventral and dorsal primary rami of these nerves to blood vessels, sweat glands and hair follicles.

Thus the VPR of T1–L3 are connected with the sympathetic trunk by both white and grey rami communicantes. All other spinal nerves are connected with the sympathetic trunk by grey rami only.

Somatic arteries

The **dorsal aorta** extends along the posterior wall of the trunk from T4–L4 where it divides into two **common**

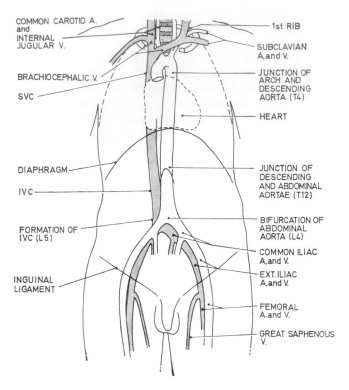

COMMON CAROTID A.
and
INTERNAL
JUGULAR V.

1st RIB

SUBCLAVIAN
A.and V.

BRACHIOCEPHALIC V.

JUNCTION OF
ARCH AND
DESCENDING
AORTA (T4)

SVC

HEART

DIAPHRAGM

JUNCTION OF
DESCENDING
AND ABDOMINAL
AORTAE (T12)

IVC

FORMATION OF
IVC (L5)

BIFURCATION OF
ABDOMINAL
AORTA (L4)

COMMON ILIAC
A.and V.

EXT. ILIAC
A.and V.

INGUINAL
LIGAMENT

FEMORAL
A.and V.

GREAT SAPHENOUS
V.

FIG. 21.10. The large arteries and veins of the trunk.

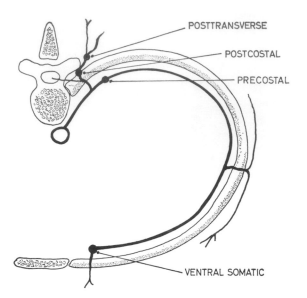

POSTTRANSVERSE

POSTCOSTAL

PRECOSTAL

VENTRAL SOMATIC

FIG. 21.11. The sites of longitudinal anastomoses between the somatic arteries.

iliac arteries (fig. 21.10). Each common iliac artery subsequently divides into an **external iliac artery** to the lower limb and an **internal iliac artery** to the pelvic cavity and perineum. The aorta lies more or less on the anterior aspect of the vertebral column and anterior to the sympathetic trunk and the spinal nerves. From the postero-lateral aspects of the aorta, somatic branches arise at regular intervals (fig. 21.9), and passing laterally and backwards behind the sympathetic trunk, become associated with the spinal nerves from T3–L4 just lateral to the intervertebral foramina. Here they divide into anterior and posterior branches which thereafter run in close association with the ventral and dorsal primary rami of the corresponding nerve. Each posterior branch gives off, in addition, a spinal branch which traverses the corresponding intervertebral foramen and takes part in the formation of the arterial plexuses which lie in the extradural space and on the surface of the spinal cord.

In early development the branches of these somatic arteries are linked by a series of longitudinal anastomotic channels (fig. 21.11). The anterior branches are joined by the precostal anastomosis in front of the posterior ends of the ribs or costal elements, and by the ventral somatic anastomosis in the anterior part of the body wall. The dorsal branches are joined by the postcostal and post-transverse anastomoses which lie in front of and behind the transverse processes respectively.

Beyond the region T3–L4 the somatic arteries are not derived directly from the dorsal aorta. Above, the somatic arteries are derived from subclavian arteries (fig. 21.10) which are arterial trunks to the upper limbs. Below they arise from the external and internal iliac arteries.

Somatic veins

In the region T3–L4 the somatic veins follow courses similar to those of the corresponding arteries. Like the arteries they are linked together in the anterior part of the body wall by a ventral somatic anastomotic channel, and each receives a spinal tributary, through the intervertebral foramen from the venous plexuses in the spinal extradural space.

The veins end in a series of longitudinal venous channels which lie lateral to the vertebral bodies (figs. 21.9 and 21.27) and drain upwards to end in the **superior vena cava** (SVC) (fig. 21.10) in the upper part of the thoracic cavity. Collectively these longitudinal channels constitute the **azygos system of veins**.

Above T3 the somatic veins drain into the **brachiocephalic veins** (fig. 21.10) which receive the venous blood from the upper limbs and head and neck and are tributaries of the SVC. Below L4 they drain predominantly into the external and internal iliac veins which are tributaries of the **inferior vena cava** (IVC) (fig. 21.10).

Body wall as a whole

Between T3 and the middle lumbar region the arrangement of the nerves, arteries and veins of the body wall is strictly segmental. However, above and below this region the simple segmental arrangement is less evident, due to the development of the upper and lower limbs.

SKELETON OF THE TRUNK

THORACIC SKELETON

The thoracic skeleton or cage surrounds and partially encloses the thoracic cavity. In the coronal plane its shape is parabolic (fig. 21.7), while in the transverse plane it is reniform, the anterior wall being convex and the posterior concave (fig. 21.33).

The anterior wall is comparatively short and is formed by the sternum (fig. 21.7). The longer posterior wall extends above and below the limits of the sternum and is composed of all the thoracic vertebrae (fig. 21.1). The lateral walls consist of the ribs and costal cartilages separated from one another by the intercostal spaces (fig. 21.7).

Below, the thoracic cavity is separated from the abdomen by the dome of the diaphragm. Above it is directly continuous with the tissues of the neck. The oblique plane of this continuity is surrounded by the first ribs and costal cartilages, the first thoracic vertebra and the upper border of the sternum, and is conveniently described as the **thoracic inlet** (fig. 22.35).

Thoracic vertebrae

In this region of the vertebral column the intervertebral discs have the same depth anteriorly and posteriorly; but the vertebral bodies are slightly deeper behind than in front, and consequently, the column is concave forwards. The twelve thoracic vertebrae increase gradually in size from above down. The upper nine are all similar whereas the lower three are atypical in certain respects.

In a typical vertebra (figs. 21.2 and 21.3), the body is roughly cylindrical, the vertebral foramen is small and circular, and the spine is long and directed downwards and backwards. The facets on the superior articular processes are flat and face backwards, upwards and a little laterally, while the similar inferior articular facets face in the opposite directions. The transverse process is directed laterally and somewhat backwards. Each side of the vertebra carries three small costal articular facets. Two of these lie on the posterolateral aspect of the body and abut against the upper and lower surfaces, while the third lies near the lateral end of the transverse process.

In the atypical thoracic vertebrae, the lower costal facets are absent on the bodies of T10, T11 and T12, and the upper costal facets are displaced backwards on to the pedicles; the costal facets are absent from the transverse processes of T11 and T12, and the inferior articular processes of T12 resemble the lumbar processes with which they articulate (fig 21.13).

Sternum

This is a flat bone, in the anterior thoracic wall (fig. 21.7). In the adult it consists of three parts named,

from above down, the **manubrium, body** and **xiphoid process**. The manubrium and body articulate at the secondary cartilaginous **manubriosternal joint**, and the body and xiphoid process at the similar **xiphisternal joint**.

The manubrium extends downwards and forwards, and its transverse diameter is greater above than below. Its upper border is marked by the wide **jugular (suprasternal) notch**, and on either side of this by a concave cartilage-covered facet for articulation with the medial end of the clavicle. Its shorter lower border articulates with the body. The forward inclination of the body is less than that of the manubrium, and the two parts thus make a very obtuse angle open backwards. The slight ridge formed by this **sternal angle** can be readily felt through the skin and is an important landmark. The body increases in width from above down throughout its upper three-quarters and subsequently becomes narrower as far as its lower end. The shape of the xiphoid process varies considerably, but usually it is roughly triangular. The lateral borders of the manubrium, body and xiphoid process articulate in various ways with the costal cartilages of the upper seven ribs.

Ribs

The twelve pairs of ribs are long curved flat bones. Each articulates posteriorly with the vertebral column and thereafter extends forwards and downwards round the chest wall before becoming continuous with a costal cartilage. The ribs become progressively longer from 1–7 and then shorter from 7–12.

The posterior end of each rib (fig. 21.8), is called the **head**, the adjacent 2 cm the **neck**, and the rest is described as the **shaft**. Neck and shaft are separated by the **tubercle** on the posterior aspect. Ribs 1, 11 and 12 exhibit features which are atypical of the series, whereas the others are very similar.

The head of a **typical rib** carries upper and lower articular facets separated by a horizontal non-articular zone. The lower facet on the rib head articulates with the upper costal facet on the numerically corresponding vertebral body, and the upper facet on the rib head with the lower costal facet on the vertebral body immediately above (fig. 21.8). This **costovertebral joint** is enclosed by an articular capsule and its synovial cavity is divided into two compartments by an intra-articular ligament which extends from the non-articular zone on the rib head to the adjacent intervertebral disc. The neck of a typical rib (figs. 21.2 and 21.8) extends laterally and backwards, anterior to the numerically corresponding transverse process. At its lateral end, a small cartilage-covered facet on the lower medial part of the tubercle articulates with the costal facet on the transverse process at the **costotransverse joint**. In the upper part of the series the costal facet lies on the anterior aspect of the transverse process and the plane of the costotransverse joint is concave forwards. On the other hand the costal facets associated with ribs 8, 9 and 10 lie on the upper surfaces of the transverse process and the plane of the joint is flat and nearly horizontal. Each costotransverse joint is enclosed by an articular capsule and is associated with a number of accessory ligaments. Two costotransverse ligaments join the neck and the tubercle of the rib to the corresponding transverse process on either side of the joint (fig. 21.2), and the **superior costotransverse ligament** is a broad sheet which extends from each rib neck to the transverse process immediately above it (fig. 21.8). The shaft of a typical rib has inner and outer surfaces, and upper and lower borders, and the lowest part of the inner surface is marked in its posterior two-thirds by the **costal groove** (fig. 21.8). From the tubercle the shaft first extends laterally, more or less in line with the neck, but it then turns, quite abruptly, into the curvature of the chest wall. This sharp bend is called the **angle** of the rib shaft, and its distance from the tubercle is proportional to the length of the whole rib.

The head of the **first rib** carries one facet and the costovertebral joint which it forms with the upper costal facet on the first thoracic vertebral body has a single synovial cavity. The neck is not associated with a superior costotransverse ligament. The angle coincides with the tubercle and the shaft subsequently follows an acute and even curvature, downwards and forwards round the thoracic inlet (fig. 21.7). Its surfaces face upwards and downwards so that its borders are described as inner and outer. There is no costal groove on the lower surface, but the upper surface carries a number of features associated with structures in the neck and upper limb (fig. 22.24).

The heads of the **eleventh** and **twelfth ribs**, carry one facet, which articulates with the single costal facet on the body and pedicle of the corresponding vertebra. There are no tubercles and no costotransverse joints. Both ribs are short and the twelfth is usually confined to the posterior wall of the trunk.

Costal cartilages

The distal end of each rib shaft is fused to the corresponding costal cartilage which thereafter continues round the chest wall (fig. 21.7). These bars of hyaline cartilage vary in length in the same way as the ribs, increasing in length from the first to the seventh and decreasing from the seventh to the twelfth rib. The first costal cartilage is fused to the lateral angle of the manubrium of the sternum and thus forms a primary cartilaginous joint between that bone and the first rib, unlike the other sternocostal joints, which are synovial. The first sternocostal joint is also unusual in being the only primary cartilaginous joint to persist into adult life; all others lie between centres of ossification, which fuse when growth

ceases. The second cartilage extends horizontally and articulates by a synovial **sternocostal joint** with twin facets on the adjacent parts of the lateral margins of the manubrium and body of the sternum. The cavity of the joint is split into two compartments by an intra-articular ligament which is continuous with the manubriosternal joint. The cartilages from the third to the seventh extend upwards and medially, the upward obliquity increasing progressively from above down. The third to the sixth articulate with the lateral margin of the body of the sternum at synovial sternocostal joints. The seventh costal cartilage articulates with the body and xiphoid process. All the sternocostal joints tend to degenerate in old age, the costal cartilage becoming continuous with the sternum, either directly or through a zone of fibrous tissue. The eighth, ninth and tenth costal cartilages also turn upwards and medially, but, becoming progressively shorter from above down, they end, short of the sternum, by articulating with the costal cartilage immediately above at the synovial **interchondral joints**. The eleventh and twelfth cartilages are very short and pointed, and they end freely, without articulation, in the lateral part of the body wall.

MOVEMENTS AT THE JOINTS OF THE THORACIC SKELETON

Vertebral movement

Changes in the form of the vertebral column are the result of small displacements of adjacent vertebrae upon one another, and although individual displacements are small, in summation their effect may be considerable. Intervertebral movement is essentially an elastic distortion of the intervertebral disc, controlled and limited by the intervertebral joints and intervertebral ligaments. Consequently the extent of movement is proportional to the moving force and when this force ceases the displaced bones recoil to their neutral relationship.

Although intervertebral movement can occur in any direction as at a synovial ball and socket joint, it is convenient to regard any particular movement as being a combination of certain cardinal movements. Thus flexion and extension describe angulations forwards and backwards by the vertebrae in the sagittal plane. Lateral flexion is angulation in either direction in the coronal plane, and rotation is a twisting of one vertebra on its neighbour about a vertical axis through the intervertebral disc.

In the thoracic region flexion, extension and lateral flexion are all somewhat limited in range by the presence of the rib cage. On the other hand rotation is comparatively free because the curvatures of the facets of the intervertebral joints form arcs of a circle which is concentric with the intervertebral disc.

Movements of the ribs and costal cartilages

In the upper seven or true ribs, the rib head lies higher than the anterior end of the corresponding costal cartilage, and the most lateral part of the rib shaft lies below the plane which traverses these two points. Movements of these ribs on the vertebral column may be regarded as occurring simultaneously about two axes of rotation. One axis extends from the costovertebral joint to the centre of curvature of the facets of the costotransverse joint; because of the obliquity of the rib, movement upwards round this axis displaces the costal cartilage and the related part of the sternum upwards and forwards (fig. 21.12a). The other axis traverses the costotransverse and sternocostal joints; elevation of the rib round this axis causes the lateral part of the shaft to move upwards and laterally (the so-called bucket handle movement) while the rib head is displaced very slightly downwards (fig. 21.12b).

Rotation of the eighth, ninth and tenth ribs at the costotransverse joint around either a transverse or an anteroposterior axis is largely prevented by the plane form and almost horizontal disposition of the articular surfaces. On the other hand, the costal cartilage is free to move laterally because of its lack of attachment to the sternum. Consequently, movement is restricted to rotation of the rib about a vertical axis traversing the costovertebral joint, such that the rib tubercle slides backwards or forwards on the upper surface of the transverse process and

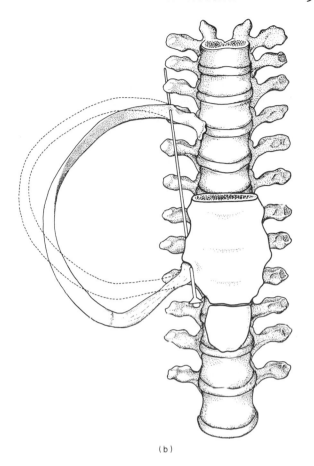

(b)

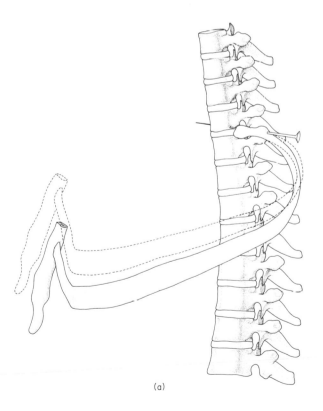

(a)

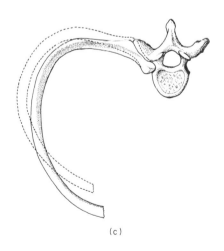

(c)

FIG. 21.12. Movements of the ribs (a) lateral view showing increase of anteroposterior thoracic diameter by true ribs (1–7) during inspiration; (b) anterior view showing increase of transverse thoracic diameter by true ribs during inspiration; (c) increase of transverse thoracic diameter by lower ribs during inspiration. The pin in (a) and (b) represents the axis of rotation in each movement.

the costal cartilage is carried laterally or medially (fig. 21.12c). In simultaneous lateral movement of the three ribs, the relationship of their anterior ends at the interchondral joints remains unchanged, but the eighth costal cartilage tends to move on to a more lateral and therefore a lower part of the seventh (fig. 21.7). The downward displacement of the eighth rib, which would thus be expected, does not occur, for in practice, lateral displacement of the eighth, ninth and tenth ribs is always associated with upward displacement of the upper seven.

The eleventh and twelfth ribs articulate with the rest of the thoracic skeleton at costovertebral joints only, and are consequently capable of small movements in any direction. This mobility is of little value.

Sternal movements

Movements between the segments of the sternum at the manubriosternal and xiphisternal joints are restricted to small angulations of one segment on another in the sagittal plane, and are always secondary to movements of the upper seven ribs.

Respiratory movements of the thoracic skeleton

Inspiration depends on an increase in the volume of the thoracic cavity by increase of one or more of its three diameters, vertical, anteroposterior and transverse. As a result air is sucked into the lungs and, incidentally, venous blood and lymph are drawn into the thoracic vessels from surrounding parts.

The vertical diameter is increased in small part by straightening of the normal concavity of the thoracic vertebral column, but predominantly by contraction of the diaphragm downwards towards the abdominal cavity. The efficiency of diaphragmatic contraction is dependent both on the stability of the ribs from which it arises and on the accommodation of the abdominal viscera which are displaced by its downward movement. Stability of the diaphragmatic origin is achieved by fixation of the eleventh and twelfth ribs by the posterior abdominal muscles and by the natural restriction of movement, in the eighth, ninth and tenth ribs to a transverse plane (see above). Accommodation for the displaced abdominal viscera is found in part by relaxation of the anterior abdominal muscles, and in part by an increase in the transverse diameter of the upper part of the abdominal cavity resulting from a passive lateral displacement of the eighth, ninth and tenth ribs by the pressure of the displaced abdominal viscera. This passive lateral displacement of the lower ribs increases the transverse diameter of the lower thorax as well as that of the upper abdomen. When the dome of the diaphragm is brought to a halt by the pressure of the abdominal contents, the costal fibres of the diaphragm act from the fixed central tendon and elevate the lower ribs.

It has just been noted that diaphragmatic contraction results both indirectly and directly in an increase in the transverse diameter of the lower part of the thorax. The transverse and anteroposterior diameters of the rest of the thorax are increased by elevation of the upper seven ribs by muscles in the thoracic wall and neck. Each rib is moved simultaneously about its transverse and anteroposterior axes and the resulting forward displacement of the costal cartilages and sternum and the lateral displacement of the rib shafts increase the anteroposterior and transverse diameter respectively. It is evident that the magnitude of these increases is always proportional to the length of the rib concerned. It follows that the forward displacement of the body of the sternum is greater than that of the manubrium and that this disparity must be accommodated by a slight increase of the sternal angle.

At birth the ribs are almost horizontal and do not achieve their adult obliquity until about the seventh year. Thus during infancy, and to a lesser degree in childhood, inspiration depends almost entirely on diaphragmatic movement.

Expiration, in quiet respiration, is produced largely by the recoil of the elastic lung tissue. The additional force required in forced expiration, as in blowing a trumpet, is derived from contraction of the anterior abdominal muscles.

ABDOMINAL AND PERINEAL SKELETON

Lumbar vertebrae

In the adult, the lumbar part of the vertebral column, composed of the five lumbar vertebrae and the corresponding intervertebral articulations, is convex forwards. This convexity increases from above down and is more pronounced in the female than the male. It is due largely to the shape of the intervertebral discs, which are thicker in front than behind.

In this region the costal element is small and is incorporated into the definitive transverse process early in development; there are therefore no ribs and no costal facets on the vertebral bodies.

The lumbar vertebrae continue the progressive increase in size noted in the thoracic region. The bodies are wider in the coronal than in the sagittal plane, the vertebral foramina are triangular and larger than in the thoracic region, and the spines are rectangular and project horizontally backwards (figs. 21.13 and 21.14). The most characteristic feature is the orientation of the facets on the articular processes. The superior facets are concave and face medially and backwards, whereas the inferior are convex and face laterally and forwards. The upper four transverse processes are long, thin and

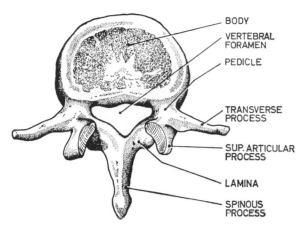

FIG. 21.13. Lumbar vertebra seen from above.

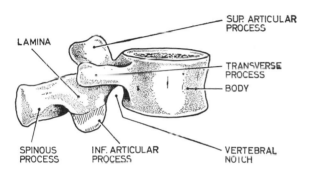

FIG. 21.14. Side view of lumbar vertebra.

These vertebrae possess two important peculiarities: short but comparatively massive costal elements are fused to the transverse processes, pedicles and bodies (fig. 21.15a); and the vertebral foramina of the fourth and

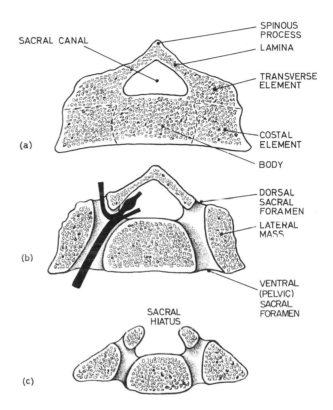

FIG. 21.15. Cross sections of sacrum: (a) through upper sacral segment, (b) between upper sacral segments, (c) between lower sacral segments.

spatulate, and their anterior surfaces are divided into medial and lateral halves by a vertical ridge. The fifth transverse process is conical and its base is continuous with the pedicle rather than with the junction between the pedicle and lamina.

The movements in the lumbar vertebral column are the same as those in the thoracic region but their individual extents are different. The range of flexion and extension is greater than in the thorax, partly because of the absence of the restricting influence of the ribs and sternum, and partly because the intervertebral discs are thicker and therefore more easily deformed. Extension is greater than flexion; flexion reduces the resting curvature and usually ends when the column is straight. Lateral flexion is also greater in the lumbar than in the thoracic region for the same reasons. On the other hand rotation is very limited in the lumbar column, because the facets on the articular processes are radial rather than circumferential to the axis of rotation which passes vertically through the intervertebral discs.

Sacrum

The adult sacrum is formed by the fusion of five sacral vertebrae which diminish in size from above down.

fifth vertebrae are incomplete posteriorly because of the absence of laminae and spines (figs. 21.15c and 21.17).

Fusion between the sacral vertebrae involves the whole of their adjacent surfaces except for that T-shaped zone on either side which is related to the corresponding spinal nerve and its ventral and dorsal primary rami (fig. 21.15b).

During fusion, the five vertebral foramina become continuous as the **sacral canal**, but the lower part of the posterior wall of this canal remains deficient at the **sacral hiatus**. From the sacral canal, four paired, T-shaped canals lead laterally through the regions originally occupied by the intervertebral foramina and subsequently open on to the pelvic and dorsal surfaces at the **ventral (pelvic)** and **dorsal sacral foramina**. Lateral to these foramina transverse and costal elements fuse completely to form the **lateral mass** (figs. 21.15b, 21.16 and 21.17).

The adult sacrum is triangular in form and presents a broad base above, a narrow blunt apex below, and pelvic, dorsal and lateral surfaces.

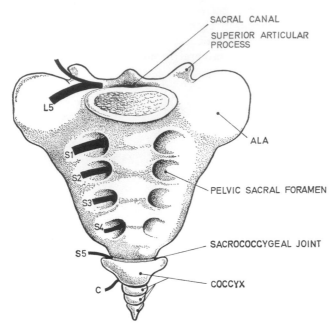

FIG. 21.16. Upper and pelvic surfaces of sacrum and coccyx. Ventral rami of the related nerves are shown in black.

On the **base** (figs. 21.16 and 21.17), the upper end of the sacral canal is surrounded by the upper aspects of the body and vertebral arch of the first sacral vertebra which resemble in form and attachments the corresponding surfaces of a lumbar vertebra. The body is surmounted by the lumbosacral intervertebral disc, the pedicles form the

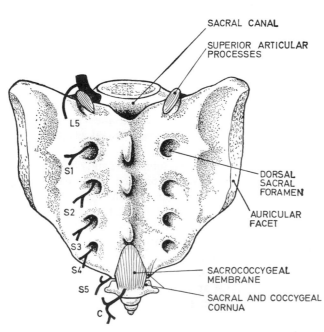

FIG. 21.17. Dorsal surface of sacrum and coccyx. The dorsal rami of the related nerves are shown in black.

lower margins of the fifth lumbar intervertebral foramina and the superior articular processes, the laminae and the spine are joined to the corresponding features on the fifth lumbar vertebra by intervertebral joints, ligamenta flava and an interspinous ligament. The smooth upper surface of the lateral mass extends laterally from the body, pedicle and articular process and is named the **ala**.

The **apex of the sacrum** is formed by the inferior surface of the fifth sacral vertebral body and is attached to the coccyx below by the sacrococcygeal intervertebral disc (fig. 21.16).

The **pelvic surface of the sacrum** (fig. 21.16) is smooth, concave in the sagittal plane and faces downwards and forwards towards the pelvic cavity (fig. 21.39). It exhibits two rows of four pelvic foramina, and each pair of foramina is joined across the midline by a ridge which demarcates two fused vertebral bodies. The upper border of the first sacral vertebral body forms a prominent ridge which lies just below the lumbosacral intervertebral disc and is named the **sacral promontory** (fig 21.22).

The **dorsal surface** (fig. 21.17) is rough, convex and faces upwards and backwards. It presents two rows of four dorsal foramina. The upper foramina are separated by a median row of tubercles which represent the spines of the fused vertebrae, while the lower foramina are separated by the sacral hiatus. The lowest parts of the lateral margins of the hiatus project downwards as two processes named the **sacral cornua.**

The **lateral surface** (fig. 21.18) is broad above where it is associated with the first three sacral vertebrae, but narrows to a mere border in its lower part. On the broad upper part, the dorsal third is rough whereas the pelvic two-thirds carry a large cartilage-covered facet for articulation with the ilium at the sacro-iliac joint. The facet is ear-shaped, the concave border being directed dorsally, and is consequently named the **auricular facet.**

Coccyx

The three or four vertebrae caudal to the sacrum are small and incomplete, and are more or less fused to form the coccyx (figs. 21.16 and 21.17). The lower two or three are mere nodules of bone, but the first consists of a body with small transverse processes and rudimentary superior articular processes, the coccygeal cornua.

The triangular coccyx is attached to the apex of the sacrum on which it is angulated forwards. The sacrococcygeal joint is formed, anteriorly, by a rudimentary intervertebral disc and posteriorly by the sacrococcygeal membrane which extends from the dorsal surface of the coccyx and its cornua, to the margins of the sacral hiatus and the sacral cornua. The intervals between these two elements represent intervertebral foramina and are traversed by the fifth sacral nerves. The tiny coccygeal nerves pierce the lowest part of the sacrococcygeal membrane and turn laterally below the coccygeal cornua.

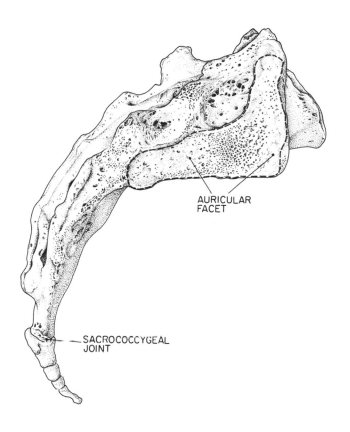

FIG. 21.18. Side view of sacrum and coccyx.

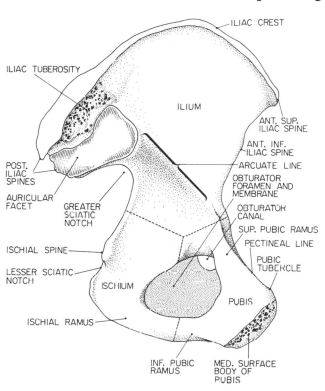

FIG. 21.19. Inner aspect of left hip bone.

Osteoligamentous pelvis

This is formed by the two hip bones, the sacrum and coccyx, and the ligaments which join these bones to one another (fig. 21.22). Anteriorly the hip bones articulate in the median plane at the symphysis pubis, and posteriorly each hip bone articulates with the upper part of the lateral surface of the sacrum at a sacro-iliac joint.

It is important to note that, despite its name, the osteoligamentous pelvis is not co-extensive with the pelvic cavity. It forms the side walls of both the pelvic cavity and the perineum and projects upwards into the posterolateral walls of the abdominal cavity proper.

HIP BONE

Each hip bone is ossified in cartilage from three primary centres of ossification (fig. 21.26) and the three regions of bone so formed are named the **ilium,** the **pubis** and the **ischium.** These remain separated by thin zones of cartilage until after puberty and, although thereafter they fuse to form the single hip bone, the corresponding regions of the adult bone retain their original names.

The general features of the inner and outer aspects of the hip bone, and the extents of its three component parts are shown in figs. 21.19 and 21.20.

The large oval aperture in the lower part of the bone

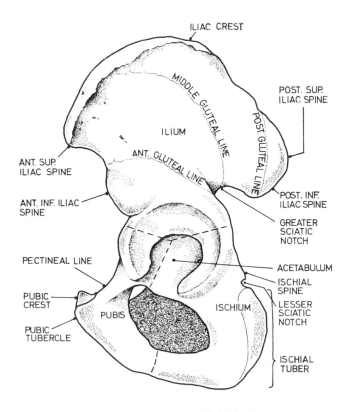

FIG. 21.20. Outer aspect of left hip bone.

is the **obturator foramen**. It is occupied by the fibrous **obturator membrane** except at its anterosuperior corner, where the pelvic cavity and the thigh communicate through the **obturator canal**.

The obturator foramen separates the pubis in front from the ischium behind. The body of the pubis lies in front of the foramen and articulates with its counterpart at the symphysis pubis. The **superior** and **inferior pubic rami** extend backwards from the body, above and below the foramen. Similarly, the comparatively thick body of the ischium lies behind the foramen and the single **ramus of the ischium** extends forwards below it. The lower boundary of the obturator foramen is thus formed by both the inferior pubic ramus and the ischial ramus, and so is called the **ischiopubic** or **conjoined ramus**.

The large cup-shaped hollow on the outer surface of the hip bone is the **acetabulum** which articulates with the head of the femur at the hip joint. It is contributed to by all three components of the hip bone, the superior pubic ramus forming its anterior part, the body of the ischium its posteroinferior part, and the ilium its posterosuperior part. The ilium forms the whole of the hip bone above the level of the acetabulum and its free upper margin is named the **iliac crest**.

Because the main function of the pelvis is the transmission of body weight, its orientations in sitting and in standing are important. In sitting, a coronal plane which passes through the anterior ends of the iliac crests traverses the acetabula. In standing, the upper part of the pelvis is farther forwards in relation to its lower part so that the anterior ends of the iliac crests and the upper border of the pubic symphysis all lie in the same coronal plane. In all descriptions of the pelvis, this is taken as the formal anatomical position.

PUBIS

The **body of the pubis** has a rough medial surface which is involved in the formation of the pubic symphysis, an outer surface which faces downwards, forwards and laterally towards the thigh, and an inner surface which faces upwards and backwards. Its upper border, the **pubic crest,** ends laterally in the distinct prominence of the **pubic tubercle**. The **superior pubic ramus** extends from the body, backwards, upwards and laterally to the anterior part of the acetabulum. A sharp ridge, the **pectineal line,** runs laterally along its upper aspect from the pubic tubercle. The **inferior pubic ramus** passes backwards, downwards and laterally, and the interval between the diverging inferior pubic rami in the articulated pelvis is described as the **subpubic angle**. The inner surface of this ramus, in the male, is usually divided by a faint ridge into upper vertical and lower everted zones.

ISCHIUM

The notable features of the **body of the ischium** lie along its posterior aspect. Below, and just behind the acetabulum, the **spine of the ischium** projects backwards and medially as a spatulate process with inner and outer surfaces. At the lower end of the body the massive, oval prominence of the **ischial tuber** faces backwards. Its surface is divided by two ridges into upper lateral, upper medial, lower medial and lower lateral quadrants. The ischial spine and tuber are separated by the smoothly rounded **lesser sciatic notch**. The inner surface of the ramus of the ischium is divided, as on the inferior pubic ramus, into upper and lower parts.

ILIUM

The **iliac crest,** S-shaped when seen from above (fig. 21.21), is the free upper border of the ilium. It ends anteriorly at

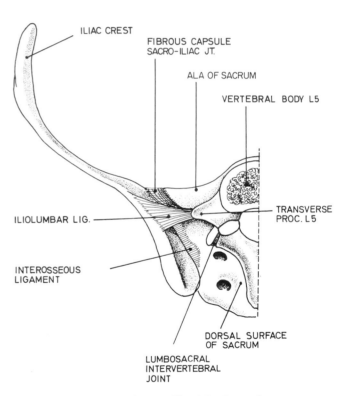

FIG. 21.21. Left sacro-iliac joint from above.

the **anterior superior iliac spine** and posteriorly at the **posterior superior iliac spine**. The anterior two-thirds is convex laterally and its outer aspect is expanded about 5 cm behind the anterior superior spine to form the tubercle of the crest. This is to be distinguished from the iliac tuberosity (see below). The posterior one-third is concave laterally and lies above and behind the dorsal surface of the sacrum.

The anterior border extends from the anterior superior iliac spine to the acetabulum and exhibits the blunt eminence of the **anterior inferior iliac spine** on its lower part. The posterior border runs from the posterior superior iliac spine to the acetabulum. Its lower part exhibits the deep and extensive **greater sciatic notch** with the **posterior inferior iliac spine** at its posterior and upper limit.

The outer surface of the ilium is demarcated from the posterior part of the iliac crest by the rough **posterior gluteal line** which diverges upwards and forwards from the greater sciatic notch. On the inner surface, the rough area of the **iliac tuberosity** separates the posterior part of the crest from the auricular surface which articulates with the sacrum. In front of these features the bone is smooth; it is crossed obliquely by the blunt ridge of the **arcuate line**, which runs from the auricular facet, downwards and forwards to the pectineal line of the pubis.

PELVIC JOINTS

The **pubic symphysis** is a secondary cartilaginous joint which lies in the median plane between the medial surfaces of the bodies of the pubic bones. Thin plates of hyaline cartilage cover the rough bone surfaces and are joined by a dense zone of fibrocartilage. The peripheral fibres of this zone extend directly on to the neighbouring aspects of the pubis while the central part of the zone frequently degenerates in middle life to form a cavity.

The **sacro-iliac joint** is a synovial joint between the auricular surfaces on the ilium and the upper two or three segments of the sacrum. Anterior to the joint is the upper part of the pelvic and lower part of the abdominal cavity while below it is the greater sciatic notch. Behind and above the joint the iliac crest and tuberosity overlap the dorsal surface of the sacrum, and the two bones are separated by a narrow deep crevice.

The plane of the joint is more or less vertical and extends backwards and medially at a small angle to the sagittal plane. In general, the articular surfaces are plane, but in detail they are covered by small reciprocal depressions and elevations. After middle age fibrous bands frequently join the articular surfaces to one another.

The joint cavity is surrounded and enclosed by a fibrous capsule which is attached to the adjoining surfaces of the ilium and the sacrum. In front and below, the capsule is thin, but behind it consists of an extremely thick mass of short fibres. These extend between the iliac tuberosity and the closely adjacent lateral surface of the sacrum and form the **interosseous ligament** (fig. 21.21).

The joint is additionally strengthened by four accessory ligaments. The **iliolumbar** and **lumbosacral ligaments** (fig. 21.21) have a common medial attachment to the conical transverse process of the fifth lumbar vertebra. The former extends laterally to the most anterior part of the iliac tuberosity whereas the latter turns downwards to blend with the fibrous capsule. The **sacrotuberous ligament** (fig. 21.22) arises from the greater part of the dorsal surfaces of the sacrum and coccyx and from the posterior border of the ilium above the greater sciatic

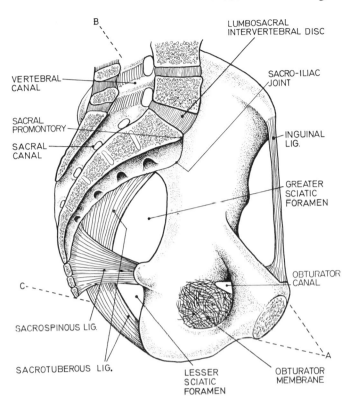

FIG. 21.22. Median section of osteoligamentous pelvis. Refer to fig. 21.19. AB and AC indicate planes of pelvic inlet and outlet in the erect posture. Details of the vertebral canal are given in fig. 21.5.

notch. The fibres extend downwards and laterally, converging rapidly as they go, and are attached to the medial edge of the ischial tuber. The **sacrospinous ligament** (fig. 21.22) is triangular. It has a broad attachment to the lateral aspects of the lower part of the sacrum and the coccyx, and extends laterally and forwards across the inner aspect of the sacrotuberous ligament to the spine of the ischium.

FORM AND FUNCTIONS OF THE VERTEBRAL COLUMN AS A WHOLE

Up to the time of birth and for some time afterwards, the shape of the vertebral column conforms to the wall of the uterine cavity and is slightly and uniformly concave forwards (fig. 21.23a). This **primary curvature** persists into adult life in the thoracic and sacrococcygeal regions. On the other hand the cervical curvature is obliterated and then replaced by an anterior convexity when the child begins to hold up its head, and a similar reversal occurs in the lumbar region when walking begins in the second year (fig. 21.23b). The formation of these **secondary curvatures** is largely due to changes in the intervertebral discs, which become thicker in front than behind. The cervical and

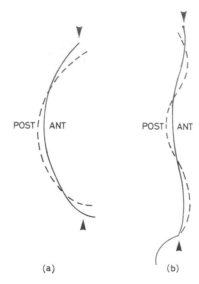

FIG. 21.23. The sagittal curvatures of the vertebral column: (a) in the infant, (b) in the adult. The interrupted lines indicate the changes in the curvatures produced by longitudinal forces.

lumbar convexities merge smoothly with the thoracic concavity, but the lumbar and sacral regions join at the abrupt **lumbosacral angle.** This is of the order of 140–150° and hence the lumbosacral intervertebral disc is wedge-shaped.

The vertebral column protects the spinal cord, permits movement between adjacent parts of the trunk and gives attachment to numerous muscles. It also supports the weight of the greater part of the body and transmits the weight across the sacro-iliac joints to the hip bones. In conformity with this function the vertebral bodies increase progressively in size from the skull to the level of the sacroiliac joints and thereafter they decrease rapidly. Similarly, the trabeculae of the spongy bone within the vertebral bodies are predominantly vertical and are larger and more numerous on the concave side, i.e. the compression side, of the relevant curvature. The readily deformable nature of the intervertebral discs under compressive stress combined with their elasticity allows the efficient absorption of the strain energy involved in sudden loading of the column. This strain energy is absorbed also by another mechanism. Any long column tends to bend under axial compression. General experience, from a superficial understanding of springs to the knowledge that it is advisable to land, after a jump, with bent rather than straight knees, tells us that strain energy is more efficiently absorbed in bending than in compression. It has already been noted that all intervertebral movement depends on distortion of intervertebral discs and is resisted elastically. Thus the strain energy of sudden loading can be absorbed by bending the vertebral column as well as by compression of the intervertebral discs. However, if the vertebral column were straight or uniformly curved, bending would distort the erect posture and the orientation of the head. The alternation of convex and concave regions through the length of the column allows bending under axial compression without disturbance of the erect posture (fig. 21.23b).

OSTEOLIGAMENTOUS PELVIS AS A WHOLE

It has been noted already that the osteoligamentous pelvis is not co-extensive with the pelvic cavity, but forms part of the boundaries of the abdominal cavity proper and of the perineum as well. The plane of continuity between the abdominal and pelvic cavities, which is called the **pelvic inlet,** extends upwards and backwards at an angle of about 50° to the horizontal (fig. 21.22). It is surrounded by a circular bony margin which is known as the **pelvic brim,** and consists of the sacral promontory, the alae of the sacrum, the arcuate lines, the pectineal lines, the pubic tubercles and crests, and the upper border of the pubic symphysis, in broad continuity with one another. The part of the osteoligamentous pelvis which lies above the pelvic brim is associated with the abdominal cavity proper and is consequently described as the **greater** (false) **pelvis,** while the part which lies below the brim is associated with the pelvic cavity and the perineum and is described as the **lesser** (true) **pelvis.** Thus the pelvic inlet is the entrance to the pelvic cavity from the abdominal cavity proper and is also the entrance into the lesser pelvis from the greater pelvis.

The lower margin of the true pelvis (figs. 21.22 and 21.41) is diamond-shaped and is formed by the inferior aspect of the pubic symphysis, the ischiopubic rami, the ischial tubers, the sacrotuberous ligaments and the coccyx. The **pelvic outlet** which is enclosed by this margin extends backwards and upwards at an angle of about 15° to the horizontal. Because the margin lies entirely in the perineum and indeed forms the boundaries of that region, the term pelvic outlet means the outlet from the true part of the osteoligamentous pelvis and not the outlet from the pelvic cavity. The two terms, pelvic inlet and pelvic outlet are important in obstetrical practice.

The cavity of the osteoligamentous true pelvis has three communications with neighbouring regions (fig. 21.22):

(1) the **obturator canal** leads into the medial part of the thigh.

(2) the aperture bounded by the greater sciatic notch, the spine of the ischium and the sacrotuberous and sacrospinous ligaments is named the **greater sciatic foramen,** and leads into the buttock.

(3) the aperture bounded by the ischial spine and tuber and the sacrospinous and sacrotuberous ligaments

is named the **lesser sciatic foramen**; it too leads into the buttock.

OSTEOLIGAMENTOUS PELVIS IN THE FEMALE

The shape of the true osteoligamentous pelvis tends to differ in the female and male subject, but it is important to note that the differences may be small. In the female the distances between the paired arcuate lines, ischial spines and ischial tubers are all greater, the sacrum is wider and shorter, and the sub-pubic angle is larger, approximating to a right angle. Furthermore the anterior concavity of the sacrum is mainly at its lower part, and the lumbosacral angle is more acute.

These differences mean that the female true pelvis is wider both anteroposteriorly and transversely, and is more cylindrical in form than funnel-shaped. The size and form of the female true pelvis can be assessed both radiographically and by vaginal examination, the more important diameters being:

(1) the distance from the back of the pubic symphysis to the sacral promontory, which is known as the obstetrical conjugate diameter and has an average value of about 11 cm,

(2) the transverse diameter of the inlet which has an average value of about 13·5 cm,

(3) the transverse distances between the ischial spines and the ischial tubers which have average values of 12·5 cm and 11·5 cm respectively.

Function of the osteoligamentous pelvis

Like other bones, those of the pelvis protect underlying structures and give attachment to muscles. However the main purpose of these bones is to transmit body weight from the vertebral column, either to the acetabula and so to the lower limbs in standing, or to the ischial tubers in sitting. Accordingly the zones within the hip bone through which these stresses are transmitted, namely the arcuate line of the ilium and the body of the ischium, are thicker and stronger than the rest of the bone. The sacro-iliac joint lies across both these lines of stress and also is a joint at which little purposeful movement is required. Consequently, like the fibrous joints of the skull and the small synovial joints in the middle part of the foot, the sacro-iliac joint is primarily a shock absorber. By virtue of the elastic deformability of its cartilaginous and collagenous tissues it absorbs a large part of the strain energy involved in stress transmission. During late pregnancy, its ligaments become more easily deformed and allow some joint movement which increases the capacity of the true pelvis; in all other circumstances its movements are of little importance. The efficiency of the joint depends on its stability and its ability to resist displacements which body weight tends to produce. This is

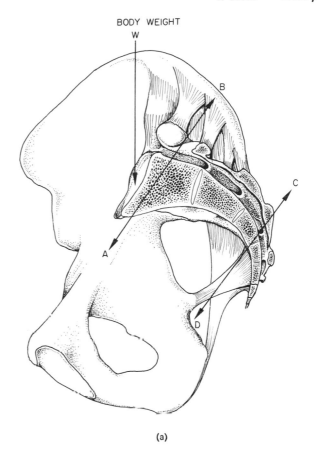

(a)

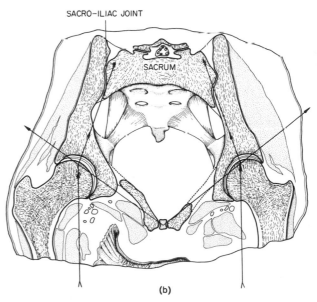

(b)

FIG. 21.24. (a) The effect of body weight at the sacro-iliac joint. Body weight, W, tends to displace upper end of sacrum forwards (arrow A); this is resisted by tension in posterior sacro-iliac ligament (arrow B). Backward displacement of lower end of sacrum (arrow C) is resisted by tension in sacrotuberous and sacrospinous ligaments (arrow D). (b) Frontal section through pelvis and hip joints showing direction of stresses operative during standing. (See text.)

achieved by the interlocking form of its articular surfaces and by the size and disposition of its ligaments. In standing, the tendency of body weight to drive the sacrum downwards in relation to the hip bones is restricted by the strong interosseous sacro-iliac ligaments, while the tendency to rotate the sacrum so that its posterior part moves backwards and upwards is controlled by the sacrotuberous and sacrospinous ligaments (fig. 21.24a). At the same time the upward pressure of the femoral head on the acetabulum is resolved into one component acting along the arcuate line towards the vertebral column, and another which tends to separate the hip bones from one another (fig. 21.24b). Actual separation is prevented by tensile stress in the pubic bones and the pubic symphysis which thus constitute a tie bar between the two acetabula.

The posture of the trunk affects the tilt of the pelvis. In standing, the angle of the brim of the pelvis is usually 50°–60° to the horizontal, and is determined by the postural pull of the abdominal, spinal and thigh muscles on the pelvis. Abnormal forward tilting of the pelvis is compensated by an increased lumbar curvature (**lordosis**). Similarly abnormal backward tilting is compensated by increasing the thoracic spinal curvature (**kyphosis**).

These abnormal postures are usually acquired during childhood and adolescence and frequently bring trouble in later life because of the excessive strain they throw on muscles and ligaments.

DEVELOPMENT OF THE SKELETON OF THE TRUNK

Each bone in the trunk is formed by ossification of a cartilage model.

VERTEBRAE

In all the **thoracic** and **lumbar vertebrae** the process of ossification is similar (fig. 21.25). Each half of the vertebral arch with the posterolateral corner of the vertebral body is ossified from a primary centre, while the rest of the body is ossified from a separate primary centre, the **centrum**. These primary centres appear about the eighth week of intrauterine life and at birth the ossified halves of the vertebral arch are still separated from one another and from the bone of the centrum by persistent zones of cartilage. The median zone is ossified during the first year and the two lateral zones during the fourth or fifth year. At this age cartilaginous epiphyses persist at the extremities of the transverse and spinous processes and on the upper and lower surfaces of the vertebral bodies. Secondary centres appear in these epiphyses about the sixteenth year. Those related to the upper and lower surfaces of the body are confined to anular peripheral

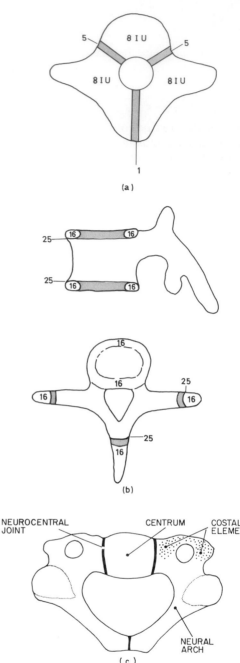

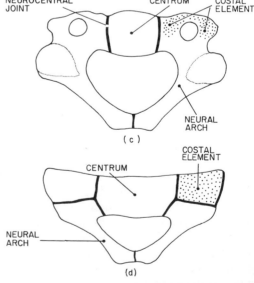

FIG. 21.25. Ossification of vertebrae, (a) at birth, (b) at about eighteen years. Numerals on the figures indicate age, in years, of appearance of ossification centre. Stippled areas are cartilaginous at birth. Leaders show time of fusion in years. I.U., age in weeks of intrauterine life. Compare with pattern in typical cervical vertebra (c) and upper sacrum (d).

zones. The secondary centres fuse with the primary at the twenty-fifth year. Thereafter the upper and lower surfaces of the vertebral body present a raised peripheral bony strip surrounding a thin central plate of persistent cartilage.

Each **sacral vertebra** is ossified from the same three primary centres as in the thoracolumbar region. In the upper three vertebrae, however, additional primary centres form in the anterior, or costal, region of the lateral mass. The primary centres appear rather later in the sacral than in the thoracic and lumbar vertebrae, between the twelfth and twenty-fourth intrauterine week.

By the ninth year the primary centres within each sacral vertebra have fused, but cartilaginous epiphyses persist on the upper and lower aspects of each body and on the lateral aspects of the lateral masses.

At puberty the hitherto separate sacral vertebrae fuse with one another except in the regions of the bodies. At about the same time secondary centres of ossification appear in the upper and lower parts of the lateral mass epiphyses, while anular secondary centres form in the upper and lower epiphyses of the bodies. These secondary centres fuse with the primary part of the sacrum at between twenty and twenty-five years of age, and it is only then, with the final fusion of the vertebral bodies, that the consolidation of the sacrum becomes complete.

Each piece of the **coccyx** is ossified from a single primary centre. The centres appear, from above down, between the ages of one and fifteen years.

HIP BONES

Three primary centres of ossification appear in the ilium in the ninth week, in the ischium in the third month and in the pubis in the fourth month of intrauterine life.

At birth, the ilium, ischium and pubis are separated, across the region of the acetabulum, by a Y-shaped, or triradiate, strip of cartilage, while the ischium and pubis are separated across the ischiopubic ramus by a second cartilaginous zone (fig. 21.26). Moreover the whole length of the iliac crest, the anterior inferior iliac spine and the ischial tuber consist of cartilaginous epiphyses.

At eight years the ischiopubic ramus is consolidated by fusion of the ischial ramus with the inferior pubic ramus, and at puberty secondary centres form in the three epiphyses and, as the os acetabuli, in the iliopubic part of the triradiate cartilage.

Obliteration of the triradiate cartilage occurs soon after puberty, but fusion of the other secondary centres with the primary part of the bone does not occur until between the twentieth and twenty-fifth years.

STERNUM

Early in development the sternum is represented by two separate and symmetrical cartilaginous **sternal plates** which fuse to form the cartilaginous sternum. One

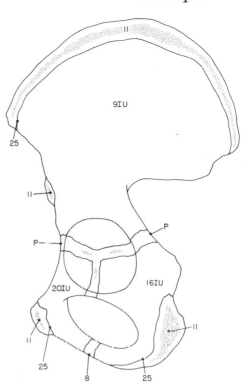

FIG. 21.26. Ossification of hip bone. Leaders show time of fusion in years. IU, age in weeks of intrauterine life. P, puberty.

primary centre of ossification appears in the future manubrium in the 24th week and four centres, one above the other, appear in the body between then and birth. The centre for the xiphoid process may appear at any time after the third year of life. The four centres in the body fuse between puberty and the twenty-fifth year. The manubriosternal and xiphisternal joints persist between the body and the manubrial and xiphoid centres.

RIBS

The primary centre of ossification in each rib appears near the angle about the eighth intrauterine week. The head, and the tubercles where they are present, are ossified from secondary centres which appear, much later than most centres of this kind, at or after the age of puberty. The primary and secondary centres fuse at about the twenty-fifth year.

Congenital abnormalities of the trunk skeleton

An appreciable proportion of the population exhibits variations in the number of vertebrae which have the characteristic features of the several regions of the vertebral column. Thus:

(1) a **cervical rib** may be associated with the seventh cervical vertebra or the first thoracic rib may be absent,

(2) a **lumbar rib** may be associated with the first lumbar vertebra or the twelfth thoracic rib may be absent,

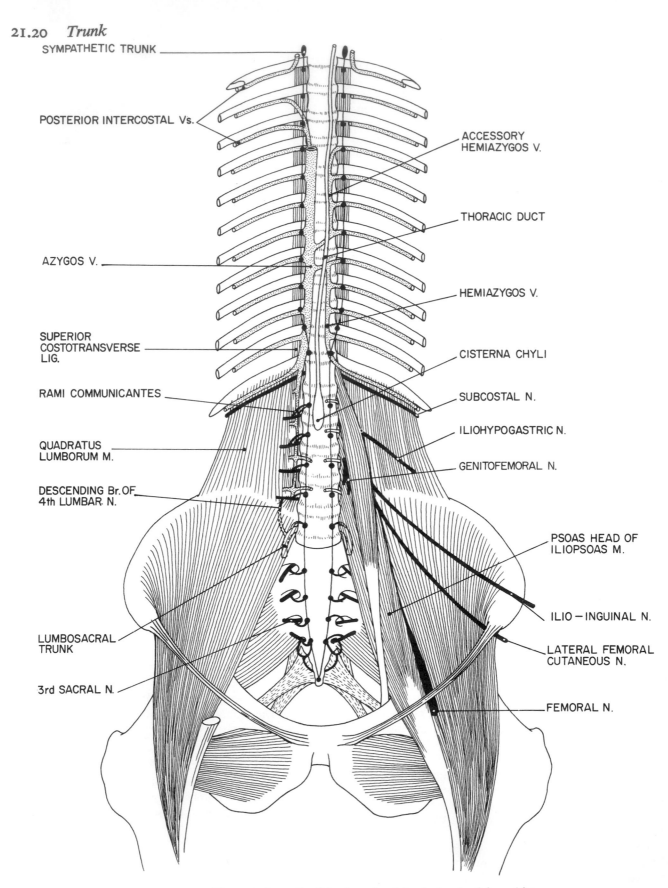

SYMPATHETIC TRUNK

POSTERIOR INTERCOSTAL Vs.

ACCESSORY
HEMIAZYGOS V.

THORACIC DUCT

AZYGOS V.

HEMIAZYGOS V.

SUPERIOR
COSTOTRANSVERSE
LIG.

CISTERNA CHYLI

RAMI COMMUNICANTES

SUBCOSTAL N.

ILIOHYPOGASTRIC N.

QUADRATUS
LUMBORUM M.

GENITOFEMORAL N.

DESCENDING Br. OF
4th LUMBAR N.

PSOAS HEAD OF
ILIOPSOAS M.

ILIO–INGUINAL N.

LATERAL FEMORAL
CUTANEOUS N.

LUMBOSACRAL
TRUNK

3rd SACRAL N.

FEMORAL N.

FIG. 21.27. The posterior walls of the thoracic, abdominal and pelvic cavities.

(3) the fifth lumbar vertebra may be partially or completely fused to the sacrum (**sacralization of the fifth lumbar**) or the first piece of the sacrum may persist as a separate vertebra (**lumbarization of the first sacral**) and

(4) the first piece of the coccyx may be incorporated into the sacrum.

In a smaller number of people, individual vertebrae are malformed. (1) One-half of a vertebra may fail to develop and the corresponding rib is usually absent. (2) In **spina bifida,** the two halves of the vertebral arch fail to fuse. Abnormalities of the sternum can usually be traced to incomplete fusion of the paired cartilaginous sternal plates. Therefore they tend to occur in the lower part of the sternum and take the form either of a central foramen in the body or of a complete division of the lower part of the body or the xiphoid into bilateral halves.

MUSCLES AND FASCIA OF THE TRUNK

These muscles fall naturally into three groups, first, those which are attached solely to the trunk skeleton, secondly those which arise from the trunk skeleton but are inserted into the bones of the lower limb and thirdly, several large superficial muscles which arise from the trunk skeleton and are inserted into the shoulder girdle and the humerus. In this chapter the first group and one member of the second (iliopsoas) are considered. These are conveniently divided, both functionally and topographically, into the pre- and postvertebral muscles, the diaphragm, and the anterolateral muscles of the thorax and abdomen. The muscles of the pelvis and perineum form a rather separate functional group and are considered on p. 21.30.

Postvertebral muscles of the trunk (sacrospinalis)

This group forms a massive band of muscle which, because it extends from the bony pelvis to the cervical region of the vertebral column, is conveniently described collectively as **sacrospinalis.** The group lies in a groove bounded medially by the vertebral spines and laminae and their associated ligaments, and in front by the transverse processes and by the ribs between the tubercles and angles (fig. 21.28). All the components of sacrospinalis share a common nerve supply from the dorsal primary rami of the spinal nerves.

The **superficial fibres of sacrospinalis** are predominantly vertical and comparatively long so that they extend over several vertebrae. They arise from the greater part of the dorsal surface of the sacrum, from the adjacent inner slope of the dorsal part of the iliac crest (p. 21.14), and from the lumbar and lower thoracic spines. Passing upwards they are attached, successively, to the spines of the thoracic vertebrae, the transverse processes of the

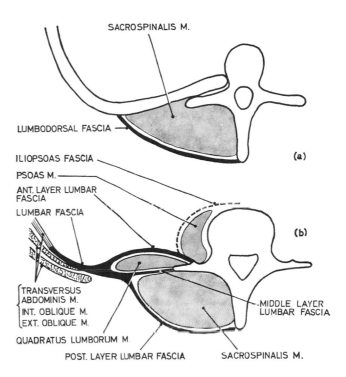

Fig. 21.28. The lumbodorsal fascia (a) in thoracic region, (b) in lumbar region.

lumbar and thoracic vertebrae, and the outer aspects of the ribs between the tubercles and angles.

The **deep fibres of sacrospinalis** are short and oblique, extending from below upwards and medially over one or two vertebrae. They arise from the posterior aspects of the lumbar and thoracic transverse processes and are inserted into the spines and laminae of higher vertebrae.

Prevertebral muscles of the trunk

Unlike the postvertebral group, these muscles are restricted to certain regions of the vertebral column. **Longus colli (cervicis)** lies in the cervical and upper thoracic regions, **iliopsoas** and **quadratus lumborum** are associated with the lumbar region.

Longus colli may be divided conveniently into three sets of fibres. The vertical set extends along the anterior aspects of the cervical and upper thoracic vertebral bodies; the superior oblique set extends, from the upper cervical transverse processes, upwards and medially to blend with the vertical fibres; and the inferior oblique set arises from the transverse processes of the lower cervical vertebrae except the seventh, and extends downwards and medially to join the vertical fibres. In the trunk itself, the vertical and inferior oblique fibres of longus colli extend downwards over the anterior aspects of the vertebral bodies as far as the fourth thoracic level (fig. 21.45a).

Iliopsoas arises in the lumbar region as separate psoas

and iliacus heads. The large, fusiform **psoas head** has multiple origins (1) from the medial halves of the anterior aspects of the upper four lumbar transverse processes (fig. 21.28), (2) from the lateral aspects of the upper four lumbar intervertebral discs and from the adjacent regions of the vertebral bodies (i.e. the highest and lowest fibres come from the twelfth thoracic and fifth lumbar bodies respectively) and (3) from four fibrous arches which extend across the concave anterolateral aspects of the upper four lumbar vertebral bodies (fig. 21.27).

The muscle passes downwards and laterally along the lateral aspects of the lumbar vertebral bodies, along the arcuate line of the ilium, and then across the superior pubic ramus, lateral to the pectineal line. Thereafter it passes beneath the inguinal ligament (p. 21.24) and enters the thigh (figs. 21.27 and 21.39).

Because of the discontinuous origin of the muscle, four separate spaces exist between the fibrous arches and the psoas muscle fibres on the one hand, and the upper four lumbar vertebral bodies on the other. These spaces form important neurovascular pathways from the prevertebral region, in front, to the intervertebral foramina behind (figs. 21.27 and 21.28).

The fan-shaped **iliacus head** arises from the inner surface of the ilium above the arcuate line. The fibres extend downwards and, converging towards the lateral aspect of the psoas head, pass with it beneath the inguinal ligament and into the thigh (figs. 21.27 and 21.39).

In the upper part of the thigh the two heads fuse to form the common tendon of iliopsoas which is inserted into the lesser trochanter of the femur.

Quadratus lumborum (figs. 21.27 and 21.28) is attached below to the iliolumbar ligament and the adjacent part of the iliac crest. Extending upwards, lateral to psoas and in the plane of the lumbar transverse processes, it becomes attached to the lateral halves of the anterior aspects of the upper four lumbar transverse processes and to the medial half of the lower border of the twelfth rib.

Deep fascia of the vertebral region

The **lumbodorsal fascia** is a collective term describing a series of interconnected fascial layers which are intimately associated with the vertebral muscles (fig. 21.28).

In the thoracic region, a single layer covers the posterior aspect of the sacrospinalis and extends from the thoracic spines medially to the angles of the ribs laterally.

In the lumbar region three layers of fascia are attached to the vertebral column and fuse into a single layer as they are traced laterally. The **posterior layer** extends from the lumbar spines across the posterior surface of sacrospinalis. Above, it is continuous with the thoracic part of the lumbodorsal fascia while below, it is attached to the sacrum and iliac crest. The **middle layer** arises from the tips of the lumbar transverse processes and extends laterally between sacrospinalis and quadratus lumborum. Above, it reaches the twelfth rib, and below, the iliac crest and iliolumbar ligament. The **anterior layer** is attached to the ridges on the anterior aspects of the lumbar transverse processes between the regions associated with psoas and quadratus lumborum, and passes laterally across the anterior surface of quadratus lumborum. Above, it reaches the twelfth rib, and below, the iliac crest and iliolumbar ligament. Traced laterally the three layers fuse at the lateral border of quadratus lumborum. The single **lumbar fascia** so formed is a thick collagenous sheet which extends laterally for two inches or so in the interval between the lateral half of the twelfth rib and the iliac crest.

The **iliopsoas fascia** is a comparatively thin layer which covers the free surface of both the iliacus and psoas heads of iliopsoas.

The **arcuate ligaments** are thickened and strengthened zones in the deep fascia of the vertebral region, which give origin to some of the muscle fibres of the diaphragm (fig. 21.34). The **medial arcuate ligament** is such a thick zone in the fascia covering the upper part of the psoas head of iliopsoas; it extends across that muscle between the body and the middle of the transverse process of either the first or the second lumbar vertebra. The **lateral arcuate ligament** is a thickening of the anterior layer of the lumbodorsal fascia over the upper part of quadratus lumborum; it extends from the middle of the first or second lumbar transverse process to the middle of the lower border of the twelfth rib.

Anterolateral muscles of the thorax

In the thoracic region the characteristic three concentric layers of the body wall are divided into intercostal segments by the ribs and costal cartilages. Each layer consists in part of muscle and in part of collagenous tissue, and the inner and middle layers are separated by a neurovascular plane.

In each intercostal space (fig. 21.29), the **outer layer** is formed by the fibrous **external intercostal membrane** which extends from the sternum to the costochondral junctions, by the **external intercostal muscle** which extends from the costochondral junctions to the rib tubercles, and thereafter by the **superior costotransverse ligament**. Each external intercostal muscle is attached to the adjacent borders of two ribs and its fibres run downwards and forwards round the chest wall.

In the **middle layer**, the **internal intercostal muscle** extends from the sternum to the rib angles, and the **internal intercostal membrane** from the rib angles to the rib tubercles. Thereafter this layer is also completed by the superior costotransverse ligament. The fibres of each internal intercostal muscle are attached to the costal groove of one rib, and extend downwards and backwards round the chest wall, to reach the upper

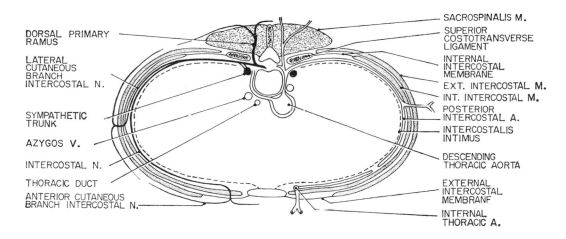

DORSAL PRIMARY RAMUS

LATERAL CUTANEOUS BRANCH INTERCOSTAL N.

SYMPATHETIC TRUNK

AZYGOS V.

INTERCOSTAL N.

THORACIC DUCT

ANTERIOR CUTANEOUS BRANCH INTERCOSTAL N.

SACROSPINALIS M.

SUPERIOR COSTOTRANSVERSE LIGAMENT

INTERNAL INTERCOSTAL MEMBRANE

EXT. INTERCOSTAL M.

INT. INTERCOSTAL M.

POSTERIOR INTERCOSTAL A.

INTERCOSTALIS INTIMUS

DESCENDING THORACIC AORTA

EXTERNAL INTERCOSTAL MEMBRANE

INTERNAL THORACIC A.

FIG. 21.29. Main relations of somatic arteries and nerves in an upper intercostal space.

margin of the rib immediately below (fig. 21.45). The constitution of the **inner layer** is very variable. It is to be regarded as a fibrous sheet which may or may not contain thin laminae of muscle fibres in its anterior, central and posterior parts. These muscle fibres are described collectively as the **intercostales intimi.**

Anterolateral muscles of the abdomen

The greater parts of the anterior and lateral regions of the abdominal wall consist of the three partly muscular and partly fibrous layers which are characteristic of the whole body wall, and the neurovascular plane lies between the inner and middle layers. Anteriorly this basic pattern is disturbed by the presence of a longitudinal muscle, the rectus abdominis.

The **rectus abdominis** (fig. 21.30) is a long flat muscle which is attached below by tendinous fibres to the pubic crest and the outer surface of the pubic symphysis. It extends through the length of the abdominal wall on to the anterior aspect of the thorax, and there becomes attached, from the lateral to the medial side, to the fifth, sixth and seventh costal cartilages and the xiphoid process. The muscle is wider above than below so that, although its medial border is vertical, its lateral border is gently curved and extends upwards and a little laterally to cross the costal margin over the ninth costal cartilage. In thin people the slight prominence of the lateral border creates a parallel groove on the skin surface, which is named the **linea semilunaris.** The muscle is usually incompletely divided into segments by three transverse **tendinous intersections,** which lie at the levels of the umbilicus and xiphoid process and midway between. Each intersection extends to the anterior surface of the muscle, but does not reach the posterior surface which is purely muscular.

The **external oblique muscle** (fig. 21.31) is the most

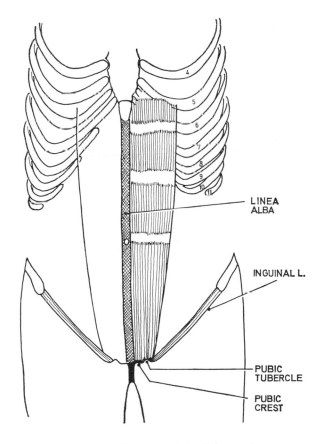

LINEA ALBA

INGUINAL L.

PUBIC TUBERCLE

PUBIC CREST

FIG. 21.30. The rectus abdominis muscle.

superficial of the three concentric, flat muscles of the abdominal wall, and it corresponds both in plane and in fibre direction to the external intercostal muscle in the thorax. It arises by eight digitations from the outer surfaces of the lower eight ribs along a straight oblique line extending from the anterior extremity of the fifth rib to

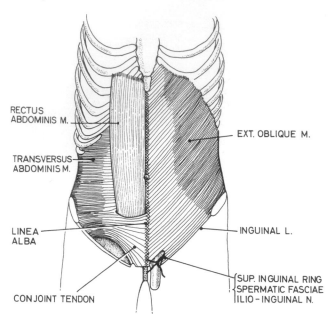

RECTUS
ABDOMINIS M.

EXT. OBLIQUE M.

TRANSVERSUS
ABDOMINIS M.

LINEA
ALBA

INGUINAL L.

CONJOINT TENDON

SUP. INGUINAL RING
SPERMATIC FASCIAE
ILIO - INGUINAL N.

FIG. 21.31. The external oblique and transversus abdominis muscles.

the twelfth costal cartilage. The posterior part of the muscle passes downwards and forwards to the anterior third of the iliac crest, so that the posterior border is free and overlies the lumbodorsal fascia (fig. 21.28). The remaining fibres extend in a parallel direction into the anterior abdominal wall. Here they give way to an extensive aponeurosis along a line which runs from the anterior superior iliac spine towards the umbilicus, and thereafter passes vertically upwards to the ninth costal cartilage.

The **aponeurosis of external oblique** continues medially in front of the abdominal and thoracic parts of rectus abdominis. Reaching the midline its greater part achieves an insertion by becoming continuous with the aponeurosis of the opposite side. The fibres of the two aponeuroses interdigitate in a linear zone which runs from the xiphoid process to the symphysis pubis and is named the **linea alba.**

The part of the aponeurosis immediately below that which reaches the linea alba splits, about 2 cm above the pubis, into two diverging parts which are attached to the pubic symphysis and the pubic tubercle respectively. The triangular aperture so formed is larger in the male than in the female, and is named the **superficial inguinal ring**. Its base is formed by the pubic crest and the diverging aponeurotic fibres which form its medial and lateral boundaries are the **crura of the ring**. The apex is directed upwards and laterally and the centre of the ring lies 1 cm above and lateral to the pubic tubercle.

The lowest part of the aponeurosis is described as the **inguinal ligament** (figs. 21.31, 21.37 and 21.38). It is curled backwards so that it presents a grooved upper sur-

face, a free posterior border, and an anterior border which is directly continuous with the rest of the aponeurosis. The ligament is attached at its lateral end to the anterior superior iliac spine, from which it extends medially and downwards. At its medial end all its anterior fibres are attached to the pubic tubercle, but its posterior fibres curve, first backwards and then backwards and laterally, to become attached to the pectineal line on the superior pubic ramus. The latter part is distinguished as the **lacunar ligament.**

The fascia lata of the thigh is fused to the under surface of the inguinal ligament (fig. 21.38), and consequently although the ligament is straight when the hip joint is flexed it is convex downwards when the joint is extended. The large space between the inguinal ligament and the hip bone is one of the major pathways through which structures may pass from the abdominal cavity to the thigh; the greater part of the space is occupied by the iliopsoas muscle (fig. 21.39).

The **internal oblique muscle** (fig. 21.32) lies deep to the

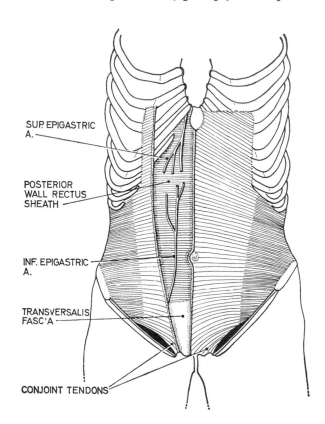

SUP. EPIGASTRIC
A.

POSTERIOR
WALL RECTUS
SHEATH

INF. EPIGASTRIC
A.

TRANSVERSALIS
FASC'A

CONJOINT TENDONS

FIG. 21.32. The internal oblique muscles.

external oblique. It is homologous with the internal intercostal muscle in the thorax and its fibres in general follow a similar direction, from behind, upwards and forwards, round the body wall. It arises continuously from (1) the lateral two-thirds of the grooved upper surface of the inguinal ligament (fig. 21.36), (2) the anterior part of the iliac crest, and (3) the outer surface of the lumbar fascia between the iliac crest and the twelfth rib (fig. 21.28). The uppermost muscle fibres are short and are inserted into the lower three costal cartilages, becoming contiguous with the anterior parts of the internal intercostal muscles of the tenth and eleventh intercostal spaces (fig. 21.32). The remaining fibres join a broad aponeurosis along a line which runs downwards from the tenth costal cartilage and gradually approaches the lateral border of rectus abdominis. This aponeurosis is described below.

The **transversus abdominis muscle** (fig. 21.31) lies deep to the internal oblique, but although it thus corresponds in position to the intercostales intimi in the thorax, its fibres are horizontal. The muscle fibres take origin continuously from (1) the lateral one-third of the grooved upper surface of the inguinal ligament (fig. 21.37), (2) the anterior part of the iliac crest, (3) the lateral edge of the lumbar fascia (fig. 21.28), and (4) the costal cartilages of the lower six ribs. Those coming from the eighth, seventh and sixth arise deep to rectus abdominis (fig. 21.31). All these fibres join an aponeurosis along a line which extends from the xiphoid process towards the midpoint of the inguinal ligament. The line is slightly convex laterally and crosses the lateral border of rectus abdominis midway between the xiphoid process and the umbilicus.

The **aponeuroses of internal oblique and transversus abdominis** both extend towards the midline deep to that of external oblique, but their form and relationship to rectus abdominis vary at different levels.

(1) The aponeuroses derived from the lowest fibres of both muscles fuse to form the **conjoint tendon** (figs. 21.36b and 21.37). This curves medially and downwards, and, after passing behind the superficial inguinal ring and in front of rectus abdominis, is attached to the pubic crest and tubercle and the medial part of the pectineal line on the superior pubic ramus.

(2) From the conjoint tendon to a level midway between the umbilicus and the pubic symphyses, the two aponeuroses fuse and, after passing in front of rectus abdominis, blend with the linea alba (figs. 21.31, 21.32 and 21.35c).

(3) Above this level the aponeurosis of transversus abdominis passes entirely behind rectus abdominis to reach the linea alba (figs. 21.31 and 21.35b). On the other hand that of internal oblique splits at the lateral border of rectus abdominis into anterior and posterior layers which cross the corresponding aspects of rectus abdominis before fusing again in the linea alba (figs. 21.32 and 21.35). The anterior layer is closely associated with the aponeurosis of external oblique, and both extend on to the thoracic part of rectus abdominis to become attached to the ribs and costal cartilages around its margins. The posterior layer is similarly associated with the aponeurosis of

transversus abdominis; the two layers are attached above to the seventh and eighth costal cartilages, while their free lower margin is named the **arcuate line.**

Diaphragm

This dome-shaped muscle separates the thoracic from the abdominal cavity (fig. 21.1). When the muscle is seen from above (fig. 21.33), it is evident that, because of the considerable forward projection of the vertebral column, it consists of extensive right and left parts, which are separated by and lie slightly above the smaller central part. The lateral parts are named the **cupolae.**

The kidney-shaped origin of the muscle from the bones and fasciae of the body wall is obliquely placed, the anterior part lying at a considerably higher level than the posterior (fig. 21.1). The fibres are inserted into an aponeurotic **central tendon** which is crescentic and convex forwards (fig. 21.33) and, since this tendon lies at the

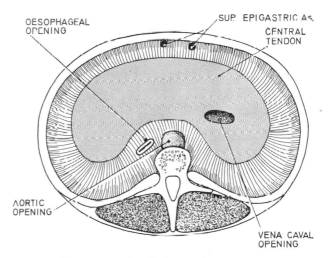

FIG. 21.33. The diaphragm from above.

summit of the diaphragm, the anterior muscle fibres are much shorter than those lying posteriorly or laterally.

It is convenient to divide the origin into three parts. The **sternal origin** arises from the posterior aspect of the xiphoid process, and the **costal origin** from the deep aspects of the lower six ribs and costal cartilages. The **vertebral origin** (fig. 21.34), arises from the medial and lateral arcuate ligaments (p. 21.22) of both sides and by two separate, fusiform, tendinous bundles or **crura** from the anterior aspect of the lumbar vertebral column. The right crus arises from the upper three lumbar bodies and the intervening intervertebral discs, whereas the left arises from only the upper two. The initially separate crura pass upwards and forwards and eventually fuse in front of the lower border of the twelfth thoracic vertebral body. The junction is coated by tendinous fibres which are described as the **median arcuate ligament.**

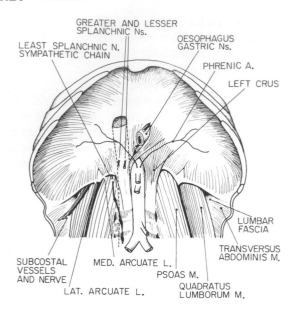

GREATER AND LESSER
SPLANCHNIC Ns.

LEAST SPLANCHNIC N.
SYMPATHETIC CHAIN

OESOPHAGUS
GASTRIC Ns.

PHRENIC A.

LEFT CRUS

LUMBAR
FASCIA

TRANSVERSUS
ABDOMINIS M.

SUBCOSTAL
VESSELS
AND NERVE

MED. ARCUATE L.

PSOAS M.

QUADRATUS
LUMBORUM M.

LAT. ARCUATE L.

FIG. 21.34. The abdominal surface of the diaphragm and the posterior abdominal wall.

The muscle fibres of the right and left halves of the diaphragm are supplied solely by the corresponding phrenic nerve (p. 22.28). Sensory fibres are provided by the phrenic nerves and, round the periphery of the diaphragm, by intercostal nerves.

In the mid-phase of quiet respiration, in the erect posture, the right cupola is a little higher than the left at the level of the eighth thoracic vertebra. In the supine position the resting level rises because of the absence of the gravitational pull of the abdominal viscera, and the thoracic volume is reduced. When the body lies on one side the lower cupola rises to a higher level, but its excursion during respiration is increased.

The diaphragm presents a number of openings in its substance (figs. 21.33 and 21.34).

(1) The small **sternocostal gap** between the sternal and costal fibres transmits the superior epigastric vessels from the thorax to the abdomen.

(2) The large median **aortic opening** lies between the right and left crura. It is obliquely placed and bordered, above, at the twelfth thoracic level, by the median arcuate ligament, and below by the second lumbar vertebral body. It contains the aorta and thoracic duct.

(3) The **vertebrocostal trigone**, present in some people, is an interval between the vertebral and costal fibres of the diaphragm which varies considerably in size.

(4) The round **vena caval opening** lies within the central tendon in the right cupola of the diaphragm, about 3 cm to the right of the midline and at about the eighth thoracic level in quiet respiration.

(5) The **oesophageal opening** lies in the vertebral part of the muscular substance of the diaphragm, above and about 2 cm to the left of the aortic opening and at the level of the tenth thoracic vertebra. The oesophagus, accompanied by the vagus (gastric) nerves, passes through the opening to join the stomach at the cardia.

Fascial envelope of the abdominal cavity

The inside of the wall of the abdominal cavity is formed by the deep surface of several muscles and their aponeuroses, by bones and by the lumbar fascia. All these elements are lined by a continuous fascial envelope. Over the muscles it is a distinct layer, over the bones it joins the periosteum, while elsewhere it blends with the lumbar fascia and the muscle aponeuroses. Different parts of the envelope are given distinct names, often corresponding to the muscle to which the part is related. Thus over the diaphragm and the iliopsoas muscles it is named the **diaphragmatic fascia** and the **iliopsoas fascia** respectively; in relation to the transversus abdominis and rectus abdominis it is described as the **transversalis fascia**, and over the quadratus lumborum it is known as the anterior layer of the lumbar fascia.

Nevertheless these layers of fascia are continuous with one another and form a single envelope lining the abdominal cavity. The envelope is separated internally from the viscera and peritoneum by a layer of fatty areolar tissue. This varies in thickness and adiposity in different people and is described collectively as the **extraperitoneal tissue**. Within the abdominal cavity it is a useful, though not an invariable rule, that the somatic nerves lie outside the fascial envelope whereas the large arteries and veins and the splanchnic nerves lie inside the fascial envelope within the extraperitoneal tissue.

Special regions of the abdominal wall

RECTUS SHEATH (fig. 21.35)

This is formed by the several tissues which encapsulate the rectus abdominis muscle and its character varies at different levels. The thoracic part of the rectus abdominis is covered anteriorly by the aponeurosis of external oblique and by the anterior layer of the aponeurosis of internal oblique. Posteriorly the muscle lies directly against the sixth, seventh and eighth costal cartilages and the corresponding external intercostal membranes. From the costal margin to the arcuate line the anterior relations of the muscle remain the same, but it is now related posteriorly to the posterior layer of the internal oblique aponeurosis, to the aponeurosis and the uppermost muscle fibres of transversus abdominis (fig. 21.32), and to the transversalis fascia. Below the arcuate line the aponeuroses of all three flat muscles pass in front of rectus abdominis, which consequently is related posteriorly to the transversalis fascia alone.

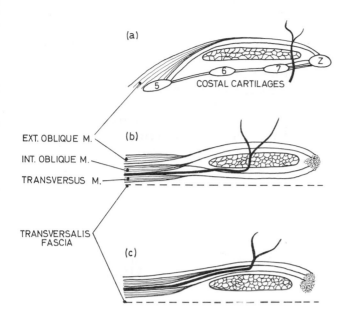

FIG. 21.35. The rectus sheath (a) above the costal margin, (b) between the costal margin and the arcuate line, (c) below the arcuate line. The thick black lines indicate intercostal nerves in (a) and (b) and the subcostal or iliohypogastric nerve in (c).

It is important to note that the tendinous intersections in the upper part of rectus abdominis (p. 21.23) are fused to the anterior wall of the rectus sheath whereas they have no attachment to the posterior wall.

INGUINAL CANAL

Development

This is an oblique passage through the abdominal wall, immediately above the inguinal ligament, traversed in the male by the spermatic cord, in the female by the round ligament of the uterus. Its biological significance is that it is the route through which the testis descends from the abdominal cavity into the scrotum, drawing after it its duct (the vas deferens), its blood vessels, lymphatics and nerves. The presence of an inguinal canal in the female as well as in the male suggests that its development is determined by factors acting during the 'indifferent' stage of gonadal development. The canal initially develops around the gubernaculum, a column of mesenchyme which extends from the developing gonad (testis or ovary) through the abdominal wall into the genital fold (scrotum or labium majus). During the last third of intrauterine life a pouch of parietal peritoneum, the **processus vaginalis**, extends into the mesenchyme of the gubernaculum, through the developing canal and into the scrotum or labium majus. It is followed, in the seventh to eighth month, by the testis; the comparable descent of the ovary is arrested in the pelvis, leaving the round ligament of the uterus (derived from the gubernaculum) as the major

content of the canal in the female. The processus vaginalis is normally obliterated in the female by full term; in the male only its distal end normally persists, as the **tunica vaginalis testis**, the innermost of the various investments of the testis.

At birth, the inguinal canal is a short, direct passage; as the pelvis increases in breadth the canal lengthens and becomes more oblique. In the adult it is about 5 cm long and extends between the superficial and deep inguinal rings. The **superficial inguinal ring** (fig. 21.36a) is an

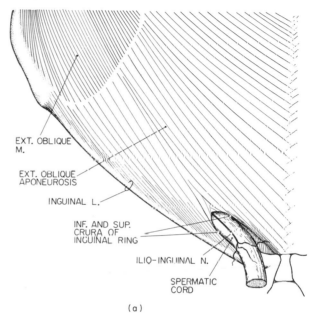

(a)

FIG. 21.36a. The inguinal region showing the superior infusional ring.

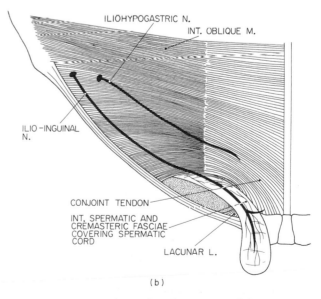

(b)

FIG. 21.36b The inguinal region after removal of the external oblique muscles. Refer to fig. 21.31.

opening in the external oblique aponeurosis. It is triangular, with its base formed by the outer part of the pubic crest (p. 21.24). From its margins, a tubular fibrous sheath, the **external spermatic fascia**, extends to invest the spermatic cord. The **deep inguinal ring** (fig. 21.36b) is an opening in the transversalis fascia (p. 21.26), and is situated at the mid-point between the pubic symphysis and the anterior superior iliac spine, 1·25 cm above the inguinal ligament. From its margins, another tubular fibrous sheath, the **internal spermatic fascia**, is given off to invest the spermatic cord (fig. 21.37). As the cord traverses the canal towards the external ring it receives from the internal oblique muscle a further tubular investment, the cremasteric fascia. This is partly fibrous, but also contains the **cremaster muscle**, consisting of fasciculi of skeletal muscle which extend in oblique loops, around the cord and testis.

The inguinal canal is a region of potential weakness in the abdominal wall, through which protrusion of abdominal contents may occur; this is known as **inguinal hernia**. Knowledge of the walls of the canal, and of its normal defence mechanisms, is important clinically.

The **anterior wall of the canal** is formed by the external oblique aponeurosis, reinforced laterally by muscular fibres of the internal oblique, which arises from the outer two-thirds of the inguinal ligament.

The **posterior wall** is formed by the transversalis fascia, reinforced medially by the conjoint tendon (p. 21.25). This is a common tendon for the lowermost fibres of the internal oblique and transversus muscles, which arise from the inguinal ligament on a plane in front of the canal, and

arch medially above the spermatic cord. The conjoint tendon descends behind the cord, to be inserted into the pubic crest and the medial part of the pectineal line (fig. 21.37). Medially, the conjoint tendon is directly continuous with the anterior wall of rectus sheath. The **floor of the canal** is formed mainly by the grooved upper surface of the inguinal ligament, whose backturned edge is firmly fused with the transversalis fascia (fig. 21.38). The medial

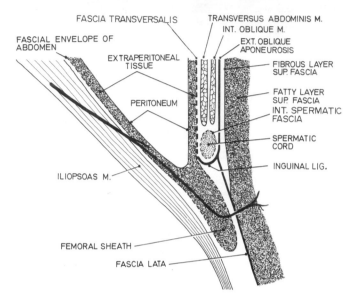

FIG. 21.38. Sagittal section showing course of genitofemoral nerve and its femoral branch in black.

end of the floor is formed by the lacunar ligament. The **roof of the canal** consists of arching fibres of the internal oblique and transversus muscles.

Several factors contribute to the defence mechanism of the inguinal canal and reduce the risk of development of an inguinal hernia:

(1) the normal obliteration of the upper end of the processus vaginalis;

(2) the obliquity of the canal;

(3) the presence of muscular fibres of internal oblique in front of the deep ring;

(4) the presence of the conjoint tendon directly behind the superficial ring;

(5) when the intra-abdominal pressure is increased by contraction of the abdominal muscles, thus increasing the risk of herniation, the arching lower fibres of internal oblique and transversus contract downwards towards the inguinal ligament, reducing the vertical height of the canal and acting as a kind of protective 'shutter'.

FEMORAL SHEATH (figs. 21.38 and 24.44)

This is a conical protrusion of the fascial envelope of the abdominal cavity into the thigh. It traverses the interval bounded in front by the medial half of the inguinal

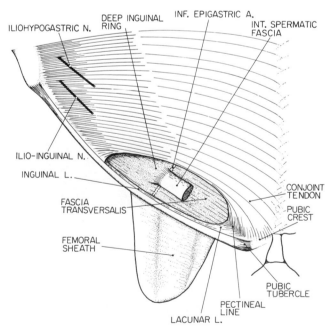

FIG. 21.37. The inguinal region after removal of the external and internal oblique muscles.

ligament, medially by the lacunar ligament, and behind by the pectineal line on the superior pubic ramus. The cavity of the sheath is divided by two sagittal septa into lateral, intermediate and medial compartments, each of which is continuous at its upper end with the abdominal extraperitoneal tissue (fig. 21.38). The lateral and intermediate compartments are largely occupied by the femoral artery and vein respectively. On the other hand the medial compartment, which is named the **femoral canal,** contains only one or two deep inguinal lymph nodes and loose connective tissue. The upper end of the canal is limited laterally by the femoral vein and is described as the **femoral ring** (fig. 21.39).

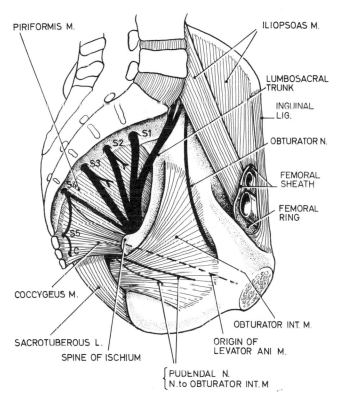

FIG. 21.39. Median section of osteoligamentous pelvis. Nerves in black. Refer to figs. 21.16, 21.19 and 21.22.

Protrusion of abdominal contents through this ring constitutes a **femoral hernia.**

Functions of the trunk muscles

Excluding the muscles of the pelvis and perineum, the muscles of the trunk have two functions. Firstly, they create pressure changes in the thoracic and abdominal cavities, including those involved in respiration. Secondly, they are concerned with displacements of one part of the trunk in relation to another, through movements of the vertebral column.

RESPIRATORY MOVEMENTS

The mechanism by which the volume of the thoracic cavity is increased in inspiration is considered on p. 21.10. It can now be appreciated that this mechanism involves several factors.

(1) Contraction of the diaphragm displaces its central tendon downwards and increases the vertical diameter of the thorax. This displacement depends on the fixation of the lowest ribs by the quadratus lumborum, and on the displaced abdominal viscera being accommodated partly by the relaxation of the abdominal muscles, and partly by the passive lateral displacement of the eighth, ninth and tenth ribs. Contraction of the diaphragm also actively raises the lower ribs.

(2) The anteroposterior and transverse diameters of the thorax are increased by elevation of the upper seven ribs. In quiet respiration this is achieved by the intercostal muscles, particularly the external intercostals. In more vigorous inspiration these muscles are augmented by the scalene and sternomastoid muscles in the neck and even, in exceptional circumstances, by muscles acting on the ribs from the fixed upper limbs.

(3) Increase in the vertical diameter of the thorax is effected through extension of the thoracic vertebral column by the sacrospinalis muscles.

Quiet expiration is a passive process which is achieved by the elastic recoil of the expanded lungs, the extended vertebral column and the distended abdominal wall. In forced expiration contraction of the oblique and transversus muscles increases intra-abdominal pressure and thereby passively raises the diaphragm. Contraction of the intercostal muscles prevents bulging of the intercostal spaces by the raised intrathoracic pressure.

Raising intra-abdominal pressure for defaecation and parturition involves the same mechanism as that of forced expiration, except that actual expiration of air is prevented by the closure of the glottis, by adduction of the vocal folds. Inspiration is brought about by descent of the contracting diaphragm; closure of the glottis then fixes the diaphragm, and thereafter the intra-abdominal pressure is raised by contraction of the oblique and transversus muscles of the abdominal wall.

SPINAL MOVEMENTS

Ignoring the effects of gravity, it is evident that in movements of the spine:

(1) thoracolumbar extension is produced by the superficial fibres of sacrospinalis;

(2) rotation is by the deep fibres of sacrospinalis;

(3) flexion is caused by the muscles of the anterior abdominal wall, particularly rectus abdominis, and to a lesser extent by iliopsoas;

(4) lateral flexion is produced by all the muscles of one side of the trunk, particularly sacrospinalis, quadratus

lumborum and the oblique and transversus muscles of the abdominal wall.

However, these actions are of little significance unless they are considered in relation to gravity.

In standing, because of the different curvatures of the lumbar and thoracic regions, the force of gravity tends to cause flexion of the thoracic column and extension of the lumbar (fig. 21.23). The maintenance of posture depends on the prevention of these displacements. It has been noted (p. 21.8) that flexion and extension both involve elastic deformation of the tissues of the intervertebral articulations. It will be appreciated, therefore, that gravitational displacement of the vertebral column in standing is prevented largely by the stresses in the deformed joint tissues, and to only a small degree by activity in the relevant muscle groups.

Deviations from the normal metastable standing position, e.g. flexion or lateral flexion, are, of course, initiated by the relevant muscle groups. Thereafter they are assisted by gravity, and are controlled and limited by a combination of elastic joint resistance and the antagonistic muscle group. Thus flexion from standing is initiated by the flexor muscles but, thereafter, gravitational flexion is controlled by both the activity of sacrospinalis and elastic joint resistance. As flexion proceeds, joint resistance increases and consequently muscular activity decreases until, in full flexion, sacrospinalis is totally inactive. On the other hand, flexion of the vertebral column when lying supine is achieved by the flexor muscles acting against both the force of gravity and elastic joint resistance.

In walking, the trailing leg exerts an upward and forward force which maintains the body's forward momentum. But, because this force is unilateral, it also tilts the trunk towards the opposite, i.e., the supported, side so that gravity tends to carry the vertebral column into lateral flexion. Some lateral flexion is necessary to carry the centre of gravity of the body, from its original central position, to a position over the single supporting foot. Once this relationship has been established, further lateral flexion must be prevented by the lateral flexor muscles of the opposite side. Thus throughout walking, each time the left foot leaves the ground, the trunk inclines towards the right and the sacrospinalis, the quadratus lumborum and the lateral abdominal muscles of the left side become active (p. 24.27).

Superficial fascia of the trunk

The trunk is completely invested by fatty superficial fascia which is directly continuous with that of the limbs and neck. Its thickness varies enormously, from a few millimetres to several centimetres, in different individuals. Over the lower part of the anterior abdominal wall, the deep part of the superficial fascia is a membranous layer.

It contains a relatively high proportion of elastic fibres and acts as a natural corset over that part of the abdominal wall against which gravity exerts the greatest force. Below, the central part of this membranous layer extends down to envelop the scrotum and penis and eventually turns backwards into the perineum (p. 21.32, fig. 21.40). Each lateral part of the same layer crosses the inguinal ligament and becomes fused to the deep fascia of that part of the thigh, the fascia lata (fig. 21.38).

On the anterior aspect of the thoracic wall the mammary gland is contained within the superficial fascia.

PELVIC CAVITY AND PERINEUM

The muscles which lie within the true osteoligamentous pelvis are associated with the pelvic cavity and the perineum.

Obturator internus (fig. 21.39) arises from the deep aspect of the obturator membrane, the immediately surrounding bone, and that part of the ilium which lies below the arcuate line. Its fibres converge like a fan on the deep aspect of the lesser sciatic foramen and, becoming tendinous, turn at right angles through the fora-

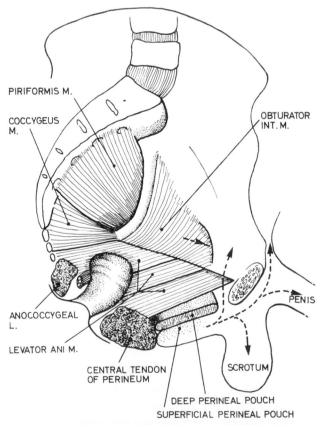

FIG. 21.40. Median section of osteoligamentous pelvis showing division into pelvic cavity and perineum. Arrows show the obturator canal, and routes from superficial perineal pouch to pelvic cavity, scrotum, penis and anterior abdominal wall. Refer to figs. 21.39 and 21.41.

men into the buttock. After being joined by two small additional heads, the **gemelli**, the tendon is inserted into the greater trochanter of the femur (p. 24.4). Functionally the muscle is concerned entirely with the lower limb.

Piriformis (fig. 21.40) arises from the pelvic surface of the second, third and fourth pieces of the sacrum, between and lateral to the corresponding sacral foramina. Its fibres pass laterally through the greater sciatic foramen into the buttock and, becoming tendinous, they are inserted into the greater trochanter of the femur. Like the obturator internus, the muscle acts on the lower limb.

The **pelvic diaphragm** is an incomplete muscular partition, convex downwards, which extends across the true osteoligamentous pelvis and divides it into the **pelvic cavity** above and the **perineum** below. It is deficient anteriorly and is traversed posteriorly by the anorectal junction.

The partition consists of two symmetrical pairs of muscles; the coccygeus muscles form its posterior part and the levator ani muscles form the remainder. Each **coccygeus muscle** (figs. 21.39 and 21.40) overlies the pelvic aspect of the corresponding sacrospinous ligament (p. 21. 15). Laterally its apex is attached to the ischial spine while medially it is inserted into the lateral margins of the lower part of the sacrum and the upper part of the coccyx. Each **levator ani** muscle has a linear origin on the side wall of the true pelvis and its fibres extend downwards, medially and backwards to reach the median plane. The line of origin (fig. 21.39) reaches from the pelvic aspect of the body of the pubis to the pelvic aspect of the ischial spine, and between these bony origins the muscle arises from a dense layer of fascia which covers the inner surface of the obturator internus muscle. The posterior fibres run parallel to and in close proximity to the lower margin of coccygeus and are inserted into the lowest part of the coccyx (fig. 21.40). The fibres immediately in front of these end in a median fibromuscular region named the **anococcygeal ligament** (figs. 21.40 and 21.41). It occupies the interval between the tip of the coccyx and the anorectal junction and extends downwards into continuity with peri-anal skin. The succeeding fibres of the levator ani become directly continuous with the corresponding fibres of the opposite side around the lateral and posterior aspects of the anorectal junction; although they are part of levator ani, they may be distinguished under the name of the **puborectalis muscle** (figs. 21.40 and 21.41). The most anterior fibres of levator ani are inserted into a second median fibromuscular region, the **central tendon of the perineum** (perineal body) which lies in front of the anorectal junction and is continuous with the perineal skin (figs. 21.40 and 21.41). Between the pubic symphysis and the central tendon of the perineum, and limited on either side by the most anterior fibres of the levator ani muscles, is a large gap in the pelvic diaphragm through which the pelvic cavity and perineum communicate (fig. 21.41).

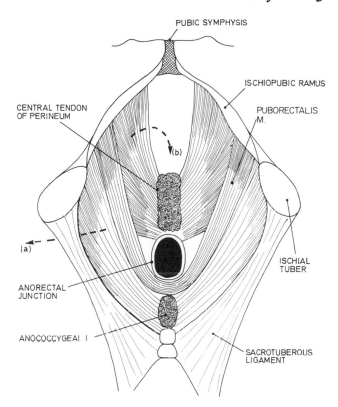

FIG. 21.41. The perineum from below showing the inferior surfaces of the levatores ani muscles. Arrows indicate exits from perineum (a) through lesser sciatic foramen into the buttock and (b) into the pelvic cavity.

Pelvic cavity

The pelvic cavity is shaped like a bowl, obliquely placed so that its inlet is directed upwards and forwards. It is in broad continuity above with the abdominal cavity proper at the level of the brim of the pelvis. Its lateral wall is formed by bone and that part of obturator internus which lies between the pelvic brim and the origin of levator ani (fig. 21.39). Its dorsal wall faces predominantly downwards and consists of the sacrum, the coccyx, the sacro-iliac joints and piriformis muscles. The short ventral wall faces upwards and backwards and is formed by the bodies of the pubic bones and the pubic symphysis. Below, the walls merge smoothly into the concave floor formed by the coccygeus and levator ani muscles.

Apart from its continuity with the abdominal cavity proper, the pelvic cavity communicates with several other adjacent regions. The obturator canal leads into the medial part of the thigh, the greater sciatic foramen into the buttock, and the median gap in the pelvic diaphragm into the perineum.

The bony and muscular walls of the pelvic cavity are lined by a layer of fascia which is continuous, through periosteum, with the fascial envelope of the abdominal cavity proper (p. 21.25). This fascia is separated from the pelvic peritoneum by extraperitoneal tissue. In the upper part of the pelvic cavity this layer is comparatively thin but below it forms an extensive zone in which the extraperitoneal parts of many of the pelvic viscera are embedded. Although different zones of this tissue vary in density and may be given distinct names, it is to be appreciated that they are only subdivisions of the continuous pelvic fascia.

Perineum

The perineum is the lowest part of the cavity of the true osteoligamentous pelvis, and lies between the pelvic diaphragm and the area of skin between the thighs. It differs from the other three divisions of the trunk in that it contains no serous cavity. It is occupied by connective tissue of various densities and is traversed by the terminal parts of the intestinal and genitourinary tracts.

In the horizontal plane it is diamond-shaped (fig. 21.41) while in coronal section its depth is greater in its lateral than in its median part (figs. 21.43 and 21.44).

The roof of the perineum (fig. 21.41) is the convex undersurface of the pelvic diaphragm and is therefore deficient anteriorly between the pubic symphysis and the central tendon of the perineum. The side walls (figs. 21.39, 21.43 and 21.46) consist of those parts of the osteoligamentous pelvis and its associated muscles which lie below the level of levator ani and coccygeus. From before back these are the lower parts of the pubic symphysis and the pubic bodies, the ischiopubic rami and the lower parts of the obturator internus muscles, the ischial tubers, the lesser sciatic foramina and the sacrotuberous ligaments. Posteriorly, the coccyx, to which the pelvic diaphragm is attached, comes into contact with the skin; in other words the roof and floor join and there is no side wall.

The floor of the perineum is skin. Posteriorly this skin lies in the lower part of the natal cleft and contains the anus; anteriorly it differs in the two sexes and so is described with the reproductive system (chap. 38 and figs. 21.42 and 21.43).

The perineum communicates with the pelvic cavity through the anterior gap in the pelvic diaphragm (fig. 21.41), and with the buttock through the lesser sciatic foramen (figs. 21.41 and 21.44).

Compartments of the perineum

The diamond-shaped perineum may be divided into anterior and posterior triangular parts by a coronal plane through the central tendon of the perineum and the anterior parts of the ischial tubers. The anterior region contains the genital and urinary tracts and is named the **urogenital triangle**. The posterior region contains the anal canal and is named the **anal triangle**.

The **urogenital triangle** is divided into several compartments by three horizontal, triangular layers of fascia lying one above the other (figs. 21.40, 21.42 and 21.43).

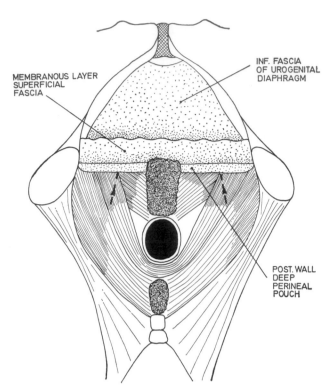

FIG. 21.42. The perineum from below. Arrows lead from ischiorectal fossae into anterior recesses. Refer to figs 21.40, 21.41, 21.43 and 21.44.

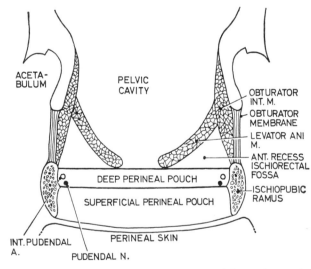

FIG. 21.43. Coronal section through pelvic cavity and urogenital triangle of perineum.

The middle and thickest layer is the **inferior fascia of the urogenital diaphragm (perineal membrane)**; above this lies the **superior fascia of the urogenital diaphragm** and, below, the **membranous layer of the superficial fascia**. The three layers are attached by their lateral margins to the upper, middle and inferior parts of the ischiopubic rami.

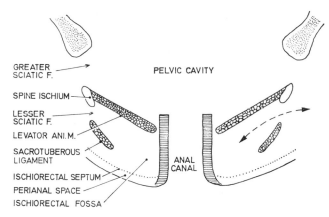

GREATER
SCIATIC F.

PELVIC CAVITY

SPINE ISCHIUM

LESSER
SCIATIC F.

LEVATOR ANI.M.

SACROTUBEROUS
LIGAMENT

ISCHIORECTAL SEPTUM

PERIANAL SPACE

ISCHIORECTAL FOSSA

ANAL
CANAL

FIG. 21.44. Coronal section through pelvic cavity and anal triangle of perineum. Arrows indicate communication of ischiorectal fossa and buttock through lesser sciatic foramen.

Posteriorly they fuse with one another and also, near the median plane, with the central tendon of the perineum. Anteriorly the superior and inferior fasciae of the urogenital diaphragm end by fusing with one another a short distance behind the lower part of the pubic symphysis (fig. 21.40). A gap is thus left between the symphysis and the fasciae. The anterior part of the membranous layer of the superficial fascia extends forwards beneath the pubic symphysis and envelops the scrotum and penis before becoming continuous with the membranous superficial fascia on the abdominal wall (p. 21.30). In the scrotum, the fascia contains involuntary muscle fibres which are inserted into the overlying skin and are named the **dartos muscle**; they contract in response to cold and fear, and wrinkle and thicken the scrotal skin. A thick septum of this fascia traverses the scrotum to reach the under surface of the penis and thereby divides the scrotum into two compartments.

The **deep perineal pouch** (figs 21.40 and 21.43) is that part of the urogenital triangle which lies between the superior and inferior fasciae of the urogenital diaphragm. It is completely separated from the surrounding regions by these two fascial layers and by the ischiopubic rami. This completely closed pouch is traversed in both sexes by the urethra and the terminal parts of the pudendal vessels and nerves, and in the male contains the bulbourethral glands.

The **superficial perineal pouch** (figs 21.40 and 21.43) lies between the inferior fascia of the urogenital diaphragm and the membranous layer of the superficial fascia. It is completely enclosed behind and on either side but anteriorly it is in direct communication with other neighbouring regions. Through the gap between the pubic symphysis and the deep perineal pouch, and subsequently through the gap in the anterior part of the pelvic diaphragm, it communicates with the pelvic cavity. Anteriorly it is in continuity with the tissues of the scrotum, the penis and the anterior abdominal wall.

On either side of the midline, and between the pelvic diaphragm, the superior fascia of the urogenital diaphragm and the obturator internus, lies a tissue space which is triangular in coronal section (fig. 21.43). Anteriorly it is limited by the body of the pubis, but posteriorly it is in continuity with an ischiorectal fossa. It is consequently named the **anterior recess of the ischiorectal fossa.**

The **anal triangle** (figs. 21.42 and 21.44) of the perineum is almost completely divided into two symmetrical parts by the central tendon of the perineum, anal canal, and anococcygeal ligament which all extend from the roof of the region to its floor, that is from the pelvic diaphragm to the skin. These lateral parts, the **ischiorectal fossae**, are wedge-shaped regions largely occupied by fatty tissue. In each fossa the medial wall consists of the pelvic diaphragm, the central tendon, anal canal, and anococcygeal ligament, whereas the lateral wall is formed by the obturator internus, the ischial tuber and the sacrotuberous ligament. The lateral wall is traversed by the lesser sciatic foramen. These walls meet above along the attachment of the pelvic diaphragm, and behind at the attachments of the pelvic diaphragm and the sacrotuberous ligament to the coccyx and sacrum. Anteriorly, the fossa is separated from the superficial and deep perineal pouches by the posterior walls of those compartments, but continues forwards at a higher level as the anterior recess. The base of the fossa is formed by the perineal skin. The fatty tissue immediately deep to this skin has a finer texture than that in the rest of the fossa and is separated from it by a thin fascial septum. This part of the ischiorectal fossa is known as the **perianal space.**

ARTERIES OF THE BODY WALL

Main arterial trunks (fig. 30.27).

The main systemic artery of the body is the aorta which arises directly from the left ventricle of the heart. In its course it undergoes several changes in direction and on the basis of these changes it is divided into three parts (fig. 21.10). The short first part, the **ascending aorta**, passes upwards, forwards and to the right, close to the anterior thoracic wall. Reaching the deep aspect of the second right costal cartilage it becomes continuous with the second part, named the **arch of the aorta**. The arch is convex upwards and passes backwards and to the left to end in contact with the left side of the fourth thoracic vertebra. It gives off three large branches from its upper surface. The **brachiocephalic artery,** after a short upward course, divides into the **right subclavian** and the **right common carotid arteries**. The **left common carotid** and the **left subclavian arteries** arise directly from the arch beyond the origin of the brachiocephalic.

Each subclavian artery turns laterally at the thoracic inlet and arches laterally over the upper surface of the first rib. Here it becomes the axillary artery which supplies the upper limb. Each common carotid artery ascends into the corresponding side of the neck.

The third part of the aorta, the **dorsal aorta**, begins as a continuation of the arch at the left side of the lower border of the fourth thoracic vertebra, and ends by bifurcating slightly to the left of the midline on the anterior aspect of the fourth lumbar vertebra. In the thorax it follows the curvature of the vertebral column and gradually shifts from its lateral to its anterior aspect. It then traverses the aortic opening in the diaphragm (fig. 21.34) and continues vertically downwards to its termination. The vessel is divisible at the level of the median arcuate ligament into the **descending thoracic aorta** and the **abdominal aorta.**

The **common iliac arteries** (figs. 21.46 and 30.27) arise at the terminal bifurcation of the abdominal aorta and run downwards and laterally. Each ends in front of the corresponding sacro-iliac joint and at the level of the lumbosacral intervertebral disc by dividing into internal and external iliac arteries. The common iliac arteries are about 5 cm long in the adult, but because their origins are to the left of the midline, the right artery is a little longer than the left.

The **internal iliac artery** (fig. 21.46) is about 2·5 cm long. From its origin it turns downwards and backwards along the side wall of the pelvic cavity and ends at the upper border of the greater sciatic foramen by dividing into a spray of branches.

The **external iliac artery** (fig. 21.46) runs downwards and forwards along the medial border of iliopsoas. It passes beneath the midpoint of the inguinal ligament and, changing its name to that of the femoral artery, enters the lateral compartment of the femoral sheath (p. 24.29).

Most of the tissues of the body wall are supplied by somatic branches arising from the major vessels named above. Many of these vessels also give off branches to the tissues of the neck, to the upper or lower limbs, or to the thoracic, abdominal, pelvic or perineal viscera, but these are considered in the appropriate sections. Moreover the muscles which, though overlying the thorax, are functionally associated with the shoulder girdle and upper limbs are supplied to a large extent from the upper limb arteries.

Blood supply of the deep tissues of the thoracic and abdominal walls

SEGMENTAL VESSELS

The **costocervical trunk** (fig. 21.47) arises from the subclavian artery in the region of the thoracic inlet, and runs backwards to the neck of the first rib. There it divides into a **deep cervical branch** which continues backwards into the cervical part of sacrospinalis, and a **superior intercostal branch** which descends into the thoracic cavity, where it represents a persistence of the embryonic precostal anastomosis (fig. 21.11). The superior intercostal artery gives off **posterior intercostal arteries** to the first and second intercostal spaces where their subsequent course corresponds to the posterior intercostal arteries arising from the descending thoracic aorta (see below).

The **posterior intercostal arteries** to the remaining intercostal spaces arise from the descending thoracic aorta (fig. 21.45). Because the descending thoracic aorta begins at the lower border of the fourth thoracic vertebra and lies to the left of the midline, the upper intercostal arteries ascend to reach their intercostal spaces, and those of the right side cross the anterior aspects of the vertebral bodies from the left to the right. Reaching its proper intercostal space each posterior intercostal artery runs laterally midway between two ribs, lying between the

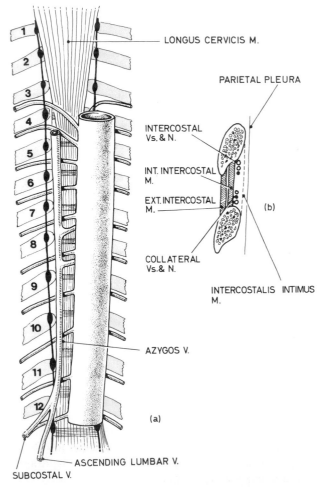

FIG. 21.45. (a) The descending thoracic aorta and its somatic branches. (b) Section of intercostal space.

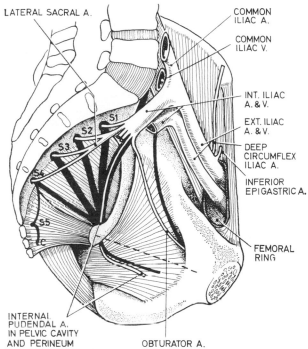

FIG. 21.46. Parietal vessels of pelvic cavity and perineum. Refer to figs. 21.39 and 21.40.

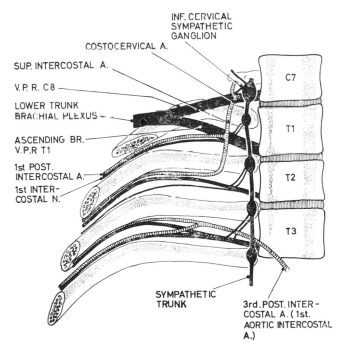

FIG. 21.47. Nerves and arteries of upper intercostal spaces. V.P.R., ventral primary ramus.

superior costotransverse ligament and the internal intercostal membrane externally, and the intercostales intimi (when present) and the pleura internally. At the rib angles it ascends into the costal groove, where it is lodged

between the internal intercostal muscle and the intercostalis intimus (fig. 21.45b), and thereafter continues in the same plane to the anterior end of the intercostal space. The lower two arteries continue forwards from the tenth and eleventh intercostal spaces into the abdominal wall where they lie between the internal oblique and transversus abdominis muscles. The posterior intercostal arteries supply branches to the tissues associated with the intercostal spaces, spinal branches which pass through the intervertebral foramina into the vertebral canal, and posterior branches which pass between the superior costotransverse ligaments and the vertebrae to reach the postvertebral tissues (fig. 21.29).

The **subcostal artery** is in series with the posterior intercostal vessels and, early in its course, gives off typical spinal and posterior branches. Running below the twelfth rib on quadratus lumborum it passes behind the lateral arcuate ligament into the abdominal cavity (fig. 21.34). It reaches and pierces the lumbar fascia and then continues round the body wall in the neurovascular plane between the internal oblique and transversus abdominis muscles. The vessel ends lateral to the rectus sheath.

The **lumbar arteries** arise from the posterolateral aspects of the abdominal aorta, in front of the upper four lumbar vertebrae, and pass laterally to reach the spaces beneath the fibrous arches of the psoas head of iliopsoas (fig. 21.27). Turning backwards deep to the fibrous arches, the arteries pass between psoas and the vertebrae to the intervertebral foramina, and there give off posterior and spinal branches similar to those of the posterior intercostal arteries. Thereafter the vessels turn laterally, behind psoas and quadratus lumborum, into the substance of the lumbar fascia, and from here they pass round the body wall in the neurovascular plane to the lateral border of the rectus sheath. The arteries give off branches to the surrounding muscles and overlying skin.

The **iliolumbar artery** arises from the internal iliac but is in series with the posterior intercostal, subcostal and lumbar arteries. It passes upwards, deep to the external iliac vessels, to the medial border of psoas where it divides into two branches. The **lumbar branch** corresponds closely to the posterior branch of a lumbar artery. It gives off a spinal twig which passes through the fifth lumbar intervertebral foramen and thereafter passes backwards into sacrospinalis. The **iliac branch** turns laterally and supplies both heads of iliopsoas.

The segmental vessels associated with the sacral part of the vertebral column are the branches of the lateral sacral artery and are described on p. 21.37.

DEEP VENTRAL VESSELS OF THE BODY WALL

The **internal thoracic artery** (fig. 21.29) arises from the subclavian artery in the thoracic inlet. It passes downwards in the anterior thoracic wall lying just lateral to the sternum and immediately external to the pleura and to the intercostalis intimus when that layer is present. At the sixth intercostal space it divides into **superior epigastric** and **musculophrenic branches**.

The vessel gives off several small branches to the thoracic viscera some of which reach the upper surface of the diaphragm. But its major branches are the **anterior intercostal arteries** which run laterally in the upper six intercostal spaces, and the **perforating branches** which pierce the anterior ends of the same intercostal spaces to reach the overlying muscles, fascia, skin and mammary glands.

The **musculophrenic artery** passes downwards and laterally towards the twelfth rib along the line of origin of the diaphragm. It distributes twigs to neighbouring parts of the thoracic and abdominal walls and the diaphragm.

The **superior epigastric artery** descends through the sternocostal gap in the diaphragm and passes into the rectus sheath behind the rectus abdominis (figs. 21.32 and 21.33). It is considerably smaller than the inferior epigastric artery and anastomoses with it between the xiphoid process and the umbilicus. It gives branches to the structures in its vicinity including the overlying skin.

The **inferior epigastric artery** arises from the external iliac immediately above the midpoint of the inguinal ligament (fig. 21.46) and passes upwards and medially in the anterior abdominal wall, in the general direction of the umbilicus. The initial part of its course is in the extraperitoneal tissues and lies to the medial side of the deep inguinal ring (fig. 21.37). It pierces the transversalis fascia below the arcuate line and continues upwards within the rectus sheath lying deep to the rectus abdominis (fig. 21.32). It gives branches to the neighbouring tissues of the body wall, but only two of these are important. A small **pubic branch** passes close beside the femoral ring, either on its lateral or its medial side, and turns downwards on to the side wall of the pelvic cavity. In about 25 per cent of individuals this branch replaces the obturator artery (see below). It is then of considerable size and its proximity to the femoral ring makes it of surgical interest. In the male a small **cremasteric branch** enters the spermatic cord through the deep inguinal ring and supplies its fascial coverings.

The **deep circumflex iliac artery** arises from the external iliac close to the inferior epigastric (fig. 21.46). Running behind the inguinal ligament to the anterior superior iliac spine it ramifies amongst the muscles of the lateral abdominal wall.

BLOOD SUPPLY OF THE SUPERFICIAL TISSUES OF THE THORACIC AND ABDOMINAL WALLS

The deep vessels described in the previous sections contribute superficial branches to the overlying superficial fascia and skin, and these tend to be located in rows

on the anterior, lateral and posterior aspects of the trunk. In addition, these superficial tissues are supplied by arteries which arise from the proximal parts of the arterial stems of the upper and lower limbs (fig. 21.48). Thus the

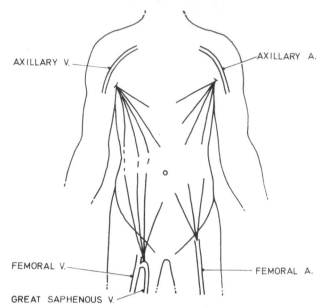

FIG. 21.48. Schematic diagram of arteries (right) and veins (left) of the superficial fascia of the trunk.

lateral thoracic artery (p. 23.35) arises from the axillary artery and runs downwards and forwards to reach the superficial fascia on the anterolateral aspect of the chest wall. Similarly, the **superficial epigastric artery** arises from the proximal part of the femoral artery and, passing over the inguinal ligament, extends upwards through the superficial fascia of the anterior abdominal wall.

The only structure of individual importance in the superficial fascia of the trunk is the **mammary gland** (p. 38. 53). It is supplied by the lateral thoracic artery, the perforating branches of the internal thoracic artery and some smaller twigs from the corresponding intercostal arteries.

ARTERIAL SUPPLY TO THE DIAPHRAGM

The diaphragm receives its blood supply in part from neighbouring arteries of the body wall, the internal thoracic, the musculophrenic and the lower posterior intercostals. In addition two phrenic arteries arise from the anterior aspect of the uppermost part of the abdominal aorta, pass laterally across the corresponding crura and ramify on the under surface of the diaphragm behind the oesophageal and vena caval openings (fig. 21.34).

ARTERIES OF THE PELVIC WALL AND THE PERINEUM

The great majority of the somatic vessels in these regions arise from the internal iliac artery opposite the upper border of the greater sciatic foramen (fig. 21.46). This vessel also gives off visceral branches and branches to the lower limb which are considered in the appropriate sections (pp. 24.38, 32.52, 38.7).

The **lateral sacral artery** represents the posterior branches of the lower segmental arteries of the body wall. It passes medially and downwards across the piriformis and the ventral primary rami of the sacral nerves towards the coccyx, and gives off four branches which pass through the pelvic sacral foramina to reach the sacral canal and the tissues on the dorsal part of the sacrum.

The **obturator artery** (fig. 21.46) runs downwards and forwards over the obturator internus and its fascia. Traversing the obturator canal it passes into the thigh and its subsequent course is described later (p. 24.38). It gives branches to the surrounding tissues including a pubic branch which ascends and anastomoses with the pubic branch of the inferior epigastric artery.

The **internal pudendal artery** runs downwards across piriformis and the ventral primary rami of the sacral nerves to the lower border of the greater sciatic foramen, through which it passes into the buttock (fig. 21.46). Here it turns downwards across the outer aspect of the ischial spine to the lesser sciatic foramen. Turning medially and forwards it passes through this opening into the perineum where it lies high on the lateral wall of the ischiorectal fossa, about 4 cm above the ischial tuber (fig. 21.46). In this position it is embedded in the fascia covering the perineal part of obturator internus, the fascial tunnel containing it being known as the **pudendal canal**. The artery continues forwards and downwards and pierces the posterior fascial wall of the deep perineal pouch (fig. 21.42). In the pouch it lies against the deep aspect of the inferior pubic ramus (fig. 21.43). The vessel gives off a few muscular twigs in the pelvic cavity and the buttock, but its main branches arise in the perineum. The **inferior rectal artery** arises in the pudendal canal and spreads medially as several branches to the anal canal and the skin of the anal triangle. In the anterior part of the ischiorectal fossa the **scrotal or labial branches** radiate forwards through the superficial perineal pouch to the corresponding areas of skin. The several branches arising in the deep perineal pouch supply structures in that region and in the superficial perineal pouch.

In addition to these three branches of the internal iliac certain other small arteries are involved in the blood supply of the pelvic cavity and perineum.

The **median sacral artery** arises from the bifurcation of the abdominal aorta. It descends along the dorsal wall of the pelvic cavity to the coccyx and anastomoses freely with the lateral sacral arteries on either side.

One or two **external pudendal arteries** arise from the femoral in the proximal part of the thigh, and, crossing the ischiopubic ramus, anastomose with the scrotal or labial branches of the internal pudendal.

VEINS OF THE BODY WALL

Main venous channels

The **axillary vein**, which receives the greater part of the blood from the upper limb, leaves the axilla to become the **subclavian vein** and this is joined in the thoracic inlet by the **internal jugular vein** descending from the tissues of head and neck (fig. 21.10). The confluence of these two large vessels at symmetrical points on either side of the midline forms the **brachiocephalic veins**, which join one another behind the first right costal cartilage to form the **superior vena cava**. Because of the eccentricity of their termination, the two brachiocephalic veins are dissimilar in course and length, that on the right being about 2·5 cm long and descending almost vertically, and that on the left being some 6 cm long and running to the right with only a slight downward inclination. The superior vena cava descends vertically to open into the right atrium of the heart.

The **femoral vein**, which carries a large part of the venous blood of the lower limb, traverses the intermediate compartment of the femoral sheath where it is joined by the great saphenous vein which drains much of the superficial fascia of the thigh and leg. Passing behind the inguinal ligament each femoral vein becomes the corresponding **external iliac vein**, and ascends along the brim of the pelvic cavity, medial to iliopsoas (figs. 21.10 and 21.46). On the right the vein begins on the medial side of the artery and later lies behind it, whereas on the left it remains medial to the artery throughout its course. The **internal iliac vein** of each side begins by the confluence of numerous tributaries at the upper border of the greater sciatic foramen and ascends to the pelvic brim behind the corresponding artery and in front of the sacro-iliac joint (fig. 21.46).

The **common iliac veins** are formed on either side by the confluence of the external and internal iliac veins (figs. 21.10, 21.27 and 21.46). On the right the origin lies behind the bifurcation of the common iliac artery whereas on the left it lies to the medial side of that vessel. Both veins extend upwards and medially and join one another, slightly to the right of the midline, on the anterior aspect of the fifth lumbar vertebral body, to form the **inferior vena cava**. The right common iliac begins behind the corresponding artery and ends on its right side, whereas that on the left extends along the medial side of the corresponding artery and then passes behind the right common iliac artery.

The **inferior vena cava** (figs. 21.10 and 21.34) passes upwards, lying slightly to the right of the median plane, in contact with the right side of the abdominal aorta and anterior to the fifth, fourth and third lumbar vertebral bodies and the fourth and third right lumbar arteries. Coming into association with the right crus of the diaphragm it begins to move forwards and to the right, becoming separated from the abdominal aorta and the vertebral column. It then continues upwards and to the right in front of the vertebral fibres of the diaphragm, and passes through the vena caval opening in the central tendon of the diaphragm. In the thorax the vein immediately opens into the right atrium of the heart.

The main venous channels described above are associated with an additional system of veins, named the azygos system, which has no direct counterpart on the arterial side.

In the **azygos system** (fig. 21.27) the **ascending lumbar vein** begins below as a branch of the corresponding common iliac vein and passes deep to the psoas head of iliopsoas. It extends upwards lying deep to these muscle fibres, in front of the transverse processes of the lumbar vertebrae and immediately lateral to the lumbar intervertebral foramina. Above it leaves the upper part of psoas in the thorax and turns medially on to the anterolateral aspect of the twelfth thoracic vertebra. Here each ascending lumbar vein is joined by the **subcostal vein** (see below) and the vessel so formed is known on the right side as the **azygos vein** and on the left as the **hemiazygos vein**.

The **azygos vein** (figs. 21.27, 21.29 and 21.45) passes upwards along the anterolateral aspect of the thoracic vertebral bodies, but separated from them by the right posterior intercostal arteries. Reaching the fourth thoracic level it arches forwards away from the vertebral column, above the root of the right lung, and opens into the posterior wall of the superior vena cava.

The **hemiazygos vein** (figs. 21.27 and 21.29) follows a similar course on the left side, where it lies behind the descending thoracic aorta and lateral to the left posterior intercostal arteries. At the eighth thoracic level, or thereabouts, it turns abruptly to the right and passing behind the aorta joins the azygos vein.

The accessory **hemiazygos vein** (fig. 21.27) runs along the left anterolateral aspect of the thoracic vertebrae from the fourth to the ninth, lying behind the aorta and lateral to the left posterior intercostal arteries. At its lower end it also turns to the right, passes behind the aorta, and joins the azygos vein.

Thus all the venous blood from the azygos system of vessels on both sides of the body eventually enters the terminal arch of the azygos vein and drains into the superior vena cava.

VENOUS DRAINAGE OF THE DEEP TISSUES OF THE THORACIC AND ABDOMINAL WALLS

The great majority of the veins involved in the venous drainage of the body wall follow courses which are similar to those of the corresponding arteries, and descriptions are required only for their terminal parts.

SEGMENTAL VESSELS

The segmental veins of the body wall correspond in name and course to the posterior intercostal, subcostal, lumbar and iliolumbar arteries, and each receives close to its termination a **posterior tributary** from sacrospinalis and the overlying skin, and a **spinal tributary** which issues from the vertebral canal through the appropriate intervertebral foramen.

The **posterior intercostal veins** lie above the corresponding arteries. Reaching the posterior end of the intercostal space (fig. 21.27) the first posterior intercostal vein of each side turns upwards in front of the neck of the first rib and in close association with the superior intercostal artery. It then turns forwards in the thoracic inlet and joins the corresponding brachiocephalic vein. The second and third veins on the left join to form the **left superior intercostal vein** which turns forwards across the left side of the arch of the aorta to join the left brachiocephalic vein.

All the remaining posterior intercostal veins drain into the azygos system. On the left the fourth to the ninth join the accessory hemiazygos, and the ninth, tenth and eleventh join the hemiazygos. On the right the second, third and fourth join and open into the beginning of the arch of the azygos vein by a common trunk named the **right superior intercostal vein**, while all the others join the azygos vein directly.

The **subcostal veins** (figs. 21.27 and 21.34) join the upper ends of the ascending lumbar veins at the commencement of the azygos and hemiazygos veins.

The **four lumbar veins** follow the corresponding arteries on to the deep aspect of the psoas head of iliopsoas (fig. 21.27). In this situation they are connected to the ascending lumbar veins. The first and second usually terminate by this connection, but the third and fourth usually continue beyond it and passing between psoas and the lumbar vertebrae, they appear from beneath the fibrous arches of psoas and join the inferior vena cava. Those of the left side pass behind the abdominal aorta.

The **iliolumbar vein** is similarly connected to the initial part of the ascending lumbar vein deep to psoas, but usually continues beyond this to join the common iliac vein.

VENTRAL VESSELS

The **superior epigastric, musculophrenic, internal thoracic, inferior epigastric** and **deep circumflex iliac veins** follow the corresponding arteries usually as venae comitantes. The **internal thoracic** drains into the brachiocephalic vein, and the **inferior epigastric** and **deep circumflex iliac** into the external iliac vein.

VENOUS DRAINAGE OF THE SUPERFICIAL TISSUES OF THE THORACIC AND ABDOMINAL WALLS

The skin and superficial fascia of the trunk are drained in large measure by the terminal tributaries of the deep veins. In addition, however, the anterolateral aspect of the thorax and the anterior aspect of the abdomen are drained by the lateral thoracic and superficial epigastric veins (fig. 21.48). The **lateral thoracic vein** is formed by the confluence of tributaries from the superficial fascia as far down as the umbilicus, and passes upwards to the axilla to join the axillary vein. The **superficial epigastric vein** is formed by tributaries from below the umbilicus. It passes downwards into the proximal part of the thigh where it joins the terminal part of the great saphenous vein (p. 24.41).

Thus the venous drainage of the superficial fascia presents a kind of watershed at the level of the umbilicus. But this watershed is not complete; many connections exist between the lateral thoracic and superficial epigastric vessels and frequently the two are continuous and form the **thoraco-epigastric venous channel**. When the venous drainage by the inferior vena cava is obstructed, the blood may return by way of the femoral, great saphenous, superficial epigastric, lateral thoracic, axillary, subclavian, and brachiocephalic veins to the superior vena cava.

VENOUS DRAINAGE OF THE DIAPHRAGM

This corresponds closely to the arterial supply. The **phrenic veins** open into the upper part of the inferior vena cava.

VENOUS DRAINAGE OF THE PELVIC WALL AND THE PERINEUM

The **lateral sacral, obturator** and **internal pudendal veins** follow the courses of the corresponding arteries, usually as venae comitantes, and drain into the internal iliac vein.

The **median sacral venae comitantes** join either the beginning of the inferior vena cava or the left common iliac vein. The two **external pudendal veins** pass laterally into the thigh and join the terminal part of the great saphenous vein.

SOMATIC LYMPHATICS OF THE TRUNK

Main lymphatic trunks

The terminal lymphatic trunks which drain into the great veins at the root of the neck are shown in figs. 21.49 and 22.35. The thoracic parts of the thoracic duct and the right bronchomediastinal trunk are described below.

The sacculated lower end of the **thoracic duct** is named the **cisterna chyli**. About 5 to 8 cm in length, it lies within the aortic opening in the diaphragm, on the right side of the aorta. It has the first and second lumbar vertebrae and the corresponding right lumbar

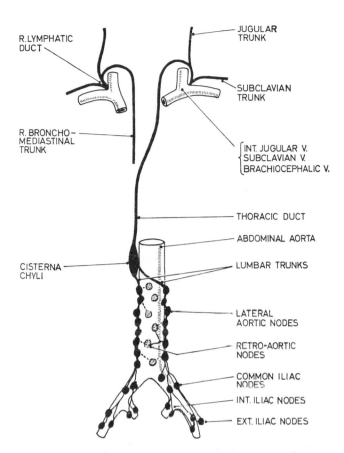

FIG. 21.49. The lymphatics of the body wall. Refer to fig. 21.27.

arteries behind it, and the right crus of the diaphragm on its right side (figs. 21.27 and 21.34). Its lower end receives the right and left **lumbar trunks** (fig. 21.49) which drain lymph from the lower limbs, the abdominal wall below the umbilicus, the genitourinary system and that part of the gut supplied by the inferior mesenteric artery; and the **intestinal trunk** which drains lymph from the territory supplied by the coeliac and superior mesenteric arteries. The upper end of the cisterna chyli is continuous with the thoracic duct.

The duct runs upwards, in front of the thoracic vertebral column, to the thoracic inlet where it opens into the junction between the left internal jugular and subclavian veins. In the lower part of its course it is slightly to the right of the median plane, between the azygos vein and the aorta, and anterior to the right posterior intercostal arteries (fig. 21.27). Approximately at the middle of the thorax it moves to the left of the midline, and lies close to the accessory hemiazygos vein and the aorta and anterior to the right posterior intercostal arteries. Above, it rests on the left border of the longus cervicis muscle and is in close association with the left recurrent laryngeal nerve.

The **right bronchomediastinal trunk** begins about the

middle of the thorax and runs upwards in close association with the azygos vein. Thereafter it continues along the right border of the longus cervicis muscle to the root of the neck.

Lymph vessels and nodes of the deep tissues of the thoracic wall

In the anterior thoracic wall, the lymph vessels run with the anterior intercostal arteries and veins and reach the **internal thoracic chain** of lymph nodes. These are placed along the course of the internal thoracic vessels, and their efferents ascend to join the right lymphatic duct or the thoracic duct in the root of the neck.

The lymph vessels of the lateral and posterior parts of the thoracic wall follow the posterior intercostal arteries and veins to reach the **intercostal** lymph nodes in the posterior parts of the intercostal spaces. The efferents from the upper intercostal nodes on the right side join the right bronchomediastinal trunk, whereas those of all the other intercostal nodes join the thoracic duct.

Lymph vessels and nodes of the deep tissues of the abdominal and pelvic cavities and the perineum

The lymph vessels from these tissues follow the corresponding blood vessels and the majority reach two long chains of lymph nodes placed along the abdominal aorta and the common, external and internal iliac vessels. The efferents of these chains are the lumbar trunks which join the cisterna chyli (fig. 21.49).

From the deep tissues of the anterior abdominal wall above the umbilicus the lymph vessels follow the superior epigastric artery and vein to reach the internal thoracic lymph nodes. From the deep tissues of the lower part of the anterior abdominal wall, the lymph vessels follow the inferior epigastric and deep circumflex iliac arteries to reach the external iliac lymph nodes.

The lymph vessels from the deep tissue of the lateral and posterior parts of the abdominal wall pass alongside the lumbar arteries and veins to the lateral aortic and retro-aortic lymph nodes. Lymph vessels from the walls of the pelvic cavity and from the deep tissues of the perineum run with the corresponding arteries and veins to the internal iliac lymph nodes.

Lymph vessels of the superficial tissues of the trunk

These lymph vessels are in communication with the deep vessels described above and throughout their course they follow closely the arteries and veins of the superficial fascia (fig. 21.48). Those from areas below the umbilicus, including the superficial tissues of the perineum, converge on the inguinal nodes at the root of the lower limb (p. 24.42). Those from areas above the umbilicus, including the mammary gland, converge on the axillary nodes at the root of the upper limb (p. 23.38).

NERVES OF THE TRUNK

The nerves of the trunk contain four functional types of fibres. **General somatic efferent fibres** are concerned solely with the innervation of voluntary muscle fibres. **General visceral efferent fibres** constitute the **autonomic system** and may be either of **sympathetic** or **parasympathetic** type. Parasympathetic fibres in the trunk are concerned only with the innervation of the viscera. On the other hand sympathetic fibres are involved in the innervation both of the viscera and certain somatic structures, namely, the involuntary muscle fibres associated with arterial walls, the dartos muscle in the superficial fascia, the arrectores pilorum muscles and the sweat glands of the skin. **General somatic afferent fibres** carry sensory impulses from many tissues in the body wall. **General visceral afferent fibres** transmit sensory impulses from viscera and from the walls of both visceral and somatic blood vessels.

GROSS FORM OF THE NERVOUS SYSTEM OF THE TRUNK

The **thoracic nerves** emerge through the intervertebral foramina of that region. Their ventral primary rami pass into the intercostal spaces while their dorsal primary rami turn backwards between the superior costotransverse ligaments and the vertebral arches into the sacrospinalis muscle (fig. 21.29). The **lumbar nerves** appear through the corresponding intervertebral foramina deep to the psoas head of iliopsoas. The ventral primary rami run laterally into the body wall whereas the dorsal primary rami turn backwards between adjacent transverse processes into the sacrospinalis muscle (fig. 21.29). The **upper four sacral nerves** leave the sacral canal through bony canals from which the primary rami emerge through the pelvic and dorsal sacral foramina (figs. 21.16, 21.17 and 21.46). The **fifth sacral** nerve emerges from the vertebral canal through an aperture which is bordered, in front, by the sacrococcygeal intervertebral disc and, behind, by the sacral and coccygeal cornua and the sacrococcygeal membrane (fig. 21.17). At this point it lies outside the pelvic cavity on the outer surface of the coccygeus muscle, and divides into its primary rami. The dorsal ramus turns backwards into sacrospinalis, whereas the ventral turns forwards, and passes through coccygeus and the sacrospinous ligament into the pelvic cavity (fig. 21.46). The tiny **coccygeal nerve** emerges from the lowest part of the vertebral canal by piercing the sacrococcygeal membrane, and the courses of its primary rami are similar to those noted in the fifth sacral nerve (figs. 21.17 and 21.46).

The **sympathetic trunks** (figs. 21.27, 21.45 and 21.50) extend, on either side of the vertebral column, from the base of the skull to the coccyx. Developmentally the

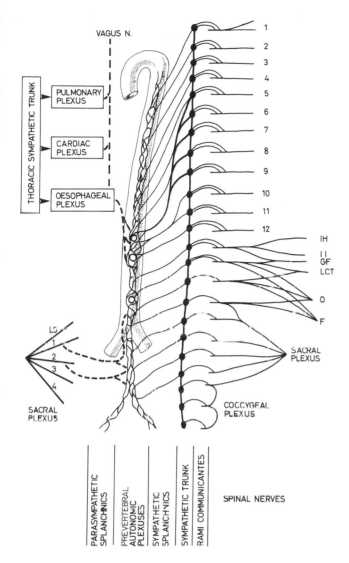

Labels in figure:

VAGUS N.

THORACIC SYMPATHETIC TRUNK

PULMONARY PLEXUS

CARDIAC PLEXUS

OESOPHAGEAL PLEXUS

1 2 3 4 5 6 7 8 9 10 11 12

IH
I I
GF
LCT

O

F

SACRAL PLEXUS

L5
1
2
3
4

SACRAL PLEXUS

COCCYGEAL PLEXUS

PARASYMPATHETIC SPLANCHNICS

PREVERTEBRAL AUTONOMIC PLEXUSES

SYMPATHETIC SPLANCHNICS

SYMPATHETIC TRUNK

RAMI COMMUNICANTES

SPINAL NERVES

FIG. 21.50. Schematic diagram of distribution of autonomic nerves to autonomic plexuses and spinal nerves.

enters the abdominal cavity by passing beneath the medial arcuate ligament (fig. 21.34). It then passes downwards, anterior to the lumbar vertebral column and the lumbar vessels, and just medial to the fibrous arches of psoas (fig. 21.27). The right trunk is partially covered by the inferior vena cava and the left trunk by the abdominal aorta. Below, the trunk passes behind the corresponding common iliac vessels and turns over the sacral promontory into the pelvic cavity. Here it extends downwards and medially on the pelvic surface of the sacrum, lying just to the medial side of the pelvic sacral foramina.

The **prevertebral autonomic plexuses** (fig. 21.50) are dense and extensive collections of autonomic nerve fibres, of both the sympathetic and the parasympathetic type, which are interspersed with autonomic nerve cells. Where the concentration of nerve cells is high, that part of the plexus is called a ganglion. In the thorax, the **thoracic aortic plexus** lies along the wall of the aorta, and additional plexuses, such as the **cardiac, pulmonary** and **oesophageal**, are closely associated with individual viscera. In the abdominal cavity the **pre-aortic plexus** extends along the anterior aspect of the abdominal aorta and its branch plexuses pass along the several branches of that vessel to the viscera with which they are associated. At the bifurcation of the abdominal aorta the pre-aortic plexus is continued downwards, in and around the median plane, as the **hypogastric plexus**. This passes anterior to the left common iliac vein and, crossing the sacral promontory, descends on the pelvic aspect of the sacrum between the sympathetic trunks. In the lower part of the pelvic cavity the hypogastric plexus divides into two symmetrical **pelvic plexuses**, which extend forwards across the pelvic diaphragm on either side of the midline pelvic viscera.

Connections of the sympathetic trunk

Preganglionic sympathetic axons arise from cell bodies in the intermediolateral grey column of the spinal cord, between T1 and L2 or L3 segments. The fibres leave the cord through the ventral roots of the corresponding spinal nerves and run from the ventral primary ramus of each of these nerves in a **white ramus communicans** to the sympathetic chain. Collectively the fibres of these white rami constitute the **thoracolumbar sympathetic outflow**. Fibres are distributed from the sympathetic trunks by several routes.

(1) Via **spinal nerves**. Every ganglion on the sympathetic trunk sends postganglionic fibres through one or more **grey rami communicantes** to the ventral primary ramus or rami with which it is associated developmentally. In the thoracic region (figs. 21.27 and 21.47) the rami (grey and white) lie in the posterior ends of the intercostal spaces and run laterally from the sympathetic trunk for a distance of about 1 cm. In the lumbar region (fig. 21.27), because of the more anterior position of the sympathetic

number of ganglia corresponds to the number of spinal nerves, but fusion of adjacent ganglia reduces the number in each region. The definitive number in the cervical region is three, in the thoracic region it is usually eleven or twelve, in the lumbar region four and in the sacral, four or five. The lower ends of the sympathetic trunks join in front of the coccyx in the single **ganglion impar**. The cervical part of the trunk is described on p. 22.33. The thoracic part of each trunk (figs. 21.27, 21.45 and 21.47) lies anterior to the heads of the ribs and anterior to the posterior intercostal vessels as they lie in the posterior ends of the intercostal spaces. It is thus lateral to the vertebral column and behind and lateral to the azygos or hemiazygos veins (fig. 21.29). In the lower part of the thorax the trunk inclines medially on to the uppermost part of the psoas head of iliopsoas (fig. 21.27), and

trunk, the rami are about three times as long, and extend backwards with the lumbar vessels deep to the fibrous arches of the psoas head of iliopsoas. In the pelvic cavity the rami are very short and run laterally from the sympathetic trunk on the pelvic aspects of the sacrum and coccyx.

(2) Preganglionic fibres pass through **direct visceral (splanchnic) nerves** which run forwards and usually downwards to reach the prevertebral autonomic plexuses (fig. 21.50). The thoracic plexuses receive branches from both the cervical and thoracic ganglia. The pre-aortic plexus receives splanchnic branches from the lower thoracic and lumbar ganglia. The contributions from the lower thoracic ganglia are three large branches, which are named the **greater**, the **lesser** and the **least splanchnic nerves** and arise respectively from T5–9, T10 and 11, and T12. They run downwards on the lateral aspect of the vertebral bodies between the azygos or hemiazygos vein and the sympathetic trunk. The greater and lesser splanchnic nerves pierce the corresponding crus of the diaphragm (fig. 21.34), while the least splanchnic passes behind the medial arcuate ligament just medial to the sympathetic trunk. The hypogastric and pelvic plexuses receive fine visceral branches from the lumbar and sacral parts of the sympathetic trunk.

(3) Postganglionic fibres run through **direct vascular branches** which pass from the sympathetic trunk to walls of many large arteries.

Parasympathetic connections with the prevertebral autonomic plexuses

(1) Several large branches arise from the ventral primary rami of S2 and 3 within the pelvic cavity and are named the **pelvic splanchnic nerves** (figs. 21.39 and 21.50). These are quite distinct from the grey rami communicantes which join the ventral primary rami to the sympathetic chain and they must also be differentiated from the visceral or splanchnic branches of the sympathetic chain which pass to the hypogastric and pelvic plexuses. The pelvic splanchnic nerves are parasympathetic in character and run directly from the spinal nerves into the hypogastric and pelvic plexuses.

(2) The **vagus** or **tenth cranial nerve** descends from the brain stem, through the neck and into the thorax and abdomen (figs. 21.50 and 22.31). It gives all the parasympathetic fibres to the thoracic autonomic plexuses and further fibres (the gastric nerves) to the pre-aortic plexus.

COURSE AND DISTRIBUTION OF THE SPINAL NERVES

Each spinal nerve carries several different functional types of nerve fibres, namely, general somatic efferent and afferent fibres, a few general visceral afferent fibres and general visceral efferent fibres of sympathetic type, inner-

vating sweat glands, and involuntary muscle fibres in blood vessels, skin and superficial fascia.

Dorsal primary rami

All the dorsal primary rami supply the sacrospinalis muscle. In addition, with the exception of those arising from the fourth and fifth lumbar and certain cervical nerves (p. 22.27) which are devoid of cutaneous fibres, they innervate a continuous strip of skin on the posterior aspect of the trunk (fig. 21.51). This extends from the posterior part of the scalp to the tip of the coccyx; it

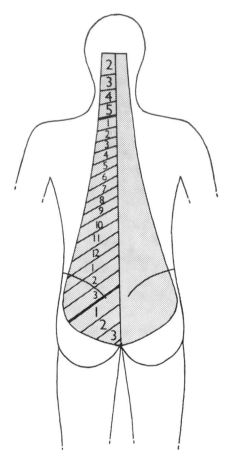

FIG. 21.51. Cutaneous distribution of the dorsal primary rami of spinal nerves.

widens progressively from above down as far as the middle of the sacrum, where it reaches the lateral aspect of the buttock, and thereafter narrows rapidly. The cutaneous branches of the dorsal primary rami exhibit a general downward inclination which becomes increasingly acute as far as L3. Those derived from L1, 2 and 3 cross the posterior part of the iliac crest and run downwards and laterally across the upper part of the buttock. Those derived from S1, 2 and 3 supply the medial part of the buttock, and those from the lowest three spinal nerves supply the skin of the natal cleft over the coccyx (fig. 21.53).

Ventral primary rami

The basically segmental distribution of the ventral rami in the trunk is modified in the first and second thoracic nerves, and in the nerves between the first lumbar and the fourth sacral, by the partial or complete incorporation of these rami into the plexuses of the upper and lower limbs. From the third to the sixth thoracic nerve each ventral ramus runs its entire course in the thoracic wall within an intercostal space (fig. 21.29). On the other hand, from the seventh to the twelfth thoracic, the ventral rami begin their course in the thoracic wall, but later emerge from the intercostal spaces into the abdominal wall.

The **ventral rami of T3–T6 are intercostal nerves**. Each extends along the length of the corresponding intercostal space (fig. 21.29) lying in the upper part of its neurovascular plane (fig. 21.45b) and immediately below the corresponding intercostal arteries and veins. Eventually it passes anterior to the internal thoracic artery and pierces the overlying tissues as a spray of anterior cutaneous twigs. The branches are as follows:

(1) A collateral branch arises from the proximal part of the nerve and follows it in the lower part of the same intercostal space to end as additional anterior cutaneous twigs.

(2) A lateral cutaneous branch arises near the angles of the ribs and follows the parent nerve to the midaxillary plane. There it pierces the overlying muscles, in vertical alignment with the corresponding branches of the other intercostal nerves, and divides into anterior and posterior parts.

(3) Motor branches to the corresponding intercostal muscles and sensory branches to the related part of the parietal pleura arise throughout the course of the nerve.

The anterior and lateral cutaneous branches given off by one of these intercostal nerves together supply a strip of skin, which is continuous posteriorly with the skin area supplied by the corresponding dorsal primary ramus. They also 'overlap' on to the skin areas associated with the nerves immediately above and below. Consequently interruption of one of these nerves does not result in an area of complete anaesthesia.

The **ventral ramus of T1** (fig. 21.47) passes behind the superior intercostal artery (p. 21.34) in the interval between the necks of the first and second ribs and there divides into a large **ascending branch** and a small **first intercostal nerve**. The latter extends round the neurovascular plane of the first intercostal space and is concerned purely with the innervation of the muscles of the first intercostal space and the related parietal pleura. Because it carries no cutaneous fibres it has neither lateral nor anterior cutaneous branches. The lateral part of the first intercostal space is related to the axilla, and is thus not directly covered by skin, whereas the skin which covers the anterior part of the space is supplied by the supraclavicular nerves which descend from the ventral rami of C3 and 4. The ascending branch passes upwards and laterally across the neck of the first rib, lateral to the sympathetic trunk and the superior intercostal vessels. Turning laterally on to the upper surface of the first rib it joins the ventral ramus of C8 to form the lower trunk of the brachial plexus, and is thereafter distributed to the tissues of the upper limb.

The **ventral ramus of T2** is atypical only in respect of its lateral cutaneous branch. This emerges through the chest wall in line with those of the succeeding intercostal nerves. However, it does not divide into anterior and posterior branches, but crosses the axilla to be distributed to the skin on the upper half of the medial aspect of the arm. Because of this distribution it is named the **intercostobrachial nerve**.

The **ventral rami of T7–T11** extend laterally as intercostal nerves along their respective intercostal spaces. Reaching the anterior ends of these spaces, however, they pass between the adjacent digitations of the diaphragm and those of transversus abdominis and enter the abdominal wall in the neurovascular plane between transversus abdominis and internal oblique. Here the nerves diverge from one another, the seventh and eighth passing upwards and medially, the ninth horizontally and the tenth and eleventh downwards and medially. At the lateral border of the rectus sheath each nerve pierces the posterior lamella of the aponeurosis of internal oblique (fig. 21.35). It then traverses the substance of rectus abdominis and the anterior wall of the sheath to reach the overlying skin as the terminal **anterior cutaneous branch**. The anterior cutaneous branch of T10 lies about the level of the umbilicus. Like the higher intercostal nerves each member of this group gives off both **collateral** and **lateral cutaneous branches**. The former run parallel to and below the parent nerves and terminate like them as additional anterior cutaneous branches. The lateral cutaneous branches emerge through the overlying muscles in the midaxillary plane, and consequently in vertical alignment with the higher lateral cutaneous branches. Thereafter they divide into anterior and posterior divisions and, in association with the corresponding anterior cutaneous branches and the corresponding dorsal primary rami, they supply continuous strips of skin extending in succession round one half of the body wall. As was noted in the thoracic wall, each strip is additionally innervated by the nerves immediately above and below it.

The lower intercostal nerves also supply their respective intercostal muscles, the three flat muscles of the abdominal wall and rectus abdominis. Throughout their course they supply sensory twigs to the adjacent regions of the parietal pleura and the parietal peritoneum.

The **subcostal nerve** is the ventral ramus of T12. It is in series with the intercostal nerves and has a similar distribution. It runs across the quadratus lumborum immediately below the subcostal vessels and the twelfth rib and, passing deep to the lateral arcuate ligament, reaches the abdominal aspect of the lumbar fascia (fig. 21.34). Piercing this fascia, it enters the neurovascular plane between transversus abdominis and internal oblique, and passes round the abdominal wall. It then passes through the overlying aponeuroses and ends as an anterior cutaneous branch. Throughout its course the nerve gives motor branches to the flat abdominal muscles and sensory filaments to the parietal peritoneum. The collateral branch of the subcostal nerve follows a course similar to those at higher levels. However, the lateral cutaneous branch is rather atypical. It pierces the internal and external oblique muscles in line with the rest of its kind, and divides into anterior and posterior parts, but many of its filaments descend over the iliac crest. Consequently the strip of skin supplied by the dorsal and ventral rami of T12 is not entirely confined to the body wall but overlaps on to the anterolateral aspect of the thigh immediately below the anterior superior iliac spine (fig. 21.52).

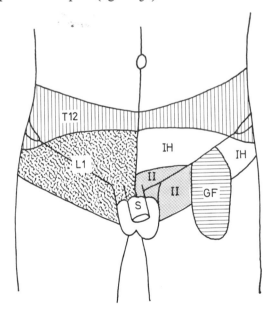

FIG. 21.52. Cutaneous distribution of the ventral primary rami of T12 and L1. IH, Iliohypogastric; II, ilio-inguinal; GF, genitofemoral; S, sacral nerves.

The **ventral rami of L1–L4** run laterally into the substance of the psoas head of iliopsoas (fig. 21.27). Within this muscle L4 gives off a descending branch which becomes incorporated into the sacral plexus (p. 21.45). On the other hand, the rest of L4 and the ventral rami of L1, 2 and 3 form the **lumbar plexus**. This plexus is comparatively simple and involves the separation of the roots into a number of divisions and the formation of branches from one or more of these divisions (fig. 21.50). The branches so formed emerge from the lateral, anterior and medial aspects of psoas.

(1) Direct motor branches arise from the roots of the plexus to the quadratus lumborum and the psoas head of iliopsoas.

(2) The **iliohypogastric nerve** derives its fibres entirely from L1. Emerging from the upper part of the lateral border of psoas, it runs outside the fascial envelope of the abdominal cavity (p. 21.26), across quadratus lumborum and the lumbar fascia (fig. 21.27). It pierces the transversus abdominis immediately above the iliac crest (fig. 21.37) and runs forwards in the neurovascular plane of the abdominal wall. It pierces internal oblique about 2 cm medial to the anterior superior iliac spine (fig. 21.36b) and finally appears through the aponeurosis of external oblique a little above the superficial inguinal ring (p. 21.24) as a terminal anterior cutaneous branch. In its course the nerve supplies the adjacent part of the parietal peritoneum and gives motor branches to the flat abdominal muscles but not to rectus abdominis. Its lateral cutaneous branch pierces the internal and external oblique muscles, in line with those of the thoracic nerves, and descends over the iliac crest, behind the lateral cutaneous branch of the subcostal nerve, to supply skin in the thigh below the anterior superior iliac spine (fig. 21.52).

(3) The **ilio-inguinal nerve** also arises solely from L1. It emerges from the lateral border of psoas immediately below the iliohypogastric nerve and passes downwards and laterally, outside the fascial envelope of the abdomen, and across the quadratus lumborum, the iliac crest and the upper fibres of the iliacus head of iliopsoas (fig. 21.27). Recrossing the iliac crest, it pierces transversus abdominis and internal oblique in rapid succession just above the anterior superior iliac spine (figs. 21.36 and 21.37) and continues downwards and medially into close association with the spermatic cord, or the round ligament. The nerve then follows the spermatic cord through the superficial inguinal ring and divides into cutaneous branches (fig. 21.31). These are distributed to the skin of the thigh below the medial end of the inguinal ligament and to the proximal part of the penis and scrotum, or the mons pubis and the anterior part of the labium majus (fig. 21.52). The ilio-inguinal nerve gives off neither a collateral nor a lateral cutaneous branch, but throughout its course distributes twigs to the flat abdominal muscles and the parietal peritoneum.

(4) The **genitofemoral nerve** is formed by contributions from both L1 and L2. It emerges from the anterior surface of psoas and, turning downwards, divides almost immediately into femoral and genital branches (fig. 21.27). Unlike the other branches of the lumbar plexus, these traverse the fascial envelope of the abdomen and come to lie in the extraperitoneal tissue (fig. 21.38). This peculiarity is associated with the fact that each branch eventually leaves the abdominal cavity within a protrusion of the fascial envelope. The femoral branch, which carries

only cutaneous fibres, descends just lateral to the external iliac artery, and follows that vessel into the lateral compartment of the femoral sheath. Passing through the anterior wall of the sheath and the overlying fascia lata, (fig. 21.38) it supplies a considerable area of skin below the central part of the inguinal ligament (fig. 21.52). The genital branch, which carries only motor fibres, descends lateral to the femoral branch. It turns forwards across the deep aspect of the inguinal ligament and passes through the deep inguinal ring into the spermatic cord, where it supplies the cremaster muscle.

The cutaneous distribution of the first lumbar nerve (figs. 21.51 and 21.52) comprises the skin areas supplied by the dorsal primary ramus and the iliohypogastric and ilio-inguinal nerves, together with the upper part of the area supplied by the genitofemoral nerve.

(5) The **lateral cutaneous nerve** of the thigh (fig. 21.27) arises from L2 and L3 and leaves the lateral border of psoas below the level of the iliac crest. It runs between iliacus and the fascial envelope of the abdomen to the anterior superior iliac spine and, thereafter, passes beneath the lateral end of the inguinal ligament into the thigh.

(6) The **femoral nerve** (fig. 21.27) is the largest branch of the lumbar plexus and draws its fibres from L2, 3 and 4. It emerges from the lateral border of psoas and descends, outside the fascial envelope of the abdomen, in the deep groove between the psoas and iliacus heads of iliopsoas. The nerve then passes deep to the inguinal ligament and enters the thigh outside and lateral to the femoral sheath. In the abdomen it supplies the iliacus. Its later course and distribution are described with the lower limb (chap. 24).

(7) The **obturator nerve** is formed by branches from L2, 3 and 4 and emerges from the medial border of psoas (figs. 21.39 and 21.46). It turns over the brim of the pelvic cavity, passing behind the common iliac vessels and lateral to the internal iliac vessels. Thereafter it extends downwards and forwards between the obturator internus muscle and its fascia, and gradually approaches the obturator vessels which lie below it. It then passes through the obturator canal into the medial part of the thigh where all its branches arise. In about 30 per cent of the population some of the fibres of the obturator nerve follow a separate course as the **accessory obturator nerve**. When present, this follows the medial border of psoas and passes into the thigh between the inguinal ligament and the superior pubic ramus.

The **ventral rami of L5, S1, 2, 3 and 4** take part, together with the descending branch of the ventral ramus of L4, in the formation of the **sacral plexus** (figs. 21.39 and 21.50).

The descending branch of L4 emerges from the medial border of psoas in close association with the obturator nerve and the iliolumbar artery, and turns downwards over the brim of the pelvis behind the common iliac vessels. The ventral ramus of L5 runs laterally from its intervertebral foramen, into the interval between the fifth lumbar transverse process and the ala of the sacrum. It then turns downwards into the pelvic cavity and joins the descending branch of L4 to form the **lumbosacral trunk**. This trunk continues downwards between the sacro-iliac joint and the bifurcation of the common iliac vessels, and then across the surface of piriformis to the lower part of the greater sciatic foramen. The ventral rami of S1, 2 and 3 emerge through the upper three pelvic sacral foramina. That of S1 is large and comparable in size to the lumbosacral trunk, that of S2 is considerably smaller and that of S3 smaller still. The three nerves pass laterally across piriformis and converge with the lumbosacral trunk on the lower part of the greater sciatic foramen. The ventral ramus of S4 is very small. It emerges through the lowest pelvic sacral foramen and gives off (like the ventral ramus of L4) a descending branch. The nerve then extends laterally to join the other roots of the sacral plexus. Close to the lower part of the greater sciatic foramen the roots of the plexus unite to form a broad band from which the branches of the plexus arise. The great majority of these branches are concerned with the innervation of the lower limb tissues (chap. 24). The branches considered below are those which innervate abdominal, pelvic and perineal tissues.

The **pelvic splanchnic nerves** are parasympathetic branches arising from the ventral rami of S2 and 3.

Muscular branches arise from the roots of the plexus, and supply piriformis (S1 and 2), coccygeus (S4) and levator ani (S4).

The **perineal branch of S4** arises from the corresponding root of the plexus and passes through the pelvic diaphragm between coccygeus and levator ani into the ischiorectal fossa. It supplies cutaneous filaments to the perineal skin around the anus and contributes to the innervation of the anal musculature.

The **nerve to obturator internus** arises from L5, S1 and 2 in the greater sciatic foramen. It first passes into the buttock where it lies on the outer aspect of the ischial spine, lateral to the internal pudendal vessels. At the lower border of the ischial spine it turns forwards through the lesser sciatic foramen into the perineum and runs into the substance of the obturator internus (fig. 21.39).

The **pudendal nerve** is formed at the lower part of the greater sciatic foramen by contributions from S2, 3 and 4 and follows the same course as the previous nerve into the ischiorectal fossa, except that it lies on the medial side of the internal pudendal vessels. Thereafter it follows the internal pudendal vessels through the pudendal canal and the deep perineal pouch (p. 21.33, figs. 21.39 and 21.43). In the pudendal canal the nerve gives off a spray of **inferior rectal branches** which follow the corresponding arteries across the ischiorectal fossa towards the anal canal. They are distributed to the musculature and lining membrane of the anal canal, and to the skin around the anus. In the same region a spray of **scrotal** or **labial branches** extend forwards into the superficial perineal pouch and supply the skin of the urogenital triangle and the distal part of the scrotum. In the cutaneous distribution of the pudendal nerve, S2 fibres are distributed anteriorly and S4 fibres posteriorly. The other branches of the pudendal nerve are concerned with the innervation of the penis or clitoris, the urethra and the muscles associated with these structures (chap. 38).

The **ventral rami of S5** and the **coccygeal nerve** are very small. Initially they lie on the outer surface of coccygeus, but passing through that muscle they enter the pelvic cavity just lateral to the coccyx. There the ventral ramus of S5 divides into ascending and descending branches which form loops with the descending branch of S4 and the coccygeal nerve respectively. These two loops constitute the **coccygeal plexus** (fig. 21.39). From the plexus, minute branches arise which pierce coccygeus and supply the perineal skin between the tip of the coccyx and the anus (fig. 21.53).

Cutaneous innervation of the perineum and scrotum
(fig. 21.53)

The skin immediately behind the tip of the coccyx is innervated by the dorsal primary rami of the lower sacral and the coccygeal nerves. That in front of the coccyx and over the anococcygeal ligament is supplied by branches of the coccygeal plexus. The skin around the anus, over the

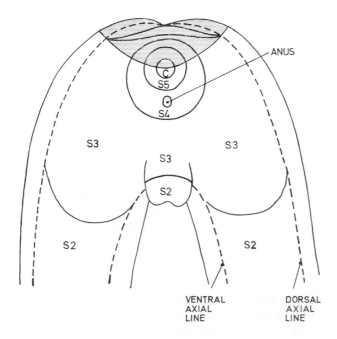

FIG. 21.53. Segmental cutaneous innervation of the perineum. Dark areas dorsal rami, white areas ventral rami.

central tendon of the perineum and over the urogenital triangle and the distal part of the scrotum is innervated by the pudendal nerve, the perineal branch of S4, and by the perineal branch of the posterior femoral cutaneous nerve (p. 24.33). These nerves are not associated with individual areas. Their distributions overlap so that successive areas from the scrotum to the anococcygeal ligament are supplied by the ventral rami of S2, 3 and 4, in that order (fig. 21.53). The proximal part of the scrotal skin is innervated by fibres from the ventral ramus of L1 through the ilio-inguinal nerve.

SURFACE ANATOMY

In clinical practice it is necessary to relate particular structures in the walls and cavities of the trunk to its skin surface. With a few important exceptions soft tissue features on the trunk, such as the nipples and the umbilicus, are too variable in position to be used for this purpose, and in practice the deep structures are usually related to bony features which can be palpated through the skin.

However three soft tissue features are of value. Unless there is a great deal of fat in the superficial fascia, the lateral border of the rectus abdominis muscle can usually be seen as a slightly curved ridge on the anterior abdominal wall. This ridge is named the **linea semilunaris** and it crosses the costal margin over the ninth costal cartilage. The position of the **inguinal ligament** can usually be seen and felt as a round ridge between the abdomen and the thigh. When the hip joint is flexed the ridge is straight, whereas when the hip joint is extended the ridge is somewhat convex towards the thigh. On the posterior aspect of the trunk, and immediately above the natal cleft which separates the buttocks, paired dimples on the skin usually mark the positions of the **posterior superior iliac spines** of the hip bones. These overlie the upper parts of the corresponding sacro-iliac joints.

Many bony features can be palpated through the skin. The **jugular notch**, **sternal angle**, **xiphisternal joint** and the **lateral border of the body of the sternum** are all readily palpable.

Most of the **ribs** and **costal cartilages** can be palpated on the anterior aspect of the thoracic wall. However, it is very important to note that the ease with which the first rib can be felt varies greatly in different individuals. Consequently, it is usual, in numbering the ribs, to begin from the second costal cartilage, which can always be identified by its relationship to the sternal angle (see p. 21.8).

When the **costal margin** is palpated the extremities of the eighth, ninth and tenth costal cartilages can usually be identified and the free end of the eleventh costal cartilage can be clearly felt, but the identification of the twelfth costal cartilage depends very much on the length of the corresponding rib.

In the lower part of the trunk, the upper border of the **pubic symphysis,** the **pubic crest and tubercle,** the **anterior superior iliac spine,** the **iliac crest** and its **tuberosity,** and the **posterior superior iliac spine** can all be felt through the skin. In the male the pubic crest and tubercle are most readily palpated by invaginating the thin skin of the scrotum behind the testis and the spermatic cord.

In the perineum, the inferior border of the **pubic symphysis,** the inferior margins of the **ischiopubic rami,** the **ischial tubers** and the **coccyx** can be palpated.

On the posterior aspect of the trunk the **spines of the thoracic and lumbar vertebrae** and the **posterior surface of the sacrum** can be identified. In numbering these features it must be noted that, although most of the cervical spines are impalpable, the highest spine which is readily palpable, in most individuals, is that of the seventh cervical vertebra.

Surface anatomy of the anterior abdominal wall

(1) The **lateral border of the rectus abdominis** is identified by the **linea semilunaris.**

(2) The muscle fibres of the **external oblique** may be demarcated from the aponeurosis by a line running from the anterior superior iliac spine towards the umbilicus and, thereafter, vertically upwards to the ninth costal cartilage.

(3) The musculo-aponeurotic junction of the **internal oblique** muscle is gently convex forwards. It begins at the tenth costal cartilage and becomes confluent with the linea semilunaris in the lower part of the abdominal wall.

(4) The aponeurosis of the **transversus abdominis** muscle begins along a line which is concave forwards, and extends from the xiphoid process to the middle part of the inguinal ligament.

(5) The **inguinal canal** is about 5 cm long and lies parallel to, and a little above, the inguinal ligament. It begins at the **deep inguinal ring** which is 1 cm above the midinguinal point, and ends at the **superficial inguinal ring,** whose centre is 1 cm above and lateral to the pubic tubercle.

(6) The **inferior epigastric artery** arises immediately above the midinguinal point and runs in the direction of the umbilicus.

Surface lines and regions of the trunk

The palpable bony points of the trunk may be used to construct two horizontal and two vertical planes which divide the body wall into regions (fig. 21.54).

The horizontal planes are the **transpyloric plane,** which lies midway between the sternal notch and the upper border of the pubic symphysis and the **transtubercular plane** which traverse the tubercles of the iliac crests. The

right and left **lateral planes** extend vertically through the midinguinal points which are the points, on the inguinal ligaments, midway between the pubic symphysis and the anterior superior iliac spines. The midclavicular planes usually lie lateral to the lateral planes. The three abdominal regions which lie between the lateral planes are named **epigastric, umbilical** and **hypogastric** from above down, while the three corresponding regions which lie lateral to each lateral plane are described as **hypochondriac, lumbar** and **iliac.**

Projection of the vertebrae on the anterior body wall

(1) The sternal notch corresponds to the lower border of T2 in the adult male and the upper border of T3 in the adult female. At birth the sternum lies at a relatively higher level.

(2) The transpyloric plane traverses the lower border of L1.

(3) The transtubercular plane cuts the upper part of L5.

(4) In standing the upper border of the pubic symphysis is level with the sacrococcygeal joint.

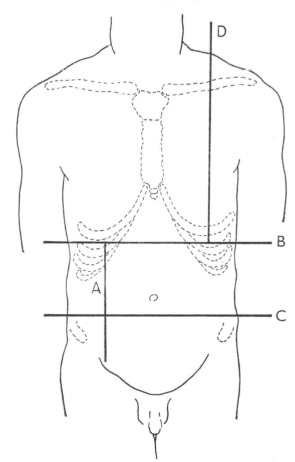

FIG. 21.54. Artificial planes which are used as surface markings for the abdomen and thorax. A, lateral plane; B, transpyloric plane; C, transtubercular plane; D, midclavicular plane.

Chapter 22
Head and neck

The head can be considered as being made up of two parts:

(1) the upper end of the central nervous system with its protective coverings. In this the neurocranium is the bony support and extends to form the bony orbit;

(2) the structures which surround and support the upper ends of the alimentary and respiratory systems. These are both derived from the gut tube of the embryo. The rigid supporting structures are the bones of the upper and lower jaws. The muscles for chewing and swallowing and for facial expression, along with their nervous and vascular supply, are built on to this scaffolding.

All these components are intimately related to each other and in a descriptive anatomical account it is not possible to separate them. Hence the region is described under the following headings:

(1) cranial cavity,
(2) face and scalp,
(3) neck,
(4) median hollow viscera,
(5) orbit (see chap. 26),
(6) middle ear and related cavities (see chap. 26).

CRANIAL CAVITY

The central nervous system is the largest single organ in the human embryo, and although its later growth lags behind that of other parts of the body, it is the most important of all the organs of the body. The head is constructed around the greatly enlarged upper end.

The subdivision of the central nervous system into brain and spinal cord at the level of the foramen magnum is arbitrary as far as its organization is concerned. This is not true, however, of the covering and protective structures which surround it. The cranium is, for all practical purposes, a rigid container. By contrast, the vertebral canal is surrounded by a series of jointed bony segments and its walls are mobile. The mobility is most marked in the cervical region immediately inferior to the base of the skull, where vulnerability to indirect violence is increased. Moreover, the interposition of soft tissues between adjacent segments of the vertebral column

allows a needle to be inserted into the subarachnoid space for the collection of cerebrospinal fluid.

The skull is formed by the interlocking of a number of bones. Those at the base are mainly ossified in cartilage, while those in the vault are entirely developed in membrane. When ossification is complete, these bones fuse to form a single structural unit. Although capable of deformation during the period of growth, the skull becomes less malleable as age advances and by the age of forty becomes virtually rigid with the fusion of the sutures.

The interior of the bony skull is identical with the cranial cavity that is identified radiographically. It is not equivalent to the cavity which encloses the brain as this is separated from the radio-opaque shell of bone by soft tissues.

A midline section of the skull reveals that its interior is not of uniform height. The base is divided into three regions or fossae by two transverse boundaries. The anterior fossa, the shallowest of the three, lies above the nasal cavity in the midline and above the orbits, which are extensions of the neurocranium. Below the middle fossa lie the sphenoidal air sinuses and the nasopharynx, with masticatory structures on either side of them. The posterior fossa is directly continuous with the vertebral canal at the foramen magnum. It is the deepest of the three fossae, and the vertical height of the cranial cavity is greatest between the vault of the skull and the foramen magnum (fig. 22.1).

The division of the interior of the basal part of the cavity into three fossae is precisely defined when the interior of the base of the skull is viewed from above. The boundaries are shown in fig. 22.2c.

Anterior cranial fossa

The floor of the fossa is not level but is depressed where it overlies the nasal cavity and bulges upwards over the orbits. It is made up of the following bones:

The **ethmoid bone** occupies the central part of the fossa and from its upper surface projects the **crista galli**, a sharp-edged midline keel of bone. On either side, the floor of the fossa is depressed and consists of the thin, heavily-perforated bone of the **cribriform plate**. Near the

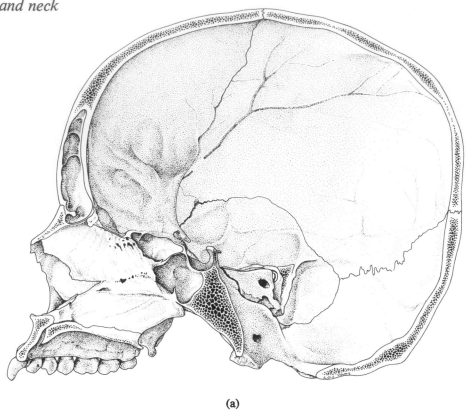

(a)

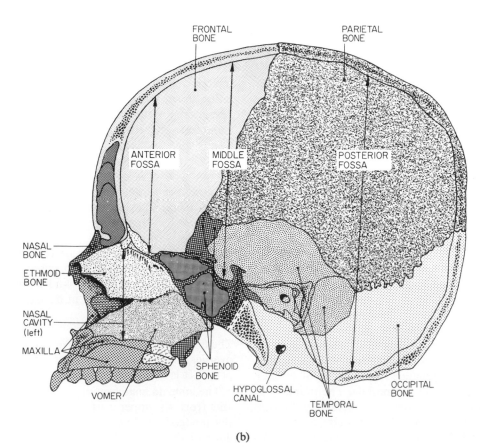

(b)

FIG. 22.1. Midline sagittal section of skull.

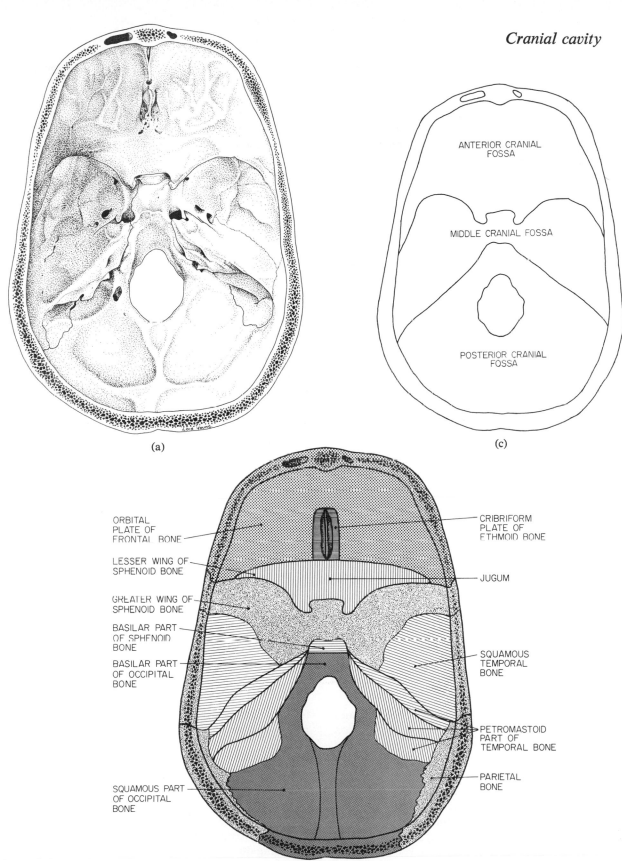

(a)

(c)

ANTERIOR CRANIAL FOSSA

MIDDLE CRANIAL FOSSA

POSTERIOR CRANIAL FOSSA

ORBITAL PLATE OF FRONTAL BONE

LESSER WING OF SPHENOID BONE

GREATER WING OF SPHENOID BONE

BASILAR PART OF SPHENOID BONE

BASILAR PART OF OCCIPITAL BONE

SQUAMOUS PART OF OCCIPITAL BONE

CRIBRIFORM PLATE OF ETHMOID BONE

JUGUM

SQUAMOUS TEMPORAL BONE

PETROMASTOID PART OF TEMPORAL BONE

PARIETAL BONE

(b)

FIG. 22.2. Interior of base of skull.

anterior end of the plate, close to the side of the crista galli, is a narrow elongated aperture, the **nasal slit**, which is larger than the other perforations of the plate. All these apertures connect directly with the nasal cavity. At the lateral edge of the cribriform plate, two fine apertures, the **anterior** and **posterior ethmoidal foramina**, run laterally between the upper surface of the ethmoid labyrinth and the medial edge of the frontal bone to the orbit.

to each other across the midline by the **jugum of the sphenoid**.

FORAMINA AND THEIR CONTENTS (fig. 22.3b).

The **nasal slit** contains the anterior ethmoidal nerve and vessels. The **foramina of the cribriform plate** transmit the nerve fibres from the olfactory mucous membrane to the olfactory bulbs. The **anterior** and **posterior ethmoidal**

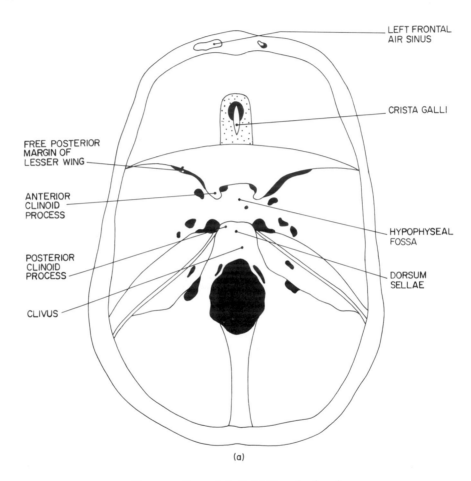

LEFT FRONTAL AIR SINUS

CRISTA GALLI

FREE POSTERIOR MARGIN OF LESSER WING

ANTERIOR CLINOID PROCESS

HYPOPHYSEAL FOSSA

POSTERIOR CLINOID PROCESS

DORSUM SELLAE

CLIVUS

(a)

FIG. 22.3. Base of skull. (a) Bony landmarks.

The **frontal bone** articulates with both the lateral and the anterior edges of the ethmoid bone, enclosing it on three sides. The two **orbital plates** form the anterolateral parts of the fossa and bulge upwards. The frontal air sinuses frequently extend into them, separating the bone of the roof of the orbit from the bone of the floor of the fossa. The part of the frontal bone which connects the two orbital plates across the midline in front of the cribriform plate and the crista galli has a sagittally-placed groove on its cranial aspect. This groove is occupied by the superior sagittal sinus.

The lesser wings of the **sphenoid bone** spread laterally along the posterior margin of the fossa and are connected

foramina contain the anterior and posterior ethmoidal nerves and vessels.

Middle cranial fossa

The raised central part of the fossa, the **sella turcica,** is comparatively short from front to back. It lies between the anterior and posterior clinoid processes and contains a concave fossa to accommodate the hypophysis and its enclosing dura mater. Lateral to the sella, the floor of the fossa slopes downwards and outwards. The two lateral regions form the greater part of the fossa and extend forwards for a short distance below the free posterior margins of the lesser wings of the sphenoid bones. Their floors are composed of parts of both temporal and sphenoidal bones and are pierced by a number of foramina. The parts of the individual bones involved are as follows:

The **body of the sphenoid bone** forms the median part of the middle fossa, including its anterior and posterior boundaries. Immediately behind the jugum of the sphenoid

of the sphenoid bone by a jagged aperture called the **foramen lacerum**. A wide suture, between the petrous temporal bone and the greater wing of the sphenoid, contains a smooth canal for the intrapetrous part of the internal carotid artery. The apex of the petrous temporal bone is marked by a notch which runs forwards, interrupting the groove for the superior petrosal sinus. This is occupied by the motor and sensory roots of the trigeminal

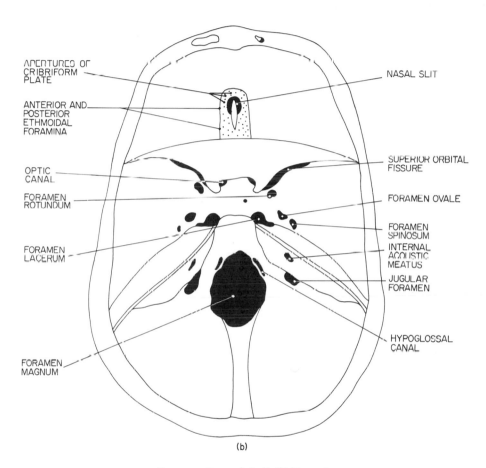

APERTURES OF CRIBRIFORM PLATE
ANTERIOR AND POSTERIOR ETHMOIDAL FORAMINA
OPTIC CANAL
FORAMEN ROTUNDUM
FORAMEN LACERUM
FORAMEN MAGNUM
NASAL SLIT
SUPERIOR ORBITAL FISSURE
FORAMEN OVALE
FORAMEN SPINOSUM
INTERNAL ACOUSTIC MEATUS
JUGULAR FORAMEN
HYPOGLOSSAL CANAL

(b)

FIG. 22.3. Base of skull. (b) Foramina

is the shallow **optic groove**; at each end of the groove, where the lesser wing unites with the body of the sphenoid, there is a rounded aperture, the optic canal. Posterior to the groove on the upper surface of the sphenoidal body is the concavity for the accommodation of the pituitary gland, and on each side there is a groove for the internal carotid artery. The **lesser** and **greater wings of the sphenoid bone** project laterally from the body of the bone and form the anterior wall and floor of the anterior half of the extensive lateral part of the fossa.

The **upper surface of the petrous temporal bone** completes the fossa posteriorly. It is separated from the body

nerve, whose ganglion lies between the petrous temporal and sphenoid bones.

Laterally, the **squamous bone** fits into the angle between the petrous temporal and the greater wing of the sphenoid bone. The suture between it and the lateral part of the petrous bone is normally obliterated by the age of five but forms a potential route for the spread of infection. In early life an otitis media may extend through it and involve the temporal lobe of the brain.

FORAMINA AND THEIR CONTENTS (fig. 22.3b)
The **optic canal** lies between the roots of the lesser wing and the body of the sphenoid bone. It is a tube

rather than a foramen which during its course may protrude into the upper lateral corner of the sphenoidal air sinus. It connects the fossa to the orbit and contains the optic nerve, its meningeal coverings and the ophthalmic artery.

The **superior orbital fissure** passes between the greater and the lesser wings of the sphenoid bone and contains the oculomotor, trochlear and abducent nerves, the three branches of the ophthalmic division of the trigeminal nerve, a sympathetic root from the internal carotid plexus and the ophthalmic veins (fig. 26.4).

The **foramen rotundum** lies immediately below the superior orbital fissure. It connects the middle fossa with the pterygopalatine fossa and contains the maxillary nerve.

The **foramen spinosum** contains the middle meningeal vessels. These run in grooves to the pterion and lambda.

The **foramen ovale** is larger than the foramen spinosum and is situated anteromedial to it. It contains the mandibular division and motor root of the trigeminal nerve, the accessory meningeal artery, the lesser petrosal nerve and emissary veins.

The **sphenoidal emissary foramen** contains only emissary veins.

The **foramen lacerum** is blocked in its lower half by fibrous tissue and cartilage. The carotid canal enters its posterolateral aspect and so connects the middle fossa with the part of the neck alongside the pharyngeal wall. The upper part of the foramen is occupied by the internal carotid artery, its sympathetic plexus of nerves and some emissary veins.

The **foramina for the greater and lesser petrosal nerves** are minute holes on the superior surface of the petrous temporal bone. They allow these nerves to run on their respective courses from the geniculate ganglion to the nerve of the pterygoid canal, and from the tympanic plexus to the otic ganglion.

Posterior cranial fossa

The floor is made up of parts of the occipital and temporal bones, with small contributions from both the body of the sphenoid and the parietal bones. The parts of the individual bones involved are as follows:

The **body of the sphenoid bone** projects downwards and backwards from the **dorsum sellae** to the middle of the sloping **clivus**, which forms the midline part of the anterior wall of the fossa.

The **occipital** bone forms the major part of the floor of the fossa and completely surrounds the centrally placed foramen magnum. Posterior to the foramen, the occipital bone extends into the flattened concave **squamous part**. A midline ridge called the **internal occipital crest** joins the posterior margin of the foramen magnum to the promi-

nence of the **internal occipital protuberance**. From this point on each side of the midline, a groove runs laterally in a horizontal plane to the parietal bone and is occupied by the transverse venous sinus. Between this groove and the posterior margin of the foramen magnum, the bone is concave for the accommodation of the cerebellum, the **cerebellar fossa**. The groove for the transverse sinus turns downwards at its lateral end to follow an S-shaped course to the jugular foramen.

The **petrous** and **mastoid temporal bones** are commonly described as a single unit, the **petromastoid**. Together they form the anterolateral wall of the fossa.

The posterior inferior angle of the **parietal bone** fits into the angle between the petromastoid and squamous occipital bone.

FORAMINA AND THEIR CONTENTS (fig. 22.3b)

The **internal acoustic meatus** penetrates and ends in the petrous temporal bone. It is connected by canaliculi with the vestibular apparatus and the cochlea, and with the stylomastoid foramen. It contains the facial nerve, the sensory and parasympathetic root of the facial nerve (nervus intermedius), the vestibulocochlear nerve and the labyrinthine vessels.

The **jugular foramen** lies inferior to the internal acoustic meatus and its shape varies even on the two sides of the one skull. Immediately below the internal acoustic meatus, the upper margin of the foramen shows a well-marked notch for the glossopharyngeal nerve. The termination of the sigmoid sinus in the superior bulb of the internal jugular vein occupies the posterior and lateral part of the aperture; the inferior petrosal sinus lies in the anteromedial angle of the opening; between these two venous sinuses lie the glossopharyngeal, vagus and accessory nerves. The vagus and both parts of the accessory nerve share the same opening in the dura mater.

The **hypoglossal canal** is below and medial to the jugular foramen and wholly within the occipital bone. A bony prominence, the jugular tubercle, overhangs and partly conceals it and separates it from the jugular foramen. It contains the hypoglossal nerve.

The **foramen magnum** is occupied by the junction of the medulla oblongata and the spinal cord, the intradural part of the vertebral artery and its branches, vertebral veins, the spinal part of the accessory nerve and the meninges.

The **mastoid emissary foramen** connects the groove for the sigmoid sinus to the retroauricular surface of the mastoid bone. The **posterior condylar canal** connects the same groove to the lower surface of the occipital bone, behind the condyle. Both of these foramina transmit emissary veins only.

The regions with which the cranial cavity is directly connected by foramina are as follows:

Connection	Foramina
Nasal cavity	Nasal slit
	Cribriform plate
Orbit	Optic canal
	Superior orbital fissure
	Ethmoidal foramina
Pterygopalatine fossa	Foramen rotundum
Infratemporal fossa	Foramen spinosum
	Foramen ovale
Neck	Carotid canal
	Jugular foramen
	Hypoglossal canal
Petrous temporal bone	Internal acoustic meatus
	Petrosal foramina
Vertebral canal	Foramen magnum

Cranial vault

The roof of the cranium is formed by the frontal, parietal and occipital bones which meet at the coronal, sagittal and lambdoidal sutures. In young adults when the individual bones are still separate, the connection between the adjacent edges of these flat bones is by a serrate arrangement of peg and socket joints, the individual components of which are about 1 mm long and sealed by fibrous tissue.

The interior of the vault is grooved in the midline for the superior sagittal sinus. The venous blood within the sinus flows backwards towards the external occipital protuberance and the groove becomes wider when traced in this direction. The bone, within and alongside the groove, is often deeply pitted, particularly in aged skulls. Such pitting marks the site of the arachnoid granulations (p. 22.9). The parietal bone is often perforated, usually near its posterior end, by emissary veins.

From either side of the vault, grooves run upwards and medially on the internal surface of the bone, breaking up into progressively finer channels. These grooves are occupied by the middle meningeal vessels. These supply only the bone and dura mater; the veins are closer to the bone than the arteries.

Structures separating the intracranial part of the central nervous system from the surface of the head

The skull develops in the fetus from a number of isolated centres of ossification which gradually grow together, separating the brain from the superficial structures of the head. Nevertheless, some communications remain between intracranial and extracranial structures. Such communications, usually in the form of small venous channels, may allow infection in superficial sites to extend across the cranial barrier and invade the cavity. The protective structures around the intracranial central nervous system comprise:

(1) skin and superficial fascia,
(2) deep fascia and epicranial aponeurosis in the scalp,
(3) skeletal muscle, e.g. in the temporal fossa and the occipital region,
(4) the periosteum of the exterior of the skull,
(5) bone of the cranium consisting of two layers of compact bone, the inner and outer tables of the skull, separated by marrow-containing cancellous bone, the **diplöe**,
(6) periosteum of the interior of the skull,
(7) the dura mater which is fused to the periosteum, except where venous spaces, the intracranial venous sinuses, occur between these two layers, and
(8) the pia-arachnoid investing the central nervous system.

Interior of the brain case (fig. 22.4)

The dura mater encloses the entire central nervous system and is separated from the pia-arachnoid by a narrow interval, the subdural space. At the foramen magnum, the cranial dura mater is continuous with the spinal dura mater. Except for a loose connection to the posterior longitudinal ligament, the spinal dura is separated from the walls of the vertebral canal by the extradural space, containing fat and the vertebral venous plexus. Movement of a vertebra has accordingly little effect on the spinal cord and its meninges. In contrast, the cranial dura mater is firmly bound to the surrounding bone and changes in the latter closely affect both the dura mater and the vascular and nervous structures connected to it.

The dura mater exhibits three major folds, the **tentorium cerebelli**, the **falx cerebri** and the **falx cerebelli**. These form incomplete partitions within the cranium and separate adjacent parts of the brain, acting as a set of baffles which prevent massive shift of the brain within the cranial cavity during movements of the head.

The partitions intersect along a line which runs downwards and backwards in the cranial cavity to end on the internal occipital protuberance. This is the position of the straight sinus. Above and to each side of the sinus are situated the two occipital lobes of the cerebrum, and below lies the superior vermis of the cerebellum. From the dura mater of the upper wall of the sinus, the falx cerebri extends upwards and forwards between the two cerebral hemispheres. From the lower surface of the posterior part of the sinus, the smaller falx cerebelli runs downwards and backwards on the wall of the posterior cranial fossa. On either side of the sinus, the two halves of the tentorium cerebelli extend laterally and forwards, enclosing the U-shaped tentorial notch.

The **supratentorial space** contains the two cerebral

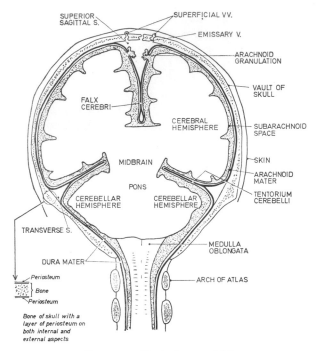

FIG. 22.4a. Tentorium and falx.

hemispheres, which are united across the midline by the corpus callosum. On the under surface of the hemispheres lie the olfactory bulbs and tracts, and the optic nerves, chiasma and tracts. Behind, above and in front of the corpus callosum, the hemispheres are separated by the falx cerebri.

The **infratentorial space** accommodates the remainder of the cranial contents. These include the brain stem, the cerebellum and all the cranial nerves from the trigeminal to the hypoglossal. Although the trigeminal nerve crosses the posterior margin of the middle cranial fossa to connect with its ganglion, it remains concealed from the other structures by the roof of the cavum trigeminale in which it lies. The cavum connects only with the infratentorial space.

The oculomotor and trochlear nerves emerge from the superficial surface of the brainstem at the level of the tentorial notch, where the supratentorial and infratentorial spaces intercommunicate. Both the nerves pierce the dura mater at that level and their position is at the natural boundary between the two spaces.

The **tentorium cerebelli** slopes upwards and inwards from its fixed peripheral margin towards its centrally placed free edge. The fixed margin extends laterally on each side of the internal occipital protuberance along the lips of the groove for the transverse sinus. Here the two layers of the dura mater diverge to form the upper and

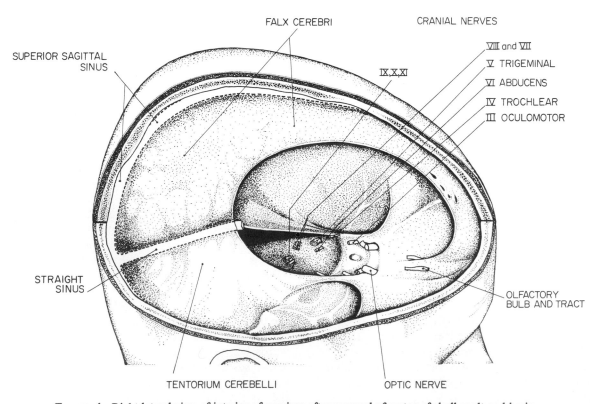

FIG. 22.4b. Right lateral view of interior of cranium after removal of sector of skull vault and brain.

lower walls of the sinus. At the lateral end of the transverse groove, the fixed margin of the tentorium continues medially and forwards along the lips of the groove for the superior petrosal sinus to the posterior clinoid process. The **cavum trigeminale** connects with the infratentorial space by its opening below the superior petrosal sinus at the trigeminal notch. The superior petrosal sinus, which lies above the opening of the cavum, and the inferior petrosal sinus which lies in the posterior cranial fossa below and medial to the opening, are continuous here with the cavernous sinus. The opening of the cavum is therefore at the apex of the angle between the converging superior and inferior petrosal sinuses.

The free anterior margin of the tentorium cerebelli forms the boundary of the tentorial notch, within which lies the midbrain and the oculomotor and trochlear nerves. This border is U-shaped and the two free ends are attached to the anterior clinoid processes. Where the free edges of the falx cerebri and of the tentorium cerebelli are continuous, the great cerebral vein pierces the dura mater to enter the straight sinus.

The **falx cerebri** at its anterior end blends with the dura mater of the anterior cranial fossa around the crista galli. Superiorly, its two layers separate to enclose the superior sagittal sinus and become continuous with the dura mater of the cranial vault. Posteriorly, its layers are continuous with the dura mater of the upper surface of the tentorium cerebelli around the straight sinus. The depth of the falx cerebri is greatest posteriorly. The inconstant inferior sagittal sinus is enclosed in its free inferior edge.

The central nervous system is connected to the dura mater by nerves and blood vessels which cross the subarachnoid space to their destinations. Changes in the relative positions of parts of the brain, due to local or general alterations in intracranial pressure, exert traction on these connecting structures. This produces clinical effects which are not directly related to the site of the primary lesion. For example, a rise in supratentorial pressure, with a downward shift of the brain stem towards the foramen magnum, often stretches the abducent nerves and so paralyses the lateral rectus muscles.

Intracranial venous sinuses (fig. 22.5)

The system of venous sinuses is extradural. Venous blood from the brain traverses the subarachnoid space and the dura mater to enter a sinus. Usually, the shortest possible route is taken and drainage is into the nearest sinus.

Some sinuses are connected to extracranial veins by emissary venous channels which occur at a number of points in the neurocranial wall. The diploic veins which are situated between the tables of the skull drain into superficial or intracranial venous channels, or into the emissary vessels which connect them. The venous

sinuses possess no valves, and since their walls are of dense connective tissue they cannot distend or collapse. Their main drainage to the exterior of the skull is through the sigmoid sinus and internal jugular vein.

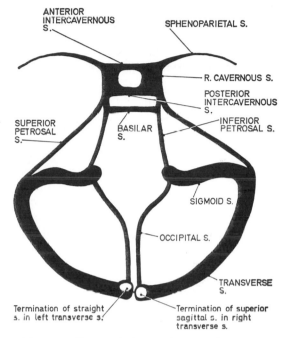

Fig. 22.5. Venous drainage of the cranial cavity.

The **superior sagittal sinus** begins at the crista galli. It may drain blood from the upper part of the nose and frontal air sinuses. As it runs backwards in the midline, it is in contact successively with the deep aspect of the frontal bone, the sagittal suture and adjacent parts of the parietal bones, and the occipital bone, following the upward curve of the vault of the skull in the attached margin of the falx cerebri. It terminates usually by turning sharply to the right to become continuous with the right transverse sinus at the internal occipital protuberance. Here also it communicates with the straight and left transverse sinuses and, if an occipital emissary vein is present, with the superficial veins at the back of the neck.

The sinus is connected with wide, laterally placed extensions called **lacunae laterales.** There may be as many as three of these on each side of the midline. The most constant overlies the upper part of the precentral gyrus of the cerebrum.

The **arachnoid villi** are concentrated along the walls of the superior sagittal sinus and around the walls of the lacunae laterales. These villi are buds of cellular connective tissue, derived from the arachnoid mater. They pierce the dural wall of the sinus and project into its lumen, where they are covered by the endothelial lining of the sinus. Each villus possesses a central channel, through which cerebrospinal fluid percolates into the sinus when pressure within the latter is low. When the intracranial venous pressure rises the villus functions as a valve, to prevent blood flowing into the subarachnoid space (fig. 25.99). Large groups of villi are described as granulations which may lie in shallow depressions on the internal surface of the skull.

The superior sagittal sinus drains the upper parts of the superolateral and medial surfaces of the cerebral hemispheres. It receives the parietal emissary vein and connections from the lacunae laterales.

The **inferior sagittal sinus** lies in the posterior part of the free inferior edge of the falx cerebri. It terminates at the anterior end of the straight sinus, where it joins the great cerebral vein.

The **straight sinus** runs posteriorly from the junction of the inferior sagittal sinus and great cerebral vein to the region of the internal occipital protuberance, where it turns sharply to the left to form the left transverse sinus. The confluence of sinuses at the internal protuberance leads to the risk of extensive intracranial bleeding following direct injury to this part. In addition to the inferior sagittal sinus and the great cerebral vein, tributaries from the adjacent surfaces of the occipital lobes and cerebellum enter the sinus.

The **transverse sinuses** follow symmetrical courses in the attached margin of the tentorium cerebelli. Each sinus terminates at the posterior end of the petrous temporal bone by turning downwards to become the corresponding sigmoid sinus. The course of each sinus can be traced on the exterior of the skull from the external occipital protuberance along the superior nuchal line to the root of the auricle.

The **sigmoid sinuses** are directly continuous with the transverse sinuses. Turning downwards, each sinus leaves the tentorial margin and follows the general line of the junction of the petromastoid and occipital bones. In the floor of the posterior fossa, the sinus turns forwards to the jugular foramen and passes through its posterolateral part to become the superior bulb of the internal jugular vein.

The transverse and sigmoid sinuses receive superficial veins from the adjacent parts of the brain. The sigmoid sinus is connected with the posterior auricular and occipital regions by the **mastoid and posterior condylar emissary veins**. The mastoid vein drains the parietal diplöe. In addition, the beginning and the end of the sigmoid sinus are connected to the cavernous sinus of the same side by the narrow superior petrosal and inferior petrosal sinuses, and the terminal part of each sigmoid sinus communicates with the confluence of sinuses by means of the corresponding occipital sinus.

The **superior petrosal sinuses** are channels lying in the anterior part of the attached border of the tentorium cerebelli. At the opening of the cavum trigeminale, each lies in the double layer of dura mater in the roof of the opening and drains adjacent parts of the brain.

The **inferior petrosal sinuses** separate the clivus from the petromastoids and leave the cranial cavity through the anteromedial part of the jugular foramina. In addition to veins from the adjacent part of the cerebellum, each sinus receives the labyrinthine vein from the internal acoustic meatus.

The **occipital sinuses** unite the confluence of sinuses to the terminal parts of the sigmoid sinuses, running as parallel channels in the attached margin of the falx cerebelli, and diverging to their separate terminations on either side of the foramen magnum.

The **cavernous sinuses** are situated on either side of the fossa for the hypophysis (fig. 22.6). This endocrine gland lies on the upper surface of the sella turcica, connected to the base of the brain by a thin stalk of neural tissue. The dura mater which condenses around it in fetal life encloses the gland to leave only a small median aperture for this connection. At the edges of the aperture for the connecting stalk, the dura mater which encloses the hypophysis is continuous with that which lines the remainder

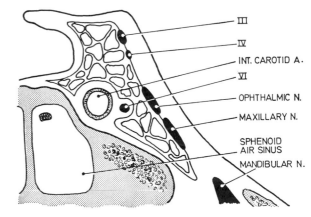

FIG. 22.6. Coronal section of cavernous sinus.

of the middle cranial fossa. But, around the aperture, between the anterior and posterior clinoid processes there is a raised area of dura mater, the **diaphragma sellae**. Separating the diaphragma and the adjacent dura mater of the middle fossa from the underlying periosteum and bone is an arrangement of venous spaces, the cavernous and intercavernous sinuses.

The cavity of the cavernous sinus is subdivided into a number of venous channels by fibrous partitions, covered by vascular endothelium. Each sinus contains part of the internal carotid artery, surrounded by its sympathetic plexus. This artery enters the sinus through the upper part of the foramen lacerum and runs anteriorly in a groove on the body of the sphenoid. On its lateral side, and also within the sinus, is the abducent nerve. Both artery and nerve are enclosed in fibrous tissue, continuous with the partitions of the sinus, and also separated from the lumen of the sinus by vascular endothelium. The artery leaves the sinus by turning upwards on the medial side of the anterior clinoid process and pierces the dura and arachnoid to enter the subarachnoid space. At this point, the thin-walled artery, well supported within the sinus by its connective tissue covering, enters a fluid-filled space where support is minimal and movement is free. Within the lateral wall of the sinus, and separated from the artery and the abducent nerve by venous channels, are the oculomotor, trochlear, ophthalmic and maxillary nerves in that order from above downwards.

The two cavernous sinuses intercommunicate across the midline by means of the anterior and posterior intercavernous sinuses, which lie on the sella turcica in front of and behind the dural sac of the hypophysis, and through the basilar sinus, which runs posterior to the base of the dorsum sellae.

Posteriorly, the cavernous sinus receives the superior and inferior petrosal sinuses and the basilar sinus. Anteriorly, it receives the ophthalmic veins, and the small sphenoparietal sinus, which runs along the posterior margin of the lesser wing of the sphenoid bone. Superiorly, the superficial middle cerebral and other cerebral veins enter the roof of the sinus. Inferiorly, it is freely connected with the veins outside the skull by means of emissary veins which pass through the foramen ovale and the foramen lacerum.

The cavernous sinus is deeply placed within the cranial cavity and yet is connected with extracranial veins by means of emissary channels. These potential routes for the extension of infection into the sinus are as follows:

(1) from the face, via the connections between the facial and ophthalmic veins at the orbital margin,

(2) from the pterygoid region, via veins in the foramen ovale and the sphenoidal emissary foramen,

(3) from the pharynx via veins which surround the intrapetrous part of the internal carotid artery.

Cranial nerves (fig. 25.33)

The point at which a cranial nerve emerges from or enters the substance of the brain is its superficial point of origin or attachment. Cranial nerves may be classified in accordance with the position of their superficial attachments as follows:

Cerebral hemispheres—I or olfactory nerve.
Junction of the midbrain and the cerebral hemispheres—II or optic nerve through the optic chiasma and tract.
Midbrain—III or oculomotor nerve and IV or trochlear nerve.
Pons—V or trigeminal nerve.

Ponto-medullary junction—VI or abducent nerve, VII or facial nerve, and VIII or vestibulocochlear nerve.
Medulla—IX or glossopharyngeal nerve, X or vagus nerve, the cranial part of XI or accessory nerve, and XII or hypoglossal nerve.
Spinal cord—the spinal part of XI or accessory nerve.

As with spinal nerves, a dural sheath becomes applied to the nerve as it leaves the skull, and blends with its fibrous tissue coverings. The deep origins of the cranial nerves within the brain and the points where they leave that organ are described in chap. 25. Here we are concerned only with their course inside the skull and their passage through the foramina.

The cranial nerves can also be classified according to their exit points from the cranial cavity.

CRIBRIFORM PLATE GROUP OF NERVES

The dura mater of the anterior fossa is tightly bound down to the margins of the foramina which exist in the ethmoid bone on either side of the crista galli. The axons of the receptor cells of the olfactory zone of the nose occupy these foramina and pierce the dural and arachnoid membranes at their upper ends. Thereafter, they cross the subarachnoid space to enter the olfactory bulbs.

The anterior ethmoidal nerves and vessels, which pass from the orbit to the nasal cavity, lie within the dura mater of the cribriform plate. More posteriorly, terminal branches of the posterior ethmoidal group of neurovascular structures supply the dura mater.

CAVERNOUS SINUS GROUP (fig. 22.6)

The **optic nerves** differ from the other cranial nerves in that they are part of the central nervous system and share the physiological and histological characteristics of that system. When injured, they are incapable of regeneration. They possess no nucleated sheath of Schwann. Their blood supply is ultimately from the same source as that of other adjacent parts of the brain, the internal carotid artery. The optic nerves lie immediately superior to the cavernous sinus. Each is enclosed in a sheath of the dura, arachnoid and pia. Cerebrospinal fluid separates the pia and arachnoid here as elsewhere, and extends as far as the back of the eyeball where the tube of dura mater blends directly with the sclera. At the point where the optic nerve emerges from the optic canal and enters the main cranial cavity, the internal carotid artery also emerges from the dura mater of the upper surface of the cavernous sinus and comes to lie on the lateral side of the nerve, between it and the anterior clinoid process. At this point, the ophthalmic artery branches off from the internal carotid, passes below the optic nerve into the canal, and enters the orbit on its lateral side, piercing the dural sheath of the nerve as it does so. Either just before or just after it becomes extradural, the ophthalmic artery gives off the central artery of the retina, which crosses the pia-arachnoid sheath of the optic nerve to enter its substance. The vena comitans of this central artery drains into one of the veins of the orbit. Increase in the cerebrospinal fluid pressure is transmitted along the optic sheath to the back of the eyeball. Thus the central retinal vein, and to a lesser extent the retinal artery, may be partially or completely occluded as they pass through the subarachnoid space of the optic nerve.

The **abducent nerve** pierces the pia mater at the ponto-medullary junction, and runs upwards and forwards on the clivus, within the subarachnoid space. Two-thirds of the way up the clivus, it pierces the arachnoid and dura and continues in the same direction as before outside the dura mater. It enters the middle cranial fossa immediately medial to the opening of the cavum trigeminale. Thereafter, it runs forward within the cavernous sinus, on the lateral side of the internal carotid artery, to the superior orbital fissure, where it passes into the orbit through the fibrous ring at the apex of the rectus cone. The major part of its intracranial course is therefore extradural.

The **oculomotor nerve** is superficially attached at the medial side of the crus cerebri of the midbrain. It runs anteriorly between the posterior cerebral and the superior cerebellar arteries, and pierces the arachnoidal and dural membranes. It continues on its course in the lateral wall of the cavernous sinus, and leaves the cranial cavity by passing through the superior orbital fissure, within the fibrous ring at the apex of the rectus cone. It divides into an upper and a lower branch just before leaving the cranial cavity.

The **trochlear nerve** arises superficially from the dorsal surface of the lowest part of the midbrain, just below the inferior colliculus, passes around the brain stem and runs anteriorly in the lateral wall of the cavernous sinus, at first below and later lateral to the oculomotor nerve. It enters the orbit by passing through the upper lateral part of the superior orbital fissure, outside the fibrous ring of the rectus cone.

The **trigeminal nerve** is the only nerve that is superficially attached to the pons. Its sensory and motor roots are attached to the brain stem at the junction of the pons and the middle cerebellar peduncle, and cross the posterior boundary of the middle cranial fossa at the trigeminal notch at the apex of the petrous temporal bone. The motor root passes below the trigeminal ganglion to pierce the arachnoid and dural meninges at the foramen ovale. It may have a dural exit separate from the sensory part of the mandibular nerve, which also passes through this foramen, a fact which may permit the preservation of the motor root in surgical destruction of the sensory fibres of the mandibular nerve. The three terminal sensory

branches of the trigeminal ganglion, ophthalmic, maxillary and mandibular, run forwards from the ganglion, each piercing the dura mater separately. The mandibular division has virtually no intracranial course. It leaves the cavity by the foramen ovale almost at the anterior margin of the ganglion, while the maxillary and ophthalmic nerves run forward in the lateral wall of the cavernous sinus. The maxillary nerve leaves the cavity at the foramen rotundum. The ophthalmic nerve, by contrast, breaks up into its lacrimal, frontal and nasociliary branches while still within the wall of the cavernous sinus. The lacrimal and frontal branches pass into the orbit through the upper lateral part of the superior orbital fissure, outside the fibrous ring of the rectus cone. The nasociliary nerve, however, enters the fissure through its lower medial part, within the ring and within the rectus cone (fig. 26.4).

INTERNAL ACOUSTIC MEATUS GROUP

The **facial nerve**, along with its autonomic and sensory root, the nervus intermedius, and the **vestibulocochlear nerve** are all attached to the brain stem at the ponto-medullary junction. The cochlear element of the vestibulocochlear nerve is the most lateral, and the motor root of the facial nerve the most medial of the entire group. All these nerves are enclosed in a tunnel of dura and arachnoid mater, and a thin layer of cerebrospinal fluid, within the internal acoustic meatus. They are accompanied by the labyrinthine artery, a branch of the basilar vessel, and its vena comitans. The nerves and the blood vessels pierce the meninges at the lateral end of the meatus and are distributed to the interior of the petrous temporal bone through a number of foramina in the lateral wall of the meatus.

JUGULAR FORAMEN GROUP

In spite of its size, the jugular foramen is almost completely obscured by its covering of dura mater. Two apertures exist in the dura mater between the inferior petrosal and sigmoid sinuses, a small one directly below the internal acoustic meatus, and a larger one a little lower down. The **glossopharyngeal nerve** occupies the superior opening, while the **vagus** and cranial and spinal parts of the **accessory nerve** share the lower one.

All these nerves, excluding the spinal part of the accessory nerve, arise from the medulla oblongata by a series of rootlets which run in the longitudinal axis of the brain stem well posterior to the olive. The spinal accessory nerve pierces the lateral aspect of the upper six segments of the spinal medulla in the same longitudinal plane as the cranial roots. Gathering into a single trunk, the spinal accessory fibres enter the cranial cavity through the foramen magnum, and hook over the intracranial part of the vertebral artery, which is running upwards and medially at that point on its way to the lower border of the pons. The spinal and cranial parts of the accessory nerve

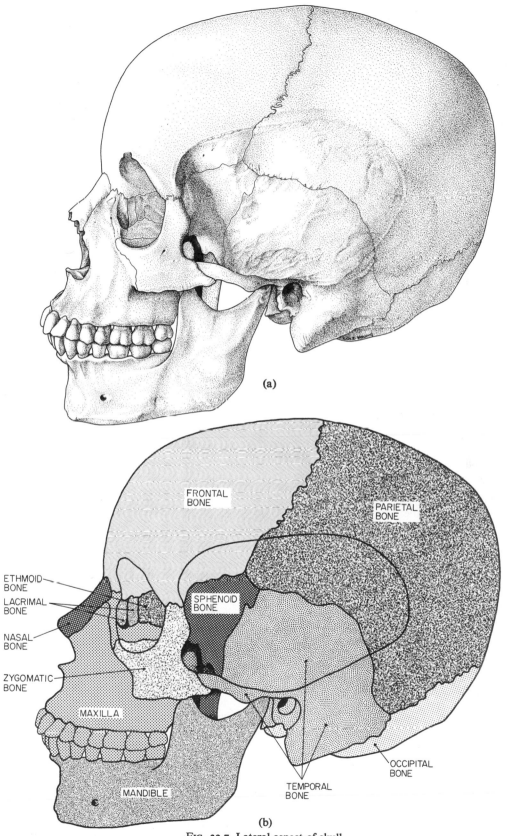

FRONTAL
BONE

PARIETAL
BONE

ETHMOID
BONE

LACRIMAL
BONE

SPHENOID
BONE

NASAL
BONE

ZYGOMATIC
BONE

MAXILLA

TEMPORAL
BONE

OCCIPITAL
BONE

MANDIBLE

(b)

FIG. 22.7. Lateral aspect of skull.

then converge upon the jugular foramen, crossing the jugular tubercle of the occipital bone to do so. Upon this tubercle, the glossopharyngeal, vagus and cranial and spinal parts of the accessory nerve are in contact with the dura mater covering the bone, in that order from before backwards. Thereafter, the glossopharyngeal nerve follows its separate route. Two sensory ganglia are found on the course of the nerve just after it pierces the dura mater, the upper one within and the lower one just below the jugular foramen. From the inferior ganglion arises the tympanic branch, which enters the middle ear through a small foramen on the undersurface of the base of the skull. It carries secretomotor fibres to the parotid gland, and sensory fibres to the middle ear and its related cavities.

After the vagus and the cranial and spinal parts of the accessory nerves pierce the dura mater, the two components of the accessory nerve separate and the cranial part joins the vagus nerve. Two sensory ganglia also occur on the vagus. The spinal accessory nerve takes a separate course to the sternomastoid and trapezius muscles.

HYPOGLOSSAL CANAL

The **hypoglossal nerve** is superficially attached to the medulla oblongata by a vertical series of rootlets, which coalesce into two trunks which often pierce the dura mater separately. Both trunks hook over the intracranial part of the vertebral artery, and leave the cranial cavity through the hypoglossal canal, forming a single trunk after piercing the dura mater.

Surface relationships of the brain (figs. 22.7 & 22.8)

The frontal poles of the **cerebral hemispheres** lie immediately above and lateral to the root of the nose and are separated from the surface of the head by the frontal

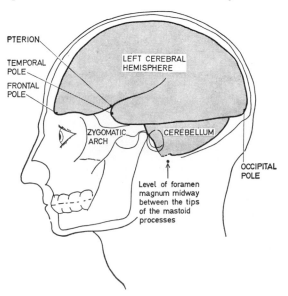

FIG. 22.8. Surface relations of the brain.

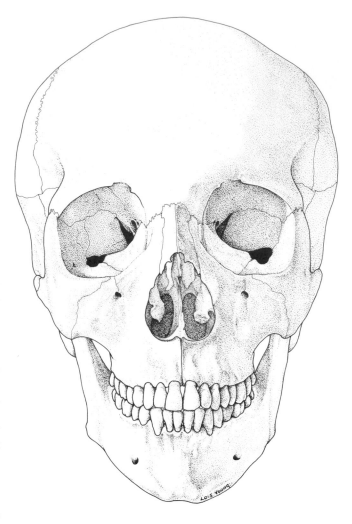

(a)

FIG. 22.9. Anterior aspect of skull.

bone and its contained air sinuses. The occipital poles are placed above and lateral to the external occipital protuberance and between them lies the terminal part of the superior sagittal sinus.

The stem of the lateral sulcus fits against the free posterior margin of the lesser wing of the sphenoid bone, and both lie opposite the **pterion**. This is a point which lies about 3 cm posterior to the frontozygomatic suture, and 1 cm above that level. It is situated at the upper end of the greater wing of the sphenoid bone on the outside of the skull. Within the cavity and opposite this point lies the anterior division of the middle meningeal vessels external to the dura mater.

From the frontal pole, the lower lateral margin of the frontal lobe follows the supraorbital margin to its lateral end and then upwards to the pterion. The temporal pole can be indicated by a line which runs, convex forwards, to connect the pterion to the upper margin of the zygomatic arch. Its most anterior point fails to reach the lateral margin of the orbit. The floor of the middle

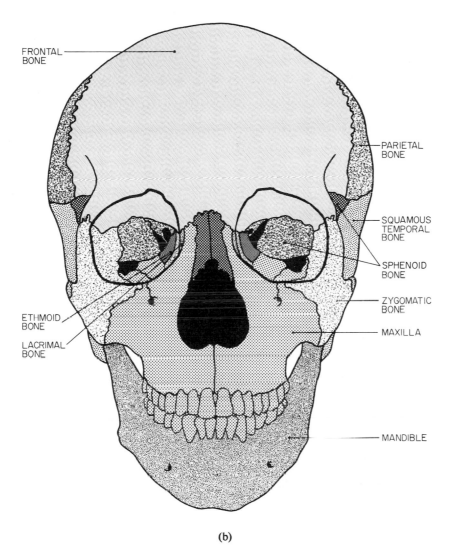

FRONTAL BONE

PARIETAL BONE

SQUAMOUS TEMPORAL BONE

SPHENOID BONE

ZYGOMATIC BONE

MAXILLA

MANDIBLE

ETHMOID BONE

LACRIMAL BONE

(b)

fossa lies opposite the upper margin of the zygomatic arch, and the inferolateral margin of the temporal lobe coincides with this level. A continuation of this line through the upper margin of the external acoustic meatus, and along the superior nuchal line to the external occipital protuberance, indicates the position of the inferolateral border of the occipital lobe. In the last part of its course it coincides in position with the transverse sinus. The upper medial margins of the cerebral hemispheres and the superior sagittal sinus correspond to adjacent parallel sagittal lines on the top of the head.

The **brain stem** is placed too deeply within the cranium to permit accurate surface marking. The anterior surface of the pons does not extend any further forward than the anterior edge of the external acoustic meatus. The junction of the brain stem and the spinal cord at the foramen magnum lies midway between the tips of the mastoid processes.

The parts of the **cerebellum** which lie in relationship to the walls of the posterior cranial fossa are the posterior and inferior aspects of the two hemispheres, and the inferior vermis which unites them in the midline. This part of the cerebellum which is in contact with the interior of the skull is therefore situated inferior to the superior nuchal line, and is separated from the skin of the upper part of the posterior surface of the neck by the insertions of the postvertebral muscles. The upper, deeper surface of the cerebellum is situated immediately below the tentorium cerebelli.

The **middle meningeal vessels** lie opposite the midpoint of the upper border of the zygomatic arch and end by dividing into a frontal and a parietal branch about a thumb's breadth above that point. The frontal division runs upwards and forwards from the point of bifurcation to the pterion, and from there upwards and backwards to the middle of the vertex. Both artery and vein frequently run in a tunnel of bone at the pterion and are easily damaged. The less important parietal division runs upwards and backwards towards the lambda, at the apex of the occipital bone.

FACE AND SCALP (fig. 22.9)

Muscles of the face and scalp

Over the face and scalp, the skin and the superficial fascia are bound to an underlying layer of skeletal muscle which becomes an aponeurosis over the vertex of the head. This layer is of uneven depth and where it is fleshy, its fibres are frequently inserted into the dermis. This musculo-aponeurotic layer produces changes in facial expression. It is derived from the mesoderm of the second or hyoid arch, and the muscle fibres in it accordingly obtain their motor nerve supply from the second arch nerve, the facial nerve. A continuous sheet of the same muscle extends into the neck as the platysma muscle.

The muscle in the face is arranged as three sphincters, one over each orbit and one around the mouth, linked by poorly defined bands. These latter features radiate on each side of the face from a point a little lateral to the angle of the mouth. All these muscles, linear and sphincter, have limited connections with the underlying bones.

The **orbicularis oculi muscle** is the sphincter muscle of the orbit and surrounds the palpebral fissure. The main sheet of the muscle, the orbital part, is attached to the medial margin of the orbit from the supraorbital notch to the region of the infraorbital foramen, and includes the medial palpebral ligament in its attachments. These fibres loop around the tarsi, but do not become attached to the lateral part of the orbital margin. Finer fibres, the palpebral part, form a layer on the superficial aspect of the tarsi, and are traversed by some of the fibres of the levator palpebrae superioris, as they pass from the orbit to the skin of the upper eyelid. The lacrimal part is deep to the rest of the muscle; it arises posterior to the naso-lacrimal sac and is inserted into the medial ends of the tarsi.

The **buccinator-orbicularis oris muscle** forms the contractile element in the lips and the cheeks. The buccinator is a sheet of muscle which continues posteriorly as the superior constrictor muscle of the pharynx. The line of junction between the two is a vertically placed fibrous intersection, the pterygomandibular raphe. Superiorly and inferiorly, the buccinator is attached to the maxilla and the mandible on the lateral aspects of their alveolar processes, at the line of reflection of the gingival mucous membrane. It blends medially with the fibres of the orbicularis oris, which form an elliptical sphincter around the lips. The oral aspect of the buccinator is lined by a thick layer of connective tissue, the inner cheek pad, which supports the stratified squamous non-keratinizing epithelium of the vestibule of the mouth. The duct of the parotid salivary gland pierces both the buccinator and the inner cheek pad to open into the vestibule of the mouth at the level of the second upper molar tooth.

The **occipitofrontalis muscle** extends from the superior margins of the orbits to the superior nuchal lines. Anteriorly, it is mainly connected to the other muscles of the face, posteriorly to bone. Laterally, it blends with a layer of deep fascia, which extends in the temporal region down to the zygomatic arch. Over the top of the skull, it is aponeurotic. Its importance lies in its intimate attachment to the overlying skin, particularly over the vertex of the skull, where there is one composite layer of skin, dense connective tissue and aponeurosis. Within this triple layer the nerves and vessels of the scalp are distributed, entering from the periphery. This permits free movement of the skin-aponeurosis as one layer, when either frontal or occipital fibres of the muscle contract. Except where the parietal emissary veins enter their foramina alongside the sagittal suture, the anatomical separation of the scalp from the underlying periosteum of the cranial vault is complete. In industrial scalping injuries and when this skin-aponeurosis layer is raised in surgical operations, the survival of the scalp flap depends on an adequate peripheral attachment.

The **platysma** is a subcutaneous sheet of skeletal muscle. It extends from the upper part of the pectoral region to the lower jaw, where it blends with the muscles around the mouth. It has an interrupted attachment on its deep aspect to the lower margin of the body of the mandible.

NERVE SUPPLY TO THE MUSCLES OF FACIAL EXPRESSION

The **facial nerve** emerges from the stylomastoid foramen, turns on to the lateral aspect of the styloid process, and enters the parenchyma of the parotid gland. Fibres pass to the posterior part of the occipitofrontalis, the posterior belly of the digastric muscle and to the stylohyoid muscles prior to its entry into the gland. Within the substance of the parotid, the remainder of the nerve breaks up into five bundles of fibres, which penetrate the secretory tissue and emerge along the whole extent of the anterior border of the gland from its upper to its lower poles. In the face, they are distributed to the muscles by numerous small branches. The presence of these motor fibres in the superficial layers of the face must be remembered during facial surgery.

In its course through the parotid gland, the main trunk of the facial nerve passes superficial to the retromandibular vein and the external carotid artery, both of which are within the gland.

When the facial nerve is paralysed, the affected half of the face is immobile and expressionless. More serious complications arise from the loss of function of the orbicularis oculi and the orbicularis oris-buccinator muscles. Paralysis of the orbicularis oculi abolishes the blinking response, so that the affected eye is totally unprotected from direct injury. Since the puncta are not kept in contact with the ocular conjunctiva, the resorption of lacrimal fluid ceases and tears flow down over the surface of the cheek. As the eyelids cannot be closed, the eye has to be turned upwards during sleep. The loss of function in the orbicularis oris-buccinator sheet prevents effective closure of the lips and occlusion of the vestibule of the mouth during chewing, which itself is unimpaired. The vestibule becomes distended with partially masticated food, which cannot be retained between the teeth, and which eventually dribbles from the affected corner of the mouth.

CUTANEOUS NERVE SUPPLY OF THE HEAD AND NECK

The nerves involved are partly cranial and partly spinal in origin. The detailed distribution of these nerves is shown in figs. 22.10 and 11.

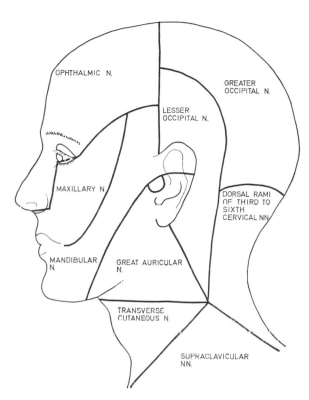

FIG. 22.11. Cutaneous nerve supply of the head and neck.

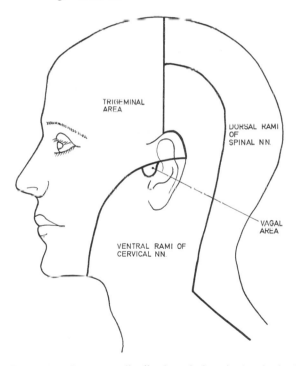

FIG. 22.10. Cutaneous distribution of trigeminal and spinal nerves.

BLOOD SUPPLY OF THE FACE AND SCALP

The arterial supply is unequally divided between the external and internal carotid arteries, the contribution of external predominating. The internal carotid artery, through its ophthalmic branch, supplies the regions which receive branches from the ophthalmic nerve. The external carotid artery supplies the skin through the following branches:

The **facial artery** runs from the anterior margin of the masseter muscle to the medial angle of the eye, supplying the lower and upper lips, the face and the side of the external nose. It anastomoses freely in its terminal part with branches of the ophthalmic artery. Blood can reach the bed of a ligated ophthalmic artery through the facial arterial route.

The **superficial temporal artery** accompanies the auriculotemporal nerve, and crosses the zygomatic arch with it, immediately in front of the ear. It is distributed to the temporal region and the scalp.

The **posterior auricular artery** is small, and supplies the region immediately behind the ear.

The **occipital artery** enters the posterior part of the scalp region at the superior nuchal line, about 25 mm from the midline, and accompanies the greater occipital nerve to the skin and superficial tissues of the posterior half of the scalp.

In the face and scalp regions, the main veins run as follows:

The **facial vein** is formed by veins from the front of the scalp which converge at the medial angle of the eye. Here the skin is very thin so the vein is usually clearly visible and is commonly termed the **angular vein**. This is one of the sites of facial-ophthalmic venous anastomosis. The main trunk of the vein runs posterior to the artery to the anterior margin of masseter communicating with the pterygoid venous plexus by means of the deep facial vein. It finally drains into the internal jugular system, often in

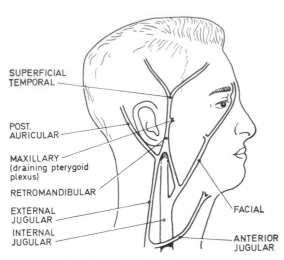

SUPERFICIAL
TEMPORAL

POST.
AURICULAR

MAXILLARY
(draining pterygoid
plexus)

RETROMANDIBULAR

EXTERNAL
JUGULAR

INTERNAL
JUGULAR

FACIAL

ANTERIOR
JUGULAR

FIG. 22.12. Veins of the neck.

common with the lingual vein. It receives the anterior division of the retromandibular vein prior to doing so.

The **superficial temporal vein** drains the area of supply of the corresponding artery and accompanies it on its course. At the zygomatic arch, it enters the substance of the parotid gland, and joins the retromandibular venous channel. This vessel leaves the parotid gland at its lower pole, and divides into a small anterior division which enters the facial vein, and a larger posterior division which constitutes the main part of the external jugular vein.

The **posterior auricular vein** joins the posterior division of the retromandibular vein to form the external jugular vein.

The **occipital vein** accompanies the occipital artery only as far as the upper part of the back of the neck, where it ends in the suboccipital venous plexus. The deep cervical vein connects the plexus to the brachiocephalic vein at the root of the neck.

Emissary veins, of which the facial-ophthalmic connection is only one example, connect the superficial veins of the scalp, face and the back of the neck to the intracranial venous sinuses.

Parotid salivary gland

The parotid gland fits into the space between the posterior border of the mandible and the anterior borders of the mastoid process and the sternomastoid muscle. Its lateral surface is smooth, and conforms to the contours of the face. It has a diamond shape with sharp upper and lower angles. These fit between the temporomandibular joint and the external acoustic meatus at the upper end, and between the angle of the mandible and the anterior margin of the sternomastoid muscle at the lower. From the blunt anterior angle of the gland, the parotid duct runs across the masseter, at

the anterior border of which it turns sharply medially, pierces the buccinator and the inner cheek pad and opens into the vestibule of the mouth.

Because the deep surface of the gland is moulded into the cleft between the mandible and the sternomastoid, it is irregular. It has an anteromedial surface, related to the masseter, the mandible and the medial pterygoid muscle, and a posteromedial surface related to the sternomastoid, the posterior belly of the digastric muscle and the styloid process. Between these two surfaces, the medial edge of the parotid gland may extend as far as the internal carotid artery and the internal jugular vein (fig. 22.17).

During prenatal growth the parotid gland comes to surround the external carotid artery, the retromandibular vein, the facial nerve, and the deep and superficial parotid lymph nodes. The external carotid artery enters the parotid from the lateral aspect of the styloid process, and soon divides in the gland into the superficial temporal and maxillary arteries. The maxillary artery runs forward deep to the neck of the mandible, and enters the pterygomaxillary fissure. The retromandibular vein, which is formed within the gland, runs superficial to the artery, while the facial nerve passes through the gland superficial to them both. The deep parotid lymph nodes form part of the deep cervical group, while the superficial ones are part of the collar chain and drain the skin of the temporal region, the forehead and the front of the auricle. The whole parotid gland is enclosed in a strong envelope of deep fascia. A superficial layer spreads upwards over the lateral surface of the gland to blend with the periosteum of the zygomatic arch and with the perichondrium of the external acoustic meatus. Another layer passes deep to the gland, blending with the periosteum of the tympanic plate and the styloid process. A thickened layer, the stylomandibular ligament, extends from the styloid process to the angle of the mandible, separating the parotid from the posterior pole of the submandibular gland and from the medial pterygoid muscle.

Masticatory apparatus (fig. 22.7)

During mastication, the maxilla, which is firmly fixed to the rest of the skull, is immobile; while the mandible is moved in relation to it by the four pairs of muscles of mastication.

TEMPOROMANDIBULAR JOINT (fig. 22.14)

Because the mandible is a single bone from the age of two onwards, the two temporomandibular joints function as a single unit; thus they may be regarded as a bicondylar joint with two cavities separated from one another by the width of the base of the skull.

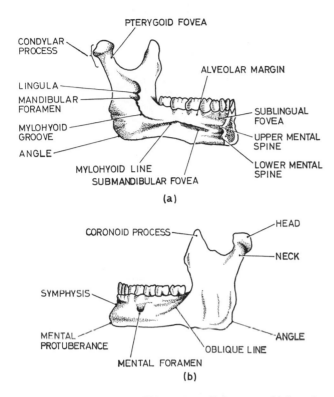

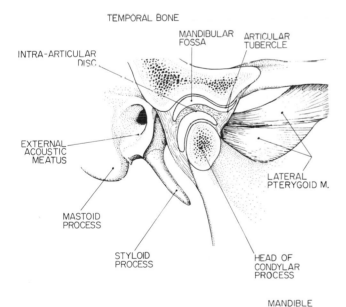

FIG. 22.13. The mandible; (a) medial aspect, (b) lateral aspect.

FIG. 22.14. Lateral view of sagittal section of right temporomandibular joint.

Each temporomandibular joint is formed by the head of the condylar process of the mandible and the mandibular fossa and articular tubercle of the squamous temporal bone. These two bony surfaces are not congruent.

The superior surface forms a wide shallow groove, facing downwards, whose anterior edge is enlarged into a ridge, the articular tubercle. The long axes of both groove and ridges run transversely. The articular upper surface of the head of the mandible is ellipsoidal and has a long axis which runs medially and slightly backwards. The neck of the mandible below it is flattened anteroposteriorly and exhibits a fossa, the pterygoid fovea, on its anteromedial aspect. The lateral pterygoid muscle, which is intimately associated with the joint both structurally and functionally, is mainly inserted into the fovea but also passes through the capsule of the joint to become continuous with the articular disc. This is an oval plate, composed mainly of dense collagenous tissue, which lies within the joint cavity. Its edge is fused with the capsule and the disc therefore divides the joint cavity into upper and lower compartments.

The capsule of the joint is attached superiorly to the margins of the mandibular fossa, except anteriorly, where it extends on to the anterior aspect of the articular tubercle. Inferiorly it surrounds the neck of the mandible. It is thickened laterally to form the **lateral ligament**, whose fibres run downwards and backwards from the lateral margin of the fossa and the tubercle to the lateral side and posterior aspect of the neck of the mandible. It has no counterpart of comparable strength on the medial aspect of the joint, since the two temporomandibular joints are separate parts of the same functional articulation. The two lateral ligaments are the widely separated **collateral ligaments** of the single mandibulocranial articulation.

The fibres of the capsule which connect the superior articular surface of the joint to the intra-articular disc are lax. Those connecting the disc to the lower articular surface are, by contrast, shorter and tighter. Movement between the disc and the squamous temporal bone is accordingly easier to achieve than movement between the disc and the mandible.

The **sphenomandibular** and **stylomandibular ligaments** are situated close to the temporomandibular joint, but have little functional connection with it. The former is the remnant of the perichondrium of the first arch cartilage of the embryo (Meckel's cartilage), and the latter is a thickening in the fascia between the parotid and submandibular glands.

MUSCLES OF MASTICATION

This group of four muscles is supplied by motor (branchial efferent) fibres of the trigeminal nerve, which reach them through its mandibular division. The muscles are derivatives of the first or mandibular arch mesoderm. The masseter lies on the lateral aspect of the plane of the mandible, the temporalis is situated in that plane, and the lateral and medial pterygoid muscles lie deep to it.

The bony arch which gives origin to the masseter is the **zygomatic arch**; it is formed by the zygomatic process of the temporal bone, the zygomatic bone itself and the zygomatic process of the maxilla. The muscles of mastication are shown in figs. 22.15 and 16 where *O* and *I* represent their origins and insertions respectively.

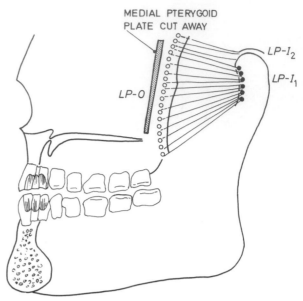

Lateral Pterygoid (*LP*)

LP-O Lateral surface of lateral pterygoid plate and the infratemporal surface of the greater wing of the sphenoid.
LP-I₁ Pterygoid fovea on the neck of the mandible.
LP-I₂ Intra-articular disc of the joint.

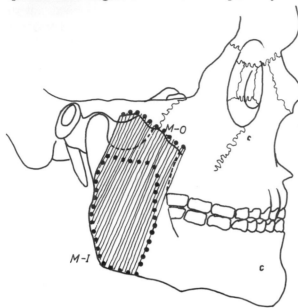

Masseter (*M*)

M-O Lower border of zygomatic arch.
M-I Lateral aspect of the ramus of the mandible.

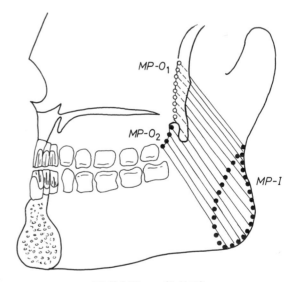

Medial Pterygoid (*MP*)

MP-O₁ Pterygoid fossa.
MP-O₂ Tuberosity of the maxilla.
MP-I Medial aspect of the angle of the mandible.

FIG. 22.16. Muscles of mastication; medial view.

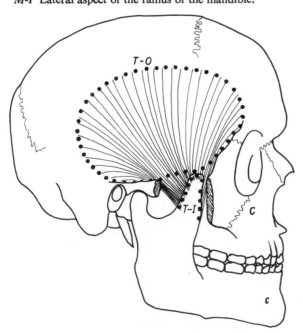

Temporalis (*T*)

T-O Floor of temporal fossa and overlying fascia.
T-I Tip and margins of the coronoid process of the mandible.

FIG. 22.15. Muscles of mastication.

MOVEMENTS OF THE TEMPOROMANDIBULAR JOINT

Movements at this joint are mainly, but not exclusively, produced by the masticatory muscles. The mouth is opened by the lateral pterygoid muscle, by the digastric, suprahyoid and infrahyoid muscles, and by gravity. In this action, two movements occur within the double joint cavity. First, the head of the mandible and the disc move together under the traction of the lateral pterygoid muscle, sliding downwards and forwards until they lie directly under the articular tubercle. Because of the direction of the fibres of the lateral ligament of the temporomandibular joint, no resistance is encountered from it. Secondly, and occurring at the end of the first movement, the head of the mandible rotates in a hinge movement on the undersurface of the intra-articular disc. The axis of the combined movements is a horizontal line passing through the mandibular foramina; traction on the inferior alveolar nerve and vessels is therefore minimized.

Apposition of the teeth, or occlusion, is achieved by the combined actions of the masseters, medial pterygoids and the temporals. Protrusion (forward thrusting) of the chin is produced by the contraction of the medial and lateral pterygoids, assisted by the masseters, while retraction is effected by the posterior fibres of the temporales. A slewing of the jaw to one side is achieved by combining protrusion by the muscles of one side of the head with retraction by the temporalis of the other.

NECK

The neck extends from the level of the lower margin of the mandible anteriorly and from the superior nuchal line posteriorly down to the thoracic inlet. The structures which lie in front of the cervical vertebrae are, however, continued upwards, deep to the mandible, as the midline hollow visceral spaces of the head, and as the laterally placed neurovascular bundles as far as the under surfaces of the middle and anterior cranial fossae. The infratemporal and submandibular regions are simply upward extensions of the neck.

The structures which form the neck can be divided into: the **central supporting structures** (the cervical vertebral column with its prevertebral, paravertebral and postvertebral muscles), the **neurovascular bundles of the head** and the superficially placed **muscle sheet** with its enclosing layers of deep fascia (figs. 22.17 and 18).

Anterior to the prevertebral muscles and between the neurovascular bundles, the hollow viscera run through the neck into the thorax.

Central supporting structures

CERVICAL VERTEBRAL COLUMN

The individual vertebrae differ from each other more sharply than do those of the thoracic, lumbar or sacral regions. They fall into the following groups:

(1) atlas-axis complex, which is modified from the basic vertebral pattern,

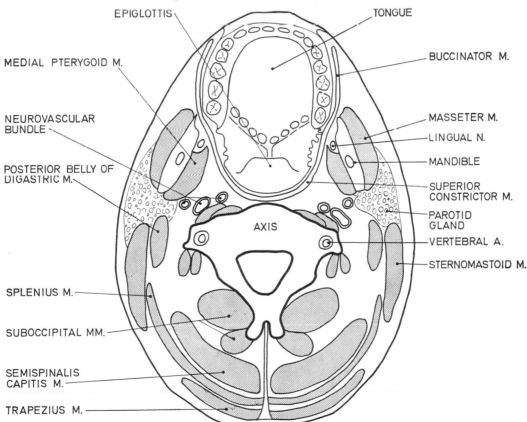

FIG. 22.17. Horizontal section of head.

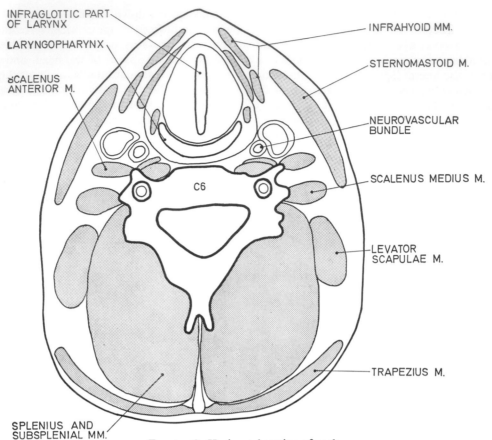

INFRAGLOTTIC PART OF LARYNX

LARYNGOPHARYNX

SCALENUS ANTERIOR M.

INFRAHYOID MM.

STERNOMASTOID M.

NEUROVASCULAR BUNDLE

SCALENUS MEDIUS M.

C6

LEVATOR SCAPULAE M.

TRAPEZIUS M.

SPLENIUS AND SUBSPLENIAL MM.

FIG. 22.18. Horizontal section of neck.

(2) typical cervical vertebrae, the third to the sixth,

(3) seventh cervical vertebra, which is transitional in form between the typical cervical and the upper thoracic vertebrae.

Atlas-axis complex

The part of the skull which surrounds the foramen magnum is a series of modified vertebrae, which have fused into a single mass. The synovial joints between this mass and the upper surface of the atlas, and between the atlas and the axis, are of the same nature.

The **atlas** (fig. 22.19) is unique in possessing no body. Instead, two lateral masses are connected by two bony arches, the posterior arch being longer and more slender. Elongated kidney shaped facets on the superior aspect of each lateral mass articulate with the occipital condyles.

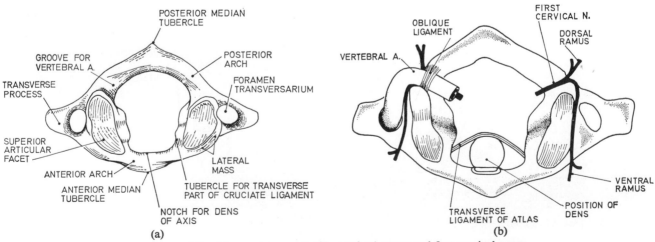

POSTERIOR MEDIAN TUBERCLE

GROOVE FOR VERTEBRAL A.

POSTERIOR ARCH

TRANSVERSE PROCESS

FORAMEN TRANSVERSARIUM

SUPERIOR ARTICULAR FACET

LATERAL MASS

ANTERIOR ARCH

ANTERIOR MEDIAN TUBERCLE

TUBERCLE FOR TRANSVERSE PART OF CRUCIATE LIGAMENT

NOTCH FOR DENS OF AXIS

(a)

OBLIQUE LIGAMENT

FIRST CERVICAL N.

DORSAL RAMUS

VERTEBRAL A.

VENTRAL RAMUS

TRANSVERSE LIGAMENT OF ATLAS

POSITION OF DENS

(b)

FIG. 22.19. Atlas (a) superior aspect, (b) vertebral artery and first cervical nerve.

On the corresponding parts of the inferior aspects of the lateral masses are circular, flattened facets, set at a slight angle to the horizontal plane, for articulation with facets on either side of the dens of the axis.

The **anterior arch** of the atlas is slightly anterior to the plane of the anterior aspects of the succeeding vertebral bodies. It unites the two lateral masses of the atlas, whose body (or, more strictly, centrum) has become separated and fused to the axis forming a pivot, the **dens** (odontoid process). There is a tubercle on the anterior aspect of the arch to which are attached the upper ends of the anterior longitudinal ligament of the vertebral column and the longus colli muscles. On the posterior aspect of this arch there is a synovial area for articulation with the dens of the axis.

The **posterior arch** is grooved on its upper surface by the vertebral artery, immediately posterior to the condyle. The first cervical nerve lies in the floor of this groove, and divides while within it. The ventral ramus turns anteriorly around the lateral margin of the condyle, while the dorsal ramus runs straight backwards in the groove. Above the nerve, the vertebral artery fills the whole width of the groove as it turns backwards and medially around the posterior margin of the condyle, before turning forwards on its medial side to pierce the posterior atlanto-occipital membrane (fig. 22.19b).

From the lateral aspect of the lateral mass projects the **transverse process**, within which is the **foramen transversarium** for the vertebral artery and its venae comitantes. The tubercle on its lateral margin is the posterior one. Neither the atlas nor the axis has a readily demonstrable anterior tubercle on its transverse process.

The transverse processes of the atlas are prominent on the lateral aspect of the neck, just below the external acoustic meatus.

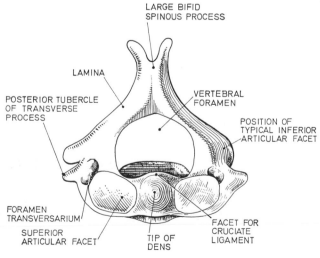

FIG. 22.20. Axis.

The **axis** (fig. 22.20) is a compound of the centrum of the atlas and the whole of the second cervical vertebra. It is further modified on its superior surface by the absence of typical articular facets, which would hinder rotation of the atlas and skull around the dens of the axis. The inferior aspect of the axis, however, exhibits none of these specialized features, and conforms to that of any typical cervical vertebra. The superior articular facets are therefore anterior to its inferior facets and consequently also to the articular facets of the other vertebrae. These superior facets correspond to those involved in the atlanto-occipital articulation. They consist of flat circular areas on either side of the dens and are inclined slightly downwards and outwards.

In contrast to the atlas, which has no true spine, the axis possesses a very strong, prominent bifid spinous process. The ligamentum nuchae is attached to the groove between the two parts of the split spinous process. When a needle is to be inserted into the cisterna magna (cisternal puncture), the palpable prominence of the spinous process of the axis is used to direct the point of the needle towards the posterior atlanto-occipital membrane.

The **occipito-atlanto-axial** joints differ from those uniting other vertebrae (p. 21.3). The movement of nodding involves the articulating surfaces of the atlas and the occipital bone. The rotary movement, however, only takes place between the dens of the axis and the anterior arch of the atlas, and involves the movement of the combined skull and atlas as a single mobile unit upon the axis and the remainder of the cervical column. Fusion of the atlas and axis virtually prevents rotation of the head.

The specialized articulations (fig. 22.21) involving the base of the skull, the atlas and the axis are therefore:

(1) atlanto-occipital.
(2) atlanto-axial.
(3) occipito-axial.

The atlas and the occipital bone are united by the two articular capsules of the joints between the condyles of the two bones, and by membranes uniting the arches of the atlas to the margins of the foramen magnum. These membranes are continuous at their edges with the capsules of the synovial joints. The anterior **atlanto-occipital membrane** is uninterrupted, but the larger posterior membrane is pierced laterally by the vertebral artery and its venae comitantes and by the emerging first cervical nerve.

The union of the atlas and the axis is also achieved by synovial joints which connect the opposed articular surfaces of the two bones. The posterior arch of the atlas is united to the arch of the axis by the **atlanto-axial membrane.** The undivided trunk of the second cervical nerve pierces this membrane, and its large dorsal ramus lies in contact with the upper surface of the arch of the axis. The posterior aspect of the body of the axis is connected to the lateral masses of the atlas by two diverging accessory atlanto-axial ligaments.

The apex of the dens of the axis is connected to the base of the skull at the anterior margin of the foramen magnum by the vestigial apical ligament. From either side of this slender structure, two much stronger **alar ligaments** radiate from the dens to the foramen magnum. Posterior to the dens the **cruciate ligament** covers the atlas and axis to reach the occipital bone. It consists of a thin longitudinal band, running from the posterior surface of the body of the axis to the anterior margin of the foramen magnum, blended with a much stronger transverse band which connects the two tubercles on the lateral masses of the atlas. This transverse band holds the dens against the arch of the atlas. Behind the cruciate ligament, the posterior longitudinal ligament extends upwards as the membrana tectoria to the anterior margin of the foramen magnum.

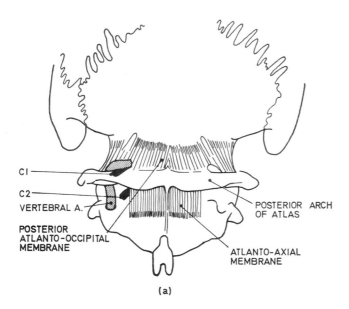

(a)

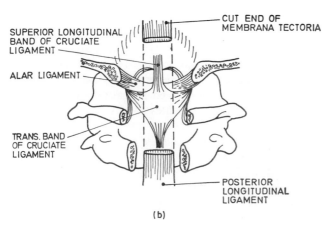

(b)

FIG. 22.21. The occipito-atlanto-axial connection; (a) posterior view, (b) internal ligaments.

Typical cervical vertebrae

The third, fourth, fifth and sixth cervical vertebrae are alike in all but minor details. Their bodies, when viewed from above or below, are kidney-shaped (fig. 22.22). The

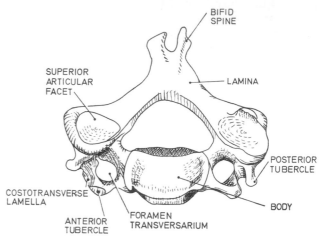

FIG. 22.22. Typical cervical vertebra.

posterolateral margins of the upper surfaces of the bodies are drawn upwards like the seat of a chair. Correspondingly, on the inferior surfaces, the posterolateral margins are bevelled off.

The pedicles project backwards and laterally from the body and, with the laminae, complete the vertebral foramen which is triangular in outline. The articular facets are supported by a short pillar of bone, which runs from the superior to the inferior articular surfaces. The upper facet faces upwards and backwards, the lower downwards and forwards.

The transverse process projects from the lateral aspect of the body and the anterior part of the neural arch of the vertebra. It contains the foramen transversarium for the vertebral artery. The lateral edge of the transverse process is drawn up into two tubercles, an anterior and a posterior united by a thin bar of bone, the **costotransverse lamella**. This bar is bent downwards in the middle and so accommodates the ventral ramus of the cervical nerve corresponding in number to the vertebra. The anterior tubercle is only present on the typical vertebrae and is most marked on the sixth where it is termed the **carotid tubercle**, since it is possible to compress the common carotid artery against it. To these tubercles are attached the longus colli, the longus capitis and the scalenus anterior muscles, whose origins are therefore restricted to the typical vertebrae. This is in contrast to scalenus medius and all the muscles posterior to it, which are attached to posterior tubercles and so arise at any level of the cervical column. The anterior tubercle and the costotransverse lamella are homologues of the ribs.

Seventh vertebra

This differs from the typical members of the series in having a long, non-bifid spine. Because this spinous process can usually be seen in the back of the neck, it is referred to as the **vertebra prominens**. The anterior tubercle of the transverse process of this vertebra, as in the atlas and axis, is suppressed. The foramen transversarium of the process is often as large as that of any other cervical vertebra, but usually only contains a vein. The general appearance is therefore intermediate between that of a typical cervical and a typical thoracic vertebra.

CERVICAL VERTEBRAL MUSCLES (figs. 22.23a & b)

Prevertebral muscles. The **longus colli** is a strip of skeletal muscle fibres and tendon, which lies on the fronts of the cervical and upper three thoracic vertebrae, immediately lateral to the anterior longitudinal ligament.

The **longus capitis** arises in common with the longus colli. Its fibres run upwards and medially on the anterior surface of the latter muscle to be inserted into the basilar part of the occipital bone, lateral to the pharyngeal tubercle. The two longus muscles form the immediate posterior relations of the midline hollow viscera and the neurovascular bundle, separated from them by the prevertebral layer of fascia.

Paravertebral muscles. These are grouped around the brachial and cervical plexuses, and the subclavian artery. The **scalenus anterior muscle**, arising from the anterior tubercles of the typical cervical vertebrae, forms the anterior wall of the cleft for the plexuses and the artery. The posterior wall is composed of the scalenus medius and posterior muscles and the levator scapulae (p. 23.6).

The course of the scalenus anterior muscle is downwards, forwards and laterally from its origin on the cervical column to the scalene tubercle on the superior surface of the first rib. Here it is inserted behind the groove for the subclavian vein and in front of the groove for the subclavian artery.

The **scalenus medius muscle** extends downwards and laterally from its extensive origin from all or most of the posterior tubercles of the transverse processes of the cervical column to the posterior part of upper surface of the first rib (fig. 22.24). The posterior fibres of the muscle extend downwards as far as the second rib, and are called the **scalenus posterior muscle.**

The prevertebral and paravertebral groups of muscles are supplied directly by the ventral rami of the cervical nerves. The longi flex the vertebral column, in opposition to the postvertebral group of muscles; the scaleni bend the cervical column, and indirectly the head, to their own side of the body. They play an important part in the elevation of the first, and to a lesser extent the second ribs, in costal respiration.

Postvertebral muscles. The posterior aspects of the laminae of the cervical vertebrae below the level of the first give attachment to an irregular series of obliquely placed muscle bundles, the **multifidus**. Superficial to these bundles, a more clearly defined layer of muscle runs obliquely from transverse processes to spines, ending at the spine of the axis. This is the **semispinalis cervicis muscle**. From the spine of the axis two muscles extend in the same plane as the semispinalis; the **inferior oblique muscle** which goes to the transverse process of the atlas, and the **rectus capitis posterior major**, which is attached superiorly between the inferior nuchal line and the foramen magnum.

The angle between the inferior oblique and the rectus major muscles is closed above and laterally by the **superior oblique muscle**, which extends from the transverse process of the atlas to the lateral part of the occipital bone. The three-cornered recess enclosed by the two obliqui and the rectus major is the **suboccipital triangle** (fig. 22.25).

The muscles of the triangle are supplied by the dorsal ramus of the first cervical nerve. The nerve breaks immediately into bundles to the individual muscles within the suboccipital triangle.

Immediately superficial to the semispinalis cervicis and the suboccipital muscles lies the **semispinalis capitis**. This is a thick, powerful structure and gives rise to the longitudinal prominence on either side of the midline of the back of the neck. It arises from the transverse processes of the upper half of the thoracic column and from the articular processes of the lower half of the cervical column, and is inserted into the medial posterior part of the infranuchal area of the occipital bone. It lies in contact with the ligamentum nuchae, but usually has no attachment to it. Other ill-defined slender muscles complement semispinalis.

The **splenius capitis** and **cervicis muscles** form a single continuous sheet which arises from the lower half of the ligamentum nuchae and the upper thoracic spinous processes and radiates upwards, laterally and forwards to be inserted into the lateral part of the superior nuchal line, the mastoid process, and the posterior tubercles of the upper cervical vertebrae. The splenius muscular sheet separates the deep postvertebral muscles from the levator scapulae, scaleni, the trapezius and the sternomastoid muscles.

All the postvertebral muscles are supplied by the dorsal rami of the cervical and upper thoracic spinal nerves. They extend the head and neck.

CERVICAL SPINAL NERVES (fig. 22.26)

The cervicothoracic enlargement of the spinal cord lies at the region of attachment of the nerves forming the brachial plexus. This enlargement commences gradually a little below the foramen magnum, reaches its greatest size at the level of the fifth cervical vertebra and tapers off at the second thoracic vertebral level.

The cervical spinal nerves are attached to the spinal cord, like all spinal nerves, by a ventral, efferent and a dorsal, afferent root. In the first cervical segment, however, the dorsal afferent attachment is very small, and may be absent since there is no cutaneous distribution of this nerve. Between the dorsal and ventral roots of the upper five or six cervical nerves, and dorsal to the ligamentum denticulatum, the rootlets of the spinal part of the accessory nerve ascend to the foramen magnum.

The cervical nerves divide into dorsal and ventral rami. In the first two of the series, the dorsal ramus is by far the larger; the remainder conform to the pattern of the other spinal nerves, with a large ventral and a small dorsal ramus. The ventral rami of the second to the fourth nerves send cutaneous branches to the side of the head, the angle of the jaw, part of the external ear and the anterior part of the neck. The fifth and succeeding cervical ventral rami supply the upper limb. The dorsal rami supply the back of the head and the posterior part of the neck as far down as the vertebra prominens with cutaneous branches derived from the second to the sixth segments only, the remaining segments having no cutaneous representation through the dorsal rami.

The prevertebral and paravertebral muscles are supplied by ventral rami, while the dorsal rami supply all

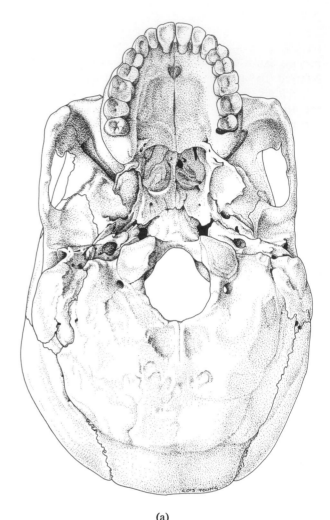

(a)

FIG. 22.23. Inferior aspect of skull.

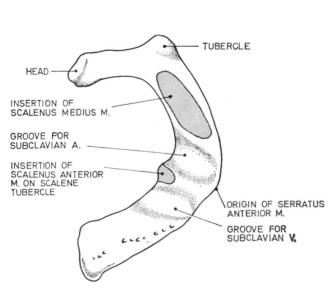

FIG. 22.24. The first rib from above.

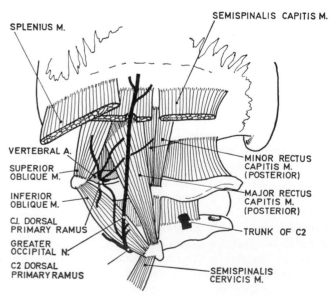

FIG. 22.25. The suboccipital triangle.

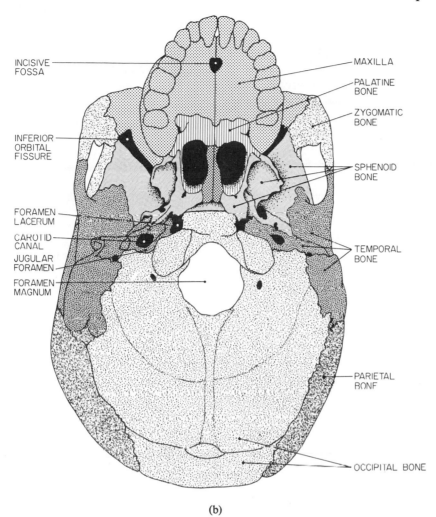

INCISIVE FOSSA

INFERIOR ORBITAL FISSURE

FORAMEN LACERUM

CAROTID CANAL

JUGULAR FORAMEN

FORAMEN MAGNUM

MAXILLA

PALATINE BONE

ZYGOMATIC BONE

SPHENOID BONE

TEMPORAL BONE

PARIETAL BONE

OCCIPITAL BONE

(b)

of the postvertebral muscles. Since any one muscle, for example, semispinalis capitis, may be supplied from a series of cervical and upper thoracic segmental nerves, defects of motor innervation become clinically obvious only when an extensive lesion exists.

The **first cervical nerve** has a very small dorsal afferent root since this nerve has no cutaneous distribution. The nerve emerges from the vertebral canal dorsal to the synovial joint of the atlanto-occipital articulation. Its ventral ramus turns forward on the lateral side of the lateral mass of the atlas to appear as a descending nerve bundle which joins the larger ventral ramus of the second cervical nerve. A large part of the ventral ramus of the first cervical nerve is distributed with the hypoglossal nerve which it joins just below the base of the skull. This is distributed to muscles of the infrahyoid group by the ansa cervicalis. The dorsal ramus of the first cervical nerve is distributed to the muscles of the suboccipital triangle.

The **second cervical nerve** pierces the atlanto-axial membrane and then divides into a large dorsal and a

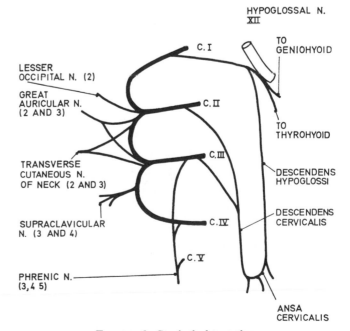

HYPOGLOSSAL N. XII

C. I

C. II

C. III

C. IV

C. V

LESSER OCCIPITAL N. (2)

GREAT AURICULAR N. (2 AND 3)

TRANSVERSE CUTANEOUS N. OF NECK (2 AND 3)

SUPRACLAVICULAR N. (3 AND 4)

PHRENIC N. (3, 4 5)

TO GENIOHYOID

TO THYROHYOID

DESCENDENS HYPOGLOSSI

DESCENDENS CERVICALIS

ANSA CERVICALIS

FIG. 22.26. Cervical plexus plan.

smaller ventral ramus. The latter is distributed partly to skin with the cutaneous branches of the cervical plexus, and partly to the adjacent muscles, including the sterno-mastoid. From the point of division, it passes forwards around the lateral aspect of the vertebral artery as it lies between the transverse processes of the axis and atlas, and joins the first and third cervical rami on the front of the vertebral column. The dorsal ramus supplies fibres to some of the postvertebral muscles, but the major part of the nerve is distributed to the skin of the back of the head as the **greater occipital nerve**. It passes below the inferior oblique muscle, crosses the suboccipital triangle, pierces semispinalis capitis and trapezius to enter the superficial fascia at the superior nuchal line.

The **ansa cervicalis** is a loop of nerve fibres which runs with the neurovascular bundle in the neck. It has two roots, a superior one derived from the trunk of the hypoglossal nerve, but containing cervical fibres only, and an inferior root of fibres from the second and third cervical ventral rami. The branches of the ansa pass to the infrahyoid group of muscles (p. 22.55).

Cutaneous branches (fig. 22.27) are derived from the interconnected ventral rami of the second, third and fourth cervical nerves. The combination of the second and third rami produces the **lesser occipital, great auricular** and **transverse cutaneous nerves.** From the third and fourth nerves are derived the **medial, intermediate** and **lateral supraclavicular nerves.**

The **phrenic nerve** (fig. 22.28) supplies the diaphragm which develops in the neck and so its efferent nerve supply comes from the fourth cervical segment, with additional fibres from the third and fifth segments. These roots

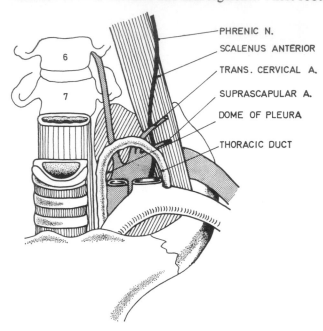

FIG. 22.28. Phrenic nerve in the neck.

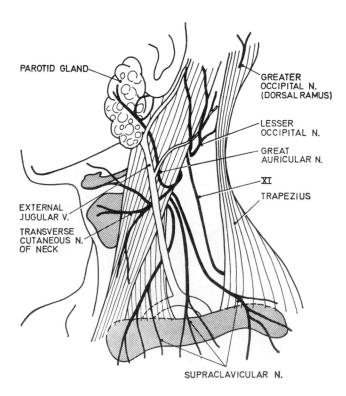

FIG. 22.27. Cutaneous branches of the cervical plexus.

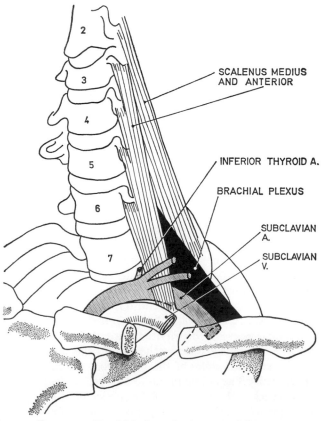

FIG. 22.29. Brachial plexus in the root of the neck.

pass on to the anterior aspect of the scalenus anterior muscle deep to its fascial covering. There they combine to form a single trunk, which passes off the medial margin of the muscle at the root of the neck to enter the superior mediastinum. An accessory phrenic nerve, composed of fibres of the fifth cervical nerve, often arises from the nerve to the subclavius muscle.

The ventral rami of the lower four cervical nerves, with some fibres from the fourth nerve as well, are distributed to the upper limb and shoulder girdle. Along with the ventral ramus of the first thoracic nerve, they form the **brachial plexus** (p. 23.30). This occupies the posterior part of the interval between the scalenus anterior and scalenus medius muscles, and the upper surface of the first rib. The subclavian artery lies anterior to the plexus in the lowest part of the interval. The combined bundle of nerves and artery passes to the axilla through the cervicoaxillary canal. This connects the posterior triangle of the neck with the apex of the axilla, and is bounded by the first rib, the clavicle and the upper border of the scapula. The subclavian vein, which completes the neurovascular bundle of the upper limb, lies slightly more anterior than the artery and nerves and is separated from them at the root of the neck by the scalenus anterior muscle (fig. 22.29).

Neurovascular bundle (figs. 22.17 and 18)

The blood vessels and nerves passing through the neck either to or from the head occupy the triangular interval between the prevertebral muscles, the midline hollow viscera and the superficial muscle, sternomastoid. They form a bundle which extends from behind the medial third of the clavicle to the base of the skull at the carotid canal and jugular foramen, medial to the lower part of the external acoustic meatus. The common carotid artery and its internal and external branches, the vagus nerve and the internal jugular vein are the major components of the bundle. The relationships of these components to each other vary at different levels of the bundle. They are together enclosed in a tubular sheath of deep fascia, the **carotid sheath**. Posteriorly, it fuses with the prevertebral layer of fascia which covers the longi and the scaleni, and anteriorly it blends with the fascia which encloses the thyroid gland.

CAROTID ARTERIES (fig. 22.30)

The **internal carotid artery** supplies the major part of the cerebral hemisphere of its own side, and communicates, by means of the circulus arteriosus (circle of Willis) at the base of the brain, with the opposite internal carotid artery, and usually with both vertebral arteries. By contrast, the **external carotid artery** supplies muscles, fasciae, skin and bone, and plays no part in the arterial supply to the central nervous system.

Although the cervical part of the course of each **common carotid artery** is practically identical, their origins differ on the two sides of the body. The right common carotid and subclavian arteries originate as the two branches of the brachiocephalic artery at the level of the upper part of the right sternoclavicular joint. The left common carotid artery arises, as does the left subclavian, from the arch of the aorta, and has a short intrathoracic course between the trachea and the left lung. It enters the neck opposite the left sternoclavicular joint. The left subclavian artery is likewise sandwiched between the superior mediastinal structures and the left lung. It enters the root of the neck medial and slightly anterior to the apex of the left lung and runs laterally in a groove on its upper surface.

The common carotid artery ascends in the neck, just under cover of the anterior border of the sternomastoid muscle, and divides at the level of the upper margin of the thyroid cartilage, opposite the lower border of the third cervical vertebra. The internal carotid artery continues in exactly the same direction as the common carotid, while the external carotid artery commences anteromedial to its internal counterpart, but progressively moves to an anterolateral position as it ascends in the neck. It becomes smaller as it is followed headwards, since it gives off a series of branches. It ends posteromedial to the neck of the mandible by dividing into the superficial temporal and maxillary arteries. By contrast, the internal carotid artery, which gives off no branches in the neck, remains the same size until it enters the petrous temporal bone through the carotid canal. At its origin

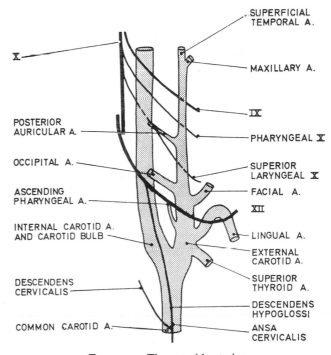

FIG. 22.30. The carotid arteries.

there is a slight dilation of its wall, the **carotid sinus**. Between the two branches of the common carotid artery is found a small group of chemoreceptor cells embedded in fibrous tissue, the **carotid body** (p. 31.27). Both the body and the sinus are supplied by the glossopharyngeal nerve through its sinus branch, to which some vagus fibres are added.

Branches of the external carotid artery

The **superior thyroid artery** supplies the thyroid gland where it anastomoses with the inferior thyroid artery (p. 22.34). A large branch, the superior laryngeal, pierces the thyrohyoid membrane to supply the larynx.

The **ascending pharyngeal artery** is a long vessel which runs up to the base of the skull and supplies the wall of the oropharynx, the nasopharynx and the palatine tonsil.

The **lingual artery** passes deep to the hyoglossus muscle to supply the tongue, the sublingual gland and the floor of the mouth.

The **facial artery** passes upwards on the lateral aspects of the middle and superior constrictors of the pharynx, before turning sharply downwards, directly opposite the bed of the palatine tonsil, from which it is separated only by the thin superior constrictor muscle. At this point, it gives off the ascending palatine and tonsillar branches. It then descends well lateral to its ascending course, lying in a groove in the posterior pole of the submandibular salivary gland, to which it gives an arterial supply. Thereafter it lies between the gland and the medial surface of the medial pterygoid muscle before it appears at the lower margin of the mandible, and turns upwards on the anterior edge of the masseter to enter the face. Its branches are distributed to the palatine tonsil, the pharynx, the soft palate, the submandibular gland and the skin and superficial muscles of the face.

The **occipital artery** arises from the posterior aspect of the external carotid at the point at which the hypoglossal nerve turns from its posterior to its lateral aspect. Its course is first below and then medial to the posterior belly of the digastric muscle. It grooves the base of the skull just medial to the mastoid notch, from which the digastric muscle arises, and then runs across the occipital bone to appear at the superior nuchal line with the greater occipital nerve and supplies the posterior part of the scalp. It gives branches to the muscles of the neck, including the sternomastoid.

The **posterior auricular artery** is a small branch whose only importance is that it gives rise to the stylomastoid branch which supplies the distal part of the facial nerve.

The **superficial temporal artery**, one of the two terminal branches, supplies the parotid gland and the temporomandibular joint behind which it passes. Thereafter it crosses the zygomatic arch and breaks up into branches to the temporal part of the scalp.

The **maxillary artery**, the other terminal branch, runs forward and medially, deep to the mandible to reach the pterygo-maxillary fissure, where it breaks up into branches to the nose, nasopharynx and palate. It gives off numerous branches in the infratemporal region. Of these, only two are of importance. The **middle meningeal artery** enters the middle cranial fossa via the foramen spinosum to supply only dura mater and bone. The **inferior alveolar artery** accompanies the inferior alveolar nerve through the mandibular foramen to the teeth of the lower jaw and to the skin of the chin and mucous membrane of the lower lip.

INTERNAL JUGULAR VEIN

The internal jugular system drains the cranial cavity and only a few of the superficial veins of the head and the neck end in it. Its course is downwards, forwards and medially from its start at its superior bulb in the jugular foramen to its end at its inferior bulb at the root of the neck, where it joins the subclavian vein to form the brachiocephalic venous trunk.

The relationship of the internal jugular vein to the axis of the internal carotid and common carotid arteries and the vagus nerve alters as it descends. As it emerges from the jugular foramen, it is posterior and very slightly lateral to the internal carotid artery, as this latter vessel is entering the carotid canal. Between the artery and the vein, the last four cranial nerves pass from the cranial cavity to the neck. The glossopharyngeal, vagus and spinal accessory nerves leave the jugular foramen anterior to the vein, while the hypoglossal nerve gains its exit medial to the others through the hypoglossal canal, and runs laterally between the vagus nerve and the internal jugular vein to the lateral aspect of the external carotid artery. The glossopharyngeal nerve turns anteriorly around the internal carotid artery, and comes to lie on its lateral aspect, where it becomes one of a group of structures separating the internal and external carotid arteries. The spinal accessory nerve turns posteriorly on one or other side of the internal jugular vein, before supplying and piercing the sternomastoid muscle. The vagus nerve descends vertically, initially between the artery and the vein, but later posterior to both of them, lying in the interval between them.

In the neck, the internal jugular vein swings on to the lateral aspect of the arterial axis, often overlapping it anteriorly, and permitting the vagus nerve to lie against the prevertebral muscles. As the vein descends it passes to a plane anterior to that of the common carotid artery, which it is accompanying at this point. The brachiocephalic vein, in which the internal jugular vein terminates, lies on a plane anterior to that of the three large branches of the aortic arch, the brachiocephalic, left common carotid and left subclavian arteries. As the venous drainage is to the right atrium, both veins deviate to the right and the right vein is often larger than the left.

The internal jugular vein receives the inferior petrosal sinus just below the base of the skull. The venous efferents from the pharyngeal plexus of veins, the facial, lingual and superior and middle thyroid veins join it in the neck.

VAGUS NERVE (fig. 22.31)

The two vagi follow similar courses from the base of the skull to the lower part of the neck. Thereafter, differences in the great blood vessels on the two sides affect the course of the two nerves.

Within the jugular foramen and for a short distance below, the vagus nerve has two elongated swellings, the superior and inferior sensory ganglia. These contain pseudo-unipolar cells concerned in the transmission of somatic sensation, taste and sensation from viscera. From the superior ganglion, a small twig is given off to the dura mater of the posterior cranial fossa, and a slightly larger one, the auricular branch, proceeds through the lateral part of the temporal bone to emerge on the lateral aspect of the skull at the tympanomastoid fissure, and supplies the skin of the external acoustic meatus and the lateral aspect of the tympanic membrane with sensory fibres, in association with fibres of the auriculotemporal nerve (fig. 22.10).

Two branches of greater importance leave the inferior sensory ganglion just below the base of the skull. These are as follows:

The **pharyngeal branch,** which passes between the internal and external carotid arteries to reach the pharyngeal plexus of nerves on the lateral aspect of the middle constrictor of the pharynx. The nerve contains mainly efferent fibres, derived from the cranial part of the accessory nerve.

The **superior laryngeal nerve,** which passes medial to both the internal and external carotid arteries to run downwards and forwards on the side of the pharynx, where it breaks up into an internal and an external branch. The former pierces the thyrohyoid membrane to supply the upper part of the larynx and the epiglottis with sensory fibres, including taste fibres to the latter structure. The external laryngeal nerve sends motor fibres to the cricothyroid muscle and to the inferior constrictor of the pharynx.

Although these two branches arise from the parent trunk of the vagus at the site of the inferior sensory ganglion, many of their fibres come from nerve cell nuclei within the medulla oblongata. True sensory fibres, the peripheral processes of the cell bodies of the ganglia, form only a proportion of these nerves.

The vagus nerve descends in the neck within the carotid sheath, coming to lie directly on the prevertebral structures a short distance below the jugular foramen, as

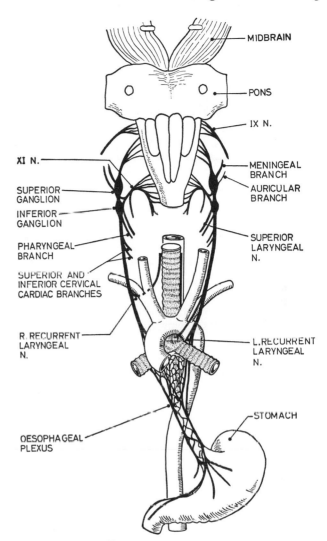

FIG. 22.31. Vagus nerve.

the internal jugular vein swings laterally on its descending course. It gives off two further branches to the cardiac plexuses.

At the root of the neck, the courses of the two vagi differ. On the right, the nerve passes anterior to the beginning of the subclavian artery and then runs downwards and backwards, inclining medially to become applied to the right lateral aspect of the trachea. As it crosses the subclavian artery, it gives off the **right recurrent laryngeal nerve,** which passes around the artery to reach the interval between the trachea and the oesophagus. There it ascends to the lower border of the cricopharyngeus muscle, on to whose deep surface it passes as it enters the larynx. On the left side, however, the vagus nerve passes from the posterior wall of the carotid sheath into the interval between the carotid and subclavian arteries, and runs downwards on to the left lateral aspect of the arch of the aorta. The **left recurrent laryngeal nerve** arises from the vagus in the thorax, passes below the aortic arch and ascends into the neck on its medial aspect, in the tracheo-oesophageal groove, to end in the same way as the right nerve.

GLOSSOPHARYNGEAL NERVE (fig. 22.32)

Like the vagus, the glossopharyngeal nerve has two ill-defined swellings on its course in the jugular foramen. These are likewise composed of sensory cells, whose peripheral processes are distributed with the branches of the nerve. From the better defined inferior ganglion, arises the **tympanic nerve** which enters the petrous temporal bone by means of a canaliculus on the crest which separates the lower openings of the carotid canal and the jugular foramen. This is a mixed nerve, containing sensory fibres from the middle ear and the auditory tube and secretomotor fibres for the parotid gland.

In the upper part of the neurovascular bundle the nerve runs laterally, anterior to the vagus and posterior to the internal carotid artery, to gain the lateral aspect of the artery. It then passes downwards and forwards between the internal and external carotid arteries, gradually sliding round the stylopharyngeus muscle which it supplies. From the anterior margin of the stylopharyngeus muscle, the nerve runs forward on the side of the pharynx, deep to the stylohyoid ligament, to break up into its terminal branches. These supply the posterior

third of the tongue and the circumvallate papillae, the palatine tonsil and its bed, and the lateral part of the soft palate. The various fibres concerned are sensory from mucous membrane, taste fibres from the posterior one third of the tongue and from the circumvallate papillae, and secretomotor fibres to the mucous and serous glands of the tongue and oropharynx. These secretomotor fibres are postganglionic parasympathetic efferents, whose cell bodies lie in a number of scattered unnamed ganglia on the course of the main nerve trunk.

In addition to these branches, the glossopharyngeal nerve gives off a sinus branch to the carotid sinus and body, and a pharyngeal branch, which distributes sensory and secretomotor fibres to the wall of the pharynx.

SPINAL PART OF THE ACCESSORY NERVE

This nerve leaves the neurovascular bundle just below the jugular foramen to reach and supply the sternomastoid and trapezius muscles (pp. 22.35 and 23.5).

HYPOGLOSSAL NERVE (figs. 22.33 and 37)

After passing between the vagus nerve and the internal jugular vein, the hypoglossal nerve slips around the external carotid artery on to its lateral aspect where the occipital artery arises. Thereafter, it runs anteriorly on the lateral aspect of the carotid artery, passing deep to the posterior belly of the digastric and stylohyoid muscles, the submandibular gland and the mylohyoid muscle, to break up into branches to the intrinsic and extrinsic muscles of the tongue. It communicates with the first and second cervical nerves at the lower surface of the base of the skull and gives a root to the ansa cervicalis.

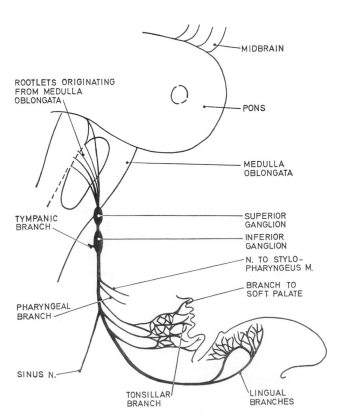

FIG. 22.32. Glossopharyngeal nerve.

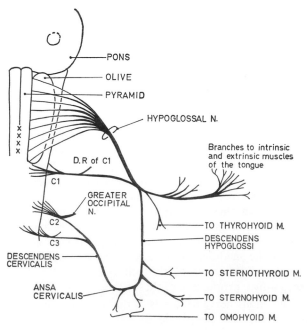

FIG. 22.33. Hypoglossal nerve.

CERVICAL SYMPATHETIC TRUNK (fig. 22.34)

All the fibres from the central nervous system to the sympathetic trunk enter below the level of the neck. The cervical part of the trunk is connected to the spinal nerves only by grey rami communicantes (p. 20.13). Usually, the cervical part consists of three ganglia, the superior, middle and inferior. The inferior cervical ganglion is, however, usually fused with the first, or the first and second thoracic sympathetic ganglia, to form a mass called the cervicothoracic ganglion.

The general position of the cervical part of the sympathetic trunk is within the prevertebral layer of fascia, on the front of the longus capitis and longus colli muscles, posteromedial to the carotid sheath. It is not, however, uniformly orientated in the vertical plane. The superior cervical ganglion, spindle-shaped and 2–3 cm long, lies on the front of the longus capitis muscle at the level of the second and third cervical vertebrae. The variable middle ganglion is often found near the inferior thyroid artery at the level of the sixth cervical vertebra. Below this, the trunk deviates laterally as it descends to the neck of the first rib, over the front of which it is continuous with the remainder of the sympathetic trunk.

All three ganglia give off grey rami communicantes, carrying postganglionic sympathetic effector neurones to the adjacent spinal nerves, with which they are distributed to blood vessels, sweat glands and erector pili muscles.

The superior ganglion gives off four, the middle ganglion two, and the cervicothoracic ganglion three or more grey rami. In addition, all three give branches to the cardiac plexuses.

Additional branches are given off by the individual ganglia as follows:

The **superior ganglion** gives branches to form plexuses around the internal and external carotid arteries and to the pharyngeal plexus of nerves. The internal carotid plexus is of particular importance as the principal route for the sympathetic supply of intracranial structures, including the eye.

The **middle cervical ganglion** forms a plexus around the inferior thyroid artery and provides an upper root to the ansa subclavia.

The **cervicothoracic ganglion** gives branches which form a plexus around the vertebral artery and provide a lower root to the ansa subclavia.

The **ansa subclavia** is an additional connecting bundle between the cervicothoracic and middle cervical ganglia, which passes in front of the proximal part of the subclavian artery, giving a plexus to that part of the vessel only. Fibres passing to the middle and superior ganglia from the second thoracic segment may utilize this route.

THORACIC DUCT IN THE NECK (fig. 22.35)

Although not a part of the neurovascular bundle, the thoracic duct is closely related to the lower part of the bundle on the left side of the root of the neck. It ascends

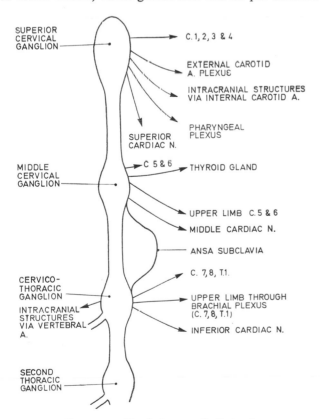

FIG. 22.34. Cervical sympathetic trunk.

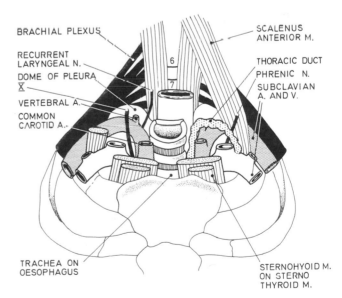

FIG. 22.35. Root of the neck.

on the left side of the oesophagus, and is therefore very deeply placed at the cervicothoracic junction. Passing upwards to the level of the seventh cervical vertebra, it turns sharply laterally between the carotid sheath and the structures immediately anterior to the vertebral column. It then passes forwards, lateral to the neurovascular bundle of the neck, to end at the junction of the internal jugular and subclavian veins. It may receive the jugular, subclavian and broncho-mediastinal lymph trunks of the left side of the body before it ends in the vein, or these may find separate entrances into the venous circulation. The corresponding three lymph trunks on the right side of the neck may also obtain separate openings into the junction of the right internal jugular and subclavian veins, or they may unite prior to doing so to form a right lymphatic duct (p. 21.39).

ADDITIONAL RELATIONSHIPS OF THE
NEUROVASCULAR BUNDLE

Between the internal and external carotid arteries at the upper part of their course are the styloid process, the stylopharyngeus muscle, the glossopharyngeal nerve and the pharyngeal branch of the vagus. The uppermost part of the external carotid artery runs through the deep part of the parotid salivary gland, which also separates it from the internal carotid artery.

On the medial aspect of the bundle lie the median hollow viscera. At the root of the neck these are represented by the trachea and oesophagus. At a higher level, the larynx and laryngopharynx and finally, extending to the base of the skull, the nasopharynx. Intervening between the bundle and the hollow viscera are the superior laryngeal nerve and its internal and external laryngeal branches, the pharyngeal branch of the superior cervical sympathetic ganglion, the pharyngeal venous plexus and the ascending pharyngeal artery.

In the neck, the neurovascular bundle is covered by parts of the infrahyoid muscles and the thyroid gland and its capsule, the sternomastoid muscle and its enclosing fascia, and the structures in the superficial fascia of the neck overlying it. Superiorly, the posterior belly of the digastric and the stylohyoid cross superficial to the bundle just below the angle of the mandible. Above that level, the bundle lies deep to the parotid gland and its enclosed structures, and to the mandible and the attached muscles of mastication.

The internal jugular vein is surrounded by the deep cervical chain of lymph nodes which begins superiorly as the retropharyngeal nodes, and which receives afferents from the collar chain and other superficial groups of nodes in the head and neck region (p. 22.56). The efferents from this series of nodes drain into the jugular lymph trunk.

SUBCLAVIAN VESSELS IN THE ROOT OF THE NECK
These are components of the neurovascular bundle of the upper limb (p. 23.39). In the neck each **subclavian artery** runs in a groove immediately anterior to the dome of the

pleura and the apex of the lung, forming a smooth curve, convex upwards. Passing through the narrow vertical slit between the scalenus anterior and the scalenus medius muscles and anterior to the brachial plexus, each artery crosses the upper surface of the first rib to enter the cervico-axillary canal. In the neck they give off the following branches:

The **vertebral artery** arises from the parent trunk well medial to the scalenus anterior muscle and runs upwards and medially behind the neurovascular bundle and enters the foramen transversarium of the sixth cervical vertebra. Thereafter, it runs upwards in the foramina transversaria of the remaining cervical vertebrae, with the ventral rami of the cervical nerves emerging posterior to it. Above the transverse process of the atlas, it turns backwards and medially, pierces the posterior atlanto-occipital membrane and enters the foramen magnum. After piercing the dural and arachnoid membranes, it runs upwards and forwards on the front of the medulla to unite with the artery of the opposite side to form the **midline basilar artery**. In its course in the neck it is accompanied by venae comitantes, which drain often as a single vertebral vein into the brachiocephalic vein. The vertebral artery is surrounded by its sympathetic plexus of nerves, derived from the cervicothoracic ganglion. Its only important branch below the foramen magnum is the **radicular branch** to the spinal cord. Within the cranial cavity, it gives off anterior and posterior **spinal branches**, which descend through the foramen magnum to supply the spinal cord.

The **internal thoracic artery** leaves the subclavian trunk just lateral to the origin of the vertebral artery and runs inferiorly to enter the thorax behind the first costal cartilage (p. 21.8).

The **thyrocervical trunk** arises from the upper surface of the subclavian artery just at the medial edge of the scalenus anterior muscle. It breaks up into three branches, two of which run laterally, anterior to the scalenus anterior muscle and the phrenic nerve, to supply structures in the posterior triangle of the neck and the scapular region. The upper of these two branches, the **transverse cervical artery**, sends a deep branch to accompany the dorsal scapular nerve, and a superficial branch which joins the spinal accessory nerve on the deep surface of the trapezius muscle. The lower branch, the **suprascapular artery**, runs laterally behind the clavicle to pass above the suprascapular ligament into the supraspinous fossa.

The third branch of the thyrocervical trunk is the **inferior thyroid artery**, which ascends on the medial edge of the scalenus anterior muscle to the level of the sixth cervical vertebra, and then turns sharply medially to enter the posterior aspect of the lateral lobe of the thyroid gland, supplying both it and the parathyroid glands. The transverse part of the inferior thyroid artery lies posterior to the neurovascular bundle of the head, but anterior to the vertebral artery and the prevertebral structures.

The **costocervical trunk** takes origin from the subclavian artery deep to the scalenus anterior muscle. It runs backwards across the apex of the lung to end at the neck of the first rib by dividing into the **superior intercostal artery,** to the first two intercostal spaces, and the **deep cervical artery** to the postvertebral muscles.

The **subclavian vein**, running anterior to the scalenus anterior muscle, is at a slightly lower level than the artery because of the inclination of the first rib. It is the terminal section of the main upper limb vein, and extends from the outer margin of the first rib to its junction with the internal jugular vein behind the medial third of the clavicle. It receives the external jugular vein, which pierces the deep fascia in the roof of the posterior triangle of the neck to join it.

Superficial structures of the neck

These structures include the sternomastoid and trapezius muscles, the deep fascial layer that splits to enclose them and which forms the roofs of the anterior and posterior triangles of the neck, the platysma muscle and the superficial vessels and nerves.

The **trapezius** and the **sternomastoid** muscles are parts of the same muscular sheet, but are usually separated by an interval, the **posterior triangle of the neck**. Occasionally, this interval may be almost obliterated, with nerves and blood vessels issuing from a narrow slit in an almost complete sheet of muscle fibres. The **trapezius** is a muscle of the shoulder girdle (p. 23.5). The fibres of insertion of the **sternomastoid** are attached along the lateral part of the superior nuchal line and the lateral aspect of the base of the mastoid process in exactly the same plane as the fibres of origin of the trapezius. The inferior attachment of the sternomastoid muscle is its origin. This consists of a tendinous attachment to the front of the manubrium sterni, and a thin musculo-aponeurotic origin from the superior surface of the medial third of the clavicle. The interval between the anterior margin of the sternomastoid and the midline of the front of the neck is the **anterior triangle of the neck**. The lower margin of the mandible forms its remaining side.

The nerve supply of the sternomastoid and trapezius muscles is mainly derived from the spinal part of the accessory nerve. This nerve runs in the deep fascia which forms the roof of the posterior triangle of the neck where it is superficial and easily damaged. Its course across the posterior triangle can be marked by joining the midpoint of the posterior margin of the sternomastoid to a point two fingers' breadths above the clavicle on the anterior border of trapezius. There is an additional supply to the sternomastoid from the second cervical nerve, and to the trapezius from the third and fourth cervical nerves.

One sternomastoid muscle acting alone turns the face to the opposite side of the body. The two acting together, can flex the neck and the head on to the trunk. But if the head is first extended by the postvertebral muscles, the sternomastoids will operate together to maintain it in forcible hyperextension. When respiration is impeded, the sternomastoids act as accessory muscles of respiration.

The deep fascia of the neck encloses sternomastoid, the spinal accessory nerve and the trapezius and forms the roof of the posterior triangle between the two muscles and the roof of the anterior triangle anterior to the sternomastoid. Between the two manubrial heads of the sternomastoids, it splits into two layers just above the jugular notch, in order to enclose the jugal venous arch, which connects the two anterior jugular veins across the midline of the neck. More superiorly, the deep fascia blends with the perichondrium of the thyroid cartilage and with the periosteum of the hyoid bone, mandible and zygomatic arch. It splits to enclose the submandibular gland anteriorly and the parotid gland posteriorly. At the attachments of the sternomastoid and trapezius muscles to the mastoid process and the superior nuchal line, it blends with the periosteum of the skull.

The superficial veins of the neck are the **external** and **anterior jugular veins**. The former begins just below the external acoustic meatus where the posterior division of the retromandibular vein joins the small posterior auricular vein (fig. 22.12). It runs vertically downwards across the lateral surface of the sternomastoid muscle, and pierces the deep fascia of the posterior triangle of the neck to enter the subclavian vein. It receives the anterior jugular, transverse cervical and suprascapular veins just before doing so.

The **anterior jugular vein** commences in the submental region and runs downwards in the anterior triangle of the neck, superficial to the infrahyoid muscles. It is connected with the vein of the opposite side by the jugal venous arch, and ends by passing behind the sternomastoid muscle to join the external jugular vein.

Infratemporal fossa and submandibular region

The mandible is separated from the wall of the pharynx and mouth by muscle, glands, blood vessels and nerves. Posteriorly, the region intervening between the ramus of the mandible and the pharyngeal wall is termed the infratemporal fossa. More anteriorly, the structures lying between the body of the mandible and the tongue are described as lying in the submandibular region. The infratemporal fossa and submandibular regions are continuous and are described together.

The lateral and medial pterygoid muscles (p. 22.20) separate the ramus of the mandible from the tensor veli palatini and superior and middle constrictor muscles of the pharynx. The two pterygoid muscles are separated by the inferior alveolar and lingual branches of the mandibular nerve which occupy the **interpterygoid plane**. This plane slopes downwards and laterally from the foramen ovale to the ramus of the mandible. The maxillary artery runs, in the majority of cases, between the lateral pterygoid muscle and the ramus of the mandible. Less frequently it lies superficial to the inferior alveolar and lingual nerve in the interpterygoid plane. The veins which drain the area supplied by this artery form a plexus around the lateral pterygoid muscle, the **pterygoid venous plexus**. From this plexus, blood is drained via the short maxillary vein into the retromandibular vein.

MANDIBULAR NERVE (fig. 22.36)

The mandibular nerve and the motor root of the trigeminal nerve frequently leave the cranial cavity by separate openings in the dura mater covering the foramen ovale. The two become united within or just below the foramen, and the motor root is distributed as a component of the mandibular nerve through some of its branches. Immediately medial to the emerging nerve, and separating it from the tensor veli palatini muscle, lies a small parasympathetic ganglion, the **otic ganglion**. Preganglionic fibres reach this ganglion from the glossopharyngeal nerve by way of its tympanic branch, the tympanic plexus in the middle ear, and the lesser petrosal

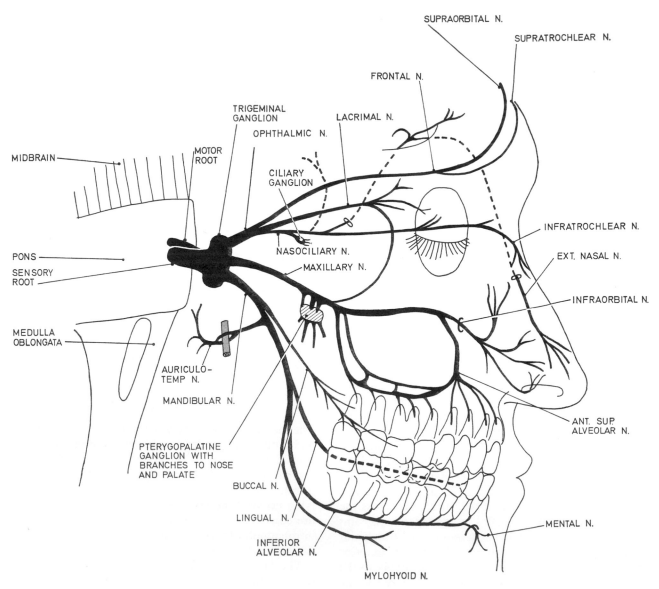

FIG. 22.36. Trigeminal nerve.

nerve. Postganglionic fibres pass to the auriculotemporal nerve, which conveys them to the parotid gland. Fibres from the mandibular nerve, such as those supplying the medial pterygoid, tensor veli palatini and tensor tympani muscles directly from the undivided trunk of the nerve, may pass through the ganglion on their way to their respective muscles.

The mandibular nerve breaks up into a small anterior and a larger posterior division. The former passes through the fibres of the lateral pterygoid muscle to end as the sensory **buccal branch** to the skin and mucous membrane of the cheek, but gives off efferent twigs to the masseter, temporalis and lateral pterygoid muscles prior to doing so. The posterior division gives rise to the **auriculotemporal nerve** which passes posterolaterally to supply the temporomandibular joint and the parotid gland. It passes behind the mandibular fossa and climbs over the zygomatic arch to enter the temporal region where it supplies the overlying skin and the upper lateral aspect of the auricle. The posterior division of the mandibular nerve then breaks up into an anterior branch, the lingual nerve, and a posterior branch, the inferior alveolar nerve.

The **lingual nerve** passes from the deep surface of the lateral pterygoid muscle on to the medial aspect of the mandibular ramus, posterior to the tendon of insertion of the temporalis. It passes below the lowest fibres of the superior constrictor of the pharynx, and comes to lie above the posterior part of the mylohyoid muscle. Here it is immediately deep to the mucous membrane of the linguogingival sulcus in the floor of the mouth. It then runs on the lateral surface of the hyoglossus muscle just above the hypoglossal nerve (fig. 22.37). The main part of the submandibular gland lies on its lateral side. The nerve turns below the submandibular duct and passes from its lateral to its medial side. It then turns upwards and forwards into the anterior two-thirds of the tongue, whose mucous membrane it supplies with sensory fibres. The lingual nerve is joined by a branch of the nervus intermedius of the facial nerve, the **chorda tympani**, a short distance below the base of the skull. This nerve leaves the middle ear and passes medial to the spine of the sphenoid, the middle meningeal artery and vein and the inferior alveolar nerve before joining the lingual nerve. The chorda tympani contains taste fibres whose cell bodies lie in the geniculate ganglion, and parasympathetic fibres to the glands of the floor of the mouth. This latter group of nerves fibres relays in the **submandibular ganglion**, which is suspended from or fused with the lingual nerve on the lateral surface of the hyoglossus muscle. The taste fibres are distributed to the oral surface of the tongue, which is its anterior two-thirds, but not to the taste buds of the circumvallate papillae, which are supplied by the lingual branch of the glossopharyngeal nerve. The parasympathetic fibres are

distributed to the glands of the tongue and to the submandibular and sublingual salivary glands.

The **inferior alveolar nerve** passes across the deep surface of the lower fibres of the lateral pterygoid muscle, lateral to the sphenomandibular ligament, and enters the mandibular foramen. It runs within the bone of the mandible in the mandibular canal, together with the inferior alveolar branch of the maxillary artery and its accompanying vein. It sends twigs to the pulp cavities of the mandibular teeth, and gives off a large mental branch near its termination. This mental branch leaves the mandibular canal by the mental foramen, and breaks up into branches which supply the skin of the region of the chin and the mucous membrane and skin of the lower lip. Before entering the mandibular foramen, the inferior alveolar nerve gives off a small motor branch, the mylohyoid nerve, which runs forwards and downwards in the mylohyoid groove on the medial aspect of the mandible, lateral to the medial pterygoid muscle. As it runs forwards, it slips between the submandibular gland and the mylohyoid muscle, supplying that muscle along with the anterior belly of the digastric.

MAXILLARY AND INFRAORBITAL NERVES
These nerves form a single trunk, the name changing at the posterior end of the infraorbital groove.

The trunk of the maxillary nerve leaves the cranial cavity through the foramen rotundum, and immediately enters the pterygopalatine fossa. Leaving the fossa by turning sharply laterally through the upper part of the pterygomaxillary fissure, it lies for a very short part of its course in the deepest part of the infratemporal fossa. From there, it turns forward into the inferior orbital fissure, and runs anteriorly in the infraorbital groove and canal to enter the superficial fascia through the infraorbital foramen. Its terminal branches are distributed to the skin of the lower eyelid, cheek, side of the nose and the skin and mucous membrane of the upper lip. The infraorbital part of the nerve is accompanied by the infraorbital branch of the maxillary artery.

Within the pterygopalatine fossa, the trunk of the maxillary nerve is connected by two pterygopalatine branches to a small mass of parasympathetic nerve cells, the **pterygopalatine ganglion**. From the inferior aspect of this ganglion a number of nerves are directed to the nasal cavity, the palate and the nasopharynx. These are mainly sensory branches of the maxillary nerve, but contain other fibres, some of which are derived from the parasympathetic cells of the ganglion. The largest of these branches is the **greater palatine nerve** which occupies the greater palatine canal and foramen, and supplies the major part of the hard palate. The **lesser palatine nerves** leave the greater palatine canal to open on to the soft palate which they supply with taste fibres, as well as the general sensory, parasympathetic secretomotor and sympathetic fibres which are present in all the other branches. The **nasopalatine** and **lateral** and **medial nasal branches** leave the pterygopalatine fossa by the sphenopalatine foramen to be distributed to the septum and lateral wall of the nasal cavity. The pharyngeal branch reaches the upper part of the wall of the nasopharynx. All these nerves are accompanied by similarly named branches of the maxillary artery and their venae comitantes (p. 22.45).

In the infratemporal fossa, a zygomatic and two or more posterior superior alveolar branches are given off. The **zygomatic nerve** enters the orbit through the lateral part of the inferior orbital fissure. It gives off the zygomaticofacial and zygomaticotemporal branches to the skin of the face, and its communication with the lacrimal nerve transmits secretomotor fibres from the pterygopalatine ganglion. The **posterior superior alveolar nerves** enter fine canaliculi in the bone of the posterolateral wall of the maxillary air sinus, and are distributed with the neurovascular bundles to the molar and premolar teeth and adjoining gum.

The **infraorbital nerve** gives off an anterior superior alveolar branch while in the infraorbital groove. This nerve runs in a bony canal, along with the corresponding vessels, across the anterolateral surface of the maxillary air sinus, passing lateral to the infraorbital foramen, to the region of the anterior nasal spine. At this point, a small twig is given off to the anterior part of the floor of the nose. The greater part of the nerve passes in the neurovascular bundles, present in the walls of the maxillary air sinus, from which branches go to the pulp cavities of the incisor and canine teeth, and to the mucous membrane lining the maxillary sinus.

The function of the pterygopalatine ganglion is to act as the relay station for preganglionic fibres derived from the nervus intermedius of the facial nerve, which are destined for the area of maxillary nerve distribution. Fibres subserving the special sense of taste, whose cell bodies are in the geniculate ganglion, are also contained among the nerve bundle passing to the pterygopalatine ganglion from the nervus intermedius, but they just pass through the ganglion. The route followed by these two sets of fibres from the facial nerve is by the greater petrosal nerve to the foramen lacerum, where they are joined by sympathetic fibres from the internal carotid plexus, and thence by the nerve trunk which occupies the pterygoid canal to the ganglion in the pterygopalatine fossa. The sympathetic fibres which join the greater petrosal nerve in the foramen lacerum are derived from the upper end of the thoracolumbar outflow and reach the cranial cavity in the form of a plexus around the internal carotid artery. These are postganglionic fibres, whose cell bodies are situated in the superior cervical ganglion in the neck.

Tongue

The tongue (fig. 22.37) is formed from the blended fibres of the extrinsic muscles, described below, and the longitudinal, transverse and vertical intrinsic fibres. Numerous serous and mucous glands are enclosed between the interlacing strands of these muscles. Their ducts open on to the dorsum and side of the tongue, which is covered with a layer of non-keratinizing stratified squamous epithelium, modified on the dorsum of the tongue into the various kinds of papillae. At the junction of the anterior two-thirds and the posterior third of the dorsum of the tongue, there is a V-shaped row of prominent sessile projections, the circumvallate papillae, so arranged that the apex of the V points backwards. Immediately behind the row of papillae is an ill-defined groove, the sulcus terminalis. At its posteriorly pointing apex, there is a slight pit, the foramen caecum, indicating the position of the thyroid diverticulum, the forerunner of the thyroid gland in the embryo.

The mucous membrane of the tongue and adjacent parts of the mouth contains **taste buds** (fig. 22.38) which

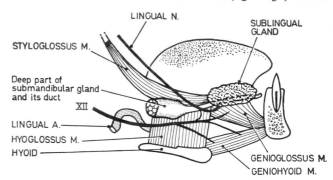

FIG. 22.37. Lateral view of the tongue.

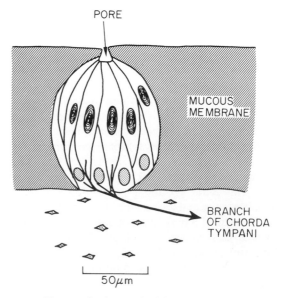

FIG. 22.38. A taste bud in the tongue.

are nests of cells sensitive to flavoured solutions. They are most numerous in the circumvallate papillae, but occur in other parts of the upper surface of the tongue and a few may be found elsewhere in the mouth and throat. The mucous membrane of the tongue posterior to the sulcus and foramen is raised and made irregular by subepithelial lymphoid tissue, the lingual tonsil.

VASCULAR SUPPLY

This is mainly derived from the lingual artery, which passes forwards from its origin from the external carotid deep to the hyoglossus muscle. It terminates as the deep artery of the tongue, and supplies the organ to its tip. The veins which drain the area are both deep and superficial to the hyoglossus muscle and drain into the internal jugular system, either directly or through the facial vein.

NERVE SUPPLY

The sensory supply to the anterior two-thirds of the tongue is derived from the lingual nerve, which also carries taste and secretomotor fibres from the chorda tympani, ultimately derived from the nervus intermedius. The circumvallate papillae and the posterior third of the tongue, the pharyngeal surface, is supplied by the glossopharyngeal nerve with fibres subserving taste sensation and with secretomotor fibres. A few fibres of the internal laryngeal branch of the superior laryngeal nerve, derived from the vagus, reach the most posterior part of the tongue. The motor supply to the intrinsic and extrinsic muscles of the tongue reaches them through the hypoglossal nerve. The palatoglossus, whose fibres blend with the posterior part of the side of the tongue, is a muscle of the soft palate, and is supplied by the pharyngeal branch of the vagus.

TASTE

It is conventional to distinguish four varieties of taste, sweet, sour, salt and bitter. In fact an animal as simple as a blowfly has only two receptors in its taste system, one for sugary material which it eats, and one for salty material which it avoids. The nerve fibres that innervate mammalian taste buds do not usually respond only to one of the varieties of taste, but to several or all of them, with varying sensitivities (fig. 22.39). In spite of this, different tastes can be discerned. Evidently the nervous system correlates the information arriving on an array of nerve fibres. In contrast to light where any colour can be mimicked by a mixture of the four primary colours, it is not possible to mimic every taste by a mixture of sweet, sour, salt and bitter.

What substances of similar taste have in common chemically is to some extent clear. Sour substances dissociate in solution to give H^+, but the tongue is not a reliable pH meter, since a solution of 2·2 mmol/l of

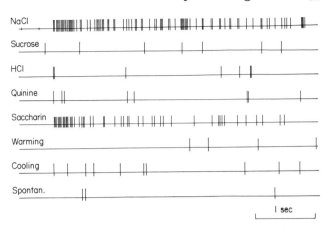

FIG. 22.39. Nerve impulses in a single fibre of a rat's chorda tympani in response to different stimuli. Note the varieties of taste which evoke responses, and that there is a slow spontaneous discharge. From Ogawa H. *et al.* (1963) *J. Physiol.* **199**, 223.

sulphuric acid (pH 2·38) tastes as sour as a solution of 10 mmol/l of succinic acid (pH 3·08). NaCl tastes purely salty and other salts produce mixed tastes. The common molecular conformation possessed by sweet substances can be defined with some precision, but not that possessed by bitter substances. Phenylthiourea and closely related compounds possess the remarkable characteristic of tasting bitter to some persons but being tasteless to others. Inability to taste it is inherited as a recessive autosomal character.

A striking increase in the sensitivity of taste is a feature of Addison's disease (p. 27.32) and is not limited to salt but extends to other varieties of taste. The increase depends on deficiency of cortisol and ceases when cortisol is given.

After the chorda tympani nerve has been cut, taste buds can no longer be found on the front of the tongue; when the nerve regenerates they re-form so that function is resumed. Hence the nerve fibres appear to have a trophic effect upon the receptor cells.

SUPRAHYOID MUSCLES AND MUSCLES OF THE TONGUE (fig. 22.40)

The **genioglossi** radiate backwards into the substance of the tongue from origins on the upper mental spines (fig. 22.13). Their fibres blend with the intrinsic muscles of the tongue on a plane which is medial to that of the styloglossus and hyoglossus muscles. Their upper edges are covered by the mucous membrane of the linguogingival sulcus, while their lower edges are in contact with the geniohyoid muscles.

The **geniohyoid muscles** arise from the lower mental spines and are inserted into the upper surface of the body of the hyoid bone on either side of the midline.

The **styloglossus** obtains an origin from the styloid

process, at the point at which it becomes continuous with the stylohyoid ligament. Its fibres gather together to form a bundle which runs forwards and downwards through the lowest part of the superior constrictor of the pharynx, to blend with the upper fibres of the hyoglossus at the side of the tongue.

The **hyoglossus** is a sheet of muscle which arises from the upper margin of the greater horn and body of the hyoid bone, and runs upwards and forwards to blend with the styloglossus and the intrinsic muscles of the tongue. It is situated lateral to the plane of the middle constrictor of the pharynx and the genioglossus, and is medial to the submandibular gland and the mylohyoid. The lingual artery and its venae comitantes lie on the medial side of the lowest fibres of the hyoglossus, while the lingual and hypoglossal nerves run across its lateral surface.

The **mylohyoid** arises from the mylohyoid line of the mandible, and its anterior fibres run downwards and medially to meet in a median fibrous raphe. The posterior fibres gain an attachment into the upper surface of the body of the hyoid bone. Associated with it, and often partly blended with it, is the **anterior belly of the digastric muscle**. Arising from a shallow depression on the lower margin of the mandible just lateral to the symphysis, the fibres of this muscle run downwards and backwards to become continuous with a tendon which unites them to the fibres of the posterior belly. This tendon is slung from the junction of the body and greater horn of the hyoid bone by a pulley formed from a loop of deep fascia. The **posterior belly of the digastric muscle** arises from the floor of the digastric notch, and is joined in its course in the uppermost part of the neck by a slender band of muscle fibres which arises from the styloid

process, and passes anteroinferiorly to reach the digastric tendon, around the sides of which it passes to its insertion on the hyoid bone. This is the **stylohyoid muscle**.

Actions of the muscles of the tongue and the suprahyoid muscles

The extrinsic and intrinsic muscles of the tongue act as a group in modifying the whole organ in phonation and in the action of guiding the food between the teeth during mastication. Protrusion of the tongue is effected by the intrinsic muscles. In the voluntary part of the act of swallowing, the tongue is drawn upwards and backwards by the combined actions of the styloglossi and mylohyoids. The digastric, stylohyoid and mylohyoid muscles raise the hyoid bone, and with it the larynx, during the second or involuntary phase of swallowing (p. 22.51).

Nerve supply of the suprahyoid muscles

The anterior belly of the digastric and mylohyoid muscles are derived from the mesoderm of the first pharyngeal arch of the embryo, and are accordingly supplied from the first arch, or mandibular, nerve through its mylohyoid branch. The posterior belly of the digastric and stylohyoid muscles are derived from second arch mesoderm and are therefore supplied by the second arch, or facial, nerve (p. 19.33).

Salivary glands of the floor of the mouth
(figs. 22.37 and 40)

The main or superficial part of the **submandibular salivary gland** is situated in the angle between the mylohyoid muscle and the inner side of the mandible. A layer of deep fascia extends upwards from the body of the hyoid bone and splits to enclose the gland and to bind it to the mandible. The two bellies of the digastric muscle, which are also enclosed within this fascial capsule, form a hammock-like arrangement for the lower edge of the gland. The inferolateral surface extends from this hammock arrangement to the lower margin of the mandible and is related to the superficial structures of the upper part of the neck. The posterior pole of the gland extends backwards beyond the mylohyoid and lies between the hyoglossus and the insertion of the medial pterygoid muscle. The ascending part of the facial artery turns laterally above the stylohyoid muscle into a groove on the posterior pole of the submandibular gland. Emerging from this groove, the descending part of the vessel runs to the lower margin of the mandible between the gland and the lowest part of the medial pterygoid muscle. Between the bone of the mandible and the lateral aspect of the gland lie several small lymph nodes, the submandibular lymphatic nodules. These are members of the collar chain of lymph nodes, and drain the adjacent parts of the face and the side of the tongue.

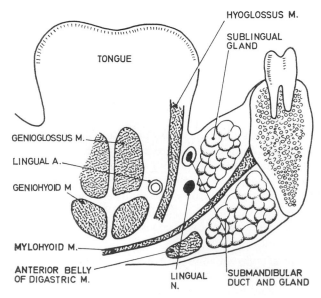

FIG. 22.40. Coronal section of the floor of the mouth.

The deep part of the gland extends forwards from the medial surface of the main mass of the structure and is accompanied by the submandibular duct. Both structures occupy the gutter between the mylohyoid and hyoglossus muscles. The duct runs anteriorly, passes medial to the sublingual gland, and discharges into the floor of the mouth by the opening in the summit of the sublingual papilla, which lies immediately lateral to the frenulum of the tongue (p. 22.48).

The **sublingual salivary gland** lies in the anterior part of the floor of the mouth, and raises a ridge in the linguo-gingival sulcus. On the summit of this ridge, a row of small apertures allows the secretions of the gland to reach the cavity of the mouth. Laterally, it is in contact with the medial surface of the mandible at the sublingual fovea, and below that with the anterior fibres of origin of the mylohyoid muscle. Its medial surface is in contact with the hyoglossus and genioglossus muscles.

MEDIAN HOLLOW VISCERA

Sections of the head and neck (figs. 22.41 and 42) show the vertical extent of the hollow viscera which lie within it. From the spheno-ethmoidal recess, which lies immediately below the cribriform plate of the ethmoid bone, a series of cavities stretches downwards to the upper part of the thorax.

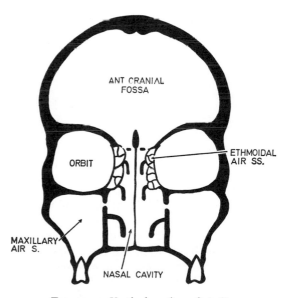

FIG. 22.41. Vertical section of skull.

The bony plate of the **hard palate** (fig. 22.43) supplemented posteriorly by the soft palate forms a horizontal dividing wall between the paired nasal cavities and the median nasopharynx above, and the mouth and oropharynx below. The septum of the nose is fused with the upper surface of this dividing wall in the midline, and the free posterior edge of the septum meets the hard and soft palates at their point of junction. The **soft palate**, in addition to its central aponeurotic support, includes fibres of skeletal muscle, and a small bundle of this is continued backwards to form the **uvula.** Both the upper and lower surfaces of the hard and soft palates are clothed with connective tissue, glands and epithelium. On the superior or nasal surface, this epithelium is of the 'respiratory', columnar ciliated type, while on the inferior or oral aspect, it is of the stratified squamous non-keratinizing type. When the narrow, transversely placed slit which connects the nasal and oral parts of the pharynx is closed by the combined action of the palatine and pharyngeal muscles, as in swallowing, the upper respiratory cavity and the lower alimentary cavity are separated completely.

The cervical part of the visceral space is divided by a vertical septum formed, in the coronal plane, by the muscles and cartilages of the posterior wall of the larynx and by the apposed walls of the trachea and the oesophagus. In front of the septum are the larynx and trachea, behind it the laryngopharynx and oesophagus. The cricoid cartilage forms the major part of the dividing wall between the larnyx and laryngopharynx. Its rigid nature and almost circular outline determines the form of the interior of the larynx, while the laryngopharynx, which is applied to the convex posterior aspect of the cartilage is a curved slit with an anterior concavity (fig. 22.18).

Nose and nasopharynx

The nasal cavities are situated on either side of a midline septum. In coronal section each forms an inverted wedge, with its base on the upper surface of the hard palate and its apex in the narrowest part of the cavity, immediately below the cribriform plate of the ethmoid bone. Each nasal cavity opens on to the surface of the face anteriorly and into the nasopharynx posteriorly. Both openings are immediately adjacent to the floor of the nose, so that during normal respiration air is directed through the lower part of the cavity. Only a small proportion of the inspired air is drawn up into the cul-de-sac lined by olfactory epithelium.

The nasopharynx is a single slit-like cavity, slightly convex anteriorly. The lateral angles of the slit lie in the pharyngeal recesses, posterior to the expanded medial ends of the auditory tubes. The posterior wall of the cavity bulges downwards and forwards because of an aggregation of lymphoid tissue, the nasopharyngeal tonsil.

ROOF OF THE NASAL CAVITIES (fig. 22.44)

The nasal cavities and the nasopharynx are placed behind the median part of the face, above the hard palate and below the median parts of the cranial fossae. The roof extends from the cartilaginous external nose, along the under surface of the nasal and frontal bones to the

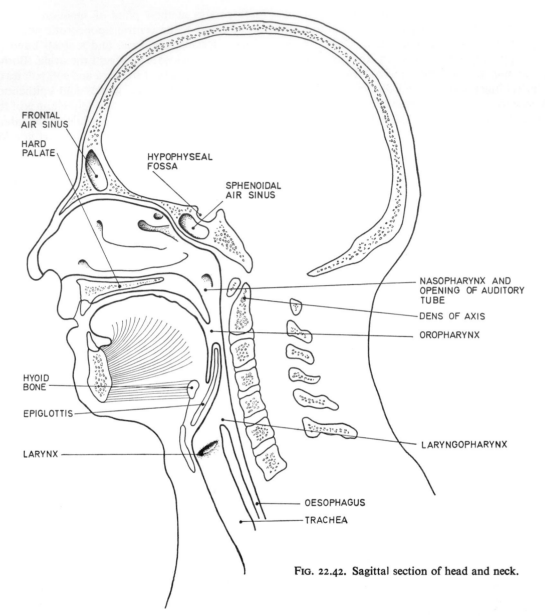

FRONTAL
AIR SINUS

HARD
PALATE

HYPOPHYSEAL
FOSSA

SPHENOIDAL
AIR SINUS

NASOPHARYNX AND
OPENING OF AUDITORY
TUBE

DENS OF AXIS

OROPHARYNX

HYOID
BONE

EPIGLOTTIS

LARYNX

LARYNGOPHARYNX

OESOPHAGUS

TRACHEA

Fig. 22.42. Sagittal section of head and neck.

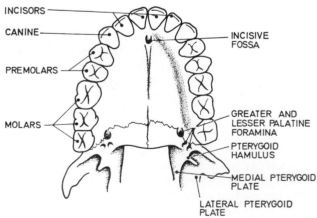

INCISORS

CANINE

PREMOLARS

MOLARS

INCISIVE
FOSSA

GREATER AND
LESSER PALATINE
FORAMINA

PTERYGOID
HAMULUS

MEDIAL PTERYGOID
PLATE

LATERAL PTERYGOID
PLATE

Fig. 22.43. The hard palate.

inferior aspect of the cribriform plate of the ethmoid bone, where it reaches its highest point and is separated from the anterior cranial fossa only by that thin, perforated lamina of bone. Injury to the bone at this point may establish a connection between the subarachnoid and nasal cavities, through which cerebrospinal fluid flows down the nose. Posterior to the cribriform plate lies the body of the sphenoid with its two enclosed air sinuses which open on each side of the midline, where the bony septum and the sphenoid articulate. The lower part of the sphenoid body, and the basiocciput with which it articulates posteriorly, continue downwards and backwards as the roof of the nasopharynx. The pharyngeal tubercle on the under surface of the basilar part of the occipital bone indicates the most posterior extent of the nasopharyngeal

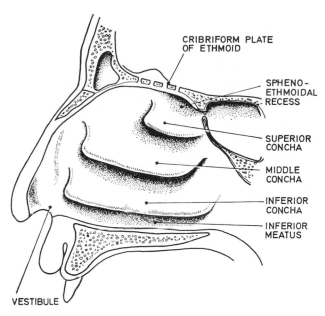

FIG. 22.44. The lateral wall of the nasal cavity.

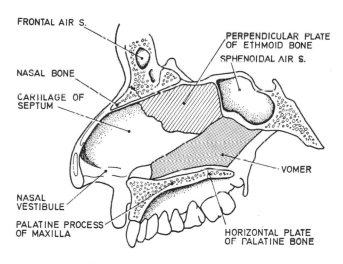

FIG. 22.45. The septum of the nose.

mucous membrane on the base of the skull and the point of its reflexion on to the muscular part of the posterior pharyngeal wall.

LATERAL WALL OF THE NASAL CAVITY (fig. 22.44)

The major part of the lateral wall of the nose is composed of the ethmoid bone above and the maxilla below. From these two bones project the delicate conchae or turbinate bones; when covered with mucous membrane, they give a characteristic appearance to the interior of the nose. There are three of these conchae in each nasal cavity, two from the ethmoid bone, but the largest, the **inferior nasal**

concha is a bone in its own right. The small superior concha projects from the medial surface of the ethmoid bone immediately below the cribriform plate. It is grooved vertically on its medial surface for the axons of the receptor nerve cells of the olfactory mucous membrane, as they converge on the cribriform plate. The space above the superior concha is the **sphenoethmoidal recess**, while that lateral to it is the superior meatus of the nose. From the lower part of the ethmoid bone, the middle concha, a much larger horizontal lamina of bone with a downward turned medial edge, projects into the cavity. The space below and lateral to it is the middle meatus. The lateral wall of this meatus is distended medially by a group of air sacs, whose thin bony walls are translucent. The prominence so produced is the **bulla ethmoidalis**. The middle ethmoidal air sinuses open on to the surface of the bulla; below and in front of it, a gap in the bone of the lateral wall of the nose, the **hiatus semilunaris**, leads directly into the maxillary air sinus. Because of the size of the inferior concha, the inferior meatus which lies below and lateral to it is the largest of the three. The only aperture in its lateral wall is the **nasolacrimal duct**.

The maxillary bone completes the antero-inferior part of the lateral wall of the nose. Posterior to the ethmoid and inferior conchal bones, the perpendicular plate of the palatine bone and the medial pterygoid lamina form the lateral wall. The nasal and frontal bones provide the anterior part of the roof and a small part of the lateral wall of the cavity, while the lacrimal bone, in the medial wall of the nasolacrimal duct, also forms a small part of the lateral wall of the middle meatus.

At the upper end of the perpendicular plate of the palatine bone, the **sphenopalatine foramen** intervenes between the central part of the edge of the plate and the body of the sphenoid bone with which it is articulating. In life, the foramen is covered with mucous membrane, deep to which the nerves and vessels from the pterygopalatine fossa pass into the lateral wall and septum of the nose.

NASAL SEPTUM (fig. 22.45)

This is composed of the perpendicular plate of the ethmoid, the septal cartilage and the vomer. The free posterior edge of the vomer, smooth and slightly concave, forms the medial boundary of the posterior nasal aperture (posterior naris, posterior choana). A groove runs downwards and forwards on each side of the vomer, from the body of the sphenoid to the incisive fossa in the anterior part of the hard palate. This lodges the nasopalatine nerve and associated blood vessels.

That part of the perpendicular plate of the ethmoid bone which is situated below the cribriform plate is grooved like the medial surface of the superior concha; these grooves also carry olfactory nerve bundles.

FIBROCARTILAGINOUS PART OF THE AUDITORY
(PHARYNGOTYMPANIC, EUSTACHIAN) TUBE

The medial part of the tube connecting the nasopharynx
and the middle ear is an incomplete roll of elastic
cartilage, with the deficiency in its anterolateral aspect
filled in with fibrous tissue. It occupies the suture
on the under surface of the base of the skull between the
posterior margin of the greater wing of the sphenoid and
the quadrate area of the petrous temporal bone. Its expanded pharyngeal end is directed medially and anteriorly
into the aperture enclosed by the upper part of the posterior margin of the medial pterygoid plate and the body
of the sphenoid bone, and is often supported inferiorly
by a spine projecting backwards from the middle of the
posterior edge of the plate. When covered with mucous
membrane, the edges of the tubal opening form a prominence in the lateral wall of the nasopharynx, the **tubal
elevation.** Posterior to its opening, the recess of the
pharynx wall extends laterally to the under surface of
the foramen lacerum, which is, of course, blocked off
inferiorly by fibrous tissue. (The bony part of the
auditory tube and the functions of the tube are considered on p. 26.26).

SOFT TISSUE LINING OF THE NOSE AND NASO-
PHARYNX

The mucous membrane of the nose and of most of the
nasopharynx consists of columnar ciliated epithelium
intermixed with goblet cells and supported by connective tissue. This latter layer contains both serous
and mucous acini, and numerous vascular spaces of a
venous nature, over and above the normal blood supply,
and sensory and secretomotor nerve fibres. In the olfactory area the epithelium contains both receptor and
supporting cells.

As well as the **nasopharyngeal tonsil** on the posterior
wall of the nasopharynx, other deposits of lymphoid
tissue occur around the openings of the auditory tubes,
the **tubal tonsils.** These collections of lymphoid tissue
form part of a ring around the upper parts of the respiratory and alimentary passages. The palatine and lingual
tonsils complete the encirclement.

The epithelial lining of the nasal cavities is continuous
anteriorly with the skin which lines the nostrils. Laterally,
it blends with the columnar ciliated epithelium of the
paranasal sinuses, and with the lining of the nasolacrimal duct. Posteriorly, it continues onwards from
the bony walls of the nose to the internal surface of
the superior constrictor muscle of the pharynx, where it is
supported by the thickened connective tissue of the
pharyngeal wall, the pharyngobasilar fascia. At a line
running around the interior of the nasopharynx from the
dorsum of the soft palate to the opening of the auditory
tube and onwards to the posterior pharyngeal wall there is
an irregular transition from respiratory epithelium to one
of a stratified squamous non-keratinizing kind.

SPACES CONNECTED WITH THE NASAL CAVITY AND
THE NASOPHARYNX (fig. 22.46)

These spaces, the paranasal air sinuses, the nasolacrimal
duct and the auditory tube, have connections with the
nasal cavity which have existed from the very earliest
phase in their development. Thus, the paranasal sinuses
develop initially as grooves in the roof or lateral wall of

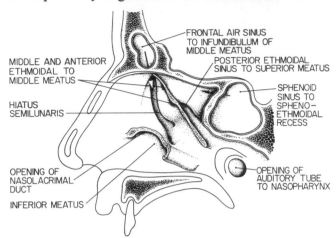

FIG. 22.46. The meatuses and the lateral wall of the nose,
showing the connections and drainage of air sinuses.

the nose. The auditory tube is part of the tubotympanic
recess which develops from the first internal pouch of the
primitive pharynx (p. 19.30). The nasolacrimal duct is
completed by the fusion of the lips of the groove separating the maxillary and frontonasal processes of the
embryonic face to enclose a canal which is drawn into
the substance of the face, with its lower end opening into
the lower part of the nasal cavity (p. 22.58).

The arrangement of the openings of these cavities and
tubes in the lateral wall of the nose and nasopharynx is as
follows:

(1) the sphenoidal air sinus opens into the spheno-
ethmoidal recess,

(2) the posterior ethmoidal air sinuses open by several
pinhole apertures into the superior meatus of the nose,

(3) the nasolacrimal duct opens into the anterior part
of the inferior meatus,

(4) the auditory tube opens into the nasopharynx,

(5) all the remaining cavities, the frontal, maxillary,
anterior and middle ethmoidal air sinuses open into the
middle meatus. The middle ethmoidal sinuses open on to
the summit of the ethmoidal bulla, while the anterior
ethmoidal group of sinuses has an aperture into the upper
anterior part of the hiatus semilunaris. The maxillary
sinus opening occupies the central part of the hiatus.
The frontal sinus, which is an extension of an anterior
ethmoidal air sac between the tables of the frontal bone,
opens by its infundibulum, which has to pass through the
ethmoidal labyrinth to do so, into the uppermost anterior part of the middle meatus of the nose.

NERVE SUPPLY OF THE NOSE AND NASOPHARYNX
(figs. 22.47 and 48)

The special sense of smell. See olfactory nerves (chap. 25).

The general sensory supply of the nose. Both the septum and the lateral walls of the nasal cavity are innervated by

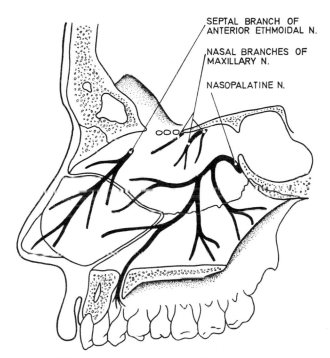

FIG. 22.47. Nerve supply of the nasal septum.

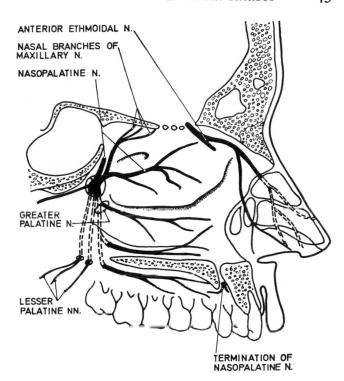

FIG. 22.48. Nerve supply of the lateral wall of the nose.

the ophthalmic and maxillary divisions of the trigeminal nerve. The ophthalmic region of supply is confined to the upper anterior part of the mucous membrane of the lateral wall and septum, while the maxillary nerve supplies the larger lower and posterior parts of both. The ophthalmic supply is derived from the **anterior ethmoidal nerve**, which goes to the lateral wall and septum, before becoming the external nasal nerve to the skin of the tip of the nose.

Most of the maxillary supply enters the nasal cavity from the pterygopalatine fossa through the spheno-palatine foramen. The **nasopalatine nerve** crosses the most posterior part of the roof of the nose to the septum, and runs downwards and forwards on the vomer, innervating the adjacent mucous membrane. Anteriorly, it penetrates the hard palate at the incisive fossa, and supplies the gum in the premaxillary region. Other shorter **nasal branches** leave the sphenopalatine foramen to supply the more posterior part of the septum, and the lateral wall in the region of the posterior ends of the superior and middle conchae. Branches of the greater

palatine, anterior superior alveolar, infraorbital nerves and pharyngeal branches of the maxillary nerve complete the innervation of the nasal cavity.

VASCULAR SUPPLY OF THE NOSE AND NASOPHARYNX
The ophthalmic area of nerve supply receives branches of the anterior ethmoidal branch of the ophthalmic artery, derived from the intracranial part of the internal carotid artery. These follow the arrangements of the nerves. The area supplied by branches of the maxillary nerve also receives branches of the maxillary artery. On the septum, the artery accompanying the nasopalatine nerve forms an anastomosis with the terminal part of the greater palatine artery, which enters the nasal cavity through the incisive fossa. They are joined by branches of the anterior ethmoidal and facial arteries. the latter entering deep to the skin of the upper lip and the vestibule of the nose. This septal anastomosis is where epistaxis is likely to occur.

The venae comitantes of these arteries drain to the sphenopalatine foramen, the nasal slit, the incisive fossa and the vestibule of the nose, following the general direction of venous flow from these areas.

Paranasal sinuses

These air-filled cavities communicate with the nose and are lined by a mucoperiosteum, consisting of ciliated columnar epithelium, lying directly on the periosteal covering of the bony walls. Nasal infections often spread into these sinuses.

The **maxillary air sinus** occupies the interior of the maxillary bone from the floor of the orbit to the hard palate, and may extend into the alveolar process, often as much as half an inch below the general level of the floor of the rest of the cavity. Its shape is roughly pyramidal, with its base in the lateral wall of the nose. The drainage exit of the sinus is, in fact, in the substance of the ethmoid bone, high up in the medial wall. Drainage is not normally dependent upon gravity, therefore, but on ciliary activity. The apex of the sinus is in the zygomatic process, and often extends into the zygomatic bone itself. The cavity may be subdivided by a number of thin bony septa.

It is by far the largest of the paranasal sinuses; the orbit lies immediately above it, the nose on its medial side, the oral cavity below it, and the pterygopalatine fossa immediately posteriorly. Posterolaterally, it faces into the infratemporal region, and anterolaterally into the face. Its most important immediately related structures are the trunk and branches of the maxillary nerve, and the terminal part of the maxillary artery and its accompanying veins. Thus, the infraorbital neurovascular group lies in its roof, the posterior superior alveolar group in its posterolateral wall, and the anterior superior alveolar group in its anterolateral wall. The greater palatine group lies inferiorly, below the hard palate, and the nerves and vessels supplying the lateral wall of the nose are related to its medial surface. It is from these nerves and blood vessels that the walls and mucous membrane of the sinus are supplied.

The **ethmoidal air sinuses** are situated between the upper part of the nasal cavity and the medial wall of the orbit. Superiorly, they are separated from the anterior cranial fossa by part of the orbital plate of the frontal bone. They are supplied by the ethmoidal arteries and nerves.

The **sphenoidal air sinuses** are paired but usually unequal in size, and occupy most of the substance of the body of the sphenoid bone (fig. 22.42). They are situated behind the upper part of the cavity of the nose, and above the nasopharynx. They are related superiorly to the pituitary and its coverings, and laterally to the cavernous sinus and its contents, particularly to the internal carotid artery (fig. 22.6). Its neurovascular supply is posterior ethmoidal in origin.

The **frontal air sinuses** penetrate the frontal bone immediately above and lateral to the root of the nose and frequently extend backwards into the roof of the orbit. They are usually asymmetrical, the dividing septum not being in the midline. The anterior ethmoidal arteries and nerves supply them.

The situations of the openings of the sinuses into the nose are summarized on p. 22.44.

Mouth, oropharynx, laryngopharynx and oesophagus

MUSCLES OF THE PHARYNX AND THE SOFT PALATE (fig. 22.49)

The pharynx, unlike the remainder of the alimentary tract, possesses a double layer of skeletal muscle in its wall, comprising an inner longitudinal and an outer

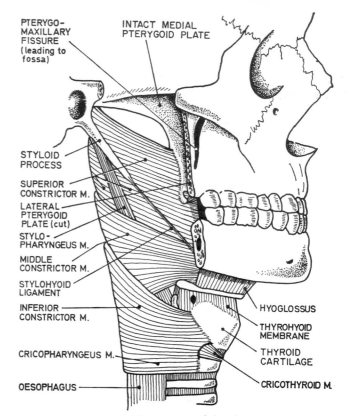

PTERYGO-MAXILLARY FISSURE (leading to fossa)

INTACT MEDIAL PTERYGOID PLATE

STYLOID PROCESS

SUPERIOR CONSTRICTOR M.

LATERAL PTERYGOID PLATE (cut)

STYLO-PHARYNGEUS M.

MIDDLE CONSTRICTOR M.

STYLOHYOID LIGAMENT

INFERIOR CONSTRICTOR M.

CRICOPHARYNGEUS M.

OESOPHAGUS

HYOGLOSSUS

THYROHYOID MEMBRANE

THYROID CARTILAGE

CRICOTHYROID M.

FIG. 22.49. Musculature of the pharynx.

circular lamella. The outer circular layer is better developed and consists of three constrictor muscles, superior, middle and inferior.

Attachments of the pharyngeal constrictors. A poorly defined median fibrous raphe stretches from the pharyngeal tubercle on the inferior aspect of the basilar part of the occipital bone down almost to the oesophagus. The three constrictor muscles are inserted into it.

The **superior constrictor** arises from the lower half of the posterior border of the medial pterygoid plate, the pterygomandibular raphe, the posterior end of the mylohyoid line of the mandible and the side of the tongue. Through the pterygomandibular raphe it is continuous with the buccinator muscle.

The **middle constrictor** arises from the lower part of the stylohyoid ligament, and the lesser and greater horns of the hyoid bone.

The **inferior constrictor** arises from the oblique line on the lateral aspect of the thyroid cartilage, from a fibrous band which connects the lower end of the line to the cricoid cartilage, and from the lateral aspect of that cartilage. Its lowest fibres are horizontal, and form the **cricopharyngeal sphincter** at the pharyngo-oesophageal junction. Its fibres are continuous with those of the other side, with no intervening raphe.

The internal longitudinal layer of pharyngeal muscle is poorly defined. It is provided by the stylopharyngeus, the palatopharyngeus and the salpingopharyngeus, in that order from anterior to posterior. The first of these three muscles commences its course outside the plane of the pharyngeal wall, while the other two are situated within it throughout their length. Their fibres blend into a single longitudinal sheet in the lower part of the wall of the pharynx.

The **stylopharyngeus** arises from the medial aspect of the base of the styloid process, and passes between the superior and middle constrictor sheets to enter the longitudinal layer of muscle. It is inserted into the posterior margin of the thyroid cartilage, and into the lamina propria of the mucous membrane of the pharynx. The **palatopharyngeus** arises from the soft palate, and blends with the posterior margin of the stylopharyngeus. It is inserted into the subepithelial connective tissue of the pharyngeal wall. The **salpingopharyngeus** arises from the posterior margin of the tubal elevation. It forms the muscular interior of the salpingopharyngeal fold. Inferiorly, it blends with the posterior margin of the palatopharyngeus, with whose fibres it is inserted.

SOFT PALATE

The central supporting structure of the soft palate is the palatine aponeurosis, formed by the union in the midline of the posterior part of the roof of the mouth of the expanded tendons of the two tensor veli palatini muscles. The remaining muscles of the soft palate are attached to either the upper or lower surface of this aponeurosis. The anterior margin of this latter structure is attached to the palatine crests of the hard palate, and to the posterior nasal spine at its posterior margin. The aponeurosis blends posteriorly with the lamina propria of the mucous membrane of the free edge of the soft palate.

The **tensor veli palatini** arises from the cartilage and fibrous tissue on the anterolateral aspect of the auditory tube, and from the adjoining bone by an attachment extending from the spine of the sphenoid to the scaphoid fossa. Its fibres pass downwards and converge on the lateral side of the inferior end of the medial pterygoid plate of the sphenoid bone. Here the muscle blends with its tendon, which turns sharply around the lower margin of the plate to pass medially to the palatine aponeurosis, with which it becomes continuous. In doing so, it passes through the buccinator muscle immediately anterior to the hamulus (fig. 22.43).

The **levator veli palatini muscle** arises from the medial aspect of the auditory tube, and from the adjoining part of the petrous temporal bone. Its fibres descend and turn medially to be inserted into the upper surface of the palatine aponeurosis. Together with the tensor and the pharyngeal end of the auditory tube, it obliterates the triangular aperture between the superior margin of the superior constrictor and the inferior surface of the base of the skull.

The **palatoglossus** is a muscular band which arises from the lower surface of the palatine aponeurosis and descends on the lateral boundary of the oropharyngeal isthmus to the lateral side of the tongue, where it blends with the musculature of that organ. It is covered with mucous membrane, and, as the **palatoglossal fold**, forms the anterior boundary of the tonsillar fossa. Posterior to that fossa, the **palatopharyngeus muscle** descends in a similar fashion, and is likewise clothed in mucous membrane forming the **palatopharyngeal fold**. This muscle arises from the soft palate, mainly by a layer of fibres which separates the levator veli palatini from the upper surface of the palatine aponeurosis, and sweeps downwards and backwards in the wall of the oropharynx.

The uvula contains a few muscle fibres, the musculus uvulae. The exterior of the pharyngeal muscles is clothed by a thin, poorly defined layer of connective tissue, the buccopharyngeal fascia. Their internal aspect is in direct contact with the lamina propria of the pharyngeal mucous membrane, the **pharyngobasilar fascia**, which is thickest in the triangular area above the upper edge of the superior constrictor muscle where it blends with the other structures filling in the deficiency.

PALATINE TONSIL (fig. 22.50)

The two palatine tonsils are the largest of the collection of lymphoid tissue which surrounds the lumina of the upper ends of the alimentary and respiratory tracts (p. 22.44). Each tonsil is situated in the lateral wall of the oropharynx between the palatoglossal and palatopharyngeal folds, above the side of the posterior third of

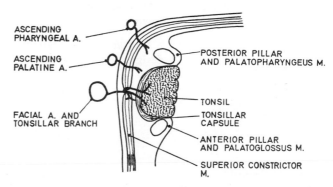

FIG. 22.50. A horizontal section of the tonsil showing its relations.

the tongue. Laterally, it is separated by a layer of strong connective tissue, the tonsillar capsule, from the superior constrictor of the pharynx, and from the loop of the facial artery which lies lateral to the muscle. It receives an arterial supply from the tonsillar and ascending palatine branches of that loop, and from the ascending pharyngeal artery.

ORAL CAVITY

The teeth and gums divide the cavity into the mouth proper and the vestibule, which lies between the gums and the cheeks. Within the cheeks is found the buccinator muscle (p. 22.16), which is covered with superficial fascia and skin externally, and lined by the dense connective tissue of the inner cheek pad and the oral mucous membrane internally. The parotid duct opens through the buccinator sheet into the vestibule of the mouth opposite the second upper molar tooth.

The mouth proper lies within the line of the teeth and gums, and is anterior to the palatoglossal fold. Its roof is formed by the hard and soft palates, and its floor by the tongue and the sulcus which separates it from the gums, the linguogingival sulcus. In this sulcus, the epithelium is raised up over the ridge of the sublingual salivary gland, and a row of about a dozen small ducts from this gland open through it. At its anteromedial end, the aperture of the submandibular salivary duct opens into the floor of the mouth alongside the midline, separated from its opposite number by a thin fold of epithelium on the under surface of the tongue, the **frenulum linguae.** The deep vein of the tongue may be seen shining through the epithelium on the inferior aspect of the organ. It is the vena comitans of the terminal part of the lingual artery.

THE TEETH

There are two sets of teeth, the deciduous (milk) dentition and the permanent dentition.

Deciduous dentition

There are twenty deciduous teeth. Each quadrant of the dental arcade contains the following:

Name of tooth	Dental designation	Date of eruption
Central incisor	A	6 months
Lateral incisor	B	9 months
Canine ('eye tooth')	C	18 months
First deciduous molar	D	12 months
Second deciduous molar	E	24 months

Permanent dentition

There are thirty-two permanent teeth, which replace the deciduous teeth. The permanent molars have no deciduous predecessors. Each quadrant of the dental arcade contains the following:

Name of tooth	Dental designation	Date of eruption
Central incisor	I	7 years
Lateral incisor	2	8 years
Canine ('eye tooth')	3	11 years
First premolar	4	10 years
Second premolar	5	11 years
First permanent molar	6	6 years
Second permanent molar	7	12 years
Third permanent molar	8	18–25 years

It must be stressed that while these dates give an approximate time and order of eruption, there are individual and racial variations. In general, eruption tends to occur earlier in girls. The times of appearance of the dentition give a measure of developmental (as distinct from the chronological) age of the individual.

On eruption, the crowns of the teeth are fully formed and do not increase in size. The roots, however, are incomplete at this stage; those of the deciduous teeth take another year for completion, those of the permanent teeth another three years. Minor changes in the relationship of the teeth to each other and to the jaws occur throughout life.

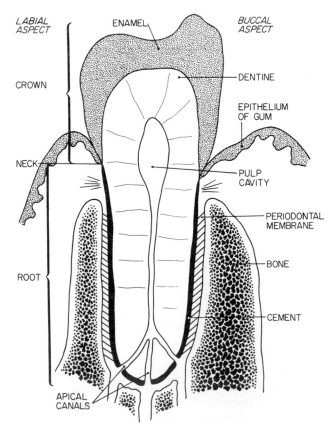

FIG. 22.51. Longitudinal section of a premolar tooth.

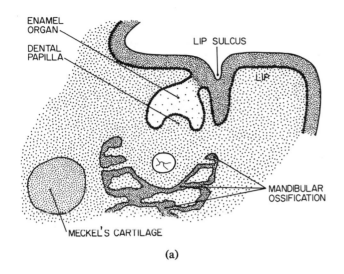

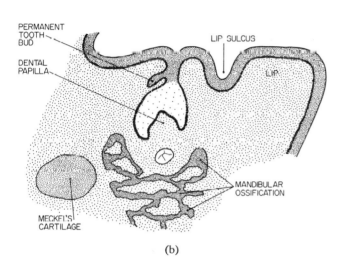

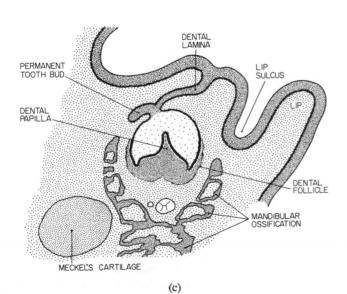

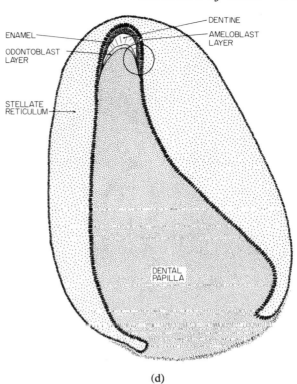

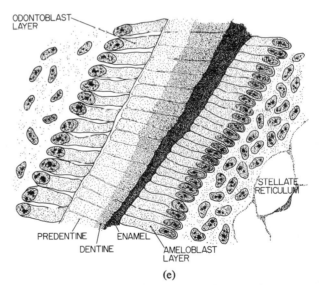

FIG. 22.52. Stages in the development of a tooth. (a) Appearance of the enamel organ; (b) formation of the permanent tooth germ from the lingual aspect of the dental lamina; (c) intramembranous bone of the mandible coalesces around the developing deciduous tooth; (d) appearance of the deciduous tooth germ in a fetus of approximately 5½ months; (e) enlargement of the region enclosed by the circle in (d).

STRUCTURE OF TEETH (fig. 22.51)

The bulk of the tooth consists of **dentine**, which is covered in the **crown** by **enamel**, in the **root** by **cement**. The enamel and cement meet at the **neck** where the mucous membrane of the gum is adjacent to the tooth. The dentine surrounds the **pulp cavity**, which is lined by odontoblasts and filled with loose connective tissue, the **dental pulp**. This contains blood vessels, lymphatics and nerves which enter and leave the root of the tooth by means of the apical canals. Survival of the tooth depends upon the integrity of the pulp.

DEVELOPMENT OF TEETH (fig. 22.52)

In the late embryo two parallel proliferations occur from the ectodermal epithelium of the mouth, close to the margins of the developing jaws. These proliferations, one buccal, the other lingual, form the **lip furrow band** and the **dental lamina** respectively (fig. 22.52a). Desquamation of surface cells transforms the lip furrow band into the **labio-gingival sulcus**, which ultimately separates the gums from the lips or cheeks. The dental lamina, on the other hand, grows into the underlying connective tissue and gives rise initially to twenty buds for the deciduous teeth (fig. 22.52b), and twenty buddings from these teeth, with twelve additional buds, for the permanent dentition.

The dental lamina continues to grow in a lingual direction and becomes dimpled, forming a series of epithelial buds, the **enamel organs**. From the lingual surface of each bud a further outgrowth occurs, the permanent tooth bud. The enamel organ becomes bell-shaped; its concavity is lined by a cuboidal epithelium, the internal enamel epithelium, and filled by a mesodermal core which forms the dental pulp and, adjacent to the internal enamel epithelium, differentiates into a layer of columnar cells, the **odontoblast layer** (fig. 22.52d). This layer initiates tooth formation by depositing predentine against the concave (internal) surface of the enamel organ. The cells of the internal enamel epithelium later differentiate into columnar **ameloblasts**, which form enamel.

The layers of dentine and of enamel increase in thickness and the odontoblasts and ameloblasts are moved further apart. As the crown of the tooth assumes its recognized form root formation begins. On the surface of the root there is deposited cement which will give attachment to the collagen fibres of the periodontal membrane.

Enamel is the hardest tissue in the body. It consists of 95 per cent inorganic material and 5 per cent water and organic material. Almost all of the solid material consists of calcium hydroxyapatite and trace elements, including fluorine. Enamel is laid down in the form of closely set hexagonal prisms. Dentine is similar to bone in constitution; it exhibits long tubules, but contains no cells. Cement is a modified form of bone.

The teeth are attached to their bony sockets by a fibrous ligament, the **periodontal membrane**, whose fibres slope towards the cement of the root, in which they are anchored. These fibres thus form a sling, which absorbs some of the force of the bite. The nerves of the periodontal membrane are of particular importance in providing proprioceptive information on the force of the bite in mastication.

OROPHARYNX AND LARYNGOPHARYNX (fig. 22.58).

The oropharynx extends from the palatoglossal folds to the posterior wall of the pharynx. Its roof is formed by the soft palate. The tonsillar bed and palatopharyngeal fold lies in its lateral wall. Its floor extends from the circumvallate papillae to the tip of the epiglottis, and includes the pharyngeal surface of the tongue with its lingual tonsil, and the median glosso-epiglottic fold which connects it to the front of the epiglottis. On either side of this fold, there is a hollow, the **vallecula**. Its posterior boundary is a poorly defined fold of mucous membrane, the lateral glosso-epiglottic fold, which sweeps around the posterior and lateral aspects of the hollow to fade away in the lateral part of the tongue.

The laryngopharynx lies between the upper edge of the epiglottis and the pharyngo-oesophageal junction. In the median part of its anterior wall lies the inlet of the larynx, bounded by the epiglottis, and the two aryepiglottic folds which spread laterally and posteriorly from its margins to converge posteriorly at the posterior margin of the laryngeal orifice. Here in each fold there are two tubercles composed of cartilage nodules covered with mucous membrane, the medial being the corniculate and the lateral the cuneiform tubercle. On either side of the laryngeal opening lie the deep pyriform fossae. Below the tubercles, the anterior wall of the laryngopharynx bulges backwards, so that its lumen is reduced to a curved slit with an anterior concavity, which gradually merges inferiorly with the oesophageal lumen.

CERVICAL PART OF THE OESOPHAGUS

This is continuous with the laryngopharynx at the level of the lower border of the sixth cervical vertebra. It is suspended from the posterior aspect of the cricoid cartilage by an upward extension of its outer longitudinal layer of muscle, which is skeletal at this level. It is placed immediately anterior to the anterior longitudinal ligament and the prevertebral muscles, and directly posterior to the trachea. The recurrent laryngeal nerves lie on either side in the tracheo-oesophageal grooves, and the thoracic duct is situated posteriorly on the left side, tucked into the interval between the left margin of the oesophagus and the front of the prevertebral structures.

ACTION OF SWALLOWING

This takes place in two stages. In the first or voluntary phase, a bolus of food is lifted upwards and backwards into the space between the palatoglossal folds by the combined action of the mylohyoid and styloglossus muscles. Respiration is restrained, and the palatopharyngeal isthmus is reflexly occluded by the coordinated action of the tensores and levatores veli palatini, which draw the soft palate upwards and backwards. The superior constrictor muscles contract to bring the posterior pharyngeal wall into contact with the upper surface of the soft palate, thus completing the occlusion of the isthmus.

In the course of the second or involuntary phase, the bolus passes through the oropharynx and laryngopharynx

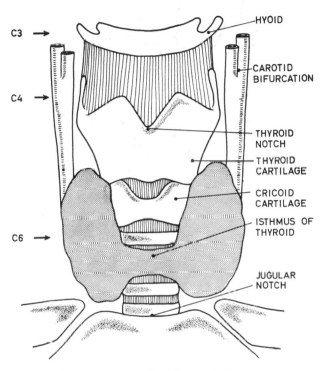

FIG. 22.53. Anterior view of the larynx.

to the upper end of the oesophagus, where it is temporarily retarded by the cricopharyngeal sphincter. During this phase, the opening of the larynx is shut off by a muscular, sphincteric mechanism. The epiglottis is drawn downwards and backwards towards the tubercles of the posterior margin of the inlet by the action of the aryepiglottici, while the thyroepiglottici widen the inlet, reducing it to a transverse slit. The food mass passes to either side of the epiglottis, pouring as two streams through the pyriform fossae. At the same time, the whole larynx is drawn upwards by the suprahyoid muscles, removing the obstruction produced by the backward pressure of the rigid posterior surface of the cricoid cartilage against the anterior aspect of the body of the sixth cervical vertebra. The food mass now collects at the lower end of the laryngopharynx, and the cricopharyngeal sphincter relaxes to permit it to pass into the oesophagus. The larynx returns to its normal position under the traction of the infrahyoid muscles and gravity.

It is usual for the lips to be closed during the act of swallowing, and it is difficult to carry out the act without this assisting factor. Non-occlusion of the jaw margins renders swallowing practically impossible.

Larynx

The larynx extends from the level of the third cervical vertebra to the lower border of the sixth, where it is continuous with the trachea. It is a semirigid structure with a framework of bone and cartilage, connected together by ligamentous sheets and bands and by synovial joints. Its lowest or infraglottic division is shaped like a nozzle pointing upwards; its rigid wall is due to the cricoid cartilage (fig. 22.53). This part of the larynx is not capable of deformation by the food bolus and is an obstacle to be overcome in the act of swallowing. The outlet of this rigid nozzle, the **rima glottidis**, can be altered in length, breadth and outline, so enabling air to be puffed or bubbled in varying quantities and at varying rates over the resonators of the oral cavity.

LARYNGEAL CARTILAGES

The support of the larynx is provided by three rigid elements, two of which are cartilaginous, while the third is bony from childhood onwards. These are the thyroid and cricoid cartilages, and the hyoid bone (fig. 22.54). The last structure represents the fused anterior ends of the second and third arch cartilages of the embryo.

The **hyoid** bone is U-shaped with the convexity of the letter forming the body and the greater horns the two free extremities. The lesser horns project upwards from the junctions of the body with the greater horns. The bone is ossified from a hyaline cartilage model, the centres appearing during the first year of postnatal life and fusing in middle age. It is subcutaneous, the deep fascia of the anterior triangles of the neck blending with the periosteum of the outer surfaces of the body and greater horns. Its deep surface is in contact with the submucosa of the pharynx, except in the midline, where it is separated from the front of the epiglottis by the loose tissue below the glossoepiglottic fold, and by the hyoepiglottic ligament.

The **thyroid cartilage** is composed of two hyaline cartilaginous laminae united anteriorly. The angle between these two plates is about a right angle in the male, and up to 120° in the female. The free posterior border of each lamina is prolonged upwards and downwards into superior and inferior horns. A raised oblique line runs downwards and forwards across the lateral surface of each lamina, converging on the inferior part of the fused anterior margins.

The **cricoid cartilage** is roughly circular in outline when viewed from above, and is in the form of a short cylinder, whose posterior wall projects above its upper margin.

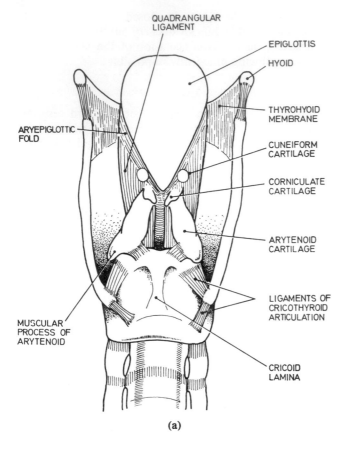

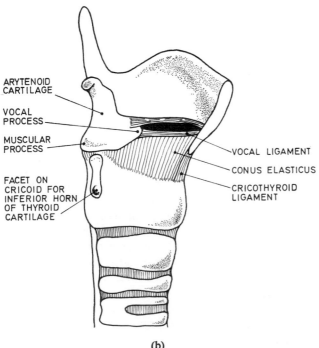

FIG. 22.54. Cartilages and ligaments of the larynx; (a) posterior view, (b) lateral view with the right half of the thyroid cartilage removed.

Facets on the lateral aspects of the cartilage articulate with the inferior horns of the thyroid cartilage, and others on the upper surface of the posterior part of the body articulate with the arytenoids. The posterior aspect of the cartilage has a midline ridge for the attachment of the upper end of the external longitudinal layer of muscle of the oesophagus, and two lateral hollows for the origins of the posterior cricoarytenoid muscles.

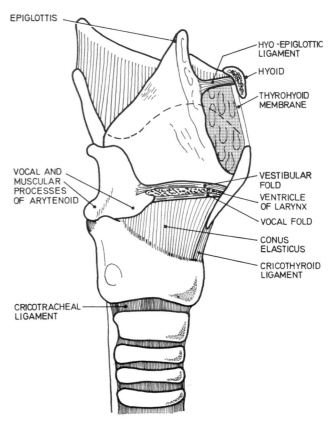

FIG. 22.55. Cartilages and ligaments of the interior of larynx, shown by removing right half of the thyroid cartilage.

On the upper edge of the posterior part of the cricoid cartilage lie the two **arytenoid cartilages**, each of which resembles a quarter of a pyramid, with an apex, a medial angle placed alongside the middle of the larynx, a muscular process which is the lateral angle, and a vocal process which points directly forwards (figs. 22.54 and 55). The vocal process is composed of non-calcifiable elastic cartilage, while the remainder is hyaline. The medial surface of the arytenoid cartilage is covered with the mucous membrane of the larynx, and the lower margins of the two cartilages form the boundaries of the intracartilaginous part of the rima glottidis. In the fresh larynx, the remaining aspects of the arytenoids are obscured by muscular and ligamentous attachments.

The **epiglottic cartilage** is composed entirely of the elastic variety and is not subject to ossification. It is attached to the posterior aspects of the median parts of the hyoid bone and thyroid cartilage by the hyoepiglottic and thyroepiglottic ligaments. Its posterior surface and upper margins, with some of the upper part of its anterior surface, are covered with mucous membrane. It is linked by a fold of mucous membrane to the apex of the arytenoid cartilage on each side of the laryngeal orifice, the **aryepiglottic folds** (fig. 22.58).

JOINTS OF THE LARYNX

The upper margin of the thyroid cartilage is attached to the posterior edge of the hyoid bone by a tough sheet of fibrous tissue, the **thyrohyoid membrane**, which passes deep to the hyoid bone to reach its upper attachment. The free posterior edges of this membrane are thickened to form the lateral thyrohyoid ligaments which contain small cartilaginous aggregations. The lateral aspect of the membrane is pierced by the internal laryngeal branch of the superior laryngeal nerve, accompanied by the superior laryngeal branch of the superior thyroid artery and its

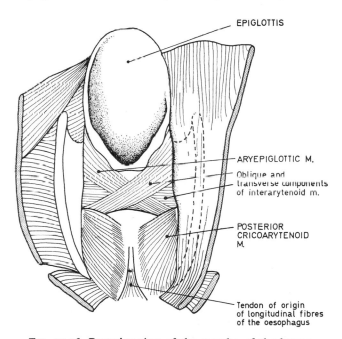

EPIGLOTTIS

ARYEPIGLOTTIC M.

Oblique and transverse components of interarytenoid m.

POSTERIOR CRICOARYTENOID M.

Tendon of origin of longitudinal fibres of the oesophagus

FIG. 22.56. Posterior view of the muscles of the larynx.

venae comitantes. These ramify in the floor of the pyriform fossa, which lies on the immediate medial aspect of the membrane. A bursa separates the upper median part of the membrane from the posterior aspect of the body of the hyoid bone. Remnants of the thyroglossal duct may be found tucked up deep to the anterior edge of the body of the hyoid bone (p. 19.32).

A band of fibrous tissue, the median cricothyroid ligament, unites the anterior parts of the thyroid and cricoid cartilages. More posteriorly and separate from it, a strong sheet of connective tissue extends from the upper

margin of the cricoid cartilage and the vocal process of the arytenoid cartilage to the posterior aspect of the fused median part of the thyroid cartilage, about halfway up its length. This is the **conus elasticus**. The upper free margin, extending from the vocal process to the back of the thyroid cartilage, is the **vocal ligament**. The space between the edges of the vocal ligaments is the anterior or interligamentous part of the rima glottidis. A few millimetres above this level a thin ligamentous band, the **vestibular ligament**, connects the lateral aspect of the arytenoid cartilage with the back of the median fused part of the thyroid cartilage a little above the attachment of the vocal ligament. It is the supporting structure of the vestibular fold, which is the upper boundary of the ventricle of the larynx.

A thin sheet of connective tissue runs from the lateral margin of the epiglottis to the anterior margin of the arytenoid cartilage blending with the vestibular ligament below and having a free superior margin in the aryepiglottic fold. This is the **quadrangular ligament** which forms part of the lateral wall of the vestibule or uppermost part of the interior of the larynx. It also forms the medial wall of the pyriform fossa.

Two pairs of synovial joints occur in the larynx. The **cricothyroid articulations**, which involve the inferior horns of the thyroid cartilage, and the lateral aspects of the cricoid, are involved in flexion-extension of these two cartilages on each other. The **cricoarytenoid articulations**, involving the bases of the arytenoid and the upper surface of the cricoid cartilages, have incongruent surfaces in most positions of the arytenoids. They are capable of permitting rotation of the arytenoids around a vertical axis, and lateral traction of these cartilages.

LARYNGEAL MUSCLES

Unlike the remainder of the intrinsic muscles of the larynx, the **cricothyroid muscle** is placed largely on the external aspect of the supporting cartilages. It arises from the anterior surface of the cricoid cartilage close to the median plane, and runs upwards and backwards to be inserted into the deep surface and inferior margin of the thyroid cartilage. Its lateral surface is partly obscured by the fibrous band which gives origin to some of the muscle fibres of the inferior constrictor of the pharynx. The muscle flexes the thyroid cartilage upon the cricoid, approximating the anterior margins of these two structures, and increasing the tension in the vocal ligament. The **thyroarytenoid muscle** (fig. 22.57) extends from the lateral aspect of the arytenoid cartilage to the posterior aspect of the median part of the thyroid cartilage. The medial fibres are placed parallel to the vocal ligament, and are connected to its lateral edge, constituting the **vocalis muscle.** The main part of the muscle draws the arytenoid cartilage towards the posterior aspect of the thyroid cartilage, opposing the action of the cricothyroid and relaxing the tension in the vocal ligaments. The vocalis portion can alter the tension within individual parts of the vocal ligament.

Continuous with the thyroarytenoid posteriorly, and connecting the posterior surfaces of the two arytenoid cartilages, is the thin **interarytenoid muscle**. The central part of its anterior aspect, between the two arytenoid attachments, is clothed with the mucous membrane of the larynx, and so forms the posterior boundary of the rima glottidis. Its posterior aspect is traversed by two slender obliquely placed muscle bundles, the oblique arytenoid muscles, which connect the muscular process of one arytenoid cartilage with the apex of the other and which are continuous with the aryepiglottici. The transverse and oblique muscles separate the backs of the arytenoid cartilages from the mucous membrane of the laryngopharynx. The transverse fibres draw the two arytenoid cartilages together, and thereby reduce the width of the aperture of the rima glottidis. The two obliqui act as part of the aryepiglottici.

The **aryepiglotticus muscle** (fig. 22.57) runs from the tip of the arytenoid cartilage, where it is continuous with the oblique muscle, to the lateral margin of the upper edge of the epiglottis. It blends with the upper margin of the quadrangular ligament. At its upper end, it is associated with muscle fibres which arise from the deep aspect of the thyroid cartilage, close to the insertion of the thyroaryte-

noids, the **thyroepiglotticus muscle**. It also is blended with the quadrangular ligament. The aryepiglotticus closes the laryngeal inlet by drawing the epiglottis and the arytenoid cartilages together, and the thyroepiglotticus assists by changing the inlet to a transverse slit.

Two muscles gain an insertion into the muscular processes of the arytenoid cartilages. The **posterior cricoarytenoid muscle** arises from the concavity lateral to the median ridge on the posterior surface of the cricoid cartilage, while the much smaller **lateral cricoarytenoid muscle** gains an origin from the upper margin of the lateral part of the same cartilage. The tendons of insertion of the two muscles therefore pull upon the muscular process of the arytenoid cartilage from opposite directions. Consequently, when acting alone, the posterior cricoarytenoid muscle abducts the vocal ligament from the midline position, while the lateral muscle reverses this action. When both the posterior and lateral muscles contract together, they oppose the action of the transverse arytenoid muscle and draw the two arytenoid cartilages apart, widening the rima glottidis, particularly its posterior intercartilaginous part.

INTERIOR OF THE LARYNX

The inlet of the larynx is covered by the same stratified squamous non-keratinizing epithelium that occurs in the oral and laryngeal parts of the pharynx. Inside the orifice this changes to a stratified columnar ciliated epithelium, as found in the nose and trachea. This epithelium is supported by connective tissue which contains serous and mucous acini, and lines the whole of the

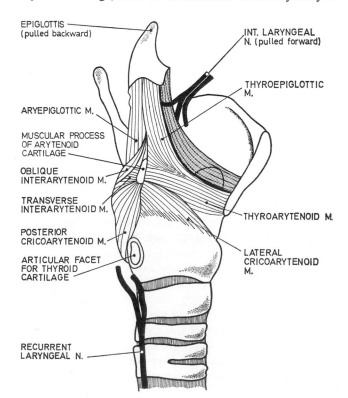

FIG. 22.57. Lateral view of the muscles of the larynx.

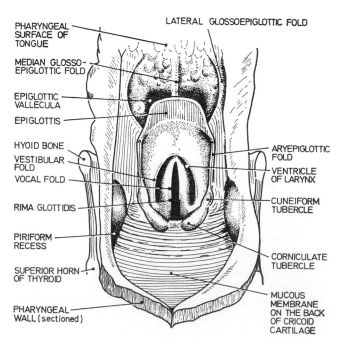

FIG. 22.58. Rima glottidis and vestibule of larynx.

interior of the larynx except over the vocal folds, where it is replaced by a stratified squamous non-keratinizing variety.

When viewed with a laryngoscope, the interior wall exhibits a transversely placed elliptical recess, the **ventricle of the larynx** (fig. 22.58). At its posterior end, the arytenoid cartilage can be seen shining through the lining epithelium. The upper lip of the ventricle is the vestibular fold, and the lower lip the vocal fold. The interior of the larynx is subdivided into a superior portion, **the vestibule**, above the vestibular folds, an **intermediate region** between the vestibular and vocal folds, including the ventricles, and an **infraglottic region** below the vocal folds.

NERVE AND BLOOD SUPPLY OF THE LARYNX

The *sensory innervation* of the mucous membrane comes from the internal and recurrent laryngeal nerves, both of which are ultimately derived from the vagus. The former supplies the region between the epiglottis and the vocal folds, while the latter innervates the region below that level and also sends fibres to the trachea. The rima glottidis is thus the dividing level between superior and recurrent laryngeal zones of innervation.

The *motor supply* to the cricothyroid muscle is obtained from the external laryngeal branch of the superior laryngeal nerve. The remainder of the intrinsic muscles of the larynx are supplied by branches of the recurrent laryngeal nerve.

The *blood supply* follows much the same course as these nerves. The superior laryngeal branch of the superior thyroid artery accompanies the internal laryngeal nerve through the thyrohyoid membrane to the upper part of the larynx. The lower part is supplied by the inferior laryngeal branch of the inferior thyroid artery, which enters the larynx along with the terminal part of the recurrent laryngeal nerve.

Structures related to the trachea in the neck

The trachea is directly continuous with the infraglottic part of the larynx, the lower margin of the cricoid cartilage being connected by the cricotracheal membrane to the first ring of the trachea. Like the oesophagus, the trachea is inclined backwards as well as downwards, following the curve of the vertebral column. This is demonstrable in a lateral radiograph. The cervical part of the trachea is clothed anteriorly and laterally by the isthmus and lateral lobes of the thyroid gland. The recurrent laryngeal nerves run in the tracheo-oesophageal grooves, and so lie posterolateral to the viscus. The common carotid arteries lie posterior to the lateral lobes of the thyroid gland, and therefore posterolateral to the trachea in the neck. The subsequent course of the trachea is described on p. 31.3.

THYROID AND PARATHYROID GLANDS (fig. 22.59)

The thyroid gland has a median isthmus and two lateral lobes. The isthmus lies across the second, third and fourth tracheal rings and blends with the two lateral lobes which extend superiorly on each side of the larynx as far as the

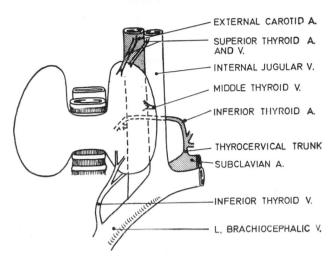

EXTERNAL CAROTID A.
SUPERIOR THYROID A. AND V.
INTERNAL JUGULAR V.
MIDDLE THYROID V.
INFERIOR THYROID A.
THYROCERVICAL TRUNK
SUBCLAVIAN A.
INFERIOR THYROID V.
L. BRACHIOCEPHALIC V.

FIG. 22.59. Blood supply of the thyroid gland.

oblique lines. The whole gland is enclosed in a capsule formed from the pretracheal fascia, which binds it to the thyroid cartilage and to the front of the cricoid cartilage. It lies in a plane which is superficial to the inferior pharyngeal constrictor and the external laryngeal nerve, and deep to the sternothyroid muscle, which is attached along with the fascial capsule of the gland to the oblique line of the thyroid cartilage. Two parathyroid glands are embedded in each lateral lobe of the thyroid gland (p. 27.24), a superior gland, parathyroid IV, and an inferior gland, parathyroid III. Sometimes, however, one or both of these parathyroids may lie free of the thyroid gland in the adjacent connective tissue and be difficult to find.

The *arterial supply* is derived from the superior and inferior thyroid arteries, which anastomose freely. The recurrent laryngeal nerve may run among or even superficial to the branches of the latter vessel and so is at risk in thyroidectomy. An additional arterial supply may be obtained from the brachiocephalic artery by its thyroidea ima branch, which supplies the region of the isthmus.

The *thyroid veins* drain by three main routes, a superior and middle to the internal jugular vein, and an inferior to the brachiocephalic veins within the thorax.

The development of these glands and other structural features are found on p. 19.30 and 27.17.

PRETRACHEAL (INFRAHYOID, STRAP) MUSCLES

This group includes both of the bellies of omohyoid and the sternohyoid, sternothyroid and thyrohyoid muscles.

Their importance lies in their close relationship to the thyroid gland.

The thyrohyoid muscle receives its nerve supply from the first cervical nerve by a branch which travels within the hypoglossal nerve. All the other muscles are supplied by fibres from the first three cervical nerves running in the ansa cervicalis. The action of these muscles is to draw the larynx downwards at the end of the second or involuntary phase of swallowing. They act as antagonists to the suprahyoid muscles. The thyrohyoid muscle draws the thyroid cartilage into the concavity of the hyoid bone during the second stage of swallowing, raising the infra-hyoid part of the larynx.

The **sternohyoid** connects the posterior aspect of the sternoclavicular joint to the medial part of the front of the body of the hyoid bone. On the lateral side of its superior attachment arises the superior belly of the **omohyoid**. This slender band of muscle runs downwards and laterally across the neurovascular bundle of the neck, where it narrows to blend with the inferior belly at a tendinous junction. The inferior belly arises from the scapula. Deep to these two muscles run the **sternothyroid** and **thyrohyoid**, both of which are rather wider than the sternohyoid. The sternothyroid connects the back of the sternoclavicular joint to the oblique line of the thyroid cartilage, and the thyrohyoid continues from this attachment to the front of the hyoid bone.

LYMPH DRAINAGE OF THE HEAD AND NECK (fig. 22.60)

The lymph nodes of the head and neck may be regarded as forming two main groups, a **chain of deep cervical lymph nodes** surrounding the neurovascular bundle in the neck, and a series of more superficial nodes arranged as a so-called **collar** at the junction of head and neck. The chain of deep cervical lymph nodes is particularly associated with the internal jugular vein. Superiorly, this chain can be traced to a small node occupying the angle between the posterior wall of the nasopharynx and the prevertebral muscles, the **retro-pharyngeal node**. Posteriorly, individual members of the deep cervical chain appear in the posterior triangle of the neck, spreading from the border of the sternomastoid muscle. One of these, the **jugulo-omohyoid node**, lies at the point at which the inferior belly of the omohyoid muscle crosses the neurovascular bundle. Among its afferent vessels are a few which come directly from the tip of the tongue. At the anterior border of the sternomastoid, where it crosses the posterior belly of the digastric muscle, is another member of the deep cervical chain, the **jugulodigastric** or **tonsillar node**, which receives afferents from the posterior third of the tongue, the tonsillar bed and the adjacent wall of the oropharynx. The efferent lymphatic vessels from the deep cervical nodes converge on the **jugular lymph trunk**, which drains into

the junction of the internal jugular and subclavian veins through the thoracic duct or right lymphatic duct (p. 21.39).

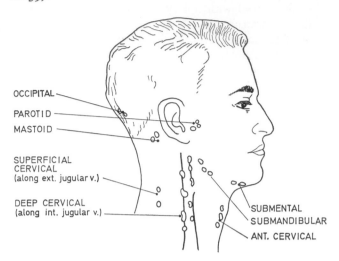

FIG. 22.60. Main groups of lymph nodes in the head and neck.

The **collar of superficial nodes** drains the superficial region of the head and also receives some deeply placed efferents. It consists of the following groups:

The **submental nodes** lie between the diverging anterior bellies of the digastric muscles, on the under surface of the mylohyoids, and drain the median parts of the tongue, gum and lower lip.

The **submandibular nodes** are wedged between the submandibular gland and the medial surface of the mandible, and drain the remainder of the lower jaw and the side of the tongue.

The **superficial parotid group** drains the upper part of the face and the temporal region. It continues downwards over the superficial aspect of the sternomastoid muscle as the superficial group of cervical nodes, which drain into the lower posterior group of deep nodes. They follow the course of the external jugular vein. The **deep parotid nodes** do not belong to the collar chain series but are members of the deep cervical group.

The **mastoid group** lies on the lateral aspect of the mastoid process, and drains the side of the head.

The **occipital group** lies on the superficial aspect of the upper fibres of the trapezius, and drains the posterior part of the scalp.

All these nodes drain into the deep cervical series of nodes. The submental group tends to send its efferent vessels to the more inferiorly placed nodes, particularly the jugulo-omohyoid.

In addition to these, there are scattered groups of lymph nodes in the anterior part of the neck, the **anterior cervical nodes**. These include the infrahyoid group on the thyrohyoid membrane, the prelaryngeal group on the cricothyroid ligament, the pretracheal nodes at the lower end of the thyroid gland, and some upper members of the paratracheal series in the tracheo-oesophageal groove. All these nodes drain into the lower deep cervical nodes.

The tongue is drained by lymph vessels which pass from its tip to the submental and jugulo-omohyoid nodes, from its lateral edge into the submandibular group, from the median part of its dorsum into submandibular and deep cervical nodes of both sides of the neck, and from its posterior third into the upper deep cervical group (fig. 22.61). The nasopharynx sends vessels into the retropharyngeal nodes. The oropharynx, including the palatine tonsil, drains mainly to the jugulodigastric node. The larynx sends vessels from its upper part, above the vocal ligament, to the infrahyoid group, and thence to the upper deep cervical nodes. From its infraglottic part, vessels pass to the prelaryngeal, pretracheal and paratracheal nodes.

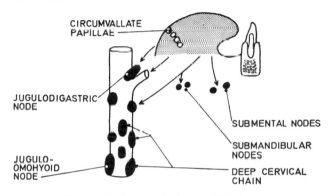

FIG. 22.61. Lymph drainage of the tongue.

The lymphatic vessels from the thyroid gland run to the upper deep cervical, pretracheal, paratracheal, lower deep cervical and anterior mediastinal nodes. Some of its vessels may bypass all nodes and end in the thoracic duct or subclavian vein. The vessels of the cervical part of the trachea end in the prelaryngeal and pretracheal nodes, and in some members of the deep cervical group. The cervical part of the oesophagus drains to the paratracheal nodes.

DEVELOPMENT OF THE FACE

The face develops from that part of the embryo which immediately surrounds the buccopharyngeal membrane. A thickening develops in the epithelium on either side of the midline of the surface of the embryo, immediately superficial to the forebrain. These are the two olfactory placodes, and they are destined to form the olfactory mucous membrane of the definitive nose. The mesoderm in the regions surrounding the placodes grows faster than that deep to them. As a result, the placodes become buried in the surface of the embryo. The depressions

thus produced are the **olfactory pits** (fig. 22.62). Between them, the mesoderm and overlying ectoderm are raised up into a **median nasal process**, whose lateral margins are the **globular processes**. Lateral to the placodes, the elevated mesoderm in similar fashion forms

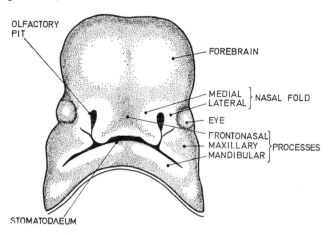

FIG. 22.62. Ventral aspect of fetal head.

the **lateral nasal processes**. The placodes sink progressively dorsally and caudally into the substance of the embryonic head, until they meet the cephalic boundary of the primitive pharynx, into which they achieve a temporary opening. This is later occluded by epithelial proliferation. The region between the primitive nostrils provided by this pair of nasal pits, and the cephalic edge of the stomatodaeum, is the rudimentary palate. This latter structure, along with the median and lateral nasal processes, together constitute the **frontonasal process**. Branches of the ophthalmic nerve grow into this process. Mesoderm proceeds to proliferate also between the ectoderm and endoderm at the sides of the stomatodaeum, forming the **maxillary process** at either lateral end of the primitive mouth. The primitive mouth is completed inferiorly by the two mandibular arches which grow forwards to fuse in the midline.

Associated with the maxillary process is the maxillary division of the trigeminal nerve, which grows into the mesoderm of the process. Similarly, the mandibular division of the same nerve, along with the motor root, grows into the mandibular arch, supplying its derivatives, including the skeletal muscle which develops from its mesoderm.

As growth continues the optic outgrowths extend laterally from the diencephalon, until they come into contact with the epithelium of the surface of the embryo at the dorsal end of the groove which separates the frontonasal and maxillary processes. The overlying ectoderm becomes invaginated to form the lens vesicle, and the eye develops at the extreme dorsal end of the maxillo-frontonasal groove.

By this time, the buccopharyngeal membrane has

broken down, and the primitive oral cavity and the pharynx are in direct continuity. The maxillary processes grow ventrally, separating the primitive frontonasal palate from the oral cavity, and the medial edges of the two maxillary processes fuse with the very narrow down-

and frontonasal processes is progressively lengthened by the ventral growth of the former, and deepened by the proliferation of mesoderm within the adjacent parts of both processes. It is designated the **nasolacrimal groove**, since the apposition of its growing lips eventually converts it into a canal, the nasolacrimal duct of the full-term fetus. Where the apposed edges fail to fuse, an oblique fissure extends from the medial angle of the eye to the lateral margin of the oral fissure of that side of the face, a condition of **cleft face**.

From the floor of the oral cavity, the tongue is developed initially from the internal aspects of the fused ventral ends of the first and second pharyngeal arches. Later, the third arch grows cranially to contribute to the posterior third of the tongue, and obliterates all traces of the second arch in doing so. In the early stages of fetal development, the tongue projects headwards, sufficiently virtually to fill the primitive oral cavity. While this situation exists, epithelially covered ridges grow medially from the oral aspects of the maxillary processes. These are the **palatine processes**. At first, their free medial edges are turned caudally. Later, as the cavity of the mouth increases in size relative to the tongue, the medial edges of these two processes meet, and their ventral ends fuse with the margins of the primitive frontonasal palate, and, dorsal to that, with each other. A septum is thus formed between the nasal and oral cavities. When the ventral ends of the frontonasal and maxillary processes fail to fuse, a false or paramedian hare lip exists (fig. 22.63). If this failure is more extensive and involves the palatine contributions of both processes, partial or complete cleft palate may result. This may be further complicated by a failure to join up with the nasal septum. In its extreme form, no roof exists to the mouth, and a median tag of tissue is suspended from the septum of the nose, just above the oral cavity.

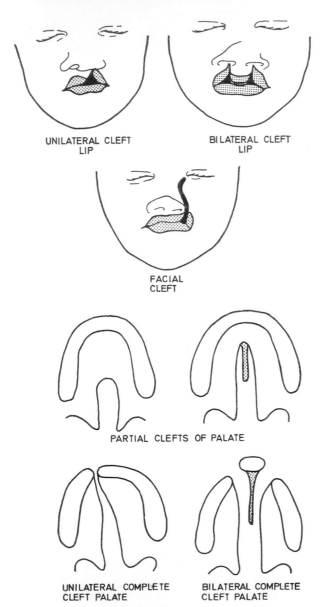

FIG. 22.63. Congenital abnormalities of the face and palate.

ward projecting portion of the frontonasal process which forms the philtrum of the upper lip. A more limited fusion takes place between the adjacent edges of the maxillary process and mandibular arch, and upon the extent of this depends the size of the definitive mouth.

The lateral part of the groove between the maxillary

FURTHER READING

MacConaill M.A. & Basmajian J.V. (1969) *Muscles and Movements*. Baltimore: Williams & Wilkins.

Sarnat B.G. (1951) *The Temporomandibular Joint*. Springfield, Ill.: Thomas.

Scott J.H. & Dixon A.D. (1972) *Anatomy for Students of Dentistry*, 3rd Edition. Edinburgh: Churchill Livingstone.

Scott J.H. & Symons N.B.B. (1971) *Introduction to Dental Anatomy*, 6th Edition. Edinburgh: Churchill Livingstone.

Truex R.C. & Kellner C.E. (1948) *Detailed Atlas of the Head and Neck*. London: Oxford University Press.

Chapter 23
Upper limb

The upper limb (fig. 23.1) is composed of the shoulder girdle, the upper arm, the forearm and the hand. In ordinary speech the distal part of the forearm is called the wrist. The hand is divided into three parts, the carpus (anatomical wrist), the hand proper (the dorsum and the palm) supported by the bones of the metacarpus, and five

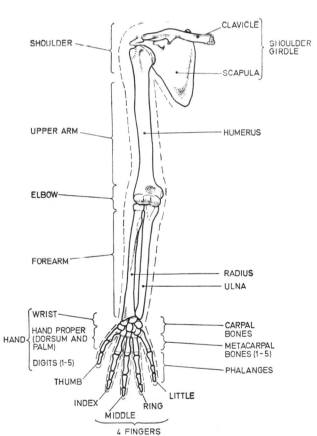

FIG. 23.1. General plan of the upper limb.

digits, the thumb and four fingers (index, middle, ring, little).

The upper and lower limbs are built on a similar plan. Each has a girdle (shoulder or pelvic) which connects it to the trunk, a single bone in the upper arm or in the thigh, two bones each in the forearm or leg, the carpus and metacarpus in the hand and the tarsus

and metatarsus in the foot and each has phalangeal bones.

There are, however, considerable functional differences between the two limbs. The pelvic girdle has no free movement, while the shoulder girdle possesses great mobility. The lower limb, specialized for simpler tasks of weight-bearing, locomotion and balance, differs from the upper limb which is a mobile system of joints and levers for positioning the hand, a delicate organ capable of the complicated tasks of exploration, gripping and manipulation. The hand is also an important sense organ; through sensory endings in its skin, muscles and joints, it provides information for the brain about the shape, size, weight, temperature and texture of handled objects. It has been said that man owes his progress to the development of the cerebral hemispheres and to his opposable thumb, since the contact between the thumb and the pulps of the other digits is necessary for delicate processes of exploration and manipulation. Even computers and automation systems require skilful hands for their production.

Any diminution in the efficiency of the hand affects our livelihood; unfortunately injuries to the upper limb and particularly to the hand are common in a mechanical age. In their treatment special care needs to be given to preserving function.

BONES, JOINTS AND MUSCLES OF THE SHOULDER GIRDLE AND SHOULDER

The shoulder girdle is made up of two bones, the clavicle and the scapula (fig. 23.2), united by the strong coraco-clavicular ligament and a synovial acromioclavicular joint, an arrangement which allows slight movement between the two bones. The girdle is attached to the axial skeleton in front by the synovial sternoclavicular joint and its ligaments, and by muscles (pectoralis minor, fig. 23.16; subclavius, fig. 23.16 and serratus anterior, fig. 23.17), whilst at the back the link is purely muscular (trapezius, fig. 23.13; levator scapulae, fig. 23.14 and rhomboids, fig. 23.14).

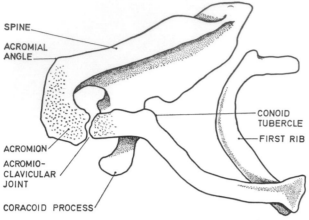

SPINE
ACROMIAL ANGLE
CONOID TUBERCLE
FIRST RIB
ACROMION
ACROMIO-CLAVICULAR JOINT
CORACOID PROCESS

FIG. 23.2. The bones of the right shoulder girdle with the first rib, seen from above.

Functionally the shoulder girdle should be considered together with the upper part of the arm, with the shoulder joint and its muscles (deltoid, fig. 23.19; supraspinatus, infraspinatus, teres major and minor, fig. 23.20; subscapularis, fig. 23.21) and with the muscle links between the humerus and trunk (pectoralis major in front, fig. 23.15, and latissimus dorsi at the back fig. 23.18).

In contrast to the pelvis, the shoulder girdles are separate from each other; this, together with the method of their attachment to the axial skeleton, gives considerable mobility to these regions, their stability depending largely on the action of the muscles.

BONES OF THE SHOULDER REGION

Clavicle (fig. 23.3)

This is a curved strut extending from the sternum to the acromion process of the scapula and holding the point of the shoulder at its proper distance from the trunk. If the strut is broken, which usually happens at the junction of the middle and lateral thirds, the shoulder falls forwards and medially.

The medial end is expanded and overrides the sternum

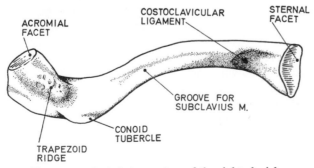

ACROMIAL FACET
COSTOCLAVICULAR LIGAMENT
STERNAL FACET
GROOVE FOR SUBCLAVIUS M.
CONOID TUBERCLE
TRAPEZOID RIDGE

FIG. 23.3. The inferior surface of the right clavicle.

where it forms the sternoclavicular joint. The suprasternal notch intervenes between the medial ends of the two clavicles. The lateral end is flattened and articulates with the acromion of the scapula. The medial two-thirds of the shaft is convex forwards, conforming with the anterior curvature of the chest wall; near the medial end of the bone the inferior surface is rough for the attachment of the costoclavicular ligament and, more laterally, it is grooved for the attachment of the subclavius muscle. The lateral third of the shaft overlies the shoulder and is flattened from above downwards. Its inferior surface is marked by a **conoid tubercle** near the posterior border and by a **trapezoid ridge** running forwards and laterally from the tubercle.

Scapula

The scapula is a triangular plate of bone whose anterior surface is applied to the posterior curvature of the chest so that it makes an angle of 30° with the coronal plane when the arm is by the side (fig. 23.4). The posterior

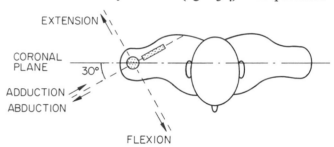

EXTENSION
CORONAL PLANE
30°
ADDUCTION
ABDUCTION
FLEXION

FIG. 23.4 The position of the scapula in relation to the coronal plane, the head of the humerus and the planes of movement of the arm.

surface is divided into **supraspinous** and **infraspinous fossae** (fig. 23.5) by the **spine** which projects backwards and continues laterally and forwards as the **acromion process**. The **acromial angle,** which can be readily palpated at the back of the shoulder, is the point where the acromion bends forwards to meet the lateral end of the clavicle. The scapula has superior, lateral and medial borders, and superior, inferior and lateral angles, the last being thickened to form the neck and head of the bone. The lateral surface of the head faces forwards and laterally (fig. 23.6) and is slightly hollowed out to form the shallow **glenoid fossa** which articulates with the almost hemispherical head of the humerus. Supraglenoid and infraglenoid tubercles are to be found respectively just above and below the rim of the glenoid fossa. The **coracoid process** projects anteriorly from the upper part of the neck of the scapula. From its vertical portion or root it bends forwards at its angle into a horizontal part which ends in its tip. The blade-like body of the scapula is covered by muscles and only the inferior angle, the lower part of the medial border, spine, acromion and the coracoid tip can be felt through the skin. With the arm

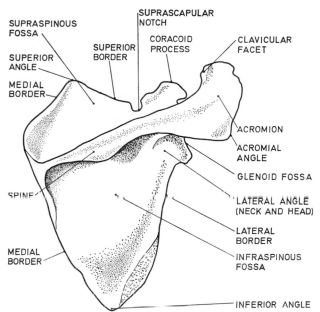

FIG. 23.5. Posterior view of the right scapula.

by the side, the root of the spine lies at the level of the third thoracic vertebral spine and the inferior angle at the seventh spine.

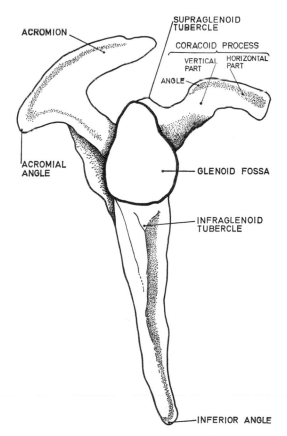

FIG. 23.6. Lateral view of the right scapula.

Humerus (fig. 23.7)

The almost hemispherical **head**, covered by articular cartilage, faces upwards, medially and slightly backwards in the plane of the scapula to meet the shallow and much smaller glenoid fossa. The head is separated from the rest of the bone by the shallow constriction called the **anatomical neck**. The **greater tubercle** is the large prominence, lateral to the head, which forms the point of the shoulder. The **lesser tubercle** on the anterior

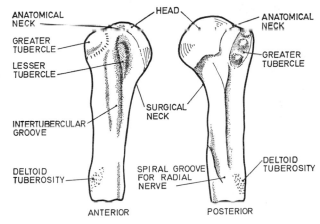

FIG. 23.7. The upper part of the right humerus.

aspect of the proximal end of the bone is separated by the intertubercular groove from the greater tubercle. The **surgical neck** is the region immediately below the head and the tubercles. The **deltoid tuberosity**, the rough V-shaped impression at the attachment of the deltoid muscle, is found around the midpoint of the lateral aspect of the shaft. On the posterior surface of the shaft a shallow groove for the radial nerve runs obliquely downwards and laterally.

JOINTS OF THE SHOULDER REGION

Sternoclavicular joint (fig. 23.8)

The shoulder girdle is united to the trunk by the muscles and by the synovial sternoclavicular joint. The large medial end of the clavicle fits into a socket formed by a notch on the manubrium sterni and by the first costal cartilage. A strong fibrous capsule surrounds the joint. Two accessory ligaments are the **interclavicular ligament** extending from clavicle to clavicle, and the **costoclavicular ligament** from the under surface of the clavicle to the upper surface of the first costal cartilage. An articular disc, attached to the clavicle above and to the first costal cartilage below, blends with the capsule and divides the joint into two compartments, medial and lateral. These ligaments and the articular disc prevent medial

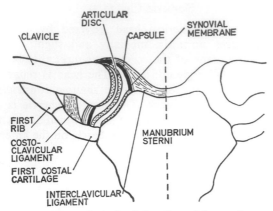

FIG. 23.8. Sternoclavicular joint. Synovial membrane is black and cartilage is dotted.

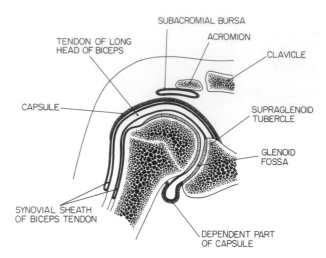

FIG. 23.10. The shoulder joint. The cavity is distended as normally only potential spaces exist. The section is in the plane of the tendon of the long head of biceps.

dislocation of the clavicle even when an impact on the shoulder is sufficient to break the bone.

Acromioclavicular joint (fig. 23.9)

This joint unites the two bones of the girdle. It has a weak capsule and usually contains an incomplete articular disc. The plane of the joint is oblique so that the lateral end of the clavicle tends to override the acromion,

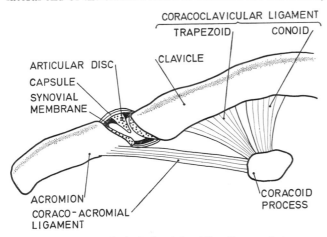

FIG. 23.9. Acromioclavicular joint. The distance between clavicle and coracoid process is exaggerated.

and the security of the joint depends on the strong **coracoclavicular ligament** which anchors the clavicle to the coracoid process. Attachments of this important ligament are the conoid tubercle and trapezoid ridge on the clavicle, and the coracoid process in the region of its angle.

Shoulder (glenohumeral) joint (fig. 23.10)

The shoulder joint which is of the synovial ball and socket variety has a very free range of movement. Neither the fit of the bones, nor the capsule and ligaments contribute much to its stability, which depends almost entirely on the surrounding muscles.

The **capsular ligament** is very loose and it presents inferiorly a dependent pouch when the arm is by the side; if the arm is immobilized in this position, the walls of the pouch may become permanently fused together, causing a stiff joint. The capsule is attached around the anatomical neck of the humerus except medially where it descends on to the surgical neck; on the scapula it is attached to a fibrocartilaginous rim called **labrum glenoidale**, bound to the periphery of the glenoid fossa. The capsule extends above to include the supraglenoid tubercle and the attachment of the tendon of the long head of the biceps muscle. The **transverse ligament** bridges across the upper part of the intertubercular groove to hold the tendon in position. The **coracohumeral ligament** runs from the lateral part of the root of the coracoid process to the anatomical neck and greater tubercle, blending with the capsule. The tendons of the rotator cuff muscles (p. 23.10) fuse with and strengthen the capsular ligament.

The synovial membrane lines the deep aspect of the capsule, covers the labrum glenoidale, surrounds the tendon of the long head of biceps and lines those surfaces of the bone within the capsule, which are not covered by articular cartilage. There are two bursae communicating with the synovial cavity; one surrounds the bicipital tendon, the other lies anteriorly under the subscapularis muscle.

The weakest part of the capsule is at the inferior aspect and this is the area which is usually torn in dislocation of the shoulder joint. The axillary nerve which lies inferior to the joint may then be injured.

Coraco-acromial arch and subacromial bursa (fig. 23.11)

These should be regarded as a functional extension of the shoulder joint. One of the commonest causes of pain

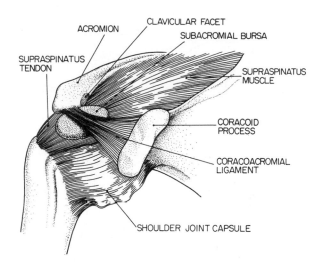

FIG. 23.11. Coraco-acromial arch and subacromial bursa. The bursa is distended.

and disability in the shoulder region is due to the disturbance of this bursal joint.

The **coraco-acromial arch** forms a shelf above the shoulder joint. It is composed of the horizontal part of the coracoid process, the coraco-acromial ligament and the acromion. The ligament is attached to the lateral border of the horizontal part of the coracoid and to the acromion in front of the acromioclavicular joint. The arch is separated from the shoulder joint by the supraspinatus tendon which blends with the superior aspect of the capsule. To ensure a smooth movement the subacromial bursa lies between the upper surface of the supraspinatus tendon and the capsule of the shoulder joint

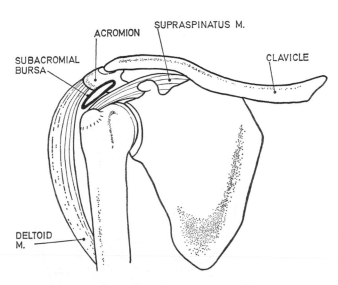

FIG. 23.12. A diagram illustrating the relations of the subacromial bursa.

below, and the arch and overlying deltoid muscle above. This bursa does not normally communicate with the cavity of the shoulder joint, but it may do so in disease or following changes due to age.

MUSCLES OF THE SHOULDER REGION

The muscles connecting the upper limb to the axial skeleton are shown in figs. 23.13–18 and consist of trapezius, rhomboids, levator scapulae, pectoralis major, pectoralis minor, subclavius, serratus anterior and latissimus dorsi. In all these figures O and I represent the origin and insertion of the muscles respectively.

The muscles of the shoulder are shown in figs. 23.19–21

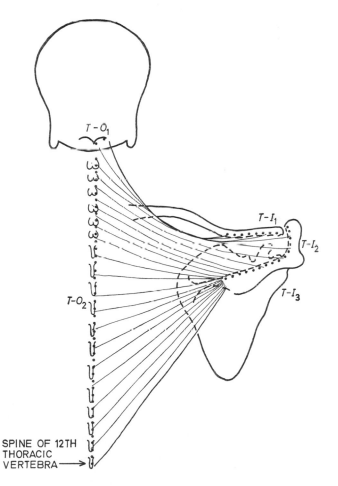

FIG. 23.13. **Trapezius muscle** (T). which lies superficial to the levator scapulae and rhomboid.

T-O_1 Medial third of superior nuchal line of occipital bone and external occipital protuberance.

T-O_2 Ligamentum nuchae, the spines of the seventh cervical and all thoracic vertebrae.

T-I_1 Lateral third of clavicle.

T-I_2 Medial border of acromion.

T-I_3 Crest of the spine of scapula.

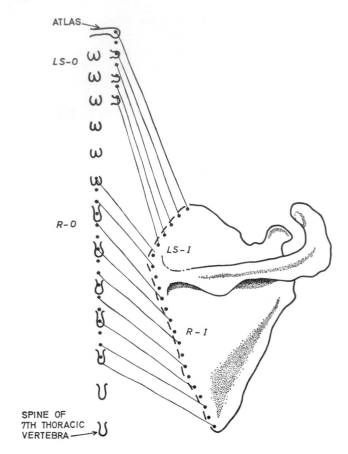

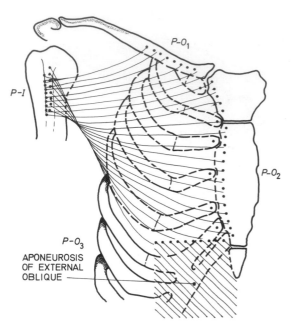

ATLAS

LS-O

R-O

LS-I

R-I

SPINE OF
7TH THORACIC
VERTEBRA

FIG. 23.14. The levator scapulae and the rhomboid muscles, which lie deep to trapezius.

Levator scapulae muscle (*LS*).

LS-O Posterior tubercles of the transverse processes of the first three or four cervical vertebrae.

LS-I Medial margin of scapula from the upper angle to the spine.

Rhomboid muscles (*R*).

R-O Lower part of ligamentum nuchae, spines of seventh cervical and first five thoracic vertebrae.

R-I Medial border of scapula from the spine to the inferior angle.

FIG. 23.16. The pectoralis minor, subclavius and coracobrachialis muscles.

Pectoralis minor muscle (*PM*).

PM-O Third, fourth and fifth ribs.
PM-I Medial border of coracoid process.

Subclavius muscle (*S*)

S-O First rib and its cartilage.
S-I Floor of groove on the inferior surface of the clavicle.

Coracobrachialis muscle (*CB*)

CB-O Tip of coracoid process.
CB-I Middle of medial border of the shaft of the humerus.

P-O₁

P-I

P-O₂

P-O₃

APONEUROSIS
OF EXTERNAL
OBLIQUE

FIG. 23.15. Pectoralis major which lies superficial to the pectoralis minor, subclavius and coracobrachialis muscles.

Pectoralis major muscle (*P*).

P-O₁ Medial half of the clavicle.
P-O₂ Manubrium and body of sternum, first six costal cartilages.
P-O₃ Aponeurosis of external oblique muscle of the abdomen.
P-I Lateral lip of the intertubercular groove.

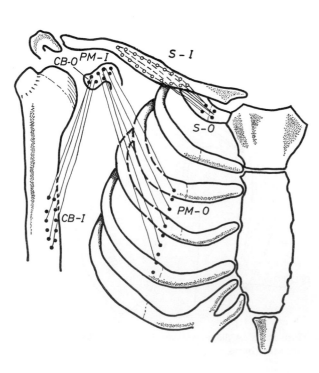

CB-O PM-I

S-I

S-O

CB-I

PM-O

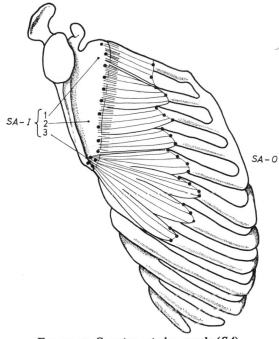

FIG. 23.17. **Serratus anterior muscle** (*SA*)

SA-O Outer surfaces of the upper eight ribs.

SA-I (1) Costal surface of the superior angle, (2) medial border, (3) inferior angle of the scapula.

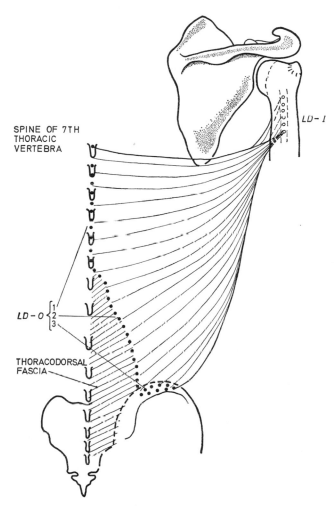

FIG. 23.18. **Latissimus dorsi muscle** (*LD*).

LD-O₁ Spines of lower six thoracic vertebrae.

LD-O₂ Through thoracolumbar fascia from the spines of the lumbar and sacral vertebrae.

LD-O₃ Posterior part of the iliac crest.

LD-I Floor of the intertubercular groove of the humerus.

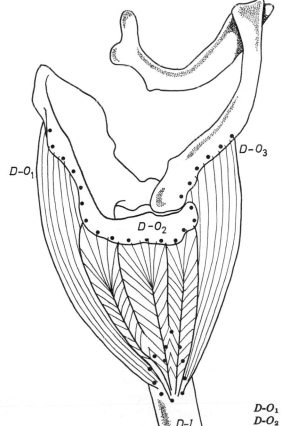

FIG. 23.19. **Deltoid muscle** (*D*).

D-O₁ Crest of the spine of the scapula.

D-O₂ Lateral border of acromion.

D-O₃ Lateral third of the clavicle.

D-I Deltoid tuberosity of the humerus.

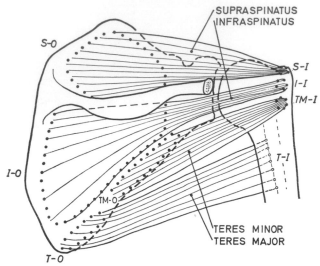

FIG. 23.20. Supraspinatus, infraspinatus and teres muscles.

Supraspinatus muscle (*S*).

S-O Walls of the supraspinous fossa, except near the neck of the scapula.

S-I Facet on the top of the greater tubercle of the humerus.

Infraspinatus muscle (*I*)

I-O Walls of the infraspinous fossa except at the neck of the scapula.

I-I Middle facet on the greater tubercle of the humerus.

Teres major muscle (*T*)

T-O Dorsal aspect of the lower third of the lateral border of the scapula.

T-I Inner lip of the intertubercular groove.

Teres minor muscle (*TM*)

TM-O Dorsal aspect of the upper two-thirds of the lateral border of the scapula.

TM-I Lowest facet on the greater tubercle of the humerus.

and consist of deltoid, supraspinatus, infraspinatus, teres major and minor, subscapularis and coracobrachialis.

MOVEMENTS OF THE SHOULDER REGION

The mobility of the structures associated with the shoulder girdle and the shoulder itself has been emphasized. Before the individual movements are described it is necessary to discuss the important concept of the **scapulothoracic mechanism**. The scapula is joined directly to the trunk only by muscles and is freely movable on the chest wall. As these muscles have much greater leverage than those acting on the shoulder joint itself, the scapulothoracic mechanism makes an important contribution to the range and power of the movements of the shoulder girdle and arm.

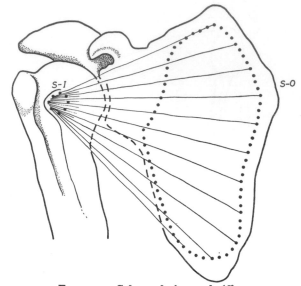

FIG. 23.21. **Subscapularis muscle (*S*).**
S-O Anterior surface of the scapula.
S-I Lesser tubercle of the humerus.

The position of the socket for the head of the humerus can be altered either by translation or rotation of the scapula on the trunk. Even if surgical fixation of the shoulder joint is carried out, increase in the movements of the scapula on the trunk preserves considerable mobility. Some movement of the scapula on the clavicle is possible in spite of the strong coracoclavicular ligament and it occurs at the acromioclavicular joint when the scapula moves on the trunk. However, the contribution of this joint to the mobility of the shoulder region does not seem to be of importance, since its surgical fixation does not cause any appreciable disability. The contribution of the sternoclavicular joint is important since with the elevation of the shoulder, the clavicle rotates in this joint until its anterior surface inclines upwards. When the lateral end of the clavicle moves forwards or backwards, downwards or upwards, the medial end moves in the opposite direction because of the strong fulcrum formed by the costoclavicular ligament.

Movements at the joints of the shoulder girdle

The shoulder girdle with the attached limb can be elevated, depressed, moved forwards and backwards. Elevation is achieved by the upper fibres of the trapezius, levator scapulae and rhomboids. It is checked by the costoclavicular ligament. Depression is achieved by subclavius, pectoralis minor and the lower fibres of the trapezius. It is checked by the articular disc of the sternoclavicular joint and by the interclavicular ligament. Serratus anterior and pectoralis minor are responsible for forward movement and trapezius and rhomboids for backward movement.

Pectoralis major and latissimus dorsi muscles, although

acting primarily at the shoulder joint, assist in the movements of the girdle, the former in the forward and the latter in the backward direction.

Movements of the arm in relation to the trunk

These occur at the shoulder girdle and at the shoulder joint itself in a well co-ordinated and synchronized manner. Abduction and adduction, by definition, occur in the plane of the scapula and flexion and extension at right angles to this plane (fig. 23.4). Circumduction is a combination of the above four movements. Rotation can occur at any given position of the arm and consists of movement of the limb around the long axis of the humerus (fig. 23.22).

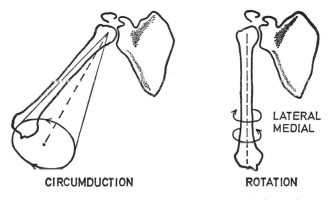

CIRCUMDUCTION   ROTATION

FIG. 23.22. Lateral and medial rotation and circumduction.

Flexion is achieved by pectoralis major, the anterior fibres of deltoid, coracobrachialis and the short head of biceps. Extension is brought about by latissimus dorsi, teres major and minor, posterior fibres of the deltoid, infraspinatus and long head of triceps. Pectoralis major, latissimus dorsi, teres major and minor are responsible for adduction. Lateral rotation is carried out by infraspinatus, teres minor, posterior fibres of deltoid and medial rotation by pectoralis major, anterior fibres of deltoid, subscapularis, latissimus dorsi and teres major. Medial rotation is stronger than lateral rotation.

The three muscles of the arm: biceps, coracobrachialis and triceps, are shown on figs. 23.16 and 23.29.

The **movement of abduction** deserves separate description because of its importance and complexity and because it is a good example of the functional co-ordination of many structures. As already indicated, abduction occurs in the plane of the scapula and only in this plane is the capsule of the shoulder joint not twisted. This is an important consideration when it is necessary to rest the joint for some time. The range of abduction is from the dependent position to above the head, approximately two-thirds of the movement occurring at the shoulder joint and one-third by rotation of the scapula. Some degree of lateral rotation accompanies abduction.

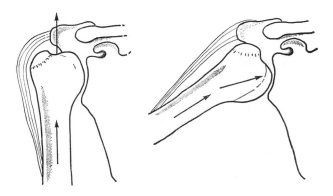

FIG. 23.23. Diagram showing the effect of the deltoid pull in early and middle range of abduction.

The joints and links concerned with the abduction of the upper limb are sternoclavicular, acromioclavicular and shoulder (glenohumeral) joints, the coracoacromial arch with the bursal joint and the scapulothoracic link.

The muscles effecting abduction are the deltoid, supraspinatus, trapezius and serratus anterior. A powerful middle multipennate portion of the deltoid abducts while the anterior and posterior fibres prevent anteroposterior sway of the humeral head in the shallow glenoid fossa.

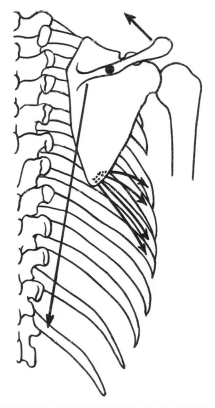

FIG. 23.24. Diagram showing the rotation of the scapula on the trunk. From Sinclair D.C. (1975) *An Introduction to Functional Anatomy*, 5th Edition. Oxford: Blackwell Scientific Publications.

Supraspinatus assists in the early stages of abduction, but together with the other **rotator-cuff muscles** (infraspinatus, teres minor and subscapularis) it has a much more important synergistic action in preventing the powerfully contracting deltoid from pulling the head of the humerus upwards out of the joint in the early stages of abduction (fig. 23.23). Later in abduction, the deltoid is at a mechanical advantage and tends to press the head into the joint. The scapula is rotated by the **trapezius** and **serratus anterior** (fig. 23.24) in such a way that the socket for the humeral head looks more and more upwards, increasing the extent of the abduction of the arm.

It is important to realize that all these muscles are involved together throughout abduction, and act in unison and balance; they differ in the degree and timing of their contribution. The so-called rhythm of abduction refers to co-ordination of the movement of the humerus on the scapula with that of the scapula on the chest wall. This rhythm is subject to individual variations, but usually some movement of the scapula can be felt in the very early stages by grasping and following the inferior angle of the scapula through the soft tissues. This movement of the scapula begins at the same time on both sides of the body when both arms are being abducted.

BONES, JOINTS AND MUSCLES OF THE ELBOW REGION

BONES OF THE ELBOW REGION

The distal end of the humerus is compressed anteroposteriorly and bent forwards (fig. 23.25). The **capitulum,** on the lateral part of the distal end, is convex for articulation with the head of the radius. The **trochlea,** pulley-shaped, is on the medial part of the distal end and articulates with the ulna; its medial lip projects lower than the lateral. The **medial** and **lateral epicondyles** are two prominences above the articular surface of the distal end; their anterior and distal aspects serve for attachment of many muscles and ligaments. Medial and lateral supracondylar ridges extend from the epicondyles proximally on to the shaft. There are three fossae above the capitulum and the trochlea between the epicondyles, two in front (**radial** and **coronoid**) and one at the back called the **olecranon fossa;** these three accommodate the proximal ends of the forearm bones in movements at the elbow joint.

The posterior and most proximal part of the ulna is called the **olecranon** and where it embraces the humerus in the elbow joint it is lined with articular cartilage (fig. 23.26). Projecting forwards and continuous with the olecranon is the **coronoid process;** its upper surface is articular and together with the olecranon forms the **trochlear notch** of ulna. On the lateral aspect of the coronoid process, facing the head of the radius, is the **radial notch.** The **tuberosity of ulna** is below the coronoid and, below the radial notch a large depression, the supinator fossa, is limited posteriorly by a supinator crest.

The radius does not overlap the humerus. The proximal end (fig. 23.26) consists of head, neck and tuberosity. The **head** is a thick disc with the superior surface concave; the distal part of the circumference of the head is narrower than the proximal; this confers stability to the joint. The **neck** is the constricted portion supporting the head; below the neck on the medial side there is a projection called the **tuberosity of the radius.**

ELBOW JOINT

The elbow joint (fig. 23.27) is a synovial joint of the hinge variety but has some characteristics of a saddle-shaped joint in that it allows some movement of the ulna on the humerus besides flexion and extension (see supination and pronation). Essentially the elbow joint is an articulation of ulna with the humerus, the radius being attached to the ulna and moving with it. Stability of the elbow joint depends on the ulna, since it does not seem to be affected by surgical removal of the head of the radius. The concave superior surface of the radius matches the round capitulum and the trochlear notch of the ulna fits the pulley shaped trochlea of the humerus. The capsule is attached,

(1) around the articular surface of the humerus including the fossae situated above it (only the lower half of the olecranon fossa),

(2) to the **anular ligament** of the superior radio-ulnar joint,

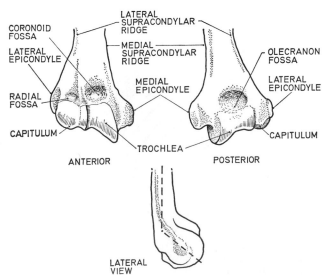

FIG. 23.25. Lower part of the right humerus. Lateral view shows the angle between the shaft and lower end.

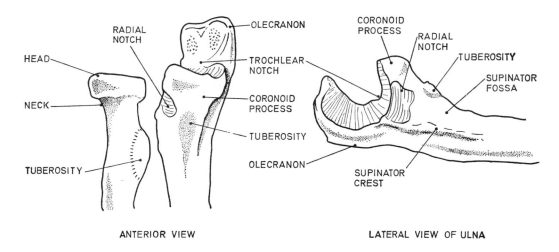

FIG. 23.26. Upper part of the ulna and radius.

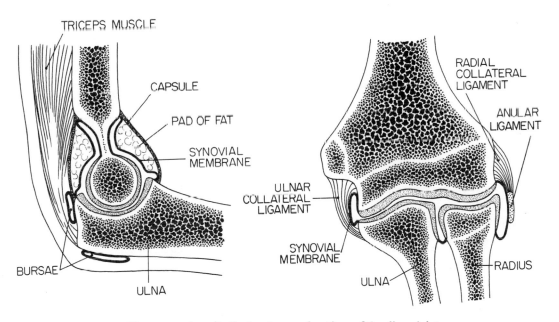

FIG. 23.27. Longitudinal and coronal sections of the elbow joint.

(3) to the olecranon, and
(4) to the coronoid process.

Being mainly a hinge joint, the anterior and posterior parts of the capsule are weak while the lateral and medial parts are strongly reinforced by **collateral ligaments.** The radial ligament extends from the lower part of the lateral epicondyle to the anular ligament and the ulnar extends from the lower edge of the medial epicondyle to the coronoid process and olecranon (fig. 22.28). The synovial cavity is continuous with that of the superior radio-ulnar joint. The synovial membrane lines the deep aspect of the capsule and those surfaces of the bone within the capsule not covered by articular cartilage. Pads of fat are

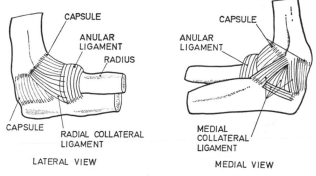

FIG. 23.28. Ligaments of the elbow joint.

interposed between the synovial membrane and the capsule in the region of the three fossae. They bulge into dead space within the joint during movement and thus may help in lubrication of the joint.

MUSCLES OF THE ELBOW REGION

Fig. 23.29 shows the attachments of the biceps, brachialis, triceps and anconeus muscles which act primarily at the elbow joint.

Acting primarily on the more distal parts of the limb, but assisting in movements at the elbow joint, are brachioradialis, pronator teres, and flexor and extensor groups of the forearm muscles (figs. 23.41–43).

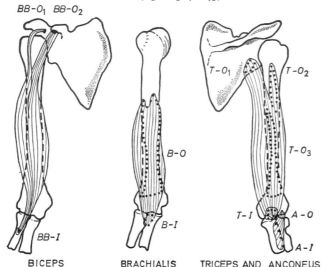

FIG. 23.29. Muscles which act primarily on the elbow joint.

Biceps brachii muscle (*BB*).

BB-O₁ Long head from the supraglenoid tubercle of the scapula.

BB-O₂ Short head from the tip of the coracoid process.

BB-I Posterior part of the tuberosity of the radius and through the bicipital aponeurosis to the deep fascia of the forearm.

Brachialis muscle (*B*) which lies deep to *BB*

B-O Distal two-thirds of the front of the shaft of the humerus.

B-I Tuberosity of the ulna.

Triceps muscle (*T*)

T-O₁ Long head from the infraglenoid tubercle of the scapula.

T-O₂ Lateral head from the back of the humerus, above the radial nerve groove.

T-O₃ Medial head from the back of the humerus, below the radial nerve groove.

T-I Posterior part of the proximal surface of the olecranon.

Anconeus muscle (*A*)

A-O Distal part of the back of the lateral epicondyle of the humerus and from the capsule of the elbow joint.

A-I Triangular area on the lateral aspect of the olecranon and the posterior surface of the ulna.

MOVEMENTS AT THE ELBOW JOINT

The main movements are flexion and extension but some contribution is made to supination and pronation, by adduction and abduction respectively of the ulna at the saddle-shaped humero-ulnar compartment of the elbow joint. Flexion is achieved by brachialis (the strongest) and by pronator teres and brachioradialis, assisted by the flexor and extensor groups of the forearm muscles attached to the front of the epicondyles. Extension is brought about by triceps and anconeus.

BONES, JOINTS AND MUSCLES OF THE FOREARM

BONES OF THE FOREARM

The shafts of the ulna and radius (fig. 23.30) face each other by their interosseous borders to which the tough interosseous membrane is attached. The shaft of the radius is convex medially in the proximal quarter and

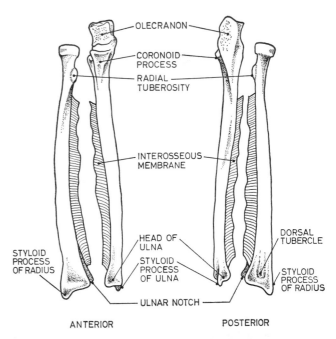

FIG. 23.30. Bones of the right forearm.

laterally in the distal three-quarters. The shaft of the ulna is subcutaneous posteriorly. The ulnar **styloid process** juts down from the posteromedial aspect of the rounded head of the ulna.

The distal end of the radius is expanded and bent anteriorly (fig. 23.31). Its **styloid process** juts down from the lateral side and the **dorsal tubercle** is the most prominent of the ridges on the back. The ulnar notch, situated on the medial side, articulates with the head of ulna.

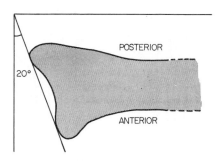

FIG. 23.31. Distal end of radius traced from a lateral radiographic view in pronation.

JOINTS OF THE FOREARM

Proximal radio-ulnar joint

The head of the radius is encircled by the anular ligament and the radial notch of ulna (fig. 23.32). The **anular ligament is a strong band** attached to the anterior and posterior borders of the radial notch of ulna forming a ring which is narrower below than above. The upper margin of the ligament is attached to the lateral epicondyle and to the lateral part of the elbow capsule. The lower

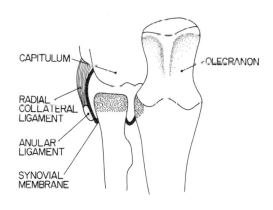

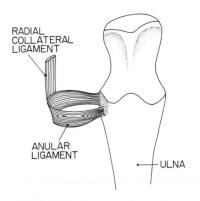

FIG. 23.32. Proximal radio-ulnar joint. Distance between bones is exaggerated.

margin of the ligament allows for rotation by being very loosely attached to the neck of the radius. The synovial membrane of the elbow joint lines the inner surface of the ligament and is reflected on to the neck of the radius.

Interosseous membrane (fig. 23.30)

The interosseous membrane is thin and strong and attached to the interosseous margins of ulna and radius. Its fibres are directed downwards and medially.

Distal radio-ulnar joint (fig. 23.33)

The head of the ulna articulates with the ulnar notch of the radius laterally and with a triangular articular

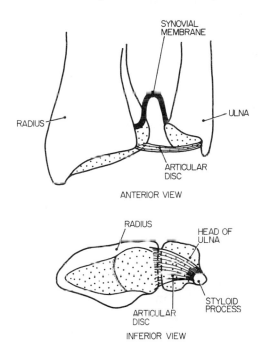

FIG. 23.33. Distal radio-ulnar joint. Distance between bones is exaggerated.

disc inferiorly. This disc is attached by its apex to the pit at the root of the ulnar styloid and by its base to the edge between the carpal and medial surfaces of the distal end of radius. Its upper surface articulates at the inferior radio-ulnar joint with the head of the ulna, and its lower surface forms part of the articular surface of the wrist joint; thus this disc separates these two joint cavities and excludes the ulna from the wrist joint.

MUSCLES EFFECTING MOVEMENTS AT RADIO-ULNAR JOINTS

The prime movers are biceps (powerful supinator, figs. 23.29 and 23.34) supinator (figs. 23.34 and 23.43) pronator teres (fig. 23.41) and pronator quadratus (fig. 23.43). Other muscles which pass obliquely across the forearm

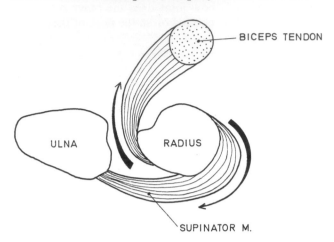

FIG. 23.34. The supinating action of supinator and biceps muscles.

contribute to these movements. These are flexor carpi radialis and palmaris longus in pronation (fig. 23.41), and extensor pollicis longus in supination (fig. 23.43).

MOVEMENTS AT THE RADIO-ULNAR JOINTS

In the supine position of the forearm its bones are parallel, while in the prone position the radius crosses the ulna (fig. 23.35). The movement of pronation starts from the supine position, carries the radius and the hand forwards around the lower end of the ulna which at the same time moves slightly back and laterally (p. 23.12). The axis of these movements passes through the centre of the radial head to the pit at the root of the ulnar styloid.

To these radio-ulnar movements, the rotation of the humerus in the glenohumeral joint should be added, medial rotation increasing the range of pronation and lateral rotation the range of supination. The glenohumeral contribution is most marked when the elbow is extended, so that the range of radio-ulnar rotation alone is best tested by fixing the flexed elbow at the side of the body. The range of radio-ulnar supination or pronation is approximately 130–140°, the rotation at the shoulder adds another 140–160° and the full combined range may reach almost 360°.

Owing to the slant of the trochlear surface of the distal end of the humerus (fig. 23.25) the arm and the forearm are not in a straight line when the limb is straightened and supinated; the angle between them, about 170°, is called the carrying angle. This angle is masked by pronation. It is therefore easier to bring the hand to the mouth

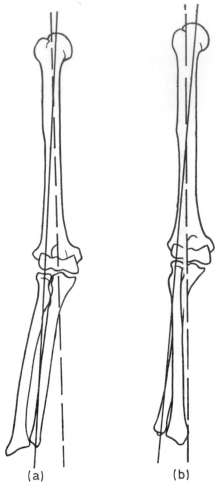

(a)   (b)

FIG. 23.35. Diagram showing (a) supine and (b) prone positions. The broken line represents the axis of the humerus and the continuous line the axis of supination and pronation. From Sinclair D.C. (1975) *Introduction to Functional Anatomy*, 5th Edition. Oxford: Blackwell Scientific Publications.

when the elbow is flexed with the forearm in mid-pronation. Moreover, in the mid-prone position, the forearm falls in line with the arm when the elbow is extended, an arrangement which gives minimal strain and maximal stability when weights are carried (fig. 23.35). When stability of the hand is required for fine manipulation, the elbow is flexed to a right angle and the forearm held midway between pronation and supination.

BONES, JOINTS AND MUSCLES OF THE HAND

BONES OF THE HAND

The bones of the hand can be considered in three parts: the skeleton of the wrist or carpus; the skeleton of the hand proper (palm and dorsum), the metacarpal bones; and the skeleton of the digits (thumb and fingers), the phalanges.

Carpus (fig. 23.36)

This is composed of eight bones in two rows which together form a transverse arch spanned by a strong tiebeam called the flexor retinaculum (fig. 23.48). The proximal surface of the carpus is convex both anteroposteriorly

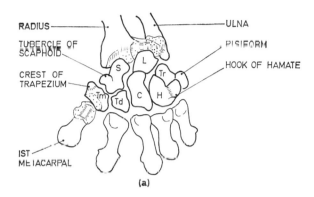

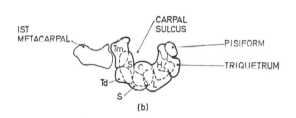

FIG. 23.36. Bones of the carpus. (a) Anterosuperior view; the bones are distracted. (b) Inferior view showing carpal arch and sulcus; S. scaphoid, L. lunate, Tr. triquetrum, H. hamate, C. capitate, Td. trapezoid, Tm. trapezium.

and from side to side. Blood supply is carried to the carpal bones with the ligaments attached to them, so it may be interrupted by injuries to the ligaments. The blood supply to the scaphoid is peculiar as the blood vessels often run from the distal to the proximal end of the bone and in some fractures the supply to the proximal part may be interrupted.

Metacarpus (fig. 23.37)

All metacarpal bones have a base, shaft and a large rounded head. The second, third, fourth and fifth metacarpal bones can be considered together. Their heads have articular cartilage on their distal and anterior surfaces. Near the posterior and proximal part of the side of the head there is a tubercle and a pit just in front of it. The shafts are curved, being concave towards the palm. The bases conform to the carpus and its arch, the metacarpal

bones being arranged like a fan diverging from the distal row of the carpal bones.

The first metacarpal has a shorter and flatter shaft than the rest; it does not lie in the plane of the palm as its broad anterior surface faces medially. Its base has a saddle-shaped articular surface which fits a similar surface on the trapezium. The setting of this metacarpal and the nature of its joint at the base are important in gripping and opposing with the thumb.

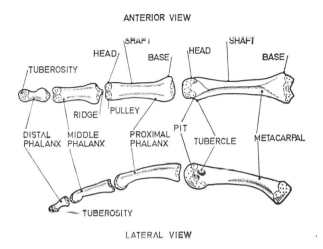

FIG. 23.37. The metacarpal and phalangeal bones of a finger.

Phalanges (fig. 23.37)

Each finger has a proximal, middle and distal phalanx. The thumb has only two; proximal and distal, they are shorter and broader than those of the fingers. Each phalanx has a base, shaft and head. All phalanges are concave towards the palmar aspect of the hand. The proximal phalanx has a concave oval facet on the base for the head of the metacarpal. The head of this phalanx has a pulley-shaped articular surface for articulation with the base of the middle phalanx, which has a median ridge fitting the groove on the head pulley. A similar arrangement exists at the distal joint. The distal phalanx has a tuberosity instead of the head.

JOINTS OF THE HAND

Wrist (radiocarpal) joint (fig. 23.38)

This is of the synovial type and ellipsoid variety. The distal end of the radius and the triangular articular disc form a socket for the convex surface of the scaphoid, lunate and triquetral bones. The triquetrum is related to the medial ligament of the joint in the anatomical position and makes contact with the socket only in

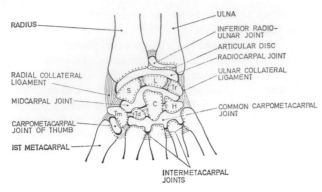

Fig. 23.38. Joints in the wrist region. Bones shown distracted.

adduction. The capsule is attached to the margins of the articular surfaces and is strengthened by anterior, posterior, medial and lateral ligaments. The medial ligament extends from the ulnar styloid to triquetrum and pisiform and the lateral one from the radial styloid to scaphoid and trapezium.

Midcarpal joint (intercarpal joints) (fig. 23.38)

Bones of the proximal row are united to the distal row by dorsal, palmar, medial and lateral ligaments. This synovial joint is of the ellipsoid variety, the same as the wrist joint; and both are concerned with the movements at the wrist.

Carpometacarpal joints (fig. 23.38)

Except for the first and fifth digits, these irregular, synovial, joints are of little importance. The carpometacarpal joint of the thumb on the other hand is important because of the mobility of this digit; the saddle shaped base of the first metacarpal fits into the corresponding saddle of the trapezium. The carpometacarpal joint of the little finger is also often almost a saddle joint, and this finger therefore has more mobility than the others at this joint.

Intermetacarpal joints (fig. 23.38)

These are between the bases of the second, third, fourth and fifth metacarpal bones. The joint between the last two is concavo-convex to allow for the mobility of the little finger.

Except for the carpometacarpal joint of the thumb and the joint between triquetrum and pisiform, the midcarpal, carpometacarpal and intercarpal joints share a common synovial cavity.

Metacarpophalangeal (MP) joints (fig. 23.39a, b and c)

These synovial joints allow flexion and extension, adduction and abduction, and some rotation. The latter movement can be observed during opposition; thus they have some features of ball and socket joints. The rounded

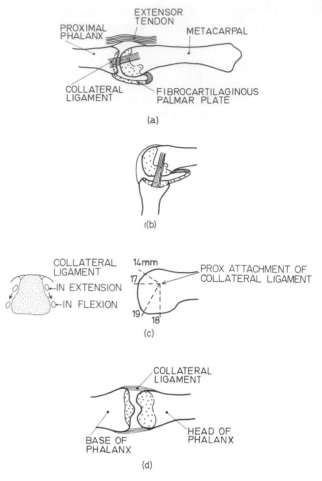

Fig. 23.39. Metacarpophalangeal and interphalangeal joints. Extended (a) and flexed (b) metacarpophalangeal joints. (c) Transverse cam and profile of metacarpal head. (d) Interphalangeal joint (palmar view).

head of the metacarpal articulates distally with the concave surface of the base of the proximal phalanx and anteriorly with the palmar ligament of the joint. The capsule is strengthened at the sides by eccentrically attached

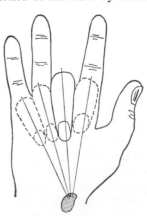

Fig. 23.40. Individual fingers in flexion point to the scaphoid.

collateral ligaments which, as can be seen in fig. 23.39b and c, become slack in extension and taut in flexion. On the dorsum the capsule is very thin as it is replaced by the expanded extensor tendon. The palmar ligament of the joint is a plate of fibrocartilage firmly attached to the proximal phalanx but connected only loosely to the meta-carpal bone. At the sides this plate fuses with the col-lateral capsule and is connected to the deep transverse

ligaments of the palm which unite the four medial meta-carpophalangeal joints.

These joints are important in the prehensile (gripping, seizing) movements of the hand. Owing to the manner of attachment of the collateral ligaments and the profile of the metacarpal head (fig. 23.39c) it is clear that if the ligaments should, through disease, become permanently shortened when the joint is in the extended position,

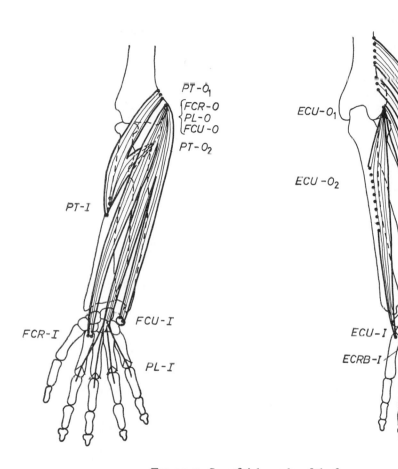

FIG. 23.41. Superficial muscles of the forearm.

Pronator teres (*PT*).
PT-O$_1$ Humeral attachment: lowest part of medial supracondylar ridge, medial epicondyle.
PT-O$_2$ Ulnar attachment: coronoid process.
PT-I Middle of lateral surface of radius.

Flexor carpi radialis (*FCR*)
FCR-O Common flexor origin on the medial epicondyle.
FCR-I Base of second metacarpal.

Palmaris longus (absent in 10%) (*PL*)
PL-O Medial epicondyle.
PL-I Flexor retinaculum and palmar aponeurosis (see later).

Flexor carpi ulnaris (*FCU*)
FCU-O Medial epicondyle, medial border of olecranon and upper part of posterior border of ulna.
FCU-I Pisiform bone.

Brachioradialis (*BR*)
BR-O Upper two-thirds of lateral supracondylar ridge.
BR-I Lateral side of lower end of radius.

Extensor carpi radialis longus (*ECRL*)
ECRL-O Distal third of lateral supracondylar ridge.
ECRL-I Base of second metacarpal.

Extensor carpi radialis brevis (*ECRB*)
ECRB-O Lateral epicondyle of humerus (common extensor origin).
ECRB-I Base of third metacarpal.

Extensor carpi ulnaris (*ECU*)
ECU-O$_1$ Lateral epicondyle.
ECU-O$_2$ Middle part of posterior border of ulna.
ECU-I Base of fifth metacarpal.

flexion of the joint is impossible and the power grip against palm is lost and against the thumb very much less efficient.

Interphalangeal (IP) joints (fig. 23.39d)

These are synovial of the modified hinge variety. At the proximal joints (PIP) the flexion-extension arc is about 110°. Extension is limited by the palmar structures. The distal joints (DIP) have 60–90° range of movement. The collateral ligaments in both joints are represented by the thickening of the medial and lateral aspects of the capsule. No active rotation occurs in these joints, but if the fingers are flexed individually, they all point to the tubercle of the scaphoid bone (fig. 23.40). This is due to the setting of the metacarpal bones in their joints, their different lengths and the arrangements within the individual digital joints.

The interphalangeal joints are more vulnerable than the MP joints owing to their superficial position between rigid bones, fibrous flexor sheaths and the skin. The PIP joints are the most important since if they are damaged, the function of the hand is seriously impaired.

MUSCLES CONCERNED WITH MOVEMENTS OF THE HAND

The flexor carpi radialis, palmaris longus, flexor carpi ulnaris, extensor carpi ulnaris, and extensor carpi radialis longus and brevis act only at the wrist (fig. 23.41).

Muscles acting on the digits and at the wrist secondarily are:

(1) on the fingers, flexor digitorum superficialis (fig. 23.42), flexor digitorum profundus (fig. 23.43), extensor

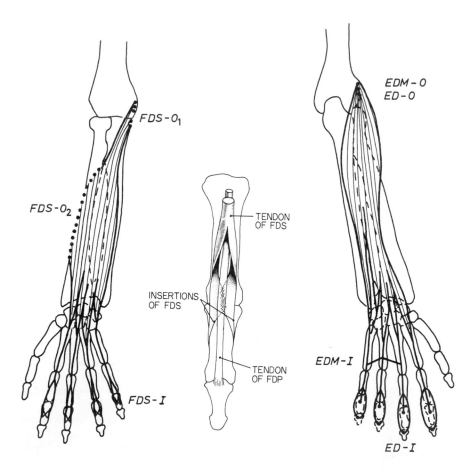

FIG. 23.42. Muscles of the forearm.

Flexor digitorum superficialis (sublimis) (FDS)

FDS-O_1 Humero-ulnar attachments: medial epicondyle of humerus, ulnar collateral ligament, medial border of coronoid process.

FDS-O_2 Upper two-thirds of anterior border of radius.

FDS-I Margins of palmar surface of middle phalanx (see insert).

Extensor digitorum (ED)

ED-O Lateral epicondyle of humerus.

ED-I Bones of the fingers and to the extensor expansion (fig. 23.54).

Extensor digiti minimi (EDM)

EDM-O Lateral epicondyle of humerus.

EDM-I Joins the tendon of ED to the little finger.

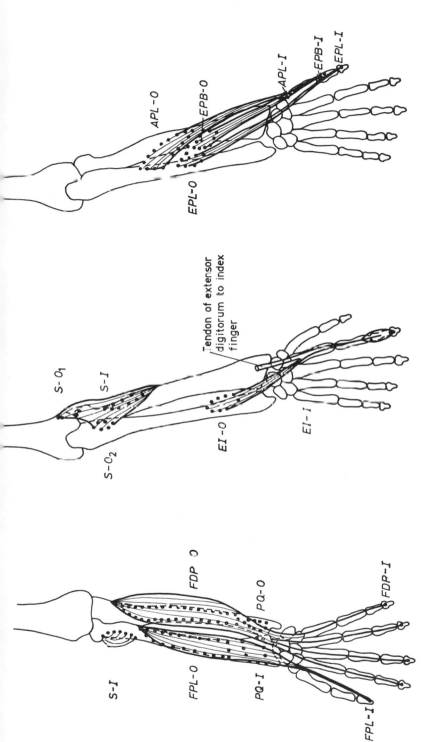

FIG. 23.43. Deep muscles of the forearm.

Flexor pollicis longus (FPL).

FPL-O Middle 2/4 of anterior surface of radius and adjoining interosseous membrane.

FPL-I Base of distal phalanx of thumb.

Flexor digitorum profundus (FDP)

FDP-O Upper two-thirds of anterior and medial surface of ulna and adjoining interosseous membrane.

FDP-I Base of distal phalanges after passing through the split in the tendon of *FDS* (fig. 23.42).

Pronator quadratus (PQ)

PQ-O Distal part of anterior surface of ulna.

PQ-I Distal part of anterior and medial surfaces of radius.

Supinator (S)

S-O₁ Superficial humeral attachments: lateral epicondyle of humerus, radial collateral ligament, anular ligament.

S-O₂ Deep ulnar attachment: supinator fossa and crest of ulna.

S-I Round the upper third of shaft of radius.

Extensor indicis (EI)

EI-O Back of lower part of ulna and adjoining interosseous membrane.

EI-I Extensor insertion of index finger (see *ED*).

Abductor pollicis longus (APL)

APL-O Posterior surface of radius, posterior and lateral surface of ulna, intervening interosseous membrane.

APL-I Base of first metacarpal.

Extensor pollicis longus (EPL)

EPL-O Middle third of posterior surface of ulna and adjoining interosseous membrane.

EPL-I Base of distal phalanx of thumb.

Extensor pollicis brevis (EPB)

EPB-O Posterior surface of radius and adjoining interosseous membrane.

EPB-I Base of proximal phalanx of thumb.

digitorum (fig. 23.42), extensor indicis (fig. 23.43) and extensor digiti minimi (fig. 23.42);

(2) on the thumb, are flexor pollicis longus, extensor pollicis longus, extensor pollicis brevis and abductor pollicis longus (fig. 23.43).

The intrinsic muscles of the fingers are palmar and dorsal interossei, lumbricals (fig. 23.44), and hypothenar

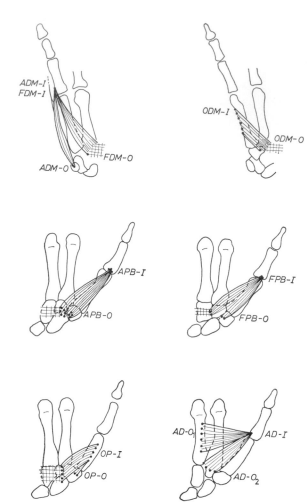

FIG. 23.45. Muscles of thumb and little finger.

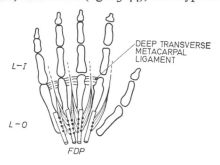

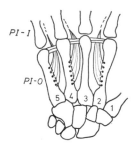

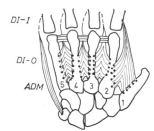

FIG. 23.44. Intrinsic muscles of the fingers.

Lumbrical muscles (*L*) of the right hand.

L-O Tendons of flexor digitorum profundus (*FDP*, fig. 23.43).

L-I Distal wings of extensor expansion.

Palmar interossei muscles (*PI*)

PI-O Palmar aspect of second, fourth and fifth meta-carpal shafts.

PI-I Almost all fibres inserted into the distal wings of the extensor expansion (like lumbricals).

Dorsal interossei muscles (*DI*)

DI-O Adjacent sides of two metacarpal bones. Abductor digiti minimi (ADM) completes the series.

DI-I Considerable variation as distal attachment is divided in variable amounts between: base of proximal phalanx, proximal and distal wings of extensor expansion.

muscles, i.e. flexor digiti minimi brevis, abductor digiti minimi and opponens digiti minimi (fig. 23.45). Intrinsic muscles of the thumb are the thenar muscles, i.e. flexor pollicis brevis, abductor pollicis brevis, opponens pollicis and adductor pollicis (fig. 23.45). The first dorsal interosseus muscle is included since it also stabilizes and adducts the thumb.

MOVEMENTS AT THE WRIST

The radiocarpal and midcarpal joints are one functional unit and flexion, extension, abduction, adduction and

Abductor digiti minimi (*ADM*).

ADM-O Pisiform bone.
ADM-I Base of proximal phalanx.

Flexor digiti minimi brevis (*FDM*)

FDM-O Flexor retinaculum and hook of hamate.
FDM-I Base of proximal phalanx of little finger.

Opponens digiti minimi (*ODM*)

ODM-O Flexor retinaculum, hook of hamate.
ODM-I Medial aspect of fifth metacarpal.

Abductor pollicis brevis (*APB*)

APB-O Flexor retinaculum, scaphoid, trapezium.
APB-I Radial side of proximal phalanx of thumb.

Flexor pollicis brevis (*FPB*)

FPB-O Flexor retinaculum and trapezium.
FPB-I Radial side of base of proximal phalanx.

Opponens pollicis (*OP*)

OP-O Flexor retinaculum and trapezium.
OP-I Whole length of radial aspect of first metacarpal.

Adductor pollicis (*AD*)

AD-O$_1$ Front of third metacarpal.
AD-O$_2$ Front of carpus and bases of metacarpal bones.
AD-I Ulnar side of base of proximal phalanx.

circumduction can take place there. The muscles mainly concerned are the radial and ulnar flexor and extensors of the carpus, abduction being performed by a combination of radial flexors and extensors and adduction by the ulnar groups of the corresponding muscles. Abduction, which occurs mostly in the midcarpal joint, is assisted by abductor pollicis longus and extensors pollicis longus and brevis. Flexion, occurring mostly in the midcarpal joint, is assisted by palmaris longus, long flexors of the digits and abductor pollicis longus. Extension, which occurs mostly in the radiocarpal joint, is assisted by the digital extensors. The extensors of the carpus act as synergists during flexion of the digits as they fix the wrist in an extended position. Lack of this synergistic action is obvious when gripping with the fingers when the wrist is markedly flexed.

MOVEMENTS OF THE HAND

All movements in the upper limb as far as the wrist obviously serve to position the business end of the limb, the hand. The movements of the hand can be arbitrarily divided into **non-prehensile**, e.g. pushing, hitting with the flat hand, karate, swimming, and **prehensile**, e.g. movements concerned with seizing and gripping. The hand is not a rigidly specialized tool and its versatility is shown by its uses as a chuck, pliers, hook and ring (fig. 23.46).

These prehensile functions of the hand are effected by (1) *opposition*, in which the pulp of the thumb is brought into contact with the pulp of any of the other digits (fig. 23.47a), (2) *power grip*, in which the object is clamped against the palm, all digital joints being involved (fig. 23.47b), (3) *precision grip*, in which the object is held by the opposing surfaces of the digits, mainly by movement at the MP joints (fig. 23.47c), and (4) *key grip* or lateral pinch grip (fig. 23.47d).

Fine movements of the individual digits are controlled mostly by the intrinsic muscles of the hand, and are used in activities such as piano playing and typing.

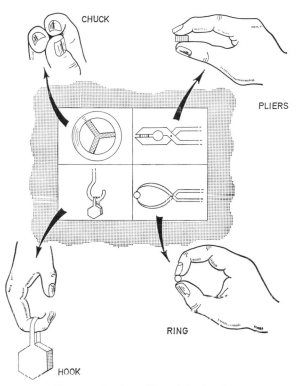

FIG. 23.46. Versatility of the hand.

For these various functions it is necessary for the bones and joints to be assembled and functioning normally and for their movements to be coordinated accurately by contraction, relaxation and fixation of the appropriate muscles. The hand is represented in the central nervous system by large motor and sensory areas.

Each type of tissue in the hand makes a special contribution to all these functions.

Skin

Without its normal mobile skin cover the hand would be absolutely useless. The blanching of the knuckles when

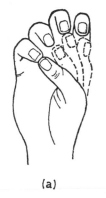

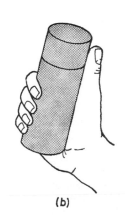

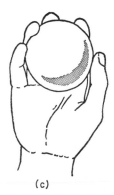

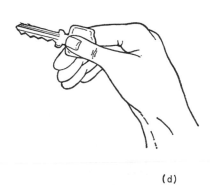

(a) (b) (c) (d)

FIG. 23.47. (a) Opposition, (b) power grip, (c) precision grip and (d) key grip.

making a fist shows that the hand is covered with just a sufficient area of skin. Palmar skin has a thick epidermis and is fixed by strong anteroposterior fibres to the deep palmar fascia (fig. 23.49); this stabilizes it on the underlying tissues for gripping. The papillary ridges on the palm increase its surface friction. In contrast the mobile skin of the dorsum allows for flexion and prehension. Any loss or contracture of the skin of the hand is disabling, particularly so over the pulp of the digits where there is a special concentration of the sensory end organs. Grafting skin cover for the pulp is of limited value, unless

it is transferred from the pulp of another digit with its blood and nerve supply.

Superficial and deep layers of the connective tissue of the hand

SUPERFICIAL FASCIA

The superficial fascia of the palmar aspect of the hand is a layer of fatty and areolar tissue arranged like sponge rubber in the spaces of a network of collagen fibres which connect the skin to the deep fascia (fig. 23.49). This serves

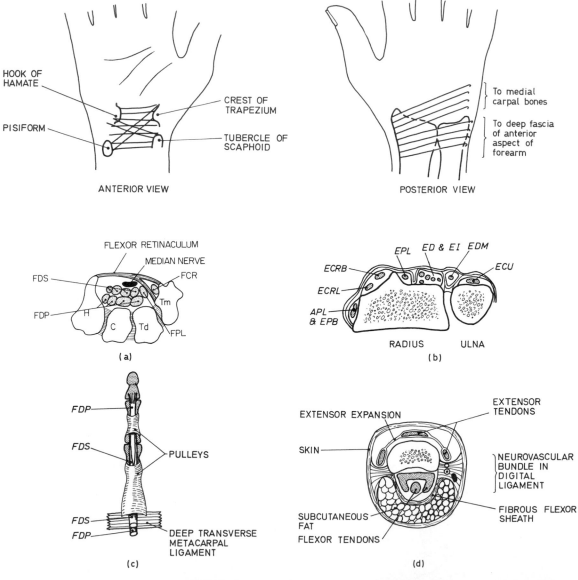

FIG. 23.48. Retaining structures in the hand. (a) Flexor retinaculum, (b) extensor retinaculum, (c) fibrous flexor sheath, (d) transverse section of the finger showing digital ligaments. *APL*, Abductor pollicis longus; *ECRB*, Extensor carpi radialis brevis; *ECRL*, Extensor carpi radialis longus; *ECU*, Extensor carpi ulnaris; *ED*, Extensor digitorum; *EDM*, Extensor digiti minimi; *EI*, Extensor indicis; *EPB*, Extensor pollicis brevis; *EPL*, Extensor pollicis longus; *FCR*, Flexor carpi radialis; *FDP*, Flexor digitorum profundus; *FDS*, Flexor digitorum superficialis (sublimis); *FPL*, Flexor pollicis longus.

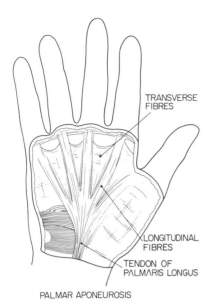

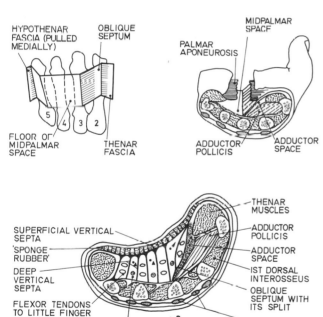

FIG. 23.49. Arrangement of the superficial and deep fascia of the hand.

as an elastic protective cushion taking the brunt of the pressure in the palm associated with the power grip. The superficial fascia on the dorsal aspect is much thinner and stretches easily.

DEEP FASCIA
The deep fascia of the hand is arranged in a specific manner for retention and gliding.

Retention
If tendons were not retained in position during grasping, they would bowstring across the hollow of the palm; this is prevented in five ways.

The **flexor retinaculum** is attached to the bones of the carpus and stretches over the transverse arch of the carpus, so forming the **carpal tunnel**, which contains nine long flexor tendons and the median nerve (fig. 23.48a).

The **palmar aponeurosis** is found in front of the tendons in the palm (fig. 23.49). It consists of two layers fused together, the superficial one being a continuation of the tendon of the palmaris longus and the deep layer continuous with the distal edge of the flexor retinaculum. The palmar aponeurosis is continuous on each side with the much thinner deep fascia covering the thenar and hypothenar groups of muscles. The palmar aponeurosis is anchored to the skin by superficial anteroposterior fibres, and to the deep metacarpal and interosseous fasciae by the deep anteroposterior fibres which form septa in the distal part of the central palm. These septa lie on each side of the long tendons and of the neurovascular bundles and lumbrical muscles. One of these deep septa extends from the shaft of the third metacarpal to the radial border of the palmar aponeurosis at its junction with the thenar part of the deep fascia. This is known as the **oblique septum**, and it is separated from the anterior surface of the adductor pollicis by a space filled with loose areolar tissue. This is the **adductor** or **thenar space**. On the medial side of the oblique septum is the **mid-palmar space** extending deep to the palmar aponeurosis as far as the hypothenar muscles. It is filled with loose areolar and fatty padding arranged around the structures and between the deep septa which separate them. The distal edge of the palmar aponeurosis divides over the level of the metacarpal heads into four slips, each of which in turn splits into three bands; a central one is continuous along the palmar aspect of the finger with the fibrous flexor sheath and one on each side is attached to the deep transverse ligament of palm.

The **fibrous flexor sheath** is attached to the sides of the proximal and middle phalanges and to the base of the distal phalanx (fig. 23.48c). It is thin over the joints and rigid opposite the shafts of the phalanges. This arrangement provides an osteofascial tunnel for the flexor tendons and prevents bowstringing in the fingers. The thumb has its own fibrous sheath attached to the sides of the proximal phalanx and to the base of the distal phalanx.

The **extensor retinaculum** is simpler as the fingers cannot be extended much beyond the straight line. An extensor retinaculum is attached laterally to the distal part of the anterior border of radius and medially to the medial carpal bones, sending an extension round the distal end of the ulna to blend with the deep fascia on the palmar aspect of the lower part of the forearm (fig. 23.48b). The septa, which extend from the retinaculum to the bony points lying deep to it, form separate compartments for the tendons.

The **digital ligaments** are sheets of connective tissue extending from the sides of the phalanges to the skin, and which contain the neurovascular bundles of the digits (fig. 23.48d).

Gliding

The sliding movements of the tendons are facilitated by the loose surrounding connective tissue, which forms a paratenon, when more or less straight line movement occurs (fig. 23.50a). Where a tendon slides round a corner or a bend the paratenon is replaced by a synovial sheath formed by substitution of the middle areolar layer of the paratenon by a space filled with a film of synovial fluid (fig. 23.50a). The position of the synovial sheaths of flexor and extensor tendons is shown in fig. 23.50b. Obviously some areas have tough and unyielding walls surrounding the tendons, e.g. fibrous flexor sheaths of the digits, carpal tunnel (fig. 23.50c) where the fit of the tendon is very tight and there is hardly any surrounding loose areolar tissue. In other areas, like the palm, the tendons move in much softer, looser spaces.

Assembly of the skeletal elements of the hand

Although the forces created in the hand during its movements are transmitted along multiple lines and surfaces, a general account of the **arches of the hand** is useful for a clear picture of its functions and their disturbances. The following arches (fig. 23.51a) can be recognized:

(1) the transverse carpal arch which is fixed and rigid,

(2) the transverse metacarpal arch traversing the metacarpal heads, the second and third of which are fixed, the first, fourth and fifth being mobile.

(3) the longitudinal metacarpal arch formed by the fixed concavity of the metacarpal shaft, and

(4) the longitudinal metacarpophalangeal and digital arch, which is mobile and continuous with the longitudinal metacarpal arch.

These arches are maintained by fibrous and muscular elements and differ considerably in the degree of their mobility. The principal **fixed axis of the hand** is continuous with the radius through the fixed carpal arch and consists of the second and third metacarpal bones, which are fixed and positioned for function by synergistic action of the radial extensor and flexor muscles of the carpus. Around the principal axis the mobile elements can be moved into many positions. These mobile elements (fig. 23.51b) are composed of,

(1) the thumb which possesses the greatest mobility,

(2) the index finger which possesses considerable independence from the other fingers, and

(3) the middle, ring and little fingers with the two medial metacarpal bones.

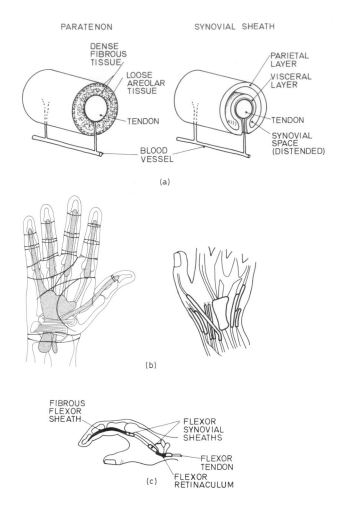

FIG. 23.50. Gliding mechanisms in the hand. (a) Paratenon and synovial sheath; (b) palmar and dorsal synovial sheaths; (c) arrangement of connective tissue around a flexor tendon. Palmar in (b) modified from Wood Jones.

Action of the muscles in the movements of the hand

Appropriate positioning of the mobile elements of the hand around its fixed axis is carried out by the integrated action of many muscles through their complicated attachments. Stressing the action of a single muscle is an oversimplification; the functional balance of all the other elements must be considered.

Before the actions of the muscles are described it is useful to consider the posture of the hand at rest. This can be seen in one's own hand. There is a moderate degree of dorsiflexion of the wrist with slight ulnar deviation. From index to little finger, there is a gradual increase in the flexion of the MP and IP joints of the fingers, and the pulp of the thumb is near the radial aspect of the DIP joint of the index.

MOVEMENTS OF THE THUMB

The functional value of the thumb is about half that of the whole hand. The notable feature is a wide range of

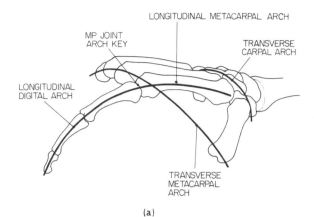

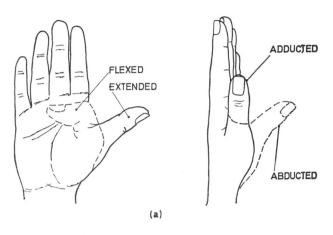

(a)

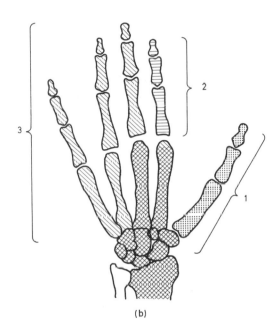

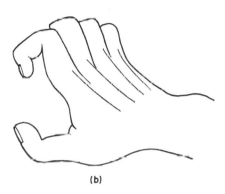

(b)

FIG. 23.52. (a) Movements of the thumb, (b) position of claw hand, the MP joints are hyperextended and the IP joints are flexed.

FIG. 23.51. Assembly of the skeletal elements of the hand. (a) Arches, (b) mobile elements (see text).

movement at the carpometacarpal joint. The movements (fig. 23.52a) are as follows.

Abduction: abductor pollicis brevis assisted by abductor pollicis longus.

Adduction: adductor pollicis.

Flexion: flexor pollicis brevis, flexor pollicis longus, opponens and abductor pollicis brevis.

Extension: extensor pollicis longus and brevis, assisted by abductor pollicis longus.

Medial rotation: opponens pollicis.

Lateral rotation: extensor muscles of the thumb.

Extension occurs together with lateral rotation, and flexion with medial rotation, as in the movement of **opposition**. The association of these movements is de-

termined by the configuration of the articular surfaces of the carpometacarpal joint of the thumb.

The muscles of the thenar compartment act, like stay ropes on a mast, in positioning and stabilizing the thumb; they bring the thumb away from the rest of the hand in readiness for gripping and pinching. In all these movements, the ability to oppose is most important. The thumb is brought into the starting position, i.e. abduction, and from there on, the composite **movement of opposition** consists of some flexion, adduction and medial rotation of the thumb. This brings the most important sensory areas of the hand, i.e. the pulp of the digits, into functional contact (fig. 23.47a). The mobile transverse metacarpal arch is produced by the thenar and hypothenar muscles. The arch is deepened and the integrated action of the long flexors, extensors and intrinsic muscles of the digits completes the opposition.

MOVEMENTS OF THE FINGERS

The normal longitudinal arch of the digit, which is so important in the final stages of opposition, is necessary for small object prehension and for the power grip. For the same reason the arch is balanced in favour of flexion (fig. 23.51a). The arch is maintained by four factors:

(1) shape of bones, i.e. concavity of palmar aspects of metacarpals and phalanges,

(2) arrangements of joints, i.e. articular surfaces present on the palmar aspects of the heads of bones,

(3) palmar structures at the IP joints and the fibrous sheaths prevent hyperextension,

(4) muscles.

A finger controlled only by long flexors and extensors cannot be kept in equilibrium. Such a finger assumes the position of clawing, with hyperextension at the MP and flexion at the IP joints (fig. 23.52b). Normally this deformity is prevented by the action of the intrinsic muscles which flex at the MP and extend at the IP joints. When these intrinsic muscles are put out of action, for instance in ulnar nerve paralysis, the 'clawed hand' is produced. The normal longitudinal arch of the finger ray therefore depends on three muscular elements, long flexors, long extensors and intrinsic muscles. The distal insertions of the long flexors have already been given. The other two require more consideration.

The extensor and intrinsic components are applied through the complicated mechanism of the **extensor expansion.** This lies in a shallow connective tissue bed, gliding immediately beneath the skin and closely related to the bones and joints of the fingers, and is therefore vulnerable. It can be visualized as a plexiform arrangement of bands and flat thin membranes sandwiched between two thin layers of connective tissue (fig. 23.53a) in which it can slide not only longitudinally but also transversely, changing the position of one band in relation to the others and also to the axes of the joints over which they act.

Extensor extrinsic component (fig. 23.53b)

The long extensor tendon at the MP level divides into three bands. Its direct continuation proceeds along the dorsum of the proximal phalanx, while the transverse (shroud) fibres embedded in the proximal edge of the hood of the extensor expansion, encircle the metacarpal head to fuse with the deep tranverse ligament of the palm. This attachment of the long extensor limits its proximal retraction. The main portion of the tendon gives a slip, variable and very often absent, to the dorsum of the base of the proximal phalanx and then continues towards the PIP joint. Before reaching it, the tendon divides into three terminal bands. A central one is attached to the base of the middle phalanx. Two lateral bands, which at first lie in the grooves over the lateral part of the dorsum of the PIP joint, converge to be attached to the base of the distal phalanx. All these elements of the extrinsic component are bound together by oblique and transverse

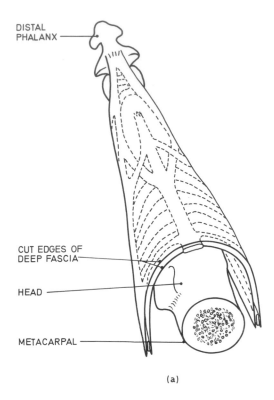

(a)

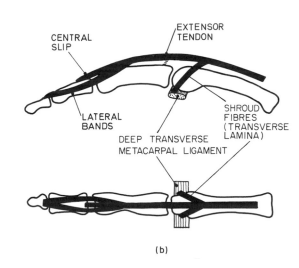

(b)

FIG. 23.53. (a) Dorsal expansion, (b) extensor extrinsic component.

fibres embedded in the flat triangular extension expansion with its hood, and proximal and distal wings (fig. 23.54c).

Intrinsic component (fig. 23.54a)

Although the **interossei muscles** are posterior to the deep transverse ligament of the palm, they lie anterior to the axis of flexion at the MP joint and so flex this joint.

The dorsal and palmar interossei both send most of their insertions into the extensor expansion, contributing, with the lumbricals, to its proximal and distal wings. They therefore extend the IP joints (fig. 23.54b). Four dorsal interossei, together with abductor pollicis brevis and abductor digiti minimi, are strong digital abductors from the axial line of the third digit, while palmar interossei are concerned with adduction towards this line (fig. 23.44).

The line of pull of each **lumbrical muscle** lies palmar to the axis of the MP joint and dorsal to the axes of the IP joints. The lumbricals therefore assist in flexing the MP joint and in extending the IP joints. They also serve as an adjustable, contractile link between the flexor and extensor systems of the fingers where their muscle spindles can function as an important nervous feed back mechanism.

Fig. 23.54b shows the combined extrinsic and intrinsic components of the extensor expansion.

Before the function of the dorsal apparatus is discussed, the **link** or **retinacular ligament** should be considered. This is a strong fibrous band extending from the palmar aspect of the fibrous flexor sheath and the adjoining bone; it passes obliquely on the palmar side of the axis of the PIP joint towards the dorsum of the finger, joining the lateral band of the dorsal expansion, dorsal to the DIP joint axis. The mechanical effect of this ligament can be seen when passively flexing the DIP joint; this causes the ligament to become taut and forces the PIP joint into flexion simultaneously and automatically (fig. 23.55a and observe on your own finger). If now the PIP joint is passively extended, the DIP joint is brought into extension as well. With this link it might be thought unnecessary to have muscles for active extension of the DIP joint, since this would be automatically accomplished by the extensor muscles of the PIP joint. However, passive extension of the DIP joint by the retinacular ligament is not complete and some active force is necessary to complete it.

When measured along the dorsum, the finger is about 2·5 cm longer in flexion than in extension. This is because of the palmar projection of the heads of the metacarpals and phalanges. Obviously this feature augments the effect of the retinacular ligament during flexion, but diminishes it when the flexed finger is extended. Complete extension at the DIP joints is due to the tension in the terminal parts of the lateral bands and follows the contraction of the muscles attached to the distal wings of the extensor expansion. This contraction relaxes the central band so that the force (A–B, fig. 23.55b) of the long extensor is transferred to the lateral bands to act on the DIP joint and complete its full extension. This resembles a servo mechanism, since the force from the long extensor has its point of application changed from the PIP to the DIP joint by the contraction of the muscles attached to the distal wings of the extensor expansion.

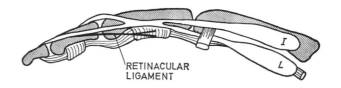

RETINACULAR
LIGAMENT

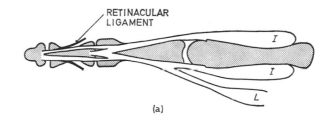

RETINACULAR
LIGAMENT

(a)

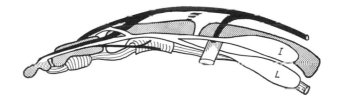

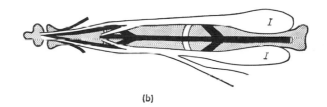

(b)

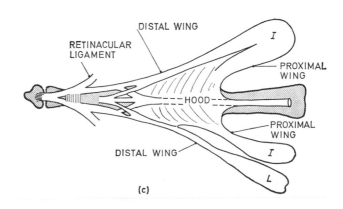

DISTAL WING

RETINACULAR
LIGAMENT

PROXIMAL
WING

HOOD

PROXIMAL
WING

DISTAL WING

(c)

FIG. 23.54. (a) Intrinsic component, (b) combined extrinsic and intrinsic components, (c) the extensor expansion spread out flat. *L*, Lumbrical; *I*, Interosseous muscle.

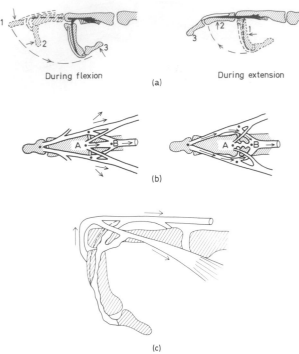

During flexion   (a)   During extension

(b)

(c)

FIG. 23.55. Mechanism of extension of the interphalangeal joints (see text).

When extending the fully flexed finger, contraction of the long extensor tendon extends the MP joint; it is also involved in the extension of the IP joints by a more complex mechanism. In the fully flexed position of the PIP joint the distal wings and lateral bands of the extensor expansion lie on the sides of the head of the proximal phalanx (fig. 23.55c). In these circumstances the pull of the extensor muscles is applied to the central slip and extends the middle phalanx at the PIP joint, and not to the lateral bands which in the flexed PIP joint are relaxed as they lie along the short cut, i.e. in the line of the shortest distance to the base of the distal phalanx. Any further pull on the lateral bands in this position shifts them more towards the palm and makes them less able to extend the DIP joint. Thus the pull on the central fibres extends only the PIP joint, but as a result of this extension the retinacular ligament partially extends the DIP joint. After extension of the PIP joint, the lateral bands have moved dorsally and the distal wing muscles now pull on them to cause the active final extension of the DIP joint.

In summary, the normal phalangeal movements are co-ordinated by the retinacular ligament, while the MP joint moves independently, being extended by extensor digitorum, extensor digiti minimi and extensor indicis, and flexed by the long flexors and intrinsic muscles.

Electromyographic studies and clinical observation show that the flexor digitorum profundus is very important in flexion of both IP joints, and it assists the intrinsic

muscles in flexion of the MP joint. Flexor digitorum superficialis is less important, coming into action when additional power is required.

FASCIAE OF THE UPPER LIMB

Superficial **fascia of the pectoral region** contains fat in which the breast is embedded. Deep fascia is attached above to the clavicle and medially to the sternum. It invests the pectoralis major muscle and is continuous below with the fascia of the abdominal wall. Beyond the inferolateral border of this muscle it is thickened to form the floor of the armpit. This **axillary fascia** is continued posteriorly on to the posterior fold of the armpit and laterally joins the deep fascial sleeve of the upper arm. Deep to the pectoralis major muscle another layer of connective tissue invests the pectoralis minor muscle. From the superomedial border of the muscle this deep connective tissue, called here the **clavipectoral fascia** (fig. 23.56), extends upwards and is attached to the inferior surface of the clavicle, where it splits to enclose the subclavius muscle. Medially the clavipectoral fascia is attached to the first costal cartilage, laterally to the coracoid process and coracoclavicular ligament. Below the pectoralis minor muscle, a continuation of this fascia passes down to join the axillary fascia and is called the **suspensory ligament of the axilla.**

The deep **fascia of the upper arm** is arranged as a strong tubular investment for the muscles. It is continuous above with the deep fascia of the shoulder and with the axillary fascia; below it is attached to the olecranon and the epicondyles of the humerus and becomes continuous with

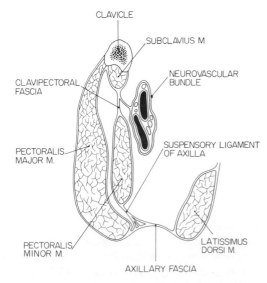

FIG. 23.56. Almost sagittal section through the axilla showing the arrangement of the deep fascia.

the deep fascia of the forearm. Two intermuscular septa extend from this sleeve to the supracondylar ridges of the humerus. The medial one, which is stronger, provides origin for the medial head of the triceps posteriorly, and for the brachialis anteriorly. The lateral septum provides origin for the medial and lateral heads of the triceps posteriorly. and for the brachialis and brachioradialis anteriorly.

The superficial **fascia in the forearm** does not present any special features, but in the hand is modified as already described (p. 23.23). A small muscle, palmaris brevis, is found in the deep layer of the superficial fascia. It extends from the medial border of the flexor retinaculum and palmar aponeurosis to the skin of the medial border of the hand. It deepens the hollow of the hand.

The deep aspect of the deep fascia provides an extensive area for the attachment of the muscles and plays an important part in the return of fluid from the upper limb by providing tough walls for the muscular compartments in which active muscle contraction can exert pressure on the venous and lymphatic channels. Being relatively impervious to fluid, the deep fascia determines the location and spread of extravasated fluids and inflammatory processes.

The muscles and the deep fascia of the upper limb form the boundaries of three important regions.

The **axilla** is the space between the upper arm and the chest wall. The narrow **cervicoaxillary canal**, at the apex of the axilla, accommodates the main nerves and vessels of the upper limb. It is bounded in front by the middle portion of the clavicle, medially by the outer border of the first rib and posteriorly by the superior border of the scapula (fig. 23.2). The anterior wall of the axilla is composed of two layers, the pectoralis major muscle and posterior to this, from above downwards, the subclavius muscle, clavipectoral fascia, pectoralis minor muscle, and the suspensory ligament of the axilla (fig. 23.56). Medially, lies the chest wall covered by the serratus anterior muscle. The posterior wall of the axilla is formed by subscapularis, latissimus dorsi and teres major muscles, while laterally the biceps and coracobrachialis muscles separate the axilla from the intertubercular groove. The floor of the space is formed by the axillary fascia which is held up by the suspensory ligament of axilla. The **axillary sheath** is the continuation of the deep cervical fascia which is drawn into the axilla through its apex around the main neurovascular bundle. Distally it fuses with the connective tissue coats of the bundle. The axilla contains the axillary vessels, lower part of the brachial plexus, its branches and numerous lymph nodes and vessels, all set in areolar tissue and fat.

The **cubital fossa** is a triangular hollow in front of the elbow. It is covered by skin, superficial and deep fascia which includes the **bicipital aponeurosis**, a flat fibrous band extending down and medially from the bicipital

tendon to blend with the deep fascia of the forearm. The floor of the fossa consists of two muscles, brachialis and supinator. It contains the brachial, radial and ulnar vessels, tendon of biceps and median nerve (fig. 23.57).

The **anatomical snuff box** lies on the lateral aspect of the wrist; it is bounded in front by the tendons of the long

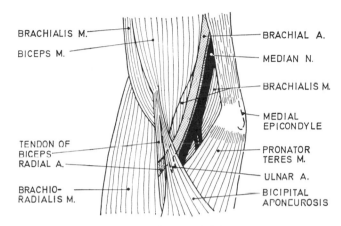

FIG. 23.57. Right cubital fossa.

abductor and short extensor of the thumb, posteriorly by the tendon of the long extensor of the thumb. In its floor the tip of the radial styloid, scaphoid and trapezium, are spanned by the lateral ligament of the wrist. The radial artery crosses this ligament in the floor of the snuff box.

NERVES OF THE UPPER LIMB

Almost all of the upper limb is supplied by the ventral rami of the fifth, sixth, seventh, eighth cervical and the first thoracic nerves which form the brachial plexus. The fifth cervical usually receives a contribution to the plexus from the fourth cervical, and the second thoracic may send fibres to join the first thoracic. There is some variation in the position of the plexus; it may be **prefixed**, i.e. when the fourth cervical contribution is large and the thoracic segment contributions small or absent. In a **postfixed plexus** the second thoracic contribution is large while the fourth cervical does not contribute and only a few fibres come from the fifth cervical.

The second thoracic always contributes to the cutaneous supply of the upper limb, not through the brachial plexus, but by an independent intercostobrachial nerve which crosses the axilla to reach the arm. The lateral supraclavicular nerves from the third and fourth cervical ventral rami supply part of the skin of the shoulder region. The skin over the upper part of the scapula is supplied from the ventral rami of the third and fourth cervical nerves

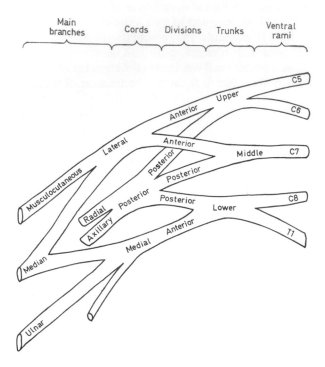

FIG. 23.58. General plan of the brachial plexus. From Romanes G.J. ed. (1964) *Cunningham's Textbook of Anatomy*, 10th Edition. London: Oxford University Press.

while that of the lower part is supplied from the cutaneous branches of the dorsal rami of the upper thoracic nerves.

Two muscles acting on the upper limb do not receive their nerve supply through the brachial plexus; trapezius is supplied from the spinal part of the accessory nerve and from the ventral rami of the third and fourth cervical nerves, and levator scapulae, which is supplied by the same cervical nerves, often also receives a branch from the plexus through the dorsal scapular nerve. The pathways of the **brachial plexus** are contained in its roots (ventral rami), trunks, divisions and cords (fig. 23.58) and they follow a complicated course through the plexus. The cords finally divide into the main nerves of the upper limb. Before that, however, branches are given off to the upper limb from the plexus itself. These are the long thoracic nerve which supplies serratus anterior, nerve to subclavius, suprascapular nerve, and dorsal scapular nerve which supplies the rhomboid muscles (fig. 23.59).

The roots and trunks are found in the neck above the clavicle, while the divisions and cords are in the axilla. The divisions lie posterior to the clavicle and the cords, with the commencement of the main nerves of the upper limb, lie below the clavicle.

The **three cords of the brachial plexus** are named **lateral, medial** and **posterior,** from their relationship to

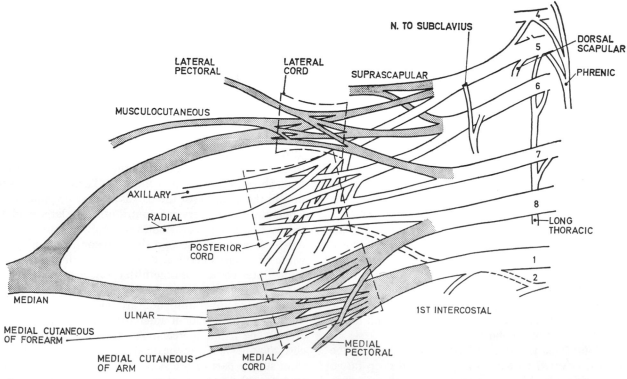

FIG. 23.59. Diagram of brachial plexus, showing the origin of its branches. Dorsal divisions are clear and ventral divisions stippled (Cf. fig. 24.48). From *Cunningham's Textbook of Anatomy*, 10th Edition.

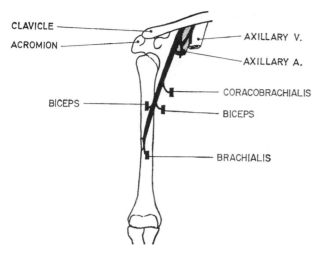

FIG. 23.60. Diagram of the musculocutaneous nerve and the muscles which it supplies. Modified from Pitres and Testut.

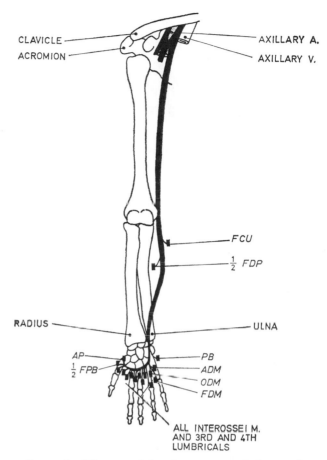

FIG. 23.62. Diagram of the ulnar nerve and the muscles which it supplies. Modified from Pitres and Testut. All interosseous muscles are supplied by the deep branch of the ulnar nerve. *AP*, Adductor pollicis; *FPB*, Flexor pollicis brevis; *FCU*, Flexor carpi ulnaris; *FDP*, Flexor digitorum profundus; *PB*, Palmaris brevis; *ADM*, Abductor digiti minimi; *ODM*, Opponens digiti minimi; *FDM*, Flexor digiti minimi.

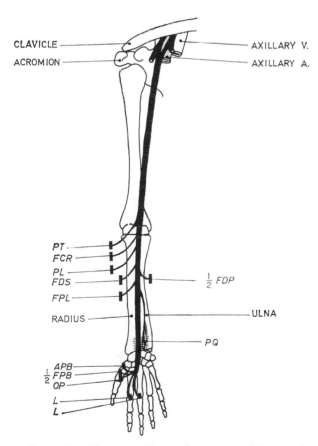

FIG. 23.61. Diagram of the median nerve and the muscles which it supplies. Modified from Pitres and Testut. *PT*, Pronator teres; *FCR*, Flexor carpi radialis; *FDP*, Flexor digitorum profundus; *PL*, Palmaris longus; *FDS*, Flexor digitorum superficialis; *FPL*, Flexor pollicis longus; *APB*, Abductor pollicis brevis; *PQ*, Pronator quadratus; *FPB*, Flexor pollicis brevis; *OP*, Opponens pollicis; *L*, lumbricals.

the axillary artery. In general, branches of the posterior cord are distributed to muscles of the posterior wall of the axilla, and of the posterior (extensor) compartments of the arm and forearm, while the lateral and medial cords are distributed to the anterior (flexor) region of the limb.

Lateral cord gives off the lateral pectoral, musculocutaneous and lateral root of the median.

Medial cord gives off the medial pectoral, medial root of the median, ulnar, medial cutaneous nerve of the arm and medial cutaneous nerve of the forearm.

Posterior cord gives off the radial, axillary, upper and lower subscapular and thoracodorsal which supplies latissimus dorsi.

The **lateral pectoral nerve** supplies the pectoralis major muscle, while the **medial pectoral nerve** supplies both pectoralis major and minor muscles.

The **musculocutaneous nerve** ($C5, 6, 7$) pierces the coraco-

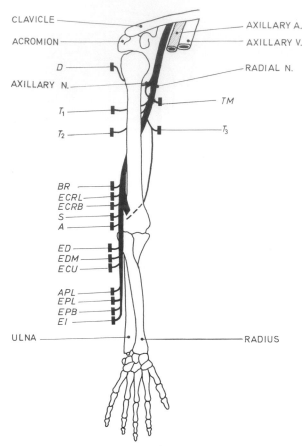

Fig. 23.63. Diagram of the axillary and radial nerves and the muscles which they supply. Modified from Pitres and Testut. *D*, Deltoid; *T*, Triceps; *BR*, Brachioradialis; *ECRL*, Extensor carpi radialis longus; *ECRB*, Extensor carpi radialis brevis; *S*, Supinator; *A*, Anconeus; *ED*, Extensor digitorum; *EDM*, Extensor digiti minimi; *ECU*, Extensor carpi ulnaris; *APL*, Abductor pollicis longus; *EPL*, Extensor pollicis longus; *EPB*, Extensor pollicis brevis; EI, Extensor indicis; *TM*, Teres minor.

brachialis muscle to supply the muscles shown in fig. 23.60. Its sensory terminal part pierces the deep fascial sleeve, just above the elbow, to become the lateral cutaneous nerve of the forearm (fig. 23.64).

The **median nerve** (C5, 6, 7, 8, T1) is formed from its lateral and medial roots; these usually join in the axilla, but may join lower. The median nerve runs with the

brachial artery, passes in the forearm between the superficial and deep muscles and traverses the carpal tunnel (fig. 23.48a) to end in the hand. Its muscular branches are shown in fig. 23.61. The anterior interosseous nerve arises from the median nerve at the upper part of the forearm and runs downwards in front of the interosseous membrane, contributing to the supply of the flexor pollicis longus and the lateral half of the flexor digitorum profundus, and supplying pronator quadratus muscle. The cutaneous distribution of the median nerve is represented on fig. 23.64.

The **ulnar nerve** (C8, T1) often receives a contribution from C7 either through the lateral cord or through the lateral root of the median nerve. It follows the course of the axillary and brachial arteries as far down as the middle of the upper arm, where it deviates from the artery by piercing the medial intermuscular septum. Then it lies posterior to the medial epicondyle, before passing medial to the elbow joint, to descend on the medial side of the forearm, between the superficial and deep muscles, to supply the hand. It crosses in front of the flexor retinaculum and divides into its two terminal branches, superficial and deep. Its muscular branches are shown in fig. 23.62 and the cutaneous distribution in fig. 23.64.

The **medial cutaneous nerves** of the arm (T1) and forearm (C8, T1), are distributed as shown in fig. 23.64.

The **axillary nerve** (C5, 6) leaves the axilla together with the posterior circumflex humeral artery inferior to the shoulder joint and divides into anterior and posterior branches, both of which pass across the back of the upper end of the humerus. Its muscular branches are shown in fig. 23.63 and the cutaneous distribution in fig. 23.64.

The **radial nerve** [(C5) C6, 7, 8 (T1)] extends from the axilla round the posterior aspect of the shaft of the humerus to the front of the lateral epicondyle just above the elbow joint, where it ends by dividing into its superficial and deep terminal branches. The muscular branches of the trunk of the radial nerve and of its deep branch are shown in fig. 23.63. The cutaneous distribution of both the trunk and its superficial terminal branch is shown in fig. 23.64.

The **thoracodorsal nerve** (C6, 7, 8) supplies the latissimus dorsi. The **subscapular nerves** (C5, 6). The upper

TABLE 23.1. Root innervation of movements.

Shoulder		Elbow		Forearm		Wrist		Fingers (long muscles)		Hand
Abduction Lateral rotation	C5	Flexion	C5, 6	Pronation	C6	Flexion	C6, 7	Flexion	C7, 8	Movements effected by intrinsic muscles T1
Adduction Medial rotation	C6, 7(8)	Extension	C7, 8	Supination	C6	Extension	C6, 7	Extension	C7, 8	

supplies the subscapular muscle, the lower supplies the lateral part of the same muscle and the teres major.

Cutaneous innervation of the upper limb is shown in fig. 23.64 and the areas of dermatomes in fig. 23.66.

Innervation of the joints of the upper limb is derived from the adjoining nerves:

(1) sternoclavicular joint by the medial supraclavicular,

(2) acromioclavicular and shoulder joints by the lateral pectoral, suprascapular and axillary,

(3) elbow joints by musculocutaneous, median, ulnar and radial.

(4) superior radio-ulnar joint by anterior interosseous and deep branch of radial,

(5) radiocarpal, midcarpal and carpometacarpal joints by the anterior interosseous, deep branch of radial and ulnar,

(6) metacarpophalangeal and interphalangeal joints by the digital branches of the median and ulnar.

The nervous control of movements at the particular joints as effected by the roots of the brachial plexus is shown in table 23.1.

Nerve supply of the hand

The **cutaneous** distribution and important variations are shown in fig. 23.65. The afferent impulses are of great importance for sensory feedback, from the skin, joints and muscles, and for protection against injury. The sensory function of the hand can be classified as:

(1) informative of position, size, shape, weight, etc. of objects,

(2) 'grip sight' for fine sensory appreciation and tactile discrimination both in precision and power grip,

(3) protective.

The **muscular** branches to the intrinsic muscles of the hand are all derived from the ventral ramus of the first thoracic nerve. They are distributed through the ulnar and median nerves; the median supplies the thenar muscles, except adductor pollicis, and two lateral lumbricals, while the ulnar supplies the rest. An important variation is the nerve supply to the flexor pollicis brevis which is usually double, from median and ulnar, but may be only from the ulnar.

The functional deficit caused by interruption of the

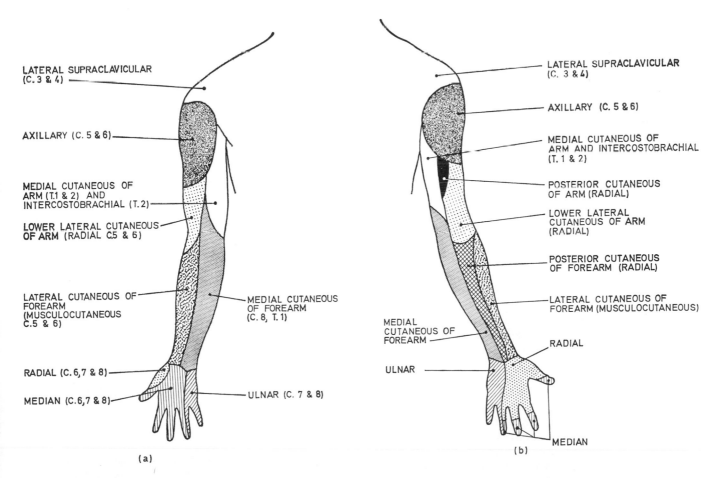

FIG. 23.64. Distribution of cutaneous nerves. (a) on the front; (b) on the back of the upper limb. From *Cunningham's Textbook of Anatomy*, 10th Edition.

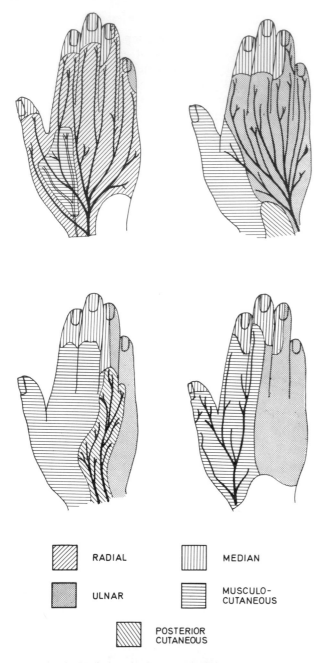

FIG. 23.65. Variations in the pattern of the cutaneous nerves to dorsum of the hand. From Grant J.C.B. (1962) *An Atlas of Anatomy*. London : Baillière.

activity of the nerves of the upper limb depends on the level of interruption. To understand this deficit knowledge of the levels at which the particular muscular branches are given off from the parent trunks is necessary. Examples of the common motor tests for the main nerves of the upper limb are given below:

(1) Radial nerve damage in the middle of the arm is tested by trying to dorsiflex the wrist or extend the metacarpophalangeal joints.

(2) Ulnar nerve damage at the wrist is tested by trying to abduct and adduct the fingers (interossei muscles).

(3) Median nerve damage at the wrist is shown when trying to abduct the thumb, as the only muscle which can carry out this movement, abductor pollicis brevis, is supplied by the median nerve.

Autonomic nerve supply of the upper limb

There are no parasympathetic fibres in the upper limb. The efferent fibres of the sympathetic system are distributed to the blood vessels, sweat glands and to the arrector pili muscles. The preganglionic fibres are derived from the lateral horn of the upper thoracic spinal cord, and they synapse in the first thoracic and inferior cervical sympathetic ganglia, and probably in the middle cervical ganglion. From these ganglia the postganglionic fibres, transmitted mostly in the lower trunk of the brachial plexus, accompany the peripheral nerves and

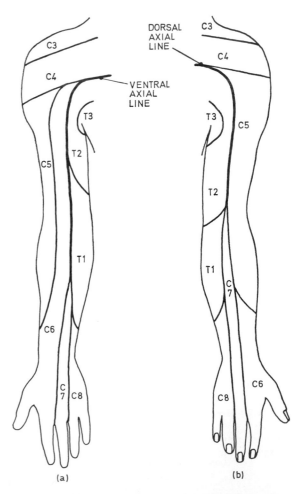

FIG. 23.66. Dermatomes of upper limb, showing segmental cutaneous distribution of spinal nerves on (a) the front, and (b) the back of the limb. From *Cunningham's Textbook of Anatomy*, 10th Edition.

are distributed in their field of supply. The vessels of the upper limb have, however, a double source of vasomotor fibres. Some of the postganglionic fibres are distributed directly, often by the ansa subclavia, to the subclavian artery to form a periarterial sympathetic plexus on the wall of the artery. It is important to note, however, that these fibres do not extend beyond the axilla and the continuation of this plexus on the arteries of the upper limb is provided by contributions from adjacent peripheral nerves.

BLOOD VESSELS OF THE UPPER LIMB

ARTERIES (fig. 23.67)

Blood for the right upper limb leaves the aortic arch through the short, wide brachiocephalic trunk which divides into the right common carotid and right subclavian arteries, the latter delivering blood to the limb. On the left side, the subclavian artery is a direct branch of the arch of the aorta. At the outer border of the first rib, on entering the axilla, the main stem of the subclavian artery changes its name to **axillary artery**. At the lower border of the teres major muscle, it is called the **brachial artery**. This vessel ends in the cubital fossa, by dividing into **radial** and **ulnar arteries**. The radial artery runs down the forearm to the lateral aspect of the wrist, where it curves round to the back of the hand before passing anteriorly through the interosseous space between the first and second metacarpal bones. Entering the palm in this way it ends by anastomosing with the deep palmar branch of the ulnar artery. The ulnar artery runs from the cubital fossa to the flexor retinaculum on the ulnar side of the forearm. It ends on the retinaculum, lateral to the pisiform bone, by dividing into the superficial palmar arch and a deep palmar branch which joins the radial to form the **deep palmar arch**. The **superficial palmar arch** lies just beneath the palmar aponeurosis. Four arteries arise from it; the palmar digital artery goes to the ulnar border of the little finger and three common palmar digital arteries divide distally into branches supplying the contiguous sides of the fingers.

The **deep palmar arch** lies deeply in the proximal part of the palm and gives off three palmar metacarpal arteries which join distally the common palmar digital arteries.

SUBCLAVIAN ARTERY

Besides being a stem vessel it supplies some upper limb structures through two branches in the neck. The **transverse cervical** is associated through its superficial branch with the deep surface of the trapezius muscle and through its deep branch with the levator scapulae, supraspinous, infraspinous and subscapular regions. The **suprascapular**, which crosses anteriorly to the brachial plexus, reaches the suprascapular notch and is distributed in the supra-

spinous and infraspinous fossae of the scapula and gives branches to the adjacent muscles and joints.

AXILLARY ARTERY

This is divided into three parts: the first, above the pectoralis minor muscle, the second, posterior to it and the third, inferior to it. The branches of the axillary artery are:

(1) one from the first part; **superior thoracic artery** is distributed to the first intercostal space.

(2) two from the second part; **thoraco-acromial** pierces the clavipectoral fascia and divides into acromial, clavicular, deltoid and pectoral branches and **lateral thoracic** descends along the inferolateral border of the pectoralis minor muscle.

(3) three from the third part; the largest, **subscapular** is distributed to the subscapular region, to the infraspinous region (through its circumflex branch), to the chest wall and the latissimus dorsi muscle, the **posterior circumflex humeral artery** passes backwards together with the axillary nerve round the back of the surgical neck of the humerus and ends under cover of the deltoid muscle, and the smallest of the three, the **anterior circumflex humeral artery** passes around the front of the surgical neck.

BRACHIAL ARTERY

This has the following named branches:
Profunda brachii artery runs with the radial nerve at the back of the humerus to divide into a radial collateral artery which accompanies the radial nerve to the front of the lateral epicondyle and a posterior descending branch which passes behind the lateral epicondyle. An ascending branch of this last artery anastomoses with the posterior circumflex humeral artery. **Superior ulnar collateral artery** runs towards the back of the medial epicondyle. **Inferior ulnar collateral artery** 'supratrochlear', gives branches both in front and behind the medial epicondyle. A small nutrient artery to the humerus is given off from the middle of the brachial artery.

RADIAL ARTERY

The branches are: **Radial recurrent artery** arises in the cubital fossa. **Superficial palmar branch** arises just above the wrist and passes into the palm, often taking part in the formation of the superficial palmar arch. **Palmar carpal branch** runs to the palmar carpal arch. **Dorsal carpal branch** is given off at the side of the wrist to the dorsal carpal arch; from the dorsal carpal arch three dorsal metacarpal arteries pass distally and near the knuckles each divides into two **dorsal digital arteries**. Each dorsal metacarpal artery communicates with the deep palmar branch and with digital palmar arteries through the intermetacarpal spaces. The dorsal digital arteries of the thumb and the radial side of the index arise independently from the radial artery. **Princeps pollicis artery** is given

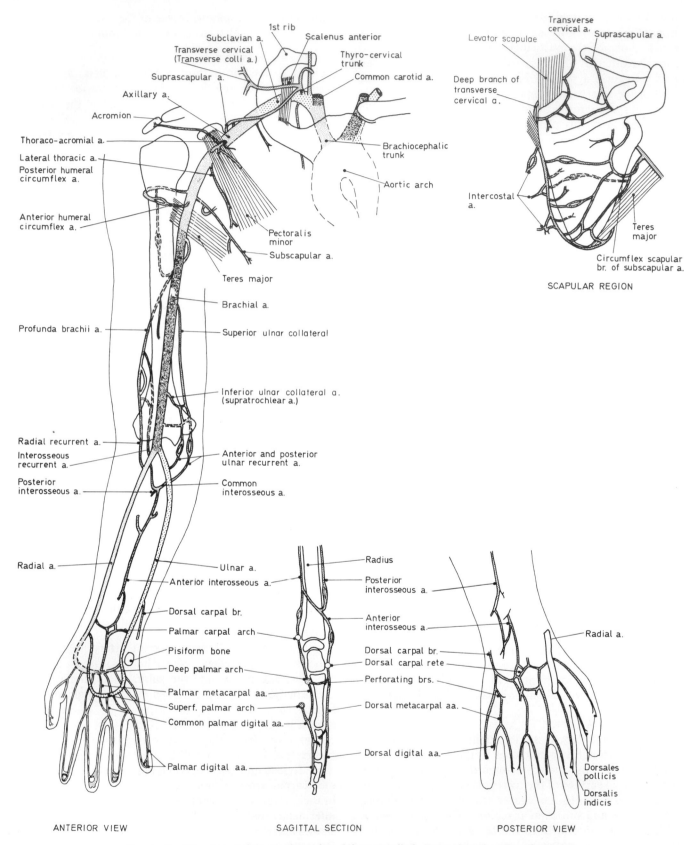

Transverse
cervical a.
Levator scapulae   Suprascapular a.

Deep branch of
transverse
cervical a.

Intercostal
a.

Teres
major

Circumflex scapular
br. of subscapular a.

SCAPULAR REGION

1st rib
Subclavian a.   Scalenus anterior
Transverse cervical
(Transverse colli a.)   Thyro-cervical
trunk
Suprascapular a.   Common carotid a.
Axillary a.
Acromion   Brachiocephalic
trunk
Thoraco-acromial a.
Lateral thoracic a.   Aortic arch
Posterior humeral
circumflex a.
Anterior humeral
circumflex a.
Pectoralis
minor
Subscapular a.
Teres major
Brachial a.
Profunda brachii a.   Superior ulnar collateral
Inferior ulnar collateral a.
(supratrochlear a.)
Radial recurrent a.
Interosseous
recurrent a.   Anterior and posterior
ulnar recurrent a.
Posterior
interosseous a.   Common
interosseous a.
Radial a.   Radius
Ulnar a.   Posterior
interosseous a.
Anterior interosseous a.
Anterior
interosseous a.   Radial a.
Dorsal carpal br.
Palmar carpal arch   Dorsal carpal br.
Pisiform bone   Dorsal carpal rete
Deep palmar arch   Perforating brs.
Palmar metacarpal aa.   Dorsal metacarpal aa.
Superf. palmar arch
Common palmar digital aa.
Dorsal digital aa.
Dorsales
pollicis
Palmar digital aa.   Dorsalis
indicis

ANTERIOR VIEW   SAGITTAL SECTION   POSTERIOR VIEW

FIG. 23.67. Diagram of the named arteries of the upper limb. From Grant's *Atlas of Anatomy*.

off in the palm and divides into two digital palmar arteries to the thumb. **Radialis indicis artery** supplies the palmar aspect of the radial side of the index.

ULNAR ARTERY

It gives the following branches: The anterior and posterior **ulnar recurrents** pass in front of and behind the medial epicondyle. **Common interosseous artery** passes to the upper border of the interosseous membrane and divides into: (1) **anterior interosseous artery** which runs in front of the membrane to the upper border of the pronatus quadratus muscle where it sends one branch to the palmar carpal arch and another perforating to the back of the forearm to join the dorsal carpal arch, (2) **posterior interosseous artery** which passes to the back of the forearm above the upper border of the interosseous membrane, supplies the muscles on the back of the forearm and ends in the dorsal carpal arch. At its origin it gives off the interosseous recurrent artery which passes to the back of the lateral epicondyle.

The **palmar carpal branch** of the ulnar artery completes the palmar carpal arch. The **dorsal carpal branch** ends in the dorsal carpal arch. The **deep palmar branch** joins the radial artery in the depths of the palm to complete the deep palmar arch.

The upper limb is provided with many anastomotic arterial communications which may open up to provide an adequate collateral circulation in case of blockage of the main arteries. These are illustrated in fig. 23.68 and may be listed as follows: scapular anastomosis; communication between the intercostal arteries in the chest wall and lateral thoracic, subscapular arteries and branches of the thoracoacromial artery; between the descending branch from the posterior humeral circumflex and the ascending branch from the profunda brachii; anastomosis around the elbow; between the muscular branches of the radial, ulnar and anterior interosseous arteries in the forearm; free anastomoses in the hand between the carpal and palmar arches, intermetacarpal communications and between the dorsal and palmar arteries in the digits.

VENOUS DRAINAGE

The main venous return from the upper limb is through the axillary vein which continues as the subclavian and brachiocephalic veins before opening into the superior vena cava. The veins of the upper limb can be divided into **superficial veins** which lie for most of their course outside the sleeve of the deep fascia, and **deep veins** which accompany the arteries inside the fascial sleeve.

Superficial veins (fig. 23.69)

The digits are drained of venous blood through anastomosing palmar and dorsal digital veins. From the palm

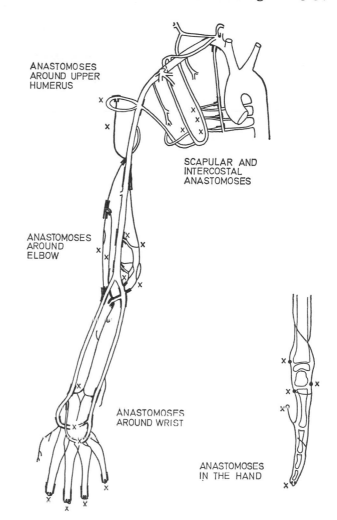

FIG. 23.68. Anastomoses. X denotes the anastomotic branches and the heavy lines the segments of the vessels which are linked.

most of the venous return goes to the dorsum, particularly through the intercapitular veins between the heads of the metacarpal bones and around the margins of the hand. The blood from the digits and the palm thus drains to the dorsal venous network (fig. 23.69) on the back of the hand. The cephalic vein issues from the radial end of this network and the basilic vein arises from the ulnar end. The further course of these veins is shown in fig. 23.69. The cephalic vein pierces the clavipectoral fascia to end in the axillary vein. The basilic vein runs to the axilla where it continues as the axillary vein.

The superficial veins of the forearm are extremely variable, but, at the elbow, the superficial veins are usually arranged as shown in fig. 23.69.

Deep veins

The deep veins, except for the axillary vein, are arranged in pairs, one on each side of the various arteries. The

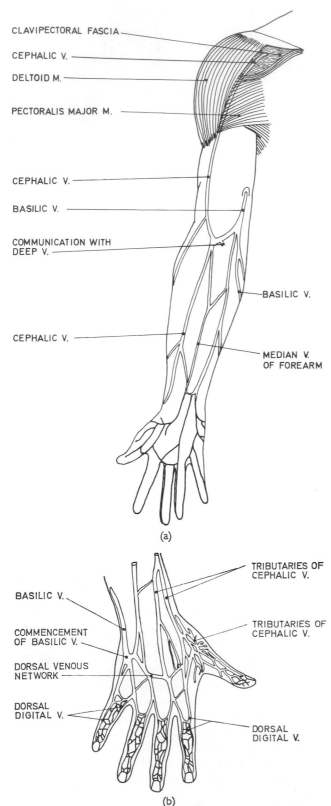

CLAVIPECTORAL FASCIA

CEPHALIC V.

DELTOID M.

PECTORALIS MAJOR M.

CEPHALIC V.

BASILIC V.

COMMUNICATION WITH DEEP V.

CEPHALIC V.

BASILIC V.

MEDIAN V. OF FOREARM

(a)

TRIBUTARIES OF CEPHALIC V.

BASILIC V.

COMMENCEMENT OF BASILIC V.

TRIBUTARIES OF CEPHALIC V.

DORSAL VENOUS NETWORK

DORSAL DIGITAL V.

DORSAL DIGITAL V.

(b)

FIG. 23.69. (a) Superficial veins on flexor aspect of right upper limb. (b) Superficial veins on dorsum of hand and digits. From *Cunningham's Textbook of Anatomy*, 10th Edition.

axillary vein, a direct continuation of the basilic vein, traverses the axilla and becomes the subclavian vein at the outer border of the first rib. Its tributaries correspond to the branches of the axillary arteries except for the thoraco-acromial which joins the cephalic vein. The axillary vein receives the brachial veins in the lower part of the axilla and the cephalic vein in its upper part.

LYMPH DRAINAGE
(fig. 23.70)

The collecting system is arranged in superficial or subcutaneous and deep layers, which remain practically separate until the main trunks of the superficial set pierce the deep fascia in the upper arm.

The palmar surfaces of the digits and the palm itself have a rich plexus of **superficial lymphatics**. Most of these drain into the vessels of the dorsum around the sides of the digits, margins of the palm and through the interdigital clefts. In their further course they accompany the main superficial veins. Some are interrupted at the superficial lymph nodes, but nearly all run to the axilla before they pierce the deep fascia.

Deep lymphatics accompany the deeper blood vessels. Most of the superficial and deep lymphatics end in the axillary lymph nodes from whence the lymph passes to the **subclavian lymph trunk**. There is also a communication between the axillary and lower deep cervical nodes and some lymph from the axilla may drain to the jugular lymph trunk. The left subclavian trunk drains into the thoracic duct and the right one joins the right lymphatic duct (p. 21.39).

Lymph nodes

Superficial nodes include cubital nodes lying a little above the medial epicondyle. Infraclavicular nodes lie anterior to the clavipectoral fascia and drain some of the shoulder area. Deltopectoral nodes lie in the groove between the two muscles and drain part of the arm and shoulder.

Small **deep nodes** may occur along the course of the deep blood vessels. **Axillary lymph nodes** (fig. 23.71) are divided into the following groups which intercommunicate freely:

Lateral, along the axillary vein.
Pectoral, in the anterior part of the axilla.
Subscapular, in the posterior part of the axilla.
Central, in the middle.
Apical, in the apex of the axilla; they convey the collected lymph to the subclavian trunk.

The axillary lymph nodes drain a large part of the

trunk (p. 21.40). Most of the lymph from the upper limb passes into the lateral group of nodes.

MECHANISM OF FLUID RETURN

The main bulk of the centripetal flow of the fluid passes from the dorsal aspect of the hand through the venous and lymphatic channels. Compression of these channels by the active contractions of the muscles within the fascial compartments creates a pumping action which maintains this backflow, its direction being determined by the valves in the vessels. In the upper limb this mechanism is particularly active in the axilla and hand. In the axilla, the veins and the lymphatics are surrounded by muscles and fasciae; thus the movements of the shoulder region facilitate the fluid return. In the hand, the veins can be emptied by repeated clenching of the fist; the venous blood and lymph are squeezed into the dorsal region of the hand where they can accumulate since the connective tissue is loose and mobile on the back of the hand. Inter-

ference with normal movement of the shoulder and hand therefore causes swelling. If a normal upper limb, even in a young person, is immobilized in a dependent position, the pumping mechanism is ineffective and swelling develops in less than 12 hours. As there is just enough skin on the hand (p. 23.22) any accumulation of fluid on the dorsum makes the skin tighter and impairs the range of flexion, so creating a vicious circle.

It is important to realize that immobilization of the shoulder and the hand has its inherent risks and if possible in injury or disease one or both of these regions should be kept mobile.

SHORT NOTES ON THE COURSE OF NEUROVASCULAR BUNDLES

Axilla

In the axilla the **axillary artery**, surrounded by the cords and branches of the brachial plexus, with the **axillary vein** lying on its medial aspect, enters the axilla at the

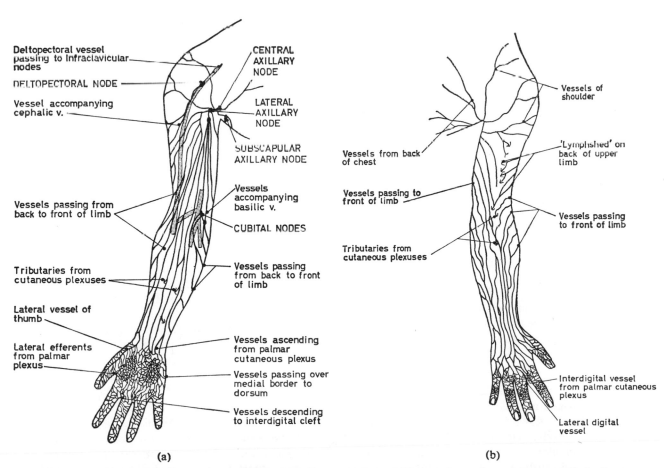

FIG. 23.70. Superficial lymph vessels and lymph nodes of (a) anterior and (b) posterior surface of the upper limb. From *Cunningham's Textbook of Anatomy,* 10th Edition.

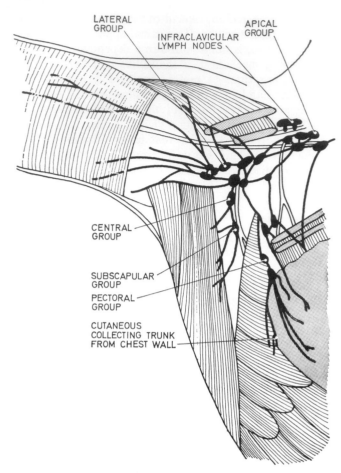

LATERAL GROUP
INFRACLAVICULAR LYMPH NODES
APICAL GROUP
CENTRAL GROUP
SUBSCAPULAR GROUP
PECTORAL GROUP
CUTANEOUS COLLECTING TRUNK FROM CHEST WALL

Fig. 23.71. Axillary lymph nodes. From *Gray's Anatomy*, 33rd Edition (1962). London : Longman

apex, but then deviates towards its lateral wall so the main neurovascular bundle in the lower part of the axilla follows the movements of the arm. However, the **axillary nerve** and **posterior circumflex humeral vessels** leave the axilla at the level of the surgical neck of the humerus, inferior to the capsule of the shoulder joint. The **radial nerve** lying behind the axillary artery enters the upper arm directed towards the back of the humerus where it is found in its groove accompanied by the **profunda brachii artery**. The **musculocutaneous nerve** having pierced the coracobrachialis muscle traverses the upper arm between brachialis and biceps muscles.

Upper arm

In the upper arm the **brachial artery** together with the **median nerve, medial cutaneous nerve of the forearm and the ulnar nerve** runs down from the lower border of the axilla along the medial aspect of the arm in the groove between the brachialis and biceps muscles. The **ulnar nerve** passes backwards, at the mid-point of the arm, pierces the medial intermuscular septum, reaches the

back of the medial epicondyle and then crosses the medial ligament of the elbow joint (fig. 23.28). The **brachial artery** with the **median nerve**, which has crossed it from the lateral to medial side, reaches its end in the cubital fossa (fig. 23.57). The **radial nerve** together with the **profunda brachii artery** traverses the spiral groove on the back of the humerus, the anterior descending branch of the artery accompanying the nerve as it pierces the lateral intermuscular septum and descends to the front of the elbow.

Forearm

In the forearm the **ulnar nerve** continues down the medial part of the forearm towards the radial side of the pisiform bone under cover of the flexor digitorum superficialis and flexor carpi ulnaris muscles, accompanied on the lateral side in its lower two-thirds by the **ulnar artery** which reaches it from its point of origin in the cubital fossa.

The **superficial branch of the radial nerve** continues from the front of the lateral epicondyle down the lateral part of the forearm under cover of the brachioradialis muscle, lying a little lateral to the middle third of the radial artery. In the distal third of the forearm it inclines backwards across the distal end of the radius to end on the dorsum of the hand. The **radial artery** begins in the cubital fossa and runs downwards and slightly lateral to the distal end of the radius where it turns posteriorly to leave the forearm by entering the anatomical snuff box, where it lies on the lateral ligament of the wrist joint. It is under cover of the brachioradialis muscle as far as the distal third of the forearm where it is covered only by the skin and fasciae and so its pulsation can be felt just above the wrist.

The **median nerve** leaves the cubital fossa by passing between the heads of the pronator teres muscle; here it crosses superficially to the ulnar artery and then runs downwards through the middle of the forearm in front of the flexor digitorum profundus and behind the flexor digitorum superficialis to which it is closely adherent. Just below the pronator teres it gives off the **anterior interosseous nerve** which reaches the wrist region lying on the anterior surface of the interosseous membrane. The **deep branch** of the radial nerve runs in front of the elbow joint, enters the supinator muscle in whose substance it winds round the lateral side of the upper part of the radius, and reaches the dorsum of the forearm between the superficial and deep muscles where it divides almost immediately into its multiple terminal branches.

Wrist

Just above the wrist, at the common site of cut wounds, the disposition of the main nerves and vessels on the palmar aspect is shown in fig. 23.72. The most lateral structure is the radial artery, as the superficial branch of

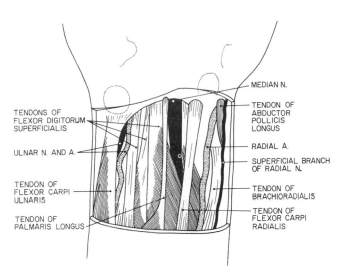

TENDONS OF FLEXOR DIGITORUM SUPERFICIALIS

ULNAR N. AND A.

TENDON OF FLEXOR CARPI ULNARIS

TENDON OF PALMARIS LONGUS

MEDIAN N.

TENDON OF ABDUCTOR POLLICIS LONGUS

RADIAL A.

SUPERFICIAL BRANCH OF RADIAL N.

TENDON OF BRACHIORADIALIS

TENDON OF FLEXOR CARPI RADIALIS

FIG. 23.72. The anterior aspect of the wrist.

the radial nerve is already on the lateral aspect of the region. The median nerve appears on the lateral aspect of the tendons of the flexor digitorum superficialis and is found between the tendons of the flexor carpi radialis and palmaris longus, superficial to the tendon of the flexor pollicis longus. The ulnar artery with the ulnar nerve on its medial side lies in the medial part of this region partly under cover of the flexor carpi ulnaris. The median nerve enters the carpal tunnel alongside the tendons of the flexor digitorum superficialis, while the ulnar artery and nerve lie anterior to the flexor retinaculum, but under cover of the palmaris brevis muscle.

Hand

In the palm, the common digital nerves lie posteriorly to the superficial palmar arch and its branches, which are immediately behind the palmar aponeurosis. Near the fingers they cross each other, the arteries lying now posterior to the nerves. The neurovascular bundles in the digits are enclosed in the digital ligaments and lie against the sides of the fibrous flexor sheaths (fig. 23.48d).

OSSIFICATION OF THE BONES OF THE UPPER LIMB

The general features and principles of ossification are discussed on p. 19.38. The diagrams below show the parts of the bones of the upper limb ossified from the primary and secondary centres and their approximate times of appearance and fusion (fig. 23.73). The variations in these times caused by genetic, nutritional and sexual factors are omitted for simplicity.

LINE OF IMPACT
(fig. 23.74)

A fall on the outstretched hand or striking a blow causes an impact which is taken mainly by the third metacarpal bone, from which it is transmitted to the capitate and scaphoid bones of the carpus. The force then passes along the radius, but in normal conditions does not reach the humerus directly as it is taken up by the obliquely disposed fibres of the strong interosseous membrane which transfer it to the ulna and so to the humerus and scapula. The impact is then partially absorbed by the muscular attachment of the scapula to the trunk, but if severe or unexpected, the bony strut of the clavicle is strained or broken.

REVERSE ACTION OF THE MUSCLES

Usually, the muscles of the upper limb act from the trunk on limb, in other words from their origin on their insertion and from their more proximal to their more distal attachments. However, there are many instances when the opposite occurs, as for example in swimming or climbing. It is important to realize this as there are circumstances in which the reverse action of the muscles can be used to assist or replace the action of one which is weakened or lost. For example, after loss of the musculocutaneous nerve and hence the action of the biceps and brachialis muscles, flexion at the elbow can be produced by the muscles in the forearm. Their reverse action at the elbow can be helped by moving their origins up the humerus surgically.

SURFACE ANATOMY

Bony landmarks

The **clavicle** is subcutaneous throughout and can be palpated from its rounded sternal end to the lateral edge of the acromial end, which is 3 cm medial to the lateral border of the acromion. If this border is followed posteriorly for about 5 cm a sharp **acromial angle** can be felt, from which the **crest of the spine of the scapula** can be traced medially towards the third thoracic spine. The **tip of the coracoid process** can be felt indistinctly on pressing backwards 2 cm below the junction of the lateral and intermediate thirds of the clavicle. The **greater tubercle of the humerus** forms the most lateral point in this region and is known as 'the point of the shoulder'. The **lesser tubercle** lies 2·5 cm lateral to the tip of the coracoid process.

Both **epicondyles of the humerus** are subcutaneous and easily palpated. The line joining them passes through the tip of the **olecranon** when the elbow is extended, but in

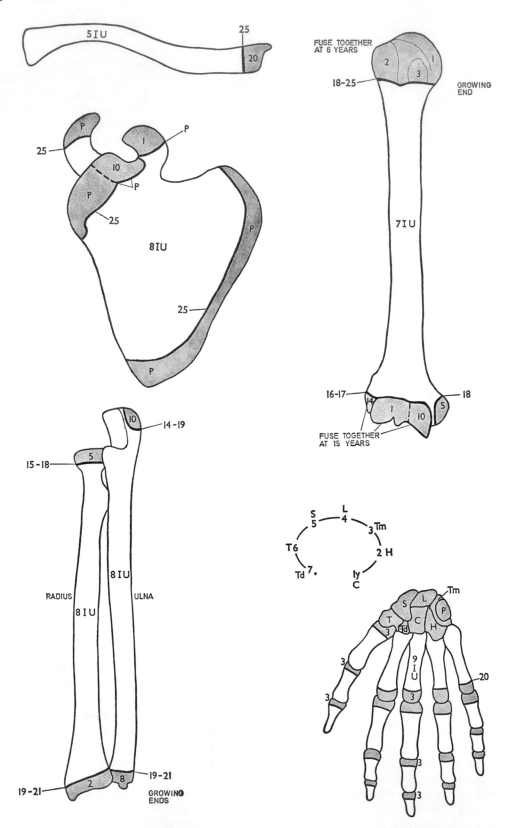

Fig. 23.73. Numbers on the bones indicate age, in years, of appearance of ossification centres. Stippled areas are cartilaginous at birth. Leaders show the time of fusion in years. IU, age in weeks of intrauterine life; P, puberty.

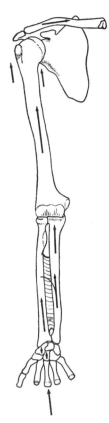

FIG. 23.74. Line of impact in the upper limb.

full flexion the tip is 2 cm distal to this line. The **head of the radius** lies 2·5 cm distal to the lateral epicondyle and its position can be verified by feeling it to rotate when the forearm is pronated or supinated. The **posterior border of the ulna** is subcutaneous throughout and can be traced from the olecranon down to the **head of the ulna** which stands out prominently in pronation. On its posteromedial aspect the **styloid process** can be felt. The **anterior border of the lower end of the radius** is felt as a distinct transverse ridge on the front of the forearm about 2–3 cm proximal to the base of the thenar eminence. The **styloid process of the radius** may be felt projecting down from the lateral aspect of the distal end of the radius and its tip is 1 cm distal to the tip of the ulnar styloid. The **dorsal tubercle of the radius** can be felt on the back of the distal end of the radius in line with the second intermetacarpal space. The four points of the attachments of the flexor retinaculum can be identified on the palmar aspect of the carpus. The **tubercle of the scaphoid** can be felt at the proximal border of the thenar eminence and the **crest of the trapezium** immediately distal to it; the **pisiform** is a prominence felt at the base of the hypothenar eminence and the **hook of the hamate** lies 2–3 cm distal and lateral to the pisiform. When the fist is made the prominences of the heads of the meta-

carpals and phalanges are easily felt and identified as the knuckles.

Soft-tissue landmarks

Most of the superficial muscles and tendons of the upper limb can be easily identified by palpation and in lean individuals can be observed particularly when in action. Some of the soft tissue landmarks are described below.

AXILLARY FOLDS

The anterior fold, formed by the lower part of the pectoralis major muscle can be gripped by the hand and palpated throughout; the posterior fold is formed by the latissimus dorsi and teres major muscles. It extends to a lower level than the anterior one. The **biceps muscle** forms a longitudinal prominence on the front of the arm. In the cubital fossa, with the elbow flexed, the **tendon of the biceps** can be felt in the middle with the sharp upper edge of the **bicipital aponeurosis** passing medially and distally. On the back of the pronated forearm with the hand clenched, a groove can be seen and palpated which extends from the lateral epicondyle towards the dorsal tubercle of the radius (see fig. 23.77). This groove overlies the **intermuscular septum** separating the radial extensors of the wrist from the digital extensors. **Tendons** near the palmar aspect of the **wrist** can be easily palpated; from the radial to the ulnar side they are: tendon of the flexor carpi radialis, then of the palmaris longus (absent in 10 per cent), of the flexor digitorum superficialis and lastly of the flexor carpi ulnaris. There are usually two distinct **creases at the wrist**; the proximal one overlying the line of the wrist joint and the distal one over the upper border of the flexor retinaculum.

Using the above mentioned bony and soft tissue landmarks the following structures can be mapped out on the surface of the upper limb.

Axillary and brachial arteries. With the arm abducted to a right angle and the forearm supinated (fig. 23.75) a line

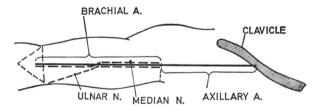

FIG. 23.75. Surface anatomy of the main neurovascular bundle.

is drawn from the midpoint of the clavicle to the midpoint of the cubital fossa. Proximal to the junction of the posterior axillary fold with the arm, this line represents the axillary artery; the rest denotes the brachial artery.

Brachial plexus. Its main elements in the upper limb are indicated by a line joining the midpoint of the clavicle to a point one finger's breadth distal and medial to the tip of the coracoid process (fig. 23.76).

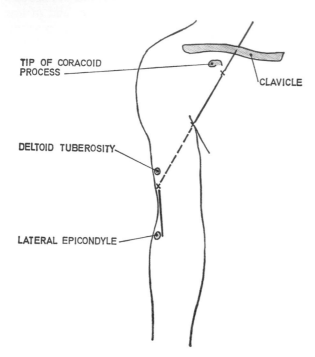

FIG. 23.76. Surface anatomy of the brachial plexus and radial nerve.

Axillary nerve. Most of its course can be indicated on the skin by a transverse line at the back of the shoulder a hand's breadth below the acromial angle.

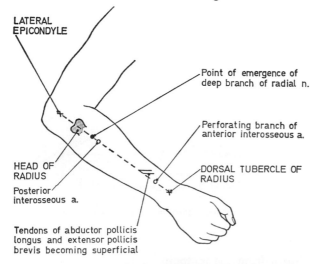

FIG. 23.77. Surface anatomy of the dorsum of the forearm.

Radial nerve (fig. 23.76). The radial nerve is represented by a line joining the following points: point of termination of the brachial plexus (see above), point of junction of

the posterior axillary fold with the arm, point at the junction of the upper and intermediate thirds of the distance between the insertion of the deltoid and the lateral epicondyle and finally the anterior aspect of the lateral epicondyle. The *deep branch of the radial nerve* appears on the back of the forearm at a point on a line joining the lateral epicondyle to the dorsal tubercle of the radius shown in fig. 23.77, which also shows other structures found along this line.

Median nerve (fig. 23.78). In the arm it follows the line

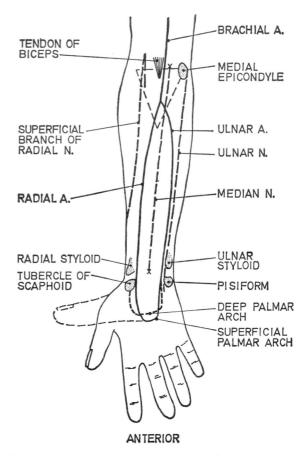

FIG. 23.78. Surface anatomy of the anterior aspect of the forearm and hand.

of the brachial artery and is found in the cubital fossa halfway between the biceps tendon and the medial epicondyle. From this point the line continues in the forearm to the point halfway between the radial and ulnar styloids. *Ulnar nerve* (fig. 23.78). In the arm it follows the line of the brachial artery as far as the midpoint of the arm: at this point it deviates to the back of the medial epicondyle; from there a line drawn to the distal and radial aspect of the pisiform represents the nerve in the forearm. *Ulnar artery* (fig. 23.78). From the point of termination of the brachial artery it joins the line of the ulnar nerve at the junction of its upper and intermediate thirds.

Radial artery (fig. 23.78). Represented by a line convex laterally from the points of termination of the brachial artery to the scaphoid tubercle.

Superficial palmar arch reaches as far distally as the lower border of the extended thumb (fig. 23.78), with the deep arch being about 1·5 cm more proximal, accompanied here by the deep branch of the ulnar nerve.

Metacarpophalangeal joints on the palmar aspect are 2 cm proximal to the digital webs, posterior to the distal

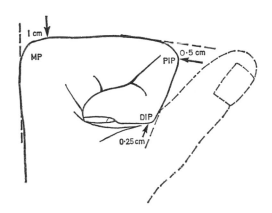

FIG. 23.79. Surface anatomy of the joints of the fingers.

transverse skin crease of the palm. The *proximal interphalangeal joints* are 0·5 cm and the *distal joints* 0·25 cm from their knuckles (figs. 23.79).

FURTHER READING

Many concepts and diagrams in this chapter are based on the following works.

HOLLINSHEAD W.H. (1969) *Anatomy for Surgeons*, 2nd Edition, vol. 3. The limbs. London: Cassell.

JAMIESON J.G. (1950) The fascial spaces of the palm. *British Journal of Surgery* **38**, 193.

JONES F.W. (1948) *The Principles of Anatomy as seen in the Hand*, 2nd Edition. London: Baillière.

KAPLAN E.B. (1965) *Functional and Surgical Anatomy of the Hand*, 2nd Edition. Philadelphia: Lippincott.

LITTLER J.W.W. (1964) *Textbook of Reconstructive and Plastic Surgery*, vol. 4, ed. Converse J.M. Philadelphia: Saunders.

LANDSMEER J.M.F. (1949) The anatomy of the dorsal aponeurosis of the human finger and its functional significance. *Anatomical Record* **104**, 1.

LANDSMEER J.M.F. (1955) Anatomical and functional investigations of the human fingers. *Acta anatomica (Basel)* **25** (Suppl. 24).

LANDSMEER J.M.F. (1963) The co-ordination of finger-joint motions. *Journal of Bone and Joint Surgery* **45-A**, 1654.

PITRES J.A. & TESTUT L. (1925) *Les Nerfs en Schemas; Anatomie et Physiopathologie*. Paris: G. Doin.

STACK H.G. (1962) Muscle function in the fingers. *Journal of Bone and Joint Surgery* **44-B**, 899.

STACK H.G. (1963) A study of muscle function in the fingers. *Annals of the Royal College of Surgeons of England* **33**, 307.

Chapter 24
Lower limb

The upper and lower limbs in man share the basic vertebrate pattern. Each is attached to the trunk by a bony girdle; the free limb consists of a single proximal bone, paired intermediate bones and a distal hand or foot (fig. 24.1). The primary function of the upper limb is to

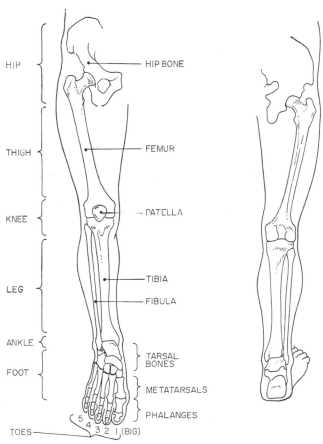

FIG. 24.1. General plan of the lower limb.

position the hand to perform its delicate skilled movements. These are made possible by the unspecialized anatomical construction of the human hand, inherited from our arboreal ancestors, and directed by a highly developed brain. The primary functions of the lower limb

are locomotion and support of the trunk in an upright posture. The human foot, by contrast with the hand, is a highly specialized organ, adapted mainly to the transfer of body weight to the ground and to its function as a lever in locomotion. In some circumstances however, for example congenital absence of the hands, the feet and brain may be trained to achieve a surprising degree of manipulative skill.

Other differences in form between the two limbs have arisen with adoption of the erect posture. In the fetal position, both upper and lower limbs are flexed upon the trunk. After birth, the lower limbs become extended and the femur undergoes medial rotation at the hip, while the leg below the knee adopts a position comparable to pronation of the forearm. Thus the anterior aspect of the knee corresponds to the posterior aspect of the elbow, and the great toe can be compared to the thumb with the hand held in full pronation.

BONES, JOINTS AND MUSCLES OF THE HIP

BONES OF THE HIP

The pelvic girdle is described on p. 21.13. The femora are the longest bones in the body. Each articulates above with the hip bone at the acetabulum, and below with the tibia and patella. Their upper ends are separated by the width of the pelvis, while their lower ends come together at the knee, so that the femora slope obliquely downwards and medially with the subject standing at attention. This obliquity is greater in the female due to the relatively broader pelvis.

Femur (figs. 24.2 and 3)

The upper end of the femur is characterized by an almost spherical head which is connected to the shaft by a long neck set obliquely into the shaft.

The head is covered by articular cartilage to form two-thirds of a sphere for articulation with the acetabulum. A depression on the head, the **fovea capitis femoris,** is for the attachment of the ligamentum teres. Through this pit a number of small blood vessels enter and supply the head to a minor extent.

The neck is relatively narrow above and expands downwards and slightly posteriorly towards its insertion into

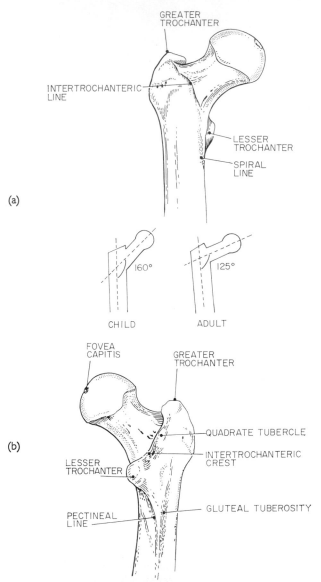

FIG. 24.2. Upper end of right femur; (a), anterior view; (b), posterior view.

the shaft at an angle of 125° in the adult and 160° in the child (fig. 24.2).

It is ridged longitudinally, and many small vessels enter it to run upwards and provide the major blood supply of the femoral head. In fractures of the neck of the femur, these vessels may be damaged, resulting in death (ischaemic necrosis) of the head.

The **greater trochanter** projects above the neck laterally to receive the attachments of the gluteal muscles. On the medial surface of the greater trochanter is the **trochanteric fossa** for the attachment of the obturator externus muscle (fig. 24.3). The greater trochanter is a useful landmark easily palpable on the lateral aspect of the hip.

The **lesser trochanter** lies below the femoral neck on the posteromedial aspect of the bone, and receives the attachment of the iliopsoas tendon. Posteriorly, the two trochanters are joined by a prominent **intertrochanteric crest.**

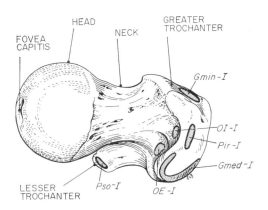

FIG. 24.3. Upper end of right femur seen from above, showing the insertions (*I*) of gluteus minimus (*G min*) and medius (*G med*), obturator internus (*OI*) and piriformis (*Pir*) to the greater trochanter. Iliopsoas (*Pso*) is inserted into the lesser trochanter. The insertion of obturator externus (*OE*) is into the deep trochanteric fossa.

This crest is partially interrupted by another tubercle, the **quadrate tubercle,** to which the quadratus femoris muscle is attached. Anteriorly, the two tubercles are joined by a less prominent ridge, the **intertrochanteric line.**

The shaft of the femur is slightly bowed anteriorly and is triangular in cross-section, with anterior, medial and lateral surfaces. The medial and lateral borders are rounded, while the sharp, rough posterior border is known as the **linea aspera.** This line receives the attachment of the adductor and other muscles and it extends from the level of the lesser trochanter down to the junction of the middle and lower thirds of the femur, where it separates into the medial and lateral **supracondylar lines** (p. 24.7).

The **pectineal line,** for attachment of pectineus muscle, passes from the lesser trochanter to the linea aspera (fig. 24.2). The **spiral line,** to which a portion of vastus medialis muscle is attached, runs below the pectineal line from the linea aspera across the medial surface of the shaft, towards the lower part of the intertrochanteric line. The **gluteal tuberosity,** a roughened longitudinal ridge on the posterior aspect of the upper femoral shaft, lies lateral to the linea aspera (fig. 24.2) and receives the attachment of the lower part of gluteus maximus.

HIP JOINT

The femoral head articulates with the hip bone at the acetabulum forming the hip joint. This is a good example of a ball and socket joint, the acetabulum partially enclosing the femoral head. Although it is less mobile than the shoulder joint, it has the greater stability necessary for weight transfer.

The **acetabulum** is a cup-shaped cavity which is deficient below at the **acetabular notch**. This notch is bridged by the strong transverse acetabular ligament. The acetabulum is deepened by a rim of fibrocartilage, the **labrum acetabulare**. This is attached round the acetabular margin and its diameter is slightly less than that of the femoral head, which it therefore grasps. The articular surface of the acetulum is horseshoe-shaped and smooth, and is covered with articular cartilage; it surrounds a rougher, non-articular area, the **acetabular fossa**.

The joint capsule is very strong and surrounds the joint on all sides. Proximally it is attached around the acetabulum, and distally it grasps the neck of the femur, reaching anteriorly to the intertrochanteric line, but posteriorly falling short of the intertrochanteric crest by about 2 cm.

There are three strong ligaments, which are special thickenings of the capsule. The strongest is the **iliofemoral ligament** which extends in front of the joint from an attachment just below the anterior inferior iliac spine to the intertrochanteric line on the femur. It is the strongest ligament in the body and has the form of an inverted Y. The **pubofemoral ligament** arises from the iliopubic eminence and from the obturator membrane; its femoral attachment is to the lower end of the intertrochanteric line extending upwards on the back of the joint. The

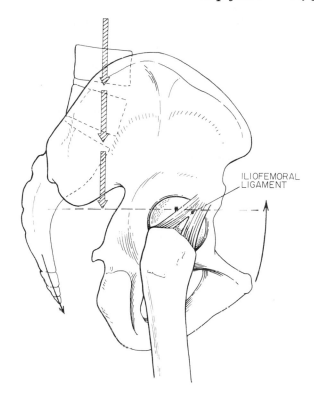

FIG. 24.4. The iliofemoral ligament resists the tendency of the pelvis to rotate.

ischiofemoral ligament is a relatively weak band of fibres which is attached to the ischium close to the acetabular margin, and spirals forwards across the back of the femoral neck to be attached to the medial aspect of the greater trochanter. Its outermost fibres contribute to the

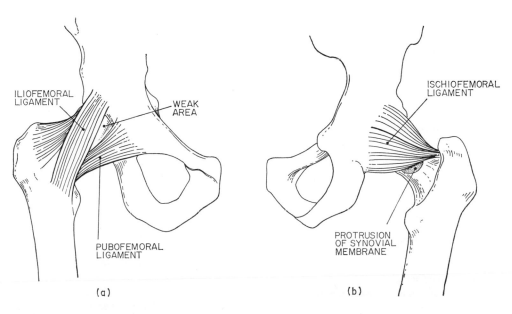

FIG. 24.5. Ligaments of the hip joint, (a) anterior, (b) posterior view.

zona orbicularis, whose fibres encircle the femoral neck on a plane deep to the other ligaments.

All three ligaments become taut when the hip joint is extended, helping to make this the most stable position of the joint. In the erect position, the trunk is balanced, at the acetabula, on the heads of the two femurs, each of which has a smooth and highly slippery surface. The maintenance of balance, the dynamic aspect of joint stability, is largely a co-operative function of the various muscle groups which act on the hip.

In the erect posture, the axis of the centre of gravity may fall at times in front of, at other times behind, the axis of flexion and extension of the hip joint. The tendency for the pelvis and, with it, the trunk to tip backwards or forwards is corrected from moment to moment by balanced activity of hip flexor and extensor muscles. Valuable support, economical of muscular work, is provided by the ligaments of the hip, all three of which resist backwards tilting of the pelvis at the hip.

The **synovial membrane** covers all parts within the joint capsule, except the femoral head and the articular surfaces of the acetabulum and of the labrum. It lines the capsule up to the line of its attachment to the femur, where it is reflected to cover the intra-capsular part of the femoral neck up to the margin of the femoral articular surface. Posteriorly it usually protrudes from under cover of the capsule, here rather loosely attached, to form a bursa beneath the obturator internus tendon. Anteriorly the synovial membrane frequently communicates with the **iliopsoas bursa** through the interval

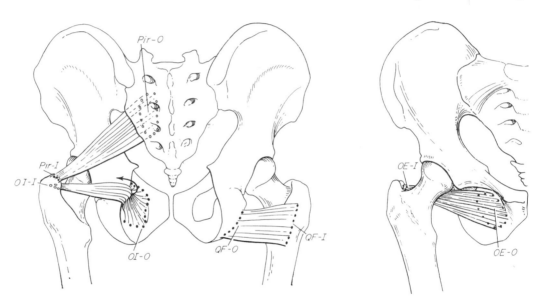

FIG. 24.6. Short lateral rotating muscles of the hip joint. *O* and *I* represent the origin and insertion of the muscles.

Piriformis (*Pir*)

Pir–O Pelvic surface of middle three pieces of sacrum.
Pir–I Tip of greater trochanter.

Quadratus femoris (*QF*)

QF–O Lateral margin of ischial tuber.
QF–I Quadrate tubercle and intertrochanteric crest.

Obturator internus (*OI*)

OI–O Internal surface of the true pelvis (see fig. 21.39).
OI–I Medial surface of greater trochanter. The tendon curves around the lesser sciatic notch and the gemelli muscles then accompany the tendon to its insertion.

Obturator externus (*OE*)

OE–O External surface of obturator membrane.
OE–I Trochanteric fossa (see fig. 24.3).

FIG. 24.7. Gluteal and tensor fasciae latae muscles.

Gluteus minimus (*G min*)

G min–O Gluteal surface of ilium between middle and anterior gluteal lines (fig. 21.20).
G min–I Anterior surface of greater trochanter (fig. 24.3).

Gluteus medius (*G med*)

G med–O Gluteal surface of ilium between posterior and middle gluteal lines (fig. 21.20).
G med–I Lateral surface of greater trochanter (fig. 24.3).

Gluteus maximus (G max)

G max–O_1 Gluteal surface of ilium behind posterior gluteal line.
G max–O_2 Posterior surface of sacrum.
G max–O_3 Sacrotuberous ligament.
G max–I_1 Gluteal tuberosity of femur.
G max–I_2 Iliotibial tract.

Tensor fasciae latae (*TFL*)

TFL–O Anterior superior iliac spine and part of ilium.
TFL–I Iliotibial tract and fascia lata.

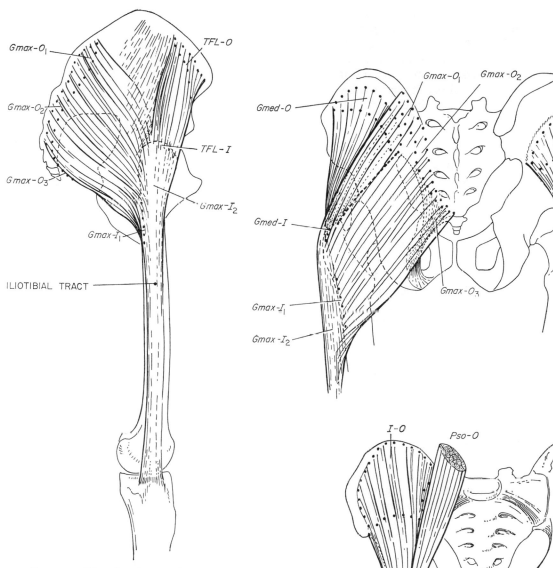

FIG. 24.7. Gluteal and tensor fasciae latae muscles. For details see facing page.

FIG. 24.8. Flexor muscles of the hip.

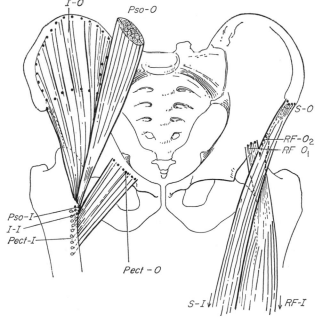

Psoas major (Pso)

Pso–1 Transverse processes, bodies and intervertebral discs of lumbar vertebrae.
Pso–1 Lesser trochanter.

Iliacus (I)

I–O Iliac fossa.
I–I With psoas as iliopsoas into lesser trochanter and area below between spiral and pectineal lines.

Pectineus (Pect)

Pect–O Pectineal surface of pubis.
Pect–1 Pectineal line below lesser trochanter.

Sartorius (S)

S–O Anterior superior iliac spine.
S–I Medial surface of tibia (fig. 24.21).

Rectus femoris (RF)

$RF–O_1$ Straight head: anterior inferior iliac spine.
$RF–O_2$ Reflected head: groove above the acetabulum
$RF–I$ With quadriceps tendon (figs. 24.17 and 19).

between the iliofemoral and pubofemoral ligaments. (fig. 24.5a). The **ligamentum teres** is a specialized part of the synovial membrane, of no mechanical significance. It is roughly conical, attached by its apex to the fovea capitis, by its base to the transverse acetabular ligament and to the margin of the acetabular fossa. It carries a few small vessels to the femoral head, of little functional importance in the adult.

MUSCLES OF THE HIP REGION
(figs. 24.6–9)

Gluteus maximus (fig. 24.7) is a large fleshy muscle, best developed in man, which acts on the hip joint through its attachment to the femur and on the knee joint through its attachment to the tibia by way of the iliotibial tract. It is a muscle of the erect position, extending the hip and completing and maintaining extension of the knee. It is active particularly in forceful extension of the hip, as in standing up from a seated position or in rising from touching the toes. The hamstring muscles (fig. 24.18) assist the gluteus maximus in extending the hip.

Gluteus medius and minimus are powerful fleshy muscles, attached proximally to the ilium, distally to the greater trochanter. Both are abductors of the hip joint. However, abduction as such is a relatively unimportant movement, and the major functional role of these muscles is in helping to balance the pelvis on the femoral head. This is especially important in walking, when their contraction in the supporting limb tilts the pelvis towards that side, allowing the free limb to swing forward (p. 24.27).

The adductor muscles are shown in fig. 24.9. They are mainly adductors and co-operate with the abductors in balancing the pelvis on the femoral heads. Fig. 24.9 makes it clear, however, that the 'hamstring' part of adductor magnus (AM-O_2I_2) is mainly an extensor of the hip.

It is important to notice that rectus femoris and the hamstrings act on both the hip and knee joints, and they can function as extensible ligaments which link movements of flexion and extension in the two joints. For example, flexion of the hip by iliopsoas is often associated with flexion of the knee; during the combined movement, the rectus femoris contracts, but maintains a more or less constant length. Similarly, extension of the hip is often associated with extension of the knee, and the hamstrings, although contracting during the combined movement, shorten only a little.

The flexor muscles of the hip (fig. 24.8) are chiefly the iliopsoas, assisted by pectineus, rectus femoris and sartorius.

The extensor muscles of the hip are gluteus maximus and the hamstrings (fig. 24.18).

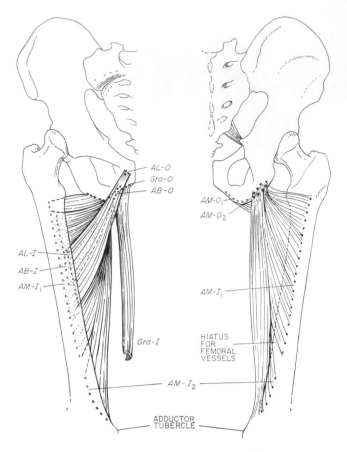

FIG. 24.9. Adductor muscles of the hip.

Gracilis (*Gra*)
Gra–O Medial margin of inferior ramus of pubis.
Gra–I Medial surface of upper end of shaft of tibia.

Adductor longus (*AL*)
AL–O Round tendon from body of pubis.
AL–I Lower part of linea aspera.

Adductor brevis (*AB*)
AB–O Femoral surface of body and inferior ramus of pubis.
AB–I Upper part of linea aspera.

Adductor magnus (*AM*)
(Adductor portion supplied by obturator nerve)
AM–O$_1$ Inferior pubic ramus.
AM–I$_1$ Linea aspera.
(Hamstring portion supplied by sciatic nerve)
AM–O$_2$ Lower lateral part of ischial tuber.
AM–I$_2$ Medial supracondylar line and adductor tubercle.

MOVEMENTS AT THE HIP REGION

These are typical of a ball and socket joint. Flexion and extension occur around a transverse axis through the centre of the femoral head. Flexion is much the more extensive and is limited by opposition of thigh and trunk when the knee is bent. With the knee straight, as in high kicking or in touching the toes, flexion is limited by tension (passive insufficiency) of the hamstrings. In flexion, all parts of the joint capsule are relaxed and dislocation of the femoral head from the acetabulum is most likely to occur with the joint in this position. Extension is limited primarily by tension in all three major ligaments in the joint capsule.

Abduction and adduction occur around an antero-posterior axis through the centre of the femoral head. Abduction is limited by tension in the adductor muscles and in the pubofemoral ligament. Adduction is limited by the abductor muscles and by the lateral limb of the iliofemoral ligament.

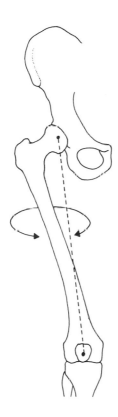

FIG. 24.10. Axis of rotation of the femur.

Rotation accurs around a vertical axis passing through the centre of the head of the femur to the intercondylar notch (fig. 24.10). In medial rotation, the femur swings forwards around this axis and in lateral rotation in the reverse direction, like a gate on its hinges. If the **line of pull** of a muscle passes anterior to this axis, it will produce medial rotation; if it passes posterior, it will produce lateral rotation.

If the neck of the femur is fractured, the thigh becomes rotated about a different axis, passing along the femoral shaft; as the line of pull of most of the rotators passes behind this axis, the thigh is rotated laterally.

BONES, JOINTS AND MUSCLES OF THE KNEE REGION

BONES OF THE KNEE REGION

The lower end of the femur articulates with the upper end of the tibia and with the patella to form the knee joint. The head of the fibula articulates with the lateral side of the lateral tibial condyle forming the superior tibiofibular joint (fig. 24.11).

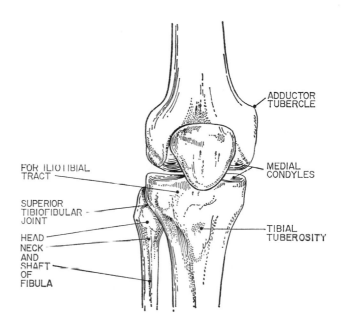

FIG. 24.11. Articulation of bones of right knee and superior tibiofibular joints.

Femur (fig. 24.12)

The shaft of the femur expands below to form the lower end of the femur. From the lower end of the linea aspera, the well-marked medial and lateral **supracondylar lines** run towards the epicondyles. The flat posterior surface of the lower end of the femur forms part of the floor of the popliteal fossa, and is known as the **popliteal surface.**

The large mass of the lower end of the femur is made up of the **medial** and **lateral condyles,** which are separated posteriorly by the deep **intercondylar notch.** Anteriorly, the condyles are joined by an articular surface known as the **patellar surface**; this articulates with the patella in all positions of the joint, except in full flexion, when the patella articulates with a facet on the medial condyle (fig. 24.12e). The anterior surfaces of the condyles lie in the line of the femoral shaft, but posteriorly they project beyond it. The **epicondyles** are small projections on the surface of each condyle. A more marked projection at the upper end of the medial condyle is the **adductor tubercle,** to which is attached the tendon of the hamstring portion

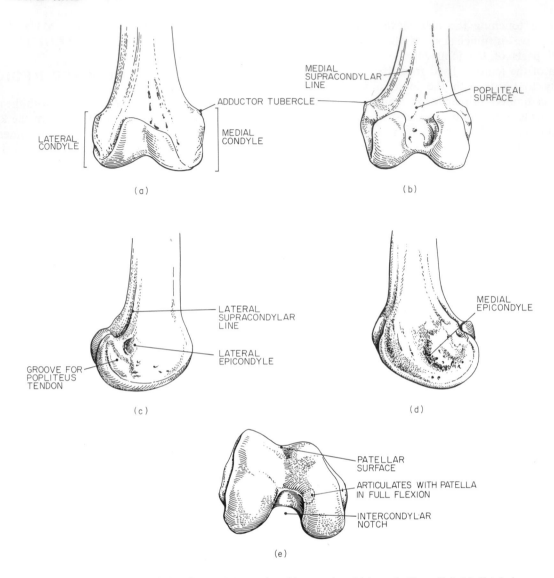

FIG. 24.12. Lower end of right femur, (a) anterior, (b) posterior, (c) lateral, (d) medial, (e) distal views.

of adductor magnus muscle. On the lateral surface of the lateral condyle, posterior to the epicondyle, there is a well marked groove for the tendon of popliteus muscle.

Tibia (fig. 24.13)

The upper end of the tibia is large and expanded to form a plateau for articulation with the lower end of the femur, and is composed principally of two condyles and the tibial tuberosity. The two **condyles** are separated by a roughened intercondylar area, to which the intra-articular structures, i.e. cartilages and ligaments (p. 24.10) are attached. The **intercondylar eminence** is a sharp projection in this region. The upper surface of each condyle is smooth and oval for articulation with the corresponding femoral condyle, the medial articular surface being slightly the larger. On the back of the medial condyle is a rough horizontal groove to

which part of the semimembranosus tendon is attached. The lateral condyle stands out from the shaft more than the medial condyle. This gives it a distal surface, on the posterior aspect of which is a circular facet for articulation with the head of the fibula. On the anterior part of the lateral surface of the lateral condyle, the attachment of the iliotibial tract creates an impression.

The **tuberosity of the tibia** is situated anteriorly where the upper end joins the shaft. The lower part of this tubercle is rough and vertically ridged, and receives the ligamentum patellae, which is separated from the upper smooth part of the tubercle by a bursa.

The shaft of the tibia is triangular in cross section, with anterior, lateral (interosseous) and medial borders. The anterior border can be felt subcutaneously in all its length running down the front of the shin. The posterior surface

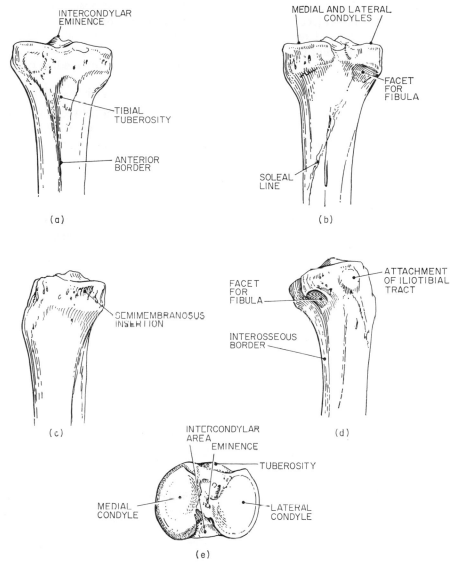

FIG. 24.13. Upper end of right tibia, (a) anterior, (b) posterior, (c) medial, (d) lateral, (e) proximal views.

has an oblique ridge near its upper end which runs downwards and medially from the region of the fibular facet. This is the **soleal line** caused by the origin of a portion of the soleus muscle.

Patella (fig. 24.14)

The patella is a roughly triangular sesamoid bone situated in the common tendon of the quadriceps muscle. Its anterior surface is subcutaneous, and roughly marked with vertical grooves. The upper three-fourths of the posterior surface articulates with the femur, and is roughly divided into medial and lateral halves by a low ridge which fits into the groove on the patellar surface of the femur. The **ligamentum patellae,** the continuation of the quadriceps tendon, is attached proximally to the lower pole of the patella, and distally to the tibial tuberosity. There is frequently a sesamoid bone or cartilage (fabella) in the tendinous origin of the lateral head of gastrocnemius, and occasionally in old people one in the medial head. These have no functional significance, but in radiographs of the knee they may be misinterpreted as loose bodies in the joint.

Fibula (fig. 24.11)

The fibula is the smaller, lateral bone of the leg, and articulates with the tibia at the superior and inferior tibiofibular joints. The upper end is composed of the head and neck, and can be palpated on the lateral side just below the knee.

A large oval articular facet for articulation with the

lateral tibial condyle is present on the proximal surface of the head. The **apex** of the fibula projects upwards posterolateral to the articular surface, and receives the attachment of the fibular collateral ligament of the knee joint.

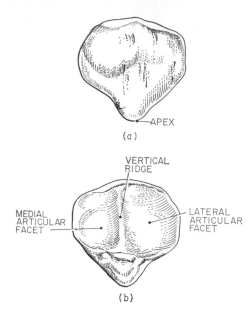

FIG. 24.14. Right patella, (a) anterior, (b) posterior.

A narrow neck connects the head with the shaft of the bone. The common peroneal nerve (p. 24.33) winds round the lateral side of the fibular neck, and can be felt against the bone in this region.

The shaft of the fibula is slender, with a slight spiral twist. It has anterior, posterior, and medial (interosseous) borders which separate the anterior, posterior and lateral surfaces. The posterior surface has a pronounced longitudinal ridge, the medial crest, which further divides it. The markings on the fibular shaft are very variable.

KNEE JOINT

The knee joint is basically a synovial joint of the simple hinge type. It is the largest joint in the body, and the presence of many intra-articular structures makes its structure complex.

As in all hinge joints the strongest parts of the joint capsule (fig. 24.15) lie on the sides of the joint, forming inextensible ligaments which prevent medial or lateral displacement. The anterior and posterior parts of the capsule are weaker to allow flexion and extension.

The capsule is thin and membranous posteriorly; anteriorly, it is largely replaced by the quadriceps tendon, patella and ligamentum patellae. It is attached to the femur around the articular margins of the femoral condyles and the intercondylar line posteriorly. Its lower attachment is to the posterior surfaces and sides of the tibial condyles and to the anterior surfaces of the condyles along oblique lines extending to the tibial tuberosity. The capsule is considerably strengthened in certain regions by expansions from surrounding muscles.

DEFICIENCIES IN THE CAPSULE

The capsule is absent between the quadriceps tendon and anterior aspect of the femur, allowing the synovial membrane to bulge upwards, forming the **suprapatellar bursa** (fig. 24.17a). Posteriorly the popliteus muscle emerges from the knee joint through a gap in the capsule (fig. 24.15e). In addition, posterior to the medial femoral condyle, there is frequently a deficiency through which the synovial membrane may communicate with bursae under semimembranosus and the medial head of gastrocnemius.

THICKENINGS AND EXPANSIONS OF THE CAPSULE

The continuation of the quadriceps tendon, extending between the lower pole of the patella and the tibial tuberosity, is called the **ligamentum patellae** (fig. 24.19).

The **quadriceps expansion** extends from the quadriceps tendon and patella to the oblique lines on the anterior surfaces of the tibial condyles (fig. 24.19). The **oblique popliteal ligament** is an extension from the semimembranosus tendon which runs upwards and laterally on the posterior aspect of the capsule (fig. 24.15e). The **arcuate ligament** is a thickening in the capsule above the deficiency through which the popliteus tendon emerges (fig. 24.15e).

EXTRACAPSULAR STRUCTURES

The **tibial collateral ligament** (fig. 24.15d) is a broad strap-like ligament extending from the medial epicondyle of the femur to the upper quarter of the anteromedial surface of the tibia. Its deep surface is closely attached to the capsule and thus to the intermediate part of the medial meniscus. The **fibular collateral ligament** (fig. 24.15c) is a strong cord-like band about 5 cm long, which extends from the lateral femoral epicondyle to the apex of the fibula. For most of its length it is quite separate from the joint capsule, with vessels and nerves to the joint passing through the gap.

INTRACAPSULAR STRUCTURES

The **menisci** or **semilunar cartilages** (fig. 24.17b) are two intracapsular structures attached to the tibial condyles. They consist almost entirely of dense collagenous fibrous tissue, with a few scattered cartilage cells. They improve the congruence between the lower femoral and upper tibial surfaces and thus permit smoother movements of the tibia on the femur during flexion and extension. They also act to a lesser degree as shock absorbers during walking. They may also contribute to more effective lubrication of the joint by dividing the synovial fluid into

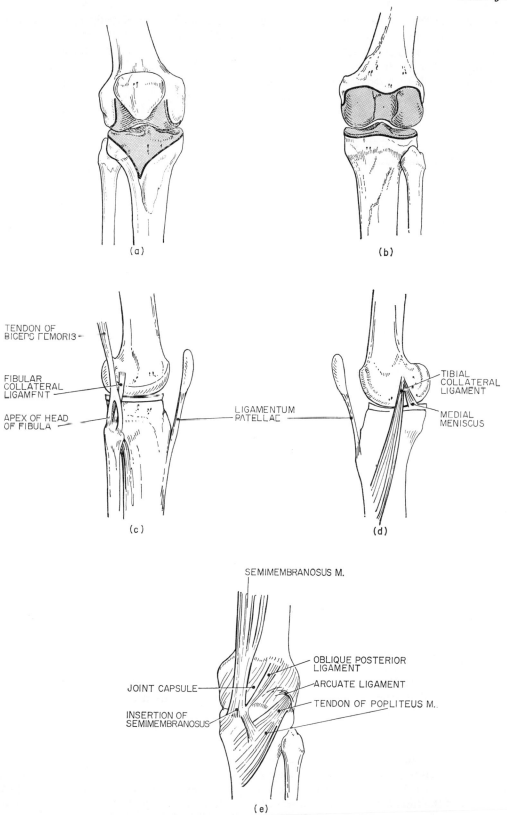

FIG. 24.15. The knee joint. The attachments of the joint capsule are shown from the front (a), and back (b). The collateral ligaments are shown in lateral (c), and medial (d) views. The ligaments on the back of the joint are shown in (e).

two wedges, one between the menisci and the tibia, the other between the menisci and the femoral condyles.

The medial and lateral menisci are attached to the tibial condyles and, being thicker at their outer margins, increase the concavities on these condyles to receive the femoral condyles. Each meniscus is curved, the medial meniscus forming a letter 'C', while the lateral meniscus forms almost a complete circle. The menisci are attached to the intercondylar eminence at their anterior and posterior horns and at their periphery to the tibial condyles by short ligamentous fibres, the **coronary ligaments.** The medial meniscus is also closely attached to the joint capsule, and particularly to the tibial collateral ligament of the knee, and is therefore less mobile than the lateral meniscus. This reduced mobility renders the medial meniscus more liable to injury during sudden rotatory strains of the knee

The **anterior cruciate ligament** passes upwards, laterally and backwards from the anterior part of the intercondylar eminence to be attached to the medial surface of the lateral femoral condyle. The **posterior cruciate ligament** passes

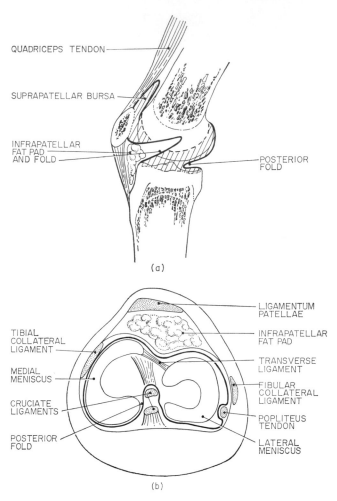

(a)

(b)

FIG. 24.17. Synovial membrane of the knee joint in vertical (a) and horizontal (b) section.

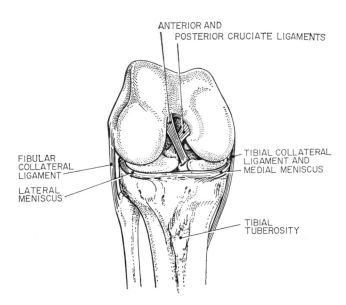

FIG. 24.16. The cruciate ligaments. The joint is viewed from the front after removing the patella and ligamentum patellae.

joint such as may occur during a game of football. The lateral meniscus moves during such strains, while the more fixed medial cartilage is subject to shearing forces and may tear, particularly towards its posterior part. The **transverse ligament** is a small ligament joining the anterior parts of the medial and lateral menisci (fig. 24.17b).

The poor coaptation of the femoral and tibial articular surfaces makes the joint potentially unstable in the anteroposterior direction. The **cruciate ligaments** (figs. 24.16 and 17b) play an important part in preventing dislocation in these directions. They are attached to the intercondylar eminence of the tibia below and pass upwards to the internal surfaces of the two femoral condyles. As they ascend they cross each other and so earn the name cruciate.

upwards, forwards and medially from the most posterior part of the intercondylar eminence to be attached to the lateral surface of the medial femoral condyle. While these two ligaments are relatively taut in all stages of joint movement, they are most taut when the knee is fully extended. The anterior ligament prevents backward displacement of the femur on the tibia, while the posterior ligament blocks anterior displacement of the femur on the tibia.

The **synovial membrane of the knee joint** lines the capsule of the joint and covers all those structures which lie within the capsule, but which do not intervene between the articulating surfaces. Superiorly it bulges above the patella, deep to the quadriceps tendon, forming the suprapatellar bursa. (fig. 24.17a). When there is an excess of fluid in the joint, e.g. in an infection or following trauma, this bursa becomes prominent and may be easily demonstrated clinically. An infrapatellar fat pad lies posterior to the ligamentum patellae and is surrounded by synovial membrane. This forms a tent-like **infrapatellar fold**, which runs upwards and backwards to be attached by its apex to the intercondylar fossa of the femur (fig. 24.17b). The relationships of the synovial membrane are shown in fig. 24.17 where it is seen that the intra-articular structures, with the exception of the menisci, are in fact extrasynovial.

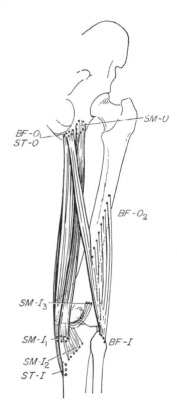

FIG. 24.18. Hamstring muscles.

Biceps femoris (*BF*)

BF–O₁ Long head: medial part of ischial tuber with *ST–O*.
BF–O₂ Short head: linea aspera.
BF–I Apex of head of fibula.

Semitendinosus (*ST*)

ST–O Medial part of ischial tuber.
ST–I Upper part of medial surface of tibia (fig. 24.21).

Semimembranosus (*SM*)

SM–O Lateral part of ischial tuber.
SM–I₁ Groove on back of medial condyle of tibia.
SM–I₂ Through fascia over popliteus to the soleal line.
SM–I₃ Oblique posterior ligament of knee joint (fig. 24.15e).

MUSCLES OF THE KNEE REGION

Extension is achieved by vastus medialis, lateralis, intermedius and rectus femoris, which combine to form quadriceps (figs. 24.8, 19 and 20). Flexion is due mainly to the hamstrings (fig.24.18), with some assistance from

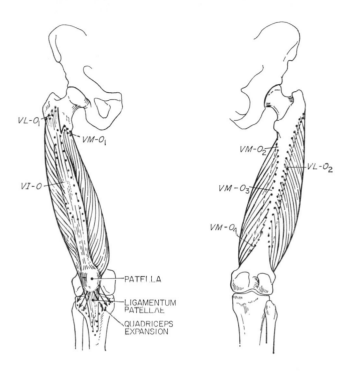

FIG. 24.19. Extensor muscles of the knee.

Vastus medialis (*VM*)

VM–O₁ Intertrochanteric line.
VM–O₂ Spiral line.
VM–O₃ Medial edge of linea aspera.
VM–O₄ Medial supracondylar line and adductor magnus tendon.

Vastus lateralis (*VL*)

VL–O₁ Anterior surface of greater trochanter.
VL–O₂ Lateral edge of linea aspera.

Vastus intermedius (*VI*)

VI–O Anterior and lateral surfaces of the shaft of femur.
With rectus femoris (fig. 24.8) they are inserted into the patella (fig. 24.17a) and thence to the tibial tuberosity as ligamentum patellae with expansions to adjoining parts of upper end of tibia.

gracilis and sartorius (figs. 24.8, 9 and 21). The calf muscles, gastrocnemius and plantaris, also assist in flexion of the knee (fig. 24.31). The popliteus is partially intra-articular and plays an important part in initiating flexion at the knee joint by laterally rotating the femur on the tibia (fig. 24.22).

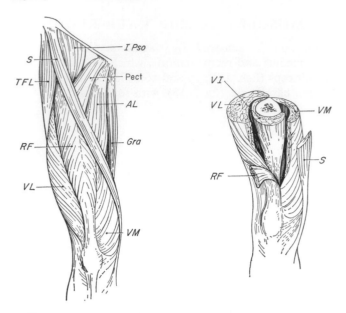

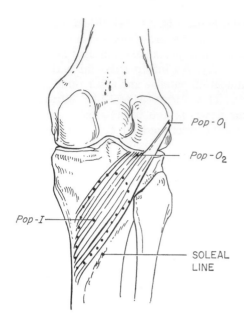

FIG. 24.20. Muscles of the thigh. In the right diagram the rectus femoris muscle has been turned forwards to reveal vastus intermedius.

FIG. 24.22. **Popliteus** (*Pop*)

Pop–O₁ Pit at anterior end of groove on lateral condyle.
Pop–O₂ Lateral meniscus.
Pop–I Posterior surface of tibia above soleal line.

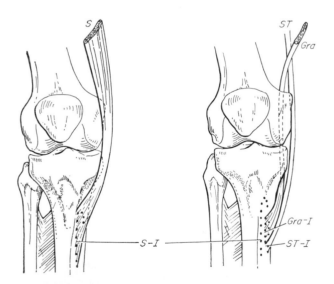

FIG. 24.21. Insertions of sartorius (*S–I*), gracilis (*Gra–I*) and semitendinosus (*ST–I*) to the anteromedial surface of tibia.

MOVEMENTS AT THE KNEE JOINT

The knee is a hinge joint and its principal movements are flexion and extension. It is not, however, a typical hinge joint, since the femoral condyles both roll and glide on the tibial articular surfaces and the axis of movement is not a fixed one. Furthermore, rotatory movements, both active and passive, can occur between femur and tibia.

When the joint is fully flexed as, for example, in the squatting position, the posterior surfaces of the femoral condyles are in contact with the posterior part of the tibial articular surfaces and of the menisci. As the knee is extended, the two femoral condyles roll parallel to each other on the tibia and its menisci. The changing radii of curvature of the two condyles are accommodated by elastic deformation of the menisci. The contact surface of each condyle with the tibia moves forwards, until the rolling of the lateral condyle is halted when a groove on its tibial articular surface comes in contact with the anterior edge of the lateral meniscus. The medial condyle continues to roll forwards, wheeling around a vertical axis which passes through the lateral condyle. This movement, which produces medial rotation of the femur relative to the tibia, is finally halted by tension of all the strong ligaments of the joint. The anterior margin of the medial meniscus now fits into a groove on the tibial articular surface of the medial condyle. The joint is now said to be 'locked' in full extension; this is the most stable position of the joint.

Before flexion of the knee from the fully extended position can begin, this medial rotation of the femur must be reversed to unlock the joint. The necessary lateral rotation of femur on the tibia is achieved by popliteus, whose tendinous attachment to the lateral femoral condyle pulls back the lateral condyle, while the muscular attachment to the posterior part of the lateral meniscus prevents this portion of the meniscus being damaged. Once this rotation has occurred, simple flexion may begin and can continue until the calf muscles come into contact with the posterior thigh muscles.

Medial rotation of the tibia on the femur, especially in the flexed knee, is due to the sartorius, gracilis and semitendinosus muscles with biceps femoris opposing this movement.

The patella increases the leverage of the quadriceps muscle in extending the knee from the fully flexed position. When this extension is proceeding, the patella is jammed hard against the femoral condyles and is immobile from side to side. When the quadriceps muscle is relaxed, the patella is freely mobile from side to side. The patella occasionally has to be removed surgically and, although the quadriceps muscle functions remarkably well in its absence, the power of knee extension never quite matches that of the normal side.

The femur makes a laterally oriented oblique angle with the tibia and so contraction of the quadriceps muscle tends to dislocate the patella towards the lateral side (fig. 24.19). This is normally prevented by the more prominent lateral margin to the patellar groove on the femur and by the medial pull of the lowest fibres of vastus medialis $(VM-O_4)$. Nevertheless lateral dislocation of the patella is more common in women as their femora are more oblique.

BONES AND JOINTS OF THE LEG

BONES OF THE LEG

The lower end of the tibia (fig. 24.23) is a continuation of the triangular shaft, which is thinnest about the junction of the middle and lower thirds of the bone and thickens

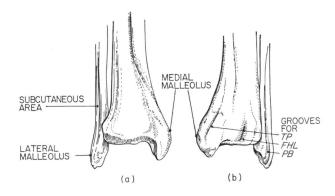

FIG. 24.23. Lower ends of right tibia and fibula, (a) anterior, (b) posterior views. *TP*, tibialis posterior; *FHL*, flexor hallucis longus; *PB*, peroneus brevis.

towards the lower end where it becomes four-sided. The subcutaneous medial surface becomes the **medial malleolus,** which is easily felt at the medial side of the ankle. The lateral surface of the malleolus is smooth and has an

articular surface, continuous with that on the distal surface of the bone, for articulation with the talus. The lateral surface is characterized by the triangular **fibular notch** into which the lower end of fibula is firmly attached by a fibrous interosseous ligament.

The shaft of the fibula continues downwards to the distal end of the bone (fig. 24.23) which is named the **lateral malleolus.** This is easily palpable and visible on the lateral aspect of the ankle joint and is pyramidal in shape. The subcutaneous lateral surface is smooth and convex, and it extends to a slightly lower level than the medial malleolus. The medial surface has a large articular area for articulation with the lateral surface of the talus, while above this there is a rough area for attachment of the interosseous tibiofibular ligament. Posterior to the articular area, a deep malleolar fossa indents the medial surface of the malleolus. The posterior surface of the malleolus is grooved for the peroneus brevis and peroneus longus tendons.

JOINTS OF THE LEG

Proximal tibiofibular joint

The head of the fibula articulates with the lateral condyle of the tibia by a small plane synovial joint. It is surrounded by a circular capsular ligament and allows only slight gliding movements of the head of the fibula when stress is applied to the ankle joint.

Interosseous membrane

The interosseous membrane, which stretches between the interosseous borders of the tibia and fibula, is similar to that in the forearm.

Distal tibiofibular joint (figs. 24.27 and 28)

This is a very strong fibrous joint. The lower ends of the tibia and fibula are held together by the thick **interosseous ligament** passing between the floor of the fibular notch of the tibia and the rough area on the medial surface of the fibula above the lateral malleolus. Three further ligaments are associated with this joint; the strong **anterior** and **posterior tibiofibular ligaments** stretch downwards and laterally from the anterior and posterior margins of the lower end of the tibia to the anterior and posterior surfaces of the lateral malleolus, and the **transverse tibiofibular ligament** passes from the posterior margin of the lower end of the tibia to the malleolar fossa on the lateral malleolus.

These ligaments maintain the integrity of the ankle joint, as they prevent the tendency for the talus to be forced upwards between the malleoli during weight bearing. If the upward force becomes too great, as in landing on the feet from a great height, the ligaments may rupture and the tibia and fibula are split apart.

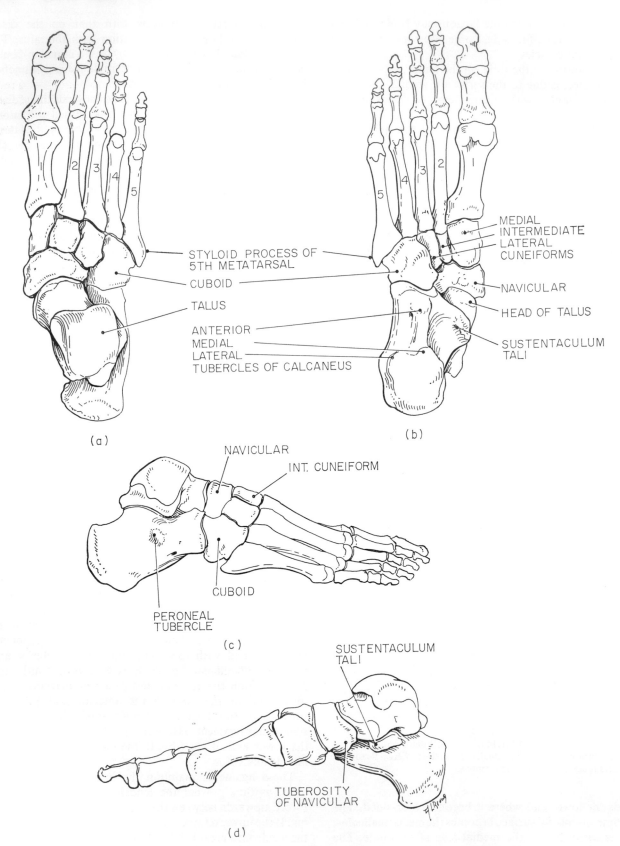

STYLOID PROCESS OF
5TH METATARSAL

CUBOID

TALUS

ANTERIOR
MEDIAL
LATERAL
TUBERCLES OF CALCANEUS

MEDIAL
INTERMEDIATE
LATERAL
CUNEIFORMS

NAVICULAR

HEAD OF TALUS

SUSTENTACULUM
TALI

(a)

(b)

NAVICULAR

INT. CUNEIFORM

CUBOID

PERONEAL
TUBERCLE

(c)

SUSTENTACULUM
TALI

TUBEROSITY
OF NAVICULAR

(d)

FIG. 24.24. Skeleton of right foot, (a) superior, (b) inferior, (c) lateral, (d) medial views.

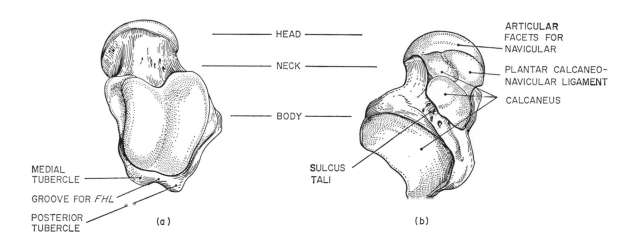

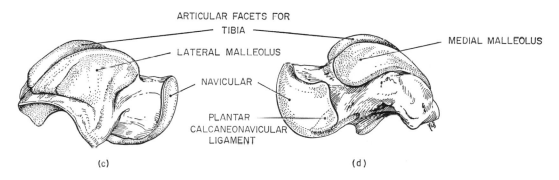

FIG. 24.25. Right talus, (a) superior, (b) inferior, (c) lateral, (d) medial views.

BONES, JOINTS AND MUSCLES OF THE FOOT

BONES OF THE FOOT

These consist of the tarsal and metatarsal bones and the phalanges (fig. 24.24).

Tarsus

There are seven tarsal bones (cf. eight carpal bones).

The **talus** (fig. 24.25) provides the link between the leg bones, tibia and fibula, and the remaining bones of the foot. It has no direct muscular attachments. The talus consists of a body and a head joined by a narrow neck. The body lies posteriorly and fits between the malleoli, articulating with them and with the distal end of the tibia superiorly. The superior articular surface tapers posteriorly and is convex anteroposteriorly and slightly concave from side to side.

A large articular area on the lateral surface articulates with the lateral malleolus and is continuous with the superior articular surface. A smaller comma-shaped facet for articulation with the medial malleolus is on the medial side and is also continuous with the superior articular surface. These three contiguous articular surfaces are known as the **trochlear surface** of the talus and are surrounded by the attachments of the capsule of the ankle joint. Like the articular surface on the distal end of the tibia, the trochlear surface is wider anteriorly.

The inferior surface is concave and articulates with the posterior articular facet on the calcaneus. The posterior margin of the inferior surface bears two projections, the posterior and medial tubercles, with a groove between them for the tendon of flexor hallucis longus.

The head of the talus is directed anteromedially. It is hemispherical and covered by articular cartilage. It articulates with the navicular bone anteriorly, the anterior and middle calcaneal facets inferiorly and the plantar calcaneonavicular (spring) ligament which lies between the navicular bone and the sustentaculum tali (fig. 24.30). Between the middle and posterior calcaneal facets is a deep groove, the **sulcus tali.**

The **calcaneus** (fig. 24.26), or heel bone, has six irregular surfaces and is roughly rectangular in shape. The posterior part of this bone forms the prominence of the heel. The **sustentaculum tali** projects from the upper part of the

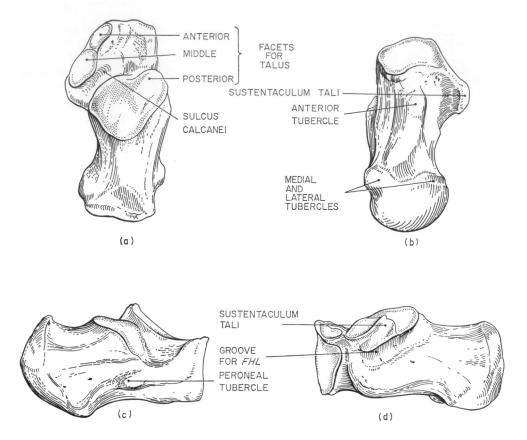

FIG. 24.26. Right calcaneus, (a) superior, (b) inferior, (c) lateral, (d) medial views.

medial surface. The lateral surface bears a short ridge, the **peroneal tubercle,** which separates the tendons of peroneus longus and brevis. Anteriorly, the calcaneus articulates with the cuboid bone. The tendo calcaneus is attached to the posterior surface in its middle third and there is a smooth area above this where a bursa lies between the tendon and the bone.

The upper surface bears three articular facets; the posterior articulates with the body of talus, and the middle and anterior articulate with the head of talus.

The middle facet lies on the upper aspect of the sustentaculum tali, and is separated from the posterior facet by a deep sulcus, the **sulcus calcanei.** This corresponds to the sulcus tali, so that when the bones are articulating, a narrow non-articular cleft, the **canalis tarsi,** is formed. This contains only fat, a few small vessels and a few weak ligamentous fibres. The main bond between the talus and calcaneus is a strong **interosseous talocalcaneal cervical ligament.** This runs between the under surface of the neck of the talus and the upper surface of the neck of the calcaneus and lies in the **sinus tarsi.**

The inferior surface is concave and ridged and bears three tubercles, the anterior tubercle, and the medial and lateral posterior tubercles.

The **navicular** bone lies between the head of the talus posteriorly, and the three cuneiform bones. Its posterior surface is concave and smooth, while its anterior surface has three facets for the cuneiforms. A prominent tuberosity arises from its medial surface, and this may be palpated about 2 cm below and anterior to the medial malleolus.

The **cuboid** bone is a large bone, described by its name, which lies on the lateral side of the foot between the calcaneus posteriorly, and the fourth and fifth metatarsals anteriorly. There is a prominent groove on the anterior part of the inferior surface through which the peroneus longus tendon passes.

The three **cuneiform** bones are wedge shaped and articulate with the navicular posteriorly, and with the bases of the first three metatarsals anteriorly. The medial cuneiform is the largest, and it is narrowest superiorly, while the intermediate and lateral bones are narrower inferiorly. The intermediate bone is shorter than the other two, so that the base of the second metatarsal lies more proximally than the other metatarsals and thus it also articulates with the sides of the medial and lateral cuneiforms. This feature complicates the operation of disarticulation through the tarsometatarsal joint.

Metatarsals and phalanges

These are similar to the metacarpal bones and phalanges of the hands (p. 23.15), but some differences are worth noting.

With the exception of the first, the metatarsals are longer and more slender than the metacarpals. The articular base of the first metatarsal is not saddle shaped. The fifth metatarsal has a styloid process projecting from the lateral side of its base which is easily palpable. The phalanges of the toes are shorter than in the fingers, and the fifth toe frequently has only two phalanges.

ANKLE JOINT

Ankle (tibiotarsal) joint (figs. 24.27 and 28)

The ankle joint is a synovial joint of the hinge variety. The trochlear surface of the talus fits between the malleoli and articulates with them and the distal surface of the tibia. The posterior tibiofibular ligament completes the socket posteriorly.

As this is a hinge joint, the medial and lateral ligaments are strong. The medial ligament is named the **deltoid ligament** on account of its shape. Proximally it is attached to the distal end of the medial malleolus and it fans out distally to be attached to the upper surface of the navicular bone, the neck of the talus, the plantar calcaneonavicular (spring) ligament, the sustentaculum tali and the medial

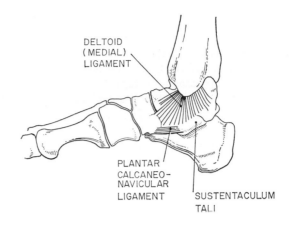

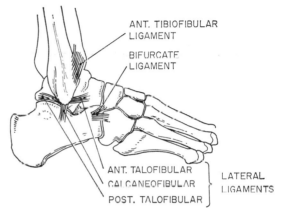

FIG. 24.28. Ligaments around the ankle.

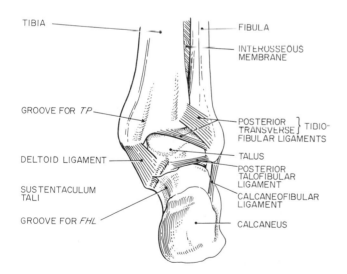

FIG. 24.27. Posterior view of the right ankle joint.

surface of body of talus. The **lateral ligament** extends from the distal end of the lateral malleolus and is divided into three parts, the posterior talofibular, calcaneofibular and anterior talofibular ligaments (fig. 24.28).

The anterior and posterior parts of the joint capsule are

relatively weak to allow the movements of flexion and extension. The synovial membrane lines the interior of the joint capsule.

Because the trochlear surface of the talus is wider anteriorly than posteriorly, this surface is gripped more tightly between the malleoli when the foot is dorsiflexed than when it is plantarflexed. With the foot in plantar flexion the slight side-to-side rocking movements of the talus contribute to abduction and adduction of the foot.

Tarsal joints

The individual tarsal joints are joints of varying degrees of complexity, at any one of which movement is relatively slight. Their summation however, results in the movements of **inversion** and **eversion**. Functionally, the most important joints in this respect are the joints between the talus above and the calcaneus and navicular below.

TALOCALCANEAN JOINT

This is a synovial joint between the concave facet on the inferior surface of the body of the talus and the posterior convex facet on the calcaneus.

THE TALOCALCANEONAVICULAR JOINT

This synovial joint is of the ball and socket variety. The head of the talus lies in the socket which is made by the navicular bone anteriorly, by the middle and anterior articular facets of the calcaneus posteriorly, and inferomedially between these two by the **plantar calcaneonavicular (spring) ligament** (fig. 24.29). This strong ligament passes

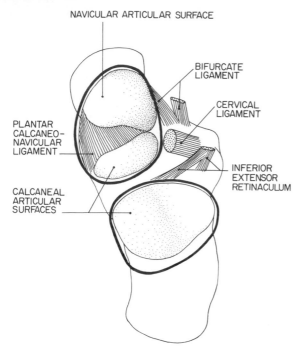

FIG. 24.29. Articular contacts of talus at the talocalcaneonavicular and subtalar joints, exposed by removal of the talus.

between the sustentaculum tali posteriorly and the tuberosity and inferior margin of navicular anteriorly. Its upper surface is articular and is covered by a thick layer of fibrocartilage.

A fibrous capsule surrounds the joint, and this is supported medially by the navicular extension of the deltoid ligament and laterally by the navicular extension of the bifurcate ligament (fig. 24.28).

Though anatomically the talocalcanean and talocalcaneonavicular joints are separate, they act functionally as the **subtalar** joint, allowing movements of the calcaneus, and so the rest of the foot, around an axis which passes from the point of the heel up through the neck of the talus (fig. 24.37).

MIDTARSAL JOINT

The articulation between the head of the talus and the navicular lies roughly in the same transverse line in the foot as the articulation between the calcaneus and cuboid. Though these articulations have separate joint cavities and capsules, they function as one unit, the midtarsal

joint; movements at this joint are additive to the movements of the calcaneus (p. 24.23) at the talocalcaneonavicular and talocalcanean joints. This is because the muscles which produce these movements of the calcaneus are all attached to the foot in front of the midtarsal joint. The midtarsal joint has three important accessory ligaments (figs. 24.28 and 30).

The **short plantar ligament** is a thick ligament which passes between the anterior tubercle of the calcaneus and the posterior ridge of the groove on the cuboid. The **bifurcate ligament** is attached posteriorly to the upper surface of the calcaneus behind its anterior margin, and bifurcates anteriorly; the medial limb is attached

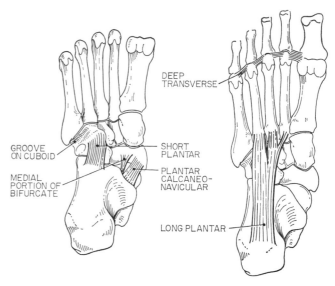

FIG. 24.30. Ligaments of the sole of the foot.

to the inferomedial aspect of the navicular, and forms part of the socket for the head of the talus; the lateral limb is attached to the upper surface of cuboid. The **long plantar ligament**, lying superficial to the short plantar ligament, is attached posteriorly to the plantar surface of the calcaneus and passes forwards to be attached to the bases of the middle three metatarsals. Some deeper fibres are attached to both anterior and posterior margins of the groove in the cuboid, converting this into a tunnel for peroneus longus tendon.

The remaining intertarsal joints do not warrant special description, other than to state that the plantar aspects of their joint capsules are always stronger than the dorsal aspects.

TARSOMETATARSAL JOINTS

These joints are relatively immobile, plane, synovial joints. The first is the most mobile, while the second, being wedged between medial and lateral cuneiforms, is the least mobile. This fact may account for the frequency with which

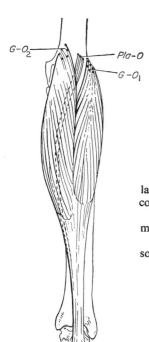

FIG. 24.31. Muscles of the calf.

Gastrocnemius (G)

G–O₁ Lateral head: upper part of lateral surface of lateral femoral condyle, and lower part of lateral supracondylar line.

G–O₂ Medial head: popliteal surface of femur above medial condyle.

G–I Tendo calcaneus in company with plantaris and soleus (*Sol* fig. 24.32).

Plantaris (Pla)

Pla–O Popliteal surface of femur above lateral condyle.
Pla–I Medial side of tendo calcaneus.

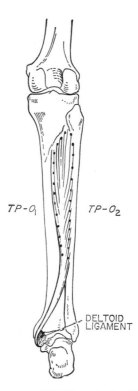

FIG. 24.33. **Tibialis posterior (TP)**

TP–O₁ Lateral part of upper two-thirds of posterior surface of tibia below soleal line.

TP–O₂ Posterior surface of fibula and interosseous membrane.

TP–I See figs. 24.34 and 38.

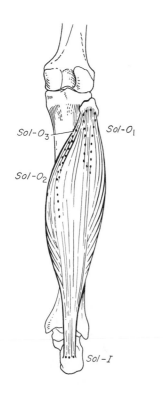
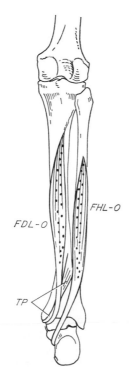

FIG. 24.32. Muscles of the calf.

Soleus (Sol)

Sol–O₁ Posterior surface of upper one-quarter of fibula.
Sol–O₂ Soleal line of tibia.
Sol–O₃ Tendinous arch between O₁ and O₂.
Sol–I Middle one-third of posterior surface of calcaneus after joining gastrocnemius to form tendo calcaneus.

Flexor digitorum longus (FDL)

FDL–O Upper two-thirds of posterior surface of tibia below soleal line and medial to *TP–O₁* (fig. 24.33).
FDL–I See figs. 24.34 and 38.

Flexor hallucis longus (FHL)

FHL–O Lower two-thirds of posterior surface of fibula.
FHL–I See figs. 24.34 and 38.

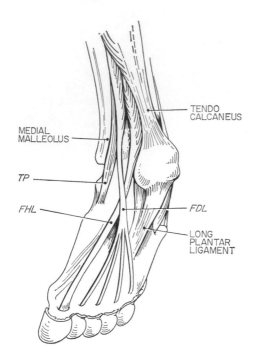

FIG. 24.34. Arrangement of tendons of deep calf muscles.

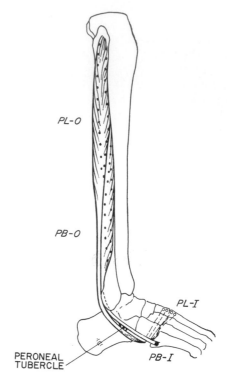

FIG. 24.36. The peroneal muscles.

Peroneus longus (PL)

PL–O Upper two-thirds of lateral surface of fibula.

PL–I Base of first metatarsal and medial cuneiform bone. Its tendon runs in a deep groove on the plantar aspect of the cuboid.

Peroneus brevis (PB)

PB–O Lower two-thirds of lateral surface of fibula.

PB–I Tuberosity on base of fifth metatarsal. Its tendon lies in a groove on the posterior aspect of the lateral malleolus.

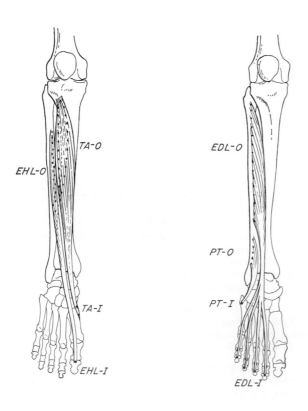

FIG. 24.35. Muscles of the anterior compartment of the leg.

Extensor hallucis longus (EHL)

EHL–O Anterior surface of fibula and adjacent interosseous membrane.

EHL–I Base of distal phalanx of big toe. This muscle lies between extensor digitorum longus and tibialis anterior and is partially concealed by them.

Tibialis anterior (TA)

TA–O Upper two-thirds of lateral surface of shaft of tibia.

TA–I Medial surface of medial cuneiform and base of first metatarsal.

Extensor digitorum longus (EDL)

EDL–O Upper two-thirds of anterior surface of fibula.
EDL–I Bones of the toes and extensor expansions.

Peroneus tertius (PT)

PT–O Lower one-third of anterior surface of fibula.
PT–I Base of fifth metatarsal.

the second metatarsal is fractured (march fracture) during relatively light exercise.

Metatarsophalangeal and interphalangeal joints

Though less mobile than the corresponding joints of the fingers, these joints resemble them closely in structure and function. The heads of the metatarsals are bound together by a deep transverse ligament which unites the plantar thickenings of all the joint capsules.

The movements at these joints are very similar to those in the hand, though the range of movement is smaller.

The big toe or hallux is considerably less mobile than the thumb, though it has similar muscle attachments. Its main functions are concerned with weight distribution and with propulsion during walking or running; hence there are sesamoid bones in the tendons of flexor hallucis brevis. Thus since stability rather than mobility is required, the deep transverse ligament of the foot connects the metatarsophalangeal joint of the hallux to that of the second toe, whereas the thumb is free of such restraint.

MUSCLES AND MOVEMENTS OF THE ANKLE

The ankle joint is essentially a hinge joint and provides mainly for the movements of dorsiflexion and plantarflexion. Dorsiflexion at the joint is produced by muscles passing to the foot anterior to the ankle joint, i.e. tibialis anterior, extensor hallucis longus, extensor digitorum longus and peroneus tertius (fig. 24.35). This movement results in elevation of the forefoot and lowering of the heel.

The opposite movement of plantarflexion is produced by calf muscles gastrocnemius, plantaris and soleus (figs. 24.31 and 32), assisted by tibialis posterior (fig. 24.33), flexor digitorum and flexor hallucis longus (fig. 24.32), and the peroneal muscles (fig. 24.36).

It has been noted already that the trochlear surface of the talus is rather broader anteriorly than posteriorly, so that in dorsiflexion, the talus fits more compactly between the malleoli; in fact dorsiflexion is limited by this locking mechanism. The joint is most stable in this position.

MOVEMENTS OF THE FOOT

Four movements may be described; adduction occurs when the foot is moved horizontally towards a line running forwards between the feet, abduction when it is moved horizontally away from this line; inversion takes place as the medial border of the foot is raised so that the sole of the foot tends to face medially, and eversion when the lateral border of the foot is raised so that the sole tends to face laterally.

Though these movements may be quite separate, adduction and inversion are frequently combined, as are ab-

duction and eversion. Inversion is produced mainly by tibialis posterior and tibialis anterior assisted by flexor hallucis longus. The principal evertors of the foot are the peroneal muscles. These muscles are all attached to the foot in front of the midtarsal joint, and the major part of these two movements occurs at the subtalar joint around an oblique axis (fig. 24.37). This can be checked by the

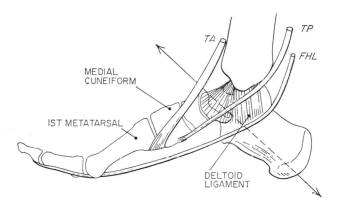

FIG. 24.37. The muscles which produce inversion, and the axis of inversion and eversion.

student if he attempts inversion or eversion while holding his own calcaneus still with the hand. Minor gliding movements at the other tarsal joints add only slightly to the range of movement achieved. The major functional importance of the inverting and everting muscles is in walking over rough ground, when they balance the body on the foot, acting 'in reverse', from their insertions in the foot to their origins in the leg.

Adduction and abduction of the forefoot are relatively limited movements, more particularly in the dorsiflexed position. Tibialis anterior and posterior are the principal adductors, assisted by the long muscles to the big toe, while peroneus longus and brevis are the important abductors. Movements of the toes are similar to but much less important than those at the fingers. The intrinsic muscles of the foot and the long flexors and extensors of the toes are shown in figs. 24.38 and 39.

In considering the movements of abduction and adduction of the toes, the line of reference passes along the second toe and not, as in the case of the hand, along the third digit. Thus the arrangement of the interossei muscles is slightly different (fig. 24.38). The plantar interossei adduct, and the dorsal interossei abduct as in the hand; however, the second toe cannot be adducted into itself and so has no plantar interossei. Since the hallux has its own adductor, there are only three plantar interossei, which pass to the lateral three toes. The hallux and the fifth toe have their own abductors. The second toe has attached to it the medial two dorsal interossei, while the lateral two muscles pass to the lateral sides of the third and fourth toe respectively.

First (superficial) layer

Abductor digiti minimi (ADM)

ADM–O Medial and lateral tubercles of calcaneus.

ADM–I Lateral side of base of proximal phalanx of the little toe.

Flexor digitorum brevis (FDB)

FDB–O Medial tubercle of calcaneus.

FDB–I Palmar surface of base of middle phalanx of second, third, fourth and fifth toes. The tendons split to allow the *FDL* tendons to reach the distal phalanx.

Abductor hallucis (AbH)

AbH–O Medial tubercle of calcaneus.

AbH–I Medial side of base of proximal phalanx of the big toe.

Second layer

Flexor digitorum longus (FDL)

FDL–O Posterior surface of tibia.

FDL–I Base of distal phalanges after passing through the split in the tendon of flexor digitorum brevis.

Flexor hallucis longus (FHL)

FHL–O Posterior surface of fibula.

FHL–I Base of distal phalanx of big toe.

Flexor digitorum accessorius (FDA)

FDA–O$_1$ Lateral edge of plantar surface of calcaneus.

FDA–O$_2$ Long plantar ligament and medial surface of calcaneus.

FDA–I Tendon of *FDL*.

Lumbricals (L)

L–O Tendons of flexor digitorum longus.

L–I Extensor expansions.

Third layer

Flexor digiti minimi brevis (FDM)

FDM–O Base of fifth metatarsal and long plantar ligament.

FDM–I Lateral side of base of proximal phalanx of the little toe with *ADM*.

Adductor hallucis (AdH)

AdH–O$_1$ Transverse head; palmar aspect of joint casules of second, third, fourth and fifth metatarsophalangeal joints.

AdH–O$_2$ Oblique head: long plantar ligament and bases of metatarsals 2–4.

AdH–I Lateral side of base of proximal phalanx of the big toe, together with *FHB*.

Flexor hallucis brevis (FHB)

FHB–O Cuboid and lateral two cuneiforms.

FHB–I Medial and lateral sides of base of the proximal phalanx of the big toe in association with adductor hallucis (*AdH*) and abductor hallucis (*AbH*).

Fourth layer

Peroneus longus (PL)

PL–O Upper two-thirds of fibula.

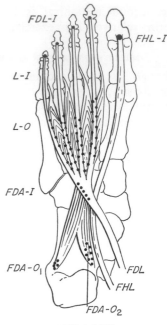
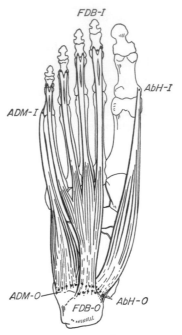

FIRST LAYER

SECOND LAYER

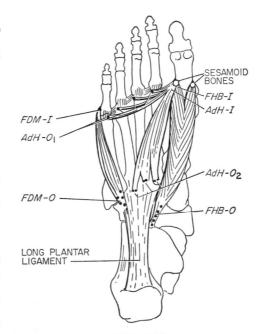
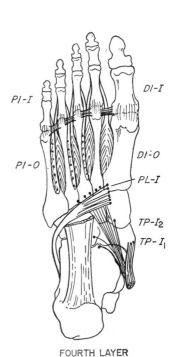

THIRD LAYER

FOURTH LAYER

FIG. 24.38. The muscles in the sole of the foot.

PL–I Base of first metatarsal and medial cuneiform bone.

Tibialis posterior (TP)

TP–O Posterior surface of interosseous membrane (fig. 24.33).

TP–I$_1$ Tuberosity of the navicular.

TP–I$_2$ All the bones of the tarsus, except the talus, and the bases of the second, third and fourth metatarsals.

Plantar interossei (PI)

PI–O Medial side of the plantar aspect of third, fourth and fifth metatarsals.

PI–I Medial side of the extensor expansions.

Dorsal interossei (DI)

DI–O Contiguous sides of metatarsals.

DI–I As shown with their centre of action at the second toe (cf. fig. 24.48).

The flexor digitorum accessorius muscle (fig. 24.38) has no counterpart in the hand. It alters the line of pull of the flexor digitorum tendons from a slightly oblique angle so that they act along the longitudinal line of the toes thus increasing efficiency, but it is probably more important in producing flexion of the toes when the long flexor muscles are at a mechanical disadvantage, in full plantar flexion of the ankle.

ARCHES OF THE FOOT

The normal foot displays a well-marked longitudinal arching which is present from birth. The medial side of the foot is normally arched more prominently than the lateral side so that there is also a transverse arch of the foot, this arch being completed by the transverse arch of the other foot when standing with the feet together.

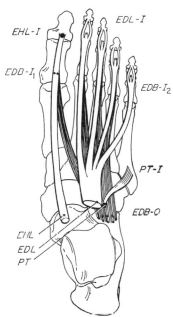

FIG. 24.39. Muscles of the dorsum of the foot.

Extensor digitorum brevis (EDB)
EDB–O Anterior part of upper surface of calcaneus.
EDB–I₁ Dorsal surface of base of proximal phalanx of the big toe.
EDB–I₂ Extensor expansions of second, third and fourth toes.

Extensor hallucis longus (EHL)
EHL–O Anterior surface of fibula (fig. 24.35).
EHL–I Dorsal surface of base of distal phalanx of the big toe.

Extensor digitorum longus (EDL)
EDL–O Anterior surface of fibula (fig. 24.35).
EDL–I Extensor expansions of second, third, fourth and fifth toes.

Peroneus tertius (PT)
PT–O Anterior surface of fibula (fig. 24.35).
PT–I Base of fifth metatarsal.

The **longitudinal arch** is in two parts (fig. 24.40); the medial longitudinal arch consists of the talus, calcaneus, navicular, cuneiforms, metatarsals and phalanges of the medial three toes. The lateral longitudinal arch consists of the calcaneus, cuboid, metatarsals and phalanges of the lateral two toes.

The **transverse arch** is most marked at the height of the longitudinal arches, namely across the distal row of tarsal bones.

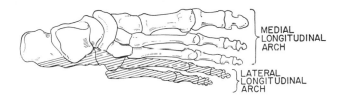

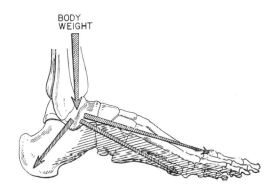

FIG. 24.40. The longitudinal arches of the foot and the directions of weight transmission.

Although the longitudinal and transverse arches form part of a unitary mechanism, there are differences in the relative importance of the factors which maintain each of them.

The integrity of the medial and lateral longitudinal arches is maintained by complementary muscular and ligamentous mechanisms:

(1) the plantar aponeurosis, flexor digitorum brevis and the long plantar ligament; the latter acts like a bowstring between the posterior tubercles of the calcaneus and the bases of the metatarsals;

(2) the plantar calcaneonavicular ligament; this completes the socket for the head of the talus and, supported below by the tendon of tibialis posterior, limits downward displacement of the head of the talus;

(3) extrinsic muscles of the foot, which may be divided into two groups; first, those which maintain an upward pull on the arches, i.e. the tibialis anterior and posterior which act on the medial arch and the peroneus brevis and tertius which act on the lateral arch; second, the long flexor tendons which function as bowstring supports, and

(4) the short muscles of great and little toes.

The integrity of the transverse arch is similarly maintained by muscles and ligaments:

(1) the transverse metatarsal ligaments and the transverse head of adductor hallucis;

(2) the dorsal interossei which bunch up the metatarsals, assisted by the oblique pull of the oblique head of adductor hallucis and of the flexor hallucis brevis, and

(3) the bowstring support of the tendon of peroneus longus.

In addition the shape of the bones is of major importance in the maintenance of the transverse arch (fig. 24.41a and b). The wedge-shaped bones, bound together by strong interosseous and plantar ligaments, may truly be likened to a stone arch. The medial longitudinal arch has also been regarded as an architectural arch, with the talus as the keystone. However, the comparison is erroneous. The articular facets of the bones which form the medial longitudinal arch are reciprocally curved and the arch is a dynamic one, becoming flatter when loaded. This is in marked contrast to a true architectural arch, which is a static arch, whose constituent wedge-shaped blocks meet at plane surfaces, and which may collapse but not flatten under load. The foot arches may also alter in active foot movement; in inversion

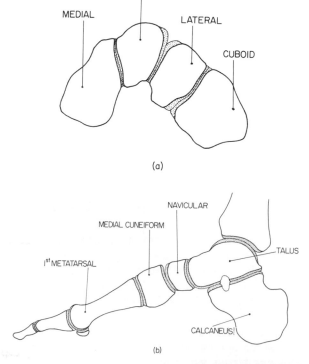

CUNEIFORMS:

MEDIAL — INTERMEDIATE — LATERAL — CUBOID

(a)

NAVICULAR

MEDIAL CUNEIFORM

1st METATARSAL — TALUS

CALCANEUS

(b)

FIG. 24.41. (a) Transverse section through tarsal bones showing how their wedge shape contributes to the transverse arch. (b) Section through medial longitudinal arch to show reciprocal curvature of articular surfaces.

the medial longitudinal arch is heightened, in eversion it is lowered.

The arches of the foot distribute the weight of the body from the tibia and hence talus to the ground over as wide an area as possible. This reduces the pressure on individual areas of the foot. The mechanism is illustrated by fig. 24.40. The jointed nature of the arches confers spring to the foot, which increases the propulsive efficiency of the foot during walking; this resilience absorbs the shock during weight transference. The arches also protect the nerves and vessels running in the sole of the foot.

MECHANISMS OF STANDING, WALKING AND RUNNING

Posture and standing

When standing erect 'at attention', the centre of gravity of the body is just in front of the second piece of the sacrum. The effective body weight thus acts along a perpendicular line from this point to the ground (fig. 24.4). This line passes just behind the hip joints and just in front of the knee joint and the ankle joint. Thus the trunk tends to fall backwards at the hip joint and forwards in front of the knee joint and ankle joint, producing extension at the hip joint and the knee joint, and dorsiflexion at the ankle joint.

These tendencies bring each of these major joints into its most stable position:

(1) the strong iliofemoral ligament of the hip joint is tightest in extension;

(2) the final phase of extension at the knee joint is accompanied by a medial rotation of the femur on the tibia, which tightens all the ligaments of the knee joint, and

(3) dorsiflexion at the ankle brings the broadest portion of the trochlear surface of the talus between the malleoli.

When standing in such a position, electromyography of the leg muscles reveals remarkably little muscular activity. However, minor alterations in the posture cause a stabilizing activity of muscles around these joints.

If the weight of an individual is taken as 24 equal arbitrary units, 12 units are transmitted through each ankle in normal standing. In each foot, 6 units are transmitted to the heel and 6 units in all to the metatarsals, 2 units to the metatarsal of the great toe and 1 unit to each of the other four metatarsals (fig. 24.42a).

The supporting area provided by the two feet in normal standing is shown in fig. 24.42b. A perpendicular dropped from the body's centre of gravity reaches the ground midway between the two navicular bones (CG) and lateral stability depends on the maintenance of that situation. Because the line of body weight falls in front of the axes of the ankle joints, there is a constant tendency for the legs to tilt forward at the ankle joints; this state of forward

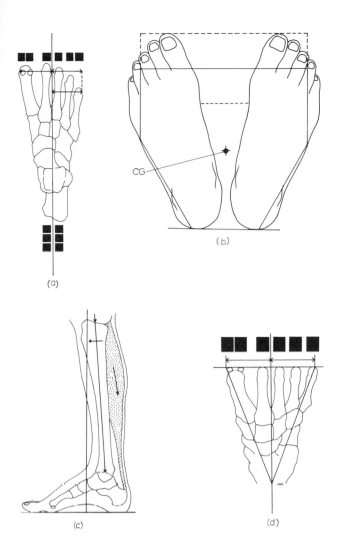

(a)

(b)

(c)

(d)

FIG. 24.42. (a) Distribution of load in normal standing on two feet. Each square represents one twenty-fourth of body weight. (b) Supporting area provided by two feet in normal standing. A perpendicular line from the body's centre of gravity reaches the ground at CG between the navicular bones and in front of the axis of the ankle joint. (c) The state of forward imbalance is maintained by contraction of the calf muscles. (d) Axis of balance and distribution of load in standing on one foot. (a), (b) and (d) after Morton.

unbalance is opposed by minimal contraction of the powerful calf muscles (fig. 24.42c).

In standing on one foot, the centre of gravity of the body is moved laterally to a point vertically above the axis of balance of the foot, which is a line drawn through the point of heel contact behind, to the interval between the second and third metatarsals in front (fig. 24.42d). Lateral stability now depends upon continuous slight balancing action of the invertors and evertors, acting through the subtalar joints.

Walking and running

During walking, one leg supports the body weight while the other leg is swung forwards. Thus each leg alternates between a swinging and a supporting phase.

The movement of walking is initiated by tilting forward the body which advances the centre of gravity and line of body weight. This forward movement is now increased by pushing off with one leg by plantar flexion at the ankle, while the other leg swings forward. This movement also pushes the body weight to the opposite side, so that it arrives over the other leg as this reaches the ground ready to enter the supporting phase.

SWINGING PHASE

The leg moves from a position behind the centre of gravity to pass in front of it so that it is ready to take up the body weight during the supporting phase. In order to prevent the foot trailing along the ground during this phase, the hip is flexed and laterally rotated, the knee is flexed, and the foot is dorsiflexed. Clearance is also assisted by tilting the pelvis to elevate the whole swinging limb; this is achieved by contracting the hip abductors, principally gluteus medius and minimus, on the side of the supporting limb. Once momentum has been achieved by the swinging limb, little muscular effort is required, and as the leg passes its supporting companion the knee extends and the foot becomes slightly plantar flexed and inverted as the heel reaches the ground for the supporting phase.

SUPPORTING PHASE

The body weight is initially taken on the heel and then passes along the outer border of the foot to be distributed across the metatarsal heads. The knee is kept extended while weight is being borne, but at the end of the supporting phase, the knee is unlocked by lateral rotation of the femur on the tibia. At the ankle joint plantar flexion gives way to active dorsiflexion, pulling the body weight over the ankle. The foot now becomes slightly everted, and 'push off' occurs by strong plantar flexion at the ankle, the final thrust being given by flexor hallucis longus as the leg moves once more into the swinging phase. When plantar flexion of the foot at the ankle produces 'push off', the entire body weight is transmitted through the metatarsals of one foot. The metatarsal of the great toe transmits 12 of the 24 units of body weight, the other metatarsals 3 units each (fig. 24.43a). A medial shift of weight stresses on the foot obviously occurs in locomotion as compared with standing; undue flattening of the medial longitudinal arch is resisted by the spring ligament assisted by the tendons of the long digital flexors of peroneus longus and of tibialis posterior (fig. 24.43b).

It will be noted that during walking many muscles act in the opposite manner to that usually described, in that the distal attachment, insertion, remains fairly static while the contracting muscle moves the proximal bone from which it arises. This reverse action of muscles is of

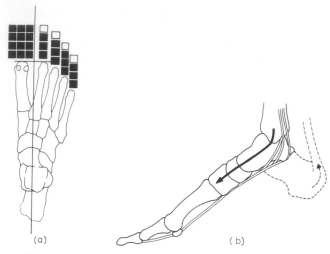

FIG. 24.43. (a) Distribution of load through metatarsals in 'push off' phase of walking. After Morton. (b) Transmission of load to front part of feet during 'push off' phase of walking.

greater importance in the lower than the upper limbs (p. 23.41).

MAINTENANCE OF BALANCE DURING WALKING

The tilting action of the pelvis during walking tends to move the centre of gravity and line of the body weight from side to side. This tilt is steadied and compensated for by contraction of the erector spinae and abdominal muscles on the side opposite to the contracting hip abductors, i.e. on the side of the swinging limb, to prevent the thorax falling over too far laterally. This tilting action is also counterbalanced by the swinging of the arms, the right arm swinging forward as the left leg is swinging. Arm swinging also contributes to the forward momentum achieved during walking.

The invertors and evertors of the foot keep the body stable on each foot during walking, another example of reverse action, and they are particularly active when walking over uneven ground. The short flexors of the toes, the flexor accessorius, interossei and lumbricals are important in improving the grip of the foot on the ground.

RUNNING

The mechanics of running are similar to those of walking. The main differences are that the trunk is inclined further forward, the movements are more powerful and exaggerated and the feet are parallel to the line of movement of the body, increasing their leverage to a maximum. There is an interval of time between 'push off' of the supporting leg and the landing of the swinging leg, so that the body is momentarily unsupported. In running the touch down is not made with the heel, but on the metatarsal heads.

FASCIA OF THE LOWER LIMB

The whole lower limb, like the upper limb, is enclosed in a sleeve of deep fascia which blends proximally with the deep fascia of the trunk. It is attached to bone along the outer lip of the iliac crest and along the pubic crest and ischiopubic ramus of the pelvis. In the leg it is attached to the anterior and medial margins of the tibia, so that the anteromedial surface of the tibia, the shin, is devoid of deep fascia.

The deep fascia maintains the smooth shape of the limb and assists the muscles in returning venous blood. From the covering sleeve of deep fascia various septa pass deeply to be attached to the long bones of the limb. These septa, the **intermuscular septa**, divide the leg into functional muscle compartments, each muscle in a group having a similar action.

Various portions of the deep fascia of the lower limb show special peculiarities which deserve more detailed description. The deep fascia of the thigh is thick, and is given the name **fascia lata.** This fascia is attached proximally to the inguinal ligament and to the whole of the outer lip of the iliac crest; it blends with the fascia on the posterior aspect of the sacrum and is attached medially to the ischial tuber and ischiopubic ramus, to the body of the pubis and to the pubic crest.

In its upper part it splits to enclose two muscles, the tensor fasciae latae anterolaterally and the gluteus maximus muscle posteriorly. These two muscles converge on and are attached to a considerably thickened portion of the fascia lata, the **iliotibial tract** (fig. 24.7). This tract commences about the level of the greater trochanter and, passing vertically down the posterolateral aspect of the thigh, it passes lateral to the knee joint to be attached to the anterior surface of the lateral tibial condyle. Gluteus maximus and tensor fasciae latae thus exert an action on the knee joint. Their pull through the tract maintains the knee in the extended position and acts most powerfully in stabilizing the knee when weight is being taken on the semiflexed knee. During this movement, which is important in walking, the tract can be felt most easily.

The fascia lata is attached distally to the patella, to the inferior margins of the tibial condyles and to the head of the fibula. Posteriorly it blends with the popliteal fascia. A defect is present over the upper part of the femoral triangle. This defect, known as the **saphenous opening**, is about 1 cm in diameter and in the adult is situated about 4 cm below and lateral to the pubic tubercle. Through this opening the great saphenous vein reaches the femoral vein. Lymphatics from the superficial inguinal nodes and superficial branches of the femoral artery also pass through the opening. A thin layer of loose fascia which covers the saphenous opening is perforated by all these structures and hence receives the name of **cribriform fascia** (fig. 24.65).

The femoral vessels, as they pass out of the abdomen into the thigh, draw with them an extension of the extraperitoneal transversalis fascia (fig. 24.44). This funnel-shaped prolongation of fascia fuses with the adventitia of the femoral vessels about 2 cm below the inguinal ligament and is known as the **femoral sheath** (p. 21.28). The femoral nerve, which is not included in the femoral sheath, lies lateral to the artery.

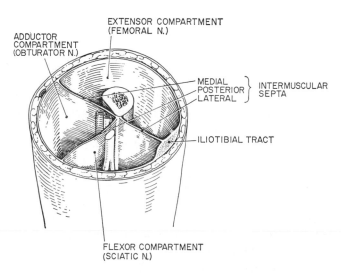

FIG. 24.44. Femoral sheath and canal.

Three **intermuscular septa** pass in from the deep fascia of the thigh to be attached to the linea aspera of the femur (fig. 24.45). The lateral intermuscular septum arises from the deep surface of the iliotibial tract. The three functional muscular compartments produced by these

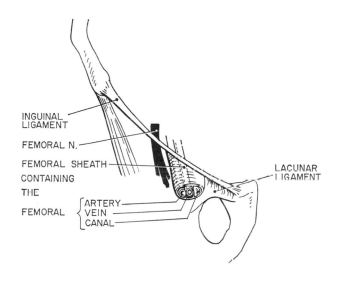

FIG. 24.45. Fascial compartments of the thigh.

septa contain respectively adductors of the hip, extensors of the knee and flexors of the knee. Note that the femoral vessels leave the adductor compartment to pass into the flexor compartment through the opening in adductor magnus.

The fascial arrangements in the leg are shown in fig. 24.46; the posterior compartment is divided into anterior and posterior subdivisions by a deep septum. This separates the superficial plantar flexors, soleus and gastrocnemius, from the long flexors passing to the foot. The tibial nerve and vessels lie deep to this layer of fascia.

The thickenings of the deep fascia which form **retinacula** at the ankle, and the associated synovial sheaths,

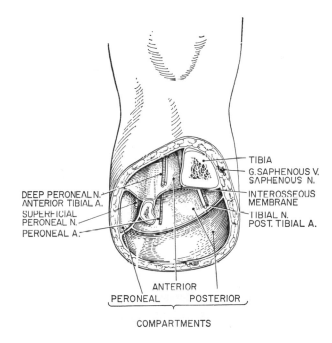

FIG. 24.46. Osteofascial compartments of the leg.

are shown in fig. 24.47. The fibrous flexor sheaths in the toes are lined with synovial sheaths and are similar to those described in the fingers (p. 23.24).

The deep fascia of the sole of the foot is similar to that in the hand. The central part is thickened and is known as the **plantar aponeurosis**. Attached posteriorly to the posterior tubercles of the calcaneus, this aponeurosis covers the flexor digitorum brevis and widens as it runs forward to divide into five slips, one for each toe. As in the hand, these slips are attached to the proximal borders of the fibrous flexor sheaths and to the sides of the metatarsophalangeal joints. In contrast to the big toe, however, the thumb does not receive a slip from the palmar aponeurosis, as this would limit its mobility. The plantar aponeurosis assists in the maintenance of the longitudinal arches of the foot (p. 24.25).

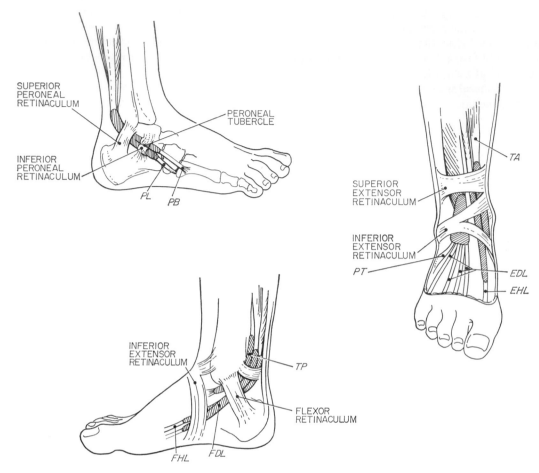

Fig. 24.47. Retinacula at the ankle.

Bursae

The important bursa at the hip joint lies between the iliopsoas tendon and the capsule of the hip joint. This often communicates with the joint through the weak area in the capsule (fig. 24.5a).

Many bursae are present around the knee and five are worth special mention:

(1) a prepatellar bursa lies between the skin and patella;

(2) an infrapatellar bursa lies between the skin and ligamentum patellae;

(3) two bursae lie between the heads of gastrocnemius and the posterior aspect of the knee joint; the bursa beneath the medial head always communicates with the knee joint;

(4) one bursa lies between semimembranosus and the knee joint and usually opens into the joint, and

(5) the suprapatellar bursa, deep to the quadriceps tendon, is a direct extension of the synovial membrane of the knee joint (p. 24.12).

When kneeling, friction between the skin and these underlying hard structures can cause inflammation; housemaid's knee is inflammation of the prepatellar bursa and clergyman's knee affects the infrapatellar bursa.

At the ankle the important bursa lies between tendo calcaneus and the upper third of the posterior surface of the calcaneus.

NERVES OF THE LOWER LIMB

The nerves supplying the lower limb arise over a wide area of the spinal cord, from the twelfth thoracic segment above to the fifth sacral segment below (fig. 24.48). The muscles are supplied entirely by the ventral primary rami of the nerves. The dorsal primary rami of the first three lumbar nerves and the sacral nerves assist in the cutaneous innervation of the limb by supplying the skin over the buttock (fig. 24.56 and 24.57).

The ventral primary rami of the lumbar and sacral regions form two complex plexuses, the **lumbar plexus** and the **sacral plexus**, which share a common nerve at L4. These are described on p. 21.44, and only the nerves which supply the limb are discussed here.

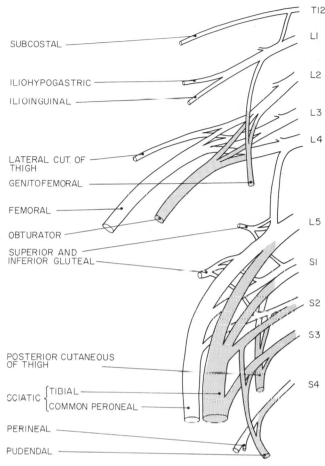

T12
L1
SUBCOSTAL
ILIOHYPOGASTRIC
L2
ILIOINGUINAL
L3
L4
LATERAL CUT. OF
THIGH
GENITOFEMORAL
FEMORAL
OBTURATOR
L5
SUPERIOR AND
INFERIOR GLUTEAL
S1
S2
S3
POSTERIOR CUTANEOUS
OF THIGH
S4
SCIATIC { TIBIAL
COMMON PERONEAL
PERINEAL
PUDENDAL

FIG. 24.48. Simplified diagram of the lumbosacral plexus, which omits small muscular branches. Dorsal divisions are clear and ventral divisions stippled (cf. fig. 23.59).

Branches of the lumbar plexus

The **genitofemoral nerve** (L1, 2) emerges on the anterior surface of psoas major near the pelvic brim and runs down to leave the abdomen on the anterior aspect of the external iliac artery. Its genital branch traverses the inguinal canal, supplying cremaster muscle, while the femoral branch supplies the skin over the upper part of the thigh (fig. 24.57).

The **lateral cutaneous nerve of thigh** (L2, 3) traverses the iliac fossa lying on iliacus to leave the abdomen by piercing the inguinal ligament near the anterior superior iliac spine. It is distributed to the skin on the lateral side of the thigh (fig. 24.57).

The **obturator nerve** (L2, 3, 4) emerges in the pelvis from behind the medial border of psoas and runs on the side wall of the pelvis towards the obturator foramen. It is accompanied in the pelvic part of its course by the obturator vessels and escapes from the pelvis through the obturator groove at the upper part of the foramen. The obturator nerve supplies the obturator externus muscle, the adductor muscles of the hip (fig. 24.55) and the hip

joint itself. A cutaneous branch often accompanies the saphenous nerve to supply the medial aspect of the lower third of the thigh, and a genicular branch descends on adductor magnus to reach the knee joint posteriorly.

The **femoral nerve** (L2, 3 and 4) is the largest branch of the lumbar plexus. It emerges from the lateral border of psoas major below the iliac crest and runs between psoas major and iliacus to enter the thigh by passing behind the inguinal ligament. As it enters the thigh it is an immediate lateral relation of the femoral artery, which separates it from the femoral vein (fig. 24.44). It runs a very short course in the thigh before breaking up into numerous branches (fig. 24.49). Twigs also supply the hip joint.

The muscular branches separate to the four components of quadriceps, to sartorius and pectineus. The nerve thus supplies the flexors of the hip joint, but not the major one, iliopsoas, and the extensor muscles of the knee. The cutaneous branches run into the medial and intermediate cutaneous nerves of the thigh and the saphenous nerve which is distributed to the medial side of knee, calf and heel (fig. 24.57).

The region of the thigh where the femoral nerve breaks up is known as the **femoral triangle,** the boundaries of which are the inguinal ligament above, the sartorius muscle laterally and the medial border of adductor longus medially (fig. 24.49). The floor of this triangle is gutter shaped and is made up of iliacus, psoas major, pectineus and adductor longus. The roof of the triangle is the strong fascia lata of the leg, and it is pierced by the great saphenous vein which joins the femoral vein in the triangle. The profunda femoris artery arises from the femoral artery in the triangle and passes posteriorly behind adductor longus.

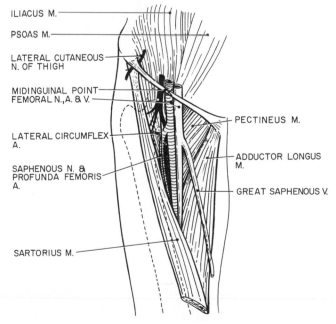

ILIACUS M.
PSOAS M.
LATERAL CUTANEOUS
N. OF THIGH
MIDINGUINAL POINT
FEMORAL N., A. & V.
LATERAL CIRCUMFLEX
A.
SAPHENOUS N. &
PROFUNDA FEMORIS
A.
SARTORIUS M.
PECTINEUS M.
ADDUCTOR LONGUS
M.
GREAT SAPHENOUS V.

FIG. 24.49. The femoral triangle. Superficial branches of the femoral artery are omitted.

The femoral vein lies posterior to its artery in the lower part of the triangle and is separated from the profunda femoris vein lying anterior to its artery by the adductor longus muscle.

The **saphenous nerve** leaves the femoral triangle at its apex on the lateral side of the femoral artery, and enters the **adductor canal** (fig. 24.50). This canal lies between the vastus medialis laterally and the adductor muscles posteriorly. It has a roof of fascia, which is covered by the sartorius muscle. The femoral artery and vein leave the canal at the opening in adductor magnus to reach the popliteal fossa. The saphenous nerve spirals round the artery, passing first on to the anterior aspect of the artery and then lying slightly medial to it. Below the adductor hiatus, the nerve is accompanied by the descending genicular branch of the femoral artery. It emerges from the canal posterior to sartorius and in front of gracilis, just

below the knee, and runs down in the company of the great saphenous vein to supply the skin of the medial side of the leg and heel. Just before it leaves the adductor canal it gives off an infrapatellar branch to the skin around the knee and to the knee joint (fig. 24.50).

Branches of the sacral plexus

The **sciatic nerve** is the largest nerve in the body and the main nerve of the lower limb (figs. 24.48 and 51). It is formed by contributions from all the ventral rami concerned in the sacral plexus; the ventral divisions of the rami eventually form the tibial nerve, and the dorsal divisions form the common peroneal nerve. The sciatic nerve leaves the pelvis below the lower border of the piriformis muscle and enters the gluteal region. There it inclines laterally across the obturator internus tendon to reach the space between the ischial tuber and the greater trochanter of the femur. It then runs downwards in the thigh on the posterior surface of the adductor magnus muscle. Intramuscular injections into the buttock should always be given into the upper outer quadrant to avoid damage to the sciatic nerve, which lies just medial to the midpoint of a line between the ischial tuber and the apex of the greater trochanter.

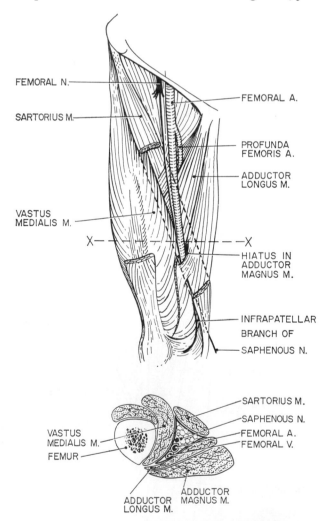

FIG. 24.50. The adductor canal. The roof, formed by the sartorius muscle, has been removed and the femoral vein is omitted for clarity. In the section through X–X shown below, the vessels and nerve occupy part of the adductor canal.

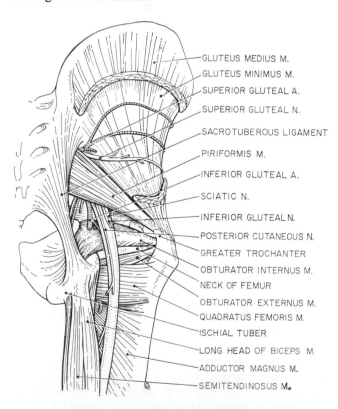

FIG. 24.51. The gluteal region after removal of gluteus maximus muscle. A portion of the gluteus medius muscle has been resected and the gemelli muscles, above and below the tendon of obturator internus, have been omitted to reveal the back of the hip joint capsule.

The sciatic nerve gives off no branches in the gluteal region, and its course in the thigh and its distribution are considered in more detail below.

The **superior gluteal nerve** (L4, 5, S1) leaves the pelvis above the piriformis muscle in the company of the gluteal artery. In the buttock it passes laterally between the gluteus medius and minimus muscles, along with the deep division of the superior gluteal artery. After supplying the hip joint and these muscles it reaches the deep surface of tensor fasciae latae in which it ends (fig. 24.51).

The **inferior gluteal nerve** (L5, S1, 2) leaves the pelvis below the piriformis, lying posterior to the sciatic nerve, and at once enters the overlying gluteus maximus muscle which is all it supplies.

The **nerve to quadratus femoris** (L4, 5, S1) passes out of the lower part of the greater sciatic foramen, and closely applied to the ischium it runs deep to obturator internus and gemelli to reach quadratus femoris. It also supplies the inferior gemellus.

The **nerve to obturator internus** (L5, S1, 2) is described on p. 21.45.

The **posterior cutaneous nerve of thigh** (S1, 2, 3) is the largest purely cutaneous branch of the sacral plexus. It enters the gluteal region along with the inferior gluteal artery and nerve and then runs downwards on the posterior surface of the sciatic nerve. Several small gluteal branches curve upwards over the lower border of gluteus maximus to supply the skin of the lower part of the buttock while a perineal branch runs forward to supply the skin of the perineum and posterior part of the scrotum. The main trunk of the nerve gives off branches to the posterior aspect of the thigh, finally becoming expended behind the knee.

The **perforating cutaneous nerve** (S2, 3) pierces the sacrotuberous ligament and lower part of gluteus maximus to supply a small area of skin in the inferomedial region of the buttock.

Course and distribution of the sciatic nerve

In the thigh, the sciatic nerve runs downwards on the posterior surface of adductor magnus. It passes deep to the long head of biceps femoris (fig. 24.52) and at a variable position in the thigh divides into its two major components, the tibial and common peroneal nerves. Unlike the other major nerves of the limb, femoral and obturator, it does not have an accompanying large artery, but a small branch of the inferior gluteal artery accompanies and supplies it.

The sciatic nerve supplies muscular branches to the hamstring muscles. With the exception of the branch to the short head of the biceps, which arises from the common peroneal part, these branches all arise from the tibial component of the nerve. The adductor magnus muscle is innervated by two nerves, the sciatic and the obturator (fig. 24.9). The sciatic nerve supplies the vertical fibres of this muscle, those attached to the ischial tuber, which act as a hamstring muscle to extend the hip, while the obturator nerve supplies the more oblique fibres to the shaft of the femur which act as an adductor muscle.

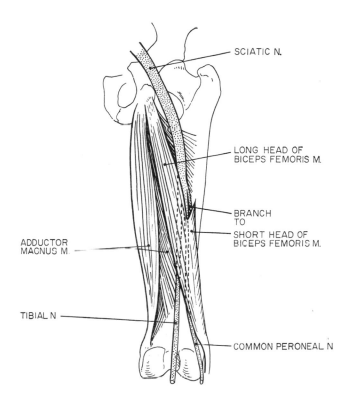

FIG. 24.52. The course of the sciatic nerve.

The two terminal branches of the sciatic nerve enter the **popliteal fossa** near its apex (fig. 24.53). This diamond-shaped fossa is situated behind the knee and lower femur, and is bounded above and laterally by the biceps femoris and above and medially by the semimembranosus and semitendinosus muscles. Its lower boundaries are formed by the two heads of the gastrocnemius muscle. The floor of the fossa is the popliteal surface of the femur and the upper part of the posterior capsule of the knee joint. The fossa is covered superficially by deep fascia of the leg, which is slightly thickened in this region, and called the **popliteal fascia.**

The **common peroneal (lateral popliteal) nerve** (L4, 5, S1 and 2) inclines laterally across the upper part of the fossa to pass superficial to the lateral head of gastrocnemius. It continues on this superficial course behind the head of the fibula and winds around the neck of this bone, where it can easily be felt and where it is particularly vulnerable to damage by ill-fitting plasters, by direct blows and by fractures of the upper fibula. Before entering the substance of peroneus longus, it gives off branches in the fossa. The lateral cutaneous nerve of the calf pierces the popliteal fascia to reach its cutaneous distribution over the lateral aspect of the upper calf. A branch descends deep to the deep fascia to join the sural nerve in the back of the calf.

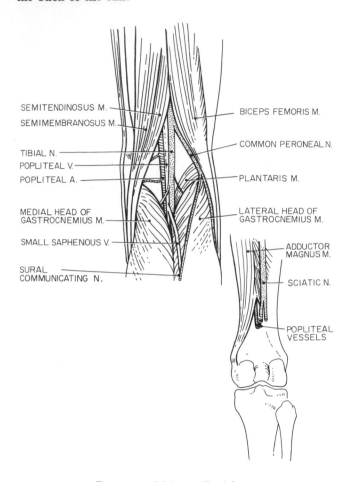

FIG. 24.53. Right popliteal fossa.

The **tibial (medial popliteal) nerve** (L4, 5, S1, 2 and 3) crosses the popliteal fossa with the popliteal vessels to leave the fossa by passing deep to the gastrocnemius. In its course through the fossa, the nerve is superficial to the vein and the popliteal artery runs deep to them both. In the lower part of the fossa, the small saphenous vein pierces the popliteal fascia to enter the popliteal vein. After leaving the popliteal fossa, the tibial nerve descends on the posterior surface of the popliteus muscle and enters the calf by passing deep to the tendinous arch between the tibial and fibular attachments of soleus (fig. 24.54). In the popliteal fossa, the tibial nerve gives off numerous branches. One cutaneous branch, the **sural nerve**, runs downwards beneath the deep fascia, which it pierces near the middle of the back of the calf, and continues to the lateral side of the foot. Branches from the upper part of this nerve pierce the deep fascia to reach the skin of the posterior part of the upper calf. Muscular branches pass

to plantaris, both heads of gastrocnemius, popliteus and soleus. Articular branches accompany the genicular arteries to the knee joint.

Nerves in the leg and foot

In the substance of peroneus longus on the neck of the fibula, the common peroneal nerve divides into superficial and deep peroneal nerves.

The **deep peroneal (anterior tibial) nerve** continues to spiral round the neck of the fibula, deep to extensor digitorum longus, until it reaches the interosseous membrane

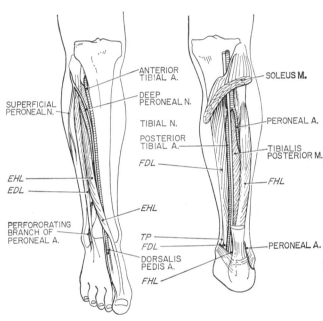

FIG. 24.54. Vessels and nerves of the leg. The tibialis anterior muscle has been removed from the anterior view seen on the left.

lateral to the anterior tibial vessels (fig. 24.54). It runs down the leg with these vessels lying between tibialis anterior medially and extensor digitorum longus and then extensor hallucis longus laterally. In the lower part of the leg the extensor hallucis longus muscle crosses superficially to reach the medial side of the nerve, so that at the ankle joint it lies between tibialis anterior and extensor hallucis longus tendons medially, and extensor digitorum longus and peroneus tertius tendons laterally.

The nerve continues forward on the dorsum of the foot lying deep to the extensor digitorum tendons to reach the first interdigital cleft, the skin of which it supplies; this is the only cutaneous branch of the deep peroneal nerve. Muscular branches pass to the long extensors, tibialis anterior and peroneus tertius in the leg and extensor digitorum brevis in the foot (fig. 24.55). These muscles dorsiflex the ankle, extend the toes, and contribute to inversion and eversion of the foot. It also sends articular branches to the ankle joint.

The **superficial peroneal (musculocutaneous) nerve** runs downwards in the substance of peroneus longus and then comes to lie between peroneus brevis and longus, which it supplies before becoming subcutaneous by piercing the deep fascia two-thirds of the way down the leg. It then passes on to the dorsum of the foot and breaks up into digital branches into the toes, supplying the dorsum of all the toes apart from the lateral side of the fifth toe (sural nerve) and the adjacent sides of hallux and second toe (deep peroneal nerve).

The **tibial nerve** runs vertically down the leg closely applied to the fascia covering the deep surface of soleus. It emerges from the cover of soleus in the lower third of the leg, and passes behind the medial malleolus lying between the tendons of tibialis posterior and flexor digitorum longus medially, and flexor hallucis longus laterally. In its course in the calf it is accompanied by the posterior tibial vessels. At a point midway between the medial malleolus and the medial prominence of the heel, the tibial nerve divides into its terminal branches, the medial and lateral plantar nerves. It supplies the muscular branches to the deep surface of soleus muscle, to tibialis posterior and to the flexors digitorum and hallucis longus. These muscles contribute to plantar flexion at the ankle, to inversion of the foot, and flexion of the toes. Through the cutaneous branches it supplies a small area of skin on the medial side of the heel. Finally it supplies the ankle joint via the articular branches.

The two **plantar nerves** supply all the small muscles in the sole of the foot and the skin of the sole. They follow the course of the plantar arteries (fig. 24.64).

The **medial plantar nerve** runs forward under cover of abductor hallucis and crosses superficial to the flexor hallucis longus and flexor digitorum longus tendons to lie on flexor hallucis brevis. It gives off cutaneous branches to the sole which pass through the interval between abductor hallucis and flexor digitorum brevis and then pierce the deep fascia of the foot. It then divides into digital cutaneous branches for the medial three and a half toes. Its muscular supply is limited to muscles close to its course i.e. abductor hallucis, flexor digitorum brevis, flexor hallucis brevis and, usually, the first lumbrical (fig. 24.55).

The remaining muscles of the foot are supplied by the **lateral plantar nerve**, which crosses the sole of the foot on the medial side of the lateral plantar artery, passing between flexor digitorum brevis and flexor accessorius to the deep surface of abductor digiti minimi. It supplies both flexor accessorius and abductor digiti minimi and sends cutaneous branches to the lateral part of the sole before dividing into superficial and deep branches under the base of the fifth metatarsal. The superficial branch sends a cutaneous branch which divides to supply the skin of the plantar surface of the little toe and the lateral part of the fourth toe. It supplies muscular branches to the flexor digiti minimi brevis and the interosseous muscles of the

fourth interosseous space (third plantar and fourth dorsal). The deep branch passes deeply into the sole and lies in the concavity of the plantar arch across the bases of the metatarsals deep to the long flexor tendons. It supplies branches to the remaining muscles of the foot and ends in the substance of the oblique head of adductor hallucis.

The general pattern of distribution of the lateral plantar nerve resembles that of the ulnar nerve in the hand, while the distribution of the medial plantar nerve resembles that of the median nerve.

Nerve distribution in the lower limb

Movements at joints are regulated by centres in the spinal cord, and fig. 24.59 illustrates the spinal segments involved in leg movements. Familiarity with this diagram and a knowledge of the action of any muscle, determines the segmental supply of that muscle. Such knowledge is of importance in localizing injury or disease in the spinal cord. The segmental nerve supply of the joints of the limb is the same as that of the muscles producing movement at the joints.

The muscular distribution of the main nerves is given in fig. 24.55 and the cutaneous nerve distribution and the segmental dermatomes are shown in fig. 24.56 and 57.

Autonomic nerve supply to the lower limb

The sympathetic nerve supply to the blood vessels, arrector pili muscles and sweat glands of the lower limb arises in the spinal cord from segments T12 to L2.

White rami pass to the sympathetic ganglia from these nerves. Branches from the ganglia pass into the aortic plexus and also back to the peripheral nerves. From the aortic plexus, sympathetic fibres accompany the iliac arteries and pass to the limb. The fibres supply only the most proximal part of the major limb artery; by far the greater part of the limb receives its sympathetic innervation from fibres carried in peripheral nerves.

BLOOD VESSELS OF THE LOWER LIMB

ARTERIES

Each limb has a single main artery which carries the blood necessary for the function of the limb (fig. 24.58). Branches of this artery supply the various muscles, bones and joints. Such a simple arrangement suffers from the disadvantage that an injury or disease of the main arterial trunk causing blockage would result in the death of the limb distal to the obstruction unless alternative pathways to the distal parts were available. Hence, many of the branches of the main arterial vessel anastomose with branches given off lower down the vessel, providing a collateral circulation.

The collateral circulation of the lower limbs is not so

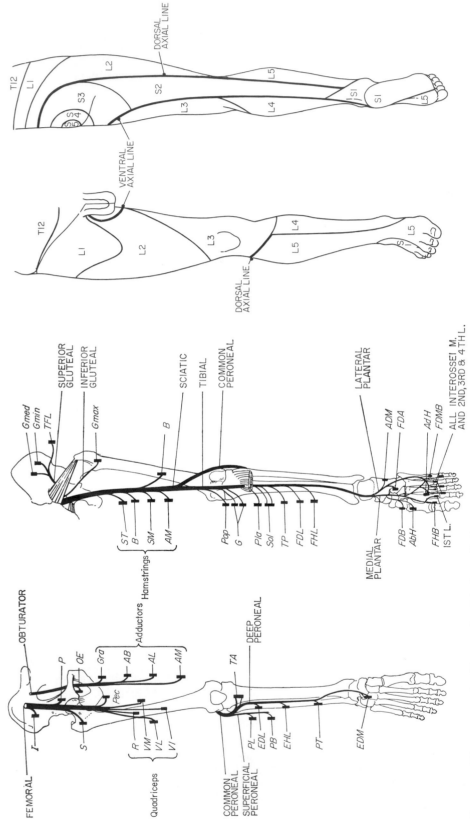

FIG. 24.56. Dermatomes of lower limb, showing segmental cutaneous distribution of spinal nerves on (a) the front, and (b) the back of the limb. From Romanes G.J. Ed. (1964) *Cunningham's Textbook of Anatomy*, 10th Edition.

FIG. 24.55. The nerve supply of the muscles of the lower limb.

I, Iliacus; *P*, Psoas; *S*, Sartorius; *OE*, Obturator externus; *Gra*, Gracilis; *Pec*, Pectineus; *AB*, Abductor brevis; *AL*, Abductor longus; *AM*, Abductor magnus; *R*, Rectus femoris; *VM*, *VI* & *VL*, Vastus medialis, intermedius and lateralis; *PL* & *PB*, Peronous longus and brevis; *EHL*, Extensor hallucis longus; *PT*, Peroneus tertius.

Gmed, min & max, Gluteus medius, minimus and maximus; *TFL*, Tensor fasciae latae; *ST*, Semitendinosus; *SM*, Semimembranosus; *B*, Biceps femoralis; *Pop*, Popliteus; *G*, Gastrocnemius; *Pla*, Plantaris; *Sol*, Soleus; *TP*, Tibialis posterior; *FDL*, Flexor digitorum longus; *FHL*, Flexor hallucis longus; *ADM*, Abductor digiti minimi; *FDA*, Flexor digitorum accessorius; *AbH* & *AdH*, Abductor and adductor hallucis; *FDB*, Flexor digitorum brevis; *FDMB*, Flexor digiti minimi brevis; *FHB*, Flexor hallucis brevis.

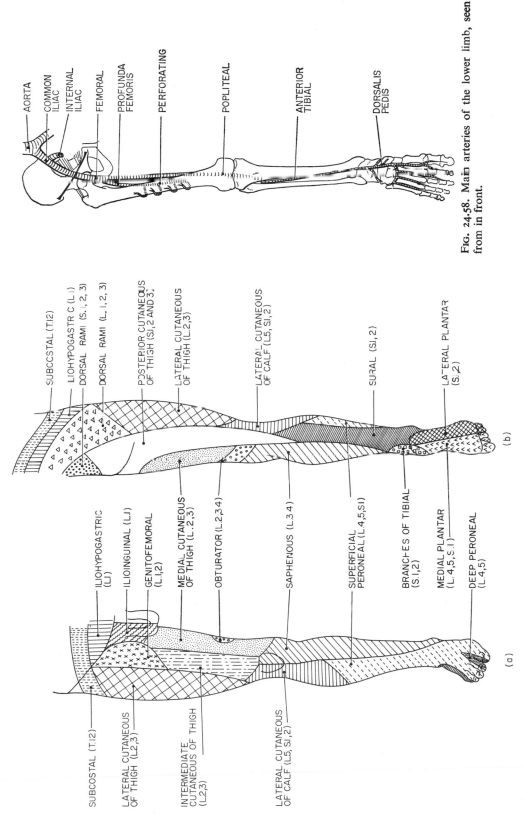

SUBCOSTAL (T.12)
ILIOHYPOGASTRIC (L.1)
DORSAL RAMI (S.1, 2, 3)
DORSAL RAMI (L.1, 2, 3)
POSTERIOR CUTANEOUS OF THIGH (S.1, 2 AND 3)
LATERAL CUTANEOUS OF THIGH (L.2,3)
LATERAL CUTANEOUS OF CALF (L.5, S.1, 2)
SURAL (S.1, 2)
LATERAL PLANTAR (S.2)

ILIOHYPOGASTRIC (L.1)
ILIOINGUINAL (L.1)
GENITOFEMORAL (L.1,2)
MEDIAL CUTANEOUS OF THIGH (L.2,3)
OBTURATOR (L.2,3,4)
SAPHENOUS (L.3,4)
SUPERFICIAL PERONEAL (L.4,5,S.1)
BRANCHES OF TIBIAL (S.1,2)
MEDIAL PLANTAR (L.4,5, S.1)
DEEP PERONEAL (L.4,5)

SUBCOSTAL (T.12)
LATERAL CUTANEOUS OF THIGH (L.2,3)
INTERMEDIATE CUTANEOUS OF THIGH (L.2,3)
LATERAL CUTANEOUS OF CALF (L.5, S.1, 2)

(a)

(b)

FIG. 24.57. Distribution of cutaneous nerves on (a) the front, and (b) the back of the lower limb. There is considerable variation in these territories and the extent to which they overlap each other.

AORTA
COMMON ILIAC
INTERNAL ILIAC
FEMORAL
PROFUNDA FEMORIS
PERFORATING
POPLITEAL
ANTERIOR TIBIAL
DORSALIS PEDIS

FIG. 24.58. Main arteries of the lower limb, seen from in front.

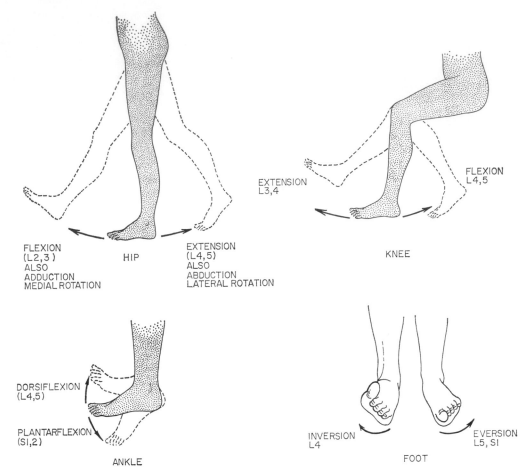

FIG. 24.59. Segmental nerves and movements in the lower limb. From Last R.J. (1972) *Anatomy: Regional and Applied*, 5th edition. Edinburgh : Churchill Livingstone

efficient as in the upper limb, but is important since in old age arterial disease and obstruction are common. It is discussed in greater detail after a brief description of the arteries of the limb.

The aorta bifurcates in the abdomen at the level of the fourth vertebra into the common iliac arteries. At the pelvic brim the common iliac artery divides into the internal iliac artery, which supplies blood to the pelvis and gluteal region, and the external iliac artery which continues along the pelvic brim, carrying the major part of the blood supply to the limb. The external iliac artery gives off the inferior epigastric artery immediately before it passes from the abdomen behind the inguinal ligament at the midinguinal point. As it enters the thigh, it is called the **femoral artery,** and its pulsations can easily be felt below the midinguinal point. The major blood supply to the lower limb is carried by the femoral artery. The gluteal region is supplied from within the pelvis by the **gluteal arteries**, branches of the internal iliac and the upper part of the adductor muscles of the thigh receive their blood supply from the **obturator artery**.

Branches from the internal iliac artery

The superior and inferior gluteal arteries both arise inside the pelvis. The **superior gluteal artery** enters the gluteal region by passing through the greater sciatic notch above piriformis, and divides into a superficial and deep branch (fig. 24.51). The superficial branch supplies mainly gluteus maximus, while the deep branch runs forward between gluteus medius and minimus. Both these divisions anastomose freely with one another, with branches of the inferior gluteal artery, and particularly with ascending branches of the medial and lateral circumflex vessels. The **inferior gluteal artery** passes out of the pelvis through the greater sciatic notch below piriformis and runs downwards posteromedial to the sciatic nerve to reach the proximal part of the thigh. It supplies numerous muscular branches to the buttock muscles and hip joint before anastomosing freely with neighbouring vessels.

The **obturator artery** is a small branch of the internal iliac artery, which leaves the pelvis through the obturator foramen. It sends a branch to the hip joint, and muscular branches to the proximal parts of the adductor muscles.

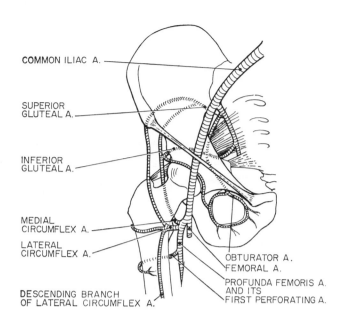

FIG. 24.60. Anastomoses around the hip joint.

By anastomosing with the profunda femoris, it contributes to the anastomosis around the hip (fig. 24.60).

Femoral artery

The femoral artery gives off four small branches below the inguinal ligament, which supply the skin of the upper

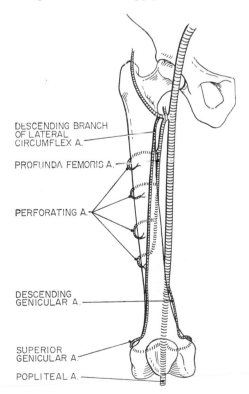

FIG. 24.61. Anastomoses in the thigh.

thigh, the scrotum and adjoining abdominal wall. It continues down the leg, carrying blood to the knee, leg and foot. It passes downwards in the adductor canal deep to sartorius muscle and reaches the back of the thigh by passing through the opening in adductor magnus (figs. 24.50 and 53). This part of the femoral artery is often called, by clinicians, the superficial femoral artery to distinguish it from the **profunda femoris artery**, a large branch of the femoral which arises 4 cm below the inguinal ligament. The profunda femoris artery passes deep to the femoral artery to reach the posteromedial aspect of the femur. It supplies many branches to the muscles of the thigh, including **perforating branches** passing through the adductor magnus to curve round the posterior surface of the femur; medial and lateral circumflex arteries are the other named branches of the profunda femoris artery (figs. 24.60 and 61). The **lateral circumflex artery** is more superficial, and supplies branches to the muscles in front of the hip joint and to vastus lateralis, and sends an ascending branch anterior to the hip joint to reach the tensor fasciae latae. The **medial circumflex artery** passes deeply into the thigh to pass medial to the femur below the hip joint, supplying muscles as it goes. It supplies branches to the hip joint and its surrounding short muscles. The branches of the profunda femoris artery play an important part in providing a collateral circulation when the flow through the femoral artery is obstructed.

POPLITEAL ARTERY

When the femoral artery passes through the opening in adductor magnus to reach the back of the thigh, it becomes the popliteal artery. The popliteal artery passes downwards lying close to the popliteal surface of the femur, where it is liable to injury in fractures of the femur. The artery then passes posterior to the capsule of the knee joint and to popliteus, at the lower margin of which muscle it ends by dividing into the anterior and posterior tibial arteries (fig. 24.54). This is about the level of the neck of the fibula. The popliteal artery gives off muscular and genicular branches (fig. 24.62) which supply the knee joint and its capsule.

POSTERIOR TIBIAL ARTERY

The posterior tibial artery is the larger of the two divisions of the popliteal artery and passes deep to soleus muscle and the fascia clothing the deep surface of this muscle (fig. 24.54). As it passes down the leg, it remains close to the tibial nerve (p. 24.34). It can be palpated easily at the ankle, halfway between the medial malleolus and the medial prominence of the heel. The artery ends at this point, dividing into the main arteries of the sole of the foot, the medial and lateral plantar arteries.

The main branch of the posterior tibial artery is the

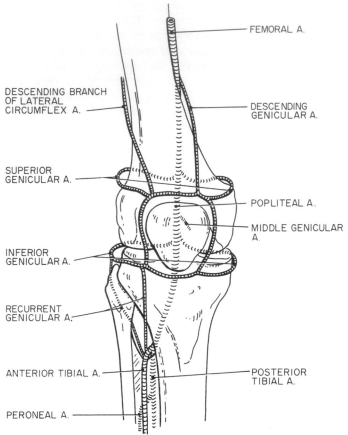

FIG. 24.62. Anastomoses around the knee, showing the genicular arteries.

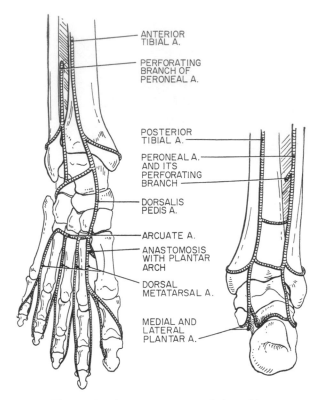

FIG. 24.63. Anastomoses around the ankle.

peroneal artery, which is given off about 5 cm below popliteus. As it passes down the limb it inclines laterally across the posterior aspect of the tibialis posterior to lie between that muscle and flexor hallucis longus in close relationship to the fibula. It gives off a **perforating branch** which passes through the interosseous membrane just above the inferior tibiofibular joint (fig. 24.63). The peroneal artery then passes behind the lateral malleolus to end as branches on the lateral side of the heel.

The posterior tibial and peroneal arteries supply branches to the muscles of the calf, to the ankle and inferior tibiofibular joints and to the tibia and fibula respectively.

PLANTAR ARTERIES

The medial and lateral plantar arteries arise from the termination of the posterior tibial artery below the medial malleolus (fig. 24.64).

The **medial plantar artery**, which corresponds to the radial artery in the hand, is the smaller of the two and runs forward along the medial side of the foot between abductor hallucis brevis and flexor digitorum brevis to end as the medial digital artery of the big toe. Near the

first metatarsophalangeal joint it anastomoses with the medial branch of the first plantar metatarsal artery. It supplies muscular branches to the two adjacent muscles, and cutaneous branches to the skin on the medial side of the foot.

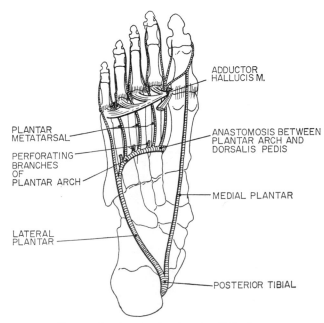

FIG. 24.64. Arteries in the sole of the foot.

The **lateral plantar artery** is much larger and corresponds to the ulnar artery in the hand. It crosses to the lateral side of the foot, accompanying the lateral plantar nerve, and passes between flexor digitorum brevis and flexor digitorum accessorius; it then runs forward between abductor digiti minimi and flexor digitorum brevis to reach the medial side of the base of the fifth metatarsal. It then passes deep, and arches across the sole of the foot, under the bases of the metatarsals, to anastomose with the dorsalis pedis artery; this portion of the artery is known as the **plantar arch**.

The lateral plantar artery gives off cutaneous branches to the sole and lateral side of the foot, and muscular branches to the small vessels of the foot. From the plantar arch arise the **four plantar metatarsal arteries**, each of which runs forward on the interosseous muscles to divide near the heads of the metatarsals into two **digital arteries** which supply the medial and lateral sides of adjacent digits (fig. 24.64). Three **perforating arteries** also rise from the plantar arch, passing through the lateral three intermetatarsal spaces to anastomose with the corresponding **dorsal metatarsal arteries**.

ANTERIOR TIBIAL ARTERY

From its origin this artery passes forwards below the popliteus muscle to reach the anterior compartment of the leg by passing over the upper border of the interosseous membrane (fig. 24.54). It runs down the leg with the deep peroneal nerve (p. 24.34). Passing in front of the ankle joint it lies between the tendons of extensor hallucis longus and extensor digitorum longus to reach the dorsum of the foot, where it becomes known as the dorsalis pedis artery. The anterior tibial artery may be palpated at the level of the ankle joint, and the dorsalis pedis may be palpated in its course over the dorsum of the foot.

The artery gives off muscular branches and two recurrent arteries supply the knee joint.

DORSALIS PEDIS ARTERY (fig. 24.63)

The direct continuation of the anterior tibial artery, this vessel begins in front of the ankle joint and runs forward over the dorsum of the tarsus. It ends by passing downwards between the heads of the first dorsal interosseous muscle to anastomose in the sole with the lateral plantar artery (plantar arch). A branch called the **arcuate artery** runs laterally deep to the extensor tendons and gives off three dorsal metatarsal arteries.

Collateral circulation of the limb

The anastomoses which provide for the collateral circulation tend to be best developed around the major joints like the hip, knee and ankle. Additionally there is an important anastomotic chain in the thigh. These are all illustrated in figs. 24.60-63. The anastomosis around

the hip is important since it allows communication between branches of the internal iliac artery, which supplies the pelvis and gluteal region, and branches of the femoral artery in the limb itself. Thus an arterial obstruction even as high as the external iliac artery does not prevent blood reaching the leg provided this anastomotic pathway is patent.

VENOUS DRAINAGE

The veins of the leg are described in two groups, the **superficial veins**, which lie in the superficial fascia, and the **deep veins**, which lie deeply, within the deep fascial stocking of the limb. The two groups are connected by **communicating veins**, which pierce the deep fascia and possess valves which normally direct blood flow from superficial to deep veins.

Superficial veins (fig. 24.65)

These veins drain the skin and subcutaneous tissues. The veins from the toes form metatarsal veins which run into a small plantar and a larger dorsal venous arch on the

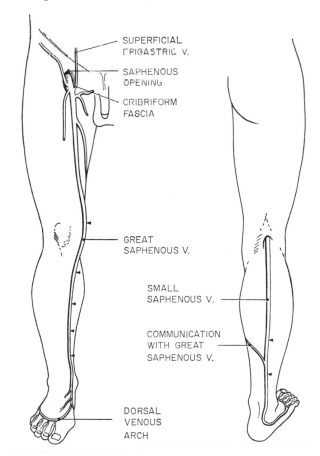

FIG. 24.65. Superficial veins of the lower limb. Many tributaries are omitted and the common sites of communication with deep veins are shown by arrows.

foot. The medial ends of these arches join the great saphenous vein, while the lateral ends join the small saphenous vein.

The **great (long) saphenous vein** ascends in the subcutaneous tissues across the medial malleolus, and as it passes up the leg with the saphenous nerve it receives further tributaries. It crosses the knee posteromedially to the medial condyle of the femur and then inclines slightly medially across the thigh. It pierces the deep fascia of the leg, at a point 4 cm below and lateral to the pubic tubercle, to enter the femoral vein. Just before it pierces the deep fascia, it receives quite large tributaries from the medial aspect of the thigh, from the lower abdominal wall and from the scrotum.

The **small (short) saphenous vein** ascends posterior to the lateral malleolus and runs upwards in the subcutaneous tissues of the calf alongside the sural nerve. It pierces the deep fascia behind the knee and enters the popliteal vein.

Deep veins

The deep veins are formed by tributaries arising in the muscles, bones and joints of the leg. The small muscular veins join to form venae comitantes which accompany the arteries, and there are no named deep veins until the venae comitantes of the anterior and posterior tibial arteries unite at the lower border of popliteus to form the **popliteal vein**, which initially lies posteromedial to the artery. As the vein ascends, it crosses posterior to the artery separating it from the tibial nerve (fig. 24.53) to lie posterolateral to it as it passes through the adductor magnus opening into the thigh and becomes the femoral vein.

The femoral vein ascends alongside the femoral artery and inclines slightly medially to become a posterior relation of the artery. The **profunda femoris vein** joins the femoral vein 5 cm below the inguinal ligament and at this point these two large veins separate the femoral and profunda femoris arteries. The femoral vein now inclines more medially, and as it leaves the thigh by passing behind the inguinal ligament to become the external iliac vein, it lies medial to the artery (fig. 24.44).

LYMPH DRAINAGE

The lymphatic drainage tends to follow the venous drainage, with the lymphatics from tissues deep to the deep fascia following the deep veins, and the lymphatics from skin and superficial tissues following the saphenous veins. The superficial lymphatic drainage is shown in fig. 24.66.

Lymph nodes

The lymphatic vessels drain into lymph nodes, which are situated in two places, behind the knee and in the groin.

The **popliteal nodes** are situated deep to the popliteal fascia. Lymphatic vessels accompanying the short

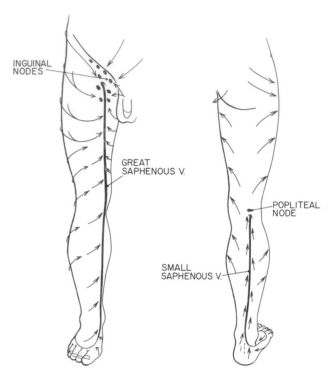

FIG. 24.66. Superficial lymphatic drainage of the lower limb.

saphenous vein enter these nodes and the lymph then passes onwards in the deep lymphatics which accompany the popliteal and femoral vein to the deep group of inguinal nodes.

The deep fascia divides the **inguinal nodes** into superficial and deep groups. The superficial nodes lie along the line of the inguinal ligament and along the upper part of the great saphenous vein. The former group receive lymph from the upper thigh, buttock and lower abdominal wall. The saphenous vein group drains the lymph from the superficial tissues of the leg. From both these groups of nodes the lymph passes through the cribriform fascia to the deep group of nodes.

The deep inguinal lymph nodes lie around the upper part of the femoral vein, and in addition to receiving lymph from the superficial nodes, they collect the lymph from all the deep lymphatics in the leg. From the deep inguinal nodes, lymphatics accompany the external iliac vein to reach the abdominal lymph nodes. Like the veins, the lymphatic vessels are supplied with numerous valves and so again muscular activity aids the upward movement of the fluid.

MECHANISM OF FLUID RETURN

In order to assist the return of blood, the limb veins are supplied with valves, which prevent reflux of venous blood towards the periphery.

In the lower limb, these valves are particularly important, since the erect posture adds a considerable hydrostatic pressure opposing return of blood to the heart. The sucking action of the thorax during inspiration and the transmitted pressure from the arteries assist the venous return, but the most important mechanism promoting venous return from the limb is the contraction and relaxation of the limb muscles.

The whole limb and its muscular compartments are surrounded by tough, relatively inelastic, deep fascia (p. 24.28). When a muscle contracts, it squeezes on the blood contained in the deep veins within the deep fascial envelope. The blood is then pushed out of the muscular compartment, and because of the arrangement of the valves in the leg veins, it must pass upwards towards the heart. When the muscle relaxes, more blood enters the muscle from the arterial side, and from veins below it. Blood also enters the deep veins during this phase from the superficial veins, via the communicating veins, which also have valves to prevent reflux into the superficial veins. Repeated muscular contractions and relaxations thus keep the venous blood flowing.

These skeletal muscles can thus be compared to a peripheral muscle pump; the soleus muscle is particularly important. Guardsmen on parade faint because they do not move their leg muscles for long periods so that blood pools in their legs, resulting in impaired venous return and hence cardiac output, and the diminished cerebral arterial flow causes the faint.

Failure of function of the venous valves in the leg results in increased pressure on valves below them which may themselves fail, creating a further increase in pressure on lower valves. Failure of the valves in the communicating veins is particularly serious as the flow of blood in these veins during muscular contraction is reversed, so that blood flows from the deep to the superficial veins, resulting in localized dilatations of the superficial veins called **varicose veins.** Blockage of the deep veins by thrombosis also produces dilatation of superficial veins.

OSSIFICATION

As for the upper limbs (p. 23.41) the diagrams in fig. 24.67 show the parts of the bones ossified from primary and secondary centres. The approximate dates given for their appearance and fusion show the usual sequence.

SURFACE ANATOMY

The length and direction of the long bones determine the basic form of the limb, which may be long, short, straight, knock-kneed or bowed. The femora slant inwards from the acetabula to the knees, and in the adult female this angulation is more marked than in the male because of the shorter length of the femur and the greater width of the pelvis. As discussed on p. 24.26 the shape of the bones in the foot is an important factor in maintaining the arches and hence the shape of the foot.

The general shape of the limb is given by the muscles within their fascial envelopes surrounding the bones. The rather stark outline which this produces is smoothed out by the layer of subcutaneous fat. In females, this layer is thicker than in males, particularly in the thighs and buttocks, giving a more rounded appearance to the female limb. In obese females excess fat deposits first appear in the buttocks and upper thighs.

The fullness of the buttock is due to the gluteus maximus muscle, and the size of the gluteal fat pad determines its final shape. The gluteal fold or buttock crease does not represent the lower border of gluteus maximus, which extends well below the gluteal fold on its way to its insertions into the gluteal tuberosity of the femur and the iliotibial tract.

The fusiform shape of the thigh is produced mainly by vastus intermedius and lateralis. The rounded muscular prominence above the anteromedial aspect of the knee is due to the lower fibres of vastus medialis. If the subject stands on one leg, with the knee slightly flexed, the iliotibial tract is easily felt, and is sometimes seen, passing to its insertion into the lateral condyle of the tibia. When the thigh is flexed, abducted and slightly laterally rotated, the sartorius muscle becomes prominent, coursing across the thigh. Posteriorly, the tendons of the hamstring muscles bordering the popliteal fossa may be seen and felt, particularly when the knee is flexed.

The shape of the calf is produced by the two heads of gastrocnemius and the underlying soleus. These muscles become tendinous forming the tendo calcaneus, which is easily seen and felt behind the ankle passing to its insertion into the calcaneus. The medial belly of gastrocnemius extends lower down than the lateral belly.

On the dorsum of the foot, the fleshy belly of the extensor digitorum brevis is felt proximally, and the tendons of tibialis anterior and the long extensor muscles can be seen and felt passing to their insertions.

Bony landmarks

The **anterior superior iliac spine** can be palpated at the anterior end of the iliac crest, and the **posterior superior iliac spine** is palpable at the posterior end.

The **pubic crest,** and the **pubic tubercle** at its lateral end can be palpated easily. The **inguinal ligament** passes between the pubic tubercle and the anterior superior iliac spine. The **midinguinal point** is that point on the inguinal ligament which lies midway between the anterior superior iliac spine and the pubic symphysis.

The **ischial tuber** is readily palpated as a thick bony mass in the lower part of the buttock, being separated from the tuber of the opposite side by a distance of one hand's

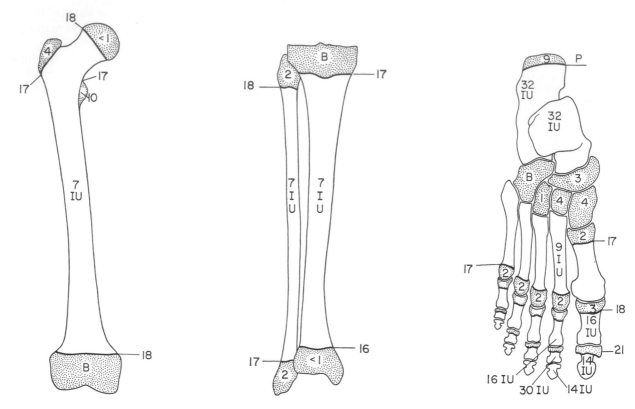

FIG. 24.67. Numbers on the bones indicate age, in years, of appearance of ossification centres. Stippled areas are cartilaginous at birth. Leaders show the time of fusion in years. IU, age in weeks of intrauterine life; B birth; P, puberty.

breadth. The **greater trochanter** of the femur is subcutaneous and hence easily palpable in the lateral aspect of the upper thigh. If a line be drawn around the side of the buttock from the anterior superior iliac spine to the ischial tuber, it crosses the tip of the greater trochanter. This is known as **Nelaton's line,** and use is made of it in diagnosing dislocation of the hip or fracture of the femoral neck.

The shaft of the femur is clothed by muscles and hence is not readily palpable.

The **condyles** of the femur and tibia are subcutaneous and easily palpated at the knee. Between the femoral and tibial condyles anteriorly, the joint line can be palpated, particularly when the knee is flexed and the **patella** lies just above the level of the plane of the knee joint.

The **adductor tubercle** of the femur is felt as a sharp prominence immediately above the medial femoral condyle. The **tibial tuberosity** is palpated at the upper border of the shin, and the **ligamentum patellae** may be felt stretching between this tubercle and the lower pole of the patella.

The **head of the fibula** is seen and felt as a posterolateral prominence below the lateral tibial condyle. The tendon of biceps femoris is inserted into the apex of the head of the fibula and is easily felt here. The **lateral ligament** of the knee may be felt and seen as a strong rounded cord, when the knee is flexed to a right angle and passively adducted. The **neck of the fibula,** with the common peroneal nerve crossing it, is palpable immediately below the head.

The anteromedial surface of the **tibia,** and its sharp anterior border, forming the shin, are subcutaneous throughout their length, and hence easily palpable.

The **medial** (tibia) and **lateral** (fibula) **malleoli** form the subcutaneous prominences at each side of the ankle. The lateral malleolus extends 1 cm lower than the medial one. The prominence of the heel is produced by the calcaneum. The **sustentaculum tali** can be palpated 2.5 cm distal to the tip of the medial malleolus, while 2.5 cm anterior to the sustentaculum the **tuberosity of the navicular** is easily felt.

The **styloid process** of the fifth metatarsal forms the prominent projection half-way along the lateral border of the foot.

Soft tissue landmarks

The **femoral artery** may be felt pulsating in the upper part of the femoral triangle, below the midinguinal point. With the thigh laterally rotated and slightly flexed, draw a line between the midinguinal point and the adductor tubercle.

The femoral artery follows a course corresponding to the upper two-thirds of this line.

The **great saphenous vein** passes through the saphenous opening in the deep fascia to join the femoral vein. This is surface marked by a point 4 cm below and lateral to the pubic tubercle.

The **sciatic nerve** enters the gluteal region at a point opposite the junction of the upper and middle thirds of a line joining the posterior superior iliac spine and the ischial tuber. It curves downwards and slightly laterally to pass into the thigh midway between the greater trochanter and the iscial tuber. The nerve therefore occupies the lower medial quadrant of the buttock.

In the thigh, the nerve runs slightly medial to the midline of the thigh, and it normally divides into its two main branches in the upper part of the popliteal fossa.

The **popliteal artery** may be represented by a line extending from a point just medial to the apex of the popliteal fossa above, to a point in the midline of the leg just below the level of the tibial condyle. The arterial pulsation may be palpated in the popliteal fossa, though this is sometimes difficult as the artery lies deep in the fossa. Palpation is facilitated by flexing the knee and compressing the artery against the popliteal surface of the femur.

The **common peroneal nerve** is easily felt at the lateral side of the neck of the fibula as it passes from the popliteal fossa into the peroneal compartment of the leg.

Pulses in the ankle and in the foot

The **anterior tibial artery** is palpable anteriorly mid-way between the medial and lateral malleoli. It lies lateral to the tendons of tibialis anterior and extensor hallucis longus, and medial to the tendons of extensor digitorum longus and peroneus tertius.

The **dorsalis pedis artery** is the continuation of the anterior tibial artery, and may be palpated on the dorsum of the foot lateral to the tendon of extensor hallucis longus until it passes into the sole of the foot between the first and second meratarsal bones.

The **posterior tibial artery** is palpable at the medial side of the ankle midway between the tip of the malleolus and the medial tubercle of the calcaneus.

The **perforating branch of the peroneal artery** can be palpated the anterior border of the lateral malleolus.

FURTHER READING

BARNETT C.H. (1961) *Recent Advances in Anatomy*, 2nd Edition. Joints and Movement, p. 404. London: Churchill.

BARNETT C.H., DAVIES D.V. & MacCONNAILL M.A. (1961) *Synovial Joints; Their Structure and Mechanics*. London: Longmans.

BREATHNACH A.S. (1965) *Frazer's Anatomy of the Human Skeleton*, 6th Edition. London: Churchill.

BRUCE J., WALMSLEY R. & ROSS J.A. (1964) *Manual of Surgical Anatomy*. Edinburgh: Livingstone.

CROUCH J.E. (1965) *Functional Human Anatomy*. London: Kimpton.

HOLLINSHEAD W.H. (1954) *Anatomy for Surgeons*, vol. 3. The Limbs. London: Cassell.

HOLLINSHEAD W.H. (1960) *Functional Anatomy of the Limbs and Back*, 2nd Edition. Philadelphia: Saunders.

LAST R.J. (1972) *Anatomy: Regional and Applied*, 5th Edition. Edinburgh: Churchill Livingstone.

MORTON D. J. & FULLER D. D. (1952) *Human Locomotion and Body Form*. A Study of Gravity and Man. Baltimore: Williams & Wilkins.

Chapter 25
Nervous system

And afterwards I showed what must be the fabric of the nerves and muscles of the human body to give the animal spirits contained in it the power to move the members; what changes must take place in the brain to produce waking, sleep and dreams; how light, sound, odours, tastes, heat and all the other qualities of external objects impress it with different ideas by means of the senses; how hunger, thirst and the other internal affections can likewise impress upon it divers ideas; what must be understood by the common sense (sensus communis) in which these ideas are received, by the memory which retains them, by the fantasy which can change them in various ways, and out of them compose new ideas, and which can cause the members of such a body to move in as many different ways as can take place in our own case apart from the guidance of the will.

Descartes, R. (1637)   *Discourse on Method.*

Descartes' achievements were formidable. He invented co-ordinate (Cartesian) geometry. He was an experimentalist who made important contributions to the physics and physiology of his time. As a philosopher he proceeded from universal doubt to his famous statement 'I think, therefore I am.' He was a dualist who distinguished radically between mind and body (or matter in general), a point of view commonly, though not necessarily correctly, held to this day. His life-long practice of pursuing his studies in bed until midday is not recommended nowadays, since domestic heating has improved immeasurably since his time.

In this passage he defines clearly most of the problems faced by the student of the nervous system; how movement is brought about, what goes on in sleep, how the special and ordinary senses work, and how hunger, thirst and imagination operate. The unravelling of these problems is a task approached by three different but complementary routes. It begins with neuroanatomy, which Descartes studied personally in animals. The neuroanatomist aims at a complete description of the structure of the nervous system, from what is seen by the naked eye to what is visible by electron microscopy; he also seeks an account of how the structure came to be what it is, how it is maintained and how it changes under various conditions. The neurophysiologist, who cannot begin without some knowledge of structure, investigates function, excelling particularly when some response can

be confidently predicted (i.e. a reflex) and fully accounted for. The psychologist enjoys the rewards of studying the full range of human behaviour; he suffers the frustration that this is rarely predictable and that its structural basis remains largely inscrutable. The present account of the nervous system is not possible without a basis in these three studies. Without neuroanatomy disease cannot be located. Without neurophysiology it cannot be understood. Without psychology its impact on the more exalted functions of the nervous system, such as intelligence, cannot be assessed.

The student should appreciate at the start the daunting complexity of the nervous system. In the grey matter of the cerebral cortex alone there are about 10 000 million individual nerve cells or neurones; in the spinal cord, each of the 200 000 or so nerve cells which supply the muscles of the limbs and trunk receives the synaptic terminations of a few thousand axonal branches from other nerve cells; the optic nerve contains about 1 million nerve fibres. These numerical indices of complexity are further reinforced by a glance at an electron micrograph of central nervous tissue (fig. 25.1) and by reflecting on the numbers of nerve cell processes, and of the connections between them, in the minute volume of tissue illustrated. In short, 'the human brain ...weighing about 1·5 kg is without any qualification the most highly organized and most complexly organized matter in the universe' (Sir John Eccles).

The form and functional activity of neurones, the structural units of the nervous system, are described in chap. 15. The next step in reaching an understanding of the nervous system requires the study of 'nervous pathways', i.e. conduction routes formed by chains of synaptically linked neurones. These pathways which, to some extent at least, are structurally and functionally discrete, are named according to their origin and termination. Thus corticospinal tracts (pathways) begin in the cerebral cortex and terminate at synapses in the spinal cord; spinothalamic tracts link the spinal cord and the thalamus. A variety of techniques are available for defining such pathways. For example, during development, pathways may myelinate at different ages and thus be transiently

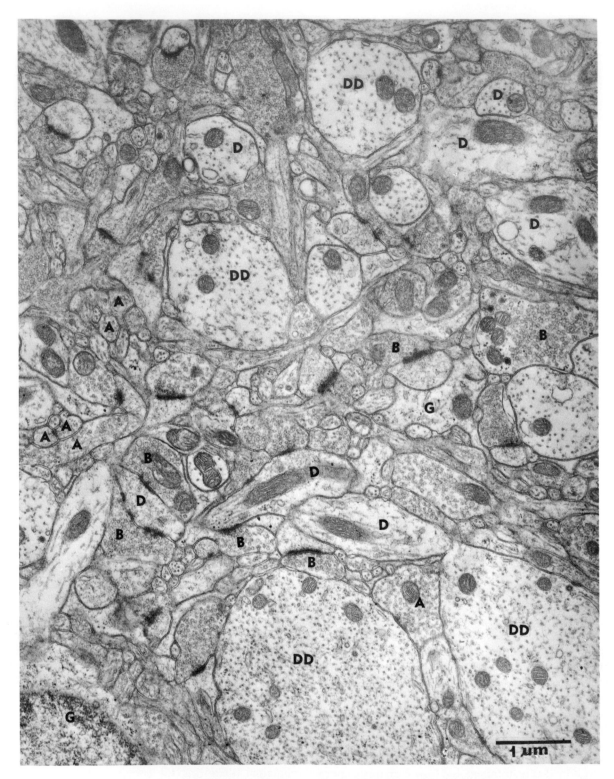

FIG. 25.1. EM of grey matter from the parietal cortex of an adult rat.
In this section, tangential to the surface, the apical dendrites (DD) of pyramidal cells are transected and between them large numbers of smaller dendrites (D), axons (A) and boutons (B) are seen. Astrocyte cytoplasm (G) is also present. The section is approximately 0.05 μm thick. Courtesy of Dr A. Peters.

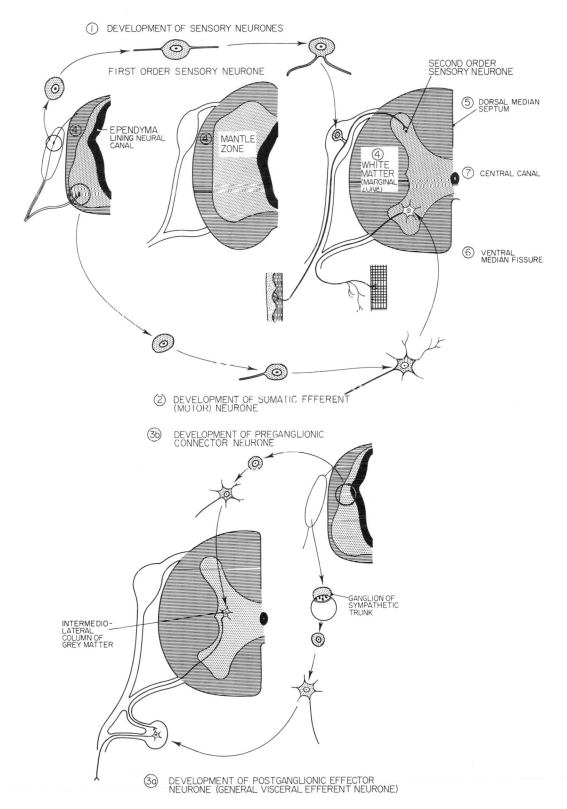

FIG. 25.2. Schematic drawing showing the main features in the development of the spinal cord and spinal neural crest. Numbers on the diagrams correspond to paragraph numbers in the text.

distinguishable in section. In adult animals, they can be transected experimentally, and the consequent degeneration of the nerve axons (vol. 2, p. 25.9) traced along their course in histological sections prepared on killing the animal after a suitable interval. Electrical stimulation can also be used to evoke traffic in a pathway, and the response can be recorded at remote points; by observing such features as the timing of the response, additional information is gained about conduction velocity and the presence or absence of intervening synapses.

DEVELOPMENT AND GENERAL PLAN OF THE CENTRAL NERVOUS SYSTEM

The simplest way of becoming familiar with the general layout of the nervous system and the rather complex terminology of its parts is to study the main steps in its development.

The brain and spinal cord, which together form the central nervous system (CNS) arise in common, in the first month of embryonic life, from the neural tube (pp. 19.6 and 10). The neural tube is initially a pseudostratified epithelium, consisting of long narrow **ventricular cells**, each of which extends through the whole thickness of the wall. The ventricular cells are stem cells, which divide mitotically to form embryonic nerve cells, **neuroblasts** and **supporting cells**. When a ventricular cell enters mitosis, its outer end retracts from the surface of the tube and its nucleus migrates towards the inner (central canal) end of the cell. After division, the inner end of each daughter cell remains attached to the luminal margin, while its outer end extends towards the outer surface of the tube and the nucleus also moves peripherally. The process of nuclear movement up to and away from, the lumen of the tube is known as **interkinetic migration**.

Some of the progeny of dividing ventricular cells migrate outward and establish the **intermediate** or **mantle zone** which consists mainly of immature neurones which do not normally divide again. Others form the (definitive) **ependyma**, the lining epithelium of the ventricular cavities of the brain and of the central canal of the spinal cord. A third group forms the **subventricular zone**, a layer of proliferating cells from which arise the macroglia (astroglia and oligodendroglia).

The **marginal zone**, the outermost zone of the neural tube, consists initially of the outer cytoplasmic parts of the ventricular cells. It forms the bed through which run the processes of nerve cells entering or leaving the spinal cord or running upwards or downwards. It corresponds, in a general way, to the white matter of the adult cord.

Each side wall of the neural tube shows a shallow longitudinal furrow facing into the neural canal; this **sulcus limitans** is a landmark of importance, since it demarcates a dorsal part of the tube, the **alar lamina**, from a ventral part, the **basal lamina**. In the adult, that part of the spinal grey matter derived from the alar lamina will be concerned with sensory function, that from the basal lamina with motor function.

In the following description of later stages in the development of the neural tube and crest, the paragraph numbers correspond to the numbers in fig. 25.2.

(1) From the neuroblasts of the neural crest (p. 19.12) the nerve cells of the dorsal root ganglia of spinal nerves develop. These are the first link in a chain of neurones which conduct sensory nerve impulses from the periphery, and are called **first order afferent** (sensory) **neurones**. They are bipolar neurones (p. 15.2); one process (peripheral) grows outwards to establish peripheral sensory terminations in skin, muscle, tendon, joint capsule etc; the other process (central) grows into the neural tube where it ends synaptically on the second link in the afferent chain of neurones, the **second order afferent** (sensory) **neurones**. These are situated in the developing grey matter of the alar lamina of the neural tube. Clusters of second order afferent cell bodies are grouped in the grey matter of the cord as **somatic afferent** (sensory) **nuclei**, and groups of these nuclei form the main mass of the dorsal grey columns of the adult cord. The nervous elements of the dorsal (sensory) root of a spinal nerve are thus seen to be derived from neuroblasts of the neural crest. Other cells from the neural crest migrate and apply themselves to the surface of developing peripheral axons, forming the Schwann cells, the source of the myelin sheath (p. 15.4).

(2) From neuroblasts in the basal lamina, **multipolar** (motor) **neurones** develop. Their dendrites ramify in the vicinity of the cell body; their axons grow away from the tube to innervate groups of skeletal muscle fibres in the limbs or trunk. Each of these **somatic efferent neurones**, with the group of muscle fibres which it innervates, constitutes a motor unit (p. 16.10). Groups of cell bodies of these neurones form **somatic efferent** (motor) **nuclei** of the ventral columns of grey matter in the adult spinal cord.

(3) **Sympathetic ganglia**, both of the paravertebral sympathetic chains and the prevertebral ganglia, e.g. coeliac and superior mesenteric, arise from young nerve cells (sympathoblasts) which migrate from the neural crest. These cells will innervate visceral structures (smooth muscle and glands) and are called **postganglionic effector neurones** (3a). They lie entirely outside the central nervous system, with which they are linked by **preganglionic connector neurones** (3b). These develop from multipolar neuroblasts in the basal lamina of the neural tube immediately ventral to the sulcus limitans. Groups of their cell bodies will form the intermediolateral columns of grey matter which extend between the 1st thoracic and 2nd lumbar segments of the adult cord.

Their axons leave the cord in the ventral roots of the corresponding spinal nerves and travel in white rami communicantes to the sympathetic trunk (p. 21.41), where many of them synapse with postganglionic effector neurones. Pre- and postganglionic sympathetic neurones are classified as **general visceral efferent**.

(4) The **white matter of the spinal cord** develops from the marginal layer of the neural tube as more and more developing fibres grow up or down within that layer.

(5) The **dorsal median septum** is formed by fusion of the apposed surfaces of the ependymal lining of the dorsal part of the neural canal, brought about by the increased bulk of the alar laminae.

(6) The **ventral median fissure** develops through the ventral expansion of the two sides of the neural tube on either side of the midline.

(7) The **central canal** of the adult cord represents the most ventral part of the neural canal.

Later development of the spinal cord

At embryonic stages, the cord extends through the whole length of the vertebral canal. It tapers gradually, to end at the level of the lowest coccygeal vertebra, and the dorsal and ventral roots of each spinal nerve run horizontally outwards to the corresponding intervertebral foramen. Here is situated the dorsal root ganglion and here the dorsal and ventral roots unite to form the spinal nerve. This simple pattern is greatly changed by three events. (1) The most caudal segments of the neural tube regress and this is paralleled by a similar loss of several rudimentary coccygeal vertebrae. (2) The cord enlarges at the levels of the brachial plexus, segments C(4)5–T1(2), which supplies the developing upper limb, and of the lumbosacral plexus, segments L2–S4, which supplies the developing lower limb; these **cervical** and **lumbosacral enlargements** reflect the greater numbers of motor and sensory neurones involved in the innervation of the limbs. (3) The vertebral column elongates rapidly after the third fetal month and its growth outstrips that of the spinal cord. The upper end of the cord is anchored to the brain. The lower end of the vertebral column extends progressively beyond the end of the spinal cord, which appears to recede up the vertebral canal. The end of the cord has reached the level of the 3rd lumbar vertebra at birth and the 1st or 2nd lumbar vertebra when growth ceases. As the lower end of the spinal cord recedes up the canal, the roots of the lumbar, sacral and coccygeal nerves are drawn out between their attachment to the cord and their point of exit through the intervertebral foramen; the leash of descending nerve roots forms the **cauda equina** (mare's tail). The dorsal root ganglion and the junction of the dorsal and ventral roots of a particular spinal nerve remain in their original position, in the appropriate intervertebral foramen (fig. 25.3 & p. 20.12).

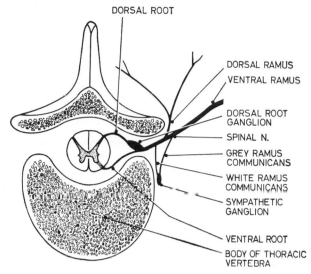

FIG. 25.3. The thoracic spinal nerve with the coverings of the spinal cord and of the nerve roots omitted.

As the spinal cord recedes, its tip becomes drawn out as the **filum terminale**. In later fetal life this contains little nervous tissue and consists mainly of fibrous tissue derived from membranes investing the cord.

The relations between the spinal cord and nerves and the vertebral column in the adult are illustrated schematically in fig. 25.4. The lack of coincidence between vertebral segments and spinal cord segments, **vertebrosegmental discrepancy**, is of clinical importance and becomes increasingly obvious as one descends the column. The relationship is complicated by the varying length of successive segments of the spinal cord. While the cord itself is not obviously segmented, either in external appearance or in internal structure, a spinal cord segment may be arbitrarily defined as the region of cord to which are attached the dorsal and ventral rootlets of a pair (right and left) of spinal nerves. In the cervical region, the correspondence between spinal cord and vertebral segments is good; in the lower thoracic region, the spinal cord segments are considerably elongated; the ten lumbosacral segments are short and correspond in vertical extent to vertebrae T11–L1 or 2. Below L1–2, the vertebral canal contains only spinal nerve roots, the filum terminale and the spinal meninges.

SEGMENTAL DISTRIBUTION OF SPINAL NERVES

The primitive segmental distribution of the spinal nerves, seen in the early embryo, is in the adult best preserved in the thoracic region, where the intercostal nerves represent typical segmental nerves (fig. 21.29). Here each dermatome (the area of skin receiving its sensory innervation from a single pair of dorsal nerve roots) takes the form of a narrow strip of skin stretching round the chest like a girdle. In the limbs this simple pattern is distorted and obscured through the formation of limb nerve plexuses

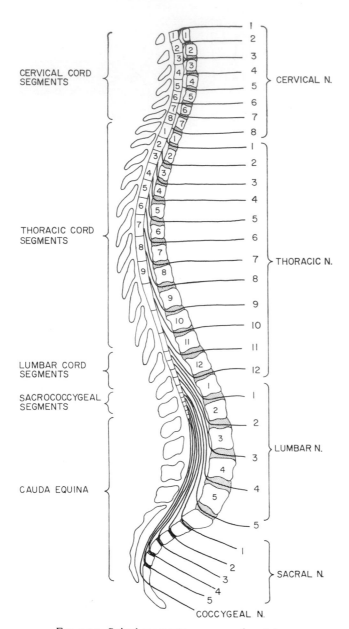

FIG. 25.4. Spinal segments, nerves and vertebrae.

and the complex axial rotation of the limbs during development (fig. 25.5). The differences in published dermatomal maps reflect not only individual variation in the pattern, but also the technical difficulties involved in determining the extent of individual human dermatomes. Thus there is substantial overlap between adjacent dermatomes, so much so that sensory deficit may not be detectable when only a single dorsal spinal root is damaged. Also the size of individual dermatomes may vary for different sensory modalities, being greater for touch than for pain and temperature.

Development of the brain
Despite a general resemblance, there are some differences

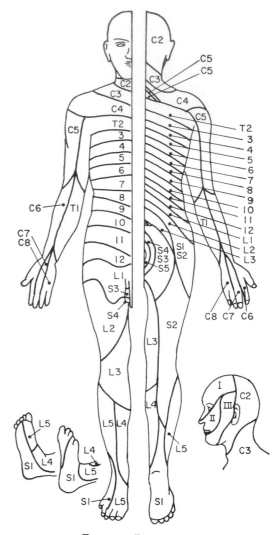

FIG. 25.5. Dermatomes.

between developing brain and spinal cord, even in the early stages.

The brain is ahead of the spinal cord in its development and grows more rapidly. It soon shows several bends or flexures, which presumably arise because it grows faster than its surroundings. These flexures demarcate three descriptive subdivisions of the brain, **fore-, mid-** and **hindbrain** (fig. 25.6a).

The sulcus limitans extends forwards only to the junction between midbrain and forebrain, and the alar and basal laminae are, therefore, recognizable only in mid- and hindbrains. Only the alar lamina is thought to be represented in the forebrain.

In the hindbrain and the forebrain the roof plate remains thin, consisting only of ependymal epithelium. These are areas in which, at a later date, the choroid plexuses develop through the invagination of the ependyma by the layer of vascular pia mater which invests the neural tube.

The neural crest forms irregularly disposed clumps rather than regular segmental masses.

The sharp segregation of grey and white matter, so characteristic of the spinal part of the neural tube, is absent in the mid- and hindbrain, where the grey matter forms nuclear groups lying in a complex network of nerve fibres with neurones and neuroglial elements, the whole constituting the reticular formation.

HINDBRAIN

The acuteness of the pontine flexure causes the lateral walls of the tube to splay apart, opening out like a book. The ependymal roof becomes diamond-shaped, like that part of the neural canal (**fourth ventricle**) which it covers. The sulcus limitans now lies in the floor of the fourth ventricle; the alar lamina lies lateral, rather than ventral, to the basal lamina. When nuclear groups develop in the hindbrain, they do so in the same general positions as in the spinal cord, i.e. motor nuclei in basal lamina, sensory nuclei in alar lamina. Their positions relative to one another have been changed, however, by the opening out of the tube. In addition to the somatic efferent nuclei, there are general visceral efferent and somatic afferent groups which are equivalent to those described in the spinal cord. The new groups are the branchial (special visceral) efferent motor nuclei which innervate the muscles of the branchial arches (p. 19.32) and the special somatic afferent nuclei of termination receiving special sense afferents (cochlear and vestibular). The pons, medulla and cerebellum are of hindbrain origin.

The **cerebellum** develops from paired thickenings of the alar laminae at the anterior end of the hindbrain; as it enlarges it overgrows the fourth ventricle, whose original ependymal roof is displaced, so that it covers only the lower end of the ventricle and forms the inferior medullary velum of the adult (fig. 25.6b). Here the choroid plexus of the fourth ventricle develops (fig. 25.7). Cells which migrate from the intermediate zone establish the surface layer of grey matter, the cortex, while others remain deeply placed and form the deep cerebellar nuclei.

MIDBRAIN

This initially shows the typical pattern of the neural tube. Its transformation to the adult condition is summarized in fig. 25.8. The neural canal narrows to form the cerebral aqueduct, and the alar laminae thicken to produce the **tectum** from which arise the **superior** and **inferior colliculi**. The basal laminae form the **tegmentum** of the midbrain and the **substantia nigra**, while the **crura cerebri** become more prominent as more descending fibre groups, **corticopontine**, **corticonuclear** and **corticospinal**, grow down the neural tube. The **cerebral peduncles** include the tegmentum and crura cerebri.

The **corticonuclear fibres** end synaptically on motor nuclei of mid- and hindbrain. Corticopontine fibres grow

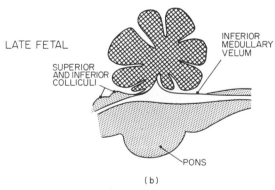

FIG. 25.6(a). The flexures of the brain and the fundamental subdivision into fore-, mid- and hindbrain; (b) a series of parasagittal sections of the hindbrain to show the developing cerebellum overgrowing the ependymal roof of the fourth ventricle.

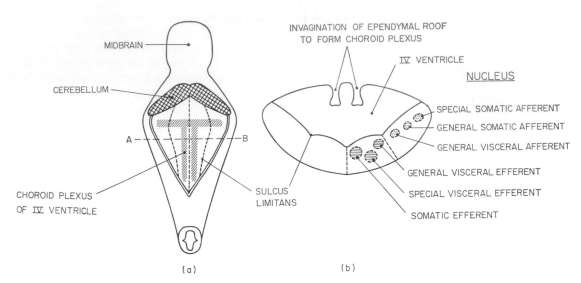

FIG. 25.7. Floor of the fourth ventricle viewed (a) from behind, and (b) in transverse section A–B.

down into the hindbrain, where they continue to lie ventrally. They end on the pontine nuclei, which have migrated ventrally far from their origin in the alar lamina. Axons of cells of the pontine nuclei enter the opposite cerebellar hemisphere via the middle cerebellar peduncle. Corticospinal fibres continue growing inferiorly on the ventral surface of the medulla, where they form the **pyramids**, and on into the spinal cord, most of them crossing in the pyramidal decussation (fig. 25.9). Just as the crura are ventral additions to the tegmentum of the midbrain, so the basilar part of the pons, comprising corticopontine, corticonuclear and corticospinal fibres and the pontine nuclei, is a ventral addition to the tegmentum of the pontine part of the hindbrain. The midbrain and hind-

brain together are often referred to as the **brain stem.** The development of the forebrain is dealt with later (p. 25.29).

SPINAL CORD

The structural plan of the spinal cord, with its central mass of grey matter, H-shaped in transverse section, and peripheral white matter, has already been illustrated (fig. 25.2). This plan shows important regional variations (fig. 25.10). The cord is larger where the nerves of the limb plexuses are attached (cervical and lumbar enlargements). The amount of white matter is greatest at high cervical levels where the full complement of both descending and ascending fibres is present. The amount of grey matter is greatest at the levels of origin of the limb plexuses, providing for the motor supply of the large bulk of limb muscles and for receipt of the large sensory input from the limbs. And, in addition to the dorsal and ventral grey columns, which are common to all levels, between levels T1 and L2 there are present the intermediolateral grey columns.

The internal organization of the spinal cord may be analysed by considering the input of nerve impulses through afferent pathways, the output through efferent pathways, and the connections of each with higher levels of the central nervous system and between each within the cord.

INPUT: AFFERENT PATHWAYS
The first neurones on the afferent pathways in a spinal nerve (first order or primary afferents) have their cell bodies in the dorsal root ganglion and enter the cord via the dorsal rootlets. Their peripheral processes end in a variety of sensory receptors (p. 25.34).

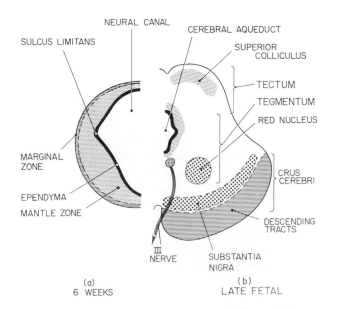

FIG. 25.8. Scheme to show the main features of the development of the midbrain.

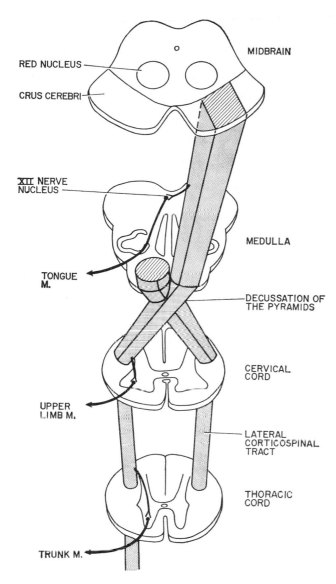

FIG. 25.9. Corticospinal tracts from the midbrain to the spinal cord.

Labels on figure 25.9: RED NUCLEUS, CRUS CEREBRI, MIDBRAIN, XII NERVE NUCLEUS, TONGUE M., MEDULLA, DECUSSATION OF THE PYRAMIDS, UPPER LIMB M., CERVICAL CORD, LATERAL CORTICOSPINAL TRACT, THORACIC CORD, TRUNK M.

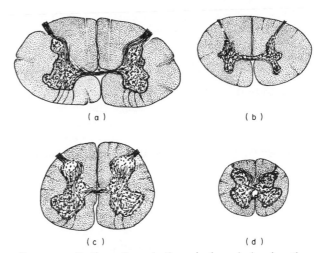

FIG. 25.10. Sections through the spinal cord showing the different proportions of grey and white matter at various levels; (a) cervical, (b) thoracic, (c) lumbar and (d) sacral.

functional and clinical importance. Fibres of the lateral division are concerned with pain and temperature sensibility, those of the medial division with touch, vibration and proprioceptive sense. On entering the cord, first order afferent fibres may make a variety of connections depending, among other things, on the sensory modality with which they are concerned. Before looking at the various possibilities in detail it is helpful to indicate the general patterns of afferent pathways, in three broad groupings: sensory, cerebellar and reflex.

Sensory pathways

This term should, strictly, be confined to those which give rise to conscious appreciation of one of the sensory

Dorsal nerve roots

Impulses generated by stimulation of the various peripheral receptors are conveyed by first order afferent neurones, whose cell bodies lie in the dorsal root ganglion, and whose central processes constitute the dorsal rootlets of spinal nerves. Each spinal nerve has several rootlets, which enter the cord in linear series at the posterolateral sulcus (fig. 25.11). Each rootlet contains a variety of nerve fibres, ranging from fine, non-myelinated (C) fibres to large, heavily myelinated (group I) fibres (p. 15.23). These are intermingled within the rootlets but, just before entering the cord, they become grouped into two divisions, a larger **medial division**, consisting of the larger fibres, and a **lateral division**, of unmyelinated and finely myelinated fibres. This segregation is of some

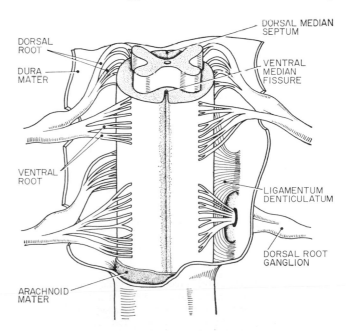

FIG. 25.11. Spinal cord and roots of spinal nerves.

Labels on figure 25.11: DORSAL MEDIAN SEPTUM, DORSAL ROOT, DURA MATER, VENTRAL MEDIAN FISSURE, VENTRAL ROOT, LIGAMENTUM DENTICULATUM, DORSAL ROOT GANGLION, ARACHNOID MATER

modalities. Each such pathway consists of a chain of three afferent neurones (first, second and third order), synaptically linked, and terminating in the cerebral cortex. They are mainly crossed pathways, terminating in the cortex of the cerebral hemisphere of the side of the body opposite to that in which the nerve traffic was generated.

Fig. 25.12 illustrates schematically the three-neurone chain. The central processes of first order neurones terminate on second order neurones, whose cell bodies lie in a **sensory nucleus** in the dorsal grey column. The axons of second order neurones cross over (decussate) in the ventral white commissure of the cord and ascend in the white matter of the cord. Fibres subserving particular sensory modalities tend to run together in more or less discrete tracts, whose position in the human cord is now fairly well charted. These tracts continue upwards through the spinal cord and brain stem, to reach the **thalamus**, a large collection of nuclei in the side wall of the forebrain (p. 25.29). Here a second relay occurs and the third order (thalamic) neurones send their axons to the **somatosensory areas** of the cerebral cortex.

That the pathway is a chain of three neurones and that it is crossed has significance. Thus, decussation leads to sensory input from the right side of the body being 'appreciated' in the left hemisphere, and that from the left, in the right hemisphere. The presence of synapses along the route is of more subtle significance; the cells in the sensory and thalamic nuclei receive not only excitatory stimuli from neurones lower in the chain, but also inhibitory stimuli from neurones both within the nuclei themselves and in the cerebral cortex. These inhibitory stimuli 'sharpen' the excitatory neuronal signals and provide for greater sensory discrimination.

Pathways to the cerebellum

These differ from the sensory pathways just described in at least three important respects. They involve a two-neurone chain, are mainly uncrossed and terminate in the cerebellar hemisphere of the same side of the body as that in which the nerve impulses are generated. The impulses do not result in conscious appreciation of sensation but are part of the automatic feedback of information from the locomotor system which allows continuous modulation of its control by the CNS (p. 25.53).

Reflex connections (fig 25.13)

All first order afferent neurones also establish one or more of a variety of reflex connections which may be on their own or opposite sides of the cord, and at their level of entry or lower or higher in the cord. Reflex connections are widespread and effected by (1) dorsal root fibres which terminate directly, or via intercalated neurones, on

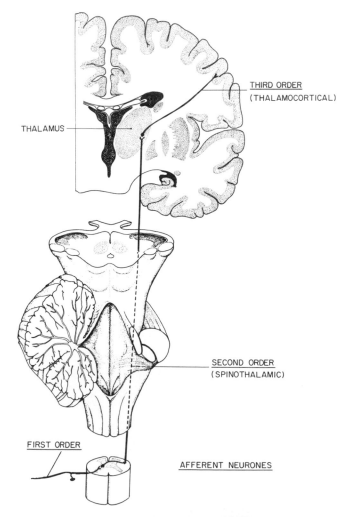

FIG. 25.12. Scheme of the three-neurone chain which forms a typical somatic sensory pathway between a sensory end organ, e.g. in the skin, and the somatic sensory cortex. The diagram shows a dorsal view of the spinal cord and brain stem, and a coronal section of the cerebral hemisphere.

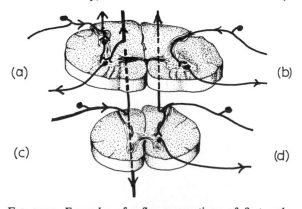

FIG. 25.13. Examples of reflex connections of first order afferent neurones; (a) collateral branch of first order neurone ends on intercalated neurone; (b) ipsilateral, segmental, monosynaptic; (c) ipsilateral, intersegmental; central process of first order neurone divides into ascending and descending branches; (d) collateral branch of first order neurone forms an intersegmental, monosynaptic connection.

motor neurones in the ventral grey column at their own level of entry, (2) axons of dorsal root fibres which divide T-wise, on entering the cord, into ascending and descending branches. These run in the white matter before terminating in the grey matter, and (3) collateral branches which arise both from root fibres, at their level of entry, and from their ascending and descending branches.

These connections provide the anatomical basis for several specifically-named reflexes, the tendon jerks (myotatic reflexes), stretch reflexes, flexor (withdrawal) reflexes, and crossed extensor reflexes, discussed in detail later in this chapter. Reflexes are classed (a) as **monosynaptic**, when the entering dorsal root fibre, or a collateral from it, ends directly on a motor neurone, and as **polysynaptic**, when there are one or more intercalated neurones; (b) as **segmental**, when they involve a single spinal cord segment, and as **intersegmental**, when more than one segment is involved.

The **proprius bundles** (fasciculi proprii) are longitudinally coursing fibres which ascend and descend in the white matter, mainly close to the grey columns. They contain axons of intercalated neurones and provide connections for intersegmental reflexes and for two-way polysynaptic links between the spinal cord and brain stem.

GREY MATTER OF THE SPINAL CORD
Afferent nuclei

Substantia gelatinosa lies beneath the apex of the dorsal grey column and extends throughout the length of the cord. It receives terminals of fibres in the lateral division of dorsal rootlets and serves, in part, as a relay on the pathways involved in pain and thermal sensibility. These are described more fully on p. 25.38.

The **thoracic nucleus** (Clarke's column) is found principally in thoracic segments of the cord (C8-L2), at the medial side of the base of the dorsal column. Its afferents are first order neurones whose peripheral processes end mainly in muscle spindles, tendon organs or Pacinian corpuscles; its axons run in the dorsal spinocerebellar tract to the cerebellar hemisphere of the same side. The nucleus therefore forms part of the uncrossed two-neurone chain which feeds back proprioceptive information from the locomotor system to the cerebellum.

The **nucleus proprius** is the more diffusely organized remainder of the dorsal grey column. It receives fibres from the medial division of the dorsal rootlets, and conveys information to the thalamus via ascending tracts of the cord involved in various sensory modalities and to the cerebellum via the ventral spinocerebellar tract. It also contains small intercalated neurones which receive traffic from the main descending motor pathway (corticospinal tract) and transmit it to motor neurones in the ventral grey column.

Efferent nuclei

The **intermediolateral grey column**, confined to segments T1–L2, is a visceral efferent (motor) nucleus. Its axons leave the cord through the ventral nerve roots and run to the sympathetic chain, forming the thoracolumbar (sympathetic) outflow of the autonomic nervous system. An equivalent group of cells is found in segments S2–S4, also occupying a position intermediate between dorsal and ventral columns, but not projecting as a 'lateral' column. Its bodies give rise to the axons of the sacral (parasympathetic) outflow and run in the pelvic splanchnic nerves. Visceral efferent nuclei provide the motor innervation of smooth muscle and glands in visceral organs in the thorax and abdomen, and elsewhere.

The **ventral grey column** has a complex pattern but, in general, shows a medial column which sends fibres to muscles of the neck and trunk, and a lateral column (confined to segments C4-T1 and L2-S3) which sends fibres to the limbs. In the lateral column, nerve cell bodies which supply muscles of the proximal part of the limb arise more ventrally and from higher segmental levels than those supplying distal muscle groups. In the cervical cord there are found, in addition, the nuclei of origin of the spinal accessory nerve and of the phrenic nerve. All the nuclei of the ventral grey column are somatic efferent nuclei, since they supply skeletal muscle of somite origin. Each constitutes a **final common path** in central control over body movement. They are commonly known as **lower motor neurones**. Lower motor neurones are the same as α motor neurones, which are so called because they are large and have thick axons in the Aα class, commonly termed simply for brevity (p. 15.23). Each receives hundreds or even thousands of synaptic terminals, among which are those of axons of **upper motor neurones**, most of whose cell bodies lie in the cortical grey matter of the cerebral hemispheres.

The ventral grey column also contains γ motor neurones, smaller, and with thinner axons in the Aγ class; these have the special function of regulating the sensitivity of muscle spindles (p. 25.18) and do not evoke contraction of ordinary striated muscle.

REFLEX ACTIVITY

Reflexes are predictable, automatic, reliable responses to preceding sensory stimuli, and mediated by the nervous system. The responses may be simple, as in a knee jerk, or very complex as in a conditioned reflex (p. 25.77). They may involve action of striated muscle, decreased or increased activity of cardiac or smooth muscle, or secretion by glands. The part of the nervous system concerned may be the spinal cord, as in a knee jerk, or higher parts, as when the pupil of the eye contracts in response to light and the midbrain is involved.

Reflexes are not necessarily all present at birth. Some develop later, like the normal plantar response (p. 25.19); others are present at birth and subsequently vanish, like the Moro startle reflex (vol. 3, p. 41.5). Voluntary movements play no part in reflexes; and a habit, arising as it does out of earlier deliberate actions, is not a reflex. Conditioned reflexes are a special type of reflex discussed on p. 25.77.

We understand the spinal reflex better because we can stand upon the shoulders of Sir Charles Sherrington (1857–1952), who shared a Nobel prize and was appointed to the Order of Merit for his 'discoveries regarding the function of the neurones'. He analysed the behaviour of the **reflex arc** which is the conducting path between a stimulus and the ensuing response. He drew comparisons between the behaviour of a nerve trunk and the behaviour of a reflex arc.

SPEED OF CONDUCTION

The reflex arc conducts more slowly; the weaker the stimulus, the more slowly it conducts. Fig. 25.14 shows

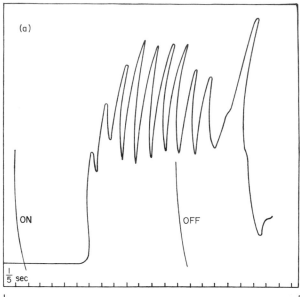

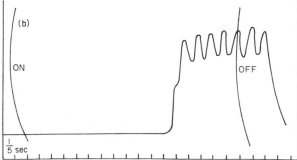

FIG. 25.14. Scratching movements of a dog in response to stimulation of skin from 'on' to 'off'. (a) stronger stimulation, (b) weaker stimulation. After Sherrington C. (1906) *Integrative Action of the Nervous System.* London: Cambridge University Press.

the scratching movements of a dog in response to electrical stimulation of its skin. Stimulation starts at 'on' and is continued until 'off'. Note the length of time elapsing from the start of the stimulus until scratching begins.

This is much longer than the time that would elapse during conduction along any large nerve fibre from the skin via the spinal cord to the scratching muscles. Is it possible that this reflex is conducted along slowly conducting nerve fibres only? This explanation is ruled out by the second part of the figure. Here the stimulus is reduced in intensity, but not in duration (note the slightly altered time scale); the delay before scratching starts is clearly greater. So the reflex arc is conducting more slowly than any but the tiniest nerve fibre and, unlike any nerve fibre, at a variable speed depending on the intensity of stimulation. The speed can be shown to vary during conduction through the spinal cord and not during conduction to or from the cord.

AFTER DISCHARGE

The response, or the muscular movement, does not end exactly when the stimulus ceases, even allowing for conduction time along the reflex arc. There may be marked after discharge prolonging the response. Fig. 25.15 records the withdrawal of a cat's leg in response to electrical stimulation of the skin, more intense than the

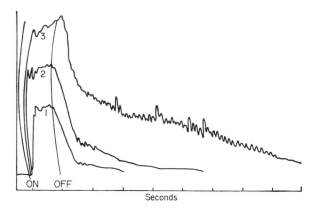

FIG. 25.15. Flexion of cat's leg in response to stimulation to skin lasting 1 sec from 'on' to 'off'. Traces 1 to 3 evoked by increasing strength of stimulus. After Sherrington.

delicate stimulation which evokes scratching. Three different intensities of stimulation were employed and three degrees of response recorded. The record was made by using levers pivoted at the right of the figure and so the time of starting stimulation is shown by an arc of a circle, marked 'on'. The interval between this arc and the start of the upswing produced by the retreating leg is the **latent period**, the gap during which conduction is occurring along the reflex arc but before the response begins. This latent period is evidently brief and clearly well below one-tenth second, especially with the higher strengths of stimulus.

The stimulus was stopped at time 'off', shown by another similar arc of a circle. But the response does not end immediately and the leg does not resume its initial position for a number of seconds, and with the highest intensity of stimulation, rhythmic jerking (**clonus**, p. 25.49) persists practically to the end of the record.

After discharge is not a feature of a nerve trunk but is shown here to occur in a reflex arc. A brief stimulus gives rise to a much more prolonged response; the spinal cord processes operate over a much longer time scale than the impulses in peripheral nerve fibres. This is true even though in the long, jerky clonus the spinal cord is not itself setting up a rhythm but is being restimulated by the incoming sensory traffic from the jerking limb.

A peripheral nerve trunk responds to a single stimulus, if this is sufficiently strong, with a single impulse. Repeated impulses are the product of repeated stimulation. But the scratch reflex is a rhythmic, repeated response in a reflex arc which can occur after a single stimulus (fig. 25.16). A single shock in the skin at the time

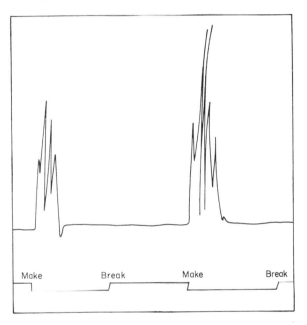

FIG. 25.16. Scratch reflexes of a dog in response to faradic stimulation of the skin. The second stimulus is stronger than the first. After Sherrington.

marked 'make' gives rise to four scratches, and the weaker shock at 'break' to none; a stronger shock then produces five scratches. The rhythm of a reflex response does not conform strictly to the rhythm of stimulation.

GRADED RESPONSES

A single nerve fibre exhibits the **all-or-none phenomenon**. When sufficiently strongly stimulated, it conveys an impulse, but it cannot convey half an impulse or a double-sized impulse. Conduction in a reflex arc shows much more gradation. Fig. 25.17 is a record of a dog's flexion reflex, in which the leg is withdrawn in response to electrical stimulation of a digit. As the strength of stimulation is increased, the response increases, but not in a linear fashion.

TEMPORAL SUMMATION

The dog's scratch reflex is difficult to elicit by any single stimulus of whatever strength. But the reflex arc concerned is capable of adding together successive stimuli; two weak stimuli, one after the other, can be successful when either alone fails. Admittedly a single nerve fibre can respond

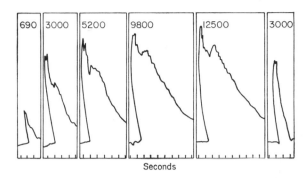

FIG. 25.17. Flexion reflex; withdrawal of a dog's leg in response to stimulation of varying intensity. Strength of stimulus is given in arbitrary units for each response. After Sherrington.

in a similar way, but only when the stimuli are a mere fraction of a millisecond apart. Enormously greater intervals can be dealt with by a reflex arc, which possesses a property termed temporal summation permitting the summing of incoming traffic spaced apart in time. In the case of the scratch reflex, the interval may be as long as 1·4 sec. In other words, if a dog's skin is stimulated at a strength insufficient to make it scratch, and the same small stimulus is repeated as long as 1·4 sec later, the second stimulus may prove effective; the spinal cord has a holding capacity of that length. The beginnings of this holding capacity can be seen when one notes how much longer an excitatory postsynaptic potential lasts than the nerve impulse responsible for it (p. 25.16). But in the case of a simple monosynaptic reflex, such as a tendon jerk (p. 25.17), the holding capacity may not extend further than about 10 msec.

SPATIAL SUMMATION

A flexion reflex can be produced when two stimuli are applied at different places on a limb, even when neither alone would be effective. Here the cord is showing an ability termed spatial summation; two stimuli at different places are being summed. So one can think provisionally of the spinal cord as a system capable of two kinds of addition: spatial summation and holding information over a period of time (temporal summation). But this is still to underestimate its capacity. It is certainly capable of evolving one response rather than another, when simple arithmetic would produce a different solution. Fig. 25.18 shows what happens when a scratch reflex is first induced alone and then what happens when it is superimposed upon a flexion reflex. The two do not add, or the trace

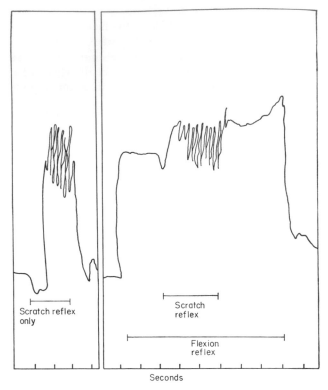

FIG. 25.18. Interaction of flexion reflex and scratch reflex in a dog. After Sherrington.

would rise off the record; instead, the new reflex displaces the old temporarily after a second or so of confusion.

ONE WAY CONDUCTION

Another distinction between a nerve trunk and a reflex arc is the 'one way only' property of the arc. When a nerve trunk is artificially stimulated in the middle of its length, impulses are generated in its fibres which proceed both ways, i.e. towards the end of the fibre, and back towards the neurone body (**antidromic conduction**). But the antidromic impulse is unable to proceed backwards round a reflex arc and reach the receptors which normally originate the reflex activity. Nor it is possible to stimulate a ventral spinal root and produce impulses in dorsal spinal roots.

FATIGUE

A healthy nerve fibre, adequately supplied with blood, is extremely difficult to fatigue and will continue to respond to stimulation much longer than a reflex arc. Fig. 25.19 shows a record of a scratch reflex being elicited by a tickle first at one point on the skin (stimulus A) and then at another (stimulus B). After some 21 sec of continuous stimulation, the rhythm and amplitude are much reduced; but it is hard to believe that the stimulated skin is the site of the fatigue since some recovery appears during the persistence of the stimulus. It is impossible to

believe that the outward path from the spinal cord or the responding muscles are fatigued, because changing the position of the stimulus restores completely the vigour of the response. The fatigue occurs in the central element of the reflex arc, i.e. in the spinal cord.

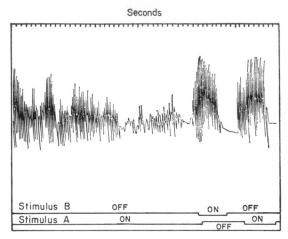

Fig. 25.19. Scratch reflex of a dog in response to stimulation at two different places on skin. After Sherrington.

Similarly, conduction through the spinal cord is much more susceptible to hypoxia and anaesthetics than conduction through nerve fibres. The higher parts of the central nervous system are even more susceptible. But it should not be assumed that fatigue is a word which has a constant physiological accompaniment. It describes human experience and needs careful interpretation. The weak link in the chain which gives way in fatigue may be one of many. For instance, if one uses a thumb muscle to press continuously and very hard, the force exerted falls off even during the first minute, because of failure of neuromuscular conduction, and then further decreases because of failure of the muscle fibres. On the other hand, during severe physical exercise, the weak link may lie outside the neuromuscular system altogether and the transport of oxygen or the availability of glucose may be deficient. Other forms of human fatigue may defeat analysis, except by those who sell popular remedies.

INHIBITION

A further property of a reflex arc is that conduction in it can be impaired by inhibition. Fig. 25.20 shows withdrawal of a cat's leg in response to electrical stimulation of the foot of the same leg, a flexion reflex. The stimulation lasts from A to C. From B to C, the other foot is stimulated as well and the reflex response is reduced. Impulses from the second foot, on reaching the spinal cord, excite second order afferent neurones on their own side of the cord, which is the opposite side from the one traversed by the reflex arc. The axons of these neurones cross the midline (fig. 25.21) and form synapses on the reflex arc.

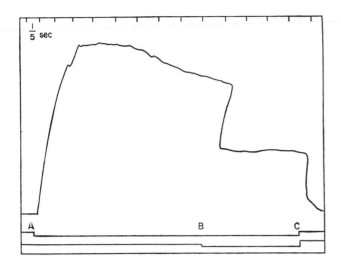

FIG. 25.20. Flexion reflex of leg. From time A to time C the foot of the same leg was being stimulated. From time B to time C the opposite foot was being stimulated also. After Sherrington.

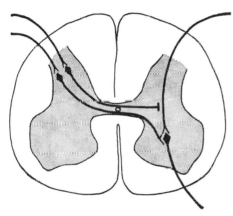

FIG. 25.21. Inhibitory pathways in a spinal cord segment.

Synaptic transmission

STRUCTURE OF SYNAPSES

Synapses are the sites where the activity of a neurone (the presynaptic element) can affect the activity of another cell (the postsynaptic element). The postsynaptic element may be another neurone or a skeletal muscle fibre; much of our knowledge of synaptic function is derived from motor end plates, where acetylcholine is the transmitter (p. 15.25).

At most synapses in the CNS an axon is the presynaptic element and it may branch many times to form a large number of terminals or boutons. The electron microscope shows these to contain many synaptic vesicles, 20–50 nm in diameter, just as at the end plate, and there is often a collection of mitochondria. The plasma membrane of the presynaptic terminal is separated from that of the

postsynaptic element by a cleft about 20 nm wide which contains dense material. The complex of pre- and postsynaptic membranes together with the cleft between them is the **synaptic junction**. Where synaptic transmission occurs, vesicles aggregate close to the presynaptic membrane and appear to discharge their contents into the synaptic cleft (fig. 25.22). The postsynaptic membrane

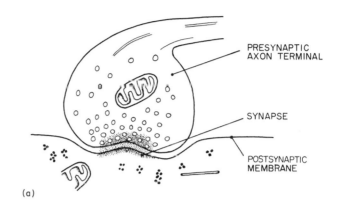

(a)

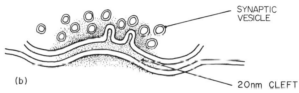

(b)

20nm CLEFT

FIG. 25.22. Generalized diagram of a synapse within the central nervous system; (a) shows the presynaptic axon terminal with its content of synaptosomes and accumulation of electron-dense material at the synaptic junction, (b) is a higher power of the synaptic region to show the 20 nm cleft and two synaptic vesicles bursting into the cleft.

facing them has a coating of dense material, the **postsynaptic density**, on its cytoplasmic side. When the postsynaptic density is prominent the synapse is termed asymmetric and such synapses, which are usually excitatory in function, have round synaptic vesicles. At the other extreme are symmetric synapses; these have a less prominent postsynaptic cleft and vesicles which are ellipsoidal when fixed in certain ways; they are often inhibitory in function. Most synaptic vesicles in the CNS have clear contents which on differential centrifugation are found in the **synaptosome fraction**. This may contain such chemicals as acetylcholine, γ-aminobutyric acid (GABA) and glycine. Other synaptic vesicles have dense granules within them and these vesicles are known to contain catecholamines. Transmission occurs by the release from the vesicles of these transmitter substances into the synaptic cleft. Excitatory or inhibitory postsynaptic potentials may then develop across the postsynaptic membranes (see below).

When an axon is the presynaptic element, the postsynaptic element may be a dendrite (axodendritic synapse), a neuronal perikaryon (axosomatic synapse) or another axon (axo-axonic synapse). A neurone may be entirely covered by such synapses, and an individual ventral horn neurone of the spinal cord, for example, may have as many as 10 000 synapses upon its surface. Parts of the neurone other than the axon may contain vesicles and be presynaptic. Thus dendrodendritic and dendrosomatic synapses are common in the olfactory bulb and the thalamus. Much less commonly a peri-karyon may be presynaptic to either another perikaryon or a dendrite. Seemingly axons are postsynaptic only to other axons, and not to dendrites or neuronal somata.

Because of the specific location of the transmitter in the synaptic vesicles of the presynaptic element, chemical synapses can only function in one direction. Also, because of the necessity to discharge the transmitter into the synaptic cleft, there is a synaptic delay of 0·5–1·0 msec.

Electrical synapses have the form of gap junctions, i.e. the plasma membranes of the two neurones are separated by a cleft of only 2–3 nm. Tiny channels may cross this narrow cleft which allows ions to pass, and transmission is by the flow of action currents. Transmission may occur in either direction and there is no synaptic delay. Electrical synapses are rare in mammalian nervous systems although they have been encountered in places such as the vestibular nucleus and other brain stem nuclei. They are very common in fish and in invertebrates, however, and it is

from these animals that our knowledge of their functioning is derived.

EXCITATORY POSTSYNAPTIC POTENTIAL (EPSP)
A microelectrode impaling a motor neurone in the spinal cord can record the changes of potential within the cell when the neurone is stimulated through an excitatory afferent nerve. After a latent period (0·5–1·0 msec) the potential rises from a resting level of -70 mV to as much as $+30$ mV, the size of the rise being dependent on the strength of the afferent stimulus (fig. 25.23). This EPSP is a depolarization analogous to the end plate potential (EPP) in the neuromuscular junction and it is probably associated with the same ionic movements. There is a critical rise, about 10–18 mV, above which a sharp secondary rise, the axon spike, occurs (fig. 25.23c); this is due to the initiation of an impulse in the axon hillock, the most excitable part of the neurone, from which the impulse leaves to travel down the motor nerve.

INHIBITORY POSTSYNAPTIC POTENTIAL (IPSP)
The stimulation of afferent nerve fibres which reflexly inhibit muscle movement produces a hyperpolarization of the membrane of the motor neurone. This increase in potential is called the inhibitory postsynaptic potential. IPSP subtracts from EPSP and makes it harder for the latter to reach a level sufficient to make the neurone fire.

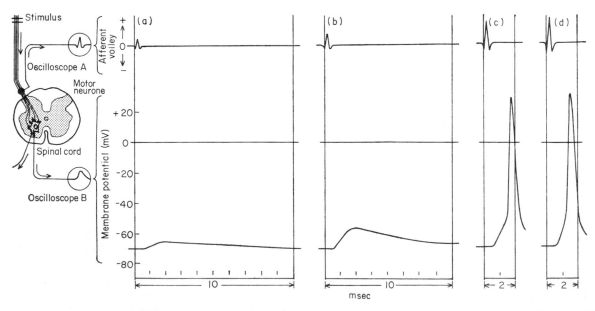

FIG. 25.23. Excitation of a motor neurone is studied by stimulating the sensory fibres that send impulses to it. The size of the afferent volleys reaching the motor neurone is displayed on oscilloscope A. A microelectrode implanted in the motor neurone measures the EPSP which appears on oscilloscope B. The size of the afferent volley is proportional to the number of fibres stimulated to fire. It is assumed that one to four fibres can be activated. When only one fibre is activated (a) the potential inside the motor neurone shifts only slightly. When two fibres are activated (b) the shift is somewhat greater. When three fibres are activated (c) the potential reaches the threshold at which depolarization proceeds swiftly and a spike appears on oscilloscope B. The spike signifies that the motor neurone has generated a nerve impulse of its own. When four or more fibres are activated (d) the motor neurone reaches the threshold more quickly. From Eccles J.C. (1965). *Scientific American* reprint No. 1001.

If anions, especially Cl⁻, are injected by iontophoresis into the neurone from which the record is being obtained, they have a marked effect on the IPSP, reducing it or even reversing it. It is probable that the IPSP acts by making the cell membrane more permeable to Cl⁻; these ions then enter the cell from the extracellular space and make the interior more negative. Fig. 25.24a shows a normal IPSP converted into a false EPSP by the injection of Cl⁻ into the neurone. Fig. 25.24b shows the injection of Cl⁻

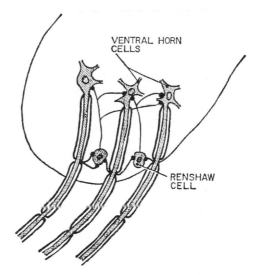

Fig. 25.25. Feedback inhibition through Renshaw cells in the ventral horn of the spinal cord.

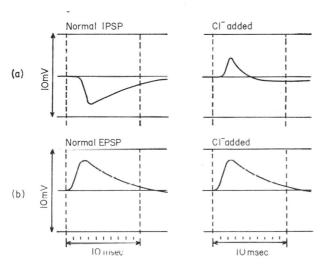

FIG. 25.24. Recording of (a) inhibitory postsynaptic potential (IPSP) and (b) excitatory postsynaptic potential (EPSP) from a motor neurone. The effect of altering the internal Cl⁻ is shown. From Eccles.

has no effect on the depolarization of a normal EPSP. IPSPs in response to a single impulse can last between 10 and 200 msec, and the contribution of any later impulses is added on if they arrive within this time. IPSP generation within the spinal cord is blocked by strychnine, hence the violent muscle spasms which occur through unrestrained excitatory processes in strychnine poisoning.

Presynaptic inhibition
Nerve impulses which have entered the spinal cord along sensory axons can be reduced in amplitude below the normal level at axo-axonic synapses with nerves carrying inhibitory impulses. As this occurs just before the impulse reaches the synapses with the motor neurones, it is called presynaptic inhibition. Afferent impulses are thus subject to suppression within the central nervous system even before they reach their destination at the end of the axon along which they are travelling. The suppression occurs over a much longer time course than inhibition operating by IPSPs.

Motor neurones may also inhibit themselves by a feedback mechanism involving cells with very short axons which lie adjacent to them in the grey matter of the spinal cord, **Renshaw cells** (fig. 25.25). Shortly after

leaving the axon hillock, the axon of the motor nerve sends off short branches which synapse with the Renshaw cell. When this cell fires, it inhibits the original motor neurone and also adjacent ones. Similar local inhibitory circuits exist in the cerebellum and in the motor cortex.

Inhibition entails delay
Inhibition always involves one or more interneurones within the spinal cord, which intervene between the afferent fibres (for instance from the opposite foot in fig. 25.20) and the reflex arc in which conduction is impaired. So inhibition, like repentance, is always late; if both feet were stimulated simultaneously, the flexor reflex would appear at full amplitude before the inhibition took effect. It seems that interneurones are essential for inhibition, because the same neurone cannot produce both excitatory and inhibitory effects at its axon's synaptic terminations. The afferent axons from a foot can bring a flexion reflex into action, an excitatory function; these same axons cannot inhibit a reflex directly, but can do so only by exciting an inhibitory interneurone or a chain of such interneurones.

Tendon jerks
These are simple reflexes of great clinical importance. The **knee jerk** can be elicited by crossing one leg over the other while sitting down, and allowing it to hang freely. When the patellar tendon is tapped sharply, quadriceps contracts briefly and partially extends the knee. This jerk is one of a whole family of tendon jerks, most readily found in the antigravity muscles. They include the **ankle jerk**, since soleus and gastrocnemius support the body when one is on tiptoe, the **biceps** and **triceps jerks**, which do the same when one hangs from one's hands or does a press-up, and the **masseter-temporalis** or **jaw jerk**. The

reflex arcs concerned, like all reflex arcs, comprise a receptor, a conducting nervous path, and an effector organ. The receptor here is a muscle spindle, a type of receptor found in all striated muscles, which is exquisitely sensitive to stretch. It also responds to vibration. Hence a blow on a bone from a tendon hammer may stimulate spindles in muscles quite far removed from the blow, and evoke apparent tendon jerks in them. Such a spread of the response is a mechanical phenomenon and not an indication of an overexcitable nervous system.

A **muscle spindle** is a complicated structure, which has a fusiform capsule of connective tissue lying parallel with the muscle fibres. It contains a few short and very slender striated muscle cells; these are the intrafusal fibres which contrast with the main mass of extrafusal fibres. The intrafusal fibres receive motor nerve terminals, but their axons come from small cells in the ventral horn of the spinal cord and although myelinated they are very much smaller (8–2 μm) than the 20–12 μm motor nerve fibres to the rest of the muscle. These motor fibres to the intrafusal muscle are known as γ-efferents because of their fibre classification (Aγ, p. 15.23). There are two sorts of intrafusal muscle fibre (fig. 25.26), and two sets of sensory

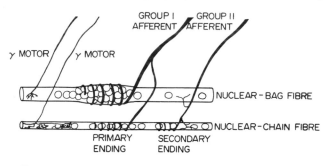

FIG. 25.26. Simplified diagram of the central region (about 1 mm long) of a muscle spindle. From Matthews P. B. C. (1971) Scientific Basis of Medicine Annual Reviews, p. 101.

endings are present on each of them. The anulospiral ending, is wrapped around the muscle cell and the other is described by its name, the flower-spray ending. The afferent fibres from the anulospiral endings are large and myelinated (20–12 μm) but those from the flower-spray endings are smaller. Large numbers of spindles lie within striated muscles, in parallel with the muscle fibres; in a human lumbrical muscle, they are about 2 mm long. When such a spindle is stretched, it generates impulses in a large, group I nerve fibre. The impulse traffic from these is relatively easy to record in animals, since the large fibres are simpler to isolate than small ones. Fig. 25.27 shows the traffic provoked, not by a brief stretch as in the knee jerk, but by sudden and maintained stretch of a muscle. The group I fibre fires vigorously at the onset of the stretch, but soon slows, though continuing to fire at higher rates than before the stretch. A steadier increase in rate of firing is recorded from the other fibre

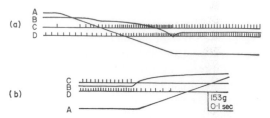

FIG. 25.27. Response of muscle spindles in anterior tibial muscle to (a) stretch and (b) release. A, muscle length; B, muscle tension; C, response of primary ending; D, response of secondary ending. From Alnaes E. *et al.* (1965) *Acta physiol. scand.* 63, 200.

which is a group II afferent from a muscle spindle, conducting more slowly.

A tendon jerk is a monosynaptic reflex, since the conducting nervous path traverses one synapse only in the spinal cord. By stimulating electrically IA fibres from a muscle and recording the impulse traffic at two stages on the reflex arc, one can time its progress. Fig. 25.28

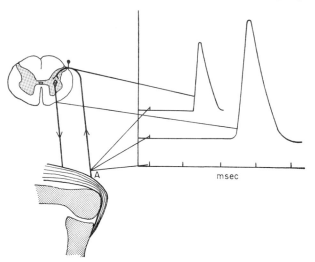

FIG. 25.28. The nervous pathway involved in a knee jerk, and the electrical recordings obtained in a cat from two sides of the path after electrical stimulation at point A. After Lloyd D.P.C. (1943) *J. Neurophysiol.* 6, 111.

shows the record of such an experiment. Here, the time taken to reach the spinal cord along the afferent nerve from the point of stimulus at A was 1·4 msec, and a further 1·1 msec saw the traffic a short distance down the efferent nerve, having passed through the cord. If the time allowed for the short distance of travel down the efferent nerve is 0·3 msec, it follows that a mere 0·8 msec elapsed during conduction through the cord and synaptic transmission. This is not long enough to cross more than one synapse. So one branch of a I afferent fibre ends at the motor neurone; in fact a branch of every I fibre ends on every, or nearly every, motor neurone of the muscle concerned. It is worth bearing in mind that other branches of the same fibre terminate in the thoracic nucleus of the spinal cord, from where traffic is relayed to the cerebellum; yet other branches pass up the dorsal columns to end in the gracile or cuneate nuclei. Conduction from afferent fibre to motor neurone occurs through the generation of an EPSP; this occurs when even a single impulse arrives and has a much longer duration than the impulse itself. If the EPSP rises sufficiently, the motor neurone fires, and the impulse then proceeds along its axon to reach the motor end plate in quadriceps.

The reflex arc of a tendon jerk crosses only one segment of the cord. The presence of a normal jerk shows that the receptors are sensitive, the relevant afferent and efferent nerves are intact, the spinal cord segment, including the motor neurones, is working normally, and the responding muscle is in order.

Stretch reflexes

A tendon jerk is elicited artificially and it is difficult to assign a clear-cut function to it. When a joint is moved passively and the new position is maintained, a rather different response, the stretch reflex, comes into play. The stretched muscles respond by increased tension, but the response is polysynaptic, may involve paths leading up to the cerebral hemisphere and down again, and depends on factors to which a tendon jerk is practically immune. For instance, the subject can affect the response, and if he intends to retaliate by pulling back when the muscle is stretched it makes the response much larger. Again, cerebellar damage may reduce a stretch reflex but not the tendon jerk at the same joint. When the tone of muscle is tested by moving a joint passively to and fro, an impression is gained of whether the stretch reflexes are normally active, i.e. whether a limb appears limp or stiff. If they are overactive, the joint is moved only with difficulty. It may suddenly give (the claspknife response). The receptors in this reflex of giving way to strong bending are the **Golgi tendon organs** (fig. 25.29), which are sprays of unmyelinated nerve terminals penetrating the tendon close to the myotendinous junction. These receptors are less sensitive (higher threshold) than muscle spindles, but feed large afferent nerve fibres (also group I).

Flexion reflexes

These act so as to withdraw out of harm's way a limb that is being hurt, and responses of this kind of reflex are shown in figs. 25.15 and 17. A human being will naturally behave in this way if he is pricked, burnt or pinched; pulling body hairs may be used in clinical testing as a stimulus. A flexion reflex is more complex than a tendon jerk. It is polysynaptic, the reflex arc traversing more than one synapse in the spinal cord, and shows greater variability.

For instance, a tendon jerk is normally confined to the muscle that is stretched; there is no response from other

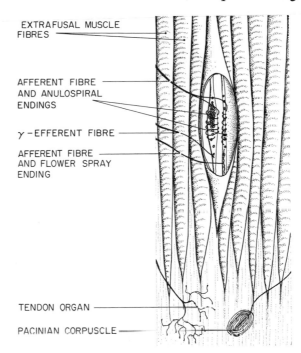

FIG. 25.29. Sensory innervation of skeletal muscle showing anulospiral and flower spray endings on intrafusal muscle fibres, and Golgi organ and Pacinian corpuscle in the tendon. Also shows motor fibre (γ-efferent) to intrafusal muscle fibre.

muscles. But a varying number of muscles may be involved in a flexion reflex. A very slight prick on one toe makes only that toe move upwards out of the way. If the prick is sharper, the movement is more extensive. The whole limb may be drawn up, and in addition, the other limb may be extended (**crossed extension reflex**). The value of such a response in helping to get the injured toe clear of trouble is obvious. So here a stimulus at one site can produce a muscular response of very variable extent, depending on how strong it is.

Again, a tendon jerk has a sharply defined latency. In a monosynaptic arc this is composed mostly of delays in the excitation of the muscle spindle by the sudden stretch of the muscle. In contrast, the latency of a flexion reflex can vary greatly; it is greatest when the stimulus is smallest and becomes less with more effective stimulation. The synaptic chain in the spinal cord conducts with variable speed.

Plantar response

When the skin of the sole of the foot is firmly stroked, so as not to tickle, yet not to hurt, especially in the area shown in fig. 25.30, the normal response is a downgoing or 'clenching' of the big toe, which in some sense attempts to grasp the source of the stroking. The abnormal or Babinski response consists in an upgoing of the toe, a dorsiflexion (sometimes ambiguously called 'extension'), together with fanning out of the other toes. In early infancy the response is normally upgoing, but before the

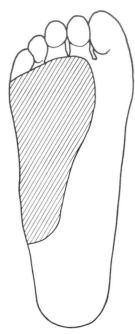

FIG. 25.30. The area on the sole of the foot over which the plantar response is best obtained. From Walshe F. (1965) *Further Clinical Studies in Neurology*. Edinburgh: Livingstone.

child walks it takes on the adult downgoing pattern. The abnormal sign is a clinical index of faulty function of the corticospinal tracts and is found also during anaesthesia and sleep. However, conversely a normal plantar response is not proof positive that the corticospinal tracts are operating normally.

Other reflexes affected by corticospinal tracts are the **abdominal** and **cremasteric reflexes**. The former takes place when the skin of the abdomen is lightly scratched; the underlying part of the abdominal wall musculature contracts, pulling over the umbilicus. The response may fail when the corticospinal tracts are interrupted; it may also fail in normal health. The cremasteric reflex consists in retraction of the testis when the skin of the medial upper thigh is stroked and this too may fail in disorders of the corticospinal paths. In both cases a difference between the two sides is much more conclusive evidence than bilateral absence of the reflexes.

Control and modification of reflexes

Even a tendon jerk is a variable phenomenon. The sensitivity of the receptor, the muscle spindle, can be altered. The intrafusal fibres, when their γ motor neurone activity causes them to contract, pull upon the receptor portion of the spindle, making it more sensitive to stretch. When the intrafusal fibre is taut, even a slight or brief pull on the whole muscle increases the activity of the spindle receptor. When it is slack, a longer or faster pull is necessary. Fig. 25.31 shows diagrammatically a muscle

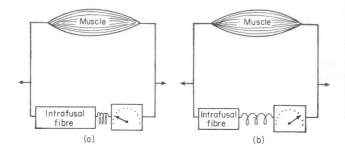

FIG. 25.31. Muscle and muscle spindle being stretched by constant force. (a) The intrafusal fibre is relaxed, and little tension is recorded by the spindle; (b) the intrafusal fibre is contracting, and more tension is recorded by the spindle.

being stretched by the same force all the time; but clearly on the right where the intrafusal fibre is short, the meter is recording a larger apparent pull than on the left where the intrafusal fibre is long. The stretching force operates virtually entirely on the muscle; negligible force is required to stretch the intrafusal fibre (operating on the little spring in the diagram). The intrafusal fibres, when they contract, contribute nothing to the tension produced by the whole muscle in which they lie.

Tendon jerks can be modified by a procedure called **reinforcement** or Jendrassik's manoeuvre; in Jendrassik's words: 'If when the patellar tendon is struck, the patient clenches the hand, or makes other violent movement, the coincident jerk is increased.' It is simple to make the subject link the fingers of his two hands together and then instruct him to pull them apart, without letting go, just before one strikes the patellar tendon. The increase in the jerk could occur because Jendrassik's manoeuvre increases γ motor neurone activity. But there is another site on the reflex arc where its condition can be altered. This is at the synapse; on the motor neurone's surface there may be no less than 10 000 synaptic knobs. Only a small number of these are the endings of afferent fibres from muscle spindles. There are also terminations from many other sources, including those responsible for voluntary movement (p. 25.45), and some of these are inhibitory. Their activity can affect the excitability of the motor neurone and hence the conduction in the tendon jerk reflex arc.

So any motor neurone serving as the efferent path of a tendon jerk can also serve as the final common path for a large number of reflexes, including complex reflexes organized from higher levels of the central nervous system than the spinal cord itself. These include tonic neck reflexes (p. 25.49) and, more complex still, conditioned reflexes (p. 25.77).

Is it possible to say how much of the behaviour of a motor neurone consists of reflex responses, and how much of directed activity or acts of free will, which are not tethered to the compulsion of reflex arcs? It is important to realize how difficult it is to make the behaviour of a reflex arc really dependable and rigorous. This ought to be most easily achieved in the simplest arc: the mono-synaptic arc of the tendon jerk. But, as Sherrington pointed out, the knee jerk as tested clinically in normal man is 'delicately variable'; to make it reasonably dependable, a standard position must be adopted and the subject's attention must not vary. Changes in many higher parts of the nervous system alter the response. Really consistent records of spinal reflexes are generally obtained in animals in which the spinal cord has been isolated from the rest of the nervous system, and so in a very real sense a reflex is a 'convenient fiction' (Sherrington). If it were possible to assemble all the reflexes there are and to assess all their interactions, one might then begin to look for a residue of behaviour which is non-reflex, the place where Mind intervenes. But no picture can be even outlined of the sum of all reflexes, and to obtain dependable reflexes at all demands careful and deliberate simplification. One cannot guess all the contents of a black box by supposing that they must all be like the one fraction that can be made understandable. Sherrington, when aged 90, wrote: 'The reflex was a very useful idea, but it has served its purpose. What the reflex does is so banal.'

Reflexes operating on smooth muscle and on glands

Efferent paths from the spinal cord run not only to voluntary muscle but also to other organs, such as the smooth muscle of blood vessels and the cells of the adrenal medulla. Reflex paths through the spinal cord end in them too. Fig. 25.32 shows a huge rise in blood pressure following electrical stimulation of a toe nerve; this occurred in a dog which had previously undergone transection of the spinal cord at the eighth cervical level

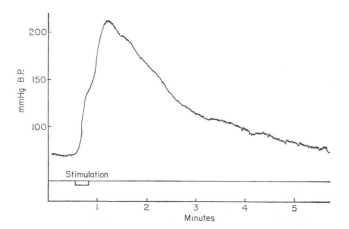

FIG. 25.32. Rise in arterial blood pressure in a dog in response to electrical stimulation of the hind leg. The dog's spinal cord has been transected in the cervical region. After Sherrington.

and the path is a spinal reflex arc. Similarly, reflexes affecting the urinary system can be organized by the spinal cord alone (p. 36.8).

Spinal cord transection

When the spinal cord is severed, no sensory impulses can pass to the brain from the region below the cut, and so nothing in the lower part of the body can be felt. This part is also incapable of voluntary movement, since the necessary paths are interrupted. But the mechanism of spinal reflexes still remains in the separated part of the cord. Immediately after a sudden transection there is a period of **spinal shock**, with absence of any activity in the separated spinal cord below the cut. The higher nervous system transmits to the spinal cord impulse traffic which is predominantly excitatory. Remove this source of excitation and all activity ceases for a time. No reconnection of the severed parts of the cord ever occurs, but reflex activity is recovered in the isolated portion.

Recovery takes a long time in man and may not be maximal for many weeks. It is much shorter in other animals. A cat recovers activity in its cord below a transection in a few hours and a frog in a few minutes. The greater the importance of higher parts of the nervous system to an animal, the more prolonged the effect of their disconnection.

In man, during spinal shock, the part of the body innervated by the spinal cord below the lesion is at first entirely flaccid. Pulling hairs and tapping tendons call forth no movement whatever, and are of course not felt by the victim. The bladder is inert and fills up; when it is sufficiently overstretched, the excess dribbles out but only a small part of its contents is evacuated.

After some days, recovery begins and cord function appears gradually, as shown by recovery of reflexes and appearance of upgoing plantar responses (p. 25.19). Flexion reflexes in response to quite trivial stimuli may be troublesome; before injury, the extensor muscle system seems to depend much on excitatory influences from higher levels of the nervous system and it never recovers proper activity; hence the victim may become bent in a flexed position. The bladder recovers reflex activity enough to empty itself fairly completely when full (the automatic bladder, p. 36.8); vascular and sweating reflexes can now be demonstrated which are being handled by the isolated part of the cord. Until these vascular responses return, whenever the victim is tilted up, pooling of blood occurs in the venous vessels in the part of the body below the injury so that a marked fall in arterial blood pressure occurs.

BRAIN STEM AND CRANIAL NERVES

External appearance (figs. 25.33 and 34)

The brain stem consists of the midbrain, pons and medulla and is the direct upward continuation of the spinal cord.

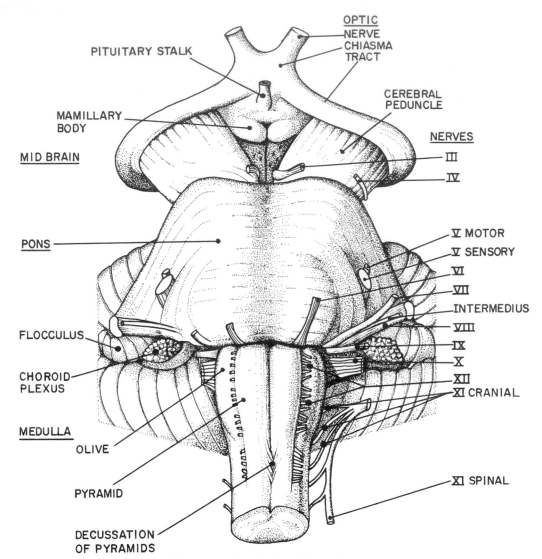

PITUITARY STALK

OPTIC
NERVE
CHIASMA
TRACT

CEREBRAL
PEDUNCLE

MAMILLARY
BODY

MID BRAIN

NERVES

III

IV

PONS

V MOTOR
V SENSORY
VI
VII
INTERMEDIUS
VIII
IX
X
XII
XI CRANIAL

FLOCCULUS

CHOROID
PLEXUS

MEDULLA

OLIVE

PYRAMID

XI SPINAL

DECUSSATION
OF PYRAMIDS

FIG. 25.33. Ventral view of the brain stem.

The boundary between the two is arbitrarily defined as the interval between the lowest rootlet of cranial nerve XII and the highest rootlet of spinal nerve CI. Bundles of fibres ascend or descend through the cord and brain stem without regard for territorial boundaries, and it is best to concentrate attention on their longitudinal organization rather than on the regional anatomy of what is basically a continuous tubular structure.

VENTRAL VIEW (FIG. 25.33)

The **cerebral peduncles** contain the **crura cerebri,** two large bundles of fibres which descend from the forebrain, form the most ventral part of the midbrain, and converge and disappear from view to run more deeply through the pons. Between them is the **interpeduncular fossa,** the front part of which shows the mamillary bodies and the pituitary stalk, which belongs to the forebrain.

The **pons** shows, on its ventral surface, transversely running bundles of fibres which enter the cerebellum through the middle cerebellar peduncle. It does not, as its name implies, form a bridge for exchange fibres between the two cerebellar hemispheres.

The **medulla oblongata** begins at the lower border of the pons and tapers gradually to its point of continuity with the spinal cord. Its median sulcus is continuous with the ventral median fissure of the cord; on either side of it is a medullary **pyramid.** This consists of descending **pyramidal (corticospinal) fibres** which run through the central part of the crus cerebri, and then more deeply through the pons to emerge at its lower border. Many of the fibres in each pyramid cross the midline as coarse bundles of fibres visible to the unaided eye, in the **decussation of the pyramids.** Dorsal to each pyramid is an ovoid surface elevation, the **olive,** produced by the underlying inferior olivary nucleus. The olive is separated ventrally from the pyramid by the preolivary sulcus and dorsally from the **restiform body** by the retro-olivary sulcus. The restiform body is a surface elevation produced by fibres entering the cerebellum in the inferior cerebellar peduncle.

Origin of cranial nerves
The names and numbers of the cranial nerves are given on p. 22.11.

Nerves III and V–XII are attached to the ventral surface of the brain stem. Although they do not repeat the regular simple pattern of origin of the spinal nerves, their attachment is not haphazard, but reflects a functional grouping.

Somatic efferent group. This consists of nerves III, IV, VI and XII. These are equivalent to, and in linear series with, the ventral rootlets of spinal nerves and, like them, supply skeletal muscles of somite origin. Nerve IV belongs to the group but emerges from the dorsal surface of the brain stem, and has to wind round the midbrain to appear ventrally.

Branchial (special visceral) efferent group. This consists of nerves V (motor root), VII (motor root), IX, X and cranial root of XI. These also arise in linear series and include fibres which supply skeletal muscle of pharyngeal (branchial) arch origin (p. 19.32) and which have no equivalent in the spinal nerves.

General visceral efferent group. This consists of the cranial parasympathetic outflow of the autonomic nervous system, which runs in nerves III, VII (nervus intermedius), IX and X.

Somatic afferent group. Almost all of these fibres from the head region enter the brain stem in nerve V (sensory root). They are equivalent to somatic afferent fibres entering the cord in the dorsal roots of spinal nerves.

Special sense afferent group. This also has no equivalent in the spinal nerves and consists of the two parts, vestibular and cochlear, of nerve VIII.

General visceral afferent fibres are carried in nerves IX and X, and special visceral afferent (taste) fibres in nerves VII (nervus intermedius), IX and X.

DORSAL VIEW (fig. 25.34)
In the intact brain, most of the dorsal aspect of the brain stem is concealed either by the cerebral hemispheres or by the cerebellum. Fig. 25.34 shows the appearance of the brain stem, separated from the forebrain and with half the cerebellum removed.

The **midbrain** shows two pairs of swellings, the **superior**

and **inferior colliculi.** Nerve IV emerges from the anterior medullary velum at the junction of midbrain and pons, and winds forwards round the midbrain. Removal of the cerebellum opens the **fourth ventricle**, which is continuous above with the narrow **cerebral aqueduct of the midbrain** and below with the central canal of the lower medulla. Its floor is formed above by the pons and below by the upper

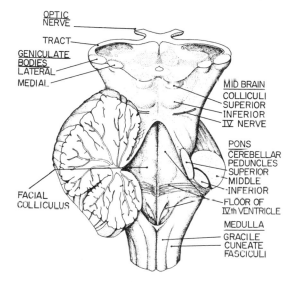

FIG. 25.34. Dorsal view of the brain stem. The right half of the cerebellum has been removed. The left half has been drawn over to the left to expose the floor of the fourth ventricle.

medulla and is divided by a midline sulcus; each half is further divided by a **sulcus limitans** into a lateral part, derived from the alar lamina, and a medial part, derived from the basal lamina.

The efferent (motor) nuclei of the brain stem are found medial to the sulcus limitans. The nucleus of VI (abducens) lies beneath the **facial colliculus** (so called because fibres of the nerve VII wind over its dorsal surface and contribute to the prominence); the nucleus of XII lies beneath the **hypoglossal triangle**, and the motor nucleus of X beneath the **vagal triangle**.

Lateral to the sulcus limitans is the derivative of the alar lamina. The lateral part of the floor of the ventricle, at its widest part, is called the **vestibular area**; this marks the position of the vestibular nuclei, the afferent nuclei of the vestibular nerve.

The roof of the ventricle is formed mainly by the cerebellum, but the remnant of the originally extensive ependymal roof is at the lower end of the ventricle, and known as the **inferior medullary velum**. This shows a single midline foramen and paired lateral foramina, which allow CSF to escape from the ventricular system, and a choroid plexus, involved in its production (p. 25.86).

On the side from which the cerebellum has been removed there are seen the cut ends of the three stalks or peduncles which attach the cerebellum to the brain stem. At present only the following features need be noted.

(1) The **superior cerebellar peduncle** carries principally efferent fibres, which run forwards away from the cerebellum, to disappear from sight at the upper end of the fourth ventricle, diving deeply beneath the inferior colliculus of the midbrain to form an important ascending link between cerebellum and cerebral cortex. Between the two superior cerebellar peduncles is the **superior medullary velum** which, like the inferior one, is mainly ependymal.

(2) The **middle cerebellar peduncle** is the largest and most laterally placed of the three. It is exclusively afferent, carrying fibres to the cerebellum from the opposite side of the pons. This is part of the important **corticoponto-cerebellar pathway**, a major descending link between the cerebral cortex and the cerebellum.

(3) The **inferior cerebellar peduncle** ascends beneath the vestibular area on the medial side of the middle peduncle, to enter the cerebellum. It carries fibres both to and from the cerebellum. A major component is the dorsal spinocerebellar tract, an uncrossed tract which links the corresponding sides of the cord and cerebellum.

The lower medulla tapers gradually into the spinal cord, which it resembles in some respects. It is traversed by a narrow central canal; its dorsal median sulcus is flanked on either side by direct upward continuations of the dorsal white columns of the cord, **gracile** and **cuneate fasciculi**; these end synaptically on cells of the gracile and cuneate nuclei (sensory nuclei of termination) which produce surface elevations (**gracile** and **cuneate tubercles**).

These surface features of the brain stem can now be related to the internal structure shown in transverse sections made at various levels (fig. 25.35).

Organization of grey matter

The simple pattern of the spinal cord, with its centrally placed continuous columns of grey matter, completely surrounded by white matter, is greatly modified in the brain stem. Indeed it might seem at first that there is no pattern at all, but rather a hopeless muddle of nuclei and fibre tracts. In fact, however, a pattern is discernible, based mainly on embryological and functional criteria.

EFFERENT NUCLEI OF CRANIAL NERVES

The motor (efferent) fibres of cranial nerves are classified as somatic, branchial and visceral (fig. 25.36). Somatic fibres supply skeletal muscle of somite origin; branchial fibres skeletal muscle of branchial origin; visceral fibres cardiac muscle, smooth muscle and glands. Two important principles should be noted at the start:

(1) Efferent nuclei of a particular group form linearly arranged, though discontinuous, columns in the brain stem. The **somatic efferent column** is a continuation of the ventral grey column of the spinal cord, while the **visceral efferent column** is a continuation of the intermediolateral grey column of the cord. The **branchial efferent column** is not represented in the spinal cord.

(2) Clear-cut segregation of afferent and efferent fibres into sensory and motor roots, corresponding to the dorsal and ventral roots of spinal nerves, is seen in only one of the cranial nerves, the trigeminal. In the others, a wide variety of pattern is seen. Some are purely afferent, some purely efferent; in some, afferent and efferent fibres run together in a single nerve trunk (e.g. nervus intermedius); the vagus contains as many as four functionally different types of fibres. The sorting out of the complex pattern of cranial nerve constituents was done mostly between 1900 and 1920 by C. Judson Herrick, a distinguished American neuroanatomist.

Somatic efferent column

This includes the nuclei of nerves III, IV and VI, collectively concerned in innervating the muscles which move the eye (extrinsic ocular muscles), and the nucleus of XII nerve, which supplies the muscles of the tongue. In lower forms these muscle groups arise, respectively, from the pre-otic and the occipital somites. This is the theoretical justification for classifying the nuclei as somatic, despite the doubt which exists about the somite origin of the tongue muscles of mammals (p. 19.35).

The position of each of these nuclei is shown in figs. 25.35, 36 & 37, which show that the nuclei form a discontinuous linear column, and that they lie close to the midline and ventral to the central canal, in the region derived from the basal lamina.

Branchial (special visceral) efferent column

This includes the nuclei of nerves V and VII, and the **nucleus ambiguus**, the nucleus common to three nerves, IX, X and cranial root of XI. They are called branchial, because they supply skeletal musculature derived from the branchial (pharyngeal) arches; for example, from the 1st arch arise the muscles of mastication (mandibular division of V); from the 2nd arch, the muscles of facial expression (nerve VII); from the 3rd arch, the stylopharyngeus muscle (nerve IX) and from the 4th and 6th arches, the musculature of the pharynx and larynx (nerves X and cranial XI). For details see p. 19.33.

These nuclei form a discontinuous linear column (figs. 25.36 and 37). However, all of them, and particularly VII and nucleus ambiguus, have migrated ventrally and laterally, away from their original position immediately lateral to the somatic efferent column. This migration occurs during embryonic development; it is reflected in the curious looped course of fibres of VII and of IX, X and cranial XI (fig. 25.36). It is suggested that the migration confers functional advantage in that it brings the nuclei closer to their main source of afferent reflex stimulation through nerve V.

Although the distinction between the somatic and

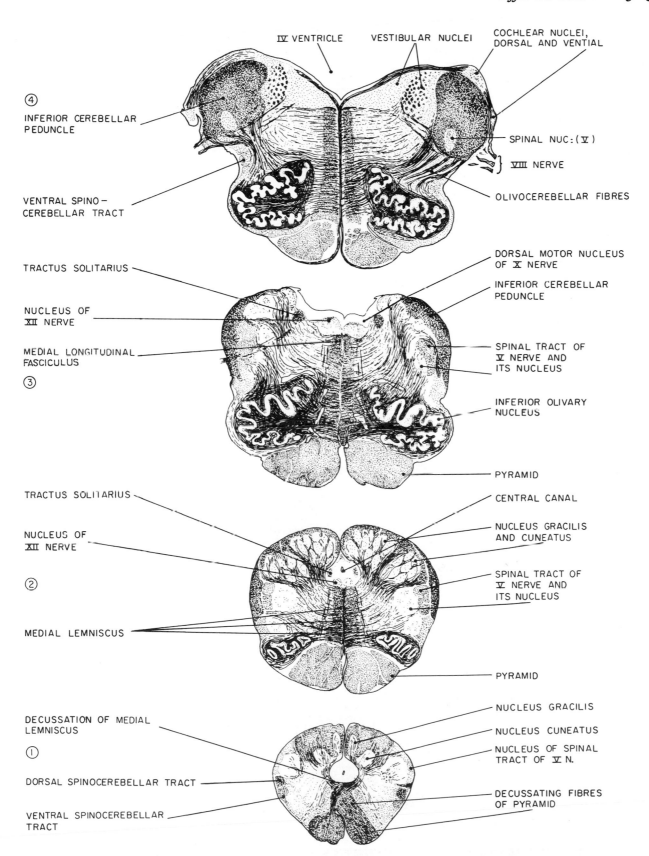

IV VENTRICLE

VESTIBULAR NUCLEI

COCHLEAR NUCLEI, DORSAL AND VENTIAL

④

INFERIOR CEREBELLAR PEDUNCLE

SPINAL NUC: (V)

VIII NERVE

VENTRAL SPINO - CEREBELLAR TRACT

OLIVOCEREBELLAR FIBRES

TRACTUS SOLITARIUS

DORSAL MOTOR NUCLEUS OF X NERVE

INFERIOR CEREBELLAR PEDUNCLE

NUCLEUS OF XII NERVE

MEDIAL LONGITUDINAL FASCICULUS

SPINAL TRACT OF V NERVE AND ITS NUCLEUS

③

INFERIOR OLIVARY NUCLEUS

PYRAMID

TRACTUS SOLITARIUS

CENTRAL CANAL

NUCLEUS GRACILIS AND CUNEATUS

NUCLEUS OF XII NERVE

SPINAL TRACT OF V NERVE AND ITS NUCLEUS

②

MEDIAL LEMNISCUS

PYRAMID

NUCLEUS GRACILIS

DECUSSATION OF MEDIAL LEMNISCUS

NUCLEUS CUNEATUS

①

NUCLEUS OF SPINAL TRACT OF V N.

DORSAL SPINOCEREBELLAR TRACT

DECUSSATING FIBRES OF PYRAMID

VENTRAL SPINOCEREBELLAR TRACT

FIG. 25.35a. Drawings of Weigert-stained transverse sections of medulla oblongata in ascending sequence.

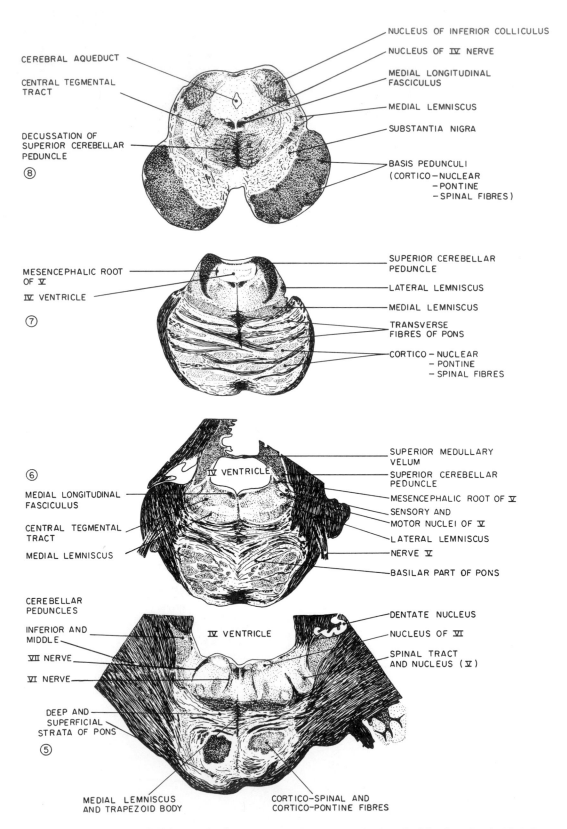

CEREBRAL AQUEDUCT

CENTRAL TEGMENTAL TRACT

DECUSSATION OF SUPERIOR CEREBELLAR PEDUNCLE

⑧

NUCLEUS OF INFERIOR COLLICULUS

NUCLEUS OF IV NERVE

MEDIAL LONGITUDINAL FASCICULUS

MEDIAL LEMNISCUS

SUBSTANTIA NIGRA

BASIS PEDUNCULI (CORTICO–NUCLEAR –PONTINE –SPINAL FIBRES)

MESENCEPHALIC ROOT OF V

IV VENTRICLE

⑦

SUPERIOR CEREBELLAR PEDUNCLE

LATERAL LEMNISCUS

MEDIAL LEMNISCUS

TRANSVERSE FIBRES OF PONS

CORTICO–NUCLEAR –PONTINE –SPINAL FIBRES

⑥

MEDIAL LONGITUDINAL FASCICULUS

CENTRAL TEGMENTAL TRACT

MEDIAL LEMNISCUS

IV VENTRICLE

SUPERIOR MEDULLARY VELUM

SUPERIOR CEREBELLAR PEDUNCLE

MESENCEPHALIC ROOT OF V

SENSORY AND MOTOR NUCLEI OF V

LATERAL LEMNISCUS

NERVE V

BASILAR PART OF PONS

CEREBELLAR PEDUNCLES

INFERIOR AND MIDDLE

VII NERVE

VI NERVE

DEEP AND SUPERFICIAL STRATA OF PONS

⑤

IV VENTRICLE

DENTATE NUCLEUS

NUCLEUS OF VI

SPINAL TRACT AND NUCLEUS (V)

MEDIAL LEMNISCUS AND TRAPEZOID BODY

CORTICO-SPINAL AND CORTICO-PONTINE FIBRES

FIG. 25.35b. Drawings of Weigert-stained transverse sections of pons (5–7) and midbrain at level of inferior colliculus (8) in ascending sequence.

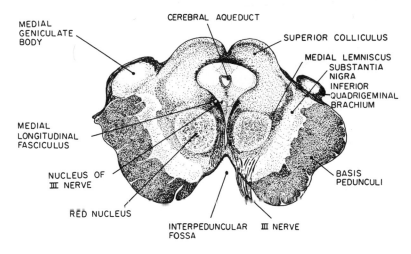

MEDIAL GENICULATE BODY

CEREBRAL AQUEDUCT

SUPERIOR COLLICULUS

MEDIAL LEMNISCUS
SUBSTANTIA NIGRA
INFERIOR QUADRIGEMINAL BRACHIUM

MEDIAL LONGITUDINAL FASCICULUS

NUCLEUS OF III NERVE

BASIS PEDUNCULI

RED NUCLEUS

INTERPEDUNCULAR FOSSA

III NERVE

FIG. 23.35c. Drawing of Weigert-stained transverse section of midbrain at level of superior colliculus.

branchial efferent groups on the basis of their position and of the developmental origin of the muscles which they supply has been emphasized, the two groups form, together, the lower motor neurones of the brain stem. They are, collectively, the equivalent of lower motor neurones of the spinal cord and form the final common path to those muscles of the head and neck supplied by cranial nerves.

Like the lower motor neurones of the spinal cord, those of the brain stem do not function in isolation, but only as parts of neuronal chains. These include descending pathways from the cerebral cortex which terminate on

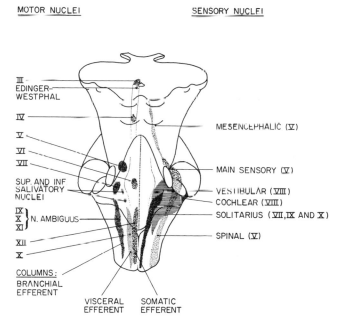

MOTOR NUCLEI   SENSORY NUCLEI

III EDINGER-WESTPHAL

IV

V

VI

VII

MESENCEPHALIC (V)

SUP. AND INF. SALIVATORY NUCLEI

MAIN SENSORY (V)

IX
X
XI
} N. AMBIGUUS

VESTIBULAR (VIII)
COCHLEAR (VIII)
SOLITARIUS (VII, IX AND X)

XII

SPINAL (V)

X

COLUMNS:
BRANCHIAL EFFERENT

VISCERAL EFFERENT

SOMATIC EFFERENT

FIG. 25.37. Cranial nerve nuclei, superimposed on outline of dorsal view of brain stem, to illustrate their arrangement in longitudinal columns.

lower motor neurones of the brain stem, and are called **corticonuclear fibres** and are equivalent to corticospinal fibres which end on spinal motor neurones. Local connections within the brain stem provide for reflex responses of muscle groups of the head and neck to a variety of afferent stimuli, a situation which is again comparable to that of motor neurones of the spinal cord.

General visceral efferent column
This consists of a discontinuous chain of nuclei, which contain cell bodies of preganglionic parasympathetic

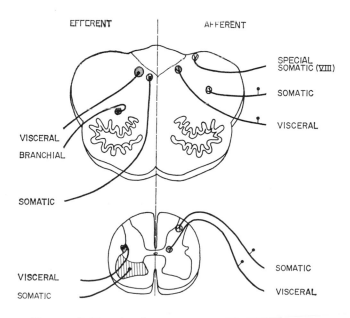

EFFERENT   AFFERENT

SPECIAL SOMATIC (VIII)

SOMATIC

VISCERAL

VISCERAL

BRANCHIAL

SOMATIC

SOMATIC

VISCERAL

VISCERAL

SOMATIC

FIG. 25.36. Functional components of cranial nerve nuclei in the medulla and the spinal nerve nuclei in the spinal cord.

neurones. It gives origin to the cranial parasympathetic outflow, the equivalent of the thoracolumbar (sympathetic) and sacral (parasympathetic) outflows from the spinal cord (p. 25.91). The position of these nuclei is indicated in figs. 25.36 and 37, but only X (dorsal motor nucleus of vagus) is easily identified in routine sections (fig. 25.35a). The cranial visceral efferent column is concerned with the motor innervation of smooth muscle in the eye (nerve III), of the salivary and lacrimal glands (nerves VII or IX) and of smooth muscle and glands in the respiratory and digestive tracts (nerve X). The activity of its neurones is influenced by descending pathways from the hypothalamus, a major integrating autonomic centre (p. 25.62), and by local connections within the brain stem, which provide for responses to a variety of afferent stimuli arising both in somatic and in visceral structures.

The larynx, pharynx and oesophagus are the site of complex reflexes mediated through nuclei in the brain stem. Mucus from the nose and saliva arrives continuously in the upper pharynx, and mucus from the lungs arrives via the larynx in the lower pharynx. Both are automatically swallowed down the oesophagus, and from time to time food and drink are swallowed in addition. During swallowing the bolus of liquid or solid is transferred in an orderly fashion (p. 32.7), and the larynx is temporarily closed so that none goes the wrong way, into the lungs by the trachea. Any that does so excites the **cough reflex** and is returned. So if this group of reflexes is impaired by disease of the brain stem or relevant cranial nerves, the patient is in danger of drowning in his own secretions which leak through the ill-closed larynx. Giving fluid by mouth makes matters worse. The correct immediate procedure is to turn the patient on his side with his head dependent to let the pooled secretions drain out of the mouth.

Besides such complex activities, quite simple reflexes are organized by the brain stem, for instance, the **corneal reflex**. If the cornea is lightly touched or even blown upon, the eyelids are immediately closed. The afferent path of this reflex is in the ophthalmic division of the trigeminal nerve, and the efferent path in the motor fibres of the facial nerve, terminating in the muscle orbicularis oculi. The link between the two paths lies in the brain stem, and there too the response becomes bilateral, since touching one cornea brings about blinking of both eyes.

AFFERENT NUCLEI OF CRANIAL NERVES
The cell bodies of first order afferents of cranial nerves lie outside the central nervous system, as is the case with spinal afferents. Their axons enter the cord and terminate on the cell bodies of second order afferent neurones. These form three separate columns, named according to the type of first order input which they receive (figs. 25.36 and 37).

Somatic afferent column
This is associated almost entirely with nerve V (trigeminal) with some minor contributions from nervus intermedius, IX and X. It consists of an elongated column of cells, extending from midpons to upper cervical spinal cord. The individual nuclei and their connections are described more fully under somatic afferent pathways (p. 25.41).

General and special visceral afferent column
This consists of a single elongated nucleus, **nucleus of the tractus solitarius**, which extends through the medulla (fig. 25.35a). It receives:

(1) special visceral afferent (taste) fibres of the nervus intermedius and nerves IX and X;

(2) general visceral afferent fibres of nerve IX, from baroceptors in the carotid sinus and chemoreceptors in the carotid body;

(3) general visceral afferent fibres of nerve IX, from the back of the tongue, tonsillar region and upper pharynx; (pain fibres of nerve IX, with a similar distribution, terminate in the spinal nucleus of nerve V, and are classed as somatic afferents);

(4) general visceral afferent fibres of nerve X, from the larynx and lower pharynx, and from those thoracic and abdominal viscera which receive their motor innervation through nerve X.

Fibres of nerves IX and X form the afferent limb of two important reflexes which occur in response to touch. (1) The **gag reflex** consists of contraction of pharyngeal muscles, retching and, if the stimulus is sufficiently powerful, vomiting with contraction of diaphragm and abdominal muscles and associated effects of autonomic stimulation, e.g. salivation, bradycardia, sweating, cutaneous vasoconstriction. (2) The **swallowing reflex** consists of contraction of muscles of the pharynx and of the entrance to the larynx and of the smooth muscle of the oesophagus via branchial and visceral efferent fibres of the vagus nerve. Both these reflexes have an important protective function.

Pharyngeal and laryngeal branches of the vagus nerve carry visceral afferents from the mucosa of the larynx and laryngopharynx. Cell bodies are in the inferior (nodose) ganglion, and the fibres terminate in the nucleus solitarius. Central connections provide for two important protective reflex actions—closure of the laryngeal aditus in swallowing and contraction of expiratory muscles against a closed glottis in coughing.

Special somatic afferent nuclei
These are the **vestibular** and **cochlear nuclei**.

There are four vestibular nuclei on each side, which lie as a group beneath the floor of the widest part of the fourth ventricle, and extend upwards into the pons and downwards into the closed medulla. They receive fibres of the vestibular nerve, whose cell bodies lie in the vestibular ganglion and whose peripheral processes end in the specialized sensory epithelia of the vestibular apparatus.

There are two cochlear nuclei on each side, dorsal and ventral, applied to the outer side of the inferior cerebellar peduncle at the level of the widest part of the floor of the fourth ventricle. They receive fibres of the cochlear nerve, whose cell bodies are in the spiral ganglion in the internal ear and whose peripheral processes end in the specialized sensory epithelium of the organ of Corti.

DEVELOPMENT AND GENERAL ANATOMY OF THE FOREBRAIN

At early stages, the forebrain forms simply the cephalic end of the neural tube, continuous with the midbrain, and lying in the midline. From its cephalic end there develop two hollow outgrowths, the **cerebral vesicles**, which will form the two **cerebral hemispheres**. These, together with the extreme cephalic end of the forebrain, constitute the **telencephalon**; the remainder of the forebrain is the **diencephalon**. The hemispheres soon overgrow the rest of the brain and conceal most of the diencephalon from view.

Diencephalon

The cavity of the forebrain is the third ventricle and various structures arise from its walls (fig 25.38).

THALAMUS

The thalamus is an ovoid thickening of the dorsal part of the side wall of the diencephalon. Its medial surface faces into the third ventricle and is demarcated below, by the hypothalamic sulcus, from the hypothalamus. As the thalami of the two sides grow they encroach on the narrow, slit-like third ventricle and may meet and fuse, forming the massa intermedia. Although often conspicuous, it is of little functional importance. The medial surface of the thalamus is limited above by the line of attachment of the thin ependymal roof of the third

ventricle. When the adult brain is sliced in the midsagittal plane, the thin roof and the small choroid plexus, which hangs from it in the cavity of the third ventricle, are usually torn away. However, the line of attachment of the roof is marked by a narrow band of fibres, the taenia thalami. Beyond the roof is the upper surface, the medial part of which faces into the transverse cerebral fissure (see fig. 25.47). This is a space between the roof of the third ventricle and the corpus callosum; it is lined by pia mater. The lateral part of the upper surface of the thalamus lies in the floor of the lateral ventricle, the cavity of the cerebral hemisphere. The lateral surface of the thalamus is adherent to the cerebral hemisphere. The developmental origins of these relations between thalamus and hemisphere are described below.

HYPOTHALAMUS

The hypothalamus develops from the lower part of the side wall of the diencephalon, below the hypothalamic sulcus; its medial surface therefore bounds the lower part of the third ventricle (fig. 25.39a). The posterior lobe of the pituitary gland develops as a downgrowth from the floor of the diencephalon (fig. 25.40). It establishes contact with an upgrowth of ectoderm (Rathke's pouch) from the roof of the primitive mouth cavity; this forms the anterior lobe. Both anterior and posterior lobes are intimately linked, structurally and functionally with the hyphothalamus.

SUBTHALAMUS

The subthalamus develops from the side wall of the diencephalon, ventral to the thalamus and lateral to the hypothalamus (fig. 25.41). It is the direct cephalic continuation of the tegmentum of the midbrain, and contains extensions of midbrain structures, such as the red nucleus, the substantia nigra, and the midbrain reticular formation, and several ascending fibre tracts which terminate in the thalamus.

EPITHALAMUS

The epithalamus lies at the roof of the caudal part of the

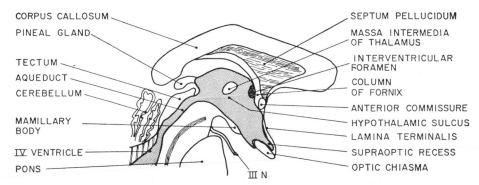

FIG. 25.38. Midsagittal section through third ventricle.

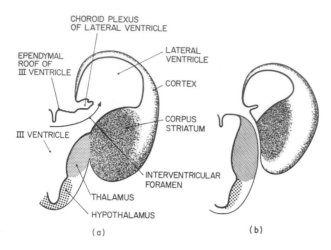

FIG. 25.39. Coronal sections of forebrain and hemisphere; (a) at the level of the interventricular foramen, (b) caudal to the interventricular foramen.

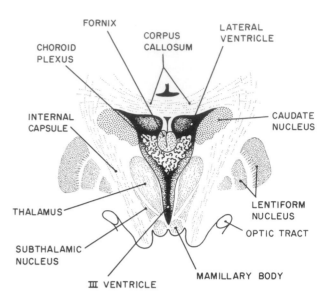

FIG. 25.41. Frontal section of the diencephalon.

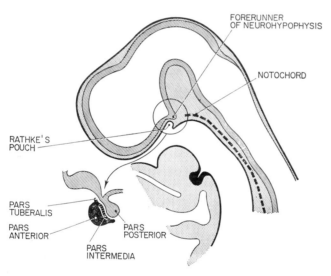

FIG. 25.40. Sagittal section to show the development of the pituitary gland.

diencephalon, above the thalamus and adjacent to the roof of the midbrain (fig. 25.38). It includes the pineal gland and the habenular nucleus (p. 25.69).

OPTIC VESICLES

The optic vesicles arise as outgrowths, one from each side wall of the diencephalon, just cephalic to the pituitary downgrowth. Their contribution to the development of the eye and the optic nerves is described on p. 26.6. The optic nerves are not typical peripheral nerves but are tracts of the brain, and the optic chiasma, which contains decussating optic nerve fibres from each eye, is an integral part of the floor of the diencephalon (figs. 25.38 and 26.10).

Telencephalon

This includes the cephalic extremity of the primitive forebrain, and the two cerebral hemispheres which develop from it.

The **midline telencephalon** is very limited in extent and is demarcated arbitrarily from the diencephalon by a line drawn between the interventricular foramen and the optic chiasma. It includes the cephalic wall of the third ventricle, a very thin coronal sheet which was originally the most cephalic part of the neural tube, a fact reflected in its name, the **lamina terminalis**. Its importance is that it provides the major route for the development of fibres which interconnect the two hemispheres and form the major cerebral commissure (p. 25.32).

CEREBRAL HEMISPHERES

Each cerebral hemisphere develops as a hollow outgrowth from the telencephalon. Its wall initially shows the usual layers and its cavity, the lateral ventricle, communicates with the third ventricle through a large **interventricular foramen**. Part of the wall of the hemisphere consists only of ependymal epithelium. This is called the **choroid fissure**; it lies, at first, in the roof of the hemisphere and is directly continuous with the thin, ependymal roof plate of the third ventricle (fig. 25.42). It marks the site of development, at a later stage, of the choroid plexus of the lateral ventricle.

The floor of the hemisphere thickens to form a deeply placed mass of grey matter, the **corpus striatum**. Cells of the intermediate zone migrate to the surface of the hemisphere where they form the **pallium**, a superficial layer of cells from which will develop the definitive **cerebral cortex**. The hemisphere grows rapidly forwards,

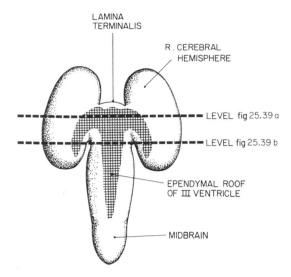

FIG. 25.42. Schematic dorsal view of developing cerebral hemispheres, to show the continuity between the thin ependymal roof of the third ventricle and the ependymal portion of the wall of the hemisphere, which will form the choroid fissure. Based on Frazer, *Manual of Human Embryology*.

dorsally and, more particularly, backwards. Hence, although it develops originally as an outgrowth of the forebrain, it comes to overlie the midbrain and, later still, the hindbrain, including the cerebellum. As the hemisphere grows and expands like an inflating balloon, the thick floor, the corpus striatum, expands more slowly than the remaining thinner wall with the result that the hemisphere gradually assumes a C-shape (fig. 25.43). The C-curvature affects not only the hemisphere as a whole, but also the lateral ventricle within it and the choroid fissure which, because of the expansion of the

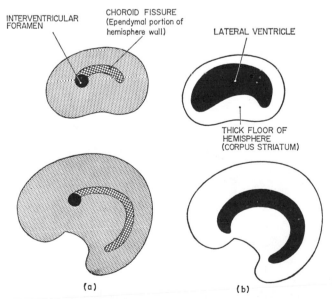

FIG. 25.43. The developing right cerebral hemisphere; (a) medial surface, (b) parasagittal sections.

hemisphere, now lies on its medial wall. Two coronal sections through the midline part of the forebrain and the two hemispheres, one passing through the interventricular foramen, the other somewhat behind it, make clear some important relationships (fig. 25.39).

First, the thin roof plate of the third ventricle is continuous on either side with the choroid fissure of the hemisphere, by way of the roof of the interventricular foramen, which is also ependymal.

Secondly, behind the level of the interventricular foramen, the hemisphere is separated by a gap from the midline part of the forebrain. This gap is obliterated, as if by adhesion between the two, although adhesion is apparent rather than real, and developing nerve fibres grow from the hemisphere to lower levels in the neural tube and in the opposite direction. These descending and ascending fibres form the **internal capsule** which cuts through the grey matter (corpus striatum) in the floor of the hemisphere, dividing it into **caudate** and **lentiform nuclei**. The internal capsule, like the lateral ventricle and the choroidal fissure, is bent into a C-shape by the curvature of the whole hemisphere. This means, of course, that the caudate nucleus also is C-shaped, with its head and body lying in the floor of the anterior horn and central part of the lateral ventricle and its tail lying in the roof of the inferior horn (fig. 25.44).

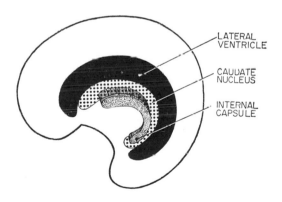

FIG. 25.44. Schematic medial view of the right cerebral hemisphere, to show the relationships of the lateral ventricle, caudate nucleus and internal capsule.

The lower part of the ependymal wall of the hemisphere becomes adherent to the thalamus. This has the result that part of the thalamus, a derivative of the midline part of the forebrain, appears in the floor of the lateral ventricle.

The anterior and posterior horns of the lateral ventricle develop as secondary extensions of the original cavity of the hemisphere. They, therefore, lack the choroid fissure, and the choroid plexus when it develops later does not extend into them.

Cerebral cortex

Mechanical factors probably play an important part in determining the complex pattern of fissures, sulci and gyri of the adult cerebral cortex. As the hemisphere grows and becomes C-shaped, the cortex which overlies the outer surface of the corpus striatum is progressively hidden from view, in the depths of the lateral fissure, by the **frontal** and **temporal opercula**, and forms the **insula** (fig. 25.45).

The cortex grows more rapidly than the deeper tissue and becomes elaborately convoluted. Folding occurs at first between areas which differ in their structure, thickness and rates of growth, e.g. between the uncus and hippocampus (archipallium) and the rest of the cortex (neopallium) and between primary motor and somatic sensory areas, at the central sulcus. These are called primary fissures. Secondary fissures are those which do not demarcate cortical areas of different structure and function.

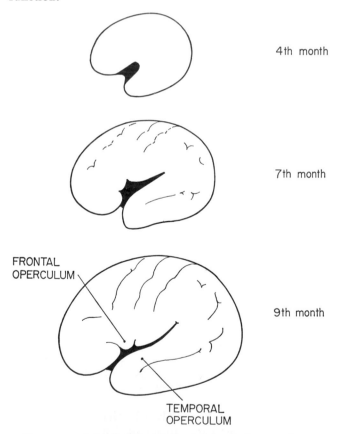

4th month

7th month

FRONTAL OPERCULUM

9th month

TEMPORAL OPERCULUM

FIG. 25.45. Lateral views of the left hemisphere to show successive stages in the formation of the frontal and temporal opercula.

CEREBRAL COMMISSURES

Several groups of nerve fibres serve to interconnect corresponding parts of the hemispheres, forming the commissures. In early stages of development the most convenient route for such commissural fibres to follow

is the lamina terminalis, and it is here that the major commissures develop (fig. 25.46a). Two of these, the **hippocampal** and **anterior commissures**, are called **archipallial** because they connect phylogenetically ancient parts of the brain. The third, the **corpus callosum**, is the largest in man, and connects phylogenetically recent cortical areas, the **neopallium**. The corpus callosum at first lies within the lamina terminalis but, as more fibres are added, it extends beyond the lamina terminalis, the more dorsal part of which becomes stretched and thinned to form the **septum pellucidum** (fig. 25.46b and c). The corpus callosum grows backwards, so that its **splenium** eventually lies close to the pineal gland, the most posterior derivative of the forebrain roof. In its growth backwards, the corpus callosum carries with it the hippocampal commissure (fig. 25.46d).

The **posterior commissure** is a bundle of fibres, running transversely in the roof of the third ventricle at its junction with the cerebral aqueduct and below the pineal gland. Its function is not known but, along with the anterior commissure, it is a landmark for stereotactic surgery.

Fig. 25.47 is a coronal section through the forebrain at the conclusion of all these changes. The space between the corpus callosum and the roof of the third ventricle is the transverse cerebral fissure; it contains pia mater (here called tela choroidea), which invaginates the ependymal roof of the third ventricle to form the choroid plexus of the third ventricle. The choroidal fissures of each lateral ventricle form the choroid plexuses there. The three plexuses are continuous with one another at the interventricular foramen, as a natural consequence of their development. The nature of choroid plexuses is described on p. 25.86.

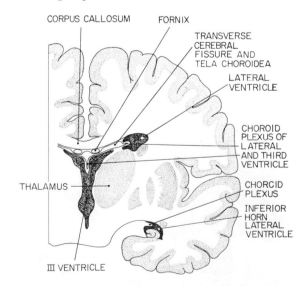

CORPUS CALLOSUM — FORNIX

TRANSVERSE CEREBRAL FISSURE AND TELA CHOROIDEA

LATERAL VENTRICLE

CHOROID PLEXUS OF LATERAL AND THIRD VENTRICLE

CHORCID PLEXUS

INFERIOR HORN LATERAL VENTRICLE

THALAMUS

III VENTRICLE

FIG. 25.47. Coronal section of the brain to show the relationships of the corpus callosum, tela choroidea and choroid plexuses of the third and lateral ventricles, cf. fig. 25.41.

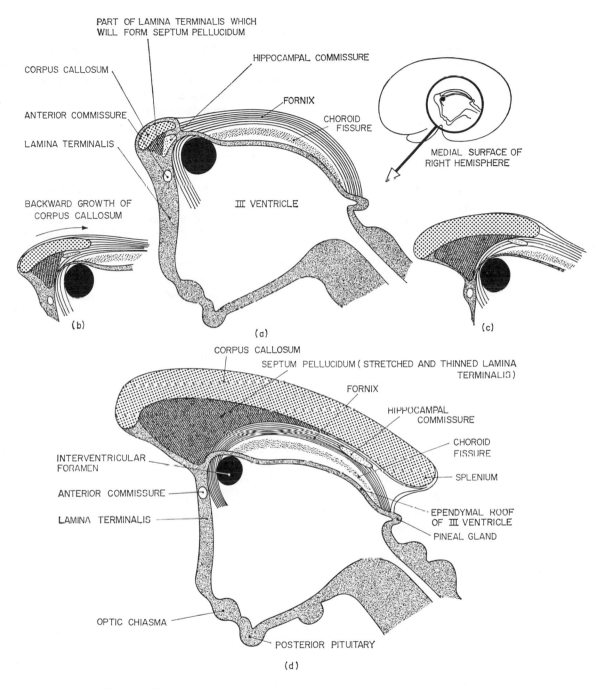

FIG. 25.46. Scheme to summarize the development of the cerebral commissures.

SENSORY SYSTEMS

Somatic sensory pathways subserve various sensory modalities which are aroused by stimulation of receptors in the skin (cutaneous sensibility), in subcutaneous tissue, fasciae and other deep connective tissue (deep sensibility) and in muscles, tendons and joints (proprioceptive sensibility). Visceral sensory pathways convey information from the internal organs and tissues to the CNS. The special senses, sight and hearing, are described in chap. 26, and smell on p. 25.69.

Receptors

The axons of first order sensory neurones may terminate in one of several types of specialized receptors, but many end in unmyelinated **free nerve endings**. These often form plexuses, especially in the skin, from which fine branches penetrate between the cells. These certainly subserve pain and, in the skin, probably touch. Large fibres which lose their myelin sheaths form free **endings on hair follicles** in the epithelial sheaths of hair roots.

At least five types of receptors which subserve cutaneous sensibility have been described.

Meissner's corpuscles (fig. 25.48a) are most abundant (as many as $50/mm^2$) in the palmar skin of the fingers, the region used in making discriminative judgements by touch. They lie in rows in the dermal papillae. Each has

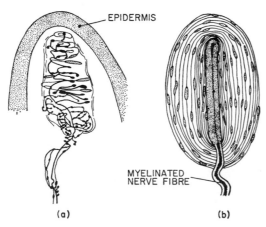

FIG. 25.48. (a) Meissner's corpuscle in a human dermal papilla and (b) a human Pacinian corpuscle.

an outer connective tissue capsule, which contains horizontally stacked, flattened laminar cells and receives several thick myelinated fibres. These lose their myelin before entering the corpuscle, and terminate on the surface of the laminar cells.

Merkel's corpuscles are disc-shaped axon terminals applied to a spherical 'clear' cell in the epidermis.

Krause end bulbs and **Ruffini terminals** are ramifications of free nerve endings enclosed in a capsule of connective tissue which is bulbous in the former and flattened in the latter.

These, together with free nerve endings and Pacinian corpuscles (see below), which are present in the dermis but not in the epidermis, respond to cutaneous stimuli. Meissner's corpuscles certainly respond to light touch and Pacinian corpuscles to pressure, but electrical recordings from single nerve fibres have not identified any of them solely with a specific sensory modality. In particular, there are no specific specialised receptors for heat or cold.

Pacinian corpuscles (fig. 25.48b) are abundant in deep structures such as the serous membranes, joints, tendons, periosteum and interosseous membrane, as well as in the dermis and subcutaneous tissue. A large myelinated axon enters the base of the corpuscle, which consists of an inner bulb of cells equivalent to Schwann cells and an outer bulb, composed of concentric layers of flattened cells derived from, and continuous with, the perineurium. Spaces between lamellae contain collagen fibres, some blood vessels and interstitial fluid. These corpuscles are involved in vibration sense and in perception of pressure on deep structures. They play an important part in deep sensibility, as may free nerve endings and Ruffini terminals. They may also contribute with muscle spindles and tendon organs (pp. 25.18 and 19) to proprioceptive sensibility.

An axon of a first order sensory neurone may divide and end in several receptors, and one receptor can be coupled with more than one fibre. Information is likely to be scrambled on entry to the cord and to require disentanglement by central processes.

TRANSMISSION OF INFORMATION FROM RECEPTORS

When a receptor has received an adequate stimulus, information passes up its nerve fibre in the form of nerve impulses and the frequency of these provides the code for the message. Does this mean that when the skin is pressed by a given weight, impulses begin to travel along the relevant fibre at a frequency corresponding to the weight and continue until the weight is taken off?

When the skin becomes warmer or cooler, does the frequency along the appropriate fibre simply change accordingly and stay at the new rate as long as the temperature is steady? Neither of these simple statements is generally true; indeed, such an arrangement would be both wasteful of energy and, metaphorically speaking, boring for the central nervous system. Stimulation of a sensory ending gives rise to a **receptor potential** which appears at the specialized end of an afferent nerve fibre, e.g. inside a Pacinian corpuscle, or in some cases at a special separate cell from which it can evoke nerve impulses in an adjoining nerve fibre, e.g. in the cochlea. A receptor potential is not unlike an EPSP (p. 25.16) and so is not an all-or-none phenomenon, but varies in electrical size and time course; it may be rapidly dissipated even though the stimulus continues, and then the firing

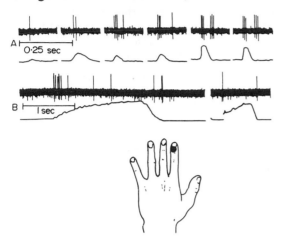

FIG. 25.49. Nerve impulses from a fast adapting human receptor at the site shown. A, a series of taps monitored on lower trace; note volleys of impulses at both 'on' and 'off' of the taps towards right end of trace. B, longer pressure, similarly monitored. Activity at 'on' and 'off', little in between, no sign of resting discharge. Modified from Vallbo Å.B. & Hagbarth K.-E. (1968) *Exper. Neurol.* **21**, 270.

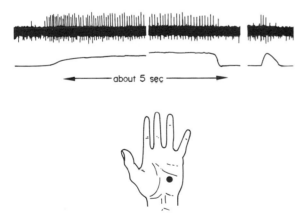

FIG. 25.50. Nerve impulses from a slowly adapting human receptor at the site shown, in response to prolonged and to briefer pressure monitored on lower trace; note that prolonged pressure produces a prolonged response with little adaptation and without 'off' discharge. Modified from Vallbo Å.B. & Hagbarth K.-E. (1968).

frequency in the nerve fibre rapidly falls away (fig. 25.49), a feature called **adaptation**; in other cases (fig. 25.50) the receptor potential is prolonged and the firing frequency falls off slowly or not at all. Receptors which adapt slowly are especially likely to show resting discharge.

Another question is whether there is a tidy separation of sensory fibres into those signalling touch, temperature and damage to tissue. The picture is not clear cut.

Most of the touch fibres are highly specific and respond to nothing else, but some, usually of the slowly adapting type, respond to temperature change too, although they are perhaps a hundred times less sensitive than the specific temperature fibres. This is less surprising when one remembers that the skin functions over a wide range of temperatures, and most biological processes are markedly affected by change of temperature.

The temperature receptors generally fire faster at the time that a change of temperature occurs; cold receptors respond in this way to a fall in temperature and warm receptors to a rise. In cats, the fall or rise can be as small as 0·2°C, which is comparable to the smallest change sensed by one's own skin. These transient, dynamic changes in frequency are superimposed on a continuous, static background discharge which depends also on temperature; the steady static background might, for instance, be 15 spikes/sec at a temperature around 38–43°C for a 'warm' fibre, or around 15–34°C for a 'cold' fibre. Hibernating animals, interestingly enough, are equipped with cold fibres reaching a maximum static discharge rate at only 4°C, which could function to awaken them if in peril of freezing. The dynamic response that signals the onset of a change may raise the rate temporarily to 150 spikes/sec. Just as touch receptors may respond with low sensitivity to temperature changes, so temperature receptors may respond to pressure, but less sensitively.

Lateral inhibition

Scrambled information passing into the cord in the axons of several primary neurones may be disentangled at the relay to either secondary sensory neurones or motor neurones by a process known as lateral inhibition (fig. 25.51). This shows the impulse traffic in an array of

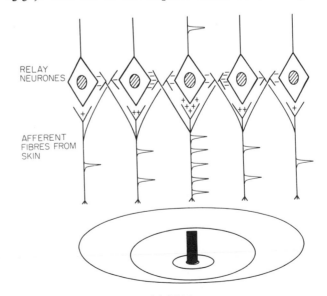

FIG. 25.51. Lateral inhibition arrangement.

cutaneous nerve fibres stimulated by a prod which deforms the skin most at the centre, but to a lesser extent for some distance round. Five impulses per unit time proceed along the centre fibre, giving five units of excitation at the central cell in the relay nucleus; similarly the adjoining fibres on each side transmit two impulses per unit time, and the outer fibres transmit one. By the lateral inhibitory paths shown, two units of inhibition from each side reach the central relay cell, from which there is a net output of one unit; the more lateral relay cells are entirely inhibited.

Thus when the strong central signal proceeds further, it indicates precisely the centre of the prodded area. The simplified diagram does not show that inhibitory effects are always delayed, because inhibitory signals have to traverse more synapses than excitatory ones. Hence the earliest of a volley of impulses normally proceeds further than its followers. Fibres from higher centres in the nervous system may also play a part in the control of this sharpening and selecting process. Lateral inhibition occurs not only in afferent and efferent nuclei in the cord, but in higher centres, e.g. thalamic nuclei and lateral geniculate nuclei, and also in the retina. If, as is usual, a system shows resting activity, the central relay cell ticks over gently without any stimulus. A gentle prod on the centre of its receptive area excites it to faster activity. But a gentle prod on the edge slows or stops the resting activity, via the inhibitory links shown. This behaviour in retinal ganglion cells is illustrated in fig. 26.19.

Such a system can withstand some loss of fibres. If the afferent fibre from the centre of the prodded area in fig. 25.51 is destroyed, two upper lateral fibres begin to fire and convey that the skin is being prodded. The message gets through, but the signals received at the centre are not so accurate. In general the nervous system is 'overwired', i.e. it contains more fibres than are absolutely necessary to convey the message, and it can continue to function after a fashion even after considerable damage, but less precisely than before. Lateral inhibitory organization is probably one reason why this is so.

Pain

Two kinds of afferent nerve fibres appear to convey information of tissue damage. One is relatively large, often confusingly described as $A\delta$ and so smaller than the $A\gamma$ fibres running to skeletal muscle (p. 15.23) and conducts at 10–20 m/sec. The other is fine and unmyelinated and consists of C fibres conducting at 1–2 m/sec. But not all fibres of these two sizes are devoted to this function; many C fibres convey information only about temperature or pressure, and are not concerned with signalling damage. It is clear that pain does not follow high rates of firing from receptors of just any kind. Touch receptors, for example, may fire at maximal rates when stimulated in entirely innocuous ways. It is also evident that not all

pain information is urgent, so that there is nothing absurd about the use of small fibres for its transmission. For example, anyone lying quite still develops bed sores in a few hours, because pressure cuts off the blood supply of the skin on which the weight rests. Normally the skin receptors presumably prevent this by prompting a change of position, but seconds are unlikely to count for what is nevertheless a most important response.

The nature of the receptors is not so certain, since it is easier to record from nerve fibres in a nerve trunk than to know exactly what receptors are at the transmitting outer ends of the fibres. The receptors for tissue damage seem to be free nerve endings without elaborate organization, though many such endings are concerned with other matters like touch and temperature. Sensitivity can vary at the periphery; it is exquisite near a boil, much lower elsewhere.

HANDLING OF PAIN INFORMATION IN THE CENTRAL NERVOUS SYSTEM

Sensitivity can also vary because of changes in the central nervous system. Those who have lost a limb may suffer from agonizing phantom pains which appear to originate in the absent limb, yet there can be no input of nerve impulses from the part to trigger the pain. In contrast, people under hypnosis undergo operations without anaesthesia and without seeming to sense pain. Lucretius (98–55 B.C.) wrote how in a battle with scythed chariots: 'such is the quickness of the injury and the eagerness of the man's mind that he cannot feel the pain'; or to come nearer home:

'For Witherington needs must I wail,
As one in doleful dumps,
For when his legs were smitten off
He fought upon the stumps.'

(Ballad of Chevy Chase)

Nerve traffic related to pain, after entering the spinal cord, passes upwards chiefly by the spinothalamic tracts, but enters these tracts through synapses where modification, recombination or suppression can occur. Efforts to trace nervous traffic related to pain alone beyond the thalamus have never been successful. The sensory areas of the cerebral cortex appear relatively unresponsive to painful stimulation of the appropriate part of the body. Nor, if these cortical areas are stimulated electrically during operations on conscious patients, is pain often produced. And damage to the cerebral cortex does not abolish pain, at any rate after the first few days.

On the other hand, it cannot be shown that any part of the thalamus is the 'pain centre' and that its removal abolishes pain. There are widespread interconnections between the region where the spinothalamic tracts end and other parts of the forebrain, the frontal cortex and limbic system for instance. Damage to the thalamus occasionally brings about a state in which pain is not so easily provoked as before, but peculiarly disturbing when it occurs; it is localized and does not yield to analgesic drugs. In contrast, if the frontal cerebral cortex is severed from the thalamus on both sides **(leucotomy)**, painful stimuli are just as easily appreciated, but the patient is much less disturbed by them than before. Pain is, it seems, the outcome of an analysis in which the final answer is not deciphered in any one part of the brain. Surgical procedures to mitigate intractable pain are described in vol. 3, chap. 57.

REFERRED PAIN

The correct interpretation of pain originating deep to the skin is a key problem in most branches of medicine. One automatically localizes precisely pain from the skin, or else learns to do so in earliest life. This precision is absent from deep pain. Several special features make its interpretation possible.

Firstly, what hurts a great deal on the skin may not hurt at all in muscles and viscera. The alimentary canal, kidneys, ureters, heart and lungs are normally insensitive to cutting or burning. On the other hand, these organs are sensitive to sudden distension or to ischaemia. In contrast, the parietal lining of body cavities (peritoneum, pleura, pericardium) is sensitive to mechanical damage.

The location of pain originating in deep tissues is often ill defined. It is sensed as in the midline when it arises from alimentary canal or heart, both of which originally developed in the midline. It also is often referred to the surface of the body corresponding to the spinal nerve roots concerned, yet the subject rarely doubts that the pain arises from some deep origin and not from the skin. This phenomenon of reference means that cardiac pain can be felt in the midline and in addition in the arms, because the afferent fibres from the heart reach the spinal cord in the roots T2 or higher, up to C5. It also means that pain arising in the pleura over the diaphragm is felt in the neck and shoulder, since the afferent fibres are in the phrenic nerve (C3–5), and on the appropriate side, since the diaphragm is not simply a midline structure. Similarly pain arising in a joint or muscle in the neck may be referred to the appropriate arm where the cutaneous branches of the same spinal root lie.

This reference is of course not simply a delusion in the patient's mind. The afferent traffic from body surface and from deeper structures converges in the nervous system. The skin surface may be hypersensitive to painful stimulation when a deep structure is also contributing a source of pain; for instance, lightly stroking the skin with a pin over an inflamed appendix may seem very painful. Conversely, pain from a deep structure may diminish if traffic from the skin surface at the corresponding root level is abolished by local anaesthesia of the skin surface. For instance, in the cervix and in the vagina above the hymen touch, heat and cold cannot be sensed, but pain can be produced by electrical stimulation of the cervix and is referred to the skin midway between the umbilicus and symphysis pubis. In Theobald's experiments, a stimulus strength above five units evoked pain, but he could abolish this by local anaesthetic infiltrated, not into the cervix, but into the abdominal skin at the site of reference. In this way stimulus strength could be increased up to ninety units without pain, but stronger stimuli produced pain in the abdominal wall which could not be abolished by local anaesthetics.

Vibration sense

The skin can detect that something pressing upon it is vibrating, and it is most sensitive to vibration at 200–400 Hz, readily applied by a tuning fork. Bone underneath the skin makes the stimulation more effective, and so vibration sense is usually tested on skin overlying bone. Fast-adapting receptors for touch and pressure are clearly able to signal such vibrations, especially perhaps the Pacinian corpuscle, which is known to produce one nerve impulse per cycle over the appropriate range of frequencies. Vibration sense is thus closely linked to the sensation of touch and pressure and, along with the sense of the position of joints, is conveyed centrally by the dorsal columns and the medial lemniscus.

Stereognosis

This word means the ability to recognize by hand, blindfold, the shapes of solid objects, e.g. of a key or a milled edged coin. It involves not only analysing complex incoming traffic from the receptors, but also actively handling the objects. Clearly it depends on the traffic being adequate for analysis; numb fingers cannot be used for recognition. But it also depends on the analysing ability of the cerebral cortex, especially its posterior parietal part, and even when the receptor system cannot be faulted, stereognosis may be defective if there is damage to this part of the cerebral cortex (p. 25.73.).

Somatic sensory pathways

Somatic sensory pathways are crossed, terminate in the somatic sensory cortex of the cerebral hemisphere on the opposite side of the body to that stimulated, and consist essentially of chains of three neurones. There are three pathways which are anatomically separate for the greater part of their course to the thalamus: the **dorsal column-medial lemniscus pathway** ascends the spinal cord in the dorsal white columns and traverses the brain stem in the medial lemniscus, the **spinothalamic pathway** lies in the lateral white column of the spinal cord and, in the brain stem, lateral to the medial lemniscus, and **trigeminothalamic pathways** ascend to the thalamus from the sensory nuclei of the trigeminal nerve.

DORSAL COLUMN-MEDIAL LEMNISCUS PATHWAY (fig. 25.52)

Large, thickly myelinated fibres of the medial division of the dorsal spinal nerve roots enter the dorsal white column of their own side and divide into ascending and descending branches. The descending branches establish reflex connections by sending collateral branches into the dorsal grey column; the ascending branches are the first link in the sensory pathway (fig. 25.13). They ascend in the dorsal white column to the upper end of the spinal cord and continue into the lower medulla where they terminate synaptically on second order sensory neurones in the gracile or cuneate nuclei. Their axons curve ventrally and medially, cross the midline in the **great sensory decussation** and turn upwards to form a prominent bundle of fibres, the **medial lemniscus**. In the medulla, this lies close to the midline in a parasagittal plane. As it ascends its orientation changes, and in the upper midbrain it lies lateral to the red nucleus in a horizontal plane. It terminates in one of the sensory relay nuclei of the thalamus, the **nucleus ventralis posterolateralis**. This contains the cell bodies of third order sensory neurones, whose axons run in the posterior part of the posterior limb of the internal capsule and terminate in the **somaesthetic cortex** (somatic sensory cortex 1) in the postcentral gyrus (areas 3, 1 and 2 of the Brodmann classification, p. 25.65).

Somatotopic localization

Nervous impulses generated in particular regions of the body are transmitted in localized parts of the pathway. This orderliness of structural organization in certain parts of the central nervous system is indeed one of its most important characteristics. It is seen in the dorsal white columns of the spinal cord, in which fibres entering from sacral nerves are situated medially and fibres entering at successively higher levels are added in successively more lateral layers (fig. 25.52). This laminar pattern is reflected in the termination of the fibres in the gracile nucleus, which receives sacral, lumbar and lower thoracic fibres, and the cuneate nucleus, which receives upper thoracic and cervical fibres. Somatotopic localization is also seen in the medial lemniscus and, most strikingly, in the pattern of termination in the somaesthetic cortex (p. 25.72).

The medial lemniscus establishes abundant reflex connections, in addition to serving as a truly 'sensory' route. For example, the ascending fibres of the dorsal white columns send collaterals into the dorsal grey column.

Both the gracile and cuneate and the thalamic relay nuclei receive descending fibres from the cerebral cortex, which may exert either excitatory or inhibitory effects on the ascending pathway. These actions may provide for more precise localization and evaluation of sensory stimuli, or may occlude undesirable or irrelevant sensory input.

The dorsal column-medial lemniscus pathway is concerned with: (1) the finer and more discriminative aspects of tactile sensibility, i.e. the ability to localize accurately the site of touch, to recognize, as separate, two touch stimuli applied close together on the skin (two-point discrimination) and to discriminate between different textures and between degrees of roughness; (2) the appreciation of the position of the body, and particularly of the limbs, in space and the recognition of active or passive joint movements (muscle and joint sense); (3) the recognition, by feel, of the shape of objects, stereognosis; and (4) vibration sense.

Discrimination and localization are not modalities of sensation and they are not conducted by the dorsal column-medial lemniscus pathway, which conducts coded nerve impulses. They are functions of the higher centres.

SPINOTHALAMIC PATHWAY (fig. 25.53)

This transmits impulses which are appreciated as sensations of heat and cold and of pain. It also provides an alternative pathway for touch sensibility, referred to as crude or coarse touch. Loss of the dorsal column pathway and dependence upon the spinothalamic pathway reduces a patient's ability in tests of tactile localization and two-point discrimination.

The first order neurones have their cell bodies in a dorsal root ganglion; their fibres are thinner than those concerned in the dorsal column-medial lemniscus pathway, and have a thin myelin sheath or none at all. They enter the spinal cord in the lateral part of the dorsal root and divide into short descending and ascending branches, which run for one or two segments in the posterolateral fasciculus before synapsing with second order sensory neurones, which lie deeply in the dorsal column. Their axons cross the midline, in the ventral white commissure, and ascend in the ventrolateral white column as the **spinothalamic tract**. Some first order fibres terminate in the **substantia gelatinosa**, a column of small, densely packed neurones situated in the dorsal grey column close to its dorsal apex. These were formerly regarded as second order sensory neurones whose axons formed the spinothalamic tract. It is now known that their axons do not travel far; some run in the posterolateral fasciculus and form short intersegmental links with the second order neurones lying deeper.

Throughout the brain stem the spinothalamic tract lies lateral to the medial lemniscus, which it accompanies to terminate in the thalamus, in the nucleus ventralis posterolateralis and, in addition, in the posterior group of thalamic nuclei. The extensive connections between the thalamus and the somatic sensory cortex make it difficult for the anatomist to exclude the cortex from a role in pain perception, but the experimental evidence from cortical ablations in man suggests that the cortex may

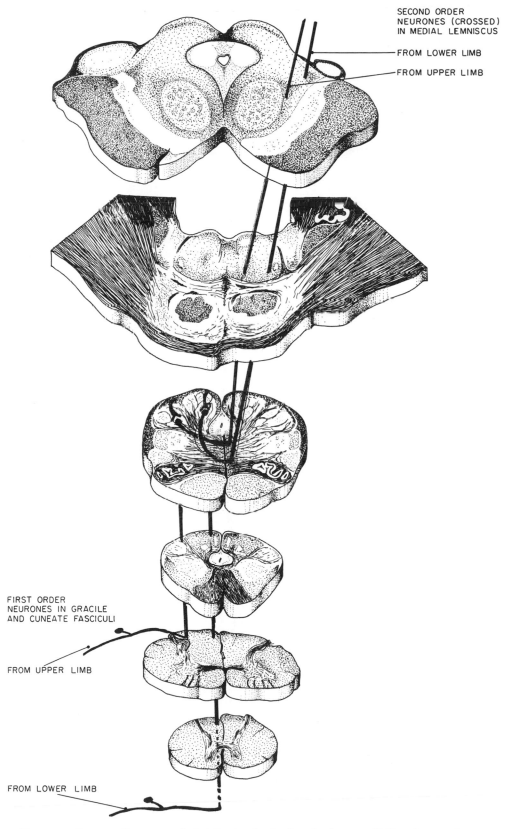

SECOND ORDER
NEURONES (CROSSED)
IN MEDIAL LEMNISCUS

FROM LOWER LIMB

FROM UPPER LIMB

FIRST ORDER
NEURONES IN GRACILE
AND CUNEATE FASCICULI

FROM UPPER LIMB

FROM LOWER LIMB

FIG. 25.52. Pattern of somatotopic localization in the dorsal column-medial lemniscus pathway.
Cf. Brain stem sections in fig. 25.35.

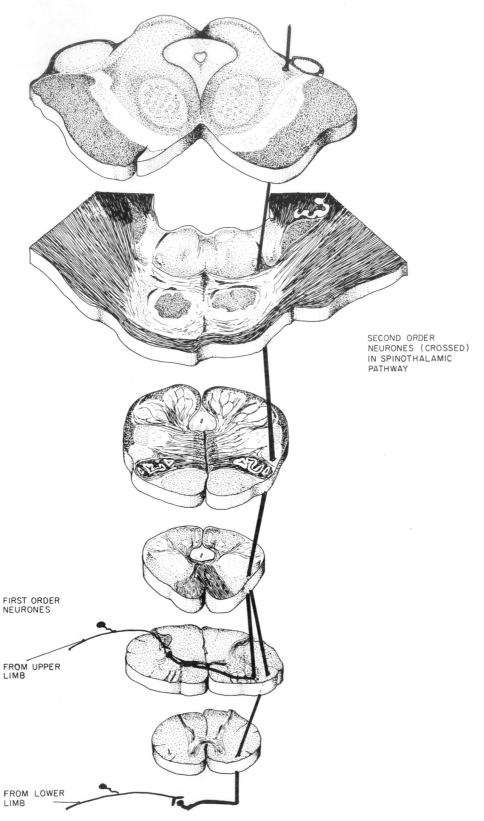

FIG. 25.53. General plan of spinothalamic pathway and pattern of somatotopic localization within it in the spinal cord.
Cf. Brain stem sections in fig. 25.35.

not be essential, and that pain may be appreciated at thalamic level.

Some clinically important features of the spinothalamic pathway should be noted:

(1) The second order fibres cross the midline only one or two segments above the level of entry of the corresponding dorsal root fibres.

(2) The site of decussation, in the ventral white commissure, exposes fibres of both sides to damage by expanding lesions beginning around the central canal of the spinal cord, e.g. syringomyelia (vol. 3, p. 34.48).

(3) Sacral fibres are situated laterally and dorsally, cervical fibres medially and ventrally in the spinothalamic tract, a pattern of somatotopic localization shown in the lower part of fig. 25.53.

(4) Fibres concerned with pain and temperature sensibility are, in general, situated dorsally to those involved with touch and pressure.

(5) Throughout its course, the spinothalamic tract is less compactly organized than the medial lemniscus, being intermingled with other ascending pathways. Moreover it gives off many collaterals to the brain stem reticular formation, providing for additional pathways to the thalamus and elsewhere.

TRIGEMINOTHALAMIC PATHWAYS

These provide for sensory input from most of the skin of the face, and of the forehead as far as the vertex, from the mucous membranes of the nasal cavities and paranasal sinuses, of the mouth, tongue and part of the pharynx, from the teeth and gums and from part of the dura mater. The cell bodies of primary sensory neurones are in the trigeminal ganglion, and their axons enter the pons in the sensory root of the nerve. Some fibres terminate, at their level of entry, in the **chief sensory nucleus** (fig. 25.54); others descend through the brain stem for variable distances, in the **spinal tract** of the trigeminal nerve and terminate in the **nucleus of the spinal tract**. About half of the entering fibres divide into one branch which terminates in the chief nucleus and another which descends in the spinal tract to end in the spinal nucleus. The chief and spinal tract nuclei are sensory nuclei and contain cell bodies of second order neurones, whose axons cross the midline and ascend as **trigeminothalamic fibres**, most of which accompany the medial lemniscus, and terminate in the thalamus (nucleus ventralis posteromedialis). This sends thalamocortical projections to the somatic sensory cortex.

There is a small group of trigeminal first order sensory fibres which are exceptional in having cell bodies within the midbrain, in the **mesencephalic nucleus** (fig. 25.35b). The peripheral processes are distributed with branches of the trigeminal nerve to end in the muscles of mastication, in the temporomandibular joint and in relation to the teeth and gums. They are important in proprioceptive

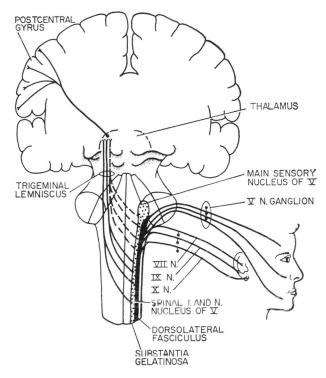

FIG. 25.54. Central sensory connections of the trigeminal nerve. Modified from Noback C.P. (1967). *The Human Nervous System*. New York. McGraw-Hill.

reflexes in chewing and in regulating the strength of the bite. Some fibres are also thought to subserve proprioceptive function in the extrinsic ocular muscles and in the muscles of the tongue and face.

There is a division of labour among the trigeminal nuclei, broadly corresponding with that described for the sensory nuclei associated with spinal nerves. The chief sensory nucleus receives neurones which are distributed to tactile corpuscles, and subserves discriminative tactile sense, corresponding in this respect to the gracile and cuneate nuclei of the dorsal column-medial lemniscus pathway. The spinal trigeminal nucleus is continuous below with the dorsal apex of the dorsal grey column of the spinal cord (including substantia gelatinosa) and it is similarly concerned with pain sensibility. Both nuclei are probably concerned with 'crude' touch.

Surgical section of the lower part of the spinal tract has been used in the attempt to relieve intractable pain in the trigeminal territory, and knowledge of the position of the tract and of somatotopic localization within it is therefore of some importance. It lies superficially and posterolaterally in the lower medulla, and ophthalmic, maxillary and mandibular fibres are arranged in that order, ventrodorsally. It is joined by somatic afferent fibres of the nervus intermedius, glossopharyngeal and vagus nerves which lie dorsally to the mandibular fibres, and terminate in the spinal nucleus. This means that all somatic sensibility subserved by cranial nerves follows trigeminothalamic pathways.

The long-standing belief that mandibular, maxillary and ophthalmic fibres end in successively lower parts of the spinal nucleus has not been substantiated.

Visceral afferent system

Visceral afferent fibres arise not only in the viscera in the strict sense, i.e. the organs of the thoracic, abdominal and pelvic cavities, but also in blood vessels of the limbs and trunk and in the mucous membranes of the back of the tongue, and of the pharynx, larynx and oesophagus. Over this extensive and varied distribution, the modalities of sensation subserved, and the types of stimuli required to produce a response, also vary greatly. Indeed in some sites the sensory modalities which can be appreciated, and one's ability to localize them, differ little from those in the skin, and the distinction between visceral and somatic is rather finely drawn. Over most of the visceral territory, however, the distinction between visceral and somatic sensibility is functionally significant and clinically important.

Just as in the somatic system, so in the visceral, the terms afferent and sensory are not synonymous. Some visceral afferents, e.g. baroceptors, are involved only in reflex responses, not consciously appreciated; most serve conscious sensibility as well as reflex function.

Most visceral afferent fibres run with the efferent fibres of nerves of the autonomic system. Their cellbodies lie in the dorsal root ganglia of spinal nerves or in the sensory ganglia of cranial nerves. After entering the cord or brain stem they terminate synaptically on cells in the visceral afferent column (fig. 25.36). The course followed by second order visceral afferent neurones is uncertain, but probably is via bilateral ascending polysynaptic pathways to higher centres.

DISTRIBUTION AND LOCAL FUNCTION
Mouth and oropharynx
The glossopharyngeal nerve provides visceral afferent fibres for the back of the tongue, the tonsillar region and the nasal and oral parts of the pharynx, which subserve the sensory modalities of touch, pain, heat and cold. Sensibility is similar to that of the skin, and has a comparable degree of localization. The nerve also provides taste fibres for the same region of the tongue; these are classed as special visceral afferents. A third group of fibres supplies baroceptor fibres to the carotid sinus and chemoreceptor fibres to the carotid body. These fibres have their cell bodies in the ganglia of the glossopharyngeal nerve; some terminate in the nucleus of the tractus solitarius, pain fibres in the spinal nucleus of nerve V (p. 25.28 & fig. 25.37).

The fibres of ordinary sensation form the afferent limb of two important reflexes, the gag reflex (p. 25.28) and the swallowing reflex (p. 25.28); both these reflexes have an important protective function. The fibres to the carotid sinus and body contribute to cardiovascular homeostatic control.

Laryngopharynx and pharynx
The vagus nerve carries visceral afferents from the mucosa of the larynx and laryngopharynx. Cell bodies are in the inferior (nodose) ganglion, and the fibres terminate in the nucleus solitarius. Central connections provide for two important protective reflexes: the sphincteric closure of the laryngeal aditus in swallowing, and forceful contraction of expiratory muscles against a closed glottis in coughing.

Alimentary canal
The alimentary canal is largely insensitive to stimuli which arouse sensations when applied to the skin, such as touch, cutting, heat and cold. It is none the less well supplied with visceral afferent fibres which generate the feelings of fullness after a good meal, distension often due to wind, and discomfort from excessive peristalsis. These fibres are also involved in reflex responses of the canal; some of them, when the stimulus is excessive, generate sensation of pain. The adequate stimulus for pain from the alimentary canal (and from other hollow viscera) seems to be the overdistension and consequent hyperactivity of the smooth muscle. Pain arising in the oesophagus may be felt substernally as a burning sensation ('heartburn'); in the stomach and duodenum as a gnawing or burning sensation in the epigastrium; in the small and large intestines as a 'colicky' or 'cramping' pain at the umbilicus and in the suprapubic region, respectively. In each case, the pain is felt as midline, regardless of the precise location of the initiating stimulus; it is, however, regarded subjectively as arising in structures deep to the body wall and should not be confused with referred pain (p. 25.37) which is often associated with disorders of the abdominal viscera. Visceral afferent fibres generating pain sensibility probably accompany sympathetic efferent fibres. Those from the stomach travel with the splanchnic nerves to the thoracic sympathetic chain and thence via white rami communicantes to spinal nerves (T5–T9), entering the spinal cord through the dorsal roots.

Heart
William Harvey was able to demonstrate to King Charles I that the heart was insensitive to touch. His patient was a young nobleman who, when a child, had a suppurating wound of the chest wall; this healed leaving a gap through which the King 'could, with his own hand, even touch the ventricles' without the young man knowing. Ischaemia is a common cause of pain generated in heart muscle. Visceral afferents travel with visceral

efferent branches of the cardiac plexus. Typically the pain is referred to the inner side of the left arm.

Respiratory system

There are abundant terminals of visceral afferent nerves in the lung—in the bronchial mucosa, in the bronchial and pulmonary arteries and in the pulmonary veins—provided mainly by the vagus nerve. They are involved in the cough reflex and in the Hering-Breuer reflex (p. 31.26). The vagal afferent fibres terminate in the nucleus solitarius whose axons run to the medullary centres involved in the cough reflex and in the regulation of respiration.

Like the gut, the lung is insensitive to stimuli which, in the skin, generate sensations of touch, heat, cold. Extensive pulmonary disease may produce little or no pain, unless it involves the endings of somatic sensory nerves (intercostal and phrenic) in the parietal pleura.

Urinary system

Visceral afferents from the kidney accompany both vagal and sympathetic efferents. Pain may arise in the kidney, as in other solid viscera, when it becomes swollen and tense within its restraining collagenous capsule.

When the ureter is obstructed, as by a calculus, powerful spasmodic contractions of its smooth muscle stimulate the terminals of visceral afferent nerves and cause ureteric colic, often a very severe pain. It is commonly referred and radiates round the body wall from the loin into the groin (p. 36.6).

The mucosa of the urinary bladder is probably insensitive to touch and to thermal stimuli, but pain is generated by overdistension and resultant overactive contraction of the smooth muscle of the bladder. The visceral afferents involved accompany the pelvic splanchnic nerves (parasympathetic) to the sacral nerves and spinal cord.

Female reproductive system

The cervix of the uterus is insensitive to cutting (e.g. in taking a biopsy) and to burning (e.g. in cauterization), but when it is dilated, in the later stages of labour, the stretching of the submucosal connective tissue generates painful stimuli in endings of nerves which accompany the pelvic splanchnics to the spinal cord.

The upper part of the vagina is almost insensitive, the lower part is supplied by somatic afferents via the pudendal nerves.

The subsequent course of sensory pathways from the thalamic nuclei is described on p. 25.61.

CONTROL OF SKELETAL MUSCLE ACTIVITY

The final link in the control of skeletal muscle by the CNS is provided by lower motor neurones of the brain stem and spinal cord. The cell bodies of these neurones are found in the somatic efferent column of the brain stem (motor nuclei of III, IV, VI and XII cranial nerves), in the branchial efferent nuclei of the brain stem (motor nuclei of V, VII and IX, X and XI cranial nerves) and in the somatic efferent column of the spinal cord.

A motor unit (p. 16.10) consists of one lower motor neurone and the muscle fibres it innervates. The fibres of one motor unit are scattered throughout a muscle and do not lie all side by side. In addition, motor units include different numbers of fibres, so that their power varies. For gentle movements, units of small power are used. To increase the strength of a movement, two procedures are possible. Either more units and those with greater power may contract or the rate of stimulation of each unit may be increased. In fact, extra units start contracting, **recruitment**, early on, and if still more power is needed, the stimulation rate rises.

The progress of a movement, unless it is very rapid, is monitored in several ways. The eyes may see what happens and joint receptors signal how the joints move. Through the γ efferent system, the intrafusal fibres of the muscle spindles can be made to contract in synchrony with the muscles in which they lie; there is evidence that this occurs in human voluntary movements, and it may keep group I afferent activity stable throughout movement (fig. 25.31). The elegance of this arrangement is that any unexpected intervening force which frustrates the movement prevents the extrafusal muscle fibres from contracting, but not the intrafusal fibres. The increased stretch of the muscle spindles then leads very rapidly to increased contraction of the extrafusal fibres, and so to correction of the movement.

The activity of a lower motor neurone is influenced by a wide variety of neuronal pathways. Some of the influences are excitatory, others are inhibitory. Some of the neuronal pathways which terminate on a spinal motor neurone are shown in fig. 25.13; those involved in segmental and intersegmental reflexes have been discussed on p. 25.11. Here we are concerned with those descending pathways which originate at levels above the spinal cord, the **supraspinal descending pathways.**

Corticospinal (pyramidal) tract

This was described by Türck in 1851 and was one of the first tracts in CNS to be discovered. Although our ideas about it have been revised radically since 1940, it is still regarded as the most important single route over which voluntary control of skeletal muscle is exercised. It was called pyramidal for no more profound reason than that its fibres constitute the pyramids of the medulla. The name is unfortunate for several reasons. First, it led people to assume that the tract originated solely from conspicuous giant pyramidal cells in the cerebral cortex. Secondly, it has helped to crystallize a concept of control of movement by two systems of fibres, one 'pyramidal', the other 'extrapyramidal', a concept which has enjoyed considerable vogue, particularly in clinical neurology, but one which now appears to be wrong. Thirdly, it does not make clear that corticospinal fibres, ending on or near spinal motor neurones, have their counterpart in the corticonuclear fibres, which terminate on motor nuclei of the brain stem; if the concept of a pyramidal system continues to be used in clinical neurology, it must include both corticonuclear and corticospinal pathways although most of the corticonuclear fibres leave the tract before it enters the pyramids. Finally, although damage to the pyramidal tract is common in clinical neurology, it very seldom involves the tract where it runs through the pyramid. Most commonly the tract is damaged in the internal capsule of the cerebral hemisphere (p. 25.49) or in the lateral white columns of the spinal cord. In each of these situations there is, inevitably, concomitant damage to other tracts, and the clinical concept of a pyramidal tract lesion (p. 25.49) must be recognized as a composite of the effects of damage to corticonuclear and corticospinal fibres and to other tracts which closely accompany these.

ORIGIN

Since each pyramid contains about one million fibres, more than half of them unmyelinated, it is not surprising that the cellular origin of some of them is still not known. Two direct methods have been used to determine their origin in experimental animals. The first, to cut the fibres in the pyramid and, after an interval, to study retrograde cellular degeneration in the brain; the second, to excise different areas of the cerebral cortex and subsequently to study fibre degeneration in the pyramids. The first method showed retrograde cell degeneration in the giant pyramidal cells of Betz in area 4 of the cortex (p. 25.65). On the strength of this observation, and in the belief that the Betz cells formed a unique population, these cells were widely held to be the main, if not the sole, origin of pyramidal tract fibres. This comfortable dogma was shaken principally by the work of Lassek, an American neuroanatomist, who found that 90 per cent of fibres in the pyramid were of small diameter (1–4 μm) and only 1·7 per cent were large (11–22 μm). He also counted all the giant (Betz) cells in area 4 and found a total of about 30 000. In a further study he excised different areas of cerebral cortex in a series of monkeys and found that, following ablation of extensive areas of frontal and parietal lobe cortex, about one-half of the pyramidal tract fibres remained. However following extirpation of area 4, almost all large fibres disappeared. As a result of this and other work, it now appears that the giant pyramidal cells are not a unique population, providing the sole origin of the pyramidal tract. They are only the largest in a continuous range of cells of varying

size which contribute to the pyramidal tract. However giant pyramidal cells are probably the most important group functionally, especially for initiating fine fast movements. But large numbers of small fibres arise not only from non-giant cells of area 4, but from area 6 in the frontal lobe, from the primary somaesthetic cortex (areas 3, 1 and 2) and from the second somatosensory area in the parietal lobe.

COURSE AND TERMINATION

From these widespread origins, fibres dive deeply into the interior of the cerebral hemisphere and run in the central part of the fan of fibres, the **corona radiata** (fig. 25.55). They then converge on the **internal capsule**, so-

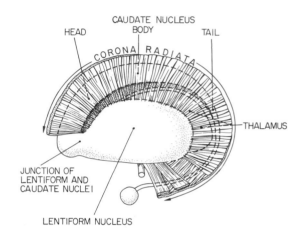

FIG. 25.55. Corona radiata showing its relation to other structures. Left cerebral hemisphere, lateral view.

called because it forms a capsule or investment for the internal surface of the lentiform nucleus. In horizontal sections through the hemisphere the internal capsule appears as a boomerang-shaped collection of fibres (fig. 25.56). Its anterior limb lies between the lentiform nucleus and the head of the caudate nucleus, its posterior limb between the lentiform nucleus and the thalamus, and the two limbs meet at a knee-like angle, the **genu**. The corticonuclear and corticospinal fibres of the pyramidal tract have traditionally been described as lying at the genu and in the anterior part of the posterior limb, but recent work places them in the posterior one-third of the posterior limb. The fibres show an orderly somatotopic arrangement. The corticonuclear fibres lie most anterior and behind them lie the corticospinal fibres; of these the most anterior terminate on upper limb motor neurones, next are those destined for trunk motor neurones, and most posterior are those descending to end on lower limb motor neurones. This part of the internal capsule receives its blood supply from the lenticulostriate arteries (p. 25.83). Bleeding from one of these arteries, or blockage by a small blood clot, is a common cause of severe neurological disturbance, because the internal

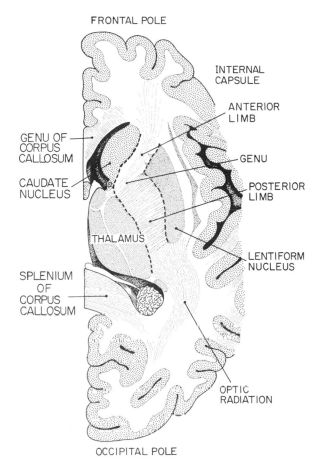

FRONTAL POLE

INTERNAL CAPSULE

ANTERIOR LIMB

GENU OF CORPUS CALLOSUM

GENU

CAUDATE NUCLEUS

POSTERIOR LIMB

THALAMUS

LENTIFORM NUCLEUS

SPLENIUM OF CORPUS CALLOSUM

OPTIC RADIATION

OCCIPITAL POLE

FIG. 25.56. Upper surface of horizontal section of right cerebral hemisphere.

capsule contains, in a very confined space, all the fibres running to and from the cerebral cortex (vol. 3, p. 34.94). It is important to be aware of the pattern of localization of different functional categories of fibres, because small lesions may produce somewhat selective neurological deficits. At the same time it is important to appreciate that the various functional categories of fibres are not sharply segregated, and therefore a lesion which damages pyramidal tract fibres in the internal capsule inevitably damages other fibres as well.

After traversing the internal capsule, the pyramidal tract enters the midbrain, where it forms a compact bundle, occupying the central part of the crus cerebri. The tract lies more deeply in the basilar part of the pons, and is no longer compact, but is broken up into coarse bundles, separated by nuclei pontis and their axons, the transverse fibres of the pons. At the lower border of the pons, the tract once more becomes a compact bundle and runs superficially on the ventral surface of the medulla where it forms the surface prominence called the pyramid. In the lower medulla most fibres (75–95 per cent) cross to the opposite side, forming the decussation of the pyramids (fig. 25.57), and then run dorsally and down-

ward to enter the lateral white column of the cervical spinal cord, where they constitute the **lateral (crossed) corticospinal tract**. This descends throughout the length of the cord, at first superficially, then, over most of the cord, more deeply placed, finally becoming superficial once more in the sacral cord. As they descend, fibres successively leave the tract to enter the grey matter, where they terminate on α or γ motor neurones in the ventral grey column, the minority directly and the majority indirectly, after relaying on intercalated neurones at the base of the dorsal grey column.

The minority of fibres which do not cross at the decussation continue into the ventral white column of the spinal cord, forming the **ventral (uncrossed) corticospinal tract.** This does not descend below midthoracic level. As it descends, it gives off fibres, many of which cross to the other side of the cord before terminating, either directly or via intercalated neurones, on α or γ motor neurones. A small minority of fibres descend from the pyramid into the lateral corticospinal tract of their own side. As most fibres cross in the decussation of the pyramids and the rest at their individual level of termination in the cord, the right hemisphere controls the left side of the trunk and left limbs and the left hemisphere controls the right side of the body. Some of the lower motor neurones which supply muscles of neck and trunk receive some uncrossed corticospinal fibres, and these muscles are therefore less affected by damage to one tract above the decussation.

Not surprisingly, the motor neurones destined for the upper limb, with its greater range and quality of dextrous movement, receive the largest share of corticospinal fibres (about 55 per cent); lower limb motor neurones receive about 25 per cent, and the trunk motor neurones about 20 per cent.

Fibres of the corticonuclear component of the pyramidal tract leave the main bundle at various levels in its course through the brain stem, and most reach the cranial nuclei after crossing, either directly or indirectly, via intercalated neurones. However, the motor nucleus of V and that of IX, X and cranial XI (nucleus ambiguus) receive bilateral pyramidal connections, so damage to the pyramidal tract in the internal capsule produces little disturbance in movements of chewing and swallowing. The upper part of the facial (VII) nucleus also receives bilateral pyramidal connections and a patient who has had a unilateral stroke is still able to raise the eyebrow and close the eye on each side (vol. 3, p. 34.62).

PYRAMIDAL MECHANISMS OF MOTOR CONTROL
Detailed though the preceding account of the pyramidal tract might seem to be, it tells us little or nothing about the part the tract plays in the control of movement. The following paragraphs summarize some general concepts essential for understanding the normal mechanisms

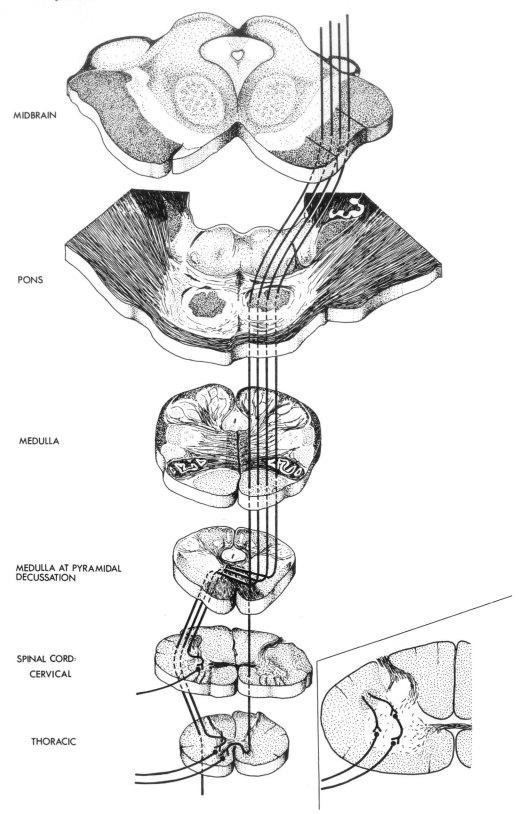

MIDBRAIN

PONS

MEDULLA

MEDULLA AT PYRAMIDAL DECUSSATION

SPINAL CORD:

CERVICAL

THORACIC

FIG. 25.57. A series of transverse sections of the brain stem and spinal cord to show in continuity the course of corticospinal neurones. Inset shows details of the mode of termination of corticospinal neurones, directly on lower motor neurones, or indirectly via intercalated neurones. Cf. Brain stem sections in fig. 25.35.

that control movement and, therefore, the effects of damage by disease.

Control through the motor cortex

Patterns of movement are not initiated in the motor cortex. Hughlings Jackson (1835–1911) long ago argued theoretically for the existence of a 'highest motor centre' in which the concept of a movement was developed and which directed the execution of the movement through the keyboard of the motor cortex. Unfortunately this brilliant insight has been ignored by some, at least, of those who have subsequently investigated the function of the motor cortex by electrical stimulation in conscious men and other animals, and who have concluded that, because movement can be elicited by electrical stimulation, this reproduces the normal activity of the brain in initiating and controlling voluntary movements. Kornhuber has recorded action potentials simultaneously at various sites over the surface of the skull before and during a voluntary movement, and found a slowly increasing negative potential over a wide area, beginning up to 850 msec before the onset of movement. This is called the **readiness potential** and is assumed to be generated by discharges of cortical neurones which excite pyramidal cells in the motor cortex. Larger action potentials were picked up over the area of motor cortex involved in the particular movement less than 100 msec before the onset of movement.

Although traditionally the motor cortex has been described as a laminated structure, from a functional point of view it is more illuminating to think of it as composed of a collection of columns or cylinder of cells, arranged orthogonally to the surface. Each of the columns contains hundreds of pyramidal cells. Fig. 25.58 shows the spread of excitation from a single somatic afferent fibre to pyramidal cells within the column, and inhibition of pyramidal cells in adjacent columns.

It is now established that impulses from muscle spindles pass along fast paths to the motor cortex and may be presumed to provide it with further information about the movement as it progresses.

The cerebellum exercises a major role in regulating the control of movement by the motor cortex. It does this by virtue of (1) the extensive input it receives from the

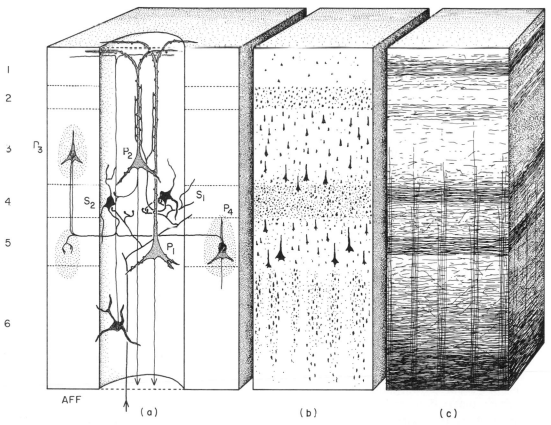

Fig. 25.58. Three complementary views of the structure of the motor cortex. (a) Columnar arrangement of cells. An afferent fibre (from the thalamus) terminates on a stellate intercalated neurone, S_1, whose axonic branches form multiple excitatory synapses on the apical dendrites of two pyamidal cells, P_1 and P_2. Pyramidal cells in adjacent columns are inhibited by afferent impulses relayed through other interneurones, S_2. (b) Laminar arrangement of cell bodies, as seen in a Nissl-stained section. (c) Arrangement of fibres, in horizontal layers and in vertical bundles. (a) After Szentagothai.

musculoskeletal system through spinocerebellar tracts and from the vestibular apparatus, and (2) the numerous reciprocal connections between cerebellum and motor cortex (p. 25.54).

Each of the preceding paragraphs emphasizes the important part played by input to the motor cortex in determining and regulating output. As Jung and Hassler have stated, 'a motor system without sensory control is a fiction, and not even a useful fiction'.

Control at spinal level

Corticospinal fibres terminate on both α and γ motor neurones. It is now clear that activation of the α motor neurone, with contraction of extrafusal fibres, is accompanied by synchronous activation of associated γ motor neurones. This ensures sensitive monitoring of the progress of the movement by the muscle spindles and adjustment to compensate for unexpected interventions (p. 25.43).

While the fibres of the pyramidal tract may terminate at lower motor neurones in the spinal cord, many do not; they end at interneurones nearby. At first sight it seems absurd that any interneurones should be interposed between the signals for action descending from the cerebral cortex to lower motor neurones. Time is lost at the synapses, though only in trifling amounts. What is gained is the better organization of movement. On flexing the elbow, for instance, one contracts brachialis and biceps, but simultaneously relaxes triceps; movements are controlled much better by the regulated slackening of antagonist muscles. This phenomenon, relaxation of antagonists when a muscle contracts to bring about a movement, is **reciprocal innervation** of the opposed muscle groups; as the impulse traffic to one muscle increases, the traffic to its antagonists is reduced. The interneurone systems of the spinal cord organize reciprocal innervation and are interposed in the pathway for voluntary movement.

Other supraspinal descending pathways

RED NUCLEUS AND THE RUBROSPINAL TRACT

The red nucleus is a conspicuous feature in sections of the midbrain (fig. 25.35c), where it appears as a large circular mass, surrounded by a 'capsule' of nerve fibres, which arise from or terminate in the nucleus. In man it consists mainly of small neurones, with a few (150–200) large, multipolar ones at its lower end. From these two groups respectively, axons with small and large diameters arise and immediately cross the midline before descending through the brain stem as the **rubrospinal tract**; this probably extends throughout the length of the spinal cord, lying close to, and intermingled with, the corticospinal tract. It terminates via intercalated neurones on α and γ motor neurones.

The red nucleus receives corticorubral fibres from the precentral gyrus and forms part of a cortico-rubro-spinal circuit through which the motor cortex influences lower motor neurones. Other connections which involve the red nucleus less directly in the control of motor activity are afferent fibres from the cerebellum and the basal nuclei and efferent fibres to the vestibular nuclei.

VESTIBULAR NUCLEI AND THE VESTIBULOSPINAL TRACT

The vestibular nuclei lie laterally beneath the floor of the fourth ventricle at its widest part. They receive central processes of vestibular neurones which convey information from the vestibular apparatus of the internal ear (p. 26.31) about movements of the head and about its position in space. From cells in the lateral vestibular nucleus, axons descend in the uncrossed **lateral vestibulospinal tract** throughout the length of the spinal cord and terminate on α and γ motor neurones. The medial vestibulospinal tract is the continuation downwards into the ventral white column of the spinal cord of the **medial longitudinal fasciculus** (fig. 25.59). This arises from

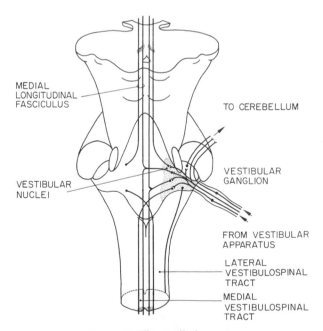

MEDIAL LONGITUDINAL FASCICULUS

TO CEREBELLUM

VESTIBULAR NUCLEI

VESTIBULAR GANGLION

FROM VESTIBULAR APPARATUS

LATERAL VESTIBULOSPINAL TRACT

MEDIAL VESTIBULOSPINAL TRACT

FIG. 25.59. The vestibular nerve.

all the vestibular nuclei and forms a conspicuous bundle of fibres found throughout the brain stem close to the midline, beneath the floor of the neural canal. The fasciculus links the vestibular apparatus with the motor nuclei of the III, IV and VI nerves and of the spinal accessory nerve; it provides for the co-ordination of movements of the head, produced by trapezius and sternomastoid muscles (spinal accessory nerve) and other muscles, and of movements of the eyes. Its downward continuation, the medial vestibulospinal tract, ends bilaterally on α and γ motor neurones of the cervical and upper thoracic spinal cord, providing for responses of muscles of the neck and upper limb to head movements and posture, **tonic neck reflexes.** When the posture of the head is altered, alterations of the whole posture of the body follow. This type of postural change may sometimes be seen in a premature baby, not yet endowed with a full repertoire of behaviour. Its limbs take up different attitudes, depending on the side to which it is induced to turn its head by the offer of a bottle (fig. 25.60). Similarly, when its head is bent back, its arms may extend and its legs flex, and conversely when its head is bent forwards. The body takes up a posture appropriate for the head's

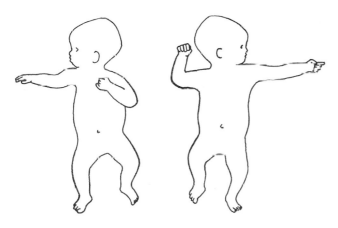

FIG. 25.60. Posture of supine baby when offered a bottle from left or right side. From Gesell A. (1938) *J. Pediat.* **13,** 455.

position on the neck. These effects are not a matter of vestibular responses alone. By suitable experiments in animals, contributions can be distinguished from the vestibule, from receptors in the neck muscles, and also from the skin surface of the body.

The lateral tract excites, and the medial tract inhibits, α motor neurones which innervate extensor musculature. The effects of the lateral tract on extensor muscle tonus contribute to decerebrate rigidity (p. 25.59). This follows transection of the brain stem above the level of the vestibular nuclei, which now act unopposed.

RETICULOSPINAL TRACTS

These arise from the pontine and medullary parts of the reticular formation (p. 25.58) and descend throughout the spinal cord, as crossed and uncrossed pathways, to terminate, probably via intercalated neurones, on α and γ motor neurones. Of the many afferent connections of

the reticular formation, those from the cerebral cortex, the red nucleus and cerebellum are probably involved in the motor functions, particularly the control of muscle tone.

TECTOSPINAL TRACT

This originates in the superior colliculus, part of the tectum of the midbrain and terminates on α motor neurones of the cervical spinal cord and provides for reflex movement of the head (neck musculature) in response to visual information received in the superior colliculus via the optic tract (p. 26.18).

Two other structures, the basal nuclei and the cerebellum, exert important influences on lower motor neurones, but mainly by indirect routes rather than through major supraspinal descending pathways. They are therefore dealt with separately, after the account of the effects of damage to the motor pathways.

Effects of damage to motor pathways

Damage to lower motor neurones involving either their cell bodies within the CNS or their axons in any part of their course to their peripheral termination, produces a characteristic group of effects; the muscles supplied are paralysed, they are flaccid (flabby when felt), they cease to show reflex responses and, after a time, they undergo atrophy or wasting.

Damage limited to the pyramids of the medulla rarely occurs, except deliberately in animal experiments. Damage due to disease or injury to voluntary paths occurs in the cerebral cortex, internal capsule, or spinal cord, where other pathways are interrupted as well as the pyramidal tract. Then, in addition to loss of movements, **spasticity** develops. The normal stretch reflexes are exaggerated; the affected limbs are stiff and resistant to efforts to bend them by external force. The activity of lower motor centres is responsible, no longer restrained by cerebral cortical activity.

When there is spasticity, **clonus** is often present. It is produced by flexing a joint (for instance, dorsiflexing the ankle joint) by external force and keeping up the flexing force. The stretched muscles respond to the tension on their muscle spindles by contracting and do so excessively, so that for a moment they remove altogether the tension upon the spindles. This allows the muscles to relax again, but the examiner's continued pressure stretches the muscle once more, and the cycle restarts. So a maintained rhythm of contraction and relaxation at about 6Hz persists as long as the examiner pushes.

In general, it is possible to distinguish damage to lower motor neurones from damage to motor paths higher up (upper motor neurones). The principal distinctions are shown in table 25.1.

TABLE 25.1. Distinctions between lower and upper motor neurone lesions.

	Lower motor neurone lesion	Upper motor neurone lesion
Voluntary movements	None by affected motor units	Gross movements are possible, especially at limb girdles
Nutrition of the muscles	Wasted and atrophic	Normal
Tone	Limp	Often spastic
Spinal reflexes	None in affected muscles	Reflexes such as tendon jerks may be very brisk; clonus may be present
Plantar response (see p. 25.19)	None, if the relevant muscles are affected	Upgoing

Basal nuclei and the extrapyramidal system

Formerly the view was widely held (and the idea still has currency) that lower motor neurones in the brain stem and spinal cord were controlled directly by two major systems of descending fibres, the pyramidal or cortico-spinal system, already described, and an extrapyramidal system. The latter was thought to arise from cells in the basal nuclei, which lie below the cortex in the cerebral hemispheres, and to descend to the spinal cord in a multi-synaptic pathway and by routes other than the pyramids (hence the name, **extrapyramidal**). This concept was fortified by the view that the extrapyramidal system was the relict of a phylogenetically ancient motor system of subcortical origin and that, in higher animals, it took care of the humbler motor chores, e.g. stereotyped, repetitive, automatic movements such as walking, leaving the more recent pyramidal system to concentrate on more discrete, precise and skilled movements such as writing, typing or playing the piano. Although there are elements of truth in this concept, detailed structural and functional studies make it clear that it represents a crude oversimplification.

BASAL NUCLEI (figs. 25.41 and 61)
The basal nuclei develop from a large mass of grey matter in the floor of the cerebral hemisphere which comes to be divided by the fibres of the internal capsule. They are large nuclei lying deep within the cerebral hemispheres lateral to the thalamus. They are the **putamen** and **globus pallidus** (which together form the **lentiform nucleus**), the **caudate nucleus**, the **amygdaloid body** and the **claustrum**.

Of these the claustrum is a thin sheet of grey matter, which lies beneath the insula (p. 25.71). Little is known about its connections. The amygdaloid body lies at the tip of the tail of the caudate nucleus; it is functionally related to the rhinencephalon.

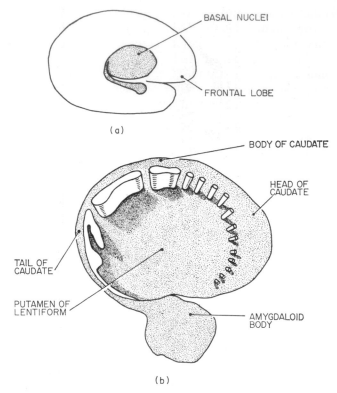

FIG. 25.61. Basal nuclei, showing (a) position and (b) component parts. Lateral view of right hemisphere.

The caudate nucleus is composed of a head, body and tail. It is separated from the thalamus by a narrow groove in the walls of the lateral ventricle. The head lies close to the midline anterior to the thalamus and bulges into the lateral wall of the anterior horn of the lateral ventricle. It is fused with the putamen inferiorly and is then separated by the anterior limb of the internal capsule from the lentiform nucleus. The body of the caudate nucleus arches over the lentiform nucleus, separated from it by the internal capsule which is penetrated at many points by cellular bridges connecting the body of the caudate and putamen. These bridges of grey matter, amongst the white matter of the internal capsule, give a striated appearance and so the caudate and lentiform nuclei are sometimes called the **corpus striatum**. The tail of the caudate curves around the posterior part of the lentiform nucleus and lies first in the lateral wall of the body of the lateral ventricle and then in the roof of its inferior horn. The **stria terminalis,** a white fibre band, accompanies the tail of the caudate to end in the amygdaloid body. This band passes from the amygdaloid region of each side and crosses at the head of the anterior commissure to follow the course of the opposite stria and ends in the opposite amygdaloid region. Some of its fibres end in the anterior hypothalamus.

The lentiform nucleus lies between the insula and internal capsule; a sheet of white matter divides it into a lateral portion, the putamen, and a medial portion of lighter colour, the globus pallidus. The external capsule separates the putamen from the claustrum.

The globus pallidus derives its name from its conspicuous pallor in sections of fresh brain and is often called simply the pallidum; it is represented in the brains of fish and amphibians, in which it forms a primitive motor centre. The caudate and putamen, usually referred to collectively as the striatum, are of more recent evolutionary origin and are best developed in mammals; their structure and connections are essentially similar.

Neuronal connections (fig. 25.62)

Corticostriatal fibres reach the striatum principally from frontal and parietal cortex. Some of the fibres traverse

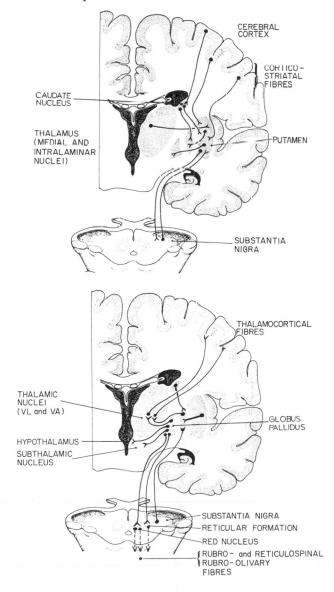

FIG. 25.62. Main connections of (a) striatum (caudate nucleus and putamen) and (b) globus pallidus.

the internal capsule, either independently or as collaterals of corticonuclear and corticospinal fibres, and are inevitably damaged, with the pyramidal fibres, by lesions in the internal capsule. Other corticostriatal fibres enter the lenticular nucleus on its outer side, via the external capsule.

The major output of the striatum is to the pallidum, which therefore retains its primitive position as the motor centre of the basal ganglia. In addition, the striatum has direct, reciprocal links with the substantia nigra, a pigmented nuclear mass in the midbrain (**striatonigral** and **nigrostriatal fibres**).

From the pallidum, fibres travel to several terminations in the diencephalon and in the midbrain.

Pallidothalamic fibres run to the thalamus, principally to the nucleus ventralis anterior, but also to the nucleus ventralis lateralis, which in turn project to the motor cortex. This completes an important **cortico-striato-pallido-thalamo-cortical circuit** which links functionally the basal nuclei and the motor cortex, where the largest fibres of the pyramidal tract originate.

Pallidohypothalamic fibres form a connection which may be of significance in the genesis of autonomic and emotional disturbances seen in some diseases of the basal nuclei.

Pallidosubthalamic fibres run to the subthalamic nucleus, which lies ventral to the thalamus at the junction of diencephalon and midbrain.

Pallidorubral fibres run to the red nucleus and **pallido-reticular** fibres to the reticular formation in the brain stem. These provide routes, via the rubrospinal and the reticulospinal tracts respectively, through which the basal nuclei might directly influence lower motor neurones of brain stem and spinal cord. However neither of these downward projections seems to be numerically important; the midbrain reticular formation contributes little to the reticulospinal tracts, and the pallidorubral fibres are said to end on large cells of the red nucleus, which number about 200 in all. More important numerically, and probably functionally, is a **rubro-olivary tract** (central tegmental bundle). This is part of a **pallido-rubro-olivo-cerebellar circuit** which links the basal nuclei and the cerebellum.

DAMAGE TO THE BASAL NUCLEI IN MAN

Parkinsonism or the shaking palsy is a common degenerative disease in old people and may arise earlier in life as a result of virus infections. The main features are involuntary movements or tremor, delay in the initiation of movements (hypokinesia) and disturbances of tone with rigidity. Lesions are often found in the basal nuclei and their connections, especially substantia nigra. However there is no close association between specific motor disabilities and the sites of the lesions either in the human disease or in monkeys with experimental lesions (vol. 3, p. 34.148). The pyramidal tract and other descending motor pathways seem unable to control skeletal muscle activity adequately when their connections with the basal nuclei are damaged.

Cerebellum

The cerebellum develops from the alar laminae of the cephalic end of the hindbrain, as described on p. 25.7, and it receives afferent fibres from several sources, including skin, muscles, tendons, joints and the vestibular apparatus. Despite this extensive input of information, the cerebellum has no role in the appreciation of conscious sensation, but provides rather for moment-to-moment regulation of the mechanisms which control movement.

In the evolution of the cerebellum there have been three major developments. In fish, it is mainly a nucleus where input from the vestibular apparatus ends, and is concerned with the maintenance of balance. This, the most ancient part of the cerebellum, is represented in man and known as the **archicerebellum**. In amphibia, reptiles and birds, the limbs send neuronal input, via spinocerebellar pathways, into a new addition, represented in man, and known as the **palaeocerebellum**. In mammals, and particularly in man, progressive development of the control of movement by the cerebral cortex is associated with the emergence of the corticopontocerebellar pathway which ends in the **neocerebellum**; this is characterized by its large size and extensive reciprocal connections with the cerebral cortex.

RELATIONS TO OTHER STRUCTURES
The cerebellum lies behind and partly above the brain stem connected to it by the **inferior, middle** and **superior cerebellar peduncles**. It forms most of the roof of the fourth ventricle and partly surrounds the lateral aspect of the pons and medulla. It is separated from the occipital lobes by the tentorium cerebelli and thus lies entirely in the posterior cranial fossa.

STRUCTURAL ORGANIZATION
The gross topography is shown in fig. 25.63. The cerebellum may be imagined as rolled up nose to tail, like a startled hedgehog. In fig. 25.64 it has been unrolled and represented schematically in a flat plane, showing only those landmarks which are essential to the appreciation of its main morphological subdivisions.

The cerebellum has a covering of grey matter, the **cortex**, which is structurally uniform and has a large number of narrow folds, the **folia**. In the midline is the **vermis**, so named from its fancied resemblance to a worm, and it is flanked by the **cerebellar hemispheres**. The **posterolateral fissure** separates the **flocculonodular lobe**

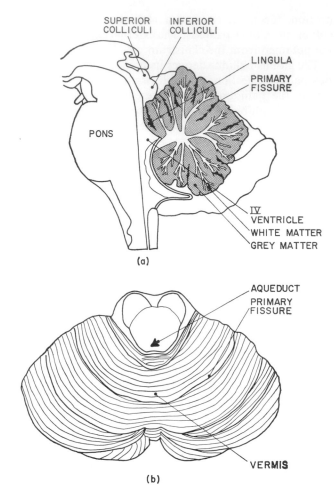

FIG. 25.63. External appearance of cerebellum; (a) sagittal section to show lobules and fissures, (b) as seen from above. Modified from *Cunningham's Textbook of Anatomy*, 10th Edition (1964). London: Oxford University Press.

(archicerebellum) from the remainder, the **corpus cerebelli**, which itself is subdivided by the badly named **primary fissure**, into **anterior** and **posterior lobes**. Most of the vermis, and of the immediately adjacent hemispheres, belongs to palaeocerebellum, and the great bulk of the hemispheres is neocerebellum. The ventral part of each cerebellar hemisphere, which may be forced through the foramen magnum by increased intracranial pressure, is known as the **tonsil** (vol. 3, p. 11.3).

Sections through the cerebellum show a central core of white matter, composed mostly of fibres running to and from the cortex, and buried masses of grey matter, the four pairs of cerebellar nuclei, **fastigial, globose, emboliform** and **dentate**.

The neuronal organization of the cerebellum is briefly as follows. Afferent fibres enter in one or other of the three pairs of stalks or peduncles which connect the cerebellum to the brain stem, and terminate mainly in the cerebellar cortex. Information leaves the cortex through

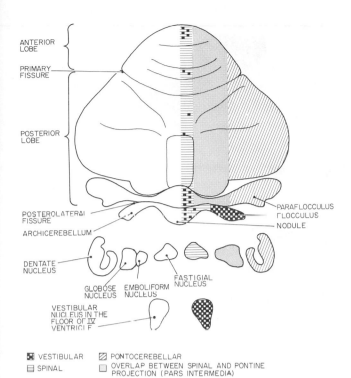

ANTERIOR
LOBE

PRIMARY
FISSURE

POSTERIOR
LOBE

POSTEROLATERAL
FISSURE

ARCHICEREBELLUM

DENTATE
NUCLEUS

GLOBOSE   EMBOLIFORM
NUCLEUS   NUCLEUS

FASTIGIAL
NUCLEUS

VESTIBULAR
NUCLEUS IN THE
FLOOR OF IV
VENTRICLE

PARAFLOCCULUS
FLOCCULUS
NODULE

◼ VESTIBULAR   ▨ PONTOCEREBELLAR
▤ SPINAL   ▢ OVERLAP BETWEEN SPINAL AND PONTINE
                    PROJECTION (PARS INTERMEDIA)

FIG. 25.64. Connections of cerebellar cortex with deep cerebellar and vestibular nuclei shown in corresponding tints. Modified from Krieg W.J.S. (1966) *Functional Anatomy*, 3rd Edition. New York: Blakiston-McGraw.

fibres which are exlusively the axons of a single cell type, the **Purkinje cells**. Their axons terminate on cells in one or other of the deep cerebellar nuclei, and from these efferent fibres leave through either the superior or the inferior peduncle and go to widespread destinations in the central nervous system.

INPUTS OF INFORMATION

Input from the vestibular apparatus

The vestibular apparatus provides information about angular acceleration of the head in the three planes and the orientation of the head in space. This information is carried to the brain stem by first order vestibular neurones, some of which enter the cerebellum either as **direct vestibulocerebellar fibres** or, after relay in the vestibular nuclei, as **indirect vestibulocerebellar fibres**. Both direct and indirect fibres enter through the inferior peduncle on their own side and terminate principally in the **flocculonodular lobe.** This is the archicerebellum which is also known as the vestibular cerebellum.

Input from the spinal cord

There are two **spinocerebellar pathways,** each with a **two-neuronal link** with the periphery. The cell bodies of the first order afferent neurones are in dorsal root ganglia and their peripheral processes terminate in many end organs; their central processes synapse on second order neurones, the axons of which enter the cerebellum principally on their own side, and terminate in the palaeocerebellar cortex.

Dorsal spinocerebellar pathway. The first order neurones end peripherally in muscle spindles, tendon organs and receptors associated with touch and pressure sensibility. Their thick, myelinated central processes enter the spinal cord through dorsal roots and ascend in the ipsilateral dorsal white column for many segments before ending in the nucleus dorsalis, an elongated afferent nucleus situated at the base of the dorsal grey horn at levels between T1 and L2. From the nucleus dorsalis, thick, myelinated fibres ascend in an uncrossed tract situated at the periphery of the lateral white column, immediately ventral to the posterolateral fasciculus (fig. 25.65). This enters the inferior cerebellar peduncle, which inclines dorsally and underlies the floor of the lateral angle of the fourth ventricle, before turning backwards at right angles to enter the cerebellum on the medial side of the middle cerebellar peduncle. Fig. 25.65 shows that the dorsal spinocerebellar tract carries impulses only from the lower trunk and the lower limb. First order neurones from equivalent endings in the upper trunk and upper limb (spinal nerves C1–T4 or 5) ascend in the ipsilateral dorsal white column for many segments and terminate on the **lateral cuneate nucleus** in the medulla, from which **cuneocerebellar fibres** enter the cerebellum through the inferior peduncle. Fibres of both tracts end in the anterior lobe and in the posterior vermis, which belong to the palaeocerebellum.

Ventral spinocerebellar pathway. Like the dorsal pathway, this is two-neuronal. Its first order neurones transmit information from the lower limb arising in Golgi tendon organs and receptors in skin and joints which are concerned in flexor reflex responses. Fibres of the second order neurones mostly cross and ascend in the contralateral white column as the ventral spinocerebellar tract, which is less heavily myelinated than the dorsal tract. On reaching the upper pons it turns dorsally and downwards to enter the cerebellum through the superior cerebellar peduncle. Many of its fibres cross (for a second time) before terminating in the cerebellar cortex. This means that information from muscles, tendons, joints and skin of one side of the body is conveyed by both dorsal and ventral spinal tracts to the cerebellum on the same side. This is in striking contrast to the somatic sensory pathways and the corticospinal motor pathways which are both predominantly crossed. The significance of this difference emerges later.

Trigeminocerebellar pathway. This enters through the inferior peduncle and serves the trigeminal territory in the same way as the spinocerebellar tracts serve trunk and limbs; it terminates in the palaeocerebellar cortex.

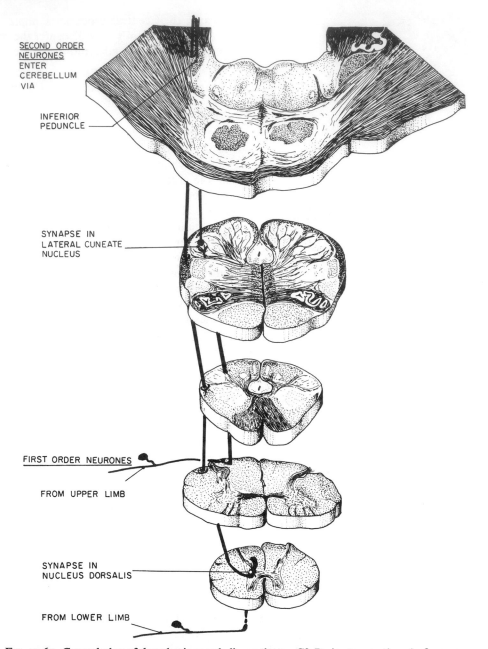

SECOND ORDER
NEURONES
ENTER
CEREBELLUM
VIA

INFERIOR
PEDUNCLE

SYNAPSE IN
LATERAL CUNEATE
NUCLEUS

FIRST ORDER NEURONES

FROM UPPER LIMB

SYNAPSE IN
NUCLEUS DORSALIS

FROM LOWER LIMB

FIG. 25.65. General plan of dorsal spinocerebellar pathway. Cf. Brain stem sections in fig. 25.35.

Input from the cerebral cortex

From extensive areas of the cerebral cortex, principally the sensorimotor areas of the frontal and parietal lobes, **corticopontine fibres** descend through corona radiata and internal capsule to enter the crus cerebri of the mid-brain, where they flank the corticospinal fibres. They terminate on cells of the pontine nuclei, from which fibres cross the midline as **transverse pontine fibres** to form the entire **middle cerebellar peduncle** of the opposite side. The prominence, in man, of all components of this **corticopontocerebellar pathway**, which terminates in the cortex of the contralateral cerebellar hemisphere (fig.

25.66), reflects the importance of the neocerebellum in the regulation of the control of voluntary movement by the cerebral cortex.

Other cerebellar inputs

Olivocerebellar fibres. The inferior olivary nucleus lies in the medulla, appearing in sections like a crumpled bag of grey matter (fig. 25.35a). It is a recent evolutionary development whose connections indicate its indirect involvement in the motor system. It receives projections from (1) the globus pallidus and red nucleus through the central tegmental tract (fig. 25.36), (2) the pre- and

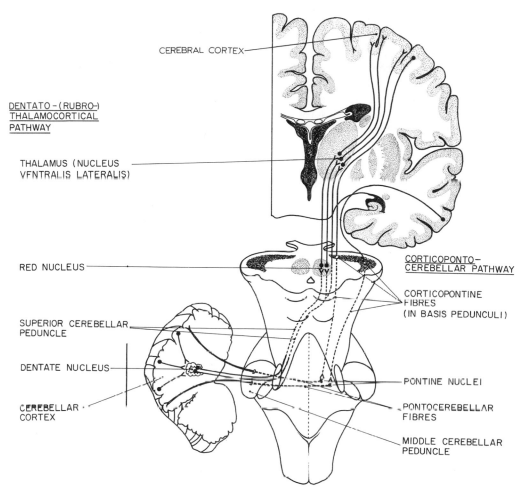

CEREBRAL CORTEX

DENTATO-(RUBRO-)
THALAMOCORTICAL
PATHWAY

THALAMUS (NUCLEUS
VENTRALIS LATERALIS)

RED NUCLEUS

SUPERIOR CEREBELLAR
PEDUNCLE

DENTATE NUCLEUS

CEREBELLAR
CORTEX

CORTICOPONTO-
CEREBELLAR PATHWAY

CORTICOPONTINE
FIBRES
(IN BASIS PEDUNCULI)

PONTINE NUCLEI

PONTOCEREBELLAR
FIBRES

MIDDLE CEREBELLAR
PEDUNCLE

FIG. 25.66. Interconnections between the cerebral cortex and the cerebellum. Brain stem, dorsal view; cerebellum, medial surface of left half; cerebral hemisphere, coronal section.

postcentral gyri through a corticoreticulo-olivary pathway and (3) the spinal cord through a spino-olivary tract, which carries information from cutaneous, muscle and tendon receptors. These tracts enter the outer surface of the inferior olivary nucleus. Olivocerebellar fibres leave the olive, cross the midline, sweep laterally and dorsally and enter the cerebellum through the inferior peduncle. Most terminate in neocerebellar cortex, but all other parts of the cortex receive some fibres.

Optic and acoustic input. This arrives through pathways from the tectum of the midbrain.

Although the evolutionary concept of archi-, palaeo- and neocerebellum as separate parts of the organ is a useful simplification, only the archicerebellum approaches autonomy with its almost exclusive vestibular connections. Fig. 25.64 shows an overlap of spinocerebellar and corticopontocerebellar terminations in the cerebellar cortex, in a band called **pars intermedia** on either side of the vermis. The lateral part of each hemisphere receives principally corticopontocerebellar connections, but, even

here, olivocerebellar projections link it with the spinal cord.

OUTPUT FROM THE CEREBELLUM

Output from archicerebellum
This is linked, through the inferior cerebellar peduncle, with the vestibular nuclei and with the reticular formation. It influences the activity of lower motor neurones through vestibulospinal and reticulospinal pathways.

Output from palaeocerebellum
Like the archicerebellum, this is linked with vestibular and reticular nuclei. In addition, it is connected, through the superior peduncle, with the red nucleus and thus can influence spinal motor neurones through the rubrospinal tract.

Output from neocerebellum
The neocerebellar cortex projects principally on to the dentate nucleus, the most recently evolved of the deep

cerebellar nuclei. This sends fibres upwards through the superior cerebellar peduncle into the midbrain, where they cross the midline (**decussation of brachium conjunctivum**, fig. 25.35b) and run upwards, round or through the red nucleus, to terminate in the thalamus (nucleus ventralis lateralis). This in turn projects to areas 4 and 6 of the cerebral cortex, i.e. to those areas principally concerned in the cortical control of voluntary movement. This crossed **dentatothalamocortical pathway** is the reciprocal of the crossed corticopontocerebellar pathway; the two pathways provide for the interaction of the cerebral cortex of one side and the cerebellar cortex of the other.

Laterality of cerebellar connections

It is a useful clinical generalization that each half of the cerebellum is concerned in the regulation of motor control of its own side of the body.

HISTOLOGICAL STRUCTURE AND NEURONAL MECHANISMS

Ramón y Cajal, a Spanish neuroanatomist of genius, at the end of the nineteenth century described in detail the neurones of the cerebellar cortex. Since 1960 their connections and functional activity have been brilliantly elucidated by Szentagothai and Eccles, among others.

The cerebellar cortex has a uniform and regular neuronal pattern (fig. 25.67a). Fig. 25.67b–g shows the principal features of the cells.

Purkinje cells are large neurones with flask-shaped bodies of diameter about 50 μm. They have a dendritic tree, elaborately branched in a plane at right angles to the long axis of the folium, and axons which run centrally to terminate in one of the deep cerebellar nuclei. Recurrent collaterals terminate in Golgi cells. There are some 30 million Purkinje cells in the cortex.

Granule cells have several short dendrites; their axons divide T-wise, and each branch (parallel fibre) runs for a distance of 2 mm or so along the long axis of the folium, making synaptic contact with the dendritic trees of some 450 Purkinje cells. There are some 30 000 million granule cells, and each Purkinje cell receives synaptic terminals from some 80 000 granule cells.

Basket cells have axons which terminate synaptically on a cluster of Purkinje cells arranged in a line at right angles to the folium. Their dendritic trees lie in the same plane as that of Purkinje cells and also form synapses with parallel fibres.

Stellate and Golgi cells are intercalated neurones which link parallel fibres respectively with Purkinje dendrites, and with granule cell dendrites.

Studies of the cerebellar cortex, by electron microscopy and by recordings from microelectrodes, have established some of the major functional neuronal circuits. Input to the cortex is through **climbing** and **mossy fibres.** Climbing fibres are thin axons, probably mainly of cells in the inferior olive. Branches of a single climbing fibre wind through, and make many synaptic contacts with, the dendritic tree of a single Purkinje cell. Most of the other afferent fibres to the cortex are mossy fibres from the spinocerebellar tract, whose branches end in globular swellings or **rosettes**. Each rosette receives synaptic terminals from several granule cells. The intracortical connections of the two types of afferent fibre are strikingly different. A climbing fibre makes synaptic contact with a single Purkinje cell, which it excites. A mossy fibre has a widely dispersed input and excites a cluster of several hundred granule cells, each of which excites a column of several hundred Purkinje cells, arranged along the long axis of a folium. At the same time columns of Purkinje cells on either side of the excited column are inhibited through the action of basket cells. During normal activity, sequential input from hundreds or thousands of mossy fibres produces in the cortex a constantly changing, overlapping pattern of areas of excitation, surrounded by areas of inhibition, of Purkinje cells. Superimposed on this pattern is the powerful focussed excitatory effect of the input from climbing fibres. The output from the cortex is through Purkinje cell axons, which form inhibitory synapses on deep cerebellar nuclei. Indeed, all cerebellar cortical neurones are inhibitory, apart from the granule cells. The final output from the cerebellum is excitatory; the cells of the deep nuclei generate spontaneous action potentials and are also excited by collaterals of both mossy and climbing fibres.

Although knowledge of these neuronal patterns is now well established, the way in which they contribute to regulation of motor control is still speculative. Szentagothai has developed the concept of **continuous dynamic loop control** (fig. 25.67a, b and c). Throughout the performance of a movement the palaeocerebellum receives input from proprioceptors in the limbs, through spinocerebellar tracts, ending as mossy fibres, and olivocerebellar fibres, ending as climbing fibres. Purkinje cell output then exerts an influence on spinal motor neurones through the deep cerebellar nuclei and vestibulospinal and reticulospinal pathways.

In the neocerebellum, there is a more complex dynamic loop. Collaterals from corticospinal neurones terminate in the pontine nuclei, whose axons end in the opposite cerebellar cortex as mossy fibres, and on inferior olivary cells, whose axons end as climbing fibres, also on the opposite side. This input is computed by the cerebellar cortex, using its store of learned motor skills, and the output of Purkinje cells is made available to the motor cortex through the dentatothalamocortical pathway. Activity of this cerebrocerebello-cerebral circuit, a round trip thought to take about 20 msec in man, continually modifies the activity of the corticospinal mechanism,

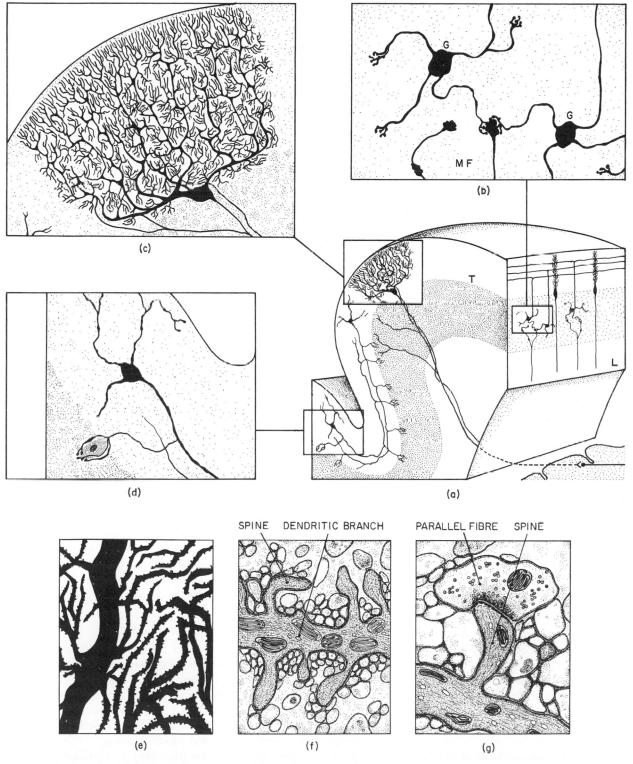

FIG. 25.67. Structure of the cerebellar cortex. (a) Three-dimensional view of part of a cerebellar folium; T, transversely cut face, L, longitudinally cut face; (b) two granule cells (G) and their synaptic connection with a terminal branch of a mossy fibre (MF); (c) a Purkinje cell, showing its dendritic tree *en face*, and climbing fibre; (d) a basket cell, with an axonal branch ending on a Purkinje cell body; (e) high power optical microscope appearance of dendritic tree of Purkinje cell, showing the spines on the surface of dendritic branches; these are synaptic organs; (f) drawing of EM showing the spines as cytoplasmic protrusions from a dendritic branch; (g) drawing of high power EM showing synapse between a spine and a parallel fibre; (e), (f) and (g) modified from Fox C.A. *et al.* (1967) *Progr. Brain Res.* **25**, 174.

which has executive control of movement, in the light of moment-to-moment input of proprioceptive information.

HUMAN CEREBELLAR DAMAGE

Firstly, conscious sensation remains unchanged. Although the cerebellum is liberally supplied with information from the sensory systems, it is not part of the arrangement for conscious sensation. So after cerebellar damage the patient sees, hears and feels, just as before. So far as can be judged, he is as intelligent as before. A rat after cerebellar damage can still get through a familiar maze; if it is too unsteady to run, it rolls through the maze.

Secondly, a man walks clumsily, with a reeling drunken gait and feet wide apart. On reaching out to grasp anything, his arm trembles, and the nearer he gets to his target, the more his arm jerks and oscillates. He is not paralysed; all his joints can be moved at will, though not as strongly as before. The movements are **ataxic**, and are also slow to start and finish. When asked to make a movement, he starts later than normal by perhaps 200 msec and is similarly slow to stop. If the damage is one-sided, the effects are much more prominent on the same side of the body. However, in the majority of our movements both sides of the body must cooperate, and so movement of the other side may suffer from lack of properly timed cooperation. Affected movements are poorly balanced, tremulous and ill organized; they seem guided on inadequate and behind time information, their progress is not smoothly controlled, and their endpoint uncertain.

Speech may be similarly affected and be slow and deliberate. Of all voluntary movements, those of the eyes are the most delicately controlled. The eyes are affected very much like the limbs. The limbs, at rest and supported, do not tremble; neither do the eyes, while gazing straight ahead. But when turned to either side on request, they move too fast and too far and are corrected by a slower reverse movement; a rhythmic to-and-fro sequence is set up. This is cerebellar **nystagmus**. The eyes move together and one is not more affected than the other, even if the limbs are more affected on one side.

The limbs are more flaccid than normal when the examiner moves them. This is **hypotonia,** since passive bending of joints is a method of assessing how much the normal 'tone' of muscles resists displacement of joints. The knee jerks (fig. 25.68) become pendular, and the legs swing to and fro after the initial jerk more than normal. A knee jerk cannot be termed voluntary; here an involuntary reflex response becomes abnormal in cerebellar disease, and the active quadriceps and its antagonist hamstrings are not properly co-ordinated to damp the swing as effectively as usual. Suppression of swinging and oscillation of this kind is evidently much more necessary for movements in air than for movements in water, which are

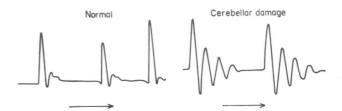

FIG. 25.68. Movement of the leg during knee jerks produced thrice in a normal person and twice in a patient with cerebellar damage. From Holmes G. (1922) *Lancet* i, 1177.

in more than one sense 'damped' by the surrounding water which prevents them from overshooting. In fact, animals with cerebellar damage swim remarkably well; a primitive fish like the lamprey possesses little in the way of a cerebellum. The effects of damage to localized areas of the cerebellum are described in vol. 3, p. 34.73.

RETICULAR FORMATION

The brain stem contains a diffuse network of nerve cells and fibres which fills the spaces between the ascending and descending pathways and is known as the reticular formation (fig. 25.69). These neurones receive connections from the main sensory pathways and can be excited by stimuli from skin, deep tissue and viscera, as well as by sound and light. It may also receive information from the cortex by connections with the corticonuclear and corticospinal tracts. Efferent fibres go to the thalamus and cerebral hemispheres and also to α and γ motor neurones in the spinal cord via the reticulospinal tract.

On first consideration the numerous connections and the diffuse arrangement of the neurones, which are not collected into definable nuclei of grey matter, might suggest only a means of jumbling information. In fact, control of four important mechanisms of the body is dependent on at least a large area of the reticular formation being intact and functional.

AROUSAL AND CONSCIOUSNESS

Severing connections of the reticular formation with the cerebral cortex in cats and monkeys can lead to a comatose condition. Conversely in a sleeping animal, stimulation of the reticular formation via implanted electrodes can change the pattern of the electroencephalogram from that characteristic of sleep and awaken it. Stimulation also alerts an animal which is awake.

The reticular formation may be considered as responsible for the unity of consciousness by providing a sieve or gate for the sensory inflow. This controls the amount of information that reaches the higher centres. Clearly at any one time it is possible to attend to only a part of the sensory information entering the brain (p. 40.13).

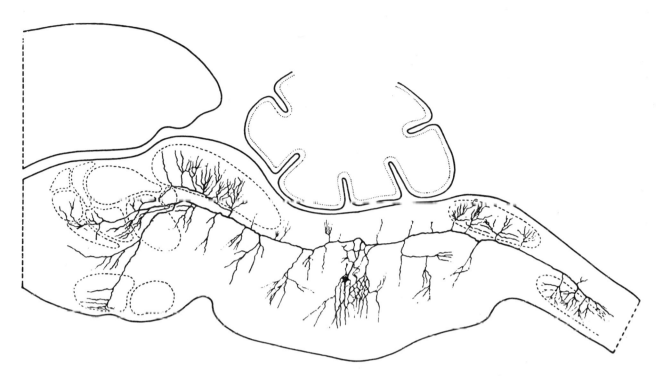

FIG. 25.69. Drawing of a Golgi-stained section of brain stem of a two-day-old rat. A single large cell in the reticular formation is shown. Its axon divides into ascending branches which give collaterals to nuclei in the brain stem and diencephalon. From Scheibel M.E. & Scheibel A.B. (1958). In *Reticular Formation of the Brain*, ed. Jasper H.H. *et al.* Boston: Little, Brown.

Partially opening or closing the gate may alter the flow and so determine the state of awareness.

CONTROL OF MUSCLE TONE

The connections of the reticular formation with motor neurones in the spinal cord lead to complex effects on spinal reflexes. Stimulation of its lateral part facilitates extensor muscle stretch reflexes, e.g. the knee and ankle jerks become more brisk. Stimulation of the more medial parts facilitates flexor reflexes. If the brain stem of a cat is transected immediately above the pons, more of the lateral nuclei than of the medial nuclei remain connected with the spinal cord. As a result there is marked increase in tone in the antigravity extensor muscles; the legs are stiff and extended and resist passive stretch. The increased activity is chiefly due to increased firing of γ motor neurones. This condition is known as **decerebrate rigidity**. In man a condition in some ways analogous to the decerebrate state in the cat may follow an acute head injury (vol. 3, p. 11.6).

CARDIOVASCULAR CONTROL

Most of the integrated responses of the cardiovascular system discussed on pp. 30.49–52 depend on an area of the reticular formation known as the **vasomotor centre**. The isolated spinal cord can maintain some tone in the

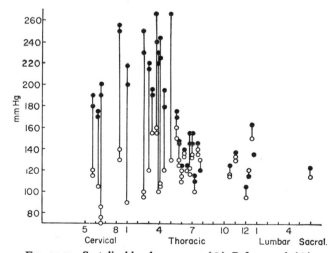

FIG. 25.70. Systolic blood pressure. (○) Before and (●) after distension of the bladder in patients with traumatic section of the spinal cord at the levels shown. When the transection is low in the cord, most or even all of the sympathetic outflow to the blood vessels is still linked to the medulla and therefore to the baroceptor system; hence when bladder distension evokes vasoconstriction in the body below the transection, there is compensatory vasodilation above the transection and little or no rise in systemic blood pressure occurs. However, when the transection is high, the path for compensatory vasodilation is blocked and a gross rise in blood pressure is seen. From Guttmann L. & Whitteridge D. (1947) *Brain* **70**, 387.

arterioles of the body and from the spinal cord at levels T1–L2 the sympathetic preganglionic fibres emerge to form the first link in the efferent path to the arterioles. Indeed, painful stimulation of the skin, or distension of a hollow viscus such as the bladder, can lead to vaso-constriction and often a reflex rise in blood pressure which can be mediated by the cord in isolation (fig. 25.70). Normally, however, an over-riding control is exerted by the medullary system, which receives information from the baro- and chemoreceptors of the carotid region (p. 30.39) and commands as efferent paths not only the the sympathetic outflow already mentioned, but also the vagus nerve which includes fibres supplying the atria. Fig. 25.71 shows that cardiovascular control is conducted

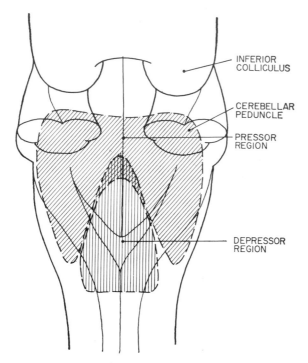

FIG. 25.71. Dorsal view of medulla and pons of the cat, after removal of cerebellum, to show the location of the cardiovascular control system. After Alexander (1946) *J. Neurophysiol.* **9**, 205.

by two regions with opposing effects, an upper and more lateral pressor region, where stimulation increases vascular tone, and a lower, more medial part, from which reverse effects arise.

RESPIRATORY CONTROL

The neural control of respiration (pp. 31.25–31) is effected by neurones in the **respiratory control area** in the reticular formation (fig. 25.72). Neurones responsible for expiration are on the whole more posterior, but are not so clearly segregated as in the cardiovascular control system, since they overlap those responsible for inspiration. The respiratory rhythm is the product of their

interaction. Sneezing and swallowing interrupt the normal respiratory rhythm, as does speech. This link clearly involves traffic from higher up in the nervous system. When the medulla is cut off from the pons and the higher parts of the CNS, it generates a jerky gasping type of rhythm, lacking the smoothness of normal breathing.

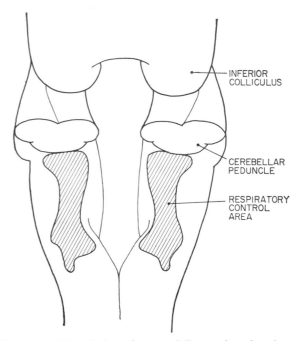

FIG. 25.72. Dorsal view of cat medulla, to show location of respiratory neurones. After Salmoiraghi G.C. & Burns B.D. (1960) *J. Neurophysiol.* **23**, 2.

DIENCEPHALON

The development and general anatomy of the diencephalon, which includes the thalamus, hypothalamus, subthalamus and epithalamus, is described on p. 25.29.

Thalamus

The thalamus lies immediately lateral to the third ventricle, separated from the posterior part of the internal capsule by the thalamic reticular nucleus and the external medullary lamina. Its relation to the surface of the brain is shown in fig. 25.73.

With the sole exception of those carrying olfactory information, all sensory pathways relay in the thalamus before terminating in the cerebral cortex.

THALAMIC NUCLEI (fig. 25.74)

The thalamus consists of many clusters of cell bodies, the thalamic nuclei. Precise demarcation of these nuclei was begun over forty years ago by Earl Walker, a Canadian

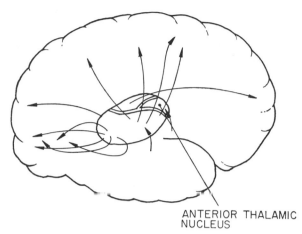

FIG. 25.73. Position and connections of the thalamus.

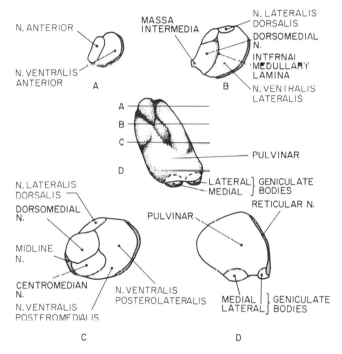

FIG. 25.74. Thalamic nuclei. A, B, C and D are cross sections at the levels shown in the central drawing, which is the right thalamus seen from above. Modified from Krieg W.J.S. (1966) *Functional Neuroanatomy*, 3rd Edition. New York: Blakiston–McGraw.

neurosurgeon, and Le Gros Clark, an English neuroanatomist. It is based on a variety of methods: descriptive study of cellular structure; study of localized areas of retrograde cell degeneration after removal of localized areas of the cerebral cortex; recording electrical responses in the thalamus on stimulation of sensory receptors or ascending sensory pathways; recording electrical responses in the cerebral cortex after localized stimulation of the thalamus, and vice versa. These methods have now shown that the thalamus cannot be subdivided into

discrete, autonomous nuclei. However, certain generalizations can be made.

A sheet of white matter, the **internal medullary lamina** lies roughly in a sagittal plane, and divides the thalamus into **medial** and **lateral nuclear groups**. Anteriorly, the lamina splits into two diverging sheets, which enclose the **anterior nuclear group**.

Functional groupings

Sensory relay nuclei. The three major sensory pathways, medial lemniscal, spinothalamic and trigeminothalamic, terminate close together in nuclei in the lateral group, which lie at the ventral part of the posterior end of the thalamus. The termination of each pathway shows precise somatotopic localization; the trigeminal pathways end medially in the nucleus ventralis posteromedialis (VPM), as does the smaller solitariothalamic pathway carrying taste information; the other two end in the nucleus ventralis posterolateralis (VPL). Moreover, termination is modality specific; stimulation of particular peripheral receptors evokes electrical responses in particular thalamic neurones. This orderly pattern is continued in the thalamocortical projection to the somaesthetic cortex.

The **medial** and **lateral geniculate nuclei** belong to the same topographic group as VPL and VPM, but have been displaced posteriorly and seem to be part of the midbrain rather than of the diencephalon (fig. 25.35). The lateral geniculate nucleus is a thalamic relay nucleus on the visual pathway, which receives fibres of the optic tract of its own side (p. 26.18). Each nucleus consists of six layers of cells; layers 1, 4 and 6 receive fibres which have crossed in the optic chiasma, while layers 2, 3 and 5 receive fibres from the eye of their own side. Corresponding points on adjacent laminae in the lateral geniculate body receive fibres from corresponding points in each retina, which have received stimuli from the same part of the opposite half of the visual field. This orderly somatotopic arrangement is continued in the geniculocalcarine tract, which terminates in the visual cortex around the calcarine fissure.

The medial geniculate nucleus is a thalamic relay nucleus on the auditory pathway (p. 26.30), and probably also receives input from the vestibular apparatus.

It is to be noted that the links between each sensory relay nucleus and a particular area of the cerebral cortex are reciprocal; the corticothalamic projections are thought to be important in enhancing acuity of sensory perception.

Motor relay nuclei. These are not involved directly in motor activity, but form part of pathways which influence the activity of motor areas of the cerebral cortex. They belong to the same lateral group as the sensory relay nuclei, but lie more anterior. The **nucleus ventralis anterior** (VA) relays impulses from the globus pallidus to motor and premotor areas (4 and 6), and forms part of the important cortico-striato-pallido-thalamo-cortical circuit. The **nucleus ventralis lateralis** (VL) relays impulses from the dentate nucleus of the cerebellum to the same areas of the cortex.

Limbic relay nuclei. These are the **anterior nuclear group** and the lateral dorsal nucleus, which belongs with them functionally but has been displaced into the lateral nuclear group. The anterior group receives a large and easily dissectable projection from the mamillary body (mamillothalamic tract) and, in turn, projects to the cingulate gyrus. It therefore forms part of the circuit which includes the hippocampus, fornix, mamillary body, thalamus and cingulate cortex, known as the limbic system (p. 25.70).

Association thalamic nuclei. These are reciprocally linked with association areas of the cerebral cortex. Two are described to illustrate some general principles.

The **pulvinar** is a large nucleus at the posterior end of the thalamus, overhanging the geniculate bodies. It belongs to the dorsal part of the lateral nuclear group, the so-called dorsal tier nuclei. It receives indirect sensory projections from the sensory relay nuclei (VLP and VPM), from the intralaminar nuclei (see below) and probably from the medial and lateral geniculate nuclei. It also receives reciprocal connections with posterior parietal, posterior temporal and occipital cortical areas, and appears to provide the anatomical substrate for integration and analysis of sensory information from a variety of sources. It is probably of importance, therefore, in the intellectual functions of the brain, and is best developed in higher primates.

The **medial nucleus** is also well developed in man and, like the pulvinar, receives fibres from other thalamic nuclei. These include the lateral nuclear group, providing somatic sensory information; the intralaminar nuclei, whose input derives from ascending sensory systems, via the reticular formation; and the midline nuclei, which receive visceral sensory input (including taste), also via the reticular formation. The medial nucleus exchanges fibres with prefrontal and orbital cortical association areas, contributing to a neuronal system thought to be involved in emotional affect or moods.

Nuclei without direct cortical connections. The **intralaminar nuclei** are so named because they lie within the internal medullary lamina. They include the centromedian nucleus, which is best developed in higher primates, including man. Their input comes principally from the reticular formation, which relays impulses from ascending sensory systems. Through other thalamic nuclei, they project to extensive cortical areas and, with them, contribute to the level of alertness and the state of awareness or consciousness.

The **midline nuclei** are a primitive group, just beneath the ependyma of the third ventricle. They receive visceral sensory input, including taste, via the reticular formation. Projections to the hypothalamus provide for autonomic responses to this input. The significance of other projections, to the medial and intralaminar nuclei, has already been indicated.

LESIONS OF THE THALAMUS

When the thalamus is damaged by disease, gross disorders of sensation or movement may follow, and also disturbances of the emotions and of personality.

Using stereotactic methods neurosurgeons can make small lesions in discrete areas of the thalamus in man. Such lesions may be of great benefit to patients. Thus lesions in the anterior nuclear group and in the anterior radiations from it are made for various mental disorders and may have profound effects on personality. Lesions in the central median nuclei of medial nuclear group influence both pain and movement, and lesions in the dorsomedial nucleus have led to improvement in patients with mental and motor disorders.

Tremor and rigidity due to diseases such as Parkinsonism may be treated by destroying portions of nuclei VA or VL of the thalamus.

Stereotactic methods, used both in patients and in experimental animals, are likely to lead to more accurate knowledge of the connections of the thalamus and their functions, and be of benefit in the treatment of disease.

Hypothalamus

This forms the lower part of the lateral wall of the third ventricle, below the thalamus, from which it is separated by the hypothalamic sulcus (fig. 25.38). Lateral to the hypothalamus is the subthalamus, and the two are continuous, below and behind, with the tegmentum of the midbrain. The hypothalamus is bounded in front by lamina terminalis and the optic chiasma. Below are the structures which form the floor of the third ventricle: the posterior perforated substance; the mamillary bodies and the **tuber cinereum**, a sheet of grey matter lying between the mamillary bodies and the optic chiasma. The **median eminence** is a funnel-shaped downward extension of the tuber cinereum; from it arises the infundibular stem, which is continuous below with the neural lobe of the pituitary gland (fig. 27.8). The median eminence is claimed by both the hypothalamus and the neuropypophysis, an indication of the close links between the two.

The hypothalamus is divisible into medial and lateral regions in the plane of the fornix, which runs through it to the mamillary body. The **medial region** consists mainly of grey matter, divided into several more or less distinct nuclear groups, with a multitude of interconnections. The **lateral region** contains much fewer neurones, which project to the medial region and other parts of the CNS, and receives most of the hypothalamic afferents.

The nuclei of the medial region include:

(1) Supraoptic and paraventricular nuclei, whose cells elaborate neurosecretory material which is carried in their axons, the supraopticohypophysial tract, to the neurohypophysis (p. 27.9).

(2) Preoptic and anterior nuclei which are connected by polysynaptic routes (including the dorsal longitudinal fasciculus and the brain stem reticular formation) with parasympathetic efferents in the brain stem and spinal cord.

(3) Nuclei of the tuberal region.

(4) Nuclei of the mamillary region. The mamillary body receives the fornix, the largest afferent bundle of the hypothalamus, and is linked to the anterior thalamic nucleus, and hence with the cingulate cortex, through the mamillothalamic tract, forming part of the limbic system (p. 25.70).

(5) The posterior nucleus which is linked by polysynaptic pathways (including the mamillotegmental tract) with sympathetic visceral efferents in the spinal cord.

AFFERENT CONNECTIONS

These come from many parts of the nervous system through routes not fully defined: from visual, olfactory, visceral (including taste) and somatic sensory systems; from the hippocampus, globus pallidus and cerebral cortex. Known routes include the fornix, the medial forebrain bundle and the dorsal longitudinal fasciculus.

EFFERENT CONNECTIONS

In addition to those already mentioned, there are links between the hypothalamus and the anterior lobe of the pituitary. The location of the nuclei which produce the various hypothalamic regulatory substances (p. 27.11) is not yet precisely known, but it seems likely that there are separate hypothalamic tracts which carry the various releasing or inhibiting factors from hypothalamic neurosecretory cells to the anterior lobe via the hypophysial portal vessels (p. 27.10).

FUNCTIONS OF THE HYPOTHALAMUS

The hypothalamus has a controlling action on the following functions:

(1) secretory activity of the pituitary gland (p. 27.7),
(2) temperature regulation,
(3) regulation of osmolality of the blood,
(4) feeding behaviour,
(5) cardiovascular regulation, and
(6) expression of emotions (p. 25.75).

Temperature regulation
Body temperature is precisely regulated by alterations in

several physiological functions (chap. 43). When hot, we move into a cooler place if possible and reduce clothing; the blood circulating through the skin increases and sweating starts. The efferent path for these reactions to heat and cold is the sympathetic outflow of the autonomic nervous system which conveys nerve fibres to sweat glands and to the skin's blood vessels. When the outflow to these blood vessels is less active, the vessels dilate. When cold, we find a warmer place and increase clothing, the skin circulation is reduced and shivers may occur. These responses can be produced by electrical stimulation within the hypothalamus. But more important, they can also be produced by local cooling and heating of the hypothalamus. Evidently the hypothalamus contains cells which sense the temperature of the blood perfusing them and bring about appropriate responses. This is not the whole story, because the temperature-regulating mechanism is certainly responsive to chilling of the skin, quite apart from any change in blood temperature. But the hypothalamus plays a cardinal role in controlling body temperature and damage here can put the regulating system out of action.

At first glance, the neuronal network in the hypothalamus ought to be easy to investigate. There might be only two types of input, one from skin, and the other from the neurones in the hypothalamus itself which sense the local temperature there. Similarly, there might be only two types of output, one to increase heat production and conservation in various ways, and the other to increase heat loss. It might be reasonable to have two chemical neurotransmitters linking the neurones on the input side, one transmitting the information from the skin and the other the information from the hypothalamic sensors; similarly there might be only two neurotransmitters on the output side, perhaps the same two.

Such hypotheses can be tested by applying likely neurotransmitters to the hypothalamic neurones. 5–HT and noradrenaline are here strong candidates. They can be applied by adding them to the cerebrospinal fluid in the lateral ventricles of an animal, to travel from there to the third ventricle and diffuse into the hypothalamus, or with more difficulty and greater precision they can be infused directly into the hypothalamus itself. Alternatively, attempts can be made to wash them out of the hypothalamus of an animal responding to heat or cold and to assay them in the necessarily tiny volume of washings. There are extraordinary species differences, but in the monkey it is clear that noradrenaline given in these ways evokes a fall in body temperature and 5–HT a rise. However, the whole neural circuitry involved in temperature regulation cannot yet be disentangled.

In fever, temperature control is set at a higher level as a result of the action on the hypothalamus of circulating pyrogens. These may be exogenous and come from pathogenic micro-organisms invading the tissues, or they may be endogenous and liberated from polymorphs by the action of micro-organisms and various immune reactions (vol. 3, p. 12.2).

Osmolality of the blood

Drinking behaviour in rats is most effectively altered by electrical stimulation of the lateral hypothalamus; this provokes prompt and vigorous drinking which results in marked overhydration if stimulation continues. In goats the hypothalamus has been shown to be sensitive to the osmolality of the blood perfusing it, and when this rises drinking is stimulated. The receptors are also stimulated by circulating angiotensin II.

The thirst following stimulation of these hypothalamic cells differs from that following damage in the nearby supraoptic region. Here cells, also sensitive to the osmolality of the blood, are found lying in immediate relation to the capillaries surrounding them, unlike the usual arrangement in the nervous system where neuroglial cells intervene between capillary and neurone. They generate the hormone ADH and release it into the circulation, either in the hypothalamus or else at the termination of their axons in the posterior part of the pituitary gland, the pars posterior. Damage to these cells results in the polyuria and the dehydration, and hence the thirst of diabetes insipidus (p. 27.17).

Feeding behaviour

For a long time the hypothalamus has been associated with the control of food intake. Localized lesions there change markedly the feeding behaviour of rats and other experimental animals. Immediately after a lesion in the ventromedial region of the hypothalamus, the animal overeats and gains weight until a plateau is reached, when overeating ceases. Less consistently a lesion in the lateral hypothalamus has the reverse effect; the animal refuses to eat and may die of starvation. These observations led to the concept of a medial satiety centre and a lateral feeding centre in the hypothalamus. But experiments on rats have indicated that the effects of damage to neurone bodies in the ventral medial nuclei are slight and that hyperphagia follows if adjacent axons traversing the region are alone damaged. Thus the neurone bodies may not be the site of control.

The nature of the sensory stimuli governing feeding behaviour is not entirely clear. After a period without food a person becomes aware of a sensation of hunger. This may be due to the large rise in plasma free fatty acids or to the small fall in plasma glucose that occur when food is not taken for a few hours. Exposure to cold may initiate feeding behaviour and extreme heat may inhibit it. Such factors may operate to regulate feeding behaviour in wild animals, but may be much less important in prosperous human communities where the incidence of obesity is high. Our feeding behaviour is largely a matter of custom and habit, and depends on appetite rather than hunger; hunger may be regarded as a physical sensation, appetite as an emotive state. Appetite depends on the quality of the food, the way it is cooked and served, and the social and physical environment in which it is eaten. Schachter has shown that in comparison to normal controls obese subjects in New York ate amounts of food that depended little on previous food intake, but more on the taste and appearance of the food and on the environment in which it was presented. The hypothalamus has a role in governing feeding behaviour, but factors involving other areas of the brain appear more important in man.

Cardiovascular regulation

The medullary vasomotor control system is able to maintain a normal arterial blood pressure even when cut off from the upper parts of the CNS. But this is not a sufficient degree of control for everyday life; for instance, during exercise an increased arterial blood pressure is maintained. This higher level is produced even in anticipation of exercise, when the need for it is foreseen. The medulla cannot organize an anticipatory response; it is quite possible that the hypothalamus can. Stimulation at some sites within it produces changes in the cardiovascular system which strongly suggest a function in regulating cardiovascular activity more effectively and flexibly than can be achieved by lower levels of the nervous system acting alone.

FUNCTION OF THE PINEAL GLAND

Rene Descartes (1596–1650), preoccupied with the idea of Animal Spirits and the analogy between them and liquids, surmised that the best place to control fluid flow in the brain would be at the pineal and posted the Rational Soul at this point. But long before, in the second century A.D., Galen thought that this part of the nervous system looked spongy, more like a gland. Experiments on rats led to the discovery that the pineal produces a hormone, melatonin, capable of antagonizing the effects of gonadotrophic hormones slowing the oestrous cycle and reducing the weight of the ovaries. Production of melatonin falls when a rat is in a constantly lit environment and an unexpected feature of the system is that the information about the amount of light seems to reach the pineal from the sympathetic chain in the neck, a strange path when one reflects how close the pineal is to the superior colliculus, itself closely linked to the retina. How far these findings in the rat relate to man is uncertain; but rare secreting tumours of the pineal in children may lead to delayed sexual development, as if too much melatonin were being released, and destructive tumours or nearby damage can give rise to precocious puberty as if melatonin release had been cut off.

CEREBRAL HEMISPHERES

The whole surface of the hemisphere consists of an external layer of grey matter, the **cortex**. This covers a mass of white matter surrounding the basal nuclei and thalamus which form the core of grey matter.

Gross anatomy

The cerebrum is divided into two hemispheres by the longitudinal fissure which is interrupted by the corpus callosum joining the two hemispheres together. Each hemisphere has a lateral, medial and inferior surface. The frontal poles project into the anterior cranial fossa, resting upon the roofs of the orbits. The occipital poles occupy the posterior part of the supratentorial compartment, resting upon the tentorium cerebelli which separates the occipital pole from the cerebellum. The temporal lobes occupy the middle fossa. The cortical area is vastly enlarged by folding, the summit of the fold being termed the **gyrus** and the space between each fold the **sulcus**. Particularly deep sulci are termed **fissures**.

The deepest and most obvious fissure apart from the longitudinal fissure is the posterior limb of the lateral sulcus separating the temporal lobe below from the parietal and frontal lobes above. This sulcus overlies a submerged portion of the cortex which is known as the insula (p. 25.71).

LATERAL ASPECT OF THE HEMISPHERES
(fig. 25.75)

The **central sulcus** separates the frontal and parietal lobes, with the precentral gyrus of the frontal lobe in front and the postcentral gyrus of the parietal lobe lying behind. It is an important landmark since the precentral gyrus forms the motor strip and the postcentral gyrus the

sensory strip. The central sulcus is recognized by its tendency to continue on to the medial side of the hemisphere. No such sulci separate the temporal lobe from the posterior part of the parietal lobe or the occipital lobes.

The **frontal lobe** which comprises nearly 40 per cent of the cerebral hemispheres is roughly divided into three horizontal gyri by two sulci, the superior and the inferior frontal sulci.

The **parietal lobe** amounting to 20 per cent of the hemispheres is divided by a horizontal intraparietal sulcus which demarcates the superior and inferior parietal lobule. The inferior parietal lobule is itself subdivided into a supramarginal gyrus which embraces the extreme end of the lateral sulcus and behind it the angular gyrus.

The **temporal lobe**, also 20 per cent of the hemispheres, is divided by two horizontal sulci, the superior and inferior temporal sulci.

The **occipital lobe** occupying about 20 per cent of the hemisphere has three sulci visible from the lateral aspect; the transverse occipital sulcus runs vertically from the intraparietal sulcus; the lateral occipital sulcus lies horizontally below it and a curved lunate sulcus lies immediately in front of the occipital pole. The calcarine sulcus can often be seen notching the occipital pole.

MEDIAL SURFACE OF THE HEMISPHERES
(fig. 25.76)

The medial surface is flat, the hemispheres being separated by the longitudinal fissure and falx cerebri. The corpus callosum forms a prominent feature and its divisions into the rostrum, genu, body and splenium can be readily recognized. The cingulate gyrus surrounds the corpus callosum separated only by the callosal sulcus. The cingulate sulcus in turn separates the gyrus from the superior frontal gyrus and superior

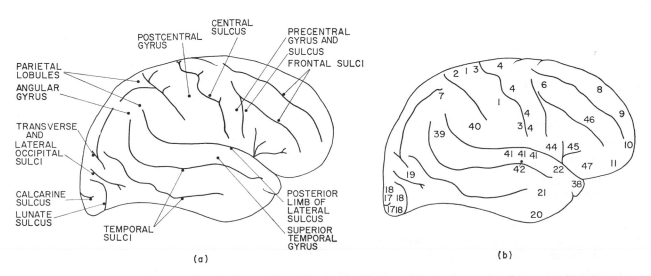

FIG. 25.75. Lateral aspect of cerebral hemisphere. (a) Sulci and gyri; (b) cytoarchitectural map showing some of Brodmann's areas.

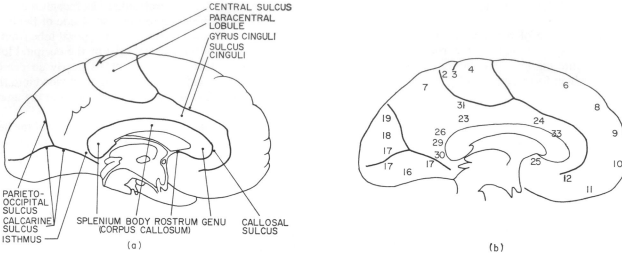

FIG. 25.76. Medial surface of cerebral hemisphere. (a) Sulci and gyri; (b) cytoarchitectural map showing some of Brodmann's areas.

parietal lobule, splitting as it passes posteriorly into the marginal sulcus which runs up, almost vertically, immediately behind the central sulcus. At the splenium the cingulate gyrus narrows and becomes the isthmus, uniting with the parahippocampal gyrus of the temporal lobe. Immediately behind the isthmus, the calcarine sulcus passes posteriorly to notch the occipital pole, the parieto-occipital sulcus branching off it to demarcate the parietal and occipital lobes. The medial surface of the temporal lobe is largely made up of the uncus and parahippocampal gyrus.

INFERIOR ASPECT OF THE HEMISPHERES (fig. 25.77)

The olfactory tract lies in the olfactory sulcus forming the lateral boundary of the gyrus rectus. Lateral to the olfactory tract lies the orbital sulcus in the shape of an H.

The inferior surface of the temporal lobe is angled towards the medial part of the hemisphere. It has a deep collateral sulcus which separates the parahippocampal gyrus medially from the rest of the surface.

Histological structure of the cortex

The neurones and fibres are arranged in parallel layers and five types of cells can be distinguished (fig. 25.78).

(1) **Pyramidal cells** are classed according to their size as giant, large or small. The axon goes to the white matter giving off collaterals which ramify in various layers of cortex whilst the apical dendrite extends towards the surface of the cortex and ramifies there. Smaller dendrites arise from the sides of the pyramidal cells.

(2) **Granule cells** have short repeatedly branching axons which extend only short distances in the cortex.

(3) **Cells of Martinotti** which have axons travelling to the surface and ramifying in the superficial layer.

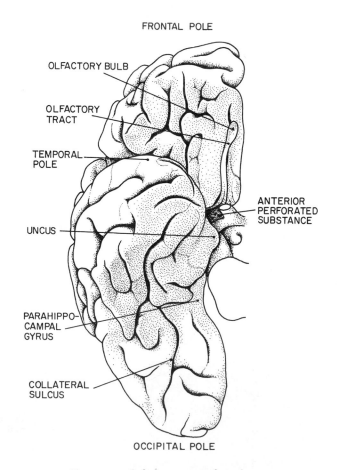

FIG. 25.77. Inferior aspect of cerebrum.

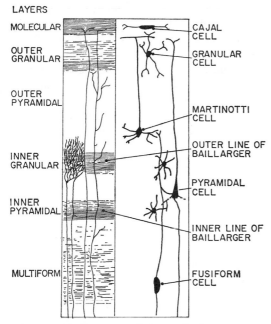

LAYERS

MOLECULAR

OUTER GRANULAR

OUTER PYRAMIDAL

INNER GRANULAR

INNER PYRAMIDAL

MULTIFORM

CAJAL CELL

GRANULAR CELL

MARTINOTTI CELL

OUTER LINE OF BAILLARGER

PYRAMIDAL CELL

INNER LINE OF BAILLARGER

FUSIFORM CELL

FIG. 25.78. Structure of the cerebral cortex.

(4) **Horizontal cells of Cajal** lie in the superficial layer and have axons which remain at the same level as their cell bodies.

(5) **Fusiform cells** lie in the deepest layer of the cortex with their axons entering the white matter.

Below a thin superficial band of white matter, the tangential layer, there are two well defined bands, the inner and outer lines of Baillarger. In the visual cortex (area 17, p. 25.66), the outer line of Baillarger is conspicuous. Apart from these gross appearances various parts of the cortex differ microscopically from one another.

In the older parts of the cortex, such as the rhinencephalon, only three layers of cells may be distinguished: the superficial molecular layer of fibres, the intermediate granular layer and a deep layer of pyramidal cells. In the neocortex six layers may be distinguished from without inwards (fig. 25.78):

(1) the molecular (plexiform) layer containing horizontal cells of Cajal and granule cells within which the terminal branches of the apical dendrites of the pyramidal cells ramify,

(2) the outer granular layer containing short axons, granule cells and small pyramidal cells,

(3) the outer pyramidal layer containing medium-sized pyramidal cells and some granular cells,

(4) the inner granular layer of small granule cells,

(5) the inner pyramidal layer of large pyramidal cells which in the motor area include the giant cells of Betz, and

(6) the multiform (fusiform) layer containing fusiform cells.

Layers 2, 3 and 4 receive most of the afferent fibres to the cortex. Layers 5 and 6 are largely efferent and give rise to the main cortical tracts.

Histological studies have led to a subdivision of the brain into different areas, which have been given numbers or letters. The best known and most generally used map is that of Brodmann (figs. 25.75b and 76b). While these histological distinctions mirror functional differences revealed by experiment or disease, there is much functional overlap in many areas.

White matter

The white matter of the hemisphere consists of three major groups of fibres:

(1) projection fibres running in both directions between the cerebral cortex and subcortical centres such as the internal capsule, the fornix (p. 25.70) and the corticostriatal fibres (p. 25.51), among others,

(2) commissural fibres of the telencephalon, which include the hippocampal commissure, the anterior commissure and the corpus callosum (p. 25.32) and interconnect corresponding parts of the two hemispheres, and

(3) association fibres, which interconnect different parts of each hemisphere.

The internal capsule, whose development is described on p. 25.44, contains fibres running to and from the cerebral cortex in a great sheet of fibres, the corona radiata, which radiates from the periphery of the lentiform nucleus (fig. 25.55). The **anterior limb** of the capsule lies between the lentiform nucleus laterally and the head of the caudate nucleus medially. The **posterior limb** lies between the lentiform nucleus laterally and the thalamus medially. The two limbs meet at a knee-like ankle, the genu (fig. 25.56.). It is to be noted (fig. 25.55) that fibres run horizontally in the anterior limb, vertically in the genu and anterior part of the posterior limb and horizontally in the posterior part of the posterior limb. Comparison of figs. 25.55 and 25.56 will show that some fibres, called **sublenticular**, lie below the lentiform nucleus and are not seen in typical horizontal sections of the internal capsule. Fig. 25.55 also makes clear the close packing of fibres in the internal capsule, and hence serious effects may follow small haemorrhages from central branches of the cerebral arteries (p. 25.83).

The anterior limb includes the **anterior thalamic radiations,** which provide reciprocal links between the thalamus and the cerebral cortex (p. 25.61), and the **frontopontine fibres** (p. 25.54).

The posterior limb includes the **corticospinal** and **corticonuclear tracts** (p. 25.44) and the **thalamocortical** part of the main somatosensory systems (pp. 25.37 and 61).

The sublenticular part of the internal capsule includes the auditory radiations, reciprocal links between the medial geniculate body and the auditory cortex; most of the visual radiations, from the lateral geniculate body to the visual cortex (fig. 25.86); and the **temporoparieto-occipitopontine fibres**, which link the cerebral cortex with the pontine nuclei.

Functions of the cerebral hemispheres

To understand the function of the cerebral hemispheres is not far from understanding the behaviour of the whole person or animal. The methods used must match the diversity of the problem and the oldest (armchair speculation aside) is to determine the effects of injury. This was being used at least as long ago as the time of Galen (129–200 A.D.), who exposed the hemispheres in the living animal and noted in a general way the consequences of pressure and of incisions. Even earlier, war wounds of the head could be observed and the symptoms analysed. Modern methods of creating accurately placed injuries employ electric currents passed through fine electrodes inserted into the brain or freezing by miniature cooling devices.

Stimulation, instead of damage, can be achieved by applying drugs or even mechanically, but electrical stimulation is less damaging and better controlled. The results of electrical stimulation require cautious interpretation. Normally neurones do not fire synchronously as they do after electrical stimulation; this is hard to confine to a single neurone in the cerebral hemispheres; so the effects of electrical stimulation can rarely be identical with normal function.

Electroencephalogram (EEG)

Electrical recording of nervous activity in the cerebral hemispheres is another method of investigation. It falls into two categories. The first employs relatively large electrodes applied to the scalp. This type of record is called the electroencephalogram (EEG). Clearly it is convenient to use since no surgical operation is involved, but inevitably it cannot do more than record the summed activity of large amounts of neural tissue between the electrodes. Accordingly, in a normal alert subject, at first glance it seems to show small random and incomprehensible fluctuations, seen in the central parts of fig. 25.79. But several varieties of rhythmic activity appear in different circumstances. Berger noted in 1924 (though he waited five years to publish it) a rhythm with a period of 8–13 cycles/sec, noticeable when a healthy subject closed his eyes and chiefly present at the occipital poles of the hemispheres. This is the **alpha rhythm** and is shown at both ends of the traces taken from Lord Adrian and from a water beetle (fig. 25.79).

Sleep removes this rhythm and may substitute others in its place (p. 25.76). An epileptic convulsion is accompanied by gross rhythmic activity, suggesting the sort of synchronous discharge of neurones which is ordinarily absent, but which can be produced, for instance, by artificial electrical stimulation applied to the cerebral hemi-

spheres; in fact, convulsions can be initiated in this way.

The precise origin of EEG rhythms can be traced to some one part of a hemisphere by recording from numerous electrode positions on the scalp and comparing the records so obtained but to explain the rhythm in detail is not simple. Their amplitude and time course bear little resemblance to those of an action potential. But they certainly depend on the integrity of the connections between the cerebral cortex and the underlying thalamus,

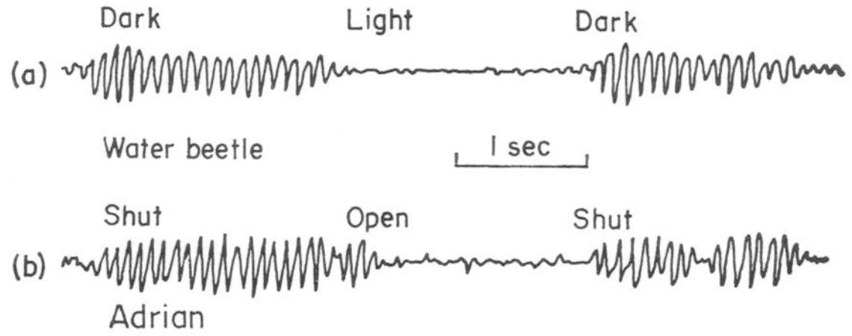

FIG. 25.79. Electrical rhythm (a) from the cerebrum of a water beetle in darkness and in light, and (b) from the cerebrum of Lord Adrian with eyes closed and open. From Adrian E.D. and Matthews B.H.C. (1934) *Brain* 57, 355.

for they are absent when these connections are interrupted. Hence they are a feature more of the complete system of thalamus and cortex than of the cerebral cortex alone.

It is obviously desirable to remove the uncertainties of the EEG by recording the activity of single neurones in the cerebral cortex. However, there are formidable difficulties in the way, chief among which is the pulsation of the cerebral hemispheres when they have been exposed by removing the overlying bone. Techniques exist for overcoming this difficulty in animals, but they are as yet barely applicable to man.

OLFACTORY SYSTEM

High in the roof of each nasal cavity there is a patch of yellow-brown epithelium in which the olfactory receptors lie. They are very numerous (the rabbit has 50 million) and each consists of a neurone with fine processes on its superficial surface and a thin slow-conducting axon running from its deep surface up through the cribriform plate of the ethmoid (p. 22.1).

Immediately above the cribriform plate the fibres penetrate the dura and enter the olfactory bulb of the brain. There they form synapses; their terminations are gathered together in groups to form conspicuous clusters or **glomeruli** (fig. 25.80) where they meet the dendrites of 'mitral' cells of the olfactory bulb. Some 25 000 single olfactory receptor axons might meet the dendrites of some 24 mitral cells in each glomerulus. The axons of the mitral cells run back to terminate in the cerebral cortex and adjacent parts of the forebrain. Besides the mitral cells, other cells in the olfactory bulb link one glomerulus to another, and one olfactory bulb to the other across the midline. So the pathway from the olfactory receptors to axon terminations in the cerebral cortex has only one synapse, and the route is more direct than that of any other type of receptor. The **olfactory bulbs** are small flattened ovoid bodies narrowing to form a flat **olfactory tract** passing backwards along the orbital surface of the frontal lobe. Each tract divides into medial and lateral olfactory striae, which diverge to enclose the olfactory trigone lying immediately anterior to the anterior perforated substance. This is so named because when the many small vessels are pulled out they leave behind perforations. Immediately behind this substance lies the optic tract (fig. 25.77).

The medial olfactory stria ascends anterior and lateral to lamina terminalis to become continuous with the grey matter of the para olfactory area and subcallosal gyrus (fig. 25.80). Fibres from the medial stria end in the olfac-

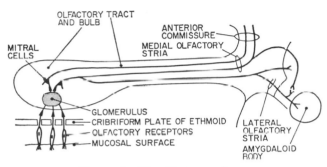

FIG. 25.80. The olfactory pathway

tory trigone and medial part of the anterior perforated substance and also in the septum pellucidum, a thin sheet of fibres stretched between the corpus callosum and fornix. A few olfactory fibres pass into the anterior commissure and end in the opposite olfactory area, but most end in the uncus which also receives the lateral olfactory striae passing to the lateral part of the perforated substance.

The uncus forms the anterior boundary of the hippocampal fissure and becomes continuous with the parahippocampal gyrus bounded medially by the hippocampal fissure and laterally by the collateral sulcus. The anterior end of the parahippocampal gyrus, the uncus and the amygdaloid with the prepyriform area (a mass of cells lying along the lateral olfactory striae) together form the **pyriform area**. The para-olfactory area, subcallosal gyrus and septum pellucidum nuclei form the **medial olfactory area**. Fibres arising in this area arch over the thalamus as **striae medullares** and end in the habenular nucleus which lies lateral to the pineal in the region of the posterior commissure. Hence they pass to the interpeduncular nucleus (lying between the peduncles) as the habenulopeduncular tract. From this nucleus fibres pass to the midbrain where they synapse with the dorsal tegmental nucleus (fig. 25.82).

From this nucleus the dorsal longitudinal fasciculus

passes caudally and connects with many cranial nerve nuclei especially those concerned with mastication (V) swallowing (V, X) and digestion (X). Other fibres pass from the habenular nucleus to the midbrain tectum coordinating olfactory and visual impulses. Thus the odour of food evokes olfactory memories and through connection with visceral neurones produces salivation and gut movement.

The **medial forebrain bundle** arises from the para-olfactory area and other parts of the medial olfactory area to end in the ventromedial nucleus of the hypothalamus.

SMELL

This is the sense of a myriad theories, but of few established facts. Any complete account requires to explain a number of interesting features. First is the immeasurably large number of odours that can be distinguished by a competent dog. These may be present in extreme dilution in the air. How many a human being can distinguish is also hard to guess. The ability to distinguish scents is little valued, except among perfumiers, and there is evidence that labourers are better at doing this than members of learned professions.

Four odours that have been recommended for testing the sense of smell are coffee, benzaldehyde (almond), tar and oil of lemon. There is nothing fundamental about these four. The merit they possess is simply that people can generally name them. Another test material is asafoetida, which possesses the advantage of smelling so unpleasant that the nose wrinkles uncontrollably.

Secondly, all smells cannot be made up by mixing a small number of components as in the case of vision. Light of any colour can be matched by an appropriate mixture of three carefully selected wavelengths and many tastes can be made up from a similar mixture of four basic tastes, sweet, sour, salt, and bitter, although it is agreed that on due reflection we can separate out the components of a taste, but not those of a colour. The huge variety of smells, on the other hand, cannot be so simply created. There is no visible difference between one olfactory receptor neurone and another which would allow them to be classified into a few simple types. Even if there were, the simple activity or silence of even, say, eight different types of receptor would in itself allow us to discriminate $2^8 - 1$ different smells, i.e. 255. This number hardly seems enough even for the disregarded human sense of smell. There must be facilities for recognizing different grades of activity in the receptors, not just its presence or absence.

Thirdly, there is some evidence that odour may influence behaviour even without being consciously recognized, let alone being clearly named. For instance, half of a batch of boxes of nylon stockings, otherwise identical, were perfumed and the whole batch exhibited for sale in a selfservice store. For every unperfumed box chosen, three perfumed boxes were chosen by customers. Yet in retrospect no customer could recall being aware of the perfume at all.

Fourthly, we soon cease to notice any smell which persists, so that the sense of smell must adapt strikingly and almost completely. 'We'll wait awhile,' the Master said, 'that thus our senses may grow used to this vile scent, and after that it will not trouble us.' (Dante, *Inferno*, canto xi, transl. Sayers).

The obvious approach to the olfactory system is to record the electrical activity of the receptor neurones while stimulating them with appropriate scents. This is singularly difficult; the neurones are small and inaccessible and their axons among the thinnest to be found in the nervous system. Besides, delivering only one kind of scent is not easy in practice. But evidence has been obtained that certain units in the frog's olfactory mucosa respond selectively to particular scents. Adrian was able to record the activity one stage further back, at mitral cell level, and show that it was more easily evoked by one of a group of five or six different odours.

Other investigators have looked for a physical or chemical basis underlying the resemblance in smell between different chemical compounds and have tried to define what it is about a molecule that determines its smell. The acid test of such an approach is its ability correctly to predict the odour of newly synthesized compounds and some success has been achieved, on the premise that there are about seven primary odours, each linked to a particular stereochemical configuration. A further line of approach is to look for individuals with impairments of smell corresponding to the varieties of colour blindness. Some ten varieties have been recognized, but recognition is not a simple procedure.

So the sense of smell can be assessed clinically only in the crudest way, but it may be a sense undervalued because it is difficult to talk about and difficult to investigate.

LIMBIC SYSTEM

In 1878, Paul Broca, a French physician, noticed how the inferior part of the cortex (the orbitofrontal area, the cingulate and parahippocampal gyri and the pyriform area) formed a rim or border (Latin, *limbus*) encircling the upper brain stem. This border together with the underlying brain stem structures soon came to be known as the limbic system. There has never been agreement as to the precise anatomical extent of the system, nor as to the scope of its functions; it is certainly involved in expression of emotions (p. 25.75). However, the term is likely to continue in use until further knowledge of the functions and connections of the structures in this area permits a more rational nomenclature.

During early development the hippocampus lies close

to the olfactory and hypothalamic region but the later development of the temporal lobe draws it down and extends its olfactory and hypothalamic connections. The fornix system (figs. 25.81 and 82) traces this development and remains as the connecting link between the hypothalamus and temporal lobe. During development the hippocampus rolls on itself to enclose the dentate gyrus, which lies between the hippocampus and parahippocampal gyrus. Although the hippocampus probably receives some direct olfactory impulses from the nearby uncus, it is not primarily an olfactory centre but it may serve as a co-ordinating or association centre for olfactory and other impulses. The hippocampus lies in the floor of the inferior horn with its bulbous anterior end grooved to resemble a paw and therefore termed pes hippocampi.

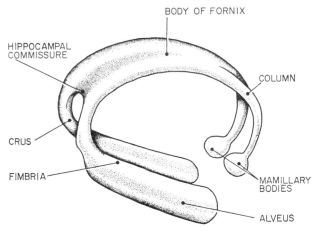

FIG. 25.81. The fornix.

Axons arising from the hippocampal cells form a thin layer of white matter, the **alveus** which covers the hippocampus and deviates to its medial side to form the **fimbria**. This is a narrow band passing backwards on the medial wall of the temporal horn to form the crus of the fornix. The two crura finally join to form the body of the fornix where fibres cross and make the hippocampal commissure. The fornix continues in the roof of the third ventricle before dividing again as the columns, which end in the **mamillary bodies** and hypothalamus.

The mamillothalamic tract arises from the mamillary bodies and ends in the anterior thalamic nucleus which in turn has connections with the cingulate gyrus. Other mamillary fibres pass to the midbrain tegmentum.

The cingulate region comprises areas 33, 24, 31, 23, the isthmus, 26, 29, 30; the para-olfactory area 25 is an anterior continuation of the cingulate gyrus, and although it extends to the frontal and parietal cortex, it is functionally part of the limbic system and therefore considered under that heading. The major connections are with the anterior thalamic nucleus through the anterior thalamic radiation, and with the mamillary bodies through the mamillo-thalamic tract. The cingulate gyrus has important and rich connections with the frontal lobe and fibres also pass in the internal capsule from the gyrus to the basal nuclei. As well as receiving impulses from the anterior thalamic nucleus it also donates fibres to it. The connection between frontal cortex, thalamus, hypothalamus and hippocampus implies that the cingulate gyrus influences autonomic function and behaviour. Surgical extirpations of the cingulate gyrus (cingulectomies) have been made for mental disorders, especially obessional states.

Closely associated with the hippocampus is the amygdaloid body which receives fibres from the medial olfactory striae. Fibres pass from the amygdala in the stria terminalis to end in the anterior hypothalamus (fig. 25.82).

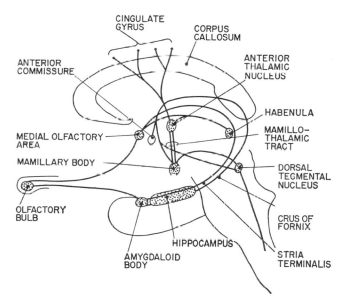

FIG. 25.82. Connections of the hippocampus and fornix (limbic system).

The **insula** is buried beneath the opercula (fig. 25.45) formed by the frontal, parietal and temporal lobes. The buried island is roughly triangular, surrounded by an indefinite sulcus. Experimental and clinical evidence show that it is related to visceral motor and sensory function. Little is known of its anatomical connections. Impulses carrying taste sensations may reach the anterior part of the insula.

TEMPORAL LOBES

Apart from its contribution to the limbic system and rhinencephalon, the temporal lobe has a major function in **auditory appreciation**. Areas 41 and 42 occupy the part of the superior temporal gyrus that is largely hidden within the lateral sulcus. The auditory radiations arise from the medial geniculate bodies and pass laterally

through the sublenticular part of the internal capsule, beneath the lower border of the insula, and enter the auditory cortex. This has many connections by association bundles with more distant parts of the brain. The auditory areas of the two sides are connected through commissural fibres in the corpus callosum. The superior temporal gyrus receives vestibular impulses and patients with lesions in this situation may have symptoms of vertigo or dizziness.

Like somatic sensation, hearing is represented on the cerebral cortex in a main auditory area. In the somatic sensory area each part corresponds to a part of the body, i.e. there is a somatotopic projection. But in the auditory area each part corresponds to part of the cochlea only in a very general sense; there is no definite 'tonotopic' projection, and so local damage to the auditory cortex does not lead to loss of high or of low tone hearing in the opposite ear. In fact, hearing differs from somatic sensation in being a much more bilateral sense. Thus damage to the auditory area in one of the two hemispheres is hard to detect at all; only when both hemispheres are affected does deafness become apparent.

Area 22 borders the auditory cortex and may be regarded as its association area. Lesions of area 22 produce word deafness or auditory receptive aphasia. Area 38 lies at the temporal pole and seems to be associated with recent memory. It has connections with surrounding cortex especially with the amygdaloid body, hippocampus and fornix.

FRONTAL LOBES

The precentral gyrus is largely occupied by primary motor cortex or area 4. Originally it was thought that only fibres originating in this area of brain contributed to the pyramidal tract, but in the human motor cortex the giant pyramidal cells in layer 5 of the precentral gyrus form only about 3 per cent of the corticonuclear and corticospinal tracts. Hence the cells of origin of the fibres in these tracts must lie either in other cells of the motor cortex or elsewhere in the cerebrum (p. 25.44).

Stimulation of a discrete area in the motor cortex in man and other primates leads usually to a specific movement of only one part of the opposite side of the body. There is certainly some localization of function, which is indicated in fig. 25.83.

The amount of cortex given to each part of the body is dependent more upon its function than its mass. Thus the hand occupies a greater cortical area than leg and trunk together whilst face, tongue and lips occupy an equally large area. All the voluntary muscles are represented with one striking exception, the external ocular muscles. These can be activated from central areas remote from area 4 and area 46 is often termed the frontal eye field since movements of the eyes are elicited by stimulation in this area.

Anterior to area 4 is a large cortical area, area 6, which possibly acts as a co-ordinator of muscle movement initiated by area 4, so that movements of many muscles produce a smooth action.

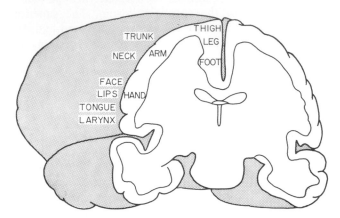

FIG. 25.83. Approximate representation of the body on the precentral gyrus. Note the position of the tongue and larynx below the face.

Damage to the main motor area of one cerebral hemisphere paralyses voluntary movements of the opposite side of the body, but there are reserve mechanisms. The face and mouth tend to have bilateral representation. Further motor areas certainly exist in animals and help to explain how relatively gross voluntary movements may be preserved, when fine movements are lost because of damage to the main motor area.

Areas 44 and 45 in the dominant hemisphere are related to speech. This should not be surprising in view of its close relationship to the motor areas of tongue and lips. This region is often called Broca's area.

Prefrontal cortex

Areas 9, 10, 11 and 12 have many connections with other parts of the brain through association bundles. Fibres from areas 9 and 10 pass to the dorsomedial nucleus of the thalamus and influence the hypothalamus. Area 10 with 47 and 53, which lies deep, also have connection with each other by commissural fibres passing in the genu of the corpus callosum and with other parts of the brain by long and short association bundles.

If one compares a human brain with a monkey's, the most obvious difference is the larger frontal lobes inside the high human forehead. But it is strangely difficult to allot a clear cut function to these lobes in front of the main motor area. They have no relation to reflexes, body posture and no sensation. The celebrated case of Phineas Gage (1848) is to the point. An iron rod was accidentally driven through the front of his skull, transfixing both frontal lobes. Yet intelligence-wise, he seemed little the worse. He was still able to carry out the tasks of road construction. But he was unfit to go on supervising his gang, which he had previously done. His character was the principal sufferer. He had become capricious, lazy and foul-mouthed. Normal social restraints were lost and natural anxieties removed.

The damage was bilateral and in the frontal lobes function is so conspicuously bilateral that damage to one side alone often produces quite elusive symptoms and signs, such as subtle character changes, until or unless it extends to involve the motor area. Probably, as in animals, the frontal lobes are specialized to play some part in learning, though not as actual stores of knowledge, and are also involved in curiosity, affection and pleasure. A monkey without frontal lobes can barely remember for 10 sec in which cup it has seen food placed. Yet in other ways it is perfectly intelligent and can lay complicated plans. Such a monkey does not care much about its faulty memory or even about excessively difficult problems, which usually upset a normal animal considerably. This indifference to disturbing situations prompted the use of surgical removal or disconnection of the prefrontal areas (prefrontal leucotomy) for the relief of extreme human anxiety or emotional tension or to produce indifference to pain. When adult life is reached and learning processes become less rapid, these emotional changes become the most prominent if the frontal lobes are damaged.

PARIETAL LOBES

The sensory or postcentral gyrus contains areas 1, 2 and 3 which are often considered together as the **somaesthetic cortex**, receiving sensations from the opposite side of the body (fig. 25.12 & pp. 25.37–41). It is overlapped, however, by areas which have been shown to be motor in function while a similar extension of the somaesthetic cortex into primary motor areas has also been demonstrated.

There is some localization of sensory function in the cortex. Thus when parts of skin are pressed or hairs are moved, the arrival of sensory traffic can be recorded in restricted areas of the cortex. The pattern in the postcentral gyrus is broadly similar to that in the motor cortex. (fig. 25.83). Thus the genitalia are represented on the bottom of the medial part of the hemisphere close to the toes.

Besides this basic arrangement, there is also evidence that the skin surface of the body is related to the front part of the somatic sensory area and the deeper tissues to the part slightly further back along the cortex. Again, the area on one hemisphere is concerned with the opposite side of the body, but the face is bilaterally represented.

So, when part of the sensory cortex is damaged, feeling may be impaired, but only in the part of the body corresponding to the cortical damage. The loss of feeling does not lead to loss of all responses. Lower levels of the nervous system are quite capable of jerking a limb away from harmful stimuli. The patient is often aware that something damaging is happening to him even though he does not know exactly where. When part of his sensory cortex is not working, the defect is far more subtle than the simple unresponding numbness that follows damage to a peripheral nerve. A test which helps is **two point discrimination**. When the skin is touched by two points, they may seem one to him when they are a greater distance apart on the affected side than on the normal side.

The mechanism of two point discrimination is not so simple as a sensory cortex 'looking' at a map of the body surface to see whether two adjoining receptors are firing or only one. Some neurones in the sensory cortex increase their firing rate when their area of skin is stimulated, but actually decrease it when a nearby area is stimulated. A neurone of this kind responds to stimulation within its area and then decreases its response when stimulation is added outside; it fires particularly vigorously if the stimulus moves out of its area into the immediately adjoining 'inhibitory' area (fig. 25.84). A further practical test of the integrity of the sensory cortex is to look for **astereognosis**; a patient holding some simple object is aware that he holds it, but cannot identify it by touch, without looking at it.

Besides the main somatic sensory area, monkeys and cats certainly have at least one subsidiary sensory area on which the body is similarly laid out but on a smaller

localization of this secondary area is rather uncertain as each neurone can be influenced by a relatively large part of the body surface, compared with a neurone in the main sensory cortex.

The somaesthetic areas of the hemisphere are connected through the corpus callosum and through long and short association bundles with many other parts of the brain. The most important connection is the sensory radiation from the nucleus ventralis posterior of the thalamus which passes in the posterior part of the internal capsule.

Speech

Speech is a feature of human beings, who have a highly-developed cerebral cortex, though even a dog can learn to obey several dozen verbal commands. It is linked with the cortex, predominantly in one hemisphere, commonly the left hemisphere in righthanded persons. Penfield of Montreal, described sites where electrical stimulation especially interfered with speech (fig. 25.85) Broca in France had long ago defined one of these areas by finding that damage there led to a disorder of speech. A patient of his who 'understood almost all that was said to him', could not speak.

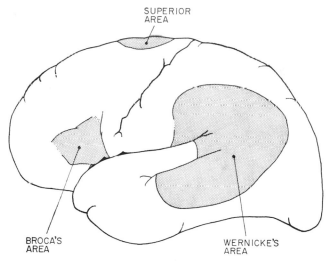

FIG. 25.85. The three speech areas shown on the left cerebral cortex. From Penfield W. & Roberts L. (1959) *Speech and Brain Mechanisms*. Princeton: Princeton University Press.

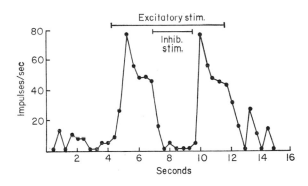

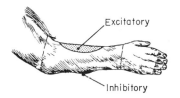

FIG. 25.84. Response of a neurone in the somatic sensory cortex of a monkey to stimulation in different areas of the forearm. From Mountcastle V.B. & Powell T.P.S. (1959) *Bull. Johns Hopkins Hosp.* **105**, 201.

scale. It lies behind the main somatic sensory area of the cortex and rather lower down the cortical surface. The

Although speech is dependent upon the co-ordination of large areas of cerebral cortex, certain parts, as has already been indicated, bear a special relationship. Although an undoubted simplification, clinical evidence tends to suggest that the region of the angular gyrus and supramarginal gyrus, namely areas 39 and 40, can be regarded as the co-ordinating centres, receiving and co-ordinating impulses received from the associative auditory areas (area 22) and visual associative areas (area 18) and projecting impulses probably through long association bundles to the expressive motor centre for speech or Broca's area (areas 44 and 45) in the dominant hemisphere.

Impairment in the use of speech can arise at many levels. For instance, the respiratory muscles, larynx, lips, tongue and palate each play a part, and so damage to nerves supplying any of these affects speech production; though the higher levels of the nervous system are marshalling the words quite normally, articulation can be faulty. Again, in speech, as in other activities, normal co-ordination of muscles depends on normal cerebellar activity. Finally, in damage to the cerebral cortex varieties of **aphasia** or inability to speak, can be distinguished by refined methods, and involve more than mere faulty articulation. Unable to marshal the right words, the patient may also be unable to read and write correctly. The various forms of aphasia are described in vol. 3, p. 34.8.

We can use either hand for most tasks and so either hemisphere can organize the movements. But for the most skilled hand movements and for the highly skilled activity of speech, little reserve capacity exists in the opposite hemisphere once these abilities have been acquired. However, a baby can transfer his future speech area to the other side if injury to one side compels him. Adults cannot achieve this and cannot usually gain much skill in fine movements with the non dominant hand. So the Ambidextral Culture Society which once existed is now in abeyance.

OCCIPITAL LOBES

These are the posterior part of the brain and have two major areas, the primary visual cortex or area 17 and a visual association cortex, area 18.

Area 17 occupies the occipital pole and in man has been pushed largely on to the medial side of the hemisphere by the greater development of the rest of the brain. It occupies the superior and inferior lips of the calcarine fissure and may extend on to the occipital poles laterally and as far forward as the parieto-occipital sulcus. It is often called the **striate area** because it contains extra fibres which widen the outer line of Baillarger into a broad white band.

Area 17 receives the visual radiations from the lateral geniculate body. Information from the superior retinal quadrant, that is from the inferior visual fields, passes to the medial half of the lateral geniculate body and thence to the superior lip of the calcarine fissure. Fibres from the superior visual field or inferior retinal quadrant relay in the lateral half of the lateral geniculate body and end in the inferior lip of the calcarine fissure. Central visual impulses from the macula end in the posterior part of area 17 whilst peripheral visual impulses pass into the more anterior part of area 17. Central vision occupies a large part of area 17, i.e. the macula is greatly magnified; peripheral vision occupies very much less. Thus there is a retinotopic projection of the information.

The visual radiations sweep mainly below the lentiform nucleus in the internal capsule. The fibres from the superior retinal quadrant pass almost directly posteriorly into the superior lip of the calcarine sulcus although the inferior retinal fibres pass forwards first looping into the anterior temporal region, before continuing posteriorly to join the superior retinal quadrant fibres and end in the inferior lip of the calcarine fissure (fig. 25.86).

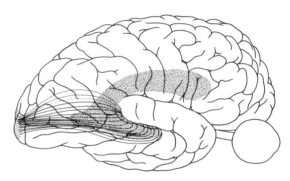

Fig. 25.86. Relation of the optic radiation (geniculocalcarine tract) to the lateral ventricle. Note particularly the fibres which loop round the inferior horn of the ventricle, within the temporal lobe. After Cushing.

After entering the visual cortex the fibres pass in the lines of Baillarger ending by synapse with cells in area 17 which connects with 18 and possibly 19 by association bundles.

The visual associative area or area 18 forms the parastriate area which lies immediately in front of area 17 and is distinguished by the absence of striation. Area 18 is richly connected with area 17 and also has a narrow strip adjoining area 17 which has many callosal fibres. The two halves of the field of view unite at the centre of gaze and along a line running vertically through it. So the two halves of the visual system, separate even in the cerebral hemispheres, must be suitably linked to create a functional whole. The link is the splenium of the corpus callosum, interconnecting the occipital poles of the hemispheres. From area 18, long association bundles connect the visual areas with the motor and sensory cortex, midbrain and tectum. Lesions of area 18 produce **visual agnosia** or the inability to recognize objects, a special form of which is **alexia** or inability to recognize written symbols, i.e. read. Stimulation of area 18 produces unformed visual images, flashes of light, colour and outline. In contrast, lesions of the temporal lobe and area 19 may result in formed images (hallucinations).

EXPRESSION OF EMOTIONS

An emotion is commonly accompanied by changes in the physical state of the body. There are many emotions and their expression varies. Charles Darwin's book *The Expression of the Emotions* (1872) is a classic and one of the first biological studies to make use of photography. There are photographs of men, women and children: suffering—with eyes closed and weeping; in low spirits and anxious—with depression of the corners of the mouth and oblique eyebrows; joyous—with head thrown back and eyes and mouth wide open in laughter; angry and defiant—with a canine tooth uncovered on one side of the mouth; helpless—with the palms of the hands turned out, elbows bent and head turned to one side; and afraid—with the lower part of the mouth and cheeks drawn down, and prominent ridges on the sides of the neck caused by contraction of the platysma muscle. Facial expression and posture serve to differentiate one emotion from another and may make it easy to recognize what a person is experiencing.

ANXIETY

Emotions are also expressed in many ways which are not specific. Some of these are listed in table 25.2 and each is commonly associated with anxiety. However they are not all present when the dominant emotion is anxiety. Indeed bodily reactions to anxiety differ markedly from individual to individual and are described more fully in vol. 3, p. 35.15. Prolonged periods of anxiety are a common experience and sometimes precede the onset of many diseases such as essential hypertension, coronary heart disease, peptic ulcer, ulcerative colitis, migraine, bronchial asthma, and chronic dermatitis. These are sometimes referred to as **psychosomatic disorders**. While it is uncertain to what extent the emotions contribute to their pathogenesis, there is no dispute that they have to be considered in interpreting their clinical features and in the management of patients.

TABLE 25.2. Physical manifestations of anxiety.

Muscular tension and trembling
Restlessness and fidgeting
Incoordination and impaired motor performance
Flushing, sweating and dry mouth
Choking feeling like a lump in the throat
Rapid breathing and hyperventilation
Palpitations, tachycardia and hypertension
Headache, fatigue, weakness and fainting
Anorexia, dyspepsia and diarrhoea
Urgency and frequency of micturition

Role of the brain

Two parts of the brain, the prefrontal cortex and the limbic system, are involved in bringing about the physical changes in emotion. Over a hundred years ago the celebrated case of Phineas Gage (p. 25.72) demonstrated that lesions involving the prefrontal cortex and underlying white matter are followed by changes in the experience and expression of emotion, both becoming blunted. Such changes, when they develop gradually, are elusive to the onlooker; it is especially distressing when degeneration of character and antisocial behaviour are interpreted as loss of moral fibre and subsequently turn out to be due to loss of nerve fibres and neurones caused by a frontal brain tumour. The limbic system was supposed at one time to be especially concerned with the sense of smell. Indeed the whole anterior pole of the brain originated in fish, which depend on smell to signal the chemical composition of the water in which they swim. Subsequently when the first mammalian brains developed, the limbic system contributed the first part of the cerebral cortex in small land animals where visual horizons were narrow and directed to the ground. Hence they presumably depended to a great extent on their sense of smell. Many mammals, notably dogs, rats and other nocturnal species, depend on smell as much as on vision when moving about. Smell is much less important in the daily life of man, although smells still retain an archaic ability to release powerful emotions, such as disgust and sexual attraction. The relation of the human limbic system to smell now seems purely historic.

Diverse and not always consistent experimental evidence links the limbic system to expression of the emotions. Lesions of the amygdaloid complex in cats, monkeys and man seem to remove any expression of rage or fear or aggressiveness. Conversely, stimulation here and in other parts of the system evokes a response which begins with dilation of the pupils, pricking up of the ears and an increase in the rate and depth of respiration. Active vasodilation occurs in muscles and vasoconstriction in the skin and gut. Pulse rate and cardiac output and arterial blood pressure rise, and the normal stabilizing effect of the baroreceptor reflexes is inhibited. Adrenaline is released into the blood stream and the animal behaves in a way suited for defence, exhibiting features of fear and rage. Similar stimulation has been carried out in the course of neurosurgical operations on patients who then reported that they felt these emotions.

Thus the limbic system takes part in important and complex reactions which are accompanied by powerful emotions of fear and rage, in the course of which the body is prepared for violent activity which has not yet begun; the usual prosaic control of cardiovascular and respiratory systems is temporarily overridden. These reactions alter the internal environment, for instance by reducing the P_{CO_2} in the blood through overbreathing.

There are sites within the limbic system, such as the lateral hypothalamus, where electrical stimulation is in itself gratifying to rats. When a stimulator connected to a pedal is implanted there the rat rapidly learns to press the pedal, and then presses it to the exclusion of all else, the stimulus itself being evidently a sufficient reward. In other sites stimulation is not attractive and rats learn to avoid it. Similar stimulation has been carried out in human beings at operation for the diagnosis or treatment of disease in this region. What they say and do is reminiscent of what might be expected from the results in rats; by stimulation the surgeon can make the patient extremely angry with him. But the responses are not entirely in agreement with the rat results.

The functions of each component within the limbic system cannot yet be described, and portions responsible for the expression of specific emotions cannot usually be defined. Yet glimpses of the arrangement are certainly discernible, e.g. in the hypothalamus where specific areas are associated with the expression of hunger and thirst.

SLEEP

Sleep can be rather clumsily defined as: 'a reversible, periodically recurring state of reduced muscular activity and sensory reactivity of an organism to the surrounding world'; the reversibility is obviously important, since sleep can be distinguished from coma by the relative ease with which the sleeper can be awakened. Beyond what common sense tells, little is known about why we need sleep in normal life. So it is impossible to calculate how many hours of it one needs. Explorers spontaneously take about eight hours when they are away from all social pressures and are pleasing themselves. Young children clearly need more and individuals vary greatly.

The requirement need not be taken in a single dose daily. In hot countries a siesta in the heat of the day is customary, except for mad dogs and Englishmen, as Noel Coward put it. Again, Oswald trained volunteers to sleep and wake on a 48 hour cycle instead of the normal 24 hours, and they grew accustomed to this. The sleep debt incurred in the first 24 hours was repaid during the second, and, unlike an oxygen debt, was not repaid in full; the extra sleep taken was not equivalent in length to the sleep lost.

No one is known to have died from lack of sleep. When people have been awake for long periods, it grows harder and harder to keep them awake and in the end practically impossible. Irritability, inattention and slowness of thought are well known consequences; delusions and liability to infective illness may be others.

Is sleep no more than a switching off of parts of the central nervous system? Since the plantar response (p. 25.19) becomes upgoing during deep sleep, it may be argued that the pyramidal tract is switched off. On the other hand, some individual neurones recorded in the pyramidal tract and the visual cortex of sleeping animals have actually been discharging more frequently than during resting wakefulness. Further, there is no apparent decrease in cerebral oxygen consumption and blood flow during sleep, although the measurements are not beyond criticism. The nervous system does not seem to be just switched off.

In fact this has long been clear. A mother, though asleep, is far more easily roused by her baby's cry than by other louder but less important noises. Pavlov painted the picture of a watchman still awake in the brain while the rest of him sleeps, and the watchman seems to be able to perform remarkable discriminations of this kind, wakening the sleeper if it is 'necessary'.

What does happen to the brain during sleep can be partly revealed by studying the electrical pattern shown in the electroencephalogram (EEG, p. 25.68). During wakefulness, there is a pattern of waves of a frequency around 10/sec and of relatively low voltage, interspersed with much random activity. When sleep begins, these waves are displaced by slower waves, of greater amplitude. Later on, perhaps after an hour of sleep, intermittent episodes of **paradoxical sleep** occur, in which the EEG waves are much reduced in amplitude. Muscle tone is also generally reduced in these episodes but rapid eye movements may occur behind the closed eyelids. However, in spite of these eye movements, the sleeper is harder to wake during paradoxical sleep than during the rest of his sleep and it is then that he dreams. Electrical changes of this type make possible experimental work to determine what brings on sleep and arousal.

In the reticular formation of the brain stem the more medial part is concerned with facilitating stretch reflexes in the flexor rather than in the extensor muscles, and with reducing vascular tone. Flexion (curling up) and a lowered vascular tone and arterial blood pressure are features of sleep. So it is not surprising that damage to this region leads to insomnia. Further, 5-HT is demonstrable in some neurones here and in the brain of animals the level is related to the amount of time they spend sleeping. Hence it is suggested that 5-HT in the brain is important in ordinary sleep mechanisms.

On the other hand, paradoxical sleep depends in animals on the integrity of the locus coeruleus, which lies in the upper pons, 'north-east' of the median longitudinal bundle; it is named blue place because some of its cells contain melanin, but the region is also rich in both noradrenaline and monoamine oxidase (MAO) which degrades noradrenaline and also 5-HT. It is thus a reasonable surmise that noradrenaline and the locus coeruleus are concerned in paradoxical sleep. Giving MAO inhibitors might be expected to raise the level of noradrenaline and increase the amount of paradoxical sleep taken by an animal. In fact, in man the use of MAO inhibitors suppresses paradoxical sleep, though not normal sleep, possibly by allowing levels of noradrenaline to rise too high. Such unexpected findings show, not that sleep is now well understood, but that it is less of a mystery than before. Growth hormone is secreted at night, often in large amounts, especially in children. More is secreted during orthodox sleep than during paradoxical sleep. Sleeping time seems well suited for growth and protein synthesis, which depend on growth hormone.

ON LEARNING AND MEMORY

Memory and learning are topics that link physiology and psychology. Many difficulties arise in translating words and figures, the natural raw material for psychological experiments on memory, into the neurophysiological events in the nervous system. Memory can be studied by comparing it to the familiar processes of note-taking, note-storing, and note-reading, i.e. what we do when we expect memory to be inadequate without aid. The comparison raises at once a string of questions: how is the note made, how long does it take to make, what form of note is it, where is it kept, how are successive notes arranged in store, is it hard work making a note, and how is it read again? Psychological aspects are discussed on p. 40.13.

A series of useful experimental plans has been devised to study memory and learning in animals. These were inaugurated by the almost legendary figure, Pavlov (1849–1936). This Russian physiologist, who was born left-handed, taught himself to be ambidextrous and became an exceedingly skilful experimental surgeon. He studied the physiology of the gastrointestinal tract until he was fifty-six and devoted the remaining thirty-one years of his life to trail-blazing experiments on the central nervous system.

In Pavlov's classical plan, the effectiveness of learning is assessed by measuring the volume of saliva produced by a dog. The pattern is shown in fig. 25.87a. The experimenter repeatedly first sounds a bell and then provides food for the dog. Salivation occurs in response to the food. The dog creates link C by learning, and will then salivate in response to the bell alone, a **conditioned reflex.** Learning is quickest if the interval between bell and food is half a second. If the experimenter breaks link A and stops providing the food but goes on ringing the bell, link C gradually becomes broken again; the animal's conditioned reflex is said to be **extinguished.** This is not the same as simple forgetting. Forgetting is the much slower loss of link C occurring when the experimenter just provides food, when needed, over a long time with no bell at all, and link B is broken.

A further experimental pattern is shown in fig. 25.87b. Here, after the bell, the animal receives a shock, causing it to withdraw its leg, and so learns to avoid the shock by lifting its leg when it hears the bell. Thus by establishing link C it breaks link D. Here again extinction can occur, if the experimenter breaks link A, and shocks can no longer be received.

Yet another pattern is shown in fig. 25.87c. The animal learns that by pressing the pedal it can obtain food, and thus the sequence is established. The dog takes the initiative in pressing the pedal; coaxing it to do this at the outset may not be easy until the reward is recognized. The process is called **operant conditioning.** The progress of conditioning may be assessed by the reliability (i.e. statistical probability) of the response, its latency, its duration or its size. Here, as in the other patterns, the experimenter generally delegates his duties to a suitable machine which provides the food whenever the dog presses the pedal, and very large numbers of variations in the pattern have been invented.

In general, the animal requires quite a number of repetitions to learn the response. This slowness may seem unintelligent, especially since it is more marked in the less

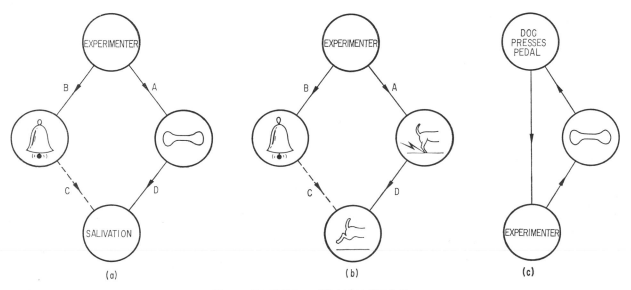

FIG. 25.87. Patterns of learning. See text.

highly developed animals. For instance, the worm is a much slower learner than the rat, and the rat slower than the monkey. We fancy we can frequently learn from a first encounter. But this is not always so apparent. A person in the position of fig. 25.87b will learn to pull his limb out of the way within half a dozen trials, and this is fast learning. But suppose he receives a light shone into his eye instead of an electric shock, not a very bright light but enough to produce constriction of the pupil, and at the same time the bell rings. His nervous system will learn in time to constrict his pupil when the bell rings, even if the light fails to shine. But it takes a great many trials to learn this, perhaps four hundred or more. Even then, the conditioned reflex is very rapidly extinguished again. This is slow learning, but by a perfectly intelligent human nervous system. Keeping out of the way of an electric shock is, of course, a defensive reaction. Pupillary constriction is not the way we protect ourselves against bright lights; it is not a defence, because the protection against bright light consists in closing the eyelids. Pupillary constriction is the 'stop', if one considers the eye as a camera, but not the shutter.

A fourth pattern of learning is peculiar and is called **imprinting**. The duckling, 16 hours after hatching, has the characteristics of the mother duck imprinted into its responses, so that it persistently follows the mother duck. The duckling is only open to imprinting during a particular brief phase of development and then has 'learnt' the appropriate responses in a lasting way. Instead of the mother duck's characteristics, some other set can be imprinted during this critical phase, and the duckling may then follow a hen or a man. This pattern seems remarkable as a variety of rapid but lasting learning, possible only during a brief phase of life; both ducklings and chicks are capable of it.

However, it can be argued that the duckling only receives the imprint because it has not previously been able, in its first 15 hours of independent life, to distinguish one moving thing from another, and that it would follow anything that moved. As soon as it is able, it identifies its mother. On this interpretation, imprinting is a feature of very early life, when the bird has little previous experience; its choice of a mother to follow is one of the first it learns to make, and rapid and durable for that reason and not because of any special, qualitatively different mechanism of learning.

A memory can take a long time to become permanently stored. The storing can be prevented entirely within the first hour or so by an electric shock to the brain of an animal or by lowering the animal's body temperature. In man, a head injury damaging the brain may extinguish the memory of all events immediately preceding the accident (**retrograde amnesia**). What is going on during storing is uncertain, but the fornix, hippocampus and mamillary body are involved, since patients with certain memory defects (the dysmnesic syndrome, vol. 3, p. 35.72) have been shown to have focal lesions involving one or more of these structures. In addition rhythmic waves may be found in electrical recordings from these sites in animals learning a conditioned reflex, and vanish again when the reflex is extinguished.

During the process of storing, a memory is available; and even when it fails to be stored, it can be recovered for a short time. A phone number read for the first time is available long enough for dialling, but usually gone beyond recall 10 sec later. This kind of short term memory is easy to test by finding out how many numbers in a sequence a patient is able to recite back again at once (p. 40.17). A person with bilateral (it has to be bilateral) hippocampal damage can perform this test tolerably well, but he fails when his permanent storage of memory is tested by finding out whether he can recall memorable events which happened after the damage to his brain, such as political changes. Yet he can recover memories stored before the damage occurred.

How is the note kept and in what form? It was at one time supposed that the note might consist in electrical activity in the nervous system. Electrical activity is continuous both when awake and asleep and in certain cases it is known to 'reverberate', i.e. pass round and round a neuronal circuit or to and fro, so that its time course may repeat itself over and over again. But if this repeated activity corresponded to long term memory, then whatever arrested or seriously interfered with the electrical activity would also disrupt memory. This is not so, because chilling animal brains, or brief convulsions, do not necessarily remove memories, even though they interrupt the sequence of electrical activity. Memory can hardly depend on continuing electrical activity.

So it may depend on permanent changes in the structure of the system. The most plausible site is at the synaptic junctions between neurones. Enormous numbers are available, and new ones could form and old ones break down. The largest mass of neurones available to a mammal is the cerebral cortex. If the connections there are the ones usually modified to create a memory, then damaging them should abolish the memories deposited in the damaged part. Synaptic links may form in response to the sum of inherited patterns of behaviour and remembered experience. There is evidence to support this view. Young rats raised in a complex environment have larger brains and more dendritic spines in their cortical neurones than those reared in a restricted environment.

There are other difficulties. An animal's cerebral cortex can be sliced through repeatedly normal to its surface, severing the connections between each piece and its neighbour, without apparently abolishing memory. So a new piece of learning is unlikely to be just the 'soldering' of a new connection in the cerebral cortex. Certainly, actual loss of cerebral cortex that is widespread enough prevents the memory being available, so that memories are closely linked to the presence of enough functioning cerebral cortex.

How far can we believe that a memory is the establishing of a new connection, not in one place in the cerebral cortex, but in many places, so that it is available in any portion of cortex? This certainly cannot be entirely true. Some simple varieties of learning do not require the presence of the cerebral cortex at all. When deprived of it, an animal is still capable of learning the simplest conditioned reflexes. It can distinguish light from darkness and learn to act upon the difference, although no one knows whether a man can do this too. Learning is a feature of the nervous system which cannot be confined to one part of it; complicated kinds of learning naturally require the most complicated part of the nervous system.

Learning can also be confined to one side of the forebrain by Sperry's fascinating 'split brain' experiments. In these, a cat or a monkey undergoes splitting of the optic chiasma from front to back. The neural connections are now such that what the animal sees with the left eye is fed to the left cerebral hemisphere, and what it sees with the

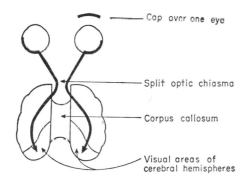

FIG. 25.88. Visual paths with split optic chiasma. After Sperry.

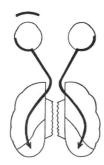

FIG. 25.89. Visual paths with split optic chiasma and corpus callosum. After Sperry.

right eye is fed to the right hemisphere. Normally what an eye sees is divided between the two hemispheres, but after chiasmal splitting this is no longer so.

After the splitting operation, one eye of the animal can

be covered, and learning can be done through the other eye; for instance, the animal can learn to find food behind a door marked with one pattern and not with another. What is seen is being fed to one hemisphere and not to the other. The next stage is to find out whether the other hemisphere has 'learnt' as well as the trained one.

This is done by splitting the corpus callosum, the bridge between the two hemispheres, and changing the eye cover from one eye to the other. The position is now as in fig. 25.89. The hemisphere not originally trained is now being tested by allowing the animal to see only with the eye feeding that hemisphere.

It turns out that the untrained hemisphere has learnt from the trained one, and in the monkey very efficiently but not so efficiently in the cat. The memory has been transferred across from one hemisphere to the other, and it is possible to show that the corpus callosum effects the transfer, because if the corpus callosum is cut at the outset, then only the trained hemisphere has 'learnt the lesson'. The other hemisphere remains unaware of it, unless, as already mentioned, the lesson is so simple as not to require the presence of the cerebral cortex.

There are a very few people without a corpus callosum, either born without it or deprived of it by operation. They naturally have an intact optic chiasma, and it is not so easy to demonstrate that they have two independent hemispheres, but it can be done. Speech is a function confined to the 'dominant' hemisphere, and so the non-dominant hemisphere cannot speak or write. Is it then totally illiterate? It seemed at one time that there must be large amounts of vacant space in the non-dominant hemisphere, and then evidence from operations on the human brain suggested that the non-dominant hemisphere might contain maps and plans, instead of the words which were the prerogative of the dominant hemisphere. Clearly our memories come to contain vast amounts of information in plan and map form, and one of Penfield's patients after operation on the non-dominant hemisphere, could never find his way home unless he could actually see the house.

In addition, evidence is now appearing that the non-dominant hemisphere does perhaps recognize words when seen. The words cannot be spoken nor written; but the hand governed by the non-dominant hemisphere can reach out to something when the same hemisphere has seen and evidently read its name.

This is just one of a number of remarkable findings which have emerged from studies on 'split-brain man'. At times, the non-dominant hand may 'go off on its own' and have to be restricted by the dominant hand. One begins to doubt whether a split brain man is singular or plural. But in no sense does he resemble a schizophrenic, in spite of the layman's interpretation of that word.

Are we then to say that a normal piece of learning depends on synaptic connections in the hemisphere which did the learning, and that similar connections are established in the other hemisphere if the corpus callosum is intact. Before pinning our faith exclusively to synaptic connections, it is worth taking a look at another type of change.

When a new memory is stored, we presume that living tissue acquires new properties. Besides the formation of new synaptic connections, there is a quite different way in which living tissue can acquire new properties. The study of immunology shows that some cells can 'learn' to recognize and respond to specific molecules in their environment. We may suppose that a neurone can respond to molecules released by axon terminals nearby and modify its RNA. Such molecules might be neurotransmitters or more complex molecules released by the passage of nerve impulses.

So memory might depend on changes in neuronal protein structure. Changes in the structure of RNA could lead to synthesis of new proteins. Such changes have recently been sought in animals after training in new tasks like climbing along a wire, or getting food with an unaccustomed paw, and do appear to occur. But this type of explanation is not necessarily an alternative to synaptic changes. Both views may in the end turn out to be complementary; synaptic change and RNA change may both play a part.

Learning, and teaching what we have learnt, is the prized tool with which men hope in their wilder dreams to break through the limitations of human genetic make up and leave their mark upon the traditions of the future. Each of us grants readily that particular feats of learning are beyond us. But we are slow to agree that all human learning must be filed on any fixed number of shelves.

About the filing system for memory traces there is little clear knowledge. Experience confirms that they are somehow filed in the same order as they are made, so that they carry a time label with them. And artificial stimulation of the temporal lobe of a human cerebral hemisphere can summon into consciousness a series of memories correct in their sequence, one following another in the same order as the related events originally occurred. It must be admitted that this resummoning of memories by electrical stimulation has not yet been demonstrated in a normal cerebral hemisphere. It is also obvious that memories are labelled in the file in many ways in addition to order of time: witness how past events are recalled when the memory is jogged by every sort of diverse association between the present and the past.

It is hard to form any estimate of how large the filing system is. Ordinarily one is aware of recollections that do not come to mind when wanted, but report for duty later on. Again, hypnosis seems to provide access to far more recollections than one is ever normally able to draw upon. Even in old age, the store is never full up, whatever one may feel like just before an examination.

The reader may be awed by the demands of his course, and the pains he has to take to remember it. Must it take great effort or special trouble to record a memory? Can learning be effortless, involuntary? Certainly, establishing a conditioned reflex is a form of learning. But it is the learning of even the lower animals; learning without understanding, learning without curiosity. It is not very different from the endless memorizing by children of scriptures that they are too young to understand, a practice which still persists in the East, but dies out when paper and print become readily available. It may lead later on to the endless memorizing of textbooks by adults.

A reader ought not to sit passively in learned books, trying to imbibe knowledge like a plant. He should prowl in them, scenting from far away the answers to questions in his mind, challenging the writer with his interest. Memories are often recorded with the utmost ease when interest gives her consent. Interest is a fickle goddess, but not too fickle to be successfully seduced. It is not enough to call loudly on the subject matter (or the teacher) to produce her. She can be lured by signs of affection, but she cannot be forced by threats or sacrifices. There comes a time to give up dogged persistence, put down the books and find another temporary mistress, till with time her feminine waywardness grows more amenable.

Finally, how is memory read back? This is just as difficult as any of the other features to explain in neurophysiological terms. The process seems rapid even when the memory is of a hoary antiquity. What is recalled carries a time label with it. All in all, memory presents problems difficult to reconcile with any one model proposed so far; it provides the facilities of an elaborate computer, but all on a mere 20 watts of power; this is the consumption of the whole brain and has to cover numerous other activities too.

MENINGES

The brain and spinal cord are covered by three membranes, the **cranial** and **spinal meninges**. The innermost is the thin and delicate **pia mater**, which closely invests them and dips into all their surface indentations. At the lower end of the cord, the pia continues as an investment of the filum terminale. Outside the pia is the **arachnoid mater**. The two membranes are referred to collectively as the **pia-arachnoid**, or as the **leptomeninges**. They develop in common from primitive mesenchymal tissue (endomeninx) surrounding the neural tube. Within this layer spaces appear and coalesce to form the **subarachnoid space**, which becomes filled with cerebrospinal fluid (CSF). In the adult, the pia and arachnoid are linked by numerous trabeculae, which indicate their common origin. The two layers, and the trabeculae, consist of a fine network of collagenous and elastic fibres. All surfaces facing into the subarachnoid space are covered by a simple squamous mesenchymal epithelium and a similar layer covers the outer surface of the arachnoid mater. This is separated from the outermost of the three meninges, the **dura mater** or pachymeninx, by the **subdural space**. As the arachnoid is held against the dura by the pressure of the CSF, the space normally contains only a thin film of fluid, but it may be distended by pus or blood.

Because the pia mater follows closely the surface contours of the brain and spinal cord, while the arachnoid is pressed against the dura, the subarachnoid space shows several localized enlargements. These are (1) the **flumina** (rivers) which overlie the cerebral fissures and sulci, and (2) the **cisterns** which overlie large surface irregularities of the brain. The **interpeduncular cistern** lies between the cerebral peduncles and the **cerebellomedullary cistern** (**cisterna magna**) in the angle between cerebellum and the dorsal aspect of the medulla. Largest is the **lumbar cistern,** which extends between the level of termination of the spinal cord (L1–L2) and the lower end of the sac of the dura mater (S2–S3).

The flumina and cisterns are continuous with the rest of the subarachnoid space, of which they are simply localized dilations. Samples of CSF may be obtained in life from the lumbar cistern by **lumbar puncture** and from the cisterna magna by **cisternal puncture**.

The subarachnoid space also contains:

(1) The main arteries, veins and their tributaries on the outer surface of the brain and spinal cord. Bleeding from these, either arterial or venous, is called subarachnoid haemorrhage and stains the CSF with blood.

(2) The cranial nerves, in that part of their course between their attachment to the surface of the brain and the point where they pierce the dura mater on their way to their exit from the skull.

(3) The dorsal and ventral roots of the spinal nerves and the dorsal root ganglia. Below the termination of the spinal cord, the cauda equina might seem to be at risk from a lumbar puncture needle, but the nerve roots fortunately are as elusive as the last pickle in the jar.

(4) The **ligamenta denticulata** (fig. 25.11) are narrow fibrous sheets, one on each side of the spinal cord, between the dorsal and ventral nerve roots. Each is continuous with the pia mater at the side of the spinal cord and is attached laterally, at intervals, to the dura mater by a series of triangular tooth-like processes. These ligaments help to anchor the spinal cord in the vertebral canal.

The dura mater is a tough, protective membrane consisting of dense, irregular, collagenous connective tissue with some elastic fibres; its internal surface is smooth, white and glistening, and covered with simple squamous mesenchymal epithelium.

The **cranial dura mater** is traditionally described as consisting of two layers, an outer periosteal layer and an inner supporting layer. The outer layer provides a periosteum (endosteum) for the internal surface of the skull;

the inner layer is reflected inwards to form supporting structures, such as the falx cerebri and tentorium cerebelli. At these and other sites of separation of the two layers are found the venous sinuses of the dura mater, described on p. 22.9. Elsewhere the distinction between the two layers is largely artificial.

The cranial dura is attached to the internal surface of the skull by fibrous strands, which penetrate the bone, and by branches of the meningeal blood vessels, which are distributed principally to the skull bones. When the dura is peeled away from the skull, these connections are torn and the exposed outer surface of the dura is rough. The dura is attached most firmly at the sutures, where it is continuous with the connective tissue of the sutural ligaments, at the foramina through which the cranial nerves leave the skull, and at the foramen magnum. These are all sites of continuity between the external periosteal covering of the skull and the internal periosteal (endosteal) layer of the dura.

At the foramen magnum, the inner layer of the dura is continued downwards into the vertebral canal as the **spinal dura mater**. This forms a sleeve-like investment for the spinal cord and for the roots of the spinal nerves and extends to the junction between the second and third pieces of the sacrum. Unlike the inner layer of the cranial dura, which is mostly fused with the periosteal layer, the spinal dura is mostly separated from the periosteal lining of the vertebral canal by an **extradural space**, which contains adipose tissue and the internal vertebral venous plexus.

Where cranial nerves and the roots of spinal nerves pierce the dura, they carry with them a short tubular prolongation of the dura, which becomes continuous with the epineurial connective tissue. The optic nerve, which develops as part of the brain, is surrounded by extensions of all three meninges, and of the subarachnoid space, as far as its junction with the eyeball.

The dura is well supplied by arteries, of which the middle meningeal is the most conspicuous. The metabolic needs of the dura itself are small; its arteries are distributed principally to the skull. When a blow on the head tears a meningeal artery (or the accompanying vein), blood accumulates between dura and skull in the potential extradural space (vol. 3, p. 11.4).

The dura is innervated principally by the trigeminal nerve. The ophthalmic division supplies the anterior cranial fossa, the anterior part of the falx cerebri and the tentorium cerebelli, a pattern of distribution which may account for the frequent association of frontal headache with lesions in the posterior cranial fossa. The maxillary division supplies the dura of the frontal part of the vault of the skull, and, with the mandibular division, that of the middle cranial fossa. The posterior fossa is innervated by meningeal branches of the vagus nerve and of the 2nd and 3rd cervical nerves.

BLOOD SUPPLY AND VENTRICULAR SYSTEM

The brain is supplied by the two internal carotid arteries and the two vertebral arteries whose external course is described on p. 22.34. The **internal carotid artery** leaves the cavernous sinus by piercing its dural roof at the medial side of the anterior clinoid process. It passes backwards below the optic nerve and then upwards, close to the lateral side of the optic chiasma, to reach the anterior perforated substance where it divides into its terminal branches, the **anterior** and **middle cerebral arteries.** The **vertebral arteries** pierce the spinal dura at the level of the atlas, enter the posterior cranial fossa through the foramen magnum. incline medially to the ventral surface of the medulla oblongata and unite at the lower border of the pons to form the midline **basilar artery.** This ascends in a shallow groove on the ventral surface of the pons and divides at the upper end of the pons into the two **posterior cerebral arteries.**

The two major arterial systems, the **internal carotid system** and the **vertebrobasilar system**, are linked on each side by a **posterior communicating artery** which unites the internal carotid and posterior cerebral arteries. The **anterior communicating artery**, which links the two anterior cerebral arteries, completes an **arterial circle** (the circle of Willis) which lies at the base of the brain, in the interpeduncular cistern (fig. 25.90). Because the com-

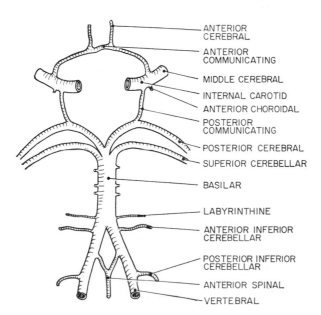

FIG. 25.90. The circle of Willis and principal arteries of the brain.

ANTERIOR CEREBRAL
ANTERIOR COMMUNICATING
MIDDLE CEREBRAL
INTERNAL CAROTID
ANTERIOR CHOROIDAL
POSTERIOR COMMUNICATING
POSTERIOR CEREBRAL
SUPERIOR CEREBELLAR
BASILAR
LABYRINTHINE
ANTERIOR INFERIOR CEREBELLAR
POSTERIOR INFERIOR CEREBELLAR
ANTERIOR SPINAL
VERTEBRAL

municating arteries are usually small, blood normally reaches each hemisphere by two separate routes, the internal carotid and the posterior cerebral. However, variations in the arterial circle are common. As examples,

the right anterior cerebral artery may be narrow at its origin and blood flow is then provided mainly through an enlarged anterior communicating artery; an enlarged posterior communicating artery may lead to the posterior cerebral functioning as a branch of the internal carotid artery. However, in an old person with arteriosclerotic narrowing of a major artery, anastomoses in the arterial circle may not be adequate to provide an adequate blood supply to part of the brain. The blood supply to the brain can be shown by arteriograms and the two major systems are illustrated in figs. 25.91 and 92.

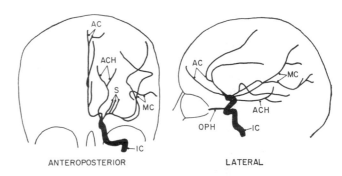

FIG. 25.91. Tracings of carotid arteriograms. AC, anterior cerebral; ACH, anterior choroidal; IC, internal carotid; MC, middle cerebral; OPH, ophthalmic; S, thalamostriate.

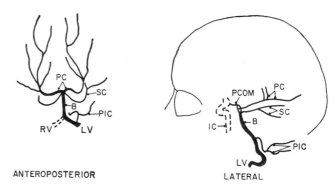

FIG. 25.92. Tracings of vertebrobasilar arteriograms. B, basilar; IC, internal carotid; LV, RV, vertebral, left and right; PC, posterior cerebral; PCOM, posterior communicating; PIC, posterior inferior cerebellar; SC, superior cerebellar.

The distribution of arteries to the brain follows a general plan.

(1) The vertebrobasilar system supplies the midbrain, pons, medulla and cerebellum and, through the posterior cerebral artery, the posterior part of the cerebral hemisphere and of the diencephalon; it also contributes to the supply of the cord through the anterior and posterior spinal arteries.

(2) The internal carotid system supplies the remainder of the brain, including the pituitary gland and the eye.

(3) Each system is distributed through two separate

sets of vessels to those parts derived from the forebrain. Small **central arteries** arise in groups from arteries within, or close to, the arterial circle; these penetrate the base of the brain and supply deeply placed grey matter, such as the basal nuclei and thalamus, and associated white matter, notably the internal capsule. **Cortical branches** of the anterior, middle and posterior cerebral arteries arise from the arterial circle and ramify on the surface of the brain, lying within the subarachnoid space.

(4) Through its cortical branches, each cerebral artery supplies its own cortical territory (fig. 25.93). The cortical

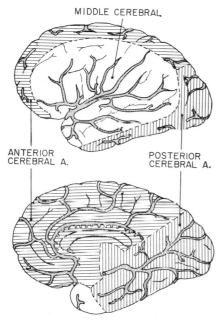

MIDDLE CEREBRAL

ANTERIOR CEREBRAL A.

POSTERIOR CEREBRAL A.

FIG. 25.93. Areas of the cerebral cortex supplied by the cerebral arteries. Above, lateral surface; below, medial surface.

territory of the middle cerebral artery includes the greater part of the motor and somaesthetic cortices, while that of the anterior cerebral artery includes the rest of these areas. The visual cortex is supplied by the posterior cerebral artery.

(5) The cortical branches form an arteriolar plexus in the pia mater, from which two types of vessel penetrate the brain at right angles to its surface; these are **cortical penetrators**, 15–50 μm in diameter, which traverse the cortical grey matter and then supply it by recurrent branches, and **white matter penetrators**, 75–150 μm in diameter, which supply the white matter as far as the ependymal lining of the lateral ventricle.

To this general outline some clinically important details may now be added.

(1) There are four main groups of central arteries. A **posteromedial group** arises from the posterior cerebral and posterior communicating arteries, pierces the brain stem

in the interpeduncular fossa (posterior perforated substance) and supplies the hypothalamus and caudal part of the thalamus. An **anterolateral group** arises from the first 2 cm of the middle cerebral artery and pierces the brain at the anterior perforated substance. This group consists of the **medial** and **lateral striate arteries** which supply the lentiform and caudate nuclei and the internal capsule. Bleeding from one or other of these arteries is one form of cerebral haemorrhage; because of the close packing of fibres in the internal capsule, even a small haemorrhage may produce serious disturbances of brain function. An **anteromedial group** arises from the anterior cerebral artery and supplies anterior parts of the basal nuclei and of the corpus callosum. A **posterolateral group** arises from the distal end of each posterior cerebral artery. Central branches also arise from the **anterior choroidal artery**, a small branch of the internal carotid which supplies the optic tract, part of the lateral geniculate body and of the optic radiation, all parts of the optic pathway; it also supplies the choroid plexus of the inferior horn of the lateral ventricle.

Although anastomoses of precapillary dimensions can be demonstrated anatomically, the central arteries behave as **functional end arteries**; if one is occluded, the nervous tissue which it supplies will die.

(2) The cortical branches of anterior, middle and posterior cerebral arteries are connected on the surface of the brain by anastomotic vessels 200–450 μm in diameter and, in the absence of complicating arterial disease, collateral circulation between the three surface territories is satisfactory. By contrast, anastomoses are inadequate between cortical penetrators and between white matter penetrators and the central arteries, which share the supply of the white matter of the hemisphere.

Blood supply to the spinal cord

Most of the blood to the cervical spinal cord comes via the vertebral arteries (fig. 25.94). The **anterior spinal**

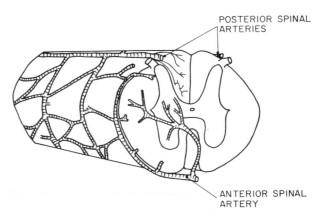

POSTERIOR SPINAL ARTERIES

ANTERIOR SPINAL ARTERY

FIG. 25.94. Sectional view of spinal cord showing blood supply.

artery is formed from branches arising from both vertebral arteries and passes down the front of the cord in the midline receiving contributions from ventral radicular arteries, especially on the roots of C7, 8 and T1 which ultimately come from branches of the subclavian arteries. The **posterior spinal arteries** are also branches of the vertebral, or sometimes the posterior inferior cerebellar artery, and these receive contributions from the dorsal radicular arteries.

Anastomoses between the anterior and posterior systems lie in the superficial part of the cord and in the pia mater. Thus both systems supply the periphery of the cord both anteriorly and posteriorly. The central part of the cord is supplied largely by the anterior spinal artery which gives off perforating branches in the ventral median fissure. The distribution of the radicular arteries to the cord varies greatly but a point of practical importance is that both ventral and dorsal radicular arteries lie on the anterior aspects of the spinal nerve roots and are hidden from view and may possibly be injured during surgical procedures. The anterior spinal artery is, in fact, an anastomotic system rather than one long artery, with the major contributions coming from the radicular arteries. Some of the more important connections arise in the cervical region, and the largest is in the lumbosacral portion of the cord, being a large artery usually arising from the tenth intercostal artery. The venous drainage follows a pattern similar to that of the arteries.

Features of the microcirculation

The relationship between capillary blood vessels and cells in the nervous system differs from that in other tissues in important respects.

First, capillaries are non-fenestrated and their endothelial cells are united by tight junctions. Also they lack nucleotidases which are involved elsewhere in active transport processes. Moreover, pinocytotic vesicles are sparse. Collectively these anatomical features constitute part of the so-called blood-brain barrier (p. 25.88).

Secondly, the extracellular space of the brain is restricted to the labyrinthine intercellular spaces, about 20–30 nm in diameter, which lie between the processes of neuroglial cells and neurones. Neuroglia constitutes about 50 per cent by volume of brain tissue, and the processes of their cells have end feet or pedicles expanded around the capillaries and neuronal elements and beneath the pia mater. The chemical composition of the extracellular fluid of the brain resembles closely that of the CSF (p. 25.87) and there is free exchange through the surface membrane formed by the pia and the glial end feet (the piaglial membrane).

Thirdly, there are no lymphatic vessels in the CNS. This may be correlated with the reduced permeability to protein of the blood capillaries of nervous tissue;

elsewhere lymphatic capillaries take up proteins from the extracellular fluid and return them to the circulation.

Venous drainage

The venous drainage of the brain can be divided into deep and superficial systems which both drain into the venous sinuses of the cranial cavity (p. 22.9).

The superficial cerebral veins have variable origins, courses and terminations but mostly drain into the venous sinus system. The dorsal part of the cerebral hemispheres, for example, sends blood into the superior sagittal sinus and the medial part of the hemispheres sends blood into the inferior sagittal sinus. The orbital surface of the frontal lobe and the anterior parts of the temporal lobe are drained by a large vein passing along the lateral sulcus and known as the **superficial middle cerebral vein**. It drains into the cavernous sinus and also joins with the **superior anastomotic vein**, draining into the parietal part of the superior sagittal sinus, and the **inferior anastomotic vein** which passes inferiorly to the transverse sinus.

The **deep cerebral veins** drain the interior of the brain (fig. 25.95). The **septal vein** is formed by small branches

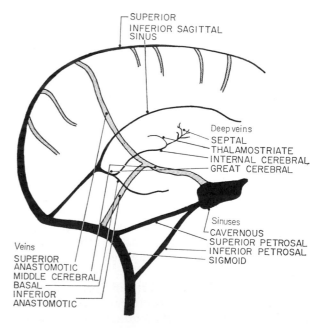

FIG. 25.95. Venous drainage of the cerebrum. Superficial veins are stippled and deep veins and sinuses are black.

draining the head of the caudate nucleus and the anterior horn of the lateral ventricle. The **thalamostriate vein** passes forwards between the caudate nucleus and thalamus draining both and then, arching backwards through the interventricular foramen, is joined by the choroidal vein and septal vein to form the **internal cerebral vein**.

The internal cerebral vein lies close to the midline in

the pia mater forming the roof of the third ventricle. It joins the other internal cerebral vein posteriorly near the pineal gland to form the **great cerebral vein** which lies beneath the splenium and curves up around it to join the inferior sagittal sinus and form the straight sinus. The **basal vein** drains the anterior and posterior perforated substance and passes backwards around the cerebral peduncle to join the great cerebral vein.

The veins draining the brain stem pass largely to the **cerebellar veins,** most of which enter by short connections into the adjacent sinuses or, as in the case of the **superior cerebellar vein,** connect with the deep cerebral veins.

The great cerebral vein therefore receives both internal cerebral veins and both basal veins. This venous system is readily demonstrated by cerebral angiography and a knowledge of its normal configuration enables the neuro-radiologist to determine whether there has been any displacement of the deep structures of the cerebral hemispheres.

Ventricular system

The brain and brain stem contain cavities, the ventricular system. Each cerebral hemisphere contains a lateral ventricle which communicates with the third ventricle through the intraventricular foramen. The third ventricle lies within the diencephalon whilst a narrow aqueduct passes through the mesencephalon to widen out as the fourth ventricle behind the pons and medulla (fig. 25.96).

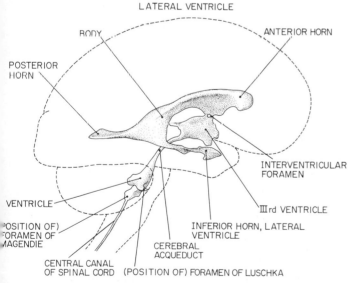

FIG. 25.96. Drawing of a cast of the ventricular system of the brain, viewed from the right side.

The **third ventricle** lies between the thalami, often interrupted by a bridge of cells, the massa intermedia, connecting the right and left thalamus (fig. 25.97). The interventricular foramen lies anteriorly near its roof, be-

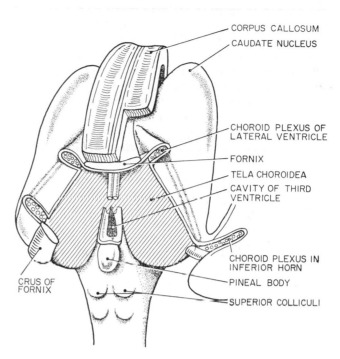

FIG. 25.97. The tela choroidea and the roof of the third ventricle. After Last.

tween the anterior tubercle of the thalamus and the anterior column of the fornix. Its anterior wall is the lamina terminalis, containing the anterior commissure above and the optic chiasma below. Above the chiasma is the supra-optic recess, below it the pituitary stalk or infundibulum. The hypothalamus forms the lower anterior portion of the lateral walls of the third ventricle. The posterior portion of the floor and walls of the third ventricle are related to the subthalamic nucleus and its fibres, and finally the floor of the ventricle reaches the mesencephalon where it joins the aqueduct (fig. 25.38).

The roof of the third ventricle is complex and contains choroid plexuses. An invagination of pia mater, **tela choroidea,** passes anteriorly beneath the splenium of the corpus callosum and the fornix and above the pineal body and the superior colliculi into the transverse cerebral fissure. It invaginates the thin roof of the third ventricle and the choroid fissure of each lateral ventricle, to form the choroid plexuses of these cavities (p. 25.30 and fig. 25.47).

The **lateral ventricle** is derived from the cavity of the primitive cerebral hemisphere (p. 25.30) and consists of a body with anterior, posterior and inferior extensions or horns.

The **anterior horn** of the lateral ventricle is roofed over by corpus callosum which curves around the tip of the horn as the genu and extends beneath it as the rostrum. The head of the caudate nucleus forms the floor and lateral boundary of the anterior horn whilst medially the two horns are separated by the septum pellucidum and the medial frontal cortex on either side.

The **body** of the lateral ventricle is triangular on transverse section and is roofed by the corpus callosum, its medial walls being formed by the septum pellucidum. Laterally lies the body of the caudate nucleus which also forms part of the floor of the body and, more medially, the thalamus and choroid plexus. The posterior horns extend from the body into the occipital lobe and the deep calcarine fissure of the medial surface of the occipital lobe forms a ridge in the medial part of the posterior horn known as calcar avis. A little above this protrusion another ridge marks the forceps major which contains callosal fibres uniting the occipital lobes.

The trigone is a triangular area in the posterior part of the body and the posterior and inferior horns (fig. 25.98).

The **inferior horn** curves downwards and forwards into the temporal lobe. The tail of the caudate nucleus forms its roof, and ends in the amygdaloid body which forms a small protrusion in the tip of the inferior horn. The hippocampal fissure forms a longitudinal projection in the medial part of the floor of the inferior horn whilst the fimbria lying in the floor and medial part of the horn

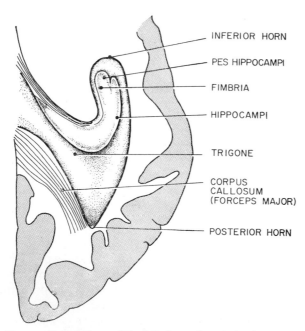

INFERIOR HORN

PES HIPPOCAMPI

FIMBRIA

HIPPOCAMPI

TRIGONE

CORPUS CALLOSUM (FORCEPS MAJOR)

POSTERIOR HORN

FIG. 25.98. Relations of the inferior and posterior horns.

close to the hippocampus passes backwards to form the fornix which joins with its fellow of the opposite side to form the body of the fornix.

The **aqueduct** connects third and fourth ventricles and is a short narrow channel lying within the mesencephalon.

The **fourth ventricle** has a diamond-shaped outline, bordered above and below by the superior and inferior cerebellar peduncles. The roof is provided mainly by the cerebellum with the superior medullary velum above and the inferior below. In the inferior velum are two lateral and one median apertures which permit CSF to escape from the ventricular system into the subarachnoid space.

A choroid plexus consists of an invagination of richly vascular pia mater into a ventricle, covered by a modified simple cubical epithelium of ependymal origin. The pial capillaries are permeable and fenestrated. The ependymal epithelium has basal infoldings of the plasma membrane, a microvillous apical border and tight junctions between the cells. The tight junctions ensure that passage of material through the epithelium is transcellular; this anatomical feature is part of the blood–CSF barrier.

Cerebrospinal fluid

The principal source of cerebrospinal fluid (CSF) is the choroid plexuses of the lateral and third and fourth ventricles. If the plexus is removed from one lateral ventricle and the interventricular foramen is blocked, that ventricle may collapse and the other lateral ventricle becomes distended by the fluid formed within it, dammed back at the interventricular foramen. It is, however, not possible to say confidently that the choroid plexus is the sole source of the fluid. It may well be that some is also formed at the ependymal lining of the ventricles. On the analogy of animal experiments, about 0·5 ml/min is produced in man by all the choroid plexuses together. The total amount of CSF in man is about 150 ml.

After secretion in the ventricles, CSF passes through the ventricular system and out from the fourth ventricle into the cisterna magna. Thence it reaches the outer surfaces of the brain and spinal cord. It is reabsorbed chiefly by a valvular mechanism in the arachnoid villi adjoining the superior sagittal venous sinus. The pressure in the sinus when one is upright is less than atmospheric pressure, but the arrangement of dura in the falx holds the sinus open, and since in the upright posture the CSF pressure is above sagittal sinus pressure, CSF can traverse the valve, along with particulate matter, and enter the venous system. But return flow of blood out from the sagittal sinus into the subarachnoid space is prevented by the valve (fig. 25.99). Similarly, much smaller valves may exist allowing CSF round the spinal cord to find its way into the adjoining veins.

Blockage of the CSF circulation can occur. If the block is within the brain, the ventricular system becomes distended with CSF (**internal hydrocephalus**). If the block is at the drainage channels (for instance, when sagittal sinus thrombosis occurs), a general rise in intracranial pressure appears. In children, in whom the skull sutures are still not firmly united, distension of the skull and separation of the sutures may ensue. The effects of hydrocephalus are discussed in vol. 3, p. 34.119.

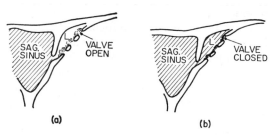

FIG. 25.99. Frontal sections of the superior sagittal sinus and adjacent lacuna lateralis showing (a) the valve open and the lacuna filled with CSF and (b) the valve closed and the lacuna filled with blood. From Welch K. & Friedman V. (1960) *Brain* **83**, 454.

SAMPLING

CSF can be removed for examination conveniently by **lumbar puncture**, which is a safe procedure except when the intracranial pressure is abnormally high. It is also possible to remove fluid, though obviously more perilously, by inserting a needle into the cisterna magna between the atlas and the occiput, and fluid can be removed from the ventricles at operation.

PRESSURE

At lumbar puncture with the patient lying on his side the CSF pressure measured in a simple manometer is normally 6–15 cm of CSF. Compressing the jugular veins produces a marked rise in the pressure (**Queckenstedt's test**) because the venous pressure increases in the cerebral venous sinuses, and the increase is communicated directly to the CSF via the cerebral veins. No rise or a trivial one is seen if the subarachnoid space is blocked by, for instance, a tumour round the spinal cord. In performing Queckenstedt's test, it is as well not to squeeze or even seem to squeeze the trachea, and it is not required to occlude the carotid arteries; firm widespread pressure on both sides of the neck but excluding the trachea is both kind and effective. The test is dangerous when intracranial pressure is high, because the medulla may become displaced down into the foramen magnum where it is subjected to pressure which impairs its blood supply.

COMPOSITION

Table 25.3 shows the normal composition of CSF. Protein is practically absent and so is any constituent of plasma adsorbed on protein, which includes for instance about half of the calcium present in blood. The absence of protein induces certain alterations in the concentrations of ions, in accordance with the Gibbs–Donnan equilibrium (p. 15.9). Is CSF then simply a filtrate of plasma, like the contents of Bowman's capsule in the kidney? This is not the case. Values for ions differ far more than the calculated Gibbs–Donnan alterations would indicate;

TABLE 25.3. Composition of cerebrospinal fluid compared with plasma in a normal subject.

Constituent	Concentration of various constituents	
	in CSF	in plasma
Na^+ mmol/l	140	142
Cl^- mmol/l	115	98
K^+ mmol/l	2·9	4·5
Mg^{++} mmol/l	1·0	0·8
Urea mmol/l	5·0	5·0
Glucose mmol/l	4·5	5·0
pH units	7·33	7·4
P_{CO_2} kPa	6·6	5·3
HCO_3^- mmol/l	22	25

there is less K^+, slightly less HCO_3^-, and more Cl^- and Mg^{++}. Glucose (un-ionized) is clearly less. The P_{CO_2} is higher and pH lower. When the composition of plasma changes, $[K^+]$ and $[HCO_3^-]$ in CSF are slow to follow, but CO_2 enters the CSF rapidly. This distinction between HCO_3 and CO_2 may be significant in the control of respiration (p. 31.28), since receptors exist on the outer surface of the medulla which are linked to the respiratory control system and respond to changes in the composition of the CSF rather than to those in the blood.

These discrepancies between CSF and plasma make it clear that CSF is not a simple filtrate and active secretion must be involved. Further confirmation is available in the fact that CSF composition and rate of formation are influenced by drugs such as acetazoleamide and ouabain which influence Na^+ transport.

A few substances reach the CSF rapidly by diffusion from the adjacent brain tissue, besides entering more gradually with the fluid secreted by the choroid plexuses. Ethyl alcohol is an instance. Others such as penicillin, even when present at a high level in blood, enter the CSF only slowly. So one pictures a blood–CSF barrier, surmounted by different substances with varying ease. Fortunately, inflammation (meningitis) lowers the barrier and penicillin then penetrates more readily into the fluid.

BIOCHEMISTRY OF THE BRAIN

The regional distribution of cell types accounts for some of the differences in the biochemistry of various areas of the brain. The neuronal cell bodies predominate in the grey matter and their dendritic processes occupy most of its volume, whereas myelinated axons and associated oligodendroglial cells are found mainly in the white matter. Much of the high respiratory activity of grey matter can be attributed to its mass of dendrites, and the relatively low oxygen uptake of white matter is explained by its high content of myelin; although glial cells and axoplasm actively respire, myelin is metabolically virtually inert.

STUDIES ON ISOLATED COMPONENTS

Because of the morphological heterogeneity of nervous tissue further elucidation of the metabolism of each cell type and their components comes from studies of isolated single cells. Ultramicro methods of sufficient sensitivity have been devised to investigate the biochemistry of individual cells from histologically identified areas of the brain. An isolated cell can be weighed (0·1 ng) on a quartz fibre balance and optical methods, which can estimate 10^{-19} moles of a substrate, allow its chemical and enzymatic composition to be determined. Thus, base composition of RNA from single nerve cells, from glial cells or even from isolated nuclei can then be determined by electrophoresis on a microscopic cellulose thread (diameter 20 μm). Using nervous tissue suspensions, neurones, astrocytes and oligodendroglial cells can also be separated by gentle centrifugation and the metabolism of each cell type has been examined. Additional information is obtained by differential centrifugation of cell free brain homogenates. The method leads to isolation of myelin, axons and subcellular components such as nuclei, mitochondria and microsomes from mixed cell populations, and enables the part played by each component in the economy of the whole cell to be elucidated (table

TABLE 25.4. Components of the neurones and their functions.

Structure	Constituents	Function
Nucleus	DNA, histones mRNA	Genetic control Ribosome synthesis
Myelin	Lipids and protein	Insulation (?)
Mitochondria	Citric acid cycle enzymes	Energy production
Synaptic endings	Acetylcholine Catecholamines	Neurohormonal transmission
Microsomes	Ribosomes, ATPase	Protein synthesis, lipid synthesis, active transport
Supernatant	Soluble enzymes	Glycolysis

25.4). The role of mitochondria in energy metabolism and of ribosomes in protein synthesis in cells of the brain is now established. Acetylcholine has been demonstrated in the vesicles of some isolated particles from synaptic endings, consistent with its role as a synaptic transmitter.

The metabolism of glial cells is probably closely linked with that of neurones. Thus, biochemical changes in neurones after physiological stimulation produce concomitant changes in the glial cell. It has been found by subjecting rats and rabbits to continual rocking movements that there is a significant increase of neuronal RNA, protein and respiratory enzyme activity in the vestibular nuclei. In contrast to these neuronal changes, RNA content and enzyme activity of the glia were found to fall. Learning and conditioning experiments result in increased synthesis of nuclear RNA in cerebral neurones with specific changes in its purine-pyrimidine base composition;

glia respond with similar but not identical base ratio changes. These experiments have focused interest on the DNA–RNA–protein system as a storage arrangement for information after molecular encoding. It appears that RNA synthesis and hence production of protein play a cardinal role in the expression of higher nervous control. This hypothesis is supported by the fact that neurones synthesize RNA and protein more rapidly than other cells and the rate of synthesis increases on stimulation; also inhibitors of protein synthesis interfere with memory in training experiments. It has been claimed that certain proteins play a key role in the consolidation of short-term memory in this process. For example, increased synthesis of a soluble acidic polypeptide (S-100) in the hippocampus is associated with training of rats. A peptide, scotophobin, has been isolated from the brain of animals trained to avoid the dark and it is alleged that the training response can be transferred by injection of scotophobin into naïve rats. However, behavioural experiments utilizing such transfer factors are difficult to control, and unfortunately there is no convincing alternative to learning the hard way.

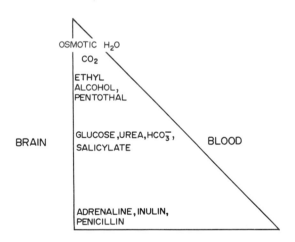

Fig. 25.100. Diagram to indicate the varying 'thickness' of the blood–brain barrier for different molecules and ions.

BLOOD–BRAIN BARRIER

Capillary endothelial cells in the developing brain are loosely joined (allowing passage of macromolecules), but with maturation tight junctions form. Hence the adult brain differs from other organs in the apparent inability of many substances to pass readily from blood to brain tissue. For example, following injection of trypan blue all the tissues except brain are stained, and while glucose is readily utilized, entry of many other substrates into the brain is apparently impeded. The failure of many drugs to penetrate into the brain has lent support to the idea that a barrier protects the brain from the action of foreign substances. The characteristics of this barrier are shown in fig. 25.100 which indicates that osmotic water and CO_2

at the top of the triangle find the barrier very thin and pass it easily, but penicillin and the substances at the bottom find it very thick and barely pass at all in health. Disease may break down the barrier, and two important consequences are that penicillin may enter the brain, and that ^{99m}Tc injected into the blood for the performance of 'brain scan' enters the brain where the barrier is deficient and its presence reveals the location of the damage. Account must also be taken, however, of the fact that the cells of the central nervous system are closely packed. Thus protein-bound dyestuffs cannot readily cross into the astrocytes which invest brain capillaries, whereas in other tissues they pass directly into the extracellular space. The concept of a single blood–brain barrier may, therefore, be incorrect in the sense that the impediment may be due not only to the tightly-sealed endothelial cells and the selective permeability of the astrocytic end feet but also to the special metabolic requirements of the central nervous system. If the cells of the nervous system do not readily oxidize free fatty acids, for example, we need no other explanation for the fact that such molecules enter the brain very slowly.

VULNERABILITY OF THE BRAIN IN FETAL LIFE

The general morphology of the brain is arranged quite early in embryological development and it is not long before the full adult population of neurones is established. The first phase of embryological development and neurone formation is of particular importance, for once the cell population is established, there is little possibility of forming fresh neurones. Growth, arborization of dendrites and formation of synaptic connections follow with the simultaneous onset of electrical activity and the appearance of respiratory enzyme activity.

The brain is therefore especially vulnerable to deprivation of nutrients and oxygen during development since demands on it are particularly great. In the adult brain myelin synthesis and the multiplication of neurones scarcely occur at all. The premature human infant may be particularly at risk because unlike the mature infant it is separated from intrauterine protection at a time of maximum development when it can be expected to be most vulnerable.

CARBOHYDRATE METABOLISM

Glucose is the main energy source for the brain. Some of the glucose is converted by glycolysis to lactate but most, about 90 g/day for the whole brain, is oxidized via the citric acid cycle. Measurements of O_2 and CO_2 consumption of brain tissue *in vitro* and also of intact human brain (p. 30.47) give a respiratory exchange ratio which approximates closely to 1·0 and are consistent with the view that the metabolism is predominantly due to oxidation of glucose at the rate given above. The level of consciousness might be thought to be correlated with oxygen and energy utilization but no gross changes have been found during sleep, mental activity or in various mental states including schizophrenia and drug induced psychosis. However, the nitrous oxide clearance method used (p. 30.38) in these studies measures whole brain blood flow and is not capable of picking up selective changes in special areas. Alterations in regional blood flow can occur as a result of increased neuronal activity; decreased flow with reduced neuronal function occurs in dementia. Since nervous tissue contains only a small carbohydrate store of glycogen of doubtful lability and availability, it is particularly dependent on maintenance of normal blood glucose concentration. Hypoglycaemia or hypoxia, even for a short period of time, result in coma and sometimes irreversible damage. The importance of carbohydrate metabolism in the brain is also apparent in the accumulation there of pyruvate and lactate associated with lack of cocarboxylase, which results from a dietary deficiency of vitamin B_1.

AMINO ACID AND PROTEIN METABOLISM

Although net uptake of many amino acids from blood to brain is restricted, some free amino acids are found in nervous tissue in relatively high concentrations and the total free amino acid concentration in brain is much higher than in most other tissues or blood plasma. Aspartic acid and glutamic acid with its amide glutamine are the most abundant. As much as 75 per cent of the intermediary glycolytic metabolites are utilized within the brain for the formation of dicarboxylic acids such as glutamic acid. Since these acids have a high rate of turnover, it is suggested that the brain is especially adapted to utilize these amino acids. Thus decarboxylation of amino acids leads to the formation of biologically active amines, for example, histamine, 5-hydroxytryptamine (5-HT), which act as local hormones (p. 27.50). Moreover, the repeated synthesis of dicarboxylic amino acids results in a conservation of amino N in the brain, thereby reducing requirements for exogenous amino acids. Proteins account for about 10 per cent of the wet weight of the brain. They are found mainly as:

(1) soluble proteins constituting the numerous enzymes and some of the hormones of the central nervous system,

(2) with lipids as lipoproteins in the insoluble membrane systems of the organ,

(3) microtubular protein in the transport system of axons (p. 15.4).

The many different types of protein in the nervous system have a wide range of metabolic activity. In general the soluble proteins undergo rapid synthesis and turnover, whereas the structural proteins are more stable. Cerebral phosphoproteins, for example, undergo very rapid exchange and may be concerned in ion transport mechanisms within the organ, but some of the protein of the myelin sheath is more stable.

LIPIDS AND THEIR METABOLISM

The brain is rich in lipid, human grey and white matter containing about 10 and 30 per cent respectively. Table 25.5 shows the distribution of lipids in nervous tissue.

TABLE 25.5. Approximate values for the lipid content of parts of the vertebrate nervous system (μmol/100mg wet tissue).

	Brain		Spinal cord	Sciatic nerve
	Cortex	white matter		
Cholesterol	2·4	9·4	18·6	4·9
Cerebrosides	0·3	4·7	9·2	1·5
Phospholipids	4·3	9·7	14·6	6·4
Sphingomyelin	0·4	1·7	3·6	1·2
Plasmalogen	0·8	4·0	—	1·3
Gangliosides	0·3	0·06	—	—

Some of this may be concerned in dynamic processes such as sodium ion transport, or provide essential co-factors in enzyme reactions, but the majority is structural. The most characteristic lipids of nervous tissue are cerebrosides (p. 10.16), galactose-containing sphingolipids; they are found in high concentration in the myelin sheath. Cholesterol and phospholipids are also present in myelin. The protein components and some of the lipids in the myelin lamellae are relatively metabolically stable but cholesterol and certain phospholipids are only loosely incorporated into the membrane structure. Experiments with labelled cholesterol show that the sterol molecules can exchange between myelin and other subcellular membranes. Lipid and protein components of membranes of subcellular particles such as mitochondria undergo turnover but at a much slower rate than in other organs.

CHEMICAL TRANSMISSION WITHIN THE NERVOUS SYSTEM

The chemical mediators of synaptic transmission in the central nervous system are more difficult to identify with certainty than those at the myoneural junction or in the sympathetic ganglion, because it is impracticable to isolate the blood leaving a homogeneous part of the tissue and measure directly the changing levels of a transmitter substance resulting from synaptic transmission. A transport system operates within the axon consisting of a hollow microtubular structure made up of 11–14 globular tubulin subunits and with the probable participation of an actomyosin-like protein (neurostenin). Packages of neurotransmitter attached to protein are thought to be rapidly transported from nerve perikaryon to the synaptic terminal by means of the microtubules coupled with the action of the contractile protein. The axon also contains slender neurofilaments.

Central presynaptic nerve endings contain granules

and vesicles as described on p. 25.15. Acetylcholine, choline acetyltransferase and acetylcholinesterase are found in the central nervous system, particularly in the motor cortex and ventral spinal grey columns, the thalamus and hypothalamus and the geniculate bodies. Acetylcholine and its associated enzymes are found in highest concentration in fractions of brain tissue containing separated nerve endings, and it has been collected from the surface of the brain in small cups in contact with the cerebral cortex of animals and from the CSF of patients who have died after generalized convulsions and epileptic fits. Microelectrodes inserted into the Renshaw cells (p. 25.17) of the spinal cord of the cat show that the cells undergo postsynaptic depolarization when the presynaptic fibres are stimulated, and acetylcholine introduced by iontophoresis through micropipettes into the neighbourhood of the cells can excite them to fire; their activity is also potentiated if the recurrent axon is stimulated electrically and acetylcholinesterase inhibitors are applied.

Besides acetylcholine other substances which are detectable in the brain show characteristics consistent with transmitter function and probably act as chemical mediators. These include noradrenaline and dopamine, 5-hydroxytryptamine, histamine, γ-aminobutyric acid (GABA), glycine and ergothioneine. Noradrenaline is found in highest concentration in the hypothalamus and the brain stem. Dopamine is found mainly in the caudate nucleus, substantia nigra and other nuclei of the midbrain. 5-HT is distributed in regions similar to those of noradrenaline, and notably in parts of the grey matter of the spinal cord, hippocampus, and pineal gland. 5-HT can be shown to be synthesized in the brain from its immediate precursors or 5-hydroxytryptophan and stored in subcellular particles. Histamine is also distributed in general like noradrenaline with highest concentration in the hypothalamus.

Brain extracts also contain the prostaglandins, and evidence suggests that they too may act as chemical transmitters. Applied iontophoretically they may excite or inhibit certain neurones and can be detected in parts of the brain, notably the cerebellum, during electrical stimulation.

Substance *P* is a polypeptide containing eleven amino acids and present in substantia nigra, the hypothalamus and the dorsal roots and columns of the spinal cord. It is also present in the intestines where it may be a transmitter for local reflexes. GABA arising from the decarboxylation of glutamic acid decreases the excitatory state in many parts of the nervous system and has been considered as a possible inhibitory transmitter. Similarly in the spinal cord there is evidence that glycine acts as an inhibitory transmitter.

The cerebellum contains little or none of the pharmacologically active substances found elsewhere in the brain, a surprising fact in view of its enormous number of synapses. Cerebellar extracts however, have been shown to contain ergothioneine, a derivative of histidine, injection of which increases the electrical activity of the cerebellum.

The metabolism and concentration of most of these substances present in different areas of the brain can be altered by numerous drugs. The drugs which cause these chemical changes also affect emotional behaviour and the personality of the patient; they include tranquillizers and mescaline. Detailed study of the mode of action of these drugs is likely to enlarge knowledge of function of these amines and other substances. This subject is more fully discussed in vol. 2, p. 5.14.

AUTONOMIC NERVOUS SYSTEM

The autonomic nervous system (ANS) has been defined as a **visceral efferent system**, concerned with the motor supply of cardiac and smooth muscle and glands. Neither the name nor the definition is fully satisfactory, but they persist because of the difficulty of finding better replacements. The ANS cannot be regarded as fully autonomous and independent of the rest of the nervous system, although much of its activity is involuntary, i.e. not consciously willed. However, the distinction between visceral and somatic is not always clear cut. Abundant afferent neurones link the viscera with the CNS and run for at least part of their course in the company of visceral efferents, but they are not usually regarded as part of the ANS and are described on p. 25.42.

Somatic and visceral efferent systems differ in their anatomical arrangements. The cell body of a visceral efferent neurone lies in a ganglion outside the CNS, but the cell body of the somatic efferent neurone lies within the CNS. The visceral efferent cell bodies are collected in the course of the nerves, forming small ganglia such as the ciliary ganglion and the otic ganglion, or are aggregated to form interconnecting masses lateral to the vertebrae (the paravertebral ganglionic trunks) or on the bodies of the vertebrae (the prevertebral ganglia) (p. 21.41). The preganglionic connector neurones which connect the CNS with the peripheral cells have their cell bodies within the lateral column of grey matter, which their axons leave to synapse at the ganglia; they are myelinated B fibres (p. 15.23) and run in the white ramus communicans (p. 21.5). Postganglionic effector neurones have fine unmyelinated fibres and run in the grey ramus communicans (figs. 20.5, 25.3 and p. 21.41). The length of the preganglionic fibre is variable. The parasympathetic or craniosacral outflow has preganglionic fibres with a long course within the somatic nerve before synapsing with ganglionic cells which are generally close to the organ innervated. Thus the postganglionic fibres are short. The sympathetic thoracolumbar outflow has relatively short preganglionic fibres and conversely often very long postganglionic fibres. Another difference between somatic and visceral neurones is that whilst somatic neurones only innervate one type of cell, namely skeletal muscle, visceral efferent neurones innervate a number of different cells such as smooth and cardiac muscle and secretory or glandular cells.

SYMPATHETIC SYSTEM (table 25.6)

This originates in preganglionic neurones emerging with the ventral roots from the first thoracic to the second lumbar segments. Their cell bodies lie in the visceral

TABLE 25.6. Origin, destination and action of sympathetic outflow.

The levels of outflow may vary in different individuals. Striated muscle in the limbs receives from the sympathetic outflow vasodilator fibres (cholinergic) as well as vasoconstrictor fibres.

Spinal nerve roots carrying outflow	Destination	Action
T1	Iris	Dilates pupils
T1–5	Head and Neck	Produces vasoconstriction and sweating
T2–9	Upper limbs	Produces vasoconstriction and sweating
T2–6	Heart	Increases rate and force of contraction
T5–9	Lungs	Produces bronchial dilation
	Adrenal medulla	Produces secretion
T6–L2	Abdominal viscera	Inhibits motility and secretion and constricts sphincters
T4–L2	Lower limbs	Produces vasoconstriction and sweating
L1–2	Genitourinary tract	Contracts seminal vesicles and uterus and relaxes bladder

efferent column, the lateral grey matter of the spinal cord and the fibres reach adjacent ganglia where they synapse or pass through them to synapse with ganglionic cells higher or lower in the paravertebral chain. The thoracic fibres, for example, ascend to the cervical ganglia which lie in the neck, and in this way a very wide area of the body is covered, although the fibres retain a rough relationship to somatic areas. For example, the upper thoracic sympathetic fibres go to the eye, innervating the pupillary muscle, and the heart and lung receive fibres originating from the second to the ninth thoracic segments. Interruption of the cervical part of the sympathetic chain of ganglia produces a condition known as **Horner's syndrome**; the pupil is smaller on the affected side, because the radial fibres of the iris are denervated, and the upper eyelid droops because levator palpebrae superioris includes a small smooth muscle element which

TABLE 25.7. Origin, route, destination and action of the parasympathetic outflow.

Origin	Leaves CNS with	Route	Ganglion	Destination	Action
Edinger-Westphal nucleus	Nerve III	With nerve III	Ciliary	Ciliary muscle	Accommodation for near vision
				Iris	Constricts pupil
Superior salivatory nucleus	Nerve VII	Greater petrosal nerve	Pterygopalatine	Lacrimal gland	Produces tears
				Nasal mucosa	Produces secretion
		Chorda tympani	Submandibular	Submandibular and sublingual salivary glands	Produces secretion
Inferior salivatory nucleus	Nerve IX	Lesser petrosal nerve	Otic	Parotid salivary gland	Produces secretion
Dorsal motor nucleus of vagus	Nerve X		Adjoining or in destination	Heart	Slows rate and conduction
				Bronchi	Produces constriction
				Alimentary canal down to proximal colon	Stimulates motility and secretion
Spinal cord sacral segments	S2–4	Pelvic splanchnic nerves	Adjoining or in destination	Distal colon and rectum	Produces contraction
				Bladder	Produces contraction
				Genitalia	Produces erection

is now denervated. In addition, the side of the head concerned is incapable of sweating and its cutaneous blood vessels are dilated because normally the sympathetic system keeps them constricted.

Table 25.6 shows the origin, destination and action of the sympathetic outflow. These fibres reach the organs innervated by the following routes.

(1) Some of the postganglionic fibres return to the spinal nerve, accompanying its various branches until it ends in its effector organ. Thus injury to a peripheral nerve may be accompanied by visceral changes, such as loss of sweating, within the distribution of that nerve.

(2) Other postganglionic fibres form discrete nerves or plexuses, often around blood vessels, following their course until they reach their terminations in other parts of the body. The postganglionic fibres arising from the superior cervical ganglion are an example, for they form a plexus around the carotid artery until they finally enter the orbit to supply the pupil.

(3) Not all preganglionic fibres end in the paravertebral ganglia, however, for in certain areas other ganglionic masses exist; the coeliac ganglion, for example, accepts preganglionic fibres from the splanchnic nerves and is a prevertebral ganglion. From these prevertebral ganglia arise postganglionic fibres which apply themselves to adjacent arteries and pass with them to various organs.

PARASYMPATHETIC SYSTEM

This arises from the brain stem and the sacral segments of the cord. The brain stem visceral efferents emerge with the oculomotor, the facial, the glossopharyngeal and the vagus nerves. Table 25.7 summarizes the origin, route, destination and action of the parasympathetic outlets.

The central connections of the autonomic nervous system have already been mentioned in the section on brain stem and spinal cord. Important connections exist with the hypothalamus via the hypothalamotegmental tract and the dorsal longitudinal fasciculus and also with the reticular system. Relatively little is known about the course of the tracts although there seems little doubt that the efferent spinal pathway is largely through the reticulospinal tracts.

DISTINCTIONS BETWEEN THE SOMATIC AND THE AUTONOMIC MOTOR SYSTEM

The transmitter substance at the motor end plate in striated muscle is acetylcholine. The transmitter in the autonomic system, however, is not everywhere acetylcho-

TABLE 25.8. Chemical transmission in the autonomic nervous system.

	Preganglionic fibres	Postganglionic fibres	Effector organs
Para-sympathetic	Acetylcholine	Acetylcholine	Heart Smooth muscle Glands
Sympathetic	Acetylcholine	Acetylcholine	Sweat glands Blood vessels to skeletal muscle (p. 30.49)
		Noradrenaline	Heart Smooth muscle Blood vessels Some glands

line. It is acetylcholine in the autonomic ganglia where the intermediate synapses of the autonomic system occur; but at the termination of the second, post-ganglionic fibre it is frequently noradrenaline (table 25.8).

So there are three distinctions between the somatic motor system and the autonomic system. (1) A synaptic junction is interposed between the CNS and the organ controlled by the autonomic system; the somatic system has no such interposed junction. (2) The transmitter in the autonomic system is not always acetylcholine. (3) The effect exerted by the autonomic system may be to reduce or slow activity or else to start it.

Visceral afferent fibres frequently accompany the efferent fibres of the autonomic system. For example, the vagus nerve contains many afferent fibres, e.g. those for the Hering-Breuer reflex (p. 31.26). Again, a peripheral nerve trunk usually contains some vasomotor efferent fibres, and so when it is cut vasodilation occurs in the skin area concerned. Painful stimulation of the skin provokes reflex vasoconstriction; the afferent path is in somatic sensory nerves, the efferent in the sympathetic outflow.

GENERAL ACTION OF THE SYMPATHETIC SYSTEM

Elements of the sympathetic part of the system can of course function in isolation from each other, but they can be thought of as a whole in some definite senses. The chief transmitter at the end organ is noradrenaline, a hormone which along with adrenaline circulates in the blood stream, especially in states of alarm or defence, because it is released by the medulla of the adrenal glands (p. 27.30). The cells of the adrenal medulla behave as neurones in sympathetic ganglia without axons, i.e. they respond to stimulation via the preganglionic fibres by secreting catecholamines into the blood stream instead of by originating nerve impulses in postganglionic fibres. When the whole system is active together the picture is one of increasing the defences of the body to protect itself: the heart rate and arterial blood pressure rise, the pupils enlarge, the bronchioles dilate, sweating occurs, hair is erected and gut mobility is inhibited.

GENERAL ACTION OF THE PARASYMPATHETIC SYSTEM

In contrast, overall parasympathetic activity corresponds roughly to the picture of an old man asleep after dinner, i.e. slow heart, small pupils, constricted bronchioles and noisy breathing, salivary secretion, vigorous peristalsis. In this case there is no circulating hormone in the blood, for acetylcholine is rapidly hydrolysed by cholinesterase in the blood stream.

FURTHER READING

ADRIAN E.D. (1947) *The Physical Background of Perception*. London: Oxford University Press.

BARR M.L. (1974) *The Human Nervous System*, 2nd Edition. New York: Harper & Row.

BATESON P.P.G. (1966) Imprinting. *Biological Reviews* **41**, 177–220.

BELLAIRS R. & GRAY E.G. (1974) *Essays on the Nervous System*. London: Oxford University Press.

BRODAL A. (1969) *Neurological Anatomy*, 2nd Edition. London: Oxford University Press.

DAVISON A.N. (ed.) (1976) *Biochemistry and Neurological Disease*. Oxford: Blackwell Scientific Publications.

DAVSON H. (1966) Formation and drainage of the cerebrospinal fluid. In *Scientific Basis of Medicine Annual Reviews*, p. 238. London: Athlone Press.

ECCLES J.C. (1973) *The Understanding of the Brain*. New York: McGraw-Hill.

ELLIOTT B. (1974). Lost bouquets (a vivid account of how it feels to lose the sense of smell). In Potter J.M. *The Practical Management of Head Injuries*, 3rd Edition, p. 86. London: Lloyd-Luke.

GREGORY R.L. (1966) *Eye and Brain*. London: World University Library.

HILTON S.M. (1965) Emotion. In *The Physiology of Human Survival*, ed. Edholm O.G. & Bacharach A.L., p. 464. New York: Academic Press.

HUBEL D.H. (1960) *The Visual Cortex of the Brain*. Scientific American Offprint No. 168.

JOHNSON R.H. & SPALDING J.M.K. (1974) *Disorders of the Autonomic Nervous System*. Oxford: Blackwell Scientific Publications.

McILWAIN H. & BACHELARD H.S. (1971) *Biochemistry and the Central Nervous System*, 4th Edition. London: Churchill Livingstone.

NATHAN P. (1969) *The Nervous System*. Harmondsworth: Penguin.

OSWALD, I. (1966) *Sleep*. Harmondsworth: Pelican.

PETERSON L.R. (1966) Short-term memory. *Scientific American* **215**, 90–95.

WALSH E.G. (1964) *Physiology of the Nervous System*, 2nd Edition. London: Longman.

WRIGHT R.H. (1964) *The Sense of Smell*. London: Allen & Unwin.

WURTMAN R.J., AXELROD J. & KELLY D.E. (1968) *The Pineal*. New York: Academic Press.

YOUNG J.Z. (1964) *A Model of the Brain*. London: Oxford University Press.

Chapter 26
Visual and auditory systems

ORBIT, EYE AND VISION

The bony orbit is an extension of the cranium which surrounds the eye, its associated muscles, nerves and vessels, and the lacrimal apparatus. It is like a hollow pyramid with the base anteriorly and the apex posteriorly. The medial walls of the two bony orbits are parallel, while the lateral walls, if projected backwards, would meet at a right angle. The anterior cranial fossa lies above the orbit, while the bone of the upper jaw, including the maxillary air sinus, lies below. Medial to each orbit are the ethmoidal air sinuses and the upper part of the nasal cavity, and lateral is the temporal fossa. The apex of the orbit communicates with the middle cranial fossa.

The following features of the bony orbit are of importance (fig. 26.1).

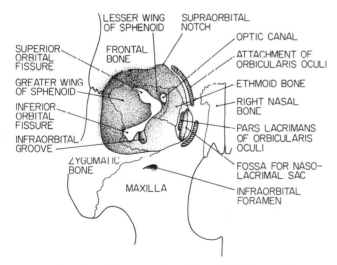

Fig. 26.1. Diagrammatic outline of the bony orbit.

(1) The **optic canal** is situated just medial to the apex of the orbit. It is a rounded aperture which transmits the optic nerve, with its meningeal coverings, and the ophthalmic artery.

(2) Immediately lateral to the optic canal is a right-angled slit. The angle points medially, and lies at the apex of the orbit. The upper limb of the slit between the roof and the lateral wall is the **superior orbital fissure**,

which links the orbit with the middle cranial fossa; the lower, between the lateral wall and the floor, is the **inferior orbital fissure**, leading into the pterygopalatine and infratemporal fossae. From the middle of the inferior orbital fissure, the **infraorbital groove** runs forwards in the floor of the orbit and continues into the **infraorbital canal**, which opens onto the face at the **infraorbital foramen**.

(3) On the upper part of the medial wall of the orbit, two small apertures, the anterior and posterior ethmoidal foramina, lead into the anterior cranial fossa.

(4) Also on the medial wall, just behind the medial margin of the orbit, is a hemicylindrical groove which lodges the lacrimal sac. It is limited behind by the posterior lacrimal crest of the lacrimal bone, in front by the anterior lacrimal crest of the maxilla.

(5) The inner surface of the bony orbit is lined by a loosely attached periosteum, which is continuous through the superior orbital fissure with the dura of the middle cranial fossa.

(6) All the space within the orbit not occupied by other structures is filled with orbital fat, which supports the eyeball and extends to the orbital septum in front, but not into the eyelids.

Soft tissue structures of the orbit (figs. 26.2, 3 and 4)
When the eyelids are closed, the orbits are shut off from the face by the dense fibrous tissue plates or **tarsi** which support the eyelids, and by the thin **orbital septum** which connects the periphery of the tarsi to the orbital margins.

The tarsi and the orbital septum are covered superficially by the orbicularis oculi muscle. From the medial ends of the tarsi, the **medial palpebral ligament** stretches in front of the lacrimal sac to be attached to the anterior lacrimal crest. A less well defined **lateral palpebral ligament** stretches to the lateral margin of the orbit.

The internal surface of the eyelids is lined by the **palpebral conjunctiva**; this is continuous at the superior and inferior fornices with the **bulbar conjunctiva**, which covers the eyeball. The stratified columnar conjunctival epithelium meets the stratified squamous epithelium of the cornea at the corneoscleral junction. When the eyelids are closed, the conjunctiva is virtually a closed sac.

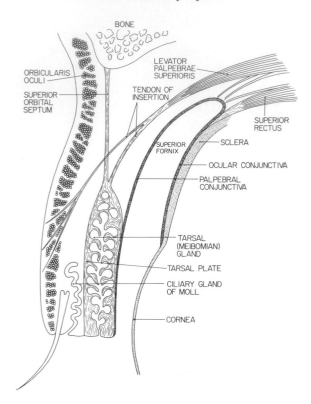

FIG. 26.2. Section of upper eyelid.

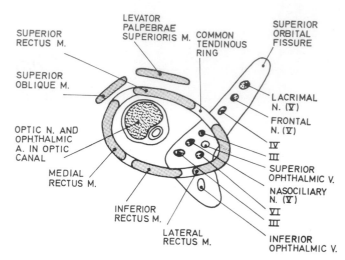

FIG. 26.4. The rectus cone and the superior orbital fissure.

The hair follicles of the eyelashes which open onto the free edges of the eyelids are interspersed with the modified sweat glands (of Moll). Embedded in the deep surface of the tarsal plates, and opening onto the free edges of the eyelids, are the large **tarsal glands** which are sebaceous glands (meibomian glands) not associated with hair follicles in man.

The **levator palpebrae superioris muscle** which raises the upper eyelid arises from the roof of the orbit just above the attachment of the fibrous ring of the recti (fig. 26.4). It is a narrow ribbon of muscle at its origin, but widens as it passes anteriorly. From its edges, expansions spread out to the medial and lateral margins of the orbit. The central part of the muscle passes anterior to the superior tarsus, partially inserting itself into its superficial surface, and spreading through the overlying fibres of the orbicularis oculi muscle to be attached more diffusely to the skin of the upper eyelid (fig. 26.2). From the deep surface of the intraorbital part of the muscle a sheet of smooth muscle fibres passes to the upper edge of the tarsus. The fibrous tissue sheath of the levator palpebrae superioris muscle blends with that of the underlying superior rectus muscle, and the resulting fibrous tissue lamella is attached to the superior fornix of the conjunctiva. As a result, elevation of both the upper lid and the fornix occurs when one looks upwards.

The skeletal muscle component is supplied by the oculomotor nerve, the smooth muscle component by sympathetic fibres derived from the internal carotid plexus.

Lacrimal apparatus

The structures responsible for the production and drainage of tears include the lacrimal gland, the conjunctival sac, the lacrimal puncta on the medial ends of the upper and lower eyelids, the canaliculi leading from them, the

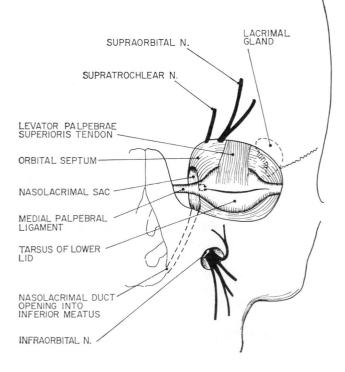

FIG. 26.3. Frontal view of the left orbit with eye closed.

lacrimal sac into which they drain and the nasolacrimal duct which carries the lacrimal fluid to the nasal cavity (fig. 26.5).

The gland is situated in a shallow fossa in the upper lateral part of the orbit, and is partially subdivided into

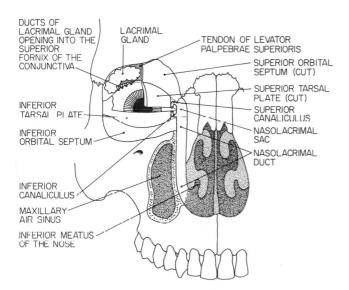

FIG. 26.5. Lacrimal apparatus of the right side. Part of the right maxilla has been cut away in order to show the course of the right nasolacrimal duct and, incidentally, reveals part of the right maxillary air sinus.

an orbital and a palpebral part by the lateral edge of the levator palpebrae superioris muscle. About twelve ducts open into the lateral part of the superior fornix of the conjunctiva. They pass within or very close to the palpebral part of the gland before they terminate. Secretions irrigate the conjunctival sac and the cornea as they flow from the upper lateral to the medial side of the sac, where they enter the lacrimal canaliculi, through the lacrimal puncta, by capillary attraction. To operate effectively, the lacrimal puncta must be closely applied to the surface of the conjunctiva. This is effected by the tone of the lacrimal part of the orbicularis oculi muscles and paralysis of the muscle, due to facial nerve damage, results in overflow of tears on the cheek. The reflex contraction of the main sheet of orbicularis oculi helps to move the lacrimal secretions across the conjunctiva and cornea. Through the canaliculi, the secretions reach the lacrimal sac in its fossa at the medial side of the orbit, and from here they pass down the nasolacrimal duct to be discharged into the inferior meatus of the nose.

The secretion of the lacrimal gland is a clear watery fluid with an electrolyte content similar to that of plasma. It irrigates the eyeball, washing out dust, microorganisms and other foreign particles. Tears contain less than 1 per cent protein, but, as Sir Alexander Fleming first reported, they contain an enzyme **muramidase**

capable of lysing many types of bacteria. Lacrimation may be caused by a variety of chemical and mechanical irritants. Secretomotor innervation is provided by parasympathetic fibres of the facial (seventh cranial) nerve.

Fascial sheath of the eyeball

The whole of the eye, except the cornea and the optic nerve and its sheath, is enclosed in a thin sheath of fascia. Anteriorly, the sheath blends with the sclera and conjunctiva at the corneoscleral junction. Posteriorly it is loosely connected to the dura mater of the optic nerve sheath, a few millimetres behind the lamina cribrosa. The **episcleral space**, containing a layer of fine connective tissue strands, most obvious posteriorly, intervenes between the sheath and the sclera. The vessels and nerves of the eyeball, and the tendons of the extrinsic ocular muscles, must traverse the fascial sheath and the episcleral space. Extensions of the sheath surround the flattened tendons of the extraocular muscles. The sheath supports the eyeball and probably moves with it, in the surrounding orbital fat. Stretching from the lateral to the medial walls of the orbit is the **suspensory ligament**. This condensation involves the fascial sheaths around the inferior rectus and the inferior oblique tendons and resembles a hammock supporting the eyeball. Provided that it is intact, even destruction of the maxilla fails to affect the position of the eye. From the medial and lateral rectus muscles triangular fascial connections blend with the bony attachments of the suspensory ligaments. These are the **medial** and **lateral check ligaments**, which limit the amount of movement of the eye. The union of the sheaths of the superior rectus and the levator palpebrae superioris with the upper part of the fascial sheath, and the union of the sheaths of the inferior rectus and oblique tendons with the suspensory ligament on the lower aspect of the eyeball, similarly limit upwards and downwards movement.

Extrinsic ocular muscles and movements of the eyeballs

The eyeball is nearly spherical and about 2·4 cm in diameter. It can be moved within the orbit by the extrinsic ocular muscles (fig. 26.6). The range of movement is about 50° in any direction away from straight forwards.

The **rectus muscles**, **superior**, **inferior**, **medial** and **lateral** are arranged round the eyeball to form the **rectus cone**. The apex of this cone is formed by a tough fibrous ring which surrounds the optic canal and the medial part of the superior orbital fissure. Each rectus muscle arises from the corresponding part of the ring and runs anteriorly to be inserted into the sclerotic coat of the eyeball about 0·5 cm from the corneoscleral junction. The cone is completed by a sheet of fine fibrous tissue which invests the recti, and connects them to each other, separating the fat within the cone around the optic nerve

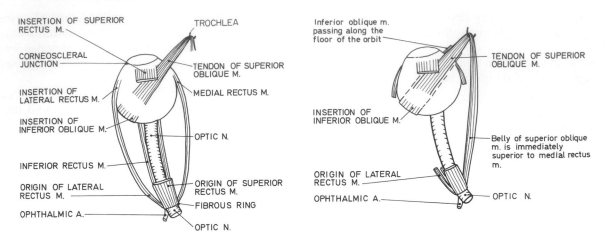

FIG. 26.6. Extraocular muscles of left eye seen from above.

from the remainder of the orbital fat; it can limit the spread of infection. Structures entering the orbit within the fibrous ring commence their course within the rectus cone. Those structures which enter outside the fibrous ring remain outside the cone.

The **superior oblique muscle** arises from the roof of the orbit, above and medial to the optic canal, and runs forwards in the upper medial corner of the orbit to a point just posterior to its medial margin. There the muscle becomes tendinous and is suspended from the frontal bone by a fibrous ring-like pulley, the **trochlea**. At the trochlea the superior oblique tendon changes direction entirely and runs backwards, laterally and downwards. It becomes flattened, and passes below the superior rectus muscle, between it and the eyeball, to be inserted into the posterior half of the upper lateral quadrant of the eyeball.

The **inferior oblique muscle** arises from the maxilla in the floor of the orbit, just lateral to the lacrimal fossa, and runs laterally. It passes below the inferior rectus muscle, but medial to the lateral rectus. It is inserted into the upper quadrant of the eyeball, mainly in its posterior half. Thus, although their routes to their respective linear attachments are different, both oblique muscles are inserted very close together on the eyeball.

The nerve supply of the extrinsic ocular muscles is as follows:

Superior rectus	
Inferior rectus	Oculomotor (third cranial) nerve
Inferior oblique	
Medial rectus	
Superior oblique	Trochlear (fourth cranial) nerve
Lateral rectus	Abducent (sixth cranial) nerve

ACTIONS OF THE EXTRINSIC MUSCLES

Starting from its basic straight forward direction, the gaze of each eye can be deviated upwards, downwards, medially and laterally. The eye can also rotate round the direction of gaze to a small extent (torsion). In medial deviation the medial rectus, and in lateral deviation the lateral rectus, can act alone. In looking upwards and downwards the situation is less simple. Owing to the oblique orientation of the orbits, the superior and inferior recti pass medial to a vertical axis running through the centre of the eyeball (fig. 26.7). So, when

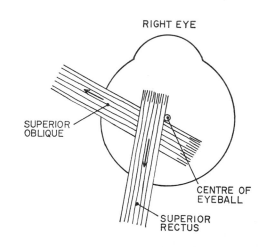

FIG. 26.7. The right eyeball seen from above to show muscle arrangements. The arrows show direction of pull.

the eyeball is in the neutral forward-looking position, the superior rectus turns the gaze upwards, but at the same time slightly inwards, and even rolls the eyeball inwards round the direction of gaze. The inward deviation can be corrected by the lateral rectus and the rolling by the inferior oblique. Thus to direct the gaze upwards requires the precise collaboration of three contracting muscles, and corresponding relaxation by their three antagonists. However, when the eye is abducted, the action of the superior rectus alone is responsible for upward gaze (vol. 3, p. 34.58).

Paralysis of extrinsic ocular muscles

The effects of paralysis (palsy) of an eye muscle or muscles can be deduced from careful study of the anatomy and from two general principles about the **diplopia** (double vision) which ensues. First, the two images come apart when the victim turns his gaze in the direction towards which the palsied muscle or muscles would have moved the eye. Second, the image which seems to him away from where he is looking belongs to the eye which has the palsied muscle or muscles. These principles are illustrated in fig. 26.8 for a right lateral rectus palsy. The

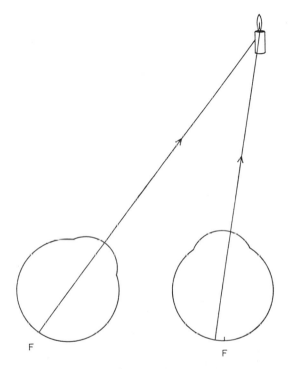

FIG. 26.8. Right lateral rectus palsy. Alignment of the eyes from above. F, fovea (p. 26.10.).

normal left eye is directed straight at the candle, whose image thus falls on its fovea. The right eye cannot turn outwards, and so the image falls to the left of its fovea, the normal position for the image of anything further to the right than the direction of gaze. So this is the image that is seen as further to the right than the other, and away from where the victim is looking. It is evident that if the victim looks to his left instead of to his right, his right medial rectus will function normally and deflect his right eye to the left, and so there will be little or no double vision in this situation.

Careful reckoning along similar lines will show that the victim of a right superior oblique paralysis will be able to shoot at partridges above his head, but not to park his car, since he will see two kerbs on his left hand side, and what is even worse, one of the kerbs will be rotated in relation to the other. The effects of more com-

plex paralyses, such as those of the whole oculomotor nerve and the four muscles it supplies, are described in vol. 3, pp. 33.15 and 34.58.

Nerve supply of the orbit

Three nerves, one motor and two sensory, enter the orbit through the lateral part of the superior orbital fissure, above and lateral to the fibrous ring of the rectus muscles. They are distributed outside the rectus cone.

The **trochlear nerve** passes medially above the levator palpebrae superioris to supply the superior oblique muscle. It contains motor and proprioceptive fibres for this muscle alone.

The **frontal** and **lacrimal nerves** are lateral to the trochlear nerve in the fissure. They are two of the terminal branches of the ophthalmic division of the trigeminal nerve. The larger frontal branch runs forwards below the roof of the orbit and divides into a small supratrochlear and a large supraorbital branch, which together supply the upper eyelid and the anterior half of the scalp. The lacrimal nerve is lateral to the frontal and runs to the lateral part of the orbit to supply the lacrimal gland, and the lateral part of the upper eyelid. It communicates in the orbit with the zygomatic branch of the maxillary nerve, so receiving from the pterygopalatine ganglion secretomotor fibres to the lacrimal gland.

A large group enters the orbit through the fibrous ring of the recti, and therefore lies within the rectus cone.

The **nasociliary nerve** is the third terminal branch of the ophthalmic division of the trigeminal nerve and, like the remainder of the nerve, is purely sensory (fig. 26.9). It

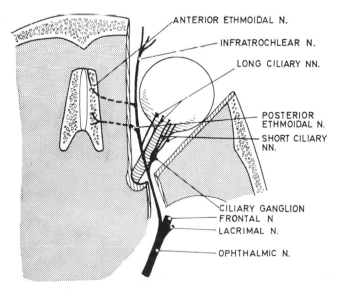

FIG. 26.9. The nasociliary nerve.

connects with the ciliary ganglion, but the fibres transmitted pass through the ganglion without interruption. Following the ophthalmic artery, it passes medially above the optic nerve, and gives an anterior ethmoidal branch which passes through the anterior cranial fossa and the nasal cavity and ends (as the external nerve) by supplying the skin of the tip of the nose. In addition to its sensory root to the ciliary ganglion the nasociliary nerve sends two long ciliary branches to the back of the eyeball. In the medial half of the orbit, it gives off a posterior ethmoidal branch to the sphenoidal and posterior ethmoidal air sinuses, and an infratrochlear branch to the skin at the root of the nose. The main trunk continues through the anterior ethmoidal foramen to be distributed with the corresponding vessels to the ophthalmic area of supply in the interior of the nasal cavity.

The **oculomotor nerve** enters the orbit as two branches, an upper and a lower, both within the rectus cone. The upper division supplies the superior rectus and the levator palpebrae superioris, the lower division is distributed to the medial and inferior recti and the inferior oblique muscles. In addition, preganglionic parasympathetic efferent fibres, originating in the accessory oculomotor nucleus (Edinger-Westphal, p. 26.13) pass through the lower division of the nerve to the ciliary ganglion, where they synapse with cells whose processes are distributed via the short ciliary nerves to the sphincter pupillae and ciliary muscles of the eyeball. The cells of the ciliary ganglion are larger than those of other autonomic ganglia, and their axons are myelinated. This is in accord with their relatively fast response to the stimuli of illumination and accommodation requirements, as compared with the speed of other autonomic reflexes.

The **ciliary ganglion** is a parasympathetic relay station for the pathway just described. It is situated on the lateral side of the optic nerve and its sole functional connection is with preganglionic parasympathetic fibres of the oculomotor nerve. Its other 'roots', sensory and sympathetic, merely use the ganglion and its short ciliary branches as a pathway to the eyeball.

The **abducent nerve** is distributed only to the lateral rectus muscle, which it supplies as it enters the orbit.

The **sympathetic supply** of the orbit is derived ultimately from the first and second thoracic segments of the spinal cord, that is to say, from the most cephalic part of the thoracolumbar outflow, and enters the cranial cavity as the internal carotid plexus. It reaches the orbit as a separate sympathetic root which passes through the apex of the rectus cone, and as a plexus around the ophthalmic artery. It supplies the dilator pupillae muscle of the eye, the smooth muscle in the levator palpebrae superioris, the vessels of the eyeball and orbit, and the strands of smooth muscle known as the orbitalis, which surrounds and constricts the veins passing through the superior and inferior orbital fissures. Paralysis of the orbital sympathetic fibres produces Horner's triple syndrome of constricted pupil (miosis), drooping upper eyelid (ptosis) and a sunken eye (enophthalmos).

Blood supply of the orbit

The **ophthalmic artery** shares the optic canal with the optic nerve and its meningeal sheaths and so enters the orbit within the rectus cone, and on the lateral side of the optic nerve. It gives a **lacrimal branch** which keeps to the lateral side of the nerve and the eyeball, and then, having crossed above the optic nerve, runs forward on the medial side of the eyeball. The distribution of both arteries is to the extraocular muscles and skin, the dura mater, part of the lacrimal apparatus and to the choroidal circulation of the eyeball. In addition, the ophthalmic artery supplies the retina, part of the nasal cavity and some of the paranasal sinuses. The important branches to the eyeball are as follows.

(1) The **central artery of the retina** is an end artery (p. 30.20) and is effectively the sole source of supply to the retina (although the photoreceptors are nourished by the choroidal circulation). Its terminal branches and their accompanying veins can be seen with the ophthalmoscope.

(2) The **ciliary arteries** supply the choroidal circulation and enter the eyeball posteriorly around the optic nerve and anteriorly just behind the corneoscleral junction. The lateral group of anterior choroidal arteries comes from the lacrimal branch of the ophthalmic artery.

The **ophthalmic veins** drain posteriorly through the superior orbital fissure to the cavernous sinus. They receive the central retinal vein and the venae vorticosae of the eyeball and all the venae comitantes from the ophthalmic arterial area, except the cutaneous ones, most of which flow into the facial vein. These latter, however, communicate with the ophthalmic veins and link the cavernous sinus to the superficial veins in the danger area of the face, above the ear-mouth line.

Development and anatomy of the eye

The eye first appears as the **optic vesicle**, a hollow outgrowth of the ventral part of the wall of the fore-brain (fig. 26.10). The wall of the vesicle has the same basic layers as the brain, i.e. ependymal, mantle and marginal, and its cavity is continuous with the third ventricle. The vesicle produces inductive substances which cross the microscopic gap between it and the surface ectoderm and induce a local thickening of the ectoderm, the **lens placode**. Invagination of the outer wall of the vesicle converts it into a two layered **optic cup**. At the same time the lens placode sinks beneath the surface forming an ectodermal cyst, the **lens vesicle**, which lies within the open mouth of the optic cup, the future **pupil**.

The following summary of subsequent development is intended to help in understanding the complexities of eye anatomy in the adult.

(1) The inner and outer layers of the cup become closely applied to one another, obliterating the original cavity of the vesicle.

(2) The two epithelial layers form: (a) in front, surrounding the pupil, the two epithelial layers of the future iris (pars iridica retinae), (b) in the deeper two thirds or so of the cup, the two epithelial layers of the retina proper (pars optica retinae) and (c) between these two areas, the two epithelial layers which line the ciliary body (pars ciliaris retinae) (fig. 26.11).

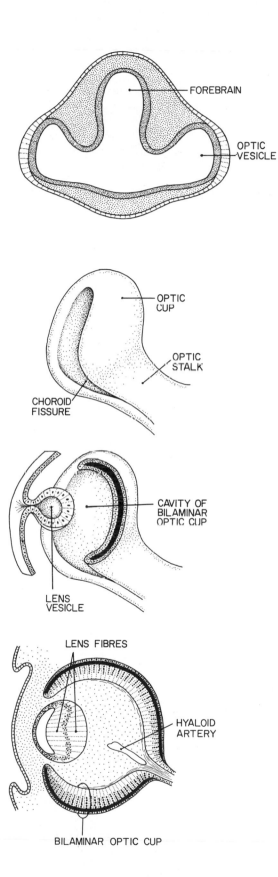

FIG. 26.10. Development of the eye.

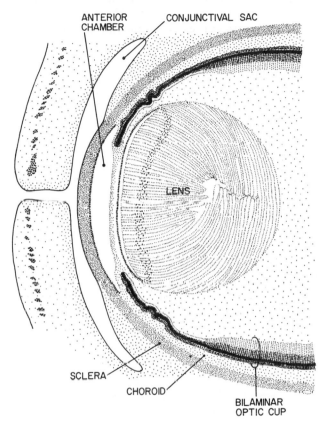

FIG. 26.11. Formation of the structure of the eye in the adult.

(3) The optic stalk, the narrowed derivative of the originally wide connection between brain and optic vesicle, provides the route by which optic nerve axons, developing from ganglion cells in the inner layer of the cup, reach the brain.

(4) That part of the cavity of the optic cup deep to the lens is filled by **vitreous humour**, a transparent jelly, largely of mesodermal origin.

(5) Condensation of mesoderm outside the cup forms an outer tough protective coat (**tunica fibrosa**), i.e. the **sclera** and the **cornea**, and an inner nutritive layer of pigmented vascular connective tissue (**tunica vasculosa**). This forms the **choroid**, the **ciliary body** and the **stroma of the iris**.

(6) The **anterior** and **posterior chambers** develop by cavitation of the mesoderm between the cornea superficially and the front of the lens and of its suspensory ligament deeply.

(7) Cells of the deep wall of the lens vesicle elongate greatly to form **lens fibres**. The epithelium of the outer wall of the vesicle persists throughout life as the **anterior lens epithelium**. New fibres are continually formed from cells at the equator of the lens.

Chambers of the eye (figs. 26.11 and 12)

The interior of the eye is divided into three chambers: anterior, posterior and vitreous. The **anterior chamber** lies between the cornea in front and the iris behind; where the iris is absent at the **pupil**, the anterior chamber is bounded by the front surface of the lens. The iris appears blue at birth in the white races of mankind, because its deep layer is pigmented, as already mentioned, and light of other colours is diffracted rather than reflected. Thus it prevents the entry of light into the eye by any path except through the pupil. Later in life the iris may remain blue; if its substance becomes more opaque, it appears grey; if pigment is deposited in its substance, or is there at birth as in negro races, it appears brown. The iris is provided with radially arranged smooth muscle fibres of the **dilator pupillae** which enlarges the pupil and is innervated by sympathetic fibres which enter the eyeball posteriorly in the long ciliary nerves. There are also circularly arranged muscle fibres of the **sphincter pupillae** which constricts the pupil and is supplied by parasympathetic fibres of the oculomotor nerve via the ciliary ganglion.

The **posterior chamber** is a narrow space behind the iris and in front of the lens and its suspensory ligament. The ciliary processes of the ciliary body project into its lateral angle.

The anterior and posterior chambers are occupied by **aqueous humour**. The **vitreous humour** consists of transparent thin jelly and lies in the vitreous chamber.

Production and disposal of the aqueous humour

The ciliary processes and posterior surface of the iris are the principal source of the aqueous humour (fig. 26.12). It is secreted into the posterior chamber and resembles an ultrafiltrate of plasma containing only 100–200 mg of protein per litre. Although the capillaries of the ciliary body, like those of the renal glomerulus and choroid plexus (p. 25.86), are fenestrated and contain blood at a relatively high pressure for capillaries (6·7 kPa, 50 mmHg), ultrafiltration is not the whole story. It fails to explain why the glucose content of aqueous humour is low, the $[Na^+]$ high, the ascorbic acid content some 12–20 times higher than that in plasma, and why carbonic anhydrase inhibitors, e.g. acetazolamide, interfere with the production of aqueous humour. There is also a potential difference of some 6–15 mV between aqueous (positive) and blood. Active secretion is evidently involved, at a rate of perhaps 2·5 μl/min. The ciliary epithelium shows elaborate infolding of apical and

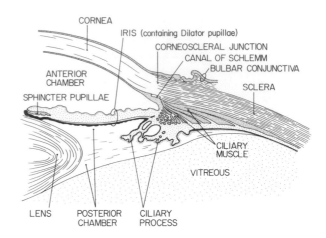

FIG. 26.12. General view of a section through the iridocorneal angle.

lateral plasma membranes, an appearance consistent with an active secretory role.

From the posterior chamber, the aqueous humour passes between the free edge of the iris and the lens into the anterior chamber. It is removed at the **iridocorneal angle** by passing through the spaces in the **trabecular meshwork** of connective tissue. These spaces, lined by mesenchymal epithelium continuous with that lining the anterior chamber, communicate with the **sinus venosus sclerae** (canal of Schlemm), an endothelially lined space in the sclera, close to the corneoscleral junction. This scleral sinus drains into veins within the sclera which join the anterior ciliary veins (fig. 26.13).

The humour clearly plays a part in the maintenance of the avascular tissues bathed by it, i.e. the lens and the cornea. It is normally at a pressure of 1·3–2·6 kPa (10–20 mmHg), which is the **intraocular pressure.** If the drainage channels are clogged or inadequate to carry the

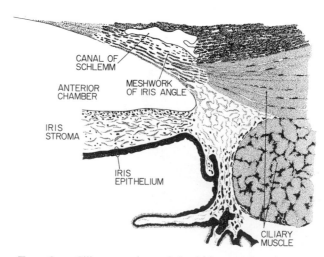

FIG. 26.13. Ciliary muscles and the iridocorneal angle.

whole amount secreted, the intraocular pressure rises. The same outcome may appear when the path followed by the humour round the margin of the pupil is blocked by inflammatory adhesions. Raised intraocular pressure, which is a feature of a condition known as **glaucoma**, can seriously damage the retina and optic nerve disc (vol. 3, p. 33.10).

Lens system

The **lens** is transparent and biconvex in shape, the front less sharply curved than the back. It consists of bundles of long thin transparent 'fibres' which are living cells; fresh fibres go on being formed very slowly throughout adult life and thus the lens continues to enlarge. The lens is enclosed in a transparent thin **lens capsule** and together they form an elastic body which becomes more globular and highly curved when released from the **suspensory ligament**, which attaches it to recesses between the ciliary processes of the ciliary body. Within the ciliary body are smooth muscle fibres, the **ciliary muscle**. Some of the fibres run circularly in a sphincter-like arrangement. Others, the meridional fibres, arise from the scleral spur, medial to the venous sinus, and run through the ciliary body to the choroid. Contraction of both groups of fibres reduces the tension in the suspensory ligament, allowing the lens to become more globular (figs. 26.12 and 13).

ACCOMMODATION

The optical system of the eye is capable of bringing entering rays of light to a sharp focus at the receptors in the retina. Most of the refraction occurs as the light passes from the outside air into the cornea, and this part does not vary, but part occurs at the lens which can change its shape and hence its refractive power. When the ciliary muscle contracts, both curvatures of the lens increase, especially the anterior curvature, and so does its refractive power. This change is accommodation. In the infant the lens is so elastic that objects can be sharply focused by accommodation when they are as near as 7 cm to the eye. A baby can see clearly the toys which he holds close to his nose, although he may look cross-eyed while he does so. The change in lens shape and in light paths during accommodation is shown diagrammatically in fig. 26.14.

By middle age the elasticity of the lens becomes much less, and the unaided eye can no longer see near objects sharply, however well the ciliary muscle contracts (**presbyopia**). Accordingly, a convex spectacle lens is used and this provides the extra refractive power for close-up vision which the eye can no longer supply. But this extra power is not required for distance vision and indeed blurs the distant scene. So when accommodation is lost bifocal lenses may be prescribed, the upper part for distant vision, the lower for reading.

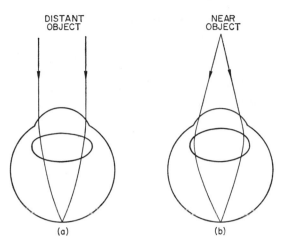

FIG. 26.14. Light paths in the (a) unaccommodated and (b) accommodated eye; note change in lens curvature.

ERRORS OF REFRACTION

A normal eye produces a sharp image at the retina when the object is at infinity, without using any accommodation at all. However, not all eyes are normal; some are too long from front to back for their refractive power, or possess too much refractive power for their dimensions. These are termed **myopic** or short-sighted and can be corrected by providing a negative, concave spectacle lens. Without the lens these eyes cannot bring the image of a distant object to a focus at the retina, but they have a 'far point'; inside the far point, an object can be sharply focused. A normal eye's 'far point' is at infinity.

Other eyes are too short, or have too little refractive power for their dimensions, and cannot provide a sharp image of near objects (**hypermetropia**, long sight). They are corrected by a positive, convex spectacle lens.

ASTIGMATISM

The curvature of the refracting surfaces, i.e. lens and cornea, is normally spherical, but if this is not so, then these surfaces may be more sharply curved, say, from above down than they are from side to side, just like the surface of a rubber ball on a table when it is pressed from above. The accommodation might then be correct for a vertical line, but incorrect for a horizontal line at the same distance; then the horizontal line would be poorly focused. This abnormality is astigmatism and is corrected by a spectacle lens which is not spherical but cylindrical. The axis of the cylinder may be oriented vertically, horizontally or at any intermediate position, according to the properties of the cornea-plus-lens refracting system. In practice, most spectacle lenses contain both a spherical and a cylindrical component in their curvatures, thus correcting both astigmatism and short (or long) sight together.

Purkinje images

The changes that occur during accommodation can be observed in the human eye by the **phakoscope**. This is a device for shining twin spots of light obliquely into the eye, one above the other. The rays from each spot follow the paths shown in fig. 26.15. A bright image of the spots

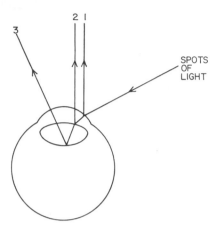

FIG. 26.15. Light paths in phakoscopy to show formation of Purkinje images 1, 2 and 3.

can be seen due to corneal reflection; this is Purkinje image 1. But by observing at a slightly different angle, another image of the two spots can be seen due to reflection at the anterior surface of the lens. It is much fainter, because the light has largely been reflected at the cornea since it has approached very obliquely. The separation of these two spots can be shown to be proportional to the radius of the curvature of the anterior surface of the lens; in other words, a more sharply curved lens means that the spots are closer together, and vice versa. Thus, by causing the subject to accommodate, one can actually observe the change in curvature of the front of the lens; the spots become closer together. With luck and a suitable subject, it is possible to find Purkinje image 3, reflected from the back of the lens, and verify that it changes little during accommodation. A further refinement is to black out one of the spots and thus confirm that images 1 and 2 are right way up, but 3 is inverted; this is a consequence of the fact that the cornea and front of the lens are convex, but the back of the lens is concave as seen from the front. We owe these observations to J.E. Purkinje (1787–1869), the Czech physiologist, who was also a distinguished histologist and gave his name to the Purkinje cells of the cerebellum and heart.

Retina

The retina can be seen in the living eye by using an **ophthalmoscope**. Very little light is reflected from the back of the eye, and what is reflected takes the same path as it took on entering; in other words, it comes

back exactly the way it went in. So the observer cannot normally see anything in the pupil of anyone's eye except reflection of light from the cornea, the 'little doll', the image of himself which originally gave the pupil its name. To see the retina through the pupil, and to see it properly, three conditions must be met. The first is a dim light, which enlarges the subject's pupil, but not pitch darkness, because then the second condition cannot be met. This is that the subject must fix his gaze on some definite point behind the observer, so that his retina keeps still; naturally the observer must keep his head out of the way of the eye not being examined. The third condition is that the observer must project light into the eye along the same axis as he himself is looking (fig. 26.16).

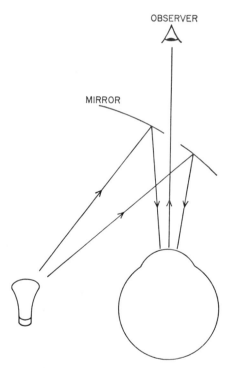

FIG. 26.16. Diagram of light paths in ophthalmoscopy.

This is done most simply by using a small mirror with a central hole in it, through which the observer looks. The light from a lamp is reflected by the mirror into the eye, and the observer's view is along virtually the same axis as the light entering the eye. Practical ophthalmoscopes usually provide their own illumination by an electric bulb in the instrument, and are used close to the subject's eye.

Thus seen (plate 26.1, facing p. 26.20) the retina is red, the colour being chiefly contributed by the underlying choroid. At its posterior pole is the **macula lutea**, a yellow oval patch about 3 mm wide which contains at its centre the **fovea**. The fovea is a depression where the retina is thinnest and where vision is most acute; it is the point on the retina where the object at which we are looking is focused, and away from this point vision becomes rapidly less effective. It 'sees' an area about 1° wide, which is twice the apparent diameter of the moon. The **optic disc** is some 3 mm to the nasal side of the fovea, and is about 1·5 mm in diameter; here the optic nerve leaves the eye. The disc is virtually flat, and of a light cream colour. The central retinal artery and vein reach the retina through the centre of the disc, where there is a depression which is not easy to see. The branches of these vessels are seen throughout the retina and supply all of it except the rods and cones, which are nourished by the separate **ciliary system** of vessels running in the choroid. The central retinal vessels and their branches have poor anastomotic connections, and a block here usually damages part or all of the retina irretrievably; though the rods and cones survive, this is not much comfort to the victim when their nervous connections are gone.

The optic disc is the **blind spot** within the retina, and is not sensitive to light; normally one is unaware of this gap in the seen world, since it is in a different position as seen by the two eyes, and each can fill in the other's gap. However, the blind spot is easy to demonstrate by closing one eye, fixing the other by looking steadily at a given point, and noting that a pencil tip becomes invisible when moved into the part of the field of view corresponding to it.

STRUCTURE OF THE RETINA

The layer of the retina which lies against the choroid is the **pigmented layer** and represents the outer layer of the original optic cup (p. 26.10). It is one cell thick, each cell heavily laden with pigment. The remainder of the retina is derived from the inner layer of the optic cup and is often loosely termed the whole 'retina', which is inaccurate both structurally and functionally. The next layer consists of the receptors for light, about 120 million rods and 6 million cones (fig. 26.17). They are not scattered at random; the cones are present alone at the fovea, where they are about eighteen times as 'thick on the ground' as they are at the periphery of the retina. There are no rods at the fovea, but they are plentiful around it and less closely packed (× 1/5) at the periphery.

Rods and cones each consist of an outer segment, a nuclear portion and a pedicle. The outer segment of a rod is cylindrical, about 24 μm long and 1 μm in diameter. The outer segment of a cone (fig. 26.18) is generally shorter and more conical, though near the fovea it may be very long and thin. The outer segments of receptor cells contain very numerous discs stacked one on top of another and shown in cross-section in fig. 26.18. It is in these discs that the photosensitive pigment (p. 26.14) is located.

The outer segment is linked to the nuclear portion by a narrow strand which by EM shows a structure almost the same as that of a cilium. This is not surprising since these receptor cells develop from ependymal cells which lined the optic vesicle and ependymal cells are commonly ciliated. The pedicle is an expansion rich in mitochondria at the base of the receptor cell, and it closely adjoins terminations of bipolar and horizontal cell processes, so that the responses of the photoreceptor can be conveyed further and analysed, in the complex links provided within the retina (fig. 26.19).

Studies with labelled amino acids indicate that the outer segments of receptors are growing all the time, and the discs nearer the nucleus move outward and are finally shed at the tip, where they can be disposed of by the pigment layer of the retina.

Inside the receptor layer is a layer of **bipolar cells**, which as their name suggests are linked synaptically to a number of rods and cones on their outer side, and on their inner side to the cells of the next layer of the retina, the **ganglion cell layer**. Ganglion cells are larger than bipolar cells, and their axons are the fibres of the optic nerve. They run from their parent ganglion cell, forming the innermost layer of the retina, to the optic disc, where they assemble as the optic nerve and leave the

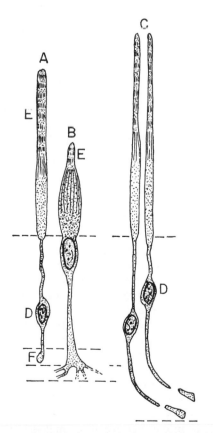

FIG. 26.17. Human rods and cones. A, rod; B, cone; C, cones in fovea centralis; D, nucleus; E, outer segment; F, central connection. After Cajal.

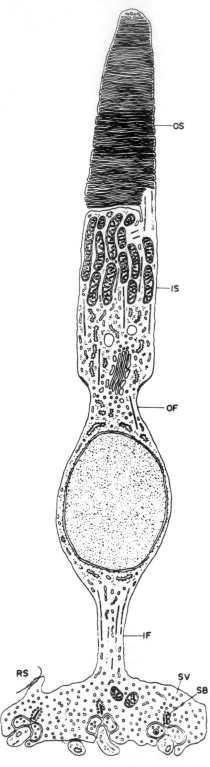

OS

IS

OF

IF

RS

SV

SB

FIG. 26.18. Fine structure of a retinal cone. OS, outer segment; IS, inner segment; OF, outer fibre; IF, inner fibre; RS, contact rod spherules; SV, synaptic vesicles; SB, synaptic ribbon. From Lentz T.L. (1971) *Cell Fine Structure*. Philadelphia: Saunders.

eyeball. They acquire myelin sheaths only on entering the nerve. In the layer of these nerve fibres lie the branches of the central retinal artery and vein. Other retinal cells such as **amacrine cells** and **horizontal cells** are present in the retina and, as shown in fig. 26.19, also play a part in controlling and comparing the information about light patterns and colours which the receptors receive. Amacrine cells derive their name from the Greek for 'no long fibre', because in Golgi preparations they appear to have no axon.

Light on its way to the receptors passes through the other layers of the retina and the retinal blood vessels, but at the fovea this is barely the case, because the blood vessels and the bodies of the bipolar and other cells are swept aside from the fovea, leaving only the minimum obstacle between the light and the cone outer segments at the fovea. Elsewhere, not only the retina but its blood vessels are in the way of the light. It seems particularly odd that one cannot see one's own retinal blood vessels where they overlie the retina. They are certainly not transparent, and are conspicuous during ophthalmoscopy. They become visible to their owner through another manoeuvre discovered by Purkinje. With the eyes lightly closed, a lit torch bulb is gently applied to the lids near the outer canthus and vibrated to and fro. The retinal vascular pattern becomes visible as black lines upon a grey ground. The explanation lies in the properties of the retina. An entirely stationary image or shadow upon the retina produces no response at all. If the retina were a photographic negative, the vessels lying on it would give rise to a contact print of their pattern. But as their shadow is normally stationary, there is no 'print' at all on the retina, which only responds when the shadow is made to move, by illuminating the eye obliquely and intensely through the (normally) opaque coat of the eye and moving the illuminating light. This is one variety of the neural process **adaptation** (p. 25.35).

Function of the iris

The iris brings about **mydriasis** and **miosis** (enlargement and constriction of the pupil). It does so in response to the amount of light entering the two eyes together and reduces the size of the pupil in bright light. Since light is assessed by both eyes together, covering one eye makes the pupil of the other eye enlarge; no wonder that many centuries ago, when vision was attributed to a visual faculty proceeding out from the eye to meet the object seen, this phenomenon was regarded as an enlargement of the outward path, to let one eye emit more visual faculty when it had to work alone.

LIGHT RESPONSE

Shining a light into either eye alone makes both constrict (**consensual reaction**). Often the constriction overshoots a little before becoming fairly steady. It can be neatly

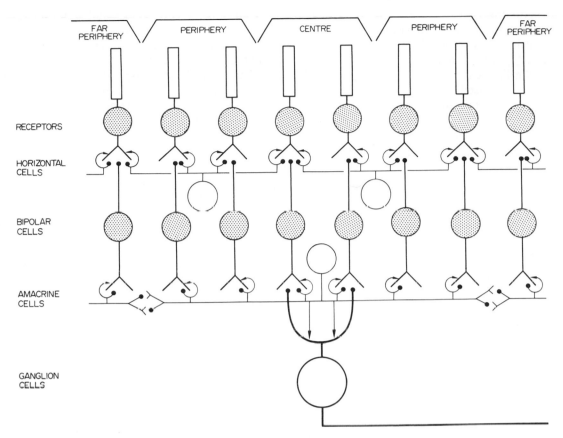

FIG. 26.19. Wiring diagram of the retina to show the connections between one ganglion cell and its associated receptors. , excitatory synapse; ↓, inhibitory synapse. Note that two-way traffic can occur at several points. From Dowling J.E. & Boycott B.B. (1966) *Proc. roy. Soc. B.* **166**, 80.

observed in one's own eye with Broca's pupillometer. With a pin make pairs of pinholes in a piece of aluminium foil 2 mm, 3 mm and 4 mm apart, set close together. Place the foil immediately in front of one eye. The pinholes are far too close to be focused and give rise to blur circles on the retina. It can be shown that the pair of circles which just touch correspond to the diameter of the pupil. If the 3 mm pair just touch, the pupil diameter is 3 mm. Now shine a light into the other eye. The consensual reaction shrinks the pupil of the eye looking through the foil, and the change will be obvious, including its time course and the overshoot.

The light response is organized by the pretectal nucleus, just in front of the superior colliculus (fig. 26.20). The afferent path is by the optic nerve and tract and is supposed to share exactly the same nerve fibres as are used in vision. Possibly the afferent fibres for the light response are different from those for vision. A stationary shadow or light patch on the retina is not seen, as already mentioned, but may be taken into account in regulating pupil size. The efferent path for constriction is by the oculomotor nerve and ciliary ganglion.

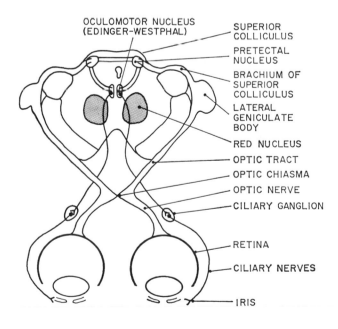

FIG. 26.20. Pupil light reflex.

In a dim light, the maximum amount is allowed to enter the eye. But in bright light, vision is more acute when the pupil is smaller, as any optical imperfections in the cornea or lens have minimal effects when only a small part of the light-carrying path is in use. Also the depth of focus is increased when the pupil is small. The depth of focus decides the distance an object can move towards the eye or away from it and still remain sharply focused without a change in accommodation. Just as in a camera, if the pupil is small and the eye 'stopped right down', there is a greater depth of focus. An eye with a large 7 mm pupil can see everything sharp from infinity to 3·1 m without any accommodation; but with a tiny 1 mm pupil it sees sharp from infinity right down to 0·6 m.

NEAR RESPONSE

The eyes make **conjugate movements** together, from side to side and up and down. In addition they make **convergent movements** (fig. 26.21) for close work, superimposed on the conjugate movements. Convergence is linked to the pupillary control system in such a way that miosis occurs with convergence. The eye gains greater depth of focus for close up work. The afferent path

includes the cerebral cortex and is not identical with the afferent path for the light response. In the Argyll-Robertson pupil described in 1869 by an Edinburgh ophthalmologist and traditionally, though not always, associated with cerebrospinal syphilis, the near response survives and the light response is lost. It is clear that this can occur because the paths are in part distinct. The Argyll-Robertson pupil is always small; there are other and more benign possible causes for a single pupil that does not react to light (vol. 3, p. 34.60).

Visual pigments

The distal segments of the rods contain rhodopsin, a light-sensitive pigment, which is purple in the dark but becomes bleached in the light. It consists of one of the isomers of retinal (vitamin A-aldehyde) coupled to opsin, a protein. Its formation from vitamin A and the protein opsin, and the changes that occur on bleaching are given on p. 10.26.

Since the vitamin is necessary for the formation of rhodopsin, it might be supposed that lack of vitamin A would lead to blindness, and especially to night blindness, since the rods are predominantly concerned with vision in poor light. As it takes many months or even years to exhaust the store of the vitamin present in the liver of a well-fed European, night blindness from this cause is seldom found in prosperous countries. It is extremely common, however, in children in many parts of Asia and elsewhere where the diet is defective in vegetables and dairy products.

As rods are plentiful in human and animal retinas, rhodopsin has long been available in quantity for examination and its absorption at various wavelengths has been measured. It is greatest for blue-green light at a wavelength of 510 nm. This can be compared with human vision in dim light. Here the sensitivity is greatest for blue-green light, although the colour of it cannot be recognized at all in such dim light. Fig. 26.22 shows the **scotopic visibility curve** of sensitivity against wavelength

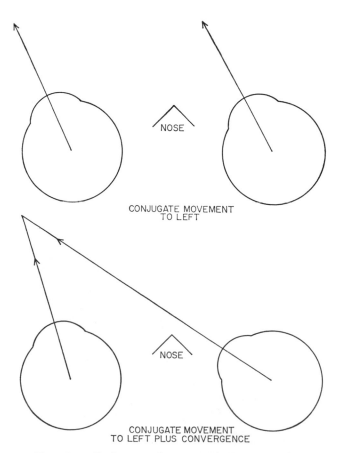

CONJUGATE MOVEMENT
TO LEFT

CONJUGATE MOVEMENT
TO LEFT PLUS CONVERGENCE

FIG. 26.21. Conjugate and convergent eye movements.

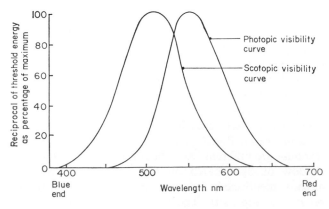

FIG. 26.22. Visibility curves for human vision.

which, when appropriate corrections are made, is the same as rhodopsin's curve. So it is difficult to doubt that vision in dim light is concerned with the rhodopsin-filled rods. Since there is only one pigment involved, the eye cannot produce any information about colour. Everything is grey by moonlight, but the lightest grey is that of objects really blue-green by daylight.

Rhodopsin is certainly not the only visual pigment. Others, similar but with different absorption curves, have been isolated in animals. So it is natural to expect that other pigments account for the **photopic visibility curve** (fig. 26.22). It is similar in shape, but displaced towards the red end of the spectrum; in daylight, yellow objects are the brightest.

COLOUR VISION

Early experiments in colour matching showed that any colour in the spectrum can be matched by some mixture of three pure spectral colours, each of a single wavelength, for instance a blue of 460 nm, a green of 530 nm and a red of 650 nm. The intensity of each of the three varies according to the colour to be matched. Admittedly often the intensity of one of the three is negative, i.e. the match is made by adding it to the colour to be matched, not to the mixture. This seems like cheating, but in the end it has turned out that a negative contribution from one colour may have a real physiological meaning (p. 26.19).

Probably the first event in the process of vision is a change in visual pigments. From three pigments, each responding differently to any colour, the information can be drawn to account for all the colour matching that normal people do. Of course, given four pigments, still more elaborate matching could be achieved, and colours could be distinguished apart which to us seem identical, though of different spectral composition.

So it is reasonable to expect three visual pigments besides rhodopsin, and to expect them in the cones. Cones are few and small compared to rods, and so the pigments have not been isolated from them. Two fruitful approaches have been made to the study of cone pigments. Rushton at Cambridge examined the tiny amount of light reflected from the human fovea, and by studying its spectral composition detected two pigments differing from rhodopsin, and probably a third. Marks, Dobelle and MacNichol at Johns Hopkins examined single monkey cones by refined spectroscopic methods; they too found evidence of three pigments.

Colour blindness of various kinds is common (8 per cent of all men and 0·4 per cent of all women). The possible varieties can be predicted from the three pigment hypothesis. Some people might have only rhodopsin and all colours would be grey to them, since they would only have rods to see with; they would be easily dazzled. A few such people have been described.

A second group might have only one pigment in addition to rhodopsin; three varieties in this group are to be expected, since any one of the three pigments might be present, but only one variety has been found, with cyanolabe only, and is very rare. A third group, **dichromats**, might have two pigments. Since any one of the three pigments might be absent, three varieties are to be expected, and three exist.

The largest group however, are the **anomalous trichromats**. Like normal people, they need mixtures of three spectral colours to achieve matches, but the intensities in the mixtures are different. This is one of the reasons why abnormal colour vision is not always obvious. Other reasons are that colour blind people can deduce a great deal from other clues. By distinguishing brightness differences they can guess colour differences, and they are aware that the top light at the traffic lights is red, but such deductions do not render them safe in fog as engine drivers or sailors. The best practical test is the **Ishihara plates** which show dots of one colour arranged as a letter or figure on a background of random dots of some other colour likely to be confused by the colour blind. Only those with normal colour vision can decipher the hidden letter or figure on all the plates.

Colour vision presents an intellectual problem which has fascinated clever minds for at least five centuries. Leonardo da Vinci, Newton, Goethe, Young (1802) and Helmholtz (1860) are among them. It is by no means entirely a theoretical problem; lighting engineering and dye technology are practical applications.

Sensitivity of vision

The dimmest light it is possible to see consists (if elaborate and approximate calculations are correct) of single quanta reaching each of several (2–14) rods. More than this has to reach the cornea, because of losses within the eyeball, but the receptors themselves appear to respond to amounts of the order of one quantum. The brightest light that can be dealt with is at least 10^9 times brighter. These extremes cannot be dealt with simultaneously. In the dark, the sensitivity becomes steadily greater as time passes, until within an hour it is maximal; most of the increase occurs within half an hour (fig. 26.23). The change is called **dark adaptation**; it raises the sensitivity ten thousandfold and is accompanied by the change in spectral sensitivity already mentioned (fig. 26.22).

The time course of the change is clearly biphasic. The first phase, levelling off after about 7 min in fig. 26.23, is probably due to change in the organization of the cones, because when deep red (which rhodopsin can't 'see' at all) is used for testing, this is all the dark adaptation that is found; the second phase is not there at all for deep red light. Again, the adaptation of the fovea itself does not seem to go any further than this first phase. In part, the changes in dark adaptation can

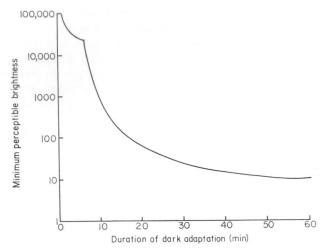

FIG. 26.23. Time course of dark adaptation. Note that the scale of brightness is logarithmic, not linear. After Kohlrausch A. (1931) *Handbuch der normalen und pathologischen Physiologie* Bd. **122**, 1450.

be regarded as due to regeneration of visual pigments previously bleached by light. The change in the organization of ganglion cell fields is mentioned on p. 26.19. Lesser degrees of adaptation occur normally in any part of the retina and allow it to have different sensitivities in different parts at the same time, a facility no camera film can offer.

Visual acuity

Whether a person can distinguish black and white patterns, such as letters, decides his visual acuity. It is impossible to measure the smallest point of light a person can see. Even if it is infinitesimal, it can be seen if it emits enough light. So instead the attempt is made to measure resolution, i.e. the ability to distinguish two points or lines close together (compare two point discrimination, p. 25.38). Foveal vision can normally do this when the space between the two lines subtends an angle of about one minute at the eye, for instance, when the space is one cm and the lines are just over 34 m away, or proportionally less if the distance is less. Really good lighting is compulsory; acuity falls off markedly in light which may seem adequate.

In practice, such a test method would be tedious. Instead, letters on a test card (Snellen chart) can be used (fig. 26.24). Each line of letters is marked with the distance at which the details will subtend one minute at the eye, and this distance is stated in metres. The top line is generally marked 60, and so should be legible at a distance of 60 m. Six metres is a practical distance for testing, and at this distance the normal eye does not need to accommodate. The acuity can then be expressed as a 'fraction'; the 'numerator' is the distance in metres at which the test is made (usually 6), and the 'denomi-

nator' is the number against the line of letters which are the smallest that can be read. Obviously this pseudo-fraction cannot be reduced by dividing top and bottom. Normal acuity is expressed as $\frac{6}{6}$. If the subject can read only the top line, acuity is poor and expressed as $\frac{6}{60}$; a more rough and ready test uses various sizes of reading type at the distance usual for reading. This is normally done using one eye at a time.

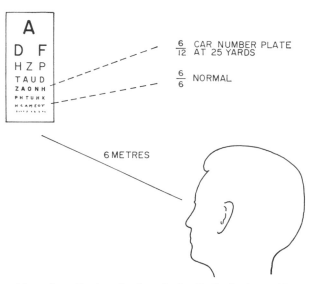

FIG. 26.24. Testing visual acuity by Snellen's charts. From Trevor-Roper P.D. (1974) *Lecture Notes on Ophthalmology*, 5th Edition. Oxford: Blackwell Scientific Publications.

The ability to distinguish a space between two lines subtending one minute at the eye is not the supreme feat of the human visual system. The images lie 5 μm apart on the retina, and as little as 1·75 μm may separate two cones. But vernier acuity enables us to observe that two lines are slightly out of alignment with each other. This can be done when the discrepancy is a mere 5 seconds of arc, one twelfth of the 'minimum separable', and a distance at the retina of only 0·4 μm. The dimensions of the receptors are given on p. 26.11. To account for vernier acuity is much more difficult than to take advantage of it by using a vernier scale.

Illumination

As already mentioned, enough light is essential for all testing of visual acuity. The recommended amount is 1076 lux, which is comparable to what a 60 watt tungsten filament lamp sheds on a surface facing towards it and 24 cm away. Even more can be used with some improvement in acuity, so long as there is no local glare. But less light than this brings real impairment of acuity. Daylight in the open air gives over ten times as much throughout most of a summer day. In industry, the same standard of illumination is needed for the finest work as is needed for testing visual acuity (table 26.1).

TABLE 26.1. Some standards of illumination recommended by the Illuminating Engineering Society, or prescribed by U.K. law.

	Lux	Approximately equivalent to a 60 watt tungsten lamp at
Fine work	1076	24 cm
School rooms	323	44 cm
General office work	215	54 cm
Legal minimum at working level		
for schools	108	78 cm
for factories	65	98 cm

Proper lighting involves other factors, such as glare and colour, too complex to discuss in detail. Colour can be used to real advantage; it ministers to morale and is an aid to safety when danger points are duly coloured. In laboratories and workshops, poor illumination leads to mistakes, inaccuracies and accidents. A well lit kitchen is also a safe and cheerful kitchen. Artificial light is never as satisfactory as daylight where patients are being examined and fails to disclose slight degrees of jaundice, because its spectral composition is different. The finest consulting rooms known to the writer provide a transparent dome admitting daylight above each examination couch.

Retinoscopy

Retinoscopy is the method of measuring the refraction of a human eye objectively. The word ought to mean looking at the retina but in fact it does not entail looking at the details of the retina at all. It contrasts with the subjective method of measuring errors of refraction which depends on placing lenses in front of the subject's eyes and requiring him to read Snellen's charts until he obtains the best possible acuity. Retinoscopy is an objective method and is useful, both for babies and for people who do not tell what they see as lucidly as the tester might wish.

The eye to be tested must not be accommodating. With an ophthalmoscope mirror 1 m from the eye, a patch of light is moved across the eye from side to side. As the eye is unaccommodated, rays emerge from it parallel (upper part of fig. 26.25). So when the light has just left the pupil, moving in the direction of the arrow, it will be followed by a 'ray of darkness'; in other words, the shadow in the pupil follows the patch of light in the same direction as the patch moves over the eye. But if a convex lens of, say, 3 dioptres is placed before the eye, the parallel rays converge one third of a metre from the eye. The dioptre is the reciprocal of the focal length of a lens in metres and offers great convenience in calculation. When the patch of light is now moved in the same fashion across the eye, the 'dark ray' (lower part of fig. 26.25) appears when viewed from the mirror to have got

ahead; in fact, the shadow is seen to chase the light patch across the pupil in the direction opposite to the actual movement of the patch.

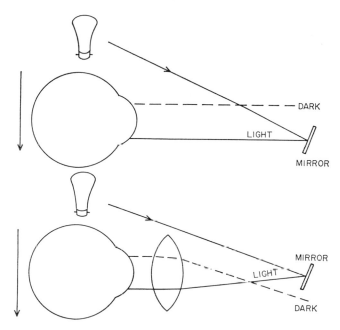

FIG. 26.25. Diagrams to illustrate retinoscopy.

Lenses are tried in succession until no movement of the shadow at all is seen. The mirror is then at the intersection of the light and dark rays shown in the lower part of fig. 26.25. If this occurs with a lens of 1 dioptre the eye is emmetropic (neither myopic nor hypermetropic) and requires no correction. If the lens has some other value, a spectacle lens is required of that value minus one dioptre. The technique is not easy to master and the principles are too complex to present fully here.

Perimetry

From fig. 26.26 it is seen that the two eyes between them when gazing straight ahead command a field of view of about 200° from side to side. Each eye separately commands rather less, because the nose blocks about 35° medially. The field of each eye can be measured separately with a perimeter, a sophisticated protractor which enables the subject to fix his gaze at its centre and the operator to test him with stimuli of varying shape and colour at measured angles from the line of gaze in any direction. The field is markedly smaller for small or poorly lit stimuli than it is for large bright ones. It should contain only one gap, the **blind spot**, where the optic nerve joins the eyeball. The perimeter is invaluable for detecting defects in the field of vision, which can be due to disease of the nervous system or of the eye.

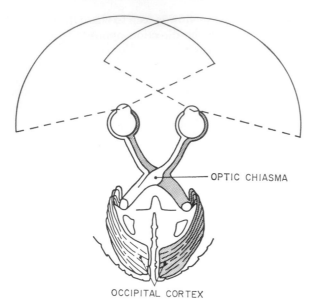

OPTIC CHIASMA

OCCIPITAL CORTEX

Fig. 26.26. The field of vision of the two eyes and the central connections of the retinae. Modified from Scott G.I. (1957) *Traquair's Clinical Perimetry*, 7th Edition. London: Kimpton.

Central nervous pathways

The intracranial part of the **optic nerve** (p. 22.11) runs backward and medially to the **optic chiasma**, where it joins its fellow from the other eye. The chiasma forms part of the floor of the third ventricle of the brain, and it lies above the diaphragma sellae, the dura mater overlying the pituitary gland.

At the chiasma the two nerves cross over, but only in part. Behind the chiasma (fig. 26.26), the re-arranged optic nerve fibres continue back as the **optic tracts**. Each tract now contains the fibres from the temporal half of the retina of the eye on its own side and the fibres from the nasal half of the retina of the eye on the opposite side. So in a sense each tract 'sees' the world on the opposite side. The world is cut in two by a vertical line through the direction of gaze; the right optic tract 'sees' the left half, and vice versa.

The pituitary gland lies below the origins of the two optic tracts from the chiasma. It can be the site of tumours and it is well worth trying to deduce what effects on vision are to be expected if such a tumour enlarges forward, splitting the chiasma, or sideways, damaging the medial sides of one or both optic tracts (vol. 3, p. 34.116).

Each optic tract continues back to the cerebral peduncle, winds round it, and terminates for the most part in the **lateral geniculate body**, but also in the **superior colliculus**. The latter is the major termination in birds, but when the cerebral hemispheres are predominant, as in man, the lateral geniculate body is the end station for most of the fibres of the optic tract. The superior colli-

culus also receives a projection from the striate area of the occipital cortex and serves as a co-ordinating organ for visual reflexes which involve head and eye movements, for instance to turn the head and the gaze towards some new stimulus which turns up in the corner of one's eye. The relevant spinal connections are mentioned on p. 25.49. Some fibres of the optic tract also run to the **pretectal nucleus** immediately anterior to the superior colliculus and below the posterior commissure. It is an important element in the path of the pupillary response to light (p. 26.13).

The lateral geniculate body is an outlying part of the thalamus and lies below the pulvinar alongside the medial geniculate body, at the level of upper midbrain. Its cells and fibres are arranged in definite layers, fibres from each retina interleaving with each other but probably remaining functionally separate. Thus binocular vision is not provided for here, but in the visual area of the cerebral cortex. The neurones of the lateral geniculate body give rise to axons which form the **optic radiation** and run to the **striate area** of the cerebral cortex in the occipital lobe. The fibres of the optic radiation follow a path just lateral to the inferior horn of the lateral ventricle, and very close to the posterior horn (fig. 25.86). This relation to the lateral horn means that damage deep in the temporal lobe may interfere with vision, a consequence at first glance not probable.

The link between retina and striate area via the lateral geniculate body is arranged so that there is a **retinotopic projection** on the striate cortex (fig. 26.27). Careful study of the arrangement will show that the central part of the visual field is greatly enlarged on the striate area and thus commands much brain space right at the posterior pole of the occipital lobes. The more peripheral parts command proportionately less brain space, and the space concerned lies deep in and also around the calcarine sulcus, disposed in such a way that the lower part of the field of view occupies the upper bank of the sulcus, and vice versa.

During the development of the brain this retinotopic projection is probably established at birth, before the eyes can be used for vision. Children with squint may lose the complete efficiency of the projection from the squinting eye and the loss may be irreparable (vol. 3, p. 33.16).

How pattern vision works

It is possible to record the electrical activity in a single ganglion cell in an animal's retina or in an optic nerve fibre, which is approximately the same thing, since the fibre is the axon of the retinal ganglion cell. It is also possible to record the activity of single neurones in the visual areas of the cerebral cortex. From such recordings a picture can be assembled of how the patterns in the seen world are analysed.

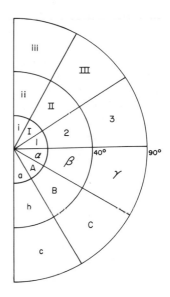

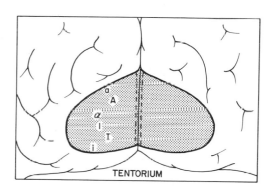

TENTORIUM

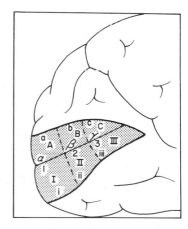

FIG. 26.27. (a) Right half of the visual field, with symbols to illustrate how it is projected (b) on the occipital pole of the left cerebral hemisphere, seen from the back, and (c) around the calcarine sulcus of the left cerebral hemisphere, seen from the medial side. These figures were derived by the careful study of the effects of head injuries in victims of World War II. From Spalding J.M.K. (1952) *Journal of Neurology, Neurosurgery and Psychiatry* **15**, 170.

Each retinal ganglion cell deals with the traffic from the receptors (both rods and cones) in a patch of the retina, a small patch at the fovea but a much larger patch at the periphery. The patch is round, and so when the sky is being looked at the cell can be thought of as 'seeing' a round portion of the sky. One might suppose that the ganglion cell would fire with vigour when the light falling on the many receptors in its patch of retina was bright, and slowly when it was dim. But the actual behaviour is more complex.

The round patch is not uniformly treated by the ganglion cell. It is divided into a circular core and an outer ring. Some ganglion cells (fig. 26.28, left) fire vigorously

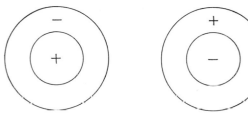

FIG. 26.28. Fields seen by retinal ganglion cells; two types of organization.

when light falls suddenly upon the inner core, but if light falls only upon the outer ring, they actually fire less than they would do in darkness. Even in darkness, the ganglion cell fires slowly. So here light can provoke a negative response.

Other ganglion cells (fig. 26.28, right) reverse this relation; light in the centre slows their firing, but in the outer ring it speeds them up. It can be deduced that illuminating the whole area, core plus outer ring together, produces little result, because the two effects cancel each other. This is perhaps hardly surprising, since a uniformly lit surface which is entirely featureless excites hardly any reaction in ourselves and gets no attention. It can also be deduced that anything moving across the patch of retina will produce a particularly brisk response in the corresponding ganglion cell, because before and after its central effect it produces the reverse; the central effect is made more prominent by what precedes and follows it.

Dark adaptation (p. 26.15) often abolishes the core-outer ring organization. The whole patch responds like its centre. The delicate balancing of core against outer ring is abandoned, and instead greater sensitivity to light over the whole patch is achieved.

The ganglion cell responds to the total amount of light reaching any part of the patch, thus performing a species of **spatial summation** (p. 25.13). Similarly, it sums the light over brief periods and responds without signalling flicker to a rapidly flickering light such as that on a cinema screen. This is **temporal summation** (p. 25.13).

In the cat, a ganglion cell's patch of retina in the most sensitive area might correspond to half a degree, which is about one quarter of the space between two knuckles when the fist is held at arm's length. In man, the patch may be a great deal smaller. The retina is not a simple mosaic of such patches, but each encroaches on the neighbours to a varying extent.

It will now be clear that the retina is much more than a camera film signalling the presence of light or darkness in any part of itself. It is part of the central nervous system, and carries out some of the necessary analysis of the information before transmitting it along the optic nerve. For instance, uniform light affects a camera film, but uniform illumination of the whole retina produces relatively little response, as already mentioned. Further, a special sensitivity to movement of light is already inherent in the traffic passing from retina to lateral geniculate nucleus.

Fig. 26.19 indicates the extreme complexity of the neural circuits within the retina and the pattern of connections which underlies the centre-surround organization. It will be noticed that some connections are reciprocal, for instance the receptors excite the horizontal cells, which in turn inhibit the receptors.

The first stages of the processes in the cerebral hemispheres can also now be outlined. One neurone there certainly does not simply receive the incoming traffic from one patch of retina. It is coupled to a number of patches which are arranged (fig. 26.29) along a straight line in the retina. So it responds to a bar of light (A in fig. 26.29) falling along the centres of the patches along this line. A bar at right angles to this (B in fig. 26.29) excites no response; it does illuminate part at least of the centres of the patches, but it also illuminates the surround, thus cancelling the response. So there can be analysis of light patterns according to the slope of lines in the outside world and this part of the analysis occurs in the visual area of the cerebral cortex. It is continued with increasing elaboration outside the primary visual area. The whole story, as yet, is by no means clear. In particular, the eyes are in incessant movement and the machinery for dealing with a picture that does not keep still and is actually deliberately moved is hardly understood.

The coding of colour information for transmission from the retina to the rest of the brain is done by some retinal ganglion cells which have different sensitivity to colour in their centres and in their surrounds. Instead of responding to white light, the centre may respond especially to red light and the surround to green, or sometimes the centre responds to yellow (red plus green) and the surround to blue. The inverse arrangements also occur. This arrangement suits the nature of light very well, since to say 'the light is red' does not mean in physical terms 'it is not white'; it means 'it is part of white, but not all of white' and this message can be derived from a combination of signals from white light detectors and other detectors which are only sensitive to part of white light.

Binocular vision

Each eye sees approximately the same world, but as already described, the world is bisected along a vertical line through the centre of gaze because of the partial crossing of the optic nerves at the optic chiasma, and subsequently one cerebral hemisphere deals with the opposite half of the seen world. So each hemisphere receives and, in effect, analyses incoming traffic from one half of each retina; the other half is linked to the opposite hemisphere.

Stereoscopic vision thus becomes possible. Both eyes are normally directed so as to see the same thing and point in the same direction; in fact, the eye muscles are controlled so that this is the case, because the central nervous system monitors the view of the two eyes and provides for eye movements that will make the view the same. The monitoring arrangement can be upset by the simple and ingenious **Maddox rod**. This is a parallel array of small red glass rods. When placed in front of one eye, it distorts the image of a spot of white light in front of the observer into a long red line. The monitoring system is evidently unable to identify the white spot and the long red line as the same picture, and so can no longer align the eyes precisely with each other. While still

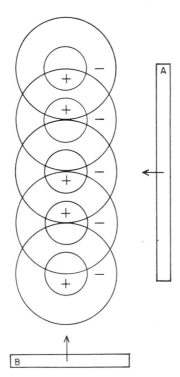

FIG. 26.29. Retinal ganglion cell fields summed in the visual area of the cerebral cortex.

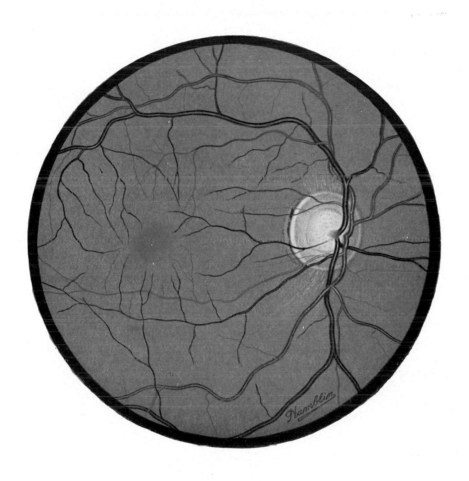

PLATE 26.1. Normal fundus as seen at ophthalmoscopy. From Last R.J. (1968)
Eugene Wolff's Anatomy of the Eye and Orbit, 6th Edition. London: Lewis.

pointing the same way approximately, they may show a 'latent squint' (**exophoria** if divergent, **esophoria** if convergent) which is not a squint, in the sense that during ordinary use the eyes point in the same direction. A latent squint of this kind is probably of no importance except perhaps where very fast responses have to be made to visual information, as by aircraft pilots.

Normally the views seen by the two eyes are made the same by appropriate eye movements, but never exactly the same. They cannot be, because the two eyes are in different places. Two photographs taken from closely adjoining positions are almost the same when correctly lined up, but never quite the same. When one looks at two such photographs in a stereoscope (simply a device enabling one eye to see one photograph and the other eye another one), one obtains an impression of depth in the picture which is otherwise absent. The impression of depth originates from the tiny differences between the two pictures. The nervous system is capable of recognizing these differences and this can be done only in the cerebral cortex, for only there does the traffic from the two eyes meet; it is still probably separate in the lateral geniculate body.

If only one eye is available, stereoscopic depth cannot be sensed. Stereoscopic vision is only one of the ways in which we can judge distance. A single eye can assess the angle subtended at the eye by any familiar object and allow for the known size of the object; it can take into account the amount of accommodation for very close objects, and compare with an extraordinary precision the angular velocities at which two objects are going past but it is still surprisingly difficult to thread a fine needle after closing one eye.

A squinting child, with eyes not pointing correctly in the same direction, loses stereoscopic depth and has double vision. But what is much worse, he often loses entirely the ability to see with one of his eyes, thus gaining single vision at the cost of a functionless eye. The reason is that if the two worlds presented to each cerebral hemisphere do not coincide as they should, then the nerve connections of one of the two eyes within the cerebral cortex, though already established at birth, and already coupled in correct alignment all the way from retina to striate area, become permanently ineffective (p. 26.18).

EAR

The ear consists of three parts, the external, middle and internal ears; these are distinguished from one another in their developmental origin, their structure and function, and to a considerable extent in the disorders which may affect them. The position and relationship of the three parts are illustrated in fig. 26.30.

The **external ear** consists of the auricle (pinna) and the external auditory meatus, a tube, part cartilaginous

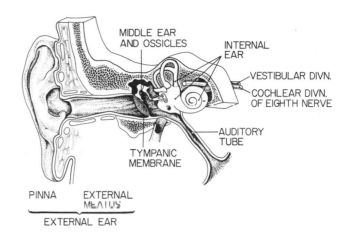

FIG. 26.30. Position and relationship of the three parts of the ear.

and part bony, lined by skin and closed at its inner end by the tympanic membrane (ear drum) which separates it from the middle ear.

The **middle ear** is a cavity within the temporal bone, lined with mucous membrane and filled with air. It communicates anteriorly with the nasopharynx by way of the auditory tube which normally allows the pressure of air in the middle ear to equilibrate with that of the atmosphere. The middle ear communicates posteriorly with the mastoid antrum and, through it, with the mastoid air cells. The auditory tube, middle ear cavity, mastoid antrum and mastoid air cells form a continuous cavity, lined by mucous membrane, into which infection may spread from the nasopharynx.

The internal ear is embedded within the petrous part of the temporal bone. It consists of a fluid-filled sac of complex form, the membranous labyrinth, encased in a shell of very dense bone, the bony labyrinth.

Development (fig. 26.31 a, b and c)

The external ear develops around the dorsal end of the first external pharyngeal groove, between the 1st and 2nd pharyngeal arches (fig. 19.53). The middle ear develops, with the auditory tube and the mastoid antrum, from the tubotympanic recess, a diverticulum from the primitive pharynx arising principally from the 1st pharyngeal pouch (fig. 19.51).

The internal ear is of dual origin. The **membranous labyrinth** develops from the ectodermal epithelium of the otic vesicle (p. 19.11), reinforced by surrounding connective tissue. It is filled with fluid, called **endolymph**. The **bony labyrinth** develops, in common with the rest of the petrous temporal bone, from the otic capsule, a layer of condensed mesoderm which early surrounds the otic vesicle, becomes cartilaginous and is subsequently replaced by endochondral bone. Some important features of the bony labyrinth are as follows.

(1) It does not exist as an entity separate from the rest of the petrous temporal bone but, because it consists of bone even denser than that which surrounds it, it may be defined artificially by dissection.

(2) It follows approximately the contours of the membranous labyrinth, the intervening space being filled by **perilymph.**

(3) In the dried skull, it communicates with the middle ear cavity by two openings (oval and round windows, fenestra vestibuli and fenestra cochleae), which are completely occluded in the fresh state by the footplate of the stapes and the secondary tympanic membrane respectively.

Outline of function

The external ear receives sound waves and transmits them to the tympanic membrane, which vibrates. These vibrations are transmitted across the middle ear cavity by a chain of small bones (the ossicles) arranged in such a way that vibrations of the drum are translated into piston-like movements of the footplate of the stapes within the oval window. These movements of the stapes set up pressure waves in the perilymph, made possible by reciprocal movements of the secondary tympanic membrane.

Pressure waves in the perilymph are transmitted to the endolymph within the **cochlear duct.** This is part of the membranous labyrinth which contains the specialized receptive epithelium of the **organ of Corti.** Its indirect stimulation by sound waves sets up nerve impulses in the cochlear division of the eighth nerve, which are eventually interpreted as sounds (p. 25.29).

The cochlear duct forms only part of the membranous labyrinth. The rest contains specialized epithelial receptors concerned with monitoring angular acceleration of the head (the **semicircular canals**) and the position of the head in space (**utricle** and **saccule**). These various organs collectively form the vestibular apparatus and are innervated by the vestibular division of the eighth nerve.

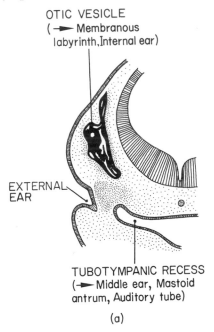

OTIC VESICLE
(→ Membranous labyrinth, Internal ear)

EXTERNAL EAR

TUBOTYMPANIC RECESS
(→ Middle ear, Mastoid antrum, Auditory tube)

(a)

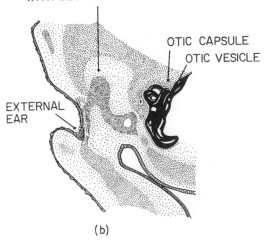

FUTURE MIDDLE EAR CAVITY WITH DEVELOPING OSSICLES

OTIC CAPSULE
OTIC VESICLE

EXTERNAL EAR

(b)

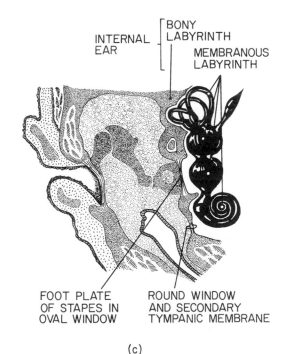

INTERNAL EAR ⎡BONY LABYRINTH
⎣MEMBRANOUS LABYRINTH

FOOT PLATE OF STAPES IN OVAL WINDOW

ROUND WINDOW AND SECONDARY TYMPANIC MEMBRANE

(c)

FIG. 26.31. (a) Frontal section through embryonic head to show position and relations of the three parts of the ear; (b) a later stage showing the auditory ossicles developing in the loose mesenchyme above the end of the tubotympanic recess, and the otic capsule developing as a mesenchymal condensation around the otic vesicle; (c) the relations of the three parts of the ear in the 3rd month of fetal life. Note that the ossicles are still embedded in loose mesenchyme. In late fetal life, this mesenchyme degenerates and the ossicles are covered by the epithelium of the expanded blind end of the tubotympanic recess.

External ear and tympanic membrane

The auricle is a plate of elastic cartilage covered with skin. This plate of cartilage is continued into the wall of the external meatus, the lateral third of which is an incomplete cylinder of the same material. Where the cylinder is incomplete, the deficiency is supplied by fibrous tissue. The remainder of the adult external meatus is part of the temporal bone, the tympanic plate forming the walls and floor, and part of the squamous temporal, the roof. The external acoustic meatus is sinuous; followed from the outside it runs medially, forwards and upwards, then inclines slightly backwards and upwards, and finally downwards and forwards to end at the tympanic membrane. This lies at an angle to the meatus, and faces downwards and forwards. Examination of the tympanic membrane with an otoscope is made easier if the examiner draws the auricle upwards and backwards, and slightly laterally.

The skin which lines both the meatus and the tympanic membrane is tightly bound to the underlying connective tissue. In the meatus, it is supplied with large coiled ceruminous glands, the source of the wax normally found in the ear. When present in excess, this wax can produce deafness. Its function is unknown, for it is certainly not protective to any noticeable extent. Sebaceous glands and hair follicles are also present in the external meatus.

NERVE SUPPLY

The afferent supply of the external meatus is derived from the auriculotemporal branch of the mandibular nerve, and from the auricular branch of the vagus. A few fibres from the facial and possibly the glossopharyngeal nerves are also found there (fig. 22.31). Infection of the geniculate ganglion of the facial nerve with herpes virus may result in severe pain in the external acoustic meatus, and blistering of the skin. The skin of the lower part of both surfaces of the auricle is supplied by the great auricular nerve (C2 and 3), the lateral side of the upper part by the auriculotemporal nerve, and the medial surface by the lesser occipital nerve (C2).

In the newborn child, the form of the external meatus is quite different. Its wall consists mainly of fibrous tissue connected medially to the slender, bony tympanic ring. The tympanic membrane is much more inclined than in the adult and, because of the undeveloped state of the tympanic plate, it lies in the plane of the base of the skull. The whole meatus is much shorter than in the adult and the tympanic membrane is thus more liable to injury during examination.

Fig. 26.32 illustrates the appearance of the living tympanic membrane as seen through an otoscope. In the adult it lies at an angle of about 55° with the floor of the meatus. The handle of the malleus, which is attached to the membrane, runs downwards and backwards; its tip

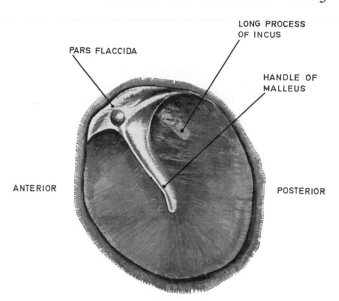

FIG. 26.32. Lateral aspects of the left tympanic membrane.

lies at the **umbo**, the most medial point on the membrane, which is concave laterally. Towards the upper end of the handle, the lateral process of the malleus projects laterally against the membrane. From its tip, the anterior and posterior tympanomalleolar folds run to the tympanic plate, bounding the flaccid part of the membrane, which consists of two apposed epithelial layers with little intervening connective tissue. The larger, tense part of the membrane consists of a sheet of connective tissue, containing radial and circular fibres, covered externally by a thin layer of modified skin and internally by a thin mucous membrane.

Middle ear and related cavities, and the ossicles
(fig. 26.33)

The auditory tube, the middle ear cavity, the mastoid antrum and the mastoid air cells are modifications of the

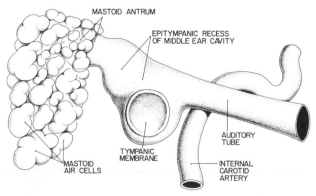

FIG. 26.33. Lateral view of the right middle ear and its extensions.

simple tubotympanic recess of the embryo. This recess is formed mainly from the first pharyngeal pouch with a contribution from the second. The series of cavities which develops from this outgrowth becomes enclosed posteriorly within the parts of the temporal bone.

The middle ear cavity lies within the lateral part of the petrous temporal bone at the medial end of the external acoustic meatus. It is some millimetres lateral to the blind end of the internal meatus, the vestibule of the internal ear intervening. A line connecting the internal and external meatuses passes through the middle ear cavity. Superiorly, the cavity is separated from the middle cranial fossa by a thin plate of bone, the **tegmen tympani**. Below the floor of the middle ear is the superior bulb of the internal jugular vein, lying in the jugular foramen. The internal carotid artery ascends within the bone which forms the anterior wall, below the opening of the bony part of the auditory tube. The terminal segment of the sigmoid sinus lies behind the lower part of the posterior wall of the cavity.

The cavity of the middle ear is a narrow vertical slit within the temporal bone, having no anterior wall above the convexity created by the internal carotid artery, since the bony auditory tube and the canal for tensor tympani are continuous with it on this aspect. Its posterior wall has the aditus to the mastoid antrum in its upper part and a small pyramidal projection for the stapedius muscle below. The part of the tympanic cavity which rises above the upper margin of the tympanic membrane is the **epitympanic recess**, which contains the greater part of the malleus and the incus.

The medial wall of the middle ear cavity is the outer wall of the bony labyrinth. A convexity occupying most of the lower part of that wall, the **promontory**, is produced by the bulging of the first coil of the cochlea. Its surface is marked by a network of fine grooves for the fibres of the tympanic branch of the glossopharyngeal nerve and sympathetic fibres derived from the plexus around the internal carotid artery. In the upper part of the medial wall a transverse ridge of bone inclines downwards at its posterior end. This marks the position of the bony canal for the facial nerve, as it passes from the geniculate ganglion to the stylomastoid foramen.

On the upper margin of the promontory, and below the facial canal, is an oval opening in the bone, the **fenestra vestibuli**, which is closed by the footplate of the stapes and its anular ligament. At the lower margin of the promontory another aperture, the **fenestra cochleae**, is closed by the secondary tympanic membrane. These two apertures lead into the **scala vestibuli** and the **scala tympani** respectively. The scalae are separate passages within the bony cochlea, which communicate with one another only at the apex of the cochlea, and which are both filled with perilymph. The perilymph is sealed off from the middle ear cavity by the structures which close off the fenestrae. At the posterior margin of the promontory is a small indentation, the **sinus tympani**, which fortuitously marks the position of the ampulla of the posterior semicircular canal of the vestibular apparatus.

MUCOUS MEMBRANE OF THE TYMPANIC CAVITY

The lining of the middle ear cavity consists of a single layer of epithelium, which varies from columnar ciliated at the opening of the auditory tube to a flattened type on the internal surface of the tympanic membrane. This epithelium is connected to the periosteum of the bony walls of the cavity by a thin layer of connective tissue which contains nerves and blood vessels. Both epithelium and connective tissue are continuous over the ossicles. The mucous membrane receives a sensory supply from the glossopharyngeal nerve, via its tympanic branch.

AUDITORY OSSICLES

The medial surface of the tympanic membrane is connected to the fenestra vestibuli by a system of small bones united by synovial joints. The upper part of this system is in the epitympanic recess, above the level of the upper margin of the tympanic membrane. This system of bony segments forms the connecting link which transmits the impulses from the tympanic membrane to the fluid-filled system of the cochlea at the fenestra vestibuli. The **malleus**, a club-shaped bone with an expanded upper end, is connected to the roof of the cavity by a superior ligament. Its lower thinner part or handle is bound to the medial surface of the tympanic membrane. At the upper margin of the tympanic membrane, the anterior ligament connects the neck of the malleus to the anterior wall of the tympanic cavity. The posterior aspect of the head of the malleus forms a true synovial joint with the body of the **incus.** The incus consists of a body and two posteriorly projecting processes, a short upper one and a longer lower one. The upper process is connected to the posterior wall of the cavity by a ligament, while the longer one articulates with the head of the third ossicle, the **stapes**. This structure is shaped like a stirrup, with a footplate bound by its anular ligament into the fenestra vestibuli.

The ossicles are thus connected to each other and to the bone of the tympanic cavity by a series of joints, all of which are involved in ossicular movement. The ligamentous attachments of malleus, incus and stapes to the bone of the cavity provide relatively fixed joints, while the joints between the ossicles are synovial and allow freer movement.

MUSCLES OF THE MIDDLE EAR

The **tensor tympani** arises from the roof and walls of the canal in which it lies, above the bony pharyngotympanic tube. As it passes to its insertion into the neck of the malleus, it turns sharply laterally around a bony spur, processus cochleariformis, at the posterior end of its canal. The tone of this muscle maintains the medial convexity of the tympanic membrane, and presses the footplate of the stapes into the fenestra vestibuli. The **stapedius** arises from the interior of the small bony pyramid on the posterior wall of the middle ear cavity, and is inserted into the head of the stapes at the point of convergence of the two limbs of the ossicle. It contracts to draw the footplate of the stapes backwards and out of the fenestra vestibuli.

The malleus develops from the first arch cartilage, the tensor tympani which is inserted into it from first arch mesoderm, and the nerve supplying the muscle is the first arch nerve, the mandibular nerve. The stapes develops from the dorsal end of the second arch cartilage, the stapedius which is inserted into it from second arch mesoderm, and the nerve which supplies the muscle is a branch of the second arch nerve, the facial nerve. The incus, which is not directly attached to either muscle, is probably of first arch cartilage derivation.

MECHANISM OF THE OSSICLES

To enable hearing to take place, the middle and inner ears together have three operations to perform:

(1) transferring a sound wave arriving through air at the ear drum into a sound wave in the perilymph,

(2) providing a means of sensing the sound wave in the perilymph, and

(3) coding what is heard as nerve impulses passing along the cochlear division of the eighth nerve to the medulla oblongata.

The perilymph is virtually incompressible, and impulses within it are absorbed by the secondary tympanic membrane. So, to transfer a sound wave in air into one in liquid, a lever system is necessary. The lever reduces the extent of movement but increases the force. Thus, a wave of given amplitude in air is changed into a wave of much smaller amplitude in perilymph. If there were no such lever system, sound in air would be able to produce hardly any wave disturbance in a liquid such as perilymph. Similarly, sound waves in water cannot produce any perceptible sound waves in air unless some device is provided to match the properties of the two media; this is one of the reasons why we cannot normally listen in to the conversation of porpoises.

The ossicles of the middle ear provide some leverage, about 1·3 : 1, but most of the leverage arises from the difference between the areas of the eardrum and the footplate of the stapes. The ratio is about 15 : 1 and so the whole middle ear system gives a ratio of 20 : 1 reduction in movement and 20 : 1 increase in force (fig. 26.34).

Extra stiffening of the middle ear mechanism is provided by the action of the two muscles, **tensor tympani** and **stapedius**. Pulling on the ossicular chain, they

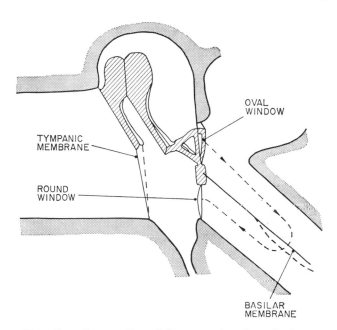

FIG. 26.34. Cross-section of the ear to show how displacement of the tympanic membrane is transmitted to the oval window, deforms the basilar membrane and then the fenestra cochleae (round window).

restrict its mobility. They are brought into action in reflexes provoked by swallowing and yawning, but especially by loud sounds. Thus, they can guard the hearing system against damage by overloading. But the reflex response to a loud noise has, like all reflexes, a latent period, in this case some 15 msec. This is a short time, but if a noise is very loud and abrupt in onset, it can slip through the reflex protection and damage the hearing mechanism before stapedius and tensor tympani can respond. Occasionally the stapedius may be paralysed by a facial nerve palsy. Then hearing on the affected side is too sensitive for comfort, and the patient suffers from **hyperacusis**, or excessively acute hearing. A loud noise may even induce pain.

FACIAL NERVE IN THE PETROUS TEMPORAL BONE

The main trunk of the nerve and the nervus intermedius enter the petrous temporal bone through the lateral end of the internal acoustic meatus (fig. 26.35). The two nerves blend to form a single trunk within the bone. Just above the vestibule of the inner ear, this trunk turns sharply backwards forming its genu. Here is situated the **geniculate ganglion**, a collection of pseudo-unipolar nerve cells mainly concerned with the sense of taste. From the ganglion, the facial nerve runs backwards in a bony canal in the medial wall of the middle ear, then downwards in its posterior wall, emerging from the base of the skull at the stylomastoid foramen (p. 22.16). Within the petrous temporal bone, it gives off branches, most of which carry fibres of the nervus intermedius, no

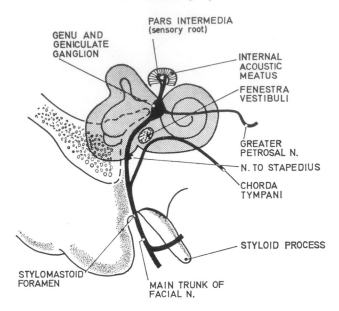

Fig. 26.35. Intrapetrous part of the facial nerve.

part of which reaches the stylomastoid foramen. At the ganglion, the **greater petrosal nerve** runs forwards to pierce the floor of the middle cranial fossa (p. 22.6). Also within the petrous temporal bone, a small branch is given off to join the fibres of the tympanic plexus, most of whose fibres are secretomotor, derived from the glossopharyngeal nerve. The **lesser petrosal nerve** leaves this plexus, incorporating the facial nerve fibres as it does so, and pierces the floor of the middle cranial fossa to lie lateral to the greater petrosal. As the facial nerve descends in the posterior wall of the middle ear, it supplies the stapedius muscle and then loses the remainder of its nervus intermedius fibres in the **chorda tympani**; this branch arises just above the stylomastoid foramen, pierces the posterior wall of the middle ear, and runs across the tympanic membrane passing lateral to the long process of the incus and medial to the handle of the malleus. It leaves the tympanic cavity by a small canaliculus in the lower part of the anterior wall. Emerging from the base of the skull, it is distributed with the lingual nerve to the tongue and to the sublingual and submandibular salivary glands.

MASTOID ANTRUM AND MASTOID AIR CELLS

The antrum lies directly posterior to the middle ear cavity, connected to it by the **aditus** in the upper part of the common wall. It lies 1–2 cm medial to its surface marking, the suprameatal triangle, which is situated above and behind the external acoustic meatus. Medially, the antrum is related to the posterior semicircular canal, posteriorly to the sigmoid sinus and above to the middle cranial fossa and the temporal lobe of the brain, only a thin plate of bone and the meninges intervening.

The extensive system of air sacs which usually fills the mastoid process opens into the periphery of the antrum. The mucous membrane of these sacs is continuous with that of the antrum, and through it with that of the middle ear cavity. Sometimes the number of mastoid air cells is greatly reduced and they may even be absent.

AUDITORY TUBE

The bony part of the auditory tube is situated immediately inferior to the canal for the tensor tympani muscle. It runs parallel and anterolateral to the intrapetrous course of the internal carotid artery, and opens into the posterior end of the suture between the posterior margin of the greater wing of the sphenoid and the quadrate area of the petrous temporal bone. Here it is continuous with the cartilaginous part of the tube (p. 22.44), which it meets at an angle of about 170°. The whole tube is lined with a pseudostratified columnar ciliated epithelium. It is normally closed, but opens on swallowing and yawning. The mechanism of opening is uncertain but probably involves the tensor and levator palati muscles.

Internal ear, hearing and equilibration

The internal ear has two components, the bony labyrinth and the membranous labyrinth, whose development and general arrangement has already been mentioned (p. 26.21).

BONY LABYRINTH

This is exposed by dissecting away the somewhat less dense bone in which it is embedded and is seen to consist of three parts (fig. 26.36). The general part is the **vestibule**, which lies immediately medial to the medial wall of the middle ear. In the dried skull, the two cavities communicate via the oval window (fenestra vestibuli); in life, the footplate of the stapes occludes this opening and its

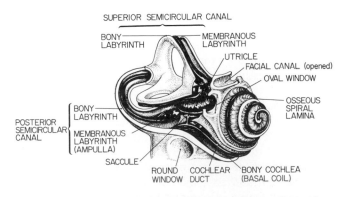

Fig. 26.36. Lateral view of the right internal ear. Parts of the bony labyrinth have been removed to show the membranous labyrinth.

movements are transmitted to the perilymph which fills the vestibule. In front of the vestibule is the (bony) **cochlea**, a spiral tube, whose first turn bulges, as the promontory, on the medial wall of the middle ear. The cavity of the cochlea is partitioned to form three tubes, each of which is similarly spirally wound around the central conical bony core of the cochlea, the **modiolus**. The central tube of the three is the cochlear duct, which is part of the membranous labyrinth, and contains endolymph. The other two, which both contain perilymph, are the **scala vestibuli**, so called because it is continuous with the vestibule, and the **scala tympani**, which communicates with the tympanic (middle ear) cavity through the round window (fenestra cochlear), closed in life by the secondary tympanic membrane. The two scalae communicate with one another only at the apex of the cochlea, through an opening called the **helicotrema** (fig. 26.37). Pressure waves generated in the

MEMBRANOUS LABYRINTH (figs. 26.36 and 38)

This is a complex system of intercommunicating sacs and tubes, filled with endolymph and partly separated from the surrounding bony labyrinth by a perilymphatic space filled with perilymph. One part of the membranous labyrinth, the **cochlear duct**, contains specialized sensory epithelium (the organ of Corti) concerned with hearing and supplied by the cochlear division of the eighth nerve; the remainder, consisting of the utricle, saccule and the three (membranous) semicircular canals, contains specialized sensory epithelia innervated by the vestibular nerve and concerned with equilibration.

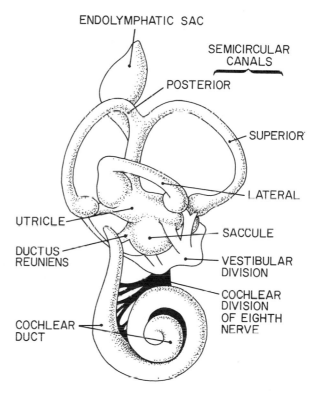

FIG. 26.38. Lateral view of right membranous labyrinth of a 30 mm human embryo. Modified from Streeter G.L. (1918) *Contributions in Embryology* v, 5.

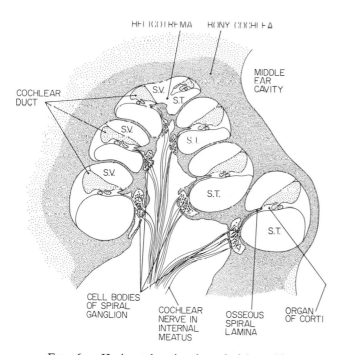

FIG. 26.37. Horizontal section through right cochlea.

perilymph of the vestibule by movements of the stapes travel into the scala vestibuli and readily traverse the thin vestibular membrane; they then deform the basilar membrane, thus reaching the scala tympani, and finally are dissipated in vibrations of the secondary tympanic membrane. The third component of the bony labyrinth is the three **semi-circular canals**. These communicate with the vestibule and are filled with perilymph. Each lies in a plane approximately at right angles to the others, and each has a dilated section, or **ampulla**, at one end adjoining the vestibule.

COCHLEA AND HEARING

The **cochlea** resembles a snail shell with the top of the shell pointing forwards and laterally (fig. 26.36 and 38). The spiral tube makes two and three-quarter turns round its bony axis, the modiolus, which is channelled to accommodate the fibres and cell bodies of the nerve cells of the cochlear division of the eighth nerve. The **cochlear** duct lies inside the bony cochlea and divides it into two tubes. Above is the **scala vestibuli** (fig. 26.39). This is continuous with the vestibule, and is separated by a thin, easily deformed vestibular membrane from the cochlear duct.

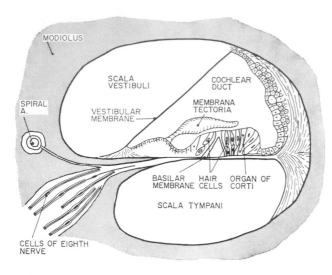

FIG. 26.39. Cross-section of cochlea showing organ of Corti and adjacent structures.

The other side of the cochlear duct is bounded by the **basilar membrane,** a highly organized sheet of radially arranged collagen-like fibres, embedded in an amorphous matrix. The inner edge of the membrane is attached to a bony ridge, the **osseous spiral lamina**, projecting from the modiolus like the slide on a helter-skelter. The outer edge is attached to the **spiral 'ligament'**, which consists of periosteal connective tissue. The basilar membrane increases in width when followed from the base of the cochlea to its apex.

Deformation of the basilar membrane by pressure waves in the perilymph of the scala vestibuli and scala tympani is sensed by two rows of hair cells in the **spiral organ of Corti,** which lies on the basilar membrane (fig. 26.39). On top of the hair cells is the soft, pad-like **membrana tectoria** which moves across the hairs when the basilar membrane is deformed, thus stimulating them. The hair cells are supplied by nerve fibres whose cell bodies lie within the modiolus of the cochlea, and form the **spiral ganglion**, the counterpart of dorsal root ganglia at spinal level. The cochlear neurones are bipolar and their central processes are the fibres of the cochlear division of the eighth nerve. This nerve also carries a few efferent fibres, which terminate on the hair cells and may have an inhibitory action on the sensory output from the cochlea.

Hearing is a very competent faculty. It can distinguish different pitches over a range of 10 octaves, from 20 to about 20 000 Hz. It can distinguish loudness over a range of 120 decibels from the softest perceptible sound to the loudest that is not actually damaging; the loudest sound is a million million times more intense than the softest. And it can distinguish the direction of a sound with a precision which is partly due to the timing ability of the two ears working together. When sound reaches

one ear 0·1 msec, or perhaps less, before it reaches the other, the difference is detectable and can be interpreted as indicating the direction of the sound.

The necessary information must be conveyed as trains of nerve impulses. The simplest way of indicating pitch would be to have one impulse per sound wave. But there is an upper limit to the frequency of impulses that a nerve fibre can carry. About 1100 Hz is the highest possible frequency and pitch can be distinguished far above this limit.

The alternative method of indicating pitch is to have one nerve fibre for a particular pitch. There are plenty of fibres, since the cochlear nerve comprises some 25 000. The available sorting device is the basilar membrane. Although not taut, it is suspended in such a way that in different parts of the cochlea it is displaced furthest by different pitches of sound. At the basal part the preferred frequency is high and at the apical part it is low.

Thus different parts of the spiral organ of Corti respond maximally to sound of different pitches. A somewhat similar effect is shown by a piano; with the pedal depressed, it selects the frequencies in a sound and the appropriate strings of the piano resonate and are heard when the sound stops. The ear, however, is not so selective; the strings are coupled together in one basilar membrane and it is not true to say that one part of the membrane vibrates in response to a note of only a single pitch. One part vibrates maximally, the rest less.

So within the eighth nerve the information about pitch is probably derived by determining which fibre in the nerve is responding maximally; this fibre is linked to the hair cells in the part of the spiral organ tuned to the frequency. Lateral inhibition (p. 25.35) in the central nervous system enables the maximally responding fibre to be singled out. Loudness can be signalled by the overall amount of traffic in the nerve. Comparison between the times of arrival of sounds at the two ears can, of course, be done only in the central nervous system.

DISORDERS OF HEARING

When the function of the middle ear is impaired, transfer of sound from air to the liquid of the inner ear is inefficient. This can happen because the external acoustic meatus is blocked by wax or because infection in the middle ear cavity has damaged the drum or locked the ossicles together. It can also happen because the footplate of the stapes has become rigidly fixed in the oval window by the process termed **otosclerosis** (vol. 3, p. 32.10).

The affected ear hears sounds arriving in the air from a tuning fork poorly. But it is possible to transfer sound waves to the liquid of the inner ear directly by applying the base of a tuning fork to the scalp and thus causing the skull to vibrate. Tested in this way, the affected ear is just as efficient as the other, or even slightly better. The normal ear, during such a test, receives a variety of sound waves by the normal route plus the bone-conducted waves. To some extent the latter are masked by the former. The damaged ear will receive only the bone-conducted waves, which are therefore clearly audible.

This is why the damaged ear seems actually to hear better when a tuning fork is applied by its base to the forehead, so that sound is being applied equally to both ears by bone conduction. The procedure is **Weber's test** and when one ear has faulty conduction from air to inner ear, the sound seems to be more in that ear than in the normal ear on the opposite side.

Simple antiquated methods of testing hearing, using just tuning forks, produce reliable and prompt information when the subject is intelligent and the examiner experienced (vol. 3, p. 32.3). More sophisticated testing can be done by **audiometry**. The instrument emits into one ear a pure tone of a selected frequency and the intensity can be altered so that the softest audible sound is measured for that frequency. When the procedure is repeated to cover the whole spectrum of audible frequencies, an **audiogram** is plotted (fig. 26.40). The plot

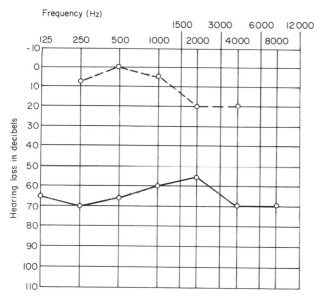

FIG. 26.40. Audiogram showing middle ear deafness; o————o bone conduction, o————o air conduction.

shows the sensitivity of the ear against normal sensitivity for every frequency. The unit is the **decibel**; one bel represents a tenfold increase in intensity, and is divided into ten decibels, so that each decibel step makes a sound 7·9 per cent more intense than it was before. A curious choice of unit on first acquaintance, but convenient because, to increase loudness by steps that seem equal to the listener, the intensity of sound must be multiplied by approximately the same factor for each step (Weber–Fechner relation).

Besides it might be supposed from the form of an audiogram that the ear is equally sensitive to sounds of any frequency. This is entirely untrue; it is far more sensitive to sounds of a frequency around 1000 Hz (about two octaves above middle C on the piano) than to sounds at the upper and lower limits of the audible range. But the audiogram compares the ear being tested with a 'standard ear' and exhibits any differences conspicuously. So it can be seen, for instance, whether a hearing loss is more marked at high frequencies than at low or confined to one small range of frequencies.

Impairment of conduction in the middle ear produces **middle ear deafness**. Damage of the cochlea, the eighth nerve or occasionally of the auditory paths in the central nervous system produces **nerve deafness**. The two can be distinguished by tuning fork tests, as already described. In addition, middle ear deafness tends to affect all frequencies of sound, but nerve deafness chiefly the higher frequencies.

Audiometry sometimes makes a further distinction possible. When the cochlea itself is at fault, then soft sounds may be heard just as well as by the normal ear or even apparently slightly better. This phenomenon is **recruitment**; it is as if the cochlea had lost its most sensitive receptors first, comparable to the rods of the retina (p. 26.15), but retained the less sensitive receptors in good order, at least until the disease progresses further. This is like 'night blindness' of the cochlea with normal vision by day. Recruitment is not normally observed when the eighth nerve or central pathways are faulty. It is a characteristic of cochlear disease.

CENTRAL CONNECTIONS OF THE AUDITORY SYSTEM (fig. 26.41)

The fibres of the cochlear portion of the eighth nerve enter the brain stem at the lower part of the pons, dividing after entry to synapse with cells in the dorsal and ventral cochlear nuclei; these lie posterior and anterior to the inferior cerebellar peduncle. Fibres from these nuclei cross the midline; those from the dorsal cochlear nucleus lie close to the ventricular floor and pass beneath the striae medullares, and those from the ventral cochlear nucleus cross at a deeper level and often relay with small cells which, together with the fibres, form the **trapezoid body**. After crossing, both sets of fibres ascend together as the **lateral lemniscus** which is formed by crossed and uncrossed fibres arising from the cochlear nuclei. The lateral lemniscus is pushed laterally and anteriorly by the formation of the superior cerebellar peduncle and reaches the inferior colliculus of the midbrain from which it is relayed to the medial geniculate body. From here fibres pass in the auditory radiation of the internal capsule to enter the auditory cortex of the temporal lobe (p. 25.71). Thus each temporal lobe receives fibres conveying impulses from both ears so

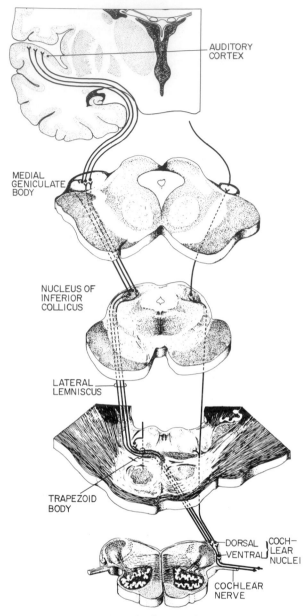

AUDITORY
CORTEX

MEDIAL
GENICULATE
BODY

NUCLEUS OF
INFERIOR
COLLICUS

LATERAL
LEMNISCUS

TRAPEZOID
BODY

DORSAL COCH-
LEAR
VENTRAL NUCLEI

COCHLEAR
NERVE

FIG. 26.41. Auditory pathways.

that lesions of the central nervous system involving the auditory pathway do not produce deafness unless both sides of the brain are involved.

Like somatic sensation, hearing is represented on the cerebral cortex in a main auditory area, and just as in the somatic sensory area each part corresponds to a part of the body, so in the auditory area each part corresponds to part of the cochlea. Thus the front end of the area is concerned with high pitched tones, the back with low pitched tones. However, hearing differs from somatic sensation in being a much more bilateral sense. Thus damage to the auditory area in one of the two hemispheres is hard to detect at all; only when both hemispheres are affected does deafness become apparent.

NOISE

Noise is no new problem; 'many a cave man must have clubbed his neighbour because of the intolerable "clink, clink, clink" of his axe-making' (Taylor). But industrial, electronic and military developments have enormously increased noise.

The intensities of audible sounds extend over a large range, from 10^{-12} W m^{-2} for the softest sound audible by the most sensitive ear to 10 W m^{-2} for the noise of a jet aircraft at 50 metres range, and still more intense sounds can occur. As mentioned on p. 26.28 these intensities are better expressed in **decibels** (dB). The aircraft's noise is 10^{13} times as intense as the minimum audible sound, and so is described as 130 dB, where the value is the exponent 13 multiplied by 10; this is so because it is given in decibels and not in the parent unit the bel, which is too large for convenience. The softest sound audible is termed 0 dB. As intensity grows, a 10 dB increase roughly doubles the **loudness**, loudness being judged by the hearer, and is thus always subjective and distinct from the physically measured intensity.

Some consequences of the decibel scale are misleading to those not familiar with the mathematical device employed. For instance, two 90 dB noises happening together make a 93 dB noise, and not a 180 dB noise. Doubling the intensity adds only 3 dB, which seems very little but obviously is not. Again, if the original 90 dB noise increases to 100 dB, the increase appears to be 11 per cent. In fact, the intensity has risen by a factor of ten and the loudness has doubled.

The physical intensity of a sound cannot properly describe its intensity for human ears, because the human ear (p. 26.29) is not equally sensitive to all frequencies of sound; very low and very high pitches are inaudible, and sensitivity varies within the audible range. In sound intensity meters an electronic network known as network A compensates for the changing sensitivity, and the unit thus measured is the **dBA**.

TABLE 26.2. Intensities of common noises and corresponding dBA values.

Sound	Intensity W m^{-2}	dBA
Peak level of 0·303 rifle at ear	10 000	160
Pop music in a youth club	0·1	110
Very noisy factory	0·01	100
Inside railway carriage	0·000 032	75
Normal conversation	0·000 0032	65
Quiet countryside	0·000 000 000 32	25

Table 26.2 shows the intensities of some common noises with the corresponding values for dBA, and makes clear the large changes in intensity that lurk behind small changes in dBA.

In practice, noise is very rarely constant for long periods, but occurs in bursts or with frequent changes of intensity. Special indices, such as the Perceived Noise Level (PNdB), have been devised which take account of changing intensities. They are used to assess aircraft and industrial noise, and to define tolerable limits. They cannot do more than show what the average person now tolerates; they cannot show what he ought to tolerate and they fail to provide for those who are more sensitive than average. Others who are less sensitive have probably become deafened. In fact the population may not show a normal distribution for sensitivity to sound, and if the distribution is skew, arithmetical average hearing is really somewhat deaf and more tolerant of noise than truly normal hearing.

Hearing loss due to noise

The din made by boilermakers riveting inside resounding boilers has long been known to damage their hearing. There are no officially recommended limits for exposure to noise at work. For instance, steady noise throughout the day should not exceed 90 dBA. Exposure to 120 dBA should never occur for more than half a minute per working day. Obviously the limits cannot be determined by human experiment. Hearing loss due to noise is doubly treacherous; first, because the noise very quickly produces an initially transient deafness and so seems to have grown less, and secondly, because any damage done in youth may only become apparent when later in life the usual changes of **presbyacusis** are added and hearing of higher frequencies grows dulled (vol. 3, p. 32.11).

It has been possible for centuries to sue the creator of an unreasonable noise in court, but only in 1972 was a Code of Practice for Reducing the Exposure of Employed Persons to Noise issued. In the same year the first award for damages for deafness due to industrial noise was made in English courts.

Other effects of noise

Even short of producing deafness, noise can block conversation, produce accidents when warnings are not heard, ruin sleep, engender ill temper and fatigue, and impair industrial productivity. In the weaving industry, notoriously noisy, ear plugs enabled a 12 per cent improvement in production to occur.

VESTIBULAR APPARATUS OF THE INTERNAL EAR

This includes those parts of the membranous labyrinth which are concerned with equilibration rather than with hearing, namely the utricle and the (membranous) semicircular canals, and possibly the saccule. These are all lined by a simple squamous epithelium except for certain areas of specialized sensory epithelium.

The **utricle** and **saccule**, which lie within the vestibule of the bony labyrinth, each have a **macula** or **otolith organ**, consisting of specialized sensory ('hair') cells and supporting cells. The 'hairs' are atypical microvilli which project into a jelly-like carpet of proteoglycans, in which are suspended the **otoliths**. These are minute crystals chiefly of calcium carbonate. Change in position of the head alters the direction of gravitational pull on the otoliths, and the resulting mechanical deformation of the 'hairs' is transduced by the hair cells into electrical energy (nerve impulses) in the fibres of the vestibular nerve which terminate on the hair cells. In crayfish larvae, iron filings have been substituted for the otoliths. Presented with a magnet, the creature makes movements appropriate to the local magnetic field. In the saccule, the hair cells lie on the side wall and may serve as detectors of low frequency vibrations.

In the ampulla of each of the semicircular ducts is a specialized sensory epithelium, covering a ridge-like thickening of connective tissues arranged at right angles to the axis of the duct. The structure is a **crista ampullaris**; in the epithelium are hair cells similar to those of the maculae; the hair cells support a dome of jelly, the **cupula**. When the head is rotated, endolymph in one (or more) of the semicircular ducts lags behind, and distorts the cupula, thus stimulating the receptors. Which ducts are involved depends on the axis round which the head is rotated.

When the fluid is at rest, the activity of most of these receptors is not zero. If it were, then distortion to one side would produce activity, but distortion to the other side would produce no change; loss of one set of semicircular canals would deprive the victim of information about three of the six kinds of spin signalled by the canals, since spin either way round, in each of three planes, makes six. What actually happens is that there is a **resting activity**. Activity is diminished by distortion of the cupula to one side and increased by distortion to the other side (fig. 26.42). When a rotation starts, it is signalled in this way. When acceleration ceases and the rotation continues at a steady rate, the cupula resumes its starting position, being elastic. At the end of the rotation, the deceleration deflects the cupula in the opposite direction and so the impulse traffic alters in the opposite direction to its first change. In fish it is possible to insert a globule of oil into the canal and watch the mechanical changes going on. The system permits us to detect rotational acceleration so slight that it takes a whole minute, starting from a stationary position, to complete the first full turn.

The response to stimulation of the semicircular canals can be evoked by rotating a person in a special chair. But it is easier to use warm or cold water syringed gently into the external acoustic meatus; this method offers the extra advantage of testing one ear at a time. The lateral part of the lateral canal protrudes a little into the middle ear cavity; when the adjacent tympanic membrane is heated or cooled and the head is tilted appropriately, the endolymph in this part of the lateral canal undergoes a change of temperature and rises or falls in relation to the rest of the endolymph. Thus the effect of rotation on the canal is mimicked.

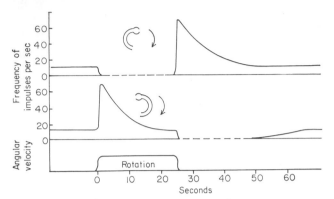

FIG. 26.42. Time course of discharge of vestibular neurones during rotation. From Adrian E.D. (1943) *J. Physiol.* **101**, 389.

The response consists in **nystagmus**, i.e. repeated movements of both eyes together slowly to one side and then rapidly back again. The direction of the nystagmus is defined as the direction of the quick movement, right or left, occasionally up or down if the head is not being held vertical. Vertical nystagmus may occur during spinning in a rotating chair. There is also **vertigo**, the sensation of rotation, often associated with vomiting. The subject also tends to misjudge the position of objects when he points to them (**pastpointing**) as if he were spinning round and round and making allowance for this.

As mentioned already, the semicircular canal system produces a resting discharge when there is no rotation. When rotatory acceleration occurs, this discharge grows or diminishes, depending on the direction of the spin. If the system on one side is damaged or removed, the effect is the same as that of rotation one way. Vertigo, nystagmus, nausea and vomiting occur and may take a month to settle down; and even then, if the damage is permanent, the control of eye movements may be deficient; the eyes may not be accurately moved to compensate for head movements.

FURTHER READING

AUTRUM H., JUNG R. *et al.* eds. (1972–) *Handbook of Sensory Physiology*, vol. VII. Berlin: Springer.

BENDER M.B. (1964) *The Oculomotor System*. New York: Harper & Row.

BRINDLEY G.S. (1970) *Physiology of the Retina and Visual Pathway*, 2nd Edition. Monograph of the Physiological Society, No. 6. London: Arnold.

DE REUCK A.V.S. & KNIGHT JULIE eds. (1968) *Ciba Foundation Symposium on Hearing Mechanisms in Vertebrates*. London: Churchill.

GREGORY R.L. (1966) *Eye and Brain*. London: World University Library.

LAST R.J. (1968) *Eugene Wolff's Anatomy of the Eye and Orbit*, 6th Edition. London: Lewis.

TAYLOR R. (1975) *Noise*, 2nd Edition. Harmondsworth: Penguin.

WERBLIN F.S. (1973) The control of sensitivity in the retina. *Scientific American* **228**, January, 70–79.

Chapter 27
Endocrine system

In the embryo, the primitive cells lining the body surfaces arc called epithelial cells. Apart from being protective, their most important function is to absorb substances from the surrounding medium which are then modified and secreted in another form. As the embryo grows, certain epithelial cells develop this function to a specialized degree and are formed into structures called glands. This is achieved by invagination of a sheet of epithelial cells as shown in fig. 27.1. They may remain connected to the epithelial surface by means of a duct through which their secretion reaches the surface, thereby localizing its site of action, or they may lose their connection with the surface and secrete their products into the blood stream, thus making them accessible to all the body cells. Glands which have a duct and secrete externally are called **exocrine glands** (fig. 27.1b), e.g. the intestinal glands, the pancreas, sweat glands, lacrimal and mammary glands. Those without a duct have an internal secretion and are called **endocrine** or **ductless glands** (fig. 27.1c). These are listed in table 27.1, together with the names of their principal secretions and common abbreviations. Endocrinology is the study of the structure and function of these ductless glands.

Some organs have both exocrine and endocrine functions, e.g. the acinar cells of the pancreas secrete digestive enzymes through the pancreatic duct into the

TABLE 27.1. The principal endocrine glands of the body and their most important secretions.

Glands	Secretions	Chemical nature
Anterior pituitary or adenohypophysis	Growth hormone (GH)	Protein, mol. wt. 21 500
	Adrenocorticotrophic hormone (ACTH)	Polypeptide, mol. wt. 4500
	Thyroid stimulating hormone (TSH)	Glycoprotein, mol. wt. 33 000
	Luteinizing hormone (LH) ⎫ gonadotrophic	Glycoprotein, mol. wt. 33 000
	Follicle stimulating hormone (FSH) ⎭	Glycoprotein
	Prolactin	Protein, mol. wt. 20 000 (sheep)
Posterior pituitary or neurohypophysis	Vasopressin or antidiuretic hormone (ADH)	Polypeptide of 9 amino acids
	Oxytocin	Polypeptide of 9 amino acids
Thyroid	Thyroxine (T4)	Iodinated amino acid
	Triiodothyronine (T3)	Iodinated amino acid
	Calcitonin	Polypeptide, mol. wt. 3600
Parathyroids	Parathyroid hormone	Polypeptide, mol. wt. 8500
Adrenals		
Cortex	Cortisol	Steroid
	Aldosterone	Steroid
	Corticosterone and many other steroids, including androgens and oestrogens in small amounts	Steroid
Medulla	Adrenaline (USA epinephrine)	Catecholamine
	Noradrenaline (USA norepinephrine)	Catecholamine
Kidneys	Renin	Protein mol. wt. 65 000
	Erythrogenin	Glycoprotein
Testes	Testosterone and other androgens	Steroid
Ovaries	Oestradiol and other oestrogens	Steroid
	Progesterone	Steroid
Placenta	Chorionic gonadotrophin (Human CG)	Glycoprotein mol. wt. 30 000
	Oestrogens	Steroid
	Progesterone	Steroid
Pancreas	Insulin	Polypeptide, mol. wt. 5800
	Glucagon	Polypeptide, a single chain, mol. wt 3500
Gastrointestinal tract		
Stomach	Gastrin	Polypeptides, mol. wts. 2000–7000
Duodenum	Secretin	Polypeptide, mol. wt. about 2700
Small intestine	Cholecystokinin–pancreozymin (CPZ)	Polypeptide, mol. wt. about 2700

duodenum, and the pancreatic islet cells secrete insulin into the blood. Although exocrine and endocrine secretions can come from the same organ, they originate from different cell types.

Endocrine glands have a characteristic morphology consisting of secretory cells surrounded by connective tissue that bears capillaries, lymphatics and nerves. The secretory cells are rich in mitochondria and secretory granules. During a phase of activity, the nuclei enlarge and the secretory granules decrease in number with the appearance of vacuoles in the cytoplasm. The posterior pituitary gland is an exception to this general arrangement as its secretions are produced in neurosecretory centres in the hypothalamus and transported along nerve fibres into the posterior pituitary gland where they are stored and released as required.

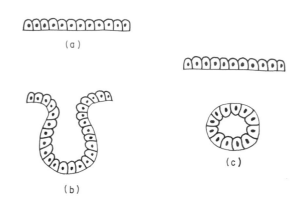

FIG. 27.1. (a) Primitive epithelial cells; (b) invaginations of epithelial cells to form an exocrine gland; (c) endocrine gland with loss of duct.

All endocrine glands have a rich blood supply into which they pour their secretions. The nerve supply to the glands appears to play little part in their function except for the adrenal medulla, posterior pituitary and hypothalamus. The importance of the lymphatic drainage as a mechanism of hormone transport is not known but is probably small.

The internal secretions of the ductless glands were first called **hormones** (Greek *hormao*, I excite) in 1905 by Starling, after he and Bayliss had isolated the hormone, secretin, from the mucosal cells of the upper gastrointestinal tract. They regarded a hormone as a substance normally produced in the cells of some part of the body and carried by the blood stream to distant parts, so acting on the organism as a whole. This definition does not describe adequately present knowledge of the diverse actions of hormones, but it is difficult to be more precise.

The hormones maintain the constancy of the internal environment by affecting such variables as water and electrolyte balance, blood glucose concentration and metabolic rate. They also regulate cell metabolism,

respiration, reproduction and neural activity. Hormones influence growth, development and ageing, and the responses to stress such as emotional disturbances, injury or infection. In certain instances their action is strictly localized, e.g. the pituitary hormone, thyroid stimulating hormone (TSH) stimulates only the cells of the thyroid gland, while others, e.g. the adrenal hormone, cortisol, affect the metabolism of most cells.

Of the hormones listed in table 27.1, those produced by the pituitary, thyroid and parathyroids, the adrenal glands and pancreas are discussed in this chapter. The placenta is also an endocrine gland, for it elaborates hormones that are necessary for the growth and function of both the pregnant uterus and the fetus. It is dealt with in chap. 38 together with the ovaries and testes. The hormones secreted by the upper gastrointestinal tract regulate the supply of the exocrine digestive secretions. The actions of these hormones are described in chap. 32. The kidney secretes two hormones; erythrogenin regulates the production of red blood cells in response to hypoxia and renin plays an important part in salt metabolism and the maintenance of blood pressure (p. 35.28).

The thymus may produce hormones which are important in the development and function of the immunological mechanisms (p. 29.41). Whether the pineal gland has an endocrine function remains obscure after many years of conjecture (p. 25.64).

STUDY OF ENDOCRINE GLAND FUNCTION

The existence of the endocrine glands has been recognized since ancient times when views on their function were purely speculative and derived mainly from the site and morphology of the glands. For example, the adrenal glands, first illustrated by Eustachius in 1563, were thought to be active only in fetal life because of their large size at birth. Subsequently they were thought to act as a support for the stomach and even to help maintain potency. The thyroid gland was first thought to be part of the vocal apparatus and then to serve as a lubricating organ for the tissues of the neck. Some physicians considered it to be only an adornment of the neck. From the seventeenth century onwards, the study of endocrinology has been more scientific.

CLINICAL OBSERVATIONS

These have been responsible for some of the most important landmarks in endocrinology and are still important today. In 1849 Thomas Addison read a paper to the South London Medical Society on 'a diseased condition of the adrenal glands which may interfere with the proper elaboration of the body generally'. This did much to dispel some of the false notions then prevailing as to the function of these glands and gave a strong impetus to further work.

Swelling of the thyroid gland (goitre) was recognized from early times to be associated in some cases with a condition now known as cretinism. It was also recognized that goitres were often endemic in populations living in certain mountainous regions. Despite this association, cretinism was still an obscure disease, even when Sir William Gull described in 1873 a similar disease, myxoedema, in adults. When thyroidectomy began to be practised at the end of the nineteenth century, it was found that symptoms resembling those seen in cases of myxoedema occurred, and this clinical observation led to the view that myxoedema and cretinism were both due to the same cause, namely loss of function of the thyroid gland.

By the beginning of this century, many of the diseases due to dysfunction of the pituitary gland had been described. For example, the condition of gigantism had been recognized, and acromegaly, characterized by overgrowth of certain parts of the skeleton, was described in 1886 by Pierre Marie. Apart from the observation that the pituitary fossa was enlarged, there was little to indicate that the pituitary gland was primarily responsible for these disorders. With the development of histological techniques, it was soon realized that acromegaly and gigantism were associated with an acidophil tumour of the pituitary gland.

PHYSIOLOGICAL AND EXPERIMENTAL APPROACH

Physiological investigations of the endocrine glands are based on studies of the effects of removing a gland and sometimes of transplanting it in the same animal. By these techniques, the effects of lack of the secretion of a gland can be observed and the status of the gland as an endocrine organ established by the demonstration that it produces its effects by humoral mechanisms independent of nervous connections.

Berthold, in 1849, demonstrated the existence of an internal secretion when he showed that transplantation of the testes of a cock to its peritoneal cavity prevented the atrophy of the comb that follows castration. Soon after, Brown–Séquard extended Addison's description of the effects of adrenal insufficiency in man, by showing that removal of these glands in animals was fatal, and that they were essential to life. Removal of the pituitary gland, hypophysectomy, in animals resulted in striking changes in which the animal failed to grow and the genital organs remained undeveloped. Changes also occurred in other endocrine organs such as the thyroid and adrenal glands which atrophied. These experiments indicated that the pituitary gland exerts a controlling influence over other endocrine organs.

Transplantation of the pituitary gland to other parts of the body was an exception to the rule about endocrine organs, since function was not restored unless the graft was replaced under the pituitary stalk. Restoration is dependent on the tissue being revascularized by vessels of the pituitary stalk called the hypophysial portal vessels (p. 27.10). In this way, it became evident that the pituitary was itself controlled by a higher centre, now known to be the hypothalamus.

The work of Houssay, in Buenos Aires in 1924, on the relationship between the anterior pituitary and the pancreas is an example of how views on the aetiology of endocrine disease were influenced by experimental studies. Before this, diabetes mellitus was thought to be a disease caused by a simple failure of the β-cells of the pancreas to secrete insulin, just as primary myxoedema resulted from inability of the thyroid to secrete its hormone. Houssay showed that after hypophysectomy an animal became very sensitive to insulin, and even small doses reduced the blood glucose dangerously. This hypoglycaemic action of insulin could, however, be prevented by injecting extracts of the anterior pituitary. He also demonstrated that in a dog from which the pancreas had been removed, the resulting diabetes could be alleviated by removing the pituitary gland. Later, Young in London gave repeated injections of anterior pituitary extract into dogs and induced permanent diabetes. It was apparent that the anterior pituitary gland produced hormones which were important in the regulation of carbohydrate metabolism and that other mechanisms, apart from simple failure of the β-cells of the pancreas, might be responsible for diabetes mellitus.

ISOLATION OF HORMONES

After observing the effects of lack of the hormones of the endocrine glands in animals, the next step was to try to make good this lack by giving extracts of gland either orally or by injection. Murray, in 1891, successfully treated a Newcastle lady, aged 46, suffering from myxoedema with an extract of sheep's thyroid gland given subcutaneously. She was subsequently given the extract by mouth, and when she died 28 years later it was estimated that she had consumed the equivalent of the thyroid glands of 870 sheep. In 1929, Swingle and Pfiffner obtained a water-soluble extract of the adrenal glands from an ox and demonstrated that daily intraperitoneal injections of this extract, together with an adequate salt intake, could maintain in health dogs whose adrenal glands had been removed, whereas without the extract the animals died. This led to the isolation, in the 1930's, of the adrenocortical hormones, which are steroids and are used in replacement therapy in patients whose adrenal glands have been destroyed and also in the treatment of many non-endocrine diseases.

In 1894, Schäfer and Oliver showed that the adrenal

medulla contained a substance which produced a rise in blood pressure. In 1901, this substance was isolated in crystalline form and called **adrenaline**; it was synthesized in 1904 and was thus the first hormone to be characterized.

A most important landmark in the history of endocrinology was the discovery of the pancreatic hormone, **insulin**, by Banting, Best and Macleod in Toronto and Paulescu in Romania in 1921. The practical importance of this hormone in the treatment of diabetes mellitus, which at that time was a fatal disease, led to the search for other hormones of therapeutic value.

One of the most recent hormones to be discovered is **calcitonin**. In 1962, Copp, in perfusion studies on dogs, produced evidence of a hormone apparently released from the parathyroid glands which lowered the blood calcium. Further experiments showed that the hypocalcaemic factor was in fact released from the thyroid gland (p. 27.24).

HORMONE ASSAYS

A natural consequence of the identification of individual hormones from the endocrine glands was the development of methods for measuring the concentration of these hormones in glands and body fluids. There are three types of assay procedure: (1) biological, (2) immunological and (3) chemical.

Biological assays

These involve the measurement of a graded or quantal effect following administration of the hormone to an experimental animal, in which the potency of the unknown preparation is compared with that of a standard preparation (p. 3.11). For example, the concentration of human pituitary gonadotrophins in the urine is assayed by injecting immature mice subcutaneously once or twice a day for 3 days with the test preparation of a urinary extract. They are killed 72 hours after the first injection and the weight of the uterus is measured; the results are compared with those obtained from mice injected with a standard preparation made from postmenopausal urine. From this comparison, the gonadotrophic activity of the test preparation can be measured (p. 38.14).

A biological assay involving radioactive isotopes is used for studying another pituitary hormone, thyroid stimulating hormone (TSH). One method depends on the discharge of radioactive iodine, ^{125}I, from the thyroid glands of mice (fig. 27.2). Mice are fed on a diet low in iodine, which ensures a high uptake by the thyroid gland of any iodine given to the animal. ^{125}I is injected intraperitoneally, and each animal is then given large doses of thyroxine which suppresses the release of endogenous TSH from the pituitary gland. Under these conditions, the thyroid hormones become labelled with ^{125}I, but as the mice are being fed large doses of thyroxine the labelled hormones remain in the gland and little radio-

activity is detected in the circulating blood, as thyroid hormone is not discharged from the gland under these circumstances. When a standard preparation of TSH, or a test preparation containing TSH, is injected intravenously, some of the hormone labelled with ^{131}I stored in the thyroid gland is discharged into the circulation. The radioactivity is measured in blood samples taken two or three hours after the injection. The increases in the blood radioactivity following the injection of the test preparation and of a standard TSH preparation are then compared.

In biological assays, in view of the variation in response which may be obtained with different strains or even the same strain of animals in one laboratory at different times of the year, it is essential that results are related to those obtained with a single standardized preparation of the material in question. To this end, an international stan-

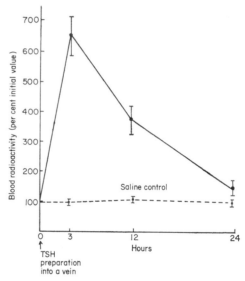

FIG. 27.2. Effect of a standard preparation of TSH on the blood radioactivity of mice (see text).

dard for TSH was established in 1955; one international unit (IU) is defined as the activity present in 13·5 mg of the standard material. International standards have been established for the bioassay of gonadotrophins, insulin and other hormones. The most sensitive assay for plasma ACTH at present is a bioassay which depends upon measurement by a redox method of the depletion of ascorbic acid from the adrenal cortex, following ACTH administration. Reducing substances such as ascorbic acid can be stained by ferric ferrocyanide in the zona reticularis of slices of guinea-pig adrenal cortex in organ culture. The intensity of staining can be measured by microdensitometry and an inverse correlation holds between the stain and the concentration of ACTH added to the medium. Such a system is capable of detecting a concentration of ACTH of 17 pg/l and is much more sensitive than the current immunoassay.

Certain tests of endocrine function used in clinical medicine are in fact a form of biological assay performed on the patient himself. For example, the measurement of plasma cortisol during insulin-induced hypoglycaemia is an index of the secretion of pituitary ACTH and an established test of the function of the hypothalamo-pituitary-adrenal axis (vol. 3, p. 23.2).

Biological assays in animals are, in general, time consuming and expensive. The animals often require removal of major endocrine glands, e.g. hypophysectomy and pancreatectomy, to increase their sensitivity to the hormone being measured and, as can be appreciated, the care of animals in such circumstances may be difficult. Bioassays may suffer also from the disadvantage that the chosen response may be influenced by hormones of different chemical structure. Provided the response being measured is sufficiently specific, the success of bioassays depends upon the careful design of the experiment and the statistical analysis of the results.

Immunological assays

On repeated injection of a pure preparation of a protein hormone into an animal the substance acts as an immunogen or antigen and produces antibodies in the animal's plasma (p.29.8); these can react with one or more binding sites on the hormone antigen. Antisera prepared in this manner can be used to detect many hormones including all the hormones of the anterior pituitary gland, insulin and parathyroid hormone. Antisera may also be raised against a hormone of low molecular weight, such as thyroxine, vasopressin or cortisol, if it is complexed with albumin.

Immunoassays depend on a reaction between a hormone labelled with ^{131}I or ^{125}I (radio-iodinated antigen) and an antibody specific to the hormone. This results in the formation of a labelled antigen–antibody complex. When, for instance, unlabelled human growth hormone (HGH) in a test preparation is added to a known amount of labelled hormone and the two mixed with antiserum, there is competition between unlabelled and labelled hormone for binding sites on the antibody.

$$\left[\begin{array}{l} {}^{125}\text{I-HGH} + \text{HGH} \\ \quad \text{(test or} \\ \quad \text{standard} \\ \quad \text{preparation)} \end{array}\right] + \begin{array}{l} \text{antibody to} \longrightarrow \\ \text{HGH} \end{array}$$

$$\begin{array}{c} {}^{125}\text{I-HGH-antibody} \\ + \\ \text{HGH-antibody} \end{array}$$

The bound and free antigen can be separated by differential precipitation, electrophoresis or paper chromatography and the ratio:

$$\frac{{}^{125}\text{I-HGH}}{{}^{125}\text{I-HGH-antibody}}$$

can be determined. The ratios obtained with the test and standard preparations are compared. The more HGH the test preparation contains, the smaller the percentage of labelled hormone bound to the antibody.

Immunological assays are potentially more specific than biological assays with the exception of the redox assay for ACTH, and can be extremely sensitive. They can be carried out on small volumes of unextracted plasma and applied to large numbers of samples at one time; they are cheaper than bioassays. One major disadvantage is that a highly purified preparation must be available for labelling with ^{125}I. It is also difficult to be certain of the purity of the preparations used and, therefore, to be sure exactly what the immunoassay is measuring. Furthermore, the antibody may be reactive with a biologically inactive portion of the hormone amino acid chain. The results of immunoassay therefore require to be checked against bioassay.

Chemical assays

Few individual hormones are now assayed by chemical methods. However the estimation of chemical groups common to several related hormones is a less specific but valuable method. Thus the fluorometric determination of 11-hydroxycorticosteroids in human plasma gives a good measure of the amount of cortisol and corticosterone in plasma, these substances being the major components of the 11-hydroxycorticosteroids. Other steroid metabolites may be less specific, for example, the 17-oxosteroids; androstenedione and testosterone are both 17-oxosteroids. Estimating this group does not distinguish between them and so is of little value in assessing the relative activity of the adrenal cortex and testes. The measurement of the catecholamines (adrenaline, noradrenaline and related products) excreted in the urine provides an index of the secretion in the body of adrenaline and noradrenaline.

HORMONE SECRETION RATE

The concentration of a particular hormone in the plasma depends upon an equilibrium between its rate of synthesis in the endocrine gland, the amount bound in the tissues, the rate of destruction by cell metabolism and the rate of loss in the urine and other excretory routes. The measurement of hormone secretion rates provides a more accurate index of the metabolic activity of an endocrine gland.

The secretion rate of cortisol by the adrenal cortex can be determined by the technique of isotope dilution. Isotopically labelled cortisol is metabolized in the same way as the patient's own cortisol, and it is excreted in the urine in the form of metabolic derivatives. A known dose of ^{14}C-cortisol is given orally to the patient. The patient's urine is then collected for a finite period of time, e.g. 48 hours. One of the metabolites of cortisol excreted in the urine, e.g. tetrahydrocortisone, is then extracted from the 48-hour collection of urine, its total amount measured chemically and its radio-activity also determined. The following formula then holds:

$$\frac{\text{Endogenous cortisol secretion}}{\text{Amount }^{14}\text{C-cortisol given to patient*}} =$$

$$\frac{\text{Urinary excretion of tetrahydrocortisone*}}{\text{Urinary }^{14}\text{C-tetrahydrocortisone*}}$$

Those variables indicated by an asterisk can be measured directly and hence the endogenous cortisol secretion rate over the period of study calculated. A similar technique may be used to determine secretion rate of aldosterone.

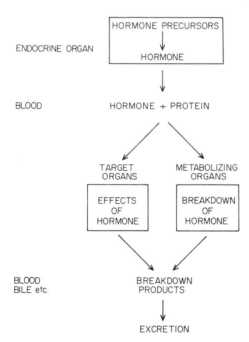

FIG. 27.3. Secretion, transport and metabolism of hormones.

Secretion, transport and disposal of hormones
(fig. 27.3)

Hormones are synthesized from precursors in the endocrine glands. Some hormones are then secreted into the blood almost as quickly as they are formed, e.g. the adrenocortical hormones. Other endocrine glands, such as the thyroid, store the hormone and secrete it over long periods of time. Hormonal secretion may follow a cyclical pattern, e.g. ovarian hormones and adrenocortical hormones. In the blood many hormones are transported wholly or partly bound to plasma proteins. Their concentration there is determined by their rate of secretion, the

rate at which they are taken up by and disposed of in the tissues and their rate of excretion.

Hormones exert their effects on the cells and tissues by a number of mechanisms only a few of which are understood. They may act by influencing enzymic mechanisms in the cells of the target organs, e.g. adrenaline increases the activity of adenyl cyclase within the membrane of sensitive cells; this, in turn raises the concentration of cyclic AMP and hence affects the phosphorylase which catalyses the breakdown of glycogen to glucose in the liver (p. 9.10). Some hormones may act by changing the permeability of membranes. In this way insulin enhances the transport of glucose and amino acids from the extracellular fluid into the cell cytoplasm. Several hormones, e.g. thyroxine and cortisol, appear to act on the cell nucleus and thereby stimulate the production of m-RNA; this may lead to the synthesis of specific enzymes which influence the direction of metabolism. Fuller accounts of the actions of individual hormones are given later in this chapter and the role of hormones in the control of metabolism is discussed on p. 14.12.

Hormones are broken down either in their target organs or in other tissues, notably the liver, to biologically inert substances. These then undergo further chemical change, referred to as conjugation, to form more soluble compounds which can be excreted by the kidney.

Control of endocrine function

A primary function of hormones is maintenance of metabolic homeostasis. This is achieved at tissue level by a complex interaction of hormones in metabolic reactions which can be either antagonistic or synergistic, e.g. growth hormone promotes protein synthesis whereas the adrenocorticosteroids promote protein breakdown in some tissues. On the other hand, growth hormone and the adrenocorticosteroids have a synergistic effect on fat metabolism, the synthesis of fat being inhibited.

At a higher level, the maintenance of homeostasis depends on a close integration between the endocrine glands and the central nervous system. The influence of the nervous system on the endocrine glands is mediated through the hypothalamus and this is well seen in the reproductive system where different conditions are necessary for ovulation in various species. In the dog and humans, ovulation is spontaneous and independent of mating. In the cat and the rabbit, however, ovulation requires the stimulus of coitus or an artificial stimulus to the vagina or cervix. In these animals, hypophysectomy prevents ovulation, thus indicating that the stimuli act through a higher centre which is probably the hypothalamus. This acts on the anterior lobe of the pituitary which in turn stimulates the ovary to liberate the ovum. Again in women it is well recognized that emotional disturbances may cause amenorrhoea. Any form of stress acts through the nervous system and has definite effects on the endocrine system, in particular on the adrenal glands, which counter the threat to homeostasis by preparing the person for 'fight or flight' through the secretion of increased amounts of adrenaline, noradrenaline and cortisol (pp. 27.31 & 35).

The hormones of the anterior pituitary gland are controlled by the hypothalamus which secretes regulatory substances, called **releasing** and **inhibiting factors** or **hormones**. These enter the portal venous system which flows from the median eminence to the anterior lobe of the pituitary. Histologically, the median eminence consists of nerve terminals, perivascular spaces and capillaries. These releasing and inhibiting substances are synthesized in areas of the hypothalamus yet to be determined and travel by axonal flow to nerve endings of the median eminence where they are stored. Their release into the capillaries of the median eminence is mediated via catecholaminergic neurones, which terminate close to the secretory terminals, although synaptic junctions are rare.

At present, seven releasing or inhibiting substances have been described (table 27.2) affecting the release of

TABLE 27.2. Hypothalamic regulatory substances

Substance	Chemical nature
Thyrotrophin releasing hormone (TRH)	Tripeptide
Luteinizing hormone/follicle stimulating hormone-releasing hormone (LH/FSH-RH)	Decapeptide
Melanocyte stimulating hormone release inhibiting hormone (MRIH)	Tripeptide
Growth hormone release inhibiting hormone (GHRIH)	Tetradecapeptide
Growth hormone releasing factor (GHRF)	?
Prolactin release inhibiting factor (PRIF)	?
Corticotrophin releasing factor (CRF)	?

TSH, LH, FSH, GH and ACTH, and inhibiting the release of prolactin and MSH, in addition to GH. It is possible that each anterior pituitary hormone is under the dual control of a releasing and an inhibiting substance. Four have been synthesized and the synthetic product has identical biological properties to the hypothalamic extract, and therefore by convention they are accepted as hormones; the chemical nature of three is as yet unidentified (table 27.2). The releasing hormones appear to increase the concentration of cyclic AMP in the anterior pituitary.

TRH is a tripeptide, pyroglutamyl-histidyl-prolinamide, which is widely used in the diagnosis of thyroid disease (vol. 3, p. 23.4). Administration of TRH also releases prolactin from the anterior pituitary gland, and it may be that TRH is the physiological prolactin releasing factor or shares part of its chemical structure.

LH/FSH-RH is a decapeptide which releases both LH and FSH from the anterior pituitary and is used clinically as a test for gonadotrophin reserve. It is also possible to induce ovulation and pregnancy in patients with unidentified hypothalamic disorders by repeated administration of the releasing hormone.

GHRIH, sometimes called somatostatin, is a cyclic tetradecapeptide, which abolishes the rise in plasma GH normally induced by exercise (p. 27.13) and lowers the high GH concentrations in the plasma of patients with gigantism or acromegaly (vol. 3, p. 23.7) when given intravenously. GHRIH also suppresses gastrin release in healthy subjects and in patients with pernicious anaemia in whom plasma gastrin is high. Suppression of the release of glucagon and insulin by the α- and β-cells respectively of the pancreatic islets has also been shown, resulting in a fall in fasting blood glucose, but a diabetic response to a glucose load. GHRIH has been found in the D cells of the pancreatic islets but its physiological role there is unknown (p. 27.49). The mode of action of GHRIH on inhibition of release of hormones from the anterior pituitary gland is not understood.

MRIH is a tripeptide which is thought to be a degradation product of oxytocin, since a microsomal exopeptidase present in the hypothalamus is capable of converting oxytocin to MRIH.

Hormones themselves exert an important influence on the nervous system. For example, the sex hormones have a role in establishing psychological behaviour patterns (p. 40.8). Diseases of the endocrine glands are also often accompanied by effects on the nervous system, e.g. the psychosis which sometimes accompanies hyperfunction of the adrenal cortex (Cushing's syndrome, p. 27.38). Hormones, however, by their influence on the hypothalamus and the pituitary gland, can regulate the rate of their own secretion by negative feedback control. Increased concentration of a particular hormone in the blood inhibits secretion of the appropriate trophic hormone from the pituitary gland within minutes, whereas a fall in the blood concentration removes this inhibition so that the secretion of the trophic hormone is facilitated; thus the level of circulating cortisol is in part controlled by a feedback mechanism by which a rise in cortisol level reduces ACTH secretion and hence cortisol output, and vice versa. The site of action of this feedback control of trophic hormone secretion includes both the pituitary and the hypothalamus and possibly even higher centres. The site of the feedback action of thyroxine, for example, is probably mainly the pituitary gland, whereas in the case of the adrenal and gonadal steroids it is thought to be the hypothalamus. This reciprocal relationship between plasma hormone level and trophic hormone secretion may become overridden under conditions of stress, for example hypoglycaemia, injury or infection in which ACTH is secreted independently of the circulating level of cortisol.

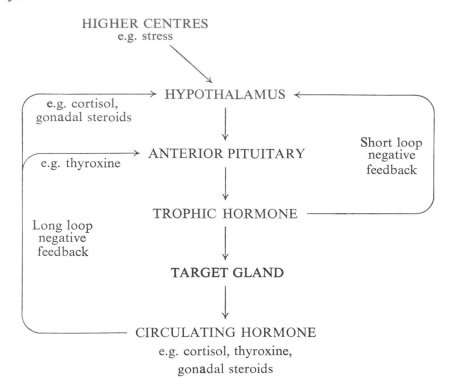

HIGHER CENTRES
e.g. stress

HYPOTHALAMUS

e.g. cortisol,
gonadal steroids

ANTERIOR PITUITARY

e.g. thyroxine

Short loop
negative
feedback

TROPHIC HORMONE

Long loop
negative
feedback

TARGET GLAND

CIRCULATING HORMONE
e.g. cortisol, thyroxine,
gonadal steroids

FIG. 27.4. Feedback mechanisms in the control of endocrine secretion.

The problem of pituitary regulation has been further complicated by the discovery that certain pituitary trophic hormones, e.g. luteinizing hormone (LH), may act on the hypothalamus to inhibit their own secretion. These observations have given rise to the idea of the 'short feedback loop' theory of pituitary control. The relationship between the hypothalamic nuclei, anterior pituitary function and circulating hormones is shown in fig. 27.4.

Structure of hormones

Hormones can be classified according to their chemical structure and are either polypeptides or proteins, steroids or phenol derivatives.

The protein hormones are complex polypeptides and include the hormones of the anterior lobe of the pituitary gland, parathyroid and pancreas. The structure of the protein hormones may vary from one animal to another so that they may exhibit species specificity with regard to their hormone activity. Thus growth hormone is partly species specific and primate pituitary glands are the only source of growth hormone effective in man. ACTH is an example of a typical protein hormone. In man it is a polypeptide containing thirty-nine amino acids (fig. 27.5).

By convention the constituent amino acids are numbered starting from the end of the molecule which has the free NH_2 group (the N-terminal end, fig. 27.6). The immunological and hormonal properties of ACTH reside in different parts of the molecule. The corticotrophin activity resides in the 9–24 amino acids. The amino acids

Ser-Tyr-Ser-Met-Glu-His-Phe-Arg-Trp-Gly-Lys-Pro-Val-
1　2　3　4　5　6　7　8　9　10　11　12　13
Gly-Lys-Lys-Arg-Arg-Pro-Val-Lys-Val-Tyr-Pro-Asp-(NH$_2$)
14　15　16　17　18　19　20　21　22　23　24　25
Gly-Ala-Glu-Asp-Glu-Ser-Ala-Glu-Ala-Phe-Pro-Leu-
26　27　28　29　30　31　32　33　34　35　36　37
Glu-Phe
38　39

FIG. 27.5. The amino acid sequence of human ACTH. The abbreviations are given in full on p. 11.2.

in positions 25–33 vary in different species of animals. When ACTH of animal origin is injected into man, it is likely to be antigenic, and may lead to allergic reactions.

Antibodies produced by preparations of parathyroid hormone may interfere with the action of the injected hormone so that continued administration of the hormone becomes ineffective. The synthesis of the biologically active part of the ACTH molecule (9–24 corticotrophin) obviates the development of any untoward immunological reactions. The hormones of the posterior lobe of the pituitary are smaller polypeptides and are not antigenic in man.

The steroid hormones are secreted by the adrenal cortex, the testes and the ovaries. Steroids have a characteristic structure described on p. 10.21. The hormones which are derivatives of tyrosine are T_4, T_3 and adrenaline.

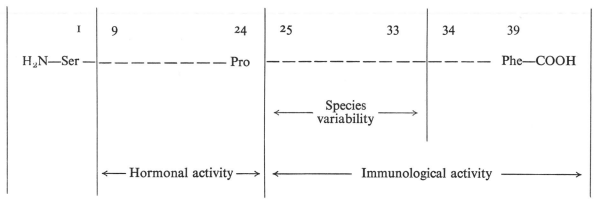

| | I | 9 | 24 | 25 | 33 | 34 | 39 | |

FIG. 27.6. Schematic representation of ACTH.

PITUITARY GLAND

Anatomy

The pituitary gland is an appendage of the ventral surface of the brain and derives its name from the Latin word, *pituita*, meaning mucus, as originally it was thought to transfer mucus from the brain through the cribriform plate of the ethmoid into the nose. It is also called the **hypophysis**, from the Greek word meaning to grow under. The gland is oval in shape, weighing about 500 mg, although it gets smaller with advancing age. It lies in the base of the skull in a depression of the sphenoid bone called the pituitary fossa or sella turcica (fig. 27.7).

The sella turcica is immediately behind the superior part of the sphenoidal air sinuses so that its floor forms part of the roof of each sinus. It is bounded laterally by the cavernous sinuses and the structures which they contain (fig. 22.6). The posterior boundary of the hypophysial fossa is a plate of bone forming the dorsum sellae (p. 22.4).

The arachnoid and pia mater blend with the capsule of the pituitary gland and so cannot be identified as separate layers in the fossa. Above, the gland is covered by a fold of dura mater, the diaphragma sellae, which thus forms the roof of the hypophysial fossa. It is pierced by the **infundibulum** which is the stalk connecting the pituitary gland to the brain. Above the diaphragma sellae is the hypothalamus and the third ventricle and slightly anteriorly is the optic chiasma. This proximity of the hypophysis to the optic pathways is of importance should the gland enlarge.

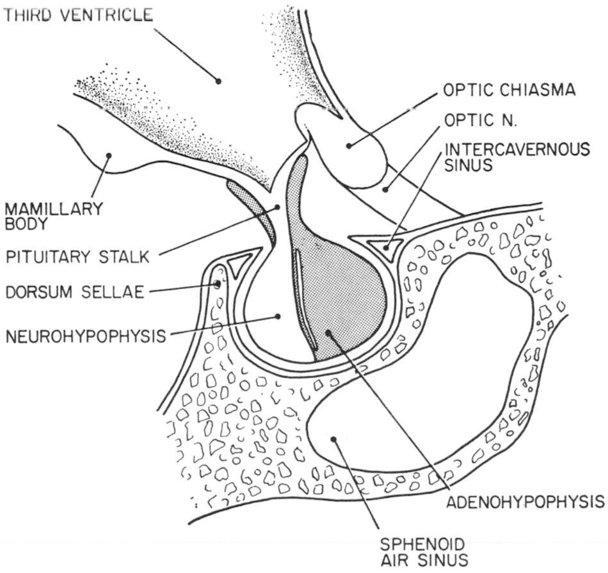

FIG. 27.7. A mid sagittal section of the pituitary gland in its fossa.

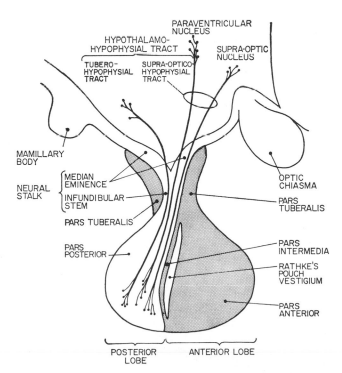

FIG. 27.8. Diagram showing the component parts of the pituitary gland and its connections with the nervous system.

The pituitary gland consists of four different parts (fig. 27.8).

(1) **Pars posterior** or **neurohypophysis** is an outgrowth of the brain to which it is attached by the infundibulum.

(2) **Pars anterior** is the main part of the organ and is glandular in structure.

(3) **Pars intermedia** is rudimentary in man but is large in some vertebrates. It lies behind the pars anterior, separated from it by a small cleft, the remnant of Rathke's pouch.

(4) **Pars tuberalis** is an extension of pars anterior and encloses the infundibulum. It is also rudimentary in man and has no functional significance.

The **adenohypophysis** consists of the pars anterior, pars tuberalis and pars intermedia.

EMBRYOLOGY

The anterior lobe of the pituitary gland is derived from the ectoderm of the primitive mouth or stomatodeum, and the posterior lobe is derived from the neuroectoderm of the floor of the forebrain.

In the roof of the stomatodeum, a diverticulum forms which remains in contact with the under surface of the brain (fig. 27.9a). The surrounding mesoderm then constricts this diverticulum, which is also known as **Rathke's pouch**, cutting it off from the stomatodeum (fig. 27.9b). The ectodermal cells of the isolated diverticulum eventually develop into those of the anterior lobe (fig. 27.9c).

Behind Rathke's pouch, a hollow neural outgrowth extends from the base of the brain towards the mouth. The distal end of this outgrowth becomes solid and forms the pars posterior. The proximal part of the outgrowth, which is also solid, becomes the infundibulum and is covered by two dorsal extensions of the anterior lobe, the pars tuberalis.

The cleft separating the pars intermedia from pars anterior is the remains of the original cavity of the stomatodeal diverticulum.

BLOOD SUPPLY

The internal carotid artery through its branches, the superior and inferior hypophysial arteries, supplies blood to the pituitary gland. The hypophysial arteries anastomose with each other on the surface of the adenohypophysis which is, therefore, richly vascularized (fig. 27.10).

The pituitary stalk or infundibulum is also supplied by a primary capillary plexus of the **hypophysial portal system**, as it is drained by a number of portal veins

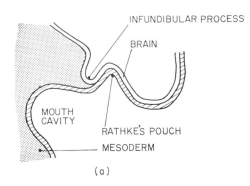

(a)

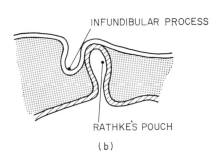

(b)

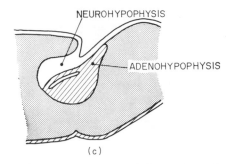

(c)

FIG. 27.9. Development of the pituitary gland.

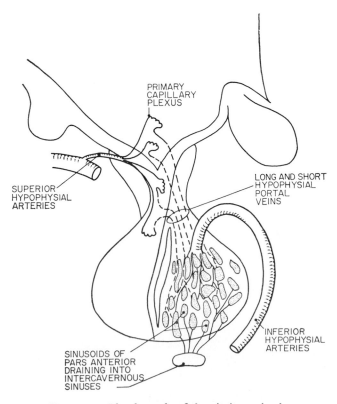

FIG. 27.10. Blood supply of the pituitary gland.

that lie on the anterior surface of the pituitary stalk. These veins are called the long and short portal veins. The long veins originate in the upper pituitary stalk and median eminence of the hypothalamus, and the short portal veins originate in the lower pituitary stalk a few millimetres below the diaphragma sellae. They penetrate the adenohypophysis and form a secondary sinusoidal plexus. The importance of this system in the hypothalamic control of the anterior pituitary has already been referred to (p. 27.7).

The venous drainage of the pituitary consists of small efferent veins which drain into intercavernous sinuses in the dura mater surrounding the gland.

NERVE SUPPLY

Although nervous influences affect the function of the anterior pituitary gland, it has no direct innervation. The neurohypophysis, however, has a well-defined nerve supply called the hypothalamo–hypophysial tract (fig. 27.8). This consists of two parts, the supraopticohypophysial tract and the tuberohypophysial tract. The former arises from the supra-optic and paraventricular nuclei of the hypothalamus and runs in the anterior wall of the infundibulum to end in the neurohypophysis. The tuberohypophysial tract arises from the nuclei in the posterior hypothalamus and descends to the neurohypophysis in the posterior wall of the stalk. The hypothalamo–hypophysial tract is situated centrally in the neural stalk, being separated from the pars tuberalis by a zone relatively free of nerve elements. A few nerve fibres from this tract may enter the pars intermedia or the pars tuberalis but it is questionable whether any enter the pars anterior.

Sympathetic nerve fibres enter the pituitary gland from the perivascular plexuses which surround the gland. They are very few in number and probably have a vasomotor function.

HISTOLOGICAL STRUCTURE

Pars anterior

The glandular cells are arranged in columns, separated from each other by sinusoids. By means of haematoxylin and eosin stains, the cells can be divided according to whether they take up or reject the stain into two main types, (1) chromophil cells and (2) chromophobe cells.

The chromophil cells are large and contain granules which stain well. They can be subdivided further according to their staining reactions into two different types of cell, (1) acidophil cells or α cells and (2) basophil cells or β cells. The acidophil cells or eosinophils are so called because they stain red with eosin and have an affinity for other acid dyes. The basophil cells stain blue with haematoxylin and have an affinity for other basic dyes (plate 27.1a, facing p. 27.20).

The chromophobe cells are smaller, do not contain

granules and stain very faintly. They are thought to be degranulated forms of the chromophil cells and are arbitarily subdivided according to size. They are regarded as resting forms of the secreting chromophil cells.

With the use of more specialized staining techniques, the chromophil cells of the anterior pituitary have been divided into a greater variety of cell types. These are designated α, $\beta 1$, $\beta 2$, $\delta 1$ and $\delta 2$. The α cells are the conventional eosinophil cells. The $\beta 1$ cell is a large polyhedral cell, usually heavily granulated, the granules being intensely PAS positive. The granules of the $\beta 2$ cells have a strong affinity for the dye aldehyde thionin, staining a blue-black colour; they are fine and tend to aggregate irregularly in parts of the cell, giving a variable staining effect. The $\delta 1$ cell is a small oval cell often found amongst the α cells. Its granules are stained by aldehyde thionin. The $\delta 2$ cell is also a small oval cell and, although PAS positive it is easily differentiated from the larger PAS positive $\beta 1$ cell.

A functional classification of the chromophil cells based on clinical evidence is shown in table 27.3.

TABLE 27.3. Classification of the chromophil cells of the anterior pituitary gland.

Staining reaction	Function	Hormone
Acidophil or α cell	Somatotrophic	Growth Hormone
	Lactotrophic	Prolactin
Basophil $\beta 1$	Corticotrophic	ACTH
$\beta 2$	Thyrotrophic	TSH
$\delta 1$	Gonadotrophic	?LH
$\delta 2$	Gonadotrophic	?FSH

The acidophil cells almost certainly secrete growth hormone since an acidophil cell tumour of the gland results in the disease called acromegaly, known to be associated with hypersecretion of growth hormone.

The $\beta 1$ cell is probably the source of ACTH, since patients with prolonged high blood levels of cortisol due either to overactivity of the adrenal gland (Cushing's syndrome) or to cortisone therapy develop a hyaline change in the $\beta 1$ cells (Crooke's hyaline change). TSH is thought to be secreted by the $\beta 2$ cells because marked hyperplasia of these cells has been observed in patients with myxoedema.

The δ cells are probably responsible for the secretion of the gonadotrophic hormones as they are not present in the pituitary glands of young children or during the last two trimesters of pregnancy. It is thought that the $\delta 1$ cell secretes LH and the $\delta 2$ cell FSH.

Pars posterior

The neurohypophysis consists of large branching spindle cells which resemble neuroglial cells. They are called pituicytes. Also in the posterior lobe of the gland are occasional mast cells and pigment cells as well as a rich network of nerve fibres and islets of basophil cells. These basophil cells have probably infiltrated from the adenohypophysis and are frequently found in the substance of the posterior lobe.

Pars tuberalis
This consists of a coarse network of nongranular chromophobe cells which have small pyknotic nuclei.

Pars intermedia
This is not sharply defined in man. It is the source of melanophore stimulating hormone (MSH) in amphibia and possibly in man.

Hormones of the anterior pituitary gland
The hormones secreted by the gland are listed in table 27.1. They are all proteins or polypeptides but TSH, FSH and LH contain carbohydrate and so are glycoproteins. Many are trophic hormones and are able to recognize their specific target cells and become attached to specific receptors on their plasma membranes.

GROWTH HORMONE (GH)
In 1921, Evans and Long showed that extracts of bovine anterior pituitary gland when injected into rats caused an increase in growth. The active principle of these extracts was finally isolated in 1945 and most of the knowledge concerning GH was originally obtained using bovine GH in animals. This preparation, however, was ineffective in man due to a structural difference between bovine and human growth hormone. HGH was isolated from human pituitaries by Li and Papkoff in 1956 and produces metabolic changes similar to those of bovine growth hormone in animals.

GH is known to be secreted by the anterior lobe of the pituitary gland since removal of the lobe in animals or a failure of secretion in children retards growth; administration of extracts of the anterior lobe or preparations of GH or HGH to such animals or children improves their growth rate. GH is elaborated by the acidophil cells of the anterior lobe. Those from primates and ruminants all have molecular weights within the range 21 000–26 000 although they differ in their composition. The amino acid sequences of HGH, prolactin and placental lactogen have much in common.

GH is necessary for maintenance of the normal rate of protein synthesis in the body with a resulting increase in size of the body tissues. At the same time, the catabolism of amino acids is decreased. As a result of the positive nitrogen balance there is a decreased urinary excretion of nitrogen. This protein-sparing effect is dependent on the presence of insulin and does not occur following destruction of the islet cells of the pancreas.

Growth hormone mobilizes the fat stores of the body and augments lipolysis with an increase in the plasma levels of free fatty acids. At the same time, fat synthesis is inhibited. The hormone when administered to the fasting subject is, therefore, ketogenic. This increase in metabolism of fat results in a low respiratory quotient.

Growth hormone also has definite effects on carbohydrate metabolism. It inhibits the oxidation of carbohydrate in the tissues so that animals fed with carbohydrate develop hyperglycaemia and glycosuria, but in starving animals it induces depletion of liver glycogen. Prolonged administration of growth hormone together with carbohydrate ultimately results in the development of diabetes mellitus.

Growth hormone is often not detectable (< 1 μg/l) in the plasma but irregular bursts of secretion take place in people of all ages, when the level may rise to 60 μg/l. On secretion its half-life in the plasma is only 25–30 min. High concentrations are found in the umbilical vein blood of the newborn. The pattern of HGH secretion in children and in adults is influenced on an hour-to-hour basis by feeding and by energy expenditure. From observations in fasting subjects, the secretion of HGH tends to occur in a series of bursts at irregular intervals throughout the day. Children may have three or four bursts of secretion at night but the reason for this is unknown.

A number of factors are, however, known to modify HGH secretion. These act by a feedback mechanism through the hypothalamus which controls the pituitary release of the hormone by means of the GHRF. Food and the consequent rise in blood glucose clear the plasma of any hormone that may be present. On the other hand,

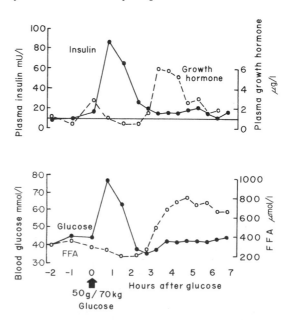

FIG. 27.11. Plasma HGH, insulin, FFA and blood glucose for 2 hours before and 7 hours following a glucose load in a 30-year-old healthy male. From Hunter W.M., Willoughby J.M.T. & Strong J.A. (1968) *J. Endocrin.* **40,** 297.

hypoglycaemia readily leads to secretion. If a normal subject is given oral glucose the rise and fall of blood glucose is shortly followed by a marked elevation of the plasma concentration of HGH. These effects are shown in fig. 27.11 where the plasma HGH concentrations in a 30-year-old healthy male have been measured for 2 hours before and 7 hours following a glucose load. The levels of free fatty acids in the plasma can be seen to follow closely the rise and fall in the plasma HGH concentration. The changes in plasma insulin are also shown and are discussed on p. 27.42.

Exercise in the fasting state also stimulates HGH secretion and fig. 27.12 shows the plasma HGH response in six normal adults during a 12·8 km walk. In addition plasma levels of FFA and glucose and values for RQ are shown. These observations indicate that HGH secretion is associated with the mobilization of depot fat to meet the energy requirements of exercise. Although exercise is a powerful stimulus, if the subject takes glucose immediately before and during the walk, the HGH rises are not seen.

Tissue growth is not completely dependent on growth hormone, being an inherent property of the tissues which is determined genetically. However, HGH appears to be necessary to support growth at normal rates and this is achieved at least in part by making available an adequate supply of fuel in the form of fat to the body.

Clinical abnormalities of HGH secretion

The first indication that the pituitary gland was concerned in the growth of the body came from clinical studies of **acromegaly** and **gigantism** which are associated with acidophil cell tumours (fig. 27.13a). Acromegaly is characterized by continuous hypersecretion of HGH with no physiological control of the plasma level. Excessive production of HGH leads to overgrowth of the membrane bones and soft tissues, especially of the hands, feet and face, giving the patient a characteristic appearance, but all organs of the body are affected. Because of the effect of HGH on carbohydrate metabolism some of the patients develop diabetes. Gigantism is due to a similar lesion occurring in younger age groups before epiphysial fusion is complete. The various parts of the body grow in proportion and the afflicted patient may attain a height of between 7 and 8 ft. The tumour responsible for these disorders may cause pressure on the nearby optic chiasma which leads to a bitemporal visual field defect (vol. 3, p. 34.56).

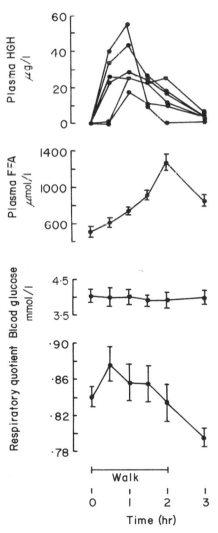

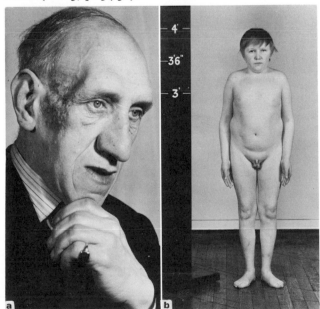

FIG. 27.12. Effect of exercise in the postabsorptive state on the levels of HGH, FFA and glucose in the plasma and on the RQ. From Hunter W.M., Fonseka C.C. & Passmore R. (1965) *Science* **150**, 1051.

FIG. 27.13. (a) Patient with acromegaly; (b) 18-year-old pituitary dwarf.

Deficiency in the secretion alone by the pituitary of HGH is rare but when it occurs gives rise to one type of **dwarfism**. Pituitary dwarfs show no deformity or mental inferiority. They grow at a reduced rate, are always small for their age and are often sexually undeveloped (fig. 27.13b).

ADRENOCORTICOTROPHIC HORMONE

Ascoli and Legnani, in 1912, found that hypophysectomy in the dog resulted in atrophy of the inner layers of the adrenal cortex. This dependence of the adrenal cortex on the pituitary gland was confirmed by Smith in 1927, who demonstrated in rats that the adrenal atrophy produced by hypophysectomy could be prevented by daily pituitary implants into the animal's tissues. It then became possible to separate this adrenal stimulating agent from pituitary gland extracts and eventually to purify ACTH.

As discussed on p. 27.8, ACTH consists of a single polypeptide chain containing thirty-nine amino acid residues. It is secreted into the circulation under basal conditions in very small quantities and is also rapidly removed. Pig ACTH injected into man has a biological half life of about 5–15 min. Because of the low secretory rate and the short half-life, the plasma content of ACTH is very low, ranging between 12–55 μg/l. There is a diurnal variation in ACTH plasma concentration which is responsible for a similar variation in the level of plasma cortisol (p. 27.37).

ACTH is necessary for the maintenance and growth of the cells of the adrenal cortex and for the regulation of their secretory activity. It stimulates the synthesis of steroids in the adrenal glands which in man results mainly in an increased secretion of cortisol as well as of corticosterone. In salt-depleted man, ACTH can also increase the secretion of the salt-retaining hormone aldosterone, but is of little or no significance in the physiological control of aldosterone secretion in salt-replete man (p. 27.38).

If animals are injected with ACTH in increasing doses, the cells of the adrenal cortex increase progressively in size and their lipid content falls. The nuclei also enlarge and the mitochondria increase in number. In addition, the ascorbic acid concentration of the adrenal cortex, which contains the highest concentration of this vitamin of any tissue in the body, is reduced and this effect is the basis of a biological method of assay for ACTH.

ACTH may stimulate steroid secretion from the adrenal cortex by activating adenyl cyclase and causing intracellular cyclic AMP concentration to rise. As a result a protein kinase is activated, and this together with ATP activates by phosphorylation a cytosolic cholesterol ester hydrolase, which hydrolyses cholesterol esters present in the lipid droplets. The cholesterol released is taken up by mitochondria for conversion to pregnenolone and hence onwards to the adrenocorticosteroid hormones (p. 27.34). The rate-limiting factor in the secretion of these steroid hormones is the supply of non-esterified cholesterol to the mitochondria.

ACTH also has effects remote from the adrenal glands. For example, in amphibians and reptiles it causes dispersal of melanin as does melanocyte stimulating hormone, MSH of the pars intermedia of the hypophysis. It is now known that this common property is due to the possession of a peptide sequence containing the same seven amino acids in both the ACTH and MSH molecules. When given in large doses to adrenalectomized animals ACTH activates adenyl cyclase in adipose tissue; the adipocyte hormone-sensitive lipase is activated and the plasma free fatty acid concentration raised. However, the physiological significance of this is in doubt. Through its action in increasing the secretion of the adrenal steroids, ACTH can also produce a fall in the blood eosinophil count (p. 27.36).

The effect of ACTH on the rate of secretion of adrenocorticosteroids is now the basis of the best method of biological assay. The response to a dose of ACTH is measured in hypophysectomized rats by analysis of the corticosteroid content of adrenal venous blood. Immunological methods of assay have been established.

The factors which influence the rate of secretion of ACTH are described fully on p. 27.7. High plasma concentrations are found after adrenalectomy in animals and in Addison's disease in man, in which the adrenal cortex is atrophied or destroyed (p. 27.32) and are due to the reduction in the concentration of circulating cortisol stimulating the β cells of the anterior pituitary. Because of the similarity of part of the amino acid chain to MSH, pigmentation of the skin commonly develops in this condition.

THYROID STIMULATING HORMONE (TSH, THYROTROPHIN)

A relationship between the pituitary gland and thyroid gland was first recognized in the nineteenth century when cretins were found to have enlarged pituitary glands at post mortem. The pituitary control of the thyroid gland was then established by the demonstration that removal of the pituitary gland in rats resulted in atrophy of the thyroid gland, which was restored to normal on administration of simple extracts of the pituitary gland. When extracts of the anterior lobe of the pituitary gland were injected into guinea-pigs, the thyroid tissue became hyperplastic. The active principle of these extracts was called thyrotrophic hormone and is now referred to as TSH; it is responsible for the maintenance of normal thyroid function. TSH has been isolated and, like LH and FSH, it consists of two sub-units. The α sub-units of TSH, LH and FSH are virtually identical and the specificity of the polypeptides is probably conferred by the β sub-units. However the β sub-units also have much in common and they may have evolved from a common ancestor. Human chorionic gonadotrophin (p. 38.47) also exists in α and β sub-units.

TSH may be assayed by a biological method (p. 27.4). This, however, lacks sufficient sensitivity to detect TSH in the majority of people with normal thyroid function. TSH can be convincingly detected by bioassay only in the plasma of patients with primary hypothyroidism and not in hyperthyroidism. Immunoassay procedures for TSH sufficiently sensitive to measure normal circulating levels in man have confirmed that the plasma TSH level is elevated in primary hypothyroidism and have shown it to be absent or reduced in hyperthyroidism.

Thyrotrophic hormone activity in the plasma appears to be located with the γ-globulin fraction of the proteins. At one time it was thought that the thyroid gland itself might inactivate TSH but it has been shown that the kidneys may play a role in its excretion. Although the biological half-life of TSH in the plasma is about 10 min, the maximum effect on iodine uptake by the thyroid gland is apparent in 12–18 hours.

The injection of TSH or extracts of the pituitary gland into the guinea-pig increases the weight of the thyroid gland. The follicles (p. 27.18) are reduced in size due to the absorption of colloid and hypertrophy of the acinar cells which assume a columnar appearance. This increase in activity of the gland is accompanied by increased secretion of thyroid hormones. Constant stimulation of the guinea-pig's thyroid gland by injection of TSH results eventually in hyperthyroidism. TSH is probably first bound to a site on the plasma membrane of the thyroid acinar cell. Once this is achieved it stimulates the oxidation of glucose and increases the RNA content of the gland and the rate of purine and nucleotide synthesis. These biochemical and morphological changes may be initiated by an increased intracellular concentration of cyclic AMP.

As discussed on p. 27.7, TSH secretion by the pituitary gland is thought to be controlled by the hypothalamus through TRH. In unanaesthetized rabbits stimulation through electrodes implanted in the hypothalamus in the region of the supraoptico-hypophysial tract increases thyroid secretion and this is due to an increase in TSH secretion. TRH was postulated to explain these findings and in 1965 this factor was isolated from sheep. Administration of synthetic TRH increases the weight of the thyroid gland, its rate of iodine uptake and plasma TSH, while section of the pituitary stalk and electrolytic lesions in the hypothalamus depress thyroid function.

The thyroid gland influences the pituitary secretion of TSH by a negative feedback mechanism. For example, TSH secretion can be depressed by the administration of thyroid hormone and is stimulated in conditions where thyroid hormone synthesis is impaired, e.g. in iodine deficiency or when congenital biochemical defects of the gland result in a compensatory hypertrophy of the gland commonly called a goitre. The main site of the negative feedback mechanism of the thyroid hormones is the anterior pituitary gland, since both *in vivo* and *in vitro* studies have shown the TSH response to TRH to be abolished by the presence of excess thyroid hormone.

GONADOTROPHIC HORMONES

In 1911, Harvey Cushing demonstrated from his observations on the effects of hypophysectomy in the dog that the gonads were dependent on the pituitary gland. It was later shown in hypophysectomized rats that the gonadal atrophy which occurred could be prevented by repeated implantation of pituitary tissue. Extracts of the pituitary gland were then found to have a similar effect on gonadal function and the hormone responsible for this effect, the gonadotrophic hormone, was detected in such extracts by Smith and by Zondek and Aschheim. In 1931, two active fractions in the crude anterior pituitary extracts were found, one having an action mainly on the growth of the ovarian follicle, and called the follicle stimulating hormone (FSH), and the other acting on the corpus luteum, and known as luteinizing hormone (LH). As LH was observed also to stimulate the interstitial cells of the testis, it is alternatively called the interstitial cell stimulating hormone (ICSH).

The physiological actions of the gonadotrophic hormones have been studied mainly in rodents. It has been difficult to get biologically pure preparations of these hormones, and FSH and LH have a synergistic action on the gonads. Despite these difficulties, however, much is known concerning the individual hormones. The main effects of these hormones and the control of their secretion are described in chap. 38.

PROLACTIN

Human prolactin is now clearly differentiated from HGH. The difficulty in separation was due to the similarity in physical, chemical and biological properties and to the very small amounts present in the anterior pituitary. As already indicated, the amino acid sequence of human prolactin has much in common with HGH and human placental lactogen. There is also histological evidence for the separation of the two hormones in the human, as immunofluorescence studies show that GH and prolactin are secreted by distinct types of acidophil cell in the pituitary.

Prolactin is essential for the development of the mammary gland during pregnancy and the production of milk by the gland following parturition. It does this in conjunction with oestrogens, progestogens, the adrenocorticosteroids, thyroid hormone and GH which are known to influence the development of the mammary alveoli and ducts during pregnancy. A luteotrophic role for prolactin has been shown in animals but there is no evidence that prolactin maintains the corpus luteum in man. In addition, bovine prolactin given to normal subjects reduces water, sodium and potassium excretion by the kidney and increases plasma osmolality probably by a direct action on the proximal renal tubules.

The estimation of plasma prolactin is by bioassay, making use of its ability to stimulate the growth and secretion of the 'crop sacs' of the pigeon, or by its mammotrophic effect on the rabbit, or preferably by immunoassay. High concentrations of plasma prolactin are found during pregnancy and lactation, in patients with hypothalamic disorders decreasing the release of prolactin inhibiting factor, and in patients taking phenothiazines which reduce the concentration of hypothalamic prolactin inhibiting factor.

HYPOPITUITARISM

Hypopituitarism arises when the anterior pituitary is wholly or largely destroyed by disease. Such patients have a lowered metabolism due to failure of TSH secretion, and suffer from the consequences of adrenocortical insufficiency from lack of ACTH and so are unable to withstand any form of stress. They are sensitive to the action of insulin and develop hypoglycaemia on fasting. If the disease occurs before puberty they fail to develop sexually from lack of FSH and LH. If it develops after puberty menstruation ceases, the sex glands atrophy and pregnancy and milk production become impossible. When the disease is severe there is muscle wasting, hypothermia and somnolence. Most of these features may be dramatically reversed by appropriate hormone treatment (vol. 3, p. 23.5).

Hormones of the neurohypophysis and posterior lobe of the pituitary gland

The neurohypophysis is a point of contact between neurological and hormonal control mechanisms. Two hormones, **vasopressin**, the antidiuretic hormone (ADH), and **oxytociu,** are synthesized in the perikaryon of nerve cells composing the supraoptic and paraventricular nuclei of the hypothalamus. The hormones, in combination with protein carrier molecules, the neurophysins, pass down the axons of the supraopticohypophysial tract in the pituitary stalk, within which they can be seen histologically as granular particles. In this way, they reach the posterior lobe where they are stored and from which they are released, together with the neurophysins, into the blood stream by exocytosis. The rate of their release is controlled by nervous impulses which originate, like the hormones, in the hypothalamus and which pass down the same axons in response to a variety of stimuli. Thus the nerve fibres of the pituitary stalk possess the dual function of hormone transport and secretomotor activity, though the final pathway of transport of the hormones to their target organs is by way of the blood stream. The

neurological and humoral components of biological control are here indissolubly interwoven and the neurohypophysis may be regarded as an entity which includes the supraoptic and paraventricular nuclei of the hypothalamus, the nerve fibres of the pituitary stalk and the posterior lobe of the pituitary gland itself.

Vasopressin and oxytocin are nonapeptides and differ in only two amino acids:

```
Gly(NH₂)              Gly(NH₂)
   |                     |
Arg                   Leu
   |                     |
Pro                   Pro
   |                     |
Cys—Asp(NH₂)          Cys—Asp(NH₂)
 |      |               |      |
 S    Glu(NH₂)         S    Glu(NH₂)
 |      |               |      |
 S    Phe              S    Ile
 |      |               |      |
Cys—Tyr               Cys—Tyr
Vasopressin           Oxytocin
```

The structural similarity between the two hormones is matched, to some extent, by overlap of biological activity, and in the discussion of their effects this point must be borne in mind. The situation is further complicated by the fact that the two hormones appear to be liberated from the posterior lobe of the pituitary simultaneously, in response to stimuli which would be expected teleologically to give rise to secretion of only one of them. It is of interest that some non-mammalian vertebrates produce one posterior pituitary principle only, to which the name **vasotocin** has been given. This hormone has the ring structure of oxytocin, the side chain of vasopressin and possesses physiological activity in mammals intermediate between the two mammalian hormones.

VASOPRESSIN

The name vasopressin was given to this hormone when it was discovered that crude posterior lobe extracts raised the blood pressure. It is now known that vasopressin raises blood pressure by direct action on smooth muscle in the arterioles but only when given in doses far exceeding those required to cause enhanced renal conservation of water (antidiuresis); the hormone has no role in the regulation of blood pressure, whereas it is paramount in the control of water excretion. The name vasopressin is, therefore, an unsatisfactory synonym for **antidiuretic hormone**, but it remains the official name for the hormone, and both names are in common use.

Mode of action

The mode of action of vasopressin upon the kidney is indicated by the observation that addition of the hormone to the fluid bathing the inner surface of a number of amphibian membranes increases their permeability to water and accelerates the flow of water across the membrane in response to an osmotic gradient. Similar experiments show also that the hormone increases the net transfer of sodium across the membrane, an effect associated with an increase in the oxygen consumption of the membrane but independent of the influence of the hormone upon permeability. In the mammalian kidney, vasopressin is believed to increase the permeability of the cells of the collecting ducts so that an increased amount of water is reabsorbed under the influence of the osmotic gradient which exists between the peritubular tissue and the collecting ducts. Thus, when the neurohypophysis is destroyed, either experimentally in animals or by disease in man, the absence of vasopressin causes large volumes of dilute urine to be produced. This condition is known as **diabetes insipidus** (vol. 3, p. 23.14). If vasopressin is given, water conservation is enhanced by increased water reabsorption, the urinary volume falls and there is a corresponding increase in the concentration of urinary solutes (p. 35.22).

The means by which vasopressin induces these changes in permeability are unknown. The hormone appears to bind reversibly to specific receptor sites where it activates adenyl cyclase with an increase in the rate of production of cyclic AMP. It is not known how this effect is related to the ensuing change in membrane permeability.

Release of vasopressin

The secretion of vasopressin is dependent upon the osmolality of the ECF. This can be demonstrated by perfusion of the internal carotid artery with hyperosmolal solutions of sodium chloride. Raising the osmolality of the plasma by 1 or 2 per cent elicits an antidiuresis which can be abolished by destruction of the neurohypophysial system. Such experiments imply the existence of osmoreceptors within the tissues supplied by the internal carotid artery, and it is probable that they are situated within the supraoptic nuclei since micro-injection of hyperosmolal solutions in this region is also an effective stimulus for the antidiuretic response.

This mechanism results in liberation of vasopressin from the posterior lobe of the pituitary in proportion to the osmolality of the ECF; a high osmolality leads to increased release of the hormone with production of small volumes of concentrated urine, and a low osmolality inhibits vasopressin release so that a large volume of dilute urine is secreted. The capacity of this system to ensure the constancy of ECF osmolality is evident.

The plasma volume is also a critical factor and when this is reduced by acute haemorrhage, antidiuresis regularly occurs, even if the plasma osmolality is low. Thus, the maintenance of plasma volume appears to take precedence over the regulation of osmolality. The nature of the receptors responsible for this effect remains obscure but it has been shown experimentally that distension of the left atrium of the heart inhibits the release of vasopressin, suggesting that atrial stretch receptors may be concerned.

Other stimuli also can influence the release of vasopressin. Alcohol, for example, produces its characteristic diuresis apparently by inhibiting the secretion of the hormone. Conversely, vasopressin release is stimulated by a number of drugs, including nicotine, morphine and ether. The activity of the two latter agents may give rise to inappropriate water retention postoperatively.

Finally, direct stimulation of the breasts or genitalia, which might be expected to lead to secretion of oxytocin, also depletes the neurohypophysial stores of vasopressin and results in an antidiuresis.

Assay

Vasopressin may be assayed biologically by measuring changes in the concentration of the urine in rats in which diabetes insipidus has been induced experimentally. Radioimmunoassays are now available and allow the determination of the hormone in concentrates of biological fluids. By their use, plasma vasopressin concentrations in mildly dehydrated subjects have been shown to be in the range 1–5 ng/l with elevations to 20 ng/l following stimulation with nicotine. The half-life of the hormone in plasma is short, approximately 10 min, the main sites of degradation being liver and kidney.

The effect of oxytocin on the contractility of the uterus and on milk secretion is discussed on p. 38.52.

THYROID GLAND

The thyroid gland is located in front of the trachea in the neck. It effects primarily the rate of metabolism by secreting into the blood the hormones **thyroxine** (T_4) and **triiodothyronine** (T_3) produced from tyrosine and inorganic iodine within the epithelial cells of its follicles. A second endocrine secretion, **calcitonin**, formed in parafollicular or C cells, influences the rate of bone breakdown. The thyroid gland stores its hormones, T_4 and T_3, bound to a glycoprotein, **thyroglobulin**, outside the follicle cell in a viscid secretion, the colloid, contained within the lumen of the follicles. Iodine required for hormone synthesis is obtained from the small amounts present in food and drink. The colloid storage may be an evolutionary adaptation which guards against periods of low iodine intake.

Anatomy

The human thyroid has two lateral lobes connected over the third to fifth tracheal rings by a broad isthmus from which may arise a small pyramidal lobe. The adult thyroid usually weighs less than 30 g but its size and shape vary with factors such as sex, age and geographic position. The gland is surrounded by a fibrous capsule from which connective tissue trabeculae invaginate the gland substance so dividing it into numerous lobules. The position and relations of the thyroid gland are given on p. 22.55 and its development is described on p. 19.31.

The gland has a rich blood supply which, in an active thyroid, may be 7 ml g^{-1} min^{-1} and so is greater than the flow through any organ except active muscle. In cretins with big goitres observed in Switzerland in the early part of this century, the inferior thyroid artery was as large as the common carotid artery. The blood supply and follicle size vary with the activity of the gland.

HISTOLOGICAL STRUCTURE

The thyroid follicle is a spherical structure composed of a single layer of cuboidal epithelial cells which surround and enclose the colloid (plate 27.1c, facing p. 27.20). A basement membrane encircles the follicle and is closely related to or even indented by the rich network of capillaries surrounding it. In the resting state the nucleus of the follicular cells is central, and only an occasional small microvillus can be seen in the EM projecting from the cell cytoplasm into the colloid. Occasional lymphoid cells, nerve fibres and lymphatic vessels are found in the interfollicular spaces. A few clear cells may be seen in the epithelial wall of the follicles but not in contact with colloid. These parafollicular cells, sometimes called C cells to distinguish them from the A cells of the thyroid follicle, produce calcitonin (plate 27.1d, facing p. 27.20). They are derived from the neural crest and come to lie in the ultimobranchial bodies. In some species, e.g. the skink (South African lizard), pigeon and chicken, these are present in the adult as distinct bodies lying alongside the trachea below the thyroid gland. Large quantities of calcitonin have been extracted from these bodies, which appear to be true endocrine glands. In man and probably in most other mammals the ultimobranchial bodies fuse with the thyroid gland, though their cells do not form true thyroid tissue. Thyroid follicles are bound together in groups of twenty to forty to form a lobule, and groups of lobules are incorporated into lobes. A single artery supplies each lobule. In an overactive gland, the follicles are small and contain little colloid surrounded by tall columnar epithelium. A resting follicle has a flattened epithelium and a large store of colloid. The ultrastructure of thyroid is considered in relation to its function on p. 27.22.

Function of the thyroid gland

The secretions of the gland, thyroxine and triiodothyronine, have a stimulatory effect on metabolism and increase oxygen consumption and thereby heat production. They are essential for normal skeletal growth and development, including metamorphosis in amphibia, and for cerebral maturation and normal mental activity. These and other physiological actions of the thyroid hormones are shown in table 27.4.

TABLE 27.4. Some actions of thyroid hormones (after Tata J.R.).

Growth promotion and development	Metabolic effects
Essential for:	
growth of many mammalian tissues,	Increase of the resting metabolic rate
maturation of the central nervous system,	Increase of cholesterol and fat turnover
maturation of bone,	Increase of protein turnover
amphibian metamorphosis,	Increase of calcium turnover
synthesis of some cell enzymes and ultrastructures.	Effect on water and ion transport

The actions of thyroid hormones are best illustrated by the study of hypothyroid and hyperthyroid states as they occur spontaneously in disease or as induced in the experimental animal.

HYPOTHYROIDISM (CRETINISM AND MYXOEDEMA)

Removal, destruction or failure of development of the thyroid gland reduce heat production due to a decrease in the metabolic rate. Oxygen consumption and carbon dioxide production may fall by up to 40 per cent and this is reflected in a subnormal body temperature, decreased respiration, slow heart rate and listless behaviour. In the newborn animal or child, growth practically ceases and such a child is known as a **cretin** (fig. 27.14a). In the tadpole metamorphosis does not occur unless the thyroid hormone is replaced. The reduced rate of bone growth produces dwarfs with immature bones and a delay in ossification, epiphyseal union and growth of cartilage. There is a delay in normal development of the reproductive system at puberty.

Thyroid deficiency in the newborn baby results in mental retardation which is permanent unless hormone therapy is begun soon after birth. In the adult hypothyroidism (fig. 27.14b) produces mental apathy, an impairment of memory, lack of concentration and increasing sluggishness and somnolence.

Primary thyroid deficiency at all ages leads to the deposition of a viscid mucinous material in the skin which becomes characteristically thick and coarse. Unlike thickening due to the accumulation of extracellular fluid (oedema) it does not pit on finger pressure and it is called **myxoedema**. The hair becomes coarse and dry and tends to fall out. In part due to the diminished metabolic demands the body weight begins to rise and there is a general loss of muscle tone. In cretins this leads to a pot belly, often with an umbilical hernia. The hypothyroid person is characteristically cold, sluggish

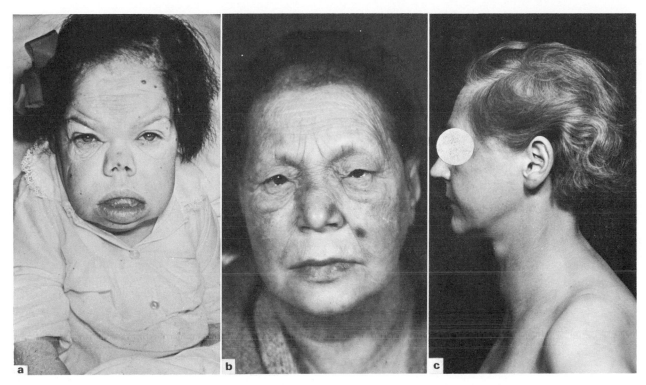

FIG. 27.14 (a) 44-year-old cretin; (b) patient with myxoedema; (c) patient with enlarged, easily visible, thyroid gland due to hyperthyroidism.

and constipated and often has a mild anaemia due to depressed marrow activity. The pulse rate is slow and the cardiac output and electrical activity of the myocardium are diminished. The concentrations of lipids and cholesterol rise in the plasma, with an increased tendency for fatty material to be deposited in the walls of the larger arteries. This may further jeopardize cardiovascular efficiency (vol. 3, p. 23.33).

HYPERTHYROIDISM

Hyperfunction usually arises spontaneously, but the onset of symptoms may follow an unusual stress such as an emotional crisis or exposure to excessive heat. The gland is often enlarged and vascular (fig. 27.14c). The condition can be induced by feeding thyroid extract or thyroxine. Oxygen consumption and heat production may be increased by up to 80 per cent. In response to the increased heat load there is vasodilation with a decreased peripheral resistance and a compensatory increased pulse rate. There is increased cardiac output due to tachycardia but no increase in stroke volume. Disordered cardiac conduction with fibrillation of the atrial muscle is a common complication. There is systolic hypertension with a raised pulse pressure. Mood changes occur, with irritability and restless behaviour, excitability and emotional instability. Altered electrical activity is seen in electroencephalograms. There is acceleration of the passage of nerve impulses with hyperactive limb reflexes. Both absorption from and movement

through the gut are accelerated and diarrhoea is often present. Characteristically the appetite is voracious. Some loss of skeletal calcium may occur with increased faecal and urinary excretion.

An increased sensitivity to the effects of circulating adrenaline and noradrenaline can be demonstrated by intravenous infusion of these substances to normal and hyperthyroid animals. The thyroid hormones potentiate the effect of sympathetic nerves on heart rate, pulse pressure, oxygen consumption, etc. The retraction of the muscles of the eyelid with pupillary dilatation commonly seen in hyperthyroidism is probably due to this sympathetic swelling and damage of the extraocular muscles, with an increase in orbital content of fat and fluid which leads to protrusion of the eye (exophthalmos).

An acceleration of intermediary metabolism takes place with increased rates of utilization of carbohydrate, breakdown of liver glycogen stores and an increased gluconeogenesis from fat and protein. While protein synthesis may actually be increased, the total body protein stores diminish with damage to muscle fibres, wasting, weakness and increased creatine excretion in urine. Fat stores are mobilized and plasma cholesterol falls for reasons that are unknown. There is progressive weight loss and finally cardiac failure develops (vol. 3, p. 23.23).

Severe hypothyroidism and hyperthyroidism lead to characteristic clinical pictures, which can often be recognized at a glance. Minor degrees of both conditions are common and are more difficult to detect. It may also be hard to decide where normal variation in thyroid function ends and disease begins.

Thyroid hormones

The hormones L-triiodothyronine (T_3) and L-thyroxine (T_4) are iodinated derivatives of L-tyrosine. Their chemical structure and synthesis are given on p. 27.21. Optical isomers exist, but only the L-forms are found in nature.

The hormones are stored in the colloid vesicles of the follicles of the gland bound to thyroglobulin. This is a

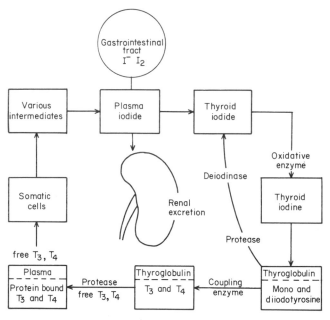

FIG. 27.15. The iodine pool. After Murray I.P.C. & McGirr E.M. (1964) in *The Thyroid Gland*, ed. Pitt-Rivers Rosalind & Trotter W.R. London: Butterworth.

complex glycoprotein, mol. wt. 650 000, which is synthesized in the follicular cells and secreted into the colloid vesicles. It consists of four polypeptide chains and contains about 4 per cent carbohydrate (mannose, galactose, glucosamine and sialic acid) and 100 tyrosine residues/molecule.

IODINE METABOLISM

Iodine occupies a unique position in human physiology as its only function is to take part in the synthesis of thyroid hormone. Dietary iodine is derived ultimately from the soil in the area from which the foodstuffs and drinking water come. A daily intake of 1.2 μmol is normally sufficient to safeguard against the development of goitre. The element enters the body in food or drink as ionic iodide, iodine or as iodine in organic combination. Most forms are reduced during digestion and are absorbed

as inorganic iodide, but some organic iodides, including thyroxine, can be absorbed from the gastrointestinal tract unchanged. Inorganic iodide is present in the blood in amounts below 0.1 μmol (10 μg)/l. The blood also contains T_3 and T_4, which are bound to protein. The level of protein bound iodine (PBI) in the blood is 0.3–0.6 μmol. Iodine is lost from the body chiefly through the kidney and to lesser extent in the faeces. The amount of iodine excreted daily in the urine depends on the dietary intake and is greater in an area where table salt is iodized or much fish consumed, and lower in areas where iodine deficiency is prevalent. T_3 and T_4 are secreted in the bile and because reabsorption from the small bowel is incomplete some iodine is present in the faeces. Most circulating hormone is de-iodinated and the iodine so released returns to the plasma iodide pool (fig. 27.15).

Inadequate dietary intake is the most important cause of iodine deficiency. Loss of iodine occurs with pregnancy, and rarely due to a familial absence of the de-iodinating thyroid enzyme. The human body contains 0.15–0.4 mmol (20–50 mg) of iodine and about a quarter of this is in the thyroid. In the adult 0.5–1.0 μmol (60–120 μg) of hormonal iodine is turned over per day, and the thyroid hormone store constitutes a 2–10 week supply.

SYNTHESIS OF THE THYROID HORMONES

T_3 and T_4 are formed by the following steps,

(1) the trapping and subsequent oxidation of inorganic iodide,

(2) the iodination of tyrosine to form monoiodotyrosine (MIT) and di-iodotyrosine (DIT), and

(3) the coupling of MIT and DIT on the thyroglobulin molecule to form T_3 and T_4.

The thyroid hormones are then stored within the thyroglobulin of the colloid or released by hydrolysis and pass into the circulation. MIT and DIT do not normally escape from the follicle cell into the circulation.

Trapping of inorganic iodide

The first step is the accumulation of iodide in the thyroid by a concentrating mechanism or **iodide pump**. This active trapping produces a concentration gradient of $25:1$ between the inorganic iodide within the cell and that in the plasma. The process requires energy and is presumably under enzyme control. The magnitude of the gradient depends on the quantity of stored iodine within the gland. Certain anions specifically inhibit the pump mechanism, e.g. thiocyanate and perchlorate. Although gastric mucosa, salivary and mammary gland share the ability to trap iodide, only the mammary gland can bind iodine in organic combination. The trapping of iodide by the thyroid is stimulated by TSH, and hence decreased by hypophysectomy or when TSH output is depressed by exogenous thyroid hormone.

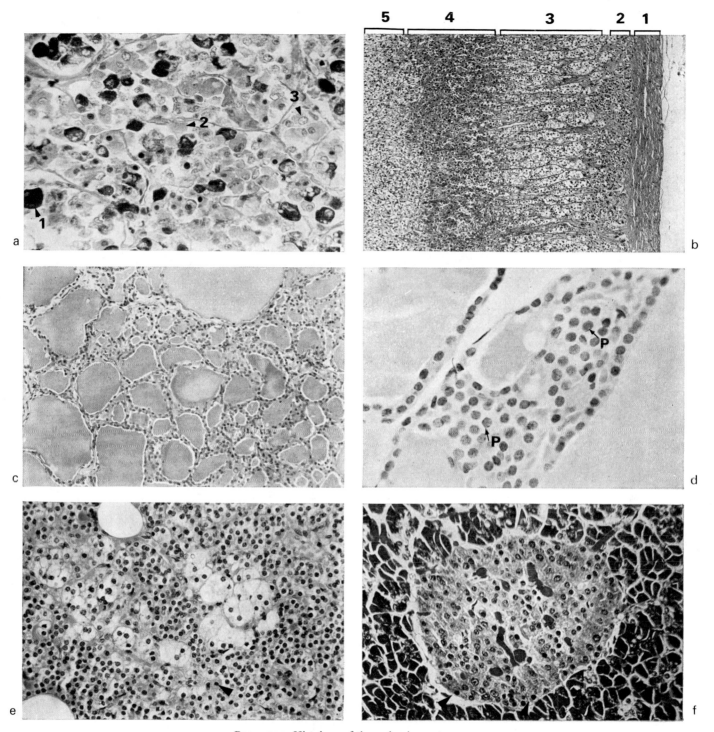

PLATE 27.1. Histology of the endocrine system.

(a) Pars anterior showing three types of secretory cell. (1) Basophil, purple; (2) oxyphil, orange; (3) chromophobe, grey-blue. Human, Slidder's Orange-G acid fuchsin ($\times 320$).

(c) Thyroid. Human, haem. & eosin ($\times 120$).

(e) Parathyroid showing many chief cells, some enlarged and vacuolated, and a few oxyphil cells (arrow). Human, haem. & eosin ($\times 240$).

(b) Adrenal cortex and medulla showing collagenous capsule (1), zona glomerulosa (2), pale cells of the zona fasciculata (3), eosinophil cells of zona reticularis (4) and medulla (5). Human, haem. & eosin ($\times 56$).

(d) Thyroid showing groups of parafollicular cells (P). Human, haem. & eosin ($\times 480$).

(f) Islet of Langerhans from the pancreas. Blue β cells are numerous, reddish α cells are less conspicuous (arrows). The rich vascularity is demonstrated. Human, Gomori ($\times 280$).

The major site of concentration of iodine is in the colloid. Autoradiographs show that injected ^{131}I is taken up by the follicle cells within 30 sec and incorporated into colloid, where binding of the ^{131}I to protein appears to take place at the periphery of the cell. Later, within minutes, the ^{131}I is distributed uniformly throughout the colloid. Iodination of thyroglobulin probably occurs at the apical cell membrane between cytoplasm and colloid. Any iodide which has not been oxidized to iodine and bound to protein can be discharged by perchlorate which does not affect bound iodine.

Formation of thyroglobulin

Nadler, working in McGill University, traced the synthesis of thyroglobulin in rats by means of autoradiographs using labelled leucine, a constituent of thyroglobulin. After 30 min the label was seen to be incorporated into protein in the follicle cell, and by 36 hours it had all passed into the colloid. This suggests that follicle cells incorporate leucine from plasma in the manufacture of thyroglobulin which is subsequently secreted into the colloid. It is possible that the continuous formation and secretion of thyroglobulin by the follicle cell is the rate-limiting step in thyroid hormone formation. The formation of T_4 and T_3 occurs within the thyroglobulin molecule following the iodination of the tyrosine residues.

Iodination of tyrosine and the formation of T_3 and T_4

The inorganic iodide (I) trapped by the thyroid is first oxidized by hydrogen peroxide, formed by autoxidation of flavoproteins. This is catalysed by an enzyme, iodine peroxidase. Iodine (I_2) formed within the follicle cell is then added to the tyrosine component of thyroglobulin to form MIT. Under the influence of iodinase, a second atom of iodine is added to form DIT. In the chick-embryo thyroid the formation of MIT can be shown to precede DIT by several hours. Subsequently coupling of

MIT and DIT occurs on the surface of the thyroglobulin molecule to produce the metabolically active iodinated hormones, T_3 and T_4. One molecule of MIT and one of DIT, in the presence of a coupling enzyme, give rise to one molecule of T_3, and two molecules of DIT to one of T_4. Approximately 80 μg of T_4 is synthesized daily by the thyroid gland. However, only 60 per cent of the 60 μg of T_3 produced each day is formed in the thyroid gland. Small amounts of ^{131}I-T_3 can be shown in the plasma of athyreotic individuals after administration of ^{131}I-T_4. The peripheral monodeiodination of T_4 by iodothyronine deiodinase, found mainly in kidney, liver and heart, accounts for the balance.

Autoradiographic techniques have shown the presence of protein-bound ^{131}I in the mouse thyroid within seconds of intravenous injection. The proportion of MIT and DIT decreases and that of T_3 and T_4 increases with time after the administration of the tracer dose.

The steps involved in the synthesis can be demonstrated by using various antithyroid substances to interfere with the successive reactions. Perchlorate prevents iodide concentration and not only blocks the active trapping process but also discharges any inorganic iodide which is not bound to protein. Although iodine combines with free tyrosine *in vitro* the iodination of tyrosine to MIT and DIT on the thyroglobulin molecule requires the presence of an enzyme system. Thiourea compounds interfere with this step in hormone synthesis.

Further understanding of the enzyme steps involved has come with the study of the genetics of thyroid disease. Goitrous cretinism is associated classically with the iodine deficiency found in the endemic goitre areas in the world. Osler, in 1897, first drew attention to a familial tendency in rare cases in nonendemic areas. Thyroid disorders arising from genetically determined absence or deficiency of one or other of the thyroid enzymes are now well established. In a tinker family group studied by McGirr

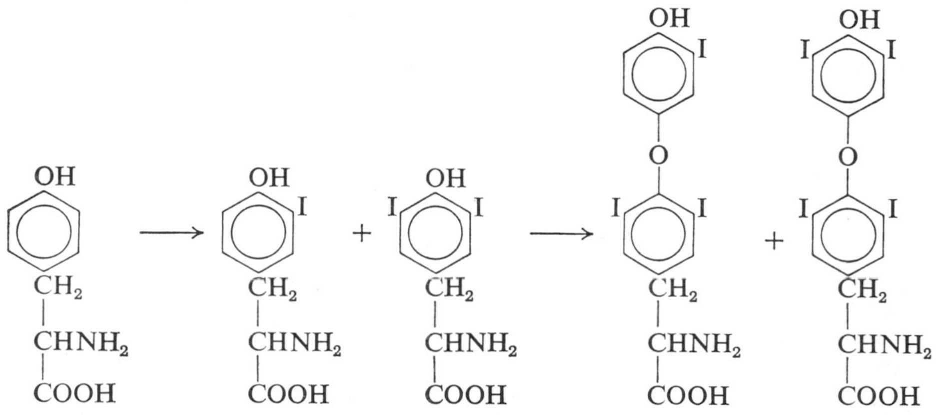

FIG. 27.16. The iodination of tyrosine to form T_3 and T_4.

and Hutchison in Glasgow, the enzyme, dehalogenase, which deiodinates MIT and DIT, was lacking. These iodotyrosines were therefore excreted in the urine with loss of body iodine and the production of an iodine-deficiency goitre (vol. 3, p. 23.40).

SECRETION OF THYROID HORMONE

When the gland is overactive due to TSH stimulation in experimental animals or in human hyperthyroidism, the stimulated cell is increased in its height and changes its

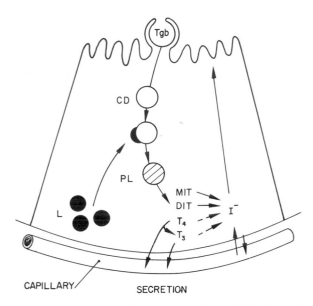

FIG. 27.17. Secretion of T_4 and T_3; Tgb, intrafollicular colloid containing thyroglobulin; CD, colloid droplet; L, lysosome; PL, phagolysosome. From Greer M.A. & Haibach H. (1974) in *Handbook of Physiology*, Section 7, Vol. III, p. 136, ed. Greep R.O. *et al.* Washington, D.C.: American Physiological Society.

shape from cuboidal to columnar. The overactivity also leads to hypertrophy of the Golgi apparatus and increased numbers of mitochondria and of microvilli, which extend into the colloid and so increase the surface area of the cell; this facilitates transport mechanisms through the cell membrane in either direction. Trapped iodine combines with the protein in thyroglobulin at the cell-colloid boundary, prior to storage or secretion of thyroid hormone. The microvilli engulf thyroglobulin into the cell as colloid droplets. The droplets then fuse with lysosomes migrating from the basal part of the cell to form phagolysosomes. Protease enzyme systems then split the thyroglobulin to release thyroid hormone into the basal cytoplasm of the follicular cell and thence into the blood capillary. A small amount of thyroglobulin escapes unaltered into the extracellular space and is removed by the lymphatics (fig. 27.17).

Protein synthesis in the cell is located in the rough-surfaced endoplasmic reticulum, where thyroglobulin formation is known to occur. In the overactive gland this area is much more prominent with increased numbers of ribosomes and many dilated cisternae. The number of mitochondria also increases in keeping with the higher rate of oxidative metabolism of the cell. Golgi bodies are thought to be the transport mechanism used by the cell to carry the manufactured thyroglobulin to the cell surface, and a carbohydrate moiety may be added to the protein molecule at this stage. At the cell surface iodine is seen to combine with the thyroglobulin which is either stored in the colloid, or hydrolysed within the cell to release thyroid hormone.

THYROID HORMONE TRANSPORT

When the thyroid hormones are secreted from a follicle cell into the capillary lumen they attach themselves to chemical groups present on the surface of plasma proteins known as binding sites. This reaction between hormone and carrier protein is reversible and continuous so that there is always a certain amount of free thyroid hormone present. Only 0·05 per cent and 0·3 per cent respectively of the total plasma concentration of T_4 and T_3 are free or unbound. The bound hormones are carried principally by **thyroxine binding globulin** (TBG) but also to a lesser extent by **thyroxine binding prealbumin** (TBPA) and albumin. The affinity of T_3 for TBG is much less than that of T_4.

The concentration of circulating thyroid hormone is largely the result of an equilibrium achieved between thyroid hormone production and tissue utilization. In euthyroid individuals concentrations of T_4 range from 75–150 nmol/l and of T_3 from 1·1–2·2 nmol/l. However, the plasma level is also dependent on changes in both free hormone and TBG. Thus in pregnancy a rise in total plasma T_4 and T_3 above the normal range occurs although thyroid function is normal. This might at first sight suggest a failure of TSH suppression, but is due to a rise in TBG which occurs in pregnancy and also after administration of oestrogen. The free hormone levels remain normal. A fall in total plasma T_4 and T_3 with normal free values may be seen when the plasma proteins fall in disease. Displacement of the hormone from its protein binding site can be caused by drugs, such as salicylates. It can be seen that it is the amount of free T_3 and T_4 circulating in the blood which determines the level of thyroid activity. This faction also seems best able to reach the target peripheral cell and to exert its effect on cell metabolism.

METABOLIC RATE OF THYROID HORMONE

The daily requirement of thyroid hormone to maintain a normal metabolic rate in a thyroidectomized adult patient is 150–400 nmol of T_4, or 100–150 nmol of T_3. A small amount is not absorbed when given by mouth, and the maintenance dose by intravenous administration would be slightly less than the above. Half the thyroxine content of blood is metabolized every 6 days, and the half-life of T_3 is 24 hours. A certain amount of conjugated thyroxine is secreted into the bile with partial reabsorption from the small intestine (enterohepatic circulation).

The thyroid hormone is conjugated and excreted with glucuronide and sulphate, deiodinated and broken down in liver and peripheral tissues to a variety of iodinated compounds of varying activity. The iodothyronines, T_4 and T_3, are deaminated to their pyruvic acid derivatives which in turn may be decarboxylated and oxidized to acetic acid derivatives. Such derivatives may have various activities of the intact hormone in relatively different degree, and some of the effects of thyroid hormone may be produced by degradation products with specific metabolic effects.

MODE OF ACTION OF THE THYROID HORMONES

T_3 and T_4 have an effect on growth, metabolic rate, water and ion transport, nitrogen balance, sterol and fat metabolism. This makes it unlikely that they act at a single metabolic control point. While it is possible that the hormones influence these different metabolic processes by affecting different cell types in different ways, there is no evidence for this. Equally, there is little evidence that the hormones exert their effects by direct interaction with any enzyme system.

If T_3 or T_4 is given to a hypothyroid animal or patient, there is a slow return to the euthyroid state, provided the dosage is adequate and maintained. There is thus a lag phase between the start of the therapy and the first observable signs of a return to normal. The first observable change found in a treated animal is an increased synthesis of nuclear RNA. Thus the activity of the nuclear RNA polymerase, which is dependent on DNA, is increased by the hormone resulting in an increased rate of synthesis of nuclear RNA. This newly synthesized m-RNA, r-RNA and t-RNA then leave the nucleus. These events are followed in time by an increased rate of synthesis of protein by the ribosomes so that there is an increased protein content of some subcellular particles and in some cases these can be shown to have increased in size or weight (fig. 27.18). It is possible to explain the lag in the rise in the basal metabolic rate of a hypothyroid patient when given thyroid hormone on the basis that enough time must elapse to permit an effect of the hormone on the nuclear DNA for increased synthesis of m-RNA, to be followed later by increased r-RNA synthesis and yet later by increased ribosomal protein synthesis. In this way the hormone may raise the concentration of the respiratory enzymes in the mitochondria and hence increase the rate of oxygen consumption by the tissues.

Thus it is likely that T_3 and T_4 exert their effect at the nuclear DNA level and, by some as yet unknown mechanism, control the transcription of information from the DNA to the m-RNA. This leads to the concept that their effect on metabolism may be exerted through the control of the amount of specific enzymes in cells by affecting the rate of enzymic synthesis. It is interesting that in the endoplasmic reticulum, RNA accumulates at a rate parallel to the rate of increase in membranous phospholipid.

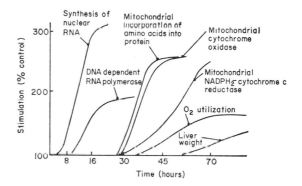

FIG. 27.18. Summary of data on the temporal relationships of RNA and protein synthesis in the liver of thyroidectomized rats following a single injection of 15–22 µg of tri-iodothyronine. Modified from Tata J.R. (1965) in *Mechanisms of Hormone Action*, ed. Karlson P. New York:Academic Press.

CONTROL OF HORMONE SECRETION

The formation and secretion of thyroid hormones are influenced and controlled in a number of ways, but TSH of the anterior pituitary is the key factor in thyroid homeostasis. Iodine is not only a constituent of the hormone but affects gland activity by change in the concentration of plasma inorganic iodide.

After a reduction in iodine intake there is a fall in plasma iodide with a progressive diminution in the iodine content of the thyroid gland. Eventually this decrease results in diminished synthesis of T_3 and T_4 with a subsequent increase in TSH production. Thyroid iodide uptake is thus increased, which prevents a further fall in the thyroid iodine content. This stimulus returns hormone synthesis to normal or T_3 may be preferentially synthesized as it contains one atom of iodine less than T_4. This functional overactivity of the thyroid is accompanied by an increase in size of the gland and is the mechanism responsible for the goitre in iodine deficiency; increased activity of the gland is required to maintain normal synthesis of hormone in the face of a continued shortage of iodine. A large excess of iodide on the other hand may partially suppress all aspects of thyroid activity with a reduction in gland size and vascularity by interfering with the actions of TSH and the formation of the iodothyronines.

Under physiological conditions the major factor determining the rate of thyroid secretion is TSH. The only other agents known to have a similar effect upon thyroid cell activity are the thyroid stimulating antibodies. Because of the manner in which these antibodies were first described they have been referred to as long acting thyroid stimulator (LATS) and LATS protector. In fact, LATS protector is a **human-specific thyroid stimulating antibody (HSTSAb)**, while LATS measured by bioassay in guinea-pig and mice is not species-specific. Human specific thyroid stimulating antibody is present in the plasma of 90 per cent of patients with hyperthyroidism associated with a diffuse goitre, whereas non-species specific thyroid stimulating antibody is only found in the plasma of the minority of hyperthyroid patients. Both types of thyroid stimulating antibody are IgG immunoglobulins. In hyperthyroidism plasma levels of TSH are reduced or undetectable, and an increase in pituitary output of TSH is not the cause of spontaneous hyperthyroidism.

In the physiological control of thyroid hormone secretion, the actions of iodide, T_3 and T_4 and TSH are closely interrelated. The rate of peripheral disposal of T_4 is another factor to be considered. Sudden exposure to cold results in increased thyroid activity dependent on the hypothalamus and abolished by T_4. In prolonged cold exposure the rate of peripheral disposal of T_4 is increased. The thyroid gland is influenced by that fraction of thyroxine which is free in serum and is not bound to carrier protein.

Calcitonin

This is a polypeptide which can be extracted from the thyroid gland or more readily from the ultimobranchial bodies of certain species (p. 27.18). It has a straight chain of 32 amino acids with a mol. wt. of 3600.

For a long time it was held that the hormonal control of plasma calcium was effected solely by variation in the rate of secretion of parathyroid hormone, which raises the calcium concentration. However, in 1962, Copp in Canada showed that in a dog given parathyroid hormone, total thyroparathyroidectomy did not lead to the expected fall in plasma calcium concentration, but to a rise. This observation led him to try the effects of extracts of parathyroid and thyroid and these experiments demonstrated the presence of a hormone in the thyroid gland, which lowered plasma calcium.

The calcitonin present in extracts can be assayed by measuring the fall in plasma calcium which occurs after injection into a rat. An immunoassay has been developed but because of limitations in methodology there is little knowledge about the levels of hormone in the blood in man. In some species, however, immunoassays have shown blood calcitonin to rise when plasma calcium is raised by oral or intravenous administration of calcium salts.

Calcitonin has important roles in the maintenance of the skeleton and in calcium metabolism in animals, but its role in man is not yet established. These and other actions are discussed together with the roles of parathyroid hormone in the next section.

PARATHYROID GLANDS

Patients with goitres which are secreting excess thyroid hormone or which are so large as to be unsightly are often treated by surgical removal of a large part of the thyroid gland. At one time it was not unusual for the patient, after a few days, to complain of tingling and numbness in the face, hands and feet, associated with muscle cramps; occasionally convulsions followed, and in some cases were responsible for the death of the patient. Probably the first person to observe these complications of thyroidectomy was Raynard, a veterinary surgeon in Lyon, who reported in 1835 that dogs often died following the removal of a goitre. He wrote: 'the most meticulous examination of the cadavers has not revealed to this day any lesion to which one might be able to attribute the death.' The parathyroid glands were discovered in 1862 by Sir Richard Owens, who first dissected them in a rhinoceros. Their anatomy in man was described in 1880 by Sandstrom, to whom their discovery is usually attributed. By the beginning of this century, it was realized that the above complications of thyroidectomy were due to the removal of the parathyroid glands. Since then surgeons have been careful to preserve the glands at operation and nowadays these features are seldom seen.

Anatomy

As a rule, there are four parathyroid glands but there may be more and, very occasionally, fewer than four. They are small, yellow, oval bodies, about 5 mm long and 4 mm wide, situated on the posterior surface of the lobes of the thyroid gland. On each thyroid lobe, there are two parathyroid glands, one being placed superiorly about the middle of the lobe at the level of the lower border of the cricoid cartilage, behind the junction of the pharynx and oesophagus (fig. 27.19). The inferior gland may be situated at the lower edge of the thyroid lobe or may lie in relation to one of the inferior thyroid veins.

The development of the parathyroid glands is described on p. 19.30. The two lower glands arise in pouch 3 together with the thymus and migrate with it, crossing over the upper two glands. As they follow the same course as the thymus in development, aberrant inferior glands are sometimes found anywhere between the angle of the jaw and the anterior mediastinum.

Most parathyroid glands lie in the capsule of the thyroid gland but they may be actually embedded in the thyroid tissue. The gland cells, however, are still separated from the thyroid tissue by a connective tissue capsule. This capsule extends into the parathyroid gland, forming trabeculae which carry the vascular and nervous supply to the gland.

HISTOLOGICAL STRUCTURE

There are two main cell types in the parathyroid glands, (plate 27.1e, facing p. 27.20). The **chief cells** (principal cells) are arranged in densely packed masses or columns supported by connective tissue and separated by numerous sinusoids. They are the more numerous and have a large centrally placed vesicular nucleus which stains poorly with haematoxylin & eosin and is embedded in a faintly staining cytoplasm.

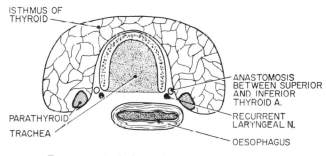

FIG. 27.19. Relations of the parathyroid glands.

The chief cells are of two types, dark and pale. The dark cells secrete the hormone of the parathyroid glands. They contain much RNA, have a prominent Golgi apparatus and can be seen on EM to possess secretory granules. Their cytoplasm contains little glycogen or lipid. The pale chief cells have little RNA and a small Golgi apparatus; their cytoplasm contains much glycogen and some lipid. Pale chief cells sometimes show cytoplasmic vacuolation and are referred to as 'water-clear' (wasserhelle) cells. This term, however, is also used for much larger vacuolated cells seen in tumours of the parathyroids, and it is probably better to reserve it for such pathological cells.

The **oxyphil cells** are larger than the chief cells. They have well marked nuclei and their cytoplasm contains many eosinophilic granules. The oxyphil cells do not appear in the parathyroid glands until a few years before puberty and become prominent only after puberty. They do not secrete the hormone, and their function is unknown. They may, in fact, stem from the chief cells and be degenerate forms. However, the eosinophilic granules seen on light microscopy are mitochondria, and their large number suggests that the cells are metabolically active.

About one-half of the substance of the normal gland is made up of fat cells; when hyperplasia of the gland occurs the fat disappears, being replaced by active tissue.

BLOOD SUPPLY

The blood supply is from the inferior thyroid arteries, derived from the thyrocervical trunks, which supply the lower and often the upper pair of parathyroid glands. Alternatively they may receive their blood supply from the anastomosis between the superior and inferior thyroid arteries. The blood supply to each gland is through a minute and delicate end artery which is, therefore, easily damaged in operations on the thyroid gland.

NERVE SUPPLY

In contrast to their rich vascular supply, the nerve supply of the glands is very poor. Branches from the superior and recurrent laryngeal nerves innervate the glands. They accompany the blood vessels and are vasomotor in function.

Functions of the parathyroid glands

By the start of this century, it was recognized that parathyroid insufficiency following thyroidectomy caused a fall in the plasma calcium, which could be relieved by subcutaneous implantation of a normal gland in the experimental animal. The parathyroid glands, therefore, became established as endocrine organs which secreted a hormone involved in the regulation of calcium metabolism. This hormone was eventually isolated by Hanson in 1923 and Collip in 1925 and called **parathyroid hormone**.

Most of our knowledge of the function of the parathyroid glands comes from studies of the effects of parathyroidectomy and the injection of parathyroid hormone. Removal of the parathyroid glands in the dog results in a fall in plasma calcium concentration and within a few days in lethargy, anorexia, vomiting and a subnormal temperature. The muscles twitch and become stiff and spastic. The hind limbs may be fixed in extension with the head sometimes held in dorsiflexion. As muscular spasms develop, the animal becomes unsteady on its feet and falls to the ground, often with convulsions. Eventually cardiac failure or paralysis of the respiratory muscles leads to death.

Thyroidectomy is still the commonest cause of parathyroid insufficiency in man and the most usual manifestation is **tetany**. The patient develops tingling, numbness and spasms which affect particularly the forearm and hand muscles; this results in pronation with flexion of the elbow and wrist together with flexion of the metacarpophalangeal joints, the interphalangeal joints being extended and the thumb and little finger being drawn towards the palm. This appearance has been called '*main d'accoucheur*'. Carpal spasm may be induced in these patients by blowing up a sphygmomanometer cuff on the upper arm to above systolic pressure (Trousseau's sign, fig. 27.20). The muscles of the larynx may also be affected by spasm giving rise to laryngeal stridor, and the abdominal muscles may be affected causing abdominal cramps. Spasm of the facial muscles can often be induced by tapping the skin over the facial nerve (Chvostek's sign).

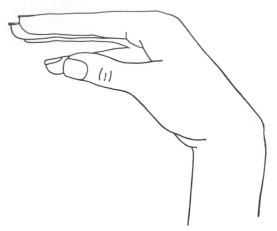

FIG. 27.20. Trousseau's sign in a patient with tetany.

PARATHYROID HORMONE

The parathyroid glands appear to secrete only one hormone. This is a polypeptide, containing about eighty amino acids. There are slight differences in the sequence and number of amino acids in the hormone of different species. Tryptic digestion or hydrolysis of the molecule shows that the physiological activity is dependent on a chain of about twenty acids.

The hormone appears to have a short half-life in the blood where its concentration may change rapidly. The polypeptide chain is split, probably in the lung, liver and kidney, and the fragments appear in the blood as inactive metabolites.

Assay

The hormone may be assayed biologically using either the dog or rat in which the parathyroid glands have been removed. The parathyroid activity of the test preparation is measured by its ability to raise the plasma calcium concentration when injected into the animal. This form of assay, however, has the usual disadvantages associated with biological assays.

An immunoassay for bovine and human parathyroid hormone has now been developed. As yet only a few laboratories have a satisfactory technique and there is only limited information about the levels in the blood under various physiological circumstances and in disease. The normal blood concentration in man is < 1 μg/l, but it is unlikely that all of this immunoreactive material is biologically active and much of it probably represents inactive polypeptide fragments. High values are present in many patients with tumours of the parathyroid glands, i.e. primary hyperparathyroidism.

REGULATION OF THE PLASMA CALCIUM

The concentration of circulating calcium is controlled within narrow limits. When determined by chemical methods, the variations in health lie between 2·12 and 2·62 mmol/l (8·5–10·5 mg/100 ml). More accurate analysis using

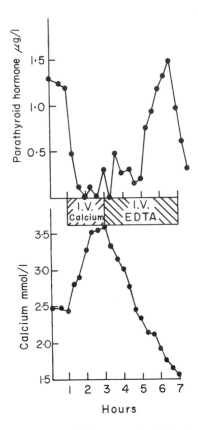

FIG. 27.21. Parathyroid hormone levels in the blood of a cow, determined by immunoassay, showing a fall when calcium is infused intravenously, and a sharp rise when the animal is given EDTA, a chelating agent that reduces the concentration of calcium in the blood. From Aurbach G.D. & Potts J.T. (1967) *Amer. J. med.* **42**, 1.

the atomic absorption spectrometer may show that the range is even narrower. Rather more than half is ionized and freely diffusible. The remainder is bound to protein, mostly to albumin or complexed with organic ions such as citrate. The amount of protein-bound calcium depends on the concentration of plasma protein and is increased by a rise in pH, but under most circumstances, the amount of protein-bound calcium in plasma remains fixed. As the determination of the ionic calcium in plasma is technically difficult, it is usual in both physiological and clinical studies to measure only the total plasma calcium. The calcium in the CSF, which is virtually free of protein, is almost all in the ionic form.

The secretions of parathyroid hormone and calcitonin are not controlled by trophic hormones of the pituitary but regulated by the calcium ion concentration of the extracellular fluid. When the calcium ion concentration is low, the parathyroid gland is stimulated to release its hormone. When the calcium ion concentration is raised, calcitonin is secreted. A clinical example is the enlargement of the parathyroid glands in response to the low plasma calcium found in severe rickets. Figs. 27.21 and 22 summarize experiments which illustrate the switching off of parathyroid hormone and switching on of calcitonin in response to rises in the blood calcium level and the switching on of parathyroid hormone secretion in response to a fall in plasma $[Ca^{++}]$.

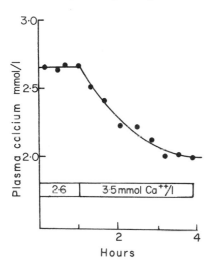

FIG. 27.22. The effect on the plasma calcium concentration of a pig with perfusion of the thyroid gland *in situ* with a solution containing a slightly higher concentration of calcium (3·5 mmol/l) than was present in the plasma (2·6 mmol/l). In the pig, the thyroid gland contains no parathyroid tissue and the fall in the level of plasma calcium in the general circulation must be due to a hormone secreted by the thyroid gland, presumably calcitonin. From Care A.D. (1965) *Nature*, **205**, 1289.

Parathyroid hormone raises the blood calcium in three ways. First and most important is a direct action on bone, mobilizing calcium. Secondly, it has a direct effect on the kidneys, increasing tubular reabsorption of calcium. Thirdly, the hormone promotes the absorption of calcium from the intestine. These three actions of parathyroid hormone are complementary, but appear independent of each other. Calcitonin lowers the blood calcium by a direct effect on bone, inhibiting its breakdown, and perhaps also by reducing renal tubular conservation of calcium.

EFFECT OF PARATHYROID HORMONE AND CALCITONIN ON TISSUES

Effects on bone

The direct action of parathyroid hormone on bone has been demonstrated by transplanting a piece of bone together with parathyroid tissue into the brain of a mouse, the two tissues being placed adjacent to each other. After 2 weeks, the bone showed the histological changes of resorption. Similar evidence has been obtained from tissue culture experiments using bone and parathyroid tissue.

The means by which the parathyroid hormone mobilizes bone calcium is not completely understood. It may increase the amount of citrate and other organic acids at the surface of bone crystal. These produce a local increase in the solubility of the bone, removing calcium and liberating it into the circulation.

The parathyroid hormone may also promote the breakdown of the bone matrix, thus liberating calcium and phosphate. It may do this by inducing depolymerization of polysaccharides in the matrix, these changes heralding the actual resorption of mineral from the bone. Thus, injections of parathyroid hormone increase urinary hydroxyproline, an amino acid largely derived from bone collagen. The hormone also causes proliferation of osteoclasts which accompanies the resorptive process and removes the collagen framework which no longer has any bone tissue to support.

Calcitonin inhibits the breakdown of bone, perhaps by stabilizing the protein matrix and by reducing the number and activity of osteoclasts. After injection of calcitonin into rats, there is a marked reduction in the urinary output of hydroxyproline.

Effects on the kidney

When parathyroid hormone is given to a parathyroidectomized animal, the first effects are on the kidney. Within minutes the urinary output of calcium and hydrogen ion is diminished and that of phosphorus and potassium increased. This is due to changes in renal tubular absorption. Later as calcium is mobilized from the bone and the plasma calcium rises, calcium excretion increases.

In man overactivity of the parathyroid glands sometimes increases the urinary output of calcium up to 7–12 mmol (300–500 mg)/day. The urine cannot easily hold such large amounts of calcium in solution and urinary stones tend to form. Overactivity of the parathyroid glands is the cause of a small proportion of the urinary stones arising in man. It is also sometimes associated with decalcification of the skeleton, which, if the disease is not treated, leads to gross skeletal deformity (vol. 3, p. 26.15).

Calcitonin has an effect similar to that of parathyroid hormone in inducing increased urinary excretion of phosphate and, by virtue of its effect on renal tubular reabsorption of calcium, increases urinary calcium.

Effect on alimentary absorption

The effect of parathyroid hormone on alimentary absorption of calcium can be demonstrated only in the presence of vitamin D. Parathyroid hormone probably stimulates the formation of 1,25-dihydroxycholecalciferol

(1,25-HCC) which then acts by stimulating calcium absorption in the alimentary tract (p. 32.45). The hormone also affects magnesium metabolism and in patients who have parathyroid insufficiency the plasma magnesium level may be low and alimentary absorption and renal conservation diminishéd. Calcitonin when injected into man does not alter alimentary absorption or the plasma magnesium.

The ionic changes in the extracellular fluid following secretion of the hormones may cause a variety of effects. A low plasma calcium increases the excitability of nerves and muscles, giving rise to tetany. A raised plasma calcium can result in cardiac dysrhythmias, thirst, polyuria, vomiting and death.

Effects at the molecular level

Little is known of the action of parathyroid hormone at molecular level. It is possible, however, by using metabolic inhibitors, e.g. actinomycin, to block the effect of the hormone on bone without altering the renal response. This suggests that the action of the hormone on the kidney, which is immediate, differs from its action on bone which includes cellular proliferation of osteoclasts.

The addition of the hormone to isolated mitochondria results in an increased uptake of phosphate, magnesium and potassium with release of hydrogen and calcium ions. As in the case of the effect on calcium absorption by the gut, the presence of vitamin D is necessary for the action of parathyroid hormone on calcium in the mitochondria, and is associated with an increase in oxygen consumption. The hormone also facilitates the entry of calcium through the plasma membrane into the cytoplasm, and it activates adenyl cyclase and increases cyclic AMP within cells. This in turn also influences the intracellular distribution of calcium. It is postulated that the hormone, by influencing the uptake and release of ions across cellular and subcellular membranes, induces changes in cellular metabolism which alter the rate of nucleic acid and protein synthesis and thus, in turn, the activity and number of bone osteoclasts.

The actions of calcitonin are immediate and are not influenced by giving actinomycin, nor dependent upon the presence of vitamin D. There are specific receptors in the kidney for calcitonin, which like parathyroid hormone probably activate adenyl cyclase.

ADRENAL GLANDS

In man, the two adrenal glands lie in the retroperitoneal space closely applied to the upper aspects of the kidneys. Each weighs about 5 g and is a composite structure comprising a central medulla and a surrounding cortex. In the lower vertebrates, however, these two components are anatomically separate and despite their intimate relationship in mammals they are totally distinct in develop-

mental origin and structure. In common with the gonads, the adrenal cortex is developed from cells of the coelomic mesothelium. Two masses of these cells form on the medial side of each developing mesonephros (p. 36.1). The first mass gives rise to the fetal cortex and the second, which envelops the first, forms the true or adult cortex.

Meanwhile, ectodermal cells derived from the neural crest migrate to form the coeliac sympathetic ganglion and some, migrating still further, invade the developing cortical tissue to form the adrenal medulla.

Anatomy

The two glands differ in shape and relations (fig. 27.23). The right adrenal is pyramidal in shape with a concave base applied to the surface of the right kidney, whereas the gland on the left is flatter and semilunar in shape. Anteriorly the left adrenal is related to the stomach, from which it is separated by the lesser sac of the peritoneum. The right adrenal is related on its anteromedial surface to

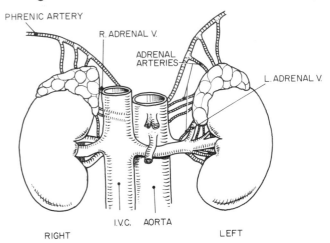

FIG. 27.23. The position and blood supply of the adrenal (suprarenal) glands.

the inferior vena cava and on its anterior surface to the liver. The upper portions of the posterior aspects of both glands are related to the diaphragm. The detailed relations of the adrenal glands vary somewhat according to the exact position of the kidneys but the glands are firmly attached to the posterior abdominal wall within their own fascial compartment so that, in the event of congenital malposition of the kidneys, the adrenals still occupy their normal situation within the abdomen, a fact of some importance in relation to adrenal surgery.

Accessory glands near the main gland usually contain both cortical and medullary tissue.

HISTOLOGICAL STRUCTURE (fig. 27.24 & plate 27.1)
The whole gland is enclosed within a fibrous capsule from which trabeculae pass inwards to support the parenchyma. In section, the distinction between the dark red central

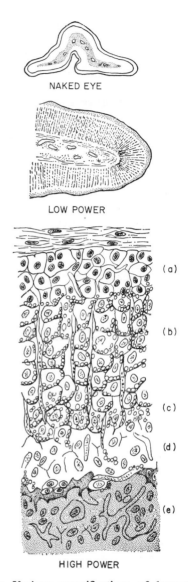

NAKED EYE

LOW POWER

(a)

(b)

(c)

(d)

(e)

HIGH POWER

FIG. 27.24. Various magnifications of human adrenal glands in section. In the section of highest magnification the cells of the zona glomerulosa (a) have small dark-staining nuclei and cytoplasm containing scanty lipid; the cells of the zona fasciculata (b) are filled with large globules of lipid, extracted during preparation for histological examination resulting in the formation of vacuoles (clear cells); at the border between zona fasciculata and zona reticularis (c) the cells are laden with lipid; the cells of the zona reticularis (d) are poor in lipid (compact cells); (e) medulla. After Ham A.W. (1965) *Histology.* London: Pitman Medical.

medulla and the surrounding pale yellow cortex is clear.

The cortex is composed of large polyhedral cells rich in lipids, particularly cholesterol and a yellow pigment from which the cortex gets its characteristic colour. These cells are arranged in three zones. The outer **zona glomerulosa** (fig. 27.24a), lies immediately under the capsule and consists of cells arranged in irregular clusters. The intermediate **zona fasciculata,** which forms the main mass of the cortex, consists of cells arranged in long radial columns while the **zona reticularis** consists of branching and anastomosing columns of cells (plate 27.1b, facing p. 27.20).

The medulla is composed of a spongework of cell columns. The cells are known as **chromaffin cells** or **phaeochromocytes** since they possess intracellular granules which stain specifically with chrome salts. In addition, small groups of nerve cells are scattered throughout the medulla. Separate aggregations of chromaffin cells (paraganglia) are found retroperitoneally and also around various organs of the body. They are probably of little physiological importance but may be the site of tumour formation (vol. 3, pp. 23.55 & 58).

BLOOD SUPPLY

The glands are highly vascular, each receiving three groups of arteries, the superior, middle and inferior adrenal arteries which are branches of the inferior phrenic artery, the aorta and the renal artery respectively. These vessels form a plexus under the capsule from which branches pass between the cortical and medullary cell columns. While the medulla receives some blood directly, most comes from capillaries that have passed through the cortex. Thus many medullary cells are bathed in blood containing a high concentration of adrenocorticosteroids. Each gland is drained by a single adrenal vein; the left one joins the left renal vein and the right one the inferior vena cava. Numerous lymphatics drain the lymph to the aortic lymph nodes.

NERVE SUPPLY

The adrenal medulla can properly be regarded as a specialized ganglion of the sympathetic nervous system and the secretory cells are richly innervated by cholinergic preganglionic sympathetic nerve fibres derived from the lower thoracic segments of the spinal cord. No nerve supply to the cortex has been demonstrated.

ADRENAL MEDULLA

In 1894, Oliver and Schäfer prepared aqueous extracts of the adrenal medulla and these administered intravenously caused a striking rise in the blood pressure of animals. Later Abel isolated **adrenaline** as a crystalline compound from the medulla and for many years this was regarded as the only medullary hormone. Not until 1949 was the second hormone, **noradrenaline,** demonstrated and it was recognized that this hormone acts also as the transmitter substance at sympathetic postganglionic nerve endings. The two hormones are both amine derivatives of tyrosine and are frequently referred to collectively as the **catecholamines,** the normal ratio of adrenaline to noradrenaline being four to one. They are synthesized from phenylalanine and tyrosine by pathways described on p. 11.23. Two types of medullary cell exist, one producing adrenaline, the other noradrenaline.

Both adrenaline and noradrenaline are stored, bound to ATP, in an inactive form in the chromaffin granules of the medullary cells, from which they may be liberated *in vitro* by lysis with hypotonic solutions. *In vivo*, release of catecholamines from the medulla by exocytosis is controlled by nervous impulses arising in the hypothalamus and conducted via preganglionic sympathetic nerve fibres. Thus, section of the nerve supply to one medulla, followed by a stimulus normally producing catecholamine release, results in selective depletion of the hormones of the gland with the intact nerve supply.

Release of catecholamines from the medulla follows such stimuli as pain, emotional disturbance, hypotension, hypoxia, hypoglycaemia, exposure to severe cold and muscular exertion. These stimuli are sometimes described as 'stress situations' (p. 27.35). The normal rate of hormone release is probably of the order of 0·1 nmol (20 ng) per kg of body weight/min and this rate may be increased one hundredfold. However, the adrenal medullae are in no way essential to life and patients may survive in good health after total bilateral adrenalectomy, if adequate substitution therapy is provided for adrenocortical function.

The adrenal medulla shares its origin with the cells of the sympathetic ganglia and of the central nervous system. Predictably, therefore, the same biosynthetic pathway exists also in brain and in the cells of the peripheral sympathetic nervous system, with one important difference; the final step, i.e. the *N*-methylation which results in the conversion of noradrenaline to adrenaline, does not occur in nervous tissue so that synthesis ceases at the stage of noradrenaline. This limitation exists also in the fetal adrenal medulla and in a proportion of adult medullary cells. Adrenaline production may, therefore, be regarded as a specialized enzymic function of a number of the medullary cells, and probably related to the fact that *N*-methyltransferase is dependent upon high concentrations of adrenocorticosteroids for its activity.

The basic unity of the sympathetic nervous system and the adrenal medullae is illustrated in fig. 27.25. Activation of preganglionic sympathetic nerve fibres results in the liberation of acetylcholine from the fibre terminals. In sympathetic ganglia, this results in the transmission of an impulse along the postganglionic neurone and the release of noradrenaline at the target organ; in the case of the adrenal medulla, a mixture of adrenaline and noradrenaline is released from the chromaffin cells directly into the blood stream. The liberation of catecholamines from the medulla is accompanied by generalized sympathetic effects in all tissues of the body provided with catecholamine receptor sites. These effects are superimposed upon those exerted by the simultaneous local release of noradrenaline from postganglionic nerve

fibre terminals. The medulla may thus be regarded as an endocrine luxury, available to reinforce and, by virtue of its unique ability to elaborate adrenaline, to modify, the effects of sympathetic nervous activity.

Actions of the catecholamines

The physiological functions of the catecholamines were summarized by Cannon in 1916 when he described the sympathetic nervous system as serving to prepare the organism for 'fright, flight or fight'. This preparation to meet the needs of stress is made by the combined effects of the catecholamines on receptors in the target organs. These receptors are divided into two main groups: the **α-receptors**, serving mainly excitatory functions such as

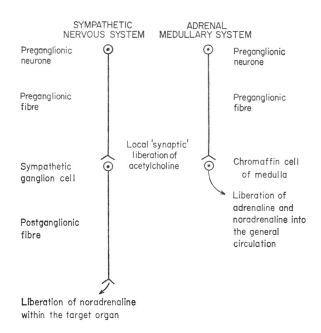

FIG. 27.25. Comparison of the sympathetic nervous system and adrenal medullary system.

vasoconstriction, and the **β-receptors**, serving predominantly inhibitory functions such as vasodilation and bronchodilation, together with one excitatory function, stimulation of the heart with resultant cardioacceleration. The nature of these receptors is not understood, but they are not dependent upon the integrity of the sympathetic nervous system; denervated tissues, indeed, demonstrate enhanced responses to the action of the hormones (Cannon's law). The usefulness and significance of the **receptor concept** is best considered in relation to the action of drugs and is discussed in vol. 2, p. 15.11.

The effects of adrenaline and noradrenaline differ both qualitatively and quantitatively. In addition, different stimuli may result in preferential secretion of one or other hormone from the medulla so that the resulting response can be expected to vary.

HEART AND CIRCULATION

Adrenaline, given intravenously at physiological rates, produces a marked tachycardia with an increase in cardiac output and an overall fall in peripheral vascular resistance. As a result the systolic blood pressure rises while the diastolic pressure falls, the mean blood pressure remaining largely unchanged. The effect of adrenaline upon vascular resistance varies in different parts of the vascular bed. Thus, in the skin and splanchnic area, adrenaline constricts the vessels, but dilates those in the skeletal muscle and, possibly, in the myocardium. All of these effects when taken together produce a lowered peripheral resistance, though individually the various effects lead to a redistribution of blood to those tissues whose requirements are likely to be high in situations of stress.

Noradrenaline stimulates the heart less than does adrenaline but greatly increases total peripheral vascular resistance. This in turn leads to a marked rise in systolic, diastolic and mean blood pressures which, by means of the carotid sinus reflex, results in a fall in cardiac output.

RESPIRATORY SYSTEM

Both adrenaline and noradrenaline increase the rate more than the depth of respiration. The minute volume increases and the P_{A,CO_2} falls. These effects are probably central in origin. Both hormones also produce peripheral effects on the respiratory system, the most important being bronchodilation. In this respect adrenaline is much more active than noradrenaline.

VISCERAL SMOOTH MUSCLE

Species differ in the effects of catecholamines on the gastrointestinal tract. In general both hormones lead to relaxation of the musculature of the gut, with the exception of the sphincter fibres, which are constricted. As a result the passage of intestinal contents is slowed.

A similar effect occurs in the case of the urinary bladder, with relaxation of the bladder wall and contraction of the sphincter.

METABOLIC FUNCTIONS

The medulla has important metabolic functions, adrenaline being about eight times more powerful than noradrenaline in this respect. The effect of adrenaline upon carbohydrate metabolism in liver and muscle is of particular interest since its biochemical basis is known. The hormone activates adenyl cyclase and so stimulates formation of cyclic AMP. The cyclic nucleotide binds to a receptor protein which acts as an inhibitor of protein kinase. The cyclic AMP-receptor complex then dissociates from the protein kinase which, now active, catalyses the phosphorylation using ATP and the inactive, dephosphorylated, phosphorylase kinase. The resulting active phosphorylase kinase then catalyses a second transphosphorylation, this time between ATP and the inactive form of the enzyme, phosphorylase b. The active phosphorylase so formed leads to the breakdown of liver glycogen with the formation of glucose-1-phosphate (p. 9.10). This compound is then acted upon by the enzyme, phosphoglucomutase, and the resulting glucose-6-phosphate then undergoes enzymic hydrolysis with the formation of free glucose which is released into the blood stream, raising the blood glucose. Muscle glycogen is also degraded by adrenaline stimulation to glucose-1-phosphate, but in the absence of glucose-6-phosphatase, hydrolysis does not occur and the hexose phosphate enters the glycolytic pathway with the production of lactic acid and free energy available for muscular work. At the same time, the protein kinase activated by cyclic AMP leads to phosphorylation of glycogen synthase with consequent reduction in its activity. Thus the adrenaline-induced increase in cyclic AMP concentration leads simultaneously to augmented glycogenolysis and reduced glycogenesis (p. 14.4).

Adrenaline and noradrenaline also accelerate the liberation of free fatty acids from the triglyceride stores of adipose tissue. This is brought about by the activation of adenyl cyclase which leads in turn to the activation of the hormone-sensitive lipase (p. 34.6). In view of the limitation of available carbohydrate stores, this supply of oxidizable substrate is of great importance, especially to the fasting animal.

SKELETAL MUSCLE

Adrenaline increases the blood supply to skeletal muscle and the quantity of hexose phosphate available to the glycolytic pathway. The hormone also increases the force of muscular contraction and delays the onset of muscular fatigue, though the mechanism for these effects is not known.

OTHER EFFECTS

Adrenaline produces pupillary dilation and activates the arrector pili muscles of the skin leading to erection of body hair. These actions have been interpreted teleologically as mechanisms to enable the animal to appear more formidable to any would-be assailant. Their importance in man, however, is small. Adrenaline also exerts marked effects upon the function of the higher centres of the central nervous system, resulting in increased wakefulness associated with sensations of anxiety and apprehension.

Metabolism of the catecholamines

Both adrenaline and noradrenaline are inactivated very rapidly in the body, so that their effects are transitory, except in circumstances which lead to their continuing liberation from the medulla. They are disposed of by two enzymes which are found widely distributed in many

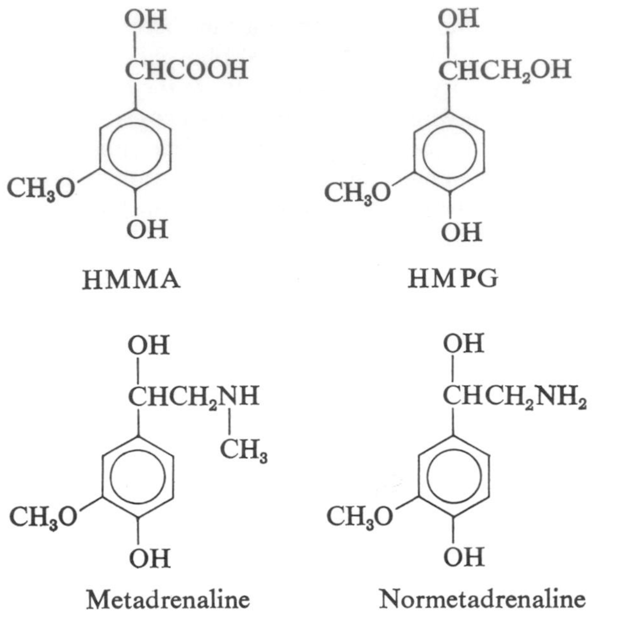

FIG. 27.26. Metabolites of adrenaline and noradrenaline in urine.

tissues of the body. These are catechol-O-methyltransferase (COMT) and monoamine oxidase (MAO). COMT catalyses the transfer of methyl groups mainly to the meta (or 3-) OH group (fig. 27.26), and MAO catalyses their oxidative deamination. Noradrenaline is also conjugated in the liver. After intravenous infusion of the hormones, approximately four per cent of the dose can be recovered unchanged from the urine, the remainder being excreted in the form of a mixture of metadrenaline, normetadrenaline, 4-hydroxy-3-methoxyphenyl glycol (HMPG) and 4-hydroxy-3-methoxymandelic acid (HMMA), products of the methylation and oxidative deamination of the hormones. HMMA can be estimated in the urine and provides an index of catecholamine production. A fuller discussion of the fate of catecholamines is given in vol. 2, p. 15.7. The diagnostic value of estimation of urinary metabolites is given in vol. 3, pp. 23.56 & 58.

ADRENAL CORTEX

Early experiments demonstrated that bilateral removal of the adrenal glands leads to a disorder of function so severe as to be incompatible with survival under normal circumstances, though it was discovered that the fatal outcome could be delayed by the administration of large amounts of sodium chloride. In the mid-nineteenth century, a similar clinical condition was described (vol. 3, p. 23.60). **Addison's disease** is characterized by weakness and muscle wasting with a low plasma sodium. There is increased urinary sodium loss which leads to a reduction in the extracellular fluid volume and a low blood pressure. The fasting blood glucose

is low. The patient is nearly always pigmented. Until modern therapy was available, the patients went downhill slowly and died. At post mortem the adrenal glands were found to have been destroyed. These observations stimulated efforts to obtain extracts from adrenal glands which would sustain life in adrenalectomized animals. In 1931, the first active extract was prepared and subsequent research has led to the identification in such preparations of almost fifty closely related chemical compounds belonging to the chemical group of steroids and known, after their tissue of origin, as **corticosteroids.** Only a few of this large number of compounds have been isolated from adrenal venous blood and it is likely that the remainder represent precursors or degradation products of the physiologically active hormones. The corticosteroids have diverse physiological functions, including the regulation of carbohydrate, protein, fat, water and electrolyte metabolism, together with the normal homeostatic responses to all forms of noxious stimulus and environmental change.

The adrenal cortex also synthesizes steroid hormones having the properties of androgens and oestrogens but the physiological importance of the glands in this respect is small, being overshadowed by the contribution of the gonads. For this reason, adrenal androgens and oestrogens are not discussed further here, but in chap. 38.

Corticosteroid hormones

The structure of the complex steroid nucleus has been described on p. 10.21. The conventional lettering of the rings and the numbering of the carbon atoms is shown again in fig. 27.27, together with the structures of the corticosteroid nucleus and of the two physiologically most important corticosteroids.

The characteristic features of the corticosteroids are the possession of a two carbon ketol side chain at position 17, representing carbon atoms 20 and 21, a ketone group at position 3 and a double bond between carbon atoms 4 and 5. The hormones also possess angular methyl groups at positions 10 and 13, representing carbon atoms 19 and 18. The corticosteroids, therefore, possess twenty-one carbon atoms in all.

Spatial isomerism occurring in the steroid nucleus is described on p. 10.21, together with the convention that groups added to the steroid nucleus are designated β if they project above and α if they project below the plane of the ring structure; β substituents are shown joined to the ring by a full line bond and α substituents by a dotted line.

In the adrenal cortex, the synthesis of the hormones occurs by means of enzyme-catalysed reactions and the stereospecificity of the enzyme systems involved ensures that the synthesis of only one of the possible isomers occurs.

In man, the physiologically important corticosteroids may, at the risk of some oversimplification, be regarded

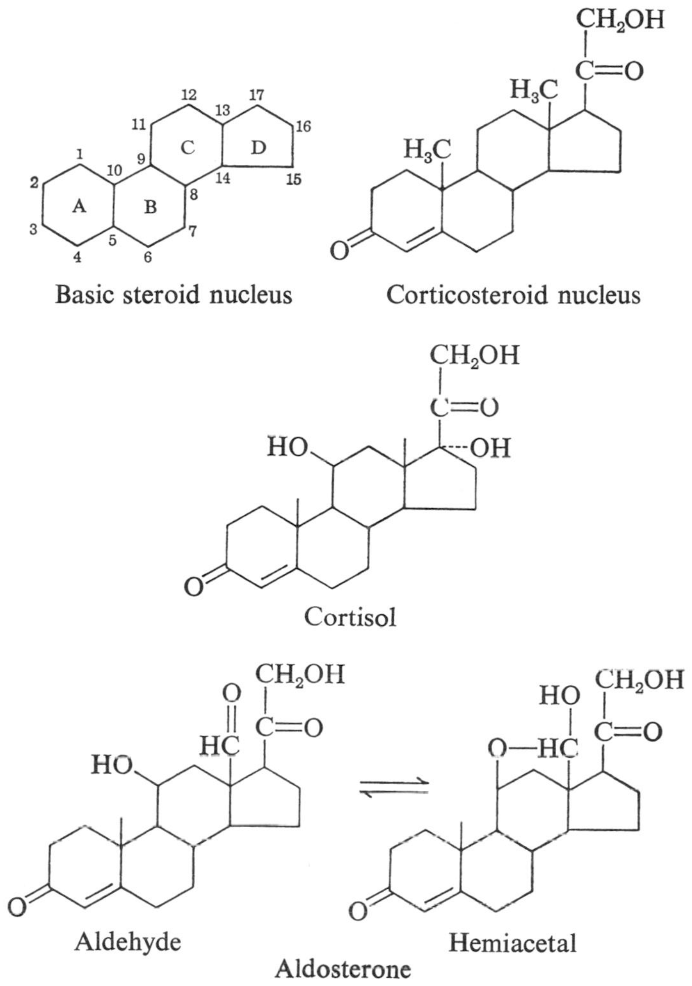

Basic steroid nucleus   Corticosteroid nucleus

Cortisol

Aldehyde   Hemiacetal

Aldosterone

FIG. 27.27. Structures of the corticosteroid nucleus, cortisol and aldosterone.

as **cortisol,** sometimes known as hydrocortisone, and **aldosterone. Corticosterone,** a steroid identical with cortisol with the exception that it does not possess the 17-hydroxyl group, is secreted in small amount in man but, although its physiological importance in certain animal species is undoubted, its significance in human physiology remains uncertain and it is not considered further here.

Cortisol possesses a hydroxyl group at C-11 together with a hydroxyl group at C-17. Aldosterone also possesses the hydroxyl group at C-11, but is unique among steroids in having an aldehyde group in place of the methyl group at C-18. By virtue of this unusual molecular configuration aldosterone exists in two forms, hydroxy-aldehyde and hemiacetal, between which an equilibrium state exists.

Biosynthesis of the corticosteroids

The corticosteroids are synthesized by the cells of the cortex from cholesterol. A summary of the pathways involved is given in fig. 27.28. The figures alongside the reaction arrows designate the number of the carbon atom at which each hydroxylation step occurs. Where appropriate, an indication of the stereospecificity is included. The final step in the synthesis of aldosterone is a dehydrogenation reaction with conversion of the C-18 alcohol to the C-18 aldehyde.

First cholesterol is converted to pregnenolone and thence to progesterone which then undergoes sequential enzymic hydroxylation to form the various corticosteroid hormones. The central position in this scheme occupied by pregnenolone and progesterone deserves special mention. Up to this point the synthetic pathway for all steroids is identical and the relative proportions of the final products, essentially cortisol, aldosterone and the sex hormones, are determined by the relative activities of the subsequent pathways. Since the activity of the enzymes involved is in part genetically determined, disorders of steroid biosynthesis can occur as congenital defects (vol. 3, pp. 23.70–73).

It is also of interest that the enzymic pathways involved appear to be distributed non-uniformly within the cortex so that different hormones are synthesized within the cells of the different cortical zones. Although conflicting evidence exists, aldosterone is probably synthesized by the cells of the zona glomerulosa, whereas cortisol is produced by the compact cells of the zona reticularis. The zona fasciculata is regarded as a non-secretory zone representing a store of steroid precursors; during periods of increased cortical activity, however, the clear cells of this zone undergo conversion to compact cells, this change beginning in the cells of the zona fasciculata adjacent to the zona reticularis. Thus the cells of the zona fasciculata may be regarded as a reserve of cortisol secretory activity which can be called upon as required.

ASCORBIC ACID AND THE ADRENAL CORTEX

The ascorbic acid content of the adrenal cortex is normally high. However, natural infections in man and experimental infections in animals reduce markedly the amount present in the gland, as do severe fatigue and the injection of ACTH. All these circumstances are associated with increased cortical secretion. Hence it is natural to postulate that ascorbic acid is associated in some way with the synthesis of cortical hormones. Possibly its role may be to exercise a tonic inhibition of steroid biosynthesis, which is reversed by the action of ACTH. Thus ACTH has been shown to deplete the cortical cells of ascorbic acid, some of which appears in adrenal venous blood before any increase in steroid production can be demonstrated. Further, *in vitro*, high concentrations of the vitamin inhibit the enzymes responsible for the 21- and 11β-hydroxylation reactions essential for cortisol synthesis.

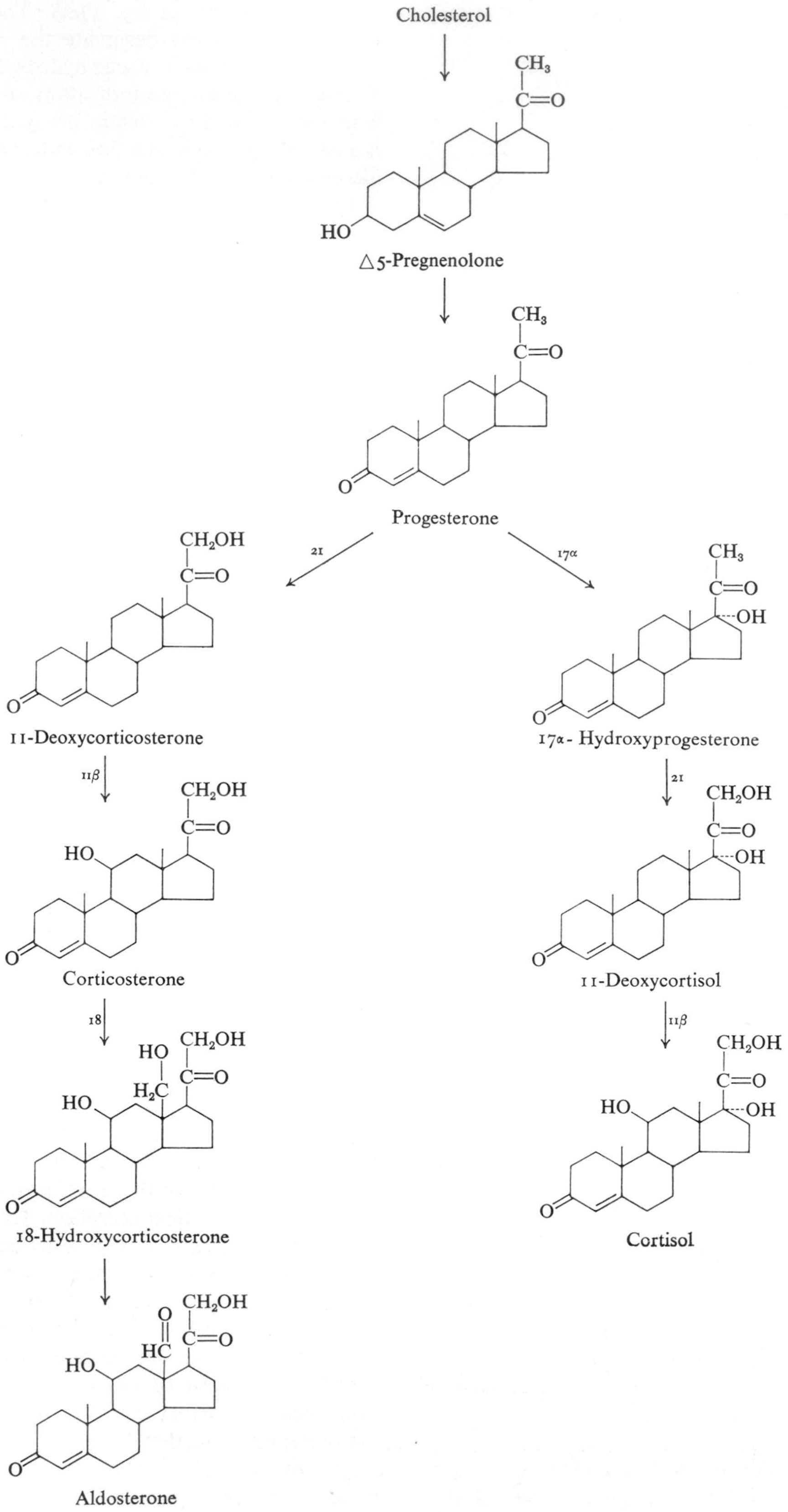

FIG. 27.28. Summary of the steroid synthetic pathway.

Actions of the corticosteroid hormones

It has been the custom to recognize two broad groups of corticosteroids, the **glucocorticoids,** regarded as exercising their principal effect upon carbohydrate metabolism and the **mineralocorticoids,** chiefly influencing electrolyte metabolism; the prototypes of these two groups were regarded as cortisol and aldosterone respectively. With increasing understanding of the corticosteroids, this arbitrary distinction becomes difficult to sustain since there is overlap in biological activity. The term glucocorticoid in particular is a misnomer because cortisol exerts perhaps its most important influences outside the sphere of carbohydrate metabolism.

CORTISOL

Cortisol given to adrenalectomized animals or to patients with Addison's disease increases the blood glucose and the urinary excretion of nitrogen; it influences carbohydrate metabolism by increasing the formation of glucose from non-carbohydrate precursors (gluconeogenesis), by promoting hepatic glycogen deposition and, possibly, by inhibiting peripheral glucose utilization. By virtue of its gluconeogenic effect, the hormone exerts a catabolic influence upon protein metabolism and amino acids are utilized for glucose synthesis and diverted from the pathway leading to protein synthesis. Although cortisol has a catabolic effect on the overall protein metabolism of the body, it has an anabolic effect on the liver, in which the incorporation of amino acids into protein is actually increased. Cortisol also modifies fat metabolism leading to liberation of FFA from the adipose tissue depots. The effect of the hormone is, however, complex since it causes mobilization of fat from some parts of the adipose tissue and deposition of fat in others. Thus, the action of the hormone results in the net availability of fatty acids for use as an energy source while at the same time exercising control upon the distribution of fat in various parts of the body.

From this point, the inappropriate nature of the term glucocorticoid becomes evident. Cortisol exerts important effects upon water metabolism by mechanisms which remain obscure. In adrenocortical insufficiency the distribution of body water is abnormal, so that extracellular dehydration and cellular overhydration may coexist. In addition, lack of cortisol results in an inability to excrete a water load. Both of these defects are specifically corrected by cortisol administration.

The hormone also exercises effects upon electrolyte metabolism; both independently and by its synergism with aldosterone, cortisol promotes retention of sodium and loss of potassium and hydrogen ions by the kidney. It also influences the distribution of sodium and potassium ions between cellular and extracellular fluid although it is much weaker than aldosterone in this respect.

Cortisol also plays an important role in the regulation of blood pressure. This effect is independent of alterations in electrolyte metabolism and appears to be a permissive action of the hormone. Thus, in adrenocortical insufficiency a state of relative refractoriness to the pressor effects of noradrenaline leads to hypotension, which is particularly marked on the assumption of the erect position. This abnormality is specifically corrected by the administration of cortisol. The corticosteroids may also contribute to the maintenance of blood pressure by a direct action upon the myocardium since it has been demonstrated experimentally that very small amounts of the hormones can increase left ventricular work.

The hormone also exerts an influence upon erythropoiesis and the anaemia of adrenocortical insufficiency is corrected by cortisol. Conversely, excessive amounts of cortisol may lead to an abnormal increase in the production of erythrocytes and polymorphonuclear leucocytes and in the number of circulating platelets. Injections of cortisol or stimulation of the cortex by ACTH lower the number of eosinophil granulocytes circulating in the blood but how this is brought about is unknown.

Cortisol also modifies the function of muscle cells and its administration corrects the muscle weakness characteristic of adrenocortical insufficiency. The hormone exerts an important influence upon the higher centres of the central nervous system, deficiency leading commonly to depression, excess to a state of euphoria. A more specific effect of cortisol upon the central nervous system is its capacity to modify the activity of the hypothalamo-hypophyseal system, resulting in the feedback mechanism decribed on p. 27.7.

The hormone exerts diverse effects upon many other organs and systems, the mechanisms and significance of which are poorly understood; high concentrations of the hormone in the blood are required before these effects are seen. Thus, cortisol reduces capillary permeability, causes dissolution of lymphoid tissue with a coincident fall in antibody synthesis, reduces the intensity of inflammatory and allergic reactions and may retard normal wound healing. Cortisol may also stabilize the membranes of lysosomes (p. 13.8). In shock and many toxic conditions lysosomes are disrupted, with release of their enzymes and these may increase the severity of the illness. Finally, cortisol has inhibitory effects upon cartilage growth, formation of bone matrix and deposition of calcium in bone.

In summary, observations of the effect upon the organism of cortisol lack or excess have demonstrated an almost bewildering variety of effects attributable to the hormone.

ADRENAL CORTEX AND STRESS

One of the most puzzling aspects of adrenocortical function is the increased secretion rate of cortisol in relation to **stress situations** of all kinds. This appears to be mediated by hypothalamo-hypophysial activity and is associated with the conversion of clear to compact cells and with as much as a five-fold increase in the rate of secretion of the hormone. Why the cortisol requirement should increase during periods of stress is unknown but failure of this mechanism impairs the resistance of the organism to the effects of the stressor. It is a not uncommon clinical experience that a patient, suffering from partial adrenocortical insufficiency but who, none the less, is capable of producing sufficient cortisol to meet the requirements of normal day to day life, is unable to increase significantly the output in response to stress. In such a patient, relatively minor stress, e.g. a brief general anaesthetic for a dental extraction, may lead to profound collapse and rapidly to death unless treatment with cortisol is given (vol. 3, p. 23.64). In a healthy person, injury such as a fracture or a surgical operation leads to an increased urinary excretion of nitrogen and potassium with retention of sodium and impaired glucose tolerance. These effects are brought about by the pituitary-adrenal system and are associated with increases in the plasma levels of ACTH and adrenal steroids. The physiological nature of these normal adaptation mechanisms and the reasons for the serious consequences of their failure in adrenocortical insufficiency remain obscure. Psychological stress is also associated with increased adrenocortical activity and raised plasma levels of ACTH and cortisol and it has been shown that the eosinophil counts of medical students fall as the time of their examinations draws near.

In circumstances in which it is not possible to measure the concentration of plasma ACTH or cortisol, eosinophil counts have been used as an indirect field test of adrenocortical activity and its relationship to stress. Thus Dr Simpson, an enthusiastic traveller, is an expert at carrying out eosinophil counts under difficult circumstances. Fig. 27.29 shows his observations on a single subject during a long and arduous sledging journey in the Antarctic. The eosinophil count fell at the start of the journey but was reduced still lower in the course of the expedition when the subject encountered great dangers.

The value to the organism of the increased cortical activity accompanying prolonged stress is not immediately obvious, though it is certain that without it we would be restricted to a very limited life. To what extent the activity is adjusted to meet the stresses and strains of everyday life is not known. Almost every degenerative disease occurring in middle age has been attributed to stress at one time or another. It is certain that some people suffer much more than others from the after-effects of either a severe psychological or physical stress. Whether this is due to excessive or prolonged cortisol responses to the stress is unknown. There is little or no evidence that such responses are either the direct or indirect cause of any disease that may subsequently arise. It is best to keep an open mind on this subject until we know much more in quantitative terms about individual responses to stresses of different natures.

Action of cortisol at the molecular level

In general, experiments in which cortisol has been added to enzyme preparations *in vitro* have yielded negative or equivocal results. However, in the intact animal the release of cortisol causes a negative nitrogen balance. This is due mainly to accelerated catabolism of protein in muscle which increases the plasma amino acid pool; lymphoid tissue is similarly affected. However in the liver, cortisol may be anabolic when it stimulates enzymes responsible for conversion of amino acids into nucleotides (fig. 27.30). The problem is to elucidate the site of action of the hormone in these reactions.

Cortisol may act by influencing a DNA-dependent RNA polymerase resulting in an increase in specific m-RNAs, which in turn increase the synthesis of certain hepatic enzymes involved in protein metabolism, e.g. 2,3-dioxygenase and tyrosine aminotransferase appear to be induced by cortisol in this way. The resulting increase in the activity of these enzymes leads to the formation of increased amounts of α-keto derivatives

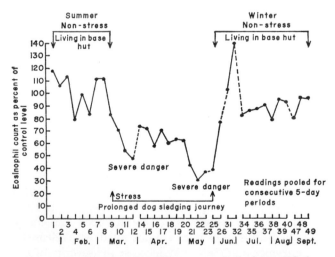

FIG. 27.29. Venous eosinophil counts made during a period of over 9 months on the leader of a British Antarctic base. During the first 'severe danger' period there were several crevasse incidents when dogs had to be rescued; also there were two occasions when his dogs charged downhill out of control in heavily-crevassed areas, since they could obtain no grip on the bare ice. In the second 'severe danger' period both tents were blown down simultaneously in the middle of the night and supplies in 50 lb (22·7 kg) boxes were blown away. Note the prolonged eosinopenia during the sledging period and return to control levels afterwards; also, since these are morning counts, they reflect the previous day's events or anticipation of the current day. From Simpson H.W. (1967) *Brit. med. J.* **i,** 530.

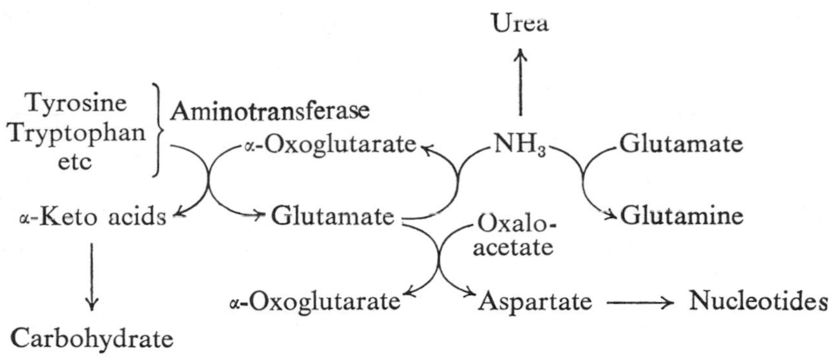

Urea

Tyrosine Tryptophan etc } Aminotransferase

α-Oxoglutarate ← NH₃ → Glutamate

α-Keto acids ← → Glutamate

Oxalo-acetate → Glutamine

α-Oxoglutarate ← Aspartate → Nucleotides

Carbohydrate

FIG. 27.30. Metabolic pathways influenced by cortisol.

and of glutamate and so enhances the rates of synthesis of liver carbohydrate, urea and nucleotides. Fig. 27.30 shows the metabolic pathways which relate these actions of cortisol to urea, carbohydrate and purine nucleotide metabolism.

ALDOSTERONE

The function of aldosterone is much less obscure. It influences electrolyte metabolism by modifying the rate of transport of sodium and potassium across membranes throughout the body. This effect has been most intensively studied in preparations of the toad bladder and in the distal tubules of the kidney. Here the hormone enhances the reabsorption of Na^+ from the tubular fluid and the excretion of K^+ and H^+ is increased. Thus in aldosterone deficiency sodium depletion and potassium intoxication result and in the presence of excess of the hormone the reverse situation occurs (vol. 3, pp. 23.67–70). Aldosterone is also known to decrease the ratio of Na^+ to K^+ in sweat and salivary secretions and to promote the reabsorption of sodium chloride and water and the secretion of K^+ by the cells of the ileum and colon.

In physiological amounts, unlike cortisol, aldosterone has little effect upon carbohydrate, protein or fat metabolism, is relatively inactive in protecting the organism against stress and does not influence the hypothalamo-pituitary axis.

Action of aldosterone at the molecular level

It is tempting to suggest that the hormone increases the uptake of Na^+ by activating or increasing the efficiency of the sodium pump. The toad bladder is an organ in which the mucosa fulfils a function comparable to the renal tubular cells in mammals and is amenable to investigations of the mode of action of aldosterone. Since a preparation continues to pump Na^+ *in vitro* for many hours an approach similar to that developed for the study of the mode of action of thyroxine at the molecular level (p. 27.23) is possible. When aldosterone is added, increased sodium transport can be detected only after a

time lag of about 1–2 hours. The aldosterone, however, is bound immediately in the cytosol and then to the cell nuclei, where it may effect changes in enzymic activities by stimulating RNA synthesis. This newly formed m-RNA may be the control factor in the synthesis of some specific enzyme involved in active sodium transport, or a specific permease which alters the permeability of the plasma membrane to Na^+. The localization of the hormone and the time course of the reactions are all compatible with this hypothesis.

Regulation of corticosteroid hormone synthesis

As the adrenal cortex contains negligible stores of the corticosteroid hormones, the regulation of the rate of steroid biosynthesis is synonymous with that of the rate of secretion of the hormones into the blood stream. In considering this regulation it is convenient to distinguish between cortisol and aldosterone, since separate mechanisms of control exist for each.

CORTISOL

The rate of utilization of the hormone may be calculated from the rate at which an intravenous dose of ^{14}C-cortisol disappears from the blood. In this way it has been deduced that in a normal unstressed human subject cortisol secretion ranges from 30–70 μmol (10–25 mg)/day, the value depending upon body weight, among other factors. Secretion is controlled by the action of ACTH, injection of which may raise the output of cortisol five or more times above the basal level. The nature of the stimulant effect of ACTH is discussed on p. 27.14. The feedback mechanism by which plasma cortisol modifies ACTH secretion is described on p. 27.7.

In normal circumstances the rate of cortisol secretion is not constant throughout the day but is highest in the early hours of the morning and lowest in the late evening (p. 47.6). This diurnal variation is a manifestation of the rhythmicity of the hypothalamus, which also determines the diurnal variation in body temperature and the menstrual cycle. It is reflected in plasma and urinary steroid concentrations and follows a diurnal variation in the production of the hypothalamic corticotrophin releasing hormone.

The influence of the hypothalamus in determining adrenocortical function also explains the increase in cortisol secretion observed under conditions of stress. The hypothalamus receives afferent impulses from many parts of the central nervous system and its activity is modified by stress in such a way that liberation of the releasing hormone is increased.

ALDOSTERONE

Aldosterone is the most potent of all of the known naturally occurring corticosteroids and by using ^{3}H-aldosterone the secretory rate of the hormone in man has been estimated as of the order of 150–500 nmol (50–200 μg)/day.

Aldosterone secretion is largely, though not absolutely, independent of ACTH and is increased by factors such as sodium depletion, potassium feeding, a fall in the plasma Na^+ to K^+ ratio and by reduction in the extracellular fluid or blood volume, all situations in which the activity of the hormone tends to restore normality.

The mechanism by which these circumstances lead to increased secretion of the hormone remains controversial. The secretory rate rises or falls with a rise or fall in plasma $[K^+]$ which influences it directly. However, the increased secretion in response to changes in Na^+ balance and extracellular fluid and blood volume can be abolished by bilateral nephrectomy. It is now thought that such stimuli lead to liberation of a protein named **renin** from the cells of the juxtaglomerular apparatus of the kidneys. Renin passes into the blood stream where it causes the hydrolytic cleavage of a circulating α-globulin with the formation of **angiotensin I**, an inactive polypeptide containing ten amino acids; this is acted upon by a converting enzyme present in lungs and plasma to form **angiotensin II**, a polypeptide containing eight amino acid residues. In addition to possessing a powerful vasoconstrictor action, angiotensin II appears to act as a specific stimulus to aldosterone production by the adrenal cortex. The significance of this renin-angiotensin system remains controversial, though it is probably an important component of the volume control system (p. 35.27).

Effects of administered corticosteroids

Corticosteroids may be administered to patients for two reasons. The first of these is the replacement of defective endogenous secretion of the hormones due either to disease of the adrenal glands themselves or of the hypothalamo-pituitary axis. The second involves the use of cortisol or of one of its natural or synthetic analogues in pharmacological rather than physiological doses. Such therapy is employed with the intention of exploiting one or other of the actions of the corticosteroids usually in relation either to their effects in suppressing inflammatory or allergic reactions or in modifying the production of cells of the haemopoietic system. The use of corticosteroid hormones in this way, while often beneficial to the primary disorder, leads to a multitude of undesirable effects. The high doses involved interfere with the normal feedback control of adrenocortical function, causing inhibition of the hypothalamo-pituitary axis and leading to consequent depression of endogenous cortisol secretion. In these circumstances sudden withdrawal of the administered steroid, or indeed the advent of a severe stress, may lead to adrenocortical insufficiency which may be so severe as to be fatal. The suppression of ACTH secretion may be prolonged. In addition other undesirable effects may appear in patients kept on high levels of exogenous steroid for long periods; these include impaired glucose tolerance, wasting of muscle and loss of total bone substance resulting from negative nitrogen balance, accumulation of sodium with secondary retention of water and progressive loss of potassium. Exactly the same effects are observed in patients with adrenocortical hyperactivity who produce excessive quantities of steroid hormones (vol. 3, pp. 23.65–67). As may be anticipated on theoretical grounds, such adrenal hyperfunction may be a reflection either of autonomous overactivity of the cortical cells themselves due to a secreting tumour which may be benign or malignant **(Cushing's syndrome)**, or of overstimulation of otherwise normal glands by excessive production of ACTH **(Cushing's disease)**.

Numerous attempts have been made to elaborate synthetic corticosteroids which would retain the desired therapeutic effects of the natural hormones without producing other unwanted and even dangerous effects. Many synthetic steroids have been produced and are used in the treatment of disease but none is free from adverse effects (vol. 2, p. 6.10).

Metabolism of corticosteroids

CORTISOL

The peripheral blood contains from 140–700 nmol (50–250 μg)/l of cortisol, the level varying with such factors as the time of day at which the specimen is taken and the weight of the subject, levels being generally higher in the obese than in lean persons. Approximately 90 per cent of this cortisol exists in bound form, a small amount attached to the red cells and a much larger quantity bound to a circulating α-globulin to which the name **transcortin** has been given. In the presence of high circulating levels of oestrogen, as in pregnancy and to a lesser extent after the consumption of the now fashionable oral contraceptives, the levels of transcortin and cortisol in the blood both rise, the latter often to abnormal values. Yet none of the expected effects of excess cortisol are observed. Conversely in hepatic disease the synthesis of transcortin by the liver cells is impaired, leading to a reduction in the circulating level of the protein with a parallel fall in the level of plasma cortisol; again, in such situations, no effect attributable to cortisol lack occurs. Such observations have led to the belief that only the unbound plasma cortisol is physiologically active, both in the exercise of corticoid activity and in participation in the feedback system.

From experiments carried out with ^{14}C-labelled cortisol, it has been estimated that the half-life of the hormone in the body approximates to 80 min.

ALDOSTERONE

In plasma, the concentration of the hormone lies normally between 1·1–2·2 nmol (400–800 ng)/l. Aldosterone is significantly less firmly bound to protein than is cortisol, a greater proportion being carried in the free state in the plasma, and hence has a shorter half-life, of the order of 45 min.

INACTIVATION AND EXCRETION OF CORTICOSTEROIDS

The inactivation of the corticosteroids occurs in the liver, the pathways involved being complex. The changes

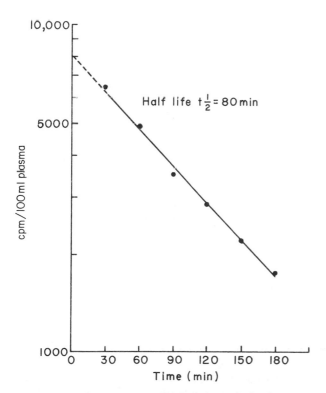

FIG. 27.31. Plasma levels of labelled cortisol after an intravenous dose of ^{14}C-cortisol. From Peterson R.E. (1959) *Recent Progress in Hormone Research* **15,** 231.

wrought in the steroid molecule are the saturation of the double bond between carbon atoms 4 and 5, and the reduction of the ketone group at carbon 3. This process is described on p. 33.11. The resulting metabolites then undergo conjugation with glucuronic acid or sulphate. These conjugated metabolites are devoid of hormonal activity and are, unlike the parent hormones, water soluble and only slightly bound to plasma proteins. The properties of the conjugates are such that they are rapidly eliminated from the body by the kidneys. In the urine they can be detected by chemical means as the 17-hydroxycorticosteroids (17-OHCS), providing a convenient and reliable method for the assessment of adrenocortical function (vol. 3, p. 23.58).

ISLETS OF LANGERHANS

Development and microstructure

The development of the pancreas is described on p. 32.57. In the 3rd month two distinct types of cell can be seen around the developing ducts. The majority remain attached to the ducts and give rise to acini of serous cells whose secretion passes into the duodenum. A minority separate from the ducts to form isolated groups of cells clustered round capillaries, the **islets of Langerhans.** These cells contain secretory granules and as early as 3 months, two types of cells, α and β, can be distinguished on the basis of the staining reactions of the granules. With Gomori's special stain (plate 27.1f, facing p. 27.20), the granules in the α-cells appear red, while those in the β-cells are light blue. Both cells secrete hormones concerned with carbohydrate metabolism, the β-cells **insulin** and the α-cells **glucagon**. At least two other cell types, C- and D-cells, have also been identified in mature islets and immunochemical techniques have shown that the D-cells contain GHRIH (p. 27.7).

At the earliest stage of development the close relationship of the β-cells to the capillaries suggests that insulin is secreted directly into the blood stream. By the fourth month islet tissue constitutes approximately one-third of the total pancreatic mass and from the 30th week onwards in an increasing number of islets, the α- and β-cells intermingle as they do in the adult. At birth the proportion of α-cells is higher than in the adult. There is evidence that GH and ACTH influence the growth of both α- and β-cells and it is likely that the relative increase in the β-cells in the adult, as compared with the fetus and newborn baby, is under hormonal control. In the adult, β-cells constitute about 75 per cent, α-cells about 20 per cent and the other cells about 5 per cent of islet cells. Thus, most of the interior of the islet is made up of β-cells which are in close proximity to the numerous capillaries, and this great vascularity led many years ago to the suggestion that they might be endocrine organs.

Islet tissue increases in size throughout childhood and adolescence and reaches a weight of about 1 g in adult life. The growth is due to an increase in both the number and size of the islets. In the first 3 years of life the number increases from about 300 000 at birth to about 1 000 000. Thereafter, the individual islets enlarge to three or four times their size at birth. Islet tissue grows more rapidly than the body as a whole during the first 2 years of life, lags behind the body between the ages of 3 and 12 years, and increases equally with the body from 13 to 21 years. It has been suggested that the incidence of diabetes at these ages may be correlated with these different growth ratios.

Ultrastructure

Figure 27.32 illustrates the sequence of events thought to occur when insulin is secreted by the β-cell in response

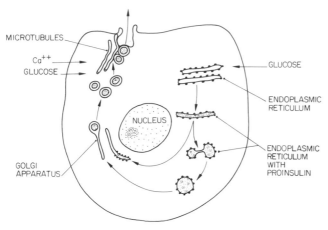

Fig. 27.32. Formation of proinsulin and secretion of insulin. Modified from Lacy P.E. (1970) *Diabetes* **19**, 895.

to glucose. This concept has been derived mainly from serial EM studies of the pancreas of the rat. Metabolism of glucose within the β-cell is the signal for the synthesis of the inactive precursor of insulin, proinsulin, within the endoplasmic reticulum. Proinsulin is transferred to the Golgi complex where it is converted to insulin. Granules of insulin, encased in smooth membranous sacs, are released into the cytoplasm and become attached to the microtubular system. The intracellular metabolism of glucose also allows calcium to enter the β-cell; this activates the microtubular system so that granules of insulin are moved to the surface of the cell, where they are released. This consists of fusing of the membranous sac of the insulin granule with the membrane of the cell and subsequent rupture, so that the granules are liberated into either the intercellular or pericapillary space where they undergo rapid dissolution. Prolonged hyperglycaemia, administration of insulin or starvation all lead to loss of granules from the β-cells.

Hormones of the islets of Langerhans

INSULIN

The discovery of insulin and its therapeutic application is one of the most dramatic stories in the history of medical science. It started in Germany in 1889 when von Mering and Minkowski removed the pancreas from a dog, which then began to pass large quantities of urine containing sugar. This condition had already been recognized in man and first named by the Greeks **diabetes mellitus** (diabetes, a syphon, or running through; mellitus, honeyed).

In 1902, Szobolew and Schultze found that if the main pancreatic ducts are ligated in animals, the pancreatic acini rapidly disintegrate but the islets persist and even increase in number and the animals do not develop diabetes. Hence they concluded that the islet cells were the source of an antidiabetic principle produced by the pancreas and that this must be an internal secretion or hormone. In 1909, de Meyer suggested the name 'insuline' for this hypothetical hormone, but it was not until 1921 that, independently and almost simultaneously, Paulescu in Romania and Banting and Best, the latter a medical student, working in Macleod's laboratory in Toronto, succeeded in extracting insulin from the pancreas. Banting, Best and Macleod shared a Nobel Prize; Banting was an imaginative genius who later turned from medical research to painting.

The Canadians succeeded where others had failed by following directly in the footsteps of Szobolew and Schultze. They used the same technique of ligating the pancreatic duct to induce atrophy of the acinar tissue and so remove the source of proteolytic enzymes, which destroy insulin in extracts of whole pancreas. They were then able to extract insulin in relatively high concentration from the islet tissue and to demonstrate that this extract lowered the blood glucose in pancreatectomized dogs (fig. 27.33). Applying the same reasoning they were also able to extract insulin from whole fetal pancreas, which contains functioning islets but has no digestive activity. Later it was found that acid and alcohol not only extract insulin but also prevent proteolytic destruction and using these it is possible to obtain insulin from whole adult pancreas.

In 1926, Abel in the USA obtained insulin in crystalline form and it was found to be a protein. In 1955, the complete chemical structure of insulin was elucidated by Sanger working in Cambridge. Finally, in 1963, Katsoyannis in Pittsburgh synthesized the hormone.

Chemical structure

The molecular weight of insulin is about 5800. It is composed of two chains of amino acid residues, an A chain of twenty-one amino acids, and a B chain of thirty amino acids, joined by two disulphide bridges. A third disulphide

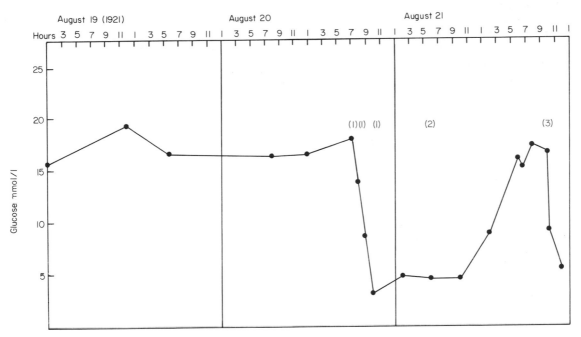

FIG. 27.33. Effect of insulin on the blood glucose level of a pancreatectomized dog. (1) Injection of extract of degenerated pancreas; (2) extract after incubation with pancreatic juice: (3) extract incubated without pancreatic juice. Redrawn from Banting F.G. & Best C.H. (1921). *J. Lab. Clin. Med.* **7**, 464.

bridge connects one part of the A chain with another part of the same chain.

Proinsulin is a polypeptide containing the A and B chains of insulin, linked end to end by an additional chain of 30 amino acids joining the terminal alanine of the B chain with the terminal glycine of the A chain. The molecule is so coiled as to facilitate the formation of the disulphide bridges between the A and B chains. When these have been built, the linking chain is split off and insulin is formed. Proinsulin is biologically much less active than insulin. The insulins from different animal species are identical in their biological and therapeutic effect but differ slightly in amino acid structure and immunologically.

Now that the structure of insulin is known it has been possible to devise experiments in which parts of the molecule are broken off by controlled enzymic hydrolysis and the residue tested for activity. Nevertheless, little is known about the relationship of the action of insulin to its chemical structure and it is not yet possible to state which amino acids make up the active centre. The following are among the more important known facts:

(1) the disulphide bridges must be intact for biological activity,

(2) the exact sequence of the amino acids within the disulphide ring of the A chain is not important for biological activity since this varies among the insulins derived from different species,

(3) the residue that remains after splitting off the eight terminal amino acids from the end of the B chain of

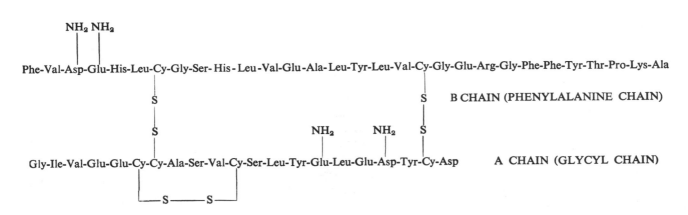

bovine insulin has only 15 per cent of the biological activity of the intact molecule,

(4) the presence of a carboxyl group from either asparagine or aspartic acid at the end of the A chain is necessary for full biological activity, but removal of this group does not bring about total inactivation.

Immunological behaviour

Insulin labelled by ^{131}I is retained for a long time in the blood stream of all subjects who have received insulin therapeutically and this is due to insulin-binding antibodies in the blood. When injected into man, beef insulin seems to be a much more potent antigenic stimulus than insulin derived from pigs which structurally resembles human insulin more closely. Furthermore, the antibody produced, although it partially neutralizes the biological effect of injected bovine insulin, shows little affinity for pork insulin. Homologous pancreatic insulin can, in some circumstances, act as a weak antigen and endogenous circulating insulin may differ antigenically from highly purified crystalline pancreatic insulin. These observations raise the possibility of autoimmune processes in disease of the pancreas. The antigenic behaviour of insulin is the basis of methods for the immunoassay of insulin.

Assay

Insulin is assayed biologically using glucose uptake or oxidation in several different preparations, such as the rat diaphragm or adipose tissue from rat epididymis. Immunological methods are also used. These methods give somewhat different results which are expressed in terms of international units. The international unit itself is based upon the hypoglycaemic effect of a standard preparation of insulin in mice (vol. 2, p. 6.16). In non-obese healthy adults the fasting level of immunoreactive insulin (IRI) lies between 10 and 25 mU/l.

TABLE 27.5. Some major physiological reactions stimulated by insulin.

On carbohydrate metabolism

Insulin lowers the blood glucose:
    (1) by promoting glycogen synthesis in liver and muscle,
    (2) by increasing cellular utilization of glucose,
    (3) by inhibiting gluconeogenesis from protein.

On fat metabolism

Insulin increases fat storage in adipose tissue:
    (1) by stimulating lipogenesis,
    (2) by inhibiting lipolysis.

On protein metabolism

Insulin increases protein synthesis:
    (1) by promoting the utilization of amino acids,
    (2) by promoting DNA and RNA synthesis,
    (3) by inhibiting protein breakdown.

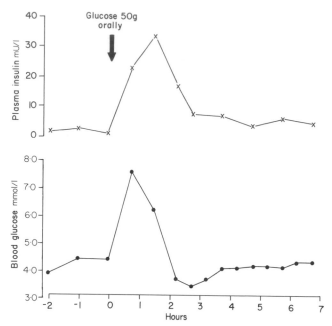

FIG. 27.34. Blood glucose and plasma insulin values in a healthy, thin, young man measured for 2 hours before and 7 hours following 50 g glucose given orally. From data of Hunter W.M., Willoughby J.M.T. & Strong J.A. (1968) *J. Endocrin.* **40**, 297.

ACTIONS OF INSULIN

Insulin is a powerful hormone whose actions affect the structure and function of every organ in the body. Not all tissues are, however, directly responsive. Among the responsive tissues muscle, liver and adipose tissue have been studied most extensively. Major physiological reactions stimulated by insulin are shown in table 27.5. In intact, fed animals, insulin is an anabolic hormone and promotes the storage of carbohydrate, protein and fat.

Under physiological circumstances insulin is secreted in response to the rising blood glucose concentration which follows a carbohydrate meal (fig. 27.34) and the best known and most readily demonstrable action of exogenous insulin *in vivo* is its ability to lower the concentration of blood glucose (fig. 27.35). This is brought about by numerous actions which fall into two groups:

(1) those increasing the rate of withdrawal of glucose from the extracellular fluid into the peripheral tissues,

(2) those decreasing the rate of addition of glucose to the extracellular fluid by the liver.

Which effect predominates depends upon a number of factors which include the route of administration. In experimental animals, the action on peripheral tissues is encouraged by rapid intravenous injection of insulin and the hepatic action by a slow injection into the portal vein. Since infusion into the portal vein more closely resembles the way in which insulin enters the circulation naturally, it is likely that the hepatic action of insulin is as important as the peripheral one in maintaining the blood glucose in the intact animal. Insulin increases the withdrawal of glucose from the ECF by direct or indirect actions on carbohydrate, fat and protein metabolism.

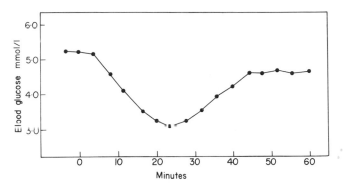

FIG. 27.35. Effect of an intravenous injection of insulin (1 unit) on the blood glucose concentration of a healthy, thin, young man. From data of Courtice F.C., Douglas C.G. & Priestley J.G. (1939) *Proc. roy. Soc. B.* 127, 41.

Effects on carbohydrate metabolism

Next to its ability to lower the blood glucose, the property of insulin that is best established is its action in **promoting glycogen deposition** in skeletal muscle. This glycogenic effect is easily demonstrated *in vitro* using thin sheets of muscle from the diaphragm of young rats (table 27.6) and this preparation has been used for the bioassay of insulin. Glycogen can be formed from glucose by isolated tissue without insulin, provided the appropriate enzyme systems

TABLE 27.6. The effect of insulin on glucose utilization and glycogen formation by the isolated rat diaphragm. The figures are averages from nine experiments. Glucose concentration in the medium was 10 mmol/l. From data of Gemmill C.L. & Hamman L. (1941) *Bull. Johns Hopk. Hosp.* 68, 50.

	No insulin	Insulin
Glucose utilization mmol/kg tissue/3 h	30	57
Glycogen deposition mmol/kg tissue/3 h	0·5	25

are present and in these circumstances the rate of glycogen formation depends on the concentration of extracellular glucose. However, for a given concentration of extracellular glucose, the rate of glycogen formation is increased by the presence of insulin. Insulin also has a glycogenic effect on adipose tissue which can be demonstrated *in vivo* (fig. 27.36). It is important to remember that this effect is related to the concentration of blood

glucose which in turn determines the amount of glucose available for deposition of glycogen. If hypoglycaemia occurs, glycogen is mobilized and enters the blood as glucose.

Insulin also **increases the rate of glucose utilization** in the tissues (table 27.6). However, glucose can be utilized in the absence of insulin. Experiments with eviscerated dogs have shown that within a certain range the rate

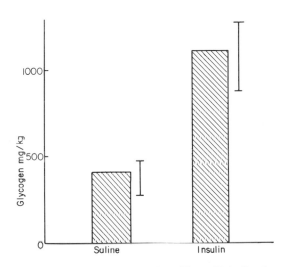

FIG. 27.36. Effect on glycogen deposition of injecting long-acting insulin (5 units) into the left groin fat of six diabetic rats compared with the effect of an equal volume of isotonic NaCl injected into the right groin. Glycogen measured 20 hours after injection. From data of Renold A.E., Marble A. & Fawcett D.W. (1950) *Endocrinology* 46, 55.

of utilization is directly related to the level of blood glucose and that raising the concentration has an effect similar to that of insulin.

The effects of insulin on the liver are complex. In the diabetic state, glucose is produced in this organ both from protein and from glycogen in large amounts and insulin **inhibits this gluconeogenesis**. This action is additional to its effect on glycogenesis and the utilization of glucose, already described, which occurs in the liver as in other tissues. Administration of insulin can markedly decrease the glucose output of the liver, as has been shown in experiments in the dog when hepatic blood flow and glucose concentrations in the arterial and hepatic venous blood have been measured simultaneously. In this way the hepatic glucose balance can be determined (fig. 27.37).

Effects on fat metabolism

Adipose tissue is the major site for the regulation of energy storage and mobilization. Insulin plays a more essential role in metabolism in adipose tissue and muscle than in liver which can perform some of its major functions without insulin. The major metabolic reactions

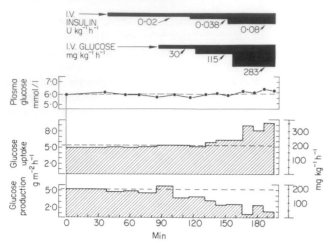

FIG. 27.37. Effects of continuous intravenous infusion of insulin on glucose production and uptake by the liver in a normal dog in the postabsorptive state; hypoglycaemia was avoided by the intravenous infusion of glucose in the amounts indicated. Modified from De Bodo R.C., Steele R., Altszuler N., Dunn A. & Bishop J.S. (1963) *Recent Progress in Hormone Research* **19**, 445.

concerned with energy storage of fat are described in chap. 10, and the metabolic roles of adipose tissue are further discussed in chap. 34. Here it is sufficient to state that in isolated fat cells and in the isolated epididymal fat pad of the rat, insulin increases not only glucose uptake but also **stimulates lipogenesis** by the conversion of glucose into triglyceride. In addition insulin **inhibits lipolysis**. It does this not only by increasing the availability of intracellular glucose and so supplying 1-glycerophosphate, but also by a direct effect on the release of FFA which is seen in the total absence of glucose (table 27.7).

Thus insulin is antiketogenic in two ways, firstly by reducing the quantity of free fatty acids delivered to the liver and secondly by increasing the rate of carbohydrate

TABLE 27.7. The effect of insulin in inhibiting the lipolytic action of noradrenaline on isolated adipose tissue. Mean values and standard deviations of observation on twenty-two rats. From data of Mahler R., Stafford W.S., Tarrant M.E. & Ashmore J. (1964) *Diabetes* **13**, 297.

	Glycerol released mmol/kg fresh tissue/h
Control (no hormonal addition)	1·34 ± 0·06
Noradrenaline (0·5 μmol/l)	4·2 ± 0·12
Noradrenaline (0·5 μmol/l) + insulin (100 mU/l)	1·72 ± 0·14

dissimilation in the liver so that the fatty acids which are delivered can be completely oxidized.

Effects on protein metabolism

Diabetes, whether produced by removal of the pancreas in animals or due to destruction of the islets by disease in man, is a wasting condition. The tissues, especially muscle, atrophy and the cell components break down and increase the amount of nitrogen and potassium in the urine. These changes can be reversed by insulin (table 27.8).

TABLE 27.8. The effect of insulin on the urinary excretion of glucose, nitrogen and potassium in a diabetic patient. During the whole period the patient was on a formula diet which provided daily protein 90 g, fat 87 g, carbohydrate 190 g and potassium 80 mmol. The figures are the mean values for 4 days in each case. Data of Baird Joyce D., Duncan L.J.P. and Passmore R. (1959).

	Glucose mmol/24h	Nitrogen mmol/24h	Potassium mmol/24h
Untreated	860	1140	84
Treated (insulin 18 units twice daily)	84	780	37

The direct effect of insulin on **stimulating protein synthesis** by muscle can be demonstrated in the isolated rat diaphragm preparation (fig. 27.38). This effect is independent of the transport of glucose or amino acids into the cell and of glycogen synthesis. Insulin appears to affect protein synthesis at three sites: (1) in the mitochondria by oxidative phosphorylation, (2) in ribosomes affecting peptide formation and (3) in the synthesis of RNA, especially m-RNA.

Mechanism of action

The discovery of the chemical structure of insulin has not yet led to an identification of the combining site on the molecule which is biologically effective, nor has any specific receptor site or sites in insulin-sensitive cells been identified. Levine has pointed out that: 'The reaction between these sites (hormone and effector) represents the primary chemical action of the hormone and all the innumerable effects of insulin observed under various conditions *in vitro* and *in vivo* should then be traceable back to this primary chemical event.' In broad terms insulin acts catalytically; minute amounts of the hormone are carried in the blood to the tissues where they permit the increased utilization of vast amounts of glucose. It has been calculated that one molecule of insulin promotes the extra utilization of 10^8–10^{10} molecules/min of glucose.

Insulin promotes all the known pathways of glucose disposal and transformation including glycogen storage, fat formation, total oxidation and the use of the hexose monophosphate pathway. Since the cell membranes must be intact for these effects to be obtained it is a reasonable hypothesis that insulin has a catalytic action on the

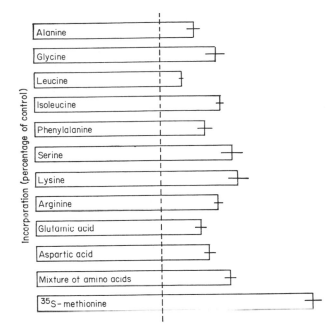

FIG. 27.38. Effect of the addition of insulin to a medium containing no oxidizable substrate on the incorporation of radio-activity from labelled amino acids into protein of the isolated rat diaphragm. The blocks represent incorporation in the presence of insulin; incorporation in the absence of insulin is shown by the dotted line; although the absolute values of these differ they have all been expressed as 100 per cent. Modified from Manchester K.L. & Young F.G. (1958) *Biochem. J.* 70, 353.

transport of glucose into the cell. Further support for this view is provided by studies employing non-utilizable monosaccharides in eviscerated experimental animals, and by measurements of the amounts of free glucose inside cells. These methods allow separation of the initial transport step from the first intracellular enzymic reaction. Moreover, it has been shown that insulin stimulates pinocytosis at the cell surface of fat cells, indicating an interaction between insulin and membrane.

However, not all mammalian tissues require insulin for maximal glucose utilization, even though the same enzyme systems for carbohydrate metabolism are universal for almost all animal cells. For example, a glucose transport system with a high degree of species specificity which does not react to insulin exists in the red blood cells. Neither glucose reabsorption by the kidney nor glucose absorption by the intestinal mucosa is affected by insulin, although in both types of cell a glucose transport system capable of raising the glucose concentration above that of the blood exists.

In what way does an insulin-sensitive glucose transport system differ from one on which insulin has no influence? Other factors such as muscular work, hypoxia and certain drugs known to inhibit oxidative processes, influence the cell surface to facilitate glucose transfer in a manner

similar to insulin. This lends support to the hypothesis that the glucose transport system in insulin-sensitive tissues is normally inhibited and that this inhibition is either temporarily removed or altered in the presence of insulin so that more glucose can enter the cell. An insulin-sensitive glucose transport system thus enables a more active and finer control to be exerted on the metabolic activity of the tissues it serves.

The glucose transport theory of insulin action can account for most of the consequences of giving insulin to man or animals, such as increased glycogenesis and lipogenesis, enhanced oxidation of glucose, decreased lipid mobilization and formation of ketone bodies and protein-sparing. However, it is difficult if not impossible to account for many other observations of the effects of insulin on this basis alone. The most important of these are as follows:

(1) It would be expected that if glucose entry could be enhanced in the absence of insulin, for example by raising the external glucose concentration in an *in vitro* system, the resulting metabolic events should be the same as those following the addition of insulin at lower concentrations of glucose. While this is broadly the case, it has been shown that insulin favours the formation of glycogen out of proportion to the other pathways and it has been suggested that insulin has a direct effect on UDP glucosyl transferase.

(2) The fact that insulin has some metabolic effects which are specific to it and independent of its effect on blood glucose means either that insulin has a variety of totally unrelated actions in the cell or that a single type of chemical reaction underlies these widely varied metabolic events.

(3) Unlike muscle and adipose tissue cells, the liver cell does not appear to possess a sugar transport system and glucose permeates freely into it. After years of controversy it now seems certain that insulin *in vivo* directly affects both the intake and the output of the liver. Table 27.9 lists some of the enzymic reactions in liver cells that have been shown to be promoted by insulin *in vitro*. These actions are difficult to account for if en-

TABLE 27.9. Actions of insulin on enzymic reactions in liver cells.

Insulin stimulates:
Deposition of glycogen – glycogen synthase
Glycolysis – glucokinase
               phosphofructokinase
               pyruvate kinase

Insulin inhibits:
Gluconeogenesis – pyruvate carboxylase
                phosphoenolpyruvate carboxykinase
                fructose-1,6-diphosphatase
                glucose-6-phosphatase

hancement of glucose transport were the only point of action of insulin.

Thus, there is at present no hypothesis which integrates satisfactorily all the diverse effects of insulin.

CONTROL OF INSULIN SECRETION

The main natural stimulus to increased synthesis and release of insulin appears to be a rise in the glucose concentration of blood perfusing the pancreas. It has been shown in the dog that the rate of insulin secretion into the pancreatic vein is a continuous function of the blood glucose concentration. An increase in the concentration of insulin in the plasma occurs in less than one minute after giving glucose intravenously. Since the cells of the islets of Langerhans are freely permeable to glucose, the concentration of glucose in the intracellular water of these cells is the same as that in the blood.

It is far from clear how glucose controls the rate of secretion of insulin but secretion does not occur in the presence of substances such as 2-deoxyglucose which block the utilization of glucose. Utilization of glucose in the islet cell seems to be the necessary stimulus for synthesis and release of insulin and it is possible that a metabolite of glucose may be the triggering mechanism. The presence of calcium, magnesium and potassium ions significantly increases the rate of secretion of insulin in response to glucose.

Other factors are almost certainly involved in the secretion of insulin in response to glucose. When glucose is ingested the concentration of insulin in the plasma does not rise as rapidly as when it is given intravenously but the insulin levels eventually become much higher in spite of lower levels of blood glucose (fig. 27.39). This suggests the possibility of an insulin-releasing factor produced by the small intestine on contact with glucose, which enters the circulation and stimulates the release of insulin from the pancreas. Glucagon (p. 27.48) has been shown to promote insulin secretion, particularly in the presence of glucose, and biologically active glucagon-like substances have been demonstrated in different portions of the intestines of many species including man. The present view is that the presence of glucose in the stomach or duodenum releases a factor, or factors, which stimulate the secretion of insulin from the islets. These alimentary factors may also affect the secretion of glucagon and thus determine the pancreatic insulin-glucagon ratio in response to variations in the amount and type of food.

Many other substances are known to increase the secretion of insulin by an immediate direct effect on the β-cells. These include other sugars, e.g. mannose, ribose and xylitol; amino acids, e.g. arginine, lysine, leucine, phenylalanine and valine; fatty acids, e.g. butyric and octanoic; hormones, e.g. ACTH and secretin; and many other substances, such as potassium, citrate, theophylline, ATP, cyclic AMP and the sulphonylurea drugs (vol. 2,

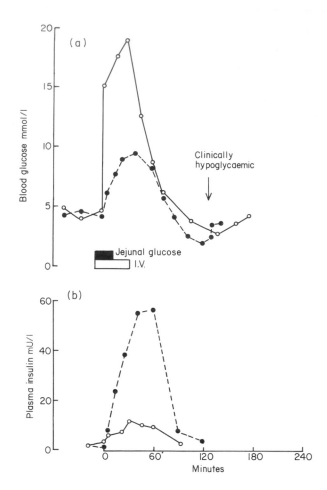

FIG. 27.39. Comparison of the effect on the blood glucose (a) and plasma insulin (b) of giving 60 g glucose intravenously (○) and into the jejunum (●) in a thin healthy young man. The intrajejunal route compared with the intravenous route causes a much smaller rise in plasma glucose, but a far greater increase in plasma insulin. From data of McIntyre N., Holdsworth C.D. & Turner D.S. (1964) *Lancet* ii, 20.

p. 6.18). Ketone bodies in physiological concentrations can also stimulate the secretion of insulin and this may be an important mechanism for protecting the organism from the development of severe keto-acidosis during prolonged fasting.

The insulin response to glucose is delayed in starvation and increased in obesity and in pregnancy. It is increased by HGH, ACTH, cortisol, thyroxine, oestrogens, many types of proteins, polypeptides and certain amino acids, particularly arginine, and by vagal stimulation. Whether the latter is of any physiological significance is not known.

Exogenous insulin decreases endogenous insulin synthesis and secretion, which is increased by giving insulin antibodies.

Zinc plays an important role in the storage and secretion of insulin. It complexes with insulin, thus rendering it less soluble. Certain glucose metabolites such as oxaloacetate, as well as other compounds, e.g. organic phosphate, cysteine, L-histidine, glycine, L-leucine and glutathione, compete with insulin for zinc and thereby promote secretion of insulin.

METABOLISM

The half-life of insulin in blood is short, probably a few minutes. Insulin is rapidly distributed throughout the body and most tissues contain some. Degradation occurs in some tissues under the influence of glutathione insulin dehydrogenase (insulinase), which catalyses reduction and cleavage of the disulphide bonds of insulin, resulting in the separation of the A and B chains of the insulin molecule. While most tissues have the capacity to destroy insulin, liver, pancreas, kidney and placenta are the most active. In man the liver removes 20–50 per cent of insulin from the blood during a single passage. Protein-bound insulin is less subject to degradation than free insulin.

HORMONAL ANTAGONISTS OF INSULIN

An insulin antagonist may be defined as any substance capable of interfering with the action of insulin. Interference by an antagonist could occur during the synthesis of insulin in the β-cell or at some point in its release into the portal circulation; an antagonist might

(1) modify or combine with circulating insulin so as to inhibit its biological activity,

(2) depress the response of the target organ, or

(3) increase the rate of degradation of insulin in the tissues with or without the increased production of inhibitory degradation products.

The known anti-insulin hormones are growth hormone and cortisol, adrenaline and thyroxine.

Growth hormone is an important physiological opponent of insulin action. It is known to be diabetogenic in the adult human subject, causing the rapid appearance of depressed responsiveness to exogenous insulin. Prolonged administration of growth hormone, however, also appears to stimulate the islet cells; this may represent a compensatory change resulting from the development of insulin antagonism. The overall effect of growth hormone is to preserve body protein and to favour the catabolism of fat to enable the body to withstand fasting.

Prolactin, like growth hormone, causes impaired glucose tolerance and even diabetes in experimental animals. During normal pregnancy, a substance sharing many immunological properties with growth hormone is produced in large amounts, probably by the placenta. Hence it has been designated placental lactogen. Little is known about its origin and biological properties but it may be responsible for the increased amounts of fatty acids and insulin in the plasma and the decreased responsiveness to insulin which are characteristic of normal pregnancy.

Following the administration of cortisol for a few days some individuals have decreased glucose tolerance, despite a raised plasma insulin level. This suggests peripheral insulin insensitivity and an early and important action of cortisol may be to decrease the peripheral utilization of glucose by inhibiting glucose phosphorylation in muscle and adipose tissue. Following this initial effect hepatic glucose release is decreased. Changes in protein, amino acid and fat metabolism are probably secondary to these alterations in carbohydrate metabolism and can be prevented by giving glucose at the same time. Cortisol also facilitates and enhances the hyperglycaemic effects of both glucagon and adrenaline.

Adrenaline also blocks insulin release. This effect seems to be mediated through stimulation of sympathetic receptors since it is abolished by administration of phentolamine, a drug which blocks α-receptors. Adrenaline also opposes the action of insulin by promoting liver glycogenolysis.

Although thyroid hormones lead to increased gluconeogenesis, proteolysis and glycogenolysis and so to increased glucose production, they also increase the secretion of insulin and glucose uptake in the periphery and promote lipid synthesis. The net result is that they do not usually exert a significant anti-insulin effect, although hyperthyroidism in man may aggravate the diabetic state.

NON-HORMONAL ANTAGONISTS

Ketone bodies and fatty acids inhibit glucose utilization by skeletal muscle *in vitro* and impair its sensitivity to insulin. In contrast these metabolites accelerate glucose utilization in adipose tissue and do not affect its responsiveness to insulin. A similar dissociation in the behaviour of these two tissues is seen in their response to growth hormone and can be demonstrated in diabetes, in hypopituitary subjects given growth hormone and in normal pregnancy, conditions where raised levels of plasma FFA are seen. It has been suggested that the anti-insulin effect of growth hormone is secondary to its lipolytic activity, and that a raised concentration of FFA in plasma is responsible for the impaired carbohydrate tolerance seen in many endocrine and nutritional disorders and represents a distinct biochemical entity, the glucose-fatty acid syndrome. Moreover in normal man a sustained elevation of plasma FFA causes impairment of carbohydrate tolerance despite adequate secretion of insulin, suggesting a decrease in peripheral sensitivity to insulin.

The B chain of insulin has been shown to inhibit the action of insulin on skeletal muscle *in vitro* and it becomes attached to the albumin fraction in plasma when it is called synalbumin antagonist. The physiological significance of this antagonism is unknown.

Glucagon

Glucagon is a pancreatic hormone, so named because on injection into an animal or man it causes a rise in the blood glucose. It has an important role in glucose homeostasis. The evidence that glucagon is secreted by α-cells of islet tissue is that it is found in pancreatic extracts obtained from animals previously treated with alloxan which produces diabetes by selectively destroying the β-cells of the islets.

Biologically active glucagon-like substances have also been identified in the gut of many species including man, and the amino acid sequences of glucagon and the intestinal hormone, secretin (p. 32.42), have much in common.

CHEMISTRY

Crystalline glucagon of high purity was obtained in 1953 and 3 years later its chemical structure was elucidated. It is a polypeptide containing twenty-nine amino acids (mol. wt. 3485). Unlike insulin, glucagon contains tryptophan and methionine but not proline, isoleucine or cystine. The absence of cystine probably explains the relative resistance of glucagon to treatment with alkali, a property used in obtaining glucagon solutions free of insulin activity. Like insulin, glucagon is antigenic and its concentration in plasma can be estimated by means of a radioimmunochemical assay method. The method is less reliable than that for insulin and subject to interference by glucagon-like substances in the gut.

ACTIONS

The initial and outstanding effect of injecting glucagon into an intact animal is to raise rapidly the plasma insulin concentration (fig. 27.40). The insulinogenic effect of glucagon is greater than that of glucose and is not dependent on a rise in the plasma glucose, although it can be strikingly increased by giving glucose simultaneously. It is likely that the effect is due to direct or indirect action on the β-cells of the islets.

Glucagon also raises the plasma glucose, provided adequate stores of glycogen are present in the liver. This is brought about by activating adenyl cyclase (pp. 9.9 & 14.12) and so increasing glycogenolysis. This action requires the presence of the adrenal cortex. Glucagon also accelerates lipolysis by a similar mechanism. Glucagon stimulates gluconeogenesis in the liver by a mechanism that is not yet clear. The effect may be secondary to the rise in hepatic cyclic AMP concentration. However, it also increases the uptake of amino acids by the liver and this may be the mechanism of the increased hepatic gluconeogenesis.

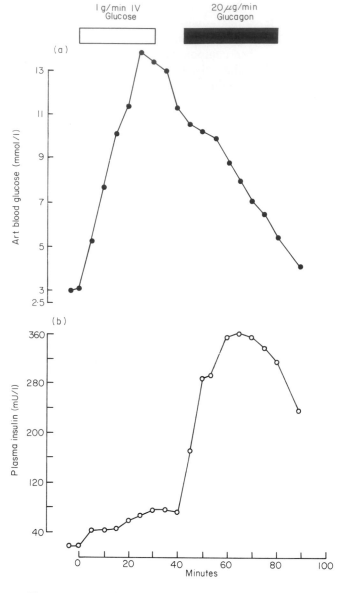

FIG. 27.40. Arterial glucose (a) and insulin (b) levels in a healthy subject during a constant intravenous infusion of glucose followed after 10 min by one of glucagon. From data of Samols E., Marri G. & Marks V. (1966) *Diabetes* **15**, 855.

CONTROL OF GLUCAGON SECRETION

The physiological role of glucagon is not clearly defined. It appears to function as the hormone of endogenous nutrient production, distributing stored glucose or free fatty acids to needy tissues and promoting the production of new glucose by the liver in situations of glucose lack. Thus experimentally induced hypoglycaemia, both acute and chronic, results in a rise in blood glucagon as do the physiological situations of starvation, both overnight or more prolonged, and exercise. Conversely, following oral

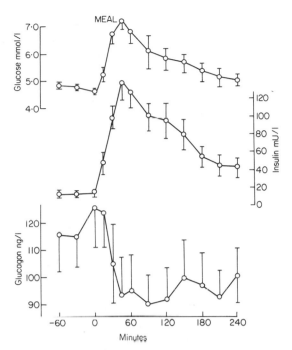

FIG. 27.41. Changes in the concentrations of plasma glucose, insulin and glucagon in response to a carbohydrate meal. Modified from Müller W.A., Faloona G.R., Aguilar-Parada E. & Unger R.H. (1970) *New Engl. J. Med.* **283**, 109.

or intravenous carbohydrate, the concentration of pancreatic glucagon in the blood falls (fig. 27.41). This reduces opposition to the hepatic storage of ingested carbohydrate. In contrast to a carbohydrate meal, a protein meal elicits an increase in both insulin and glucagon secretion. However, when both carbohydrate and protein are consumed together, protein-induced glucagon secretion is abolished.

Glucose homeostasis and the 'glucoregulatory' hormones

The term glucoregulatory hormones has been applied by Unger to insulin, growth hormone and glucagon. Their main function is to regulate the metabolic mixture and control the concentration of glucose in the blood. Adrenaline and cortisol also play a part in glucose homeostasis under normal conditions and especially when the glucose supply to the brain is actually threatened under abnormal conditions, for example, those associated with disease or experiment. A number of enteric hormones including cholecystokinin-pancreozymin (CPZ), secretin, gastrin and glucagon-like substances affect the secretion of both insulin and pancreatic glucagon and are therefore almost certainly of importance in the utilization as well as the absorption of nutrients. However, their exact physiological role in carbohydrate metabolism has not yet been defined. It appears that insulin is the hormone of glucose abundance, concerned with the storage of ingested glucose in fat and muscle. The cells of insulin-sensitive tissues are encased in a lipid membrane which under basal conditions is highly impermeable to glucose. In times of glucose abundance insulin is released and glucose entry into the cell is enhanced.

There are several 'anti-storage' hormones secreted in conditions of glucose lack. These include the glycogenolytic hormones, glucagon and adrenaline which act as a first line of defence in hypoglycaemia by releasing from liver intact preformed glucose molecules from storage. Adrenaline also suppresses insulin secretion. Hormones concerned with gluconeogenesis, particularly glucagon and cortisol, support the limited supply of preformed glucose by synthesizing new glucose from non-glucose precursors, and growth hormone spares glucose in conditions associated with glucose lack. Since during exercise muscle cells are capable of utilizing glucose even in the absence of insulin, growth hormone is of particular importance in this situation. Growth hormone prevents glucose wastage for muscle energy in two ways; by a direct action on cellular glucose metabolism, and by mobilizing FFA as an alternative and competitive substitute.

Unger has proposed that the α-and β-cells should be regarded as a single functional unit which controls the movement of exogenous and endogenous nutrients into and out of certain cells in accordance with the energy needs of the organism and the availability of exogenous nutrients. Glucagon and insulin have opposite actions on their common target tissues. The production of glucose in the liver by increased glycogenolysis and gluconeogenesis is stimulated by glucagon and inhibited by insulin. Lipolysis in adipose tissue is increased by glucagon and reduced by insulin, the latter hormone at the same time increasing lipogenesis. If the concentration of glucagon is high relative to that of insulin, then hepatic glucose production is high due to increased glycogenolysis and gluconeogenesis from glucose precursors such as amino acids; if the concentration of glucagon is low relative to that of insulin, then hepatic glucose production is low due to decreased glycogenolysis and gluconeogenesis and amino acids will be spared for protein synthesis. The enteric hormones fit into this concept by giving the islets of Langerhans advance warning about the size and nature of the incoming nutrient load. There is evidence that secretin is the glucose-responsive signal from the gut to the islets of Langerhans increasing the secretion of insulin and reducing that of glucagon. On the other hand, CPZ may be the protein- and amino acid-sensitive intestinal hormone, the function of the protein-induced increase in blood glucagon being to prevent hypoglycaemia from the aminogenic insulin secretion.

A brief reference has also already been made to the detection of GHRIH in the D cells of the pancreas (p. 27.7). The discovery that GHRIH inhibits both glucagon and insulin release as well as that of gastrin adds greater complexity to an already complex series of interactions.

LOCAL HORMONES

This chapter has been concerned so far with hormones which, as described by Starling and Bayliss (p. 27.2), are carried in the bloodstream from their sites of production to their target organs. However, control of many activities within the body is effected by chemical substances which act on tissues or cells in the immediate neighbourhood of their site of formation. Such local hormones are not dependent on the circulation. Knowledge of how they act has developed more slowly and is less complete than that of substances secreted by the endocrine glands. It has been acquired by the use of methods and techniques shared by physiologists and pharmacologists.

Dale in 1933 referred to pharmacologically active substances of the tissues as 'local chemical excitants', and to the study of their formation, storage, liberation, actions and destruction as 'autopharmacology'. The term is apt because it signifies the production by tissue cells of substances acting like drugs. When these molecules are released in response to a stimulus, they act at specific receptor sites on contiguous or nearby effector cells. Table 27.10 lists substances known to act as local hormones which are sometimes called autacoids. These substances are each discussed more fully in vol. 2.

The concept of chemical messengers between cells in close proximity followed the discovery of pressor activity in extracts of adrenal gland and the identification and synthesis of the main active principle, adrenaline. There was a striking analogy between the effects of adrenaline and stimulation of sympathetic nerves. This led to the theory that sympathetic nerves worked through the release of a substance with the actions of adrenaline (p. 27.30). Likewise, it was proposed that vagal inhibition of the heart was due to the release of a chemical substance with the actions of the drug muscarine, and subsequently shown to be acetylcholine (p. 15.26). Catecholamines are endocrine hormones, but they are also produced and act locally. Further, locally produced hormones, e.g. histamine or angiotensin, may diffuse into the circulation and have systemic effects.

METHODS

The idea of local hormones prompted the development of methods for the analysis of the effects of tissue extracts. The most important is the organ bath, introduced in 1904 by Rudolf Magnus of Utrecht. This technique makes it possible to test an extract for activity by its effect on isolated preparations. Much use has been made of guinea pig ileum, uterus and vas deferens, rat stomach, duodenum and uterus, rabbit atrium, cat papillary muscle, chick oesophagus, hen rectal caecum, frog abdominal muscle and leech dorsal muscle. Assays on such preparations and on blood pressure, usually of the anaesthetized cat, provide sensitive tests for the detection and classification of pharmacological activity. Since crude extracts contain many active principles, specific tests are applied for the identification of known pharmacologically active substances which might be present in an extract. Among these, tests based on drug antagonism are important (vol. 2, chap 3). For example, the following evidence indicates that an extract is likely to contain acetylcholine.

(1) Activity is destroyed in the presence of alkali or plasma cholinesterase.

(2) On intravenous injection, the extract causes an immediate but transient fall of blood pressure; eserine potentiates the response, and atropine blocks it.

TABLE 27.10. Local hormones.

Known substances	Occurrence	Actions	Chemical description
ORGANIC BASES			
Acetylcholine	Central and peripheral nervous systems; red blood cells, placenta.	Alters permeability of cell membranes to Na^+, K^+, Ca^{++}.	An ester of acetic acid and choline.
Histamine	Found in most tissues, usually in mast cells; also in nettle and wasp stings.	Dilates microcirculation, contracts smooth muscle, stimulates gastric secretion and is a mediator of anaphylactic reactions.	An aminoethyl derivative of imidazole.
Noradrenaline	Central and peripheral nervous systems; adrenal medulla and chromaffin cells.	Haemodynamic control; mobilizes fat and carbohydrate; temperature regulation (via CNS).	An aminoethanol derivative of catechol.
Dopamine	Central nervous system; chromaffin cells.	Control of skeletal muscle tone and hypothalamic releasing factors.	An ethylamine derivative of catechol.
5-Hydroxytryptamine (5-HT, serotonin)	Argentaffin cells, blood platelets and central nervous system.	Contracts smooth muscle, variable effects on blood vessels, chiefly vasoconstrictor; temperature regulation via CNS.	An ethylamine derivative of hydroxyindole.

POLYPEPTIDES

Bradykinin and other kinins — Kallikreins are enzymes in tissues and body fluids which combine with kininogens (α_2-globulin) in plasma to release kinins. — Contract smooth muscle, dilate vessels of the microcirculation and act directly on the adrenal medulla to release catecholamines. — Nonapeptide.

Angiotensin — Juxtaglomerular cells secrete renin which combines with angiotensinogen (α_2-globulin) in plasma to release angiotensin I; this is rapidly converted to angiotensin II, the active agent. — Contracts smooth muscle, constricts arterioles and acts directly on adrenal glands to release aldosterone and catecholamines. — Angiotensin I is a decapeptide; angiotensin II is an octapeptide.

Substance P — Nervous system, sensory pathways; gut, muscularis mucosae. — Dilates vessels of the microcirculation and lowers BP; contracts smooth muscle and stimulates peristalsis. — Hendecapeptide.

AMINO ACIDS

γ-Aminobutyric acid — Found in CNS, chiefly in the brain stem. — Inhibits EPSP; antagonized by picrotoxin. — Produced by glutamic acid decarboxylase.

Glycine — High concentration in grey matter of the spinal cord. — Inhibits EPSP; antagonized by strychnine.

Glutamic acid / Aspartic acid — Occur in all parts of CNS. — Increase EPSP.

PURINE DERIVATIVES

Adenosine — Found in all cells. — Slows heart rate, dilates coronary vessels, lowers BP, relaxes smooth muscle and promotes leucocytosis. — Nucleoside.

NUCLEOTIDES

ATP — Found in all cells. — Released on stimulation of sympathetic nerves to gut; ? transmitter of 'purinergic' nerves; dilates vessels of the microcirculation and relaxes smooth muscle. — Nucleoside triphosphate.

$3':5'$-cyclic AMP — Found in all cells. — Intracellular 'second messenger'. — Formed from ATP by adenyl cyclase

LIPID SOLUBLE SUBSTANCES

Prostaglandins (PG) — Found in most tissues; richest mammalian source is human seminal plasma. — Variable effects on smooth muscle and blood vessels, depending on PG; contract the uterus; diuretic action by inhibiting sodium absorption; temperature regulation in pyrexia. — Derivatives of prostanoic acid: PGE_2, $PGF_{2\alpha}$, PGA_2, PGC_2 etc.

Lysolecithin — In most tissues there is an enzyme lecithinase A which removes one fatty acid from lecithin to form lysolecithin. The enzyme is also present in snake venoms. — Formed in the anaphylactic reaction; contracts smooth muscle and is strongly haemolytic. — A glycerylphosphorylcholine.

OTHER SUBSTANCES

Slow reacting substance-A (SRS-A) — Formed in tissues during anaphylaxis. — Contracts smooth muscle; detected by its effect on human bronchial muscle. — Has the properties of an organic acid but is unstable.

Leucotaxine — Formed in tissues in inflammatory reactions. — Chemotaxis of leucocytes; dilates and increases permeability of vessels of the microcirculation.

Pyrogen (endogenous) — Released from leucocytes in inflammatory reactions. — Raises 'set-point' of thermal control in hypothalamus.

Lymphokines — Released from T-lymphocytes in tissue immune reactions. — Mimic the delayed hypersensitivity reaction (p. 29.23)

Chalones — Epidermis and other tissues. — Delay DNA synthesis and mitosis. — Water-soluble.

Table 27.11. Studies carried out to differentiate SRS-A (table 27.10) from other substances. After Mongar J.L. and Schild H.O. (1962) *Physiol. Rev.* **42**, 226.

Preparation	SRS-A	Prostaglandin	Bradykinin	Substance P	5-Hydroxy-tryptamine	Histamine
Guinea pig ileum	+	+	+	+	+	+
Rabbit intestine	+	+	+			
Rat colon	o	+				o
Guinea pig uterus	o	+				+
Rat uterus	o	+	+		+	−
Human bronchioles	+	o	o	o		+
Cat trachea	o				+	
Rabbit blood pressure	o	−	−	−	−	+
Cat blood pressure	o	+				−

+, Contraction of smooth muscle or rise of blood pressure; −, relaxation of smooth muscle or fall of blood pressure; o, no effect observed.

(3) Estimates of potency in parallel assays, e.g. blood pressure, dorsal muscle of leech and frog rectus abdominis, agree within the limits of error.

If it can be shown that the activity is unlikely to be due to artefact or any known substance with similar action, e.g. histamine or 5-hydroxytryptamine (5-HT), then there is presumptive evidence that the extract contains an unknown active principle. Table 27.11 shows studies carried out to differentiate SRS-A (table 27.10) from other active substances in tissues. Most of the known pharmacologically active substances in tissues have been discovered in this way.

Chemical and other methods are then joined to the pharmacological in an attempt to separate the active substance from other substances in the extract. Spectrophotofluorimetry, isotope dilution assays, electron capture in a carrier gas, radioimmunoassay and gas liquid chromatography combined with mass spectrometry are now available. Nevertheless, pharmacological methods continue to be important since there is no other way of detecting an active substance of unknown structure in an extract, and they provide the leads in the discovery of active substances in the tissues. When such a substance has been defined in terms of its pharmacological properties, it should be possible to purify it and establish its chemical identity.

HOMEOSTASIS AND PHYLOGENY

The hormones of the endocrine glands and local hormones of the tissues, especially of the nervous system, may be regarded as complementary systems of communication for the regulation and control of activities in the body. Whereas the endocrine hormones, being distributed in body fluids, exert a continuing influence on all cells, the local hormones mediate responses close to where they are formed or released; both are necessary for homeostasis.

A further relationship between the two systems lies in their phylogeny. Thus the endocrine hormones only appeared with the evolution of vertebrates, whereas local chemical excitants are found in plants, bacteria, protozoa, molluscs and arthropods. The endocrine system, it seems, has been superimposed on a more primitive system of communication, with which it co-operates.

FURTHER READING

CATT K.J. (1971) *An ABC of Endocrinology*. London: Lancet Publications.

CHARD T. & EDWARDS C.R.W. (1972) The hypothalamus and posterior pituitary. In *Modern Trends in Endocrinology*, vol. 4, p. 102, ed. Prunty F.T.G. & Gardiner-Hill H. London: Butterworth.

COUPLAND R.E. (1965) *The Natural History of the Chromaffin Cell*. London: Longmans Green.

GARREN L.D., GILL G.N., MASUI H. & WALTON G.M. (1971) On the mechanism of action of ACTH. *Recent Progress in Hormone Research* **27**, 433–478.

GREENWOOD F.C. (1967) Immunological procedures in the assay of protein hormones. In *Modern Trends in Endocrinology*, vol. 3, p. 288, ed. Gardiner-Hill H. London: Butterworth.

GREEP R.O. *et al.*, eds. (1972–1975) *Handbook of Physiology*, Section 7. Endocrinology. Vol. I. Endocrine pancreas. Vol. III. Thyroid. Vol. IV, parts 1 & 2. Pituitary gland. Vol. VI. Adrenal gland. Washington, D.C.: American Physiological Society.

GUYTON A.C. & McCANN S.M., eds. (1974) *MTP International Review of Science*. Physiology Series One, vol. 5. Endocrine physiology. London: Butterworth.

HARRIS G.W. & DONOVAN B.T., eds. (1966) *The Pituitary Gland*, vols. 1–3. London: Butterworth.

HIRSCH P.F. & MUNSON P.L. (1969) Thyrocalcitonin. *Physiological Reviews* **49**, 548–622.

LACY P.E. (1970) Beta cell secretion—from the standpoint of a pathobiologist. *Diabetes* **19**, 895–905.

McCann S. McD. & Porter J.C. (1969) Hypothalamic pituitary stimulating and inhibiting hormones. *Physiological Reviews* **49**, 240–284.

MacIntyre I. ed. (1972) *Clinics in Endocrinology and Metabolism*. Vol. 1, no. 1. Calcium metabolism and bone disease. Philadelphia: Saunders.

Oakley W.G., Pyke D.A. & Taylor K.W. (1975) *Diabetes and its Management*, 2nd Edition. Oxford: Blackwell Scientific Publications.

Pak C.Y.C. (1971) Parathyroid hormone and thyrocalcitonin: their mode of action and regulation. *Annals of the New York Academy of Sciences* **179**, 450–474.

Unger R.H. (1972) Glucagon and diabetes mellitus. *Advances in Metabolic Disorders* **6**, 73–98.

Chapter 28
Blood

The first accounts of the functions of the blood were concerned with its role in disease; an excess of phlegm as set out in the Hippocratic code or plethora as held by Erasistratus were both indications for bleeding and purging in early therapeutics. Galen added astrological reasons for blood letting and largely due to his great influence medical progress was halted for 1500 years. Then, in the sixteenth and seventeenth centuries the authority of the teachings of the Church and Medicine were challenged. Harvey described the circulation of the blood and the Dutch microscopist, van Leeuwenhoek, gave an accurate account of the red blood corpuscles as seen by the microscope. The discoveries of Boyle, Lower, Priestley and Lavoisier all led to an understanding of the respiratory process and Liebig many years later showed that a compound of iron within the red cell was capable of binding, reversibly, oxygen and carbon dioxide. The white corpuscles had been seen in the blood in the mid-eighteenth century. One hundred years later William Addison, a general practitioner in Malvern, observing diapedesis in inflammation, identified pus cells with granulocytes and emphasized their protective and reparative function. Addison is believed also to have been the first to see blood platelets and suggest that they had a role in coagulation. Hewson in 1771 described coagulation of the blood as being due to coagulation of the plasma. In 1845, Buchanan showed the role of fibrin in coagulation and at about the same time Virchow, in introducing the concept of thrombosis and embolism, suggested that fibrin is present in the blood as fibrinogen which requires activation. The marrow was not recognized as the site of production of red cells and other blood cells until 1868. In 1878, Ehrlich revolutionized haematology by the application of dye staining techniques for studying the blood and marrow cells.

Although Thomas Sydenham was using iron, as iron filings steeped in cold Rhenish wine, for the treatment of severe anaemia in the seventeenth century, iron was not known to be present in blood until 1747. This discovery led to the rational use of iron for the treatment of iron deficiency. Pernicious anaemia was described by Thomas Addison, who was no relation to William, in 1849, but its successful treatment had to wait until 1926 when the therapeutic effect of eating liver was discovered by Minot and Murphy in America. Later experiments of Castle demonstrated malabsorption of a food factor in consequence of a gastric defect and revealed the mechanism of production of this previously pernicious and fatal disease. As recently as 1948, Castle's extrinsic factor was identified as vitamin B_{12}; not long previously, folic acid had been isolated and synthesized and had also been shown to be an essential haematinic principle.

CELLS IN THE CIRCULATING BLOOD

The blood is a complex fluid which on standing or centrifugation separates into a pale, slightly opalescent yellowish liquid, the plasma, and a deposit of cells or formed elements. The blood cells are of three types, red cells or **erythrocytes**, white cells or **leucocytes** and platelets or **thrombocytes**. The deposit of the centrifuged blood is almost entirely red cells; above the red cells lies a thin layer of white cells and platelets, the buffy coat. It was this white layer, seen to be greatly increased in some diseases, that attracted so much attention among early physicians.

The number of the different blood cells per unit volume of blood remains constant within narrow limits in health. The cells can be counted under the microscope when dilutions of blood are placed in a special glass counting chamber, comprising a ruled area of known dimensions in a trough of known depth. The number of cells is expressed per litre of blood. Nowadays, much of the blood cell counting in large hospital laboratories is done semi-automatically in an electronic cell counter. Each cell, in a suitable dilution of blood, is drawn through a narrow jet orifice and is counted and sized according to the change in resistance it produces in an electrical circuit. In some instruments each cell causes light scatter.

The size, shape and characteristics of blood cells are studied by making thin smears of undiluted blood on glass slides which are subsequently stained with one of the Romanowsky stains. There are several of these, e.g. Leishman, Giemsa, May–Grünwald, Wright, but all combine a basic dye, methylene blue, and an acidic dye, eosin, together with methyl alcohol for preliminary fixation of the blood film. They produce a wide range of shades between blue and red and are necessary for studying the maturity of the cells, details of their nuclei and, in some of the white cells, the granules in the cytoplasm.

Red blood cells

The red cells are by far the most numerous of the blood cells; for every white cell there are about 500 red cells and about 30 platelets. The mature red blood cell measures approximately 7 μm in diameter and appears as a biconcave disc with no nucleus. It is strongly acidophilic on staining because of its content of the red iron-containing compound haemoglobin. The penultimate stage of erythrocytic maturation in the bone marrow (p. 28.4), the **reticulocyte**, appears transiently and in only small numbers in the peripheral blood accounting for <2 per cent of the mature red cells. Romanowsky stains containing methyl alcohol or other fixative agents cause reticulocytes to exhibit a faintly blue colour due to the diffuse precipitation of the last traces of RNA; the reticulocyte is however more easily recognized if it is stained with cresyl blue. Cresyl blue is a lipophilic dye and such dyes are believed to act by coagulating endoplasmic reticulum to produce the filaments by which the reticulocytes are recognized.

White blood cells

There are three varieties of white cell, the polymorphonuclear leucocyte or polymorph, the lymphocyte and the monocyte. The **polymorphs** are about 10–12 μm in diameter. In the adult, they account for approximately two thirds of the circulating white cells. When stained, the nucleus is a deep purplish blue and composed of coarse chromatin. It is divided into a number of lobes, usually 3 or 4, joined by thin strands; this segmentation has led to the term polymorph. The other feature of these cells is the numerous granules in the cytoplasm; the staining reactions of the granules allow a further division of the polymorphs into three types, the neutrophils, the eosinophils and the basophils (plate 28.1, between pp. 28.14–15). Neutrophils usually account for more than 90 per cent of the polymorphs; they are recognized because they contain numerous small faintly purplish granules. The eosinophils and basophils have relatively fewer but coarser granules which stain distinctly reddish-orange and blue-black respectively. Approximately 1 per cent of the polymorphonuclear leucocytes in the blood of female subjects show a nuclear appendage like a drumstick or tennis racquet. This is believed to be another form of the nuclear sex chromatin body, the inactive X chromosome (p. 12.21), which lies against the nuclear membrane in somatic cells in females.

The mature **lymphocyte** as seen in the circulation has a deeply basophilic nucleus with densely clumped chromatin, which is usually round or at most slightly indented. The most numerous cells, small lymphocytes, with a diameter of 5–10 μm, have very little pale blue cytoplasm, and a slightly eccentric nucleus. Large lymphocytes differ only in that they have more cytoplasm and may be up to 20 μm in diameter. It has been said that large lymphocytes are younger forms of small lymphocytes but this is uncertain. A few azure granules are not uncommon in the cytoplasm of the lymphocyte; they differ from polymorph granules in that they do not stain with peroxidase stains.

The **monocyte** is the largest of the circulating white cells, measuring 16–22 μm in diameter, and the least numerous. It possesses an abundant grey-blue cytoplasm with ground glass appearance. The nucleus has a stringy chromatin structure and tends to be indented, lobulated or otherwise mis-shapen. A few fine azure granules and an occasional vacuole are commonly present in the cytoplasm.

Platelets

Platelets are the smallest elements in human blood, their average diameter being 2–4 μm. When viewed by conventional light microscopy in a wet preparation they are colourless, rounded or oval, refractile bodies, though *in vivo* they are probably disc-shaped. Under dark field illumination they look translucent and granular. If they are stained by one of the Romanowsky dye techniques they show a pale blue cytoplasm and a central cluster of purplish granules. Like the red cells, they have no nucleus.

STANDARD MEASUREMENTS AND NORMAL VALUES IN STUDIES OF THE BLOOD CELLS

Red blood cells

The red blood cell count (RBC) ranges from $4 \cdot 5$–$6 \cdot 5 \times 10^{12}$/l in men and $3 \cdot 9$–$5 \cdot 6 \times 10^{12}$/l in women. Erythrocytosis denotes a raised red cell count. In the stained blood film the normal erythrocytes are spoken of as **normochromic**, due to a normal complement of haemoglobin, and **normocytic,** i.e. of normal size and shape. In disorders of the blood there may be variations in size of red cells, i.e. anisocytosis, or in shape, i.e. poikilocytosis. Small cells are said to be **microcytic** and large ones **macrocytic.** When a red cell has less than the normal complement of haemoglobin, it is described as **hypochromic**. The cells never have an excess concentration of haemoglobin.

Measurement of the haemoglobin (Hb) content of the blood is of enormous importance in clinical practice. It is achieved by converting the haemoglobin into a derivative, usually cyanmethaemoglobin, oxyhaemoglobin, acid haematin or alkaline haematin, which is then compared colorimetrically with a standard. The normal haemoglobin content of the blood in the adult ranges from 13·5–18·0 g/dl in men and 11·5–16·4 g/dl in women. When the haemoglobin level is low, as happens if the number of red cells per unit volume of blood is reduced or the haemoglobin content of the red cell is reduced, the individual is said to have **anaemia**.

When blood is centrifuged in a tube under standard conditions, the height of the column of red cells is the **haematocrit** or **packed cell volume** (PCV). Normally the PCV is measured in a thick walled tube of 2.5 mm bore (Wintrobe tube) which is spun in a special centrifuge of 15 cm radius for 30 min at 3000 rev/min (1000–1500 g). Alternatively, the blood may be drawn into a special capillary tube which is then sealed at one end, placed in the head of a microhaematocrit centrifuge and spun at 12 000 g for 5 min. PCV is expressed as the proportion of the column occupied by the packed cells. Normal values in health are 0·40–0·54 in men and 0·36–0·47 in women.

Having obtained the Hb value, the RBC and the PCV, it is possible to derive for the erythrocytes, the mean cell volume (MCV), the mean cell haemoglobin (MCH) and the mean cell haemoglobin concentration (MCHC). These indices, which are extremely useful in diagnosis are obtained as follows:

$$\text{MCV (fl)} = \frac{\text{PCV}}{\text{RBC count}}, \text{ normal range } 75\text{--}95$$

$$\text{MCH (pg)} = \frac{\text{Hb} \times 10}{\text{RBC count}}, \text{ normal range } 27\text{--}32$$

$$\text{MCHC (g/dl)} = \frac{\text{Hb}}{\text{PCV}}, \text{ normal range } 30\text{--}36$$

In modern electronic cell counters MCV is measured directly and PCV is derived from RBC and MCV.

A raised MCV occurs in macrocytosis and is a typical finding in anaemias due to deficiency of vitamin B_{12} and folate (p. 28.9). A low MCV and a low MCHC are typical of anaemia due to iron deficiency since in this condition the red cells tend to be smaller than normal and have a deficient content of haemoglobin.

The circulating **blood volume** remains stable in health and is more related to body size than any other factor. The volume of the circulating red cells (the red cell mass) in males is 29·5 ml/kg, s 3·5; the plasma volume is 40·0 ml/kg, s 5·0; in females the red cells mass is lower, 25·5 ml/kg, s 3·5, and the plasma volume 39·0 ml/kg, s 5·0. The red cell mass is naturally low in anaemia; when it is raised the patient is said to have **erythraemia.** The plasma volume is increased in cardiac failure and for reasons not understood in pregnancy and in patients with marked enlargement of the spleen.

Because there tends to be more plasma in the capillaries than in the larger blood vessels, possibly due to axial flow of the cells in small tubes with layering of the plasma along the walls, the **body haematocrit,**

$$\frac{\text{red cell mass}}{\text{red cell mass} + \text{plasma volume}}$$

tends to be lower than the haematocrit for venous blood. The body/venous haematocrit ratio in health is 0·91, s 0·026.

White blood cells

The total white blood cell count (WBC) in the adult is in the range 4·0–11·0 × 10^9/l. Reduction of the white cell count, **leucopenia,** occurs for example in marrow failure and sometimes when the spleen is markedly enlarged, an effect known as hypersplenism. Increase of the leucocyte count is seen in most bacterial infections and after injury and is termed **leucocytosis.** White cell counts as high as 50 × 10^9/l may be encountered in acute infections; much higher counts are typical of the malignant diseases of the white cell-producing tissues, the leukaemias.

Using a Romanowsky stained film, the proportions of the various types of white cell can be established. The range of values for the differential white cell count in adults is as follows:

Neutrophils, 2·5–7·5 × 10^9/l	(40–75%)
Lymphocytes, 1·0–4·5 × 10^9/l	(20–45%)
Monocytes, 0·2–0·9 × 10^9/l	(2–10%)
Eosinophils, 0·1–0·4 × 10^9/l	(1–6%)
Basophils, 0–0·2 × 10^9/l	(<1%)

Reference is made to the differential white cell count in children on p. 42.2.

Platelets

The total platelet count is in the range 150–400 × 10^9/l. Low values, **thrombocytopenia,** are encountered for example in marrow failure and when the marrow is involved in diseases such as leukaemia, in hypersplenism and when the platelets are destroyed abnormally rapidly in the circulation. Thrombocytopenia usually has no ill effect until the platelet count falls below 40–50 × 10^9/l. At this level there tends to be spontaneous bleeding into the skin and mucous membranes, a condition known as purpura (vol. 3, p. 21.45). An increase of platelets, **thrombocytosis,** occurs transiently after injury, surgical operations and after splenectomy.

Erythrocyte sedimentation rate (ESR)

When blood is treated with an anticoagulant and allowed to stand in a tube, the cells sediment slowly. The rate of sedimentation is increased by changes in the proportion of the various plasma proteins, particularly if there is elevation of the concentration of fibrinogen and γ-globulin, and by some anaemias. The red cells aggregate in rouleaux like piles of draughts, probably because of changes in the surface charge of the cells; rouleaux formation is exaggerated in some diseases and this too accelerates the sedimentation rate.

An increased sedimentation rate is not diagnostic of any one disorder but is a good non-specific indicator of disease and is often used for this purpose in clinical practice. Serial estimation of the ESR is also valuable in following the progress of an illness. In the widely used Westergren method, blood anticoagulated with sodium citrate is allowed to stand in a 200 × 2.5 mm graduated glass tube and the fall of the blood cell column is measured after 1 h. The normal ESR is less than 10 mm in healthy young males but usually slightly higher in females.

ORIGIN OF THE CELLS OF THE BLOOD

Blood cell production (haemopoiesis) in the fetus begins in the blood islands of the yolk sac and at this stage no distinctive cell type can be identified. The first recognizable cell is a primitive red cell precursor, a large cell with abundant cytoplasm. By the end of this first or mesoblastic period, definitive erythropoiesis is established and the various stages in maturation of the developing red cells can then be recognized; granular cells and megakaryocytes, which are the precursors of platelets, also begin to appear. By the end of the second month of intrauterine development blood cell production has become established in the liver. Between the 2nd and 5th months lymphopoiesis and a small amount of erythropoiesis develop in the spleen. From about the 5th month, as the placental circulation is established, the myeloid tissues of the bones increasingly take over the manufacture of red blood cells, white cells and platelets, and the lymph nodes become active with the spleen in lympho-

poiesis. These various stages in the fetus are illustrated in fig. 28.1.

The thymus has a special place in lymphopoiesis. This organ is active in lymphocyte production in the embryo and from it the other lymphoid tissues of the body may be seeded. Although the peripheral lymphoid tissues are fully organized around the time of birth or shortly afterwards, the thymus continues to exert an effect on them, particularly in regard to immunological competence (p. 29.25).

At birth and during the first few years of life the marrow of practically all the bones is red and actively cellular. In the first year of life, fat cells begin to appear between the blood cells, in the marrow of the long bones and as age advances the active marrow gradually recedes from the distal parts of the skeleton till at the end of the growing period active red marrow is found mainly in the flat bones, the skull, ribs, sternum and bones of pelvis; the other sites of red marrow are the vertebrae and the upper epiphyses of the humerus and femur.

Multipotential mesenchymal cells capable of returning to fetal and childhood patterns of haemopoiesis remain throughout life in the fatty yellow marrow of the long bones, in the liver, spleen and lymph nodes, and to a small extent in the adrenal glands and intestinal wall; this potentiality for producing blood cells may be reawakened when there are increased demands for them, e.g. after haemorrhage and in certain disease states, e.g. haemoylsis and leukaemia.

DEVELOPMENT, FUNCTION AND FATE OF THE BLOOD CELLS

The description of the development of blood cells, particularly the erythroid series, has been confused by the use of different terminologies. The original nomenclature introduced by Ehrlich is used below and appropriate common alternatives are given in parenthesis.

Studies of normal and abnormal development of the blood cells depend on examination of the bone marrow. Marrow can be obtained easily by needle puncture and aspiration from the medullary cavity of certain bones, e.g. the shaft of tibia in infants, the spines of lumbar vertebrae in older children and the body of the sternum and ilium in adults. It is best examined as smears using Romanowsky stains.

A primitive stem cell can be distinguished morphologically in the bone marrow and in the liver, spleen and lymph nodes when these are haematopoietically active. This cell, which is the common parent of all blood cells, is large, about 20–30 μm in diameter with abundant pale, slightly basophilic cytoplasm. The nucleus is also large, usually filling about one half of the cell diameter; it is pale and basophilic showing a finely reticular

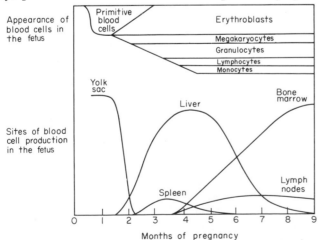

FIG. 28.1. The stages of development and the relative importance of the different sites of blood cell production in the fetus. From Wintrobe M.M. *et al.* (1974).

chromatin pattern and containing one or more nucleoli. Nucleoli, present only in very primitive blood cells, are seen in the nucleus as areas of well demarcated paler staining. The term **blast cell** is often applied to nucleolated cells and implies that the cell is of very early type; normoblasts and megaloblasts, cells concerned in normal and abnormal erythropoiesis, do not contain nucleoli in the later stages of their maturation and are exceptions to this rule.

Red blood cells

Erythropoiesis after normal full term birth occurs exclusively in the bone marrow in health and red cell precursors normally account for one third to one tenth of the bone marrow cells. In children increased demands for red cells are met by using extramedullary sites; extramedullary haemopoiesis, however, is very rare in the adult. The first distinct erythroid cell is the **proerythroblast** (pronormoblast); it is a cell of about 15 μm in diameter in which the nucleus leaves only a small rim of deeply basophilic cytoplasm. The nucleus still shows nucleoli or nucleolar remnants and contains thick strands of chromatin which may be clumped.

The time taken for the maturation process in the normal marrow from proerythroblast through the ensuing stages of normoblast to fully developed erythrocyte is 7–10 days. This is achieved at first by mitotic division and then by progressive diminution in cell size. The nucleus is seen to become progressively more compact and dense (pyknotic), the cytoplasm becomes less blue and more pink due to reduction and disappearance of RNA on the one hand, and the synthesis of haemoglobin on the other. The present view is that the nucleus disintegrates and is largely absorbed within the cell and only the indigestible remains are extruded. In the next stage, strands of endoplasmic reticulum still remain which stain with cresyl blue. These are the reticulocytes (p. 28.2). When these strands have finally disappeared the red cell is fully mature. The endoplasmic reticulum is so altered by fixation when Romanowsky dyes are used that reticulocytes appear diffusely blue.

The **normoblasts** are spoken of as early (basophilic), intermediate (polychromatic) and late (acidophilic or orthochromatic). These terms are used arbitrarily and are based on cell diameter which decreases gradually from 15 to 10 μm, and on changes in colour which take place in the cytoplasm. The early normoblast has cytoplasm which is still basophilic; in the intermediate stage it has a faintly purple colour as haemoglobin begins to appear; by the late normoblast stage the full complement of haemoglobin is present. The nucleus shrivels and becomes homogeneous (pyknosis), appearing in the late normoblast stage like an ink spot (plate 28.1, between pp. 28.14–15).

Comparison between red blood cells of lower vertebrates and those of mammals shows gradual evolutionary improvement in their efficiency as oxygen-carrying vehicles. According to Wintrobe the small cells of mammals are more efficient oxygen carriers than the large cells of the lower vertebrates and their biconcave form is believed to be the optimum shape for the rapid and even diffusion of gases to all parts of the cell. Although not easily measured, the total surface area of the circulating erythrocytes appears to be much greater than the total surface area of the body. About one-third of the erythrocyte is haemoglobin; this is probably the highest concentration which does not interfere with reaction rates. Moreover the absence of a nucleus in the mature red cell leads to great reduction in its energy requirement as compared with other cells.

The precise structure of the red blood cell and the forces which preserve its biconcavity are poorly understood. It is a flexible elastic envelope which has a complex protein and lipid ultrastructure. Only about 2 per cent of the haemoglobin content of the red blood cell is near the plasma membrane and the remainder is uniformly distributed throughout the cell.

HAEMOGLOBIN

Haemoglobin is formed by the developing erythrocyte; in health, synthesis is virtually confined to the normoblasts, about 80 per cent being at the intermediate normoblast stage. Under normal conditions approximately 6 g of haemoglobin are formed per day in the adult and this productive capacity can be increased six or sevenfold after haemorrhage or haemolysis. Haemoglobin has a molecular weight of 65 000. The globin part consists of 574 amino acids and the arrangement and sequence of these amino acids is genetically determined.

Globin is made up of two identical half molecules, each of which in the normal adult contains two different polypeptide chains, the α and β chains. Hence **haemoglobin-A**, the normal adult form, is sometimes designated $\alpha_2\beta_2$. In the early stages of fetal development **haemoglobin-F** is predominant and is designated $\alpha_2\gamma_2$. The γ chains differ from the β chains in their structure and by virtue of containing isoleucine, which is absent from haemoglobin-A. Haemoglobin-F has a higher affinity for oxygen than haemoglobin-A and in the 20-week fetus more than 90 per cent of the haemoglobin is Hb-F. At birth this has fallen to 55–85 per cent and thereafter it is usually rapidly replaced by haemoglobin-A. A third form, **haemoglobin-A₂**, also occurs normally; this is designated $\alpha_2\delta_2$; again there is a difference from the normal amino acid sequence of the β chain. The maximum proportion of haemoglobin-A₂ in the blood in health is not more than 2–3 per cent.

The haemoglobin molecule comprises globin and four haem groups, each of which is a porphyrin ring structure made up of four pyrrole rings joined by methene bridges and containing a chelated iron atom. Haem is also part of the structure of myoglobin, the cytochromes, peroxidase and catalase. The four haem groups of haemoglobin lie in pairs on the surface of the molecule in pockets formed by the polypetide chains (fig. 11.11).

The stages of the synthesis of haem-containing compounds and of haemoglobin are illustrated in fig. 28.2. This shows that the basic building-blocks are succinyl-CoA from the citric acid cycle and glycine. The condensation is catalysed by δ-aminolaevulinic acid (ALA) synthase with pyridoxal phosphate as coenzyme. The precise nature of the reactions from porphobilinogen onwards has not been established. However, it is known that the porphyrin I and III series of isomers are synthesized in parallel.

Only the porphyrin III series is required for the production of haem; the porphyrin I series has no function and is excreted in the urine and faeces. An enzyme that catalyses the insertion of iron into protoporphyrin has been localized in the mitochondria. Haem is first formed from iron and protoporphyrin and then globin is added.

Haem influences the rate of Hb synthesis since it stimulates globin synthesis, while free haem limits its own production by inhibiting ALA-synthase. Conversely, barbiturates and other drugs which are metabolized by enzymes containing haem, promote haem synthesis in the liver by stimulating ALA-synthase. In the porphyrias, a group of inborn errors of porphyrin synthesis (vol. 3, p. 47.19), uroporphyrinogens of both series may be produced in excess, oxidized to uroporphyrins and excreted with varying quantities of other porphyrins, intermediates and metabolites. Lead poisoning and certain liver disorders (vol. 3, p. 47.19) also cause secondary abnormalities of porphyrin synthesis and excretion.

The main function of haemoglobin is the transport of the respiratory gases and this is fully described on p. 31.18.

METABOLISM OF THE RED CELL

The red blood cell is the site of numerous metabolic activities, most of which are concerned with maintaining the integrity of the cell membrane and preserving optimum osmotic conditions in the cell against steep ionic gradients. Many enzymes and intermediary products without known function are, however, present in the mature red cell, suggesting that it may have functions other than the transport of respiratory gases.

The normoblast is able to synthesize DNA, RNA, lipid, haem and proteins; it has an electron transfer system, a functional citric acid cycle, and the hexose monophosphate and Embden–Meyerhof pathways. In the circulating non-nucleated erythrocyte most of these activities have been lost; the source of energy is glucose which has to be transported across the red cell membrane and only two energy producing reactions are retained; about 90 per cent of the glucose utilized is degraded anaerobically to lactate by the Embden–Meyerhof pathway and the remaining 10 per cent is accounted for aerobically by the hexose monophosphate pathway. The operation of the hexose monophosphate pathway yields $NADPH_2$ and this is *inter alia* used in glutathione reduction and in preserving the cell against the effect of oxidant compounds.

The red cell also contains significant amounts of 2,3-diphosphoglycerate (2,3-DPG) which is formed from 1,3-DPG (a constituent of the glycolytic pathway) by diphosphoglyceromutase. 2,3-DPG is reversibly bound to the β-chains of deoxygenated Hb, so stabilizing it that the affinity of Hb for oxygen is lowered. The effect of this on O_2 transport is described on p. 31.20.

Several studies indicate the wearing out of some enzyme systems as the cause of cell ageing. Measurement of the red blood cell survival time by different techniques shows that its life span is 110–120 days; the oldest cells are removed and replaced at the rate of about 1 per cent of the total red cell mass/day. Precisely what happens to the effete red cell is still not known. Sudden haemolysis in the circulation and phagocytosis by macrophages are not proved and one theory is that the cell is gradually fragmented at the end of its days, before being cleared from the circulation by the mononuclear phagocytic system. Deficiency of one of several critical enzymes may lead to marked shortening of the red cell life span (haemolytic disease) either by premature ageing or by making the cell more susceptible to damage from environmental influences. Deficiency or defect of the enzyme glucose-6-phosphate dehydrogenase is common in Negro and Mediterranean peoples, being transmitted by a sex-linked recessive type of inheritance. This enzyme is concerned with $NADPH_2$ production and affected patients are liable to suffer bouts of haemolysis on exposure to certain drugs, e.g. the antimalarial drug primaquine, and sulphonamides and after eating the fava bean (favism). Other enzyme deficiencies now known to be implicated in congenital haemolytic anaemias are pyruvate kinase, glutathione reductase and diphosphoglyceromutase (vol. 3, p. 21.34).

Methaemoglobin

Normal haemoglobin (ferrohaemoglobin) is constantly being oxidized into methaemoglobin (ferrihaemoglobin), a derivative which does not combine with O_2 and therefore does not contribute to oxygen transport. In health, methaemoglobin is reduced to the functional ferrous state as soon as it is formed and normal blood contains only traces. Two pathways are involved; the first and more important depends on the action of methaemoglobin reductase I (diaphorase I) in the presence of $NADH_2$ generated in the Embden–Meyerhof pathway; the second depends on methaemoglobin reductase II

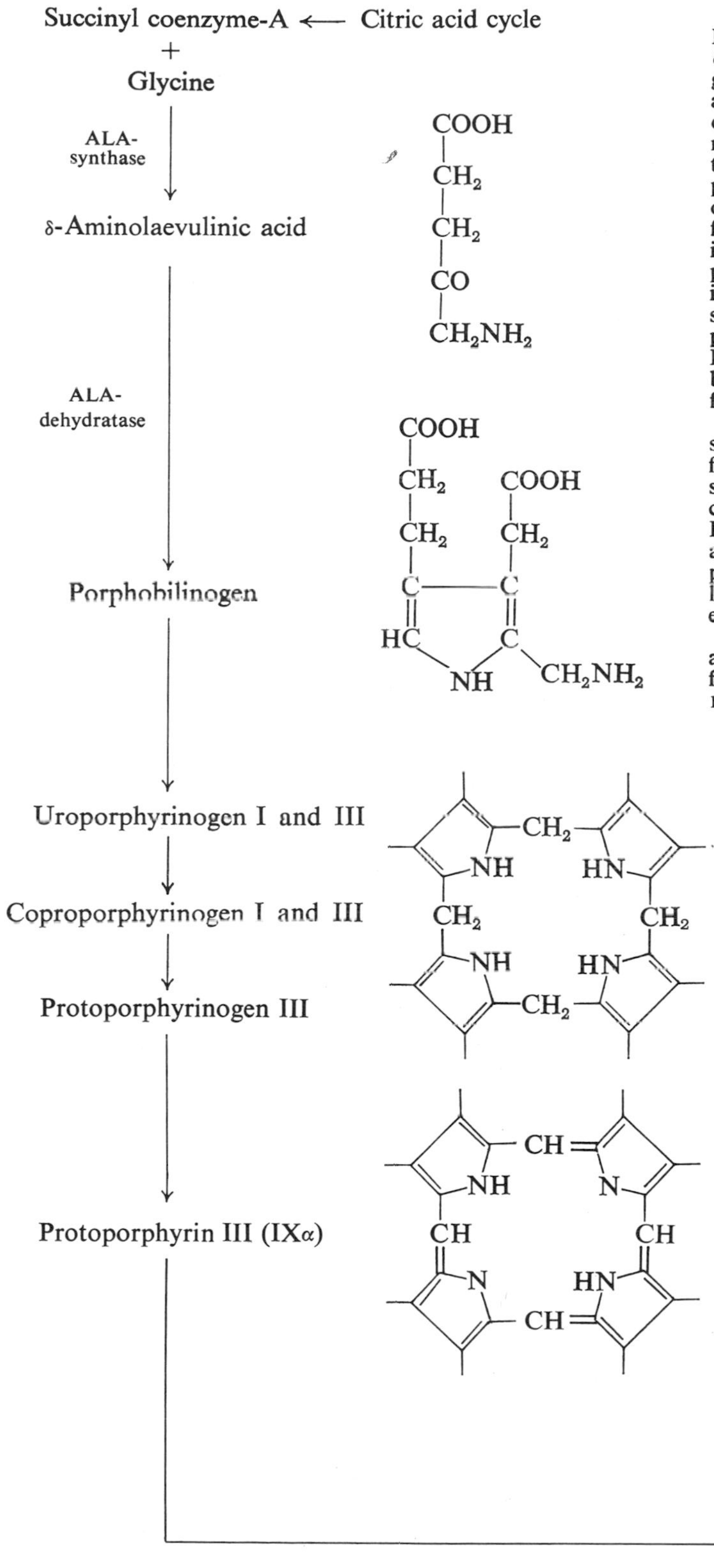

Succinyl coenzyme-A ⟵ Citric acid cycle
+
Glycine

| ALA-synthase

↓

δ-Aminolaevulinic acid

| ALA-dehydratase

↓

Porphobilinogen

↓

Uroporphyrinogen I and III

↓

Coproporphyrinogen I and III

↓

Protoporphyrinogen III

↓

Protoporphyrin III (IXα)

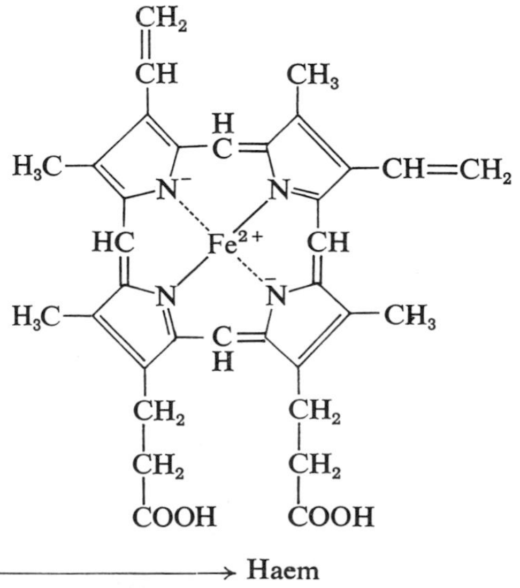

FIG. 28.2 Steps in the synthesis of haem. In the mitochondria δ-aminolaevulinate synthase catalyses the condensation of glycine with succinyl coenzyme A to give δ-aminolaevulinic acid (ALA). ALA-dehydratase then catalyses the formation of the pyrrole derivative porphobilinogen (PBG) from two molecules of ALA. Four molecules of PBG polymerize with the elimination of 4 NH₃ to give cyclic tetrapyrroles called porphyrinogens and porphyrins. The tetrapyrrole ring is less oxidized in the initially formed porphyrinogens, having fewer double bonds, but the sidechains in the correspondingly named compounds are the same. Two series of tetrapyrrole isomers (I and III) occur naturally; these differ only in the order of the sidechains which are omitted from the sketch formulae of porphyrinogen and porphyrin. Protoporphyrin, the immediate precursor of haem, belongs to series III, it is sometimes called protoporphyrin IXα. In the normal biosynthesis series III predominates, with a little series I found as by-products.

Normally all uroporphyrinogen (I and III), in which the sidechains of the precursor PBG are unchanged, undergoes further metabolism by decarboxylation of the acetic acid sidechains to give coproporphyrinogen I and III. Most of the coproporphyrinogen III is converted to protoporphyrinogen III by formation of vinyl radicals from two of the propionic acid sidechains. Protoporphyrinogen is oxidized to protoporphyrin, into which a ferrous ion is incorporated to give haem. The iron is bonded to the porphyrin nitrogens both electrostatically and covalently.

All coproporphyrinogen I and a small proportion of III are oxidized to coproporphyrins I and III and excreted. The faeces contains about 300 µg each day and the urine about 150 µg.

⟶ Haem

(diaphorase II) and NADPH$_2$ generated in the hexose monophosphate pathway of glycolysis.

Methaemoglobinaemia is a rare but important clinical entity. Not only does it inactivate part of the normal oxygen-carrying capacity of the blood, but it also interferes with oxygen dissociation from the remaining ferrohaemoglobin. Methaemoglobinaemia occurs in the following circumstances:

(1) if the individual is exposed to drugs or chemicals which increase the normal autoxidation of haemoglobin; these are mainly aromatic compounds;

(2) when there is inherited deficiency of methaemoglobin reductase I, and

(3) when there is inheritance of one of several variants of haemoglobin, known collectively as Hb-M, whose methaemoglobin derivatives seem to be peculiarly resistant to the normal intracellular reducing mechanisms (vol. 3, p. 47.20).

SUBSTANCES ESSENTIAL TO ERYTHROPOIESIS

Protein

Amino acids are required for the synthesis of the globin component of haemoglobin and for the construction of the red cell stroma. When the supply of amino acids is limited, priority appears to be given to the synthesis of haemoglobin. In consequence, in starvation and in children with protein deficiency (kwashiorkor) severe anaemia (Hb < 8 g/dl) is seldom found. Minor degrees of anaemia are common, in part due to haemodilution from an increased plasma volume, which frequently occurs in these conditions, and in part due to deficiency of other haematinic substances.

Iron

Iron is required for red cell formation because of its essential place in the haemoglobin molecule. The dietary sources of iron are described on p. 5.8. It will be remembered that a good mixed diet provides about 215–270 μmol (12–15 mg)/day, most of which is unabsorbed and lost in the faeces. Of this dietary iron an adult male has to absorb about 18 μmol (1 mg)/day, or slightly less than 10 per cent to balance the iron that is lost from the body, mainly in desquamation, and women have to absorb about twice this amount to meet the additional loss in menstruation, pregnancy and lactation (p. 5.8). The need for iron is increased in the growing child because of his expanding red cell volume and muscle bulk.

Factors which have been shown to determine the amount of iron absorbed are the rate of erythropoiesis and the state of the body stores of iron. More iron is absorbed when erythropoiesis is active and the body stores are depleted than when erythropoiesis is suppressed and the body stores are full.

Iron is transported in the plasma bound to a β_1-globulin, **transferrin**, and the level of iron in the plasma in health is of the order 14–28 μmol/l (80–160 μg/100 ml). This iron is mostly derived from the breakdown of haemoglobin and amounts to about 25 mg/day. The plasma transferrin is normally not fully saturated; the amount of transferrin available for transporting iron can be measured and is spoken of as the total iron-binding capacity (TIBC). Information regarding the plasma iron and degree of saturation of the TIBC is of value in the elucidation of some anaemias and diseases of iron overload.

The body stores contain enough iron to replace about one-third of the circulating haemoglobin in the event of haemorrhage. This iron, mostly in the form of ferritin, larger agglomerates being in the insoluble form haemosiderin, is concentrated in the macrophages of liver, spleen and bone marrow. The normal distribution of iron in the body is given in table 28.1.

TABLE 28.1. The disposition of iron in the adult. From Drabkin D. L. (1951) *Physiol. Rev.* **31**, 245.

	Approximate percentage of total iron
Circulating haemoglobin	75·0
Iron in body stores	20·0
Myoglobin	5·0
Haem enzymes	<0·5
Transferrin	<0·1

The absorption of iron from the alimentary tract is discussed on p. 32.45. An active transport mechanism is involved and the upper small intestine is the main site. The capacity to absorb iron is often inadequate to meet physiological needs, particularly if the diet is poor in respect of iron-containing foods. Hence anaemia due to iron deficiency is common in women and children in all countries. On the other hand adult males seldom suffer from iron deficiency unless there is chronic loss of blood, e.g. from an ulcer or other lesion of the gastrointestinal tract or the presence in the bowel of blood-sucking parasites, e.g. hookworms or schistosomes, such as are common in many tropical countries.

The person with iron-deficiency anaemia complains of weakness, tiredness and breathlessness, symptoms that are common to all anaemias. Diagnostic changes are found in the peripheral blood, where there is a subnormal Hb level, reduced MCH and MCHC and low plasma iron level; in the blood film the red cells vary in size and shape and are mostly hypochromic and microcytic. If body tissues, e.g. liver or bone marrow, were to be examined for iron they would be found to be grossly depleted.

Iron-deficiency anaemia gives rise to much ill-health. Fortunately it can be treated easily by removing the cause and by giving iron compounds, e.g. ferrous sulphate, medicinally.

Vitamin B$_{12}$ and folic acid

The nutritional properties of these two vitamins are discussed on p. 5.17. Despite their importance, particularly in relation to nucleic acid synthesis, the only proven functions of these two vitamins are that vitamin B$_{12}$ is concerned with the *de novo* synthesis of labile methyl groups from one-carbon precursors such as glycine and formate (p. 11.27) while folic acid is concerned with one-carbon metabolism and transmethylation (p. 11.27).

Vitamin B$_{12}$ is the extrinsic factor which Castle described in 1929. The chemical structure (p. 7.14) shows it to be a porphyrin ring like haem but containing cobalt. An alternative name for the pure substance is **cyanocobalamin**. Related substances both naturally occurring and semisynthetic without the cyano group have been described; these are spoken of as cobalamins or corrins. The term vitamin B$_{12}$ is now used to describe all naturally occurring cobalamins with physiological activity.

Vitamin B$_{12}$ is synthesized exclusively by microorganisms. For all practical purposes, animal protein forms our only dietary source; pure vegetarians (vegans) get vitamin B$_{12}$ in their food only in tiny amounts from contaminating moulds. The recommended dietary intake is 2·2 nmol (3 μg) daily which provides a large margin of safety; the daily requirement is less than 1/nmol (1·3 μg). In physiological amounts vitamin B$_{12}$ requires the action of **intrinsic factor** for its absorption. Intrinsic factor is a glycoprotein, which is secreted by the glands in the body and fundus of the stomach; it modifies the vitamin B$_{12}$ complexes in the food to a form suitable for assimilation but the precise mechanism of action is unknown. Vitamin B$_{12}$ is absorbed mainly in the ileum and is stored mainly in the liver. Studies with ^{58}Co vitamin B$_{12}$ indicate that in the liver it has a biological half life of about 1 year; this explains why patients after total gastrectomy, in which all intrinsic factor-bearing tissue has been removed surgically, may take several years to develop clinical vitamin B$_{12}$ deficiency. In the plasma vitamin B$_{12}$ is mostly bound to globulin. The normal level is 125–735 pmol/l (170–1000 ng/l).

Folic acid is widely disseminated in nature both in the plant and animal kingdom. The main dietary source is probably green leafy vegetables; it was first isolated from spinach leaves in 1941 (*folium*, a leaf), hence its name. Its chemical formula (p. 7.13) shows it to be pteroylglutamic acid (PGA) and therefore chemically related to the pterins, pigments in butterfly wings. PGA is normally present in food as polyglutamates. These and all related compounds of folic acid with biological activity are collectively referred to as **folates** or, in the USA, as **folacin**. Folates in the food are converted to free folic acid by a conjugase (γ-L-glutamyl carboxypeptidase) present in the epithelium of the small intestine.

Unlike vitamin B$_{12}$, PGA has no mediating absorptive mechanism and is assimilated mainly from the upper part of the intestine. Absorbed PGA is converted into the coenzyme tetrahydrofolic acid (THF), a reaction brought about by folate reductase.

THF is the active derivative of folic acid in the body; its N^5 and N^{10} atoms are the binding sites for one-carbon radicals. The main compound in the plasma and tissues to which all other one-carbon derivatives may be reversibly transformed is N^5-methyl THF and its concentration in the blood is 6–60 nmol/l (3–20 μg/l). The recommended intake of folate is 600 nmol (200 μg) daily. In contrast to vitamin B$_{12}$ the stores are sufficient for only a few weeks; the minimum requirement is about 150 nmol (50 μg) daily.

Two one-carbon derivatives of THF have particular application in clinical practice. The first, N^5-formimino THF, is formed from the intermediate compound formiminoglutamic acid (FIGLU) in the conversion of histidine to glutamic acid. In folate deficiency, this conversion cannot take place and FIGLU may accumulate in the body and appear in the urine. The second, N^5-formyl THF (folinic acid) is used occasionally as a therapeutic substance; certain drugs act as antagonists to folate reductase and to N^5-formyl THF and folinic acid may be needed to combat their adverse effects (vol. 2, p. 29.8).

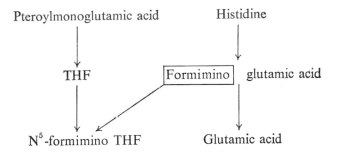

FIG. 28.3. The main stages in the production of 5–formimino tetrahydrofolic acid and its relationship to the conversion of histidine to glutamic acid. THF = tetrahydrofolic acid.

Deficiency of either vitamin B$_{12}$ or folate, due to dietary inadequacy, failure of alimentary absorption or increased metabolic requirement, produces a characteristic change in the blood known as **megaloblastic anaemia**. In the bone marrow the nucleus of the erythroid precursors matures more slowly than the cytoplasm, giving rise to abnormal cells, megaloblasts, which appear to be larger than normoblasts at a corresponding stage of development and show a nucleus with a characteristic spotted thrush breast appearance. In vitamin B_{12} and folate deficiency the red cells in the peripheral blood are reduced in number and tend to be macrocytic and, provided there is no concomitant iron deficiency, they have their normal complement of Hb. This means that when the absolute indices are calculated, the MCV usually exceeds 95 fl but the MCHC is in the normal range. In addition, vitamin B_{12}, but not folate, is essential for the integrity of myelin. Hence profound vitamin B_{12} deficiency can lead also to a specific neuropathy which affects mainly peripheral nerves and later to a patchy degeneration in the spinal cord, particularly in the dorsal and lateral columns (vol. 3, p. 21.27).

In Europe, the commonest cause of megaloblastic anaemia is **pernicious anaemia** due to vitamin B_{12} deficiency. This is seen mainly after the age of 40 years and has an inherited basis. The cause is malabsorption of vitamin B_{12} due of failure to secretion of intrinsic factor consequent on atrophy of the gastric mucosa. Megaloblastic anaemia due to folate deficiency is seen in the later stages of pregnancy when the requirement for folate to meet fetal demands may outstrip the nutritional supply. In many parts of Asia and Africa megaloblastic anaemia due to a dietary deficiency of folate is common.

Pyridoxine

A very rare anaemia showing signs of impaired utilization of iron for haem synthesis responds to administration of pyridoxine. It is believed to be due to interference with the porphyrin synthesis to haem at about the porphobilinogen stage where pyridoxal phosphate is implicated as a coenzyme (fig. 28.2).

Trace metals

There is no evidence in man that deficiency of any mineral other than iron can cause disturbance of erythropoiesis. However, veterinary studies indicate that certain elements in trace amounts are essential for normal blood production. Copper in particular seems to be important since copper deficiency in swine leads to an anaemia which is probably due to interference with iron absorption and red cell synthesis; there is also reduction in the red cell life span. Cobalt deficiency gives rise to a macrocytic anaemia in ruminants but this is because vitamin B_{12}, synthesized in the rumen, depends on an adequate supply of cobalt.

OTHER FACTORS INFLUENCING ERYTHROPOIESIS

Erythropoietin

At the beginning of this century two French workers, Carnot and Deflandre, postulated the existence of a humoral control of erythropoiesis on the basis of experiments in rabbits. This was ignored for the next 40 years mainly because the work could not be confirmed and it was believed that hypoxia was the chief stimulus to an increased rate of erythropoiesis. However, a number of unconnected observations resuscitated the humoral hypothesis; for example, it was shown that hypoxia actually inhibited erythropoiesis in tissue culture and that if one of a pair of parabiotic rats, i.e. rats with a shared circulation, was exposed to an atmosphere of low oxygen tension, both animals showed the same increase in marrow activity. Subsequently it was shown that the plasma from hypoxic, anaemic and cobalt treated animals was capable of enhancing erythropoiesis in other animals. The erythropoietic factor, named erythropoietin, is a glycoprotein. It is formed mainly in the kidneys, possibly by the action of erythrogenin on one of the α-globulins in normal plasma (p. 35.29). It is assayed *in vivo* by measuring the uptake of ^{59}Fe by developing red blood cells of mice, or *in vitro* by the uptake in various tissue cultures.

The mechanism by which erythropoietin promotes erythropoiesis is unknown but it probably acts on stem cells destined to form proerythroblasts. Biochemical studies show that the synthesis of DNA and RNA is increased; its action is inhibited by actinomycin and it may therefore increase the formation of messenger-RNA.

Observations on the levels of erythropoietin in the plasma in man in various blood diseases are conflicting. This may be due to variation in the sensitivity of the assay techniques used, to the consumption of erythropoitin by an active marrow and to renal excretion. However, the titre of erythropoietin is usually found to be raised in all severe anaemias except that associated with chronic renal damage. Some tumours of the kidney, liver and uterus are also associated with raised concentrations and with increased numbers of circulating red blood cells (erythraemia).

Age and sex

The newborn infant has higher values for PCV than at any later time in life (p. 42.2). After birth there is gradual reduction in Hb, RBC and PCV due to replacement of the larger fetal macrocytes of short life span by adult type red cells and atrophy of erythropoietic tissue in the liver. The peripheral blood values continue to fall slowly until the infant is 2–3 months old. Thereafter marrow activity gradually increases and there is a progressive rise in Hb level until puberty when normal adult figures are reached. After the sixth decade there is commonly a slight decline in Hb and PCV. This is an inconstant finding and is probably due to malnutrition and iron deficiency rather than to any diminution in marrow activity from ageing.

During the reproductive period the Hb, RBC and PCV in the female tend to be about 90 per cent those of males. This difference between the sexes may be a hormonal effect but is more likely to be due to the difficulty which the female has in maintaining iron balance consequent on menstruation; it is not present before the menarche, or after the menopause.

A 15 kg child has about the same amount of bone marrow as a 70 kg adult but since the blood volume increases greatly during growth the rate of production of blood cells is much higher in childhood and adolescence than in later life.

Exercise and emotion

A transient increase in the concentration of circulating erythrocytes following strenuous muscular exercise and in emotional states such as fear and rage has long been recognized. In the dog this can be attributed to the discharge of blood of high haematocrit value from the spleen under the influence of adrenaline. In man, however, the blood changes are not easily explained since the spleen does not form a reservoir of red cells as in some animals. Cold baths in man are said to have a similar effect and it seems likely that the finding results from redistribution of cells in the circulation due to vasoconstriction in some regions, e.g. the skin, and vasodilation in others.

Physical changes in environment

No consistent effect on erythropoiesis has been observed from changes in environmental temperature, climate or season. Hypoxaemia associated with a low barometric pressure does, however, within certain limits consistently increase the rate of erythrocyte production as measured by the rate of iron turnover in the plasma and red cells using radioactive iron techniques and the erythrocyte concentration in the blood. Healthy individuals show this effect within hours when ascending to altitudes above 2000 m and the effect is maximal within 7–14 days. On the basis of the animal studies already mentioned these blood changes are believed to be due to erythropoietin. Natives residing at high altitudes have a rate of erythropoiesis about 30 per cent above normal. Since the red cell survival time is unchanged the Hb and PCV in the blood and the red cell mass are increased.

When a person who has been at a high altitude descends to sea level the rate of red cell production gradually returns to normal in about a month.

Very severe hypoxaemia ultimately has a suppressive effect on erythropoiesis. Hurtado found that this occurred when the arterial oxygen saturation fell below 60–70 per cent, a degree of hypoxaemia comparable with that obtaining at altitudes above 6000 m.

Endocrine factors

Deficiency of thyroid, adrenocortical and anterior pituitary function either from disease or surgical removal of secreting tissue produces mild anaemia which responds to the appropriate hormone. In Cushing's syndrome, a mild erythraemia may be a feature. Thyroxine, cortisol, androgens and prolactin promote erythropoiesis experimentally and oestrogens cause a fall in Hb, RBC and PCV probably by haemodilution from expansion of the plasma volume. The effect of hormones on blood cell production is complex. Not only do their actions appear to be inter-related but also they have indirect effects by altering nutrition and metabolic rates.

Degradation of haemoglobin and metabolism of bile pigments

The precise stages of haemoglobin catabolism are still uncertain; the initial reactions are, however, extravascular in the mononuclear phagocytes. It is believed that globin splits off and that the iron protoporphyrin ring of haem is opened by oxidative breakage of one of the joining methene bridges. Iron is next removed. Each day about 25 mg of iron is released to be mostly reutilized at once for new haemoglobin synthesis. The residual pigment is biliverdin, the main bile pigment in birds and amphibia. In man, reduction converts most of this to bilirubin.

Haemoglobin is released in small amounts into the plasma where it binds with haptoglobins. The haemoglobin-haptoglobin complex is then cleared from the plasma by the mononuclear phagocytes and the haemoglobin is thought to be metabolized as described. This is the only function so far ascribed to the haptoglobins.

After bilirubin is formed by the cells of the mononuclear phagocytic system (about 200 mg/day in the adult) it is transported in the plasma bound mostly to albumin. This albumin-bound bilirubin does not pass the glomerular filter. It appears in excessive amounts in the blood when there is increased catabolism of haemoglobin as occurs in haemolytic disorders. In the liver cells, bilirubin is converted to water soluble forms and excreted in the bile. Most is conjugated with glucuronic acid into bilirubin diglucuronide, a small amount into monoglucuronide; a fraction of the bilirubin may also be converted into a sulphate.

In the intestine bilirubin is converted to stercobilinogen. Studies with ^{15}N glycine have shown that not all stercobilinogen is derived from haemoglobin. This is of great academic interest and of some clinical importance. The amount is of the order of 10–15 per cent in health and as high as 30–40 per cent in some diseases, for example pernicious anaemia. The observation may indicate that haem, not utilized for haemoglobin, and porphyrins other than haem, are also metabolized to bilirubin. The metabolism of bilirubin is described on p. 33.13.

White blood cells

GRANULOCYTE SERIES

After birth, the production of the granulocytic white

cells takes place only in the red marrow where the proportion of granular to erythroid precursors is between 3:1 and 10:1.

The first stage of development is the **myeloblast** (plate 28.1, between pp. 28.14–15), a cell of 11–18 μm in diameter with a large nucleus, of fairly homogeneous chromatin containing 2–4 nucleoli, in a small amount of foamy cytoplasm. The next cell is the **promyelocyte**, a somewhat larger cell than the myeloblast, still with nucleoli in the nucleus and a few azurophilic granules in abundant cytoplasm. The **myelocyte** is a smaller cell with a round nucleus. It does not possess nucleoli and, like the mature polymorphs (p. 28.2), shows numerous cytoplasmic granules which are clearly identifiable using Romanowsky stains as eosinophilic (bright orange), basophilic (blue-black) and neutrophilic (faint purple). Mitosis does not occur after the myelocyte stage. The **metamyelocyte** shows commencing indentation of the nucleus producing a kidney shaped or horseshoe appearance leading to the lobulation seen in the next stage of maturation, the **polymorphonuclear granulocyte**. The time taken for maturation of a granulocyte in the bone marrow prior to its release into the circulation is believed to be of the order of 3–4 days. A mature polymorph is actively motile when studied in wet preparations. Pseudopodia form in the cytoplasm and the nucleus is capable of great distortion particularly in the neutrophils.

The survival time and fate of granulocytes is not well established. Probably only a small proportion, less than 5 per cent of the total number of granulocytes, are present in the blood at any one time. There is evidence that a large pool exists, mainly in the bone marrow, from which they can be rapidly discharged, giving an abrupt rise in the white cell count. This may occur with physiological stimuli such as exercise and after adrenaline injection. Radioactive labelling indicates that most granulocytes spend only a few hours in the circulation, but their total life span is probably 6–11 days, most of which is spent in storage pools. Although immature granular cells may enter and leave the circulation, it is likely that when granulocytes pass into the tissues they never return.

There is always a proportion of non-viable granulocytes in the circulation and probably these are removed by macrophages in marrow, liver, spleen and lymph nodes. Granulocytes are lost in performing body defence functions and some pass regularly into the lungs, saliva and alimentary tract.

LYMPHOCYTES

Much new information about the origin and function of lymphocytes has been derived from studies in immunology and so is discussed in detail in chap. 29.

Lymphocytes are probably all ultimately derived from stem cells in the bone marrow. These migrate to the thymus and lymphoreticular organs such as the lymph nodes, tonsils, periarterial pulp of the spleen and Peyer's patches of the intestine, where they proliferate and develop into mature lymphocytes.

The first recognizable lymphocyte precursor, known as the **lymphoblast**, is similar to the myeloblast in appearance. Then follows the **prolymphocyte**, a cell approximately 15 μm in diameter with nuclear chromatin somewhat coarser than that of the lymphoblast and still showing nucleoli or nucleolar remnants.

MONOCYTES

These cells are produced mainly in bone marrow. The parent cell, the **monoblast**, is like the myeloblast and lymphoblast, a cell of about 15 μm in diameter with a large nucleus, containing 2–3 nucleoli, filling much of the cell cytoplasm. Intermediate cells showing nucleolar remnants are recognized in the maturation process; they are sometimes termed **promonocytes**. The next identifiable cell is the monocyte (p. 28.2). Production rates, life span and fate of monocytes are not known.

The blood monocyte is a circulating form of the tissue macrophages that exist mainly in the liver, spleen and lymph nodes and together form the mononuclear phagocytic system (p. 29.2). It is phagocytic and the fact that it adheres strongly to glass and plastic is one useful distinction between monocytes and lymphocytes. The cell membrane has receptor sites for IgG and for C_3 complement. Monocytes are identified *in vitro* usually by a rosetting technique with red cells previously treated with IgG or IgM plus complement (p. 29.11).

METABOLISM OF WHITE CELLS

When blood is centrifuged, the white cells separate as a layer on top of the red cells. By using a centrifuge tube shaped like a dumb-bell, it is possible to harvest a concentrate of leucocytes. The metabolic activities of such a suspension can be studied in the same manner as any other tissue. Much less is known about the metabolism of leucocytes than of tissues like muscle and liver, because only small amounts can be obtained from a sample of blood by this method. However, the introduction of whole blood cell separators has made it possible to obtain much larger samples and it is probable that in clinical practice studies of the metabolism of leucocytes will be made much more frequently in the future.

Leucocytes have been shown to contain glycogen, present in the cytoplasm of granulocytes, and they possess all the enzymic mechanisms for the degradation of carbohydrates both aerobically and anaerobically. Leucocytes obtained from malnourished children contain amounts of oxaloacetate, pyruvate, lactate and ATP which are significantly less than normal and this may be interpreted as evidence of impaired glycolysis.

So far two practical applications of analysis of leucocytes have been developed. Firstly their content of ascorbic acid is usually over 140 nmol (25 μg)/10^8 cells in a well nourished person, but may be less than one tenth of this when the dietary vitamin C is inadequate, and undetectable in scurvy. Secondly, alkaline phosphatase, present in normal granulocytes, tends to be low or absent in abnormal cells and this measurement is useful in the diagnosis of myeloid leukaemia.

It has not yet been possible to make adequate preparations of the different leucocytes for quantitative measurements of their constituents.

FACTORS INFLUENCING THE NUMBER OF CIRCULATING LEUCOCYTES IN HEALTH

No specific nutrient is essential to the production of white cells as is iron for haemoglobin and red cells. However, vitamin B_{12} and folic acid play some part in normal leucopoiesis since severe deficiency of either leads to leucopenia which responds to their administration.

The role of the spleen in white cell production is obscure. There is evidence for its having a remote effect on the release of white cells and platelets from the bone marrow and the existence of a splenic hormone has been postulated. When a normal spleen is removed in man, e.g. after injury, there is a rise in the leucocyte count in the blood, due mainly to neutrophils, which normally lasts for 2–3 weeks.

In the newborn infant the white cell count is usually in the region of $15.0 \times 10^9/l$ in the first 24 hours of life. After 48 hours and for the first months the count is $10.0–12.0 \times 10^9/l$; thereafter the normal white cell count is less than $10.0 \times 10^9/l$. Lymphocytes are more numerous than polymorphs until about the age of 4 years; then the number gradually diminishes until adult proportions are reached.

The white cell count may fluctuate during the day and also vary from day to day but there is no consistent pattern. Environmental changes cause variable effects; hypoxia at high altitudes produces a neutrophil leucocytosis but unlike the effect on the red cells this is transitory. Strenuous exercise, pain and severe emotional disturbance such as fear or rage produce a rise in the white cell count lasting at most a few hours, mainly due to a rise in the number of neutrophil polymorphs. In these circumstances the total count can exceed $30.0 \times 10^9/l$. The effect is seen in the absence of the spleen and occurs within minutes; it is almost certainly due to mobilization of white cells from the bone marrow. Since adrenaline and cortisol affect the white cell, many of the physiological variations in the blood picture may be hormonally induced. Adrenaline produces first a polymorph leucocytosis and lymphocytosis and a later rise due to neutrophil increase accompanied by lymphopenia and eosinopenia. Noradrenaline appears to have no effect on circulating white cells. Cortisol causes neutrophil leucocytosis, lymphopenia and eosinopenia.

Since the main functions of the leucocytes are concerned with body defence, the most striking changes in the total white cell count and the relative proportions of the different white cells are seen in infections and inflammations.

FUNCTIONS OF LEUCOCYTES

Leucocytes are one of the agents in the body's defence against infection. Granulocytes and monocytes are able to destroy or remove particles and micro-organisms; lymphocytes are concerned with the formation and distribution of antibodies. These functions are discussed in chapter 29. Leucocytes may well have transport functions and the presence of many cytoplasmic enzymes suggests that numerous activities are still to be recognized.

Towards the end of the last century Metchnikoff had suspected the role of phagocytosis, i.e. the ingestion of a particle by a living cell, as one of the main defence mechanisms. He showed the accumulation of mobile cells about a thorn placed under the skin of a starfish larva. Microscopic observation has shown that in phagocytosis by leucocytes the cytoplasm in contact with the foreign particle first flows round the particle at the site of contact and engulfs it; this is probably what happens with large and elongated bacteria. The particle sinks into the cytoplasm without there being any observable flow around it.

The neutrophil polymorphs and monocytes are the most active phagocytic cells, the neutrophils being the first defence against infection; monocytes as tissue macrophages are involved usually at a later stage (p. 29.6). Eosinophils and basophils are less adept at this operation and lymphocytes are not phagocytic. Most phagocytosis occurs extravascularly in the tissues. Aggregation of leucocytes at the site of bacterial infection or invasion by foreign particles is one of the earliest changes that can be seen microscopically. Apart from its motility, there is clearly some attracting force directing the leucocyte. This phenomenon, known as chemotaxis, has received much attention but its mechanism is obscure. In addition neutrophil polymorphs may release substances which help to generate the local response to infection or injury and the more general responses affecting the circulating leucocytes and the body temperature.

Because eosinophils are normally more abundant in tissue fluid than in blood and are found particularly in the bowel wall, the respiratory tract and skin, they are thought to be concerned with the degradation and removal of protein. They are most numerous in allergic reactions and parasitic infections. Histamine has been demonstrated to have a chemotactic effect on eosinophils.

Basophils contain physiologically active substances such as histamine, heparin and 5-hydroxytryptamine (5HT).

Platelets

Platelets are produced from megakaryocytes which lie outside the blood sinusoids of the bone marrow. The megakaryocytes are large, up to 180 μm in diameter, and when mature have a multi-lobed nucleus and a markedly granular, light blue cytoplasm (plate 28.1, between pp. 28.14–15). From their periphery processes develop which penetrate between the vascular endothelial cells lining the blood sinusoids and enter the blood stream. Platelets are believed to be formed when the ends of these processes are broken off into the blood.

Platelets are metabolically active, being rich in enzymes, particularly those concerned with glycolysis, oxidation, transamination and dehydrogenation, and they contain a particularly high concentration of ATP. They are rich in phospholipid and in potassium and they contain virtually all the blood 5HT. Phospholipid and 5HT play an important part in blood coagulation.

Studies in man, using radioactive isotopic labels, e.g. ^{51}Cr, suggest that platelets have a life span of 8–11 days. There is good evidence that in normal man minute clots are continually being formed and dissolved, resulting in the random destruction of platelets, but death by senescence may also occur. The platelet life span can be artificially increased in a variety of ways as, for example, by the intake of a low fat diet, or by giving certain drugs, such as anticoagulants, and it can be shortened by smoking. Reduction of the platelet life span is also often associated with disease states. One of the most important functions of the platelet is the part it plays in haemostasis.

HAEMOSTATIC MECHANISMS

Haemostasis is one of the most important protective mechanisms in the body and controls bleeding in the face of injury. Most of the early information concerning haemostasis arose from studies on the formation of a visible blood clot *in vitro* and in damaged vessels. More recently much has been learned from the study of diseases in which haemostasis is defective.

When a blood vessel is severed, the damaged end contracts and retracts; the diameter of the end of the cut vessel is thereby reduced. The damaged vascular endothelium undergoes a functional change and becomes water wettable. Platelets adhere to this damaged endothelium and to the exposed subintimal collagen fibres. They release ADP which causes further platelets to aggregate to the site of the injury. In this process they change their shape from that of a disc to a sphere. The platelet aggregate thus formed seals the cut end of the vessel. At this stage, aggregation is a potentially reversible process. Normally it is rapidly followed by a further change in the platelets known as viscous metamorphosis. This consists of an irreversible fusion of the platelet aggregate into an amorphous mass, probably

due to the action of thrombin on fibrinogen contained within the platelets. The platelets then discharge their content of 5HT which further enhances vascular contraction, and of phospholipid which is concerned in the early stages of the clotting mechanism (vol. 2, p. 26.2).

The process of vascular contraction and retraction and the formation of a platelet plug together constitute the **initiation phase** of haemostasis and may stop blood flow from the damaged vessel. In capillaries, where the hydrostatic pressure is low, this mechanism alone may be adequate. It is reinforced by extrinsic pressure of the clot and by the normal turgor of the tissue. In larger vessels, however, where hydrostatic pressure is higher, the platelet plug is inadequate to stop the flow of blood. The contraction and retraction of the vessel wall soon passes off and a more secure and permanent plug is needed. A **blood clot** is produced by the conversion of circulating fibrinogen into an insoluble matrix of fibrin, in which blood cells are entrapped. This is known as the **maintenance phase**. Whole blood obtained by venepuncture and placed in a clean glass tube takes 5–10 min to clot at 37°C. A similar delay *in vivo* would explain the need for the initiation phase. Insoluble fibrin is formed from its soluble protein precursor fibrinogen through the action of the proteolytic enzyme thrombin. It follows that

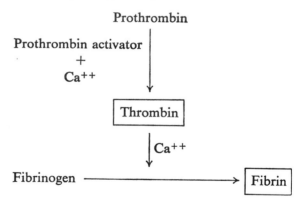

FIG. 28.4. The final two stages of the clotting mechanism.

thrombin cannot be present in intact blood except perhaps in trace amounts. It is formed from an inactive soluble blood protein precursor, prothrombin. The final two stages of the clotting mechanism can therefore be written as in fig. 28.4. These reactions, first propounded by Morawitz as long ago as 1905, still hold good today.

In 1947, Owren in Norway clearly identified an additional factor in the normal clotting process and since then many others have been discovered. These are now known by Roman numerals assigned by an International Committee on Blood Clotting Factors. A full list of the factors together with synonyms is given in table 28.2; some use is still made of the older or original names.

The reactions illustrated in fig. 28.4 are explosive in

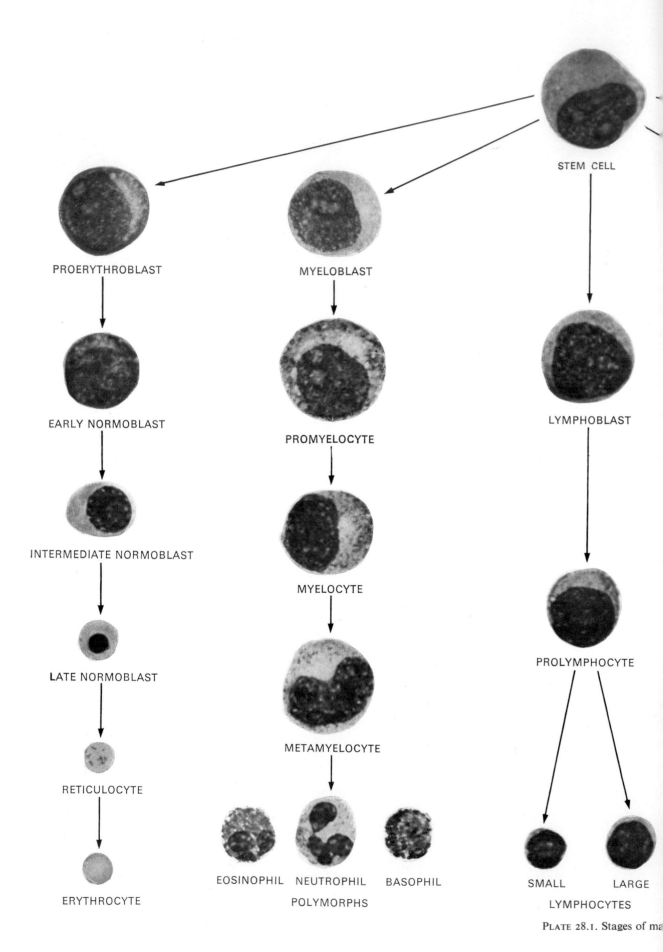

STEM CELL

PROERYTHROBLAST

MYELOBLAST

EARLY NORMOBLAST

PROMYELOCYTE

LYMPHOBLAST

INTERMEDIATE NORMOBLAST

MYELOCYTE

LATE NORMOBLAST

METAMYELOCYTE

PROLYMPHOCYTE

RETICULOCYTE

ERYTHROCYTE

EOSINOPHIL   NEUTROPHIL   BASOPHIL

POLYMORPHS

SMALL   LARGE

LYMPHOCYTES

PLATE 28.1. Stages of ma

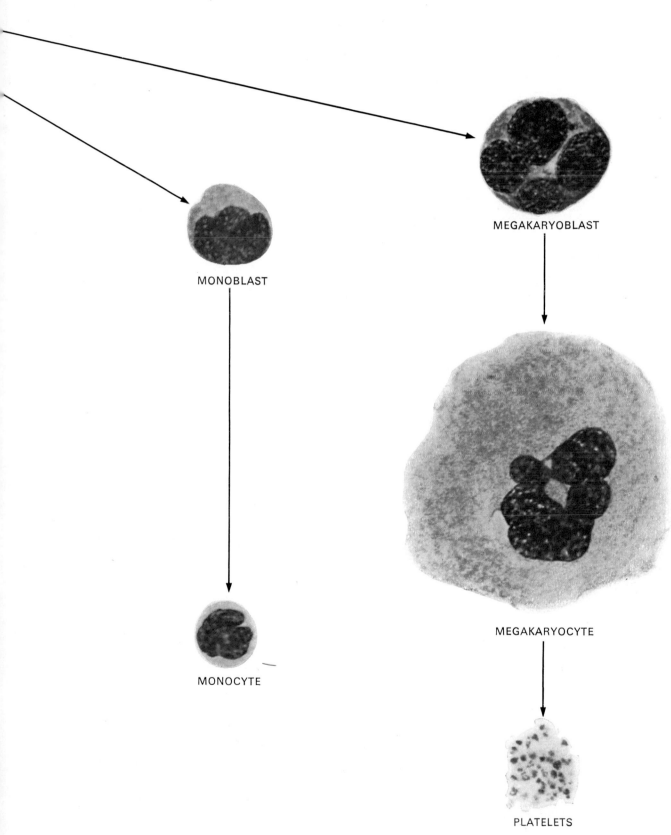

MONOBLAST

MEGAKARYOBLAST

MONOCYTE

MEGAKARYOCYTE

PLATELETS

ormal blood cells.

TABLE 28.2. International nomenclature of clotting factors.

Factor	Common synonyms
I	Fibrinogen
II	Prothrombin
III	Thromboplastin, tissue juice
IV	Calcium
V	Accelerator globulin, proaccelerin, labile factor
VI	No longer used
VII	Proconvertin, stable factor, autoprothrombin I
VIII	Antihaemophilic factor (AHF), antihaemophilic globulin (AHG), antihaemophilic factor A.
IX	Christmas factor, plasma thromboplastin component (PTC), antihaemophilic factor B.
X	Stuart–Prower factor
XI	Plasma thromboplastin antecedent (PTA), antihaemophilic factor C
XII	Hageman factor, contact factor
XIII	Fibrin stabilizing factor (FSF)

their intensity once the necessary concentration of **prothrombin activator** (thromboplastin) has been achieved. The greater part of the time taken for the blood to clot is taken up in the first stage during which the activator is being formed. There is some dispute about the precise nature of these early events in intravascular clotting but Macfarlane has put forward the attractive hypothesis that all the clotting factors are involved in a chain reaction or 'cascade of enzymes'. The exact order of their action is still uncertain but it is believed that the process is initiated when Factor XII comes into contact with a foreign surface or an area of damaged tissue. Active

Factor XII (Factor XIIa) then activates Factor XI, i.e. the proenzyme is converted into an enzyme, which in turn activates Factors IX, VIII, X and V in a similar manner. Platelet phospholipid (platelet cofactor 3), which is released by damaged platelets, also takes part in the reaction. Calcium ions are required in this stage when prothrombin activator is being formed, as in the later two stages. Hence substances which remove calcium ions as insoluble salts, e.g. oxalates, or convert them to non-ionized organic salts, e.g. citrate, are anticoagulants. Sodium, potassium and ammonium oxalate, sodium citrate and disodium or dipotassium ethylenediamine tetraacetate (EDTA or sequestrene) are frequently added to whole blood for this purpose. Heparin, which acts by blocking the action of thrombin and of active Factor X (Factor Xa) may also be used.

The intravascular (intrinsic) clotting mechanism is the principal system involved in haemostasis. A separate extravascular (extrinsic) clotting mechanism also exists in the tissues. This is brought into play by tissue damage due to either trauma or inflammation. The main function of this extrinsic mechanism is probably to produce a fibrin barrier which helps to localize infections. The final two stages are the same in both the intrinsic and extrinsic clotting mechanisms, but the initial stage of the latter is a more rapid process due to the fact that tissue juice is almost a complete prothrombin activator in its own right. This extrinsic clotting mechanism is also illustrated in fig. 28.5.

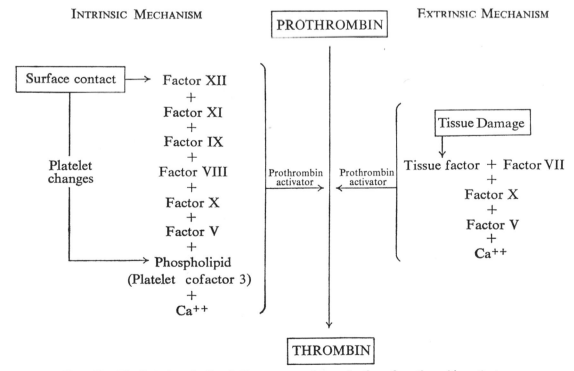

FIG. 28.5. The first stage in the clotting process; the production of prothrombin activator.

The conversion of fibrinogen to fibrin is not as simple as represented in fig. 28.4. Thrombin is now believed to split fibrinogen into one major component, fibrin monomer, and several minor polypeptide components. The major components then polymerize, under the influence of Factor XIII and calcium ions, into fibrin threads that give stability to the blood clot (fig. 28.6).

$$\text{Fibrinogen} \xrightarrow{\text{Thrombin}} \text{Fibrin monomer}$$

$$\text{Fibrin monomer} \longrightarrow \text{Fibrin polymer}$$

$$\text{Fibrin polymer} \xrightarrow[\text{Ca}^{++}]{\text{Factor XIII}} \text{Fibrin}$$

FIG. 28.6. The conversion of fibrinogen to fibrin.

The catalytic production of thrombin in the clotting process at the site of injury could theoretically result in retrograde spread of the fibrin clot throughout the vascular tree were it not controlled. This is achieved partly by the inactivation of thrombin by the newly formed fibrin and partly by the lytic influence of the **fibrinolytic system** (fig. 28.7).

The active enzyme in this system, **plasmin**, is proteolytic but possesses a preference for fibrin as substrate. It is formed from an inactive soluble blood protein precursor, plasminogen, by the action of plasminogen activator; this is found in many tissues including vascular endothelium and in body fluids and is released locally into the blood at the site of vascular injury.

Intact blood contains at least two **antiplasmins**, one fast and the other slow acting. Their neutralizing capacity is great enough to cope with the conversion of the total blood plasminogen if this should be activated slowly. Plasminogen is avidly adsorbed by fibrin, but antiplasmins cannot enter the interstices of the clot. When activator from the damaged vascular endothelium diffuses into the clot matrix, it converts the plasminogen to plasmin which acts unopposed on the fibrin and controlled lysis of the clot ensues. No free plasmin is found in the general circulation.

Occasionally in pathological states there is a rapid release of plasminogen activator into the general circulation. The plasminogen content of blood is so quickly converted to plasmin that the fast acting antiplasmin component is overwhelmed and free plasmin is present in the blood. This fibrinolytic state leads to severe bleeding. Bleeding usually becomes aggravated not only from progressive destruction of the clotting factors V and VIII by the free plasmin but also because fibrinogen degradation products tend to inhibit the polymerization of fibrin monomer. This situation arises rarely after open heart surgery, in malignant disease and as a complication of pregnancy. It can also be induced by the action of certain drugs.

It seems probable that the sequence of reactions, platelet aggregation, coagulation and fibrinolysis, occurs continuously at myriads of sites throughout the body where minute vascular damage has followed the occult trauma of everyday life.

In haemostasis, the fibrin clot is in a state of dynamic equilibrium, there being a fine balance between coagulation and fibrinolysis until the reparative process is well advanced. The fibrinolytic system then becomes temporarily dominant at the site of injury and the fibrin matrix is lysed, thus aiding in recanalization of the vessel.

It is clear that any disturbances in the delicate balance of the dynamic haemostatic mechanism pose a threat to the survival of the organism. Indeed in some patients an overactive clotting mechanism with a normal fibrinolytic system can cause thrombosis. The term **thrombosis** is used for coagulation which occurs inside an intact vessel in flowing blood.

The haemostatic mechanism is so complex that no single or simple test can be used to assess adequately its function. A major defect anywhere in this mechanism usually results in clinical symptoms, for example easy bruising or prolonged bleeding after minor injury. The bleeding may also occur in unusual sites, e.g. into joints, and may result in permanent deformity or abnormality of function. Sometimes, as in haemophilia, the defect is genetically determined so that there may be a history of a similar abnormal bleeding tendency in some of the patient's relatives. When the defect is mild, the patient's history and clinical examination may not be significantly abnormal and laboratory tests become of prime importance. These can be divided into two groups, those which

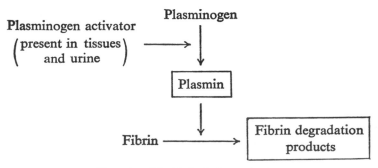

FIG. 28.7. The fibrinolytic mechanism.

measure vascular and platelet functions and those which measure the clotting and fibrinolytic mechanisms. The first group includes determination of the bleeding time, Hess test for capillary fragility and the platelet count. The second group includes measurements of the whole blood clotting and lysis times, the 'one stage' prothrombin time and more complicated procedures which measure specific parts of the clotting and fibrinolytic processes or measure the actual concentrations of the various factors present.

BLOOD GROUPS

In 1666, Richard Lower, a Cornishman, described to the Royal Society experiments in which he transfused blood from one dog to another. In the next year he demonstrated the transfusion of blood into a man before the Society. During the next 200 years these experiments were occasionally repeated, but they often resulted in a disastrous and fatal reaction in the recipient and were abandoned after a notorious legal action for murder in France. No satisfactory explanation for these accidents was found until 1901, when Landsteiner discovered the first blood group system in man.

Mode of inheritance of blood groups

Human blood groups are inherited characters involving antigen-antibody systems. The antigens are carried on the surface of the blood cells and are genetically controlled and first appear in the fetus. The antigen molecule has a chemical structure containing an amino acid complex which is capable of stimulating antibody formation, combined with a polysaccharide residue which usually confers specificity on the molecule.

There are at least nine principal human blood group systems, designated ABO, Rhesus (Rh), MNSs, P, Kell, Lutheran, Duffy, Lewis and Kidd, but only the ABO and the Rh systems are of major clinical importance. Each parent contributes a gene or a linked combination of genes for each of these blood group systems to the child. Each individual, therefore, possesses a pair of genes or a pair of linked genes, one from each parent, for each blood group system.

With the exception of those of the more recently discovered Xg system, where the genes are carried on the sex chromosome X, all the blood group genes are carried somewhere on the twenty-two pairs of autosomes and are independent of one another; indeed it has been shown that most of them must be carried on different chromosome pairs.

ABO blood group system

This was the first blood group system to be discovered. Landsteiner, in 1901, published his classical experiments in which he showed that the population could be divided into three groups which he named A, B and O and to which he later added a fourth, AB. People in groups A, B or AB carry the respective antigen or antigens on the surface of their red blood cells, whereas those in group O possess neither of the antigens. Each individual has, in his serum, the naturally occurring antibodies named anti-A (α) and anti-B (β) to the red cell antigens that he lacks. The antigen frequency of the British population has been determined. These antigen frequencies vary even in different parts of Great Britain; for instance, the frequency of group A decreases and that of group O increases from South to North. Different distributions occur in other parts of the world and the frequencies of the antigens in populations are of value in anthropological studies (table 28.3).

TABLE 28.3. Antigen frequency of ABO blood groups in the British population.

Blood group	Antigen present on red cell surface	Antibody (agglutinin) normally present in serum	Antigen frequency (%)
A	A	Anti-B	42
B	B	Anti-A	9
AB	AB	Neither	3
O	Neither	Anti-A and Anti-B	46

Every person has a pair of chromosomes each of which carries the A, B or O gene and therefore the population can be divided into four phenotypes and six genotypes (table 28.4).

BLOOD GROUP ANTIBODIES

Blood group antibodies are usually found in the γ fraction of the plasma globulins. They may either occur naturally or be acquired (immune antibodies) as a result of stimulation of the patient's antibody system from exposure to foreign red blood cells carrying blood group antigens which he normally lacks, e.g. in incompatible blood transfusion. Immune antibodies arising from exposure to foreign red cells are described as **isoantibodies**. Occasionally immune antibodies may arise spontaneously in a patient against his own blood group antigens in certain infections, diseases of lymphoid tissue and for reasons

TABLE 28.4. ABO phenotypes and genotypes

Phenotype	Genotype
AB	AB
A	AA
	AO
B	BB
	BO
O	O

unknown; such antibodies are spoken of as **autoantibodies**. The immune antibodies are usually IgG (7S) globulins and are of much smaller molecular weight than the natural occurring antibodies which are normally IgM (19S) globulins.

The naturally occurring blood group antibodies cause clumping together or agglutination in NaCl suspension of the red blood cells carrying the corresponding antigen; they are known as **complete antibodies**. Most immune antibodies, however, whilst combining with the specific antigen in 150 mmol/l NaCl do not produce visible agglutination of the red cells *in vitro* until protein, e.g. albumin, is added; such antibodies are spoken of as **incomplete antibodies**. A diagrammatic representation of the possible modes of action of complete and incomplete antibodies is given in fig. 28.8. In clinical practice incomplete antibodies can be detected by prior treatment of the red cells with a proteolytic enzyme such as papain which exposes the antigen to the action of the antibody in 150 mmol/l NaCl or by the antiglobulin (Coombs') technique (vol. 2, p. 23.2).

Most naturally occurring antibodies react optimally with the appropriate red cell antigens *in vitro* at room temperature, whereas immune antibodies react optimally at 37°C. Sometimes sera from apparently healthy people contain agglutinins in low titre which react strongly in the cold (4°C) but which are usually inactive at body temperature; they are called **cold agglutinins**. Pathological cold agglutinins are sometimes found in association with certain diseases such as mycoplasma pneumonia (vol. 3, p. 18.32). Such agglutinins may be of clinical significance because they have a wide thermal range of activity and are still active at body temperature.

A AND B SUBGROUPS

There are several subgroups of group A of which the most important are A$_1$ and A$_2$. Subgroups of B are very rare. About 20 per cent of group A people belong to group A$_2$ and the same percentage of group AB people belong to group A$_2$B: the other 80 per cent belong to groups A$_1$ or A$_1$B respectively. The A$_2$ antigen is much weaker than A$_1$ and reacts less well with anti-A sera; this is very important in blood group testing and in the cross-matching of blood. It is imperative that no anti-A serum is considered suitable for typing unless it gives a strong agglutination reaction with group A$_2$ as well as with A$_1$ cells. The naturally occurring anti-A and anti-B agglutinins vary in potency in individuals of the same blood group. They are absent at birth and do not become detectable until between the 3rd and the 6th months of life.

In addition to these naturally occurring complete anti-A and anti-B antibodies, immune or incomplete anti-A or anti-B antibodies may be acquired. This can arise after transfusion with blood incompatible in respect of the ABO system, or in a pregnant woman whose own blood is group O but whose fetus is of groups A or B, through escape of fetal red cells across the placenta into the maternal circulation. These immune antibodies, being IgG globulins of relatively low molecular weight, readily cross the placenta, whereas the natural antibodies do not because of their high molecular weight.

Rhesus (Rh) system

This was the second major blood group system to be discovered and resulted from the work of Landsteiner and Wiener who, in 1940, found that a rabbit antiserum prepared against Rhesus monkey red cells also agglutinated about 85 per cent of Caucasian human red cells; they called these cells Rh positive red cells. The other 15 per cent were said to be Rh negative cells. There are three principal Rh antigens which are said to be linked

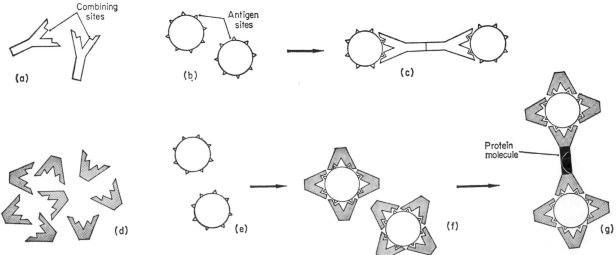

FIG. 28.8. Diagrammatic mode of action of complete and incomplete red cell antibodies: (a) complete antibody, (b) red blood cell, (c) agglutination, (d) incomplete antibody, (e) red blood cell, (f) antigen sites blocked, no agglutination, (g) addition of protein molecules, agglutination.

because they are found on one chromosome. The alleles (p. 39.3) are known as Dd, Cc and Ee. D is clinically the most important antigen because it is the most potent and accounts for more than 90 per cent of all reactions due to Rh blood group incompatibility. The existence of d antigen is assumed but so far remains unproved.

Whilst variants of most of these antigens are known, the main one of clinical importance is D^u. Red cells carrying this antigen are not agglutinated by all anti-D sera and can therefore be falsely grouped as d. When injected into a D negative person, D^u red cells behave like the D antigen and stimulate the production of normal anti-D antibody.

Naturally occurring antibodies in this system are rare and nearly all are acquired by isoimmunization of an Rh negative (d) person, such as a pregnant woman, by her Rh positive (D) fetus (see below) or by an incompatible Rh positive (D) blood transfusion or by autoimmunization in certain haemolytic states. Antibodies to the antigens C, c, E and e can also be formed.

For laboratory purposes most Rh antisera are obtained from the blood of female patients immunized during pregnancy or from volunteers deliberately immunized. Whilst potent anti-D sera are plentiful, others such as anti-C and anti-e are less common and antiserum to the d antigen has not yet been discovered. This latter fact complicates the problem of Rh genotyping, and differentiation of the homozygote DD from the heterozygote Dd can be made only on a probability basis from family studies, though the effect *in vivo* of DD is greater than that of Dd. This, however, is an oversimplification of the problem in that it is also not possible to identify single linked gene complexes using an antiserum and each individual has two of the linked gene combinations making up his genotype, one from each parent. Thus genotypes CDe/cDE and CDE/cDe cannot be differentiated by antisera typing even though all the antisera needed are available. The probable genotype is best deduced from the frequency with which each occurs within a particular phenotype and in conjunction with family studies.

Cold antibodies and the Ii system

As mentioned above, some sera contain non-specific cold isoagglutinins of no clinical importance. Occasionally, however, cold autoagglutinins may develop, sometimes complicating infection but often without known cause, and be of clinical significance. These autoantibodies can usually be detected in the plasma as well as attached to the patient's red blood cells. Often they are non-specific and react with the patient's own red cells and with practically all otherwise compatible donor cells. Sometimes the cold antibody is clearly specific for the I antigen. This minor antigen system is of particular interest in that fetal red cells, and those of the newborn, contain mostly the allele i and negligible I activity; the latter becomes fully potent only at the age of 18 months. The I antigen is so common in adults that it is almost universal and is sometimes referred to as a public antigen. The ii genotype is extremely rare in adults (less than 0·02 per cent). Hence cold antibodies with anti-I activity are detected *in vitro* if they agglutinate practically all red cells from adult subjects but not fetal red cells.

Leucocyte and platelet systems

The antigens of the ABO system are not confined to red blood cells but are also present in white cells and in platelets. In 1952 Dausset detected a further immunogenic leucocyte system consisting of more than 30 independent antigens now known as the HL-A system (human leucocyte A system). Experimental and genetic observations suggest that these antigens are present on two loci of the human chromosome; only one allele is present at each locus so that an individual never possesses more than four alleles. HL-A antigens are also present on platelets and most tissue cells.

Medical application of blood groups

In clinical medicine their importance is due to the fact that profound damage to donor red blood cells can occur when a blood group antigen carried on the cell reacts with an appropriate antibody. Such an antigen-antibody reaction can usually produce red cell destruction from agglutination or haemolysis or both. The effect of isoantibodies is seen in haemolytic transfusion reactions and haemolytic disease of the newborn; autoantibodies are the cause of autoimmune haemolytic disease (vol. 3, p. 21.36).

Only the ABO and Rh blood group systems contribute significantly to isoantibody incompatibility in the giving of blood transfusions. With improved laboratory techniques and increased care in grouping and cross matching the blood of both patient and donor, reactions are now uncommon. However, repeated transfusions can lead to isoantibody incompatibility affecting the rarer blood groups and particular care is needed in the selection of blood for patients who require repeated transfusions of blood.

Whenever possible before a transfusion, both donor and recipient blood should be tested in a well equipped blood transfusion or haematological laboratory (vol. 3, p. 51.8). If this is impracticable, this is no contraindication to a transfusion which may be life saving. However, in all circumstances, compatibility of donor and recipient blood with respect to ABO groups must be assured. An approximate 5–10 per cent suspension of the donor red cells is made by diluting the donor blood, taken direct from the transfusion bottle, with the supernatant plasma or in NaCl (150 mmol/l). One drop of this suspension is mixed on an opalescent tile or glass slide with two drops of the patient's heparinized plasma. The tile or slide is gently rocked and if no visible agglutination is seen after 5 min, the donor blood is compatible, but only for the ABO system. This procedure should only be followed in an emergency. Compatibility testing is fully described in vol. 3, p. 51.8.

Blood groups are useful genetic markers in identifying blood stains and in paternity disputes and also in anthropology. Besides the ABO system the HL-A system appears to be the only genetic system which is of major importance in human organ transplantation.

Haemolytic disease of the newborn

This is nearly always due to Rh incompatibility between the mother and her fetus and 90 per cent of cases are caused by the D antigen. If an Rh positive (D) fetus is conceived by an Rh negative (d) mother she may become immunized by the periodic escape of fetal red cells across the placental barrier into her circulation. The immune anti-D antibody which she produces, being an IgG antibody globulin, crosses the placenta into the fetal circulation where it can cause haemolysis of the fetal red cells. Haemolytic disease of the newborn is rarely encountered in a first pregnancy, possibly because immunization of the mother, if it occurs, does so most frequently towards the end of gestation and during delivery. However, once the mother is immunized, the risk to a further Rh positive fetus may increase with each succeeding pregnancy. Fetal-maternal ABO incompatibility minimizes the risk of maternal Rh immunization because it helps the mother to remove and destroy fetal cells escaping into her circulation before the Rh antigen becomes effective; reliance is no longer placed on this chance and the injection of potent anti-D sera is used to effect a more certain protective action in all Rh negative (d) mothers who at delivery are found to have Rh positive (D) cells in their circulation. This protection is now being given to more and more Rh negative (d) mothers who are delivered of an Rh positive (D) baby or fetus (vol. 3, p. 43.26).

Very rarely haemolytic disease of the newborn can be due to one of the other blood group systems.

FURTHER READING

BECK W.S. ed. (1973) *Hematology.* Harvard Pathophysiology Series, vol. 1, Cambridge, Mass.: M.I.T. Press.

BIGGS R. (1976) *Human Blood Coagulation, Haemostasis and Thrombosis,* 2nd Edition. Oxford: Blackwell Scientific Publications.

BOORMAN K.E. & DODD B. (1970) *An Introduction to Blood Group Serology,* 4th Edition. London: Churchill Livingstone.

DACIE J.B. & LEWIS S.M. (1968) *Practical Haematology,* 4th Edition. London: Churchill.

DE GRUCHY G.C. (1970) *Clinical Haematology in Medical Practice,* 3rd Edition. Oxford: Blackwell Scientific Publications.

HARDISTY R.M. & INGRAM G.I.C. (1965) *Bleeding Disorders: Investigation and Management.* Oxford: Blackwell Scientific Publications.

—— & WEATHERALL D.J. eds. (1974) *Blood and its Disorders.* Oxford: Blackwell Scientific Publications.

MCDONALD G.A., DODDS T.C. & CRUICKSHANK B. (1970) *Atlas of Haematology,* 3rd Edition. London: Churchill Livingstone.

MOLLISON P.L. (1972) *Blood Transfusion in Clinical Medicine,* 5th Edition. Oxford: Blackwell Scientific Publications.

RAPAPORT S.I. (1971) *Introduction to Hematology.* New York: Harper & Row.

WICKRAMASINGHE S.N. (1975) *Human Bone Marrow.* Oxford: Blackwell Scientific Publications.

WILLIAMS W.J., BEUTLER E., ERSLER A.J. & RUNDLES R.W. (1972) *Hematology.* New York: McGraw-Hill.

WINTROBE M.M., LEE G.R. *et al.* (1974) *Clinical Haematology,* 7th Edition. Philadelphia: Lea & Febiger.

Chapter 29
Lymphoreticular organs and tissues

The body has to dispose of particulate matter, e.g. dust and bacteria, which enter the tissues mostly through the respiratory and alimentary tracts and at sites of abrasions or injury to the skin. It also has to dispose of dead cells, notably erythrocytes, and the macromolecular complexes which are formed in certain diseases. All of these may be engulfed by cells, a process known as **phagocytosis**. Many types of cell may have phagocytic ability under certain circumstances. However two types are mainly responsible, the **microphages** and the **macrophages**. The microphages are the polymorphonuclear leucocytes described on p. 28.2.

Macrophages are mononuclear cells derived from stem cells in the bone marrow. They circulate in the blood as monocytes (p. 28.2) and enter the tissues where they have varying degrees of mobility. The body macrophages are known collectively as the **mononuclear phagocyte system.**

Macrophages are distributed diffusely throughout the body, but are most concentrated in certain sites within organs which are composed mainly of **lymphoid tissue**. This tissue is concerned with the production of lymphocytes, the cells responsible for the **immune responses** of the body to foreign proteins. Its main organs are the lymph nodes, spleen, thymus and specialized regions of the alimentary tract. Lymphocytes are derived from stem cells in the bone marrow distinct from those which give rise to macrophages.

The tissues react to the presence of foreign proteins, known as **antigens,** in two ways, called the **cellular** and **humoral immune responses.** In cellular responses, the immune reaction is mediated by the lymphocytes themselves, while in humoral responses protective substances, **antibodies,** are secreted into the blood stream by new lymphocytes. Antibodies are globulins which react with specific antigens to form **antigen-antibody complexes.** As a result, the antigen is removed in one of various ways, e.g. precipitation and phagocytosis (vol. 2, p. 22.14).

In the lymphoid organs, and also in some other tissues, notably the bone marrow and liver, in which the lymphoid component is slight or absent, there is a well-developed structural supportive framework of reticulin fibres, reticular cells and endothelial cells, these last forming the lining of blood or lymphatic sinusoids. The reticular and endothelial cells have slight phagocytic powers, but highly phagocytic cells of the mononuclear phagocyte system are found 'fixed' in the sinusoids, and also as freely moving forms in other parts of these organs.

Organs showing this intimate anatomical and functional relationship of lymphoid tissue and reticular and endothelial cells are known as **lymphoreticular organs;** these therefore include lymph nodes, spleen, thymus, bone marrow and epitheliolymphoid tissue of the alimentary tract, and the proportion of lymphoid tissue, structural reticular tissue and mononuclear phagocytes varies in individual organs. Thus in the lymph nodes all these components are highly developed, while in the thymus the mononuclear phagocyte system is poorly represented.

The term reticuloendothelial system was introduced in 1912 by the famous German pathologist, Aschoff. He considered it to include reticular and endothelial sinusoid tissue, macrophages and lymphoid tissue. The term quickly became established in textbooks. Aschoff defined the system as consisting of those cells in the body that actively take up vital dyes. Inasmuch as macrophages take up dyes much more avidly than reticular and endothelial cells, it was never a precise descriptive term. However, its continued use appeared justified by the view, now known to be mistaken, that reticular cells were stem cells from which macrophages and lymphocytes were derived in the tissues, as well as erythrocytes and microphages in the bone marrow. It is now firmly established that these various cells do not have a common origin but arise from different stem cells. Since 1970 the term reticuloendothelial system has been redefined so as to include only reticular and endothelial cells, and this definition distinguishes it from the mononuclear phagocytic and lymphoid systems. Aschoff's use of the term has been so firmly entrenched for 60 years, that it is unlikely to disappear quickly. Inevitably students will find that some authors use the term with the modern definition, whilst others retain Aschoff's. This confusion can be prevented by avoiding the use of the term 'reticuloendothelial' and referring simply to reticular and endothelial cells and to the structural reticulin fibres.

In this chapter, these three related cell systems are discussed, together with the immune mechanisms of the body, under the following headings:

Structural cells
Mononuclear phagocyte system
Nature of the immune response
Lymph nodes and epitheliolymphoid tissue
Lymphocytes and the immune response
Spleen
Thymus

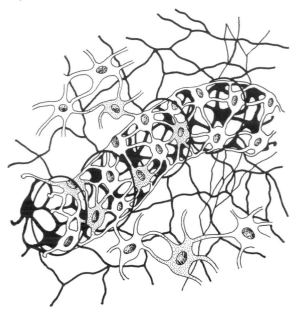

FIG. 29.1. A three-dimensional network of supporting reticulin fibres associated with stellate reticular cells. In places condensations of reticulin and greater numbers of cells create demonstrable channels or sinusoids. Their walls are fenestrated and imperfectly lined by flattened endothelial cells.

STRUCTURAL CELLS

Reticular cells are of mesenchymal origin. They are large, often stellate cells and are closely associated with reticulin fibres which they probably produce (fig. 29.1). Reticular cells and fibres form the structural framework of channels and sinusoids which carry fluids through the parenchyma of many organs, notably the lymph nodes, spleen and liver.

Sinusoids have also an internal or luminal layer of endothelial cells which is often incomplete or fenestrated (fig. 29.1). Endothelial and reticular cells often cannot be distinguished from each other under the light microscope, and are then best referred to by the non-committal term **littoral** or **lining cells**. Reticulin fibres too can be seen and identified with certainty when special silver impregnation techniques are used, and the EM shows clearly some of their distinguishing characteristics (fig. 29.2). Thus some reticulin fibres can be seen to be ensheathed by long cytoplasmic processes of the stellate reticular cells.

The endothelial cells, unlike the reticular cells, rest on a prominent basement membrane which supports them and everywhere separates them from the reticular cells and fibres (plates 29.1, facing p. 29.10 and 29.2d & e, facing p. 29.42).

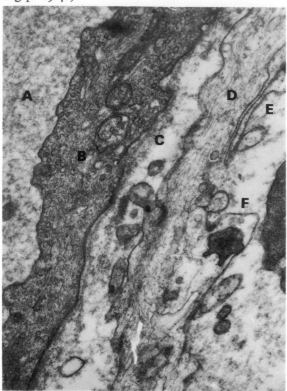

FIG. 29.2. Structure of a sinusoid wall showing the relationships of an endothelial cell, basement membrane and a reticular cell. The lumen (A) is defined by the endothelial cell (B) which is backed by a basement membrane (C). The reticular fibre (D) is distinguished by its fibrillary nature and appears partially ensheathed at (E) by the cytoplasm of a reticular cell (F). (E.M. × 20 000) Courtesy of Dr. I.I. Smith.

MONONUCLEAR PHAGOCYTE SYSTEM

Monocytes belong to a system of cells which arise in the bone marrow and are transported in the blood as monocytes; they migrate into many tissues where they form free and fixed macrophages, and where they carry out both phagocytic and immunological functions. These are summarized as follows:

(1) removal of effete cells as exemplified by the destruction of worn-out red blood cells by the macrophages in sinusoids of the spleen and bone marrow,

(2) uptake and handling of materials important to the economy of the body, such as iron and fat, by the Kupffer cells of the liver,

(3) removal of denatured proteins such as fibrin and macromolecular complexes from the circulating blood by splenic and other macrophages,

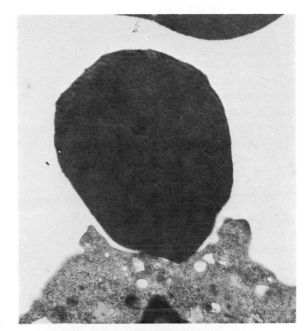

a

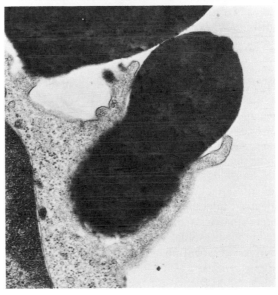

b

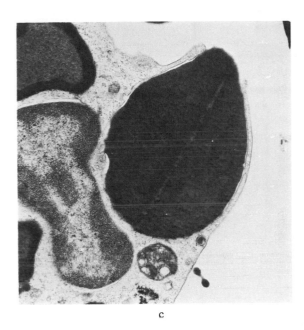

c

FIG. 29.3. Phagocytosis by adherence and membrane flow, showing (a) attachment, (b) engulfment and (c) endocytosis (E.M. (a) × 13 750; (b) × 18 750; (c) × 12 500).

(4) phagocytosis and destruction of micro-organisms and particulate substances which find their way into the tissues and then into the lymph and blood, and

(5) co-operation with the lymphoid system to produce a state of immunity to bacteria, viruses, fungi, protozoan and metazoan parasites, and perhaps to neoplastic cells.

Phagocytosis

Phagocytosis is the ability to ingest, concentrate and retain foreign matter, including certain dyes which may be injected during life. Phagocytic cells take up such material with differing degrees of avidity and there are marked differences in the uptake of particulate and of soluble material.

During the phagocytosis of a particle three stages can be recognized (fig. 29.3). First the particle adheres to the macrophage membrane (attachment). Secondly anular

lips of cytoplasm develop around the zone of contact; this is followed by a flow of cytoplasm and membrane encircling the particle (engulfment). Thirdly the edges of the lips approach each other and finally fuse; the particle then lies in a phagocytic vacuole (endocytosis) where it may be digested.

When phagocytes are observed in tissue culture, movement is seen to consist of the formation of a thin cytoplasmic veil, the leading edge of which advances leaving behind a nuclear mound (fig. 29.4). The cytoplasmic veil contains few organelles and has a ruffled border. If the leading edge meets a particle, it rises up and smothers it; the particle is then ingested without obvious preliminary adherence. This is known as surface phagocytosis. Heavy particles or those that can be trapped against a fixed surface may be dealt with in this way *in vivo*.

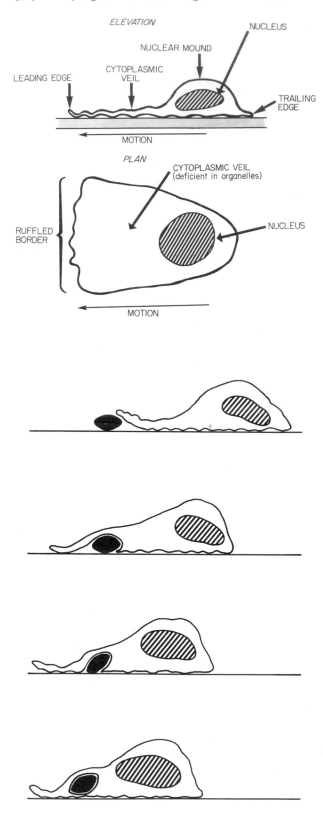

FIG. 29.4. Surface phagocytosis (for explanation see text).

BLOCKADE OF PHAGOCYTOSIS

Excessive uptake of particulate matter by phagocytes soon leads to a state of phagocytic blockade in which no more can be ingested. Most materials used experimentally to demonstrate phagocytosis, e.g. carbon particles and saccharated iron oxide, are colloidal and stabilized by solutions of substances such as gelatin. Blockade by particles may be specific not only for the particles but also for the stabilizing agent. Thus phagocytes blocked by carbon may still take up saccharated iron oxide. Likewise, after successful blockade residual phagocytic capacity for the same material may be demonstrated if it is suspended in a different stabilizing agent.

Blockade is probably due to depletion of opsonins; these are substances which stimulate phagocytes to ingest particulate material and include immunoglobulins and other plasma proteins and surface acting agents. In some experiments groups of cells can be found which have taken up little carbon although their neighbours are replete, suggesting that individual cells vary in their susceptibility to blockade.

SITES OF PHAGOCYTIC ACTIVITY

Sites where mononuclear phagocytes may be found can be divided into those in the lymphoreticular organs and those in other organs.

Phagocytes of lymphoreticular organs

The spleen and lymph nodes filter large volumes of fluid through their sinusoids and the phagocytes present in the sinusoids remove particulate and other matter. While still attached to the sinusoid these fixed cells phagocytose adequately, but when suitably stimulated by foreign particles they divide, round off and become motile in the sinusoidal lumen; these 'free' macrophages greatly increase local phagocytosis (fig. 29.5).

Splenic phagocytes. The spleen is rich in phagocytic cells and weight for weight takes up more injected particulate material from the blood than the liver. Splenic phagocytes are found in the sinusoids and in the cords of Billroth in the red pulp (p. 29.27) and may be fixed or freely motile. In addition, there are specialized phagocytes in the Malpighian bodies (p. 29.26) where they make intimate contact with maturing lymphocytes, an activity important to the immune responses. The structure of the spleen, which allows blood to percolate through sinusoids rich in phagocytic cells, makes it a very effective filter.

In some conditions where the red blood cells or platelets are abnormal, the spleen may be removed surgically because it traps and destroys too many of them. Iron from breakdown of haem is stored not only in the sinusoidal macrophages but also in the endothelial cells, a notable exception to their usually poor phagocytic powers.

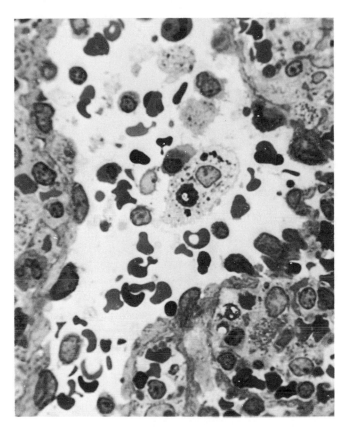

FIG. 29.5. A branching splenic sinusoid. Plump oval nuclei of sinusoidal endothelium (littoral cells) protrude into the lumen. Note the large central macrophage; its nucleus is pale and the cytoplasm contains a dark, red blood cell with central pale spot. In the sinusoid there are red blood cells, irregular in shape, and some lymphocytes. Light microscopy: araldite-embedded section stained by toluidine blue (× 840).

Lymph node phagocytes. Sinusoidal phagocytes clear the lymph of particulate matter. In addition specialized dendritic cells are found in intimate contact with lymphocytes and their precursors in the cortex and the follicles, where lymphocytes are produced. These cells play a part not only in removing dead lymphocytes but also in stimulating the production of new lymphocytes with specific immune properties after retaining and processing antigen (p. 29.18). Tingible body macrophages are germinal centre phagocytes which contain the remains of ingested nuclei of dead lymphocytes which are demonstrable by basic stains such as haematoxylin.

Thymic phagocytes. Macrophages are present in the dense lymphoid tissue of the cortex and medulla. Their chief activity is to ingest the large numbers of lymphocytes which normally die during thymic lymphopoiesis. They do not usually phagocytose particulate matter since the thymus is not richly provided with lymphatic sinusoids and is not primarily a filtering organ. However, they can be induced to take up particles or bacteria injected experimentally directly into the thymic parenchyma.

Bone marrow phagocytes. These deal with the iron essential to erythropoiesis. Effete red blood cells are removed by phagocytes in the splenic, hepatic and marrow sinusoids. Iron from degraded haemoglobin is stored temporarily in the phagocytes as the iron-protein complex ferritin, and is incorporated later into new red blood cells forming in the marrow. Ferritin is stored in the hepatic and splenic macrophages and the iron is returned to the marrow in the plasma bound to the protein transferrin. In the marrow, specialized macrophages or **nurse cells** take up transferrin from the plasma and store the iron before passing it on to the dividing erythroblasts.

The nurse cells also take up the nuclei extruded by immature erythrocytes at the late normoblast stage of erythropoiesis.

Phagocytes of other organs

Liver phagocytes. The Kupffer cells are the largest single group of phagocytic cells in the body. They form part of the lining of blood sinusoids of the liver and are continually shed and replaced by monocytes from the circulation (p. 32.38). In health they play an important role in clearing the portal blood of chylomicrons and bacteria. They also take up fragments of red blood cells. Kupffer cells which become laden with debris may be shed into the hepatic vein and pass to the lungs, ending up either in the pulmonary lymph nodes or in the bronchial secretions.

Pulmonary phagocytes. The lung contains many phagocytic cells, as may be seen on examination of lungs removed from miners, city dwellers or heavy smokers, when large accumulations of dust or carbon pigment are found in the alveolar macrophages (p. 31.6). In pneumonia and in chronic venous congestion of the lungs due to heart failure, red blood cells may enter the pulmonary alveoli, and macrophages may be seen ingesting and digesting them. Their remnants may persist within the macrophages as golden brown granules of haemosiderin (plate 29.2f, facing p. 29.42).

Phagocytes of the central nervous system. The small cells called microglia (p. 15.6) are probably derived from blood monocytes, since developmentally they are found in the brain only after it has become vascularized. They enlarge and become phagocytic when the brain tissue is damaged. Their function under those circumstances is to remove dead nerve cells and glial tissue. In infections of the brain and meninges, most of the mononuclear phagocytes found in the CSF originate from monocytes in the circulating blood which gain entry through the permeable walls of inflamed blood vessels.

Serosal and connective tissue phagocytes. In synovia and serous sacs, i.e. pleura, peritoneum and pericardium, phagocytes are attached to the lining membrane and are called synovial and serosal cells. Connective tissues always contain free macrophages, derived from blood monocytes and sometimes called tissue histiocytes.

Miscellaneous phagocytes. Sinusoidal or endothelial macrophages similar to Kupffer cells are found in the adrenal and pituitary glands. The mesangial cell of the renal glomerulus may be a specialized phagocyte (p. 35.7). A few macrophages are found in all tissues except cartilage and enamel.

MACROPHAGES AND INFLAMMATION

Macrophages appear in the tissues in large numbers, as a response to damage, infection or the presence of foreign matter. Such agents stimulate an acute inflammatory response with dilation and increased permeability of the local microcirculation. First, large numbers of polymorphs pass between the endothelial cells of the small blood vessels and enter the extracellular spaces (vol. 2, p. 21.8). Although highly phagocytic for particulate and bacterial matter, they are short-lived. Later they are joined by macrophages which complete the scavenging process by taking up the dead polymorphs, tissue debris and bacteria.

SOURCE OF MACROPHAGES

The monocyte is the developmental source of all the specialized macrophages found in different sites. Nevertheless, due to special local conditions certain tissue macrophages show marked differences from the circulating monocyte. In some instances, e.g. the microglia and the alveolar macrophages, the phagocytes are long-lived and resemble the cells of the local tissue. Local macrophages of this type maintain their numbers and phagocytic power in health largely by division *in situ*. Occasional replenishment also takes place from circulating monocytes. Although in the blood the proportion of monocytes to other leucocytes is small, their absolute number is large and more than adequate to supply the normal needs.

In prolonged inflammatory states, e.g. resolving pneumonia, the local macrophages are supplemented by exudation of large numbers of monocytes into the alveoli from the capillaries. Production of monocytes by the bone marrow is greatly increased to offset the losses. Eventually the exuded macrophages may die and be phagocytosed by fresh waves of macrophages or they may return to the circulation to be scavenged in the spleen.

In specific chronic inflammations, e.g. tuberculosis, the macrophages in the lesions are derived from monocytes, locally arrested by substances released in the immune response (p. 29.18). These macrophages may undergo transformation into epithelioid cells and syncytia known as giant cells (vol. 2, p. 21.16). Foreign body reactions also bring about giant cell formation.

The old idea that macrophages can arise in the later stages of inflammation, by transformation of local tissue cells, e.g. reticular cells, fibroblasts, lymphocytes and endothelial cells, is no longer held.

RELATIONSHIPS OF PHAGOCYTES

Fig. 29.6 sets out the types of cells with phagocytic potential and their relations with associated groups of cells. All are derived embryologically from mesenchyme.

The prime example of a structural cell with some phagocytic powers is the reticular cell. These cells are self-replicating and cannot be replenished from stem cells. There are two classes of non-structural phagocytes.

Microphages. These are the smaller phagocytes and consist solely of the polymorphonuclear leucocytes, which do not divide and have a short life. They are replenished entirely from stem cells which mature within the bone marrow. They are usually confined to the blood stream and appear in the tissues in large numbers only in acute inflammation.

Mononuclear phagocytes (macrophages). These are the most active phagocytic cells and fall into three groups.

Free circulating macrophages are monocytes and their precursors in the blood, and contribute to its phagocytic powers. They are more important as the source of macrophages in local inflammatory states (exudate macrophages) and as replenishments of tissue and fixed sinusoidal macrophages elsewhere.

Tissue macrophages are motile and found not only in the lymphoreticular organs but also in many other organs and tissues in health. They are often loosely referred to as 'macrophages', 'phagocytes' or 'histiocytes'. Their numbers are maintained both by self-replication *in situ* and by contributions from the free circulating macrophages.

Fixed sinusoidal macrophages are highly phagocytic cells, closely associated with the sinusoids of the spleen, liver and lymph nodes. Effete forms are probably shed into the circulation and destroyed in the spleen. They are replenished from circulating monocytes.

DIFFERENTIATION OF LITTORAL CELLS

Three types of cell, the reticular cell, the endothelial cell and the sinusoidal macrophage, line the sinusoids of lymph nodes and spleen, and the term littoral cells includes them all. It is difficult to distinguish them in sections stained with haematoxylin and eosin, and some of the criteria which separate them are now summarized.

Reticular cells possess the following distinguishing properties. (1) They have a constant close association with reticulin fibres which their cytoplasm often ensheaths (fig. 29.2). (2) Unlike macrophages, they lack cell membrane receptors for immunoglobulins (p. 29.11). (3) Like macrophages, but unlike endothelial cells, their cytoplasm is metallophilic when treated with silver carbonate basic stains. (4) Although weakly phagocytic, they do not round off or separate from the reticulin

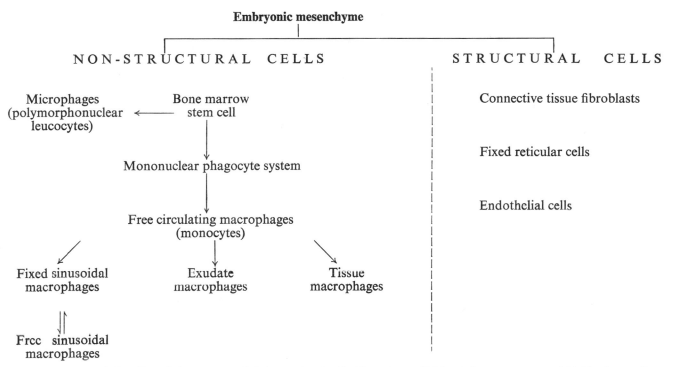

Fig. 29.6. Interrelationships of phagocytes and their associated cells. The primary division is into non-structural highly phagocytic cells and structural cells of little or no phagocytic power. The non-structural phagocytes include the short-lived microphages and long-lived macrophages. The varieties of macrophage form a family of cells, the mononuclear phagocyte system. When requirements for macrophages outstrip the local mitotic rate, reinforcements come first from the blood monocytes and later from the marrow stem cells. Of the structural cells, the fibroblast is not now regarded as capable of becoming phagocytic and the fixed reticular cell is only feebly so.

network to become free macrophages, nor do they serve as a parent cell for them. (5) They do not act as stem cells in lympho- or haematopoiesis.

Unlike the reticular cells and macrophages, endothelial cells have cytoplasm which is not metallophilic with silver carbonate. Experimentally they are not actively phagocytic, although splenic endothelial cells are exceptional and take up iron. Electron micrographs show attachment to a basement membrane.

Sinusoidal macrophages may be shown by EM to occupy interstices between endothelial cells and to thrust their actively phagocytic cytoplasm into the luminal stream of lymph or, in the spleen and liver, of blood. Leashes of cytoplasmic microfibrils are associated with their phagocytic and motile powers. They are distinguished from reticular cells by being unattached to reticulin and by having surface receptors for immunoglobulin and complement.

DISTINGUISHING MONONUCLEAR PHAGOCYTES AND LYMPHOCYTES

A glance at plate 28.1 shows that the monocyte and small lymphocyte are easily distinguished in blood films. Unfortunately, in paraffin sections of inflamed tissue cytoplasmic shrinkage makes the distinction difficult. In these circumstances macrophages and lymphocytes can be distinguished readily only if there is obvious phagocytosis of haem pigment, nuclear matter or dust pigment. When phagocytosis is not evident the larger cytoplasmic to nuclear volume of the macrophage may be helpful, but often it is not possible to differentiate the two types of cell; it is then permissible to use the collective descriptive term 'small round cell'.

For more exacting investigative purposes, two other criteria are useful. (1) Macrophages are rich in intracellular enzymes, e.g. acid phosphatase, non-specific esterase and leucine aminopeptidase, which are absent from lymphocytes. (2) Cytophilic antibodies, which react with antigen only after they have become bound to cell surfaces, passively confer the capacity to bind antigen on mononuclear phagocytic cells but not on lymphocytes.

NATURE OF THE IMMUNE RESPONSE

Phagocytosis, followed by intracellular digestion, affords immediate short term protection against infection. Long term protection depends on the immune response. This commonly begins with the uptake and processing of foreign matter by macrophages, followed by reactive changes in the lymphoid tissue with the production of cells which form antibodies. The process of immunization is greatly assisted by the close relationship of the phago-cytic sinusoidal macrophages and the sites of lympho-poiesis and antibody production.

Since it is impossible to understand the structure and function of the lymphoid system without some knowledge of immunology a brief introduction to the subject is given here. It is considered in greater detail in vol. 2.

The immune response is a protective reaction of the body to the presence within it of a foreign protein, known as an **antigen.** There are several different responses of a protective nature which the host may make, and these differ from antigen to antigen. Some of the responses, e.g. phagocytosis, are non-specific and evoked by many different antigens, but those of greatest interest, i.e. humoral immunity and cell-mediated immunity, are capable of a very high degree of specificity, directed exclusively against a particular antigen.

SPECIFIC IMMUNITY

After the first exposure to an antigen, specific immunity takes two to three weeks to develop; this is the **primary response.** The immunological memory of the host allows it to be recalled quickly on a second exposure to the same antigen, often with enhanced vigour; this is the **secondary** or **accelerated response.** In specific immunity directed against a particular antigen, the first stage is often uptake and handling of the antigen by phagocytes. Depending on the exact nature of the antigen, one of two types of specific immunity then develops as a result of activation of lymphocytes or their precursors by antigen-primed phagocytes. These types are called **cell-mediated immunity** and **humoral immunity.**

Specific cell-mediated immunity

Cell-mediated immunity is produced by antigen-primed phagocytes activating a subpopulation of small lympho-cytes, known as **T lymphocytes** because they or their precursors are thymus-derived and thymus-dependent, in the sense that their functions are depressed following thymectomy. T lymphocytes are morphologically indis-tinguishable from another subpopulation, the **B lympho-cytes,** but the two can be distinguished by a number of laboratory tests, many of them making use of their unique immunological properties.

The result of activation by antigen is to produce gene-rations of T lymphocytes which can 'home' via the blood to regions of antigen exposure. The protective effect involves a local infiltration not only of lymphocytes, but also of macrophages derived from blood monocytes.

The T lymphocyte system, suitably activated, protects the body against virus infections, fungal infections and tuberculosis and ensures the rejection of skin and other grafts transplanted to antigenically different partners.

Specific humoral immunity

Humoral immunity depends on the synthesis of specific globulins, i.e. **immunoglobulins** (Ig), known as **anti-bodies,** which circulate in the blood stream (p. 33.2). These are the immunological effectors which neutralize invading antigens specifically and protect the host from their effects. When antibodies are produced as a result of natural infection or by injection of antigen into man or laboratory animals, the serum containing the specific antibodies is known as an antiserum.

Antibody arises by activation of the B lymphocytes or their precursors either by antigen or by antigen-primed macrophages. The B lymphocytes transform into morphologically different cells, blast cells, **immuno-blasts,** (plate 29.1b & f, facing p. 29.10) and **plasma cells** (fig. 29.7), which synthesize antibody in large amounts. Plasma cells are ovoid with eccentric nuclei and a pale perinuclear halo. Their cytoplasm is rich in endoplasmic reticulum, the RNA of which accounts for the basophilic staining with haematoxylin and eosin. Thus their structure indicates their powers of protein synthesis.

B lymphocytes produce only very little Ig, but sufficient to be detectable by refined techniques and to differentiate them from the T lymphocytes on which none can be detected.

In some infectious diseases, effective immunity is achieved by a combination of cell-mediated and humoral immunity.

Complement

In 1895 Bordet showed that some antigen-antibody reactions took place only in the presence of normal serum from any of several species of animals. This property of serum was said to be due to a factor which was called com-plement. Complement is now known to be composed of at least nine major components, referred to as C_1, C_2, C_3, etc. They are proteins and are present in non-activated form in the plasma of all mammals. Activation is achieved by immunoglobulins and antigen-antibody reactions as well as by products of micro-organisms; as a result of a number of sequential reactions several sub-stances are produced which facilitate most, if not all, immunological reactions, promote an inflammatory response and enhance phagocytosis. Their mode of action and role in disease are the subject of much current research and are more fully discussed in vol. 2.

Lymphocytes

The term lymphocyte literally means the 'cell found in lymph' and it is the predominant cell in thoracic duct lymph. There, as in the blood, 80–90 per cent of the lymphocytes are small (5–10 μm), and the remainder are medium or large (up to 15 μm). The distinction is of im-portance; small lymphocytes recirculate and do not

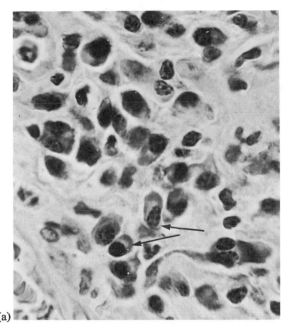

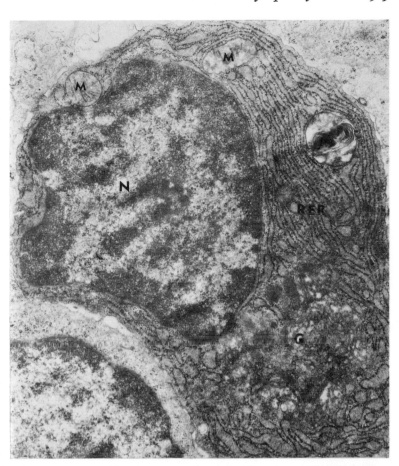

FIG. 29.7. Plasma cells. (a) A light microscopic field containing a number of plasma cells, the two most typical indicated by arrows. The clumped pattern of nuclear chromatin is seen (× 1000). (b) An electron micrograph from a rat lymph node. The nucleus (N) is eccentrically placed; the cytoplasm is packed with rough-surfaced endoplasmic reticulum (RER). There is a large Golgi region (G) and a few mitochondria (M). Glutaraldehyde fixation, araldite embedding (× 6750).

(b)

proliferate, while large lymphocytes do not recirculate, can proliferate rapidly and develop into small lymphocytes.

By light microscopy the small lymphocyte is featureless with a large nucleus and a narrow rim of cytoplasm. It lacks visible cytoplasmic granules but large lymphocytes on staining with pyronine often show cytoplasmic RNA. The EM shows that small lymphocytes have a few mitochondria, a Golgi apparatus and a small amount of smooth endoplasmic reticulum. Large lymphocytes may have numerous ribosomes in the cytoplasm. Lymphocytes have few cytoplasmic fibrils, in contrast to motile macrophages.

RECIRCULATION OF LYMPHOCYTES

Nearly all the lymph enters the blood via the thoracic duct. The lymphocytes then pass from the blood into the white pulp of the spleen or into lymph nodes. In the spleen they circulate through the white pulp and later enter the sinusoids and return to the circulation. In lymph nodes they pass through specialized postcapillary venules to enter the cortex. They then return to the blood via the efferent lymphatics and the thoracic duct lymph.

The recirculation through lymph nodes and spleen is important since it distributes immunologically competent cells and ensures their adequate exposure to antigen trapped by the macrophages in the organs. By this means, also, a large part of the lymphocyte population of the lymph nodes and spleen is replaced every few hours.

ORIGIN AND DIFFERENTIATION OF LYMPHOCYTES

All lymphocytes are derived from precursors, known as stem cells. In the fetus these first appear in the liver, but after birth they arise only in the bone marrow. Some of these precursors enter the thymus by way of the blood stream, undergo division and give rise to the T lymphocytes which then migrate to the peripheral lymphoid organs to populate their T lymphocyte areas. Others give rise to the thymus-independent or B lymphocytes. These were named B lymphocytes when it was discovered that in birds they were differentiated in the bursa of Fabricius. It was once thought that the mammalian equivalent of the bursa was the epitheliolymphoid tissue present in the walls of the gut, most markedly as Peyer's patches (p. 29.15). This view has not been confirmed and it is uncertain in what organ or organs mammalian stem cells differentiate into B lymphocytes (p. 29.16).

METHODS OF STUDYING LYMPHOCYTE FUNCTION

While light and electron microscopy have elucidated the structure of the lymphoid organs they fail to distinguish B and T lymphocytes, whose rapid and simple detection by immunological means has so greatly added to knowledge of immunology. These and other important discoveries were made by the following techniques.

Thoracic duct drainage

Cannulation and drainage of the thoracic duct allows the various cells in the lymph to be studied and identified, and pure preparations of types of lymphocyte can be prepared. The effect of injecting these cells into animals can be studied under various conditions. Drainage permits the investigation of the effects on the body of depletion of components of lymph.

Radiolabelling

Lymphocytes obtained by drainage can be labelled with ^{3}H- or ^{14}C-nucleosides or amino acids, which are incorporated in their RNA and proteins respectively. Such labelled cells can then be injected into an animal and their fate and distribution in various tissues and organs studied.

Neonatal thymectomy

The thymus gland can be excised in neonatal mice. The study of such animals established the presence of a thymic-dependent lymphoid system responsible for specific cell-mediated immunity, and identified specialized thymus-dependent sites of lymphoid tissue. If the excised thymus is enclosed in a chamber with walls permeable to fluids but not to cells and the chamber grafted into the animal, atrophy of the thymus-dependent regions does not occur; this suggests that the thymus produces a trophic hormone which plays a role in the differentiation of thymus-dependent lymphocytes.

Bursectomy

The bursa of Fabricius can be removed in birds, in the embryo within the eggshell. This technique established the existence of a lymphoid system dependent upon the bursa, controlling the development of B lymphocytes, which produce antibody.

Autoradiography

This technique, described on p. 13.3, is used to study the patterns of cell migration and to identify sites in lymph nodes where B or T lymphocytes are concentrated; it also allows the localization of antigen in primary and secondary responses to be studied.

Mitogenic agents and transformation

Substances collectively called **mitogens** can induce lymphocytes *in vitro* to enlarge, synthesize protein and divide into lymphoblastic forms sometimes known as immunoblasts. This phenomenon, known as **trans-**

formation, is used to explore the functional and class-specific attributes of lymphocytes. With mitogenic agents, e.g. plant lectins, and some bacterial lipopolysaccharides, transformation is not complete and the cells do not differentiate into fully immunocompetent cells capable of inducing cellular immunity or producing antibody. Mitogenic agents may be non-specific or specific for B or T cells.

In contrast, antigens transform only those B or T lymphocytes which have receptors for them and react to them. The resulting dividing cell lines give rise to specific effector cells.

Antigens are responsible for the immune responses leading to allograft rejection (transplantation antigens). They are represented on the donor's cells, including the lymphocytes. When two subjects are incompatible immunologically, a mixture of donor and host lymphocytes shows the phenomenon of transformation. Mixtures of cells from compatible subjects do not show such transformation.

Other agents of largely unknown biological significance such as human transfer factor (p. 29.23) can induce transformation.

Detection of antibody

Immunofluorescent techniques (p. 13.4) are used to study antibody formation by cells or groups of cells, e.g. transforming B lymphocytes.

Haemolytic plaque formation is used in the study of the production of haemolytic antibody against red blood cells. Agar plates containing fresh blood cells are covered with a suspension of the cells under test and antibody release is detected by the zones of haemolysis which surround those groups of cells which form antibody.

Skin grafts

Skin grafted from one individual of the same species to another is almost always rejected unless the donor and host are immunogenetically identical, e.g. litter mates in an inbred strain. Such graft rejection, the **host versus graft reaction**, is a valuable experimental tool in the study of the cellular immune response. It is used as an index of cellular immune competence in experiments on T lymphocyte and thymic function.

Reconstitution experiments: cell transfer

In the technique of reconstitution, procedures such as thymectomy, bursectomy, irradiation and administration of immunosuppressive drugs are used, separately or in combination, to deplete animals of their immunologically competent cells. Known, precisely defined, fractionated cell populations or tissues from other compatible animals are then transferred or grafted to the prepared animals. The nature and degree of immune

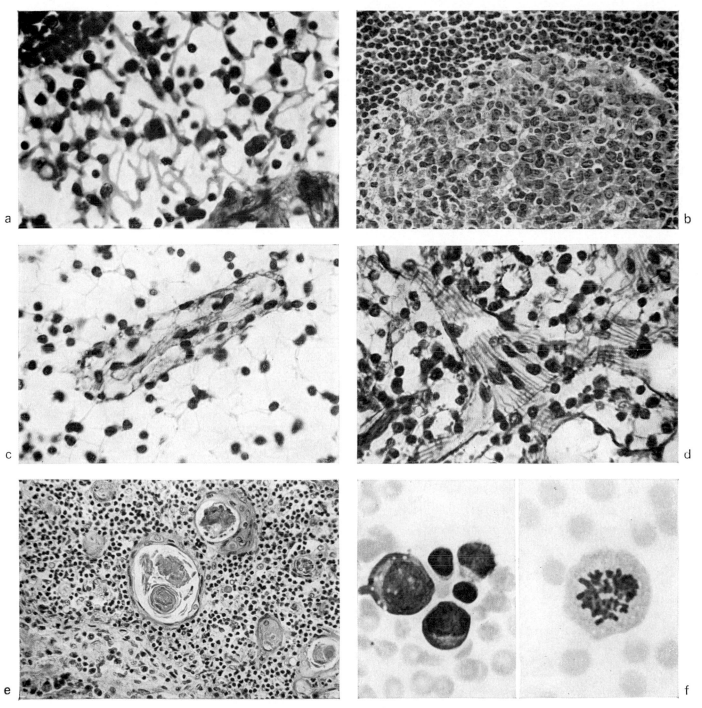

PLATE 29.1. Histology of the lymphoreticular tissues.

(a) Loose tissue in a medullary lymphatic sinusoid. Note the stellate reticular cells with their slender processes. Occasional macrophages show erythrophagocytosis. Masson trichrome (× 650). Courtesy of the late Dr. H.S.D. Garven.

(c) The prominent ellipsoid of the cat. Note the slender central capillary and loose surrounding sheath of reticular cells. Perfused spleen, haem. & eosin (× 500). Courtesy of the late Dr. H.S.D. Garven.

(e) Thymic medulla to show Hassall's corpuscles. Note the large pale medullary epithelial cells which surround them. Haem. & eosin (× 300). Courtesy of Dr. A.M. MacDonald.

(b) Germinal centre of lymph node. A zone of densely staining small lymphocytes surrounds the lighter staining germinal centre with its lymphoblasts and large lymphocytes. In the centre of the field a lymphoblast is in the metaphase stage of mitosis. Haem. and eosin (× 475).

(d) The endothelial cells (stave cells) of a splenic sinusoid which is beginning to branch into two. Perfused spleen, haem. & eosin (× 700). Courtesy of the late Dr. H.S.D. Garven.

(f) The 'blast' or pyroninophil transformation of the lymphocyte; the cell on the right is in mitosis (× 1200). Courtesy of Dr. Elizabeth Boyd.

reconstitution can be gauged by standard immunological challenges testing, for example, B or T lymphocyte responses.

Such experiments demonstrate that bone marrow contains stem cells of both thymic-dependent and thymic-independent lymphoid systems.

Graft versus host reaction

This reaction, described on p. 29.24, is an extension of the technique of cell transfer. By appropriate immunogenetic choice of host and donor, it is possible to ensure that the graft cells survive; immunologically competent T cells in the graft then react to certain of the host's antigens. The resulting graft versus host reaction leads to infiltration of the tissues of the host with dividing grafted lymphoid cells and stimulated host macrophages which produce a fatal wasting disease.

Antigenicity of the lymphocyte

Lymphocytes carry surface antigens specific for each class, i.e. B or T. The best known is the Thy 1 antigen on the surface of T lymphocytes in mice, formerly known as the θ antigen, but T and B lymphocytes in man probably also carry antigens specific for their own classes.

The antigenic differences between T lymphocytes of different strains of mice are sufficient to allow potent antisera to the Thy 1 antigen to be raised. By treatment with antiserum and complement, lymphoid cell populations can be selectively depleted of T lymphocytes, and used in the study of the cellular reactions to antigen.

Surface receptors

Lymphocytes and other immunologically active cells often possess surface receptors capable of binding antigens and immunologically active intermediates, such as complexes of antigen and antibody or of antigen, antibody and complement. Thus lymphocytes are known to carry receptors for the C3 component of complement, the Fc portion of IgG (vol. 2, p. 22.11) and antigens.

The study of lymphocyte receptors is likely to make substantial contributions to the understanding of lymphocyte function, but at present its chief value lies in the practical determination of lymphocyte class (B or T), since by using several detector systems, binding patterns specific for the two classes emerge.

Perhaps the best example of surface receptor binding is the highly specific reaction of B lymphocytes with antigen. The cells which bind the specific antigen concerned are called **antigen-reactive cells.** The phenomenon of antigen-binding causes transformation and initiates the humoral response. Antigen-reactive cells are found also in the T cell lineage and undergo transformation, in this case to initiate cellular immune reactions.

The nature of the receptors is not well known, although the B cell receptor for antigen probably consists of minute amounts of specific immunoglobulin on the cell surface.

Receptor properties can be exploited experimentally; for example, a radioactive antigen can be administered to kill the cells which bind it (antigen suicide).

The technique of **coated red cell rosetting** allows receptors for antigens and for immunologically active intermediates to be demonstrated *in vitro*. Red blood cells coated with appropriate substances, e.g. immunoglobulin or complement, can be seen to form a striking rosette surrounding a lymphocyte (fig. 29.8). A subclass of B lymphocytes of rats, mice and man binds IgG-coated red blood cells from most species, since the coating rather than the origin of the red cell is the important factor. Spontaneous red cell rosetting is seen when, for example, human T lymphocytes bind washed sheep red blood cells, and guinea-pig thymocytes spontaneously bind rabbit red blood cells. The significance of binding reactions of uncoated red blood cells is not known.

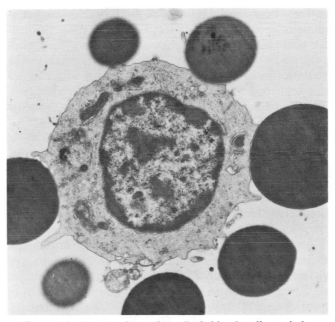

Fig. 29.8. Rosette formation. Red blood cells entirely surround and adhere to a central lymphocyte to form a rosette. (EM × 6000).

Methods for distinguishing B and T lymphocytes by receptor and other studies, and a summary of the two classes are given in table 29.1.

EXPERIMENTAL PREPARATION OF B AND T LYMPHOCYTES

B lymphocytes can be separated from T lymphocytes by virtue of their surface antibody. Suspensions of mixed T and B cells are separated by passing the cells through a column of beads coated with anti-immunoglobulin antibody. The beads are made of glass, plastic or of sepharose (a synthetic sugar polymer). B cells with

TABLE 29.1. Distinguishing characteristics of T and B lymphocytes.

Technical method	Characteristic	T lymphocyte	B lymphocyte
Rosetting with complement-coated red cells	Surface receptors for complement	−	+ + +
Rosetting with IgG-coated red cells	Surface receptors for IgG (Fc fragment)	±	+ +
Immunofluorescence or radioimmunolabelling	Surface immunoglobulins	−	+ + +

Microscopy of lymphocyte cultures	Transformation
	    by phytohaemagglutinin
	    by lipopolysaccharide
		
		+
		−
			
			−
			+

Autoradiography, thoracic duct cannulation, lymphocyte labelling	Distribution
	    in lymph nodes
	    in Malpighian corpuscles
	    in thoracic duct lymph
		
		Paracortex
		Periarteriolar sheath
		75%
			
			Cortex
			Peripheral white pulp 25%

Organ ablation	Sites of maturation	Thymus	Bursa of Fabricius in birds
Immunofluorescence with heterologous antisera	Specific human lymphocyte antigens (HL-A)	HL-T	HL-B

surface immunoglobulin stick to the anti-immuno-globulin-coated beads, while T cells pass through the column. In this way a pure preparation of T lympho-cytes can be obtained. The B lymphocytes stuck to the column can be recovered by washing or by digestion of the sepharose beads with dextranase. B lymphocytes may be prepared by destruction of T cells in a mixed suspension, using a specific cytotoxic anti-Thy 1 or anti-thymocyte antiserum. Subsequent separation of viable cells gives pure B lymphocyte suspensions. Techniques dependent on the formation of rosettes of complement-coated red blood cells around B lymphocytes have also been used to separate T and B lymphocytes. The complement-coated red cells adhere to the surface of the B lymphocytes forming a rosette (fig. 29.8) but not to the T lymphocytes. When the suspension is centrifuged on a density gradient, the B lymphocytes with their rosettes of red cells settle rapidly to the bottom, leaving a top layer of T lymphocytes. In this way fairly pure suspensions of both B and T lymphocytes can be prepared from a single sample of blood, spleen or lymph node. Nearly pure populations of circulating B or T lymphocytes can be produced in X-irradiated thymectomized animals by injecting either T lymphocytes, lymph node cells or bone marrow (B lymphocytes and their precursors). The injected cells proliferate and result in animals with only the T or B lymphocytes.

LYMPH NODES AND EPITHELIO-LYMPHOID TISSUE

The lymphatic system consists of myriads of tiny lymph-atic capillaries which form plexuses in most tissues, an important exception being the central nervous system. Numerous afferent lymphatic vessels drain into the lymph nodes, through which the lymph percolates and leaves by efferent lymphatic vessels (fig. 29.9). These carry the lymph to other nodes or groups of nodes and ultimately return it to the blood via the thoracic duct.

In the nodes the lymph is filtered and may acquire additional lymphocytes, macrophages and antibodies.

Lymph nodes are distributed widely throughout the body, and knowledge of the lymphatic drainage is of clinical importance since regional involvement of the lymph nodes is often a clue to the site of infection, and malignant tumours often spread along the lymphatic channels to involve the lymph nodes.

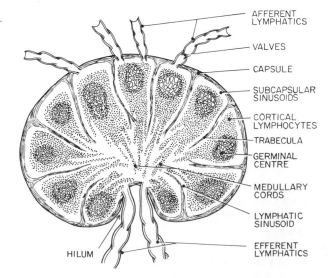

FIG. 29.9. Transverse section of a lymph node.

Structure of lymph nodes (figs. 29.9 and 10)

Lymph nodes are pale grey, and vary in size from a pinhead to a large bean, which they resemble by having flattened sides and a concave hilum. Each node is surrounded by a fibrous capsule which sends a delicate tracery of supportive fibrous trabeculae into the interior. The trabeculae are widely fenestrated and in sections routinely stained are seen only as thin sheaths of connective tissue around the blood vessels which they invest.

The interior of the lymph node can be divided into four zones (fig. 29.10).

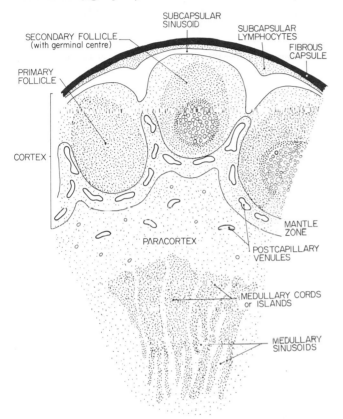

FIG. 29.10. The zones of the lymph node. The cortex extends from the capsule to include the mantle zone of the deep cortex. The mantle zone shown here between two heavy lines is a histologically vague zone, not delineated from the underlying paracortex; it is defined functionally by the localization of recirculating B lymphocytes (p. 29.9). Postcapillary venules are concentrated in the paracortex. Lymphocyte production in the paracortex is not follicular but diffuse; it occurs in numerous small foci of lymphoblasts and macrophages (not shown). Note the medullary lymphocytic islands between the rich plexus of sinusoids conveying lymph to the efferent lymphatics.

(1) The **peripheral zone** contains round dense aggregates of lymphocytes known as **follicles** and the reticulin fibres are less condensed than in the medulla. Except in very early life, follicles contain central paler areas consisting of lymphoblastic cells known as **germinal centres** (plate 29.1b, facing p. 29.10). Follicles in which there are no germinal centres are called **primary follicles**; those containing germinal centres are called **secondary** or **germinal follicles.**

(2) The **mantle zone**, also known as the marginal zone, is morphologically ill defined. It lies on the deep aspect of the follicles where the lymphocytes are more loosely packed and contains plasma cells, macrophages and a few capillary blood vessels. It differs functionally from the underlying paracortex by its resistance to lymphocyte depletion following thymectomy. It is here that antibody-producing plasma cells are most prominent in the immune response.

The peripheral zone containing the follicles and the mantle zone together make up the **cortex** which is predominantly a B cell zone.

(3) The **paracortex** lies between the cortex and the medulla and is devoid of follicles. It contains postcapillary venules and is populated predominantly by macrophages and T lymphocytes and a few scattered lymphoblastic precursors.

(4) The **medulla**, the deepest zone, is centred on the hilum and is made up of interconnecting cords of densely packed lymphocytes of both B and T type. The medullary cords are surrounded by sinusoidal spaces which are much less rich in lymphocytes and are crossed by the processes of many reticular cells. The lymph percolates through these sinusoids on its journey to the hilum.

Afferent lymphatic channels converge upon the convex surface of the node, penetrate the capsule and pour their lymph, usually through valved openings (fig. 29.11), into the **subcapsular sinusoid.** This is a potential space made up of loose reticular and endothelial tissue; it runs immediately under the capsule of the node and can be best seen when it contains only a few lymphocytes (fig. 29.10). Sinusoids run radially from it into the cortex and eventually join the loose plexus of sinusoids in the medulla. From the medulla one or two large efferent vessels carry the lymph away from the node.

Lymph always flows from the large area of the capsule with its numerous afferent lymphatics to the narrow area of the hilum with its few efferent lymphatics, in keeping with the principle that lymphatic channels decrease in number but increase in calibre as they travel towards the thoracic duct.

A neurovascular bundle supplies each node. It enters through the hilum and the main blood vessels run in connective tissue trabeculae for a short distance before ramifying in the cortex. Thence drainage is to a system of postcapillary venules from which lymphocytes migrate from the blood stream into the node. This migration offsets the large number of lymphocytes which are lost to the node in the efferent lymph. The recirculation of the lymphocyte is considered in detail on p. 29.9.

SINUSOIDS

The subcapsular, cortical and medullary sinusoids are made up of loosely arranged stellate reticular and endothelial cells, supported on a reticulin scaffolding and continuous with the endothelium of the lymphatic vessels

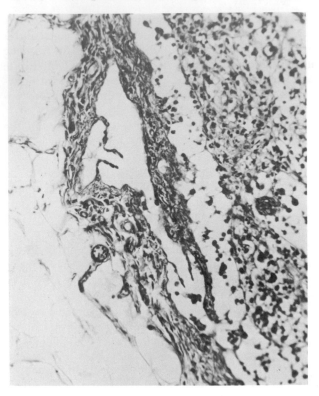

FIG. 29.11. Lymphatic valves. The tenuous valvular flaps of a small efferent vessel joining a major one are seen above left. Further down the course of the main lymphatic cleft another pair can be seen. Note the expanded subcapsular sinusoid immediately to the right of the capsule; fine reticulin threads traverse it but it is relatively free of cells in contrast to the cortical lymphoid tissue on the extreme right (× 210). Courtesy of the late Dr. H.S.D. Garven.

which penetrate the capsule. Their fenestrations provide pathways of least resistance for the lymph flow, but lymph is free to percolate back and forth into adjacent lymphoid masses and in this way lymphocytes enter the lymphatic sinusoids.

Phagocytic cells frequently bridge across the lumen of the sinusoids which often contain free macrophages. In plate 29.1a, facing p. 29.10, a macrophage which has ingested a red blood cell can be seen. Small numbers of extravasated red blood cells are normally present in the tissues and gain access to the lymphatics; after bruising, many extravasated red blood cells pass to the local lymph nodes where they are phagocytosed by macrophages which later show haemosiderin in their cytoplasm.

The number of free macrophages in the sinusoids is increased by inflammatory or antigenic stimulation. In such circumstances the subcapsular and other sinusoids become packed with large round macrophages, together with numbers of neutrophil polymorphs which have migrated in with the lymph from the inflamed region. Polymorphs are not prominent in healthy sinu-

soids. Plasma cells are also sparse in unstimulated nodes, but easily found in an inflamed or reactive node. Details of the changes seen in such nodes are given on p. 29.18.

The calibre of the sinusoids varies and they are often difficult to see, particularly in an unstimulated node which is handling little lymph, or when reactive lymphopoiesis is so brisk that expanding cortical follicles have obliterated them (fig. 29.17b). They are seen most easily when dilated in moderately reactive nodes, e.g. nodes on the lesser curvature of the stomach draining a chronic peptic ulcer. In a Masson's trichrome preparation, the delicate processes of the littoral cells can be easily demonstrated in well expanded sinusoids. Elsewhere in the node the reticular cells of the scaffolding are obscured by the density of the lymphocytes, although reticulin fibres can readily be shown by silver impregnation.

Functions of the lymph node

The lymph node serves the following defensive and immunological functions. (1) It filters the afferent lymph containing normal or inflammatory cell debris and bacteria, which are then exposed to the macrophages. (2) It is a centre where macrophages trap and process antigens, and direct the immune responses. (3) It is a centre for lymphocyte production following antigenic stimulation. The cellular immune response is mediated through T lymphocytes of the paracortex. The humoral immune response involves B lymphocytes of the cortex and their transformation into plasma cells which produce antibody.

SYNTHESIS OF ANTIBODY

Lymph nodes produce antibody in response to local antigen and release it into the circulation. If an antigen is injected into the limb of an animal, cannulation of the local lymphatics shows that antibody is absent from the afferent channels of the regional lymph nodes but present in high concentration in their efferent channels. This suggests strongly that antibody is formed in the lymph nodes, but falls short of absolute proof since the antibody may have been formed elsewhere and gained the efferent lymphatics via the blood supply to the node. Conclusive proof of the synthesis of antibody within the lymph node comes from an experiment based on the 'double antigen technique' (fig. 29.12).

Using the hind limbs of a rabbit, antigen A is injected into one foot and antigen B into the other. After a suitable interval the efferent lymphatics of the popliteal lymph nodes are cannulated and the concentration of antibody against A and B measured on each side. The efferent lymphatics contain high levels of antibody against the antigen which their nodes receive, and scarcely any against the one injected into the opposite limb. In the

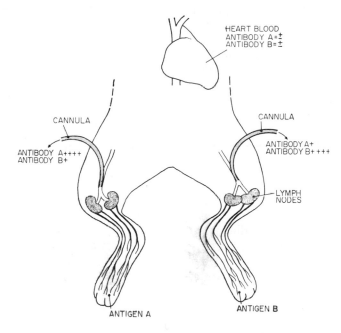

FIG. 29.12. The double antigen technique to show that antibody is produced in the lymph nodes which drain sites of local antigen injection.

blood, the antibodies against antigens A and B are present in concentrations too low to account for those in the efferent lymphatics by mere diffusion; the distribution of antibody can be explained readily only by its production in the local lymph nodes.

Epitheliolymphoid tissue

Lymphoid tissue is not always organized into lymph nodes but may lie directly under mucosal surfaces. Sites where such large aggregations occur are the tonsillar ring in the mouth and pharynx, and Peyer's patches of the small intestine and the appendix. Small aggregations, amounting perhaps to a solitary follicle, with or without an active germinal centre, occur in the mucosa of the rest of the alimentary tract and in the urinary and respiratory tracts. The lymphoid tissue in the gut wall, often referred to as gut-associated lymphoid tissue, contains large germinal centres. The corona of surrounding lymphocytes is prominent and frequently shows marked eccentricity, forming a cap overlying the luminal aspect of the germinal centre. Around the periphery of the lymphoid follicles, antibody-forming plasma cells are often numerous.

None of the epitheliolymphoid collections has a fibrous capsule or a subcapsular sinusoid as in a lymph node. The lymphatic sinusoids which traverse their lymphoid parenchyma begin blindly and connect with a plexus of lymphatic capillaries in the underlying connective tissue which convey lymph to the regional nodes.

BURSA OF FABRICIUS

The idea that certain lymphoid organs are responsible for the production of pure populations of B and T lymphocytes is an attractive one which has found many adherents. The thymus has been known for some time to be the source in the fetus and newborn animal of T lymphocytes essential to cell-mediated immunity, but the source of B lymphocytes is still controversial. Most studies of their origin have been done on birds, in which they are clearly dependent on the bursa of Fabricius. If the bursa is removed *in ovo*, the chick has no antibody-forming B lymphocytes. Like the mammalian gut epitheliolymphoid tissue, the bursal lymphocytes are closely associated with the overlying epithelium which is raised

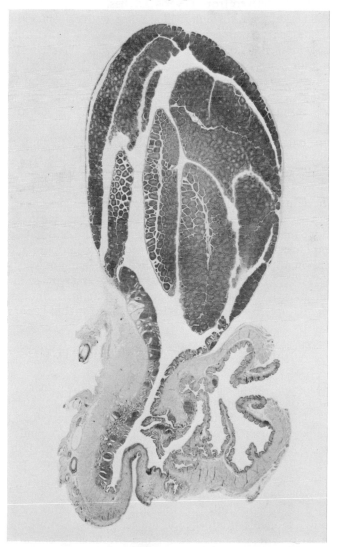

FIG. 29.13. Bursa of Fabricius. A longitudinal section shows the bursa, above; the lumen is continuous through the narrow bursal canal with the gut, below right. The longitudinal plicae of the bursal epithelium contain numerous polygonal packets of lymphocytes ($\times$ 4). Courtesy of Dr. J.G. Campbell.

into folds (fig. 29.13). Large follicles are also present in the bursa and their contained lymphoblasts take up ^{3}H-thymidine, especially if it is introduced into the lumen. The labelled cells and their progeny rapidly seed, particularly to the spleen, and on antigenic stimulation yield antibody-forming cells.

In rabbits, the appendix is rich in lymphoid tissue of a type similar to that in the bursa in birds. Lymphoid cells in the appendix can be labelled with ^{3}H-thymidine by direct instillation, as in the bursa of birds. A cap of labelled small lymphocytes subsequently appears over the epithelial aspect of the germinal centre and some of these cells later migrate to lymph nodes and spleen. They are, however, greatly diluted with similar unlabelled cells, probably derived from Peyer's patches.

The gut wall, through which many antigens enter the tissues, is very rich in lymphoid tissue. This probably provides most of the B lymphocytes which seed the mantle zones of the lymph nodes and the peripheral white pulp in the spleen. Stem cells from bone marrow may enter germinal centres of gut-associated lymphoid tissue where, possibly under the influence of antigen from the gut, they develop into B lymphocytes; they then circulate to lymph nodes, where they multiply further. Germ-free animals do not develop germinal centres in the lymph nodes and spleen.

An alternative view is that bursa-equivalent tissue in the adult mammal is in the bone marrow. This is supported by the fact that in rodents up to 30 per cent of bone marrow cells are B lymphocytes. These cells have a rapid turnover, recirculate and seed to lymph nodes and spleen where they apparently die. Some immunologists now regard the liver in the fetus and bone marrow in the adult as the bursa-equivalent tissue of mammals, but it is premature to suggest that the evidence for this is conclusive.

LYMPHOCYTES AND THE IMMUNE SYSTEM

Lymphocytes are formed in the thymus, bone marrow and cortex of lymph nodes by the division and maturation of lymphoid stem cells. These primitive cells are found chiefly in the germinal centres, where they undergo mitosis. Around the germinal centre there are young medium and small lymphocytes which push the older ones out towards the periphery of the lymphoid follicle.

When the lymphoid tissue is destroyed by X-rays, it can be reconstituted by injecting cell preparations not only from spleen and lymph nodes, but also from bone marrow. Bone marrow therefore presumably contains lymphoid stem cells which enter the circulation and gain access to the lymphoid organs, where they differentiate into lymphocytes.

In a young animal development of the peripheral lymphoid tissue depends upon the presence of a function-ing thymus (p. 29.40). Lymphoid tissue of a late embryo and newborn animal consists of loose sheets of lymphoid cells and primary follicles. These soon acquire germinal centres by exposure to natural antigens, which reach them via the lymphatics of organs in contact with the environment, e.g. the gut and the lungs. Animals kept in a germ-free environment show only a few rudimentary germinal centres. Thymectomy in the newborn animal leads to marked lymphopenia and hypoplasia of lymphoid tissue in which the size and number both of primary follicles and of germinal centres is much reduced; there are severe defects of cellular immunity and some diminution in antibody formation.

Life span of lymphocytes

Tritiated thymidine is rapidly incorporated in the DNA of dividing large lymphocytes but very poorly into small lymphocytes. Large lymphocytes appear to have a short life since they mature rapidly into small lymphocytes. The latter are formed infrequently and since their numbers are fairly constant, they must have a long life. Continuous transfusion of the rat with tritiated thymidine labels only 50 per cent of the small lymphocytes after 1 month and even after 3 months not all are labelled. In man the average life of the small lymphocyte is about 100 days, but some probably live very much longer, possibly for years. Thus at any one time only a small percentage of circulating small lymphocytes is newly formed.

Circulation of lymphocytes (fig. 29.14)

The number of cells which enter the blood from the lymph nodes via the thoracic duct each day is ten to fifteen times the total number in the blood at any given time, so there must be a compensatory loss from the blood stream. Losses of blood-borne lymphocytes from the surface of the alimentary and respiratory tracts are small, so lymphocytes must somehow circulate from the blood stream back into the lymphatic system. The afferent lymphatics carry relatively few lymphocytes, and the number in the nodes always remains substantially unchanged. The outpouring of lymphocytes from the efferent lymphatics must therefore be made good within the node. This constancy of number and distribution is maintained by small lymphocytes in the blood re-entering nodes through the unusually tall endothelium of the postcapillary venules of the cortex (plate 29.2d & e, facing p. 29.42, and fig. 29.15).

In animal experiments, external drainage of the thoracic duct eventually abstracts fewer and fewer small lymphocytes from the system, but the numbers draining away per day increase if viable compatible lymphocytes are given by intravenous injection. Administration of tritiated thymidine shows that virtually no lymphocyte regeneration goes on during the course of the experiment. If labelled lymphocytes are injected, about 80 per cent

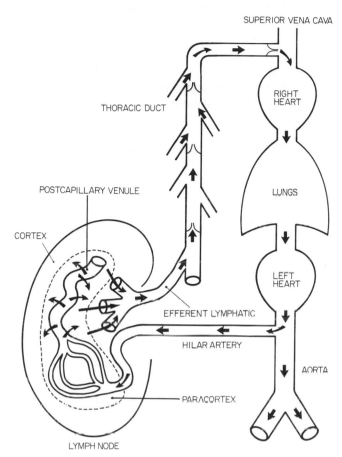

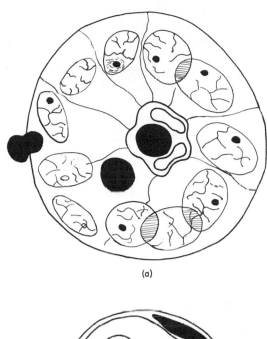

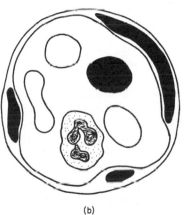

FIG. 29.14. Circulation of lymphocytes. Both B and T lymphocytes travel to the lymph nodes in the hilar artery and subsequently emigrate into the lymphoid tissue via the endothelium of the postcapillary venules. There they mingle with lymphocytes of the cortex (B areas) and paracortex (T areas). Simultaneously, equivalent numbers of lymphocytes leave in the efferent lymphatics so that a balanced flow through the node is maintained. The circulation is completed by the ultimate return of the efferent lymphocytes to the blood stream via the thoracic duct which is the main entrance of lymphocytes to the vascular system.

FIG. 29.15. Comparison of a lymph node postcapillary venule with a comparable vessel from connective tissue. (a) A postcapillary venule; this has tall endothelium and a small lumen, here occupied by two red blood cells and a lymphocyte. In sections where circulating cells are absent, the lumen often appears obliterated by the cytoplasm of opposed endothelial cells. Note the multiplicity of overlapping nuclei which are very large and pale with prominent nucleoli. In routine sections the cytoplasmic boundaries of the endothelial cells are indistinct and the endothelium often appears as an abundant eosinophilic syncytial band. A lymphocyte is shown migrating outwards through the cytoplasm of the endothelial cells. (b) A capillary venule from connective tissue; this has, by contrast, a wide lumen with flattened dense endothelial nuclei and thin cytoplasm.

appear in the thoracic duct. These findings indicate that migration of lymphocytes from blood to lymph node can balance the loss from the node without the need for appreciable lymphopoiesis.

The few medium and large lymphocytes which reach the thoracic duct daily do not appreciably lessen when the duct is drained, and so differ markedly from the small lymphocytes. They owe their continuing presence in the efferent lymph to uninterrupted production in the lymph nodes. They do not recirculate appreciably to the lymph nodes via the postcapillary venules.

Autoradiography, after injection of labelled lymphocytes into the blood, shows striking accumulations of label in lymph nodes, Peyer's patches and spleen, and these are the sites where lymphocytes return from blood to lymph. The label is not seen in the thymus, which is excluded from the circulation of the lymphocyte.

As well as keeping the number and distribution of the lymphocytes constant, their circulation has important immunological implications; chiefly it provides a corps of diversely reactive lymphocytes which enable antigens localized in one or a few regional nodes to encounter specifically responsive cells.

B lymphocyte system

Primary follicles in the cortex of the lymph node are the domain of the B lymphocytes. Around the follicles in the mantle zone there is an ill defined mesh of reticulin, also containing B lymphocytes; this is one of the sites where plasma cells develop in the humoral immune response (p. 29.9). The mantle zone is in contact with the underlying paracortex which permits easy exchange and contact between the B cells of the follicle and the T cells of the paracortex.

Follicles in Peyer's patches and the tonsils differ from those in the peripheral lymph nodes in the class of immunoglobulin produced by their B cell derivatives. Those of the gut produce IgA which is of low molecular weight, associated with the protection of surfaces and found in tears, saliva and other secretions. Those of the peripheral system produce high molecular weight IgM and low molecular weight IgG.

The detailed functional events of the primary and secondary immune response in lymphoid tissue are dealt with on p. 29.20. Suffice it to say here that after secondary antigenic stimulation, i.e. a second or subsequent encounter with an antigen, the primary follicles acquire germinal centres made up of large, pale, mitosing lymphoblasts and they are then known as germinal follicles. Because the normal animal is subject to repeated antigenic stimuli, primary follicles of the lymph nodes usually acquire germinal centres shortly after birth. In the adult most of the lymphoid follicles are therefore germinal follicles, but there may be a few newly formed primary follicles which have not yet taken part in a secondary immune response. The apparent absence of germinal centres from many follicles in a single histological section may give a false impression of the frequency of primary follicles since the section may not pass through the germinal centre, especially if it is small or eccentric. Serial sections are needed to estimate the incidence of primary follicles.

As germinal follicles form, the lymphocyte population of the mantle zones increases, making the zone prominent. However only a minority of lymphocytes found in the mantle zone are derived from the germinal follicle; the majority come from the blood stream by recirculation.

REACTIVE LYMPH NODE

Immunological stimulation leads to the development of the reactive lymph node. A reactive node usually drains an abscess site, ulcer or other focus of inflammation. Much antigen-containing lymph enters the node and dilates the subcapsular and radial sinusoids. Many macrophages appear in the sinusoids and in acute infections polymorphs may be seen. In primary humoral responses most of the immune activity and plasma cell production occur in both cortex and medulla, but the humoral response to many natural infections is essentially

secondary and there is considerable increase in the number and size of the follicles with much germinal centre activity. In cell-mediated responses there is increased paracortical activity and cellularity. Understandably the nodes become much bigger due to the cortical and paracortical hyperplasia; this and the increased lymph flow make their capsules tense and give rise to pain. Enlarged reactive subcutaneous lymph nodes are easy to detect clinically by palpation because of their size and their tenderness on pressure.

Underlying these gross changes are the responses of the B lymphocyte (immune-antibody) and T lymphocyte (immune-cellular) systems.

B LYMPHOCYTE (HUMORAL) RESPONSES

Primary response

When an antigen enters the tissues, most of it is rapidly taken up by macrophages of the subcapsular sinusoids and medulla of local lymph nodes (fig. 29.16 a). Here the antigen-bearing macrophages influence surrounding lymphocytes which are thought to have an intrinsic, genetically determined ability to react with specific antigens for which they happen to carry receptors. Virgin lymphocytes probably produce minute amounts of immunoglobulins containing receptors for one antigen or a very limited number of related ones. Those lymphocytes which are responsive to the antigen processed by or retained on macrophages transform into lymphoblastic forms, undergo mitosis and finally give rise to plasma cells which produce specific antibody of the same class and specificity as that on the lymphocyte from which they are derived. Such macrophage-centred lymphocyte transformations and plasma cell production are confined largely to the regions of antigen localization in the medullary sinusoids and superficial cortex in and around the subcapsular sinusoids. Although these changes can be detected in the cortex during the primary response, there is no marked lymphocyte proliferation or follicular enlargement.

There are three main functions of the primary response: (1) avoidance of immune tolerance, (2) production of antibody and (3) preparation for secondary and subsequent (anamnestic) responses.

Avoidance of tolerance. Tolerance is the failure of an animal to make the expected immune response following exposure to an antigen. It can be induced by injecting the antigen in certain special circumstances (p. 29.24) and may last for lengthy periods during which specific antibody formation to the specific antigen is undetectable. Thus tolerance may arise when there are large numbers of circulating B lymphocytes with low affinity for antigen which can take up antigen from the circulation but not in amounts sufficient to stimulate their transformation to antibody-forming cells. The sheer numbers of such cells may abstract so much of the avail-

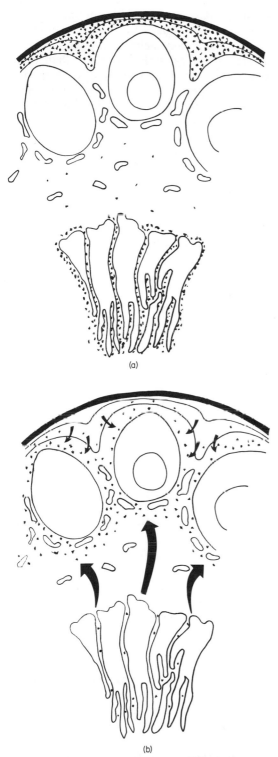

(a)

(b)

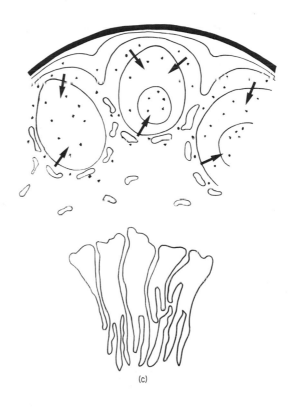

(c)

FIG. 29.16. Movements of antigen in a lymph node. Primary response. (a) Antigen injected for the first time is taken up mainly in the subcapsular and medullary sinusoids. (b) The antigen shift begins by migration of antigen from the sites of initial localization to the perifollicular zones; not only is the distribution of antigen changed but the total amount is reduced by phagocytic digestion. (c) Finally, further migration takes antigen into the middle of the primary follicles and into the germinal centres of existing secondary follicles.

able antigen that little remains to evoke a response in the minority of lymphocytes which do have sufficient affinity and sensitivity to react. The result is the state of tolerance.

Tolerance is avoided when there is good antigen trapping and concentration without exposure of free antigen to excessive numbers of lymphocytes. The primary response is well suited to meeting those requirements, since it takes place in regions of the lymph node where antigen trapping by macrophages is good, but which are outside the main traffic area for recirculation of the lymphocytes. The number of lymphocytes successively exposed to antigen is thus kept down to proportions which help to discriminate against tolerance but favour an immune response.

Production of antibody. In the primary response, trapping and processing of antigen by the macrophages appears to be essential, at least for particulate antigens. The antibody response takes place largely outside the main area of lymphocyte circulation. Perhaps for both of those reasons the antibody response is rather feeble.

In the primary response the first antibody produced by plasma cells is of high molecular weight and of the IgM class, as opposed to the low molecular weight IgG which appears later in the primary response and also characterizes the secondary response. The IgM secreted by the plasma cells leaves the lymph node in the efferent lymph and reaches the blood stream where it may neutralize antigen elsewhere in the body. Formation of IgM antibody gradually increases during the response. The primary response lasts 10–14 days, but the antibody produced may linger for some weeks.

Preparation for the secondary response. In the natural sequence of immune responses, repeated exposures to antigen lead to primary, secondary and anamnestic responses, and each stage prepares the way for the succeeding one. Thus the primary response ensures that the secondary response is sensitive, rapid and intense. This is effected by certain unspectacular events during the primary response which ensure (1) optimum sites for a future secondary response and (2) the priming of cells in these sites to produce a sensitive and rapid response. Among those events is the **antigen shift** in which there is a marked movement of antigen from the medulla and subcapsular sinusoids first into the macrophages of the mantle zone of the follicles and later into the primary follicles or germinal centres themselves (fig. 29.16 b and c).

The reasons for the shift are twofold. First, antigen-containing medullary and other macrophages may migrate actively, and secondly some antigen which is still circulating (perhaps, at this stage, combined with antibody) may be taken up *de novo* by macrophages in the mantle zones of follicles. Although only speculative, there is a possibility that IgM antibody formed early in the primary response (and perhaps complexed with antigen and complement) may become fixed to groups of macrophages, which serve as a recognition mechanism, encouraging further deposition or shift of antigen to them. The final step takes antigen into the centre of the follicle. In the absence of any lymphatic channels in the follicles, another mode of transport is needed. The processes of the local dendritic macrophages span relatively great distances; antigen passes along them and diffuses through the germinal centre while remaining bound to the surface of the cells. It may pass from one cell to another along intertwining dendritic processes. At this stage of the primary response the amount of antigen in the node is usually small and concentration on the dendritic processes may help it to exert its effect on surrounding lymphocytes. Proliferative changes in the lymphoid tissue around the macrophages in the follicles and surrounding regions are not marked at this time. However, localization of antigen there, especially in the form of complexes with IgM antibody and possibly complement, sequesters B lymphocytes from the circulation and increases the local population. Surrounding lymphoid tissue is now better able to respond to future encounters with antigen.

Macrophages of the mantle zone are particularly well placed to trigger a secondary response, for they lie directly in the pathway of recirculating lymphocytes and thus maximum contact with trapped antigen is ensured. The antigen shift during the primary response is an important determinant of the site and sensitivity of future secondary responses.

During the primary response the germinal centres do not enlarge, and there is no significant increase in the lymphoblasts or production of 'memory cells'. These findings are in keeping with the transient nature and short memory of the primary response. Secondary responses have to be stimulated before the primary response has entirely decayed, if maximal antibody production is to occur.

Secondary response

The secondary response in the lymph node is marked by rapid production of immunoglobulin of low molecular weight, i.e. IgG. Morphologically, the changes associated with the reactive node appear and new follicles with active germinal centres form in the cortex (fig. 29.17).

Particulate antigen or soluble antigen complexed with preformed antibody which reaches the node is avidly phagocytosed by the macrophages in the medulla and plays no further part in the response. Antigen is retained also by dendritic macrophages of the mantle zone which were active in processing antigen in the primary response.

Later, mitotic activity of the central lymphoblasts in the follicles enlarges the germinal centres with the production of memory cells. Plasma cells do not usually appear within the germinal centres. Heightened sensitivity of lymphocytes and redistribution of antigen during the primary response are probable reasons for the speed and site of the secondary response.

Significance of primary IgM production for the secondary response. The production of IgM antibodies during the primary response is probably central to the antigen shift and to the ensuing cellular reactions of the secondary response. IgM is retained in trace amounts in lymph nodes for prolonged periods, both free and as antigen-antibody complexes bound to surfaces of dendritic

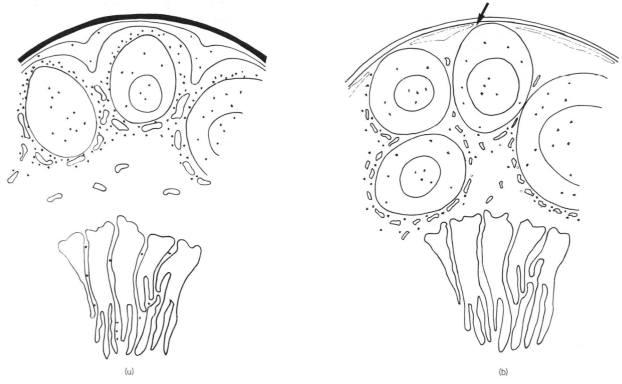

(a) (b)

FIG. 29.17. Antigens and the secondary response. In the early secondary response antigen is taken up by the lymph node much as in the early primary response (fig. 29.16 a). In the later stages the pattern differs as follows. (a) There is rapid localization of antigen in all areas primed by the antigen shift of the primary response, i.e. the perifollicular and mantle zones, inner follicles and germinal centres. Antigen is lost from the other areas, not by a redistribution or shift, but by rapid catabolism by macrophages. As much as 98 per cent of the antigen can be destroyed, leaving only 2 per cent in the cortex. (b) Later, stimulation of primary follicles and existing germinal centres by antigen-retaining dendritic macrophages takes place with much lymphoblastic mitosis, formation of new germinal centres and enlargement of existing ones. Memory cells are generated and are the basis of future anamnestic responses. The arrow indicates the compressed subcapsular sinusoids.

macrophages in the follicle and surrounding regions. The cell-bound IgM acts as a sensitive recognition and concentrating system for lymph-borne antigen. It may also allow very small amounts of antigen to trigger a secondary response in lymphocytes surrounding the IgM-bearing dendritic macrophages. The important role of preformed IgM in the formation of germinal follicles is seen in experiments where a primary injection of antigen in animals pretreated with specific IgM can mimic a secondary immune response with generation of germinal centres in the node.

Changes in the mantle zone. Germinal centres are not essential for antibody production, and are concerned largely with memory cell production later in the response. In germ-free animals the secondary response begins in the mantle zone before significant germinal centre production is under way. B and T lymphocytes of all shades of immunological specificity pass through this zone and the adjacent paracortex during their recirculation from peripheral blood. There they have the opportunity to interact with antigen which has been con-

centrated on the surfaces of macrophages of the zone. The number of transforming lymphocytes and plasma cells found around the macrophages of the mantle zone during the secondary response testify to its importance.

Changes in the follicles. Later in the secondary response and paving the way for future anamnestic responses, changes take place around the antigen-bearing dendritic macrophages within the follicles. Mitotic division of lymphoblasts increases their numbers and contributes to the production of germinal centres. In germ-free animals with only primary follicles, lymphoblastic divisions give rise to germinal centres for the first time; in adult animals they enlarge existing centres or may create new centres in primary follicles. In the reactive centres many of the proliferating cells die and are phagocytosed by macrophages. The nuclear remnants, which shrink and stain intensely with haematoxylin (pyknosis), make the macrophages which ingest them conspicuous.

Changes in the centres of the follicles during the secondary response are interpreted as producing **memory** cells which can respond to specific antigen long after serum antibody titres have fallen to insignificant levels; this is known as the **anamnestic response**. In the germinal centres continuous cell production and cell death take place, with phagocytosis of dead cells. The lymphoblasts divide in close contact with antigen-retaining macrophages which ensure their immune specificity. The mitotic potential and 'memory' can be retained almost indefinitely by asymmetric mitotic divisions (fig. 29.18). The final product, the small lymphocyte, is long-lived.

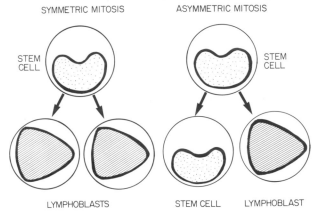

SYMMETRIC MITOSIS   ASYMMETRIC MITOSIS

STEM CELL   STEM CELL

LYMPHOBLASTS   STEM CELL   LYMPHOBLAST

FIG. 29.18. Lymphoid cell production is usually by symmetric maturation division, mitotic potential declining as the small lymphocyte is approached. Occasional asymmetric mitotic divisions help to retain mitotic potential by producing one daughter cell which is a stage more mature, and another identical to the progenitor. The process is here illustrated at the level of lymphoblast production from stem cells.

In addition, the high rate of cell death and tingible body formation is interpreted as elimination of cells not suited to the host's immunological needs, perhaps because they are aberrant or of weak specificity.

New germinal centres and the lymphocytes which they produce are initially 'clonal' in the sense that their cells are all immunologically similar and respond only to the specific antigen which evoked the germinal centre. It could therefore happen that the lymph node or group of lymph nodes richest in a given antigen might not contain a single centre capable of specific reaction. However, as the lymphocytic progeny of germinal centres can enter the efferent lymph and join the circulating lymphocyte pool, their immune specificity is soon distributed throughout the entire lymphoid system.

The generation of memory cells at a time in the secondary response when antigen is becoming scarce, due to the rise in high affinity antibody, guarantees the specificity of the future response and increases its sensitivity, so favouring good anamnestic reactions.

T lymphocyte system

In lymph nodes T lymphocytes are localized in the paracortex into which recirculating B and T lymphocytes pass after traversing the tall endothelium of the post-capillary venules. After entering the paracortex, B lymphocytes migrate to the mantle zones of the cortical follicles, but T lymphocytes remain in the pool of T lymphocytes in the paracortex. This pool is continuously turning over by migration into the efferent medullary sinusoids. Efferent lymph contains a high proportion of T cells and thoracic duct drainage depletes the lymphocytes in the paracortex much more than those in the cortex. Neonatal thymectomy causes severe hypoplasia in the paracortex and also some diminution in the number, size and reactivity of the cortical follicles, for reasons given later (p. 29.40).

Antigens differ in the kind of response which they evoke; some stimulate mainly B cell activity and some mainly T cell activity. Most antigens however provoke a mixed B and T cell response. T cells in the paracortex of lymph nodes respond to antigens by entering the circulation and homing to sites of antigen entry, where they produce local cellular infiltrates and are the basis of the cell-mediated immune responses.

DELAYED HYPERSENSITIVITY REACTION

This reaction is a form of immunological hypersensitivity mediated by cells, and distinct from antibody-dependent hypersensitivity. It is highly specific for the sensitizing agent and can be transferred to compatible hosts by thoracic duct lymphocytes from previously sensitized animals.

The reaction underlies all forms of T cell immunity which are recognized in human disease processes. Important examples are bacterial allergy, the basis of diagnostic skin tests, contact dermatitis and some auto-immune diseases. The latter are discussed in vol. 2, p. 23.7, but brief accounts of diagnostic skin tests and the sensitization of skin to various chemicals are given below.

Diagnostic skin tests

Some specific antigens when introduced into the skin of a previously sensitized individual, produce a red, indurated zone after 24 hours which usually persists for at least 48 hours. The reaction depends upon circulating immune or 'sensitized' lymphocytes which home to the antigen injection site; since it is specific, it can be used as a test to discover whether or not a patient has been previously exposed to a particular antigen, and is the basis of the well known tuberculin test (vol. 2, p. 22.18) in which a positive response indicates previous infection by *Mycobacterium tuberculosis*.

Skin sensitization

In common with all cellular immune responses, delayed hypersensitivity has three stages of development, (1) stage of sensitization, (2) generalization of the response and (3) the effector stage. These are best illustrated by the events in experimental contact dermatitis.

Stage of sensitization. Experimentally, the most frequently used contact sensitizing agent is dinitrochlorobenzene (DNCB). Contact with it induces sensitivity in a high proportion of normal animals. When painted on the ear of a guinea-pig it penetrates the epidermis and its basement membrane and reaches the dermis. There it combines with tissue proteins and gives them antigenic specificity. Substances with this property are known as haptens (vol. 2, p. 22.5). The antigen then migrates via dermal lymphatics to local lymph nodes which enlarge and undergo reactive hyperplasia. Macrophages in the medulla and paracortex may take it up. Later lymphoblasts proliferate greatly in the paracortex and appear in small groups, many showing intense pyroninophilia (see below). The number of small lymphocytes in the paracortex increases, the postcapillary venules are distended with lymphocytes and the lymph sinusoids are packed with small lymphocytes flowing out of the node towards the thoracic duct. Plasma cells are not produced.

The localization of the cellular response to DNCB in the paracortex, together with the fact that this zone is depleted of lymphocytes by thoracic duct drainage and neonatal thymectomy, provides strong circumstantial support for the view that the T cells and their precursors are confined in the lymph node to the paracortex.

T lymphoblasts of the paracortex, like B lymphoblasts of the reactive cortex, are rich in polyribosomes. Hence they are pyroninophilic when stained by the methyl green and pyronin method and are called 'large pyroninophilic cells'. Electron microscopy of lymph nodes reacting by both cellular and humoral mechanisms can distinguish the two classes of lymphoblast. Those of the cortex which differentiate into B lymphocytes and plasma cells possess much rough endoplasmic reticulum, fitting them for their ultimate role of antibody formation. Those of the paracortex lack rough endoplasmic reticulum, in keeping with the essentially non-secreting 'cellular' role of their T lymphocyte progeny.

Generalization of the response. As the response develops, many newly formed lymphoid cells and their precursors pass into the circulation. At the same time skin sensitivity gradually increases so that smaller concentrations of DNCB than were required for the original sensitization bring about a red, inflamed zone of persistent contact dermatitis after 12 to 24 hours. After the initial exposure to DNCB, it takes one to three weeks for the process of sensitization to develop.

Experiments on the transfer of delayed hypersensitivity by thoracic duct lymphocytes, extracted during the course of a local lymph node reaction, show that populations rich in lymphoblastic forms are the most potent. Preparations of macrophages from sensitized animals are not effective. In addition, animals immunized against DNCB-

protein combinations by a schedule which gives good antibody formation cannot subsequently be induced to show skin sensitivity. Indeed, administration of such an immune serum abolishes temporarily established skin sensitivity. The blocking effect of antibody on delayed hypersensitivity reactions is probably due to unequal competition for antigen between T cells of feeble affinity and antibody of high affinity.

Effector stage: delayed response. The effector stage of the response is the sequence of events which follows interaction in the skin between sensitized T lymphocytes and DNCB molecules after the second application. It culminates in the lesion of contact dermatitis. Histologically the skin reaction consists of three components, (1) oedema of the dermis and overlying epidermis, (2) capillary dilation and hyperaemia and (3) local accumulations of lymphoblastic (pyroninophilic) cells, monocytes (macrophages) and many small lymphocytes.

Sensitized lymphocytes, on contact with the antigen at the site of a delayed response, release effector chemicals known as lymphokines and, in man, transfer factor.

Lymphokines

Lymphokines are chemical mediators or local hormones (p. 27.50) which together or separately can mimic the delayed hypersensitivity reaction by direct action on the tissues. They include **skin-reactive factor** which causes local capillary hyperaemia, **mitogenic factor** which causes transformation and mitosis in small lymphocytes entering from the blood, **cytotoxic factor** which causes cell death or arrest of mitosis, **permeability factor** which increases the permeability of the microcirculation and oedema, **leucotaxic factor** which encourages macrophages and polymorphs to migrate and **migration inhibition factor** (MIF). MIF plays a well defined part in delayed hypersensitivity reactions. It inhibits spontaneous movement of macrophages from point to point but not their phagocytic activity. Macrophages which have emigrated from permeable vessels meet MIF released from the antigen-reacting lymphocytes. They are thus prevented from migrating out of the reactive zone and hence exert all their phagocytic effect locally.

It is interesting to reflect on the different ways in which the two classes of specific immune response appear to influence macrophages. In cell-mediated responses, MIF concentrates the non-specific phagocytic activity; in humoral responses, specific antibodies enhance phagocytes by acting as opsonins for antigens (vol. 2, p. 22.14), and cytophilic antibody may become attached to the cell membrane of macrophages, specifically increasing their avidity for antigen.

Transfer factor

In man (but not demonstrably in animals), a second class of mediator, quite distinct from the lymphokines, is released from sensitized lymphocytes on contact with antigen. It is known as transfer factor, is extractable from previously sensitized human lymphocytes and has a molecular weight of about 10 000. Unlike lymphokines which are ultimate effectors in the tissues, transfer factor is a sensitizer which makes virgin lymphocytes behave as if primed by antigen for a delayed hypersensitivity response. Transfer of sensitivity by the factor is rapid and detectable within hours, presumably because transfer factor bypasses the early stages in antigenic sensitization. As lymphocytes already sensitized can release the factor on contact with antigen at the site of a local response, virgin lymphocytes arriving at the site can be sensitized more rapidly, and the response may thus be enhanced and prolonged.

CELLULAR RESPONSE TO GRAFTS

Grafting, other than the 'natural graft' of the fetus in pregnancy, is a process alien to nature; thus the skin taken from one animal and grafted on to another of the same species, i.e. an allograft, is rejected except in special circumstances. After an interval of 8–21 days the graft dies, leaving a necrotic mass of tissue which is infiltrated with lymphocytes, macrophages and large pyroninophilic cells. This phenomenon depends on incompatibility antigens.

Although members of the same species have many antigens in common, successful grafting of skin between unrelated individuals is rarely possible, since each individual possesses tissue antigens not found in the other which are likely to evoke an immune response. Only by choosing identical twins or by using highly inbred animal strains or by radical immunological interference can allografts be made to survive. The most frequently used experimental system consists of a graft of skin, which has no appreciable content of immunologically competent cells. Since this piece of graft tissue is rejected by the host this is called a **host versus graft reaction.**

It is also possible to make grafts by intravenous injection of preparations of lymphocytes, i.e. immunologically active cells. Usually, when there is gross incompatibility and the dose of cells is small, they are rapidly destroyed in the spleen by a host versus graft reaction. However it is possible by resort to a genetic subterfuge to ensure (1) that the donor lymphocytes are not destroyed by the host and (2) that the host possesses antigens not present in the injected lymphocytes. Two different inbred strains of animal are crossed. By Mendelian laws the resulting first filial (F_1) generation is bound to possess histocompatibility antigens not present in one or other of the parents. If lymphocytes are now taken from either parent and injected into the F_1 animal they find themselves exposed to antigens which they do not possess, during their continued circulation

in the host. To those essentially 'foreign' antigens, the donor lymphocytes respond by proliferating and mounting a cellular immune attack upon the tissues of the host, the **graft versus host reaction.** The grafted or donor cells survive in the F_1 host because, coming from one of the parents, their antigens are represented in the F_1 host's constitution. They are not, therefore, recognized as foreign.

The graft versus host reaction has easily recognizable signs such as splenic and lymph node enlargement, and is useful because it allows known, defined, parental cell populations to be tested for their immune competence in an F_1 animal. The graft versus host reaction leads to infiltration and destruction of the tissues of the host with proliferation of lymphocytes and pyroninophilic cells. Host macrophages can also participate in the destructive reaction. Damage to the liver, lungs, kidneys and lymphoid system is severe, the latter leading to intercurrent infections and wasting similar to that found in the lymphoid atrophy which follows thymectomy of the newborn (p. 29.40); it is sometimes known as runt disease. As an experimental system the graft versus host reaction is superb; it allows exact selection of graft cells which may be separated into different populations and almost endlessly refined, labelled, fractionated, extracted, chemically treated or degraded. Its extreme experimental flexibility provides highly accurate information about cellular competence and allows precise control over the exact antigenic differences between graft donor and host.

The host versus graft reaction also provides useful information about the range of cellular types involved in the effector side of a cellular immune reaction. However, it is rather more limited in the information which it yields about cellular immune competence. The body recruits different types of cells in the response, and distinguishing their nature and ultimate source can be difficult. Nevertheless the host versus graft system allows the histological study of the complete range of cellular types involved in rejection, and their host origin may be confirmed by a chromosomal marker or by isotopic labelling followed by autoradiography. Some examples of variations on the basic host versus graft system which confirm the importance of the lymphocyte and its pyroninophilic derivatives are as follows.

(1) Lymphocytes from an animal which has already rejected a graft, usually within 8–10 days, accelerate rejection of a similar graft, perhaps in 2 to 3 days, in another animal with which they are compatible.

(2) Allografts applied immediately after birth in small rodents induce the state called tolerance which allows similar allografts to be accepted in adult life. If, however, injections of thoracic duct lymphocytes from a normal compatible animal are given to a tolerant animal with an accepted allograft, rejection follows.

(3) In tissue culture systems, lymphocytes from

animals which have rejected grafts exert a marked cytotoxic effect on cultured graft fibroblasts.

Cellular immunity as a helper of humoral immunity

Many observations in experimental immunology suggest that T cells co-operate with B cells in antibody production. Direct demonstration of such a **helper effect** has been obtained in experiments with thymectomized irradiated mice. When such animals are partially reconstituted with bone marrow, which provides only B cells, they do not form antibody in response to injected sheep erythrocytes. However, when they are reconstituted with a mixture of T and B lymphocytes from normal lymph, they give a good response to the antigen.

The transformation of B lymphocytes to cells which produce antibody requires the presence of antigen on their surface; indeed, the mechanism involves the chemical cross-linking of linear protein receptors on the cell membrane. Specific antigen provides a suitable link, as do a few non-specific materials such as phytohaemagglutinin. It is in providing the necessary concentration of antigen, especially in circumstances of relative scarcity, that both T cells and macrophages come to the assistance of B cells.

T cells make up a high proportion of the circulating lymphocytes and collectively they possess a wide range of receptors, especially for the minor determinants of antigens which are mainly destined to stimulate B lymphocytes through their major determinants. T cells can thus capture a wide range of antigens and in their recirculation come into co-operative contact with B cells. Events thereafter are speculative and there are three possibilities.

(1) T cells may interact directly with B cells.

(2) T cells may transfer their antigen for concentration and storage to macrophages, especially to those with specific surface cytophilic antibody from previous immunization; macrophage-mediated stimulation of B cells or memory cells follows.

(3) T cells may interact with B cells on the surface of macrophages; a T cell may be visualized as holding the antigen and presenting it to the B cell while replenishing itself, as required, with antigen stored on the surface of the macrophage.

In addition, B cells can be transformed directly without other cellular mediators by certain soluble antigens, e.g. pneumococcal polysaccharide, antigen-antibody complexes and endotoxins. The body provides numerous versatile routes to B cell transformation and antibody production.

SPLEEN
Anatomy

The spleen is a solid, encapsulated, deep red organ. It is suspended by a medial pedicle in the upper left part of the abdomen where it lies in contact with and below the diaphragm, concealed anteriorly by the greater curvature of the stomach and the left colic (splenic) flexure.

Its weight varies from 50 to 250 g. It is about 12 cm long and 6 cm wide, and its long axis lies under the posterior part of the tenth rib, from which it is separated, in turn, by the pleural cavity, left lung, diaphragm and peritoneal cavity (fig. 29.19). Its inferior and superior borders lie along the eighth and eleventh intercostal spaces respectively, and it is thus protected posteriorly by the thoracic cage.

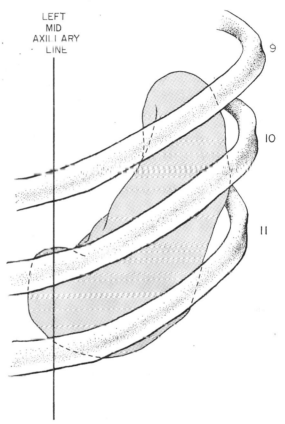

FIG. 29.19. Relations of the spleen to the thoracic cage.

The spleen has a smooth convex posterior diaphragmatic surface and a visceral surface which has a central hilus for the passage of the splenic artery and vein (fig. 29.20). The visceral surface is directed medially and is indented by the kidney posteriorly and by the stomach and colon anteriorly. The posterior end of the spleen may reach the left adrenal gland.

The borders of the spleen are formed at the junction of the diaphragmatic and visceral surfaces. The inferior border is related to the renal area and the superior to the gastric. The superior border is readily defined by the presence of a few notches which assist in the proper orientation of the excised spleen. Due to its position in the body the anterior end corresponds to the junction of the gastric and colic areas and extends forwards as far as the midaxillary line where it is in contact with the

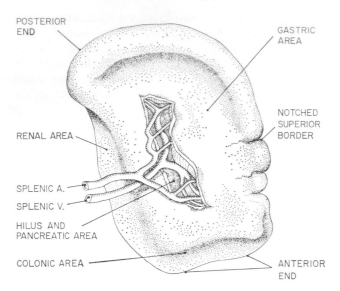

FIG. 29.20. Visceral surface of the spleen.

phrenicocolic ligament, which supports the adjacent colic flexure. Medially the spleen is attached, at the hilus, by two peritoneal folds derived from the dorsal mesogastrium (p. 32.58). The posterior fold, the lienorenal ligament, runs from the left kidney and carries the splenic vessels and the tail of the pancreas, which makes a shallow concavity within the hilus. The anterior fold, the gastrolienal ligament, runs from the greater curvature of the stomach and carries the short gastric and left gastroepiploic vessels.

In health the spleen is not palpable clinically, and it must be enlarged by at least 50 per cent before it is detectable through the abdominal wall. It is protected from minor trauma by the thoracic cage, but in crushing injuries or in severe anterior blows to the left hypochondrium its capsule may rupture, and fatal haemorrhage into the peritoneal cavity may ensue. The spleen which is enlarged by infection and protrudes below the costal margin is prone to rupture from minor trauma. In parts of the world where enlargement of the spleen due to malaria is common, assailants may contrive to rupture their victim's spleen by a swift blow with a small blunt instrument concealed in the hand.

Sometimes accessory spleens or spleniculi are found, usually attached to the hilus, but occasionally more remotely, e.g. in the root of the gastrolienal ligament. Although a harmless congenital aberration, it is important to search for spleniculi at operations for splenectomy aimed at relieving such conditions as haemolytic anaemia (vol. 3, p. 21.32). If they are present and not removed, they undergo compensatory hyperplasia and achieve a size and functional activity comparable to that of the spleen itself, thus vitiating the purpose of the operation.

The splenic artery, the largest branch of the coeliac artery, is described on p. 32.51. It is a markedly muscular

artery and has a rich innervation in its adventitia. In this way it resembles the carotid artery. Close to the hilus the artery divides into several branches which enter the capsule and pass into the organ along the trabecula. The splenic vein drains into the hepatic portal system and not into the vena cava (p. 32.52). Like the rest of the portal venous system it is devoid of valves, and this intensifies venous dilation when there is portal hypertension (vol. 3, p. 20.20).

Histological structure

Under the low power of the light microscope, and even with the naked eye, the two basic components of the splenic parenchyma can be made out (plate 29.2b & c, facing p. 29.42, and fig. 29.21). The **red pulp** forms the continuum of the organ and owes its deep red colour to

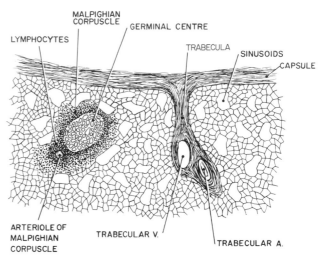

FIG. 29.21. Diagram of a section of the spleen. Not all Malpighian corpuscles contain germinal centres.

large numbers of thin-walled, blood-filled venous sinusoids. The **white pulp** is made up of numerous ovoid white nodules of lymphoid tissue about a millimetre in diameter, known as **Malpighian corpuscles** or splenic lymphoid follicles. In man, the spleen is bounded by a fibroelastic capsule from which trabeculae run radially into its interior, especially near the hilus, where they serve to distribute the major intrasplenic vessels, nerves and lymphatics. In certain species, e.g. the cat and dog, the capsule and trabeculae contain smooth muscle which contracts the spleen and makes the blood in its sinusoids available to the circulation in times of need, e.g. in shock, haemorrhage or hypoxia.

The lymphatics of the spleen are confined strictly to the capsule and trabeculae. As in the thymus, the lymphoid tissue of the spleen is of the dense type devoid of an organized lymph circulation.

The red pulp consists mainly of red blood cells and

white cells of both lymphoid and myeloid series, contained in endothelium-lined sinusoids whose shape depends on the plane of histological section. The mode of connection of the venous sinusoids to the capillaries of the spleen and to its venules is considered later (p. 29.29). In the interstices between these sinusoids silver impregnation stains reveal a reticulin scaffolding with macrophages which may show ingested red blood cells or iron

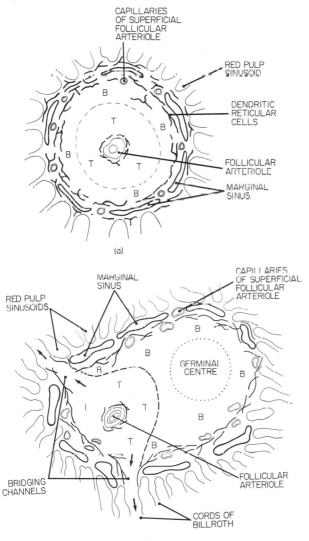

FIG. 29.22. The Malpighian corpuscle. (a) A small Malpighian corpuscle without a germinal centre. T represents T lymphocytes which form a cuff around the follicular arteriole. They are imperfectly segregated from the B lymphocytes which surround them. The ill-defined marginal sinus and capillaries of the follicular arteriole run round the follicle in a band of loose reticulin tissue, rich in phagocytes (not shown). (b) A Malpighian corpuscle after stimulation by circulating antigens to produce a germinal centre. The follicular arteriole is now markedly eccentric. Note the distribution of T and B lymphocytes. The bridging channels are gaps in the peripheral reticulin band; they are normally present and allow lymphocytes, chiefly T cells, to emigrate into the cords of Billroth.

pigment. White blood cells are present also, and in times of active antibody formation plasma cells can be very numerous. These richly cellular regions are called the **cords of Billroth**. Billroth was a professor of surgery in Vienna from 1867–94 and the operations on the stomach which he devised are still performed (vol. 3, p. 19.39). He was a friend of the musician, Brahms. The term 'cord' reflects their appearance in longitudinal sections, where they can sometimes be seen as linear strands coursing between two flanking sinusoids. However, it is best to visualize the cords as loose reticular tissue which not only invests the sinusoids but completely fills those parts of the red pulp not occupied by them.

The cords of Billroth communicate with the lumina of the sinusoids through deficiencies in their walls. This allows blood cells and intravenously injected particulate matter to pass into the cords where there are many active phagocytes. Phagocytosis by the endothelium of the sinusoids is poor, but active macrophages are to be found free in the sinusoidal lumina. In the fetus and newborn child, and in certain pathological states of the adult, extramedullary haemopoiesis occurs in the cords.

The Malpighian corpuscles form eccentric cuffs around the branches of the splenic arteries shortly after they leave the trabeculae. The lymphoid cuff does not end abruptly but tails off along the course of the vessel as a narrow sheath for an appreciable distance (periarteriolar lymphoid sheath). As human blood is normally free of foreign antigens and infecting organisms there is little call for antibody production, and the lymphoid aggregates do not show germinal centres. However, in times of active immunization or infection, reactive germinal centres appear. They form eccentrically, avoiding the artery.

The white pulp has a supporting scaffolding continuous with that of the red pulp, but as in the follicle of the lymph node, the reticular cells are concealed by the density of the lymphocytes and their precursors, and in this site fail to take up much particulate matter.

The distribution of the T and B lymphoid cells in the Malpighian corpuscles and their relationship to vascular structures is summarized in fig. 29.22. Fig. 29.23 is a photomicrograph showing a **marginal sinus** at the periphery of a follicle.

Blood flow within the spleen (fig. 29.24)

The splenic artery branches into trabecular arteries, each of which supplies a definite region of the spleen; they are end arteries with little mutual anastomosis and hence blockage of one of them causes death (infarction) of that part of the spleen supplied (vol. 2, p. 26.8).

The arteries and arterioles of the spleen, in contrast to those of other organs, frequently show in normal individuals hyaline thickening of their walls, a feature which increases markedly with age.

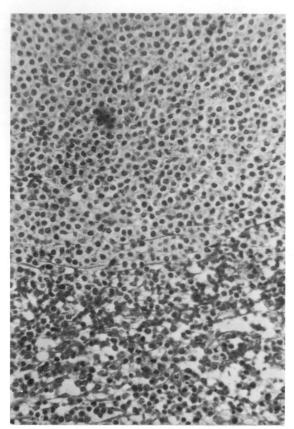

FIG. 29.23. Marginal sinus at the periphery of a Malpighian corpuscle. The lighter staining lymphocyte population of the corpuscle is seen at the top. Below, partially delineated by thin reticulin threads, is the loose reticular tissue, in which parts of the marginal sinus are seen as small spaces (× 200).

The trabecular arteries soon part company with the trabeculae, usually at an acute angle, and course directly through the red pulp. The small terminal trabeculae thus contain only small veins, returning blood from the red pulp.

After leaving the trabecula the artery acquires a slender sheath of lymphoid tissue supported in a basket-work of reticulin. Soon the lymphoid sheath expands (eccentrically to the artery) into the ovoid Malpighian corpuscle. The artery is now known as the **follicular artery**. It traverses the follicle, to which it gives off branches. On leaving the follicle the artery, now only some 40–50 μm in diameter, runs through the red pulp branching into a family of short straight **penicillar arteries** which tend to radiate from their source like the spokes of a wheel. Each penicillar artery branches into two or three small vessels which have lost their internal elastic lamina and muscularis to become capillary in nature. Many of the capillaries acquire structures known as ellipsoids.

The Malpighian corpuscle receives its blood supply from branches of the follicular artery running principally in the superficial zone and also from **postellipsoidal**

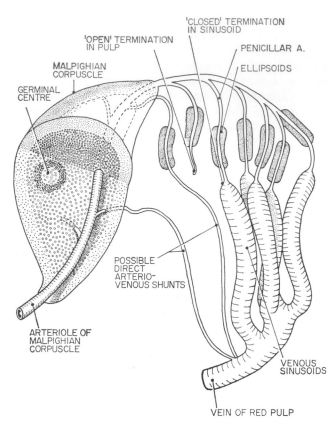

FIG. 29.24. The splenic circulation.

capillaries which return to the surface of the corpuscle after their short course in the red pulp.

The endothelium of the arterioles and capillaries which traverse the lymphoid tissue of the spleen is of the unusual 'high' variety found also in the postcapillary venules of the lymph node paracortex (fig. 29.25).

ELLIPSOIDS

Ellipsoids are short, elliptical sheaths of loosely laminated reticulin, phagocytic cells and lymphocytes, and surround many of the first capillary branches of the straight penicillar arteries (plate 29.1c, facing p. 29.10, and fig. 29.24). They are not prominent structures in man, but are well developed in the cat and fowl where they are best seen in perfused spleens from which the cells have been washed out. The sheaths are poorly innervated and, as they have no smooth muscle, do not act as sphincters to control blood flow into the red pulp. However, they are highly phagocytic and, together with the cords around the marginal sinuses, they are among the first regions of the spleen to take up injected particles. The walls of the central capillaries of the sheath are probably fenestrated, allowing blood and particles to percolate past the phagocytes in its reticulin. After taking up particles, the phagocytes migrate into the red pulp, and the ellipsoids become depleted of macrophages.

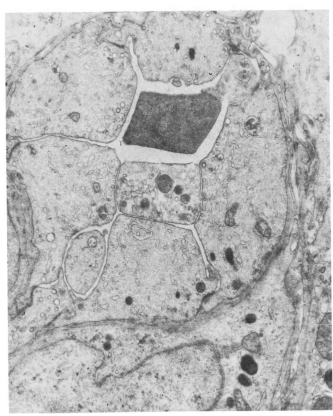

FIG. 29.25. Splenic arteriole. Note the tall endothelium and narrow lumen containing one red blood cell. The large cell surrounding the endothelium at the bottom of the field is a pericyte which identifies the vessel as arteriolar rather than capillary (EM × 4800).

After a few days they are repopulated, probably by mitosis of residual macrophages. The ellipsoid thus provides one of the mechanisms for rapid removal of particulate antigens from the splenic circulation. The post-ellipsoidal capillaries run into the red pulp, where there is uncertainty about their precise termination. They may open into the sinusoids (closed circulation) or into the cords of Billroth (open circulation) and this controversy is discussed after the description of the venous sinusoids.

VENOUS SINUSOIDS

The venous sinusoids drain the blood to the trabecular veins; their walls are made up of longitudinally arranged strap-like endothelial cells (fig. 29.26) with prominent nuclei which protrude into the lumen. These cells are only feebly phagocytic. They are retained by circumferential bands of reticulin, continuous with the reticular mesh-work of the cords of Billroth, and between the cells are potential small openings or fenestrae. The arrangement is like the staves and hoops of a barrel, and the cells are known as **stave cells**. It is not easy to demonstrate the reticulin fibres and the stave cells simultaneously, but plate 29.1d, facing p. 29.10, shows a longitudinal

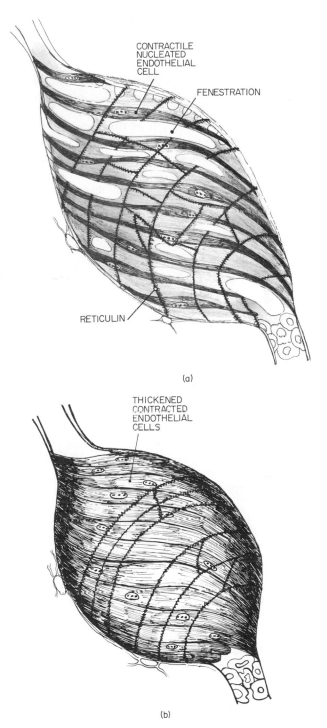

FIG. 29.26. The splenic venous sinusoid. Note the circumferential bands of reticulin (the ladder pattern seen in fig. 29.27) arranged like the hoops of a barrel. The endothelial cells, known as stave cells, run side by side lengthwise in a spiral of long pitch. (a) Open state; the intracellular microfilaments of the stave cells are relaxed, the spiral is relatively unwound and spaces between the cells allow the passage of blood cells through the fenestrated basement membrane into the cords of Billroth. (b) Closed state; contraction of the microfilaments winds up the spiral and closes the interspaces.

section of a venous sinusoid which is beginning to branch into two. The long slender striae in its wall are the bodies of stave cells with large, dark nuclei arranged along their length. A silver reticulin preparation (fig. 29.27) shows that the reticulin fibres run mainly around the sinusoids, giving the appearance of a ladder. The **stave cells**, which are not demonstrated in this type of preparation, run the length of the sinusoids roughly at right angles to the rungs of the reticulin ladder and wind around it in a helix (fig. 29.26). They are not in close contact with their neighbours, so that the endothelial lining of the sinusoid is potentially incomplete.

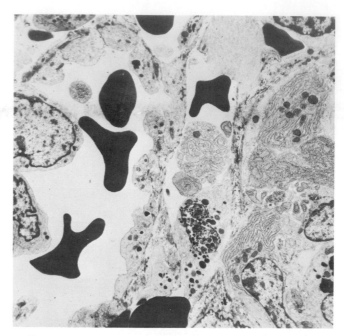

FIG. 29.28. Splenic sinusoid and cord of Billroth. The sinusoid is in transverse section and occupies the left of the picture; the fenestrae between the stave cells are tightly closed. A large nucleus of a stave cell is seen on the extreme left; these nuclei often protrude into the lumen. The cord of Billroth is on the right and it contains parts of three red cells, a fragment of macrophage cytoplasm containing dense granules (lower centre) and plasma cells (extreme right), identified by their skeins of endoplasmic reticulum (EM × 1500).

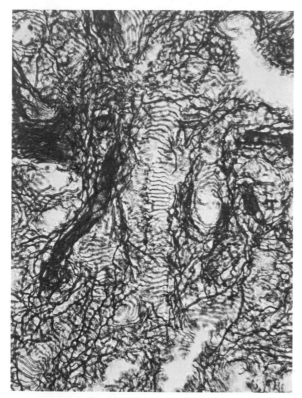

FIG. 29.27. Reticulin structure of splenic sinusoids. Thick section of a washed spleen stained by silver impregnation for reticulin. Centrally a long sinusoid appears as the rungs of a ladder. The resemblance stems from hemi-section of the circumferential reticulin bands which run round the sinusoid like the hoops of a barrel (fig. 29.26). Note many other sinusoids or parts of sinusoids mostly in elliptical or, occasionally, transverse section (× 300).

Electron microscopy (figs. 29.28 and 29.29) has provided useful detail about the structure and likely function of the sinusoids. Stave cells are attached to a fenestrated basement membrane and, at the point of attachment, there is an electron-dense zone called the basal plate which anchors dense leashes of contractile microfilaments running through the cytoplasm of the cells. When the filaments contract they shorten the cells, making them plumper, and so seal off the fenestrae. On relaxation the sinusoid lengthens and the fenestrae open, allowing red

blood cells to pass into the cords of Billroth, and *vice versa*. It seems probable that the pressure gradient between the capillary and venous ends of the sinusoid expels plasma and red blood cells into the cords of Billroth at the arterial end. They re-enter the venous end of the sinusoids after percolating slowly past the active cordal macrophages which remove any effete red blood cells. Collapse of the sinusoids is prevented both by their content of blood and by surrounding reticulin hoops. Shunting of blood through the cords is dependent upon the opening of the fenestrae of the sinusoids, which thus have some control over both phagocytosis and the amount of blood stored in the cords. In times of antigenic stimulation, lymphocytic transformation takes place in the cords and plasma cells become prominent in them. Plasma cells are rarely seen in the lumina of the sinusoids.

The course of the circulation in the spleen can be demonstrated by injecting latex particles or nucleated avian erythrocytes into the splenic artery. These fill the capillaries, enter the cords of Billroth and, rather later, reach the venous sinusoids. If, however, the splenic vein is injected, the venous sinusoids fill and the cords to a lesser extent, but the arteries do not. These findings, carried out under somewhat unnatural conditions, only suggest that

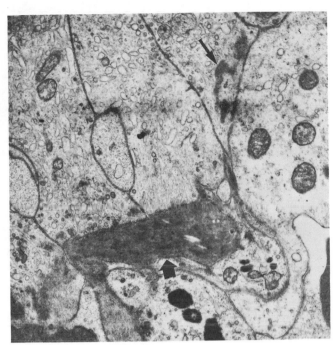

FIG. 29.29. Two stave cells, with a cell end sandwiched between them, resting on a dense segment of basement membrane shown by the broad arrow. To the right and above, the basal region of a stave cell contains a strand of electron-dense matter which is a basal plate, shown by a thin arrow. The microfilaments which are inserted into it are too fine to be resolved (EM × 4000).

postellipsoidal capillaries discharge into the cords of Billroth rather than into the venous sinusoids. Nevertheless the concept of such an open circulation has for some time challenged that of a conventional closed circulation, in which the postellipsoidal capillaries are in continuity with the venous sinusoids.

The present consensus is that most of the postellipsoidal capillaries are continuous with sinusoids, but a few empty directly into the pulp.

Phagocytosis in the spleen
Reference has already been made to the considerable phagocytic activity of the spleen (p. 29.4).

UPTAKE OF INERT MATTER
Inert particles, e.g. Indian ink or saccharated iron oxide, percolate into the marginal sinuses of Malpighian corpuscles and thence into the adjacent cords, where they are taken up by macrophages within half an hour of injection (fig. 29.30). In this way the corpuscles can be outlined. The ellipsoids also take up particles well. Thereafter a gradual shift of particles takes place into the macrophages of the red pulp where they are scattered.

UPTAKE OF ANTIGENS
With antigenic matter, whether soluble or particulate, initial uptake in both primary and secondary responses is

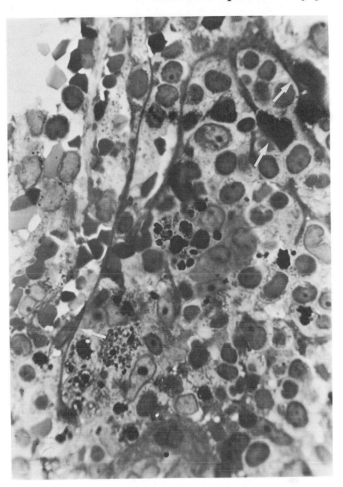

FIG. 29.30. Phagocytosis in the spleen. High power picture of a cord of Billroth showing carbon particles inside macrophages. Note also the dense linear reticulin threads with associated reticular cells (arrowed) (× 560).

similar to that of inert particles. The marginal sinuses and the ellipsoids take a major share, but redistribution to the red pulp is not prominent. Indeed the migration of antigen tends to be in the opposite direction, with much antigen subsequently appearing within the lymphoid tissue.

IMMUNE RESPONSES
In primary immunization there are diffuse reactive changes along the edges of the periarteriolar lymphoid sheaths, presumably initiated by antigen-bearing macrophages. Large pyroninophil cells appear among the lymphocytes of the inner or follicular aspect of marginal sinuses but do not aggregate to form germinal centres; plasma cells appear to differentiate from them. Large pyroninophil cells and plasma cells are found also around the arterioles emerging from Malpighian corpuscles and in the red pulp, immediately adjacent to marginal sinuses. After secondary antigenic stimulation germinal centres form in the B cell zone of the Malpighian

corpuscles (fig. 29.22) arising round antigen-bearing dendritic macrophages. They probably represent a vigorous local lymphocyte transformation, triggered by macrophage antigen reacting with the enhanced amounts of specific antibody present on the surface of previously immunized lymphocytes. The focus of transformed lymphocytes constitutes the typical germinal centre with mitotic figures among its lymphoblasts and ultimately tingible bodies (p. 29.5).

Germinal centres are seldom seen in Malpighian corpuscles of 'resting' spleens but are commonly found where there is a chronic blood stream infection, thrombocytopenia or autoimmune haemolytic disease. The follicular cells which transform into antibody-forming cells are, of course, B cells whose precursors come from the bone marrow.

Many germinal centres have a dense rim of small lymphocytes around the periphery. Labelling experiments show that only a few of these are derived from the lymphoblasts of the germinal centre; the lymphocytes produced locally are much diluted by blood-borne cells.

Circulation of lymphocytes through the spleen

Unlike lymph nodes, the spleen has no lymphatic channels, but blood lymphocytes do not simply pass straight through the splenic vessels from artery to vein. As already shown, they have excellent opportunities to circulate among the lymphocytes of the Malpighian corpuscles and the cords, and also to change places with them. Thus periarteriolar T cells can be depleted by thoracic duct drainage, presumably by emigration via the capillaries or marginal sinuses into the venous outflow. Furthermore the high endothelium in the capillaries of the Malpighian corpuscles is similar to that in the lymph nodes where it is associated with immigration of lymphocytes from vessels into the parenchyma. Hence the spleen seems well equipped for vascular emigration and immigration of lymphocytes, i.e. for recirculation.

Autoradiography of isolated rat spleens perfused with labelled lymphocytes shows that both T and B cells congregate around the periphery of Malpighian corpuscles (fig. 29.31). T cells migrate into the periarteriolar lymphoid sheath and after a stay of some 5–6 hours return probably via gaps in the reticulin band around the follicle (bridging channels), to the red pulp. B cells migrate into the corpuscle and gather around the T cell zone but do not enter the germinal centre. The transit time for B cells is about 24 hours, some four times greater than T cell transit time, which possibly accounts for the much higher B/T ratio in the spleen than in the thoracic duct.

Certain immunological advantages stem from the recirculation of antigen-reactive lymphocytes. In an immune response, they may be stimulated by antigen-

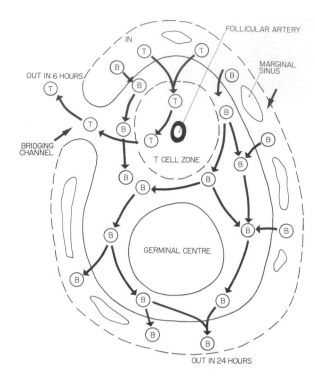

FIG. 29.31. Circulation of B and T lymphocytes through the Malpighian corpuscle.

processing macrophages during their passage through the periphery of the Malpighian corpuscle. Cells so stimulated probably cease to circulate and are sequestered within their appropriate B or T cell zones in the Malpighian corpuscles, presumably in 'immunoblastic' form. Concomitantly, a marked fall in lymphocytes reactive to the specific antigen is demonstrable in the thoracic duct.

The passage of the B cells through the margin of the T cell zone may be related to the need for T cell cooperation with B cells in the formation of antibody to certain antigens (p. 29.25).

Splenic function

The functions of the spleen can be divided conveniently, if somewhat arbitrarily, into the functions of the red and white pulp.

RED PULP
Phagocytosis and scavenging

The function of the phagocytes of the cords of Billroth is to remove from the circulation stray bacteria, cellular debris and effete erythrocytes, leucocytes and platelets. Macrophages showing erythrophagocytosis, or bearing golden-brown granules of haemosiderin which give the Prussian blue reaction for iron, can be seen in the spleen of a normal individual. Phagocytosis in the spleen assumes great importance in diseases associated with excessive destruction of erythrocytes or platelets or with marked hyperlipoproteinaemia. In these circumstances the macrophages multiply and the spleen gradually enlarges. Splenic enlargement is commonly found, for example, in countries where malaria is endemic, for in this disease the malarial parasite lives in and destroys red blood cells.

Antigen trapping and lymphoblastic transformation

The spleen acts as a focal point both for lymphocyte circulation and for antigen trapping. The chance of response to antigens present in the circulation is thus greatly enhanced. In many species almost all the antibody production after intravenous antigen administration is in the spleen. During immunization foci of transforming lymphocytes and antibody-forming plasma cells are found in the cords.

Extramedullary haemopoiesis

In the embryo, and in lesser degree in the newborn, many tissues other than the bone marrow, especially the spleen and liver, are actively haemopoietic. The marrow gradually emerges as the sole haemopoietic organ and, after a few weeks, haemopoiesis in the spleen is negligible, though the potential for it remains.

Extramedullary haemopoiesis often persists in haemolytic disease of the newborn (vol. 3, p. 45.13). In adults it is nearly always due to extensive disease of or damage to the bone marrow, with compensatory haemopoiesis from circulating marrow stem cells which mature in the spleen and liver instead.

Circulatory reserve

In man a healthy spleen weighs up to 250 g and its content of blood does not amount to more than 1 or 2 per cent of the blood volume. The spleen is not, therefore, an important reservoir of blood. However, in many animals the spleen is relatively much larger, and its volume is reduced by muscular contraction of the capsule brought about by sympathetic nerves and by release of adrenaline. In this way blood in the sinusoids may be expelled into the circulation to meet increased demands in vigorous exercise or after haemorrhage.

WHITE PULP

The lymphoid tissue of the Malpighian corpuscles has the following functions.

(1) It traps blood-borne antigen in the macrophages of the cords flanking its marginal sinuses.

(2) It transports the trapped antigen to its lymphoid interior either by phagocytic migration or perhaps by dendritic passage.

(3) It is the main site where immature T cells exported from the thymus collect. In mice, T cells have been shown to mature here into fully immunocompetent cells which later join the circulatory pool of lymphocytes.

(4) It provides both cellular and humoral immune responses to trapped antigens. The exact site and pattern of the lymphoblastic transformation depends upon immunological experience (primary or secondary exposure) and on the type of response (cellular or humoral).

Effects of splenectomy

Removal of the spleen, either in experimental animals or in otherwise healthy patients when it has been ruptured by trauma, has no dire effects in the long run, but certain changes are detectable.

(1) Partial removal is followed by a rapid regeneration of the retained part or of accessory spleens until approximately the former weight is restored.

(2) Within hours of total splenectomy there is a marked increase in the circulating leucocytes and platelets which lasts for many weeks. The effect is attributed to withdrawal of a humoral agent which may inhibit the release of neutrophils and platelets from the marrow. In parabiotic animals with a common circulation, splenectomy in one partner has no effect, but splenectomy in both induces leucocytosis.

(3) In some animals, e.g. the cat, the loss of a store of blood corpuscles diminishes tolerance to haemorrhage, shock, hypoxia and exercise.

(4) After the spleen has been removed, its haemodestructive functions are carried out mainly by the liver and bone marrow.

(5) There is an increased risk of infection after splenectomy. In animals, the production of antibodies to certain intravenously injected antigens is reduced. In man splenectomy is followed by increased risk of pneumococcal infection.

THYMUS

The thymus is necessary for the development and maintenance of the lymphoid system especially in the newborn and young animal. It is the first lymphoid organ to develop, and it secretes a humoral factor which is essential for lymphopoiesis both in its own cortex and in the developing lymph nodes and spleen. It makes an important contribution to the pool of immunologically competent cells. Without its thymus, the young animal succumbs to chance infection because of the failure of peripheral lymphoid development. The major activities of the thymus are in the neonatal and growth periods; after puberty it undergoes involution, with some loss of lymphocytes, gradual fibrosis and shrinkage.

Anatomy

The thymus is situated in the neck and anterior mediastinum and reaches its greatest size in the child at about 9 years of age. At this time it is a bilobed triangular mass which represents the embryological fusion of bilateral downgrowths of the third branchial pouch (p. 19.30). It extends downwards from its apex, close to the lower border of the thyroid, to its base which is level with the fourth costal cartilage (fig. 29.32). In the neck it lies between the trachea and the origins of the sternohyoid and sternothyroid muscles. In the thorax it lies between the great vessels and pericardium posteriorly and the sternum anteriorly. According to an ancient view of Galen it serves as a cushion set between the violent pulsations of the one and the bony hardness of the other.

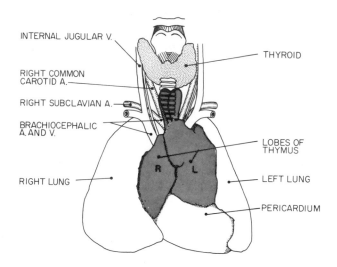

FIG. 29.32. Relations of the thymus in early childhood.

In man the thymus is often regarded as having its greatest weight relative to the body as a whole at birth (10–15 g/3·5 kg). In fact, the ratio is greatest (10 g/2 kg) around the 28th week of embryonic life, reflecting the intense activity of the thymus in developing the lymphoid system at this time. During the remainder of life its weight in relation to the body weight declines, although its absolute mass increases until it reaches a maximum of 30–40 g at the age of 8–10. During involution around puberty its mass declines markedly until, in the adult, it can be difficult to recognize the involuted thymus among the fibro-fatty tissue of the anterior mediastinum.

The blood supply of the thymus is derived from branches of the internal thoracic artery and of the superior and inferior thyroid arteries. The venous drainage is chiefly by tributaries of the left brachiocephalic vein and of the thyroid veins.

Although a lymphoid organ, the thymus is not concerned with the filtration of lymph, and it does not have the subcapsular and radiating sinusoids of a lymph node. Lymphatic channels exist in its cortex and medulla, but they are few and not easy to find; small lymphatic vessels are present in its septa and capsule. These lymphatics drain ultimately to the deep cervical, tracheobronchial and internal thoracic groups of lymph nodes.

The thymic nerve supply consists of extremely fine branches of the vagi and sympathetic trunks. Branches from the phrenic nerve and the ansa cervicalis supply its capsule but not its parenchyma.

Histological structure (figs. 29.33 and 29.34)

The lobes of the thymus are made up of many lobules up to 2 mm in diameter; these have a capsule of loose connective tissue, a cortex densely packed with lymphocytes and a lightly staining medulla where lymphocytes are much less numerous. It is probably better to refer to lymphocytes found within the thymus as **thymocytes** for, as will be seen, they show important functional differences from the peripheral T lymphocytes. The lobules have a roughly pyramidal shape with truncated apices directed centrally, and are separated from one another by deep capsular septa which carry the vessels and nerves.

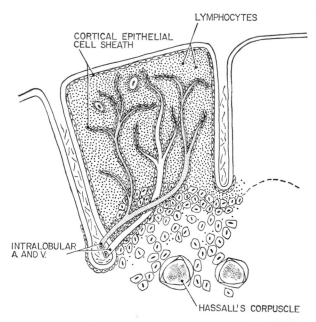

FIG. 29.33. Diagram of thymus showing cortex, medulla, blood supply and the epithelial framework or sheath.

The medulla is a central continuous structure which ramifies into each lobule and is made up of large pale eosinophilic cells. Electron microscopy shows that these form a continuum bounded by a prominent basement membrane wherever it is in contact with connective tissue. Accordingly, the medullary cells are regarded as epithelial cells. They are the probable source of a humoral factor which may stimulate lymphopoiesis in the thymus.

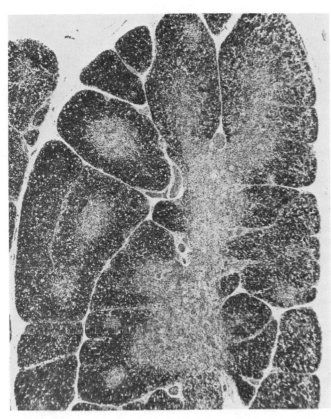

Fig. 29.34. Infant thymus. The pyramidal superficial lobules, demarcated by pale clefts, are well shown. Note the density of the cortex, due to the high concentration of lymphocytes and the relative pallor of the medulla. Medullary peninsulae penetrate into the roots of the cortical lobules. In certain planes of section they appear as round areas and can be mistaken for germinal follicles, which are absent from the infant thymus (× 20).

Oval, lightly staining myoid cells are scattered through the medulla; they contain speckled nuclear chromatin like that of fibroblasts. EM shows myosin filaments in their cytoplasm. Their function is obscure.

It was once considered that the normal human thymus did not contain lymphoid germinal centres, though these may be numerous and prominent in the presence of certain autoimmune diseases. It is now agreed that germinal follicles are not present before about 5 years of age. Thereafter their prevalence depends on the source of the thymuses examined. Those obtained at autopsy in cases in which there may have been stress involution of the thymus confirm the traditional view that germinal centres are absent. However, up to 50 per cent of thymuses from cases of sudden death, in which stress involution has not occurred, contain undoubted germinal centres. Thymic biopsies from children undergoing operation for congenital heart disease confirm these findings. Hassall's corpuscles, present in the medulla, are described on p. 29.39.

Branches of the major arteries travel deeply in the interlobular clefts and eventually penetrate the lobules usually on their deep or central aspects, to become the intralobular arterioles (fig. 29.33). These run in the corticomedullary zone and give off small branches which radiate outwards in the cortex. Their capillaries anastomose freely and drain into the cortical radial veins which run back to the corticomedullary zone to join the medullary vein; this runs beside the interlobular arteries. In man, and in most species with a highly lobulated thymus, the peripheral cortical capillaries drain also to a superficial plexus of capsular veins.

EMBRYOLOGICAL DEVELOPMENT

The thymus in man develops from the third branchial pouch at about the sixth week of gestation (p. 19.30). Initially the bilateral thymic outgrowths are composed of buds of endodermal epithelial cells; these buds are detached from the branchial pouch by about the tenth week and migrate to the upper anterior mediastinum, where they fuse in the midline to form the definitive thymus. At about the ninth week the first lymphocytes are found in the central portions of the epithelial buds. They may be derived from mesenchymal remnants lying within the developing thymus or from haematopoietic tissue in the yolk sac.

The next phase is one of rapid growth of both epithelium and lymphocytes, with the establishment of a clearly defined cortex and medulla. By the twelfth to fifteenth week Hassall's corpuscles appear, the lobulated structure is established, and during the remainder of gestation the organ rapidly enlarges by the production of lymphocytes, the cortex in particular becoming bigger and more densely cellular.

Lymphocytes appear in the thymus at a stage when very few can be found in the circulation or in peripheral lymphoid masses. Later the lymph nodes acquire a large part of their lymphoid cell population from the thymus and up to the 25th week of gestation nearly all the splenic and circulating lymphocytes are of thymic origin. The reticular structure and phagocytic cell populations of lymph nodes and spleen develop independently of the thymus, and these are already present by the time circulating thymic lymphocytes are produced.

THYMIC CORTEX

The framework of the cortex is an epithelial structure not readily seen in histological sections because of the density of the tightly packed thymocytes. The epithelium radiates out from the medulla into the cortex in sheets which divide the lobule into numerous compartments where the thymocytes are produced (fig. 29.33). Like the cells of the medulla, the cortical epithelial cells are probably of endodermal origin. Around the radial vessels the epithelium forms loose sheaths which electron micrographs show to be separated from the vessel wall by a narrow perivascular space. The sheath probably acts as a partial barrier to the passage of blood-borne antigens into the thymus. At the periphery of the lobule the epithelium lines the inner aspect of the capsule and completes the epithelial spongework in which the thymocytes divide.

The epithelial cells of the thymus are different from the reticular cells which form the scaffolding of peripheral lymphoid tissue. They are most probably endodermal derivatives, not mesenchymal, and they are not phagocytic. They form a continuous sheet which, seen on electron microscopy, has the characteristics of an epithelium (fig. 29.35). Intracellular tonofibrils are present, and desmosomes link adjacent cells into a sheet which is bounded by a prominent basement membrane wherever it comes in contact with connective tissue or blood vessels. The epithelial cells do not produce reticulin and when they do gain support from adjacent reticulin fibres they are separated from them by a basement membrane.

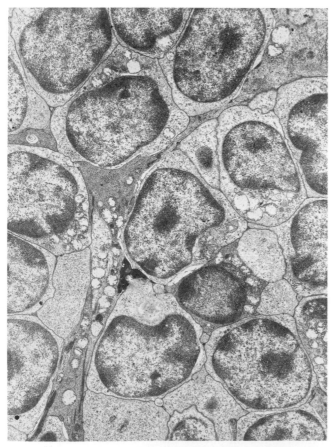

FIG. 29.35. Thymic epithelial cell framework. Numerous thymic lymphocytes are divided into three groups (uppermost, lower left, lower right) by a thin Y-shaped plate or framework of contiguous thymic epithelial cells, distinguishable by their relatively dense cytoplasm (EM × 12 500). Courtesy of Dr. R.F. Macadam.

Phagocytosis in the thymus

Phagocytosis is not marked in the thymus. In the adult rat, thymic uptake of labelled bovine serum albumin is poor and this is in striking contrast to the avid and prolonged retention of the antigen in the macrophages of the spleen. However, in certain species some antigens are retained by the thymic macrophages in amounts which would stimulate production of germinal centres in any other lymphoid organ. Then the failure to form germinal follicles may be due partly to a scarcity of reactive B lymphocytes to transform into germinal centre lymphoblasts, and partly to defects in the processing of antigens by the macrophages. This relative incompetence of thymic macrophages is suggested by experiments in which germinal centres appeared in the medulla when certain antigens were injected directly into the thymus. Possibly the high concentration of antigen overcame the inertia of the processing mechanism.

The medullary origin of the thymic germinal follicles is shown by the observation that most of the follicles are surrounded by a halo of Hassall's corpuscles which have been displaced peripherally by the follicular medullary growth (fig. 29.36). Germinal follicles do not appear

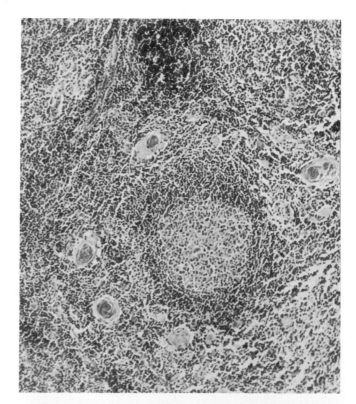

FIG. 29.36. A germinal follicle in the thymic medulla of a patient with myasthenia gravis. The newly formed follicle is surrounded by several Hassall's corpuscles, an arrangement which reveals its origin from a focus in the medulla (× 105).

in the cortex. The medullary production of germinal centres may well reflect the main thymic site of antigen-processing macrophages and available blood-borne B cells. Those few soluble antigens which are relatively well taken up by the thymus are localized most strikingly in the medulla.

Cortical thymocytes

Thymocytes differ from peripheral T and B lymphocytes in their very high and constant rate of production, in their high death rate and in being protected from antigenic stimulation within the thymus.

STEM CELLS FOR THYMIC LYMPHOPOIESIS

In the embryo, stem cells for thymic lymphopoiesis probably come from either the yolk sac or blood islands in the sinusoids of fetal liver. In young and adult animals, graft experiments show that they come from the bone marrow via the circulation.

Bone marrow cultured aseptically on nutrient agar gives colonies of proliferating cells (colony-forming units) which arise in a proportion of roughly one for every thousand seeded cells. Each colony is a group of stem cells undergoing mitosis, and under different conditions they differentiate along erythroid, granulocytic and lymphoid pathways. They are multipotent and can repopulate the bone marrow, the peripheral lymphoid tissue and the thymus of lethally irradiated animals. Although their properties are very different, stem cells in their resting state resemble small lymphocytes. They are about 8 μm in diameter, with little cytoplasm and an indented nucleus. During the earlier stages of most maturation pathways they enlarge markedly. In the marrow they are long-lived and divide slowly, and hence are relatively resistant to radiation or cytotoxic drugs.

MATURATION OF THYMIC LYMPHOCYTES

Production of thymocytes is confined largely to the cortex, not in organized germinal follicles as in the lymph node, but diffusely from lymphoblastic stem cell derivatives. Division takes place in the interstices of the epithelial framework, and proximity to the epithelial cells is necessary for certain of the maturation changes.

In young animals, the cortical mitotic rate is five to ten times greater in the thymus than in the lymph nodes. Mitosis occurs most frequently in the subcapsular zone and along the course of the radial vessels, especially in their peripheral segments. In addition the subcapsular region contains large vacuolated macrophages which are surrounded by dividing lymphoblasts. Although these macrophages are present in most species, they are especially prominent in the mouse, where they are known as chromolipid or PAS cells. The name reflects their content of yellow insoluble lipid which stains with the PAS method and is a degradation product of phagocytosed effete lymphocytes. The chromolipid cells are thought to encourage local lymphopoiesis by secreting soluble metabolites which stimulate dividing lymphoid precursors. When lympholysis and subsequent phagocytosis of dead lymphocytes is brisk, e.g. after cortisol administration, chromolipids accumulate and colour the cortex yellow. Some of the macrophages containing chromolipid migrate to the medulla and become incorporated in Hassall's corpuscles.

Experimentally the majority of lymphocytes present in the thymus are not immunologically competent. Indeed about 95 per cent die without ever leaving the organ; these may be unsuitable cells not selected for further maturation. The remaining 5 per cent undergo maturation in two stages, both of which are thymus-dependent.

First stage of maturation (T_1 cells)

The first stage takes place within the thymus and leads to the export of thymocytes known as T_1 cells, which are immunologically virgin and incompetent (fig. 29.37). This stage depends upon the presence of the thymic epithelial framework and may be mediated by a humoral factor. The presence of the epithelium is essential to the induction of certain surface antigens in the thymocyte population. In the mouse, the commonest experimental model, two distinct antigens are acquired by the newly formed T_1 cells; one, the thymic leukaemia antigen (TLA, p. 29.38), is unique and specific to thymic lymphocytes from strains of mice with a high incidence of leukaemia, and the other, the Thy 1 antigen, is present also in skin and brain (see later).

Before they leave the thymus, and presumably immediately afterwards, T_1 thymocytes have poor immune properties; when injected into irradiated animals with skin allografts, they do not produce graft rejection. Most of the thymocytes destined to leave the thymus in the T_1 state have not yet undergone antigenic stimulation. When they reach the T cell areas of the Malpighian corpuscles of the spleen, via the blood stream, they tend to remain there, not participating in the recirculation of lymphocytes until they reach full immunocompetence as described below.

Second stage of maturation (T_2 cells)

After export to peripheral T cell areas, chiefly in the spleen, the second stage of maturation takes place. It involves the gradual loss of TLA antigen, but Thy 1 antigen remains demonstrable on the lymphocytes.

When full immunocompetence is gained, the cell, now known as a T_2 cell, differs from a recirculating T cell only in that it has not yet met an antigen to which it can react. It now has the potential to make a contribution to the responses to new antigens which the body

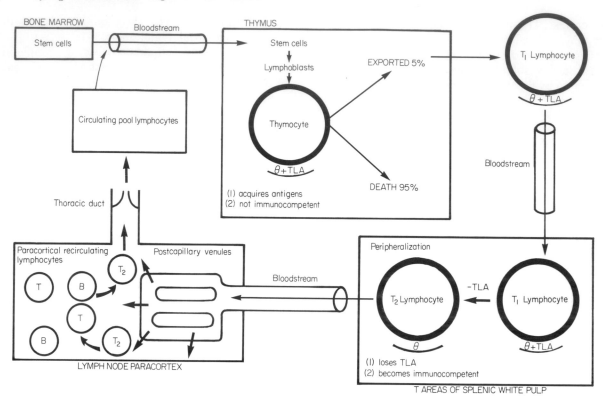

FIG. 29.37. Origin and maturation of the T lymphocytes of the mouse to full immunocompetence. $\theta = $ Thy I

may meet. T_2 lymphocytes join the recirculating T cell pool and are virtually indistinguishable from T lymphocytes.

Evidence for the differentiation of lymphocytes into T_1 and T_2 classes

The basis for the differentiation of the thymic lymphocytes into T_1 and T_2 cells comes from experiments on mice. The Thy I antigen was discovered in these animals when antisera prepared against brain tissue cross-reacted with similar antigens in skin and thymocytes. Further work established two classes of Thy I antigen called Thy I.I (θCH$_3$) and Thy I.2 (θAKR); the suffixes CH$_3$ and AKR in the old θ nomenclature served to identify two in-bred strains of mice in which the antigen is found. Antisera against Thy I.I can be prepared by immunizing AKR mice with CH$_3$ mouse thymus, and similarly antisera against Thy I.2 can be made by immunizing CH$_3$ mice with AKR mouse thymus. The discovery of distinct forms of Thy I antigen within the same species was of great experimental value, since it was possible to use the two strains of mice to produce potent cytotoxic anti-Thy I sera devoid of the species-specific antibodies which would be present in antisera prepared, for example, from rabbits immunized with mouse thymocytes.

Cytotoxicity tests showed that anti-Thy I sera were equally lethal to suspensions of thymocytes and of peripheral T lymphocytes. Pretreatment of peripheral lymphocyte suspensions with sublethal doses of anti-Thy I sera also abolished their competence in graft rejection and graft versus host reactions. The Thy I antigen is clearly common to all thymus-derived lymphocytes both in the thymus and circulating in the periphery.

The thymic leukaemic antigen (TLA) was discovered during investigation of the antigenic differences between strains of mice with a high and a low incidence of spontaneous leukaemia. The finding that the incidence of leukaemia in strains at high risk could be reduced by thymectomy led to immunological studies of thymocytes from different strains. Thymocytes from mice at high risk were found to possess TLA which is absent from those at low risk.

Studies on lymphocyte antigenicity are important because antisera prepared against Thy I and thymic leukaemia antigens can be used to demonstrate antigenic differences in the newly formed T_1 cells, T_2 cells and in mature T lymphocytes. TLA is found only on thymocytes in the thymus and not on immunocompetent T cells in other lymphoid organs or circulating in the blood, whereas all carry the Thy I antigen.

The present hypothesis is that the thymus in mice produces thymocytes which are not immunologically competent and which commonly bear both Thy I and TLA antigens (T_1 cells). Such cells are not found in the peripheral lymph nodes but are identifiable in the T cell areas of the spleen, where they often show reduced amounts of TLA. Cells carrying both antigens are not found in the thoracic duct lymph and hence are not present in significant numbers circulating in the pool; after leaving the thymus, they are presumed to migrate to the spleen and to remain there, gradually losing their TLA and becoming fully immunocompetent T_2 cells. They then join the circulating pool of T lymphocytes although they have not yet responded to antigenic stimulation.

Immunological environment of thymocytes

The lack of immunological commitment of thymocytes implies that they have been reared in an immunological environment different from that of the B and T lymphocytes of the peripheral lymphoid tissue. Failure to stimulate immune reactivity among thymic lymphocytes is partly relative and due to the small amount of lymph filtration through the organ and the virtual absence of antigen-trapping macrophages. Immunocompetent B and T lymphocytes from the circulation gain access to the thymus via ordinary capillaries and do not recirculate in a way comparable to that in the lymph nodes. Furthermore a **haemothymic barrier** restricts some blood-borne antigens to the perivascular space and excludes them from the thymic parenchyma.

REGULATION OF THYMIC LYMPHOPOIESIS

Mitotic activity in the thymic lymphoid population is between four and ten times that in the lymph nodes or spleen. The high rate is of some constancy and not readily altered by external stimuli. Indeed, mitosis continues at a high rate during natural involution. The numbers of thymocytes, and hence the size of the thymus, must therefore depend also upon other influences e.g. (1) the rate of influx of marrow stem cells, (2) the rate of cell death within the thymus, and (3) the rate of export of lymphocytes to the periphery.

In fetal life the rate of mitosis and entry of marrow stem cells more than balance the rate of lymphocyte loss to the periphery. The thymus therefore enlarges and its weight in relation to body weight is greatest during this period. At birth, there is a sharp increase in the rate of export of lymphocytes, probably due to the enhanced need for immunocompetent peripheral lymphocytes. The thymus to total body weight ratio declines.

In early adult life, although mitotic activity remains high, the rate of cell death in the thymus increases and there may be decreased production of stem cells in the marrow. The thymus to total body weight ratio continues to decrease very rapidly at involution.

Although it is easy to assemble such crude balance sheets for thymocyte numbers and thymic size, the ultimate control of the responsible factors remains obscure.

It is likely that the thymus has considerable autonomy and that its cellular traffic is regulated intrinsically. The most telling evidence for this is the process of involution which no extrinsic agent can induce prematurely, nor arrest once it is under way. Further evidence for thymic autonomy is that thymic grafts behave as they would in their donor and not according to the thymic state of their host. Thus, neonatal thymus grafted into a young adult whose thymus is undergoing involution repopulates normally, while the host thymus continues to involute.

Thymic medulla

MEDULLARY EPITHELIAL CELLS

The medulla is composed mainly of large epithelial cells. They tend to aggregate together and in man it is probable that the Hassall's corpuscles are, at least initially, the result of their fusion. The epithelial cells show certain similarities in medulla and cortex. However, in mice, PAS-staining inclusions are prominent in those of the medulla, but insignificant in those of the cortex. When lymphopoiesis is rapid the inclusions are small and few, and when it is poor they are large and numerous. These changes suggest that mouse epithelial cells have secretory activity and store and release a substance with lymphopoietic activity.

HASSALL'S CORPUSCLES (plate 29.1e, facing p. 29.10)

Hassall's corpuscles are formed continuously in the embryonic and postnatal thymus and are especially prominent during involution. They are formed only in the medulla, probably by the aggregation of medullary epithelial cells.

The corpuscles begin in the medulla as single epithelial cells which undergo degenerative changes. The nuclei become intensely basophilic, swollen and indistinct, and large crescentic perinuclear vacuoles appear. The cytoplasm meanwhile becomes deeply eosinophilic and small basophilic granules of keratohyaline develop. Other epithelial cells approach, assume a crescentic shape and apply themselves to the central cell as shown in fig. 29.38 a. The nucleus of the central cell then disintegrates and the resultant vacuole enlarges to engulf some of the nuclear fragments; as it expands it compresses the cytoplasm and the keratohyaline granules against the cell membrane. At about the same time the surrounding cells fuse to form a syncytium, closely applied to the distended cytoplasmic membrane of the central cell (fig. 29.38 b and c). New cells become applied to the periphery of the corpuscle, while others enter the vacuole through its cell membrane (fig. 29.38 d and e) where they and their keratohyaline granules may be digested. Such 'intrusion' of cells may be repeated many times until the central vacuole becomes distended by fluid and ruptures. In keeping with their known attraction to sites of protein digestion, eosinophil leucocytes migrate into the ruptured cyst. Hassall's corpuscles become progressively larger with age, and their centres fill with amorphous debris

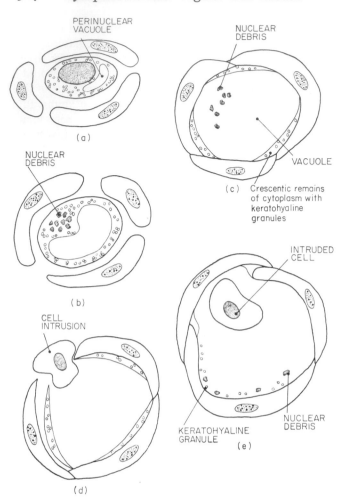

FIG. 29.38. Stages in the formation of Hassall's corpuscles.

and eosinophilic hyaline lamellae. Nuclear fragments and keratohyaline granules are prominent and only the peripheral cells retain a normal nucleus.

The Hassall's corpuscles probably destroy effete thymic macrophages which migrate to the medulla with their loads of lymphocytic nuclear debris. When the number of such macrophages increases, as in times of involution or cortisone-induced lympholysis, the number and size of the corpuscles also increase.

In EM of the human thymus, cytoplasmic organelles of a type associated with secretion may be seen in the epithelial cells of Hassall's corpuscles, together with numerous small, spheroidal secretion granules. Secretory granules or apparatus cannot be found in the medullary or cortical epithelial cells. As Hassall's corpuscles are avascular structures and surrounded by an avascular zone, these findings are in keeping with the medullary origin of a thymic humoral factor which has an inductive intrathymic function (p. 29.41).

Thymic function in the newborn

In the embryo, lymphocytes appear first in the thymus, and many experiments have illustrated its leading part in the development of the lymphoid system. If the thymus is removed from newborn mice, they continue to grow for 3 to 4 weeks but thereafter develop a fatal wasting disease with loss of weight, severe respiratory and other infections and, most important, a marked lymphopenia and hypoplasia of the lymph nodes, spleen, tonsils and Peyer's patches in the intestine. The appearances are similar to those of the runt disease which occurs in animals undergoing a graft versus host reaction (p. 29.24). There is no doubt that the failure to thrive is due to frequent infections, since the animals live much longer if they are treated with antibiotics or reared in a germ-free environment. The increased susceptibility to infection reflects a defect of cellular immunity due to the failure of thymic lymphocytes to reach the lymphoid system which, in turn, does not develop fully. Failure of cellular immunity may be confirmed by observing the behaviour of skin allografts (p. 29.24). In a normal animal a skin allograft excites a local inflammatory response in which the host's lymphocytes mount an immune attack on the graft tissue and bring about rapid rejection. A thymectomized newborn animal fails to reject an allograft and indeed may accept a xenograft from an unrelated species, e.g. the rat.

The immune defects which follow thymectomy in the neonatal mouse are fundamentally those of the lymphocyte-mediated immune cellular reactions. However, in the atrophic lymphoid tissues, germinal follicle formation also may be absent or rudimentary, possibly due to the loss of the helper effect of the T cells. The number of plasma cells is not seriously diminished and antibody production against some antigens, e.g. pneumococcal polysaccharide or endotoxin of *Escherichia coli*, is not greatly reduced.

A more positive approach to thymic function may be made by studying attempts to reverse the effects of thymectomy in neonatal animals.

RESTORATION BY CELLULAR SUSPENSIONS

Preparations of genetically compatible lymphocytes can restore the depleted lymphoid tissues, circulating lymphocytes and the cellular immunity of thymectomized neonatal animals. Complete restoration, limited only by the life-span of the injected lymphocytes, is possible by the use of suspensions from lymph nodes, spleen and thoracic duct of normal animals, but thymocytes have no such ability.

RESTORATION BY THYMIC GRAFTING

Compatible thymus grafts implanted in thymectomized neonatal animals restore their lymphoid organs and immune state after 3 or 4 weeks. After implantation the graft takes some time to acquire an adequate blood supply and during this period most of its lymphocytes die.

Thereafter the epithelial frame of the graft gradually becomes restocked with healthy lymphocytes. Meanwhile, the peripheral lymphoid tissues, which the graft saves from atrophy, acquire increasing numbers of lymphocytes and by the fourth week are restored to normal. To find out the origin of the new lymphocytes in the graft and in the peripheral lymphoid tissue, grafts can be used bearing a marker chromosome which allows cells of the host and graft to be distinguished. In this way lymphocytes which have restocked both the thymic graft and the peripheral lymphoid system can be shown to have originated almost entirely in the host. Since the lymphocytes of the graft die off rapidly, the relatively hardy epithelial framework of the graft may be in some way responsible for the reappearance of the new population.

MECHANISMS OF THYMIC LYMPHOPOIESIS

In a thymectomized animal, the effect of the epithelial framework of a thymic graft in restocking the graft itself and the peripheral lymphoid tissues with lymphocytes has two possible explanations.

(1) It could act directly to induce marrow stem cells in its interstices to mature into thymocytes, which are then exported to the periphery for further development.

(2) It could secrete thymic humoral factor (thymosin) which may promote lymphopoiesis by acting on stem cells both in the graft and in the host's peripheral lymphoid tissues.

To resolve this controversy it is best to begin by considering an experiment which appears to favour the production of a humoral factor. Thymic grafts can be enclosed in a cell-tight 'millipore' capsule before implantation so that their cells cannot enter the tissues of the host. Such grafts restore, at least partially, the peripheral lymphoid development and immune function in thymectomized neonatal mice. This experiment along with the histological appearances of a secretory cycle in medullary epithelial cells (p. 29.34) has been taken as evidence for a thymic humoral factor which promotes lymphopoiesis from marrow stem cells in the periphery. However, this interpretation has two weaknesses. First, no humoral factor has been isolated from the thymus and characterized. Second, it fails to take account of an established property of inductive systems, namely that induction of changes in one tissue by another can take place across a millipore membrane. The effect may well be humoral in the sense that a filter-passing agent carries the inductive stimulus or information; yet the amount of the agent which is effective may be too small to be detectable and incapable of remote effects after dilution in the blood stream. Such an agent could be described as a local hormone (p. 27.50), not acting on peripheral lymphoid tissue, but able to induce lymphopoiesis from stem cells in the vascularized zone around the millipore capsule,

followed by migration of maturing lymphoid cells to the periphery.

At present it is best to regard the effect of thymic grafts and, by extrapolation, the function of the normal thymus, as directly inducing stem cells within their epithelial framework. Experiments have shown that thymic grafts devoid of medullary epithelium are less effective. Inductive potential may depend on the secretion of a membrane-passing agent of low potency secreted chiefly by medullary epithelium.

EFFECTS OF IRRADIATION ON THYMIC GRAFTS

Induction of lymphopoiesis by thymic grafts in the newborn thymectomized mouse is separable into two components. One is radioresistant and is concerned with the production of thymocytes and T_1 cells; the other is radiosensitive and in some way determines the ultimate ability of the T_1 cells to mature into immunocompetent T_2 cells after leaving the thymus.

Thymic function in the adult

The adult animal has a fully developed lymphoid system and thymectomy does not give rise to severe wasting infections as in the neonate. In fact, it has little evident effect upon growth, reproduction, resistance to infection or longevity. Nor can changes be detected in humoral antibody formation or homograft rejection in the period soon after thymectomy. However, 6–9 months thereafter the adult animal loses weight and there is a fall of about 30 per cent in circulating lymphocytes. Although outwardly healthy, the animal has an impaired cellular immune response to antigens not met previously.

THYMIC FUNCTION IN THE IRRADIATED ADULT ANIMAL

Total body irradiation of sufficient dose kills an animal by destroying the haemopoietic bone marrow, but it can be kept in moderate health by injection of compatible bone marrow. This acts by providing stem cells which mature in the irradiated animal and repopulate it with blood cells and lymphocytes. If, however, the animal is thymectomized before it is irradiated, restoration of haemopoiesis is unaffected but the lymphoid tissues fail to regenerate and the cellular immune response is lost. The restoration of lymphopoiesis and of cellular immunity in the irradiated adult is therefore dependent upon the thymus, which must still retain lymphopoietic and inductive potential. Furthermore, since the thymus shares the total body irradiation, these effects must be relatively radioresistant, in keeping with the known radioresistance of the relatively hardy epithelial framework. The persistence of thymic lymphopoiesis in adult life and the poor cellular response to new antigens after thymectomy suggest that the function of the adult thymus is to maintain a small steady supply of highly selected virgin T lymphocytes, which can mature in the periphery.

EXPERIMENTAL B ANIMAL

Young adult irradiated, thymectomized animals kept alive by injections of marrow cells are known as B animals, for they have no T cell function but their B lymphocyte and plasma cell system is relatively intact. They provide a valuable experimental model for studying the functions of T cells from genetically compatible donors *in vivo* under different experimental conditions, without interference from host T cells.

INVOLUTION OF THE THYMUS

During the growth of the embryo and the young animal, the supply of T lymphocytes is assured by a relatively large and active thymus. By adolescence the peripheral lymphoid tissues are fully developed, amd most of the important antigens have been enountered and immunity to these established.

Along with the reduced demands upon it, the thymus becomes a barely recognizable fibro-fatty tag which contains many Hassall's corpuscles surrounded by a few intensely pyknotic lymphocytes. The stimulus to involution probably comes from within the thymus itself, possibly by a decline in inductive power of the epithelium or in secretion of its humoral factor. As the gland involutes there is a loss of lymphocytes, and also shrinkage of the epithelial framework of both cortex and medulla. The epithelial cells form cords and islands which may become cystic or contribute to the enlarging size and number of the Hassall's corpuscles. Their place is taken by adipose and fibrous tissue. These changes of involution are irreversible.

Natural involution must be distinguished from the atrophy induced by adrenocorticosteroids given medicinally. In contrast to natural involution, the effects of cortisol are confined largely to lympholysis with accompanying collapse, but not permanent loss, of the epithelial framework. The changes are reversible when the hormone is withdrawn. Atrophy of a similar type is found in stress situations such as burning, severe infection and prolonged illness. The weight of the thymus of young adults dying in these circumstances is less than in individuals who have died suddenly.

Thymus in disease

AUTOIMMUNE DISEASE

In autoimmune disease the immune defences, both humoral and cellular, are stimulated by the individual's own antigens and mount a self-destructive attack. Either abnormal cells, competent to react with 'self' antigens, appear in the body, or antigens, normally concealed, are released and stimulate a normal immune system.

Both mechanisms might be encouraged if the thymus failed to destroy lymphocytes of self-reactive type, or rendered the lymphoid system hyperreactive to 'self' antigens through its humoral factor. Certainly the thymus is involved in some way in autoimmune disease, for it shows proliferative changes in many of them, most markedly in myasthenia gravis (vol. 3, p. 34.31). Thus germinal follicles commonly appear, and occasionally a benign thymic tumour or thymoma may arise, either alone or along with germinal follicles in the parent thymus.

IMMUNOLOGICAL DEFICIENCY DISEASES

These are a group of hereditary diseases in which there are defects of humoral or of cellular immunity. All are rare and often an affected child does not survive long. They are listed and classified according to the immunological defect in vol. 2, p. 23.11. The thymus is often abnormal in these conditions; in Di George's syndrome it is aplastic or dysplastic and the child fails to thrive, so that the disorder is analogous to that following thymectomy in neonatal mice.

THYMUS AND MALIGNANT NEOPLASMS

Many neoplastic cells, especially those induced by chemical carcinogens and tumour viruses, contain antigens which are foreign to the host. It is thought therefore that the immune response may play some part in preventing the emergence of a malignant tumour, e.g. carcinoma. Animals which have been thymectomized show an increased susceptibility to tumours. Thus, after applying a carcinogen the interval before the development of neoplasia is shortened and the number of tumours is increased. It seems likely that the loss of the thymus diminishes the host's ability to deal with new 'tumour' antigens. It is possible also that the increased susceptibility to carcinoma in old age in human beings may depend ultimately on the waning of thymic function.

Summary of functions of the thymus

(1) In the newborn the thymus is necessary for the development of the peripheral lymphoid tissues. In its absence, lymphoid aplasia, lymphopenia and a failure of cellular immunity lead to wasting and death from infection. By adolescence the lymphoid system is fully developed and the thymus then involutes.

(2) In the adult the involuted thymus ensures the supply of virgin, immunologically uncommitted lymphocytes. Removal leads, not to severe illness, but only to a diminished response to new antigens.

(3) These two functions are achieved by the formation of thymocytes, under the influence of the medullary epithelium from stem cells supplied by the bone marrow; this may be mediated by an intrathymic humoral factor (thymosin). The thymic effect on peripheral lymphoid

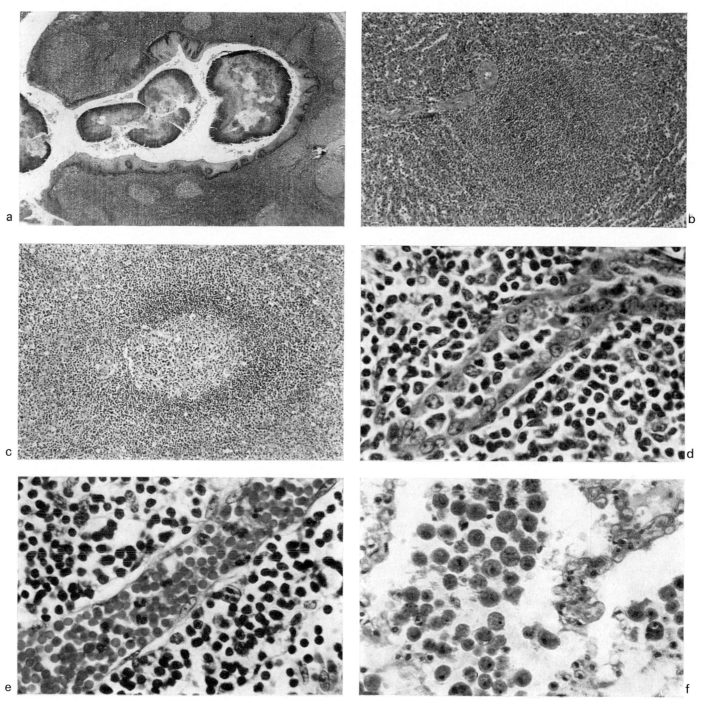

PLATE 29.2. Histology of the lymphoreticular tissues.

(a) Tonsil. The lymphoid tissue is closely apposed to the overlying squamous epithelium which is continuous with the buccal epithelium. The surface forms numerous deep epithelium-lined crypts, one of which is shown. The crypts contain pellets of bacteria and moulds. These ultimately appear on the surface as yellow spots and are expelled into the mouth causing a foul taste or odour. Colonization by bacteria provides a strong antigenic stimulus, probably responsible for the many germinal centres. Haem. & eosin (×25).

(c) Malpighian corpuscle with germinal centre. In times of antibody production germinal centres develop in the follicles. They appear as central zones of lymphoblasts surrounded by a slightly compressed zone of lymphocytes. The small eccentric arteriole is to the right of the follicle. Haem. & eosin (×100).

(e) A postcapillary venule from connective tissue. Note the elongated, sparse nuclei, flattened against the sides of a wide lumen. Haem. & eosin (×600).

(b) Malpighian corpuscle in the spleen. This is a condensation of lymphocytes which do not appear well demarcated from the red pulp. The eccentric arteriole is at the bottom right of the follicle. Haem. & eosin (×100).

(d) A postcapillary venule in a lymph node. Note the tall endothelium with large, vesicular nuclei which are crowded and protrude into the narrow lumen. Lymphocytes migrate through the endothelial cells from the circulation into the paracortex. Haem. & eosin (×600).

(f) Mononuclear phagocytes migrate into alveolar spaces from capillaries of the alveolar wall in response to infection or intra-alveolar exudation of red blood cells. Many of the phagocytes here contain rusty brown, granular pigment which is haemosiderin from ingested red blood cells. The phagocytes are large, with pale nuclei. Occasional double nuclei can be seen. Haem. & eosin (×425).

tissue may be produced by this substance carried in the blood stream.

(4) The thymus exports immature T_1 lymphocytes to the spleen where they acquire the full competence of T_2 cells and the ability to join the circulatory T cell pool from which they reach the lymph nodes.

(5) The thymocyte population is maintained autonomously by the thymus, which regulates the rates of both cell formation and cell death, and also determines the onset of natural involution.

(6) By providing T cells for 'immune surveillance', the thymus protects to some extent against experimentally induced neoplasia. However, it may play an inductive role in certain leukaemias.

(7) The thymus often shows pronounced germinal follicle formation in autoimmune diseases and may initiate some of them.

(8) The thymus is responsible for the restoration of cellular immune competence in animals rendered experimentally tolerant to antigens.

FURTHER READING

ELVES M.W. (1972) *The Lymphocytes*, 2nd Edition. London: Lloyd-Luke.

GOOD R.A. & FISHER D.W. eds. (1971) *Immunology: Current Knowledge of Basic Concepts in Immunology and their Clinical Application*. Stamford, Connecticut: Sinauer.

GREAVES M.F., OWEN J.J.T. & RAFF M.C. (1974) *T and B Lymphocytes. Origins, Properties and Roles in Immune Responses*. Amsterdam: Excerpta Medica.

HUMPHREY J.H. & WHITE R.G. (1970) *Immunology for Students of Medicine*, 3rd Edition. Oxford: Blackwell Scientific Publications.

STUART A.E. (1970) *The Reticulo-Endothelial System.* Edinburgh: Livingstone.

VAN FURTH R. ed. (1971) *Mononuclear Phagocytes.* Oxford: Blackwell Scientific Publications.

VAN FURTH R. ed. (1975) *Mononuclear Phagocytes in Immunity, Infection and Pathology*. Oxford: Blackwell Scientific Publications.

WEIR D.M. (1973) *Immunology for Undergraduates*, 3rd Edition. Edinburgh: Churchill Livingstone.

YOFFEY J.M. & COURTICE F.G. (1970) *Lymphatics, Lymph and the Lymphomyeloid Complex*. New York: Academic Press.

Chapter 30
Cardiovascular system

Since the time of the Roman physician Galen, coherent accounts of how the animal body works have started with notions of the relation of the blood to the heart and the pulse beat and recognized their importance for life. The central role of the circulation, which was dimly realized in the Graeco-Roman and even in the Chinese, Hindu and Egyptian cultures, was made explicit in Harvey's small volume *De Motu Cordis*, published in 1628, itself a landmark in the development of procedure in natural science.

Harvey made measurements of the blood volume, and by showing that the output of the heart could exceed the total blood volume, proved the existence of a circulation. The function of the veins and their valves was demonstrated and confirmed the conclusion that the blood must circulate continuously in the body. The demonstration by Malpighi (1661) and by van Leeuwenhoek (1703) of the capillaries connecting the arteries and veins, which were unknown to Harvey, completed the cycle of the circulation.

Current concepts of the function of the body continue to give the circulation of the blood a central role. The function of the cardiovascular system can be regarded basically as that of transport. Claude Bernard's '*milieu intérieur*' is maintained by and depends on a sequence of inter-relationships between events in cells, in fluid bathing the cells, in blood and in nerves, and in the external environment. Animals of more than a few million cells in size require a circulatory system to carry oxygen, carbon dioxide, nutrients and metabolites.

Functions of the circulation

OXYGEN TRANSPORT

The cells of the adult human require, in the resting state, some 200–250 ml/min of oxygen, all of which must be transported from the lungs to the cells throughout the body. To do this requires an output of blood from the heart of about 5 l/min. At rest most oxygen is required by the brain and by the liver, and relatively little by the muscles (p. 4.9). During severe exercise the oxygen requirement rises to 4 or more l/min, most of the increase being used by the exercising muscles. More of the oxygen carried by the arterial blood is removed in the tissues under these circumstances, but this factor alone allows only a two or threefold increase of the oxygen supply, and there must also be a large increase in blood flow to the exercising muscles. The cardiac output in fact may rise six or sevenfold to 30 or more l/min. Thus, in one minute, the heart may pump round the circulation a volume five times the total blood volume and supply a volume of oxygen equal to the total blood volume to the tissues.

Extremely hard exercise of this type cannot, however, be continued for more than a minute or two. The oxygen consumption of the body during normal activities is discussed in chap. 4. Table 30.1 repeats some of the findings.

TABLE 30.1.

Activity	O$_2$ used ml/min	O$_2$ used mmol/min
At rest	224	10
Standing	375	17
Walking	400–1000	18–45
Light work and exercise	750–1250	33–56

An adult usually complains of undue shortness of breath on effort if he is unable to increase his oxygen transport above 1000–1250 ml/min or treble the output of his heart on exercise. Such increases are sufficient to allow a man to earn his living in a light job and to enjoy light recreations and sport.

The cardiovascular system adjusts its rate of blood flow rapidly within these wide limits in response to metabolic need. Not only is the total heart output varied widely but the distribution of blood flow to the tissues, i.e. to muscle, skin, brain, liver and kidneys, can change greatly depending on local metabolic demand.

CARBON DIOXIDE TRANSPORT

The same considerations apply to carriage in the blood of carbon dioxide produced by the cells of the body. The amounts transported are comparable to the values for oxygen and vary according to metabolic activity, and a large excess carrying capacity is available in the form of changing blood flow.

NUTRIENTS AND METABOLITES

All the nutrients utilized by cells, including inorganic ions, glucose, amino acids, fatty acids, triglycerides and phospholipids, are transported via the blood stream. In contrast to oxygen, however, the utilization of these substances in the tissues is never so rapid as to be limited by the blood flow; in other words, the arteriovenous difference in the concentration of these substances is relatively small. Cell metabolites other than carbon dioxide, e.g. water, lactate, urea and creatinine, are transported by the blood stream and removed from it by the kidneys.

HEAT EXCHANGE

Many tissues of the body, particularly the brain, heart and viscera, function satisfactorily only within a narrow temperature range, and the central body temperature is stabilized closely around 37°C. An oxygen usage of 250 ml/min in the resting subject on an average diet means production of heat within the body of about 300 kJ/hr. About half of this heat is produced in the liver and brain and is distributed to other parts of the body via the blood stream. In exercise, heat is removed from the exercising muscles by the venous blood. Stabilizing the body temperature means that loss of heat at the surface of the body must be regulated in relation to ambient temperature. Excess heat is transported to the skin surface in the blood stream to be lost to the exterior by conduction, convection, radiation and evaporation (chap. 43).

Parts of the circulation

As though in response to the requirements mentioned above, the circulation is adapted to supply a widely varying volume flow of blood. A further adaptation is that this supply is fed into the distributing system of vessels under a stable head of pressure. There are obvious advantages in such an arrangement; it limits the tension which the walls of the blood vessels must withstand and thus permits stability of the vessels without unnecessary thickness of the wall. The brain is particularly sensitive to oxygen lack, and survives deprivation for hardly more than 3–4 min. Without a stabilized blood pressure the supply to the brain would constantly be endangered, particularly in erect animals such as man.

As a closed hydraulic system, the circulation consists of a pump, which is the heart, and a system of tubes, the blood vessels. After the neonatal period, there are in fact two pumps and two distributing systems of tubes, the **systemic** and **pulmonary circulations**, connected to each other in series. The two pumps, the left and right ventricles respectively, lie adjacent to one another in the heart, but the streams of blood passing through the right and left sides of the heart do not mix either within the heart or in the blood vessels (fig. 30.1).

The energy required to propel the blood through the circulation is supplied by the heart muscle. The mass of muscle in the heart of man is 250–400 g and the capacity of each of the pumping chambers or ventricles is about 100–150 ml. In addition to supplying energy the heart gives direction to the blood flow. The heart develops in the form of a folded tube, which contracts rhythmically, expelling its contents at each beat (p. 19.14). Valves are the non-muscular structures which allow flow to occur in only one direction. Finally, regulation of heart action is necessary to maintain constant input and output pressures and to vary the output according to requirement; various neural and humoral feedback mechanisms are involved in this regulation.

The systemic circulation may, from a functional point of view, be divided into:

(1) a distributing system consisting of the aorta and its major arterial branches,

(2) a variable resistance system consisting of the medium and small arteries and arterioles,

(3) a capillary system for the interchange of substances with the extracellular fluid of the tissues and

(4) a collecting and reservoir system of small and large veins, venae cavae and right atrium.

The pulmonary circulation similarly begins with the main pulmonary artery and ends in veins draining into the left atrium. Since the two circuits are in series, the volume flow through them must be equal if measured over any period longer than a few seconds. Pressures in the distributing systems of the two circuits are very different, however, being some five times greater in the systemic than in the pulmonary. The latter is much the shorter circuit and offers much less resistance to the blood flow; also the effects of gravity are smaller than in the widespread systemic circulation.

The distribution of the blood at rest in the different components of the circulation in an adult is given in Table 30.2. It is clear that the venous components contain over 50 per cent of the blood, but changes in the distribution can be brought about by alterations in cardiac function and in vascular tone or elasticity.

Symbols and units

As with any hydraulic system, basic quantities are required to describe the system and measure its performance. These are as follows.

Volume is the blood contained in the whole system and its various segments.

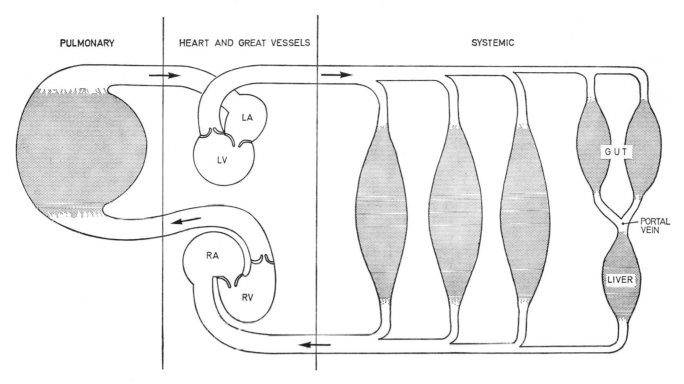

PULMONARY   HEART AND GREAT VESSELS   SYSTEMIC

FIG. 30.1. Schematic design of the circulation. The systemic circuit consists of parallel vessel systems, e.g. cerebral, muscular, renal, splanchnic. LV, RV, left and right ventricles; LA, RA, left and right atria.

TABLE 30.2. Distribution of the blood at rest in the components of the adult circulation

	Volume of blood ml
Aorta	130
Large arteries	500
Arterioles	100
Capillaries	300
Venules	1200
Veins	1300
Venae cavae	170
Heart and lungs	1300

Flow means volume flow, not velocity, and is conventionally expressed in ml/min or l/min.

Pressure is usually measured as the height to which a column of water or mercury in an open U-tube rises when connected to a cannula inserted into the vessel. This height is not affected by the bore of the manometer tube, and conventionally pressures are stated in terms of the height of the balancing column of mercury or water. Such heights, of course, can be measured only with reference to some zero level which, conventionally, is taken as heart level. Since the specific gravity of mercury is 13·6, a pressure of 1 mm mercury = 1·36 cm water. As it is the height of a column of fluid that is measured, it is convenient to record pressure in cm of water or in

mmHg. The SI unit of pressure, the pascal (Pa), is not generally used in recording blood pressures in man. Conversion of mmHg to kPa is calculated by multiplying by 0·133.

From measurements of volume, flow and pressure, the following derived quantities can be calculated.
Compliance (distensibility) = volume/pressure (m³/Pa).
Elastic resistance = pressure/volume (Pa/m³).
Resistance = pressure/flow (Pa m⁻³ s⁻¹).
Work = pressure × volume (J).

Since the main function of the circulation is to pump blood round the body, the most important measurements connected with it are the output of the heart into the distributing system and the pressure at which this supply is distributed. Second in importance is the input or filling pressure, which must be controlled within narrow limits, and third are measurements of blood flow through various organs and tissues, some of which are endangered by even a brief interruption of their blood supply.

Cardiac catheterization

The circulation in the heart and great vessels is studied in man by the technique of catheterization of vessels. A small flexible tube is inserted into a vein or an artery in the arm or leg, and the tip of the tube is advanced under radiological vision into the chambers of the right or left heart. Through these tubes pressures may be recorded and blood samples withdrawn for measurement of oxygen content; indicator dyes for measuring cardiac output and radio-opaque solutions for visualizing parts of the circulation may be injected through such catheters. This technique was first employed in 1929 by Forssman, who passed a catheter from his own antecubital vein into his right atrium. We owe the initial development of the technique to André Cournand of New York (1942). Cardiac catheterization is a safe procedure which has an established place in medical diagnosis. Some modern catheters incorporate a number of devices in their tips, such as pressure and flow transducers, which permit more accurate measurements. There is a very slight risk of severe disturbances of the cardiac rhythm. For this reason catheters should not be passed on healthy subjects, except under special circumstances and by experienced operators.

HEART

The heart lies in the centre of the thoracic cavity, above the diaphragm, behind the sternum, and flanked on each side by the lungs and pleurae. The posterior mediastinum,

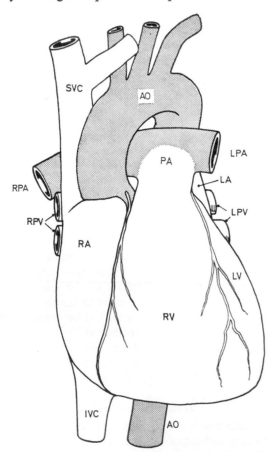

FIG. 30.2. Heart and great vessels in frontal view. LV, RV, left and right ventricles; LA, RA, left and right atria; PA, PV, pulmonary artery and veins; SVC, IVC, superior and inferior venae cavae; AO, aorta.

containing the oesophagus and descending aorta, separates the heart from the fifth to eighth thoracic vertebrae. Above are the aorta and pulmonary arteries and the two main bronchi into which the trachea divides.

The four **chambers** of which the heart consists, **right**

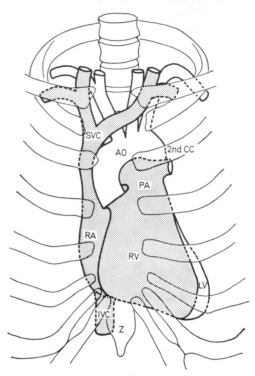

FIG. 30.3. Heart and great vessels in frontal view, in relation to thoracic cage; Z, xiphoid process; 2nd CC, second costal cartilage; other symbols as in fig. 30.2. The apex beat is usually felt in the 5th intercostal space in the mid-clavicular line.

and **left atria**, and **right** and **left ventricles**, lie as shown in figs. 30.2–30.6. The right ventricle lies anterior to the left and therefore its profile cannot be seen in an anteroposterior view of the heart. The left ventricle, the most muscular of the four chambers, lies posteriorly and to the left of the right ventricle. The left atrium lies at the posterior aspect of the heart almost in the midline of the body. The right atrium lies anterior to the left atrium and to the right of the right ventricle and forms the right border of the heart in the anteroposterior view. All four chambers are in approximately the same horizontal plane.

The connections of the heart to the main blood vessels are as follows. The two **venae cavae**, superior and inferior, which return venous blood from the systemic circulation, enter the right atrium from above and below and form most of its upper and lower walls. The **coronary sinus** is the main vein draining the heart muscle and also enters the right atrium. Having passed through the tricuspid valve and been pumped onward by the right ventricle the blood leaves the heart through the **pulmonary artery**.

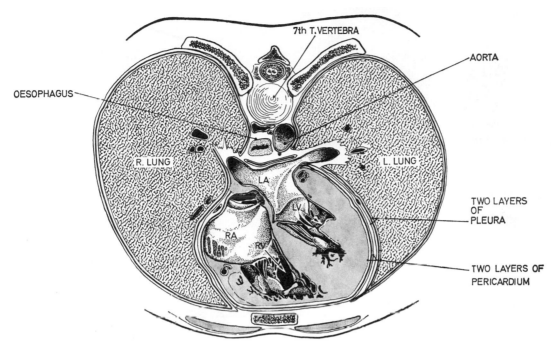

FIG. 30.4. Transverse section of thorax at heart level. LA, RA, LV, RV, left and right atria and ventricles. From *Cunningham's Textbook of Anatomy*, 10th Edition (1964) London: Oxford University Press.

This vessel crosses anterior to the root of the aorta and passes posteriorly and to the left of the aorta before dividing into a right and left branch. The **right pulmonary artery** passes to the right beneath the aortic arch and enters the hilum of the right lung. The **left pulmonary artery** continues to the left to supply the left lung.

The pulmonary venous blood returning from the lungs comes to the left atrium in four **pulmonary veins**, two on each side. These veins lie inferior to the respective pulmonary arteries, and enter the left atrium on its lateral walls. This blood, oxygenated from its passage through the pulmonary circuit, is passed through the mitral valve into the left ventricle and then ejected into the **aorta** from which branches distribute it to the whole systemic circuit. The root of the aorta lies posterior to the pulmonary artery, and the aorta follows an arching course, upwards, posteriorly and inferiorly, first to the right of the main pulmonary artery, then superior to the right pulmonary artery and left main bronchus and finally inferiorly in the posterior mediastinum anterior to and to the left of the vertebral bodies.

The relative positions of the chambers of the heart and the great vessels communicating with them are important, as are the projections they make on the cardiac outline, seen in radiographs of the chest (fig. 30.6). In the posteroanterior view the right heart border is made up of the superior vena cava, the ascending aorta and the right atrium. The left border is formed by, from above downwards, the aortic arch, the main pulmonary artery, a small portion of the left atrium known as the left

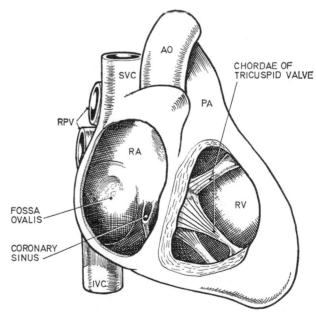

FIG. 30.5. Right heart chambers with portions of wall removed. From *Cunningham's Textbook of Anatomy*, 10th Edition (1964) London: Oxford University Press.

atrial appendage, and the left ventricle. In the lateral view the right ventricle and pulmonary artery are in front, and the left atrium forms the posterior border of the heart (fig. 30.7). In clinical practice it is sometimes helpful to examine the outline of the heart with the patient angled at 45° to the screen. These are called oblique views and are shown in fig. 30.7c & d.

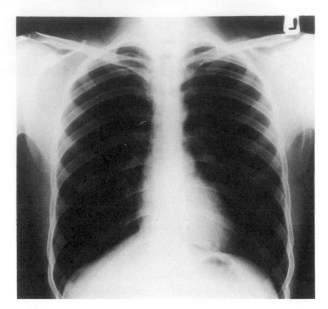

FIG. 30.6. A radiograph of the normal chest. Several of the structures shown in fig. 30.7 are easily seen. They include the ascending aorta, the pulmonary artery, the left ventricle, the right atrium and the shadow in the superior mediastinum showing the superior vena cava.

Of the two separate streams of blood being pumped through the heart, the right stream, from the right atrium to the pulmonary artery, spirals round the left stream flowing from the left atrium to the aorta. This is partly due to the geometrical shapes imposed on the ventricles by their differing functions. The main core of muscle in the heart is the left ventricle, which is roughly cylindrical in shape. The right ventricle on the other hand is thin walled, triangular in the frontal projection, and rather flattened antero-posteriorly.

Because of the oblique position of the heart in the chest, when the atria enlarge in disease they do so into the right side of the thorax. When the left ventricle enlarges it does so into the left hemithorax. When the right ventricle enlarges it does so in an anteroposterior plane.

The heart is a muscular organ. All muscles require some attachments if their contractions are to be translated into work. Some of the heart muscle is arranged in a circular form, in the wall of the left ventricle, and it therefore forms its own origin and insertion. The rest of the heart muscle spirals around the ventricles and works through its attachment to the fibrous stroma surrounding the four valve rings (fig. 30.8). The valves of the heart are set close together and in roughly the same oblique plane, with the ventricles on one side and the atria and great vessels on the other. When a ventricle contracts it does so concentrically, shortening its diameter, and also longitudinally, shortening its length by pulling on its attachment to the valve rings.

The circular layer of muscle lies innermost in the two

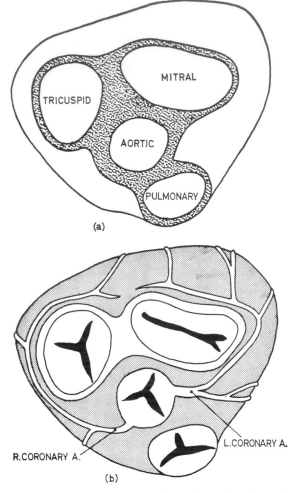

FIG. 30.8. (a) Diagrammatic section at level of atrioventricular groove to show from above the valve rings constituting the fibrous framework of the heart. (b) As in (a), with addition of valves and coronary arteries. The pulmonary and aortic valves are anterior to the mitral and tricuspid valves.

ventricles, a thick layer in the left ventricle and a thin one in the right. Outside this are two oblique or spiral layers, arranged at right angles to one another and tending on contraction to pull the ventricular chamber towards the valve rings, or vice versa (fig. 30.9). That the latter movement is important may be seen by examining the heart radiographically, as it is beating; if a contrast medium is injected, the valves can be seen to move with contraction as do the cavities of the ventricles. Indeed, the silhouette of the heart appears remarkably immobile while it is contracting despite the volume of blood being ejected from it with each beat. The explanation lies partly in the reciprocal volume changes in the atria and ventricles; as the ventricles contract the atria fill with blood and as the ventricles fill the atria contract.

The differences between the left and right ventricles are related to the different conditions under which they work. The left ventricle works against a pressure five

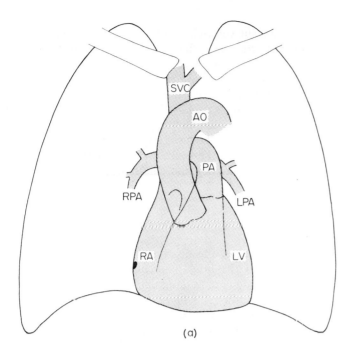

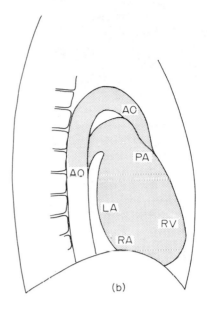

(a)

(b)

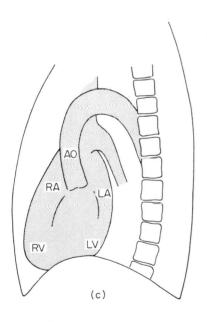

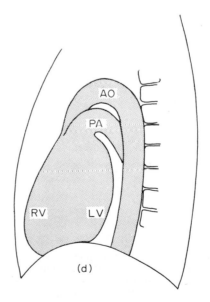

(c)

(d)

FIG. 30.7. Radiographic appearances of the heart.

(a) Posteroanterior view in which the right border of the heart is composed of the superior vena cava (SVC), the ascending aorta (AO) and the right atrium (RA). The left border of the heart is formed by the aortic arch (AO) and the first part of the descending aorta, the pulmonary artery (PA) and its main left branch, and the left ventricle (LV).

(b) Right anterior oblique view in which the anterior border is formed by the ascending aorta (AO), the pulmonary artery (PA), and the right ventricle (RV). The posterior aspect is formed by the descending aorta (AO), the left atrium (LA), and the right atrium (RA).

(c) Left anterior oblique view in which the anterior border is formed by the ascending aorta (AO), the right atrium (RA) and the right ventricle (RV). The posterior aspect is formed by the left atrium (LA) above and the left ventricle (LV) below.

(d) In the left lateral position the shadow is formed by the aorta (AO), the pulmonary artery (PA) and below them the ventricles (RV), (LV).

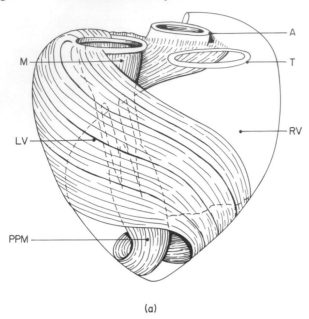

(a)

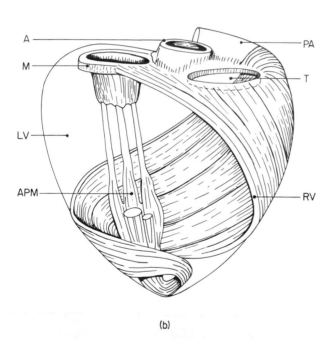

(b)

FIG. 30.9. (a) Posterior view of left spiral muscle. Origin from portions of the left A-V ring; insertion, mainly through the posterior papillary muscle and the posterior leaflet of the mitral valve to the left A-V ring. (b) Posterior view of right spiral muscle. Origin mainly from the right A-V ring; insertion, mainly through the anterior papillary and anterior leaflet of the mitral valve to the left A-V ring. A = aortic valve ring; M = mitral valve ring; PA = pulmonary artery valve ring; T = tricuspid valve ring; LV = left ventricle; RV = right ventricle; APM and PPM = anterior and posterior papillary muscles. Modified from Robb J.S., Hiss J.G.F. & Robb R.C. (1935) *Amer. Heart J.* **10**, 288.

times greater than the right. Its cylindrical shape is mechanically the most efficient for pumping against pressure.

The right ventricle, on the other hand, bears the brunt of the transient fluctuations in volume of venous blood returning to the heart. Its shape and relatively poor muscularity give it a high compliance so that beat-to-beat variations in venous return are smoothed out as the blood is passed on to the low-pressure pulmonary circuit. Before birth both ventricles work in parallel, against the same impedance, and their wall thickness is about the same. The difference in thickness develops in infancy and childhood.

Pericardium

The surface of the heart muscle is continually moving relative to the other contents of the thorax. Like the lungs, the heart is contained within a serous cavity, the pericardium, which allows free movement. The development of the pericardium from the early coelomic cavity is described on p. 19.14. In the adult, the pericardium has an outer fibrous layer which encloses the whole heart, and parietal and visceral layers of the serous sac; the fibrous layer blends with the tunica adventitia of the great vessels close to the heart. The central tendon of the diaphragm is fused to the inferior surface of the fibrous pericardium. In front it is attached to the sternum by weak fibrous bands, but the lungs and pleural cavities separate most of its anterior surface from the thoracic wall. The thymus gland occupies a variable portion of the space anterior to the pericardium.

The serous pericardium which lines the fibrous sac is reflected on to the heart at the points where the great vessels pierce the fibrous layer. The visceral serous layer covers the heart completely and is separated from the parietal layer by a thin film of fluid. The potential cavity of the pericardium has two recesses, the **transverse sinus** which passes behind the aorta and pulmonary trunk, and the **oblique sinus** which passes up behind the left atrium between the openings of the four pulmonary veins (fig. 30.10). In inflammation of the pericardium excess of fluid may accumulate within the serous cavity.

The visceral layer of serous pericardium forms the outermost part of the **epicardium**. Between it and the myocardium, the coronary vessels and cardiac autonomic nerves course over the muscle. These are normally embedded in a layer of subepicardial fat. The inner layer of epicardium is fixed to the external surface of the heart muscle.

The inner surface of the heart muscle also has a smooth low-friction lining which allows the blood to flow smoothly within the chambers. This is the **endocardium**, which has an inner endothelial lining and supporting elastic and collagenous tissue. It also covers the valves and is continuous with the endothelial lining of the great vessels.

Valves

Two pairs of valves, one at the inlet and the other at the outlet of the ventricles, are necessary to give direction to the flow of blood through the heart. The inlet valves, or **atrioventricular valves**, are the larger in size and allow forward flow to occur with almost no resistance. The **tricuspid valve** is at the inlet of the right ventricle, and the **mitral valve** at the inlet of the left. The outlet or semilunar valves are the **pulmonary valve** for the right ventricle and the **aortic valve** for the left.

Valve mechanism is complex. The valve cusps are passive structures which float into apposition and separate again in response to minute pressure differences and eddies in the flow of blood. On the left side of the heart they have to withstand high pressures when closed,

and they combine delicacy of structure with efficiency better than any model made by man.

All the valves, except the mitral, have three cusps; the mitral has two. When forward flow is occurring these cusps drift apart widely to allow unimpeded flow of blood. When forward flow slows and finally stops, the drop in pressure rapidly closes the valve cusps and there is no backflow. This action is caused by the flow patterns which form on the downstream side of the valves, a series of vortices (whirlpools) forming in either the arterial sinuses or the cavity of the ventricle (fig. 30.11). The arterial sinuses are dilations immediately downstream from the cusps of the aortic and pulmonary valves. They are essential for formation of the vortices which they trap, thus permitting wide opening of the valve cusps and

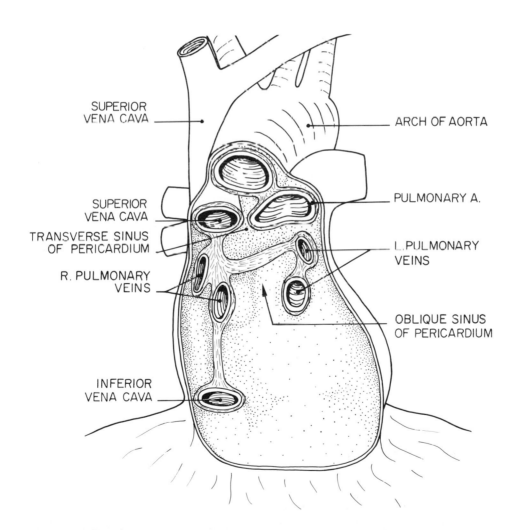

FIG. 30.10. View of posterior pericardium with the heart removed to show pericardial reflections. Note that all the veins are contained within one reflection and all the arteries in another, leaving the oblique sinus between the veins and the transverse sinus between the arteries and the veins. Modified from Warwick R. & Williams P.L. eds. (1973) *Gray's Anatomy*, 35th Edition. London: Longman.

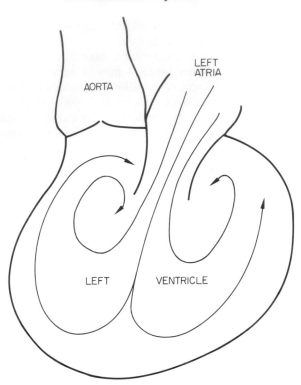

FIG. 30.11. Flow patterns around mitral valve showing vortices formed in the cavity of the left ventricle.

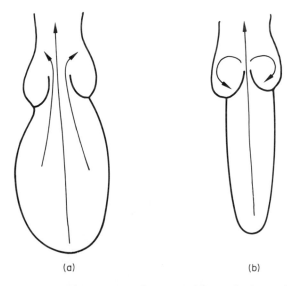

(a) (b)

FIG. 30.12. Flow patterns in LV and aorta in (a) early systole and (b) late systole showing development of ring vortices in coronary sinuses initiating closure of aortic valve. After Bellhouse.

efficient closure (fig. 30.12). Thus, during ventricular relaxation the aortic and pulmonary valves support the column of blood which has been pumped into the corresponding arteries, and the mitral and tricuspid valves prevent blood from being pumped backwards into the atria when ventricular contraction occurs. Clearly the

semilunar and atrioventricular valves act reciprocally, one set being open when the other is closed and vice versa.

The **aortic valve** has two posterior and one anterior cusp; they open when pressure in the left ventricle exceeds that in the aorta and, during the rapid phase of ejection, blood vortices form behind the valve leaflets in the three sinuses. The leaflets are held in a stable position by their trapped vortices. After the peak of systole, blood flowing through the valve decelerates. This causes the cusps to move towards a closed position. By the end of systole the cusps are almost in apposition, and only a tiny amount of backflow is required to shut the valve completely. The commissures of the valve are the junctions of adjacent cusps at their bases near the valve ring.

The **mitral valve** has a large anterior or aortic cusp and a smaller posterior or mural cusp. The cusp margins and the ventricular surface of the cusps are attached to fine cords (chordae tendineae) which are in turn attached to two papillary muscles. The chordae from the adjoining halves of the adjacent cusps are linked to the same papillary muscle. These muscles spring from and form part of the ventricular myocardium and share in ventricular contraction. Their function is through the chordae to hold the valve cusps in apposition during ventricular contraction. Damage to papillary muscles or to chordae results in leakage of blood backwards into the left atrium during systole (mitral regurgitation).

When the left ventricle relaxes and pressure within it falls below left atrial pressure, the mitral valve opens widely and blood rushes into the ventricle. Almost immediately, however, ring vortices form behind the two cusps, especially the anterior cusp, and as flow through the valve decelerates these vortices gain strength and

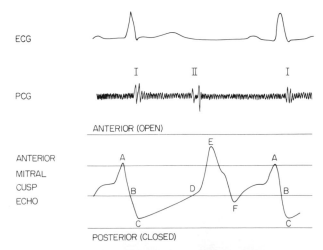

FIG. 30.13. Simultaneous electro- and phonocardiogram (ECG & PCG) with M-shaped echocardiogram of anterior cusp of mitral valve. The valve is closed at C. It opens widely at DE, but tends to close again during diastole. (F). Following atrial systole valve reopens widely (A) before closure (AC). Horizontal lines are 1 cm apart.

partially close the valve in mid-diastole. Atrial contraction in the latter portion of diastole reopens the valve slightly, but again the valve is nearly closed before the onset of ventricular contraction which merely completes the closure.

Function of the right-sided valves is similar although the forces generated are much less.

It is possible to visualize the double movement of the anterior cusp of the mitral valve by ultrasound, in which a beam of sound is projected from the skin surface towards the heart, and the time delay of reflected echoes indicates the depth of structures below the skin (fig. 30.13).

In the case of the left ventricle the inlet and outlet valves (mitral and aortic) are situated side by side, and in fact only the anterior cusp of the mitral valve separates the inflow and outflow tracts (fig. 30.14).

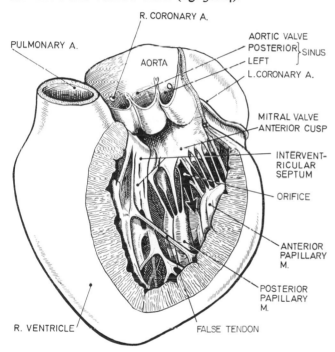

FIG. 30.14. The relation of the aortic valve to the anterior cusp of mitral valve; the arrow represents the direction of flow through the mitral valve. From *Cunningham's Textbook of Anatomy*, 10th Edition (1964) London: Oxford University Press.

Cardiac muscle

HISTOLOGICAL STRUCTURE

The myocardium consists of specialized muscle fibres separated by intercalated discs (p. 16.8). These discs offer a low resistance to the flow of electrical current so that excitation spreads throughout the muscle mass without the delay imposed by cell membrane resistance. Fibrovascular septa contain collagen, fibroblasts and blood vessels. In addition there are a few elongated cells, the nuclei of which contain a central longitudinal dense bar of chromatin, known as Anitschkow cells; they are phagocytic and probably derived from myocardial cells; they may give rise to the Aschoff cells of rheumatic carditis (vol. 2, p. 30.11).

In addition to the contractile elements, the heart contains non-contracting elastic components arranged both in series and in parallel with the contractile elements. Their internal elasticity modifies the actin-myosin contraction in relation to the development of tension and this takes place in a manner which is poorly understood.

The factors which govern the contraction of a strip of cardiac muscle may be analysed *in vitro* (p. 30.41) in terms of loading, developed tension, and speed and extent of shortening, while the pumping action of the heart as a whole may be measured in terms of pressures generated, volume flow and ventricular work (p. 30.3).

SUPPLY OF ENERGY

Under normal conditions cardiac metabolism is exclusively aerobic. The heart possesses only a small store of O_2 and polarographic measurements show a rapid fall of Po_2 to about 2 kPa within 30 sec of arterial occlusion. The large amount of myoglobin in heart muscle does not provide a store of O_2 but it facilitates diffusion of O_2 within the cells, where the diffusion constant is higher than in skeletal muscle. When the supply of O_2 to the heart is cut off or reduced, metabolism can continue at a lower level by anaerobic pathways.

The heart is a lipid-consuming organ and glucose is used relatively less than in skeletal muscle. Free fatty acids are the chief source of energy. They are derived from plasma free fatty acids and triglycerides and, in exercise, from myocardial stores of triglyceride. Keto-acids and lactate are additional important substrates which supply energy for ATP formation. The myocardium extracts more O_2 from its blood supply than other organs normally do; blood in the coronary sinus, which is the venous blood from the heart muscle itself, contains only about 3 mmol/l of O_2 whereas mixed venous blood contains about 7 mmol/l.

The nutrients enter the sarcoplasm from the blood where they are broken down to acetyl coenzyme A. Glucose is oxidized by the Embden–Meyerhof pathway and free fatty acids by β-oxidation. The oxidation of glucose via the hexose-monophosphate shunt does not normally occur in cardiac muscle. Lactate is taken up from the blood into the myocardial sarcoplasm and is oxidized to pyruvate by lactate dehydrogenase. The reverse conversion of pyruvate to lactate occurs in anaerobic circumstances only.

METABOLIC RATE

In an adult man at rest, coronary blood flow is about 220 ml/min. The arterial venous oxygen difference is about 120 ml/l, higher than in any other tissue. Oxygen consumption is therefore about 26 ml/min or 10 per cent of the resting metabolism. Oxygen requirement varies with heart rate, with developed tension and with the contractile state of the myocardium (p. 30.47). In severe exercise O_2 consumption may rise to 150 ml/min.

ELECTRICAL ACTIVITY

The action potential of the cardiac muscle cell is more complex than that of skeletal muscle or nerve (p. 15.16) and more subject to chemical control. It consists of four phases: **depolarization, plateau phase, repolarization** and **pacemaker activity** (fig. 30.15).

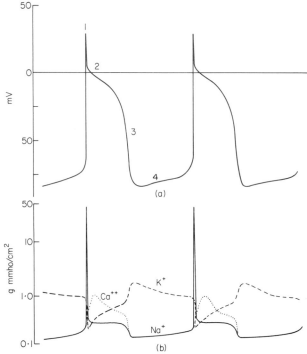

FIG. 30.15. (a) Action potential and pacemaker activity in a Purkinje cell; (b) corresponding changes in membrane conductance. Modified from Noble D. (1974) in *Recent Advances in Physiology*, Number 9, p. 47, ed. Linden R.J. London: Churchill.

Depolarization may result from impulses spread from an adjacent cell or occur automatically as described below. During the plateau phase (compare skeletal muscle and nerve), a second stimulus is inactive and the cell is said to be refractory. The absolute refractory period is about 0·15 sec in atrial cells and 0·30 sec in ventricular cells. During repolarization (or termination of the plateau), the cell is relatively refractory but strong stimuli can produce depolarization. The sinuatrial (SA) node, Purkinje cells and sometimes atrial cells possess pacemaker activity (or diastolic depolarization). Transmembrane potential follows a rising (less negative) course until it reaches a threshold value at which depolarization is initiated. In contrast, ventricular cells have no pacemaker activity and the transmembrane potential remains constant in diastole.

These phases are dependent on changes in membrane conductance (g) for the ions Na^+, K^+ and Ca^{++} which govern inward and outward currents through the cell membrane. Depolarization is accompanied by a rapid, brief rise in g_{Na^+} together with a fall in g_{K^+} which is more sustained. The plateau phase is continued by a slow rise in g_{K^+} and also by a secondary inward current of Ca^{++}. The plateau is terminated by inactivation of the Ca^{++} current and by delayed activation of g_{K^+}. In those cells which show pacemaker activity this is mediated by a slow fall in g_{K^+}.

Four types of cardiac cells are distinguished. Those of the sinuatrial node are spontaneously active due to pacemaker potential. Their membrane potential does not fall below -60 mV. Atrial cells have a large resting potential (-80 mV), a short plateau, and usually no pacemaker activity. Purkinje cells usually exhibit pacemaker activity which is operative at a large transmembrane potential (-70 to -90 mV). Ventricular muscle cells have a high plateau with positive transmembrane potential and exhibit no pacemaker activity.

The threshold potential (approximately -50 mV in the case of the SA node) is that at which g_{Na^+} suddenly increases, resulting in cell depolarization. The pacemaker may accelerate either because the Na^+ threshold is lowered (more negative) or because g_{K^+} is decreased, since this increases the slope of the pacemaker potential. This is the cause of the increase in heart rate with β-adrenergic stimulation. Acetylcholine produces temporary cardiac arrest because it increases g_{K^+} and thus abolishes pacemaker activity. The more proximal the automatic cell within the conducting tissue, the steeper is its pacemaker depolarization and hence the faster its rate of spontaneous discharge. Normally the faster proximal rhythm is propagated to the more distal cells causing them to depolarize before they would have done spontaneously.

A feature of cardiac action potentials is the role of the secondary inward current of Ca^{++} which provides a mechanism for maintaining the plateau independent of a high conduction velocity, and which offers a link between excitation and contraction. The inward movement of Ca^{++} may initiate contraction by releasing the large intracellular stores of Ca^{++} contained in the sarcoplasmic reticulum.

CO-ORDINATED CONTRACTION

The heart propels blood by alternately relaxing and contracting; it relaxes to allow the blood to flow in from the atria and contracts to expel the contents of the ventricles into the distributing systems. It is essential that contraction should occur in an ordered sequence and in a brief space of time. If contraction becomes uncoordinated, parts of the heart muscle contract and relax in an apparently haphazard manner, known as **fibrillation.**

Ventricular fibrillation causes the flow to stop in the circulation. Not only must there be nearly simultaneous contraction of all parts of the ventricles, but the atria too must contract at the appropriate time in the cardiac cycle, i.e. to complete ventricular filling just before ventricular contraction occurs and to assist closure of the mitral and tricuspid valves.

The spread of the electrical impulse is assisted by the branching arrangement of heart muscle fibres, and in small hearts such as that of the mouse this alone is sufficient to ensure co-ordinated contraction. In larger mammals including man, however, contraction would be so slow as to be ineffective without an additional fast conducting system, conducting the electrical impulse rapidly throughout the muscle mass. This system was described by the Czech physiologist Purkinje in 1839. The **Purkinje fibres** consist of specialized muscle cells, distinguishable histologically by their high glycogen content and electrically by a characteristic action potential (fig. 30.16). Some

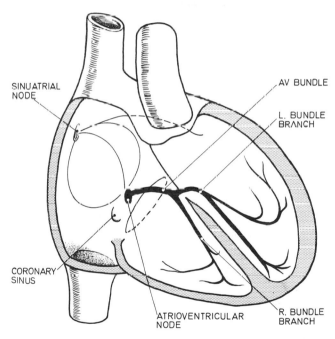

FIG. 30.16. Heart chambers opened to show specialized atrial and ventricular (Purkinje) conducting tissue.

of these fibres form cords of tissue known as **false tendons**, which cross the ventricular cavity (fig. 30.14).

Excitation must spread through the heart from a source which provides stimulation repetitively. As mentioned above, all cardiac muscle fibres have their own spontaneous rate of discharge or rhythmicity. The part of the heart with the highest spontaneous rate, therefore, provides the source of excitation of the whole heart, and this pacemaker is normally the **sinuatrial (SA) node**. It is situated high in the wall of the right atrium near the entrance of the superior vena cava. The SA node con-

sists of a small group of specialized muscle cells embedded in connective tissue and surrounded by a rich plexus of sympathetic and parasympathetic nerve endings.

From the SA node (fig. 30.16) the excitation wave spreads through the right and left atria. Transmission through the atria to the atrioventricular node occurs mainly in three muscle bands, one of which gives a branch to the left atrium. The velocity of the depolarization wave is relatively slow, 0·5–1 m/sec.

Situated low in the right atrium, near the opening of coronary sinus and tricuspid valve, is another group of cells with a specialized conducting function, the **atrioventricular (AV) node**. This structure is the starting point of the specialized fast-conducting Purkinje fibres. These fibres are collected together in the AV bundle of His (1893) which passes from the AV node into the upper portion of the interventricular septum, and constitutes the only muscular connection between the atria and ventricles. Conduction in this specialized muscle tissue is 4–5 m/sec.

High in the interventricular septum the bundle divides into left and right branches. The left bundle divides further into anterior and posterior branches. These branches arborize in the inner part of the walls of the corresponding ventricles. The false tendons provide a fast conduction pathway to the papillary muscles and adjacent areas of the ventricular wall.

ELECTROCARDIOGRAM

Spread of depolarization and repolarization through a muscle mass is accompanied by measurable electrical potentials which, since the body is a conductor, may be recorded by electrodes placed on the skin. The electrocardiogram (ECG) is a recording of the potentials which accompany cardiac activity and the various stages of spread of excitation through the heart may be followed in the ECG (fig. 30.17).

It is thus possible to identify from the ECG various stages of conduction, depolarization and repolarization in the heart and to note abnormalities. The relationship between the ECG and the individual cell action potential should be appreciated. The ECG represents the aggregate or resultant electrical activity of millions of individual cell action potentials, each of which has an amplitude and a direction.

The discharge of the SA node causes no deflection on the ECG. Atrial depolarization, however, is recorded as a deflection which is conventionally labelled the P wave. It occupies 0·05–0·1 sec. The next deflection, or complex of deflections, corresponds to ventricular depolarization and is labelled the QRS complex. Ventricular depolarization is normally complete in 0·12 sec. It starts approximately 0·1 sec later than the start of the P wave of atrial depolarization, and this interval, the **PR interval,**

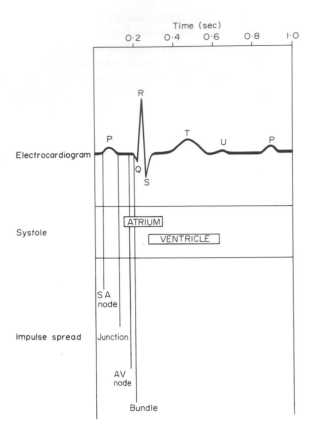

FIG. 30.17. The electrocardiogram, contraction (systole) of atria and ventricles, and spread of the electrical impulse through the heart from the SA node (pacemaker). P, deflection due to atrial depolarization; Q, initial downward deflection of ventricular activity; R, an upward deflection during ventricular depolarization; S, downward deflection following an R wave; T, deflection which may be either upward or downward following the QRS complex and due to ventricular repolarization; U, a deflection of unknown cause that sometimes follows the T wave.

measures the time required for the following events to take place:

(1) the passage of the atrial depolarization wave to the vicinity of the AV node,

(2) the delay imposed by slow-conducting junctional tissue surrounding the AV node, and

(3) the rapid spread of excitation via the AV bundle and its branches to the start of ventricular depolarization.

Most of the PR interval is occupied by delay in the junctional tissue.

Ventricular depolarization is rapid and is followed by an interval corresponding to the plateau of the action potential during which the muscle remains depolarized, the S-T interval. For this reason the S-T segment is iso-electric. The T wave represents the spread through the ventricle of the repolarization wave, associated with relaxation of the muscle contraction. Atrial repolarization

is usually not visible in the ECG as it is overlapped and obscured by the QRS complex.

Normally the SA node is the portion of the heart with the highest spontaneous rate of discharge, and therefore forms the pacemaker of the cardiac cycle. If the rate of discharge of the SA node is depressed, the portion of the heart with the next highest spontaneous discharge rate becomes the pacemaker, usually the AV node. **Sinus rhythm** is then replaced by AV **nodal rhythm**.

Again, if disease or drugs depress conduction through the AV bundle, the PR interval lengthens and a state of atrioventricular block exists. Impulses may fail altogether to be transmitted from atrium to ventricle, and the final or **complete stage of block** results in the ventricles beating independently of the atria at their own, much slower, spontaneous rate of discharge (20–40 beats/min).

Depolarization normally spreads rapidly through the ventricles in an ordered sequence, occupying less than 0·12 sec. (fig. 30.18). This is the effect of the rapidly

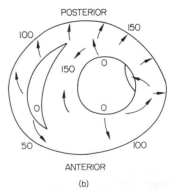

(a)

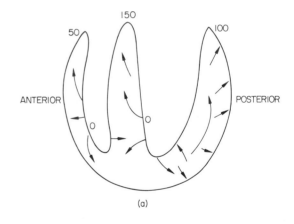

(b)

FIG. 30.18. Cross-sectional views of the canine heart; (a) coronal and (b) horizontal projections, indicating the sequence of excitation of the myocardium. Numbers indicate interval in msec after earliest excitation. The segments of the myocardium excited last are the posterior free walls of the two ventricles and the uppermost part of the interventricular septum. Modified from Scher A.M. (1965). In *Physiology and Biophysics*, ed. Ruch T.C. & Patton H.D., 19th Edition. Philadelphia: Saunders.

conducting Purkinje fibres. Damage to one or other of the branches of the bundle, left or right, results in delayed activation of the left or right ventricles respectively. In this condition, which is called **bundle branch block**, the QRS complex is increased in duration ($\geqslant$0·12 sec).

The Purkinje fibres, particularly those in the false tendons, cause ventricular depolarization to start in the immediate subendocardial area of both ventricles near the apex, including the papillary muscles (fig. 30.18). The sequence of depolarization, and therefore of contraction, follows approximately the line of the original tube from which the ventricles developed, so that blood is moved from the inflow region near the atrioventricular valves to the outflow regions near to the aortic and pulmonary valves. An abnormal beat can give rise to a reduced stroke volume both by a slower spread of activa-

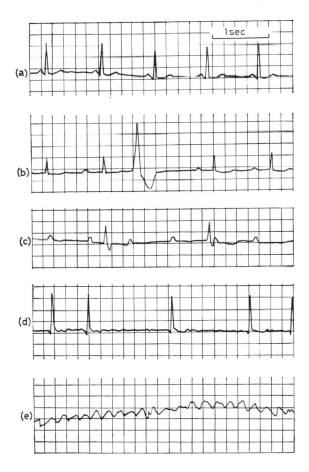

FIG. 30.19. Electrocardiograms illustrating some common disorders of rhythm. (a) Normal sinus rhythm; (b) prolonged PR interval (0·32 sec) and one ectopic (premature) beat, i.e. an irregular beat arising not from the normal pacemaker but from an abnormal irritable focus elsewhere in the myocardium; (c) complete AV block, atria and ventricles beating independently at 80 and 33/min respectively; (d) fibrillation or uncoordinated activity affecting atria only and (e) fibrillation affecting the whole heart.

tion and by a sequence of depolarization and contraction which does not assist forward pumping.

The importance of co-ordinated contraction has been emphasized. Uncoordinated, haphazard contraction, **fibrillation**, destroys the effective pumping action of the affected chambers. Fibrillation affecting the atria is a common and not usually serious condition; fibrillation of the ventricles is a terminal and rapidly fatal condition unless properly treated. The electrocardiographic record of fibrillation is a rapid totally irregular series of waves usually with no recognizable pattern (fig. 30.19d and e).

The electrocardiogram is one of the most important methods yielding information about the heart in clinical medicine. It allows the following aspects of cardiac activity to be assessed:

(1) the heart rate, at rest and under varying conditions,

(2) the rhythm, including the site of the pacemaker and any disturbances of the normal sequence of depolarization or disease of the conducting tissue,

(3) relative increase in the muscle mass, e.g. hypertrophy or overdevelopment of one or more of the four cardiac chambers,

(4) damage to portions of the heart muscle, usually caused by cutting off of blood supply (myocardial infarction),

(5) disturbances of the electrolyte composition of the intracellular fluid or reduction in oxygen tension in the heart muscle and

(6) inflammation of the pericardium or accumulation of fluid within the pericardial space.

CARDIAC CYCLE

By measuring simultaneously pressures and volumes of the heart chambers and recording the sounds of valve closure and the electrical phenomena of the ECG, it is possible to build up an accurate picture of how the electrical and mechanical events of the heart beat are related to one another in time. Pressure, sound and electrical potential present no difficulty, but recording of volume is not so easy. At first it was possible only in animals and involved opening the chest and enclosing the ventricles in a displacement recorder or plethysmograph. Now dimension gauges may be implanted within the heart; the ventricular cavity in man may be visualized by injecting radio-opaque substances and by taking radiographs in rapid succession in two planes at right angles to one another.

It is convenient to use the ECG as the reference for timing the other events.

PRESSURE CHANGES (figs. 30.20 & 21)

It is not difficult to remember the intracardiac pressures if certain facts are recalled:

(1) venous or input pressure in both circuits is low

in relation to the horizontal level of the atria (only a few mm Hg);

(2) a valve offers almost no resistance to the forward flow of blood, and when it is open pressures in the chambers on both sides of it are almost equal;

(3) the peak pressure in the systemic arterial system is approximately 100–150 mm Hg and in the pulmonary arterial system about one-fifth of this value.

Apart from the difference in pressure mentioned in (3) above, the pattern of pressure change is the same in the two sides of the heart, so it is convenient to consider only one, the left atrium, left ventricle and aorta, separated by the mitral and aortic valves.

The Q wave of the ECG signals the onset of ventricular contraction. Up to this point the atrium and ventricle have been in communication, the mitral valve being open, and pressures almost equal in these two chambers. When the ventricle contracts, pressure immediately rises within it and blood is prevented from being forced backwards into the atrium by closure of the mitral valve. Except in conditions such as atrial fibrillation or AV block, when ventricular systole is not preceded by a correctly timed atrial contraction, the mitral valve is closed before the onset of ventricular systole.

The rate of rise in pressure in the left ventricle (dP/dt) is very rapid and may reach values of above 2000 mm Hg/sec. When the pressure exceeds that in the aorta the aortic valve, which has hitherto been held closed, is opened and the blood in the left ventricle is expelled into the aorta. Ejection lasts as long as ventricular contraction persists, but is fastest in early systole.

The T wave of the ECG signals the repolarization of ventricular muscle which accompanies its relaxation. Pressure therefore falls in the ventricle, ejection stops, and since the aortic pressure now exceeds ventricular pressure blood would flow backwards into the ventricle were it not prevented from doing so by the aortic valve which is closed finally by the reversal of the pressure difference. Pressure in the ventricle falls rapidly. As soon as it falls below that in the atrium, the mitral valve, which has remained closed during the whole of ventricular

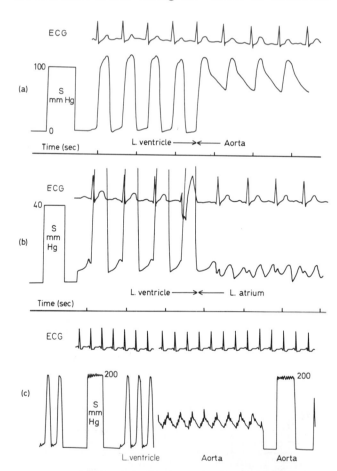

FIG. 30.21. Pressure in LV recorded in man through fine tubes. Note standard pressures (s) on the left. (a) The tube is withdrawn through the aortic valve into the ascending aorta. Note that in systole, pressure in LV and aorta is the same. (b) The tube is withdrawn through the mitral valve into LA. Note that in diastole, pressure in LV and LA is the same. (c) A patient in whom the aortic valve is narrowed by disease. Note high pressure in the LV and the pressure gradient between LV and aorta in systole.

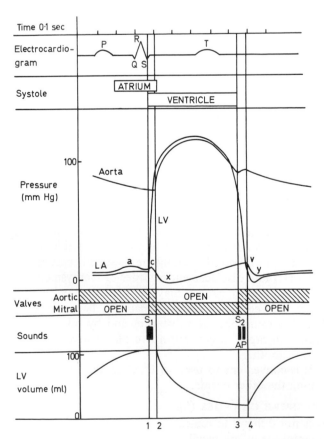

FIG. 30.20. Relationship of electrical and mechanical events and heart sounds in the cardiac cycle.

contraction, opens, blood flows in from the atrium to refill the ventricle and the pressures in the two chambers, now in communication, are again almost equal.

The P wave, which signals the contraction of the atria, is really the first event of the cardiac cycle following discharge of the SA node. Atrial contraction occurs in the latter part of the period of ventricular filling and adds a final boost to the filling of the ventricle, just before it contracts.

The period of ventricular contraction, occupying about four-tenths of the whole cycle at a resting rate of 70–90 beats/min, is known as **systole** and the period of relaxation or filling, occupying the remainder, is known as **diastole**. Ventricular contraction can be subdivided into phases:

(1) isovolumetric contraction, the brief period at the start when both valves are shut, and pressure is rising in the ventricle without change in its volume,

(2) rapid ejection phase, when blood is being pumped into the aorta more quickly than it is running off into the peripheral circulation, and aortic pressure is therefore rising, and

(3) slow ejection phase, when ejection is continuing but it is exceeded in rate by the run-off from the aorta into the periphery and aortic pressure is therefore falling.

The behaviour of the valves provides the guide to the pressure and flow events. As the valves are entirely passive structures their movement is determined by the lateral pressure acting upon them. When flow across the valve decelerates, the pressure exerted by the vortices behind the cusps begins to close them, and this process accelerates so that closure occurs at precisely the moment of zero flow and before flow begins to reverse. When the normal vortex formation cannot occur, as with a mitral or tricuspid valve with a grossly enlarged ventricle, then closure is due to a reversal of pressure gradient and flow, with a subsequent slight leak or incompetence; this method of closure occurs with most artificial heart valves used to replace damaged valves in patients. The valves open when a slight pressure gradient, sufficient to overcome the inertia of the blood, has built up across the valve. In practice the crossover points of the pressure tracings indicate the times of valves opening and closing to within a few milliseconds.

Left atrial pressure changes are small and amount to only a few mm Hg (fig. 30.20). The **a wave** is caused by atrial contraction and therefore follows the P wave of the ECG. The **c wave** is a small deflection immediately following the QRS complex. It is caused by the mitral valve shutting while blood still flows into the contracted atrium. The **x descent** occurs as the ventricle contracts and draws the mitral valve away from the atrium, thus lowering the pressure within it. Simultaneously the atrium is relaxing. The slow rise of pressure in the atrium as it fills from the pulmonary veins forms the **v wave**. Flow for-

ward into the ventricle is prevented because the mitral valve is shut. The **y descent** is the fall in atrial pressure as blood rushes into the ventricle when the mitral valve opens.

VENTRICULAR PRESSURE AND VOLUME RELATIONSHIPS

The ventricle fills and empties alternately and both parts of this cycle have an early rapid phase and a later slow phase. The only brief intervals during which the volume of the ventricle is constant are the isometric contraction period and the period of falling pressure after the aortic valve closes and before the mitral valve opens. The volume of blood ejected during systole from the left ventricle into the aorta is the **stroke volume** (60–100 ml). The **output of the heart** per minute is clearly the product of the stroke volume and the heart rate per minute. Not all the blood contained in the ventricle is ejected; a variable part of the ventricular volume remains behind (20–50 ml). This is the **residual volume**. When lying at rest the residual volume is relatively large. On standing or on exercise it is smaller.

Fig. 30.20 shows left ventricular pressure and volume simultaneously. By plotting pressure against volume throughout one cardiac cycle an anticlockwise loop can be obtained (fig. 30.22) from which the **external systolic work** of the left ventricle may be derived, i.e. the product

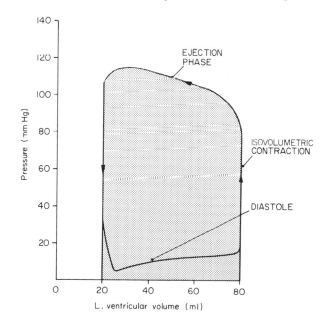

FIG. 30.22. Left ventricle pressure volume loop.

$$\text{Systolic work} = \int_{V_d}^{V_s} P\,dV$$

of stroke volume and the pressure to which that volume is raised by ventricular contraction.

SOUNDS

Valves open inaudibly. When they shut, however, vibrations are set up in the blood; these are transmitted through the chest and can be heard by the ear applied to the chest or indirectly through a stethoscope, or can be recorded by a microphone on the surface of the skin.

There are two audible sounds associated with valve closure. The first is related to closure of the mitral and tricuspid valves and occurs, therefore, after the QRS of the ECG when ventricular pressure starts to rise and exceeds atrial pressure. It is normally difficult to distinguish by ear the mitral and tricuspid components of the first sound since they are so close together in time, but in fact mitral closure occurs slightly earlier. The first sound is usually best heard at the cardiac apex.

The second sound is related to aortic and pulmonary valve closure. It occurs after the T wave of the ECG, at the cross-over points of left ventricular and aortic or right ventricular and pulmonary arterial pressures. Here, distinction of the aortic and pulmonary components is usually possible, the aortic being earlier. Deep inspiration increases right ventricular filling momentarily and prolongs right ventricular ejection, thus widening the degree of splitting of the aortic and pulmonary components and making their identification easier. The second sound is best heard to the left of the upper sternum.

A third sound may sometimes be heard in health. It is common in exercise, in pregnancy and in young persons. It may also occur in heart failure when the ventricles are dilated. It is soft and low pitched and occurs during the most rapid phase of ventricular filling. It is probably associated with changes in the formation of the vortices.

Sounds associated with valves opening almost always denote an abnormality of the valve. The flow of blood through the heart in systole and diastole is usually silent. **Murmurs** are vibrations caused by turbulence or a series of vortices in the blood stream and may be created in any part of the circulatory system, but most commonly in the heart. They indicate disease of valves, abnormal constrictions or communications in the central circulation, or reduced blood viscosity as in anaemia.

Innervation of the heart

The frequency and strength of the heart beat is regulated through the autonomic nervous system. Both sympathetic and parasympathetic autonomic fibres are present in the cardiac plexus of nerves which surrounds the origin of the great vessels at the base of the heart. The **sympathetic supply** is derived from T2–T4 and travels via the middle cervical and cervico-thoracic ganglia and the first four ganglia of the thoracic sympathetic chain. In order to remove completely the sympathetic control of the heart it is necessary to remove the cervicothoracic ganglia and the upper four thoracic sympathetic ganglia. The postganglionic fibres ramifying in the cardiac plexus supply the SA node in profusion, and also the whole cardiac muscle. The neural transmitter is predominantly noradrenaline and the cardiac effects of sympathetic

stimulation can be blocked by the β-adrenergic blocking drugs.

The vagus nerve provides the **parasympathetic supply**. The fibres branch in the cardiac plexus and then supply the SA node and both atria. There is no sure evidence of parasympathetic fibres supplying ventricular muscle. The neural transmitter is acetylcholine, and the cardiac effects of vagal stimulation can be readily reversed by atropine. Normally both sympathetic and parasympathetic impulses reach the heart continuously.

The effects of autonomic nerve stimulation on the heart are threefold:

(1) on the rate of discharge of the SA node, consequently controlling the heart rate. Sympathetic stimulation increases and parasympathetic decreases the heart rate. Studies of simple cardiac muscle fibres show that the increase in heart rate on sympathetic stimulation is due to increased rate of membrane depolarization during diastole of the cells in the SA node. As a consequence the threshold for action potential discharge is reached sooner (fig. 30.23). In contrast vagal nerve stimulation renders

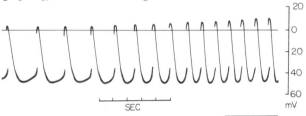

Fig. 30.23. Effect of sympathetic stimulation on pacemaker flow in sinus venosus of frog heart. Stimulation (20/sec) indicated by breaks in solid reference line at bottom of tracing. Note increase in slope of pacemaker potential, amplitude, and overshoot of action potential as heart rate increases. No change in level of 'resting' potential. From Hutter O.F. & Trautwein W. (1956) *J. gen. Physiol.* **39**, 715.

the resting potential more negative and slows the rate of spontaneous depolarization. Persistent vagal stimulation abolishes pacemaker activity in the SA node causing the condition known as vagal or sinus arrest.

(2) on the speed of conduction of excitation within the heart. The junctional tissue surrounding the AV node is particularly affected. Here parasympathetic stimulation decreases the excitability of the junctional tissue and results in slower transmission. Strong stimulation may produce AV block (p. 30.15).

(3) on the speed of contraction of the cardiac muscle and the tension developed by the fibres for a given degree of initial stretching. Under sympathetic influence the rate of rise of pressure within the ventricle is increased and the residual volume decreased without any increase in the filling of the heart in the presystolic phase. This may be looked on in another way. If we construct a length-tension diagram for a particular muscle fibre this will be reproducible provided that the neurohumoral *milieu* is unchanged. When catecholamine concentration

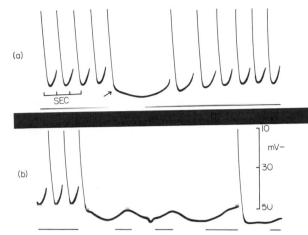

(a)

SEC

10
mV–
30
5U

(b)

FIG. 30.24. Effects of vagal stimulation on transmembrane potential of pacemaker fibre in sinus venosus of spontaneously beating frog heart. Record in (a) shows vagal stimulation at rate of 20 pulses/sec, as indicated by break in solid line at bottom of tracing. At arrow, note beginning of hyperpolarization of membrane and inhibition of pacemaker action potential. Several seconds after vagal stimulation ceases, membrane slowly depolarizes to a level at which action potentials are again generated. Record in (b) shows effects of intermittent (20 sec) stimulation on same fibre as shown in (a). Note hyperpolarization of membrane during vagal stimulation and slow return (depolarization) toward threshold when stimulation is discontinued. Note also escaped beat at beginning of fourth stimulation period. From Hutter O.F. & Trautwein W. (1956) *J. gen. Physiol.* **39,** 715.

is increased by sympathetic stimulation, however, the length-tension curve is shifted to the left, i.e. for a given degree of initial stretch a greater tension is developed in contraction. This important mechanism operates not only on ventricular contraction via the sympathetic system, but also in the atria through both sympathetic and parasympathetic influences, the former enhancing and the latter diminishing the strength of atrial contraction. The effect of increasing atrial contraction is to augment the flow of blood into the ventricle late in diastole (atrial supplementation), thereby raising the pressure within the ventricle and the degree of stretch of the myocardium before contraction. Sympathetic stimulation may therefore increase contractility in two ways, (1) by acting directly on the ventricle and moving its length-tension curve to the left, and (2) by increasing atrial contractility and hence increasing the initial stretch of the ventricular muscle fibres.

Ionic effects

The classical experiments of Ringer and Locke showed that an excised heart would only continue to beat if the medium perfusing it contained Na^+, K^+ and Ca^{++}. This is to be expected from the theory of action potentials. The Nernst equation (p. 15.9) relates the membrane potential to concentrations of these ions and the per-

meability of the cell membrane to them. A decrease in the transmembrane potential increases the readiness with which contraction occurs but weakens the contraction. An increase in potential impairs depolarization and decreases the duration of contraction.

Potassium has a greater effect on both electrical and mechanical activity than sodium. Potassium deficiency renders the resting potential less negative and the characteristic changes are low voltages in the QRS complex, flattening in the T wave, prolongation of the QT interval and the appearance of an additional positive deflection after the T wave, called the U wave. A high external $[K^+]$ is also associated with a decrease in the transmembrane potential and rapid repolarization with tall T waves and increased excitability. The effects of changes in $[Ca^{++}]$ are complex and cannot be explained simply in terms of membrane potential changes. However, it is known that the effects of low $[K^+]$ can be mitigated by reducing $[Ca^{++}]$ and those of a high $[K^+]$ by raising $[Ca^{++}]$. It is for this reason that Ca^{++} is often given intravenously in conditions associated with increased plasma $[K^+]$ (vol. 3, p. 49.30).

Tension

In any elastic spherical or cylindrical chamber the wall tension measures the force which would tend to separate the edges of a slit made in the wall. This important concept is related to the work done by the muscular walls of the heart or blood vessel to contain the blood within the vessel, and to the energy required. Also the thicker the wall, the greater the wall tension.

The relation between transmural pressure (TMP) in a chamber of radius (R) and the circumferential tension in the wall (Tc) is given by the law of Laplace.

$$Tc \propto R \times TMP$$

The larger the size of the ventricular cavity the more tension must be present in its walls to generate the same pressure within. Thus, when there is a high residual volume in the heart, the latter functions less efficiently.

ARTERIES

The systemic arteries provide a branching system of tubes taking the blood from the left ventricle and distributing it throughout the body. The pulmonary arteries similarly distribute the output of the right ventricle to the lungs; they are shorter, thinner walled, and contain blood under lower pressure than the systemic arteries.

In addition to the conduit function, arteries have a storage function. The output of the ventricles is discontinuous, occurring in ventricular systole only. The discontinuous blood flow from the heart is converted into a relatively smooth flow through the small blood vessels of the peripheral circulation. The effect of this is to conserve energy in accelerating the blood column and to reduce the pressures which the small vessels have to withstand. The arterial system, particularly the aorta, stores blood during systole and gives it up again during diastole so that the run-off of blood into the peripheral circulation is continuous. This function resembles that of a smoothing capacitor in an electrical circuit.

Structure

Arteries branch repeatedly and when their diameter is less than 0·1 mm they are called **arterioles**. Junctions between the branches are called **anastomoses** and they may occur between arteries and arterioles. In most organs these anastomoses ensure an adequate blood supply when one vessel is temporarily or permanently occluded. Occasionally anastomoses are absent or few in number, so the supply depends on a single vessel which is called an **end artery**. The central artery of the retina is a good example of an absolute end artery, but it should be apparent that as the number of anastomoses is reduced, functional end arteries increase.

Arteries are elastic tubes which are circular in cross-section because of the tension being equally distributed round their walls. These are composed of three coats or tunics.

(1) **Tunica intima** is the endothelial inner lining which provides a smooth, low friction, inner surface in contact with the blood stream.

(2) **Tunica media** is a thick middle layer composed of smooth muscle and elastic fibres intermingled and arranged both lengthwise and circumferentially.

(3) **Tunica adventitia** is an outer layer of fibrous collagenous tissue.

The elastic tissue provides for the storage function by stretching and relaxing according to the pressure within the artery. The smooth muscle under autonomic nervous control regulates the diameter of the artery. The fibrous elements serve to limit the amount of stretch and prevent the wall rupturing under a surge of pressure (fig. 30.25).

The amount of elastic tissue in the walls of arteries varies with the vessel. Near the heart, the aorta and its large branches contain a large amount which is scattered through the whole thickness of the tunica media. These vessels are often called **elastic arteries**, and they dilate to accommodate the stroke volume. The remaining muscular arteries also have some elastic tissue but it is usually confined to the inner and outer aspects of the tunica media. At the junction of the tunica intima and media there is a perforated sheet of elastic tissue, the **internal elastic lamina**. Amongst the inner layers of fibrous tissue forming the tunica adventitia, there are discrete longitudinal elastin fibres called **external elastic lamina**. The adventitia and media are thinner in small arteries and the external elastic lamina is present only in large arteries. The internal elastic lamina, however, is present even in small arterioles. The pulmonary arteries have such thin walls that they are readily confused with veins. The relative constituents of the

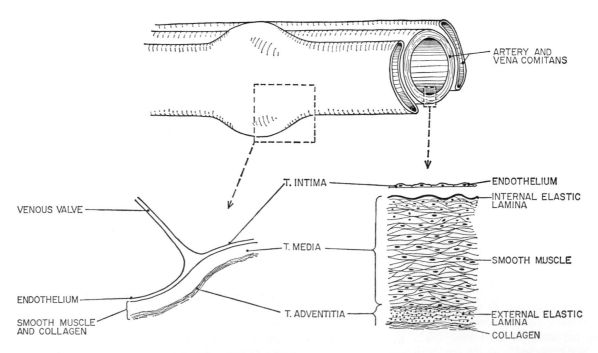

FIG. 30.25. The structure of a small, muscular artery and its accompanying veins. The tunica adventitia of the veins and artery are continuous with each other so that pulsation within the artery compresses the veins and so forces the venous blood towards the heart.

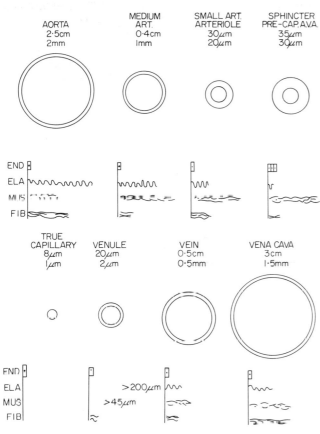

FIG. 30.26. The size, thickness of the wall and relative amount of the main constituent tissues of different blood vessels. The first figure below the vessel named represents the luminal diameter; the figure below this indicates the wall thickness. End = endothelial lining cells; Ela = elastic fibres; Mus = smooth muscle cells; Fib = collagen fibres. After Burton A.C. (1954) *Physiol. Rev.* **34**, 619.

different tissues in the blood vessels are shown in fig. 30.26.

Small arteries and arterioles are nourished by the blood they contain but such diffusion supplies only the inner layers of large arteries. The outer part of the walls of these vessels contain capillaries supplied by arterioles known as **vasa vasorum**.

Distribution

The **aorta** is the principal systemic artery (fig. 30.27). It starts at the aortic valve ring, passes in an arch upwards, backwards and finally downwards, crossing the pulmonary artery and left bronchus. The descending aorta lies anterior and to the left of the vertebral bodies and extends to the level of the fourth lumbar vertebra where it divides into the common iliac arteries. At its origin it is about 2·5 cm in diameter. Its main branches are:

(1) two coronary arteries which supply the heart,
(2) the brachiocephalic, left subclavian and left com-

mon carotid arteries which supply the head and arms,
(3) the intercostals which supply the trunk,
(4) the coeliac, superior and inferior mesenteric arteries which supply the stomach, intestine, liver, spleen and pancreas,
(5) the renal arteries which supply the kidneys,
(6) the left bronchial artery which supplies the lungs, the right usually arising from the 3rd intercostal artery, and
(7) the gonadal arteries which supply the testes or ovaries.

The common iliac arteries, into which the aorta divides, supply the pelvis and lower limbs.

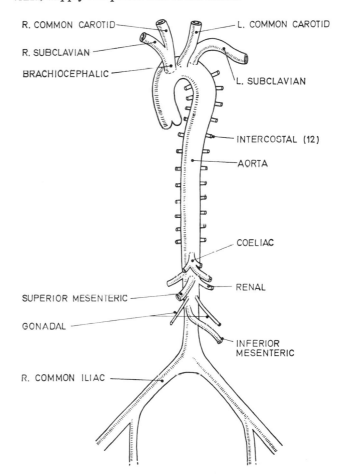

FIG. 30.27. Main branches of the aorta.

The **pulmonary artery** starts at the pulmonary valve, passes backwards and slightly upwards for 5 cm and divides into right and left main branches. The right passes under the aortic arch and into the hilum of the right lung, there dividing into upper, middle and lower branches going to the corresponding lobes. The left main branch passes backwards and to the left into the hilum of the left lung where it divides into upper and lower branches.

Blood flow in arteries

Except for part of the microcirculation, the flow of blood in vessels is pulsatile in nature; for this reason the relationships between pressure and flow, particularly when it is also borne in mind that the vessels have walls which are both elastic and viscous, are mathematically complex. However it is not necessary to know the oscillatory flow theory of haemodynamics in order to understand the dynamics of the circulation; many facts of importance may be understood by a knowledge of the much simpler steady flow theory, in which only mean pressures and flows are considered.

LAPLACE THEOREM

The French mathematician Laplace studied the relationship of pressure across an elastic surface to the tension in it and its curvature and obtained the equation

$$P_I - P_O = T\left(\frac{1}{R_1} + \frac{1}{R_2}\right)$$

where
P_I = pressure inside
P_O = pressure outside
T = wall tension

and R_1 and R_2 = greatest and least radii of curvature. The left-hand term ($P_I - P_O$) is the transmural pressure (TMP).

This theorem has several applications in the circulation and three important ones are considered.

Efficiency of cardiac pumping

For a sphere $R_1 = R_2$ and the equation becomes TMP $= 2T/R$; it can be shown that over a period of time the pressure work, which produces the cardiac output, is equal to the tension work, which is directly related to myocardial oxygen consumption divided by the ventricular radius. An increase in cardiac output produced by greater filling, i.e. an increase in heart size, requires a greater increase in oxygen consumption than one produced by greater emptying.

Curved vessels and aneurysms

If a curved vessel such as the aortic arch is viewed from the inside, the outer curvature appears convex and the inner concave. Hence R_1 is positive and R_2 is negative. As the pressure is the same in both situations, the wall tension is greater on the inner aspect of the arch than on the outer. A cross-section of the aorta confirms this point, for the aortic wall is thicker on the inside of the arch than on the outside. In the circle of Willis there are zones of increased wall tension at the angles where the cerebral vessels originate, and these are the site of aneurysms, pathological dilations, which may rupture in some patients.

Critical closing pressure

For a straight tube the relationship becomes TMP $=$ T/R. In the capillaries and small vessels the surface tension at the interface between blood and intima becomes an important factor. Unlike the tension in a vessel wall, which is a function of length of fibres, surface tension is a constant. Therefore a radius occurs below which an equilibrium is not possible and the vessel will collapse. This is known as the critical closing pressure. There is also a critical opening pressure at which the vessel will reopen; this is always greater than the critical closing pressure.

BERNOULLI THEOREM

This is one of the oldest theorems in hydrodynamics; although it assumes a perfect fluid with no frictional losses, which cannot occur in practice, it still has many useful applications. It states that the total sum of fluid energies at any point must be constant. In the general application to the circulation the lateral pressure plus the kinetic energy of flow are constant and equal to the fluid energy. In mathematical terms

$$P + \tfrac{1}{2}\rho V^2 = k$$

where
P = lateral pressure
ρ = specific gravity of fluid
and V = velocity of flow

Because of this, pressure measurements in the circulation, especially if there is jetting of blood, must take account of the direction in which the needle or catheter is facing. If only lateral pressure is measured it is possible for blood apparently to flow from lower to higher pressure where a marked reduction in flow diameter occurs. If a vessel dilates there will be conversely an increase in lateral pressure; this occurs in aneurysms and tends to increase their size.

LAMINAR AND TURBULENT FLOW

Fluid flowing along a uniform tube at a fixed rate does so in laminar form, i.e. the stream can be looked upon as an infinite number of concentric laminae or layers sliding upon one another, the innermost or axial layer having the highest velocity of flow, and the outermost layer, touching the lining of the tube, having the lowest velocity. A velocity profile can be drawn for the whole diameter of the tube (fig. 30.28). The energy utilized in propelling

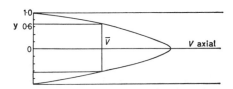

FIG. 30.28. The velocity profile in steady laminar flow.

$$V = \frac{P_1 - P_2}{4Lr}\,(R^2 - r^2)$$

V, velocity of any lamina at radius (r) from axis; L, length; η, viscosity; R, radius of tube. The average velocity ($\overline{V}$) can be shown to be half the axial velocity. $y = r/R$. From McDonald, D. A. (1974) *Blood Flow in Arteries*, 2nd Edition. London: Arnold.

the fluid along the tube is required to overcome the internal friction of one layer on another. At a given viscosity, flow continues to be laminar as long as the product of velocity and diameter does not exceed a critical value. This is determined by the Reynolds number, Re

$$Re = \frac{VD}{v}$$

where V = mean velocity, D is diameter and v is kinematic viscosity (i.e. viscosity/density). For steady flow, if Re exceeds 2000, laminar flow breaks up and becomes turbulent, i.e. forms eddies, jets and whorls. Once turbulence is established the energy required rises disproportionately to any increase in flow and the lateral pressure exerted on the tube also rises. Vibrations are set up which may be detectable as sound. For pulsatile flow, as the frequency, i.e. heart rate, increases, the velocity profile becomes more flat until an almost uniform velocity distribution occurs across the tube. This condition is known as plug flow and this type of laminar flow is what occurs in most of the circulation. As the frequency increases the flow pattern becomes more stable and a higher Reynolds number is required before turbulence occurs. Turbulent flow rarely occurs in the normal human circulation, except perhaps in the aorta under conditions of severe exercise, although the peak Reynolds number in the ascending aorta at rest may be about 7000 rising on exercise to over 12 500.

POISEUILLE EQUATION

In a given rigid tube the physical factors upon which the volume flow of fluid depends are the pressure difference between the two ends (P_1–P_2), the radius of the tube (r), the length of the tube (l) and viscosity (η) of the fluid in question. The French physiologist Poiseuille related these factors thus:

$$Flow = \frac{\pi r^4(P_1 - P_2)}{8\eta l}$$

Since resistance (R) is $\dfrac{\text{Pressure difference}}{\text{Flow}}$, the equation may be stated

$$R = \frac{8\eta l}{\pi r^4}$$

This equation illustrates the important fact that while flow is related linearly to pressure drop and inversely to length and viscosity, it is related to the fourth power of the radius; i.e. doubling of the radius, other things being equal, increases the flow sixteenfold. It follows that quite a large variation in flow may occur with a scarcely perceptible change in the diameter of the tube. The Poiseuille equation is valid for non-distensible tubes and continuous flow; its application to the human circulation

is no more than approximate, yet the principles involved are worth careful consideration.

OSCILLATING FLOW THEORY

The principles dealt with in the preceding sections need some modification when pulsatile flow is considered. Two new non-dimensional qualities should be mentioned, both of which take the frequency of the pulsation into account. These are the Strouhal number, which is defined as

$$St = \frac{f.R}{V}$$

where
f = frequency
R = radius
V = mean velocity of flow,

and Womersley's α, which is defined as

$$\alpha = R\sqrt{\left(\frac{2\pi f}{v}\right)}$$

where
R = radius
f = frequency
v = kinematic viscosity.

These are related to each other by the Reynolds number for

$$\alpha^2 = \pi . Re.St$$

The importance of St and α is that as they increase, so does the Reynolds number at which turbulence occurs increase. Within the circulation stable flow patterns can persist at Reynolds numbers over 10 000. It is of interest that for the aorta the value of α shows little variation in animals ranging in size from a mouse to an elephant. A further consequence of increasing values of St and α is that for flow in a tube the velocity profile changes from the parabola seen with steady flow, to a flat profile with merely a zone of high shear adjacent to the wall. Therefore in much of the circulation the velocity is uniform across most of the vessel.

In place of resistance, the term for pressure gradient/flow in pulsatile flow is impedance. The impedance has two components, resistance, which is due to frictional forces as with steady state flow, and reactance, which is due to inertial forces. The three are related by an equation of the form,

$$Z = \sqrt{(R^2 + I^2)}$$

where
Z = impedance
R = resistance
I = reactance.

In the circulation both resistance and reactance show frequency dependence, so that the impedance of a vessel increases with an increased heart rate.

The pattern of flow in systemic arteries changes with distance from the aortic valve. The output of the heart is discontinuous; at the root of the aorta with each systole there is a rapid forward flow during ejection of blood, followed by standstill, or even some backward flow, during diastole. Progressively along the aorta this markedly pulsatile pattern of flow becomes damped by the storage function of the aorta, and in the smaller arteries flow is much more continuous, though still roughly like sine waves (fig. 30.29). If one were to time an actual corpuscle, or a dye particle, it would take some seconds to travel from the heart to the periphery. In the aorta it would move forward in jerks with each heart beat, as has been recorded by cinematography.

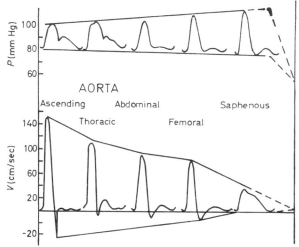

FIG. 30.29. Pressure and flow pulses in the dog in arteries at increasing distances from the heart. Pulse pressure increases while flow oscillation decreases markedly. From McDonald, D.A. (1974) *Blood Flow in Arteries*, 2nd Edition. London: Arnold.

ARTERIAL PRESSURE PULSE

As seen in Poiseuille's equation the motive force propelling blood along the arteries is a pressure drop. Pressure measured in the aorta or in a peripheral artery has a roughly triangular or saw-toothed oscillation. With ejection of blood into the aorta from the heart, there is a rapid rise of pressure, as input into the arterial system exceeds the run off into the periphery. With slowing of ejection, pressure tends to fall again, and this continues after the aortic valve has closed, as flow continues from the aorta into the periphery. The point of closure of the aortic valve is marked by the **dicrotic notch**; this is a small transient rise of pressure as blood tending to fall back into the heart is rapidly decelerated by the closing aortic valve (fig. 30.29).

The peak pressure is termed the **systolic pressure** and the lowest point the **diastolic pressure**. The difference between the two is the **pulse pressure**. The mean pressure throughout the cardiac cycle may be found by planimetry, but may be approximated by the formula:

$$Pm = Pd + \tfrac{1}{3}(Ps - Pd)$$

since the wave form is nearly triangular. P, pressure; m, mean; s, systolic; d, diastolic.

This pressure pulse, starting in the root of the aorta, travels down all the branches of the arterial tree (fig. 30.30). The velocity of the pulse wave, which is to be distinguished both from the velocity of blood flow, and also from volume flow of blood, is some 4–5 m/sec. The wave form changes somewhat as the wave travels distally. There is a progressive delay corresponding to the velocity of the pulse wave. Energy is used in propelling the blood

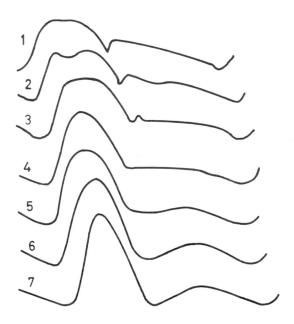

FIG. 30.30. Arterial pulses in the dog at various points (1–7) at increasing distances from the heart to the periphery. Note the change in wave form and the delay in arrival of the pulse wave. From McDonald, D.A. (1974) *Blood Flow in Arteries*, 2nd Edition. London: Arnold.

along the vessel, and therefore there is a small fall in the mean pressure along the arterial tree. Because of the geometry of the branching system, secondary waves are formed at points of branching which are reflected backwards along the arteries and which summate with the forward travelling wave. This explains why the pressure in a peripheral artery may show a higher systolic peak than does the central aortic pressure (fig. 30.29).

RELATION BETWEEN PRESSURE AND FLOW IN ARTERIES

Blood flows along the vascular tree as a result of an energy gradient. At any point in the vascular system the total energy has three components

$$E = P + \rho gh + \tfrac{1}{2}\rho V^2$$

P is the potential energy stored as pressure; ρgh is gravitational energy due to height above or below a reference point; $\tfrac{1}{2}\rho V^2$ is kinetic energy due to the velocity of the blood. When we make pressure measurements using a catheter-manometer system, we may ignore the second or positional term, since whatever the catheter position within the vascular system all pressures are recorded as they would be at the level of the manometer zero. As already indicated, if the needle or catheter orifice is orientated towards or away from the blood-stream, the kinetic energy may affect the pressure re-corded, but the kinetic component is very small in the normal circulation, and may be considerable only in certain abnormal situations, such as jet formation at a narrowed or stenotic orifice of a valve. Hence if we record a difference in lateral pressures between two points in the circulation, we may infer an energy gradient and blood will flow unless obstructed from high to low pressure. If pressure pulses are measured simultaneously at two points a fixed distance apart along a vessel, the instantaneous pressure difference between the two points can be estimated by subtracting the distal from the proximal pressure at each instant (fig. 30.30). The in-stantaneous flow along the segment of artery is a function of this pressure difference. Paradoxically, it can be shown that if flow and pressure are measured simultaneously at a point in the vessel, the peak of flow slightly precedes

the peak of pressure and, further, if the pressure at a point upstream is also measured, the peak of pressure difference precedes the peak of flow.

METHODS OF MEASURING PRESSURE

A simple liquid manometer in the form of a U tube filled with water or mercury is sometimes used as a pressure-measuring device, connected on one side by tube and cannula to the lumen of the vessel. Because of its inertia such a system is useful only for measuring rela-tively static pressures, or where a mean pressure value only is required. The wave form of pressure pulses in the cardiovascular system contains frequencies as high as 30–40 Hz, and to obtain a faithful record it is neces-sary to use a system which responds without distortion to frequencies higher than this, i.e. the system must have a high natural frequency. Such systems generally employ electromanometers; these are pressure trans-ducers which operate by transforming minute displace-ments of a metal membrane into changes of electrical resistance or current flow in a bridge circuit and these are amplified and recorded. The frequency response of the

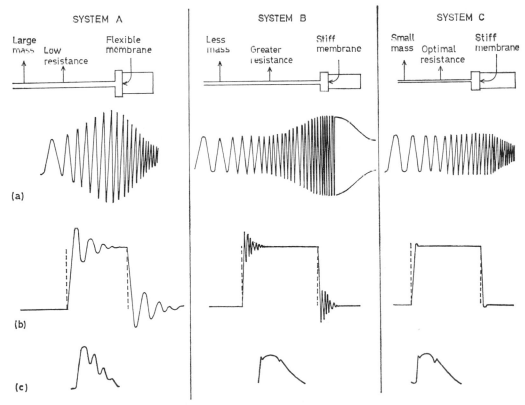

FIG. 30.31. The dynamic response characteristics of pressure recording systems, showing the effect of damping, i.e. increasing the frictional resistance of the system to match the frequency response of the measuring gauge; (a) frequency response, (b) square wave response, (c) pulse wave record.
System A is sensitive to changes in pressure but poorly damped and is unsuitable for recording intra-vascular pressures. System B is partially, and system C critically damped, i.e. the output is uniform over a wide frequency range. C reproduces intravascular pressures accurately. From Rushmer R.F. (1961) *Cardiovascular Dynamics*. Philadelphia: Saunders.

whole system, catheter, transducer, amplifier and recorder must be carefully studied either by exposing it to pressure oscillations at increasing frequency, when the point at which the accuracy of response falls off can be determined, or by studying the response to an instantaneous pressure change. A system which has an inadequate dynamic frequency response yields a record which is overdamped, i.e. the true peaks are ironed out. On the other hand, the system may respond excessively to pressure oscillations so that overshoots and spurious oscillations of pressure appear in the record. Such a system is underdamped. Damping may be introduced either by a small narrow segment in the catheter system or electronically in the amplifier. Where systems with catheters are being used it is usually necessary to work at critical damping (fig. 30.31), but for haemodynamic research it is often desirable to work at low damping in order to align accurately simultaneous pressure and flow recordings, and in these circumstances systems are

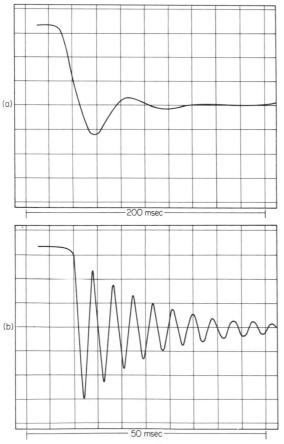

FIG. 30.32. Response of pressure transducer systems to a square (instantaneous) pressure change; (a) a system with a low frequency response and optimal damping; (b) a system with a high frequency response and low damping. Either system would be accurate for pressure wave forms in the cardiovascular system, but a system as in (b) is required if the pressures are to be related accurately to other events such as an ECG. Note the different time scales.

required which have a high frequency response. This may be tested by applying a square wave pressure change and observing the frequency of the damped oscillation produced (fig. 30.32). The results required are the undamped natural frequency of the system and the damping factor. Critical damping, at which the highest range of accurate waveform reproduction relative to the natural frequency of the system is obtained, occurs when the damping factor $\beta \simeq 0.7$. The latter is obtained from the magnitude of the overshoots which occur in response to a square wave change, and the rate at which the new equilibrium position is reached. In a system with critical damping, $\beta \simeq 0.7$, for accurate cardiovascular measurement the system should have an undamped natural frequency (f_0) greater than 35 Hz. Where β is less than 0.2, which is required for accurate alignment and timings of different signals, f_0 should be greater than 150 Hz. Using conventional manometers with catheters attached, this is very difficult to obtain, but pressure transducers on the tips of catheters allow accurate measurement with low damping to be made on patients.

The method of measuring systolic and diastolic arterial pressure in clinical use is the **sphygmomanometer**, introduced by Riva-Rocci in 1896. It consists of an inflatable cuff 13 cm wide, which is wound round the upper arm, the airfilled bag of the cuff being connected to a mercury manometer. The air pressure in the cuff is raised by means of a hand pump until it is well above the expected systolic pressure in the artery. The cuff pressure then exceeds the intra-arterial pressure at all times, and the brachial artery collapses and blood flow stops within it. The cuff is then allowed to deflate gradually. Below the true systolic pressure the artery reopens, allowing blood to flow, but until the diastolic pressure is reached it opens for only a portion of the cardiac cycle and blood goes through intermittently. Below diastolic pressure the artery remains open continuously, and blood flow continues without interruption.

In order to detect when blood flow in the artery is intermittent, the brachial artery distal to the cuff is auscultated with a stethoscope. Intermittent jets of blood coming down the vessel at high velocity result in vibrations in the vessel wall audible as a slapping or cracking sound. The pressure in the cuff below which this sound begins to be heard is therefore the systolic pressure, and the pressure at which it becomes muffled and disappears is the diastolic pressure. This method is usually accurate to within 5 mmHg. In peripheral arteries, e.g. dorsalis pedis, the systolic pressure can be measured using an ultrasonic velocity detector instead of a stethoscope.

The sphygmomanometer measures the pressure, relative to atmosphere, in the brachial artery, which is approximately at heart level. In using methods involving direct recording through needles or catheters it is important to specify the zero reference level which is being used; this is generally the level of the middle of the thorax in the lying subject and the manubrium sterni in the erect. Pressures measured at any point in the arterial system, for example in the foot in a standing subject, are approximately the same if measured with reference to the same zero level. In absolute terms, however, i.e. using a zero level at the point of measurement, the pressure in a foot artery is greater than that at heart level by an amount corresponding to the hydrostatic pressure of the intervening column of blood.

VOLUME FLOW IN ARTERIES

This may be measured in a variety of ways.

(1) It may be computed from a knowledge of differential pressures measured at fixed distances apart, and the diameter of the vessel.

(2) An electromagnetic flow meter may be applied to the vessel. If the vessel is placed in a magnetic field, between the poles of a magnet, flow along the vessel sets up a potential difference between the electrodes placed on the vessel wall in the diameter at right angles to the direction of the field. This potential difference is a function of volume flow.

(3) An ultrasonic flow meter consists of an ultrasound generator and a receiver placed alongside or near to the vessel. The usual method now makes use of the Doppler principle, where the frequency of sound reflected back from the erythrocytes is changed in proportion to the velocity of flow, as can be observed in the change of note as a train passes at high speed. Ultrasonic flow meters can give a direct measure of volume flow when placed on an exposed intact vessel, or used percutaneously can measure flow velocity. Two advances in ultrasonics are the use of a percutaneous flow meter to assess myocardial contractility by estimating the peak velocity and acceleration of blood in the ascending aorta, and the use of electronic gating to measure the velocity of individual laminae of blood within the circulation and thus determine the velocity profile.

VEINS

The veins form a collecting system for blood returning from the periphery to the heart. In general, they follow the same pattern of distribution as the arteries and frequently run alongside them. The final destination of the venous blood from the systemic circulation is the right atrium of the heart, and from the pulmonary circuit the left atrium. The main exception to this is the venous drainage of the stomach, spleen and small and large intestine, which is carried by the portal vein not directly to the heart, but first to the liver. After passage through the liver the blood returns to the heart via the hepatic vein.

Structure

Like arteries, veins have three coats in their walls. There is, however, very much less muscle and elastic tissue and the wall is much thinner in proportion to the diameter of the vessel. They have the same smooth endothelial lining as arteries. Owing to the structure of their walls veins are much more distensible, more easily collapsed or compressed and less well adapted to holding high pressures within them than arteries (figs. 30.25 & 30.35).

At intervals on the long veins, particularly in the limbs, the endothelial lining is pulled out to form cup-shaped valve cusps, similar in design to the semilunar valves of the heart. These valves permit uni-directional flow only, i.e. towards the heart. This is a functionally

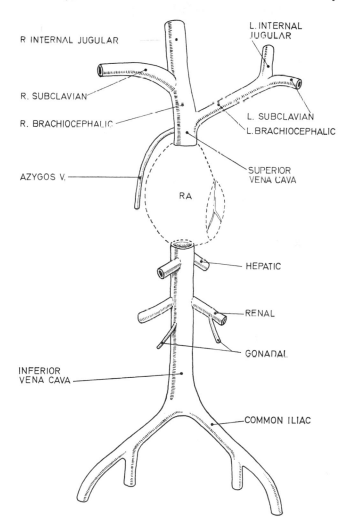

FIG. 30.33. Venae cavae and main tributaries.

useful arrangement in that veins, having thin walls, are readily compressible by surrounding muscle. During muscular activity there is alternating compression and relaxation of the tissues surrounding the veins; one-way valves allow the muscles to act on the veins as a pump and thus expedite the flow of blood back towards the heart, the **muscle pump**.

Distribution

The central venous system is shown in fig. 30.33. Veins from the head and neck, the jugular veins, join on each side the subclavian veins from the upper limbs to form brachiocephalic veins which unite in the superior vena cava. This main vein from the upper half of the body is joined by the vena azygos and vena hemiazygos from the chest wall, and ends in the right atrium.

The inferior vena cava, which drains the lower half of the body and ends in the right atrium, is formed by the junction of the two common iliac veins and is joined by the renal and hepatic veins before passing through the diaphragm and into the right atrium. The portal vein is formed by the junction of the splenic and superior mesenteric veins and enters the liver at the porta hepatis.

The pulmonary veins are four in number, two on each side, draining the upper and lower parts of the lung and passing directly via the hilum of the lung into the left atrium.

Functions of veins

The veins provide low resistance conduits for transport of blood to the heart from the periphery. In addition, they perform a reservoir function for the circulating blood volume. The bulk of the blood volume is contained in the veins and venules which thus represent the **capacity vessels** of the circulation. As we shall see later, the neural regulation of the compliance of this system plays a part in circulatory homeostasis.

Innervation

Veins are supplied with autonomic sympathetic nerves to the smooth muscle in their walls. Venoconstriction can be demonstrated in response to sympathetic stimulation.

Venous blood flow

Flow in veins is much less phasic than in arteries and more continuous. However, the flow rate fluctuates with the pulse beat, as can be seen in the pulsations in retinal veins or demonstrated by cinematography of particles travelling in the inferior vena cava.

Velocity of flow in a vein is less than in the corresponding artery because of the greater cross-sectional area, though overall volume flow must be the same. Flow in the central veins, the cavae, varies to some extent with respiration. When the intrathoracic pressure falls on inspiration, and intra-abdominal pressure rises, blood tends to be drawn into the thorax by virtue of the increased pressure difference; conversely, on expiration the intrathoracic pressure rises and blood flow slows. Forced expiration sufficient to raise the intrathoracic pressure considerably may diminish or arrest the return of blood to the thorax temporarily; the flow of blood in the superior vena cava is particularly affected (p. 30.51).

Venous pressure

The pressure in the venous system generally must be lower than that in the capillaries, and yet be high enough to fill the right atrium and ventricle and thus maintain cardiac output. When measured against a zero reference point at the horizontal level of mid-atrium the venous pressure is in health found to be remarkably constant at a few mmHg (< 5). The pressure at any point in the venous system is approximately the pressure at the zero level plus any difference in hydrostatic pressure between the zero level and the point of measurement. Thus in the erect posture, if there is no muscle movement venous pressure in the foot is over 100 mmHg, while pressure in the head veins is negative.

The **transmural** or distending pressure is the pressure difference between the inside of the vessel and the tissues surrounding it. Veins are distended when the pressure within exceeds both the tissue pressure surrounding them and the elastic tension of their walls. They are then circular in cross-section, visible or palpable if near the surface of the body, and constitute a reservoir of blood. When the pressure within them is less than the tissue pressure and wall elasticity, veins are undistended, though blood flow continues in them. They are flattened or elliptical in cross-section, and poorly visible even when lying just below the skin. This difference provides a simple method of gauging roughly the central venous pressure. The subject lies with the head and chest inclined at an angle of 30° to the horizontal. In this position the external jugular veins, if distended, are easily visible, as may be pulsation in the internal jugular vein. The height to which they are filled above mid-chest level may be estimated and indicates the general level of venous pressure in the body (fig. 30.34). This manoeuvre is valuable clinically in patients with heart failure with a raised central venous pressure.

The pressure changes in the atrium described on

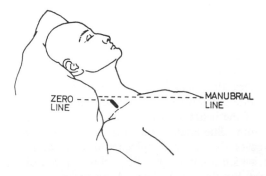

Fig. 30.34. Method of estimating central venous pressure from level of filling of neck veins.

p. 30.16 are transmitted to the jugular veins and may be recorded by a suitable transducer. When in heart failure the central venous pressure is raised, these pulsations may be seen by the naked eye and any abnormality in the size or frequency of the waves may help in assessing disorders of cardiac rhythm. For example, 'a' waves are absent in atrial fibrillation and 'v' waves are very large in tricuspid regurgitation.

Veins are low resistance channels and only a small pressure gradient exists along the major ones. Pressure in the venules, however, may be as high as 10 mmHg. above that in the veins at the same reference level. Because their walls are thin, veins are easily occluded by pressure. If in a limb a single vein is compressed, the blood by-passes the occluded vein by parallel or collateral venous pathways. If, however, a cuff is placed round the limb and inflated to a pressure of 40 mmHg, flow in the vein stops. However, arterial flow continues and blood accumulates in the veins beyond the cuff. The rate at which it accumulates is the same as the rate of arterial inflow. This is the principle of the method of measuring flow by venous occlusion plethysmography. If the cuff pressure is maintained for more than a few seconds, the venous reservoir becomes filled, and pressure in the veins rises and finally exceeds the cuff pressure when blood again flows through the compressed veins and further trapping of blood ceases.

The general level of venous pressure is remarkably constant. It may be raised by manoeuvres which increase the pressure within the thorax, e.g. coughing, retching or blowing up a balloon. Failure of the heart to transfer all the blood presented to it on the input side to the output side also raises venous pressure. A sudden excess of circulating blood volume may also raise venous pressure, but compensatory mechanisms which keep the venous pressure normal are remarkably effective (p. 30.50). In general, the relationship of venous pressure and capacity is regulated by the tone of the veins, i.e. the degree of tension in the smooth muscle in their walls.

The pressure-volume diagram for a segment of vein

may be contrasted with that of an artery (fig. 30.35). Increased tone in the vein shifts this curve downwards; the vein is less compliant and less distensible. For the venous system as a whole, wide variations in the volume of blood in the system may be accommodated by alterations of venous tone operating on the basal venous compliance, without alteration of the level of central venous pressure. This is important since the filling pressure of the heart, as such, is one determinant of cardiac performance.

CAPILLARIES

The part of the circulation of the greatest complexity, and about which the least is known, is the capillary network where the primary functions of the circulation, exchange of gases, nutrients, metabolites and heat, take place within the tissues. In general, the capillaries consist of fine tubes, approximately 7 μm in diameter, the same order of size as the red blood cell. Their walls are one cell thick and arranged in a network throughout every tissue of the body except the cornea and cartilage. Blood from an artery passes through the arterioles, which have relatively muscular walls, and then flows comparatively slowly through the capillary network. However, the capillaries are not in the direct route from arterioles to venules. The arterioles give way to vessels discontinuously coated with muscle cells; these are called metarterioles and appear to be preferential channels to the venules. Capillaries branch from the metarterioles and the flow of blood through them is controlled by one or two muscle cells, the precapillary sphincter at their origin. The metarterioles, capillaries and draining venules are known as the **microcirculation** (fig. 30.36). The capillaries within the liver and spleen are sinusoidal (p. 29.27).

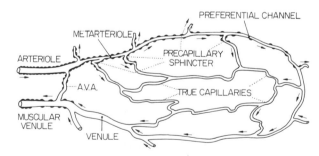

FIG. 30.36. The pattern of the microcirculation. The discontinuous smooth muscle is indicated in the vessel wall. From Zweifach B.W. (1949) *Trans. 3rd Macy Foundation Conference on Factors Affecting Blood Pressure*, p. 17.

Histological structure

Capillaries contain no muscle and their walls consist of a single layer of endothelial cells on a basement membrane. They are long in relation to their diameter, appear to have no innervation, though the arterioles and precapillary

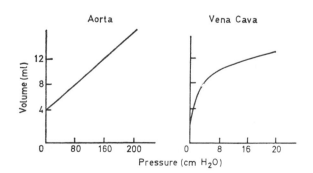

FIG. 30.35. Comparison of pressure/volume relationships of short equal lengths of aorta and vena cava.

sphincters are innervated with autonomic nerves, as are the venules. Controversy has surrounded the question of whether adjacent cells of the capillary wall are separated by a ground substance; probably they are not and are in close approximation one to another (fig. 30.37).

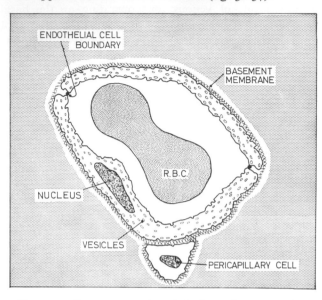

FIG. 30.37. Transverse section of single capillary shown by electron microscopy. Red blood cell shown for comparison.

The spatial arrangement of the capillaries varies with the tissue concerned. In muscle they are arranged longitudinally among the muscle bundles. In skin they appear as loops or arches coming up towards the surface, bending over and returning to the deeper tissues. In mesothelial structures like the pleura or peritoneum they form a horizontal network. One of the earliest and most important observations about the network was that it appears to be unstable or inconstant in that one capillary can be seen to transmit blood at one time and to close shortly afterwards; different capillaries open and close in turn. This varies with the metabolic activity of the tissue. The Danish physiologist Krogh observed in microinjection studies of muscle capillaries with India ink that in active muscle the capillary count or number of capillaries open per unit cross section area increased many times over that in muscle at rest. Another observation was that in the capillary circulation there sometimes occurs a separation of plasma and blood cells. Some capillaries appear to transmit only plasma while others allow blood cells to pass.

Gas exchange

All the respiratory gas exchange of the body occurs through capillary walls. In the lung capillaries oxygen diffuses into the blood and carbon dioxide out; the reverse process, quantitatively identical, takes place at the systemic capillary walls. Blood entering the capillary network from the arterioles is virtually identical in gas pressure and content with the blood leaving the lungs; its composition is shown in table 30.3. At the other end of the capillary network, in the venules and veins, the

TABLE 30.3. The oxygen and carbon dioxide content of blood.

	Arterial blood	Mixed venous blood
Oxygen		
Content (ml/ l)	200	150
Saturation (per cent)	97	75
Partial pressure (kPa)	13·3	6·0
Carbon dioxide		
Content (ml/l)	500	540
Partial pressure (kPa)	5·3	6·0

composition has altered to a variable extent, depending on metabolic activity of the tissue and flow rate of the blood, in that oxygen pressure and content have fallen and carbon dioxide pressure and content have risen. The aggregate of values from venous blood from all over the body is the mixed venous blood which may be sampled only from the right ventricle or pulmonary artery. Its composition is also shown in table 30.3.

The exchange of O_2 and CO_2 through the capillary wall between the blood plasma and the tissue fluid occurs by diffusion through the cell cytoplasm.

Movement across the capillary wall

The chemical composition of interstitial fluid is closely similar to that of blood plasma as regards small molecules and the small differences in ionic composition are in accord with the Gibbs-Donnan equilibrium. Furthermore, changes in the ionic concentration of these molecules in the blood perfusing the tissue result in an almost instantaneous similar change in interstitial fluid concentration. It is apparent that the tissue fluid and blood plasma are virtually one space as regards ions and small molecules such as sodium, potassium, chloride, bicarbonate, urea, glucose and water and that the capillary wall offers no barrier to their passage.

Large molecules such as proteins pass with difficulty through the capillary wall under normal conditions and the tissue fluid contains very little of them. However, because of the vast area of exchange and flow of blood perfusing it, the amount of protein exchanged per day is a significant quantity, and has been estimated at 60–200 g, i.e. about a quarter of the plasma protein. Under conditions of damage resulting in increased permeability of both capillaries and venules, large amounts of protein may escape into the tissue fluid. Proteins return to the circulation via the lymphatics rather than by reverse passage through the capillary wall.

Red blood cells do not normally pass the capillary wall. White blood cells, which are capable of active movement, may be seen escaping into the tissue spaces through the capillary walls (**diapedesis**).

The mode of transfer of plasma constituents is uncertain. It was previously believed that pores existed in the intercellular ground substance of the capillary wall through which substances could diffuse freely. Electron microscope studies failed to reveal any such structures, but did show the presence of vesicles of fluid in the cytoplasm of the capillary endothelial cell, and these structures may be the main route for transfer of molecules across the capillary wall (fig. 30.37).

Capillary pressure

Direct measurement of pressure within a single capillary by micropuncture is difficult technically. The values which have been obtained in the capillaries of the nailfold are about 30 mmHg. The validity of these measurements is, however, uncertain, in that they are in the larger capillaries and may be unrepresentative of the whole network. Most data about capillary pressure are based on indirect evidence. The important hypothesis of Starling (1895) depends on the fact that protein is present in the fluid on one side of the capillary wall and not on the other. This protein exerts a colloid osmotic pressure (COP) which is of the order of 25 mmHg. This force tends to attract fluid into the capillary and must be balanced at equilibrium by an equal hydrostatic pressure forcing fluid out. This transmural hydrostatic pressure must be the difference between pressures within and without the capillary wall, i.e. capillary pressure minus interstitial fluid pressure.

The full Starling hypothesis is therefore:

$$P_{capillary} - P_{tissue} = COP_{plasma} - COP_{interstitial\ fluid}$$

where P is hydrostatic pressure and COP colloid osmotic pressure.

In interstitial fluid COP is negligible. A value could therefore be assigned to $P_{capillary} - P_{tissue}$. In those days as a result of micropuncture experiments it was thought that interstitial pressure was about 5 mmHg above atmospheric pressure so that average capillary pressure would be 30 mmHg. It is now known that interstitial pressure is normally slightly less than atmospheric pressure, so that average capillary pressure is approximately 20 mmHg. This important observation regarding pressure in the interstitial spaces was the work of Guyton, who implanted small perforated spheres in animal tissues so as to permit pressure measurement without mechanical distortion.

A further important corollary of the Starling hypothesis is that since hydrostatic pressure falls from the arteriolar end to the venular end of the capillary the average value applies only at a midway point. Proximal to this point there is a net balance favouring outward movement of fluid and distally an inward movement. The concept was

thus of a circulation of fluid leaving the capillary for the tissues at one end and returning to it at the other.

This general relationship between hydrostatic and osmotic pressure has since been validated by Landis in America in the case of a single capillary, and by Pappenheimer and others in studies on perfused tissues although slight modification is needed to take account also of lymphatic drainage.

Control of the capillary circulation

Regulation of the flow through the capillaries must be adapted to two partially distinct functions. The primary function is that of exchange of substances to meet metabolic demands, and here it is clear that the critical factor is not the total volume of flow through the tissue capillaries, but the surface area of the capillary walls through which exchange takes place.

Secondly, since the capillaries are in series with the whole circulation, their regulation cannot be independent of the requirements of the circulation as a whole. As we shall see, the regulation of the arterial blood pressure depends partly on control of the arteriolar resistance, i.e. the state of constriction of the arterioles, which in turn affects blood flow through the capillary network.

The obvious possibility of conflict between the demands of these two functions has led to a search for mechanisms allowing independent control of the functions in the capillary circulation. The scheme of control envisaged at present, for which there is much experimental evidence, involves two mechanisms.

(1) The arteriolar resistance is controlled by contraction of smooth muscle in the walls of the small arterioles. This governs the overall flow through the capillary bed.

(2) The precapillary sphincters, smooth muscle fibres controlling the mouths of capillary channels, determine by opening or closing the number of capillaries through which the blood circulates, i.e. the capillary exchange area. If many sphincters are closed the blood flows through the main capillary channels, few in number and relatively large. If the sphincters relax blood is diverted through a much denser network of channels and comes intimately in contact with the metabolizing tissues.

The small arterioles and precapillary sphincters appear to be resistances both in series and in parallel.

In general, the arteriolar resistance is much more under neural control than is the precapillary. The latter is influenced mainly by locally produced vasodilator metabolites which readily diffuse through the tissues and cause the sphincters to relax. This occurs in conditions of metabolic demand such as exercise, local heating, and reactive hyperaemia following a period of arterial inflow occlusion. Although the metabolites primarily affect the precapillary sphincters, they diffuse around the arteriolar resistances, causing them to relax also.

The differences in control are reflected in differences in the histological structure of the vascular smooth muscle. Where neural control predominates there is an abundance of nerve fibres and the cell membranes of the smooth muscle cells are separate; where humoral control preponderates, nerve fibres are scanty or absent and there are numerous areas of partial fusion of the cell membranes of adjacent smooth muscle cells, similar to that seen in the intercalated discs of the myocardium, referred to as nexus formation. Within the different areas of the circulation both types of arrangement may be demonstrated, but the neural type is the major contributor in the arterioles and venules and the humoral in the microcirculation.

Neural control of the arteriolar resistance is via the sympathetic supply. Sympathetic vasoconstriction takes place reflexly in response to a variety of stimuli, e.g. pain, cold, or a drop in blood pressure which excite baroreceptors in the carotid sinus. Sympathetic tone may be reduced by general body heating or by section of sympathetic nerves. The vasodilation in these circumstances is less than the vasodilation produced by metabolites, and is not associated with opening up of large numbers of capillaries. Finally, in some tissues, especially muscle, there are special sympathetic vasodilator cholinergic fibres which on exercise or even anticipation of exercise cause arteriolar dilation.

The two resistances, arteriolar and precapillary, interact to some extent; a metabolic stimulus locally first causes precapillary dilation and then opens the arteriolar resistances. Severe arteriolar vasoconstriction may result in ischaemia and accumulation of metabolites to such an extent that the vasoconstriction is modified and relieved. This mechanism provides the basis for the phenomenonon of **autoregulation of flow** which applies widely in the terminal circulation and which is made possible by the presence and interaction of two balancing control systems.

In a few areas of the body there are communicating channels between arteries and veins of larger size than capillaries (**arteriovenous anastomoses**) which allow blood to bypass the capillary circulation to a large extent. The best authenticated sites for these shunts are in the skin of the hands and feet and in the wall of the stomach.

The effects of various stimuli on the peripheral circulation are now summarized.

(1) Local heat produces a marked local vasodilation both of skin vessels and muscle vessels, while cold contracts vessels locally.

(2) Generalized body heating such as to raise central body temperature results in a release of sympathetic constrictor tone and generalized vasodilation, affecting particularly the skin vessels. Chilling of the body results in reflex vasoconstriction.

(3) Muscular exercise results in a marked local vasodilation in the exercising muscles. Flow may increase

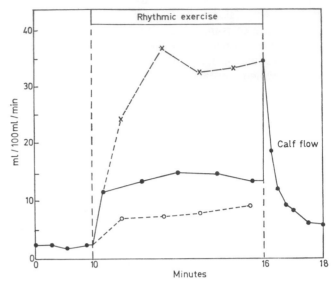

FIG. 30.38. Blood flow in the calf during rhythmic exercise consisting of a few seconds of sustained contraction, alternating with a few seconds of relaxation; ●, mean rate of flow, average results in seven subjects; ×, rate of flow measured during a few seconds' relaxation between contractions; ○, rate of flow measured during a few seconds of sustained contraction. From Barcroft H. & Swan H.J.C. (1953) *Sympathetic Control of Human Blood Vessels*. London:Arnold.

from resting values of 1–2 ml/100 ml tissue/min to over twenty times this value (fig. 30.38).

(4) If blood supply is cut off for a period of time from an area of the circulation by arterial occlusion, release of the occlusion is followed by a large increase in blood flow over the control value which persists for almost as long as the period of occlusion lasted. This is **reactive**

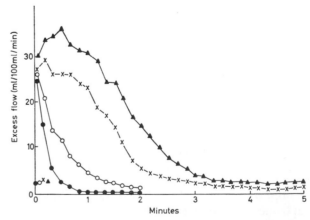

FIG. 30.39. Reactive hyperaemia following different periods of circulatory arrest. The averaged results of six experiments in which ●, 2-minute; ○, 5-minute; ×, 10-minute; and ▲, 15-minute periods of arrest were applied. The respective resting levels, indicated by the symbols at the left of the curves, have been subtracted. From Patterson G.C. & Whelan R.F. (1955) *Clin. Sci.* **14**, 197.

hyperaemia. It is probably caused by accumulation of vasodilator substances (fig. 30.39); the nature of these is unknown but suggestions include adenosine, acetylcholine, histamine and hydrogen and potassium ions. Hypoxia of the vessel wall may also play a part.

(5) The effects of catecholamines on the circulation are complex and vary from one tissue to another. They are described in detail in vol. 2, p. 15.13. In brief, circulating catecholamines, adrenaline and particularly noradrenaline, cause vasoconstriction and elevate the blood pressure. Adrenaline, however, has a powerful action on muscle blood vessels, causing them to dilate.

LYMPHATIC SYSTEM

In a 65 kg man the exchange of fluid across the capillaries throughout the body into the interstitial fluid amounts to about 20 l/day. This moves in both directions and the great bulk is returned to the circulation through the walls of the capillaries and venules. About 2–4 l/day, however, is returned to the circulation by a circuitous route through the lymphatic system and is known as **lymph.**

Lymphatic vessels

The lymphatic system consists of lymphatic capillaries, larger lymphatic vessels and lymphatic trunks. Lymph passes from the interstitial fluid into the lymphatic capillaries which are found in specially large numbers near blood capillaries. They possess round blind ends and open into irregularly dilated thin-walled channels which anastomose freely. The wall of the lymphatic capillary is composed of a single layer of endothelial cells with very little basement membrane. Lymph passes from the capillaries into larger vessels most of which form a network surrounding blood vessels. The walls of these vessels are composed of three layers similar to those of veins but are thinner and the different components less distinct. The lymphatic vessels run from the limbs and all the organs of the body, including the lungs, and unite to form larger trunks; these join finally to form the right bronchomediastinal trunk and thoracic duct which open into the venous system at the junction of the internal jugular and subclavian veins (p. 21.39). The lymphatic vessels contain valves and these together with the muscle pump in the limbs and the low venous pressure within the thoracic veins, especially on inspiration, assist its drainage.

During their course lymphatic vessels pass through accumulations of lymphoid tissue called lymph nodes which are scattered in large numbers throughout the body and especially in the prevertebral region, the mesentery, the axillae and groins. The structure and function of lymph nodes are given on p. 29.12. They contribute lymphocytes to the lymphatic fluid which leaves the nodes by efferent lymphatic vessels.

Composition and function of lymph

The composition of lymphatic fluid draining the limbs is similar to that of interstitial fluid and contains less than 10 g/l protein. Lymphatic fluid draining the intestine and liver, however, has a protein concentration of 30–60 g/l.

The volume of lymph from different regions of the body varies with the protein content of the interstitial fluid. When this is small, e.g. in the resting limb, lymphatic flow is small. When it is larger, as in the case of lymph draining the liver and intestine, the flow is larger. The lymphatic capillaries are much more permeable to macromolecules than are the blood capillaries so that protein molecules which escape from the latter are taken up into the lymph channels. This is due to the thinness of the basement membrane in the lymphatic capillaries and to the fact that the endothelial cells are less firmly attached to each other. Pinocytosis may also play a part. In this way the lymphatic system operates as an overflow drainage system of interstitial fluid and plasma proteins which have escaped from the blood capillaries. Lymph draining the intestine also contains lipid and other substances absorbed from the gut while lymph from the kidney contains some of the sodium and water absorbed by the renal tubules.

PERIPHERAL CIRCULATION AS A WHOLE

The functional aspects of the vascular system as a whole are best considered in a simple system of an artery, the capillaries supplied by that artery and the venous drainage from the system. Such a self-contained unit might represent the circulation through an organ such as a kidney or a lung, or a part of the body such as a limb. If smaller units than this are considered the situation may become complicated by collateral circulation, i.e. sharing to a greater or lesser extent of the blood supply among adjacent arterial territories by communications between them at arteriolar or capillary level. In such circumstances one unit of venous drainage is derived from several arterial supply units. If, however, a part of the body is chosen where the blood entering by the artery is identical with that leaving by the vein, a study may be made of the whole circulatory territory as shown in fig. 30.40.

Volume flow (in m³/sec) is the same for each of the five verticals shown in the diagram.

Area of cross-section (m²) varies, however, being relatively small at the arterial and venous ends and very large in the capillaries. In the case of the whole systemic circulation in a dog, for example, the aortic cross-section was estimated to be 0·8 cm² while the total capillary cross-section was 625 cm². This is a functional adaptation

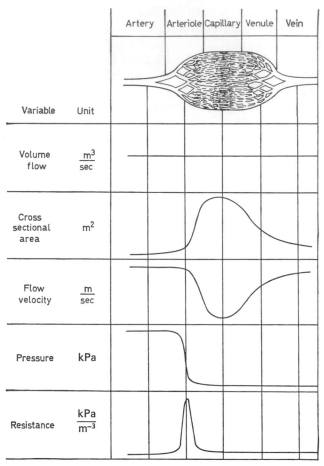

Variable	Unit	Artery	Arteriole	Capillary	Venule	Vein
Volume flow	$\dfrac{m^3}{sec}$					
Cross sectional area	m^2					
Flow velocity	$\dfrac{m}{sec}$					
Pressure	kPa					
Resistance	$\dfrac{kPa}{m^{-3}}$					

FIG. 30.40. Schematic diagram of a single circulating system and the relation of its physical variables.

in that the surface area relative to the volume flow is small in the case of the supply and drainage vessels and large in the case of the small vessels where exchange of nutrients occurs.

Flow velocity (m/sec) is inversely proportional to the cross-section ($m^3/sec \div m^2 = m/sec$). Peak flow velocity in the aorta in man may exceed 100 cm/sec, while in the capillaries it is only about 0·07 cm/sec. This affords a relatively long time for metabolic exchange to take place. In using the term blood flow, it is volume flow that is generally understood rather than flow velocity.

Pressure (kPa or mmHg). Flow always occurs down a pressure gradient, i.e. pressure is higher at the arterial than at the venous end. Fig. 30.29 shows the pattern of pressure through the system, the main drop in pressure occurring at arteriolar level. In other words, the arterioles constitute the main resistance to flow.

Resistance of any segment of the circulation is the ratio of pressure drop ($P_1 - P_2$) along the segment to volume flow (F).

$$R = \frac{P_1 - P_2}{F}$$

Since in our model F is the same at all verticals, resistance is proportional to change in pressure, dP, i.e. to the slope of the line P in fig. 30.40. It is highest, therefore, where the pressure shows the greatest fall, at the arteriolar level.

Overcoming resistance requires the use of energy which is dissipated as heat. Under normal circumstances this is the greater part of the energy loss due to impedance. Movement of all kinds implies loss of energy and this is true for both liquids and solids. In a vessel with blood flowing through it, friction does not occur only at the inner surface of the vessel wall, as one might suppose, but throughout the thickness of blood. Flow takes place most rapidly in the centre of the stream, velocity falling progressively as the wall is approached until finally the layer of fluid in contact with the vessel wall is virtually motionless. In this way coaxial layers of blood may be thought of as sliding forward upon each other, the central core having the highest velocity. A velocity profile for steady flow is shown in fig. 30.28. The shearing stress of one layer or lamina upon another uses energy and accounts for frictional loss.

The definition of resistance given above is a general one applying to any vessel or system of vessels. One may calculate, for example, the resistance of the femoral artery, or of an organ such as the kidney or lung, or indeed the resistance of the systemic or pulmonary circuits; in the latter cases the flow is, of course, equal to the cardiac output.

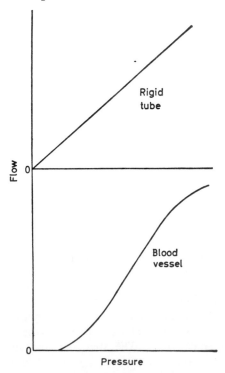

FIG. 30.41. Pressure-flow diagrams for a rigid tube and for a blood vessel *in vivo*.

In a rigid physical system, such as a hollow tube, the relationship between flow and pressure is a straight line (fig. 30.41), and the line passes through the origin. Resistance is proportional to the slope of the line and is the same under all conditions. In the case of living elastic vessels, however, this relationship is only approximately true. A typical pressure-flow diagram (fig. 30.41) shows a sigmoid curve with a positive intercept on the pressure axis. A certain threshold pressure is required to start flow, which then increases rapidly as the vessel expands, but finally the vessel resists further stretching and increase in flow tends to level off with further increase in pressure. This type of pressure-flow diagram is characteristic of living vessels. It implies that resistance alters to some extent with different perfusion conditions, and that a resistance value calculated for an observed flow and pressure is valid only within a certain range of pressures and flows. The threshold value of pressure, or the critical closing pressure, is the point at which the walls of the smallest vessels become unstable, the lumen of the vessel closes and flow stops.

In practice, resistance is derived from the ratio of pressure to flow. What are the physical factors in any given system whose resistance is being measured which affect the observed values? The answer is given in the Poiseuille equation (p. 30.23) for conditions of uniform flow in nondistensible systems. These conditions are not precisely fulfilled in the circulation, and so too much accuracy cannot be expected from such predictions. Calculation of resistance, which cannot be measured directly, as a ratio of pressure to flow is, however, useful in a variety of circumstances. Changes in blood flow in a limb, for example, may occur from three causes:

(1) alteration in the nervous control of the blood vessels,

(2) direct effects on the blood vessels due to circulating hormones or to local heat or metabolites, and

(3) alteration in the pressure of blood $(P_1 - P_2)$ perfusing the limb.

In the first two cases a change occurs in the resistance of the vessels, while the third case represents a passive change in flow without any alteration in resistance. In analysing the effects of drugs or other forms of treatment it is necessary to distinguish between these possibilities, and a first step is to see by calculating resistance values whether any actual vascular change has been produced.

Another situation where reliance on measurements of pressure alone or flow alone is misleading is in certain forms of congenital heart defect in which, owing to abnormal communications in the heart, pulmonary blood flow and systemic blood flow may be widely different. In these circumstances high pressure in the pulmonary artery might be due either to a very large flow through lung vessels of normal resistance, or to a high resistance to flow through damaged lung vessels, the actual flow level being normal or low. In the former case surgical treatment is of great benefit; in the latter case it is often lethal. With all the reservations due to the approximate nature of the estimate, a resistance value, taking into account the two variables of average pressure and flow, is of great value in some patients.

As an example of how the total systemic peripheral resistance (PR) may be calculated, suppose that in a patient measurements of mean arterial pressure and left atrial pressure are 100 and 5 mmHg respectively and of cardiac output 5 l/min. Then

$$\text{PR} = \frac{(100-5)\ \text{mmHg}}{5\ \text{l/min}}$$
$$= 19\ \text{mmHg l}^{-1}\ \text{min}^{-1}$$

To convert this figure into SI units, $1\ \text{mmHg} = 133$ Pa or $133\ \text{Nm}^{-2}$, 1 litre $= 10^{-3}\text{m}^3$ and $1\ \text{min} = 60$ s. Hence

$$1\ \text{mmHg l}^{-1}\ \text{min}^{-1} = 133 \times 10^3 \times 60\ \text{Nm}^{-5}\ \text{s}$$
$$= 8 \times 10^6\ \text{Nm}^{-5}\ \text{s}$$
$$\text{and PR} = 19 \times 8 \times 10^6 = 152 \times 10^6\ \text{Nm}^{-5}\ \text{s}$$

If it is possible to measure **instantaneous** flow and pressure, a value for impedance rather than resistance may be calculated. One can then treat the problem not on the analogy of a d.c. circuit assuming a steady pressure and flow, but as a problem in a.c. theory to which the situation more closely approximates, since both pressure and flow are oscillatory. The ratio of oscillatory pressure to oscillatory flow is termed **vascular input impedance** (hydraulic impedance). The pulsatile signals are decomposed by Fourier analysis into their harmonic components. For each harmonic, the pressure value is divided by the flow to give a modulus of impedance, and the phase angle of flow is subtracted from that of pressure. Input impedance is thus expressed as a set of values of the modulus and the phase at each frequency. Using this approach, more accurate values for energy production and distribution in the heart and circulation may be obtained.

Resistances in parallel

The branching of the aorta and arteries divides the systemic circuit to supply different organs and tissues in parallel. Besides organs like the brain and kidneys which have an obvious individual blood supply, more widespread tissues such as skin and muscle may be regarded as individual organs since their vessels, and control of these vessels, are similar. Diagrammatically, therefore, the systemic circuit may be represented as in fig. 30.1, the parallel flows being cerebral, coronary, renal, splanchnic, muscular and cutaneous.

Clearly the output of the heart is the sum of the flows through the individual circuits:

$$F = f_1 + f_2 + f_3 + \cdots$$

What is the relation of the individual resistances to the total systemic resistance? The arterial and venous pressures are approximately the same for all, so each term in the equation may be divided by $(P_1 - P_2)$ or P.

Hence
$$\frac{F}{P} = \frac{f_1}{P} + \frac{f_2}{P} + \frac{f_3}{P} + \cdots$$

But
$$R = \frac{P}{F} \quad \text{and} \quad \frac{F}{P} = \frac{1}{R}$$

Hence
$$\frac{1}{R} = \frac{1}{r_1} + \frac{1}{r_2} + \frac{1}{r_3} + \cdots$$

In other words the resistances of the parallel circuits are individually greater than the resistance of the whole system.

Methods of measuring blood flow

CARDIAC OUTPUT OR PULMONARY BLOOD FLOW
The methods in use all illustrate important general principles of the circulation.

Fick principle
The principle is that if a substance is added at a constant rate to the blood stream flowing past a point, the volume rate of flow is inversely proportional to the increase in concentration of the substance in the downstream blood. Such a naturally occurring substance is oxygen which is added to the blood as it passes through the lungs. If the rate of oxygen uptake is measured (ml/min) and, simultaneously, the concentrations of oxygen (ml/l) in the blood arriving at and leaving the lungs, the cardiac output is:

$$F(\text{l/min}) = \frac{O_2 \text{ consumption (ml/min)}}{\text{Arterial} - \text{venous } O_2 \text{ concentration (ml/l)}}$$

Oxygen consumption is measured by collecting expired air and analysing it for oxygen content. Arterial blood is sampled, at a constant rate and during the same time interval, from the left side of the heart or from a peripheral artery. Mixed venous blood is similarly sampled from the pulmonary artery.

The disadvantages of this direct Fick method are as follows:

(1) it requires catheterization of the pulmonary artery, since venous samples obtained upstream from this point are not fully mixed and so are not representative of the body as a whole;

(2) since it takes time to measure oxygen uptake (usually 2 min or more) the method is applicable only to steady-state conditions and is unsuitable for following rapid changes in output;

(3) since blood sampling is at a constant rate, while blood flow in the vessels is phasic with the cardiac cycle, a small sampling error may be introduced.

Indicator dilution methods
If a quantity (Q) of an indicator is injected into a current with a steady flow (F) and the concentration (C_t) of the indicator at a point down stream measured at intervals of time (t), then the amount of indicator passing the sampling point during an interval Δt is $FC_t \Delta t$. Then

$$Q = F \sum C_t \Delta t$$

and
$$F = \frac{Q}{\int_0^\alpha C_t \, dt}$$

The denominator is the area under the line obtained by plotting C against t.

The first use of an indicator to measure flow in the circulation was in 1893 when Stewart injected isotonic saline and measured changes in conductivity. The method did not come into clinical use until after the introduction by Hamilton in 1932 of dyes as indicators. Other indicators that have been used in man for estimating either cardiac output or flow in individual organs include radioisotopes and heat or cold. The technique of thermodilution was introduced in 1954 by Fegler in the Physiology Department at Edinburgh. For results to be valid the indicator chosen must mix uniformly and rapidly with the bloodstream, and it must not leave before sampling is complete.

For determining cardiac output, the dye most commonly used is indocyanine green. It is injected into a peripheral vein or, if the heart has been catheterized, the right atrium or ventricle; sampling is from an arterial catheter, usually in the brachial artery. Fig. 30.42 shows plots of dye concentration against time. When flow is fast, peak concentration is high and the appearance time short compared with when it is slow. With most indicators the disappearance slope of the primary curve is distorted by a secondary wave caused by indicator in the blood reappearing at the sampling site after circulating through the body (fig. 30.42). To correct for this distortion the upper undistorted portion of the disappearance slope, which forms an exponential curve, is used to predict the subsequent course of the primary curve had there been no recirculation. This can be done by plotting the data semilogarithmically when the disappearance slope starts as a straight line which is projected to the base line. In the thermodilution technique a bolus of isotonic NaCl or glucose at room temperature is injected by catheter into the superior vena cava; the resulting changes in temperature are recorded by a thermistor probe in the pulmonary artery. A constant is used to correct for heat gained by the bolus during its passage through the catheter. Since the cooled blood is rewarmed in small systemic vessels, recirculation peaks are absent and recirculation is probably slight. Although the use of cold as an indicator does not strictly meet the second condition mentioned above, thermodilution is as accurate as other methods of determining cardiac output.

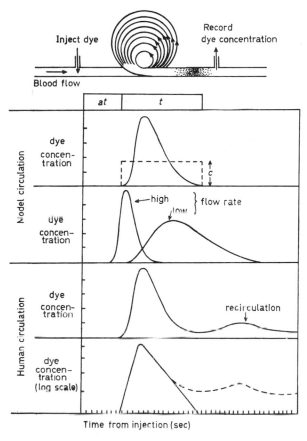

Fig. 30.42. Cardiac output by the indicator dilution method. *at*, appearance time; *t*, transit time; *c*, mean concentration. *c* × *t*, area under primary curve. Output = dye injected (mg)/*c* × *t*. Note the method of allowing for recirculation by extrapolating a logarithmic plot of dye concentration.

Its advantages are (1) sampling without blood withdrawal, (2) simple electrical calibration of the sensing device and (3) minimal recirculation.

Respiratory methods

The Fick method may be applied to figures for CO_2 output and A–V difference instead of O_2 uptake. The CO_2 content of arterial and venous blood may be calculated from partial pressures of the gas in arterial and venous blood. In arterial blood the P_{CO_2} equals, for practical purposes, that of alveolar air, which can be readily measured. An estimate of the mixed venous P_{CO_2} can be made by using the lungs as an aerotonometer. The subject rebreathes different mixtures of CO_2 and O_2 each for about 15 sec; when P_{CO_2} of the mixture is unchanged by the rebreathing, it represents that of the mixed venous blood. The advantages of the method is that no needles or catheters are required and it can be readily applied during muscular exercise. However, the subject needs to be trained in the experimental procedure. For these reasons the method is more useful to physiologists than to clinicians.

Whole body plethysmography

The rate of uptake of N_2O by the lung capillary blood may be used to measure pulmonary blood flow or cardiac output. An ingenious method of doing so is to enclose the subject in a whole body plethysmograph, together with a bag of a N_2O and O_2 mixture from which he breathes. The atmospheric pressure within the plethysmograph decreases due to the reduction in gas volume as the N_2O is dissolved in the pulmonary capillary blood flow and, from a knowledge of the partition coefficient of N_2O in blood and gas, the cardiac output can be calculated.

Other methods

The use of an electromagnetic flow meter in the ascending aorta or the pulmonary artery records instantaneous blood velocity. By integrating such a signal and from a knowledge of the vessel diameter, it is possible to estimate stroke volume and hence cardiac output.

By modification of the echocardiogram (p. 30.27) incorporating the Doppler principle, a transducer placed on the skin and directed longitudinally in the axis of aortic arch can record the velocity of blood in the aortic arch and hence the stroke volume can be estimated.

By passing a small high frequency current through tissue and measuring the voltage generated thereby, the electric flow impedance of tissue may be measured. Short oscillations occur due to changes in blood volume. Electrodes placed on the neck and abdomen allow the impedance of the thorax to be recorded. During the cardiac cycle small impedance changes occur, and from these a stroke volume index may be calculated.

ORGAN OR LIMB BLOOD FLOW

Plethysmography

Volume flow of blood in the limb may be measured by a venous occlusion plethysmograph or volume recorder. This consists of a rigid container filled with air or water into which the limb is sealed; volume changes in the limb are recorded as displacements of the air or water from the container by a float recorder system. The limb is first raised above heart level so that the veins are undistended. If the venous outflow is occluded for a few seconds by a proximal cuff suddenly inflated to 60 mmHg, which does not interfere with arterial inflow, the limb swells at a rate equal to the rate of arterial inflow. Since arterial inflow and venous outflow are normally equal, the rate of swelling measures the volume flow. Blood flow is expressed in ml/100 ml tissue/min. Most of the blood flow to the hand or foot goes to skin, and in the forearm or calf to muscle. Plethysmograph records with a cuff over the wrist are used to measure changes in cutaneous blood flow. When flow to the hand is excluded by raising the pressure in a cuff at the wrist above the arterial pressure, a plethysmograph on the forearm measures muscle blood flow.

In the case of the forearm or calf a close approximation to the changes in volume may be given by circumferential measurements recorded by a mercury-in-rubber strain gauge.

Clearance methods

The rate of flow can be calculated if a tissue is saturated via the bloodstream with some diffusible exogenous substance until equilibrium has been reached. The flow is then derived from the relationship between the changes with time in the arterial (Ca) and venous (Cv) concentrations and the partition coefficient between blood and tissues. For example, ^{133}xenon breathed in for a short fixed period of time may be used. To determine cerebral or coronary blood flow, internal jugular venous or coronary sinus blood must be sampled.

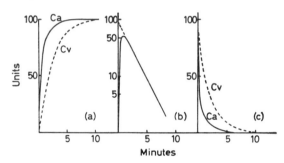

FIG. 30.43. Arterial and venous concentrations of ^{133}Xe. (a) Saturation curves; (b) Ca–Cv plotted on a log scale; (c) desaturation curves. The slope of (b) is proportional to blood flow.

Fig. 30.43 shows the rise in Ca and Cv while the subject breathes the xenon. Cv rises slowly to equal Ca when the tissue studied is fully saturated with the gas. When the subject stops breathing the gas, the curves again diverge. The area between the curves for Ca and Cv, in either case, represents the denominator of the equation below, which gives a measure of flow in ml/100 ml of tissue/min.

$$F = \frac{100 \times Cv \times S}{\int_0^{15} (Ca - Cv)\, dt}$$

Although this method is theoretically sound it is cumbersome to use and simpler but less accurate methods are now generally employed.

Radioactive isotope scanning and other methods

If a rapidly diffusible exogenous substance is injected into a tissue, it is carried away by the blood stream. The amount or concentration of the substance decreases exponentially, i.e. at a rate changing at each moment according to the concentration remaining. Thus the rate of decrease is at first rapid but then gradually slows. Exponential curves fall in a straight line when plotted semilogarithmically, and the slope of this line is therefore an index of the rate of removal and hence of the blood flow in the tissues. Fig. 30.44 shows the rate of removal of ^{24}Na injected into muscle, and how it alters with reactive hyperaemia.

Many other similar methods have now been devised for studying the relative blood flow in organs. A substance which is naturally taken up by the organ is labelled with a radioactive isotope of similar properties and half-life and given by intravenous or intra-arterial injection. The most commonly used isotope is ^{99m}Tc. Serial gamma camera pictures may show abnormalities in the regional dis-

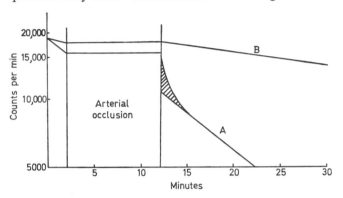

FIG. 30.44. Clearance of ^{24}Na from gastrocnemius muscle as measured by external counting. A, normal subject; B, patient with impaired arterial circulation. Note reactive hyperaemia after arterial occlusion.

tribution of the substance by the circulation or delayed clearance of the substance by the blood flow. Organs whose blood flow may be studied in this way include the brain, the heart, the liver, the kidneys and the lungs.

In animals, inert microspheres can be injected into the circulation and their distribution in the different organs is measured at autopsy; this distribution provides an estimate of their relative blood flows.

CONTROL OF THE CIRCULATION

The basic principles of the operation of the circulation are twofold:

(1) a relatively stable perfusion pressure, and
(2) wide variations in flow both as regards the cardiac output and its distribution to different organs and tissues under circumstances of varying demand.

Four main systems are involved. These are (1) control of the local circulation, (2) control of the blood and extracellular fluid volume, (3) control of the blood pressure and (4) regulation of cardiac output. The local control of circulation, for example, on exercising muscles, has already been discussed (p. 30.32). The mechanisms possible for the preservation of the blood volume and of the volume of the ECF by renal activity are described on p. 35.22. Clearly the remaining two mechanisms are not independent but interact with each other, since blood pressure, for example, cannot be altered without altering either output or peripheral resistance. For purposes of illustration, however, they may be isolated and examined individually.

Control of blood pressure

The familiar closed loop negative feedback principle operates to control blood pressure. The misalignment detector consists of stretch receptors situated in the tunica media and adventitia of the main arteries of the body, the aortic arch, brachiocephalic artery, pulmonary artery and carotid arteries. In man the main site of the receptors is the carotid sinus, which is a dilation situated at the junction of the external and internal carotid arteries; the wall of the artery is thinner here than more distally and contains more elastic fibres. The importance of stability of pressure at this site is obvious for animals adopting the upright position.

These pressure-receptors or **baroreceptors** are stimulated by tension in the wall of the vessel which in turn is increased by pressure within the vessel. Thus a rise of intra-arterial pressure increases the rate of discharge in afferent nerve fibres from the receptors, and a fall in pressure decreases the rate. However the rate of firing depends not only on the absolute tension in the receptor but also directly on the rate of change. The afferent fibres from the carotid sinus travel via the glossopharyngeal nerves and those from the aortic arch in the vagus nerves to the centres in the upper medulla which are concerned with the nervous control of the heart and blood vessels. This control is mediated predominantly by parasympathetic nerves in the case of the heart and by sympathetic constrictor or dilator nerves supplying arterioles and venules in the case of peripheral resistance. Control of the heart is exercised as regards rate through the sinuatrial node. An increased discharge rate of the baroreceptors results in a depressor response, i.e. inhibition of sympathetic vasoconstrictor activity and parasympathetic cardiac slowing (fig. 30.45).

Blockade of the baroreceptor nerves by local anaesthetic results in a large though temporary increase in blood pressure and heart rate. Stimulation of the baroreceptors by local pressure on the carotid sinus slows the heart and lowers blood pressure. A few individuals have a hypersensitive carotid sinus mechanism. In them, even light pressure on the carotid sinus, e.g. with a tight collar, may induce reflex cardiac arrest and unconsciousness.

What is the norm of blood pressure towards which the baroreceptor mechanism adjusts? Fig. 30.46 shows the range of values in a group of male subjects aged 40–44 years. With age there is a gradual rise in pressures, which mainly affects the systolic component. To some extent this increase in pulse pressure with age reflects decreasing compliance in the arterial system, i.e. impaired storage function. Like any other biological variable, blood pressure has a fairly wide frequency distribution in the population. In western societies arterial pressure tends on average to rise with age. This tendency is not present in primitive peoples. There is no arbitrary dividing line between normal and abnormal pressures, although statistically the higher pressures carry a less favourable life expectation and life assurance companies allow for this. Table 30.4 gives an indication of the limits of pressure beyond which treatment should be considered.

Table 30.4. Upper limits of blood pressure which are considered normal, related to age, in western society (mmHg). These pressures, if found consistently, are abnormally high. At any age, pressures consistently below 100/60 are abnormally low.

Age	Systolic	Diastolic
20	150	90
30	150	95
40	160	95
50	160	95
60	170	100
70	170	105

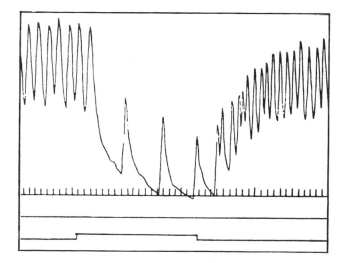

FIG. 30.45. Tracing of the blood pressure of a dog. The time marker shows 0·5 sec intervals. Over the period shown in the lowest trace, the carotid sinus nerve was stimulated, causing bradycardia and hypotension. From Hering, H.E. (1927) *Die Karotissinusreflexe*. Dresden: Steinkopff.

The baroreceptors, although the most important, are not the only controlling mechanism of the blood pressure. There are chemoreceptors situated in the aortic bodies and in the carotid bodies. These are very vascular smooth structures consisting of wide sinusoids lined by cells sensitive to changes in Pa,O_2, Pa,CO_2 and pH. In general, afferent inputs increase as Pa,O_2 falls or Pa,CO_2 or

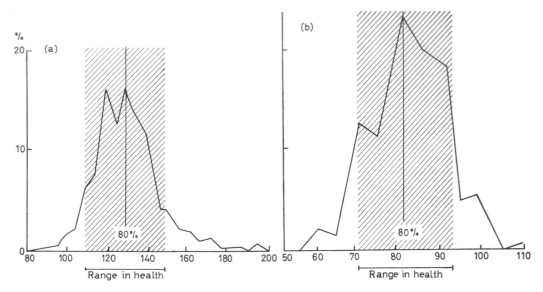

FIG. 30.46. Range of (a) systolic and (b) diastolic arterial pressures in males aged 40–44 years. The vertical line is the median and the shaded area represents 80 per cent of the population. Modified from Rushmer, R.F. (1961) *Cardiovascular Dynamics*, 2nd Edition. Philadelphia: Saunders.

arterial [H⁺] rises, the response being greatest when both changes occur together. They play a more important role in the control of ventilation than of the circulation and are described on p. 31.27. The cardiovascular response consists of bradycardia resulting from increased parasympathetic activity and peripheral vasoconstriction resulting from increased sympathetic activity which tends to elevate blood pressure.

Sympathetic impulses responsible for vasoconstriction and cardiac acceleration arise from the lateral portions of the medullary centre; the medial portion of the centre transmits inhibitory impulses to the lateral part and its activation results in bradycardia. The medullary centre also receives fibres from the reticular substance in the pons, the mesencephalon, the diencephalon and the cortex.

Emotions, particularly fear or excitement, can cause large rises of blood pressure, and it is frequently difficult in normal individuals to measure the true resting blood pressure simply because the circumstance of having the pressure measured raises it. Pain and cold are other stimuli which regularly cause a pressor response and operate through cortical pathways on the medullary and diencephalic vasomotor centres. A vasoconstrictor path from the motor cortex also bypasses the medullary centre and stimulates the lateral horn cells of the spinal cord, activating sympathetic preganglionic neurones.

The extent to which man is dependent on the baroreceptor mechanism for maintenance of consciousness in the upright posture and indeed for life itself is illustrated by the cases in which this control breaks down. When a person changes from a lying position to a standing one, the effect of gravity is to pool a large proportion of the blood volume in the veins in the lower part of the body. This would continue if there were not a re-adjustment via the baroreceptors of the tone or compliance of the venous capacity vessels and of the arteriolar resistance.

In many elderly people and often in patients after prolonged bed rest, this control mechanism is imperfect and postural hypotension, i.e. a drop in blood pressure on standing, is surprisingly common and accounts for many falls and fainting attacks. In young people, sudden emotional stimuli of an unpleasant nature may produce fainting by inhibiting vasoconstrictor tone, but only as a rule in the upright posture. The situation is rapidly restored if the subject is allowed to lie flat, and only becomes dangerous through injudicious attempts by bystanders to hold the individual upright.

Despite these mechanisms for controlling pressure, which can be demonstrated acutely, and despite the long term stability of blood pressure, continuous records of pressure in a given individual show quite large diurnal variations with minimal values during sleep and maximal values during emotional stress or exercise (fig. 30.47).

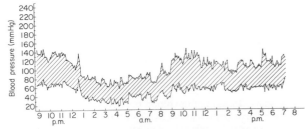

FIG. 30.47. Variations in blood pressure over 24 h in a normal, healthy adult. Courtesy of Dr. John Irving.

AUTONOMIC VASOMOTOR NERVES

What is the efferent pathway from the vasomotor centre in the medulla to the smooth muscle of the arterioles? The cardiovascular control or vasomotor centre is situated in the floor of the fourth ventricle of the brain, thence fibres pass down the cervical cord in the lateral columns to all the thoracic and upper two lumbar segments. There they synapse with the connector cells of the sympathetic which lie in the lateral horn of the grey matter of the cord. From the connector cells the preganglionic fibres leave the cord in the ventral roots of segments T1–L2 and then enter all the mixed somatic spinal nerves. There is no parasympathetic supply to the peripheral vascular system.

The sympathetic supply of the heart (T2–T4) synapses in all three cervical ganglia and postganglionic fibres reach the heart via the cardiac branches of the sympathetic chain and the parasympathetic supply via the vagus.

Sympathetic constrictor tone is constantly present. Section of the cord below the medulla cuts off such tonic impulses and results in a fall of blood pressure. When the blood pressure is chronically elevated in disease, the activity of the baroreceptors seems to be normal, but set at a higher level of response. Drugs used to lower high blood pressure reduce vasoconstrictor tone. They have widely different sites of action between the vasomotor centres and the smooth muscle of the peripheral arterioles.

Regulation of cardiac output

Of the three interdependent variables, cardiac output, blood pressure and peripheral resistance, in a given individual the blood pressure is the least variable. The continual changes in the circulation in response to environment and activity consist largely in a changing inverse relationship between cardiac output and peripheral resistance. The mechanisms by which these two variables can be altered in the body are considered first, and subsequently the ways in which they are adjusted to give rapid changes in local circulations.

The cardiac output is the product of heart rate and stroke volume. Heart rate depends on the automatic discharge of the sinuatrial node which in turn depends on the slope of the diastolic potential in phase 4 of the transmembrane action potential of its cells (p. 30.12). This inherent rate of the cardiac pacemaker may be increased by heat as in fevers or slowed by hypothermia. Like other metabolizing tissues it is responsive to the effects of thyroid hormones. However, rapid changes in rate are brought about by two extrinsic factors. Circulating catecholamines increase the rate of automaticity. Of far greater importance are the sympathetic and parasympathetic nerves which act on the sinuatrial node. In healthy individuals the heart rate is principally governed by the amount of parasympathetic tone acting on the

node. Its removal by blocking with atropine causes a great increase of heart rate while removal of sympathetic tone by drugs which block β-adrenergic receptors (vol. 2, p. 4.12) results in only a modest reduction of rate.

The great range of heart rates which are accomplished by changes in neural stimulation indicates that this is the principal means of increasing cardiac output, for example, in exercise. In severe exercise, cardiac output can increase by a factor of five to six times in a trained athlete, but less in an untrained individual. In both, the heart rate may increase almost threefold, but although stroke volume may double in the trained individual much smaller increases occur in the average person. The difference in stroke volume depends on the extent of shortening of the myocardial cells with depolarization. The arrangement of the contractile elements of the cell which bring about this shortening is discussed on p. 16.4. What factors regulate the extent of shortening of the cells of the ventricular myocardium, and hence the stroke volume?

FRANK–STARLING LAW OF THE HEART

In 1895 the German physiologist Frank, using the isolated frog heart, found that within wide limits there was a step-wise relationship between diastolic filling and pressure, and the magnitude of both the isotonic and the isometric heart beat. Fifteen years later Starling, using canine heart and lung preparations in which diastolic pressure, heart rate and aortic pressure could be controlled independently, found this relationship was true for the mammalian heart. In 1915 he summarized the direct relationship between end-diastolic fibre length and ventricular work in the statement, 'the energy of contraction is a function of the length of the muscle fibres.' This is now known as the Frank–Starling Law of the Heart.

In muscle dynamics stretching of muscle is referred to as the **preload**. The stretch of the muscle in the experimental system is equivalent to the diastolic volume of the ventricle and this in turn is related to the filling or end-diastolic pressure, which is more readily measured. This Frank–Starling relationship of increased work done by contracting muscle with increased preload underlies all cardiac responses in the healthy individual, though its effects may be obscured by other simultaneous adjustments. It provides an immediate myogenic response to changes in filling of the ventricles which may occur from one heart beat to another, as well as forming part of the response to exercise or other longer term changes. The physiological basis of this regulation is the degree to which the thick and thin elements overlap and therefore the number of interacting sites between actin and myosin molecules.

Strictly speaking the **afterload** put upon the left ventricle of the heart, which is the force which it has to develop in contracting, is the tension in the wall of the

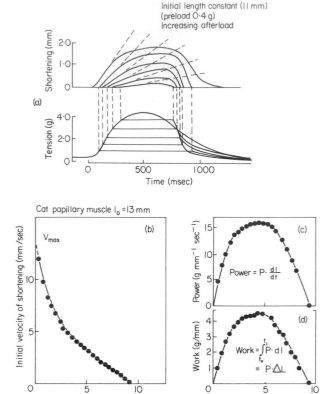

FIG. 30.48. Experiments with cat papillary muscle to show tension/velocity relationship of myocardium. When a papillary muscle with a constant preload is stimulated against increasing afterload (a) the initial velocity of shortening, indicated by the tangents in the upper trace, decreases. When velocity is plotted against load (b) a hyperbola, similar to that for skeletal muscle, is obtained, but unlike skeletal muscle the maximum value can only be obtained by extrapolation. When either power (c) or work (d) is plotted against load, it can be seen that there is a maximum value and if load is increased further, power and work decrease, as in skeletal muscle. After Henderson A.H.

are concerned with the rate of force generating processes at the contractile sites, and are referred to as changes in **contractility**. It would be of great value to be able to measure contractility, since many clinical problems are concerned with the failing heart and its therapy. Yet the problem of finding a variable which accurately reflects changes in contractility independent of pre- and afterload changes is still unsolved. Indices which have been proposed include the maximum rate of circumferential shortening of the left ventricle measured from cineradiographs, the maximum rate of rise of pressure in the ventricle before ejection, dP/dt_{max}, and more recently the maximum ejection velocity of blood leaving the ventricle V_{max}, and its maximum rate of acceleration dV/dt_{max}. All of these are reduced in the failing heart and enhanced by stimulation of β-adrenergic receptors. Enhancement of contractility is referred to as a **positive inotropic effect**.

Calcium ions and their availability in quantity in the vicinity of contractile proteins are known to be an important factor in myocardial contractility. Electrical excitation of the cell membrane results in movement of Ca^{++} from the T- tubules and lateral cisternae of the sarcoplasmic reticulum and this calcium is bound by troponin component C, one of the regulating proteins on the actin filaments. This binding removes the troponin barrier to the interaction of myosin and actin. The cross-

ventricle during ejection of blood. In the experimental situation (fig. 30.48) both the extent and the velocity of shortening diminish as the afterload is increased. In the human body, if we exclude changes in the volume or shape of the ventricle (see Law of Laplace, p. 30.22), the afterload may be represented by the aortic pressure, more precisely the mean aortic pressure during systolic ejection. Hence, in addition to the positive feedback operation of the Frank–Starling Law, there is a negative feedback arrangement in which rises in aortic pressure are compensated by reductions in stroke volume.

When changes in both preload and afterload are controlled, stroke volume is still subject to change, notably in response to β-adrenergic receptor stimulation (neural or humoral), but also with changes of metabolic substrate or ionic environment and in the not fully understood clinical condition of myocardial failure. These changes

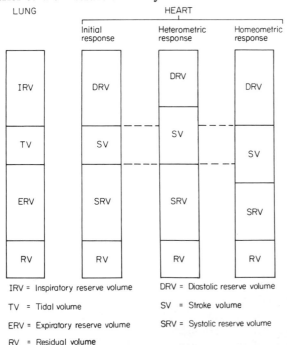

FIG. 30.49. The divisions of ventricular volume, showing the analogy to lung volumes and the difference between heterometric and homeometric responses. Heterometric responses result in an increased stroke volume by encroaching upon the diastolic reserve volume, i.e. greater filling; in a homeometric response the systolic reserve volume is encroached upon, i.e. greater emptying.

bridges are activated and the concurrent splitting of ATP produced in mitochondria provides energy for the muscle contraction (p. 16.8). Withdrawal of Ca^{++} from the region of the myofibrils in the sarcoplasmic reticulum initiates muscle relaxation.

There is some evidence that heart failure in man is associated with decreased availability of Ca^{++} at the contractile site and that the beneficial effects of digitalis are due to reversing this deficit (vol. 2, p. 8.3). There is evidence also that the positive inotropic effects of noradrenaline may be mediated by cyclic AMP promoting increased movement of Ca^{++} across the cell membrane.

HETEROMETRIC AND HOMEOMETRIC REGULATION

Even with a maximum contraction the ventricle is unable to expel all the contained blood, and therefore has a residual volume. The stroke volume at rest is capable of being increased either by greater diastolic filling or by greater systolic emptying of the ventricle. The heart may thus be regarded as analogous to the lung (p. 31.14); it possesses (1) a residual volume, (2) a stroke volume, corresponding to the tidal volume, and (3) a diastolic and systo-

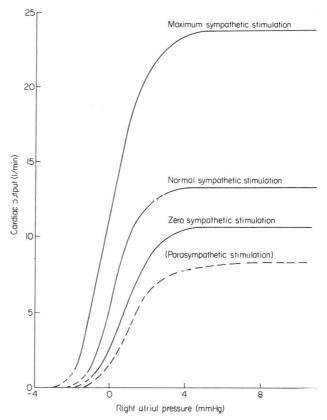

FIG. 30.51. Effect of changing level of autonomic nerve stimulation on cardiac output. At each level there is a different Frank–Starling curve; thus for every variable, such as arterial pressure, blood pH, plasma [Ca^{++}] etc., rather than one there is a family of Frank–Starling curves.

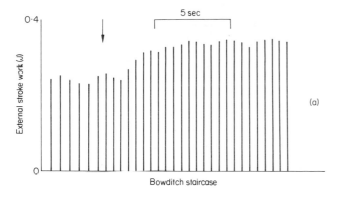

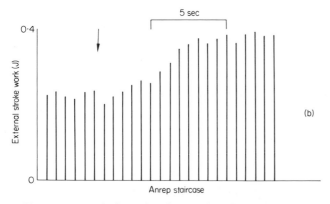

FIG. 30.50. Beat by beat plot of external stroke work showing staircase effect of autoregulation of heart *in situ* to (a) change in heart rate from 100 to 130/min (Bowditch staircase) and (b) change in afterload by increasing aortic systolic pressure from 130 to 170 mmHg (Anrep staircase).

lic reserve volumes, corresponding to the inspiratory and expiratory reserve volumes respectively (fig. 30.49). The mechanical problems of increasing the flow in a single cycle with optimum efficiency are similar in the two systems. In these terms the Frank–Starling law describes an increase in stroke volume brought about by encroaching upon the diastolic reserve volume. Because a change in end-diastolic volume involves a change of initial fibre length, this is termed a **heterometric response**. The Frank–Starling Law which arises from an intrinsic property of myocardium, is a special case of the response and is referred to as **heterometric autoregulation**.

Starling first demonstrated that for the intact heart, rather than there being a single cardiac function curve relating end-diastolic volume to cardiac output, any change in an intrinsic factor such as the level of catecholamines produced a different curve. Sarnoff and his colleagues, in the 1950s, confirmed this but also showed that changes in response to heart rate (Bowditch staircase) or afterload (Anrep staircase), which take several beats to occur, are accompanied by a change in the cardiac function curve (fig. 30.50), so that rather than one there is a family of curves (fig. 30.51). A move from one to another represents a change in contractility and is accompanied by slight but significant changes in the myocardial content of monovalent and divalent cations.

If we return to the Laplace Law it can be seen that the most efficient method of increasing stroke volume is by increasing contractility so that the end-diastolic volume remains constant, but there is better systolic emptying. As such a change does not involve a change in initial fibre length it is referred to as a **homeometric response**; where there is a change in rate or afterload, this response is an intrinsic property of the myocardium and is then referred to as **homeometric autoregulation.**

The heart usually effects its responses predominantly by a homeometric mechanism. However, this takes several beats to occur and the initial response is always heterometric. This is well illustrated by considering either the Bowditch or Anrep staircase beat by beat. The initial response is heterometric and moves along the existing cardiac function curve, but then as the homeometric autoregulatory responses occur the heart moves to a new cardiac function curve and the diastolic volume returns to approximately its initial value (fig. 30.52).

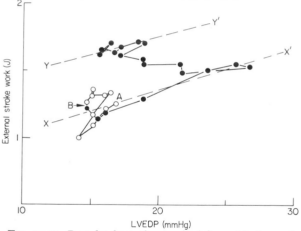

FIG. 30.52. Beat by beat changes in left ventricular end diastolic pressure and left ventricular external stroke work in response to a change in afterload (Anrep staircase). The record starts at point A and afterload was increased at B. The initial response was heterometric and moved up the existing Frank–Starling curve (X–X′), but after 8 beats a change in contractility occurred due to homeometric autoregulation, so that finally LVEDP had returned almost to the initial level but the ventricle had moved onto a higher Starling curve (Y–Y′).

The heterometric mechanism is the immediate response to any change in the heart load, and maintains the balance of output between the two ventricles, but the homeometric response occurs within 10 to 20 beats and so optimizes the efficiency of the heart as a pump. In cardiac failure there is often a loss of the homeometric response and the patient must then rely on the heterometric response and alterations in heart rate to achieve the necessary cardiac output.

REGULATION OF THE PERIPHERAL RESISTANCE

The rates of blood flow to different organs, whose sum constitutes the cardiac output, vary greatly in their resting levels and in the extent to which they can increase above the resting level. The kidney, for instance, has a very large blood flow which varies little in health. Skin and skeletal muscle have a low resting flow which can increase many fold. In every case, however, the regulation of resistance to flow and hence of the rate of blood flow lies in the state of contraction or relaxation of the smooth muscle of arteriolar walls and the factors which control this can be stated generally.

Like the tissues of the heart, vascular smooth muscle cells possess the property of automaticity, with the result that a steady basal rate of contraction maintains a level of tone even in muscle isolated from neural or humoral stimuli. Bayliss discovered that increased stretching of vascular smooth muscle by pressure within the vessel resulted in an increased rate of contraction of the muscle, thus increasing resistance to flow locally. This constitutes a local negative feedback mechanism although, if applied to the organism as a whole, the effect would act positively to increase blood pressure as well as resistance. It seems that this myogenic factor is balanced by an effect of local substances, probably metabolites, which relax smooth muscle, so that local underperfusion of tissues (ischaemia) causes a relaxation of the arterioles and an increased blood flow. The balance of these forces, metabolic and myogenic, is the basis for the considerable degree of **autoregulation** of perfusion which many tissues show. The metabolic stimulus to vasodilation is particularly considerable in the case of working skeletal muscle.

Superimposed upon the intrinsic control of local resistance to flow is the extrinsic mechanism of autonomic nerve impulses from the central nervous system, predominantly sympathetic but parasympathetic in the case of the salivary glands. Sympathetic adrenergic fibres, acting upon α-adrenergic receptors in the vascular smooth muscle, maintain a varying degree of vascular tone in different organs, while in the case of skeletal muscle there is evidence also of sympathetic cholinergic fibres which relax smooth muscle and are concerned in the large muscle vasodilation of exercise.

CIRCULATION THROUGH SPECIAL AREAS

The arrangement of the systemic circulation into a number of parallel resistances has already been noted (p. 30.35). Each of these differs in some special respects from the others, and is described separately. In addition, the pulmonary circulation, which is in series with the systemic, has several distinctive features.

Pulmonary circulation

The flow of blood through the lungs is in normal circumstances equal to the systemic flow or cardiac output. The methods for measuring it are therefore the same as for the cardiac output. The pulmonary intravascular pressures can be measured by catheterization of the main pulmonary artery; here the systolic and diastolic pressures are approximately 20 and 10 mmHg above left atrial zero reference level. The mean pulmonary venous pressure may be obtained by wedging the catheter in a pulmonary artery branch. It is approximately 5–10 mmHg and is closely similar to the mean left atrial pressure. The left atrial pressure may be measured directly by puncturing the interatrial septum from right side to left with a hollow needle introduced inside a cardiac catheter.

Anatomically, the branches of the pulmonary artery follow the distribution of the bronchi throughout the lungs. The structure of the main pulmonary arteries is similar to that of the aorta but the wall is much thinner. There are no muscular arterioles normally in the pulmonary circuit and only a small amount of smooth muscle is present, mainly in the precapillary vessels.

The features of the pulmonary circulation are as follows:

(1) a very large blood flow in relation to the weight of the lungs;

(2) a low pressure gradient (5–10 mmHg) driving the blood through the lungs. Thus there is a very low vascular resistance in the pulmonary circulation, which is only about one-eighth of the systemic resistance;

(3) a short pathway through the lungs in relation to the blood flow, and, compared with the systemic circulation, a low blood volume;

(4) great passive distensibility of the vessels, so that in conditions of increased flow the vascular resistance falls further. Thus a fourfold increase in flow on exercise may be accommodated without significant rise in pulmonary artery pressure, and

(5) the pulmonary arteries and veins are end vessels, i.e. they supply one segment of lung exclusively, without collateral supply.

Pulmonary blood flow is distributed to a vast network of capillaries which perfuse the respiratory exchange area of the alveolar walls. The pulmonary capillaries are wider and shorter than most others and their total surface area has been estimated at some 60 m², rising to 90 m² with exercise. Exchange takes place through two cell layers, the alveolar epithelium and the capillary wall (p. 31.5). Blood passes from one end of the pulmonary capillary to the other in less than 1 sec and in that time gas equilibration is complete. By measuring the instantaneous rate of uptake of N_2O by the blood in the pulmonary capillaries, using the body plethysmograph (p. 30.37), it can be demonstrated that pulmonary capillary blood flow is highly pulsatile with the heart beat, the peak flow occurring in late systole.

How is the blood distributed within the lung? The head of pressure under which the lung is perfused is relatively small. In the upright subject the hydrostatic pressure difference from the zero reference at atrial level to the top of the lung accounts for nearly all the available perfusion pressure, and hence blood flow is minimal at the apices of the lungs. Studies in which uptake of radioactive gas has been measured in three zones of the lung show that perfusion is poor in the upper zones and best in the lower zones in the upright subject. On recumbency this gradient disappears.

Arterial blood leaving the lungs is almost fully oxygenated (oxygen saturation 97 per cent). If some of the pulmonary blood flows through poorly ventilated areas of the lung, gas exchange cannot take place and arterial blood then contains an admixture of unchanged venous blood. That this does not occur despite the variations known to take place in the number of functioning alveoli implies that perfusion and ventilation are locally matched by some regulating mechanism. The ventilation/perfusion ($\dot{V}/\dot{Q}$) ratio is of central importance in understanding gas exchange in the lungs in disease and is discussed at length in vol. 3, p. 18.12. Probably the low Po_2 in poorly ventilated alveoli causes local vasoconstriction, thus shutting off perfusion. This mechanism has been observed in part of one lung, in both lungs, and after removal of the autonomic nerves to the lung vessels. Indeed, this local regulation seems to be the main vasomotor control in the lungs. Unlike the systemic circulation, marked reflex effects do not occur and autonomic denervation has little or no effect. The local hypoxic control, however, explains how in collapse or pneumonia of segments of lung, blood flow is shut down, and therefore unoxygenated blood is largely prevented from getting through to the pulmonary veins and so to the arterial side.

In addition to the pulmonary artery blood flow, the bronchi and bronchioles are supplied also via the bronchial arteries from the aorta. This supply is normally about 1 per cent of pulmonary blood flow. The venous drainage is via the pulmonary veins.

There are adrenergic vasoconstrictor fibres present in the lung and, although nervous regulation of pulmonary vascular resistance is small, it seems likely that these fibres play a part in controlling the capacitance vessels of the lung, especially the pulmonary veins. The pulmonary blood volume is highly variable, from 200 to as much as 1000 ml, of which only some 70–100 ml are in the pulmonary capillaries. The mobilizable fraction of the pulmonary blood volume acts as a reservoir for the left side of the heart and buffers short-term variations in stroke volume. Venous baroreceptors are present at the junction between the pulmonary veins and the left atrium, stimulation of which results in tachycardia, in contrast to the action of arterial baroreceptors.

Prolonged exposure to high altitudes results in many adaptive changes in the pulmonary circulation. These include an increased capillary blood volume and altered diffusion characteristics, blunting of the chemoreceptor reflex response to hypoxia, and increase in pulmonary vascular resistance with the development of muscular and elastic thickening of the pulmonary arteries and right ventricular hypertrophy secondary to the raised pulmonary artery pressure (p. 46.3).

Coronary circulation

The heart receives its blood supply from three coronary arteries, the right, left anterior descending and circumflex arteries. They lie in the epicardial fat and supply terminal branches which penetrate the myocardium (fig. 30.53).

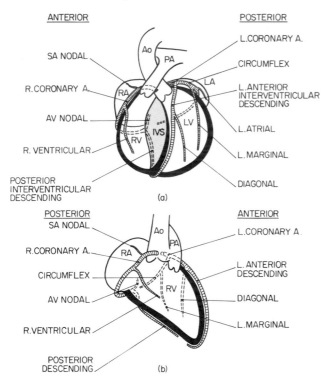

FIG. 30.53. Right and left coronary arteries; (a) left anterior oblique view; (b) right anterior oblique view.

The **right coronary artery** arises in the anterior coronary sinus of the aortic root and runs in the atrioventricular groove between the right atrium and right ventricle to the diaphragmatic surface of the heart. At the crux of the heart, where the four chambers meet, it makes a right-angled turn and becomes the posterior descending artery which runs in the intraventricular groove towards the cardiac apex. The right artery gives branches to the sinuatrial node and to the right ventricle. At the crux it gives off the small but important AV nodal artery and, as the posterior descending artery, supplies a variable area of the posterior wall of the left ventricle and intraventricular septum.

The other two arteries, the left anterior descending and

circumflex, start as a common trunk, the **left coronary artery**, which arises in the left posterior coronary sinus and runs for about 1 cm before dividing. The **anterior descending artery** runs to the cardiac apex in the groove between the left and right ventricles, supplying a large part of the anterior and, through its diagonal branch, the lateral wall of the left ventricle; its septal perforating branches supply much of the intraventricular septum. Because of its liability to atheromatous occlusion near its origin, it has been sardonically termed *l'artère de veuves*. The smaller **circumflex artery** runs in the left AV groove towards the crux of the heart. It often gives a large marginal branch to the lateral wall of the left ventricle and, in about 15 per cent of hearts, it provides the posterior descending artery.

The importance of the coronary arteries is that the heart muscle cannot survive deprivation of its blood supply for more than a few minutes without suffering severe damage or death, and in the normal heart there are few communicating branches between one artery and another which might provide a collateral supply in the event of occlusion of one artery. Narrowing of the lumen of one or more coronary arteries leads to hypoxia of a portion of the heart muscle, especially under conditions of exertion. A sudden occlusion, e.g. by a thrombus, often leads to death of a large area of muscle. This causes a myocardial infarct (vol. 3, p. 16.38) which is responsible for many heart attacks.

Venous drainage of the territory of the left coronary artery, mainly the interventricular septum and left ventricle, occurs through the coronary sinus which opens into the right atrium near the tricuspid valve. The **coronary sinus** is a wide channel which represents the left horn of the embryonic sinus venosus (p. 19.20). It lies in the atrioventricular groove on the inferior aspect of the heart. The **great cardiac vein** begins at the apex of the heart and ascends in the anterior interventricular groove until it reaches the atrioventricular groove which it follows around the left margin of the heart to open into the beginning of the coronary sinus. The sinus also receives the middle cardiac vein from the inferior interventricular groove and a small cardiac vein from the right atrioventricular groove. Some of the right coronary artery blood returns via the anterior cardiac veins which open directly into the right atrium. A small amount of the venous drainage occurs directly into the ventricles via small venae cordis minimae.

Any increase in output of the heart calls for increased energy expenditure by the myocardium. All this energy has to be supplied as free fatty acids, lactate and glucose by the coronary artery blood, since the heart can run into metabolic debt for only a brief period. Hence increased cardiac output is dependent on increased coronary flow and the coronary circulation is frequently the limiting factor in exercise tolerance.

Coronary blood flow may be measured by the clearance method (p. 30.38), but this technique is of little value in clinical medicine and values may be normal even in cases of severe coronary artery disease. This is because the distribution of affected areas is patchy, and because of their poor perfusion they tend not to take up the gas, and hence not to participate in the clearance measurement.

The identification of sites of narrowing or block by coronary arteriography is of greater clinical importance. Methods have now been devised for recording regional myocardial perfusion using radioactive isotopes. A gamma-emitting diffusible indicator such as ^{43}K or ^{201}Tl injected intravenously is taken up by heart muscle, an image of which can then be obtained by gamma camera. Areas of poor perfusion may be observed. On the other hand tetracycline, a commonly used antibiotic, when labelled with ^{99m}Tc is taken up by infarcted muscle and appears as a 'hot spot'. When the coronary arteries are catheterized for coronary arteriography an injection of isotope-labelled albumin microspheres 6–8μm in diameter may be given. The spheres are trapped in the minute vessels and for a period of some hours allow recording by gamma camera of the distribution of blood flow in the coronary circulation. These methods are being developed and may become useful clinically in suspected heart disease.

Continuous measurement by electromagnetic flowmeter of flow in the left coronary artery shows that, as might be expected, inflow into the myocardium almost ceases during ventricular systole owing to compression of the vessels by the surrounding muscle. Flow in the coronary circuit, particularly the left, therefore takes place predominantly during diastole. For this reason, a major determinant of myocardial perfusion is the level of diastolic pressure in the root of the aorta. A relatively slow heart rate is advantageous to an athlete on two grounds; long diastolic pauses lead to good coronary perfusion, and fewer contractions mean less cardiac work. Since the tension within the left ventricular wall increases from the epicardial surface towards the ventricular cavity, the blood supply to the innermost layers of muscle, the subendocardial layers, is the most precarious.

Control of coronary blood flow is not well understood. The venous blood in the coronary sinus is fairly fully deoxygenated, even in the resting state, and the arteriovenous difference for O_2 may be as much as 15 ml/100 ml. Hence increased oxygen can only be supplied by increased flow rather than by increased extraction of oxygen.

Coronary blood flow rises on exercise, and with hypoxic respiration. Autonomic stimulation affects profoundly the performance of the heart and thereby coronary flow. It is difficult, therefore, to detect separate coronary vasoconstrictor or dilator effects. Sympathectomy does not increase coronary blood flow. Local control via metabolites and hypoxia seems to be the main determinant of coronary flow in health.

OXYGEN REQUIREMENT OF THE HEART MUSCLE

The factors which may limit maximal exercise in normal people are discussed on p. 45.6. One is the maximum work output of the heart. Increased cardiac output is accompanied by an increase in the heart rate, but the latter is limited by the refractoriness of various heart tissues and a further increase is dependent on preloading and on contractility. Studies on the intact heart have shown that increases in contractility produced by catecholamines or stimulation of β-adrenergic receptors are bought at the cost of a large increase in oxygen consumption and therefore depend on a good coronary blood flow. People with impairment of coronary supply often first develop symptoms when there is strong sympathetic stimulation, e.g. during exercise or in response to emotion.

Other factors which influence oxygen consumption (per unit volume of myocardium) are the heart rate and the tension generated with each beat in the left ventricular wall (or its approximate equivalent, the aortic pressure in systole). External work against increased pressure, as when the blood pressure is abnormally high or the aortic valve obstructed, requires a greater oxygen consumption than the same amount of external work in response to increased stroke volume.

Cerebral circulation

The brain is an area of relatively high and constant metabolism which is particularly vulnerable to interruption of oxygen supply. The cerebral circulation is adapted to meet these needs.

The whole blood supply of the brain is derived from the internal carotid and vertebral arteries and is described in chap. 25.

The oxygen consumption of the brain is about 20 per cent of the whole body resting oxygen consumption, some 50 ml/min in an adult man. Blood flow is normally of the order of 750 ml/min for the whole brain.

The stability of the brain's blood flow depends on four special features:

(1) The volume of the cranial contents, together with the contents of the spinal theca, is virtually fixed. A sudden postural change, such as standing on one's head, abruptly creates a higher arterial pressure in the intracranial arteries, because there is now a vertical column of blood running up from brain to heart. But these arteries can distend only slowly, because they are surrounded by brain tissue and CSF, within a virtually indistensible cavity, and free space can only be secured by displacing venous blood out of the cranial cavity. The venous blood may well show the same rise in pressure as is seen in the arterial system, for the same reason, and in addition the major intracranial venous sinuses (though not the cerebral veins) are so tethered as to be incapable

of being squashed flat. Hence venous blood may not be readily displaced.

(2) These same anatomical features, however, imperil the cerebral circulation if any rise in CSF pressure occurs. Cerebral veins tend to become occluded, and the circulation thus arrested. But there is a reflex which increases the peripheral resistance of the whole systemic circulation enough to raise the systemic arterial pressure and to secure adequate perfusion of the brain even in the face of considerable rises in intracranial pressure. The sensor is probably the circulatory control region itself in the medulla, and the efferent path is the same as that of the baroreceptor reflex.

(3) Since brain blood flow changes so little with any change in function, the autonomic system seems to have no important vasomotor role within the skull, although some vasomotor innervation does exist.

(4) Brain O_2 consumption and CO_2 production are normally steady, yet they cannot continue unchanged in the face of a low Po_2 or a high Pco_2 in the entering arterial blood. Either of these markedly increases cerebral blood flow, and there are corresponding reductions in flow when arterial Po_2 is abnormally high, as when breathing pure O_2, or when arterial Po_2 is low, as during voluntary hyperventilation.

It may be that these are direct responses of the cerebral arterioles, and are the basis of local regulation of cerebral blood flow; in that case hypoxia and hypercapnia occur in a part of the brain, not from change in the arterial blood reaching the brain, but from a local increase in neuronal activity, and evoke a local increase in blood flow. Increase in Pco_2 or decrease in Po_2 of the arterial blood, as occurs clinically in chronic lung disease, causes an increase in cerebral blood flow. Breathing high concentrations of oxygen or voluntary hyperpnoea reduces cerebral blood flow.

Renal circulation see p. 35.14 and Splanchnic circulation see p. 32.54.

Skin circulation

The skin represents the largest specialized organ in the body. Its vascular supply, which is described on p. 37.10, is governed not so much by the needs of its own metabolism but by its functions in regulating body temperature by losing or conserving heat. Under normal resting conditions a lightly clothed person in a room at 20°C has a skin blood flow in the region of 5–10 ml min^{-1} 100 ml^{-1} tissue. This value is greater per unit volume than muscle, and less than brain, heart or kidney. The skin blood flow is, however, sensitive to minor changes in sympathetic tone and varies widely from < 1 ml min^{-1} 100 ml^{-1} tissue with vasoconstriction to

> 100 ml with vasodilation in a hot bath. Skin blood flow is controlled in a variety of ways.

Local metabolism. When this is increased, for example by heating, locally produced metabolites cause arteriolar dilation and increased blood flow. The most important example of this is **reactive hyperaemia**. Following occlusion of arterial inflow, e.g. by a tourniquet, anoxia develops in the skin and metabolites accumulate. When the circulation is restored there is an immediate large increase in flow which subsides gradually as the metabolites are swept away.

Sensory nerves in the skin give off branches which arborize around the local skin vessels. Sensory stimulation results in local vasodilation via these antidromic impulses, the **axon reflex**. This mechanism persists after proximal section of the sensory nerve, proving its independence of central reflex pathways. The **triple response** to scratching the skin demonstrated by Lewis consists of:

(1) a white reaction, i.e. white streak caused by vasoconstriction due to direct stimulation,

(2) a red reaction or flare caused by vasodilation due to an axon reflex, and

(3) a wheal, an elevated central area due to histamine release and capillary damage with extravasation of fluid.

Sympathetic nervous control of skin vessels is highly active and sensitive. Sympathetic constrictor tone is marked in the limbs and vasodilation is brought about by inhibition of this constrictor tone. The parasympathetic system is not involved. Another mechanism exists in addition in areas rich in sweat glands. Sweat gland activity, stimulated by the sympathetic, is accompanied by local production of bradykinin, which is a potent smooth muscle relaxant and this causes further local arteriolar vasodilation (vol. 2, p. 14.4).

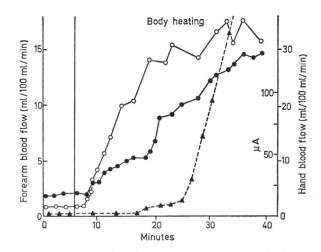

FIG. 30.54. Forearm (●) and hand blood (○) (ml/100 ml/min) before and during indirect body heating. ▲, current (μA) flowing through the forearm skin as an index of sweat gland activity. From Roddie I.C., Shepherd J.T. & Whelan R.F. (1957), *J. Physiol.* **136**, 489.

Mild pain, a sudden noise or a cold stimulus immediately causes reflex skin vasoconstriction. Radiant heat applied to the trunk causes reflex skin dilation. Body heating such as in a warm bath results in warm blood reaching the temperature control centre in the medulla which in turn inhibits sympathetic constrictor tone and increases skin blood flow (fig. 30.54). Blocking or section of the sympathetic nerve supply to a limb results in a large increase of skin blood flow, the hand being hot and, through inhibition of sweating, dry. *Hormones* also affect the skin circulation. Adrenaline and noradrenaline both cause vasoconstriction. Oestrogen dilates mildly. Of the posterior pituitary hormones oxytocin dilates the vessels while vasopressin causes a marked skin vasoconstriction, if given in pharmacological doses, but its role in the circulation is doubtful.

Skeletal muscle circulation

A 65 kg man has about 30 kg of skeletal muscle. In the resting state blood flow through muscle is some 2–4 ml min^{-1} 100 ml^{-1} tissue, so that skeletal flow represents about one-fifth of the cardiac output. Under conditions of exercise, however, blood flow to muscle can be expanded to 30–40 ml/100 ml tissue/min.

The artery supplying a muscle usually enters the muscle belly and breaks up into branches which run lengthwise within the muscle, these in turn giving rise to arterioles and capillaries which lie longitudinally between the muscle fibres.

When muscle contracts, the tension rises within and this cuts off the blood flow. During sustained strong contraction, therefore, an oxygen debt is built up and metabolites accumulate. Pain then develops in the muscle from sensory receptor stimulation. On release of the tension reactive hyperaemia occurs. During rhythmic contraction of muscle, flow stops during the contractions and is maximal during the short relaxation periods.

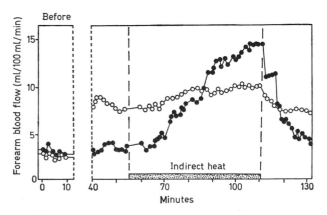

FIG. 30.55. A comparison of the effect of body heating on the blood flow through the nerve-blocked (○) and intact (●) forearm of one subject. From Roddie I.C., Shepherd J.T. & Whelan R.F. (1957), *Clin. Sci.* **16**, 67.

Muscle blood flow is controlled through the following mechanisms.

(1) Local control is effected by accumulation of metabolites and is believed to be dominant and represents a form of autoregulation.

(2) Sympathetic vasoconstrictor tone is present in muscle blood vessels; sympathectomy doubles muscle blood flow (fig. 30.55).

(3) Sympathetic cholinergic vasodilator fibres are also present, controlled not by the pressor centre but by the hypothalamic area. They are stimulated mainly during exercise. Fainting due to strong emotional stimuli is precipitated by muscle vasodilation resulting from discharge of these fibres.

(4) Adrenaline, but not noradrenaline, causes a large vasodilation in muscle vessels.

Cardiac output and its distribution

Measurements of regional blood flow have been made by many observers by the methods described on p. 30.36. Results naturally vary depending on the subject and to a lesser extent on the technique used. The data are, however, sufficiently consistent for the figures given in table 30.5 to be representative of normal men.

The effect of exercise on the cardiac output is discussed on p. 45.9, and of ageing in vol. 2, p. 36.8.

TABLE 30.5. An estimate of the distribution of the resting cardiac output in a normal man.

Organ	Weight g	Blood flow ml/min 100 g	Blood flow Total ml/min	Cardiac output %
Liver (including Splanchnic area)	1500	100	1500	30
Brain	1400	50	700	14
Kidneys	300	400	1200	24
Heart	350	63	220	4·4
Skeletal muscles	30,000	2	600	12
Remainder (by difference)			780	15·6
			5000	100

INTEGRATED RESPONSES OF THE CARDIOVASCULAR SYSTEM

Posture

When the subject changes from horizontal lying position to erect standing, the intravascular pressures, referred to atmospheric pressure, change. Pressure in the feet is higher by a hydrostatic factor affecting arteries, capillaries and veins. However, perfusion pressure, i.e. arteriovenous pressure difference, is unaltered. Following movement of water across the capillary wall, pressure rises in the tissue spaces to balance the capillary pressure, and if the subject stands immobile for any length of time swelling of the feet occurs. Rhythmic muscular contraction of the legs pumps venous blood towards the heart by virtue of the venous valves and thus tends to keep venular and capillary pressure low. Veins in the upper part of the body are collapsed and pressure in them approximately equals tissue pressure. A negative pressure relative to atmosphere exists in the CSF and venous sinuses of the brain.

In order to counteract pooling of blood in the capacity vessels of the lower body and to maintain blood pressure at the carotid sinuses, reflex vasoconstriction occurs affecting arterioles, venules and veins. Similar reflex changes affect the heart. The rate of the heart increases slightly and the heart size, both in systole and diastole, decreases. In other words, although the stroke volume is not increased, the end systolic volume is smaller. Central venous pressure is unchanged and cardiac output is slightly reduced.

As regards regional flow, blood flow through the upper zones of the lungs is decreased through diminished perfusion pressure. Brain circulation is little affected because of the syphon effect, but renal blood flow shows a small reflex diminution.

Exercise

The response to exercise is mainly dependent on neural control mechanisms. It is extremely rapid, and in many instances is evoked before exercise starts by the mere anticipation of exercise. The response of cardiac output to increasing exercise is shown in fig. 45.12. The immediate increase in output is accounted for mainly by a rise in heart rate, though in more severe exercise stroke volume also rises greatly. Central venous pressure generally falls at the start of exercise. The total cardiac response is due to sympathetic stimulation increasing rate and contractility.

As stroke volume increases, systemic blood pressure usually shows a widened pulse pressure as might be expected, the systolic rising in severe exercise to as much as 200 mmHg. The diastolic pressure usually rises a little. Since cardiac output increases up to fivefold in severe exercise in a trained athlete with little increase in systemic or pulmonary arterial blood pressure, it follows that both systemic and pulmonary vascular resistances fall. Considerable redistribution of regional blood flow takes place. Sympathetic stimulation reduces renal, splanchnic and skin blood flow, though with sweating, skin flow in certain areas may increase, overriding the constrictor tone. The exercising muscles show an enormous vasodilation, partly due to local metabolic causes and also through the activity of sympathetic cholinergic fibres. In prolonged exercise there is a demonstrable rise in the haemoglobin concentration and packed cell volume of the blood, mainly through extravasation of water by capillary filtration in exercising muscles. This circulation of fluid outside the vascular system is shown by the greatly increased lymph flow.

Exercise may also take the form of the development of tension in muscles without shortening, so called isometric exercise. Sustained hand grip, holding heavy objects, and resisting movements as in press-ups are examples. If it is of any severity, such exercise is accompanied by marked cardiovascular response including a rise in heart rate, blood pressure and cardiac output with little change in peripheral vascular resistance. Heart output changes are largely mediated by increased contractility and there is, consequently, a great increase in myocardial oxygen demand. Hence such forms of exercise may be dangerous for patients with impaired coronary blood supply.

Altitude

Exposure to high altitudes (>3000 m) results in circulatory changes. The Po_2 of the inspired air and consequently of the arterial blood is low and respiration and cardiac output are reflexly stimulated. Heart rate increases and a relative muscle vasodilation occurs. Other effects of acclimatization to altitude are described in chap. 46.

Blood volume changes

The normal blood volume is about 70 ml/kg or 4–5 litres. Sudden increase in the circulating blood volume as by rapid infusion of 1–2 litres of fluid evokes remarkable compensatory changes. If the fluid contains little or no colloid most of it rapidly passes out of the intravascular space and dilutes the body water. If it has a colloid osmotic pressure comparable with that of blood most stays in the intravascular compartment. Venous pressure tends to rise only after large volumes have been added; the capacity vessels can dilate to accommodate large volumes without rise in pressure. Stimulation of atrial stretch receptors may result in inhibition of production of aldosterone and antidiuretic hormone, thus promoting diuresis (p. 35.22).

When a healthy individual donates 500 ml of blood, the compensatory readjustments within the circulation are so rapid and complete that there are no detectable effects although occasional reactions are psychologically produced.

Sudden loss of 1–2 litres, however, as in an accident, burns, or gastrointestinal haemorrhage, results in changes due to the loss of circulating volume, and to the body's efforts to compensate for it. When fluid is lost from the intravascular compartment, which is under elastic tension throughout, the immediate physical result is a drop in the intravascular pressure. The compensatory changes which occur have the effect of maintaining pressures, both arterial and venous, and of restoring the circulating blood volume.

(1) Baroreceptor reflexes are stimulated and produce a sympathetic discharge. This has four effects:

(a) peripheral systemic vasoconstriction occurs in all areas except the brain and heart; initially the venous capacitance vessels are first constricted and this is followed by arteriolar constriction.

(b) the heart rate is increased,

(c) sweating occurs and the skin is cold, pale and moist,

(d) renal blood flow is drastically reduced and urine output may cease.

(2) Beyond the arteriolar constriction, capillary pressure falls, and the remaining blood is diluted by interstitial fluid which to some extent restores the lost circulating volume. This is shown in lowering of the packed cell volume, haemoglobin content and specific gravity of the blood.

(3) Volume control mechanisms described on p. 35.22 are set in operation; these include the secretion of ADH, renin, aldosterone and cortisol.

Though blood pressure may be well maintained, underfilling of the arterial side of the circulation results in a lack of distension in the arterial walls and an easily compressible soft pulse. Sweating occurs through sympathetic discharge, and may cause unwanted skin vasodilation. If muscle vasoconstriction is intense it may be overridden by local dilator mechanisms. Compensatory changes, which are adequate in the horizontal position, may fail on sitting or standing, when venous pressure, cardiac output, blood pressure and brain perfusion pressure may fall in rapid sequence and fainting occur.

When blood loss is severe and blood volume is not restored by transfusion, then compensatory changes are inadequate to maintain systemic blood pressure above a level needed to support tissue perfusion. Continuing anaerobic activity in the poorly perfused areas of the body results in metabolic acidosis, shown by a falling pH of the arterial blood and increased pulmonary ventilation. A state of **clinical shock** is said to exist. Loss of blood volume is an important but not the only cause of shock; a similar state of shock occurs in acute heart failure and in severe infections in which the responsible haemodynamic mechanisms are different (vol. 3, p. 3.1).

Temperature changes

Local heat. If heat is applied to a part of the body the result is a local vasodilation unaffected by reflex effects. The skin becomes red and hyperaemic and the large flow removes heat from the part so that local temperature does not rise as rapidly as it would if the circulation were stopped. This is thus a protective mechanism.

Exposure to a hot environment. The exposure of the body to a hot environment results in a great increase in skin blood flow which assists heat loss at the body surface. This vasodilation occurs in three ways:

(1) reflexly, through radiation falling on the skin surface,

(2) through warm blood reaching the thermoregulatory centre in the medulla; this causes inhibition of sympathetic constrictor tone in the skin vessels, and

(3) by sympathetic cholinergic stimulation of sweat glands which, in addition to wetting the body surface and causing heat loss by evaporation, produce bradykinin which causes further arteriolar dilation in the skin.

The great fall in vascular resistance evokes an increase in cardiac output, to maintain blood pressure.

Local cold. If a moderate degree of local cold is applied to a finger, local vasoconstriction occurs. With exposure to severe cold ($<4°C$), however, the phenomenon of **cold vasodilation** occurs and the finger becomes red and feels warm. This is a fluctuating vasodilation which is independent of nerve supply.

Exposure to a cold environment. General exposure to cold results in skin vasoconstriction and piloerection (goosepimples), as a consequence of central increase in vasoconstrictor activities. Blood pressure may rise, and cardiac output fall, i.e. there is a rise in peripheral resistance. Muscle tone is increased and shivering takes place.

When temperature homeostasis can no longer be maintained and central temperature falls, a condition of **hypothermia** is said to exist. Direct effects on the heart include (1) depression of the SA node, giving slowing of the heart (2) depression of conduction giving varying degrees of heart block and (3) finally ventricular fibrillation may occur below 30°C.

Increased intrathoracic pressure

When intrapulmonary and intrathoracic pressures are raised as in the **Valsalva manoeuvre**, where the subject takes a deep breath and blows against the closed glottis, or transiently in coughing, the pressure increment is applied to every intrathoracic structure including the vessels. Venous return to the thorax is therefore impeded and if pressure is maintained, cardiac filling falls and stroke volume and pulse pressure also fall. The carotid sinuses produce fewer afferent impulses, and therefore reflex sympathetic vasoconstriction and cardioacceleration occur. On release of the Valsalva manoeuvre and return of blood to the heart, the increased peripheral resistance results in a transient overshoot of blood pressure which in turn causes cardiac slowing. This normal pattern of response is obliterated when the venous pressure is abnormally high, since there is then an adequate reservoir under pressure to maintain cardiac filling. A prolonged Valsalva manoeuvre or bout of violent coughing may cause fainting through reduction of cardiac output.

Headward acceleration

One of the effects of exposure to acceleration exceeding

the universal I *g* is that the blood becomes abnormally heavy, twice as heavy as normal in the case of acceleration at 2 *g*. Thus to support a column of blood 13·6 cm high a pressure of 10 mmHg is required at 1 *g* (normal), 20 mmHg at 2 *g*, 40 mmHg at 4 *g* and so on.

Acceleration as in a centrifuge thus causes very high pressure in the lower limb vessels and stresses the body's power to resist pooling of blood in the limbs. Above 4 *g* an antigravity suit must be worn to prevent pooling. Blood pressure rises to maintain pressure at the carotid sinuses. Loss of vision and unconsciousness occur when the cerebral blood flow falls through lack of adequate perfusion pressure, and the retinae and visual cortex become anoxic.

Mental activity

Mental activity such as performing arithmetical tests is not associated with increased brain metabolism or increased cerebral blood flow (p. 30.47). It does, however, cause certain changes in circulation, all presumably mediated by centrally produced changes in sympathetic activity. Heart rate and cardiac output increase, and there may be a surprising increase in blood pressure. Muscle blood flow also increases, probably through activity of sympathetic vasodilator fibres.

Control of the circulation

Many of the circulatory readjustments in response to changes in posture, activity or environment occur so smoothly and precisely that it is difficult to detect that a change has occurred. In the language of control theory, misalignments are corrected almost before they can be measured. This adds to the difficulty of separating the sites of receptor and effector activity in circulatory control. Broadly speaking, however, certain features of circulatory regulation are apparent.

(1) There is a strongly autonomous local regulation of blood flow in the peripheral tissues. This control can in general override the central circulatory control.

(2) The two pumps which provide the energy of the system are input-sensitive, so that their outputs are precisely matched and venous pressure in both the systemic and pulmonary circuits is stabilized.

(3) A central nervous control, composed of a complex of reflex arcs and servomechanisms, modify the overall resistance to flow of the vessels and the volume and pressure of the venous return, and also the rate and contractility of the heart.

These three aspects of the circulation are all indispensable and damage to any one of them by disease results in a separate and sometimes serious disability.

FURTHER READING

Astrand P.-O. & Rodahl K. (1970) *Textbook of Work Physiology*. New York: McGraw-Hill.

Barcroft H. (1963) Circulation in skeletal muscle. In *Handbook of Physiology*, Section 2, Circulation, vol. II, pp. 1353–1385, ed. Hamilton D.F. Washington, D.C.: American Physiological Society.

Bergel D.H. ed. (1972) *Cardiovascular Fluid Dynamics*, vols. 1–2. New York: Academic Press.

Bing R.J. (1965) Cardiac metabolism. *Physiological Reviews* **45**, 171–213.

Braunwald E. (1974) Regulation of the circulation. *New England Journal of Medicine* **290**, 1124–1129; 1420–1425.

Burton A.C. (1962) Physical principles of circulatory phenomena; the physical equilibria of the heart and blood vessels. In *Handbook of Physiology*, Section 2, Circulation, vol. 1, pp. 85–106, ed. Hamilton D.F. Washington, D.C.; American Physiological Society.

——. (1965) Hemodynamics and the physics of the circulation. In *Physiology and Biophysics*, ed. Ruch T.C. & Patton H.D., 19th Edition, chap. 27. Philadelphia: Saunders.

Evans J.R. ed. (1964) *Structure and Function of Heart Muscle*. American Heart Association Monograph No. 9. *Circulation Research* **XV**, suppl. II.

Folkow B. & Neil E. (1971) *Circulation*. London: Oxford University Press.

Greenfield A.D.M. (1963) The circulation through the skin. In *Handbook of Physiology*, Section 2, Circulation, vol. II, pp. 1325–1351, ed. Hamilton D.F. Washington, D.C.: American Physiological Society.

Guyton A.C. (1963) Venous return. In *Handbook of Physiology*, Section 2, Circulation, vol. II, pp. 1099–1133, ed. Hamilton D.F. Washington, D.C.: American Physiological Society.

Hamer J. ed. (1973) *Recent Advances in Cardiology*, 6th Edition. Edinburgh: Churchill Livingstone.

Landis E.M. & Pappenheimer J.R. (1963) Exchange of substances through the capillary walls. In *Handbook of Physiology*, Section 2, vol. II, pp. 961–1034, ed. Hamilton D.F. Washington, D.C.: American Physiological Society.

Linden R.J. (1963) The control of output of the heart. In *Recent Advances in Physiology*, ed. Creese R., 8th Edition, p. 330. London: Churchill.

——. (1965) The regulation of the output of the mammalian heart. In *Scientific Basis of Medicine Annual Reviews*, pp. 164–185. London: Athlone Press.

—— ed. (1974) *Recent Advances in Physiology*, Number 9. Edinburgh: Churchill Livingstone.

McDonald D.A. (1974) *Blood Flow in Arteries*, 2nd Edition. London: Arnold.

Maseri A. ed. (1972) *Myocardial Blood Flow in Man: Methods and Significance in Coronary Disease*. Proceedings of an International Symposium. Turin: Minerva Medica.

Mellander S. & Johansson B. (1968) Control of

resistance, exchange and capacitance functions in the peripheral circulation. *Pharmacological Reviews* **20**, 117–196.

REEVE E.B. & GUYTON A.C. eds. (1967) *Physical Bases of Circulatory Transport; Regulation and Exchange.* Philadelphia: Saunders.

SCHER A.M. (1965) Electrical correlates of the cardiac cycle. In *Physiology & Biophysics*, ed. Ruch T.C. & Patton H.D., 19th Edition, chap. 30. Philadelphia: Saunders.

Chapter 31
Respiratory system

Respiration consists of the utilization of oxygen and production of carbon dioxide by living cells, and the means by which the cells exchange these gases with the atmosphere. The basic process is the same throughout the animal kingdom. The atmosphere contains O_2 at a higher partial pressure than that inside the cells. The direction of transfer of each gas is determined by the pressure between atmosphere and cell.

Fig. 31.1 shows the functional arrangement of the respiratory system in man. An open airway ABCD is separated from a closed blood circuit BCFE by a membrane BC across which O_2 and CO_2 can diffuse. Another membrane FE separates the blood from the tissue cells G. The air at A has an O_2 pressure of about 20 kPa (150 mmHg) and a CO_2 pressure of almost zero. The capillary blood at E has pressures of about 5·3 and 6·1 kPa (40 and 46 mmHg) for O_2 and CO_2 respectively. These differences in partial pressure between A and E impel O_2 and CO_2 in opposite directions. By itself, this would be an impossibly slow process owing to the distances

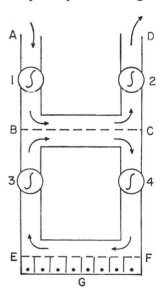

FIG. 31.1. Functional arrangement of the respiratory system. For symbols see text. Pumps 1 and 2 are the muscles of respiration. Pumps 3 and 4 are the right and left ventricles described in the previous chapter.

entailed. Pumps (1, 2, 3, 4), which circulate both gas and blood, increase the speed of gas-transport enormously, and only at the membranes does the transfer of O_2 and CO_2 depend solely on diffusion.

An account of respiratory mechanisms and their operation therefore covers the following topics:

(1) structure of the respiratory system,

(2) mechanics of breathing,

(3) pulmonary ventilation,

(4) carriage of gases in the blood,

(5) distribution of blood and gas in the lungs and its diffusion, and

(6) control of respiration.

STRUCTURE OF THE RESPIRATORY SYSTEM

The respiratory system consists of the lungs, the passages which convey air to and from the lungs, the muscles of the trunk which do the work of breathing and the pleural cavities which permit these movements.

The upper respiratory passages are considered as part of the head and neck (chap. 22). A description of the thoracic and abdominal walls, including the respiratory muscles, is given in chap. 21. The thoracic cavity contains the two lungs and pleural cavities separated by structures near the median plane. These structures form the **mediastinum**, which is the space between the sternum and the bodies of the thoracic vertebrae; it extends vertically from the inlet of the thorax to the central tendon of the diaphragm and is divided into:

(1) the middle mediastinum containing the heart and pericardium,

(2) the anterior mediastinum, the narrow cleft between the middle mediastinum and the sternum,

(3) the posterior mediastinum carrying the oesophagus, descending thoracic aorta, azygos veins and thoracic duct as they pass behind the heart, and

(4) the superior mediastinum lying behind the manubrium and containing the trachea, oesophagus, arch of the aorta, great veins and thymus.

The two phrenic nerves, running from the brachial plexus to the diaphragm, pass on the lateral sides of the parts of the superior and middle mediastinum in contact with the parietal pleura.

Pleural cavities

On each side of the mediastinum, there is a serous cavity with a smooth lining of simple squamous epithelium. These are the two pleural cavities and the lungs invaginate their medial walls, like fists pressed into the sides of almost empty balloons (fig. 31.2). The invagination is so complete that the space between the two layers of pleura is reduced to a narrow gap. The inner or visceral

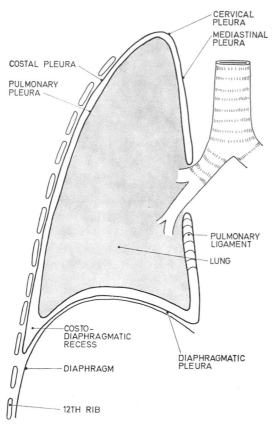

FIG. 31.2. A schematic coronal section through the right lung and pleural cavity.

layer covers the lung as the pulmonary pleura, while the outer or parietal layer is attached to the walls of the thorax. When the thorax expands during inspiration, the volume contained by the parietal pleura increases and the air drawn into the lungs causes them to expand within the pulmonary pleura. Thus, with each breath, the pulmonary pleura slides on the parietal layer and a thin film of fluid between the two layers provides the necessary lubrication.

The extent of the parietal pleura determines the maximum possible distension of the lungs. The parietal pleura is named according to the structures which it covers, i.e. there are mediastinal, diaphragmatic, costal and cervical parts (fig. 31.2). The **costal pleura** lines all the ribs, costal

cartilages and intercostal spaces down to a line which connects the xiphisternal joint, eighth rib in the mid-clavicular line, tenth rib in the mid-axillary line and twelfth thoracic vertebra. Along this curved line (fig. 31.3), the pleura is reflected on to the diaphragm, so forming a narrow gutter known as the **costodiaphragmatic recess**. This is filled by lung only at the end of a deep inspiration. The posterior parts of the pleural cavities descend below the medial part of the twelfth ribs, where they are clinically important as posterior relations of the kidneys. The costal and mediastinal parts of the pleura join along the line of reflexion posterior to the sternum.

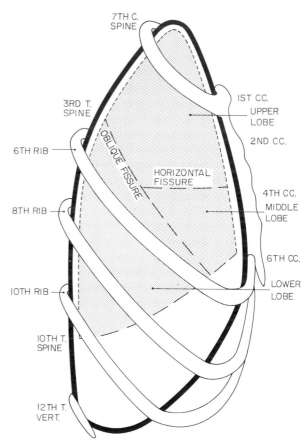

FIG. 31.3. The relation of the right lung and pleura to the thoracic wall.

These reflexions are in the midline except behind the manubrium where they diverge towards the sternoclavicular joints. Also, below the fourth costal cartilage on the left side, the heart and pericardium prevent the sternal reflexion reaching further medially than the left edge of the body of the sternum.

The **mediastinal pleura** passes on to the lung as the pulmonary pleura at the root of the lung. A thin pleural fold, which extends from the root of the lung almost to the diaphragm, is known as the pulmonary ligament (fig. 31.2). The structures covered by the mediastinal pleura are obviously different on the two sides. On the left side, it is applied to the arch and descending thoracic aorta, the pericardium in front of the lung root and the oesophagus close to its opening through the diaphragm. The right mediastinal pleura has only the azygos vein and the vagus nerve intervening between it and the trachea; in front of the trachea the superior vena cava descends to enter the pericardium at the level of the upper part of the root of the lung. As on the left side, the area below and in front of the lung root is related to the pericardium which, on the right side, contains the atrium. On both sides the pleura extends backwards around a broad groove on the sides of the vertebral bodies to join the costal pleura.

The outlines of the mediastinum are easily seen on postero–anterior radiographs of the thorax, since it is flanked by the radiolucent air-containing lung tissue (fig. 31.5a). Normally only the larger pulmonary vessels, containing blood, are sufficiently dense to cast a shadow, but the walls of the largest bronchi are occasionally seen near the root of the lung. The introduction of radio-opaque material into the bronchial tree outlines the walls clearly and so allows the pattern of branching to be demonstrated.

The **cervical pleura** forms a dome-like projection into the neck through the thoracic inlet. It can be outlined on the surface by a curved line which ascends 2·5 cm above the medial third of the clavicle. The cervical pleura is strengthened by a sheet of connective tissue which runs from the transverse process of the seventh cervical vertebra to the inner margin of the first rib and costal cartilage. The subclavian artery arches in front of the cervical pleura as it passes from the superior mediastinum to the upper surface of the first rib.

The costal and diaphragmatic pleurae are supplied with somatic sensory branches from the intercostal and phrenic nerves. Pleural pain is felt in areas of the trunk wall and shoulder supplied by the same segments of the spinal cord giving origin to these nerves. The lowest part of the whole pleural cavity is the costodiaphragmatic recess in the mid-axillary line.

Lungs

The lung has an apex which occupies the dome of the cervical pleura and so can be examined clinically by auscultation and percussion above the medial third of the clavicle. The concave base rests on the diaphragm, and the sharp lower border, around the periphery, projects into the costodiaphragmatic recess. The sides of the lung conform to the shape of the pleural cavity; a thick posterior part fits into the broad groove at the side of the thoracic vertebrae and a convex lateral surface is separated by the pleura from the ribs, costal cartilages and intercostal spaces. The anterior border is a thin process pointing towards the midline. In the centre of the medial surface the **root of the lung** is surrounded by a sleeve of pleura

which is formed by the continuity of the pulmonary and mediastinal pleurae. Within the root, the pulmonary veins are near the front, the main bronchus is at the back and the pulmonary artery is in the centre. Small bronchial arteries, numerous lymph nodes and vessels and the pulmonary nerve plexuses are scattered in the connective tissue around these larger structures.

Since the volume of the lungs changes with each breath, it is impossible to define accurately their surface marking. The upper part of each lung is always in contact with the cervical, mediastinal and upper costal pleura. During inspiration the lower part expands downwards so that it occupies more and more of the costodiaphragmatic recess. At the mid-point of quiet respiration, the lower border of the lung can be marked on the surface by a line joining the tenth thoracic vertebra, the eighth rib in the mid-axillary line, the sixth rib in the mid-clavicular line and the sixth costal cartilage where it joins the sternum. The roots of the lungs also move downwards with respiration and on standing erect; at rest, the roots are behind lines joining the sternal ends of the second and fourth costal cartilages.

The two lungs are not identical because the heart and pericardium bulge more into the left side of the thorax and the right dome of the diaphragm, covering the liver, is higher than the left dome. Hence the right lung is shorter, broader and slightly larger than the left. Both lungs are divided into lobes by fissures which are lined with pulmonary pleura and which plunge into the substance almost as far as the hilum. An oblique fissure runs from the third thoracic vertebra at the back, crosses the axilla and ends at the lower border of the lung opposite the sixth costochondral junction (fig. 31.3). The **lower lobes**, below this fissure, therefore include all the base and most of the thick posterior parts of the lung. On the left side the **upper lobe** is not usually divided again, but on the right a horizontal fissure runs from the oblique fissure at the axilla to the fourth costal cartilage at the sternum. This fissure produces a **middle lobe** which has a triangular surface directed to the anterior wall of the chest. The upper lobes are also mainly related to the anterior surface and constitute the apices of both lungs.

To the left of the lower half of the sternum, the heart and pericardium press towards the chest wall. Hence, the anterior border of the left lung is attenuated and forms a tongue-like process, the **lingula.** In this region the reflexion of the pleura does not reach the mid-line and the lingula only partially fills the pleural pocket. So below the left fourth costal cartilage, the pericardium is separated from the chest wall only by two layers of pleura.

Air passages

The trachea (fig. 31.4), about 12 cm long, runs from the cricoid cartilage of the larynx, at the level of the sixth cervical vertebra, to its bifurcation at the level of the fifth thoracic vertebra. Its course is not vertical, since the upper end is just under the skin of the neck and the lower end is only just anterior to the vertebral column. The anterior and lateral walls of the trachea contain sixteen to twenty C-shaped rings of cartilage, while the posterior wall consists of smooth muscle, the trachealis muscle. The cartilaginous rings are joined together by fibroelastic tissue so that the trachea is both flexible and extensible, in accord with respiratory and neck movements. The oesophagus lies behind the whole length of the trachea; near the cricoid cartilage and at the bifurcation it lies slightly to the left of the trachea. The inferior (recurrent) laryngeal nerves ascend in the grooves between the trachea and oesophagus; on the left side this nerve hooks around the arch of the aorta to reach the groove, while on the right the loop is around the subclavian artery. In the neck the isthmus of the thyroid gland crosses in front of the third, fourth and fifth tracheal rings with the lateral lobes of the gland clasping the sides of the trachea. As the thyroid is attached to the trachea and larynx by the pretracheal fascia, it moves during swallowing. The inferior thyroid veins descend in front of the trachea below the isthmus. Anterior to these veins and the thyroid, the strap muscles, sternothyroid and sternohyoid, separate the trachea from the deep fascia of the neck and jugular venous arch. The neurovascular bundles of the neck lie on the lateral sides of the trachea.

In the thorax, the arch of the aorta, its branches, the left brachiocephalic vein and the thymus gland intervene between the trachea and the manubrium of the sternum. The left lung and pleura are held away from the trachea by the arch of the aorta and its left subclavian branch, but the apex of the right lung is separated from the trachea only by the pleura, the arch of the vena azygos and the right vagus nerve. Hence, with a stethoscope, breath sounds from the trachea can be heard clearly over the right apex. The bifurcation of the trachea is surrounded by lymph nodes and the pulmonary nerve plexuses.

In the **main bronchi** the rings of cartilage are similar to those of the trachea. The right bronchus deviates only a little from the line of the trachea, but the left makes a more acute angle and is longer than the right bronchus. The left bronchus passes under the arch of the aorta and in front of the thoracic descending aorta to reach the root of the left lung. It passes immediately in front of the oesophagus where it can arrest the swallowing of a large object. The pulmonary trunk and the left pulmonary artery branch in front of the left bronchus. The right bronchus passes almost directly into the root of the lung, with the right pulmonary artery in front of it. Before reaching the lung, the right bronchus divides into an upper lobe bronchus and a descending bronchus which pass above and below the pulmonary artery respectively.

The lungs and air passages are supplied by the bronchial arteries as far as the terminal bronchioles.

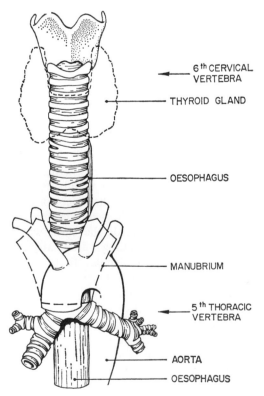

FIG. 31.4. The course and main relations of the trachea.

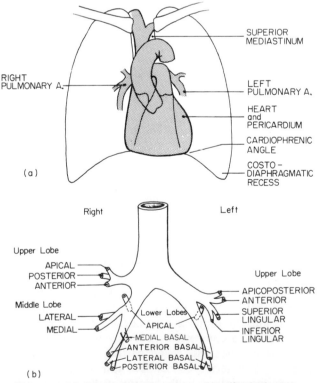

FIG. 31.5 (a) Postero-anterior view of mediastinal structures, and (b) the main lobar and segmental bronchi.

LOBAR AND SEGMENTAL BRONCHI (fig. 31.5b).

Within the lung the bronchi branch repeatedly to form a tree of tubes carrying air to all parts of the organ. The pulmonary arteries branch with the bronchi, so these structures form an elastic scaffolding within each lung. The larger branches of the bronchi supply discrete segments of lung tissue. Fig. 31.5b shows the usual pattern of branching and each named branch leads to a **broncho-pulmonary segment**. The tributaries of the pulmonary veins run in the septa between the segments. Hence the bronchopulmonary segment, although a self-contained

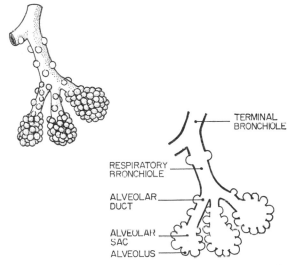

FIG. 31.6. The conducting and respiratory portions of the lung.

unit of lung tissue, does not form a completely separate vascular unit. Furthermore, although it constitutes a third order of lung organization, it is not necessarily served by a third order bronchus. With dichotomous branching of the bronchus the diameter of the bronchial tube diminishes and when the lumen falls to about 1·0 mm in diameter the tube is known as a **bronchiole**. Further division of the bronchioles continues until the last division produces the **terminal bronchioles** (fig. 31.6).

All the tubes mentioned so far have relatively thick walls and they form the **conducting portion of the lung**; the air contained in this portion does not exchange gases with the blood and this volume of air corresponds to the 'anatomical dead space' (p. 31.17). Beyond the terminal bronchiole, a thinner walled tube, the **respiratory bronchiole**, has alveoli protruding from its wall; this is the beginning of the **respiratory portion of the lung**, which consists of the alveolar ducts, alveolar sacs and alveoli.

Histological structure (Table 31.1)

Gaseous interchange occurs in the respiratory portion of the bronchial tree, i.e. the **alveolar ducts and sacs** and the **alveoli** which lead from the respiratory bronchioles.

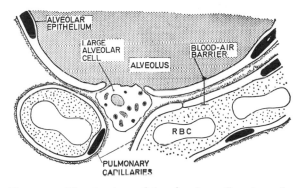

FIG. 31.7a. The structure of the alveolar wall as shown by EM.

The total area of the surface available for exchange is about 70 m² and it is lined largely by simple squamous alveolar epithelium. The alveoli are surrounded by a meshwork of pulmonary capillaries. Thus, the blood-air barrier consists of the alveolar wall and a capillary endothelium (figs. 31.7a and b); both these layers are thin and the whole barrier is less than 1 μm thick. Each alveolus is a small cavity with its mouth opening into an alveolar sac but the lumina of alveoli may also communicate with each other through pores in their walls.

TABLE 31.1. The histology of the respiratory tract.

	Diameter mm	Epithelium	Goblet cells	Clara cells	Compound glands	Cartilage	Smooth muscle	Elastic tissue
Conducting portion								
Trachea	25	Pseudostratified ciliated columnar	+	−	+	+ +	+	+ +
Large bronchi	11–19	,, ,, ,,	+	−	+	+ + +	+	+ +
Small bronchi	3–6	,, ,, ,,	+	+	−	+	+ + +	+ +
Bronchioles	1·0	Simple ciliated columnar	+	+ +	−	−	+ + +	+ +
Terminal bronchiole	0·65	,, ,, ,,	−	+ + +	−	−	+ +	+
Respiratory portion								
Respiratory bronchioles	0·45	Simple cubical	−	−	−	−	+	+
Alveolar ducts	0·45	Simple squamous	−	−	−	−	+	+
Alveolar sacs	0·40	,, ,,	−	−	−	−	+	+
Alveoli	0·25–0·3	,, ,,	−	−	−	−	?	+

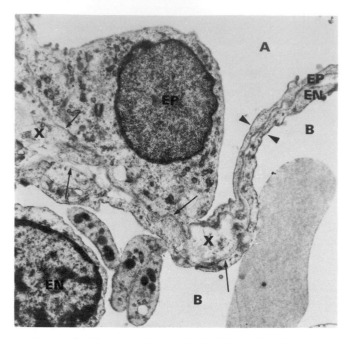

FIG. 31.7b. Electron micrograph of rat lung. The alveolar space (A) is lined by a simple flattened epithelium (EP) and the capillary (B) by endothelium (EN) each of which has its own basement membrane (arrows) between which is the interstitium (X). In its thinnest parts the air blood barrier (arrowheads) consists of attenuated epithelium and endothelium which share a common fused basement membrane and there is no interstitial space. Three platelets and an erythrocyte are seen in the capillary. (× 6000). Courtesy of Dr. B. Corrin.

These pores probably allow the collateral passage of air and this may prevent collapse in segments of lung when the lumen of a small bronchus is plugged. Almost all alveoli abut on other alveoli and it is customary to speak of an **interalveolar septum** where the two alveolar walls lie back to back, sandwiching the capillary meshwork between them. Occasionally **large granular alveolar cells**, sometimes called septal cells, are present and may be responsible for the synthesis of surfactant (p. 31.11) and phospholipids (p. 31.31).

The whole substance of the lung, apart from the bronchial tree and its associated vessels, is composed of alveoli. The alveolar sac is the expanded end of an alveolar duct, three or four of which arise from each respiratory bronchiole. This bronchiole is lined by simple non-ciliated cubical epithelium, which probably does not permit gaseous exchange.

During its passage from the nostrils to the respiratory bronchioles, the air is filtered, moistened and warmed. The process starts in the conchae of the nasal cavities, with their richly vascularized mucosa, and continues throughout the length of the conducting portion of the lung. Particulate matter is removed by the lining of this portion through cilial activity and mucous secretion. The trachea has a pseudostratified ciliated columnar epithelium with goblet cells and numerous mucous and serous glands with ducts opening through the epithelium. The mucous secretions provide a sticky slimy layer which traps the particles; the mucus and its contents are moved upwards by the action of the cilia, pass through the larynx and are swallowed. If secretions are increased in quantity due to inflammation, they form **sputum**. Coughing is an explosive expiration which propels secretions towards the larynx. The pseudostratified epithelium of the trachea is capable of regeneration when damaged.

The lining is similar, with the same functions, in the lobar and segmental bronchi. But as the liability to cell damage and the necessity for replacement diminish the epithelium becomes thinner with fewer undifferentiated regenerating cells. In the bronchioles the epithelium is reduced to a single layer of columnar ciliated cells; there are no compound glands so the only secretion is the mucus from the goblet cells in the epithelium itself. Goblet cells are not present in the smaller bronchioles, but the cilia continue as far as the terminal bronchioles and fine particles carried down to the terminal bronchioles are usually coughed up. Cells known as **alveolar macro-**

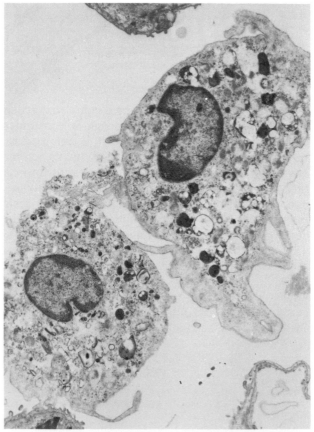

FIG. 31.8. Two alveolar macrophages free in the air space. The dense cytoplasmic inclusions are lysosomes and the vacuoles are due to phagocytosis. (× 3975). Courtesy of Dr. B. Corrin.

phages, rich in lysosomes, are found free in the alveolar lumen and are sometimes known as dust cells (fig. 31.8); their origin is uncertain, but they may come from monocytes, alveolar epithelial cells or histiocytes present in the interalveolar septum. They are phagocytic and ingest and destroy bacteria and other particles. They may pass up the bronchial tree and be ejected by coughing but some pass into the lymphatics and enter the lymph nodes at the hilum of the lung. The black, carbon-loaded lymph nodes in the lung of an adult city dweller contain inhaled particles which have escaped the protective process. Even heavily laden glands contain only a minute proportion of the particles inhaled during a lifetime. Another specialized cell is the **Clara cell**. These are found in the terminal bronchioles and have the histological characteristics of secretory cells; it has been suggested that with the large alveolar cells they also secrete surfactant.

Patency of the airway

Patency of the airways is ensured by the presence of rigid supports in the walls of the larger passages. Thus the nostrils are kept open by the nasal cartilages, the cavity of the nose is surrounded by bone and the larynx by cartilage. The trachea and main bronchi are braced by the incomplete rings of cartilage and the lobar and segmental bronchi have almost contiguous plates of cartilage in their walls. Occasional cartilaginous plaques are found in the walls of smaller bronchi but the bronchioles depend on the elastic tension of the surrounding lung substance to keep them patent.

The diameter of the bronchial tree is controlled by smooth muscle under autonomic nervous control. The circular smooth muscle around the terminal and other small bronchioles is arranged in a geodetic spiral; thus muscular contraction both narrows and shortens the bronchioles, in co-operation with the similarly arranged elastic tissue, in the expiratory phase. In the bronchi, smooth muscle lies internal to the cartilaginous plaques and in the trachea it is mainly longitudinally disposed in the posterior wall. In these larger tubes the smooth muscle assists the elastic tissue in keeping the tubes straight and taut in all stages of breathing. There is some muscle in the walls of the respiratory bronchioles and alveolar ducts but the main control is in the larger tubes.

The elasticity of the lung substance and bronchial tree provides the expiratory force in quiet breathing. Because there is normally no air between the two layers of the pleura the lung is held out against the chest wall against the pull of the elastic tissue towards the hilum (p. 31.10). If air is allowed to enter the pleural cavities (pneumothorax), the lung collapses on to its hilum by the traction of its own elastic tissue. The elastic fibres of the larger bronchi and trachea are arranged in two sheets, one inside and one outside the layer of muscle and cartilage. The inner layer keeps the mucosa corrugated in longitudinal folds. The alveoli and alveolar ducts also have an investment of elastic tissue.

Geometry of the bronchial tree

The geometry of the air passages has important functional implications. Counting the two branches of the trachea as the first 'generation', the terminal bronchioles are approximately the 16th generation. The respiratory bronchioles comprise the next three generations and the alveolar ducts and sacs the 20–23rd. In some parts of the lung the alveolar sacs are reached after fewer divisions.

In the first 5 or 6 generations the total cross-sectional area of the conducting airways is hardly changed from that of the trachea, yet these airways occupy more than half the total length. From the 7th generation (128 siblings) onwards, the airways shorten markedly and, although they continue to diminish in calibre, there are now so many of them that their combined cross-sectional area increases rapidly. In terms of area, the bronchial tree can be thought of as a trumpet with a long stem and wide mouth.

Resistance to air flow is offered mainly by the first 5 or 6 generations, because they are collectively so much longer and narrower than the rest. Narrowing of these airways by disease therefore markedly increases resistance. The deeper airways, on the other hand, contribute relatively little to resistance because they are collectively short and wide; instead, they affect the distribution of inspired gas to different alveolar regions. By constriction and dilation they help to keep, in health, a balance between ventilation and blood flow at alveolar level. In disease, patchy narrowing of these airways may seriously upset distribution and gas exchange. In asthma, widespread narrowing of airways affects both resistance and distribution.

Nerves and lymphatic tissues

The ganglion cells and nerve fibres of the **pulmonary nerve plexuses** extend along the walls of the bronchi. Parasympathetic fibres are derived from the vagus nerves and sympathetic fibres are added from the upper four thoracic segments. Apart from the motor supply to the smooth muscle, secretomotor fibres are distributed to the glands of the bronchial tree and sensory fibres from stretch receptors in the lung pass through the plexus to serve reflex control mechanisms.

The **lymphatic tissues** are widely distributed throughout the respiratory tract. The pharyngeal, palatine and lingual tonsils form a ring of lymphoid tissue around the entrance to the system. Numerous lymph vessels follow the bronchial tree to drain into the bronchopulmonary lymph nodes at the divisions of the larger bronchi. In turn, these drain into the tracheobronchial nodes at the bifurcation, from which the efferent vessels form the mediastinal lymph trunks. A superficial lymph plexus under the pulmonary pleura communicates with the lymph vessels in the lung substance.

DEVELOPMENT OF THE TRACHEA AND LUNGS

The epithelium of the lungs, trachea and larynx is developed from the endoderm of the ventral wall of the foregut. A longitudinal laryngotracheal groove appears in the ventral wall and later its lips begin to fuse at the caudal end. The fusion is not complete as the open upper end remains as the entrance to the larynx. Thus, a caudally projecting diverticulum is formed which lies on the ventral side of the developing oesophagus. The end of this diverticulum branches to form the two lung buds, which produce the definitive lung by growth and progressive branching.

The pleural cavities are derived from the primitive coelom and so they were originally continuous with the pericardium and peritoneum. The growth of the lungs causes the pleural cavities to enlarge into the chest wall until they almost surround the pericardium (fig. 19.24).

RESPIRATORY FUNCTION

SYMBOLS AND UNITS

In 1950, respiratory physiologists introduced a set of symbols given in table 31.2 with which they developed ideas about the factors which determine respiratory exchange. As a result, the subject is much more precise and scientific. The symbols are now widely used by physiologists and also by physicians and anaesthetists.

The SI unit of pressure is the pascal (Pa) which is defined as the pressure exerted by a force of 1 newton acting on 1 square metre ($N\,m^{-2} = kg\,m^{-1}\,s^{-2}$). Pascal (1623–62) was one of the first members of the Paris Academy which was founded at about the same time as the British Royal Society. He carried out experiments showing that air had weight, a revolutionary idea at that time. Pascal was a devout Catholic and also a master of epigrammatic writing. His book *Pensées* is one of the great religious works of the world.

One mmHg equals 0·133 kilopascals (kPa) and the standard atmosphere, 760 mmHg, equals 101·3 kPa. It would be sensible to re-define the standard atmosphere to equal 100 kPa. This would have far-reaching effects, especially when gases concerned in metabolism are expressed in volume units at STPD. Since 1 mole of an ideal gas has a volume of 22·4 litres at STPD, this problem is avoided by expressing amounts of metabolic gases in molar units. This practice is often but not always followed in this book; when quantities of gases are given in volumes and STPD is either stated or implied, 760 mmHg is the defined atmosphere.

TABLE 31.2. Symbols used in respiratory physiology.

Gases

Primary symbols		*Examples*	
V	gas volume		
$\dot{V}$	gas volume/unit time	$\dot{V}_{O_2}$	O_2 consumption/min
P	gas pressure		
F	fractional concentration in dry gas		
D	diffusing capacity		
T	transfer factor: this is an alternative term for D		
R	exchange ratio (respiratory quotient)	$R = \dot{V}_{CO_2}/\dot{V}_{O_2}$	

Secondary symbols			
I	inspired gas	F_{I,O_2}	O_2 concentration in inspired gas
E	expired gas	$\dot{V}_E$	ventilation rate/min
A	alveolar gas	P_{A,CO_2}	partial pressure of CO_2 in alveolar gas
T	tidal gas	V_T	tidal volume
D	deadspace gas	$\dot{V}_D$	deadspace ventilation rate/min
B	barometric	P_B	barometric pressure

Blood

Primary symbols			
Q	volume of blood		
$\dot{Q}$	blood-flow/unit time		
C	concentration of gas in blood phase	C_{a,O_2}	O_2 in arterial blood
S	saturation of Hb, per cent		

Secondary symbols			
a	arterial blood	P_{a,CO_2}	partial pressure of CO_2 in arterial blood
v	venous blood	$S_{\bar{v}O_2}$	O_2 saturation in mixed venous blood
c	pulmonary capillary blood	$\dot{Q}_c$	pulmonary capillary blood-flow/min
va	venous admixture	$\dot{Q}_{va}/\dot{Q}_t$	venous admixture as a fraction of total flow, i.e. of cardiac output
s	venous shunt	$\dot{Q}_s/\dot{Q}_t$	venous shunt as a fraction of cardiac output

In addition, we have:

f = respiratory frequency in breaths/min.

STPD = Standard temperature (0°C) pressure (101·3 kPa; 760 mm Hg) and dry.

BTPS = Body temperature and pressure and saturated with water vapour.

Lung volumes and ventilation rates are expressed at BTPS, because they 'exist' in the body at this temperature and pressure.

− Dash above a symbol denotes a mean value.

· Dot above a symbol denotes a time-derivative usually 'per minute'.

In respiratory physiology the chemical symbol N_2 includes the inert gases as well as nitrogen, unless otherwise stated or implied.

MECHANICS OF BREATHING

During respiration the lungs and thorax expand and contract rather like bellows. This requires the performance of mechanical work against forces which resist these movements. The truth of this statement is obvious to anyone who has undertaken vigorous physical exercise, and we speak appropriately of 'laboured breathing'. Discussion of respiratory mechanics requires the use of physical terms, such as force, pressure, work and energy.

A **frictional force** is set up when one body moves over another, and its magnitude is determined by the nature and extent of the apposed surfaces. It does not exist until the moving force is applied, and opposes it. During the flow of liquids and gases, friction is set up between their molecules and between these and the wall of the conducting vessel.

Elasticity, a property of solid materials, may be defined as resistance to deformation. When a particular body, made of a given material, is being considered, the term **elastance** is used. Thus the elasticity of steel is constant, but the elastance of a steel spring depends upon its length, number of coils, diameter and gauge. Elastance, for practical purposes the more useful unit, is the stretching or compressing force which must be applied to a particular body to produce unit change in length. In a perfectly elastic body, equal increments in force cause equal increments in length (Hooke's Law). No material is perfectly elastic and there is always a limit to the range over which the law applies. The reciprocal of elastance is **compliance**, which expresses the 'stretchability' of a body as change in length per unit change in stretching force.

When an elastic body is stretched or compressed, work has been done since a force has acted over a distance. This work is stored in the body as potential energy which can be expended in doing work as the body returns to its original state. The work done in winding the spring of a clock is stored as energy, which is then expended as work against the frictional forces between the clock's moving parts. The energy of a deformed spring suddenly released is dissipated as heat and sound.

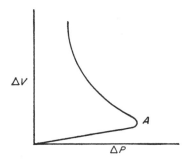

FIG. 31.9. Pressure-volume diagram during inflation of a rubber balloon.

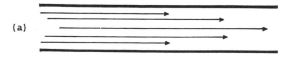

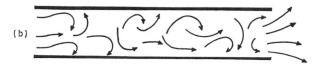

FIG. 31.10. (a) Laminar flow. Axial flow is faster than peripheral flow. (b) Turbulent flow.

Although rubber is elastic, the relation between the pressure and volume within a rubber balloon does not conform to an elastic pattern. Anyone who has blown up a balloon knows that there is first a stage in which resistance to inflation increases steeply; when the balloon reaches a certain size the resistance 'gives' and inflation then becomes easier. A 'pressure-volume diagram' (fig. 31.9) shows first the steep increase in pressure with volume, due to elasticity, but at the inflection (A) the pressure within the balloon (the deforming force) actually falls as more air is introduced. Similarly, the pressure inside small soap bubbles is greater than that in big ones, and is in inverse ratio to their radii. Structurally, the lungs could be compared to clusters of tiny balloons and so might be expected to behave like a balloon or soap bubble on inflation. In fact they do not, but resemble a stretched spring.

Flow of gas through tubes is laminar at slow speeds, but at faster rates of flow molecular collisions set up eddies and the flow is then turbulent (fig. 31.10). Laminar flow obeys the Poiseuille equation (p. 30.23). The difference in pressure of the gas between the entry and exit of the tube is directly proportional to flow rate. The pressure/flow ratio is analogous to voltage/current in electricity, and expresses resistance to flow. For laminar flow, resistance is inversely related to the fourth power of the radius of the tube. For turbulent flow, the pressure-difference is proportional to the square of the flow rate and resistance inversely related to the fifth power of the tube's radius. Flow is usually partly laminar and partly turbulent, and pressure-difference is related to flow raised to the power n, where n lies between 1 and 2.

Physiological experiments cannot be controlled as precisely as physical ones, and while the laws of physics hold in biological systems no less than on the physicist's bench, the inability to allow for every variable makes physiology a relatively inexact science. The terms and concepts of physics are, however, useful in describing and understanding many physiological processes.

FORCES AND PRESSURES ACTING ON THE THORAX AND LUNGS

Movements of the chest during the respiratory cycle are opposed by two kinds of forces which must be overcome by contraction of the respiratory muscles. These forces are (a) elastic and (b) non-elastic or 'viscous'.

Elastic forces

When a hole is made in the chest wall of a fresh cadaver, the lungs collapse and the thorax expands, air entering the space formed by separation of the pleural membranes. These movements are due to elastic recoil of the lungs and chest. At the end of a quiet expiration, with the glottis open and the respiratory muscles relaxed, the elastic forces of the lungs and thorax are just balanced; the lungs then contain about 3 litres of air. The elastic forces of the lungs, if unopposed, would empty them; those of the thorax would expand them to correspond with a lung volume of about 4 litres. At lung volumes greater than this, the elastic forces of the thorax act inwards, towards their neutral position at about 4 litres. In apposition, the lungs and thorax form an elastic system on which work must be done by the respiratory muscles.

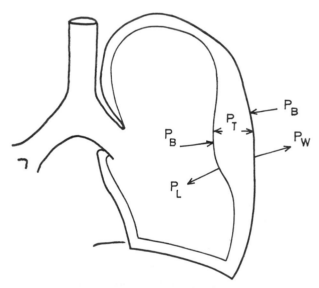

FIG. 31.11. The genesis of intrathoracic pressure (see text). P_B, Barometric and alveolar pressure; P_T, Intrathoracic pressure; P_L, 'Lung pressure' due to elasticity of lung; P_W, 'Chest wall pressure' due to thoracic elasticity with or without muscular forces.

INTRATHORACIC (INTRAPLEURAL) PRESSURE

Imagine that a small amount of air has been introduced between the pleural layers, and that the pressure in this space is P_T (fig. 31.11). The pressure outside the thorax is atmospheric, P_B, and when the airway is open and there is no flow of air into or out of the lungs the pressure within the lungs is also P_B. The retractile, elastic force of the lungs, when expressed per unit pleural surface area, becomes the 'lung pressure', P_L. The 'chest wall pressure', P_W, is derived from thoracic elasticity, with or without additional forces applied by the respiratory muscles. When no movement of air is taking place, and the airway is open, the pressures shown in fig. 31.11 must balance. Thus:

$$P_L + P_T + P_B = P_W + P_T + P_B \qquad (1)$$

Therefore

$$P_L = P_W$$

If we consider only the pressures acting on the visceral pleura, then under the same conditions these also balance. At two degrees of inflation, therefore:

$$P_1L + P_1T = P_B \qquad (2)$$

and

$$P_2L + P_2T = P_B \qquad (3)$$

Now if P_2L is greater than P_1L, as it would be at a greater lung inflation, P_2T must be less than P_1T. In other words intrathoracic pressure falls with inspiration. Further, since P_L is never zero, P_T is always less than P_B in the static condition with an open airway. The intrathoracic pressure is sometimes described as 'negative', which is confusing and inexact, because pressure is never negative; 'subatmospheric pressure' is a better term.

Under normal conditions the pleura does not contain air. Because the lung has weight, the intrapleural pressure increases by about 25 Pa (0.25 cm H_2O) per cm distance from the apex towards the base in the erect position, and from front to back when supine. At the end of a normal expiration, the apical intrapleural pressure is about -1 kPa (-10 cm H_2O) and the basal -0.25 kPa (-2.5 cm H_2O), relative to atmospheric pressure. During a normal inspiration, intrapleural pressure falls further by about 2.5 kPa. Intrapleural pressures rise towards atmospheric with advancing age, due to loss of the lung's elastic recoil (equations 2 and 3). The changes in pressure recorded from an oesophageal balloon reflect the fluctuations in intrapleural pressure fairly accurately, but cannot reflect the absolute pressures.

Sometimes P_T may exceed P_B. During forced expiration P_T may have to be raised above P_B to propel air towards the mouth at high speed; this is achieved by contraction of the expiratory muscles so that P_W acts forcibly inwards. Again, even in the static condition, P_T can be raised above P_B by an expiratory effort against a closed glottis. A violent coughing attack, for instance, may raise P_T 27 kPa (200 mmHg) above P_B. Some wind instruments, notably the trumpet and oboe, require a high mouth pressure but a low volume flow of air; here the experts learn suitable tricks with soft palate and buccinator to avoid having to perform a continuous Valsalva manoeuvre (p. 30.51).

PRESSURE-VOLUME CHARACTERISTICS OF THE LUNG

The pressure tending to inflate the lung (the **transpulmonary pressure**) is $P_B - P_T$ (fig. 31.11). The pressure opposing inflation (P_L) is due to the elastic recoil of the lung. The relation between lung volume and transpulmonary pressure gives information about the elastic recoil. Fig. 31.12 shows the relationship between transpulmonary pressure (represented by oesophageal pressure) and lung volume during two breaths of different sizes, each taken from the normal expiratory position (FRC, p. 31.14). With bigger breaths the relationship is curved and is sigmoid if inspiration starts from the deepest possible expiration (RV, p. 31.14), although it obviously differs from that for a rubber balloon (fig. 31.9). The expiratory curve does not quite follow the inspiratory but describes a hysteresis loop, which becomes narrower as the duration of breath-holding at each point (here 3 sec) increases. With a smaller breath, more representative of quiet breathing, there is little hysteresis and the pressure-volume line is almost straight.

Elastance of the lungs, usually termed **elastic resistance**, is given by the change in transpulmonary pressure divided by the change in lung volume. For the smaller breath in fig. 31.12, this is about 0·3/0·6, or 0·5 kPa/l (5 cm H_2O/l). **Compliance** of the lungs, the reciprocal of elastance, is in this case 2 l/kPa (0·2 l/cmH$_2$O). These units are not physically exact; a spring's elastance is expressed as force divided by length, or $N\ m^{-1}$, whereas pulmonary elastance reduces to $N\ m^{-2}\ m^{-3}$, i.e. $N\ m^{-5}$. Since compliance is the slope of the volume/pressure line, it thus depends upon both the degree of inflation of the lungs and whether it is measured over an inspiration or expiration. Compliance is also related to total lung capacity (TLC, p. 31.14).

Elastic work is given by the area under the pressure-volume curve, and has the units pressure × volume, or in absolute units $N\ m^{-2} \times m^3$. These reduce to $N\ m^{-2} \times m^3$ or force × length.

PRESSURE-VOLUME CHARACTERISTICS OF THE THORAX

If, instead of transpulmonary pressure in fig. 31.11, we were able to measure the effective distending pressure i.e. **transthoracic pressure** of the lungs and thorax combined, we could gain information about thoracic elasticity. To do this it is necessary to substitute an external source of energy for the respiratory muscles. The body is enclosed up to the neck in an airtight box (body respirator) inside which the pressure is varied by means of a pump. The muscles of respiration must be relaxed completely, either voluntarily or, since this is very difficult, by curarization. The difference between the pressure in the box and the atmospheric pressure is the transthoracic

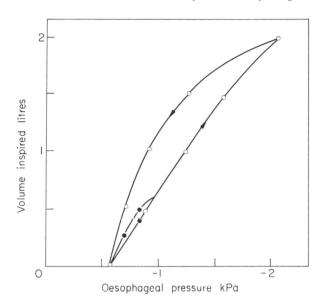

FIG. 31.12. Pressure-volume graph during inspiration and expiration of 0·6 litres (●) and of almost 2 litres (○) from functional residual capacity. Arrow up, inspiration. At each point shown, the breath was held for 3 sec, with the glottis open, before the oesophageal pressure was measured. Notice the hysteresis effect, especially in the case of the deeper breath. Redrawn from Mead J., Whittenberger J.L. & Radford E.P. (1957) *J. appl. Physiol.* **10**, 191.

pressure. Thoracic elastic resistance is the difference between the resistance of the lungs and thorax combined (obtained from a pressure-volume diagram like fig. 31.12) and the resistance of the lungs alone. The measurement of thoracic elastance is obviously difficult but, fortunately, it is not often required in clinical practice.

COMPONENTS OF PULMONARY ELASTICITY

Why the lungs behave more like a spring than a balloon or soap bubble is obscure, but is presumably related to pulmonary structure. The elastic properties of balloons are confined to their walls, corresponding in the lung to the pleura. On the other hand, the lung's elastic fibres form a system of branching springs, connecting the pleura with the hilum and also operating at right angles to this radial direction, parallel to the pleural surface. This may explain the difference in behaviour.

The honeycomb structure of the pulmonary elastic tissue ensures, in health, that not only the lung as a whole but each alveolus is endowed with the appropriate retractile capacity. This helps to equalize respiratory excursions in different parts of the lungs. Local destruction of elastic tissue in disease leads to grossly uneven ventilation.

Surfactant

Lining each alveolus is a liquid film, and surface tension exists in the interface between this film and the alveolar gas. The surface force tends to collapse the alveolus; the smaller the alveolus the greater should this tendency be, to judge from the ability of a small soap-bubble to blow up a big one connected to it. This behaviour of soap bubbles, however, depends on the fact that surface tension is independent of surface area. The surface tension of the liquid lining the alveoli, on the contrary, diminishes as the area gets smaller, thus reducing the tendency to collapse. This property is due to the presence in alveolar fluid of a lipoprotein known as surfactant. As surfactant appears in fetal lungs in increasing quantity during the last trimester of pregnancy, a deficiency of it may be one of the causes of failure of the lungs to expand in the newborn (vol. 3, p. 45.5).

Non-elastic forces

Movement of air through the conducting passages and sliding of parietal and visceral pleura over each other set up frictional forces which must be overcome during the respiratory cycle.

In fig. 31.13, change in lung volume is plotted against change in intrathoracic pressure (transpulmonary pressure with a minus sign) from measurements made continuously throughout a single respiratory cycle. The hysteresis effect is much magnified. V_0 and B represent the static points at expiration and inspiration respectively. The line joining them forms a wide loop with upstroke and downstroke (V_0AB and BCC′V_0). During inspiration, P_T falls considerably before pulmonary volume increases much, and during expiration the initial rise in P_T occurs without much change in lung volume. Changes in volume lag behind those in pressure. A pressure difference between mouth and alveoli must be established before air will move; friction must be overcome. Work

against friction is given by the area V_0ABV_0 for inspiration and V_0BCC′V_0 for expiration. The total inspiratory work, elastic plus frictional, is equal to the area V_0ABV_1V_0. This must be supplied by the inspiratory muscles. At volume V_1 the elastic work, V_0BV_1V_0, is stored in the elastic tissue and is available to do frictional work during expiration. Of the stored energy, V_0BCV_0 is used to provide expiratory frictional work, while the remainder (BV_1CB) is 'wasted' elastic energy which appears as heat. The remaining frictional work of expiration, V_0CC′V_0, has to be performed by the expiratory muscles.

In quiet breathing, the low airflow requires little frictional work and the loop V_0ABCC′V_0 is correspondingly slender; C′ may, indeed, lie to the left of the line V_0V_1. In this case all the expiratory frictional work can be provided by the stored elastic energy and the expiratory muscles do no work. Expiration is passive. But area BV_1CB is bigger, representing a bigger waste of elastic energy.

For a breath of 500 ml needing a change of 0·25 kPa in intrathoracic pressure, the elastic work done is half the rectangle $\Delta P \Delta V$, i.e. 0·5 × 500 × 0·25 ml·kPa. This reduces to 0·0625 N m or Joules (J). At 16 breaths/min, the elastic work is 1 J/min. A 100-watt electric light bulb consumes 6000 J of energy/min. Clearly the respiratory muscles contribute very little to the energy crisis.

Not all the frictional work V_0ABCC′V_0 is expended in moving air; some of it is used in moving viscera. Techniques have been devised by which the non-elastic resistance to breathing (termed, unhelpfully, **pulmonary resistance**) may be broken down into two components; (a) resistance to airflow or **airway resistance** and (b) resistance due to visceral displacement.

RESPIRATORY FREQUENCY AND RESPIRATORY WORK

Pulmonary ventilation rate, or simply **ventilation** ($\dot{V}E$) is defined as the volume of gas expired from the lungs per minute, and is expressed at BTPS. $\dot{V}E$ is slightly less than the inspired rate ($\dot{V}I$) because usually more O_2 is taken from the inspired gas than CO_2 added to it ($R < 1·0$). **Tidal volume** (V_T) is obtained by dividing $\dot{V}E$ by the respiratory frequency (f). At rest, $\dot{V}E$ is about 6 l/min, V_T about 500 ml and f about 12/min, but there is much variation in these figures.

In fig. 31.13, tidal volume (V_T) is ($V_1 - V_0$). If this is doubled, area V_0BV_1V_0 will increase four times; if trebled, inspiratory elastic work per breath (WEL) increases nine times. That is,

$$W_{EL} \propto (V_T)^2 \qquad (4)$$

Let $\dot{V}E$ remain constant while V_T is doubled; f must be

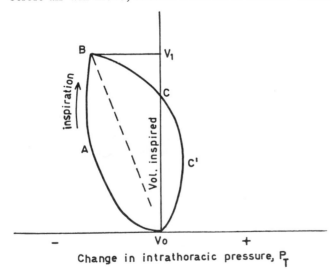

FIG. 31.13. 'Dynamic' pressure-volume diagram of lungs. Redrawn from Cooper E.A., *Behaviour of Respiratory Apparatus*, Medical Research Memorandum 2. London: National Coal Board.

halved. If V_T is trebled, f must fall to one-third, and so on. That is,

$$\dot{V}_T \propto \frac{1}{f} \tag{5}$$

The elastic work per min is equal to elastic work per breath multiplied by the respiratory frequency. Thus, from equation 4,

$$\dot{W}_{EL} \propto (V_T)^2 \times f \tag{6}$$

Substituting V_T from equation 5, we have:

$$\dot{W}_{EL} \propto \frac{1}{f} \tag{7}$$

In fig. 31.14 $\dot{W}_{EL}$ is plotted against f at constant $\dot{V}_E$

Consider now what happens to frictional work when V_T and f are reciprocally altered, $\dot{V}_E$ remaining constant. If f doubles, half as big a V_T traverses the airway in half the time; the mean flow rate, $\dot{V}$, is the same. For laminar flow,

$$(P_2 - P_1) \propto \dot{V} \tag{8}$$

Now work equals pressure-change × volume-change, and work/min against flow-resistance equals pressure gradient × flow rate. For frictional work/min,

$$\dot{W}_{FR} \propto (P_2 - P_1) \times \dot{V}$$

From equation (8)

$$\dot{W}_{FR} \propto \dot{V}^2 \propto \dot{V}_E^2 \tag{9}$$

and since $\dot{V}_E$ by definition is constant, $\dot{W}_{FR}$ in this analysis is independent of f.

We should therefore expect that for a given $\dot{V}_E$, since only $\dot{W}_{EL}$ changes with f (equation 7), respiratory work would be minimal when f is high. Physiologically, however, the 'choice' of frequency involves a rather different problem; it is to choose a $\dot{V}_E$, a V_T and a frequency which provides an **alveolar ventilation** ($\dot{V}_A$) appropriate to the needs of the moment. In the next section it will be seen that

$$\dot{V}_E = \dot{V}_A + V_D \times f$$

Then, from equation (9)

$$\dot{W}_{FR} \propto (\dot{V}_A + V_D \times f)^2$$
$$\propto \dot{V}_A^2 + 2\dot{V}_A \cdot V_D \cdot f + V_D^2 \cdot f^2 \tag{10}$$

Equation (10) shows that for a given $\dot{V}_A$ and V_D, frictional work increases as a square function of f. Moreover, at constant $\dot{V}_A$, $\dot{W}_{EL}$ does not decrease quite so fast with increasing f as equation (7) would suggest, since $\dot{V}_E$ has to rise gradually. The situation is in fact quite complex. But we might expect that for a given alveolar ventilation $\dot{W}_{EL}$ should decrease and $\dot{W}_{FR}$ increase, with increasing frequency, in curvilinear fashion as shown in fig. 31.14.

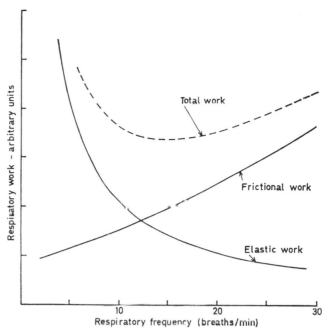

FIG. 31.14. The relation between respiratory frequency and respiratory work.

Adding elastic and frictional work, there should be an optimal frequency at which total respiratory work is minimal. Experiment bears this out, although there is a short range of frequencies over which total work changes little. The natural respiratory frequency falls within this range. How the adjustment is made is not understood, but respiratory work seems to be a factor in regulating the balance between V_T and f. A disease which alters elastic or frictional work is commonly accompanied by the appropriate shift in respiratory frequency.

RESPIRATORY WORK DURING EXERCISE

During exercise the following relationships probably apply:

$$\dot{W}_{EL} \propto (\dot{V}_E)^2 \tag{11}$$

$$\dot{W}_{FR} \propto (\dot{V}_E)^2 \quad \text{for laminar flow} \tag{12}$$

$$\propto (\dot{V}_E)^3 \quad \text{for turbulent flow} \tag{13}$$

From fig. 31.13 it has been shown that as $\dot{W}_{FR}$ increases less elastic energy is wasted during expiration; area $V_0ABCC'V_0$ approaches more and more closely to the total work per breath, $V_0ABV_1CC'V_0$. Thus at high $\dot{V}_E$ respiratory work is accounted for almost entirely by the frictional work, and equation 11 can be ignored. Combining equations 12 and 13, for all values of $\dot{V}_E$ found in exercise, we have approximately:

$$\dot{W}_{FR} \propto (\dot{V}_E)^n \tag{14}$$

where n lies between 2 and 3.

Experiments in which $\dot{V}$E increased up to 120 l/min have shown a value for *n* of 2·12. This figure suggests that in the normal airway the flow of gas remains to a large extent laminar even during exercise, a tribute to good aerodynamic design.

OXYGEN COST OF BREATHING

A muscle's O_2 consumption is a good index of the work it is performing. Respiratory work can be expressed in this way. O_2 uptake has been measured in resting subjects, at each of several ventilation rates during voluntary overbreathing. Fig. 31.15 shows the result. In health, $\dot{V}O_2$ increases by 0·5–1·0 ml/min for every l/min increase in $\dot{V}$E. The increase tends to grow as $\dot{V}$E rises,

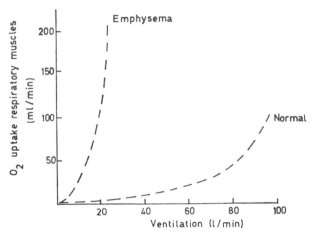

FIG. 31.15. O_2 uptake of respiratory muscles at different ventilation rates in normal subjects and in patients with pulmonary emphysema. Redrawn from Campbell E.J.M., Westlake E.K. & Cherniack R.M. (1957). *J. appl. Physiol.* **11**, 303.

consistent with equation 14. However, it remains relatively trivial; in heavy exercise $\dot{V}O_2$ rises from a resting value of 250 ml/min to over 2500 ml/min, while $\dot{V}$E increases from 6 to 50 l/min and the O_2 cost of breathing rises by only 20 ml/min (fig. 31.15). This calculation assumes that the O_2 cost of breathing is the same, at a given $\dot{V}$E during exercise, as at rest; this cannot be verified, but is probably valid.

The O_2 cost measures total respiratory work, including that done on the thoracic cage and viscera. The upper graph in fig. 31.15 shows how greatly respiratory work can increase when the lungs are abnormal, and in these conditions it may account for a significant part of total O_2 used and limit the ability to exercise.

PULMONARY VENTILATION

Ventilation of the lungs is the first step in the supply of O_2 to the tissues and the last step in the excretion of CO_2. The O_2 stores of the body are very small, and pulmonary ventilation must supply the body's needs from

minute to minute if life is to continue. As an excretory organ the lung is of great importance and eliminates as CO_2 more than fifty times as much acid as the kidneys. These functions entail, in a resting subject, a daily ventilation of 8000–10,000 litres, from which about 360 litres of O_2 are taken and to which about 300 litres of CO_2 are added. All these figures may be doubled for a heavy worker.

SUBDIVISIONS OF LUNG VOLUME

The volume of air in the lungs and airways varies widely during respiratory movements. At the deepest possible inspiration they contain, in a healthy young man, some 6 litres. This is the **total lung capacity** (TLC). TLC is conveniently subdivided into four primary 'volumes' (fig. 31.16). At the end of a quiet expiration about 3 litres of air remain. Only 1 litre of this can be expelled by a

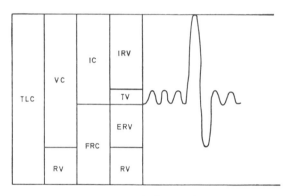

FIG. 31.16. The lung volumes.

deep expiration; this is the **expiratory reserve volume** (ERV) and the volume which remains, 2 litres or so, is the **residual volume** (RV). Starting again at the end of a quiet expiration, an average quiet inspiration draws in rather less than 500 ml; this is the ventilatory ebb and flow, or **tidal volume** (TV or VT). In addition to this it is possible to take in a further 3·5 litres, the **inspiratory reserve volume** (IRV), before TLC is reached. ERV, TV and IRV together make up the **vital capacity** (VC) while ERV and RV form the **functional residual capacity** (FRC). The **inspiratory capacity** comprises TV and IRV.

These volumes and capacities may be grossly altered in pulmonary disease and their measurement may help in diagnosis. Apart from RV, they are easily measured by means of a recording spirometer; this is a cylindrical bell floating in water, suspended by its dome from a pulley leading to a counterweight and kymograph pen; the internal air space is connected to a wide tube through which the subject respires. Vertical movements of the pen are proportional to respired volumes. RV cannot be measured directly and a dilution technique is used

(p. 1.2). A known volume of helium can be used as a marker, or the N_2 contained in the lungs can be washed out, by breathing pure O_2, and estimated by analysis. FRC and thus RV can also be measured by an application of Boyle's Law using a whole body plethysmograph.

Forced expiratory volume (FEV)

When recording ERV, TV and IRV, no stipulation is made as to speed of performance. VC is taken as the biggest volume which can be expired, in three attempts, from full inspiration, or (with greater reproducibility in healthy individuals) as the average of three technically satisfactory attempts. In clinical work the 'timed vital capacity' or FEV is useful. This is the biggest expiration which can be made in a given time; usually 1 sec but sometimes 0·75 sec is chosen. In 1 sec a healthy young subject can expire 80 per cent or more of his vital capacity; this figure falls with increasing age. Obstruction of the airway reduces the FEV_1/VC ratio (vol. 3, p. 18.10).

Maximal voluntary ventilation (MVV)

This is measured from a short spell of forced, voluntary hyperventilation, usually 15 sec. Stipulating frequency, e.g. forty breaths per min, MVV_{40}, improves reproducibility. Normal values lie in the range 100–150 l/min. MVV and FEV are related and tend to vary together in disease.

VENTILATION OF THE LUNGS

Partition of ventilation

Not all the inspired air takes part in respiratory exchange, for some of it travels no further than the conducting airway at each inspiration. This wasted volume is the **respiratory deadspace** (V_D). About 20–35 per cent of $\dot{V}_E$ is expended in ventilating the nose, mouth, pharynx, larynx, trachea and large and medium bronchi. The rest ventilates the alveolar units and exchanges O_2 for CO_2 with the pulmonary capillary blood. This part of $\dot{V}_E$ is the **alveolar ventilation** ($\dot{V}_A$).

This concept is an oversimplification. First, since many of the small conducting passages contribute significantly to respiratory exchange, it is impossible to set precise anatomical limits to the deadspace. Secondly, the alveolar ventilation is not distributed evenly to all alveoli, even in health (p. 31.23), and we must distinguish overall alveolar ventilation from regional alveolar ventilation. The subject of deadspace is complex and simplifying assumptions are necessary. At the outset the deadspace can be regarded as a clearly demarcated zone in which gas is conducted but not exchanged, and we can assume that inspired gas is evenly distributed to the alveoli where gas is mixed and exchanged but not conducted. Qualifications of this simple model will be introduced later.

Respiratory deadspace

Fig. 31.17 depicts different stages of a respiratory cycle. Just before the start of inspiration (a), the alveoli and

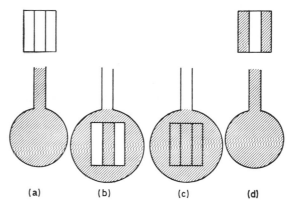

FIG. 31.17. Stages of a single respiratory cycle (see text).

deadspace are full of alveolar gas, i.e. gas which has undergone respiratory exchange. Three 'units' of atmospheric air are waiting to enter the lungs. At (b) these have been inhaled; two of them have reached the alveoli, washing in before them the alveolar gas which previously occupied the dead space, and one inspired unit now occupies the dead space. The two units which have reached the alveoli now undergo respiratory exchange and become two units of alveolar gas (c). The unit in the deadspace remains unaltered in composition. At (d) the three units have been expired; two are now alveolar gas (the 'expired portion of the alveolar gas') and one is unaltered inspired air ('deadspace gas'). Mixed, the three units are the 'expired gas'. Alveoli and deadspace are again full of alveolar gas.

Let the concentration by volume of any gas x in the inspired gas be F_{Ix}, in the alveolar gas F_{Ax} and in expired gas F_{Ex}. Let the volume of the expired portion of the alveolar gas be V_A, of the tidal volume V_T and of the deadspace V_D. Then the volume of x in expired gas = volume of x in deadspace gas plus volume of x in expired portion of alveolar gas

$$V_T \times F_{Ex} = V_D \times F_{Ix} + V_A \times F_{Ax}$$

But

$$V_A = V_T - V_D$$

Therefore

$$V_T \times F_{Ex} = V_D(F_{Ix} - F_{Ax}) + V_T \times F_{Ax}$$

Solving for V_D,

$$V_D = V_T \times \frac{F_{Ex} - F_{Ax}}{F_{Ix} - F_{Ax}} \qquad (15)$$

Equation 15, the **Bohr Equation**, is a classical one in respiratory physiology. It tells us that if we can measure tidal volume and the concentration of any gas in the inspired, expired and alveolar gas, then the volume of the deadspace can be calculated. The only real problem is how to obtain a sample of alveolar gas for analysis. This will now be considered,

Composition of expired gas

When expiration starts, the first gas to emerge is inspired air from the deadspace. As expiration proceeds, the emergent gas changes to alveolar gas. The transition is not abrupt, because of the way one gas follows another along a tube. Smoke blown along a narrow glass tube has a spike-shaped 'front', because during laminar flow, the velocity of the stream is greatest at the centre and least at the circumference (fig. 31.10). The CO_2 content of expired gas thus shows not a sudden change from inspired to alveolar levels (fig. 31.18, OFDBC) but an S-shaped curve (OABC). This may be shown by fractional sampling and analysis of successive portions of expired gas, or from the record of a rapid, continuous analyser such as the infra-red CO_2 analyser or the mass spectrometer. The curve has three phases: (1) the inspired gas phase (2) the mixing phase and (3) the alveolar plateau in which CO_2 content is almost constant.

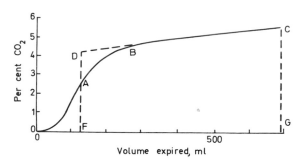

FIG. 31.18. CO_2 concentration curve in relation to volume of air expired. Modified from Aitken R.S. & Clark-Kennedy A.E. (1928) *J. Physiol.* **65**, 389.

The presence of phase (2) means that a volume some three times greater than V_D must be expired before one can be sure of obtaining alveolar gas, unmixed with deadspace gas. The composition of alveolar gas itself gradually changes as expiration proceeds, as shown by the gentle upward slope of the alveolar plateau. The causes of this change are as follows: (1) the continued addition of CO_2 to alveolar gas from mixed venous blood during expiration, (2) the presence of an increasing CO_2 concentration from the mouths to the deeper parts of the alveolar units, so-called stratified (or series) inhomogeneity and (3) uneven distribution of gas and blood to the alveoli, so-called parallel inhomogeneity, which is present in health but of special importance only in certain diseases of the lung.

In fig. 31.18, all the recorded CO_2 comes from alveolar gas. Assuming the extrapolation BD of the line CB is

justified, and drawing FD so that area OFAO equals ABDA, the expired gas can be thought of as composed of volume OF of inspired gas and volume FG of alveolar gas, i.e. OF is the deadspace. The mean CO_2 content of the expired portion of alveolar gas is $(DF+CG)/2$. This is the CO_2 concentration used to derive equation 15 and when substituted in it must yield a value for V_D equal to OF.

The above discussion is limited to CO_2 but, with modifications, applies to O_2 or to foreign gases introduced into the inspired gas. It shows one way of determining alveolar gas composition, but the method needs special apparatus.

Direct sampling of alveolar gas

HALDANE–PRIESTLEY METHOD

A piece of smooth-walled rubber hose (fig. 31.19), about 2.5 cm in diameter and about 150 cm long, is fitted with a mouthpiece. Near the mouthpiece a small hole is made in the hose, into which the end of an evacuated gas-sampling tube fits snugly. The subject sits wearing a nose-clip, breathing otherwise naturally and holding the hose. At the end of a normal expiration the command 'Blow' is given. The subject quickly raises the mouthpiece to his lips and, without inspiring, blows as rapidly and deeply

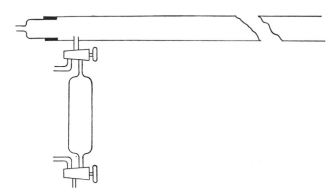

FIG. 31.19. Haldane–Priestley alveolar gas sampling tube.

as he can into the hose. At the limit of expiration he seals the mouthpiece with his tongue, holds his breath, and signals to the observer who quickly opens the tap of the sampling tube for a second or two. Gas from the proximal end of the hose, and therefore from the alveoli, enters the sampling tube and can be analysed.

END-TIDAL SAMPLING

This is usually done by means of an automatic device which takes a few ml of gas from the end of each expiration. A cumulative sample may be collected over a set period or the end-tidal gas may be fed into a continuous rapid analyser. Tidal volume must exceed 450 ml before end-tidal gas is truly alveolar (fig. 31.18).

These methods are empirical but in healthy subjects, and in appropriate circumstances, they give values for alveolar P_{CO_2} in close agreement with the P_{CO_2} of arterial blood. They have the advantages of ease and great analytical accuracy, and avoid the need for arterial puncture.

P_{CO_2} of arterial blood

For present purposes it can be assumed that, since alveolar gas is in CO_2 pressure equilibrium with end-pulmonary-capillary blood, the P_{CO_2} of arterial blood is equal to mean alveolar P_{CO_2} (see below for an account of partial pressures). In health, arterial P_{CO_2} is the same (within experimental error) as the alveolar P_{CO_2} derived from Haldane–Priestley or end–tidal sampling. In certain lung diseases when the distribution of gas and blood to the lungs is markedly uneven, arterial P_{CO_2} is higher than mean alveolar P_{CO_2} and direct alveolar samples are unrepresentative of either. In these circumstances arterial P_{CO_2} becomes the basic measurement for calculation of deadspace and alveolar ventilation, and arterial puncture or catheterization, which properly carried out is a safe procedure, is necessary.

Volume of the respiratory deadspace

The derivation of the Bohr equation assumes a dead-space equal to the volume of the conducting airway at the instant when expiration begins (fig. 31.17). X-rays show that the bronchi dilate and elongate during inspiration and shorten and narrow during expiration. Deadspace varies, according to the inspiratory level, from approximately 120 to 180 ml.

Under some conditions, the value obtained for V_D depends upon the indicator gas used to measure it. The main differences are seen between the respiratory gases (O_2 and CO_2) and the non-respiratory gases (such as N_2 H_2 and He). In exercise and hyperventilation, the non-respiratory gases yield a V_D corresponding to the inspiratory position of the chest, much the same as at rest. On the other hand, O_2 and CO_2 deadspaces may increase to 600 ml or more. This increase could not all be accommodated in the conducting airway, and represents an extension of deadspace into the alveolar units. The extension is termed **alveolar deadspace** and its functional nature is recognized by the term **physiological deadspace** used when V_D is measured with O_2 or CO_2. The non-respiratory gases, on the contrary, yield under all conditions a value for V_D much closer to that obtained by anatomical methods (plaster casts, direct measurement) and the non-respiratory gas V_D is referred to as **anatomical deadspace**.

The genesis of alveolar deadspace is too complex to be discussed fully, but at least two factors are involved. First, non-uniformity of gas concentration within a single alveolar unit (stratified inhomogeneity) is more likely to occur with gases which are rapidly transferred across the alveolar membrane, that is O_2 and CO_2, than with the non-respiratory gases, and in exercise rather than at rest. Secondly, non-uniformity of gas concentration between different alveolar units, arising from non-uniform distribution of gas and blood to the alveoli, also affects O_2 and CO_2 much more than the non-respiratory gases.

Measured physiological deadspace increases with the end-inspiratory position of the chest, and therefore with tidal volume. It also increases with body size, with age, and with respiratory frequency. An increase in frequency allows less time for diffusion up and down the alveolar ducts; stratified inhomogeneity (p. 31.15) is increased and this has the effect of increasing deadspace. In healthy adults deadspace, sitting, is related to age (yr), height (cm), tidal volume (ml) and frequency by the equation:

$$V_D = 0{\cdot}930 \times age + 1{\cdot}725 \times height$$
$$+ 0{\cdot}267 \times V_T - 1291/f - 213$$

Functions of the respiratory deadspace

The walls of the deadspace moisten and warm inspired air, which is saturated with water vapour before it reaches the alveoli. All the heat lost from the respiratory tract at rest (and quite possibly during heavy exercise) comes from the blood perfusing the walls of the deadspace, and none from the pulmonary capillary blood. This process is impaired by mouth breathing and especially by the operation of tracheostomy.

The deadspace also minimizes the results of uneven ventilation. The alveoli which fill first, during inspiration, are usually those with the highest ventilation in relation to blood flow. Since the deadspace is full of alveolar gas at the start of inspiration, these alveoli receive a greater initial share of alveolar gas before inspired air reaches them. In this way their share of inspired air is comparable to that of less well-ventilated alveoli.

RELATION OF ALVEOLAR VENTILATION $\dot{V}_A$ TO ALVEOLAR GAS PRESSURES

Partial pressure of a gas in a mixture of gases

The partial pressure of a gas in a mixture of gases is proportional to the concentration by volume of the gas in the mixture, and the sum of partial pressures of the constituent gases is equal to the pressure of the mixture. Thus, for alveolar gas:

$$P_{A,O_2} + P_{A,CO_2} + P_{A,N_2} + P_{A,H_2O} = P_B \qquad (16)$$

and

$$P_{A,CO_2} = (P_B - 6{\cdot}25) \times F_{A,CO_2} \qquad (17)$$

Gas analysis yields concentrations of dry gas, and the vapour pressure of water at body temperature is

6·25 kPa (47 mm Hg). Equations 16 and 17 ignore the small differences between P_B and alveolar pressure due to the movements of the chest.

Partial pressure of a gas in a liquid

If a liquid be exposed to a gas which is soluble in it, molecules of the gas diffuse into the liquid. An equilibrium is reached when the pressure of the gas in the liquid equals that in the gas phase. If the gas phase contains a mixture of soluble gases, equilibrium will be reached according to the gaseous partial pressures. We may thus speak of the partial pressure of a gas in a liquid.

$\dot{V}_A$ and alveolar gas composition

CARBON DIOXIDE

When atmospheric air (which contains hardly any CO_2) is breathed, all the CO_2 in expired gas must come from alveolar gas. The CO_2 output per min ($\dot{V}_{CO_2}$) equals the volume of alveolar gas expired per min ($\dot{V}_A$) multiplied by its concentration of CO_2.

$$\dot{V}_{CO_2} = \dot{V}_A \times F_{A,CO_2} \qquad (18)$$

When $\dot{V}_{CO_2}$ is constant, therefore,

$$F_{A,CO_2} \propto 1/\dot{V}_A \qquad (19)$$

But F_{A,CO_2} is proportional to P_{A,CO_2} (equation 17). Therefore

$$P_{A,CO_2} \propto 1/\dot{V}_A \qquad (20)$$

Equation 20 shows that when $\dot{V}_A$ is doubled, P_{A,CO_2} is halved, and vice versa, provided that CO_2 output is unchanged. This situation is very like the renal elimination of urea; when urea output is constant, halving the urea clearance doubles the blood urea concentration. By analogy, $\dot{V}_A$ is sometimes termed **alveolar clearance**.

OXYGEN

The corresponding 'clearance equation' for O_2 is a little more complicated because F_{I,O_2} is greater than F_{A,O_2}. Another difficulty is that R is usually less than 1, which makes inspired $\dot{V}_A$ a little greater than expired $\dot{V}_A$. Assuming $R=1$, the equation for O_2 corresponding to equation 20 is

$$(P_{I,O_2} - P_{A,O_2}) \propto 1/\dot{V}_A \qquad (21)$$

The discerning student will see that what we are really doing by doubling $\dot{V}_A$ is halving the difference between inspired and alveolar gas pressures, and that this applies to both O_2 and CO_2.

Steady and changing states of $\dot{V}_A$

In the above calculations it has been assumed that $\dot{V}_A$, P_{A,CO_2}, P_{A,O_2}, $\dot{V}_{CO_2}$ and $\dot{V}_{O_2}$ are steady. When $\dot{V}_A$ is suddenly altered, equilibrium is temporarily upset and some time elapses before a new steady state is reached.

Changing states in respiratory physiology are of interest and importance, but are too complex for discussion here.

CARRIAGE OF GASES IN THE BLOOD

OXYGEN

O_2 is held in blood in two forms, physical solution and chemical combination.

DISSOLVED O_2

At 37°C, 1 ml of blood dissolves 0·023 ml of O_2 when P_{O_2} is 101 kPa (760 mm Hg). Breathing air, P_{a,O_2} is about 13·3 kPa (100 mm Hg) and $P_{\bar{v}O_2}$ about 5·3 kPa (40 mm Hg). The volume of O_2 dissolved in 100 ml of arterial blood is thus $0\cdot023 \times 100 \times 13\cdot3/101 = 0\cdot30$ ml, and in 100 ml of mixed venous blood $0\cdot023 \times 100 \times 5\cdot3/101 = 0\cdot12$ ml. Breathing pure O_2 washes N_2 out of the alveoli and raises P_{A,O_2} (and P_{O_2} in end-pulmonary capillary blood) to atmospheric minus the partial pressures of CO_2 and H_2O ($101 - 5\cdot3 - 6.25 = 89\cdot5$). 100 ml of end-pulmonary capillary blood then contain $0\cdot023 \times 100 \times 89\cdot5/101 = 2$ ml of O_2 in solution, i.e. 1·70 ml more $O_2/100$ ml in solution than when breathing air. These facts are important in considering venous-to-arterial shunts, because the extra O_2 in solution is available to oxygenate some of the shunted haemoglobin.

COMBINED O_2

Red blood cells contain a conjugated protein, haemoglobin (Hb), in which the prosthetic group haem is bound to the protein globin. Hb can combine reversibly with O_2 to form oxyhaemoglobin (HbO_2), which is so unstable that the amount present in any given blood sample depends on the P_{O_2} with which the blood is in equilibrium. Haemoglobin free from bound oxygen is called deoxyhaemoglobin. Normal blood contains about 14·5 g/dl of Hb and the maximal amount of oxygen with which it can combine is about 20 ml/dl. This quantity, which excludes physically dissolved O_2, is called the **oxygen capacity** of the blood. The actual volume of O_2 bound as HbO_2 in 1 dl of a blood sample is called the **oxygen content** (C_{O_2}); C_{O_2} expressed as a percentage of oxygen capacity is the **oxygen saturation**, S_{O_2}.

Experimentally, it is known that 1 g Hb contains 3·4 mg or 61 μmol Fe which forms part of the molecule of haem. The same weight of Hb can combine with 1·38 ml or 61 μmol O_2, i.e. one molecule of oxygen for each atom of iron. Molecular weight determinations, however, show that a molecule of haemoglobin must contain 4 atoms of iron and can therefore combine with 4 molecules of oxygen. It is thus not surprising that the simple equation

$$Hb + O_2 \rightleftharpoons HbO_2 \qquad (22)$$

cannot account for the sigmoid oxyhaemoglobin dissociation curve obtained when So_2 is plotted against Po_2. Inspection of the curve (fig. 31.20c) shows that to increase So_2 from 0 to 20 requires a greater rise in Po_2 than is needed to change So_2 from 20 to 40 or from 40 to 60. In other words, it is much more difficult to introduce the first oxygen than the later molecules.

The explanation depends on the fact that the Hb molecule consists of four subunits, two α- and two β-polypeptide chains, each with one iron-containing haem molecule, and all held together in quaternary structure by electrostatic and other forces (p. 11.11, fig. 11.8). The quaternary structures of Hb and its various derivatives, however, are not identical, That of deoxyhaemoglobin is unique, and more compact than that of oxyhaemoglobin and other derivatives. The deoxy- and oxy-structures are often called T (tight) and R (relaxed). Reaction of deoxyhaemoglobin with the first oxygen must involve disruption of the T structure. Once this stage is passed,

the molecule is in a more flexible and structurally undefined state, more receptive to oxygen, until the final stage is reached when the R-structure is established.

These considerations do not arise with the reactions of myoglobin, the oxygen combining pigment of muscle. Mgb is monomeric, containing only one molecule of haem, and the oxymyoglobin dissociation curve is hyperbolic (fig. 31.20c).

The T structure of deoxyhaemoglobin is chiefly maintained by a small number of electrostatic bonds involving protonated histidine and arginine residues with carboxylate anions in other polypeptide regions. In the R-structure (oxyhaemoglobin) the groups concerned are no longer sufficiently close to one another for the bonds to be stable and the hydrogen ions are liberated. This explains how oxyhaemoglobin as a stronger acid than deoxyhaemoglobin. It is easy to see that increase in $[H^+]$ facilitates transition to the deoxyhaemoglobin structure and therefore oxygen release.

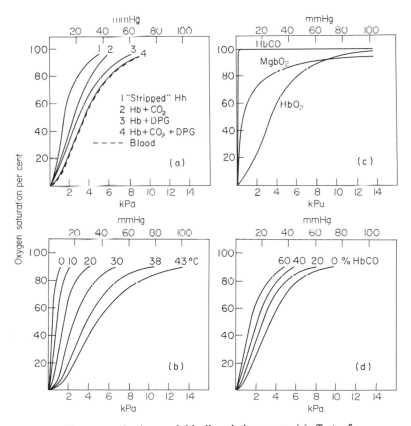

FIG. 31.20. Oxyhaemoglobin dissociation curves: (a) effects of CO_2 and 2,3-DPG, (b) effect of temperature, (c) comparison with carboxyhaemoglobin and oxymyoglobin, and (d) effect of carbon monoxide on dissociation of the remaining oxyhaemoglobin. (a) redrawn from Kilmartin J.V. & Rossi-Bernardi L. (1973) *Physiol. Rev.* **53**, 884; (b), (c) and (d), from Roughton F.J.W. (1964) in *Handbook of Physiology*, Section 3, Vol. I, p. 767. Washington: American Physiological Society.

R structure (oxy)

$\uparrow\downarrow$

T structure (deoxy)

In the conventional graphic system the dissociation curve is displaced to the right (fig. 31.20). This is the well known Bohr effect, through which increasing $[H^+]$ lowers the equilibrium So_2 at constant Po_2, thus making oxygen more readily available to the tissues.

A rise in CO_2 has similar consequences, due mainly to the direct acidifying effect of CO_2, although the formation of carbamino compounds has a subsidiary effect, perhaps by destabilizing the quaternary structure of oxyhaemoglobin (fig. 31.20a). A rise in temperature also moves the curve to the right (fig. 31.20c).

The mature normal human red cell contains 2,3-diphosphoglycerate (2,3-DPG) in molar concentration roughly equivalent to that of haemoglobin, about 5 mmol/l red cells. 2,3-DPG stabilizes the T structure of deoxyhaemoglobin by fitting into a space between the two β-chains, where it is held firmly by electrostatic bonds. In oxyhaemoglobin the R structure cannot spatially accommodate the 2,3-DPG molecule. The presence of 2,3-DPG therefore also shifts the dissociation curve to the right, and it is significant that its concentration increases when glycolysis is accelerated, as in hypoxia. During prolonged O_2 lack, therefore, HbO_2 gives up its oxygen more readily for the same value of Po_2. In blood from healthy men P_{50} (Po_2 corresponding to half saturation) may vary up to 25 per cent, and this may reflect differences in 2,3-DPG concentration (fig. 31.20a).

All these factors affect the curve in a similar way, which can be almost exactly duplicated by multiplying the Po_2 scale by arbitrarily chosen factors. This apparently reflects a similarity in mechanism, in that all the effects, with the possible exception of temperature, operate through increasing the stability or facilitating the formation of deoxyhaemoglobin. Since H^+, 2,3-DPG and to some extent CO_2 are all ligands bound in various ways to deoxyhaemoglobin, there is an analogy between their effects on the relationship between Hb and O_2 and allosteric control of activity in some important enzyme systems (p. 14.5).

Fetal blood has a higher affinity for O_2 than adult blood; its dissociation curve lies to the left of the adult curve. On the other hand, a dialysed solution of fetal haemoglobin (HbF, p. 28.5) has the same curve as one of adult haemoglobin and both lie a little to the left of the curve for fetal blood. 2,3-DPG exerts less influence on HbF than on adult Hb and this appears to be the main reason why fetal blood behaves differently. In addition, fetal erythrocytes when incubated in N_2 generate 2,3-DPG much more slowly than adult cells. The difference in P_{50} between fetal and adult blood is not great in man, about 2·6 and 3·6 kPa respectively, but is greater in other species, e.g. sheep and goat. The higher O_2 affinity of fetal blood favours the transfer of O_2 across the placenta, but must hinder transfer to the fetal tissues.

Haemoglobin is normally being continuously oxidized to methaemoglobin in which the iron is in the ferric state, but for reasons given on p. 28.6 is only present in normal blood in trace amounts. However, methaemoglobin can be produced in the blood in functionally significant amounts by many drugs and poisons, mainly aromatic compounds, and for other reasons. Because methaemoglobin cannot form a compound analogous to oxyhaemoglobin, its presence in blood not only reduces the oxygen capacity, but also moves the oxyhaemoglobin dissociation curve for the remaining Hb to the left, increasing the difficulty with which oxygen can be supplied to the tissues.

Physiological implications of the HbO_2 and $MgbO_2$ dissociation curves

The steep part of the HbO_2 curve (fig. 31.20c) is directed, not towards the origin, but towards a Po_2 intercept of about 1·33 kPa (10 mmHg). This means that So_2 can fall to very low values before Po_2 becomes negligible; thus a useful diffusion gradient of Po_2 between tissue-capillary and tissue-cell is preserved to the point of almost maximal desaturation. It also means that Hb rapidly picks up O_2 as Po_2 rises; at 6·6 kPa (50 mmHg), So_2 is already about 80 per cent. The $MgbO_2$ dissociation curve, on the other hand, has no lower tail and rises steeply from the origin; this favours a transfer of O_2 to Mgb, at low Po_2, which is presumably useful when the blood supply to the muscle is reduced intermittently by its contractions. The addition of CO_2 to blood in the tissue capillaries increases the yield of O_2 at a given Po_2 (shift of the curve to the right) and the converse effect occurs in the lungs. The liberation of heat and lactic acid in exercising muscle also helps reduction of HbO_2.

Oxygen stores of the body

Little O_2 is readily available in the body to meet an emergency. A 70 kg man can draw on only about 90 mmol or 2 l of which about 500 ml is in the lungs, 1200 ml in the blood and 300 ml in the tissues, including $MgbO_2$. Some of this store is used during exercise when the O_2 content of venous blood falls. At all times, therefore, life is almost immediately dependent upon a continued supply of O_2 from the environment.

CARBON MONOXIDE

This gas is very poisonous because the affinity of Hb for CO is very much greater than for O_2. Carboxyhaemoglobin ($Hb_4 (CO)_4$) saturation is related to Pco by a dissociation curve (fig. 31.20d) which is almost identical with the HbO_2 curve but for a lateral 'compression' of 200–250 times. Blood equilibrated with a mixture of CO and O_2 combines with both, but preferentially with CO, as follows:

$$[HbCO]/[HbO_2] = M.Pco/Po_2 \qquad (23)$$

The constant M lies between 200 and 250 in different people. Let $Po_2 = 13.3$ kPa (100 mmHg) and $[HbCO] = [HbO_2]$. Then $Pco = 67$ Pa (0.5 mmHg) approximately. An alveolar and arterial Pco of this order is reached if 0.1 per cent CO in air is breathed; yet this minute concentration is enough eventually to half-saturate circulating Hb with CO. Heavy smokers commonly have a Sco of 5 per cent or more.

The effects of Po_2 and Pco are not simply additive, for CO actually alters the HbO_2 dissociation curve (fig. 31.20d). Combination of Hb with CO increases the affinity of the remaining Hb for O_2, and release of O_2 in the tissues is greatly hampered. Reduction of the O_2 capacity by anaemia does not affect the HbO_2 dissociation curve except indirectly by stimulating an increase in 2,3-DPG concentration. 'A person whose blood is half-saturated with CO is practically helpless, but a person whose haemoglobin percentage is simply diminished to half by anaemia may be going about his work as usual' (Haldane). This effect of CO is important if exercise is undertaken, and many a patient poisoned with CO has been discharged, apparently recovered, from hospital casualty departments, only to collapse in the street.

CARBON DIOXIDE

DISSOLVED CO2

One litre of plasma at 37°C dissolves 0.251 mmol of CO_2 for every kPa of Pco_2; the plasma of normal arterial blood thus contains $0.251 \times 5.33 = 1.34$ mmol of dissolved CO_2 per litre, compared with about 25 mmol/l in combination.

COMBINED CO2

This exists in blood in two forms, bicarbonate and 'carbamino-CO_2'. When CO_2 dissolves in water or plasma, the following reactions occur:

$$CO_2 + H_2O \rightleftharpoons H_2CO_3 \qquad (24)$$
$$H_2CO_3 \rightleftharpoons H^+ + HCO_3^- \qquad (25)$$

The equilibrium constant of equation 24, the ratio $[CO_2]/[H_2CO_3]$, is about 700. This means that a solution of CO_2 forms very little H_2CO_3. The enzyme carbonic anhydrase greatly speeds the reaction in either direction but does not affect the equilibrium constant. However, equation 25, by removing H_2CO_3, favours the combination of more CO_2 in equation 24. H_2CO_3 is a weak acid and dissociates very little (though about twenty times as much as acetic acid); thus equation 25 cannot get very far unless one of its products is removed by yet other means. This is achieved by the blood buffers, which remove H^+. The possession by blood of carbonic anhydrase, and of buffers which bind H^+, is the chief reason why blood is a better carrier of CO_2 than water would be.

'Carbamino-CO_2' is a compound of CO_2 with Hb (but not with HbO_2) through an amino group:

$$Hb-NH_2 + CO_2 \rightleftharpoons Hb-NHCOO^- + H^+ \qquad (26)$$

H^+ formed in the forward reaction is buffered by the buffer systems described on p. 6.4.

Bicarbonate reacts with added H^+ as follows

$$HCO_3^- + H^+ \rightleftharpoons H_2CO_3 \qquad (27)$$
$$H_2CO_3 \rightleftharpoons H_2O + CO_2 \qquad (28)$$

The forward progress of these reactions in blood depends upon the excretion of CO_2 through the lungs.

Of the **blood proteins**, Hb is quantitatively a more important buffer than plasma proteins. Haemoglobin contains many more histidine residues than plasma proteins. The imidazole groups in these residues provide by far the greater part of the buffering action of haemoglobin in blood at pH 7.4.

The imidazole group of histidine is peculiar in that deoxygenation of HbO_2 favours H^+ acceptance and oxygenation of Hb favours H^+ donation. Oxyhaemoglobin (pK 6.7) is a stronger acid than reduced haemoglobin (pK 7.9) and so the pH in the erythrocytes tends to be raised when oxygen is given off in the tissues. This facilitates the buffering of carbonic acid and so the uptake of CO_2 by the red blood cells (fig. 31.21). These imidazole groups are responsible for the link between oxygenation and buffer activity. This link allows the exchange of O_2 and CO_2 in the tissues and lungs to take place with a smaller change in $[H^+]$ than would otherwise occur.

Uptake and release of CO2 by blood

Fig. 31.21 summarizes the reactions which take place during the uptake and release of CO_2 by blood. Added CO_2 diffuses freely through the capillary and red blood cell (RBC) membranes. Disposal of CO_2 is more rapid in the RBC than in plasma. This is because (1) the RBC is rich in carbonic anhydrase, which speeds reaction 24, whereas plasma contains none of this enzyme; (2) Hb can form carbamino-CO_2; (3) the concentration of Hb is about twice that of the plasma proteins and it has a larger buffer capacity than plasma protein, and the removal of H^+ favours both reactions in the RBC. Consequently much more HCO_3^- is formed in the RBC and since the RBC membrane is freely permeable to HCO_3^-, this ion diffuses from the RBC into the plasma. This resolves the chemical gradient but creates an electrical one. Since the RBC membrane is, in effect, impermeable to cations, K^+ cannot accompany HCO_3^- into the plasma. Instead, the electrical gradient is resolved by the diffusion of Cl^- from plasma to RBC; this is the **chloride shift**.

The sequence of reactions during the uptake of CO_2 is determined by the pressure difference of CO_2 between tissue cells and RBC. In the lungs the gradient is reversed; red blood cells in mixed venous blood have a higher P_{CO_2} than alveolar gas. The reactions follow the direction of the pressure gradient, rather as a ball might run in alternate directions down a see-saw. Their speed is remarkable. During exercise, each RBC spends much less than 1 sec in a pulmonary capillary, yet 100 ml or more of CO_2 is transferred from each litre of blood. Drugs which inhibit carbonic anhydrase may interfere with CO_2 transport.

Distribution of CO_2 in blood

Table 31.3 shows arterial and venous contents of CO_2; the difference between these is the CO_2 carried from tissues to lungs. Three points deserve notice: (1) three-

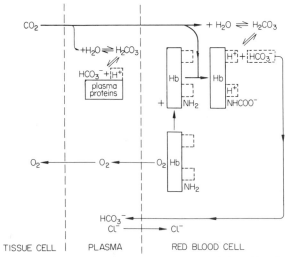

FIG. 31.21. Uptake of CO_2 from tissue cells into blood.

quarters of the total arterial or venous blood CO_2 is held in the plasma; (2) two-thirds of the carried CO_2 is held in the plasma (but most of it owes its appearance there to a reaction in the red cells); (3) most CO_2 in plasma is carried as HCO_3^-, but in red cells as carbamino-CO_2.

CO_2 dissociation curves of blood

A graph relating C_{CO_2} to P_{CO_2} of blood or plasma is a CO_2 dissociation curve (fig. 31.22). Four features need comment.

(1) Deoxygenated blood takes up more CO_2 than oxygenated blood at the same P_{CO_2}. This is due to the greater capacity of deoxygenated Hb for buffering and carbamino-CO_2 formation.

(2) All the CO_2 contained in blood is released when P_{CO_2} is reduced to zero. This contrasts with the behaviour of a simple bicarbonate solution which evolves only half its CO_2, leaving half as carbonate. In blood, H^+ is freed from protein as the blood becomes more alkaline, driving equations 24 and 25 (p. 31.21) to the left.

TABLE 31.3. Distribution of CO_2 (mmol) in 1 litre of arterial (A) and venous (V) blood, and venous-arterial differences (transported CO_2). The plasma is taken as 600 ml and erythrocytes as 400 ml. Values rounded to one decimal place. Modified from Davenport, H.W. (1958). *The ABC of Acid-Base Chemistry*, Chicago University Press.

	A	V	V−A
Dissolved			
Plasma	0·7 }1·0	0·8 }1·2	0·1 }0·2
Erythrocytes	0·3	0·4	0·1
Bicarbonate			
Plasma	15·2 }19·5	16·2 }20·6	1·0 }1·1
Erythrocytes	4·3	4·4	0·1
Carbamino			
Erythrocytes	1·0	1·4	0·4
Total CO_2	21·5	23·2	1·7

(3) Although the curves are hyperbolic, they are fairly straight over the physiological range of P_{CO_2}. This is quite different from the HbO_2 dissociation curve.

(4) The dissociation curves for 'true plasma' in fig. 31.22 have much the same slope as those for whole blood. This is because whole blood was equilibrated with CO_2, and the plasma then separated; the difference from the blood curves reflects simply the greater CO_2 content of plasma compared to cells. When plasma is separated from red blood cells and then equilibrated with other P_{CO_2}, a less steep dissociation curve is obtained, and crosses the 'true plasma' curve at the P_{CO_2} of the blood at the time of separation. The flatter curve for separated plasma reflects its inferior buffering capacity and inability to make carbamino-CO_2.

The difference between the CO_2 capacities of deoxygenated and oxygenated blood, at a given P_{CO_2}, helps in the exchange of O_2 and CO_2. More CO_2 can be transferred for a given fall or rise of P_{CO_2} when Hb is simultaneously oxygenated or deoxygenated. This is the **Haldane effect.**

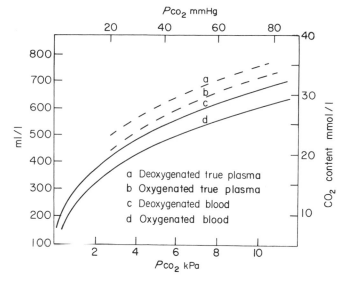

FIG. 31.22. CO_2 dissociation curves of blood and plasma. 'True plasma' is plasma separated from the red cells at the same P_{CO_2} at which CO_2 content is measured. Redrawn from Bock A.V., Field H. & Adair G.S. (1924) *J. biol. Chem.* **59**, 366.

Application of the Henderson–Hasselbalch equation

As described on p. 6.4, this equation is expressed for CO_2 as follows

$$pH = \log \frac{1}{[H^+]} = \log \frac{1}{K'} + \log \frac{[Bicarbonate]}{0.225 \times P_{CO_2}}$$

$$= pK' + \log \frac{[CO_2] - 0.225 \times P_{CO_2}}{0.225 \times P_{CO_2}} \qquad (29)$$

P_{CO_2} is expressed in kPa; $[CO_2]$ is the total CO_2 content of plasma as determined by analysis; [Bicarbonate] is $[CO_2]$ minus the concentration of dissolved CO_2. pK' is a constant which has had to be empirically determined by direct measurement of pH and $[CO_2]$ in plasma at a known P_{CO_2}. At $37°C$, pK' averages 6.10. Knowing this, we can calculate any one of pH, $[CO_2]$ or P_{CO_2} if the other two are measured. However, pK' varies slightly but significantly with change in pH and in temperature, and quite possibly when the plasma is chemically abnormal.

DISTRIBUTION OF GAS AND BLOOD WITHIN THE LUNGS

In the preceding sections it has been assumed that alveolar ventilation and blood flow are evenly distributed throughout the lungs. This is not the case, even in health; in pulmonary disease, distribution may be very uneven (vol. 3, p. 18.12).

VENTILATION

As intrapleural pressure increases from apex to base in the erect position (p. 31.10) transpulmonary pressure decreases. Thus alveoli at the apices of the lungs operate in a higher range of their pressure-volume curve than those at the bases. Fig. 31.23 illustrates this. The change in transpulmonary pressure is similar, during a respiratory cycle, at the apex and base; consequently, during normal breathing the basal regions of the lung receive a bigger share of the tidal volume because they lie on a steeper part of their curve than do the apices. The ventilation per unit volume of lung is therefore greater at the bases than at the apices in the erect position; the ratio is about 2 to 1 during quiet breathing.

The distribution of ventilation between upper and lower zones is, however, affected by the lung volume at which breathing takes place. If a person exhales from full inspiration TLC (fig. 31.16), to residual volume (RV), a point is reached at which airways at the lung bases begin to close. The reason for this is illustrated in fig. 31.23b. During expiration intrathoracic pressure rises (becomes less 'negative') and, since the pressure is always higher at the bases of the lungs, these regions reach the bottom of their pressure-volume curve before the upper regions do. When this happens, their airways close and further deflation cannot occur. Conversely, during inspiration from RV, the first part of the inspirate goes to the upper zones and the basal regions do not begin to fill until the 'closing volume' is exceeded. From then on, the bases receive proportionally more air than the upper zones, because their pressure-volume curve is steeper.

In young people, closing volume is less than FRC and basal airways thus remain open during normal breathing. Closing volume increases, however, with age (fig. 31.23c). Over the age of 45 years, closing volume exceeds FRC in the supine position (because FRC falls on lying down) and over 65 even when sitting or standing. In these circumstances the lung bases receive a reduced ventilation and arterial P_{O_2} falls because of venous admixture effects.

BLOOD FLOW

Diastolic pressure in the pulmonary artery is about 1.3 kPa (13 cm H_2O, or 12 cm blood). The adult lung is about 30 cm high. The pulmonary artery enters the lung about 13 cm from the apex. In the erect position, therefore, the diastolic pressure at the extreme apex must be at or below atmospheric and certainly below the critical closing pressure in apical vessels (p. 30.22). At the bases, diastolic pressure is approximately 3 kPa (29 cm blood). There is thus a tendency for apical vessels to close during part of the cardiac cycle, while basal vessels remain open throughout. Below the apex, blood flow occurs only when capillary pressure exceeds alveolar pressure (the 'Starling resistor' effect). Thus blood flow is greater in the dependent parts of the lungs. The ratio is about 5 to 1 between base and apex.

VENTILATION/PERFUSION RATIO

If the bases are twice as well ventilated and 5 times as well perfused as the apices, it follows that the ratio between ventilation and blood flow is about 2·5 times higher at the apices than at the bases. This ratio, the **ventilation/perfusion** ($\dot{V}/\dot{Q}$) **ratio**, is of central importance in an understanding of gas exchange in the lungs. A $\dot{V}/\dot{Q}$ ratio of infinity (ventilation but no perfusion) would cause a lung region possessing it to behave like deadspace. A

ratio of zero (perfusion but no ventilation) would be tantamount to a shunt of venous blood to the arterial side of the circulation. The distribution of $\dot{V}/\dot{Q}$ around a mean value leads to two effects, the appearance of **alveolar deadspace** (p. 31.17) and the appearance of a shunt-like situation. The combination of true anatomical venous shunt and the shunt-like effect of $\dot{V}/\dot{Q}$ variation is termed

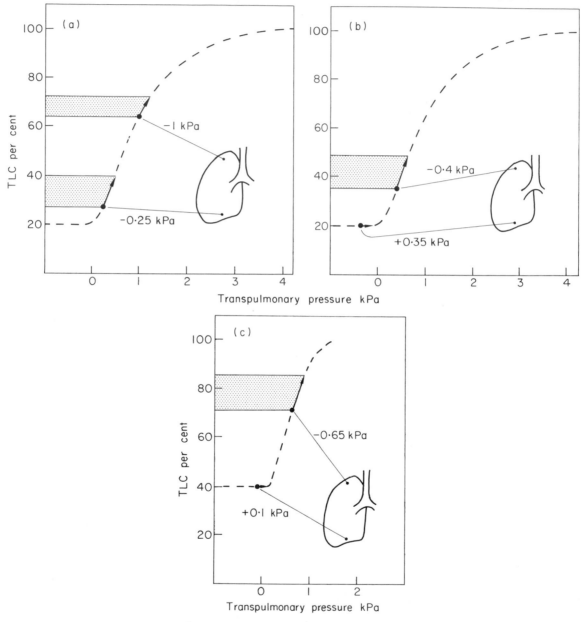

FIG. 31.23. Pressure-volume curves: (a) normal inspiration at age 30, (b) inspiration from residual volume at age 30, and (c) normal inspiration at age 70 years. In each case per cent TLC indicates the percentage of total capacity of any lung region which is filled at a given transpulmonary pressure. Two regions of lung, at apex and base respectively, are depicted. Redrawn from Milic–Emili J., Henderson J.A.M. & Kaneko K. (1968) in *Form and Function in the Human Lung*, p. 66, ed. Cumming G. & Hunt L.B. Edinburgh: Livingstone.

venous admixture. Both deadspace and venous admixture can be measured and form the best available indices of disturbances of $\dot{V}/\dot{Q}$ relationships which occur in many pulmonary diseases (vol. 3, p. 18.15).

True anatomical arteriovenous shunt in the sitting position amounts to roughly 1, 2 and 3 per cent of cardiac output at ages 25, 45 and 65 years. $\dot{V}/\dot{Q}$ variation contributes another 1 per cent to venous admixture in air-breathing subjects. Cyclical airway closure during ordinary breathing in subjects aged more than 60 years adds another 1·5 per cent to venous admixture.

ALVEOLAR-CAPILLARY DIFFUSION

Exchange of O_2 and CO_2 between alveolar gas and pulmonary capillary blood is accomplished by physical diffusion across the alveolar membrane. The rate at which a gas diffuses through a permeable medium is (1) proportional to the partial pressure difference across which diffusion occurs, (2) inversely proportional to the thickness of the medium, (3) proportional to the solubility of the gas in the medium and (4) inversely proportional to the square root of the molecular weight of the gas. At rest, at the beginning of a pulmonary capillary, the P_{O_2} gradient between alveolar gas and mixed venous blood is 13·3–5·3 = 8 kPa (60 mm Hg). The P_{CO_2} gradient in the opposite direction is only 6·1–5·3 = 0·8 kPa. Yet CO_2 is so much more soluble than O_2 in the alveolar membrane that it diffuses twenty times faster, attaining complete partial pressure equilibrium well before the end of the capillary is reached. Almost complete equilibrium is reached in healthy subjects, at rest at sea level; the P_{O_2} difference between alveolar gas and end-pulmonary capillary blood is less than 0·1 kPa (1 mm Hg). Under conditions of exercise at high altitude, diffusion of O_2 may be a limiting factor in gas transport and an alveolar-capillary P_{O_2} difference can be shown to develop (vol. 3, p. 18.17).

Diffusion is of importance at other points in the pathway of oxygen transport. Movement of molecules in the gas phase in the alveoli occurs by diffusion (p. 31.17). After an O_2 molecule has crossed the alveolar-capillary membrane, it must diffuse through the plasma and the red blood cell membrane before coming into contact with Hb and combining with it. The overall process of gas transfer can be expressed in terms of the **diffusing capacity (D)**. This is defined as the ratio between the rate of gas uptake and the mean pressure difference between alveolar gas and pulmonary capillary blood,

$$D_{gas} = \dot{V}_{gas}/P(A-\bar{c})_{gas} \qquad (30)$$

Diffusing capacity can thus be thought of as the conductance of the lungs for the gas in question. In practice, difficulties in the calculation of mean capillary P_{O_2} have

led to the use of CO, the capillary pressure of which is almost negligible, as a convenient test gas.

As we have seen, resistance to diffusion lies not only in the alveolar wall but also in the plasma. The total diffusing capacity can therefore by divided into two components in series which, being conductances, sum in the same way as electrical resistances in parallel

$$\frac{1}{D_L} = \frac{1}{D_M} + \frac{1}{\theta . V_c} \qquad (31)$$

D_L is the total diffusing capacity, D_M is the 'membrane' diffusing capacity and V_c is the pulmonary capillary blood volume. θ is a factor expressing the affinity of Hb for either O_2 or CO. In healthy people, $1/D_M$ and $1/\theta . V_c$ are approximately equal, and this emphasizes the importance of the latter part of the pathway for diffusion.

CONTROL OF RESPIRATION

NEURAL CONTROL

The respiratory muscles are supplied through a motor pathway consisting of upper and lower motor neurones. The upper motor neurones controlling respiratory movements originate in the reticular substance of the brain stem, predominantly from its lower end, in the floor of the fourth ventricle; they descend the cord in the lateral and ventral columns. The brain stem may be divided above, but not below, this level without abolishing (but not without distorting) respiration, and the 'respiratory centre' was assigned to this position. However, the whole of the reticular formation shows rhythmic electrical activity of a frequency corresponding to the respiratory cycle, even when all afferent impulses to it are blocked, and a 'respiratory centre' cannot be localized precisely; normal respiration requires that the whole reticular substance be functionally intact. The unstable, oscillatory circuits which the reticular substance contains may be left for the enjoyment of neurophysiologists.

We may, therefore, think of the respiratory control region as a 'black box' occupying a large part of the brain stem, generating spontaneous, rhythmic, inspiratory and expiratory impulses which may be modified by much information reaching the black box from outside. The rest of this section is concerned with these afferent stimuli and the effects they produce.

Impulses from other parts of the central nervous system
Breathing may be modified voluntarily, and pathways from the pyramidal and extrapyramidal systems to the respiratory centre are implicit in this fact. The over-breathing which accompanies excitement or anxiety is presumably mediated by these pathways. The neural component of the increased ventilation in physical exercise (p. 31.27) may consist partly of an irradiation

effect in which impulses 'spill over' from the cortico-spinal tracts to involve the respiratory control region, but other factors are concerned. The coordination of respiratory movements, particularly during speech, depends on the cerebellum.

Impulses from the lungs

At least seven different types of receptor organ exist in the tracheobronchial tree, alveolar walls, pleura and pulmonary vessels, and numerous reflexes can be elicited by various pulmonary manipulations; the answer to the question of which receptors serve which reflexes remains confused.

PULMONARY STRETCH REFLEXES

In many animals, an imposed and maintained inflation of the lungs delays the onset of the next spontaneous inspiratory effort (inflation reflex) and an imposed, maintained deflation increases the frequency, or force, or both, of spontaneous inspiratory efforts (deflation reflex). These two reflexes, discovered first by Breuer and known as the **Hering-Breuer reflex**, are mediated by vagal afferents. Although they seem well designed to prevent overinflation and to help decide the balance between tidal volume and frequency, there is some doubt as to their functional importance in man. They appear strong in small babies. In adults, vagal blockade does not appreciably alter tidal volume, frequency or functional residual capacity. On the other hand, when a CO_2 mixture is given during vagal blockade, ventilation increases wholly by an increase in tidal volume, frequency remaining constant; with vagi intact, both tidal volume and frequency increase.

When, in disease, the lungs become abnormally 'stiff', a relative increase in frequency and fall in tidal volume are commonly seen, especially when there is a demand for extra ventilation. It is hard to exclude the participation of pulmonary stretch-receptors in bringing this about.

The so-called paradoxical reflex, consisting of a brief spontaneous inspiratory effort in response to an imposed inflation, is of uncertain relevance in man although it has been demonstrated in very young babies. In animal experiments the afferents for the paradoxical reflex travel in the vagus nerve. Under normal circumstances the reflex could be concerned in the production of periodic sighs which are a feature of ordinary breathing. During surgical operations when ventilation has been reduced by premedication with opium alkaloids, inflating the lungs by a short compression of the anaesthetic bag often produces a deep, gasping inspiration.

COUGH REFLEX

Two types of stimuli elicit the cough reflex, and appear to act through different receptor organs. Mechanical irritation causes coughing most readily when applied to the larynx, posterior wall of the trachea, and bronchial branchings of the first degree, in order of decreasing sensitivity. Chemical irritants induce coughing via receptors in the smallest air passages, the trachea and large bronchi being relatively insensitive.

The afferent nerves for both types of reflex are contained, probably entirely, in the vagus nerves. The reflex is potentiated by deep inspiration, probably by stimulating the same receptors. The cough reflex is highly organized; it consists of a deep inspiration, closure of the glottis, contraction of expiratory muscles (causing intrapulmonary pressure to rise), and finally opening of the glottis to allow an explosive discharge of air and the dislodging of secretions or foreign matter from the trachea. Intrathoracic pressure during violent coughing may exceed 27 kPa (200 mm Hg). Peak air-flow during expulsion may reach 6 l/sec and air velocity 250 m/sec. Bronchi are narrowed during expulsion by direct compression. A slower bronchial constriction also follows the inhalation of irritants and is presumably due to reflex contraction of bronchial muscle. The central connections serving the cough reflex are ill defined; there is little evidence of a 'cough centre'.

Impulses from the respiratory muscles

The diaphragm and the intercostal muscles contain muscle spindles, and Golgi tendon organs are present in the diaphragm. These structures must have functions but at present these are largely speculative. Proprioceptive stimuli from the respiratory muscles may be concerned in the appreciation of respiratory work, the adjustment of tidal volume and respiratory frequency to minimize work (p. 31.13) and the respiratory adjustments to imposed resistance to air flow.

Impulses from the systemic circulation

Baroreceptor reflexes from carotid sinuses and aortic arch probably include a specific respiratory component; baroreceptor stimulation is said to depress breathing. It is, however, difficult to separate these responses from those due to concomitant carotid body effects and to secondary effects of induced circulatory changes. In man, there is no evidence that specific baroreceptor respiratory reflexes are important.

Temperature changes

A rise in body temperature causes hyperventilation, especially in animals which do not lose heat by sweating. The effect seems to be mediated partly by a reflex from warmed skin and partly by a rise in temperature of the blood. There are connections linking the heat regulating centre in the hypothalamus with the respiratory 'centre'.

The hyperventilation due to heating is very variable; it is limited by the fall in $P\text{CO}_2$ which ordinarily results. In fevers the position is complicated by the greater production of CO_2 due to increased metabolism, and ventilation is correspondingly stimulated.

Cooling may have several effects. If shivering results, ventilation increases. Sudden cooling of the skin, as by a cold shower, causes a prompt inspiratory response, followed by hyperventilation and a rise in end expiratory level (FRC). Prolonged cooling of the body, as in hibernation, is accompanied by a fall in ventilation; since metabolic CO_2 production falls still further, a mild respiratory alkalosis results.

Because of the change in the dissociation constant of water as temperature falls, a rise in pH is necessary to preserve cellular neutrality. Hibernating animals show about the right change in blood pH to balance the degree of cooling namely 7·4 at 37°C, 7·6 at 30°C and 7·8 at 20°C. pH of the cells is about 0·6 unit below that of blood (p. 6.5).

Impulses from exercising muscle

Crossed circulation experiments have shown that repeated contraction of limb muscles increases ventilation even when they have no vascular connection with the central or peripheral respiratory chemoreceptors. The effect is therefore presumably mediated by nervous pathways. Afferent impulses from muscle spindles may be concerned. The increase in ventilation which occurs in muscular exercise almost certainly includes such a 'neural' component.

Other impulses

Any sensory impression may modify breathing in the conscious animal; the response may be partly reflex, but emotional and other factors acting through the reticular formation may also be involved. In the anaesthetized animal, stimulation of a somatic sensory nerve often alters breathing, but here it is not possible to say that a sensory modality is concerned.

Impulses from specific respiratory chemoreceptors

These impulses serve the chemical control of breathing, dealt with in the next section. There are two main receptor groups.

The **carotid bodies** and **aortic bodies**, supplied with afferent fibres by the glossopharyngeal and vagus nerves respectively, are the **peripheral chemoreceptors**. They consist of small nodules of pink or reddish-brown tissue, composed of bands and islands of specialized receptor cells supported by connective tissue and separated by numerous sinusoids through which some 20 ml of blood per g of tissue flows each minute, a very rich blood supply. The aortic bodies regress during childhood and their functional importance in man is debatable. The carotid bodies are of great importance. They lie in close relation to the bifurcation of the common carotid artery on each side, and receive blood via branches of the occipital or ascending pharyngeal branches of the external carotid artery.

The adequate stimulus for the carotid bodies is a fall in Pa_{O_2} in or around the receptor cells. The response to hypoxia is potentiated by acidosis of the perfusing blood, due either to a primary rise in $[H^+]$ or a rise in blood P_{CO_2}. The carotid bodies are also stimulated by a fall in the blood flow through them. Changes in the oxygen content of arterial blood, with no change in P_{O_2}, as in anaemia and CO poisoning, do not stimulate them.

Metabolic poisons that lower cellular ATP stimulate the carotid bodies. Many of these drugs, like hypoxia, increase lactic acid formation, but some inhibit glycolysis. Hence lowering of cellular ATP is more likely to be the common mechanism of stimulation than lactic acid production. Stimulation of the carotid bodies by hypoxia, or electrical stimulation of the carotid body nerve, leads to an increase in ventilation. Denervation or removal of the carotid bodies in man abolishes the ventilatory response to hypoxia.

Since only a tiny fraction of the human race has ever lived at altitudes which call for a ventilatory response to hypoxia as a condition of survival, it may be asked why the carotid and aortic bodies still have this function. The answer may be found in the interaction between CO_2 and hypoxic responses (p. 31.28). The response to CO_2 is more prompt when hypoxia is present, and this rapid component is mediated by the peripheral chemoreceptors. Hypoxia appears to form a variable background on which CO_2 acts in regulating ventilation, thus allowing great sensitivity and specificity in ventilatory adjustments.

The carotid bodies have an efferent nerve supply from cervical sympathetic nerves and receive impulses from the brain stem in response to movements of the limbs. Such efferent discharges may modify the afferent return from the peripheral chemoreceptors and adjust the threshold for chemical stimuli.

The **central chemoreceptors** were originally thought to be the nerve cells of the respiratory centre itself. It is now known that intracranial receptors exist outside the centre. Of these, the best defined lie in the region of the lateral recesses of the fourth ventricle, close to the roots of the eighth, ninth and tenth cranial nerves. Perfusion studies have shown that these receptors are sensitive to change in $[H^+]$. A fall in pH of the perfusate, without change in its P_{CO_2}, causes an increase in ventilation. Surprisingly, an increase in P_{CO_2} without change in pH slightly reduces ventilation. Independence of P_{CO_2} and $[H^+]$ can be achieved in the perfusate by appropriately adjusting its HCO_3^- concentration; normally, of course, a rise in P_{CO_2} of cerebrospinal fluid (CSF) reduces its pH, and a fall increases it.

The CSF bathes the intracranial chemoreceptors and changes in its composition play an important part in ventilatory control. Normally, CSF (like intracellular fluid) is slightly acid with respect to arterial blood; its P_{CO_2} is about the same as jugular venous blood, its $[HCO_3^-]$ slightly lower than arterial blood, and its pK higher than blood. The blood-CSF barrier is freely permeable to CO_2 but much less, or selectively, so to HCO_3^- and H^+. A rise of blood P_{CO_2} is thus quickly reflected in the CSF. Since HCO_3^- cannot immediately leave the CSF and is its only buffer, CSF $[H^+]$ rises, stimulating respiration. Subsequently, over a few hours, provided P_{CO_2} remains fixed, the $[HCO_3^-]$ in CSF rises, restoring pH nearly to normal and causing a secondary reduction in ventilation. The stabilization of CSF pH makes a prolonged increase in P_{CO_2} less and less effective in increasing ventilation.

At altitude, the fall in blood P_{O_2} causes, through the carotid bodies, an increase in ventilation and a fall in P_{CO_2} in blood and CSF. CSF $[H^+]$ falls and this opposes the increase in ventilation. Subsequently there is a secondary decrease in $[HCO_3^-]$ in CSF and its $[H^+]$ rises towards normal, removing the inhibition of ventilation. There is thus a secondary increase in ventilation and a further fall in P_{CO_2}. This process continues for several days until a new equilibrium is reached, and is part of the acclimatization to altitude (p. 46.2).

When blood $[H^+]$ is changed by a primary change in blood $[HCO_3^-]$ e.g. by the administration of $NaHCO_3$ or NH_4Cl, a different sequence is followed. For example in NH_4Cl-induced acidosis blood $[HCO_3^-]$ falls promptly, but CSF $[HCO_3^-]$ does not. Since acidaemia stimulates ventilation, P_{CO_2} falls in both blood and CSF and there is thus an alkaline shift in CSF $[H^+]$, which offsets the rise in ventilation to some extent. More slowly, CSF $[HCO_3^-]$ falls in adaptation to this decreased $[H^+]$ just as in the case of altitude hyperventilation; CSF pH is again stabilized near the normal value and ventilation augmented.

It is not understood how CSF $[HCO_3^-]$ changes in response to altered P_{CO_2} but much less to a primary change in blood $[HCO_3^-]$. Active transport of $[HCO_3^-]$ at the blood-brain barrier is possible; it is known that K^+, Ca^{++} and Mg^{++} are stabilized in CSF by this mechanism. Alternatively, the regulation of CSF $[HCO_3^-]$ may take place at the interface between CSF and brain.

The central chemoreceptors are not influenced exclusively by the composition of the CSF, but respond significantly to acid-base shifts in the blood. The maintenance of an increased ventilation during NH_4Cl-induced acidosis, at a time when CSF is temporarily more alkaline, requires that there be receptors sensitive to blood changes. Probably both central and peripheral chemoreceptors can respond in this way.

CHEMICAL CONTROL

We now turn to the chemical regulation of breathing in the human subject. This is achieved by the integrated action of peripheral and central chemoreceptors, and is one of the most vivid examples of a negative feedback system in biology. Through it, a change in P_{CO_2}, P_{O_2} or pH of the body fluids produces a ventilatory response which tends to counteract the change.

Ventilatory response to CO_2

When a subject inhales a mixture of CO_2 in air or oxygen, his ventilation increases (fig. 31.24). When inspired P_{CO_2} is increased from 2 to 6·6 kPa (15 to 50 mmHg), ventilation rises from just under 10 to over 60 l/min. If alveolar P_{CO_2} is measured as well, this is found to increase by less than 2 kPa for a 4·6 kPa increase in P_{I,CO_2}. Both $\dot{V}$ and P_{A,CO_2} increase more and more rapidly as P_{I,CO_2} rises.

Fig. 31.25 is more informative. The curved lines in this figure are derived from equation 20 (p. 31.18), modified as follows:

$$(P_{A,CO_2} - P_{I,CO_2}) \propto 1/\dot{V}_A \qquad (32)$$

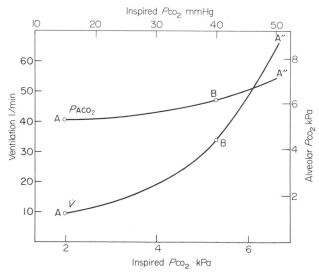

FIG. 31.24. Effects on alveolar P_{CO_2} and ventilation of increasing inspired P_{CO_2} from 2 to 6·6 kPa (15 to 50 mmHg).

When air is breathed, $P_{I,CO_2} = 0$ and we have equation 20. If we further assume that $\dot{V}_E$ is proportional to $\dot{V}_A$, we have

$$(P_{A,CO_2} - P_{I,CO_2}) \propto 1/\dot{V}_E \qquad (33)$$

In words, if ventilation is halved we double the difference between alveolar and inspired CO_2 pressure; if we double the first we shall halve the second, and so on, provided that CO_2 output remains constant (see p. 31.18). The left-hand curve in fig. 31.25 shows this relationship between $\dot{V}_E$ and P_{A,CO_2} when $P_{I,CO_2} = 0$ and the CO_2 output is normal. We can now draw curves for P_{I,CO_2} values of 1·3, 2·7 ... 6·6 kPa simply by moving the left-hand curve appropriate distances to the right. In fig. 31.25, point A represents $\dot{V} = 9\cdot5$ l/min, $P\text{A,}co_2 = 5\cdot4$ kPa (40·5 mmHg), $P\text{I,}co_2 = 2$ kPa; these are the values at the left-hand ends of the curves in fig. 31.24. If now we raise

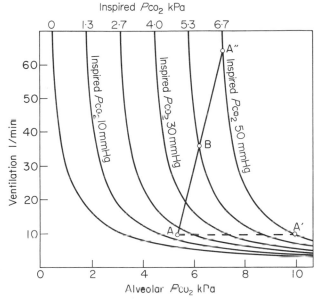

FIG. 31.25. Graph of ventilation in relation to alveolar Pco$_2$. Each curved line shows the values for $\dot{V}$ and $P\text{A,}co_2$ at a particular inspired Pco$_2$, assuming CO_2 output to be constant. A, B and A″ are plotted from corresponding points in fig. 31.24 and a line joining these points is the CO_2 response line, showing the effect on ventilation of increasing inspired Pco$_2$. If $\dot{V}$ did not increase, $P\text{A,}co_2$ would rise to point A′.

$P\text{I,}co_2$ to 6·6 kPa, the new $\dot{V}$, $P\text{A,}co_2$ point must lie somewhere on the curve representing this $P\text{I,}co_2$. If $\dot{V}$ did not increase, A would move to A′ and $P\text{A,}co_2$ would increase by 4·6 kPa; the entire increase of $P\text{I,}co_2$ would be passed on to the alveolar gas. On the other hand, a rise of $\dot{V}$E to 64 l/min brings A to A″, and the rise of $P\text{A,}co_2$ is halved. The increase of $\dot{V}$E has protected the alveolar gas, and thus the arterial blood, from the effects of a change in the environment.

Further comparison of figs. 31.24 and 31.25 shows that the values of $\dot{V}$E and $P\text{A,}co_2$ for an inspired Pco$_2$ of 5·3 kPa (B in fig. 31.24), when plotted at B in fig. 31.25, fall on a straight line joining A and A″. The same would be true for a pair of values taken from fig. 31.24 at any given inspired Pco$_2$. In other words, the rise in ventilation due to an increase in the CO_2 stimulus is proportional to the rise in alveolar Pco$_2$. The slope of the line ABA″ is a measure of the ventilatory sensitivity to changes in CO_2. A healthy adult's ventilation increases by 15–30 l/min for every 1 kPa (2–4 l/min for every mmHg) increase in $P\text{A,}co_2$; this rise is fairly constant from one day to the next in the same subject but varies a good deal from

one subject to another. At inspired CO_2 concentrations below 2 per cent the correspondence is not very close, but above this concentration the linear relationship suggests that ventilation is governed precisely by the level of alveolar or arterial Pco$_2$.

So far we have considered only steady states of ventilation; each CO_2 mixture has been breathed long enough for $\dot{V}$E and $P\text{A,}co_2$ to become steady (this takes about 20 min). Ventilatory responses during changing states, e.g. the transition from one mixture to another, are complex. In general, the ventilatory rise lags about 2 min behind the change in arterial Pco$_2$ and is more closely related in time to change in jugular venous Pco$_2$. This in itself suggests an intracellular site for the true CO_2 stimulus, because venous blood is in Pco$_2$ equilibrium with the cells it drains.

Very high inspired CO_2 concentrations produce general anaesthesia, and the ventilation, having risen to high levels, begins to fall. This effect is seen when arterial Pco$_2$ reaches 11–13 kPa.

Effects of overbreathing

Overbreathing lowers the alveolar and arterial Pco$_2$; in normal speech end-tidal Pco$_2$ may be reduced to around 4 kPa (30 mmHg) by the end of a long sentence. Acute reduction of Pco$_2$ causes alkalaemia and this may affect the plasma [Ca^{++}] with a consequent increase in the excitability of muscle and nerve (p. 27.25). If a normal person deliberately overbreathes, he may first notice tingling in the fingers, and tetany, a paroxysmal contraction of muscle (typically in the forearm, giving the so-called 'main d'accoucheur' (fig. 27.20), may follow. Cerebral vasoconstriction is another important effect of overbreathing (p. 30.48).

Ventilatory response to lack of oxygen (hypoxia)

Fig. 31.26 shows a magnified part of fig. 31.25. The line AB is the CO_2 response line, relating the change in ventilation to the change in alveolar Pco$_2$ as the inspired Pco$_2$ changes from 2·7 to 4·7 kPa. We shall assume that points A and B were plotted from an experiment in which alveolar Po$_2$ was kept constant at 13·3 kPa (100 mmHg). If the experiment is now repeated with the same inspired CO_2 pressures, but with reduced inspired O_2 concentrations so that alveolar Po$_2$ is kept at 6·6 kPa, we find, at each inspired Pco$_2$, a higher ventilation and a lower alveolar Pco$_2$ than before. Point A moves along the inspired Pco$_2$ line to A′ and point B to B′. The new CO_2 response line is A′B′. The distances AA′ and BB′ are such that, when BA and B′A′ are produced to the left, they intersect at $\dot{V} = 0$. We may say that the reduction of alveolar Po$_2$ from 13·3 to 6·6 kPa has increased the ventilatory sensitivity to CO_2, since a given rise in alveolar Pco$_2$ now causes a greater increase in ventilation. On the other

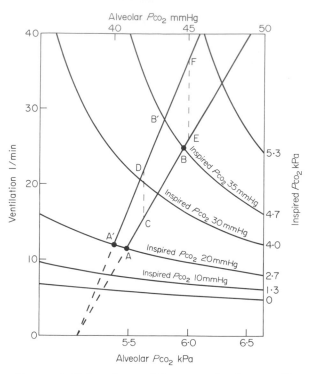

FIG. 31.26. Enlarged part of fig. 31.25, showing one CO_2 response line AB at a PA,O_2 of 13·3 kPa (100 mmHg), and another, A′B′ at a PA,O_2 of 6·6 kPa. Hypoxia increases the 'sensitivity' to CO_2 but leaves 'threshold' unchanged.

hand, the threshold to CO_2, the alveolar PCO_2 below which ventilation is theoretically zero, has not been changed by hypoxia. Conversely, it is equally true to say that CO_2 increases the sensitivity to hypoxia; the rise in ventilation due to the hypoxia at an alveolar PCO_2 of 5·6 kPa (CD in fig. 31.26) is 6·5 l/min, but at 6 kPa (EF) it is nearly 11 l/min.

As the hypoxic stimulus increases, the line A′B′ in fig. 31.26 becomes steeper. A limit (calculated from experimental data) is reached at an alveolar PO_2 of 3 to 4 kPa, when A′B′ would become vertical, that is, infinite CO_2 sensitivity. It might be thought that increasing alveolar PO_2 above the normal air-breathing value of 13 kPa would have no effect, but in fact the line AB becomes slightly less steep. This means that, when air is breathed, there is a slight but significant hypoxic stimulus and that it is necessary to breathe high O_2 mixtures in order to abolish it. At an alveolar PO_2 of 33–40 kPa practically no hypoxic stimulus remains.

Very severe hypoxia (asphyxia) results in cerebral damage and respiration is depressed. Short periods of hypoxia down to alveolar PO_2 levels of around 5 kPa (37·5 mmHg) can be tolerated, however, and it is between 5 and 9 kPa that the respiratory effects of hypoxia have chiefly been demonstrated in man. We may suppose that arterial PO_2 is some 0·5 to 1·5 kPa lower than alveolar.

Chronic, tolerated hypoxia, as in the acclimatization to altitude, produces more complex changes than does acute hypoxia. These have been discussed under chemical chemoreceptors (p. 31.27) and also in chap. 46.

Ventilatory response to H+

An increase in arterial PCO_2 due to inhalation of CO_2 mixtures is accompanied by a rise in [H+] in both cells and plasma, and it is probably by this effect that it causes a rise in ventilation. But [H+] can be increased in other ways. The ingestion of 8 g of NH_4Cl daily by a healthy subject produces, in a few days, a marked extracellular acidosis. This is accompanied by a shift of the CO_2 response line to the left, that is, the CO_2 threshold is reduced while CO_2 sensitivity remains the same (fig. 31.27). It is as though the ventilation, during acidosis, has two components: (1) the $\dot{V}$ appropriate to the alveolar PCO_2 and (2) an extra $\dot{V}$ contributed by the increase in [H+]. Unlike the response to hypoxia, which interacts with the CO_2 stimulus, the combination of an H+-ion stimulus and a CO_2 stimulus seems to be simply additive.

Integration of chemical stimuli

The carotid bodies are stimulated by CO_2 and there is growing evidence that they mediate rapid responses to changes in blood PCO_2. They can respond even to fluctuations in PCO_2 which occur within the space of one breath. Timing is important; a rise in PCO_2 which

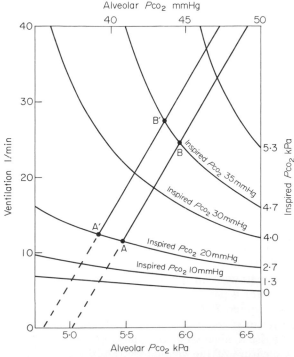

FIG. 31.27. Graph similar to fig. 31.26, but showing the effect on the CO_2 response line AB of metabolic acidosis induced by NH_4Cl. The new line A′B′ is parallel to AB. Thus 'sensitivity' to CO_2 is not altered, while 'threshold' is reduced.

reaches the carotid bodies at or just before the start of an inspiration results in a bigger breath. Some degree of hypoxic stimulus (even that present during air-breathing) is apparently necessary for this response to occur; breathing oxygen prevents it. The central chemoreceptors are concerned with slow, prolonged changes in P_{CO_2}. The whole ventilatory drive due to hypoxia appears to be mediated via the carotid bodies; after their denervation, hypoxia depresses ventilation. The carotid bodies may play a part in the response to H^+ other than that resulting from CO_2.

Ventilatory response to rise in body temperature

The rise in ventilation when the body is heated has been mentioned. This effect seems to be mediated by an increase in sensitivity to CO_2, without change in threshold. The response to hypoxia *per se* is unaffected when the increase in CO_2 responsiveness is allowed for.

Control of ventilation during muscular exercise

The causes of the rise in ventilation during exercise are not yet fully understood. It seems probable that the rise can be largely accounted for in terms of the stimuli already discussed, but that individually these vary in importance according to the intensity and duration of the exercise.

(1) The **neural stimulus** is presumably involved in the abrupt rise in ventilation which occurs as soon as exercise begins. Irradiation from corticospinal pathways, or reflexes originating in muscle spindle afferents, have been invoked as mechanisms. The neural drive to respiration appears to increase according to the intensity of exercise.

(2) The **CO_2 stimulus.** Measurements of arterial P_{CO_2} during exercise give varying results. Pa_{CO_2} tends to rise in mild to moderate exercise and to fall in severe exercise, with marked lactic acidosis. However, there is little doubt that the combined stimulus from CO_2 and H^+ is increased during all but the mildest exercise.

(3) The **lactic acidosis** of exercise is an obvious cause of an increase in ventilation, and becomes progressively more marked above an O_2 uptake of 1.5–2.0 l/min during walking up increasing gradients.

(4) Hypoxia has occasionally been noted during severe exercise in healthy subjects breathing air, though usually arterial P_{O_2} remains remarkably constant. When 50 per cent O_2 is substituted for air in heavy exercise, ventilation falls somewhat. During exercise, breath-to-breath fluctuations in alveolar and arterial P_{CO_2} are increased in amplitude, and ventilation may thus be augmented by the mechanism discussed above. This is an hypoxic response only in the sense that some hypoxic stimulus is a necessary background.

(5) **Body temperature** rises during exercise, and we have seen that heating increases ventilatory responsiveness to CO_2.

The five factors discussed above are partly additive, but hypoxia and rise in temperature both interact with the CO_2 stimulus, causing a disproportionately great ventilatory response. This fact has often been overlooked by those who find a significant portion of the ventilatory rise unaccounted for.

Control of ventilation during sleep

The response to CO_2 is depressed during normal sleep; the CO_2 threshold is slightly increased and the CO_2 sensitivity decreased. The degree of respiratory depression parallels the depth of sleep as judged by the electroencephalographic pattern. Breathing air, Pa_{CO_2} may increase during deep sleep to 7 kPa and slight hypoxia may be present. How sleep affects the ventilatory response to hypoxia has not been fully investigated.

Conversely, any influence which increases wakefulness also increases ventilation. Ventilation, indeed, seems to be part of a 'package deal' delivered by the reticular formation, and it is probably idle to suppose that ventilation can be depressed or increased specifically. CO_2 itself, as we have seen, acts in high concentration as a general anaesthetic; in lower concentration it is an 'arousal' agent and at still higher concentration it causes convulsions. At rest, breathing air, ventilation is often not well correlated with alveolar or arterial P_{CO_2}; this may be because the so-called 'waking drive' to respiration supports ventilation at this level, making it relatively independent of CO_2.

NON-RESPIRATORY FUNCTIONS OF THE LUNGS

Although the major role of the lungs is respiratory, they have diverse and complex other activities. The lungs participate in the production of several vasoactive substances. Lung tissue contains a high concentration of the prostaglandin $PGF_{2\alpha}$ which it synthesizes. It inactivates prostaglandin E_1. Mast cells (p. 17.4) are plentiful and the lung is the richest source of histamine in the body; it is also capable of removing it from the blood. Most of the 5-hydroxtryptamine in the blood is contained within platelets (p. 28.14) and the lungs are an important store of megakaryocytes. In addition, over 90 per cent of this vasoactive substance as well as bradykinin (p. 27.51) can be removed by the lungs in one circulation. The conversion of angiotensin I to angiotensin II (p. 35.27) also takes place largely within the pulmonary circulation. Cofactors which promote the formation of thromboplastin and plasminogen activator are also produced in large amounts. These substances may contribute to maintaining the system responsible for the delicate balance of the haemostatic mechanism (p. 28.14). Finally, the mammalian lung can synthesize fatty acids, hydrolyse triglycerides and form phospholipids; these functions are probably carried out mainly in the large alveolar cells and the Clara cells. The phospholipids may act to lower the surface tension in the alveolar membrane (p. 31.11).

FURTHER READING

CARO C. G. ed. (1966) *Advances in Respiratory Physiology.* London: Arnold.

CAMPBELL E.J.M., AGOSTONI E. & DAVIS J.N. (1970) *The Respiratory Muscles: Mechanics and Neural Control*, 2nd Edition. London: Lloyd–Luke.

COMROE J.H., JR. (1974) *Physiology of Respiration*, 2nd Edition. Chicago: Year Book Medical Publishers.

COTES J.K. (1975) *Lung Function*, 3rd Edition. Oxford: Blackwell Scientific Publications.

CUMMING C. & HUNT L.B. eds. (1968) *Form and Function in the Human Lung.* Edinburgh: Livingstone.

FENN W.O. & RAHN H. eds. (1964–1965) *Handbook of Physiology*, Section 3, Vols. I & II. Washington: American Physiological Society.

GUYTON A.C. & JONES C.E. eds. (1974) *MTP International Review of Science.* Physiology Series One, vol. 1. London: Butterworth.

HALDANE J.S. & PRIESTLEY J.G. (1935) *Respiration*, 2nd Edition. Oxford: Clarendon Press.

KAO F. (1973) *An Introduction to Respiratory Physiology.* Amsterdam: North-Holland.

KILMARTIN J.V. & ROSSI-BERNARDI L. (1973) Interaction of haemoglobin with hydrogen ions, carbon dioxide and inorganic phosphates. *Physiological Reviews* **53**, 836–890.

PERUTZ M.F. (1973) Haemoglobin as a model of an allosteric protein. *Symposia of the Society for Experimental Biology*, **27**, 1–3.

—— (1970) Stereochemistry of cooperative effects in haemoglobin. *Nature* **228**, 726–739.

WEIBEL E.R. (1963) *Morphometry of the Human Lung.* Berlin: Springer.

WEST J.B. (1974) *Respiratory Physiology.* Oxford: Blackwell Scientific Publications.

—— (1976) *Ventilation/Blood Flow and Gas Exchange*, 3rd Edition. Oxford: Blackwell Scientific Publications.

Chapter 32
Gastrointestinal system

'On the 1st August 1825, at 12 o'clock, midday, I introduced through the perforation between the ribs, into the stomach of Alexis St. Martin, the following articles of diet, suspended by a silk string . . . a piece of high seasoned à la mode beef, a piece of raw salted lean beef, a piece of raw salted fat pork, a piece of stale bread, and a bunch of raw cabbage. The lad continued his domestic employments about the house. 2 o'clock p.m.: withdrew and examined them: found the cabbage, bread, pork, and boiled beef all cleanly digested and gone from the string: the other pieces of meat but very little affected.'

This classical experiment was performed 150 years ago by William Beaumont on Alexis St. Martin, who was wounded in the stomach by a load of duck shot and was left with a fistula which failed to heal. It demonstrated the ability of the stomach to secrete a powerful digestive fluid for the breakdown of food. Equally remarkable is the resistance of the wall of the gut to its own digestive secretions, although the patient who suffers from peptic ulcer may testify that this resistance is not absolute.

The breakdown of food in the stomach is only one of many processes by which its constituents are assimilated into the body from the gut. The types of food in the diet vary greatly between individuals, depending on factors such as availability, economics, religious and social taboos and personal taste. In general about 500 g of solid matter and 2·5 litres of water are ingested each day. This passes down the hollow muscular tube of the gastrointestinal tract and appears at its lower end, after an interval of 24 to 48 hours, as faeces containing about 30 g of solids and 100 ml of water.

In this chapter we shall consider (1) the anatomy of this tube as it may be seen in the dissecting room or operating theatre, (2) the histology of the gut and the glands which manufacture the digestive juices, together with an account of the control mechanisms which ensure that each of the glands produces its secretion when the food reaches the appropriate place in its passage down the canal, (3) the processes of absorption by which the small molecules produced by the action of the digestive enzymes are transported from the lumen of the canal across the wall and into the veins and lymphatics, (4) the mechanisms by which the food is moved along the tract, (5) the blood supply of the digestive system and (6) the embryology of the tract.

General organization and function of the alimentary canal

The alimentary canal is a long fibromuscular tube stretching from the mouth to the anus, lined with an epithelium which in places is specialized for secretion and for absorption. The wall is composed of four concentric layers, (1) mucosa, (2) submucosa, (3) muscularis externa, (4) serosa or adventitia, shown in fig. 32.1.

The lining or **mucosa** consists of a surface epithelium, a lamina propria of supporting connective tissue and an inner thin layer of smooth muscle, the muscularis mucosae. The epithelium varies in different parts of the gut and is often richly glandular. Its surface is lubricated by a viscous adhesive layer of mucus. The lamina propria is a loose connective tissue layer which contains many capillaries where the epithelium is glandular. The muscularis mucosae is a thin sheet of smooth muscle with some elastic fibres; it causes local movements and folding of the mucosa and is innervated by sympathetic fibres.

The **submucosa** is a denser connective tissue layer with large blood vessels and contains a nerve plexus with parasympathetic ganglion cells which innervate the overlying mucosal glands. The plexus is especially prominent where the mucosa is very glandular, e.g. the stomach.

The main muscle coat, or **muscularis externa** is generally composed of an outer longitudinal and an inner circular layer of smooth muscle. In parts of the gut however, such as the oesophagus, stomach and colon there are local modifications of this arrangement.

Much of the alimentary canal is covered with a **serosal layer**, mostly peritoneum. This layer consists of a smooth simple squamous epithelium (mesothelium) with underlying loose connective tissue. Blood vessels and nerves supplying the gut often travel in this layer before entering the muscle coat. In parts where there is no serosa, loose

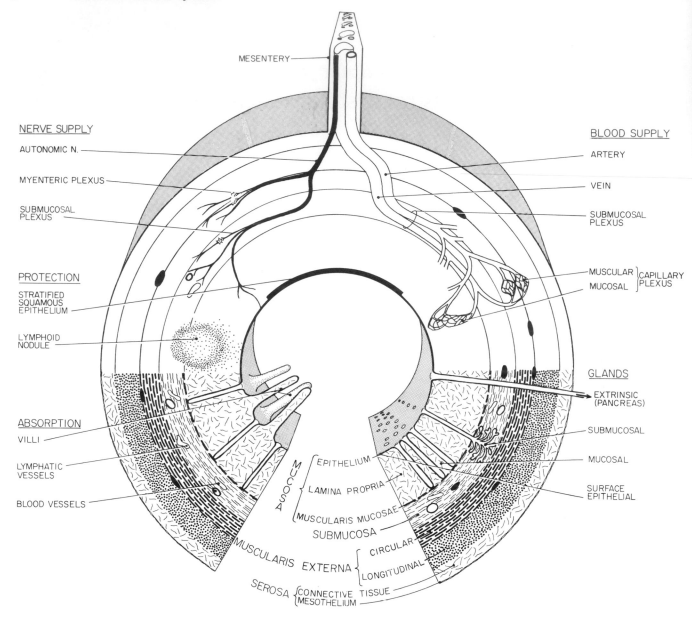

NERVE SUPPLY

AUTONOMIC N.

MYENTERIC PLEXUS

SUBMUCOSAL PLEXUS

PROTECTION

STRATIFIED SQUAMOUS EPITHELIUM

LYMPHOID NODULE

ABSORPTION

VILLI

LYMPHATIC VESSELS

BLOOD VESSELS

MESENTERY

BLOOD SUPPLY

ARTERY

VEIN

SUBMUCOSAL PLEXUS

MUSCULAR } CAPILLARY
MUCOSAL } PLEXUS

GLANDS

EXTRINSIC (PANCREAS)

SUBMUCOSAL

MUCOSAL

SURFACE EPITHELIAL

MUCOSA { EPITHELIUM
LAMINA PROPRIA
MUSCULARIS MUCOSAE

SUBMUCOSA

MUSCULARIS EXTERNA { CIRCULAR
LONGITUDINAL

SEROSA { CONNECTIVE TISSUE
MESOTHELIUM

FIG. 32.1. Layers of the wall of the alimentary tract.

connective tissue forms an **adventitious coat** which merges with the surrounding connective tissue.

The **intrinsic blood supply** varies in different regions of the gut, but is very rich in segments with high secretory or absorptive activities, such as the stomach or small intestine. Generally the arteries approach the gut at right angles to its long axis, enter the serosa or adventitia and after supplying the muscularis externa pierce it to gain the submucosa. Here the arteries form a plexus which supplies branches to the capillary beds of the overlying muscularis mucosae, glands, and lining epithelium. Veins drain these capillaries into a large venous submucosal plexus, which is the site of the splanchnic pool in which blood stagnates in some forms of shock and serious infection. The veins from the submucosal plexus follow the path described for the incoming arteries.

The **nerve supply** consists of parasympathetic preganglionic, sympathetic postganglionic and general visceral afferent fibres. These run in the serosa for a variable distance before entering the muscularis externa where they form the **myenteric plexus of Auerbach**. This contains many parasympathetic ganglionic cells which are motor to the muscularis externa. Other nerve fibres leave the serosa and form a **submucosal plexus of Meissner** containing parasympathetic ganglion cells which are secreto-motor to the mucosal glands. The sympathetic fibres are vasoconstrictor to the vessels of the gut and the para-sympathetic fibres are vasodilator. Sympathetic fibres innervate the muscularis mucosae. The general visceral afferent fibres begin as free endings in the mucosa, and also in the muscle where they act as stretch receptors (fig. 32.20).

GENERAL FUNCTIONS OF THE ALIMENTARY CANAL

The gut has a large secretory capacity because in addition to the many intrinsic glands within its walls there is the extrinsic group consisting of the major salivary glands, liver and pancreas. Many litres of fluid are secreted into the lumen of the gut daily, most of which is reabsorbed. This physiological recirculation of fluid fails in alimentary diseases which cause vomiting or diarrhoea and may lead rapidly to disturbances in water and electrolyte balance. Secretion in the main occurs in the upper part of the alimentary tract and absorption occurs mostly in the middle zone, chiefly but not exclusively in the small intestine.

A few minutes after a meal food begins to leave the stomach, which is usually empty three hours later. On leaving the stomach the food passes fairly rapidly through the small intestine. Within about three to four hours the unabsorbed remnants begin to reach the colon and the residues of the various meals taken each day lie in the descending colon till expulsion. Defaecation usually takes place once per day, but the variation is great and it is not abnormal for it to occur three times per day or to be withheld for up to three days.

The muscle of the alimentary tract regulates the passage of the contents to allow adequate time for digestion and absorption. Mastication is a voluntary movement and swallowing can be initiated voluntarily so the oral and pharyngeal muscles are all striated, and the oesophagus contains both striated and smooth muscle. From the stomach to the anus there is only smooth muscle, except for the external anal sphincter which is again striated.

MOUTH, SALIVARY GLANDS, PHARYNX AND OESOPHAGUS

The gross anatomy of the mouth and pharynx are described on p. 22.46.

Salivary glands

The oral cavity is lubricated by saliva, which is secreted by numerous glands. Many of these are small glands in the lining mucosa of the oral cavity and pharynx including the soft palate, but the bulk of the saliva comes from the three pairs of major salivary glands, the parotid, sub-mandibular and sublingual, which lie outside the oral. mucosa. Their gross anatomy is described on pp. 22.18 and 40. The salivary glands are composed of varying proportions of serous and mucous acini, the former producing salivary amylase (ptyalin), salts and water, and the latter mucus.

The **parotid gland** is the largest and is a pure serous compound tubulo-acinar gland. A fibrous capsule sends septa into the gland dividing it into lobules. The acini are composed of typical zymogenic (serous) cells (p. 18.6) and drain into intercalated ducts lined with a low cubical epithelium; these unite and form intralobular ducts lined with cubical epithelium which is striated because of basal infoldings (p. 13.14), indicating active transport. Thus the primary secretion of the acinar cells is modified as it traverses the striated ducts. On leaving the lobules these ducts become lined with columnar epithelium and lie in the interlobular septa with the vessels and nerves. The main parotid duct emerging from the gland has many goblet cells in its mucosa.

The nerves in the interlobular septa contain both parasympathetic postganglionic fibres from the otic ganglion (p. 22.36), which are secretomotor and end in close relation to the acinar and duct cells, and sympathetic fibres that accompany the arteries into the gland and are mainly vasoconstrictor.

The **submandibular gland** (fig. 32.2) is a mixed compound tubulo-acinar gland composed mostly of serous acini. The mucous acini are often surmounted by groups of serous demilunes (p. 18.7). The duct system is similar to that of the parotid, but the striated ducts are longer and therefore especially prominent.

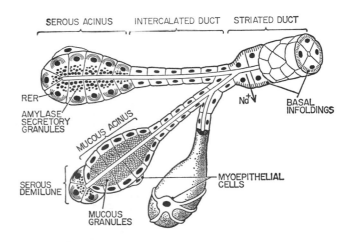

FIG. 32.2. High power diagram of acini and a striated duct in the submandibular salivary gland. RER, rough surfaced endoplasmic reticulum.

The **sublingual gland** is also a mixed compound tubulo-acinar gland but is mainly mucous. Although there are few pure serous acini, many of the mucous acini display serous demilunes. The parasympathetic secretomotor fibres of both the submandibular and sublingual glands come from the submandibular ganglion (p. 22.37).

SALIVARY SECRETION

Food in the mouth is broken up by chewing, moistened and mixed with the saliva. Since the food is present for only a short time before swallowing, there is little opportunity for digestion, but the salivary amylase continues to act after the food has passed to the stomach. The flow varies greatly from about 0·2 ml/min from the resting glands up to 4·0 ml/min with maximum secretion. In man an estimate may be made of the volume of saliva secreted in a given time by collecting the juice in dry dental swabs and weighing.

Composition of saliva

The constituents of saliva can be studied by cannulating the ducts of the glands and collecting their secretion. In this way it has been shown that different types of saliva are formed by the different pairs of glands. These types of secretion are related to the histological structure of the glands and whether they contain mainly mucous or serous cells. The secretion from the parotid glands is watery and contains a high concentration of amylase. The submandibular glands secrete a viscous fluid, containing a variable amount of amylase and mucus, while the sublingual secretions contain little amylase, but a great deal of mucus and are therefore very viscous. The saliva secreted in response to a meal is of course a mixture of these different secretions. The concentrations of ions vary according to the rate of secretion (fig. 32.3). An estimate of daily secretion is given on p. 32.44.

Saliva is always hypotonic and at maximum rates of se-cretion has about two-thirds of the osmolality of the plasma; under these conditions $[Na^+]$ is about 80 mmol/l and $[K^+]$ 20 mmol/l. When the secretory rate is slow, there is a transport of Na^+ from the striated ducts into the surrounding capillaries and $[Na^+]$ may fall to 20 mmol/l or less. This mechanism is under aldosterone control. The chief anion is HCO_3^-, which may be present at a concentration of over 50 mmol/l.

Functions of saliva

Salivary amylase initiates the breakdown of starch and glycogen to maltose and a small amount of glucose. It is active over a wide pH range, with an optimum at 6·9. The high mucus content of saliva lubricates the mouth and pharynx and without it swallowing is impossible. By dissolving solids such as sugars it intensifies the taste of food; this may have important consequences for the secretion of other digestive juices. Since little digestion takes place in the mouth, it is not surprising that no absorption of nutrients occurs there. The thin mucosal barrier, however, allows some drugs to be absorbed directly from the mouth into the blood stream.

Control of salivary secretion

This is nervous and there is no chemical or hormonal mechanism since ingested food is present in the mouth for so short a time. In fact, secretion usually increases above the resting rate before food actually enters the mouth, particularly if the food is appetizing, when its sight and smell 'make the mouth water'. This response to a stimulus which is appreciated by the subject is a conditioned reflex, which has to be 'established' and is not automatically inbuilt (chap. 25). The continuation of salivary secretion after food has been taken into the mouth is due to an unconditioned reflex. A mechanical stimulus, the contact of food on the mucosa of the mouth, leads to afferent impulses passing via the glossopharyngeal and lingual

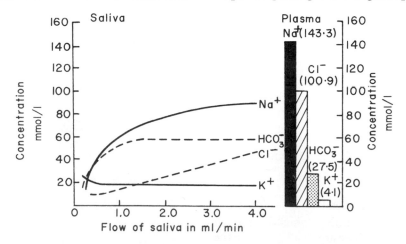

FIG. 32.3. Average composition of the parotid saliva of three young women as a function of the rate of secretion. From Thayson J.H., Thorn N.A. & Schwartz, I.L. (1954) *Amer. J. Physiol.*, **178**, 155.

nerves to a secretory centre in the medulla; efferent impulses pass via autonomic nerves to stimulate the effector organs, the salivary glands. This mechanical stimulation can be demonstrated by the increase in secretion observed when the subject chews tasteless foam rubber or paraffin wax; flow is much greater, however, when the taste of the food is appreciated. Chemical stimuli have a greater effect on salivary flow than purely mechanical stimuli, though the nervous pathways are probably the same.

Studies of the events following stimulation of the nerves to the glands in experimental animals help to explain this control. Electrical stimulation of the parasympathetic nerves, e.g. chorda tympani, of the cat causes marked vasodilation, increasing blood flow 4–8 times; the oxygen consumption of the glands also increases showing that secretion is an active process, and a copious flow of saliva follows. Injections of small quantities of acetylcholine into the arteries supplying the glands have similar effects, as would be expected since the nerves are cholinergic. While acetylcholine exerts a direct secretory and vaso-dilator effect, when released at the parasympathetic nerve endings, it liberates an enzyme called **kallikrein** from the glandular tissue; this acts on plasma globulins to form the polypeptide **bradykinin** which is an active vasodilator. This vasodilation may be responsible for some of the increase in secretion. If the sympathetic nerves are similarly stimulated, there is a vasoconstriction and the glands secrete a viscous saliva containing a great deal of mucus; injection of noradrenaline into the arterial supply has the same effect. The sympathetic nerves affect mainly the mucous cells of the submandibular and sublingual glands.

When a meal is eaten, both the sympathetic and para-sympathetic efferent pathways of the reflexes operate and the saliva is a mixture from the three pairs of glands.

CHEWING

As the food is chewed, small quantities are separated by the teeth and tongue and passed into the oropharynx to be swallowed and passed down the oesophagus to the stomach. Chewing food is partly a voluntary and partly an involuntary process. Contrary to the teaching most people receive as children, the extent to which food is chewed has a negligible effect on digestion. Chewing breaks up the food and mixes it with saliva, thereby facilitating swallowing. Each portion of food entering the mouth is broken up voluntarily to start with, but the contact of the food on teeth, gums and palate produces a reflex opening of the jaw which is followed by contraction of the muscles closing the jaw. Thus an involuntary rhythm is produced. The extent of chewing depends on the type of food, e.g. soft foods are chewed for a shorter time than hard foods,

and it is easily modified by external influences such as conversation.

Oesophagus

The oesophagus begins in the neck, just behind the cricoid cartilage, and is continuous with the lower end of the pharynx. It is a long fibromuscular tube which descends through the thorax, where it lies in the posterior mediastinum, and pierces the diaphragm to enter the abdomen. After a short abdominal course of about 2 cm it ends at

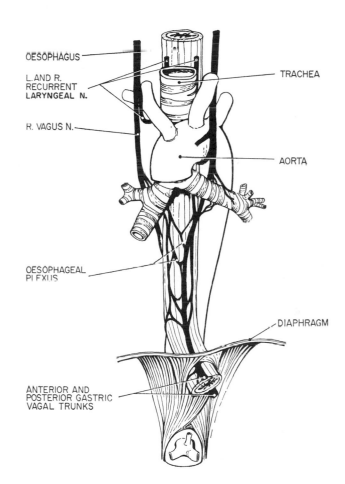

FIG. 32.4. Anterior view of oesophagus. Note relations to trachea, left main bronchus, aorta, diaphragm and the vagus nerves.

the gastro-oesophageal junction or **cardia**, the entrance to the stomach (fig. 32.4).

The oesophagus is related anteriorly first to the trachea and then to the left main bronchus and the left pulmonary artery, and the pericardium separates it from the left atrium. Enlargement of the atrium may compress the oesophagus and rarely causes difficulty in swallowing (dysphagia). The normal oesophageal lumen, in radiographs taken after swallowing a radio-opaque substance, shows slight indentations opposite these structures (fig. 32.5), and another on its left side caused by the arch of the aorta. Posteriorly the oesophagus is related closely to the lower cervical vertebral bodies, and so disease of the latter may also cause dysphagia. In the thorax the oesophagus is separated from the vertebral column by the meso-oesophagus, a double sheet of pleura containing oesophageal vessels from the aorta. On lateral radiographs, the space between the oesophagus and vertebrae appears as the retro-oesophageal window. On approaching the diaphragm the oesophagus swings

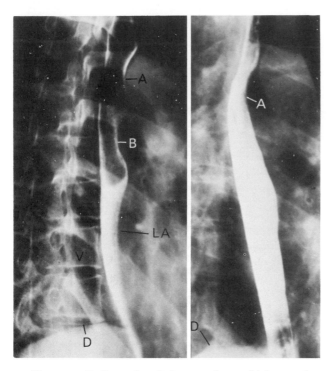

FIG. 32.5. Radiographs of the oesophagus (right anterior oblique view); barium swallows. The impressions of the aorta (A), left main bronchus (B), and left atrium (LA) show clearly on the left photograph. The oesophagus on the right is well filled and shows the aortic and cardiac impressions. Vertebra (V), diaphragm (D). Courtesy of Dr. C.K. Warwick.

forwards and to the left before piercing the left dome 2 cm to the left of the midline, at the level of the 10th thoracic vertebra.

Because the oesophagus in the mediastinum is surrounded by loose connective tissue which permits it to distend during swallowing, perforation of the oesophageal wall may lead to a spreading infection of the mediastinum, which is commonly fatal.

The vagus nerves descend behind the lung roots and then surround the oesophagus as a plexus (fig. 32.4). Near the diaphragm this oesophageal plexus forms anterior and posterior gastric trunks which lie on the corresponding surfaces of the oesophagus, and accompany it into the abdomen.

There is an important porta-caval anastomosis at the lower end of the oesophagus, which is described on p. 32.53.

HISTOLOGICAL STRUCTURE (figs. 32.6 and 7)
The oesophagus is lined with a tough non-keratinizing stratified squamous epithelium similar to that of the pharynx. A few simple mucous glands lie in the mucosa at both ends of the oesophagus and the submucosal nerve plexus is inconspicuous. The oesophageal glands proper are tubuloacinar mucous glands found in the submucosa. During swallowing the oesophagus is also lubricated by the mucus from salivary, nasal, and bronchial secretions.

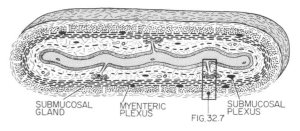

FIG. 32.6. Oesophagus T.S. The basic structure is typical of the alimentary tract.

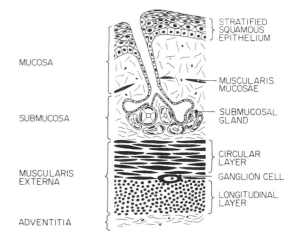

FIG. 32.7. Oesophagus T.S. This higher power view shows the tough stratified squamous epithelium and the main oesophageal mucous glands in the submucosa.

The muscle coat has the typical two layers, which consist of striated muscle in the upper third, both striated and smooth muscle in the middle third and only smooth muscle in the lower third. The inner circular coat is no thicker in the lower third of the oesophagus although there is a lower physiological sphincter above the cardia. The lower oesophageal sphincter plays a major role in preventing reflux of the gastric contents into the oesophagus. The angle of entry of the oesophagus, the gastric mucosal folds around the cardia which form a valve-like rosette, and the muscle fibres of the right crus of the diaphragm which enclose the oesophagus, each play a minor role.

The cervical and thoracic oesophagus have an adventitia, except where related to pleura, but the intra-abdominal portion is covered by peritoneum.

There is the usual myenteric nerve plexus with parasympathetic ganglion cells which innervate the smooth muscle. The striated muscle is supplied by the vagus, fibres coming directly from the nucleus ambiguus and similar to those which innervate the branchial striated muscle of the pharynx.

SWALLOWING

Swallowing involves both voluntary and reflex movements.

Small amounts of food are separated from the bolus being chewed and passed to the pharynx, as described on p. 22.50 (the voluntary phase).

A reflex phase is then initiated by the contact of food with the pharynx, soft palate and epiglottis. Impulses from these receptor sites pass via the glossopharyngeal nerves and the superior laryngeal branch of the vagus to the **deglutition (swallowing) centre** in the medulla. Here the motor response is co-ordinated and efferent impulses pass via the vagi and other nerves to the muscles responsible for the passage of food to the oesophagus. At the same time, contraction of other muscles prevents the bolus from entering the larynx or nasopharynx or passing back into the mouth.

After reaching the oesophagus the bolus is conducted along its length by peristalsis. A wave of contraction of the wall produces a pressure gradient which forces the bolus along the tube. The co-ordination of this movement depends on the parasympathetic myenteric plexuses present in the oesophageal wall. The bolus is thus passed towards the stomach, and impulses from the vagi relax the cardia and food enters the stomach. This is also assisted by the pressure built up in the terminal part of the oesophagus by repeated waves of peristalsis. The conduction of the food from the pharynx to the stomach is the only function of the oesophagus; no digestion and no absorption take place.

The motility of the oesophagus is easily studied in man. The subject swallows open-ended tubes through which water is perfused, and the intraluminal pressures are recorded. Typically three fine tubes are swallowed together, their distal apertures about 5 cm apart. As the subject swallows, a pressure wave may be recorded passing along the oesophageal lumen; that it is a propagated 'wave' may be deduced from its arrival opposite each tube in sequence. If the lowermost tube is placed in the most distal part of the oesophagus this zone is found to relax momentarily before the wave of contraction (fig. 32.8) reaches it. Respiratory variations are superimposed on the general pressure patterns. If such a multiple tube

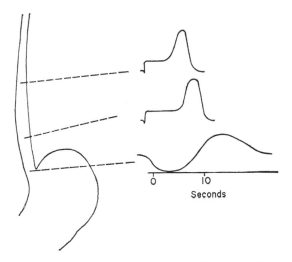

FIG. 32.8. Pressures in the lower part of the oesophagus during swallowing.

system is swallowed the length of the oesophagus and withdrawn upwards again, high pressure zones are detectable in the lowermost and uppermost areas. The lower sphincter prevents reflux of acid from the stomach into the oesophagus. The relaxation required at the upper zone before peristalsis is initiated in the oesophagus, and that at the lower end which enables the food to pass through the cardia, are reflexly induced.

Swallowing may be studied by observing the passage of radio-opaque barium along the oesophagus using cine-radiography in man and animals. The time taken for food to reach the stomach from the mouth is about 5 sec, of which the transit time along the oesophagus is about 2 sec.

ABDOMINAL VISCERA OF ALIMENTARY SYSTEM

The major portion of the alimentary tract and its two main accessory glands, the liver and pancreas, are within the abdominopelvic cavity. Because of its great length the tract follows a devious course between the lower end of the oesophagus and its termination at the anus. The digestive organs are anterior to those of the genitourinary system which lie against the posterior abdominal wall.

The general disposition of the gastrointestinal tract is shown in fig. 32.9. The stomach, which starts just beneath the diaphragm on the left of the midline, sweeps down and to the right across the midline to join the duodenum at the pylorus. The C-shaped duodenum returns to the left side and becomes continuous, behind the stomach, with the jejunum and ileum. The latter are very convoluted, filling much of the lower part of the abdominal cavity and are attached to the posterior wall by the mesentery. The ileum ends in the right iliac fossa at the ileocaecal

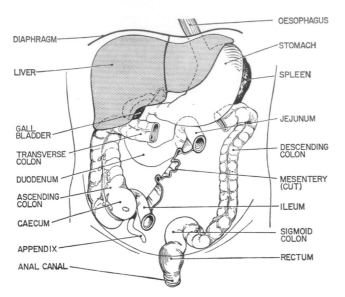

FIG. 32.9. General disposition of gastrointestinal tract. The greater omentum, most of the small intestine and part of the transverse colon have been removed.

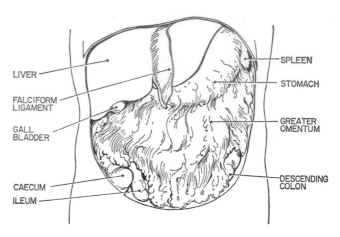

FIG. 32.10. Anterior view of abdominal contents. The greater omentum obscures much of the alimentary tract, but the stomach, ileum, caecum and descending colon are visible.

valve. The large intestine begins as the caecum, which is the blunt cul-de-sac below the level of the valve, and gives off the vermiform appendix. Above, the caecum is freely continuous with the colon which ascends to the liver, where it turns medially at the hepatic flexure and runs transversely across the abdomen to the spleen, passing in front of the duodenum and pancreas but behind the stomach. From the splenic flexure the colon descends to the left iliac fossa, and then curves medially to enter the true pelvis. There it descends in front of the sacrum and joins the rectum, which ends at the anal canal. The liver is a large solid organ occupying the right hypochondrium beneath the diaphragm. The pancreas, omitted from fig. 32.9, stretches from the concavity of the duodenum across the posterior abdominal wall to the spleen (figs. 32.29 and 32.51).

PERITONEUM

Early in development the peritoneal cavity appears as a split in the lateral mesoderm which then forms two layers of peritoneum, the **parietal layer** lining the wall of the abdominal cavity, and the **visceral layer** covering the gut and its mesenteries (p. 19.14). This simple arrangement of the mesenteries is much modified before the adult state is reached, so that the adult organs are related differently to the peritoneum (fig. 32.12). The kidneys, for example, lie behind the parietal layer on the posterior abdominal wall and are therefore termed **retroperitoneal.** Much of the duodenum is also retroperitoneal because its mesentery has fused with parietal peritoneum (p. 32.58). The

jejuno-ileum however is completely covered with visceral peritoneum, except for the thin linear attachment of the mesentery. It is important to appreciate that the peritoneal cavity is a potential space, containing only a thin film of fluid which lubricates the apposed surfaces, and that it does not contain abdominal viscera such as the small intestine. The basic relationships of peritoneum and gut can be simulated with a balloon for the peritoneum, and a pencil for the gut (fig. 32.11). If the pencil is laid along the balloon and gradually pressed down, it in-

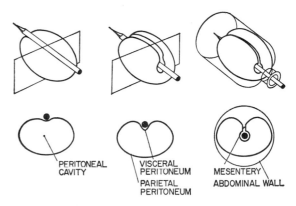

FIG. 32.11. Model of peritoneum. The balloon represents the peritoneum and peritoneal cavity and the pencil a portion of gut.

vaginates the balloon and various typical relations are established. Without pressure the pencil is 'retroperitoneal', but as pressure is applied, it becomes covered on three sides (cf. the ascending or descending colon), and with further pressure a mesentery is formed (cf. jejunum). Observe that the pencil (gut) is not inside the balloon (peritoneal cavity), unless the balloon bursts. Similarly, the peritoneal cavity is empty, and does not contain viscera. Finally, if the manoeuvre is repeated with the balloon and pencil, within a bottle representing the abdominal walls, one can appreciate that both the pencil (gut) and the balloon (peritoneum) are within the cavity of the bottle (abdominal cavity), but the cavity of the balloon (peritoneal cavity) is empty.

The peritoneal cavity is a closed one in the male, but in the female it communicates with the exterior via the openings of the uterine tubes (p. 38.2). Thus in the female an ascending infection of the genital tract may involve the peritoneum.

A mesentery is a double layer of peritoneum containing blood vessels, attaching a viscus to the parietal peritoneum. The largest is that of the jejuno-ileum, which is known as the **mesentery.** Others sometimes have the prefix 'meso' followed by the organ to which they are attached, e.g. mesocolon, or mesoappendix. Some peritoneal sheets are somewhat arbitrarily termed ligaments or folds. The latter usually have a free edge, but many ligaments also have free edges. Such peritoneal structures possess elasticity, which gives attached and related organs a high degree of mobility and allows the changes in shape, size and position

of the hollow gut as ingested food and drink is stored, digested, absorbed and moved down the tract.

The peritoneal cavity extends from beneath the diaphragm down to the pelvic floor. Although a continuous cavity, it is partly subdivided into several compartments, in which abnormal fluids such as pus or blood may accumulate and be localized to a greater or lesser degree. Thus a knowledge of these compartments or spaces is of value in predicting the spread of disease from a particular organ, or alternatively of deducing the probable source of a collection of fluid in a given site (vol. 3, p. 19.85). There are two important compartments called the **greater** and **lesser sacs.**

The simplest way to understand the peritoneal cavity is by a manual exploration of the abdomen. We shall now do this in imagination, looking first at the relations and attachments of neighbouring viscera and then try to appreciate the general features of the peritoneum.

EXPLORATION OF THE PERITONEAL CAVITY
On reflecting the anterior abdominal wall with its parietal peritoneum, the peritoneal cavity is entered.

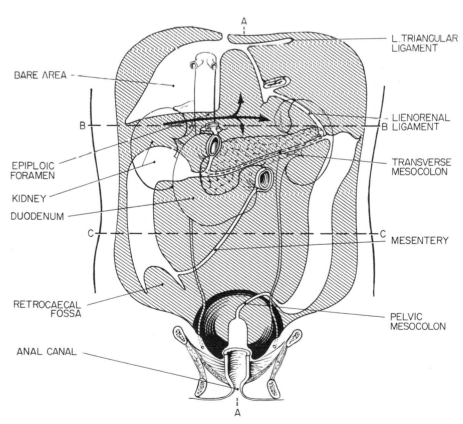

FIG. 32.12. Peritoneal relations of the posterior abdominal wall. The liver, spleen and most of the gut have been removed. Compare with fig. 32.9.

Without disturbing the viscera one can see (fig. 32.10) the liver, stomach, and the **greater omentum** which is a flattened pouch of peritoneum hanging down from the greater curvature of the stomach anterior to the jejuno-ileum. Inferior to the omentum, coils of ileum are apparent and the caecum occupies the right iliac fossa. If the greater omentum is lifted upwards over the stomach, its attachment to the antimesenteric border of the transverse colon is exposed (figs. 32.12 and 32.13). Examination of the transverse colon reveals that it is mobile because it is slung by a mesentery, the **transverse mesocolon,** from the posterior abdominal wall. Near the middle of this mesocolon, the jejunum starts. The jejunum and ileum follow a very convoluted course, but they are attached to the posterior abdominal wall by their sheet-like mesentery, which begins to the left of the midline inferior to the transpyloric plane, and runs obliquely down to the right iliac fossa where the ileum joins the caecum (figs. 32.9 and 32.12).

The caecum has a variable peritoneal relationship, but the lower end is usually completely invested and hangs free. The ascending colon is covered completely except where it rests directly on the posterior abdominal wall. The transverse colon has already been examined but note again that it is mobile as it has a mesocolon except at the two flexures.

The descending colon is bound to the posterior abdominal wall in the same fashion as the ascending colon.

The sigmoid colon is more mobile, and is attached by a mesocolon to the posterior and left side wall of the true pelvis. The upper part of the rectum is related in front and laterally to peritoneum but gradually it loses this coat as it descends towards the pelvic floor and becomes outside the peritoneum like the anal canal (fig. 32.38).

In the upper abdomen, the **lesser omentum** is a double layer of peritoneum which runs from the right border (lesser curvature) of the stomach upwards to join the liver on its inferior or visceral surface. Traced superiorly towards the diaphragm behind the left lobe of the liver, it is found to have no free upper margin because it is reflected on to the diaphragm from the oesophagus (fig. 32.12). Following it towards the duodenum, note that it arises not only from the stomach but also from the proximal part of the duodenum and has a free right margin which leads up to the porta hepatis. The latter is so-called because it is the door of the liver where the two hepatic bile ducts and major vessels leave and enter the liver.

From the left side and inferior border of the stomach another sheet, the greater omentum, runs posteriorly and eventually reaches the posterior abdominal wall. Begin at the oesophagus and confirm that the greater omentum is attached to the diaphragm and has no free upper border. Proceeding inferiorly, now run the right hand posteriorly and leftward again and you encounter the spleen (fig.

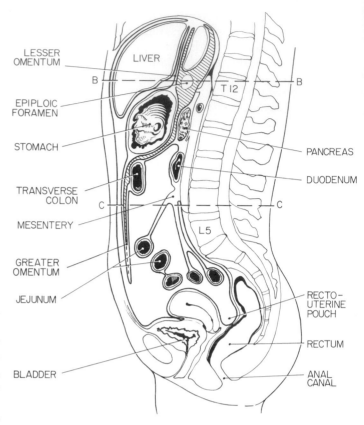

FIG. 32.13. Median sagittal section through the peritoneal cavity, with viscera intact. Section is in plane A of fig. 32.12.

32.14) which is invested in the peritoneum of the left leaf of the greater omentum. Palm the spleen in the right hand so that the fingers are behind it and the thumb anterior, and feel between finger and thumb the narrow attachment of the spleen to the omentum (fig. 32.14). At this level the greater omentum is divided by the splenic attachment into an anterior portion, the **gastro-splenic ligament**, and the **licnorenal ligament** which passes dorsally to fuse with the parietal peritoneum over the kidney on the posterior abdominal wall.

To check that the greater omentum is a thin sheet, lift it upwards and cut a hole through the mesocolon from below (avoiding damage to vessels). Now gently insert the left hand through the hole up behind the stomach, grasp the spleen in the right hand, and feel that only the thin membrane of the lienorenal ligament separates the right fingertips from the left hand, and similarly the gastrosplenic ligament lies between the right thumb and left hand. Inferior to the spleen, the omentum hangs down from the lower border (greater curvature) of the stomach like a flattened pouch (figs. 32.10 and 32.15).

The greater omentum has free lateral and inferior borders where the anterior wall of the pouch curves

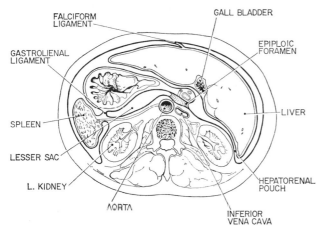

FIG. 32.14. Horizontal section of the peritoneal cavity. Plane B of figs. 32.12 and 13.

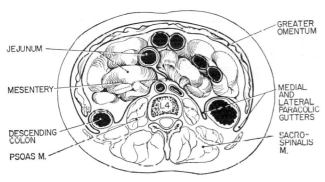

FIG 32.15. Horizontal section of the peritoneal cavity. Plane C of figs. 32.12. and 13.

backwards to form its posterior wall. The latter ascends and is attached to the transverse colon in the adult (fig. 32.13). In the embryo it rested on the superior surface of the colon and mesocolon before being reflected on to the parietal peritoneum over the pancreas, but fusion of its posterior surface to the adjacent surface of the mesocolon and colon moved its attachment to the adult position (fig. 32.70).

Push the right hand through the hole in the mesocolon and feel downwards into the pouch of the greater omentum; frequently it will be found that the cavity is obliterated by fusion of the adjacent walls.

The peritoneal relations of the liver are complex and are shown in figs. 32.16 and 32.17. The two layers of the lesser omentum separate and enclose the liver, before leaving its superior and posterior surfaces as the **coronary ligament** which ascends to the diaphragm (fig. 32.67). The liver develops in the ventral mesentery of the foregut between the stomach and the diaphragm (p. 32.57).

There are several important **subdiaphragmatic spaces** which lie between the diaphragm and the liver. To understand them, the peritoneal reflections on the liver must be traced out although not committed to memory. First

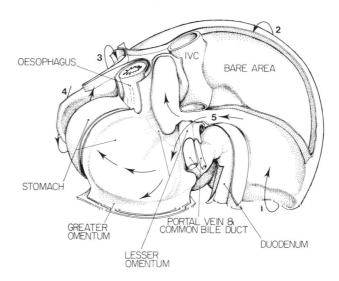

FIG. 32.16. Posterior oblique view of liver demonstrating the subdiaphragmatic spaces and peritoneal relations of the liver and lesser omentum. The oesophagus grooves the posterior surface of the left lobe and enters the stomach. The latter curves downwards to the right, posteroinferior to the liver, suspended from it by the lesser omentum.

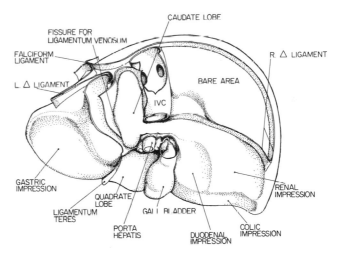

FIG. 32.17. Posteroinferior view of liver to show its peritoneal attachments and major relations.

pass the left hand into the **subhepatic space** which is posteroinferior to the right lobe of the liver and anterior to the right kidney (arrow 1 in fig. 32.16). Next slide the other hand backwards above the right lobe (arrow 2) into the **right subdiaphragmatic space.** The **bare area,** which is devoid of peritoneum, and where the liver and diaphragm are in direct contact, separates the hands. Slide both hands to the right and they meet around the free border of the **right triangular ligament.** Withdraw the hand from the hepatorenal pouch, and pass it above the left lobe of liver (arrow 3) to the **left triangular ligament.** The hands are now on either side of the **falci-**

form ligament, which runs from the liver to the diaphragm and anterior abdominal wall as far down as the umbilicus. The lower free border is thickened because it contains the fibrous remnant of the umbilical vein, the **ligamentum teres** of the liver. This goes from the umbilicus to the fissure for the ligamentum teres which is the boundary between the left and the quadrate lobes (fig. 32.17). Remove both hands and now place the left hand in the **left subdiaphragmatic space** (arrow 3), and slide the other up behind the left lobe of liver in front of the lesser omentum (arrow 4); the fingertips are separated by the thin left triangular ligament. Now trace the attachment of the lesser omentum downwards from the back of the left triangular ligament, along the fissure for the ligamentum venosum to the porta hepatis (figs. 32.16 and 32.17). Notice that the omentum lies almost in the coronal plane and passes deeply into the fissure for the ligamentum venosum on the anterior aspect of the caudate lobe (fig. 32.17). Place the left hand in the hepatorenal pouch (arrow 1) and slide the forefinger medially along its upper limit (arrow 5) until it enters a narrow aperture, the **epiploic foramen** or entrance to the lesser sac.

The epiploic foramen is bounded anteriorly by the lesser omentum with the bile duct, hepatic artery, and portal vein within its free border. Posteriorly, the inferior vena cava ascends retroperitoneally on the posterior abdominal wall. The caudate process of the liver is above the foramen and inferiorly the hepatic artery runs forwards from the coeliac artery before ascending to enter the lesser omentum (fig. 32.42).

The **lesser sac of peritoneum** lies behind the stomach, and separates it from the structures on the posterior abdominal wall (fig. 32.14). It extends as the upper recess behind the lesser omentum and caudate lobe (fig. 32.13) and inferiorly for a variable distance as the inferior recess into the greater omentum. The narrow epiploic foramen is the only communication with the greater sac. In health it is only a potential space, but in disease may be filled with fluid, e.g. a gastric ulcer (vol. 3, p. 19.44) may perforate through the posterior stomach wall and pour irritant gastric contents into the sac.

The **greater sac of peritoneum** is the remainder of the peritoneal cavity, including the pelvic portion. It is partly subdivided into various compartments by the abdominal organs and their peritoneal attachments. We have already seen that there are subdiaphragmatic spaces between the liver and diaphragm and these may become the site of an abscess (fig. 32.16). The ascending and descending colons project from the posterior abdominal wall so that there are **paracolic gutters** alongside them which may determine the spread of infection from various organs (fig. 32.15). For example, pus from a perforated appendix may, in the recumbent patient, track along the right lateral paracolic gutter to form a subdiaphragmatic abscess in the subhepatic space.

The greater omentum and mesocolon form a large flap which divides the greater sac into **supracolic** and **infracolic** compartments which are in free communication via the lateral paracolic gutters.

The greater omentum varies in size between individuals, and may contain an enormous amount of fat. In local inflammation of the peritoneum there is often a sticky exudate to which the omentum adheres, and this helps to localize the infection. The omentum is brought sooner or later to such sites because it is constantly being moved passively by the muscular activity of viscera as they fill and empty, and by the respiratory and postural movements of the diaphragm and abdominal walls.

STOMACH

Once food has been swallowed it leaves the oesophagus and enters the stomach via the cardia. The stomach is a large fibromuscular bag with a capacity of $\frac{1}{2}$–1 litre, which stores the food and passes it on to the duodenum when required. The stomach also secretes gastric juice (Greek *gaster*, stomach) which partly digests the stored contents.

Gross anatomy

The stomach lies in the upper part of the abdominal cavity, inferior to the diaphragm and liver, and is separated from the posterior abdominal wall only by the lesser sac. The stomach begins at the **gastro-oesophageal junction** or **cardia** and extends down and right to end at the

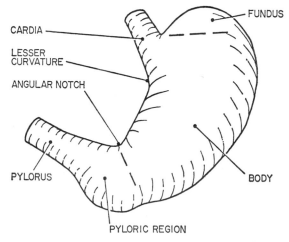

FIG. 32.18. Stomach.

gastroduodenal junction or **pylorus** (Greek *puloros*, a gatekeeper), opposite the intervertebral disc between the bodies of L.1 and L.2, 2 cm to the right of the median plane (fig. 32.9). The stomach has an anterior and a posterior surface, and two blunt lateral borders, known as curvatures (fig. 32.18 and 32.19). The whole stomach bulges downwards and to the left, so the short right

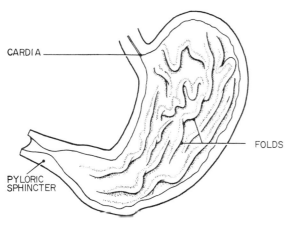

FIG. 32.19. Interior of stomach.

border is known as the **lesser curvature,** and the left as the **greater curvature.** The **fundus** is the portion of the stomach that is superior to the cardia, and usually contains a bubble of swallowed air. An oblique line running from an angular notch on the lesser curvature to the greater curvature divides the remainder into a main middle segment known as the **body,** and the **pyloric region** or **antrum.** There is an important functional distinction between body and antrum, but the division between body and fundus is arbitrary and the gastric regions defined histologically are more useful.

The stomach is attached to adjacent structures by the lesser and greater omenta which contain the gastric blood vessels and nerves. The lesser omentum runs upwards to be attached to the visceral surface of the liver

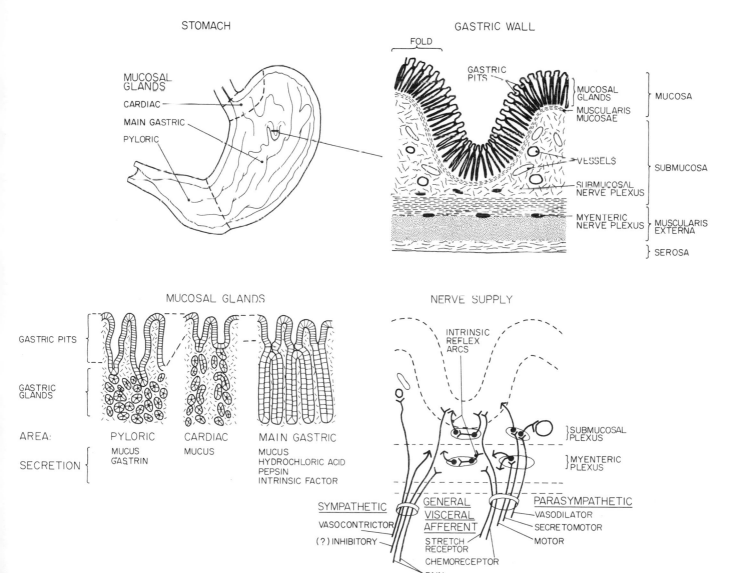

FIG. 32.20. Histology of the stomach. This composite diagram shows its regional variations and nerve supply.

and diaphragm. The greater omentum stretches from the greater curvature posteriorly to the posterior abdominal wall and transverse colon. The stomach is attached to neighbouring structures mainly by the oesophagus which is tethered as it passes through the diaphragm. The lesser and greater omenta are loose and so permit mobility. For instance the pylorus may descend by as much as 5 cm below the transpyloric plane on inspiration, sliding on the loose extraperitoneal connective tissue which holds it to the posterior abdominal wall. The shape of the stomach is also variable, tending to reflect the shape of its owner in a long thin person, but in the stocky person it is more oblique. The shape and position also depend on the degree of filling, posture, the tone of the abdominal muscles and on respiration. The greater curvature may descend to the level of the true pelvis in a thin erect individual. The tone of the muscle is also affected by emotion, and 'the heart sinking into one's boots' is more likely to be the stomach!

The anterior relations therefore vary according to its particular position, but include the greater sac and the left lobe of liver, left dome of diaphragm, and below these the anterior abdominal wall. Posteriorly, the stomach is separated by the lesser sac from the posterior abdominal wall and associated structures, including the diaphragm, the left adrenal gland, the pancreas and splenic artery, the transverse mesocolon and the left kidney (figs. 32.12 to 32.14). These structures, together with the gastric surface of the spleen, form the so-called **stomach bed**.

The inner surface of the empty stomach is covered with irregular rugae, but these folds largely disappear on filling. Over the curvatures there are several longitudinal folds which are more permanent. When fluid is sipped it flows rapidly down the lesser curvature and into the duodenum within these folds. On palpating the intact stomach the walls are felt to thicken at the pyloric sphincter and, in the living, the prepyloric vein is a useful surgical guide to the pylorus.

Histological structure
The mucosa of the stomach is covered by many small pits which lead to gastric glands. Simple tall columnar epithelium covers the surface and dips down to line these gastric pits (figs. 32.20 and 32.21). The epithelial cells contain many mucous granules above the nuclei, but in contrast to goblet cells they never become distended with mucus. The entire surface of the stomach secretes an alkaline sheet of mucus which adheres to and protects the epithelium. The lamina propria is very vascular, but is reduced to thin strands between the close packed glands, especially over the acid-bearing area of the stomach. The muscularis mucosae is very thick in the human stomach. The submucosa contains many large blood and lym-

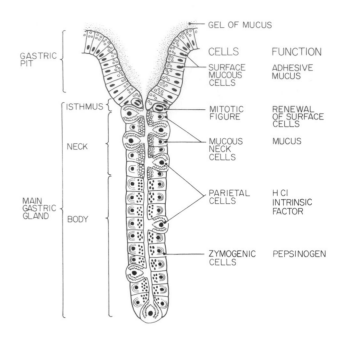

FIG. 32.21. Main gastric glands. These tubular glands are composed of zymogenic, parietal and mucous neck cells, and more primitive cells near the gastric pits which undergo mitosis.

phatic vessels and a prominent submucosal nerve plexus with ganglion cells, which are secretomotor to the glands.

The smooth muscle coat is in three layers, a complete middle circular one which thickens to form the pyloric sphincter, an incomplete outer longitudinal coat confined mostly to the curvatures, and an inner oblique layer which extends from the cardia to the greater curvature.

The gastric mucosa contains three types of gland, which occur in different areas.

GLANDS OF THE CARDIA
These cover an area about 4 cm in diameter centred on the oesophageal orifice. Here the mucosa has gastric pits joined by short branched tubular glands with mucus-secreting cells, but very few parietal cells.

MAIN GASTRIC GLANDS
These form the acid secretory area which amounts to 70–80 per cent of the mucosa. They are also called fundic glands, but as they are present in most of the body of the stomach as well as in the fundus, main gastric glands is a preferable term. The pits are relatively short and receive simple straight tubular glands, each with an isthmus, neck and body (fig. 32.21). **Mucous cells**, in the neck of the gland, are low columnar with some cytoplasmic basophilia below the nucleus and many PAS positive

mucous granules above. **Mucous neck cells,** positioned at the neck of the gland, contain many mucous granules. **Chief, zymogenic** or **pepsin-producing cells** form most of the gland body. On the luminal side they contain secretory granules and at the base the cytoplasm is intensely basophilic. Their structure is similar to that of other zymogenic cells (p. 18.6). The secretory granules contain **pepsinogen,** the inactive form of the proteolytic enzyme **pepsin,** and precursors of other gastric enzymes. The **parietal** or **oxyntic cells** are believed to secrete HCl, and also intrinsic factor which facilitates the absorption of vitamin B_{12} (p. 28.9). These large cells, with eosinophilic cytoplasm and a central nucleus, are abundant in the neck and isthmus of the gland. In the body of the gland their position on the wall of the gland gives them the name parietal; the secretion passes between adjacent cells to reach the lumen (fig. 32.21).

The parietal cell has a unique system of intracellular canaliculi. These are deep invaginations of the apical cell membrane, which branch as they extend down into the cell. The cell membrane lining the canaliculi has many microvilli, which augment the secretory surface area (figs. 32.22 to 32.24). Abundant mitochondria with close-packed cristae occupy as much as 40 per cent of the cytoplasm. This accounts for the exceptionally high metabolic rate of the parietal cell, which concentrates H^+ one millionfold, i.e. from 40 nmol/l to 40 mmol/l. The smooth endoplasmic reticulum is extensive, and the cells release their contents into the lumen of the gland by a reverse of pinocytosis. The parietal cell is rich in zinc, which is a component of the enzyme carbonic anhydrase. This enzyme catalyses the production of H_2CO_3 (p. 32.18).

Argentaffin cells (p. 32.25) are found in the mucous membrane of both the pylorus and body of the stomach.

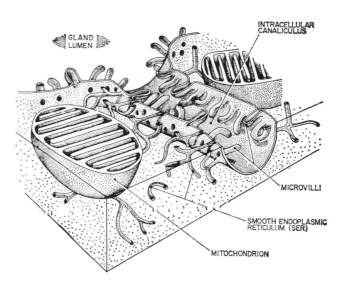

FIG. 32.23. Parietal cell, showing rectangular area in fig. 32.22.

PYLORIC OR ANTRAL GLANDS

These occupy about 15 per cent of the gastric mucosa, approximately over the pyloric region already defined. The surface cells and pits are similar to those of the other two areas, except that the gastric pits are as long as the glands (fig. 32.20). The latter are branching coiled tubular mucous glands. Rounded **gastrin cells** (G Cells) containing secretory granules (fig. 32.25) that lie scattered between the bases of mucous cells in the pyloric glands have been identified by the fluorescent antibody technique as the source of the hormone gastrin (p. 32.19).

Cell renewal of gastric epithelium

Mitotic figures are visible in the isthmus of the gastric glands, and in the mucous neck cells. The surface cells are shed at a high rate, but are replaced by fresh cells which arise in the isthmus and move upwards on to the surface. Both in animals and man complete renewal occurs every few days. The renewal rate of zymogenic and parietal cells is undetermined, but is very much slower. Experimentally, destruction in animals of a circumscribed area of gastric mucosa is followed by rapid spread inwards from the wound margins of a thin sheet of epithelium. This covering sheet is formed by division of cells in the isthmuses of the glands around the wound. Downgrowths from this sheet form new glands, which initially are composed solely of mucous neck cells, but later differentiate to form typical main gastric glands with the normal complement of parietal and zymogenic cells. The healthy gastric mucosa has therefore good powers of repair and regeneration.

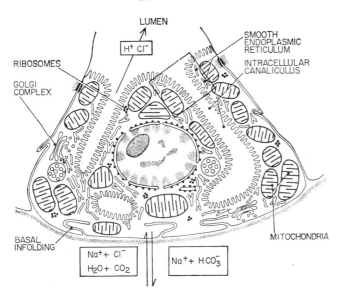

FIG. 32.22. Parietal cell.

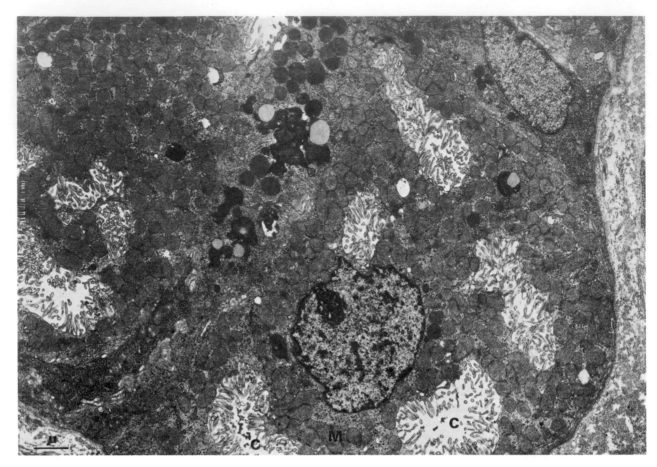

FIG. 32.24. Human gastric parietal cell, showing abundant mitochondria (M) which occupy most of the cytoplasm, and intra-cellular canaliculi (C). (× 6840). Courtesy of Dr. Katherine Carr.

Functions of the stomach

The stomach is not indispensable for life, though digestive disturbances may follow its removal (gastrectomy). Its main function is to act as a reservoir, in which a semi-solid mass known as **chyme** is formed from the ingested food. The strongly acid gastric juice kills or restricts the growth of many bacteria. Digestion proceeds in the stomach until the chyme passes on to the intestine, but little absorption takes place in the stomach, except for water and alcohol.

METHODS OF STUDY

Unlike the salivary glands, the gastric secretory glands cannot be cannulated directly and the study of gastric secretion is therefore more difficult because indirect methods must be used. In man, the most common methods involve passing a tube down the oesophagus into the stomach, so that the secretion may be aspirated and analysed. In early studies, either a 'test meal' (usually a somewhat unappetizing gruel) or an injection of histamine was given to stimulate secretion, and samples of gastric juice drawn off for study. Both methods were limited in their usefulness, as after a test meal the samples were contaminated with food, and histamine is an artificial stimulus which may not produce a normal secretion. Both tests have now been supplanted by injections of synthetic pentagastrin, which simulates the action of the natural gastric hormone (p. 32.20).

In experimental animals, more accurate studies can be made and these have given us most of our knowledge of the control of gastric secretion. In a dog, a small pouch, separate from the main stomach, can be made and brought out through the abdominal wall at a surgical operation. Such a dog can remain in excellent health for many years. Gastric secretion can be stimulated in various ways and uncontaminated samples collected from the pouch without disturbance to the animal. The pouch may be made in such a way as to leave its nerve supply intact (Pavlov pouch) or deliberately denervated (Heidenhain

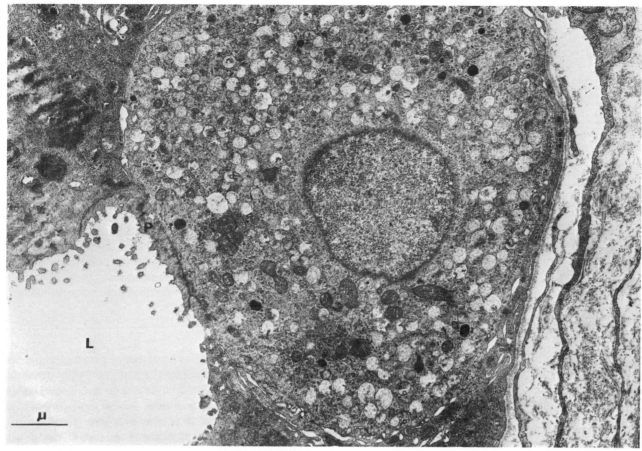

FIG. 32.25. Gastrin cell in pyloric region of human stomach. This cell does not reach the lumen (L), from which it is separated by a thin process (P) of a neighbouring cell. The gastrin secretory granules are numerous, small and appear either pale or dark. Mitochondria are scanty. (× 11 210). Courtesy of Dr. Katherine Carr.

pouch) (figs. 32.26). In addition to such pouches, an oesophageal fistula may be made, together with a gastric fistula, so that food eaten emerges from the neck and does not enter the stomach, i.e. sham feeding. Such a preparation is used to study the effects of ingested food before it reaches the stomach (fig. 32.27). The dog must, of course, be given its normal food requirements through the gastric fistula.

COMPOSITION OF GASTRIC JUICE

The principal constituents are acid, mucus and digestive enzymes.

Acid secretion

The parietal cells secrete a fluid approximately isosmotic with plasma, in which the concentrations in mmol/l of the main electrolytes are about $[H^+]$ 153, $[K^+]$ 7 and $[Cl^-]$ 160. The concentrations of electrolytes in the secretions of the other cells are approximately $[Na^+]$ 160, $[Cl^-]$ 120 and $[HCO_3^-]$ 40 mmol/l. The $[H^+]$ of the mixed juice usually lies between 70 and 130 mmol/l,

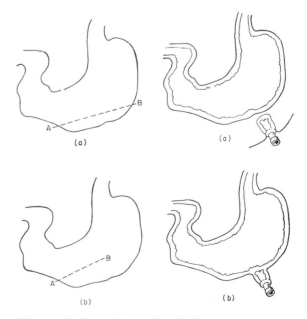

FIG. 32.26. Stomach pouches (a) denervated (Heidenhain) pouch and (b) innervated (Pavlov) pouch. A–B line of gastric incision.

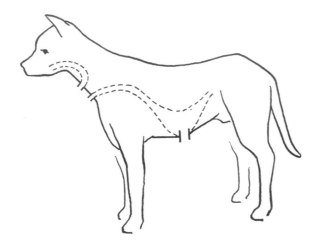

FIG. 32.27. A dog used for 'sham feeding'.

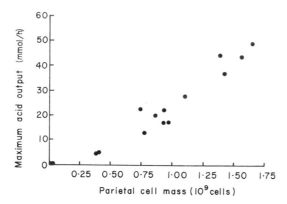

FIG. 32.28. The relation between gastric acid secretion and parietal cell mass. From Card W.I. & Marks I. (1959) *Clin. Sci.* **19**, 147.

about pH 0·9–1·5, and depends on the number of parietal cells present. These cells have been counted in stomachs removed surgically and their number correlated with maximum acid secretion (fig. 32.28). It has been calculated that this amounts to 20mmol/h10^9 cells. The number of cells, known as the **parietal cell mass,** varies widely. Low values for acid secretion are found in some healthy people, presumably due to congenitally few cells, and in certain diseases, e.g. pernicious anaemia, when the cells are destroyed by an abnormal immune mechanism (vol. 3, p. 21.24).

How the parietal cells manage to secrete a fluid with [H$^+$] more than one million times that of the blood is an old, largely unsolved problem of ion transport. The potential difference across the mucosal surface of the resting fundus of the stomach is about -60 mV and is slightly less in the secreting one. Since the [Cl$^-$] in gastric juice is about 60 mmol/l higher than in plasma, Cl$^-$ must be transported actively from the plasma against an

electrochemical gradient and the pump responsible is an electrogenic one (p. 18.9). However, when a sheet of mucosa containing parietal cells is placed in a salt solution free of Cl$^-$, the negative PD is abolished and it becomes positive; this indicates the presence of a second electrogenic pump responsible for H$^+$ transport. It is believed that in the intact parietal cell both pumps operate together. The H$^+$ are derived from the ionization of carbonic acid which is formed within the mucosal cells from CO_2 and H_2O under the influence of carbonic anhydrase. The HCO$_3^-$ which are formed in equal number are passed from the cells into the venous blood.

Consistent with the above outline are the old observations that at the height of gastric secretion there is a rise in urinary pH, the **alkaline tide,** and a fall in RQ, due to retention in the body of this reabsorbed HCO$_3^-$.

Loss of the gastric secretions by repeated vomiting leads to water and electrolyte disturbances; the patient becomes dehydrated, deficient in sodium and potassium and develops metabolic alkalosis.

Mucus secretion

Gastric mucus contains a number of proteoglycans. These have a high carbohydrate content (75–85 per cent) made up of sialic acid, *N*-acetylglucosamine, *N*-acetylgalactosamine, galactose, mannose, fucose and glucose. Side chains of specific disaccharides give some of these glycoproteins the properties of A and B blood group antigens. For example the sugar group acetylgalactosamine-fucose-galactose-acetylglucosamine is specific for group A, and galactose-fucose-galactose-acetylglycosamine for group B. The presence of antigens A and B on gastric mucus may have a protective action on the mucous membrane, since persons of blood group O, in whom they are absent, are more susceptible to duodenal ulceration than persons of other blood groups.

The mucus itself may also protect the stomach wall against the enzymes and acid. One component forms a gel which is partially adherent to the stomach wall and provides a barrier which might delay the diffusion of acid chyme. The extent to which mucus actually neutralizes gastric acidity is probably small.

Glandular mucoproteins also contain the intrinsic factor (p. 28.9). Doses of vitamin B$_{12}$ as small as 4–12 mmol (5–15 μg) when given orally with a mucoprotein fraction are rapidly absorbed and produce a striking response in the blood picture of patients with pernicious anaemia.

Enzymes

The chief enzyme present is **pepsin**. In many animals and in the human infant there is also **rennin**, which in the presence of calcium ions curdles the proteins of milk. Gastric juice may also contain traces of lipase.

Pepsin attacks many proteins, but only at a few points on the molecule. Protein digestion, therefore, does not proceed further than the polypeptide stage in the stomach. The stomach is not an important organ for enzymic digestion in man or for absorption. Indeed digestion often proceeds surprisingly well in patients after a total gastrectomy. The main role of the stomach is as a temporary store which allows food to be swallowed faster than it can be passed into the small intestine.

CONTROL OF GASTRIC SECRETION

The rate of secretion of gastric juice is determined by the interplay of excitory and inhibitory influences, both nervous and hormonal. The acidity of the stomach content is the product of the rate of H^+ secretion and the buffering capacity of the stomach contents. The latter includes swallowed saliva, the non-acid component of gastric secretion (largely from the pyloric antrum), re-gurgitated duodenal content and food. Quantitatively the most important of these is food.

Most of the experimental work on which early knowledge of the control of gastric secretion is based was, of necessity, carried out on animals. However some direct evidence is available in man. Reference has already been made to Alexis St. Martin, who had a fistula as the result of a gunshot wound. Beaumont noted that his gastric secretion increased when he was angry and hostile, and decreased when he was afraid or depressed. Similar results were seen by Wolf and Wolff in their study of Tom, an American who had a surgical gastric fistula provided after his oesophagus closed as a result of drinking excessively hot clam chowder! Another similar patient closed off his oesophagus by drinking a caustic solution. Carlson's observations on this subject confirmed that the fasting stomach secretes acid and that chewing food, even though it does not enter the stomach, induces gastric secretion.

The rate of secretion varies too with the type of food intake. In man, soup and meat extracts produce copious and prolonged secretion. It is less with carbohydrates and fat. Maximal rates, comparable to maximum stimulation of the stomach by gastrin, are achieved by meat meals.

For descriptive purposes control of gastric secretion is divided into three phases; cephalic, gastric and intestinal, according to the site at which the various stimuli act. This is somewhat artificial as the three phases not only follow one another in sequence, but to some extent proceed simultaneously.

Basal secretion

In man some acid is secreted under circumstances in which there appears to be no obvious stimulus. This is termed the resting or basal secretion and amounts to between 1·3 and 4·2 mmol/h of H^+. In some healthy individuals, however, no acid secretion may be detected.

Cephalic or psychic phase

Secretion is evoked before food reaches the stomach, in response to the unconditioned reflex stimulus of taste, and to the conditioned stimuli set up by the sight and smell of food, and noises associated with the preparation and serving of a meal.

The effectiveness of these stimuli is related to the individual's preferences for food and his appetite. The afferent pathways of these reflexes lie in the visceral afferent fibres from the mouth and afferent fibres from the cerebral cortex to the vagal nucleus. The efferent pathway lies in the vagus nerves, the preganglionic fibres of which terminate in the submucosal plexus in the stomach wall (fig. 32.20). Postganglionic fibres arise from the plexus to innervate the parietal cells in the body of the stomach and the gastrin-producing cells (G cells) of the pyloric antrum. Thus excitation of the vagus nerve in the cephalic phase leads to the direct stimulation of acid and pepsin secretion, and indirect stimulation by gastrin liberated from antral G cells. The duration of the cephalic phase is variable and may last up to about an hour.

Experimentally, this phase may be demonstrated by sham feeding when secretion can be shown to occur even though the food never reaches the stomach. Such secretion is abolished by section of the vagus nerve.

Gastric phase

When food reaches the stomach, stimuli acting through normal (unconditioned) pathways evoke acid and pepsin secretion. Two types of reflexes are involved in the response: long vagovagal reflexes in which both afferent and efferent fibres lie in the vagus nerves, and short local reflexes which lie entirely within the stomach wall. *Vagovagal reflexes.* Distension of the body of the stomach excites stretch receptors and stimulates acid secretion via vagal efferents, when all gastrin-producing areas have been removed surgically.

Local reflexes. The hormone, gastrin, is liberated into the general circulation when foods and the products of their digestion, particularly polypeptides, come into contact with the mucosa of the pyloric area, and when there is distension of the antrum. This local reflex is mediated by the submucosal plexus.

Gastrin is a polypeptide of 34 amino acids (G-34) which is converted into a heptadecapeptide (G-17) which contains the 17 N terminal amino acids of G-34 and has the following chemical composition:

Pyro-Gly-Pro-Try-Leu-Glu-Glu-Glu-Glu-

1 2 3 4 5 6 7 8 9

-Glu-Ala-Tyr-Gly-Try-Met-Asp-Phe-NH₂

10 11 12 13 14 15 16 17

Pyro = pyroglutamyl

Two forms of gastrin exist. Gastrin II differs from gastrin I only in that the OH group on the tyrosine molecule at position 12 on the chain is sulphonated. The terminal tetrapeptide, Try-Met-Asp-Phe-NH₂, stimulates acid secretion in the same manner as the whole molecule though it is less potent. A pentapeptide containing these 4 amino acids and alanine has been synthesized and is used under the name of **pentagastrin** to test gastric function. Gastrin is present in the circulation mainly as G-34 but there is some G-17 and also a form with 13 amino acids. The release of gastrin is dependent on the pH of the solution bathing the antral mucosa. It is largely inhibited when the pH falls to between pH 2 and pH 3 as a result of acid secretion.

There is also a second type of local reflex present in the wall of the body of the stomach. It is demonstrated by distension of a vagally denervated stomach, with all the gastrin-bearing areas removed by surgery, when a very small acid secretion occurs. When distension is carried out during infusion of a just threshold dose of gastrin, the rate of acid secretion is considerably increased.

Intestinal phase

Stimuli acting from the small intestine are also capable of continuing secretion already started by the cephalic and gastric phases. There is evidence that a hormone, **intestinal gastrin,** is produced in the duodenum and jejunum both by the action of digestion products and by distension.

Inhibitory mechanisms

Towards the end of the meal, when the buffering capacity of the food in the stomach is saturated, the pH of the contents falls and when this reaches between pH 2 and pH 3 gastrin secretion is greatly reduced. This appears to be due to a direct effect on the G cells.

The duodenum is also an important site from which signals arise to inhibit activity. The inhibitory mechanisms are not only active in reducing the secretion of acid and pepsin but also in slowing the rate of emptying of the stomach. Thus they prevent the duodenum from being overloaded and protect its delicate mucosa from damage. Nervous and hormonal mechanisms are involved, but the precise nervous pathways and the nature of the humoral agent, **enterogastrone**, have not been established. Though the precise mechanisms are still unknown the stimuli which cause inhibition are not; these are the

presence of acid, fat and hyperosmolal solutions in the duodenum.

Several hormones are known to inhibit gastric secretion and the release of gastrin but it is not known whether they are present in the circulation in sufficient concentration to inhibit gastrin release. They include glucagon, calcitonin, secretin and growth hormone releasing inhibiting factor.

The prostaglandin PGE₂ has also been isolated from human stomach tissue and it inhibits gastric secretion; its physiological role is uncertain but it may act as a local hormone.

Interactions of parietal cell stimulants

In man both parietal and chief cells can be activated by acetylcholine (vagal stimulation), gastrin (and pentagastrin) and histamine. However, it is not known whether or not histamine plays a physiological role and the relation between gastrin and vagal effects is complex.

Atropine, a drug which blocks the action of acetylcholine liberated at nerve endings, inhibits not only secretion by vagal stimulation but also that by histamine and gastrin. Similarly the use of metiamide which blocks the histamine (H₂) receptors in the stomach (vol. 2, p. 14.18) not only inhibits secretion induced by histamine but also that induced by both vagal stimulation and gastrin. These observations suggest that both histamine and acetylcholine receptors are needed for each of the three stimulants of gastric secretion. Whether gastrin is needed for histamine and vagal secretion is unknown as no way is known to block the action of gastrin.

Some experimental evidence supports the theory of the interdependence of vagal activity and gastrin. In the dog and cat, vagal stimulation liberates gastrin, and gastrin is also required for the vagal effect on parietal cells. However the relationship in man is unknown.

One other important effect of gastrin is a trophic one. Hyperplasia of gastric mucosa, an increase in the number of parietal cells and increased capacity to secrete acid can be induced experimentally in rats by repeated ingestion of pentagastrin, and surgical removal of the antrum causes parietal cell atrophy. In man also surgical removal of the antrum reduces maximal secretory acid output but this may be prevented by giving pentagastrin continuously during the first week after antrectomy. Whatever role gastrin secretion plays in modulating parietal cell secretion, these observations suggest that it is an important determinant of parietal cell mass.

GASTRIC MOTILITY

When a meal is eaten the stomach relaxes within seconds of swallowing and before the food enters the stomach. This receptive relaxation is probably induced by a vagal reflex as the result of swallowing and its function is to accommodate the increased volume in the stomach and at the same time to keep the intragastric pressure low. The meal distends the stomach and stimulates contractions in its wall. These **peristaltic waves** are rings of muscular contractions which sweep down the long axis of the stomach towards the pylorus. They begin in the fundus near the cardia and sweep over the pyloric portion carrying a small bolus of gastric content before them. The bolus then reaches the pylorus which is normally open, and food begins to pass through. As the wave of contraction passes towards the sphincter, this begins to contract and the narrower pyloric canal offers increasing resistance to the passage of the bolus. Because of the resistance the peristaltic contractions produce a pressure spike, forcing the remainder of the bolus to traverse the pyloric canal; then the sphincter closes and the duodenal bulb contracts, pushing the bolus into the second part of the duodenum. Thus the pyloric antrum, the pylorus and the first part of the duodenum act as one unit called the **gastroduodenal pump.**

Once food enters the stomach, peristaltic waves begin with a frequency of 3–4 per minute and continue until the stomach is empty. Under normal circumstances the stomach contents pass into the duodenum phasically, that is as discrete boluses of food. The study of stomach emptying is difficult using ordinary meals, because it is impossible to aspirate a representative sample of its contents. Consequently special meals of a liquid nature have to be used.

EMPTYING OF THE STOMACH

Gastric emptying can be studied using test meals of varying composition, e.g. barium sulphate, bread and water, solutions of simple carbohydrates and inorganic salts. These meals are either simple aqueous solutions or of such a consistency that they can be aspirated from the stomach through a polythene tube. A meal is introduced into the stomach, left there for a given time and then what remains is removed by suction. From the volume recovered the amount leaving the stomach is calculated. As the pattern of emptying of any individual remains unchanged over several days, experiments are carried out in which test meals of identical composition are given on a number of days. The meal is left for periods which vary on the different days, and the amount recovered in each experiment is plotted against the time after instillation. By this technique the pattern of emptying meals of differing volume and composition can be studied.

Effect of the volume of the meal
There are linear relationships between the square root of the volume of the meal remaining in the stomach and the time which elapses after administration. This may be explained by the law of Laplace (p. 30.22) which states that the transmural tension in a curved chamber is proportional to its radius. If the stomach is considered as a cylinder, its radius is proportional to the square root of its volume. The larger the volume in the stomach, the greater its radius and hence the tension in its wall. The increased tension leads to greater excitation of the smooth muscle either by direct action or reflexly through the intrinsic nerve plexus or the extrinsic nerve supply, the vagus.

Effect of fats, acid and osmolality
The presence of fat in a meal, the osmolality and the acidity of the stomach content entering the duodenum exert a restraining influence on stomach emptying. In the case of acid the emptying of the stomach is controlled in such a way that only so much acid leaves the stomach in unit time, and this is independent of pH. When test meals are made up of solutes of different concentrations and left in the stomach for a constant period of time, then there is a linear relationship between the volume of the meal recovered and the concentration of the solute. Such a wide range of solutes show this effect that probably only one type of receptor exists which responds to a common property, i.e. the osmolality of the solution reaching the duodenum. The conclusion is that there exist in the duodenum receptors sensitive to fats and acids, and to changes in osmotic pressure which, acting through either neural or hormonal pathways, slow gastric emptying.

SMALL INTESTINE

The small intestine starts at the pylorus and ends at the ileocaecal junction, where it joins the large intestine. The major part of digestion and absorption occurs in this long and much convoluted region of the gut. The small intestine consists of the **duodenum** which is short and fairly fixed, and the much longer, more mobile and more convoluted **jejunum** and **ileum**, which are suspended by the mesentery from the posterior abdominal wall (fig. 32.9).

Gross anatomy

DUODENUM
The duodenum is the short, wide C-shaped segment which begins at the pylorus to the right of the median plane, and curves around the head of pancreas on the posterior abdominal wall, to end at the duodenojejunal flexure to the left of the median plane (fig. 32.29). It is divided into four parts. The **first part** runs from the pylorus to the right,

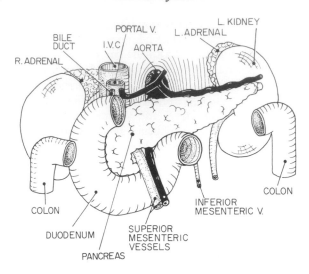

FIG. 32.29. Anterior aspect of duodenum and pancreas. The spleen has been removed.

upwards, and backwards to end by turning downwards abruptly to become the second, descending part. The first part has a 'free' portion continuous with the stomach which gives attachment to the right extremity of the lesser omentum above and the right margin of the greater omentum below. This means that its posterior surface faces the lesser sac, but its anterior surface faces the greater sac. Across the potential space of the lesser sac, the duodenum is related to the head of pancreas, and an ulcer penetrating the pancreas is an all-too-common complication of a chronic duodenal ulcer. The 'fixed' portion is covered with peritoneum on its anterior and superior surfaces. Above it is related to the epiploic foramen and posteriorly to the bile duct, portal vein and gastroduodenal artery (p. 32.34).

The **second part** descends on the pelvis of the right ureter and psoas major posteriorly, and is covered anteriorly with peritoneum except where crossed by the transverse colon. The bile duct and main pancreatic duct enter the second part by a single opening on the posteromedial wall. The **third part** sweeps leftward across the median plane lying in front of the inferior vena cava, aorta and psoas major muscles. Anteriorly it has a peritoneal coat except where crossed by the descending superior mesenteric vessels which occasionally cause duodenal obstruction. The short **fourth part** ascends on the left psoas major and turns forwards to end at the duodenojejunal flexure. The root of the mesentery is attached to its anterior surface.

The first part of the duodenum feels thin, but the remainder has thick walls because of tall circular mucosal folds. A small projection on the posteromedial wall of the mucosal surface of the second part, the duodenal papilla, contains the short dilated terminal part of the combined pancreatic and bile ducts known as the

ampulla of Vater. An accessory pancreatic duct usually enters the duodenum about 2 cm proximal to the main duct.

Radiologically the duodenum is C-shaped, but the first part is almost vertical, and conical like a dunce's cap (fig. 32.30). This **duodenal cap** lies above the narrow pylorus and is often deformed or abnormally immobile in patients with duodenal ulcer.

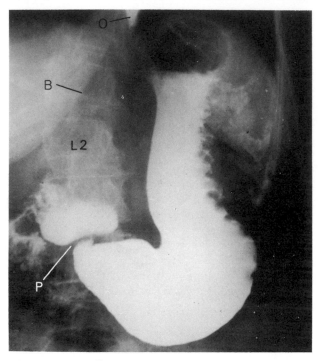

FIG. 32.30. Radiograph of the stomach and duodenum (anteroposterior view). The patient is upright a few minutes after a barium meal. The duodenum is beginning to fill. Oesophagus (O), pyloric sphincter (P), breast shadow (B) and 2nd lumbar vertebra (L2). Courtesy of Dr C.K. Warwick.

JEJUNUM AND ILEUM

A long and deep **mesentery** attaches the jejunum and ileum to the posterior abdominal wall (fig. 32.9) and gives them their mobility. The root of the mesentery begins at the duodenojejunal flexure at the lower border of the body of the 2nd lumbar vertebra, to the left of the midline, and descends obliquely to the right for 15 cm before ending in front of the upper part of the right sacro-iliac joint. But the free border of the mesentery, where the two constituent peritoneal layers separate to enclose the gut, is much longer, as the jejunum and ileum are about three metres in length. The transition between the two is gradual and the division quite arbitrary, although there are distinct differences between the proximal jejunum and the distal ileum.

When compared with the ileum, the jejunum is broader, more vascular and therefore redder, and has thicker walls because of the high circular folds on its luminal surface. The ileum has sparse and low circular folds but has distinctive patches of lymphoid tissue, **Peyer's patches,** in its wall opposite the mesentery.

Another valuable distinguishing feature between the jejunum and ileum is the pattern of the arteries in the mesentery adjacent to the gut; at the jejunum the supplying arteries form a single arcade, but the arcades increase in number as the gut is followed distally, so that beside the ileum there are three or four vascular arches. The jejunal arteries are easily seen because the fat in the mesentery does not quite reach the gut, but the ileal arteries are often obscured by the fat which may even infiltrate the gut wall.

Many of the differences just discussed are minor, and the surgeon presented with a small loop of intestine protruding through a limited incision in the abdominal wall puts a hand on either side of the root of the mesentery and then slides them towards the gut, which untwists the mesentery and reveals its polarity.

The complex high circular folds of the jejunum produce a typical feathery appearance on a barium meal radiograph, whereas the lower and sparse folds of the ileum give a smooth outline (fig. 32.31).

Although the small intestine appears to lie at random, it is generally confined within the inverted U of the colon, with the jejunum above and to the left, and the ileum in the hypogastric region and true pelvis. The terminal ileum ascends out of the pelvis into the right iliac fossa where it joins the caecum.

Meckel's diverticulum is a remnant of the proximal portion of the vitello-intestinal duct (p. 32.56) and is found in about 2 per cent of the population. It is located on the anti-mesenteric border of the ileum, and is usually within 40 cm of the ileocaecal sphincter although, rarely, this distance may be as much as 100 cm. Its mucosa is usually ileal, but in up to 50 per cent of cases contains some ectopic gastric mucosa. The clinical importance of Meckel's diverticulum lies in the fact that gastric mucosa secretes hydrochloric acid which may lead to ulceration and this is occasionally the cause of obscure digestive symptoms. An infected diverticulum may simulate appendicitis.

ABSORPTIVE AREA OF THE SMALL INTESTINE

Determining the normal length of jejunum and ileum has been aptly compared to measuring a worm, because the difficulties are similar, namely that the length varies widely according to the tone of the intrinsic muscle and the tension on the two ends. At autopsy the measurement is usually about 7–8 metres, but this is an overestimate of the length in life. Results obtained by means of indwelling radio-

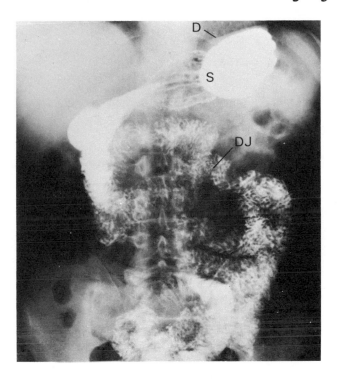

FIG. 32.31. Radiograph of stomach and small intestine (anteroposterior view), half an hour after a barium meal which has now entered the jejunum and proximal ileum. Their mucosal folds give the feathery appearance. The stomach lies almost transverse because patient is supine. Duodeno-jejunal flexure (DJ), diaphragm (D) and stomach (S). Courtesy of Dr C.K. Warwick.

opaque intestinal tubes in man suggest that the small intestine is only about 3 metres long. The **convolutions** allow the gut to be about 20 times as long as its mesenteric attachment. A second factor that increases the surface area is the presence of **circular folds** on the mucosal surface of the gut wall (fig. 32.32). These folds begin in the second part of the duodenum, reach a maximum in the jejunum, and diminish in the ileum to become sparse near its termination. Thirdly, the surface of these folds is covered with **villi,** finger-like processes of mucosa 1 mm long, which project into the lumen of the gut. Finally, the epithelial lining of the villi is composed largely of columnar absorptive cells which have a brush border. This border consists of tiny **microvilli** (p. 13.14) which further increase the surface area twentyfold. Together the convolutions, circular folds, villi and microvilli result in a total surface area of approximately 20–40 m².

Histological structure

The structure of the small intestine is related to its main function which is absorptive. This is facilitated by having a large surface area.

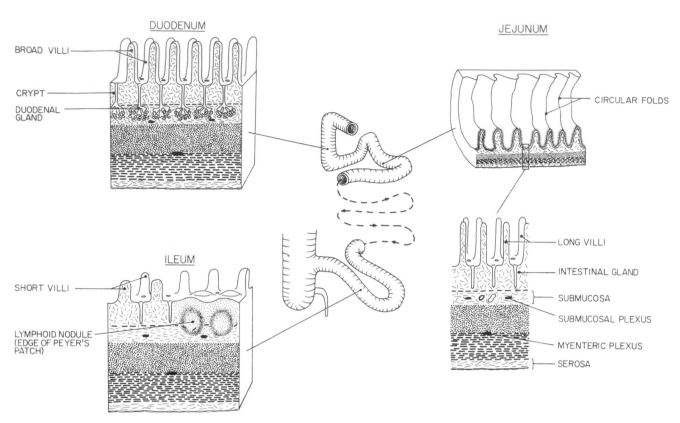

FIG. 32.32. Small intestine showing regional variations. The circular folds and the height and numbers of villi all diminish towards the ileum. Aggregated lymphoid nodules characterize the lower ileum.

JEJUNUM

This is described first because it typifies the structure of the small intestine. The jejunal wall feels thick because of the permanent circular folds, and the mucosa forms villi and intestinal glands (crypts of Lieberkühn).

Intestinal villus

The villi of the jejunum are tall, slender and close-packed (figs. 32.32 and 32.33). They are the absorptive units of the small bowel and defective villi may be a cause of malabsorption. The delicate lining epithelium is only one cell thick, which facilitates absorption. The lining is supported by the lamina propria, a loose cellular connective tissue with many lymphoid cells and occasional lymphoid nodules, which forms the core of each villus and fills the interstices between the crypts.

The submucosa is typical, with extensive vascular and nervous plexuses, and the muscular coat has a prominent myenteric nerve plexus. The jejunum is completely enveloped by a serosa except where attached to the mesentery.

Columnar **absorptive cells** cover most of the villus and engage in absorption by a variety of active and passive transport mechanisms (p. 18.7). This tall columnar cell (fig. 32.34) has a basal nucleus, a supranuclear Golgi complex, and scattered short profiles of rough and smooth surfaced endoplasmic reticulum as well as many free ribosomes. There is a brush border over the apical surface of the cell. This border, across which all absorption probably occurs, is bounded by a thick and asymmetric cell membrane which is rich in several enzymes including alkaline phosphatase. At the bases of the microvilli many invaginations may represent pinocytotic vesicles, which could be involved in the absorption of certain substances. Laterally the cell membranes of adjacent cells are firmly attached to each other near the lumen by junctional complexes (p. 13.12). The terminal web is a meshwork of fine filaments, lying parallel to the free surface, which are attached to the intermediate zone of the junctional complex. This web probably has a mechanical function, stiffening the apical part of the cell. Lateral to the nucleus the cell membranes are irregularly folded and provide a variable intercellular space which is utilized during fat and fluid absorption (p. 32.44).

The **goblet cells** are the other main component of the lining epithelium and are typical mucus-secreting cells.

Intestinal glands (*crypts of Lieberkühn*)

Straight tubular glands open between the bases of the villi (fig. 32.32). The epithelium is composed mostly of proliferating stem cells and developing absorptive and goblet cells. Clusters of **Paneth cells** lie at the base of the gland, and isolated argentaffin cells are wedged between the bases of gland cells (fig. 32.33). The Paneth cell is a typical zymogenic exocrine cell, with large eosinophilic secretory granules in its upper third, while basally there is an extensive rough endoplasmic reticulum. The secretory granules are discharged in response to food entering the small intestine, but their nature is unknown. The cells are unusually rich in zinc which may indicate that the secretory granules are a metalloprotein enzyme. There are only about a dozen Paneth cells in each crypt, but because of the enormous number of crypts the total mass of Paneth cells is large. **Argentaffin cells** are so named because they contain secretory granules which stain strongly with silver salts. These granules fill the cell, but the Golgi complex is on the basal side of the nucleus facing the capillaries, which gives a clue that the argentaffin cell is not exocrine but endocrine, and the granules are now known to be rich in 5-hydroxy-tryptamine. These cells are widely distributed throughout the gut, but are particularly numerous in the ileum and appendix where they may give rise to tumours (vol. 3, p. 19.72).

Epithelial turnover in the small intestine

The presence of large numbers of mitotic figures in the crypts, and the fact that at the tips of villi the epithelial cells often appear degenerate and heaped upon one another suggests that there is a constant formation of cells within the crypts and loss of epithelium from the tips of the villi. If mice are killed after receiving a single dose of radio-active thymidine, which is taken up during mitosis, the movement of cells which divided shortly after the injection of thymidine can be traced. In mice killed within an hour of injection, labelling is confined to the crypts; after 24 hours labelled cells are observed over the upper parts of the crypts and the basal portions of the villi. After 48 hours few labelled cells remain at the apices of the villi. Therefore complete renewal of villous epithelium occurs every two days in mice. In all mammals including man the villus is a dynamic organ existing in a delicate state of equilibrium, in which a rapid loss is balanced by a cor-

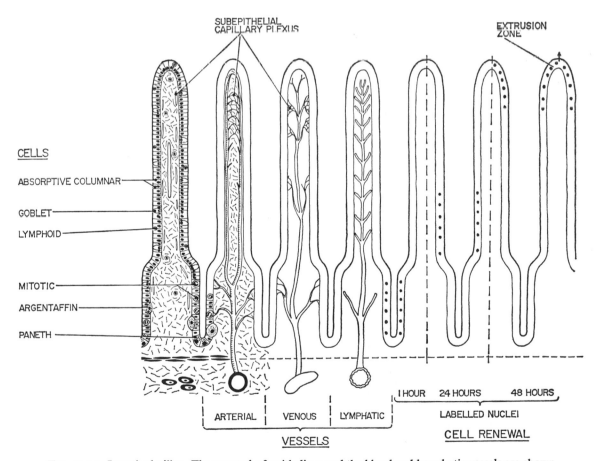

FIG. 32.33. Intestinal villus. The renewal of epithelium and the blood and lymphatic vessels are shown.

respondingly high rate of epithelial cell renewal. Disturbance of such a system would produce rapid change, and in animals blocking of mitosis by X-rays or antimetabolic drugs causes collapse of the villi within a few days. In diseases such as gluten enteropathy (vol. 3, p. 19.60) where the villi are severely reduced or absent, there is a disturbance of this equilibrium. The population of absorptive cells is reduced due to flattening of the villi, and even the remaining cells may be abnormal in that they lack their full complement of enzymes.

Blood supply and lymphatic tissue

The lamina propria carries the villous blood supply, which comes from a branch of the submucosal arterial plexus, then ascends in the long axis of each villus and supplies a widespread **subepithelial capillary plexus** (fig. 32.33). Venules from the latter end in the submucosal venous plexus and thereafter the venous drainage is typical of the gut. The lymphatics draining a villus are numerous and join a **central lymphatic** or lacteal (fig. 32.33) which descends in the villous core to a submucosal

plexus and this in turn drains to the extrinsic lacteals of the intestines. Smooth muscle fibres from the muscularis mucosae, lying parallel to the central lacteal, shorten the villus rhythmically during digestion and may have a pumping action on the lacteals which speeds the passage of the lymph. The lymphatics often contain droplets of fat as they are the main pathway for lipid absorption (fig. 32.34).

DUODENUM

The wall of the first part of the duodenum feels thin because it lacks circular folds. The villi, however, begin immediately at the pyloroduodenal junction and are leaf-shaped. The crypts also begin at the junction and resemble those of the jejunum. Additional glands, which developed as downgrowths from the crypts and invaded the underlying muscularis mucosae to lie within the submucosa, are a distinguishing feature of the duodenum. These **duodenal (Brunner's) glands** are numerous in the first part and diminish towards the end. They are branched, coiled glands which secrete alkaline mucus into the duodenum

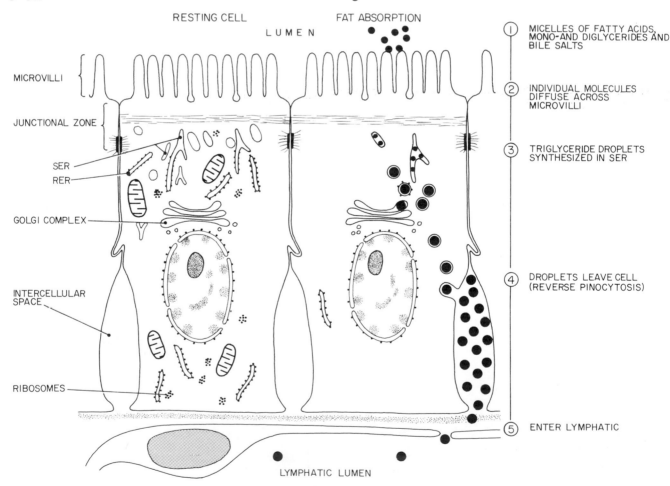

FIG. 32.34. Fat absorption across the columnar epithelial cells of a villus (p. 32.43).

and thus reduce the acidity of the gastric chyme. Duodenal contents are made alkaline by the large amounts of pancreatic juice secreted into the second part. However, in the presence of a large acid secretion this local defence mechanism may prove inadequate and, as might be expected, it is in the first part of the duodenum that peptic ulceration may develop.

ILEUM

The general structure of the ileum is similar to that of the jejunum and the transition between them is gradual. The bulk of absorption occurs in the jejunum, although there is some regional specialization, e.g. vitamin B_{12} is only absorbed in the distal part of the ileum. The villi of the ileum are less numerous and contain more goblet cells but fewer columnar absorptive cells than those in the jejunum.

Lymphoid tissue

Small lymphoid nodules, 0.5–3 mm in diameter, are found in the lamina propria throughout the small intestine. They become more numerous as one goes down it and in the ileum may form conspicuous clusters. These may be several centimetres in length and extend into the submucosa and overlying epithelium, and are known as Peyer's patches. Whereas in mammals the intestinal lymphoid tissue is spread diffusely along the length of the small intestine, in birds it is concentrated into a single organ, the bursa of Fabricius. As described on p. 29.15, removal of the bursa is a powerful experimental tool and its use led the way to the discovery of the importance of the intestinal lymphoid tissue in the defence mechanism of the whole body.

An account of the absorptive functions of the small intestine is given on p. 32.42.

LARGE INTESTINE

The large intestine begins at the ileocaecal sphincter and ends at the anus (fig. 32.9). It consists of the following parts:

(1) caecum and vermiform appendix,
(2) ascending colon and hepatic flexure,
(3) transverse colon and splenic flexure,
(4) descending colon,
(5) sigmoid or pelvic colon,
(6) rectum,
(7) anal canal.

The proximal half, as far as the splenic flexure, absorbs water and electrolytes from the fluid chyme which enters through the ileocaecal sphincter. The distal colon, beyond the splenic flexure, stores the formed faeces until they are excreted.

As the name implies, the large intestine is usually wider than the small intestine. But this is not always true, and commonly the descending colon when empty after defaecation is narrower. Several other features characterize the large intestine. The **taeniae coli** are three whitish longitudinal muscle bands which start at the base of the appendix and run along the caecum and entire colon to the upper end of the rectum, where they spread out to form two broad bands of muscle, one on the anterior, the other on the posterior, wall of the rectum. The tension of these muscle bands puckers the large intestine and, with the activity of the circular layer of muscle, forms **haustra** or sacculations (fig. 32.31). The appendices epiploicae are little fat-filled pouches of peritoneum that are scattered over the surface of the large intestine.

Gross anatomy

CAECUM

The caecum is a wide cul-de-sac of gut below the **ileocaecal sphincter** (fig. 32.35), lying in the right iliac fossa. Commonly it is completely invested in peritoneum and hangs free, but sometimes two vertical folds connect it to the posterior abdominal wall creating a **retrocaecal fossa** (fig. 32.12). Occasionally this recess extends upwards behind the ascending colon to become the retrocolic recess.

VERMIFORM APPENDIX

This worm-shaped appendage is developmentally the apex of the caecum (p. 32.59), but in the adult it opens on the posteromedial wall of the caecum inferior to the ileocaecal sphincter (fig. 32.36).

The appendix is less than 1 cm thick and usually 6–8 cm long, but length may vary from 2–20 cm. The **meso-appendix** is a peritoneal fold derived from the left layer of the mesentery which crosses posterior to the ileum to reach the base of the appendix. A second, bloodless fold joins the antimesenteric border of the ileum to the

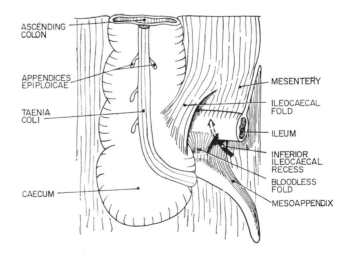

FIG. 32.35. Caecum and appendix

caecum, anterior to the mesoappendix. These two folds enclose the **inferior ileocaecal recess.**

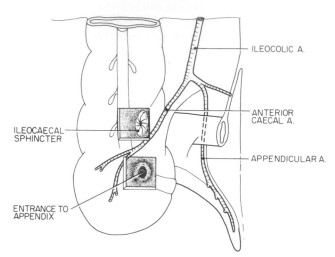

ILEOCOLIC A.

ANTERIOR
CAECAL A.

ILEOCAECAL
SPHINCTER

APPENDICULAR A.

ENTRANCE TO
APPENDIX

FIG. 32.36. Blood vessels of caecum and appendix.

The **superior ileocaecal recess** lies anterior to the terminal ileum and the bloodless fold, but behind a third fold which carries the anterior caecal artery from the mesentery to the anterior aspect of the caecum.

The appendix is freely mobile as the narrow mesoappendix exerts little restraint, and may adopt any position centred on its attachment to the caecum. In Wakeley's famous studies of 10 000 cases the commonest position was **retrocaecal** or **retrocolic** (61 per cent), while of the remainder about one third were **pelvic**. Less than 5 per cent of the total were either subcaecal or related to the ileum. Gravity probably explains the high incidence of pelvic appendices, but the preponderance of retrocaecal cases may indicate that the appendix is less free than commonly described. It may lie within one of the three peritoneal recesses, which tends to localize infection in appendicitis.

Often the best method of finding the appendix surgically is to trace the anterior taenia down the ascending colon over the caecum to its beginning at the base of the appendix. The variable position of the appendix results in equally variable relations. A pelvic appendix may come into relation with the ureter in either sex, and with the ovary and uterine tube in the female. An inflamed retrocolic appendix may cause few symptoms other than diarrhoea due to irritation of the colon.

ASCENDING COLON

The ascending colon is continuous with the upper end of the caecum and extends up as far as the right lobe of the liver. Peritoneum covers its front and sides, but behind it lies on the posterior abdominal wall (fig. 32.12). A peritoneal fold, the right phrenicocolic ligament, connects the hepatic flexure to the diaphragm, but the flexure is not completely fixed in position and descends with the liver during inspiration. The colon has only limited mobility as it usually lacks a mesentery.

The **right lateral paracolic gutter** separates the colon from the abdominal wall, and the **right medial paracolic gutter** is occupied by coils of jejunum above and ileum below (fig. 32.15). Anteriorly it is in contact with the anterior abdominal wall or is covered by the omentum or small intestine (fig. 32.10).

The ascending, transverse and descending parts of the colon all possess the characteristics of the large intestine, namely haustra, taeniae and appendices epiploicae, but the haustra are most pronounced on the transverse colon (fig. 32.37).

TRANSVERSE COLON

The transverse colon begins at the hepatic flexure low in the right hypochondrium and arches across the abdomen to the splenic flexure high in the left hypochondrium (fig. 32.9 and fig. 32.37). Since the vertical parts of the colon lie in the **paravertebral gutters** well posterior to the vertebral bodies the transverse colon curves forwards as well as downwards (fig. 32.15). The splenic flexure is more acute than the hepatic, and is almost in a sagittal plane so that its two limbs are superimposed in an anteroposterior view of the abdomen.

Peritoneal relations. These are complex and are more readily understood after its development has been described (p. 32.59). The first few centimetres or hepatic flexure has peritoneal relationships similar to the ascending colon, being invested completely except posteriorly where it lies directly on the right kidney and second part of duodenum (fig. 32.29). Antero-superiorly the flexure is in contact with the liver and gall bladder. Medial to the duodenum the transverse colon acquires a mesentery, the mesocolon, which is fixed along the entire anterior surface of the pancreas. The posterior wall of the greater omentum is attached to the antimesenteric border of the transverse colon. During development the pouch-like dorsal mesogastrium expands downwards over the upper surface of the transverse colon and mesocolon. The adjacent layers of peritoneum fuse so that in the adult the omentum, which is derived from the mesogastrium, is attached to the colon and not the posterior abdominal wall (figs. 32.13 and 32.69).

Visceral Relations. The posterior surface of the transverse colon faces into the infracolic compartment of the greater sac of peritoneum (fig. 32.13) and lies on the third part of duodenum, the mesentery containing the superior mesenteric vessels, and the first few coils of jejunum (fig. 32.9). The anterior surface faces into the cavity of the greater omentum which is part of the lesser peritoneal sac, and is related to the posterior surface of the stomach. Observe that at both ends of the mesocolon the lateral borders of the greater omentum are attached vertically to the anterior

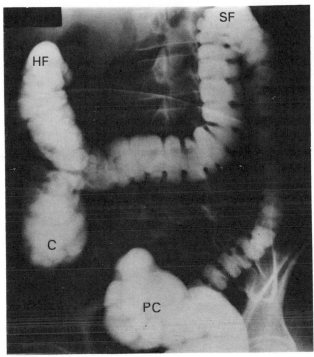

FIG. 32.37. Radiograph of large intestine (left anterior oblique view). A barium enema fills large bowel. The appendix is not visible. The splenic flexure (SF) is opened out because of oblique view and it is higher than the hepatic flexure (HF), caecum (C), pelvic colon (PC). Courtesy of Dr C.K. Warwick.

surface of the mesocolon and transverse colon, so that the flexures are outside the lesser sac. The splenic flexure is related to the diaphragm anteriorly and the spleen posteriorly (fig. 32.9).

DESCENDING COLON

The descending colon runs down from the splenic flexure on the posterior abdominal wall, crosses the iliac crest to enter the left iliac fossa and curves medially to end at the brim of the true pelvis, where it becomes the sigmoid colon. Peritoneum covers its sides and front, but its posterior wall rests on the structures in the posterior abdominal wall. The left phrenicocolic ligament is a peritoneal fold running from the diaphragm to the splenic flexure which fixes the position of the flexure and partly supports the spleen. The descending colon is fairly fixed.

The **paracolic gutters** are similar to those of the ascending colon. The omentum and jejuno-ileum cover it anteriorly, except in the iliac fossa where it may be related directly to the abdominal wall (fig. 32.10).

The descending and sigmoid colon constitute a storage unit which gradually fills with formed faeces from the proximal colon, and after an interval of some hours is emptied rapidly during defaecation. Obviously the size of the normal descending colon varies considerably; in a constipated patient it may be distended with hard faeces,

because although normally there is negligible absorption of water from the faeces beyond the splenic flexure, further absorption does occur when faeces remains in the storage unit for long periods. In a thin constipated person, the descending colon can be palpated.

SIGMOID COLON

The sigmoid colon is mobile and convoluted, and has a mesentery. The root of the mesocolon forms an inverted V attached first along the pelvic brim and then on the front of the sacrum (fig. 32.38). As part of the faecal storage unit, the sigmoid colon varies in size; when empty it may lie entirely within the true pelvis. In the pelvis the sigmoid colon occupies the pararectal fossae between the rectum and lateral pelvic walls, and the rectovesical or rectovaginal fossa anteriorly. As it fills it rises out of the pelvis usually posterior to the coils of terminal ileum.

RECTUM

The rectum, following the sigmoid colon, starts opposite the third piece of the sacrum and follows its curve through the posterior part of the pelvis to the pelvic floor. The rectum turns sharply backwards as it pierces the pelvic diaphragm at the junction with the anal canal (figs. 32.13 and 32.38).

The rectum has a broad band of longitudinal muscle anteriorly and posteriorly and lacks sacculations and appendices epiploicae; its dilated midpiece is the ampulla. The internal surface of the rectum is smooth except for three narrow crescentic transverse folds which project into the lumen, and serve as useful landmarks. The sites of these 'valves' are visible on the external surface as indentations.

The rectum is usually empty, but fills with faeces prior to defaecation. This stretches the rectal wall and reflexly stimulates the visceral muscle which contracts and expels the faeces. Thus the rectum has a function different from that of the storage unit described previously. The upper part of the rectum is enclosed in peritoneum except where it

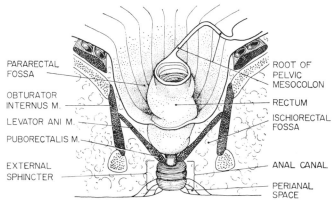

FIG. 32.38. Coronal section of rectum and anal canal.

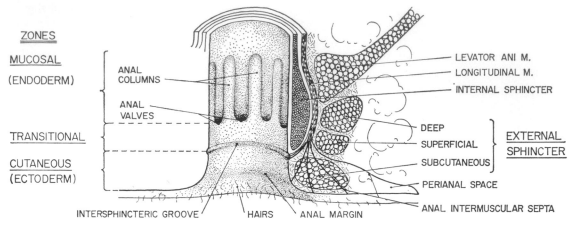

ZONES

MUCOSAL
(ENDODERM)

ANAL COLUMNS

ANAL VALVES

TRANSITIONAL

CUTANEOUS
(ECTODERM)

LEVATOR ANI M.
LONGITUDINAL M.
INTERNAL SPHINCTER

DEEP
SUPERFICIAL
SUBCUTANEOUS

EXTERNAL SPHINCTER

PERIANAL SPACE

ANAL INTERMUSCULAR SEPTA

INTERSPHINCTERIC GROOVE   HAIRS   ANAL MARGIN

FIG. 32.39. Coronal section of anal canal.

rests posteriorly on the areolar tissue covering the sacrum and emerging roots of the sacral plexus. Laterally, coils of the ileum or sigmoid colon may occupy the pararectal fossa. Lower down the rectum is extraperitoneal, and is related laterally to the sloping upper surfaces of the levator ani muscles. The pelvic nerve plexus passes forward on either side of the rectum between it and the levator ani (fig. 32.55), carrying the nerve supply to bladder, and may be damaged in operations on the rectum. Anteriorly the rectum is related to coils of ileum and in the female to the uterus, rectovaginal pouch, posterior fornix of vagina and cervix uteri, and in the male to the rectovesical pouch, bladder, seminal vesicles, and the prostate.

ANAL CANAL

The terminal 3 cm of the gut is the anal canal which runs downwards and backwards from the lower end of the rectum to the anus. The angle between the rectum and anal canal is controlled by the **puborectalis muscle** (p. 21.31). This is the most medial portion of levator ani, and arises from the pubis, passes around the side of the rectum and unites with its fellow to form the puborectalis 'sling'. The normal tone of this voluntary muscle pulls the angle forwards exerting a sphincteric action on the gut.

The lining of the canal shows regional variations (fig. 32.39). The **anal (rectal) columns** are longitudinal ridges over the **mucosal zone** on the upper half of the canal. They contain the venous plexuses of the superior rectal vessels and are therefore a dark plum colour in life. The anal valves join the bases of adjacent anal columns enclosing little pockets, the anal sinuses. The valves are probably the remnants of the anal membrane (p. 32.59) and their upper sinuous border is the **pectinate line**. The **transitional zone** below the pectinate line is shiny and bluish white. Near the lower end of the canal it gives way to the **cutaneous zone** which is lined with dull white or brownish skin.

Anal sphincters

The anal canal is guarded by a complex sphincteric mass composed of the puborectalis sling and the internal and external anal sphincters (fig. 32.39).

The **external sphincter**, composed of skeletal muscle, surrounds the anal canal throughout its entire length. It is in three parts. The subcutaneous part encircles the lower half of the canal. The superficial part consists of fibres which arise from the central tendon of the perineum and arch around the canal to insert into the anococcygeal ligament which connects the anus to the tip of the coccyx. The deep part surrounds the upper third of the canal and merges with levator ani. The circular layer of muscle in the rectum thickens at its lower end to form the **internal anal sphincter**, which is accordingly smooth involuntary muscle, and encircles the upper two-thirds of the anal canal.

The longitudinal muscle coat of the rectum becomes increasingly fibro-elastic as it passes down the anal canal between the external and internal sphincters. Finally it splits into **intermuscular anal septa** which attach to the intersphincteric groove medially, fanning out laterally, piercing the subcutaneous sphincter to insert into the perianal skin. The longitudinal coat is not sphincteric.

Relations of the anal canal

The **ischiorectal fossa** is the large fat-filled space lying lateral to the anal canal, below the levator ani muscle and medial to the ischium and obturator internus muscle (p. 21.32). The semi-fluid fat allows the rectum and anal canal to distend easily during defaecation. Infection may spread into the fossa from the adjacent anal canal, forming an ischiorectal abscess, which may attain a large size before causing pain, because the fossa is readily distended. A **perianal space** surrounds the lower end of the anal canal. It is limited laterally by the most lateral of the intermuscular septa, and medially by the wall of the anal canal below the site of attachment of the most medial intermuscular septum. This space contains the subcutaneous sphincter and some loculated fat, and inflammation in it causes considerable tension in these septa and is therefore very painful.

Histological structure of the large intestine

COLON AND CAECUM

The colon lacks circular folds and villi so that the mucosa is fairly smooth. It is pitted with **intestinal glands** which resemble those of the small intestine but have a much higher proportion of goblet cells, and normally lack Paneth cells. Numerous mitotic figures in the glands form new cells which pass upwards and renew the surface epithelium every few days. The absorptive cells have a microvillous brush border that is less developed than that of the small intestine. The lamina propria contains some lymphoid nodules and lies on the muscularis mucosae. The submucosa is less vascular than that of the small intestine, and the submucosal nerve plexus is smaller.

The muscle coat consists of two parts, a circular coat which is complete, and an outer longitudinal coat which is thickened locally to form the three taeniae coli (fig. 32.25). Between these longitudinal bands it is thin or even incomplete. The myenteric plexus lies within the muscle coat. As far as the splenic flexure, the parasympathetic component of this plexus is derived from the vagus and beyond that from the pelvic splanchnic nerves.

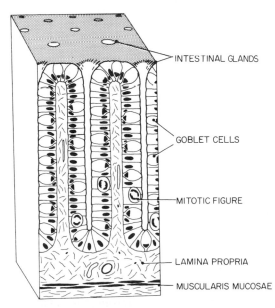

FIG. 32.40. Colon. The mucosa has a flat surface and simple tubular mucous glands.

The serosal coat of peritoneum varies along the colon, being practically complete where there is a mesentery as in the transverse or pelvic colon. The appendices epiploicae are little fat-filled projections of the serosal coat scattered over its surface.

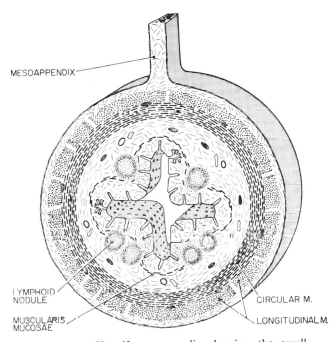

FIG. 32.41. Vermiform appendix showing the small lumen and abundant lymphoid nodules.

VERMIFORM APPENDIX

The appendix is a narrow blind sac with a small lumen which in youth is often irregular in outline due to folds, but with age it becomes more rounded as the underlying lymphoid tissue undergoes involution. The mucosa is similar to that of the small intestine, but has no villi. Only a few goblet cells are identifiable in the epithelium lining the glands; occasional Paneth cells and more numerous argentaffin cells are present at the base of the glands. These cells are present in the mucosa of the stomach and intestines, but are abundant in the terminal ileum and appendix, where argentaffin tumours are more frequent (vol. 3 19.72). Many lymphoid nodules lie in the lamina propria and give rise to a stream of lymphocytes which infiltrate the surface epithelium (fig. 32.41). The submucosa contains the deeper parts of the lymphoid nodules, and these split the muscularis mucosae. A submucosal nerve plexus is present. The inner circular coat is thick, and the outer longitudinal coat, unlike that of most of the large bowel, is complete because the taeniae coli as they are traced down the ascending colon and on to the caecum converge on the base of the appendix.

The serosa presents no special features, and is complete except over the mesoappendix.

RECTUM AND ANAL CANAL

The structure of the rectum is similar to that of the colon except that the taeniae spread out and form a broad longitudinal coat on the anterior and posterior walls of the rectum. Over the rectum and upper third of the anal canal, the mucosal epithelium is a typical colonic epithelium with many goblet cells and straight tubular mucous glands, but it becomes a stratified columnar epithelium for a short distance before becoming keratinized stratified squamous epithelium typical of true skin over the lower third of the canal.

Anal glands open between the anal columns on the posterior wall of the anal canal. Their secretory acini usually lie in the submucosa but may extend through the internal sphincter into the substance of the external anal sphincter. Infection of these glands is an important cause of ischiorectal abscess and fistula (vol. 3, p. 19.120).

Intestinal secretion

The secretions from the mucosa of the small and large intestines are increased by the direct mechanical stimulation from the presence of food. In the duodenum the secretion is mainly of mucus, whereas in the jejunum, ileum and colon, an isotonic fluid is secreted which is slightly alkaline. Some enzymes present in these secretions have come from the cells shed from the villi.

The most important secretions into the small intestine are from the pancreas and the liver and these organs and their contribution to the function of the alimentary tract are now described.

LIVER AND BILIARY SYSTEM

The liver is the largest gland in the body, and occupies the right hypochondrium (fig. 32.10). It is an important organ of intermediate metabolism and this role is described in chap. 33. It also has an exocrine secretion, the bile, which is conveyed to the duodenum by the biliary system (fig. 32.43).

The liver accounts for 5 per cent of total body weight at birth, and is largely responsible for the protuberant abdomen of infancy. As the growth rate slows during childhood there is a corresponding decline in metabolism and the liver becomes proportionately smaller until in the adult it is $2\frac{1}{2}$ per cent of body weight (1500 g).

The liver is soft because of its vascularity (one-fifth of liver volume is blood) and friable because of a very low connective tissue content. Lacerations of the liver are therefore dangerous because they bleed profusely and are difficult to repair; try stitching two halves of a table jelly together with needle and thread.

The friable nature of the liver is altered radically by embalming, but the hard liver of the cadaver is useful as it records permanently, in the form of surface impressions, the relations of neighbouring structures. These relations approximate to those in a living supine patient who has expired deeply.

Gross anatomy

The liver is wedge-shaped and is divided somewhat arbitrarily into four lobes by certain external features. The main division into a large right lobe and a smaller left lobe is marked by the **falciform ligament** on the anterior surface, and on the visceral and posterior surfaces by the fissures for the **ligamentum teres** and **ligamentum venosum**. The falciform ligament carries the ligamentum teres in its free border and is therefore continuous round the lower border of the liver with the fissure for the ligamentum teres, which in turn ascends on the visceral aspect of the liver to end at the left end of the porta hepatis. Superior to the porta hepatis the fissure for the ligamentum venosum is the boundary between the two lobes (fig. 32.17). The quadrate lobe is an integral part of the right lobe bounded by the inferior border of liver, gall bladder bed, porta hepatis, and fissure of the ligamentum teres. The caudate lobe also belongs to the right lobe, and appears on the posterior surface of liver between the groove for the inferior vena cava and the fissure for the ligamentum venosum. It is connected to the main mass of the right lobe superficially by the caudate process, which forms the roof of the epiploic foramen (figs. 32.17 and 32.42).

The **portal vein,** carrying blood from the gut, enters the liver at the **porta hepatis** (fig. 32.42). It divides repeatedly within the liver into small branches which finally enter an anastomosing system of sinusoids. In the hepatic circulation 80 per cent of the blood is portal, and the remaining 20 per cent arrives in the hepatic artery. The **hepatic artery** also divides repeatedly within the liver, sending branches with those of the portal vein to the sinusoids. The sinusoids therefore contain mixed venous and arterial blood, which percolates past the hepatic parenchymal cells or hepatocytes before entering the central veins. These central veins are tributaries of the hepatic veins, which drain blood from the liver into the inferior vena cava (figs. 32.44 and 32.45).

The lobes are useful topographically, but are neither vascular nor biliary units. For example, although the right lobe is much bigger than the left, the main left and right **hepatic ducts** that emerge from the porta hepatis have the same diameter, showing that the left hepatic duct drains half the liver tissue. The cleavage plane between the two drainage areas passes from the groove for the inferior vena cava and gall bladder bed posteriorly, to cut the anterior surface to the right of the falciform ligament, and therefore the left duct receives the bile from part of the right lobe and the entire left lobe. These two halves of the liver have been further subdivided into about a dozen segments. Each segment drains into a tributary of the

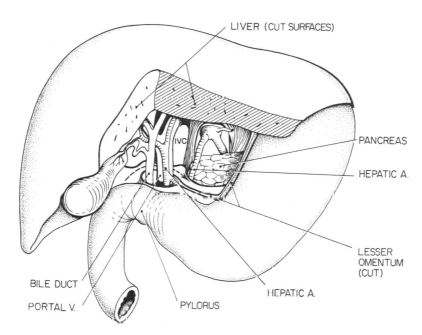

LIVER (CUT SURFACES)

IVC

PANCREAS

HEPATIC A.

LESSER
OMENTUM
(CUT)

BILE DUCT

PORTAL V.

PYLORUS

HEPATIC A.

FIG. 32.42. A portion of liver has been resected to reveal the three structures in the free border of the lesser omentum. The broken arrow passes through the epiploic foramen.

hepatic ducts and is supplied by a corresponding branch of the hepatic artery and of the portal vein, and is both a biliary and vascular unit. These **liver segments** are not easily defined, because they are not surrounded by connective tissue septa, but as they are fairly constant in position their discovery has been of value to surgeons who can now perform local resection of certain segments with only minimal damage to adjacent hepatic tissue. Some of the liver segments cannot be removed separately, because they contain vessels or ducts going to other segments, which would therefore be damaged. In practice, therefore, several segments may have to be removed along with the diseased one, in order to leave only undamaged liver with an intact circulation and duct system.

POSITION AND RELATIONS

The bulk of the liver lies in the right hypochondrium, under cover of the lower ribs which protect it, but it also extends to the left across the epigastrium in the substernal angle (fig. 32.10). In the cadaver, the upper surface of the liver reaches to the 5th right rib, crosses close to the xiphisternal junction and is inferior to the 5th left rib. This cadaveric position is somewhat higher than that of the living supine patient who has expired fully. The inferior border passes obliquely from the left across the substernal angle to intersect the right costal margin at the right margin of the rectus abdominis and then continues under cover of the ribs a little above the costal margin. On inspiration the liver descends with the diaphragm, bringing the entire lower border inferior to the costal margin.

The upper, lateral, anterior and posterior surfaces of the liver together form a smooth convex area which is moulded by the overlying diaphragm. The intraperitoneal subdiaphragmatic spaces intervene between the liver and diaphragm (fig. 32.16), but over the bare area the liver is devoid of peritoneum and in contact with diaphragm, upper pole of right kidney, and adrenal gland (fig. 32.12). The right pleural cavity and lung are important relations above the diaphragm, as disease may spread from the liver to the thorax. The lower ribs are also significant because fractured ribs may lacerate the underlying liver. Anteriorly the liver is related near the midline to the anterior abdominal wall. The extensive visceral surface is in contact with many structures, the left lobe with the oesophagus, stomach and lesser omentum, and the quadrate lobe with the first part of duodenum; finally the right lobe rests on the right kidney and hepatic flexure of the colon, separated only by the potential space of the hepatorenal pouch (fig. 32.17). It must be emphasized that these relations are only a rough guide to the changing ones in the living patient. In the upright posture, for example, a full stomach may descend by as much as 10 cm and then the pylorus and the first part of the duodenum are no longer related to the liver.

Anatomy of the biliary system

The biliary system or apparatus includes the ducts of the liver, which convey bile from within the liver to the duodenum, and the gall bladder which stores and concentrates bile.

The intrahepatic ducts collect the bile as it is formed into many tiny channels; these converge and form larger but fewer ducts until finally two main hepatic ducts emerge at the porta hepatis. These intrahepatic ducts are described more fully with the histology of the liver (p. 32.36).

The extrahepatic biliary system consists of the following structures (fig. 32.43):

  (1) right and left main hepatic ducts,
  (2) common hepatic duct,   (4) gall bladder,
  (3) bile duct,   (5) cystic duct.

The right and left main hepatic ducts, each draining half the liver, unite below the porta hepatis to form the common hepatic duct. This passes down in the free border of the lesser omentum for a few centimetres before receiving the cystic duct and becoming the bile duct. The bile duct leaves the lesser omentum and descends posterior to the first part of duodenum and then becomes embedded in the

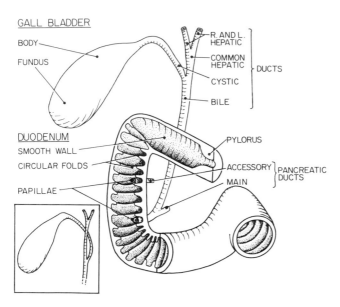

FIG. 32.43. Extrahepatic biliary apparatus. The smaller diagram shows a variation in which the cystic duct descends on the left side of the common hepatic duct before joining it.

back of the head of pancreas; there it curves laterally towards the posteromedial wall of the second part of the duodenum which it pierces obliquely to end on the duodenal papilla (figs. 32.29 and 32.43). Near its termination the bile duct joins the main pancreatic duct to form the **hepatopancreatic ampulla**, the ampulla of Vater, before opening into the duodenum.

There are many important relations of the biliary system. The common hepatic and bile ducts lie in the lesser omentum lateral to the hepatic artery and anterior to the portal vein. Hepatic lymph nodes, which surround the

biliary ducts near the porta hepatis, when enlarged by disease, may compress the ducts and obstruct the flow of bile. The bile duct is an immediate posterior relation of the first part of the duodenum and is occasionally involved in duodenal peptic ulceration. In this situation it is accompanied by the gastroduodenal artery and remains anterior to the portal vein.

GALL BLADDER

The silvery blue and pear-shaped gall bladder is found against the visceral surface of the liver along the right boundary of the quadrate lobe. The lower end, the **fundus**, is expanded, and the middle part, the **body**, tapers above to form the **neck**. The neck joins the stalk of the pear, the cystic duct, which ascends to the porta hepatis and then curves abruptly downwards into the lesser omentum, where it descends along the right side of the common hepatic duct for two or more centimetres before fusing with it.

The upper surface of the body of the gall bladder is in contact with the liver but peritoneum covers its sides and inferior surface (figs. 32.17 and 32.42). The fundus is invested completely in peritoneum and projects freely beyond the lower border of the liver, where it is related to the anterior abdominal wall, at the junction of the right costal margin and the lateral border of the rectus abdominis. Inferiorly the gall bladder rests on the duodenum and transverse colon. The position varies in the living, but in a recumbent patient the fundus descends below the costal margin on inspiration, and can then be palpated through the anterior abdominal wall if the gall bladder is distended.

The normal gall bladder is radiotranslucent but can be outlined by injecting into the bloodstream organic iodine compounds which are radio-opaque and are excreted in the bile. Its position varies with posture and respiration, and is lower in thin individuals. A normal fundus may be as high as the transpyloric plane or below the right iliac crest.

Variations of the biliary ducts
The biliary ducts are so variable that it is arguable whether a normal pattern can be described. Although of no physiological significance, some of these variations are important surgically. For example, the cystic duct must be tied and cut to remove the gall gladder; so if the cystic duct passes behind the common hepatic duct and then descends on its left side for some distance before joining it, the common hepatic duct may be tied in error (fig. 32.43).

Structure of the liver
The liver consists mainly of hepatocytes (glandular epithelium) and blood-filled sinusoidal capillaries, with little connective tissue.

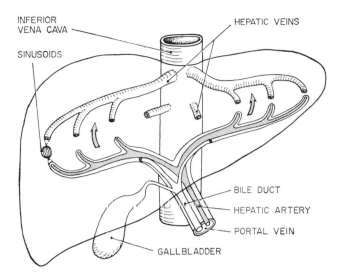

FIG. 32.44. Hepatic circulation. The liver receives a dual blood supply from the portal vein and hepatic artery. These two vessels end in the sinusoids that drain via the hepatic veins into the inferior vena cava.

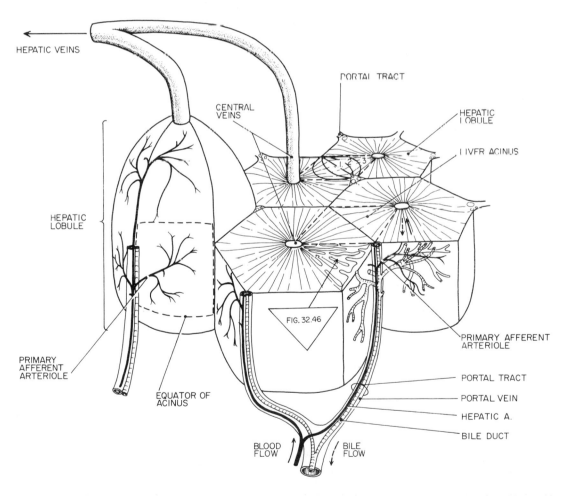

FIG. 32.45. Hepatic lobule. On section the liver parenchyma forms hexagonal or polygonal areas each with a central vein. Portal tracts lie between the areas. A classical lobule and a liver acinus are outlined.

The three structures which go through the porta hepatis are the hepatic bile duct, the portal vein and the hepatic artery (fig. 32.44). These three all divide progressively within the liver substance, but remain associated with each other and form the **portal tracts**, which are easily visible on the cut surface of the liver with a hand lens. The tributaries of the hepatic veins run separately within the liver, between the portal tracts, and are seen as isolated structures. The liver of the pig is often used to illustrate the basic structure of the liver because adjacent portal tracts are joined by fibrous septa, which divide the tissue into lobules. At the centre of each hexagonal or polygonal lobule is a tributary of the hepatic vein, the **central vein**.

Several portal tracts lie at the periphery of a single **hepatic lobule**, and each consists of a large branch of the portal vein, a smaller branch of the hepatic artery, a tributary of the hepatic bile ducts, and some lymphatic vessels, all embedded in collagenous connective tissue (fig. 32.45 and plate 32.1, facing p. 32.40). The blood vessels of the tract give off branches which pass between adjacent lobules and ramify into little vessels which enter the sinusoids. The sinusoids therefore carry mixed blood, part venous and part arterial, which flows into the central vein (plate 32.1). The sinusoids are surrounded by branching and anastomosing sheets of hepatocytes, to which they bring the products of digestion via the portal vein and oxygen via the hepatic artery. In man and other mammals there are no fibrous septa and the outlines of the lobule are not so clear.

The classical concept of a hepatic lobule is based on the venous drain at the centre, and has helped to explain the distribution of damaged areas within diseased livers in many instances, but sometimes only parts of a lobule are affected or adjacent parts of two lobules are damaged. The existence of a smaller unit, the **acinus**, is now established. This is the mass of tissue supplied by a **primary afferent branch** of the portal vein and hepatic artery. Each small portal tract gives off three branches which leave the connective tissue of the tract and running between the adjacent hepatic lobules, divide into terminal branches which enter the sinusoids of the lobules. Fig. 32.45 shows that the acinus is an irregular structure with a broad equator where the vessels enter, and two narrow extremities which end on two central veins. The fresh blood enters the centre of the acinus and then diverges, passing along the sinusoids towards each central vein. These sinusoids are surrounded by sheets of hepatic epithelial cells. The entire acinus can be divided arbitrarily into three zones. Zone 1 receives the fresh blood supply, while zone 3 receives blood that has percolated along the sinusoids and lost oxygen and other substances to the adjacent epithelial cells of zones 1 and 2 (fig. 32.47). The concept of zones is of value in interpreting liver disease; for example zone 3 is the most susceptible to hypoxia and this gives rise to a pattern of

damage which was inexplicable on the classical view of liver structure. Conversely certain toxic substances, carried in the hepatic artery or portal vein, might be expected to act on zone 1 as they reach it first (vol. 2, pp. 25.13 & 33).

HEPATIC EPITHELIUM (HEPATOCYTES)

This is arranged in the form of sheets one cell thick, which are fenestrated and branch and anastomose with each other. In general the sheets converge on the central vein,

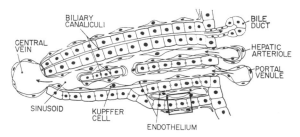

FIG. 32.46. Half a liver acinus. Blood enters the sinusoids at the equator of the acinus and percolates past the plates of hepatocytes to enter the central vein. The hepatocytes secrete bile into the intercellular network of canaliculi which drain into biliary ductules. Rectangular area is shown in high magnification in fig. 32.48.

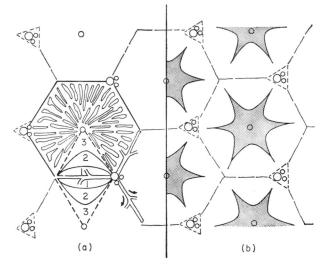

FIG. 32.47. (a) The acinar zones, (b) zonal necrosis of liver acini, showing the pattern produced by death of cells in zone 3 of acini.

and the spaces between them are filled with sinusoids. Each hepatocyte has two surfaces that face sinusoids and several surfaces that are in contact with other hepatocytes. The bile which is formed by the hepatocytes runs in intercellular channels within the sheets towards the equator of the acinus to enter ductules which unite to form the tributary of the bile duct in the adjacent portal tract. Thus the flow of blood in the acinus is from the equator to the central vein, whereas the flow of bile is in the opposite direction.

The hepatocytes (figs. 32.48 and 13.17) where they face the sinusoids are covered with microvilli, which project into a narrow extravascular space between them and the sinusoidal endothelium (the space of Disse). Because the sinusoids are fenestrated and lack a continuous basal lamina, this extravascular space contains plasma which directly bathes the plasma membranes of the hepatocytes. Fluid is removed from the extravascular space by the lymphatics which end blindly in the connective tissue of

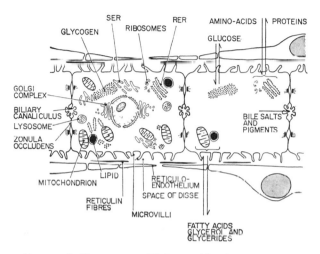

FIG. 32.48. Hepatocytes. High magnification view of rectangular area in fig. 32.46. Two surfaces of the hepatocyte face a sinusoid across the space of Disse. The remaining surfaces are contiguous with adjacent hepatocytes and are grooved to form a biliary canaliculus. The cytology and main functions are indicated. SER and RER represent smooth and rough endoplasmic reticulum.

the portal tracts. The liver is the largest single producer of lymph, which is rich in protein. The products of digestion which are brought in the portal blood, as well as the oxygen in the arterial blood, cross the extravascular space and the absorptive surface of the hepatocyte. In addition many substances formed within the cell are secreted in the opposite direction into the sinusoid. The lateral surfaces of the cell, which are contiguous with adjacent hepatocytes, have near their middle a groove which together with the similar groove in the neighbouring cell forms a cylindrical channel, the **biliary canaliculus.** The walls of these canaliculi also have microvilli and their membranes are rich in ATPase suggesting that some of the bile constituents are actively transported. The bile canaliculi form an anastomosing and branching system in which the flow of bile is away from the central vein towards the periphery of the lobule or equator of the acinus where it enters biliary ductules.

Hepatocytes have an extensive and dispersed rough endoplasmic reticulum. The Golgi complex lies between the nucleus and the biliary canaliculus, i.e. between the nucleus and the exocrine secretory surface as in other exocrine cells. Glycogen is stored in clusters of granules which are 50 nm in diameter and so larger than the ribosomes (plate 32.1, facing p. 32.40). There is an extensive smooth endoplasmic reticulum consisting of a network of interconnected tubules. This is diminished when the glycogen store is depleted by starvation, but expands on refeeding and glycogen granules first appear in close relation to it. Lipid droplets are present in normal hepatocytes and may increase in disease. Mitochondria are scattered throughout the cell. Lysosomes, first discovered in the hepatocyte, lie near the biliary canaliculi and vary in appearance according to whether they contain altered mitochondria, foreign material or granular debris (p.13.8). Hepatocytes in zone 1, where blood supply is richest and aerobic metabolism predominates, contain many mitochondria and so have a high content of succinic dehydrogenase and cytochrome oxidase. In contrast, the cells in zone 3 have fewer mitochondria but a more extensive rough endoplasmic reticulum and are presumably more active in protein synthesis. Such differences between the cells of each zone, together with their differing blood supply, may account for their differences in susceptibility to noxious agents.

CONNECTIVE TISSUE

The liver has a tough fibrous tissue capsule, which invests the vessels and the hepatic ducts as they enter the liver. In a reduced form it continues to support the portal tracts as they branch so that even the smallest tracts lie in a little collagenous tissue. A little connective tissue also surrounds the central vein (plate 32.1). The lobule is supported by fine reticular fibres lying in the space of Disse. In cirrhosis of the liver fibroblasts lay down large amounts of collagen which forms scars; the lobular architecture of the liver is destroyed and there is interference with its blood flow.

EPITHELIAL TURNOVER

The number of mitotic figures in the adult liver is very low, but the response of the liver to reduction of its mass is prompt and effective. In rats 80 per cent of the liver can be removed experimentally and complete restitution occurs by proliferation of new cells. The most active and earliest site of proliferation is in zone 1, where the blood supply is richest. The ability of the human liver to recover from damage to the cells by disease or injury is great and may be of the above order.

SINUSOIDS

Like other sinusoids, those of the liver are lined with cells which are potentially phagocytic. Most of these cells appear as endothelial cells with flattened nuclei, but a small number have rounded nuclei and long radiating processes of cytoplasm which give them a stellate shape. These are the Kupffer cells which are rich in lysosomes. Intravenous injections of dye particles increase the proportion of endothelial cells which appear as typical phagocytic Kupffer cells; this suggests there is only one cell type in the wall of the sinusoids. Normally these cells do not destroy effete red blood cells, as this process is confined to the sinusoids of the spleen. But if the spleen is removed, then the liver sinusoids assume this function.

In fetal life the liver is an active site of erythropoiesis, but this normally ceases about birth. Stem cells persist in the liver, and in certain diseases these may cause erythropoiesis in the adult liver.

Histological structure of the biliary system

BILIARY PASSAGES

In the portal tracts the bile ducts are lined with a clear cubical epithelium and some goblet mucous cells are found in the larger ducts.

The extrahepatic ducts have a simple columnar epithelium with some goblet cells and sparse mucous glands. There is a thin coat of smooth muscle consisting of an inner circular and outer longitudinal layer, similar to that of the rest of the gut. This muscle is innervated by the vagus and when in spasm causes the excruciating pain of biliary colic. The bile duct has several longitudinal mucosal folds when empty, as it is very distensible.

GALL BLADDER

This stores and concentrates hepatic bile. The mucosa has many irregular folds and is extremely vascular (fig. 32.49).

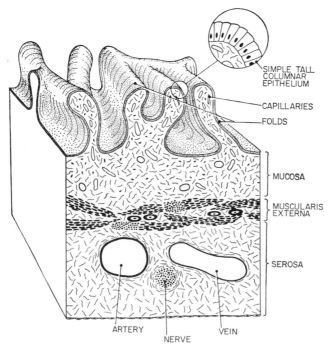

FIG. 32.49. Gall bladder. The mucosa is much folded and has a simple tall columnar epithelium.

The simple tall columnar epithelium, which concentrates the bile by absorption of salts and water, has **inferolateral folds** and a poorly-developed microvillous border (fig. 32.50). The former is of interest, because it is similar to that of the large intestine which also absorbs water and ions. There are a few mucous glands near its neck, which, together with the scattered glands and goblet cells already described, form the mucous component of the bile.

There is no muscularis mucosae, but there is a thick and vascular lamina propria. The muscular coat consists of loose bundles arranged in ill-defined longitudinal and transverse layers. The serosa is thick with many large vessels and nerves. Although these include vagal branches that are motor to the gall bladder, the main stimulus to contraction is the hormone CPZ (p. 32.42).

FILLING OF THE GALL BLADDER

The bile duct is a wide distensible tube, containing little smooth muscle, except at its lower end where it is surrounded by a well-developed **biliary sphincter** (fig. 32.51). There is an other around the hepatopancreatic ampulla, the **sphincter of Oddi**. The third part of this complex is the pancreatic duct sphincter, which is often poorly developed or absent.

Bile is continuously secreted by the liver, but is required in the intestine to complete its digestive function only periodically when food is ingested. During the interdigestive phase, the tone of the sphincter of Oddi is high and bile is diverted up the cystic duct into the gall bladder which relaxes to accommodate the inflow of bile. Here it is concentrated by a process of selective reabsorption until about one tenth of its volume remains (table 32.1).

TABLE 32.1. Approximate composition of hepatic and gall bladder bile. From Wrong O.M. *et al.* (1970). In *Biochemical Disorders in Human Disease*, 3rd Edition: ed. Thompson R.H.S. & Wootton I.D.P. Edinburgh: Churchill Livingstone.

	Hepatic bile mmol/l	Gall bladder bile mmol/l
Na^+	150	150
K^+	10	12
Cl^-	95	17
HCO_3^-	22	10
Bile anions	20–30	150–210
Osmolality mosmol/kg	285	285

In experiments in which hepatic bile was introduced into the gall bladder of a dog, its volume decreased at a rate of 16 per cent per hour. Concentration of sodium salts and bilirubin increased, but those of chloride and bicarbonate decreased. The bile salts and bilirubin recovered were identical with those first introduced, so that the increase in concentration was due to a reduction in volume. In addition, hepatic bile, gall bladder bile and plasma remained isosmotic at all times, and the pH of the bile in the gall bladder fell.

By using an *in vitro* gall bladder preparation into which simple salt solutions of various compositions can be introduced, it has been shown that concentration of the gall bladder contents is due to the active transport outward into the blood of Na^+, Cl^- and HCO_3^- in isotonic proportions. It is an active process because transport occurs against a concentration gradient (there is virtually

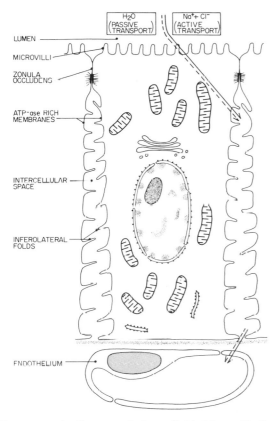

FIG. 32.50. A diagram of the gall bladder epithelium, showing lateral infolding.

no potential difference across the gall bladder wall) and is abolished by cyanide and under anaerobic conditions.

Two questions arise from these observations:

(1) How does the transport of Na^+, Cl^- and HCO_3^- and water in isotonic proportions occur? It has been proposed that the ions are actively transferred across the gall bladder and water follows passively on the osmotic gradient so created. If this is so, why do the ions not simply diffuse away into the blood before water can follow? A model has been proposed (fig. 32.50). The gall bladder cells are united solely at their apical poles (zona occludens) with the side membranes of the two adjacent cells forming a long narrow channel, open only at the basement membrane. Na^+ is transported actively at the closed end of this channel, a region rich in mitochondria, where it is pumped continuously into the inter-

cellular space. Water follows passively and osmotic equilibrium is achieved before the transported fluid reaches the basement membrane. Evidence in support of this theory is that the lateral intercellular spaces are distended when cells are transporting fluid, but closed when transport is inhibited.

(2) Why do the contents of the gall bladder remain isotonic? As the contents of the gall bladder become more concentrated the number of particles per unit volume remains constant. This is due to the remarkable property of the bile salts to form micelles, molecular aggregates with which the sodium combines to form fewer osmotically active particles.

Two other substances are also secreted in the bile which are only sparingly soluble in water. These are cholesterol and lecithin, which are held in solution by the bile salts in micelles. The amount of cholesterol which can be held in solution is determined by the relative amounts of bile salt and lecithin present in the micelle. As cholesterol is near its saturation point, disturbances of the equilibrium between salt and lecithin may lead to the precipitation of cholesterol and the formation of gall stones. This is discussed on p. 33.7 and in vol. 3, p. 20.39.

CONTROL OF BILIARY SECRETION

The secretion of bile from the liver is increased by vagal and inhibited by sympathetic stimulation. However, these influences are relatively unimportant when compared with other factors. Diversion of bile to the exterior, through a fistula, results in a reduction of the volume of the bile secreted due to the interruption of the enterohepatic circulation of the bile salts (p. 33.14).

The most important stimulants of biliary secretion are the bile salts themselves, and for this action they are termed **choleretics**. Secretin and cholecystokinin-pancreozymin, two polypeptide hormones released from the duodenal mucosa (p. 32.42), also act as choleretics though less so than the bile salts.

EMPTYING OF THE GALL BLADDER

Within half an hour of taking a meal the gall bladder contracts, the biliary sphincters relax and bile pours into the duodenum. Both nervous and hormonal mechanisms are involved. The nervous stimuli occur as part of the cephalic phase and are mediated by the vagus. Then, when acid chyme enters the duodenum from the stomach, cholecystokinin-pancreozymin is released from the mucosa into the bloodstream and causes the gall bladder to contract, i.e. the hormone acts in this instance as a cholecystagogue. In clinical practice the concentrating action of the gall bladder may be tested by the administration of iodine compounds. These are secreted by the liver and, if the gall bladder is functioning normally, they are concentrated and become radio-opaque allowing the organ to be visualized by X-rays. The contraction of the gall bladder stimulated by cholecystokinin can also be examined on radiographs under the same conditions.

PANCREAS

The second main accessory digestive gland is the pancreas. This mixed exocrine and endocrine gland is elongated, and stretches across the posterior abdominal wall from the duodenum to the spleen. The exocrine tissue forms the great mass of the gland and secretes the pancreatic juice into the duodenum. The endocrine tissue consists of the tiny spherical **islets of Langerhans** which account for less than 1 per cent of the whole. Their structure and function are described on p. 27.39.

Gross anatomy

The pancreas is a soft, lumpy organ with a large head, long body and tapering tail. The head lies within the concavity of the duodenum, and inferomedially gives off the uncinate process which passes behind the superior

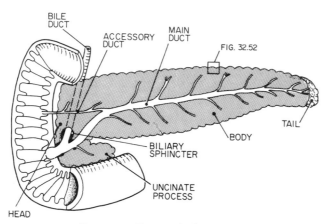

FIG. 32.51. Pancreatic duct system.

mesenteric vessels (figs. 32.29 & 51). The body extends leftwards from the upper part of the head across the vertebral column and on to the left kidney, where the tail turns forward into the lienorenal ligament to end at the hilum of the spleen.

The head and body of the pancreas are retroperitoneal and their posterior surface is directly related to several important structures. The head of the pancreas rests on the bile duct and inferior vena cava, and its neck on the origin of the portal vein. The body lies on the aorta and the left adrenal, renal vein, and left kidney. The splenic vein is also a posterior relation of the body of pancreas and the tortuous splenic artery runs along the upper border. The tail is surrounded by peritoneum as it lies in the lienorenal ligament. As the pancreas is retroperitoneal

the anterior surface is covered by peritoneum, but the root of the transverse mesocolon is attached horizontally along the anterior border. Above this border, the pancreas is related to the lesser sac and stomach, and below it to the greater sac, small intestine and mesocolon or, if the latter is shallow, the transverse colon (fig. 32.13).

The **main pancreatic duct** begins at the tail and runs towards the head, receiving large oblique interlobular tributaries along its course (fig. 32.51). At the head, the main duct turns first caudally and then to the right to join the bile duct. The upper portion of the head is drained separately in most instances by the **accessory pancreatic duct** which runs horizontally and opens into the duodenum proximal to the main duct.

Histological structure (fig. 32.52)

The exocrine pancreas is a compound tubulo-acinar gland, enclosed in a very delicate fibrous capsule, through which the glandular lobules are readily observed. The capsule sends septa into the gland which divide it into lobules.

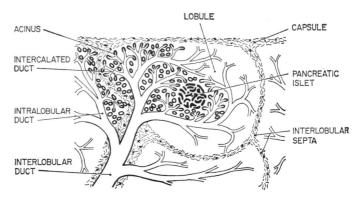

FIG. 32.52. Pancreas. This low power diagram shows the typical features of an exocrine gland. The scattered islets or endocrine portion of pancreas constitute only 1 per cent of the total mass.

The lobule is made up of many acini, each draining into an intercalated duct. The acinar cells are excellent examples of zymogenic (enzyme-secreting) cells (fig. 32.53). They are grouped around the lumen, into which they discharge their secretory granules. The lumen often appears to be filled by one or more cells with clear cytoplasm. These centro-acinar cells are the flattened epithelial cells at the start of the intercalated duct, which is partly invaginated into the acinus. The intercalated ducts unite forming the intralobular ducts, which are shorter than those of the salivary glands, and therefore appear to be less numerous. The intralobular ducts join interlobular ducts in septa alongside the incoming vessels and nerves. The larger interlobular ducts enter the main duct obliquely, in a herring bone pattern. The duct epithelium increases in height as the ducts become larger and in the main duct is a tall columnar epithelium with a few mucous glands.

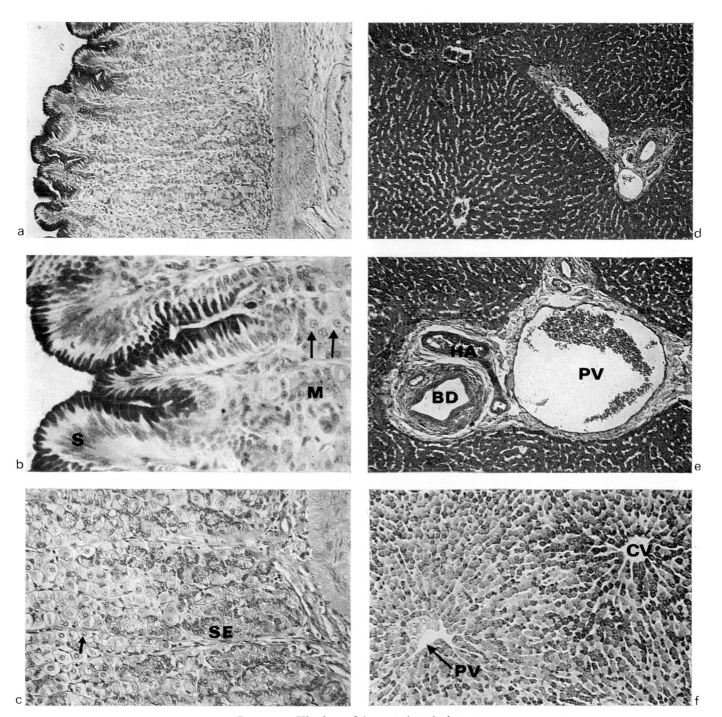

PLATE 32.1. Histology of the gastrointestinal tract.

Body of stomach (dog). PAS, haem. & aurantia. The lumen of the stomach is to the left in these photographs, and is visible in (a). (Cf. fig. 32.21.)

(a) Main gastric glands. Mucus in surface and mucous neck cells is red, parietal cells are yellow, and the serous pepsin cells have a blue cytoplasm.

(b) Gastric pits and upper portion of main gastric glands. Surface cells (S), parietal cells (arrows) and adjacent mucous neck cells (M).

(c) Base of gland. Serous cells (SE) predominate, but parietal cells (arrow) are also visible.

Liver (cat). Haem. & eosin.

(d) A liver lobule with central vein occupies the lower left quadrant and several portal tracts lie above and to the right.

(e) A portal tract with large portal vein (PV), branch of bile duct (BD) and obliquely cut branch of hepatic artery (HA).

Liver (cat). PAS & haem.

(f) The stored glycogen in the hepatocytes is stained purple. The small portal tract in the left of field contains a branch of the portal vein (PV) which opens into several sinusoids. In the right half of the field, sinusoids converge upon and terminate at a central vein (CV).

Nerve and blood supply

There are many nerve fibres and parasympathetic ganglion cells in the interlobular septa which accompany the larger ducts. Postganglionic fibres end on the acini and islets. The sympathetic component is small and distributed mainly to the vessels. Visceral afferent fibres run with the sympathetic fibres.

The pancreas is a vascular organ with a rich capillary bed. The endocrine islets are particularly well supplied, so that a vascular injection makes the islets appear as berries on the stalks of their supplying vessels.

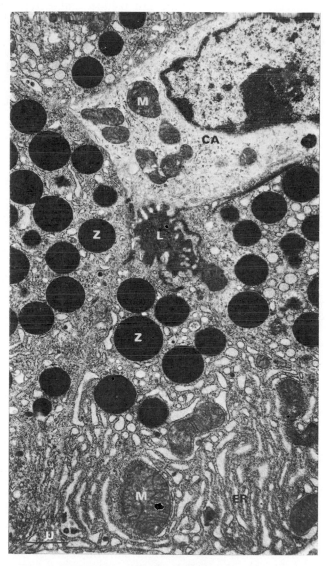

FIG. 32.53. Exocrine pancreas (guinea-pig). This view of an acinus shows the central lumen (L) surrounded by several exocrine acinar cells rich in granular endoplasmic reticulum (ER), mitochondria (M), and numerous secretory zymogen granules (Z). The lumen contains secreted zymogen. A single centro-acinar cell (CA) with pale cytoplasm containing several mitochondria (M), also abuts on the lumen. (× 11 250). Courtesy of Dr. Katherine Carr.

Pancreatic secretion

The exocrine secretion of the pancreas, the pancreatic juice, is secreted by the serous acinar cells and passes into the duodenum through the two pancreatic ducts. Experimentally, the secretion may be studied in the dog by providing the animal with a duodenal fistula which is carefully positioned opposite the main pancreatic duct. A cannula can then be passed through the fistula into the duct, and pancreatic juice collected for study. Between observations, the pancreatic juice flows normally into the duodenum, and the animal is not deprived of the digestive functions of the secretion.

COMPOSITION OF PANCREATIC JUICE

Juice collected from the duct of the gland, as described above, is found to be isotonic with plasma, but much more alkaline; $[HCO_3^-]$ is about 85 mmol/l. The constituents of the fluid are given in table 32.2. An estimate of the daily secretion of electrolytes is given on p. 32.44. The inactive enzyme precursor **trypsinogen** is converted to the active **trypsin** by the enzyme enterokinase, which is liberated from unidentified cells of the duodenal mucosa. Trypsin also acts on the precursor **chymotrypsinogen** to form the active **chymotrypsin.** The elastase, amylase and lipase are secreted by the pancreas in the active form without precursors.

TABLE 32.2. Composition of pancreatic juice.

Enzyme precursors	Trypsinogen, chymotrypsinogen
Active enzymes	Elastase, amylase, lipase
Cations	Sodium, potassium, calcium
Anions	Chloride, bicarbonate
pH	7·5–8·0

FUNCTIONS OF PANCREATIC JUICE

The secretion has several functions.

(1) The alkalinity aids in the neutralization of the acid chyme passing into the duodenum from the stomach. This is an important function, since the enzymes of the pancreatic juice act optimally in an alkaline medium.

(2) Trypsin, when formed from its precursor trypsinogen, converts the proteins ingested to polypeptides and amino acids. The enzyme has its optimum pH at 8·0–9·7.

(3) Chymotrypsin, when formed from chymotrypsinogen, has the action of curdling milk.

(4) The amylase breaks down polysaccharides, mostly to disaccharides.

(5) The lipase converts neutral triglycerides to di- and monoglycerides and free fatty acids.

CONTROL OF PANCREATIC SECRETION

Like gastric secretion, the flow of digestive juice from the pancreas is controlled by both nervous and hormonal mechanisms and can be similarly classified into cephalic, gastric and intestinal phases.

Cephalic phase

A cephalic phase of pancreatic secretion similar to that described for the stomach is present. The secretion which is initiated is small in volume but rich in enzymes.

Gastric phase

When food enters the stomach it acts as a stimulus and initiates further secretion of enzyme by reflexes similar to those operating in the gastric phase of gastric secretion. Distension of the body of the stomach excites stretch receptors in its wall to initiate a vagovagal reflex, the efferent fibres ending in relation to acinar cells. This reflex, like that of the cephalic phase, stimulates the release of pancreatic juice rich in enzymes but with little electrolyte. Gastrin also stimulates enzyme release, and so all stimuli responsible for gastrin release also affect enzyme secretion by the pancreas.

Intestinal phase

When acid enters the duodenum, a hormone **secretin** is liberated from the mucosa of the small intestine into the portal blood. When this reaches the pancreas through the arterial supply, it stimulates the centro-acinar cells to secrete water and electrolyte containing a high concentration of bicarbonate ion, but little enzyme activity.

The presence of digestion products, in particular peptides and fatty acids, liberates a second hormone from the mucosa, **cholecystokinin-pancreozymin (CPZ)**, which stimulates the secretion of enzymes from acinar cells.

Thus after a meal, cephalic, vagovagal reflexes and gastrin act on the pancreatic acinar cells to mobilize enzymes. Acid produced simultaneously in gastric secretion enters the duodenum in the acid chyme and liberates secretin, which causes a watery secretion and washes out the mobilized enzymes. CPZ released by the chyme in the upper small intestine continues to stimulate the secretion of the enzymes of pancreatic juice.

Secretin was the first hormone to be discovered, on January 16th, 1902 by Bayliss and Starling, but it was nearly 70 years later before it was isolated in a pure form and synthesized. It is a strongly basic peptide with a mol. wt. of 3055 and 27 amino acids with the following structure:

His-Ser-Asp-Gly-Thr-Phe-Thr-Ser-Glu-Leu-
-Ser-Arg-Leu-Arg-Asp-Ser-Ala-Arg-Leu-Gln-
-Arg-Leu-Leu-Gln-Gly-Leu-Val-NH$_2$.

Secretin has been located in vesicles in the intestinal mucosal cells by immunological methods and electron microscopy.

The most potent releaser of secretin is acid in the duodenum. The pH threshold for release is 4·5. Acid is increasingly effective as the pH is lowered to pH 3; below this the amount of secretin release is related only to the length of the gut acidified.

CPZ is a polypeptide of 33 amino acids and mol. wt. 3919; the sequence of the terminal four amino acids is identical to that of gastrin and the molecule has the following structure:

Lys-Ala-Pro-Ser-Gly-Arg-Val-Ser-Met-Ile-
Lys-Asn-Leu-Gln-Ser-Leu-Asp-Pro-Ser-His-
Arg-Ile-Ser-Asp-Arg-Asp-Tyr-(SO$_4$)-Met-Gly-
-Try-Met-Asp-Phe-NH$_2$.

CPZ is a single hormone with the two major functions of causing contraction of the gall bladder and secretion of pancreatic enzymes. Fatty acids with a chain length of C$_{10}$ or greater and certain neutral L-amino acids release CPZ; the amount released, as in the case of secretin, is dependent upon the length of gut exposed to the releasing agent.

During normal digestion secretin and CPZ interact, each augmenting the other's action on the pancreas.

ABSORPTION FROM THE GASTROINTESTINAL TRACT

Table 32.3 shows the quantities of different nutrients that may be eaten in a day and eliminated in the faeces. In

TABLE 32.3. An estimate of the different amounts of nutrients that may be eaten in a day and excreted in the faeces.

	In the diet	In the faeces
Protein (g)	100	6
Fat (g)	100	4
Carbohydrate (digestible) (g)	400	4
Dietary fibre (g)	4	4
Sodium (mmol)	170	8
Potassium (mmol)	65	12
Calcium (mmol)	25	20
Iron (μmol)	260	240
Total solids (g)	about 600	about 20

addition about 7 litres of digestive juices with their electrolyte and protein contents enter the gut and also the epithelial lining is shed into the gut, digested and largely absorbed. Clearly the intestines perform most of their absorptive functions efficiently.

Absorption is dependent on many physical factors, e.g. the area of the absorptive surfaces, concentration gradients, osmotic and intraluminal pressures. However for the most part, nutrients are actively transported from the lumen into the portal blood.

Ethanol is the only important nutrient apart from water which crosses the cells by simple diffusion. Consequently it may be absorbed by all parts of the intestines. The remainder of the nutrients are absorbed in the small intestine, in which digestion is virtually complete. Here absorption is favoured by the large surface area of plasma membrane.

Absorption of carbohydrates

Starch and other dietary polysaccharides are broken down by the amylases in the saliva and pancreatic juice mostly to disaccharides. After a meal of starch very little monosaccharide is found in the lumen, yet only monosaccharides are found in the portal venous blood. The breakdown of disaccharides is effected within the brush border of the columnar cells. The enzymes responsible and their activity can be determined in biopsy samples, obtained by snipping off small pieces of mucosa with an instrument which can be swallowed by man. Table 32.4 gives the enzymic activity found in such sam-

TABLE 32.4. The enzymic activity of human jejunal mucosa (units/g protein)

Enzyme	Substrate	Activity	
		mean	range
Maltase	Maltose	593	310–1120
Sucrase	Sucrose	173	70–325
Isomaltase	α-limit dextrins Isomaltose	159	65–268
Lactase	Lactose	107	39–258

ples. The monosaccharides are then actively transported across the cell and enter the portal blood. The different sugars compete for transport mechanisms and so are absorbed at different rates. The fastest rates are for galactose and glucose, followed by fructose, mannose, xylose and arabinose in diminishing order. The rates of absorption reach a maximum at high concentration. If the concentration of disaccharides in the lumen is high, hydrolysis proceeds faster than the transport mechanism can move hexoses into the blood; under these circumstances monosaccharides return temporarily to the lumen.

The nature of the transporting systems in the mucosal membrane is not known accurately nor how they are coupled to a source of energy; they depend on the presence of Na^+, which may affect the supply of energy from ATP. Absorption is inhibited by phloridzin which also inhibits the uptake of glucose by the cells of the renal tubules.

A deficiency of disaccharidases may arise in congenital or acquired disease, when carbohydrates are not completely digested, but pass into the large intestine where they are fermented by bacteria and cause diarrhoea. Owing to congenital lactase deficiency, some infants can-

not tolerate milk and can be reared only on artificial milks containing other carbohydrates.

Absorption of lipids

Dietary fat leaves the stomach in the form of coarse undigested oily drops. In the duodenum these are emulsified by the action of the bile salts with the formation of particles not exceeding 0·5 μm diameter, which are susceptible to the action of pancreatic lipase. Hydrolysis does not go to completion; a mixture of di- and mono-glycerides with some free fatty acids is formed. The presence of conjugated bile salts makes the fatty acids more soluble in water. A clear micro-emulsion of molecular aggregations or **micelles** is formed in the lumen; each micelle consists of bile salts into which the lipids enter. They are absorbed by diffusion across the microvilli. Within the epithelium lipid droplets are enclosed in vesicles of the smooth and rough surfaced endoplasmic reticulum. Triglycerides are reformed, esterification taking place with free fatty acids, some of which reach the cells from the blood stream (p. 10.15). Large droplets, **cylomicrons,** are formed at the edges of the mucosal cells near and around the Golgi apparatus; these are 0·5 to 1·0 μm in diameter and consist of over 80 per cent triglyceride with a little cholesterol and a small envelope of phospholipid and a specific protein (p. 10.5). These enter the intercellular spaces and ultimately the lymph capillaries through pores and then pass along the larger lymph vessels and the thoracic duct to enter the general circulation (fig. 32.34).

In ruminants, protozoa living in the rumen ferment the carbohydrate present in grass with the formation of short-chain fatty acids. These are absorbed and pass in the portal blood to the liver. The only fats in human diets which contain significant amounts of short-chain fatty acids are dairy fats (table 10.2). These may pass direct to the liver in the portal blood, but this route is of little significance in man.

Fat absorption is nearly complete in the small intestine. If, on a normal intake, more than 6 g of fat appear in the faeces (a daily average over 5 days), then steatorrhoea is present and a diagnosis of malabsorption can be made.

The fat-soluble vitamins are absorbed with the lipids in the micelles but, if there is steatorrhoea, the vitamins are not absorbed. The body contains only a small store of vitamin K and signs of deficiency, such as subcutaneous bleeding, arise in two or three weeks in patients who may be jaundiced and have steatorrhoea owing to a failure of bile flow. Evidence of vitamin D deficiency and, rarely, of vitamin A deficiency occurs in patients with chronic steatorrhoea.

Absorption of protein

Pepsin and trypsin break down the dietary proteins in the lumen to a mixture of amino acids and peptides. After a meal rich in protein, the level of amino N in the blood rises from a fasting value of about 3 mmol/l to about 6 mmol/l in $1\frac{1}{2}$ to 2 hours and returns to normal in 3 to 4 hours. There are quantitative difficulties in accounting for protein digestion and absorption entirely in the form of amino acids. Studies of a few dipeptides and tripeptides provide evidence that peptide units are also taken up by the brush border and hydrolysed there, but more information is needed before it is possible to account for the absorption of all the protein in a meal.

Free amino acids are absorbed by active transport involving oxidative metabolism. As in the case of the renal tubules, different transport systems may exist for different groups of amino acids. Neutral forms are transported at 10 times the rate of basic amino acids, and the L forms are also absorbed more rapidly than are D forms, though apparently the two isomeric forms compete for the same transport system.

Absorption is normally very effective and less than 10 per cent of the dietary N is lost in the faeces.

Absorption of water and electrolytes

Table 32.5 gives an estimate of the large quantities that enter the alimentary tract daily. Of this no more than 2 per cent of the water, 2 per cent of the sodium and 10 per cent of the potassium appear normally in the faeces.

TABLE 32.5. Estimates of quantities of water and Na^+, K^+ and Cl^- entering the human intestine daily (Parsons D.S. (1967) *Proc. Nutr. Soc.* **26**, 47).

	Volume ml	Concentration mmol/litre			Electrolyte load mmol/24 h		
		Na^+	K^+	Cl^-	Na^+	K^+	Cl^-
Saliva	1500	30	20	35	45	30	52
Gastric juice	3000	50	10	150	150	30	450
Bile	500	160	5	50	80	3	25
Pancreatic juice	2000	160	5	30	320	10	60
Internal load	7000				595	73	587
Dietary intake	1500				170	65	110
Grand total	8500				765	138	697

The net flux of water and electrolytes (the amounts secreted minus the amounts absorbed) between the gut lumen and the blood differs greatly in different parts of the tract. In the mouth there is a large salivary secretion, but no absorption; in the stomach there is a large secretion with little absorption; in the duodenum and upper jejunum the two processes are almost equal; the jejunum and ileum are the main sites of absorption, which is completed in the colon.

The bulk of the fluid in the alimentary tract comes from the digestive juices, which are approximately isosmotic with plasma; the dietary load may be either hypertonic or hypotonic. Hence there is no consistent osmotic gradient to facilitate absorption and fluid can be absorbed against an osmotic gradient. A basic mechanism exists for the transport of Na^+ and K^+ through the epithelial cells, which are functionally asymmetrical. Water probably accompanies the ions passively. The nature of the sodium pump is unknown, but active transport is probably achieved by a pump at the basal and lateral borders; ions which enter passively at the luminal border leak across the cell down an electrochemical gradient set up by the cell pumps. Whether Cl^- and HCO_3^- ions follows passively is not known, but probably active transport also takes place. The ions and water enter the intercellular spaces (fig. 32.34) and are then passed into the circulation.

The transport of Na^+ and K^+ is influenced by aldosterone in a manner similar to its action in the renal tubules, and the transport mechanisms for sugars and amino acids are linked in some way to the transport of sodium.

Water absorption can be explained solely as a consequence of active transport of ions. Most of the water passes into the portal venous blood and only a small portion into the lymphatics.

Certain ions, e.g. SO_4^{--} and Mg^{++}, are not readily absorbed; these hold water in the intestines and prevent absorption, and thus have a purgative action. Many natural waters contain these ions in small amounts and such mineral waters have acquired a great reputation. Perhaps the most famous came from a well near London and contained the original Epsom salt. Its owner made a fortune from the smart society of the seventeenth century.

Absorption of water-soluble vitamins

The amount of these vitamins available for absorption may be modified by the action of intestinal bacteria. In laboratory rats it is not difficult to alter the bacterial flora in the gut so that they either synthesize or utilize significant amounts of vitamin. Such synthesis of vitamins may be of practical use in animal husbandry. In a healthy man eating ordinary diets, the amount of available vitamins is probably not significantly altered by the intestinal flora, but when the bacterial flora is increased, as may happen in disease, this may not always be so. The bacteria are more likely to decrease than to increase the supply of any vitamin. Bacteria in the small intestine deconjugate bile salts and thus inhibit micelle formation and absorption of lipids. The absorption of water soluble vitamins may also be impaired for reasons unknown.

Vitamin B_{12} is entirely dependent on a specific mucoprotein secreted by the stomach (intrinsic factor, p. 28.9) or its absorption. The vitamin is probably absorbed largely, though not entirely, in the lower half of the ileum, but how the intrinsic factor operates at this site to permit the absorption of a few micrograms across the epithelium is not known.

By contrast with vitamin B_{12}, free folic acid is rapidly absorbed from the jejunum and anaemia responding to injections of folic acid not infrequently occurs in disease of the small intestine.

Tests are available for assessing the absorptive capacity for these vitamins (vol. 3, p. 21.9). In the case of folic acid, the subject is given the same dose of the vitamin on two occasions separated by an interval of a few days. On one occasion the dose is given by mouth and on the other by injection. The amount of vitamin or of one of its metabolites excreted in the urine is measured and, if absorption is defective, is much lower with the oral test. For testing vitamin B_{12} absorption, it is possible to give a small dose of the vitamin labelled with ^{57}Co and ^{58}Co and to measure the amount of radio-activity appearing in the faeces. In health over 50 per cent of an oral dose is absorbed.

Absorption of minerals

Calcium and iron and probably also the other dietary minerals and trace elements (p. 5.9) differ from the nutrients already discussed in that the major portion of the dietary intake is excreted in the faeces and only a little absorbed. Further excretion of these substances by the kidney either does not take place (iron) or is limited (calcium). The minerals, if present in excess in the body, tend to form organic complexes which accumulate in the tissues and give rise to pathological states. These are fortunately rare. These facts suggest that the amount of a mineral present in the body is controlled by a mechanism which regulates intestinal absorption. No such control mechanism exists for other nutrients and any dietary excess is absorbed and either subsequently excreted in the urine (e.g. the N in protein, sodium and vitamin C) or stored (e.g. triglyceride and fat soluble vitamins). Here only the absorptions of calcium and iron, which are the two most important dietary minerals, are discussed.

CALCIUM

Of the calcium present in most western diets, about 70 to 80 per cent is lost in the faeces (p. 5.6). However in eastern diets there is usually much less calcium (table 5.4), but the faecal losses are relatively smaller and the amounts absorbed are sufficient to allow the development and maintenance of healthy bone. Active and growing children absorb relatively more calcium than do adults. Calcium absorption thus appears to be related more closely to the physiological need than to the dietary intake. About 15 per cent of the calcium in the faeces comes from the intestinal secretions. This has been shown by using two isotopes of calcium, one given by mouth and one intravenously. Vitamin D is the most important factor influencing calcium absorption and in its absence this is negligible. It promotes the synthesis of a calcium-binding protein, responsible for transporting calcium across the epithelial cells of the mucosa. Parathyroid hormone may also promote absorption.

IRON

Dietary aspects of this are discussed on p. 5.8, where it is stated that absorption is related to requirements and raised from the normal level of about 10 per cent of the dietary intake up to 20–30 per cent when the need for iron for haemoglobin synthesis is increased, e.g. by severe haemorrhage. An early hypothesis sought to account for this control of iron absorption by reference to the fact that during absorption iron may be incorporated into the storage substance ferritin (p. 5.8). It was suggested that either the rate of formation of ferritin or the rate of removal of iron from it might be the controlling step in absorption: either lack of iron in the body fluids or local hypoxia caused by anaemia might stimulate iron release from ferritin and thus promote absorption. Experimental evidence has failed to support this theory. More recent alternatives have not yet been adequately tested, although the basic fact that iron absorption is generally related to the need for haemoglobin synthesis remains unassailed. Studies with ^{59}Fe have shown that iron may be absorbed against a concentration gradient and a transport mechanism involving oxidative metabolism must exist.

MOTILITY IN THE DIGESTIVE TRACT

Very varying rates have been reported for the passage of food down the gastrointestinal tract. In general when an opaque barium meal is followed, the passage is often slower than would be indicated by following the appearance and disappearance in the blood of the products of digestion after a normal meal. If a person taking a normal daily diet eats his food in 3–4 meals of about equal size and evenly spaced throughout the day, food begins to enter the small intestine a few minutes after the start of a meal; all may have left the stomach after 2–3 hours. The remnants that are not absorbed begin to reach the large intestine in about one hour and little remains in the small intestine after 4 hours. Digestion and absorption are probably complete for some time before the next meal is taken.

Most of the remnants that reach the large intestine are evacuated in the faeces between 24 and 48 hours later, but studies using dyes or radioactive markers show that some usually continues to appear in the faeces for 5 days and occasionally later. Transit time depends on the amount of indigestible fibre (p. 5.1) in the diet. It has been shown to be about twice as rapid in Africans eating diets based on unrefined cereals with plenty of coarse vegetables, compared with Europeans eating typical diets of refined cereals and a smaller intake of vegetable foods. It has been suggested that this prolonged transit time is responsible for the prevalence of cancer of the large intestine being much higher in Europeans than in Africans.

Food is moved along the tract by the contraction and relaxation of the muscular walls and sphincters, which also assist in breaking up the food, and mixing it with the digestive juices.

MOTILITY IN THE SMALL INTESTINE

Three distinct types of movement in the small intestine together serve to break up food particles, mix them with the secreted juices and move the food along the tract. The three types are called segmentation, peristalsis and pendular movement.

Segmentation is a series of rhythmic movements, of alternate constriction and relaxation of the gut (fig. 32.54),

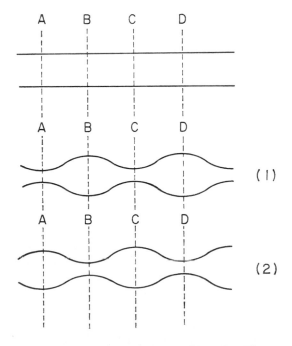

FIG. 32.54. Segmentation in the small intestine. The segments at A and C first contract (1) and then relax (2). At B and D relaxation (1) occurs followed by contraction (2).

occurring at the rate of about 7/min in man. The alternating constriction and relaxation of each portion of intestine mixes and breaks up the food, but does not cause any movement of the food along the tract. Segmentation is apparently myogenic in origin, since it can be seen even

after total nerve block which cuts off impulses from both the extrinsic and intrinsic innervation. Both the frequency and the amplitude of the waves are usually greater in the upper intestinal tract than in the lower, as breakdown and mixing are of greater importance in regions where secretion of digestive juice is greatest.

Peristalsis is a type of motility already mentioned in connection with the oesophagus and stomach. Two types are distinguished in the small intestine, under experimental conditions, ordinary peristalsis and peristaltic rush. The former consists of slow waves of contraction preceded by relaxation, and in man the waves move at about 2 cm/sec but fade out after a short distance. This type of movement was first described by Bayliss and Starling, and has been called the 'law of the intestines' or the 'myenteric reflex'. The peristaltic rush is of more doubtful physiological significance and attributed by some to experimental artefact. It is similar to ordinary peristalsis but the waves of relaxation and contraction are longer, and move at about 25 cm/min. Both types can move the food along the gut but have little or no effect on breaking up the food or mixing it. Peristalsis depends on local reflexes in the intrinsic plexuses, probably initiated by local distension, since it is abolished by the application of cocaine or stripping the mucosa, but not by section or blocking of the extrinsic nerves.

Pendular movements are waves of contraction sweeping backwards and forwards over the intestine and cause mixing of the food rather than its propulsion. Like peristalsis, they depend upon the integrity of the intrinsic nerve plexuses.

The ileocaecal sphincter is normally closed, but opens as peristaltic waves reach the site. Like the pyloric sphincter, it appears to be opened by the pressure exerted by the peristaltic wave and not by nervous activity. Intestinal contents probably enter the colon passively down the pressure gradient.

MOTILITY IN THE LARGE INTESTINE

Two types of movement occur in the large intestine, propulsive and non-propulsive. The former consists of the contraction of one segment, with relaxation of the succeeding segment, and is therefore similar to peristalsis in the small intestine. A mass contraction affecting the left colon occurs before defaecation. The non-propulsive movement is not as clear-cut as segmentation, but also results in a churning up of the gut contents. Approximately 24 hours after the ingestion of a meal mass peristalsis moves the faeces into the rectum and defaecation normally follows soon afterwards.

Defaecation

This is a reflex activity, but is under conscious control and normally occurs only when time and circumstances are suitable. The stimulus to the reflex is distension of the wall of the rectum, which gives rise to afferent impulses in the pudendal and pelvic splanchnic nerves. These travel to the S2–4 spinal segments. From there efferent impulses pass back along the splanchnic nerves causing contraction of the colon and relaxation of the internal anal sphincter. The external anal sphincter is under voluntary control. During the process the levator ani contracts and lifts the anal canal over the descending faecal mass. Usually evacuation is assisted by an increase in intra-abdominal pressure caused by contractions of the diaphragm and abdominal muscles.

MISCELLANEOUS REFLEXES

Several reflexes have been demonstrated whereby food in one part of the digestive tract may influence the motility of other parts either by stimulating or by inhibiting muscle contraction.

The **gastro-ileal reflex** is evoked when food is present in the stomach, when the distension it causes leads to increased motor activity in the ileum. The **gastrocolic reflex** is a similar stimulus to the colon and is particularly active after the first meal of the day. The **ileogastric reflex** is evoked when food products distend the ileum and gastric motility and emptying are inhibited.

In all these reflexes, the extrinsic and intrinsic nerve plexuses are concerned.

Vomiting

This is a reflex which may be caused by a wide variety of stimuli. These include irritation of the gastric mucosa by food or drugs, tactile stimulation of the throat, intestinal distension, compression or irritation of abdominal viscera, impulses from the vestibular apparatus (e.g. sea sickness), and by any severe pain or unpleasant emotion.

Impulses from many sites pass to a **vomiting centre** in the medulla, and give rise to a co-ordinated response. There is normally a deep inspiration with closure of the larynx, elevation of the soft palate and relaxation of the oesophagus and stomach. This is followed by forceful contraction of the abdominal muscles, together with expiration, which causes pressure on the walls of the stomach, and gastric contents are expelled. In prolonged vomiting, the duodenum may also contract, thus reversing the normal gastroduodenal pressure gradient, and its contents enter the stomach to be expelled with the gastric vomitus. Vomiting is usually, but not invariably, accompanied by feelings of nausea, and widespread autonomic activity, causing sweating, salivation and tachycardia.

Bacterial flora

Large numbers of bacteria are taken in with the food, but the secretions of the upper alimentary tract are bacteriostatic and bacteriocidal. The upper part of the small intestine in consequence has a limited bacterial flora and may even be sterile. The colon has a large bacterial flora (vol. 2, p. 18.87), which tends to pass into the small intestine through the ileocaecal sphincter. Thus the lower part of the small intestine may contain a number and variety of organisms. If motility in the small bowel is impaired, bacteria spread upwards and may become prolific in the whole tract.

Gas in the bowel

There is normally a gas bubble of up to 100 ml of swallowed air in the stomach. This passes quickly through the small intestine and becomes apparent only where there is delay in its transit as in obstruction of the intestinal tract. The gas reaching the colon contains less O_2, since some of it is absorbed via the intestinal mucosa, and more CO_2. In the colon gases are produced by fermentation and a healthy person may pass up to 1 litre of flatus daily. This contains little O_2 (about 10 per cent), some N (50 per cent) and hydrogen sulphide and methane. Hydrogen may be formed and absorbed and excreted in the expired air where a concentration above 20 p.p.m. may indicate abnormal fermentation in the gut.

NERVE SUPPLY

The autonomic nervous system supplies the digestive tract from the mid-oesophagus to the anus, except for the striated muscle of the external anal sphincter. Although the parasympathetic and sympathetic divisions provide a dual innervation to the gut, normal digestion is almost completely controlled by the parasympathetic nerves, aided by the gastrointestinal hormones (p. 32.42). The nerves contain large numbers of general visceral afferent fibres which have their peripheral endings in the mucosa and muscle coat of the gut wall. They carry to the central nervous system impulses which are involved in visceral reflexes and which may be appreciated as various forms of visceral sensibility.

PARASYMPATHETIC INNERVATION

The vagus nerves supply the gut from mid-oesophagus to the beginning of the splenic flexure and the pelvic splanchnic nerves supply the remainder of the gut from the splenic flexure almost to the anus (fig. 32.55).

The parasympathetic fibres in both the vagi and the pelvic splanchnics are preganglionic and synapse on intrinsic ganglionic cells found in the myenteric and submucosal plexuses of the gut wall (p. 32.2). The postganglionic fibres of the myenteric plexus are motor to the main visceral muscle coats and those from the submucosal plexus are secretomotor to the glands.

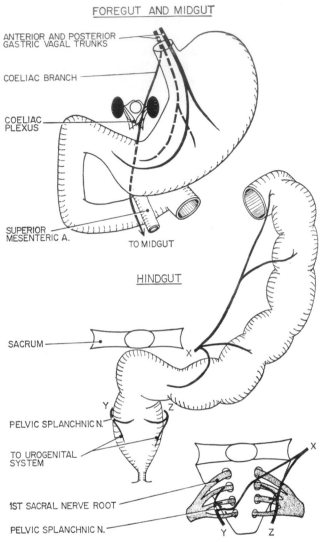

FOREGUT AND MIDGUT

ANTERIOR AND POSTERIOR
GASTRIC VAGAL TRUNKS

COELIAC BRANCH

COELIAC
PLEXUS

SUPERIOR
MESENTERIC A.

TO MIDGUT

HINDGUT

SACRUM

PELVIC SPLANCHNIC N.

TO UROGENITAL
SYSTEM

1ST SACRAL NERVE ROOT

PELVIC SPLANCHNIC N.

FIG. 32.55. Parasympathetic innervation. The lower figure shows the origin of the pelvic splanchnic nerves, X, Y and Z.

Vagus

In the thorax, the left and right vagi form an oesophageal plexus round the lower half of the oesophagus. This plexus ends as the **anterior** and **posterior gastric vagal trunks,** which descend on the corresponding surfaces of the oesophagus as it pierces the diaphragm (fig. 32.4), where they are cut during abdominal vagotomy undertaken for the relief of peptic ulcer.

The anterior vagal trunk is derived mainly from the left vagus, because the stomach rotates during development (p. 32.56). It divides at the cardia to be distributed to the foregut and its derivatives, anterior wall of stomach, liver, biliary system and pancreas.

The posterior vagal trunk divides into gastric branches which supply the posterior gastric wall. It has a large **coeliac branch** which passes inferomedially and retro-

peritoneally on the left crus of the diaphragm to the coeliac plexus, which surrounds the coeliac artery at its origin, and descends through it to the superior mesenteric plexus, at the origin of the superior mesenteric artery. The parasympathetic fibres are then distributed from this plexus and run with the arteries to the small intestine and the large intestine proximal to the splenic flexure.

Pelvic splanchnic nerves

These are derived from S2,3 and 4 segments of the spinal cord and constitute the sacral parasympathetic outflow. They emerge from the pelvic sacral foramina and pass in two directions. First, many run ventrally into the pelvic plexus (fig. 32.55) which lies on the side of the rectum. The fibres continue through this plexus and are distributed to the rectum and upper half (mucosal zone) of the anal canal. The second group ascend out of the pelvis across the superior rectal artery and its sigmoid branches, and fan out to innervate the splenic flexure, and descending and sigmoid colon. The pelvic splanchnics are therefore distributed to the hindgut, from the splenic flexure to the anal canal, which is the segment of gut responsible for defaecation.

General visceral afferent fibres in parasympathetic nerves.

The parasympathetic nerves to the gut contain, in addition to the parasympathetic (general visceral efferent) fibres, very large numbers of sensory fibres (fig. 32.20). As the major efferent control of the gut is parasympathetic, it is perhaps to be expected that the afferent nerves should use these pathways. For example, the fibres from the stretch receptors in the wall of the rectum that initiate reflex defaecation (p. 32.46) travel to the sacral cord in the pelvic splanchnic nerves.

SYMPATHETIC INNERVATION

The sympathetic nerve fibres for the abdomino-pelvic gut arise in the thoracic spinal cord, pass through the sympathetic trunk, and enter the three **thoracic splanchnic nerves** which descend into the abdomen and end in the **prevertebral ganglia** (p. 21.41). The latter ganglia send nerves which follow arterial pathways to the gut. The lumbar sympathetic ganglia send fibres to supply the more caudal part of the gut.

The preganglionic fibres traverse the sympathetic trunk without interruption and synapse in the prevertebral ganglia. The long postganglionic fibres leave the ganglia and run to the gut, where they are distributed via the myenteric and submucosal plexuses mainly to vessels, and possibly to visceral muscles (fig. 32.20).

Prevertebral plexuses and ganglia

These form a continuous network of sympathetic nerve

fibres and ganglion cells over the ventral surface of the abdominal aorta, and continue down into the pelvis, in front of the sacrum, but are divided somewhat arbitrarily into the coeliac, mesenteric, hypogastric and pelvic plexuses.

The large **coeliac plexus** surrounds the coeliac artery and contains a well defined ganglion 1 cm in length on either side of the artery on the crus of the diaphragm. The preganglionic fibres for the abdominal part of the foregut and its derivatives travel to the coeliac plexus in the thoracic splanchnics and synapse in the coeliac ganglion. The postganglionic fibres emerge from the ganglion and accompany the branches of the coeliac artery to the stomach, part of the duodenum, liver and biliary system, and pancreas.

The **superior mesenteric plexus,** around the origin of the superior mesenteric artery, contains a smaller ganglion, and arises by numerous branches from the coeliac plexus above. The preganglionic fibres for the midgut pass with those for the foregut as far as the coeliac plexus, where some synapse, and then all travel to the superior mesenteric plexus where the remainder synapse. Postganglionic fibres are distributed with the arteries to the gut from the caudal part of the duodenum to the splenic flexure.

The **inferior mesenteric plexus** contains many small groups of ganglionic cells. It lies at the origin of the inferior mesenteric artery, and is formed mainly from above by the downward continuation of the superior mesenteric plexus. Postganglionic fibres from the plexus go to the splenic flexure and descending colon.

The **hypogastric plexus** is the downward continuation of the inferior mesenteric, and as it passes in front of the sacrum it is sometimes called the presacral nerve. This plexus contributes to the bilateral pelvic plexuses.

The **pelvic plexuses** are large and lie within the true pelvis on both sides of the rectum, extending forwards on to the posterior aspect of the urogenital organs. These plexuses also get branches from the lumbar sympathetic ganglia (fig. 32.56). They innervate the pelvic viscera, including the sigmoid colon, rectum and mucosal zone of the anal canal.

General visceral afferent fibres in sympathetic nerves

Although the parasympathetic supply is accompanied by afferent fibres concerned with normal digestion, those subserving visceral pain are carried along with the sympathetic nerves. The lower half of the anal canal, which is of ectodermal origin (fig. 32.39 and p. 32.57), is supplied by somatic pain fibres via the inferior rectal branch of the pudendal nerve (p. 21.45) and is consequently much more sensitive than the endodermal upper half of the canal. This fact is pertinent in the treatment of haemorrhoids by injection (vol. 3, p. 19.119).

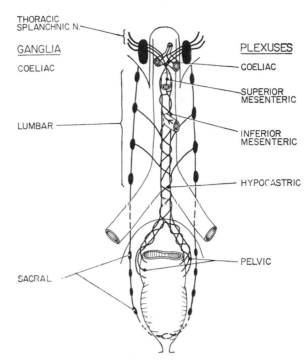

FIG. 32.56. Sympathetic innervation. The sympathetic supply from the prevertebral plexuses and lumbar sympathetic trunk accompany the arteries to the gut. Afferent fibres subserving pain also run in these nerves.

Abdominal vagotomy

This surgical procedure eliminates completely the psychic secretion of acid gastric juice and pepsin, but the effect on mucus production is variable. The vagus nerve also affects hormonal responses, and it is usual in man to find that the secretory response to food and also to gastrin and histamine is reduced by vagotomy. Gastric emptying may also be delayed, but this is most obvious if there is narrowing of the pyloric region or of the duodenum, as a result of advanced peptic ulceration. There is little disturbance of small intestine motility but some subjects suffer from intermittent diarrhoea. Increased segmentation has been recorded, attributed to asynchronous discharge of local neural reflexes in the bowel wall, or to stagnation with subsequent production of the motor amines, such as histamine and 5-hydroxytryptamine. Little is known about the effect on human physiology of the interruption of the afferent vagal pathways; in the dog the abdominal vagi have 35 000 fibres of which only 10 per cent are motor and 90 per cent serve a largely undetermined sensory role.

Sympathectomy

At one time operations to divide the splanchnic nerves were carried out in the hope of reducing blood pressure by relaxing arterioles of the splanchnic vascular territory. The blood flow through the abdominal viscera is, however, not increased by this procedure which merely promotes pooling of blood. Little change in secretion or motility has been observed, but pain from certain viscera may be reduced or abolished.

ABDOMINAL PAIN

Abnormal contractions of the intestinal tract or its appendages can cause pain. The response is probably initiated by abnormal tension in the bowel wall or mesentery. Very severe pain arises when there is obstruction of ducts such as the biliary and pancreatic ducts. On the other hand, the pain arising from the colon is less intense and often poorly localized in the lower abdomen. Stimuli from the viscera give rise to painful sensation by afferent impulses travelling to the cord with the sympathetic nervous system. Pain from various viscera is, therefore, appreciated on the basis of segmental distribution of this system, with inversion of the direction of conduction. Fibres carrying pain impulses from the oesophagus reach the upper levels of the cord, where they overlap with the cardiac fibres (T1–4), thus explaining why oesophageal and cardiac pain are so confusing clinically. The stomach and intestines have their segmental representation in the splanchnic nerves, mainly T7–T9 for the stomach, bile and pancreatic ducts, T9–11 for the small intestine, and T9–L2 for the proximal colon. The distal colon and rectum have afferent fibres accompanying the sympathetic nerves.

Pain is not always necessarily felt in the appropriate segmental levels, but may be referred to segments above and below. Though commonly referred to the cutaneous segments, it may be felt also along the deep distribution of spinal nerves. This is characteristic of pancreatic and biliary pains (T7–T9), which are often felt in the back, near the scapula. Though pain from abdominal viscera is often felt bilaterally, this is not always the case, and some viscera rarely give rise to pain involving the whole segment; gall bladder pain is more often felt on the right of the midline.

In most disease states, visceral pain is soon supplemented or even supplanted by the more commanding pain of irritation of the exquisitely sensitive parietal peritoneum. This is innervated by the somatic nervous system, and pain is now experienced as sharp localized pain, in the immediately overlying surface area. Here too there is variability; the pain of peritoneal irritation is almost unbearable when the peritoneum is diffusely irritated (e.g. when a perforated peptic ulcer leaks acid into the peritoneal cavity). It is severe when the peritoneum in the lower abdomen or under the diaphragm is irritated, but less so when the deeper pelvic or posterior parietal peritoneum is disturbed.

The viscera are however relatively insensitive; hence there is no pain when they are handled and cut at operations in which the abdominal wall has been opened under local anaesthesia.

BLOOD SUPPLY AND LYMPHATIC DRAINAGE

The blood supply of the gut is a rich one, and accounts for about one quarter of the cardiac output at rest. The supply in secretory or absorptive areas, such as stomach and small intestine, is higher than in motor and excretory areas, such as oesophagus and rectum. The vessels reach the intestinal part of the alimentary tract in its mesentery, but in the case of the stomach the folds of peritoneum between the greater and lesser sacs serve as a second means of access. Both the mesentery and these folds serve as pedicles, in which run the arteries, veins, nerves and lymphatics. The veins in the main accompany the arteries at first but diverge to form the portal system in the region of the pancreas. The intestinal lymph ultimately drains to the cisterna chyli and flows into the thoracic duct.

Arterial supply

The primitive foregut, midgut and hindgut each receive a branch from the dorsal aorta which runs ventrally in the dorsal mesentery to reach the gut (p. 32.60). In the adult the relationships of the primitive mesentery have altered, but the three unpaired visceral branches of the abdominal aorta remain as the coeliac, superior and inferior mesenteric arteries.

COELIAC ARTERY

This artery of the foregut supplies the gut from the lower part of the oesophagus down to the duodenum as far as the entrance of the bile duct, and also the biliary system, liver and pancreas. The spleen, although not functionally associated with the alimentary system, develops close to the stomach and is also supplied by this artery.

The coeliac artery is a very short wide branch of the abdominal aorta; it arises just below the aortic opening in the diaphragm and divides into left gastric, hepatic and splenic arteries (fig. 32.57).

The **left gastric artery** is the smallest of the three coeliac branches; it runs up on the diaphragm and hooks forward near the gastro-oesophageal junction, in the superior gastropancreatic fold, to enter the lesser omentum and descend along the lesser curvature of the stomach, supplying it. It also gives off oesophageal branches.

The **hepatic artery** passes ventrally in the floor of the epiploic foramen and runs up in the lesser omentum where it gives off the cystic artery to the gall bladder and enters the liver at the porta. Although sometimes there is an accessory hepatic artery from the left gastric, usually the hepatic is the sole arterial supply to the liver and it is an end artery. The **cystic artery** is also an end artery. The **gastroduodenal branch** of the hepatic descends behind the duodenum and gives branches to the lesser and greater curvatures, and to the duodenum and head of pancreas.

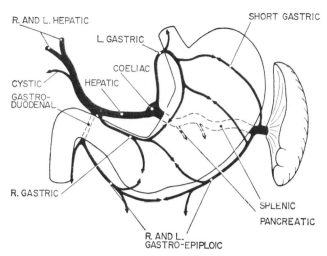

FIG. 32.57 Coeliac artery.

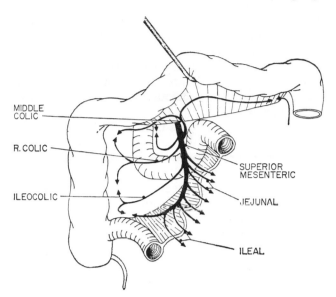

FIG. 32.58. Superior mesenteric artery.

The **splenic artery** is the largest branch of the coeliac, and is the sole supply to the spleen and the major supply to the pancreas. Passing to the left, it follows a wavy course along the upper border of the pancreas, behind the lesser sac, and then accompanies the tail of the pancreas into the lienorenal ligament to enter the hilus of the spleen. The splenic gives off short gastric branches to the fundus of the stomach and a large **left gastro-epiploic artery** which follows the greater curvature and supplies both the stomach above and the omentum below.

The various gastric arteries form rich anastomoses on and in the wall of the stomach, so that one or more major branches may be tied without fear of ischaemia.

SUPERIOR MESENTERIC ARTERY

The midgut artery supplies the gut from the duodenum caudal to the duodenal papilla down as far as the splenic flexure of the colon (fig. 32.58). As this includes nearly all the small intestine actively engaged in absorption, it is the largest of the three gut arteries. In addition it furnishes some branches to the pancreas. The superior mesenteric artery arises about 1–2 cm below the coeliac, behind the pancreas and descends anterior to the left renal vein, uncinate process and third part of duodenum to enter the root of the mesentery which it follows to the right iliac fossa. Large **jejunal** and **ileal branches** run in the mesentery to the small intestine, and a small branch ascends between the duodenum and head of pancreas supplying both, and anastomosing with a similar descending branch from the gastroduodenal artery. The large intestine is supplied by branches which arise from the right side of the vessel as it lies in the mesentery and pass retroperitoneally to the caecum, ascending colon, and hepatic flexure. The lower of these, the **ileocolic**, gives off the anterior caecal artery (fig. 32.36) and the **appendicular artery** which is an end

artery. The **middle colic artery** arises from the superior mesenteric just below the pancreas and passes forwards into the transverse mesocolon to supply the transverse colon as far as the splenic flexure.

INFERIOR MESENTERIC ARTERY

The hindgut artery is much the smallest of the three main arteries as it supplies a shorter and less active region of the gut, extending from the splenic flexure to the anal canal (fig. 32.59). The inferior mesenteric artery comes off the

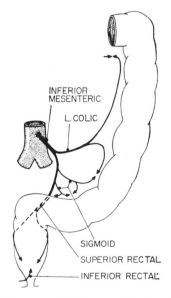

FIG. 32.59. Inferior mesenteric artery.

aorta a few cm above its bifurcation and passes caudally and to the left where it enters the true pelvis medial to the left ureter and becomes the **superior rectal artery** which descends in the pelvic mesocolon and supplies the rectum. The **left colic artery** ascends from the left side of the inferior mesenteric artery and passes to the upper part of the descending colon. Several **sigmoid arteries** arise lower down and supply the remainder of the descending colon and sigmoid colon.

The various colic arteries from both the superior and inferior mesenteric vessels characteristically divide into two divergent branches as they approach the gut, and each branch then runs parallel to the gut and anastomoses with the corresponding branch of the adjacent artery. The linkage of these branches forms the **marginal artery** which establishes an anastomosis around the colon.

INTERNAL ILIAC ARTERY

Through its inferior and middle rectal branches this large systemic artery supplies the anal canal and forms anastomoses with the superior rectal artery.

Venous drainage

The intestinal portal system of veins drains a wide area, including the entire alimentary tract from the lower end of the oesophagus to the upper part of the anal canal, and the spleen, pancreas and gall bladder (fig. 32.60).

The portal vein carries all this blood to the liver within which it divides repeatedly into a plexus of vessels, larger than capillaries, termed sinusoids. The liver sinusoids empty into tributaries of the large hepatic veins which emerge from the back of the liver and immediately enter the inferior vena cava (fig. 32.44).

A portal venous system (Latin *porta* = a door) is one which has a vascular plexus interposed on its pathway to the heart, and is a mechanism for carrying substances in the blood directly from one site to another without dispersing them into the general circulation. The intestinal portal system is the largest and is simply referred to as the portal system, but the hypophysial portal veins are another example (p. 27.10).

PORTAL VEIN (fig. 32.60)

This starts at the union of the superior mesenteric and splenic veins behind the neck of the pancreas and passes upwards to the porta hepatis where it divides into right and left branches before entering the liver with the corresponding branches of the hepatic artery, and the hepatic ducts. In its course it lies behind the duodenum, gastroduodenal artery and bile duct, and then runs up in the lesser omentum, anterior to the epiploic foramen, but posterior to the common hepatic duct and hepatic artery.

The **inferior mesenteric vein** corresponds to the artery of the same name, and drains the same area of gut extending from the splenic flexure to the anal canal. Its tributaries are also similar to the branches of the artery and are not described, except for the **superior rectal vein**. This

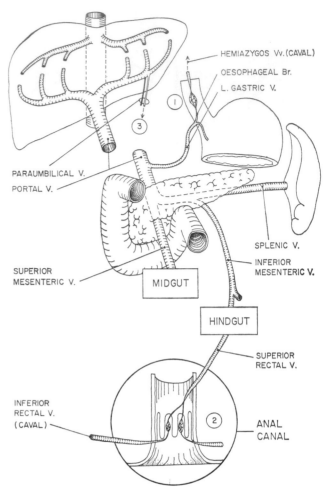

FIG. 32.60. Portal venous system. The three major portacaval anastomoses are at the (1) oesophagus, (2) anal canal and (3) umbilicus.

vein drains part of the anal canal, the rectum and the sigmoid colon. It is formed from venous plexuses within the anal columns and in the walls of the rectum. The superior rectal vein then accompanies its artery upwards, and becomes the inferior mesenteric vein as it leaves the true pelvis. The inferior mesenteric vein ascends retroperitoneally and lateral to the inferior mesenteric artery to join the splenic vein.

The **superior mesenteric vein** is a very large vein which corresponds to the artery of the same name and accompanies it from the right iliac fossa upwards in the root of the mesentery. It crosses anterior to the third part of duodenum and uncinate process of pancreas, before ending in the portal vein. It drains the midgut from the second part of the duodenum to the beginning of the splenic flexure, by tributaries which accompany the branches of the artery.

The **splenic vein** drains the entire spleen, most of the pancreas, and some of the stomach. The arterial and venous patterns are similar for both the midgut and hindgut but the venous drainage of the foregut differs somewhat from the arterial supply. The details are not given, but it should be noted that the splenic vein accompanies the splenic artery over much of its course, and drains a similar area, except that it is joined by the inferior mesenteric vein behind the body of the pancreas. The remainder of the blood from the foregut, pancreas, and gall bladder enters the portal vein by several tributaries including the **cystic vein** from the gall bladder and the left gastric vein. The **left gastric vein** follows a course similar to the left gastric artery and receives oesophageal tributaries from the lower end of the oesophagus (fig. 32.60).

PORTA-CAVAL ANASTOMOSES

The tributaries of the portal vein anastomose in certain sites with adjacent caval veins which return blood to the heart through either the superior or the inferior vena cava.

Little blood passes through these porta-caval anastomoses in health, but the portal system of veins has no valves, and therefore should the pressure within the portal system rise abnormally, e.g. due to liver disease, then blood may flow in the reverse direction out of the portal area through these anastomoses. The porta-caval anastomoses dilate and may rupture causing haemorrhage.

The main sites are:

(1) An **oesophageal venous plexus** in the wall at the lower end of the oesophagus drains downwards into the (portal) left gastric vein via its oesophageal tributaries, but also anastomoses above with oesophageal veins that pass to the (caval) hemiazygos system and enter the heart by the superior vena cava (p. 21.38). When dilated these mucosal veins are liable to be damaged during swallowing and bleed into the lumen of the oesophagus (vol. 3, p. 19.78 & 20.27).

(2) **Plexuses in the anal columns** of the anal canal drain upwards to the (portal) superior rectal vein but also anastomose with the inferior rectal veins which join the (caval) internal iliac veins (p. 21.38). Dilation of these venous plexuses causes local bulges of the mucosa known as 'haemorrhoids', which are likely to be damaged during defaecation and bleed (vol. 3, p. 19.118 & 20.11).

(3) Small veins accompany the ligamentum teres from the umbilicus to where it joins the left branch of the portal vein (p. 32.12), and so connect the portal vein to the **veins of the anterior abdominal wall**. The latter, when dilated, radiate from the umbilicus and have a striking appearance known as the caput Medusae.

(4) Many parts of the gut, such as the ascending colon, are devoid of peritoneum posteriorly where they rest directly on the **posterior abdominal wall**. Here, where areas of portal and caval venous drainage meet, there are many small porta-caval anastomoses.

Lymphatic drainage

Generally, lymph enters lymphatic vessels in the mucosa and other layers of the gut wall and passes into the peripheral group of lymph nodes adjacent to the gut. Their efferent vessels then accompany arterial branches back towards their origin from the aorta, sometimes entering a group of intermediate lymph nodes before reaching the proximal nodes which surround each of the three main arteries to the gut, at their origins from the aorta. The proximal nodes, which are the coeliac, superior mesenteric, and inferior mesenteric nodes, form two trunks which enter the **cisterna chyli** (p. 21.39). The **intestinal trunk** is formed by the efferent vessels from the coeliac and superior mesenteric nodes and therefore carries lymph derived from the stretch of gut between the lower end of oesophagus and the splenic flexure, and from the spleen, pancreas, liver and biliary system. The inferior mesenteric nodes are a component of the left para-aortic nodes which form the **left lumbar trunk,** and convey lymph from the more distal part of the gut as far down as the anal canal. *Stomach.* The lymph from the stomach drains as shown in fig. 32.61 to the coeliac glands. The lymphatics in the oesophagus communicate with those draining upwards into the thorax.

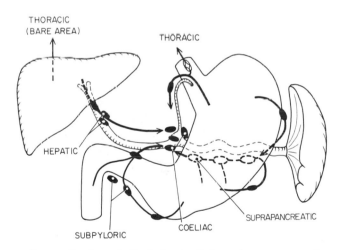

Fig. 32.61. Lymphatic drainage of stomach, pancreas and liver.

Liver. Most of the lymphatics emerge at the porta hepatis and enter hepatic nodes or pass direct to the coeliac group. Another group leaves the bare area of the liver and drains into the thoracic nodes.

Pancreas. This drains to the pyloric and the suprapancreatic nodes and then to the coeliac nodes.

Small intestine (fig. 32.62). The three groups of nodes form almost continuous chains alongside the arterial branches of the superior mesenteric artery that supply the small intestine. The lymphatic vessels of the jejuno-ileum are

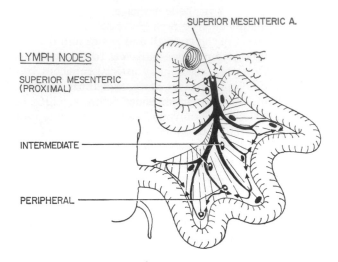

FIG. 32.62. Lymphatic drainage of small intestine.

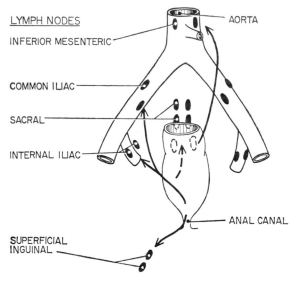

FIG. 32.63. Lymphatic drainage of rectum.

referred to as lacteals because they appear milky when they contain absorbed fat after a meal.

Large intestine. Numerous paracolic nodes are distributed along the large intestine. As the lymphatics follow the arteries, those proximal to the splenic flexure end in the superior mesenteric nodes, and those distal to the splenic flexure go to the inferior mesenteric nodes.

Rectum and anal canal (fig. 32.63). Some lymphatics from the rectum drain upwards to inferior mesenteric nodes but others pass laterally to internal and common iliac nodes, and yet a third group pass dorsally to nodes on the sacrum. Below the pectinate line the anal canal drains across the perineum to the superficial inguinal nodes.

Blood flow

The Fick principle (p. 30.36) can be applied to measure blood flow to the area drained by the portal vein (the splanchnic flow) in man in the following manner. The dye bromsulphthalein, BSP, is excreted exclusively by the liver; if a solution of the dye is infused intravenously at a rate sufficient to keep the concentration in the blood constant, then the rate of clearance of the dye by the liver can be calculated. From a catheter passed from an arm vein through the right atrium, hepatic venous blood can be sampled and the concentration of the dye in it determined. Knowing now the concentration of dye in the blood entering and leaving the liver and the amount of dye removed, the flow rate can be calculated. In man at rest it is about 1500 ml/min or 30 per cent of the cardiac output.

The capacity of the splanchnic vascular bed is large and the big veins, the spleen and the liver sinusoids act as a store of blood which can be shunted readily to other parts of the body, e.g. during muscular exercise. This is brought about by the constrictor action of the sympathetic nerves and by adrenaline. In a cat, the sympathetic nerves can be stimulated, causing visible contraction of the spleen, blanching of the gut and emptying of the large veins; at the same time a marked rise of systemic blood pressure may be recorded. The subsequent vasodilation is brought about by removing constrictor tone and there are no vasodilator nerves. Perhaps in man as much as 1 litre of blood may be removed from the splanchnic circulation by this mechanism.

At rest about one-fifth of the liver's blood supply comes from the hepatic artery and four-fifths from the portal vein. However, whereas the hepatic arterial blood is about 97 per cent saturated with oxygen, the portal venous blood is only about 60 per cent saturated in the post-absorptive state and probably less during digestion. Hence the hepatic artery supplies oxygen to the liver at a higher pressure than the portal vein; if the artery is injured or tied at an operation, fatal liver damage follows. On the other hand the portal vein can be anastomosed into the inferior vena cava in experimental animals (Eck's fistula), without serious impairment of liver function. Porta-caval anastomosis is sometimes carried out in man to relieve portal hypertension (vol. 3, p. 20.18).

The mean pressure in the hepatic artery is about 100 mm Hg and in the portal vein about 5 mm Hg. Hence any increase in the capillary resistance to the portal flow, as may be caused by fine scarring of the liver due to past infection or chronic poisoning, may cause a marked rise in portal venous pressure. This leads to congestion of all the organs whose veins drain into the portal system and the subsequent enlargement of porta-caval anastomoses (p. 32.53).

The arteries supplying the wall of the whole gut anastomose freely. Hence, only if there is obstruction to one of the large branches does the nutrition of the gut suffer.

There are also many arterio-venous anastomoses, which facilitate the transfer of the blood from the gut to other organs when there is splanchnic vasoconstriction.

EMBRYOLOGY

The basic plan of the alimentary tract is established by the fourth week, when the lateral, head, and tail folds (p. 19.7) have incorporated the endodermal roof of the secondary yolk sac into the embryo, forming the gut. The definitive yolk sac opens only into the midgut (fig. 32.64). Cranially the midgut communicates

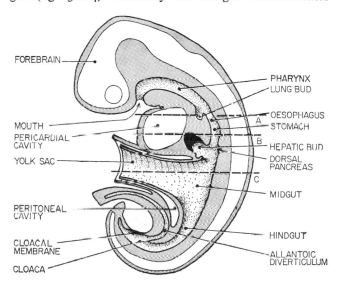

FIG. 32.64. Alimentary tract of 4-week embryo (4 mm). In this median sagittal section the secondary yolk sac communicates freely with the midgut, which in turn opens into the fore- and hindgut. The hepatic bud is present. The buccopharyngeal membrane has broken down, but the cloacal membrane is intact.

with the tubular foregut, the junction being marked by the hepatic diverticulum. The buccopharyngeal membrane (p. 19.13) has just broken down, so the foregut is continuous with the ectodermal stomatodaeum. Caudally the midgut opens into the tubular hindgut, which ends in a large chamber, the cloaca, which is shared with the urogenital system (pp. 36.1 and 38.58). The cloaca joins the mesonephric ducts posterolaterally, gives off the allantoic diverticulum ventrally, and is closed caudally by the cloacal membrane.

The endoderm differentiates eventually into epithelia, which form the lining of the gut and of the glands that arise as outgrowths of the endodermal gut, the liver and pancreas. The remaining layers of the gut wall are derived from the splanchnopleuric mesoderm, which enclosed the endodermal tube as a result of the folding and splitting of the lateral mesoderm (fig. 19.18).

DEVELOPMENT OF FOREGUT

At the end of the fourth week the foregut extends cranially from the hepatic diverticulum to the stomatodaeum. It consists of a branchial portion which gives rise to the buccal cavity, pharynx and the upper part of the oesophagus, and a postbranchial part which forms the rest of the oesophagus, stomach and duodenum as far down as the hepatic diverticulum (bile duct). The muscle of the branchial part is striated and supplied by the nerves of the branchial arches; in contrast the postbranchial portion has smooth muscle supplied by autonomic nerves.

The embryology of the branchial portion is given on p. 19.29. The postbranchial portion is slung from the dorsal wall of the embryo by a broad but shallow mesentery, which connects ventrally with the pericardium above and the septum transversum below. The lung bud descends in the mesentery ventral to the gut (figs. 32.64 and 32.65), and the pericardioperitoncal canals run on either side of the oesophagus to end in the peritoneal cavity inferiorly.

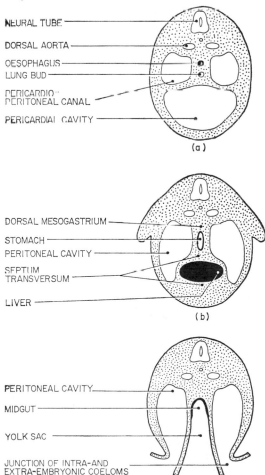

FIG. 32.65. Horizontal sections through alimentary tract at 4 weeks. These sections are through planes A, B and C of fig. 32.64.

Oesophagus. At four weeks the oesophagus is very short, but then it grows rapidly. Occasionally the laryngotracheal groove (p. 31.8) fails to separate completely from the ventral aspect of the gut, resulting in an abnormal opening between the oesophagus and trachea, through which ingested milk may enter the lungs. Frequently in such cases the oesophagus below the fistula has no lumen (i.e. atresia).

Stomach. A slight fusiform swelling of the foregut caudal to the oesophagus denotes the beginning of the stomach (fig. 32.64). This broadens anteroposteriorly (fig. 32.65) and the posterior border grows rapidly forming the greater curvature. Simultaneously the anterior border rotates towards the right, converting the original left side to the anterior surface (fig. 32.66). This

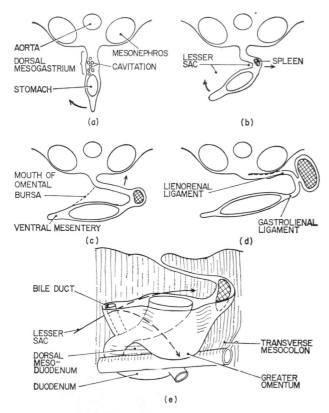

FIG. 32.66. Development of stomach and lesser sac. (a) The lesser sac forms initially by cavitation within the dorsal mesogastrium. (b) It increases as the stomach broadens ventrodorsally and rotates to the right. (c and d) With further growth the lesser sac becomes bounded by the mesogastrium which contains the spleen on the left, and ventrally by the stomach and ventral mesentery. (e) A stereogram of the developing lesser sac.

rotation explains how the left and right vagus nerves emerge from the oesophageal plexus as the anterior and posterior gastric trunks respectively.

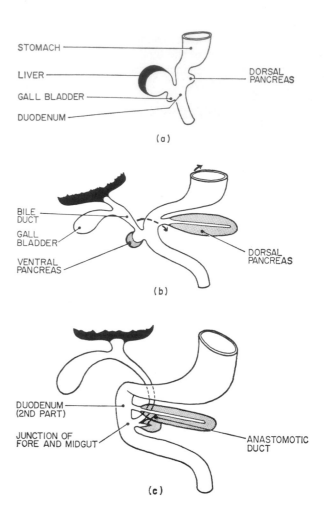

FIG. 32.67. Three stages in the development of the pancreas and biliary apparatus.

Duodenum. The foregut caudal to the stomach grows and loops ventrally. The hepatic diverticulum arises from the apex of the loop and marks the lower end of the foregut. The whole loop becomes the duodenum, which is therefore part foregut and part midgut (figs. 32.67 and 32.68).

DEVELOPMENT OF MIDGUT

The connection of the yolk sac to the midgut narrows in the fourth week, forming the vitello-intestinal duct (fig. 32.68). Cranially the midgut becomes the caudal half of the duodenum, but the major portion elongates into a long loop towards the umbilicus that is attached at its apex to the vitello-intestinal duct. The cranial limb of the loop grows more rapidly and becomes coiled, while the caudal limb develops a bulge near the vitello-intestinal duct, the primordial caecum. Thus the coiled proximal limb becomes the jejunum and most of the ileum, and the caudal limb the terminal ileum, caecum and proximal colon. The vitello-intestinal duct atrophies in the sixth week, but occasionally persists as Meckel's diverticulum (p.

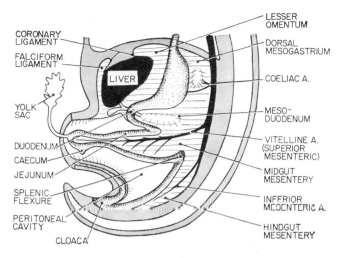

FIG. 32.68. Sagittal diagram of embryo showing mesenteries. In this 10 mm embryo the vitello-intestinal duct has narrowed, and the midgut loop has herniated into the intra-umbilical coelom. The growth of the liver into the septum transversum has formed a ventral mesentery consisting of the lesser omentum and the coronary ligament.

32.23). Rarely the entire duct may remain so that the intestinal contents leak from the umbilicus, or it may remain as a fibrous cord stretching from the ileum to the umbilicus. The caecal swelling becomes conical and later the apex of the cone lengthens to form the appendix, so that at birth the appendix arises from the apex of the caecum. Postnatally, further growth brings the base of the appendix to the posteromedial aspect of the caecum.

DEVELOPMENT OF HINDGUT

The hindgut extends from the midgut to the cloacal membrane. The cloaca becomes divided by the downgrowth of

the urorectal septum into the rectum behind and the urogenital sinus in front. The part of the cloacal membrane which closes the rectum ruptures during the eighth week and the rectum then opens on to the ectodermal anal pit. Subsequently this pit deepens to form the lower ectodermal part of the anal canal, whereas the upper part is endodermal.

Imperforate anus results from a persisting anal membrane. Failure of the urorectal septum causes very serious fistulous communications between the gut and the urinary system, or vagina in the female. Atresia of the rectum may be associated with deficiency of the muscular anal sphincter.

DEVELOPMENT OF THE LIVER AND PANCREAS

The liver arises from a diverticulum at the junction of the foregut and midgut that grows ventrally into the septum transversum and divides into two primary branches (fig. 32.67). The stem of the diverticulum is soon joined by the ventral pancreatic bud, and becomes the bile duct. The caudal primary branch differentiates into the cystic duct and gall bladder, and does not divide further, but the cranial branch divides repeatedly and proliferates forming the remainder of the biliary system and hepatocytes. These consist of sheets of cells which invade the septum transversum and encounter the vitelline veins to transform them into a system of sinusoids (p. 19.18 and fig. 32.69). The fibrous and haemopoietic tissue of the liver is derived from the mesenchyme of the septum transversum.

The liver grows quickly so that at nine weeks it weighs 10 per cent of the whole embryo, and fills most of the abdominal cavity. The rapid growth is partly due to erythropoiesis within the liver (p. 28.4). The liver is 5

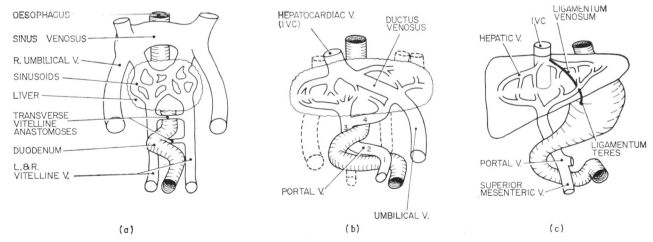

FIG. 32.69. Development of hepatic circulation. Three ventral views showing how the growing liver incorporates the vitelline veins and taps the umbilical veins, and how the portal vein forms in the region of the duodenum.

per cent of body weight at birth and declines to less than half that in the adult.

The pancreas develops from gut endoderm by two separate diverticula. The ventral one arises in common with the hepatic diverticulum, so that the main pancreatic and bile ducts share a common entrance into the duodenum in the adult. The dorsal pancreas arises more cranially, and grows into the dorsal mesentery (fig. 32.67). Growth changes within the duodenum cause the ventral pancreas and hepatic diverticulum to swing to the right around the gut until they abut on the right surface of the dorsal pancreas. The pancreatic primordia fuse, so that the ventral outgrowth ultimately forms the inferior part of the head and uncinate process and the dorsal pancreas the remainder of the organ. The developing duct of the dorsal pancreas joins a tributary of the ventral duct so that the latter then becomes the terminal portion of the main duct (cf. figs. 32.67 and 32.51). The terminal part of the dorsal duct usually separates off as the accessory duct from the newly developed main duct, and drains the upper part of the head into the duodenum more cranially.

The rotation of the bile duct around the duodenum explains its dorsal relationship to the first part of the duodenum and the head of pancreas in the adult (fig.32.51).

Development of the mesenteries

By the end of the fourth week the gut is a midline structure which is suspended by a shallow median dorsal mesentery (fig. 32.64). Above the septum transversum, the oesophagus lies within a broad mesentery which contains the lung bud and attaches ventrally to the pericardium (fig. 32.65). The thick septum transversum has not yet become the ventral mesentery which connects the foregut and anterior abdominal wall. Subsequently, much of the gut deviates from the median plane, and certain parts of the mesentery increase in depth or fuse with the dorsal wall and are obliterated. The mesenteries are considered from above down.

MESO-OESOPHAGUS

This is a broad mass between the dorsal wall and the pericardium and contains the oesophagus and the lung bud. It forms the connective tissue of much of the mediastinum and associated pleura and the entire oesophagus except for its epithelium.

MESOGASTRIUM

The dorsal mesogastrium is in the median plane, but changes within it establish the lesser sac of peritoneum. Cavitation within its right side marks the beginning of the omental bursa (fig. 32.66). This cavity enlarges by active growth of the mesentery, which thins and bulges to the left. The rotation of the stomach to the right (p.

32.56) brings it to the anterior wall of the bursa, which is limited to the left and dorsally by the mesogastrium, but opens at the right into the general peritoneal cavity. The spleen develops in the mesogastrium and distends its left layer of peritoneum. The left surface of the mesogastrium fuses with the dorsal abdominal wall, to become attached over the left kidney, and runs to the spleen as the lieno-renal ligament, and from the spleen to stomach as the gastrosplenic ligament (cf. figs. 32.66 and 32.14). Caudally the mesogastrium hangs down as a double fold from the greater curvature of the stomach over the developing transverse colon (fig. 32.70). The most posterior layer of the fold fuses with the adjacent mesocolon and colon, bringing its attachment to the antimesenteric border of the colon. This more caudal portion of the mesogastrium is the future greater omentum (cf. figs. 32.70 and 32.13).

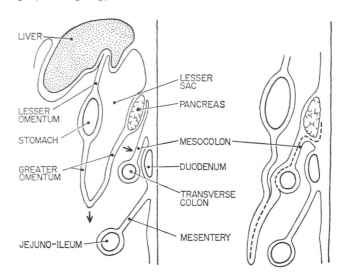

FIG. 32.70. Sagittal section through lesser sac. The dorsal mesogastrium projects caudally as a pouch which overhangs the transverse colon. This pouch is the greater omentum and fusion of its posterior wall with the adjacent transverse colon and mesocolon brings its attachment to the colon (compare fig. 32.13).

At four weeks the foregut is close to the lower part of the septum transversum (fig. 32.64), but as the embryo lengthens the septum becomes separated from the gut and thins forming the ventral mesentery which stretches from the foregut to the diaphragm and anterior abdominal wall (fig. 32.68). The liver has already distended the midportion of this mesentery (fig. 32.65), so that the thin part connecting the foregut to the liver is the lesser omentum, and the part joining the liver to the diaphragm is the coronary ligament. The free border of the latter part which carries the left umbilical vein from the umbilicus to the liver is the falciform ligament. Later cavitation of the septum transversum between the two organs establishes the sub-diaphragmatic spaces and reduces the area within the coronary ligament to the definitive bare area (fig. 32.17).

The cavitation in the dorsal mesogastrium extends cranially between the oesophagus and right lung bud as the pneumato-enteric recess and this part becomes cut off by the closure of the diaphragm. The lower part persists as the upper recess of the lesser sac, which lies between the diaphragm posteriorly and the liver in front; it is bounded on its right side by the caval fold which carries the inferior vena cava from the dorsal abdominal wall to the liver. Rotation of the stomach swings the lesser omentum into the coronal plane. It forms the anterior wall of the upper recess of the lesser sac, and its free right border bounds the entrance to the lesser sac, the epiploic foramen (fig. 32.66).

The lesser sac of the peritoneum therefore communicates with the greater sac or general peritoneal cavity via the epiploic foramen, and arises by changes in the dorsal mesogastrium and ventral mesentery. The inferior recess, derived from the omental bursa, is the large part that lies behind the stomach and within the greater omentum, while the upper recess is behind the lesser omentum and liver.

MESODUODENUM

Growth of the duodenum caused it to loop ventrally, and the pancreas develops within the mesoduodenum (figs. 32.67 and 32.68). On reduction of the physiological hernia the returning colon displaces the duodenum to the right, pressing it and the mesoduodenum against the right half of the posterior abdominal wall where the adjacent peritoneal layers fuse making the duodenum and most of the pancreas retroperitoneal (figs. 32.12 and 32.72.)

MIDGUT MESENTERY AND ROTATION OF MIDGUT

As the midgut grows, its mesentery deepens, so the gut forms a long loop towards the umbilicus (figs. 32.68 and 32.71). The fast growing liver comes to fill most of the abdominal cavity, so that in the sixth week the mobile midgut is pushed out into the umbilical coelom. This **physiological herniation** lasts about six weeks, until the liver becomes relatively smaller when the midgut returns to the abdominal cavity. As the gut continues to grow within the umbilical coelom, the cranial limb of jejuno-ileum becomes very coiled, and the caecal swelling on the caudal limb enlarges. Simultaneously the midgut loop rotates anticlockwise through 90° around the axis of the superior mesenteric artery.

Little is known of the factors that initiate the reduction of the hernia, but the relative decline in the size of the liver and increase in size of the abdominal cavity probably both contribute. The jejuno-ileum returns first, because the caecal swelling hampers the return of the caudal limb, and enters the lower left abdomen. The coils of jejuno-ileum displace the hindgut with its mesentery to the left against the posterior abdominal wall, where later the adjacent peritoneal layers fuse, binding both the splenic flexure and descending colon to the posterior abdominal wall (figs. 32.71, 32.72 and 32.12). The caecum and caudal limb return later and a further anticlockwise rotation through 180° brings them cranial to the jejunum and ileum. They enter above and to the right of the jejunum and ileum, with the caecum inferior to the liver. The colon pursues a straight course from the caecum to the splenic flexure. This rotation has brought the midgut colon ventral to the duodenum, and hence the superior mesenteric artery emerges ventral to its third part. Subsequently the liver rises away from the caecum

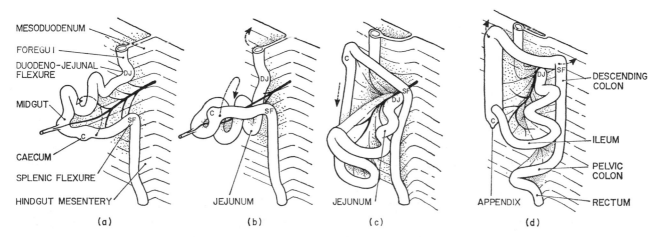

Fig. 32.71. Herniation and rotation of midgut. (a) The midgut loop herniates into the umbilical coelom in the median plane. (b) The caudal and proximal limb rotated anticlockwise. (c) Further rotation and withdrawal of the hernia brings the proximal limb (jejuno-ileum) against the hindgut. The caudal limb (caecum and colon) presses the duodenum into the right posterior abdominal wall. (d) The caecum descends from the subhepatic position.

and the ascending colon grows in length. The mesentery of the ascending colon is obliterated by fusion with the posterior abdominal wall in a similar fashion to that of the descending colon, but the transverse colon retains its mesentery.

The jejunum and ileum also retain their deep mesentery which permits mobility in the adult (cf. figs. 32.72 and 32.12).

MESENTERY OF HINDGUT

The development of the abdominal hindgut mesentery has been described. The pelvic mesentery persists in part as the pelvic mesocolon, but the mesentery of the rectum diminishes so that the rectum rests directly on the sacrum. The most caudal part of the rectum and anal canal are outside the coelom and so extraperitoneal.

The primitive dorsal mesentery of the gut is much modified since it grows in depth, fuses with the parietal peritoneum of the posterior abdominal wall, and deviates from the midline. There are two consequences of the fact that fusion occurs at a late stage of development. First, the gut remains ventral to the urogenital system on the posterior abdominal wall, and secondly the planes of fusion are natural cleavage planes that are not crossed by any major vessel or nerves, because the vessels reach the gut in the dorsal mesentery and their general pattern is established long before fusion occurs. These planes are therefore of practical value to the surgeon who can reopen them without fear of damaging vessels or nerves. For example, the lower end of the bile duct, which descends embedded in the back of the pancreas (p. 32.34), can be exposed by incising the peritoneum around the convexity of the duodenum and reflecting it ventrally and medially, which reverses the developmental fusion of duodenum and posterior abdominal wall.

The extensive fusion and obliteration of the gut mesentery is associated with an upright posture. In common with other recent evolutionary changes, it shows marked variation. A quarter of the population have a persistent mesentery on either the ascending or descending colons. More rarely, the duodenal mesentery may remain. Such faulty fixation of the gut, by allowing excessive mobility, predisposes to twisting of the gut or volvulus.

Varying degrees of incomplete rotation may occur, ranging from the extremely rare type of non-rotation where the jejuno-ileum is on the right side of the abdomen, and the entire colon on the left, to the less severe varieties such as a subhepatic caecum. In the latter condition rotation stops at a late stage, but the caecum remains under the liver and there is no ascending colon. Complete reversal of rotation is very rare and is usually associated with similar reversal of the other abdominal and thoracic organs.

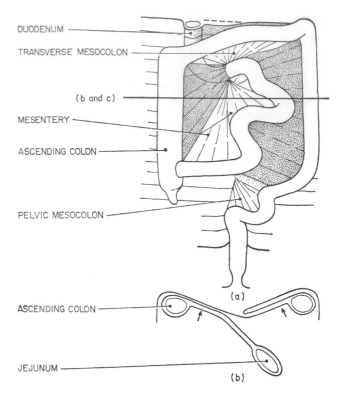

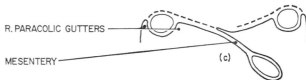

FIG. 32.72. Fixation of gut. (a) After withdrawal of the midgut from the umbilical coelom, parts of the mesenteries (shown in stipple) adhere to the parietal peritoneum on the posterior abdominal wall and fix the gut (b) before and (c) after fixation.

Umbilical hernia is a common condition that results from incomplete closure of the umbilicus by the developing anterior abdominal wall.

Development of blood vessels

Three unpaired visceral arteries arise from the dorsal aorta and enter the dorsal mesentery to reach the foregut, midgut, and hindgut respectively (fig. 32.68). The **coeliac artery** of the foregut encounters the opening of the omental bursa as it runs ventrally within the mesogastrium, and sends its branches around the margins of the entrance. The vitelline artery of the midgut originally supplied the yolk sac, but its distal portion which accompanied the vitello-intestinal duct atrophies with the yolk sac, leaving the proximal portion to become the **superior mesenteric artery**. The **inferior mesenteric artery** supplies the hindgut as far as the proctodaeum, which forms the lower part of the anal canal and receives a paired somatic segmental vessel, the inferior rectal artery.

The paired **vitelline veins** draining the yolk sac accompany the vitello-intestinal duct to the midgut, and then ascend in the mesentery on either side of the duodenal loop, and enter the liver. They emerge from the liver and end in the sinus venosus of the heart (p. 19.17).

The vitelline veins form transverse anastomoses near the duodenum, and a plexus of sinusoids within the liver (fig. 32.69). The decline in the yolk sac circulation results in the disappearance of the vitelline veins distally, but the differentiation of a new vessel, the superior mesenteric vein, in the dorsal mesentery brings more blood to the proximal part of the system. This vein develops on the left surface of the caudal limb of the duodenal loop, which as the duodenum swings to the right (p. 32.59) becomes its ventral surface, and delivers blood into the left vitelline vein that follows a direct route into the liver. This direct channel becomes the **portal vein**, and consists of (1) part of the left vitelline vein (2) the transverse anastomosis within the duodenal loop (3) the proximal segment of the right vitelline vein and (4) another anastomotic vessel (fig. 32.69). The remainder of the vitelline system caudal to the liver atrophies.

INTRAHEPATIC CIRCULATION

The vitelline veins within the septum transversum are transformed by the ingrowing sheets of hepatocytes into a continuous system of liver sinusoids (p. 32.36). These sinusoids are therefore filled from the branches of the portal system, and drain cranially via efferent veins from the liver into the vitelline veins. After the disappearance of the left hepatocardiac segment of the vitelline vein (p. 19.17) these efferent veins, which are the future hepatic veins, converge on the right hepatocardiac vein. The latter forms the terminal segment of the inferior vena cava (fig. 19.31).

The vitelline veins therefore form the portal vein and its branches, the liver sinusoids, the hepatic veins and the uppermost part of the inferior vena cava.

The more laterally placed umbilical veins also become involved by the growing liver. First, the liver sinusoids tap the umbilical veins and provide a more direct route to the heart (fig. 32.69). Later, as the placental flow increases, a large shunt is established in the liver to by-pass the slow sinusoid circulation. This **ductus venosus** connects the definitive (left) umbilical vein with the right hepatocardiac vein. The umbilical vein ascends in the free border of the ventral mesentery between the umbilicus and the liver. After birth the fibrous remnant of the umbilical vein persists as the ligamentum teres. The ductus venosus also fibroses after birth but remains as the ligamentum venosum joining the upper end of the ligamentum teres to the inferior vena cava.

FURTHER READING

CODE C.F. ed. (1967–68) *Handbook of Physiology*, Section 6. Alimentary canal. Vols. 1–5. Washington, D.C.: American Physiological Society.

CREAMER B. (1967) Turnover of the epithelium of the small intestine. *British Medical Bulletin* 23, 226–230.

DA COSTA L.R. (1971) Small-intestinal cell turnover in patients with parasitic infections. *British Medical Journal* 3, 281 283.

DAVENPORT H.W. (1971) *Physiology of the Digestive Tract; an Introductory Text*, 3rd Edition. Chicago: Year Book Medical Publishers.

JAMES W.P.T., ALPERS D.H., GERBER J.E. & ISSELBACHER K.J. (1971) The turnover of disaccharidases and brush border proteins in rat intestine. *Biochimica et Biophysica Acta* 230, 194–203.

KANAGASUNTHERAM R. (1957) Development of the human lesser sac. *Journal of Anatomy* 91, 188–206.

LECHAGO J. & BENCOSME S.A. (1973) Endocrine elements of the digestive system. *International Review of Experimental Pathology* 12, 119–201.

McCOLL I. & SLADEN G.E. eds. (1975) *Intestinal Absorption in Man*. New York: Academic Press.

PAVLOV I.P. (1910) *The Work of the Digestive Glands*, 2nd English Edition, translated by W.H. Thompson. London: Griffin.

ROUILLER C. ed. (1963) *The Liver*, vol. 1, chaps. 1–8. New York: Academic Press.

TONER P.G., CARR KATHERINE E. & WYBURN G.M. (1971) *The Digestive System; an Ultrastructural Atlas and Review*. London: Butterworth.

Chapter 33
Metabolic functions of the liver

The liver holds a key place in the metabolism of the body. Some processes are carried out exclusively or predominantly in the liver; others are shared in varying degree with other tissues; these latter are discussed here only when the liver makes a quantitatively important contribution to their total metabolism. The following list summarizes the principal topics:

(1) The liver's role in metabolism.

(2) Detoxication or inactivation of endogenous and exogenous substances and enzyme induction.

(3) Formation and secretion of bile.

(4) Chemical tests commonly used to investigate liver function.

Since about 80 per cent of the blood flow to the liver comes via the portal vein and only 20 per cent from the hepatic artery, hepatocytes carry out their metabolic functions at a lower Po_2 than most cells in other organs. Further, hepatocytes in zone 3 of the acinus near the hepatic veins receive oxygen at a lower Po_2 than those in zone 1 near the portal tracts, because their blood supply is deoxygenated during passage through zones 1 and 2. Some degree of enzymic localization is related to these differences in oxygenation. Thus cells in zone 1 have relatively high concentrations of succinate dehydrogenase, cytochrome oxidase, ATPase and alkaline phosphatase. Those in zone 3 are rich in diaphorase, $NADH_2$ and $NADPH_2$ reductases, 3-hydroxybutyrate dehydrogenase, lactate dehydrogenase, glutamate dehydrogenase and esterase. Zone 2 has intermediate properties. Morphologically, differences are also present, mitochondria being more numerous in the cells of zone 1 and microsomes in cells of zone 3. The remarkable regenerative capacity of the liver is described on p. 32.37 and in vol. 2, p. 27.1.

Nitrogen metabolism

The liver is active in protein synthesis, in the interconversion of amino acids and in the formation of urea as the main nitrogenous end-product of amino acid and protein metabolism in animals.

Amino acids for the hepatic synthesis of protein are derived partly from dietary and partly from endogenous protein. The liver is important in the utilization of any amino acids present in excess of immediate need. Protein is stored only to a limited extent and any excess of individual amino acids over those required for protein synthesis is partly offset, for the non-essential amino acids, by interconversions catalysed by the hepatic aminotransferases (p. 33.2).

The mechanism of protein synthesis is discussed on p. 12.13. The relationship between protein synthesis and nucleic acids was investigated initially on micro-organisms, especially *Esch. coli* which do not contain an endoplasmic reticulum. More recently hepatocytes have been used extensively for investigating the role of the endoplasmic reticulum in protein synthesis (p. 13.17).

The rough endoplasmic reticulum (RER) of the hepatocytes is the main site for the synthesis of protein in the liver. Disorganization, dilation and disruption of the hepatic RER may be caused by several agents, e.g. carbon tetrachloride and actinomycin D, one effect of which is to impair the synthesis of protein. One consequence of administering these poisons, obvious histologically, is the accumulation of lipid in the hepatocytes, due to diminished production of the apolipoproteins needed to transport triglycerides from the liver as very low density lipoproteins (VLDL) in plasma. A wide range of drugs, and also obstruction to the outflow of bile, may increase the formation of certain hepatic enzymes; this is discussed on p. 33.10 under enzyme induction.

The synthesis of proteins by the liver depends on an adequate supply of dietary protein. It is influenced by hormones such as cortisol and thyroxine which both stimulate the formation of albumin, although the precise way in which each exerts its effects on hepatic RNA synthesis, and thereby on protein synthesis, appears to be different. Many studies of protein synthesis by the liver have been based on measurements of albumin production which accounts for about 50 per cent of the hepatocyte's capacity for synthesizing protein.

PLASMA PROTEIN SYNTHESIS

Table 33.1 lists many of the proteins present in plasma and summarizes several of their properties. Albumin is

Table 33.1. Properties of some of the plasma proteins.

Name of protein	Plasma concentration (normal values) g/l	Molecular weight	Half-life days	Comments
Albumin	40	69 000	20	Important in maintaining plasma volume and distribution of extracellular fluid. Has several transport functions; minor role as a buffer.
α_1-globulins				
$\quad$ α_1-antitrypsin	3	45 000	6	Antiproteinase
$\quad$ α_1-acid glycoprotein	0·8	45 000	—	Function unknown
$\quad$ HDL (high density lipoproteins)	3·5	200 000	—	Lipid transport
α_2-globulins				
$\quad$ Ceruloplasmin	0·4	160 000	4	Copper transport
$\quad$ Haptoglobins	1·2	100 000 (Hp 1–1)	—	Several phenotypes. Glycoproteins that bind haemoglobin, and which may thus help to conserve iron.
$\quad$ α_2-macroglobulin	3·0	800 000	—	Antiproteinase; also possible transport function.
$\quad$ VLDL (very low density lipoproteins)	1·5	10 000 000	—	Lipid transport
β-globulins				
$\quad$ Transferrin	2·5	90 000	11	Iron transport
$\quad$ Hemopexin	1·0	80 000	—	Binds haemoglobin
$\quad$ C_3 (β_{1C}-globulin)	1·2	185 000	—	Third component of complement (vol. 2, p. 22.16)
$\quad$ C_4 (β_{1E}-globulin)	0·4	240 000	—	Fourth component of complement
$\quad$ Plasminogen	0·7	140 000	—	Fibrinolysis (p. 28.16)
$\quad$ Fibrinogen	4·0	350 000	3	Fibrin formation
$\quad$ LDL (low density lipoproteins)	4·0	2 300 000	—	Lipid transport
Immunoglobulins				
$\quad$ IgA	2·5	170 000	6	Antibodies, each group having somewhat different functions (Vol. 2, p. 22.19). They mainly move as γ-globulins on zone electrophoresis, but some migrate as β-globulins or as α_2-globulins (fig. 33.11).
$\quad$ IgD	0·02	160 000	3	
$\quad$ IgE	Trace	190 000	2	
$\quad$ IgG	10	155 000	24	
$\quad$ IgM	1·0	950 000	5	

quantitatively by far the most important and it is synthesized exclusively by the hepatocytes. Studies with ^{131}I-human albumin show that the half-life of this protein is about 20 days. Since the plasma volume is about 3 litres, and the plasma albumin concentration is about 40 g/l, the liver must normally synthesize about 3 g albumin each day.

Most of the other plasma proteins, including many of the coagulation factors (fibrinogen, prothrombin and Factors V, VII, IX and X) and several transport proteins, e.g. ceruloplasmin and transferrin, are synthesized exclusively or almost exclusively by the hepatocytes. The formation of prothrombin and Factors VII and X depends on a supply of vitamin K. Immunoglobulins provide an exception to the generalization that hepatocytes are mainly responsible for synthesis of plasma proteins; they are produced by cells of the lymphoid system.

TRANSAMINATION AND DEAMINATION

Any amino acids present in excess of the immediate needs of the body are metabolized by reactions which have the following general form:

$$\text{L-amino acid} + \text{2-oxoglutarate} \rightleftharpoons \text{2-oxoacid} + \text{L-glutamate}$$

This reaction involves the transfer of a 2-amino group from the amino acid to 2-oxoglutarate and is catalysed by an aminotransferase (alternatively called a transaminase). The 2-oxoacids are further metabolized by various pathways depending on their structure (chap. 11); some 2-oxoacids can contribute to gluconeogenesis, as discussed below. Regeneration of 2-oxoglutarate is effected by glutamate dehydrogenase, which catalyses the reaction

$$\text{L-glutamate} + \text{H}_2\text{O} + \text{NAD (or NADP)} \rightleftharpoons \text{2-oxoglutarate} + \text{NH}_3 + \text{NADH}_2 \text{ (or NADPH}_2\text{)}$$

There are several aminotransferases, most of which can be detected in other organs, e.g. kidney and muscle. Glutamate dehydrogenase is also present in other organs but the liver is one of the most active sites of transamination and deamination.

Aspartate and alanine aminotransferase have each been studied extensively in disease. These enzymes contain pyridoxal phosphate and catalyse reactions involving L-aspartate and L-alanine respectively. Alternative names for these enzymes still used widely clinically are glutamic oxaloacetic transaminase (GOT) and glutamic pyruvic transaminase (GPT) respectively. Aspartate and alanine aminotransferase are present in many different tissues.

Examples of aminotransferases that are found only in hepatic tissue are ornithine, asparagine and glutamine oxoacid aminotransferases; these are also proteins containing pyridoxal phosphate. They catalyse the following reactions:

L-ornithine + 2-oxoacid $\rightleftharpoons$
$\qquad$ L-glutamate-γ-semialdehyde + L-amino acid
L-asparagine + 2-oxoacid $\rightleftharpoons$
$\qquad$ 2-oxosuccinamate + L-amino acid
L-glutamine + 2-oxoacid $\rightleftharpoons$
$\qquad$ 2-oxoglutaramate + L-amino acid

Collectively, the aminotransferases deaminate most of the naturally occurring L-amino acids. A consequence of all these reactions is that ammonia is formed in the liver from the deamination of amino acids present in excess of immediate requirements for protein synthesis. Ammonia may also be derived from glutamine and asparagine by the action of the hydrolytic enzymes glutaminase and asparaginase. Ammonia is also carried in the blood to the liver, after production by similar reactions occurring in other tissues, notably the kidney (p. 35.32).

SYNTHESIS OF UREA

Ammonia is a toxic product of nitrogen metabolism, and the liver is the main site for its conversion into the end-product, urea, which is much less toxic. The reactions which result in the synthesis of urea are often referred to as the ornithine cycle and are associated with the names of Krebs and Henseleit. These reactions are shown diagrammatically in fig. 33.1. The cycle can go only one way because the hydrolytic reaction catalysed by arginase is virtually irreversible.

In this sequence of reactions, the first synthetic step involves the transfer of the carbamyl group from carbamyl phosphate to the 5-amino group of ornithine. This is catalysed by ornithine carbamyl transferase, an enzyme which occurs in high concentrations in liver and in much smaller amounts in a few other tissues. The enzymic mechanism for formation of carbamyl phosphate is not completely understood, but synthetic carbamyl phosphate can replace it in the reaction with ornithine. The naturally

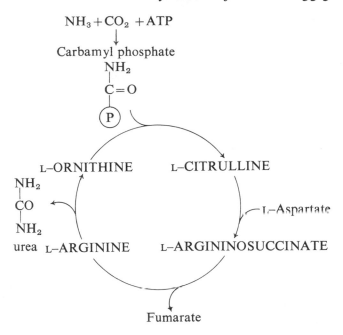

FIG. 33.1. The ornithine cycle and the synthesis of urea. The cycle is unidirectional as the hydrolytic step catalysed by arginase is irreversible, but all the other reactions can be reversed under suitable conditions.

occurring compound is formed, in the presence of *N*-acetylglutamate, from NH_4^+ and HCO_3^- by the enzyme carbamate kinase, which requires ATP and Mg^{++}. The role of *N*-acetylglutamate in this reaction is unclear and the intermediate formation of carbamic acid is assumed in the following description of events.

$$NH_4^+ + HCO_3^- \rightleftharpoons NH_4HCO_3 \rightleftharpoons NH_2COOH + H_2O$$

$$NH_2COOH + ATP \underset{Mg^{++}}{\rightleftharpoons} NH_2COO\text{℗} + ADP$$

The synthesis of carbamyl phosphate is, in practice, largely irreversible and the above representation of its formation oversimplifies the process in at least two respects. Firstly, *N*-acetylglutamate probably functions as an activator in the reaction and, secondly, the overall stoichiometry of the synthesis requires two molecules of ATP.

In the next synthetic step citrulline condenses with aspartic acid, in the presence of ATP and Mg^{++}, to form argininosuccinic acid; the ATP is converted to AMP and inorganic pyrophosphate. Argininosuccinate synthase catalyses this reaction and the product is then split reversibly to arginine and fumaric acid by argininosuccinate lyase. The hydrolytic reaction catalysed by arginase gives rise to ornithine and urea.

There is an alternative, though quantitatively less important, route for the formation of ornithine from arginine, catalysed by glycine transamidinase.

$$NH_2 \quad H_2N \qquad\qquad H_2N \qquad\qquad NH_2$$

Glycine   Arginine   Guanidoacetate   Ornithine

All the enzymes of the ornithine cycle occur in other tissues, but the high concentrations of each in the liver accounts for this organ's unique role in the synthesis of urea in mammals. The essentially cyclical nature of the process can be shown by the continuous production of urea for as long as NH_4^+, HCO_3^- and an energy source to provide ATP are available, with only catalytic amounts of intermediates such as ornithine and citrulline being used. The net reaction of the ornithine cycle (omitting energy transformations) is as follows.

$$NH_4^+ + HCO_3^- + \text{L-aspartate} \rightleftharpoons$$
$$\text{urea} + \text{fumarate} + 2H_2O$$

After total hepatectomy in experimental animals or severe liver failure in man, the concentration of amino acids in blood rises and the amount in the urine increases; this type of aminoaciduria is often called overflow aminoaciduria. There is also a fall in blood ammonia and urea concentrations unless there is concomitant renal failure.

Carbohydrate metabolism

The liver plays an essential part in carbohydrate metabolism and in maintaining blood glucose concentration, which is normally kept within fairly close limits. Glycogen, the storage form of carbohydrate, is found in higher concentrations in liver than in muscle. The body's capacity to store carbohydrate is limited and any glucose absorbed from the diet in excess both of this capacity and of immediate requirements for oxidative metabolism is converted to fat and stored as such. Like adipose tissue, the liver is an important site for conversion of carbohydrate to lipids, although other tissues, e.g. muscle, also contain the enzyme systems required for synthesis of fatty acids from acetyl coenzyme A (acetyl CoA).

The synthesis and breakdown of glycogen are described on p. 9.9. The rapidity with which glycogen can be broken down to glucose, and the efficiency of gluconeogenesis, which takes place most actively in the liver, both contribute to the maintenance of the blood glucose concentration if the dietary intake of carbohydrate is restricted. Normally the adult human liver contains about 100 g glycogen, on which the body can draw immediately to maintain the blood glucose concentration. If dietary carbohydrate is insufficient, gluconeogenesis helps to replenish the stores of liver glycogen, and several hormones include among their activities the promotion of gluconeogenesis.

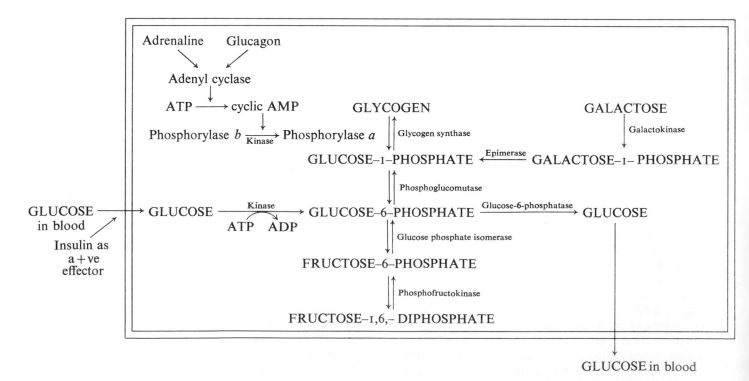

FIG. 33.2. Simplified scheme of reactions involved in the uptake and release of glucose by the hepatocyte. The scheme shows the points of action of insulin, adrenaline and glucagon; these controlling influences are discussed in detail in chap. 14.

GLUCONEOGENESIS

This process involves the net formation of glucose from compounds that are intermediates, or which can be converted into intermediates, in either the glycolytic pathway (p. 9.7) or the citric acid cycle (p. 9.16). For instance, those amino acids which after deamination form pyruvate, oxaloacetate or 2-oxoglutarate, either directly or indirectly as a result of further metabolism of their corresponding 2-oxoacids, can give rise to glucose by reversal of the glycolytic pathway in the liver. Gluconeogenesis can lead to glycogen deposition in the liver or to the release of glucose into the blood. Alanine, serine, cysteine, aspartate and glutamate are glucogenic amino acids.

The liver can also synthesize glucose from glycerol, formed during the breakdown of neutral fats and phospholipids. Glycerol enters the glycolytic pathway through the action of glycerokinase and glycerolphosphate dehydrogenase. It is the only component of fat which has been shown to give a net synthesis of glucose or glycogen in man; experiments with ^{14}C-fatty acids demonstrate incorporation of isotope into glucose and glycogen but, on balance, these experiments do not show any net synthesis of these compounds from fatty acids.

The liver is the main organ responsible for converting galactose, fructose and various pentoses (all normal dietary constituents) into glucose. Fig. 33.2 provides a simplified summary of the processes involved in glycogen storage and gluconeogenesis in the liver.

HORMONAL CONTROL OF GLUCOSE METABOLISM

Several hormones influence glucose metabolism, and fig. 33.2 indicates the main sites where their effects are exerted. Insulin is the most important, its principal effect on carbohydrate metabolism being to lower the blood glucose concentration; insulin exerts these effects by promoting the uptake of glucose by some tissues as well as by inhibiting glycogenolysis and gluconeogenesis. The other hormones, glucagon, adrenaline, growth hormone and the glucocorticoids, all tend to increase the blood glucose concentration either by promoting the breakdown of glycogen, or by stimulating gluconeogenesis, or by interfering with the uptake of glucose by the tissues.

Many of these hormones exert their effects on carbohydrate metabolism indirectly, by stimulating adenyl cyclase thereby leading to a localized increase in cyclic AMP (p. 14.12). Cyclic AMP acts as the intermediate, or second messenger, whereby adrenaline and glucagon produce hyperglycaemia as a result of increased glycogen breakdown in the liver. The degradation of glycogen to glucose-1-phosphate is catalysed by phosphorylase, an enzyme that is normally present in the liver in an inactive form. Inactive phosphorylase (phosphorylase *b*) is converted to the active enzyme (phosphorylase *a*) by a specific kinase which requires cyclic AMP as cofactor.

The action of adrenaline or glucagon in promoting glycogenolysis is brought to an end either by the breakdown of cyclic AMP to adenosine-5'-monophosphate, or by the action of phosphorylase phosphatase on phosphorylase *a*; this latter enzyme splits off inorganic phosphate from phosphorylase *a* with the production of inactive phosphorylase *b*.

These explanations of the molecular effects of hormones do not apply to the control of glucose metabolism exerted by insulin, although insulin probably mediates another of its actions, in decreasing lipolysis, by reducing the concentration of cyclic AMP in adipose tissue. It also seems unlikely that insulin exerts its effects on glucose metabolism by controlling the activity of hexokinase, an explanation which was at one time thought to be correct. Instead it seems probable that the main action of insulin is to regulate the synthesis of a membrane-linked transport system for glucose (p. 14.13).

Lipid metabolism

The principal dietary lipids of metabolic importance in man are triglycerides, phospholipids and esters of cholesterol. These are mostly or at least partly digested prior to absorption, the efficiency of the digestive process depending on the formation of a fine emulsion of these water-insoluble molecules. The liver contributes to fat digestion and absorption by providing bile, the bile salts acting both as emulsifying agents and as activators of pancreatic lipase. After absorption some of the lipid enters the portal circulation and some goes via the lacteals and the thoracic duct to the systemic circulation and the fat depots.

The liver metabolizes lipids, whether brought to it from the gut or from the fat depots as a result of lipid mobilization. Synthesis of triglycerides and phospholipids takes place in the liver, using free fatty acids (FFA) actively extracted from the plasma. The liver also synthesizes fat from carbohydrate (mainly glucose) and amino acids when the amounts of these available in the blood exceed the requirements of other tissues. Triglyceride synthesized in the liver is transported in the plasma mainly as pre-β-lipoprotein (VLDL) to the storage sites in adipose tissue.

OXIDATION OF FATTY ACIDS AND
FORMATION OF KETONE BODIES

Breakdown of long-chain fatty acids in the liver occurs in a series of stepwise reactions which result in the eventual overall production of several molecules of acetyl CoA and one molecule of acetoacetyl CoA (p. 10.8). For instance, the breakdown of stearic acid may be represented as follows.

$$CH_3(CH_2)_{16}COOH \longrightarrow CH_3COCH_2CO.SCoA +$$

Stearic acid   Acetoacetyl CoA

$$+7CH_3CO.SCoA$$

Acetyl CoA

The liver normally converts acetoacetyl CoA to two molecules of acetyl CoA by the action of acetyl CoA acetyl transferase.

$$\text{Acetoacetyl CoA} + \text{CoA} \xrightarrow[\text{Acetyltransferase}]{\text{Acetyl CoA}} 2 \text{ Acetyl CoA}$$

Acetyl CoA then takes part in a number of different metabolic processes, normally being oxidized to CO_2 and water via the citric acid cycle. When further oxidative metabolism of acetyl CoA in the liver is impaired, breakdown of fatty acids leads almost exclusively to the production of acetoacetate from which are derived, by further metabolism, 3-hydroxybutyrate and acetone (fig. 33.3). These three compounds are collectively called ketone bodies although 3-hydroxybutyrate is not in fact a ketone.

The reactions involved in the production of acetoacetate by the liver are shown in fig. 33.3. In the quantitatively more important process, two molecules of acetyl CoA first condense to give acetoacetyl CoA by a reversal of the action of acetyl CoA acetyltransferase, and acetoacetyl CoA then condenses with a further molecule of acetyl CoA to give a molecule of β-hydroxy-β-methylglutaryl CoA (HMG CoA). The presence of the enzyme HMG CoA synthase is needed and the molecule of HMG CoA is subsequently split by HMG CoA lyase, with the formation of acetoacetate and regeneration of one molecule of acetyl CoA. Another enzyme, localized in the liver, can hydrolyse acetoacetyl CoA to acetoacetate, but this is a relatively minor pathway.

The liver can only metabolize acetoacetate to a limited extent, except by reduction to 3-hydroxybutyrate. Nonenzymic decarboxylation of acetoacetate can also occur, giving rise to acetone (fig. 33.3). In bacteria the decarboxylation of acetoacetate is catalysed by acetoacetate

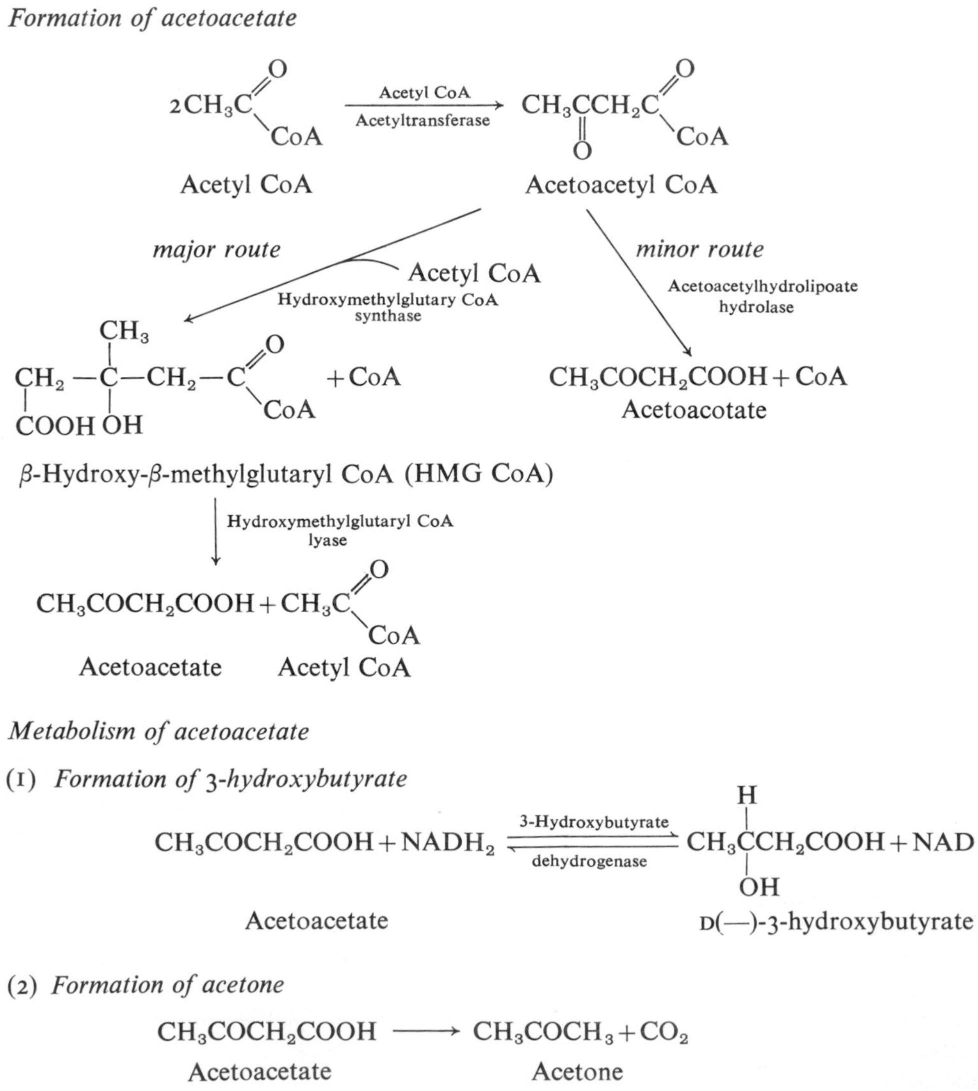

Formation of acetoacetate

FIG. 33.3. Formation of ketone bodies by the liver.

decarboxylase, but the enzymic formation of acetone has not yet been demonstrated in mammals. Acetone is quantitatively the least important of the three ketone bodies and the decarboxylation of acetoacetate which results in its formation apparently occurs slowly and spontaneously under physiological conditions.

Acetoacetate and its derivatives are normally present in blood and urine in small amounts, but when these quantities increase sufficiently to give a well-marked nitroprusside reaction (vol. 3, p. 23.82) the condition of ketosis is said to exist. Ketosis is associated with a respiratory quotient below 0·75, which reflects a predominance of fat metabolism. This state may develop in healthy individuals after a period of 36–48 h starvation at rest, and its onset during starvation is promoted by any factor which raises the metabolic rate, e.g. after vigorous exercise, severe cold, a difficult childbirth or fever. The limited ability of the liver to metabolize ketone bodies and the increased amounts accumulating in starvation may in fact be beneficial at a time when the surplus of exogenous glucose is curtailed, since ketone bodies are a fuel which can be utilized immediately by both skeletal and cardiac muscle and also by brain.

Ketosis may be very severe in patients with uncontrolled diabetes mellitus. Then, high concentrations of ketone bodies in the blood (ketonaemia) give rise to a metabolic acidosis and, owing to the limited capacity of the extrahepatic tissues to metabolize these compounds, as much as 25–50 g ketone bodies may be excreted daily in the urine (ketonuria). Acetone is volatile and is partly excreted in the expired air. Both acetoacetate and 3-hydroxybutyrate are moderately strong acids having pKa values of 3·8 and 4·8 respectively, and contribute to the development of the metabolic acidosis which is a common feature of uncontrolled diabetes mellitus. Apart from causing acidosis, it is not known whether or not these acids are toxic in any other way.

CHOLESTEROL SYNTHESIS AND METABOLISM

Cholesterol is synthesized in the liver from acetyl CoA and HMG CoA is an intermediate (p. 10.22); this is normally the main route of HMG CoA metabolism instead of being broken down to acetoacetate (fig. 33.3).

In blood, cholesterol is mostly esterified (about 70 per cent) and circulates as lipoprotein, the protein serving to maintain the lipid in colloidal solution. The enzyme that is mainly responsible for the esterification of cholesterol is lecithin-cholesterol acyltransferase (LCAT), an enzyme which is synthesized in the liver and is then secreted into the plasma where it exerts its reaction; some esterification may also take place in the liver itself. High density lipoprotein (HDL) is the substrate with which human LCAT shows highest activity, and it would appear that most of the esterified cholesterol present in plasma

is formed on HDL by LCAT. Esterified cholesterol is then transformed to low density lipoprotein (LDL) and very low density lipoprotein (VLDL). Some esterified cholesterol may be formed directly by LCAT on LDL, but LDL is not as good a substrate for LCAT as HDL. The extent of hepatic esterification of cholesterol varies with the species and with the nature of the diet; the hepatic enzyme is more important in rats than in man, and shows greater activity in rats fed a high cholesterol diet than in rats that have been starved. The reaction catalysed by plasma LCAT is described on p. 10.18.

A major pathway for the metabolism of cholesterol in the liver leads to the formation of the primary bile acids, cholic acid and chenodeoxycholic acid; alterations to the cholesterol molecule involve the insertion of additional hydroxyl groups in the nucleus at C_7 and C_{12} for cholic acid, and C_7 for chenodeoxycholic acid, and the oxidation of the side-chain (fig. 33.4). Approximately four times more cholic acid is formed than chenodeoxycholic acid in man, and these compounds are then conjugated by the liver with glycine or taurine, mainly the glycine conjugate in man. The salts of these conjugates are secreted into the bile; they have marked lipid-solubilizing or detergent-like properties and play an important part in the digestion and absorption of fat from the intestine.

A portion of the cholic acid and chenodeoxycholic acid conjugates is lost in the faeces but over 95 per cent is normally reabsorbed from the intestine and subsequently re-excreted in the bile, thereby giving rise to an enterohepatic circulation of primary bile acid conjugates. A further portion of these conjugates is hydrolysed in the large intestine and the liberated cholic and chenodeoxycholic acids are metabolized there to form the secondary bile acids, called respectively deoxycholic acid and lithocholic acid. These secondary bile acids are partly lost in the faeces but are also partly absorbed from the intestine and subsequently conjugated by the liver before being excreted into the bile. An enterohepatic circulation of secondary bile acids is thereby also established. Quantitatively, the primary bile acid cholic acid, as its glycine conjugate, forms the major single fraction of the bile salts in human bile.

CHOLESTEROL AND GALLSTONE FORMATION

Cholesterol is almost insoluble in simple aqueous solution, but the cholesterol content of normal bile is about 10 μmol/l. Most of this cholesterol, after passage into the intestine, is reabsorbed and re-enters the body's metabolic pool. Some is re-excreted into the bile, thereby giving rise to an enterohepatic circulation of cholesterol. The presence of bile salts in bile, by themselves, is insufficient to retain all the cholesterol there in solution, but the combination of bile salts and lecithin greatly increases the capacity for solubilizing cholesterol. These studies, mainly based on model systems, showed that it

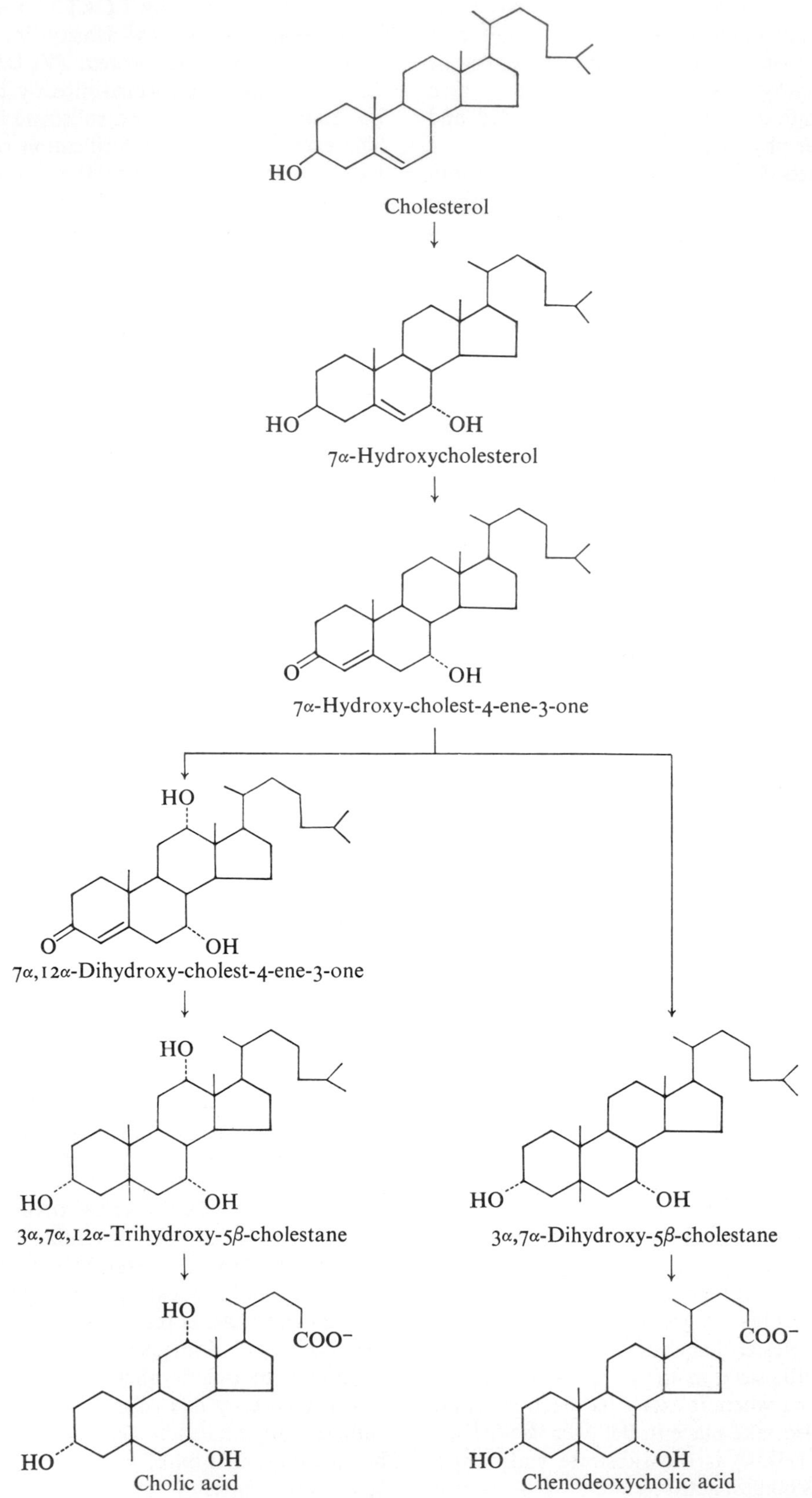

FIG. 33.4. Outline of the pathway for the conversion of cholesterol to cholic acid and chenodeoxycholic acid.

was possible for an aqueous system containing cholesterol, phospholipid and bile salts to exist as a solution, as a liquid-crystalline phase, or as a combination of these. These results have been applied to further studies, on hepatic bile and gallbladder bile, to determine the conditions which might lead to precipitation of cholesterol and hence to the commonest types of gallstone formation.

Hepatic bile and gallbladder bile differ in their composition in several respects. Hepatic bile is more dilute than gallbladder bile, and it contains proportionally less bile salt but proportionally much more cholesterol. Normally, it would seem that crystallization of cholesterol from the supersaturated solution present in hepatic bile does not occur because the process of initiating crystallization is too slow. However, in the gallbladder, stasis combined with the presence of the supersaturated solution (hepatic bile) may be sufficient in some patients to lead to the appearance of microcrystals and so on to gallstone formation. The body pool of bile salts may also be reduced in these patients.

Attempts have been made to develop a method of predicting the tendency for crystals of cholesterol to form in bile. These have usually been based on plotting in different ways data for the molar concentrations of bile salts, lecithin and cholesterol in artificial mixtures or in samples of hepatic bile or gallbladder bile. One frequently used method involves plotting these data as triangular coordinates (fig. 33.5). These studies have only

limited predictive capability, and chemical estimations on specimens of bile are not useful in the routine investigation and treatment of patients with gallstones. Factors which promote the crystallization of cholesterol from bile continue to be incompletely understood. Nevertheless, these studies have led to the possibility of dissolving gallstones by giving chenodeoxycholic acid by mouth. This increases the body's pool of bile salts, and may make the bile undersaturated in respect of cholesterol, although an alternative explanation of its action is that it decreases the rate of secretion of cholesterol into bile.

Vitamin metabolism

The liver contains the body's main stores of fat-soluble vitamins A, D, E and K. It is also concerned with their absorption from the intestine, since this is promoted by the presence of bile salts. Water-soluble vitamins are stored by the liver, particularly vitamin B_{12} and folic acid, and the liver contains the various enzyme systems which metabolize tryptophan to nicotinic acid.

Storage of vitamins becomes especially important in the face of dietary deficiency and influences the ability to survive this period of deficient intake. The normal hepatic stores of vitamins A, D and B_{12} are sufficient to meet the body's needs for over a year, whereas signs of deficiency of the other water-soluble vitamins and of vitamin K may develop much more quickly. As a result of its antioxidant properties, vitamin E protects the stores of A and D in the liver from destruction by oxidation.

The liver requires vitamin K for the synthesis of prothrombin, Factor VII and Factor X. These clotting factors are normally synthesized exclusively in the liver and failure in supply of vitamin K, e.g. due to dietary insufficiency or failure to absorb it, or interference in its utilization, e.g. due to drugs such as salicylates or indanedione derivatives, results in prolongation of the blood clotting process.

The liver not only stores vitamin D but is the organ in which the first hydroxylation, one of the stages in the metabolism of the vitamin to its active form, takes place. This first hydroxylation step results in the formation of 25-hydroxycholecalciferol (25-HCC) from cholecalciferol (vitamin D_3) (p. 10.26).

The liver is a rich source of the enzymes which synthesize a range of coenzymes and prosthetic groups, NAD, NADP, FMN, FAD, thiamine pyrophosphate, pyridoxal phosphate, from members of the vitamin B group. Enzymes concerned with these various reactions are as follows:

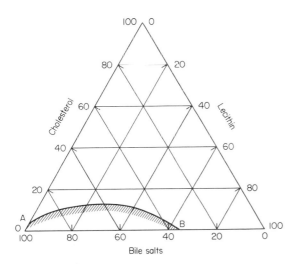

Fig. 33.5. Relative molar proportions of biliary lipids and bile salts plotted on triangular coordinates. Any point within the triangle represents a combination of three components totalling 100 per cent. Bile with a composition above the curved line A–B would precipitate cholesterol rapidly. Bile with a composition within the shaded area below the line might lead to precipitation of cholesterol in the presence of nucleating factors such as micro-organisms, mucoproteins or calcium salts. Modified from Admirand W.H. & Small D.M. (1968) *J. clin. Invest.* **47**, 1043.

$$NMN + ATP \rightleftharpoons NAD + pyrophosphate$$
NMN adenyltransferase

$$NAD + ATP \longrightarrow NADP + ADP$$
NAD kinase

$$Riboflavin + ATP \longrightarrow FMN + ADP$$
Riboflavin kinase

$$FMN + ATP \underset{\text{FMN adenyltransferase}}{\rightleftharpoons} FAD + \text{pyrophosphate}$$

$$\text{Thiamine} + ATP \xrightarrow[\text{Thiamine pyrophosphokinase}]{}$$

Thiamine pyrophosphate + AMP

$$\text{Pyridoxal} + ATP \xrightarrow[\text{Pyridoxal kinase}]{} \text{Pyridoxal phosphate}$$

+ADP

Alcohol metabolism

Ethanol is rapidly absorbed from the gut and diffuses throughout the total body water and also into the urine and expired air. The kidneys and lungs do not actively excrete it. The amounts lost by these routes are small and are proportional to the concentration in the blood. Ethanol is not metabolized by resting or active muscle. The organ mainly responsible for metabolizing ethanol is the liver, where over 90 per cent of ingested alcohol is oxidized. The oxidation provides approximately 30 kJ/g, so a daily intake of 100 g ethanol can provide about half of an adult's resting energy requirements; the alcoholic content of various beverages is given on p. 5.25.

The liver possesses an alcohol dehydrogenase which acts on ethanol and NAD to produce acetaldehyde and $NADH_2$. An aldehyde dehydrogenase converts the aldehyde into acetyl CoA, which then enters the citric acid cycle or is metabolized in other ways, e.g. cholesterol or fatty acid synthesis. Alcohol dehydrogenase is the enzyme which is mainly responsible for the metabolism of ethanol in man; it has a fairly wide range of specificity and can, for instance, also oxidize methanol and ethylene glycol. Since the serious toxic effects of these latter substances are attributable to the products of their metabolism, it is reasonable to treat patients who have ingested methanol or ethylene glycol by giving them ethanol, so as to delay their metabolism to potentially toxic compounds.

Ethanol can also be oxidized by a microsomal enzyme oxidizing system (MEOS). Normally this system is responsible for metabolizing only a small percentage of ingested ethanol in man. However, it shows many of the characteristics of the hepatic drug-metabolizing enzyme systems discussed below. Chronic ingestion of ethanol increases the activity of (i.e. induces) MEOS, a system which is capable of oxidizing not only ethanol but also other drugs, notably barbiturates. There are some inter-species differences in the effects of chronic administration of ethanol, but the changes in man include (1) an increase in the smooth endoplasmic reticulum in the liver, (2) increased activity of the hepatic MEOS, (3) increased rate of metabolism of ethanol and of other drugs such as barbiturates, (4) increased synthesis of cholesterol and production of lipoproteins, and (5) increased activity of δ-aminolaevulinate synthase (ALA synthase); this last effect may explain why ethanol may precipitate attacks of porphyria (vol. 3, p. 47.23).

Ethanol ingestion can lead to hepatic injury (vol. 2, p. 25.35; vol. 3, p. 20.16) and in addition to adaptive responses such as the induction of MEOS. The effects of chronic ingestion on the hepatocytes are reversible, at the stage described as fatty liver, but this can progress to necrosis of hepatocytes and inflammation leading on to fibrosis and cirrhosis. The effects of ethanol ingestion are not entirely predictable, being influenced for instance by the nutritional state. Acute over-indulgence can lead to inhibition by ethanol of the hepatic MEOS and thus interfere with the metabolism of various drugs, giving rise for instance to potentiation of barbiturate action.

Inactivation of drugs and poisons

Many drugs and substances with pharmacological activities taken in the diet are metabolized in the liver by processes which involve oxidation, reduction, methylation or conjugation reactions. Most of these reduce the pharmacological activity of the compound and make the molecules more polar, thereby increasing their solubility in water and facilitating renal or biliary excretion. Many poisons give rise to liver damage and disturbances of lipid metabolism. These include chlorinated hydrocarbons, e.g. carbon tetrachloride and chloroform, various aromatic compounds, e.g. dinitrophenol, trinitrotoluene and paracetamol, and inorganic poisons, e.g. phosphorus and arsenites. Histologically, droplets of fat can be demonstrated in the liver during the acute phase of poisoning and the liver may become enlarged and fatty; with large doses of poison, death (necrosis) of hepatocytes may occur on a large scale with serious failure of the liver's metabolic activities. The effects of poisons on the liver may be more marked if the nutritional state is poor, as may occur with protein malnutrition or chronic alcoholism. Starvation by itself has little demonstrable effect on the liver other than to cause reduction in glycogen and protein content and diminution in size. When fatty change occurs, the fat is mainly brought to the liver from the fat depots and accumulates because of interference with its normal metabolism (vol. 2, p. 25.33).

ENZYME INDUCTION OF DRUG-METABOLIZING ENZYMES

The drug-metabolizing systems in the liver are mainly concentrated in the smooth endoplasmic reticulum (SER) of the hepatocytes and the liver microsomal system has been shown to be the site of these enzymes. The enzymes exhibit characteristics that depend on species, sex and age. Thus the activity of certain enzymes may be low in the microsomal fraction of the liver in one species but high in another species. Also the activity of a particular enzyme may be high in the liver of males but low in the liver of females of the same species. Again, the activity of an enzyme in the SER may be high in adult animals but only just detectable or even undetectable in the newborn. These facts indicate the need for caution in interpreting results obtained in animals, especially if these results are being extrapolated to man. For instance, marked sex differences in the ability to detoxicate foreign compounds have not been shown in man.

Normally the SER in hepatocytes is small in amount but may be markedly increased after repeated administration of many drugs and poisons. There is an accompanying rise in the activity of the hepatic enzymes involved in the metabolism of these compounds; these often convert the foreign substance to a more polar metabolite, which can be conjugated with glucuronic acid, sulphuric acid or glycine and then excreted in the bile or urine. This process of enzyme induction occurs in response to the administration of any one of several hundred foreign compounds, when given individually to animals.

The term 'enzyme induction' is meant to convey the concept of an increased amount of active enzyme at some specific site. Thus the administration of certain polycyclic hydrocarbons, steroid hormones, barbiturates, azo-dyes, amines, sedatives, tranquillizers, alkaloids, anticonvulsants, muscle relaxants, hypoglycaemic agents, insecticides, food additives and other compounds all produce in time an increase in hepatic enzymes which are involved in the catabolism of the compound administered. These enzymes include various hydroxylases or oxygenases, *N*-dealkylases, *O*-dealkylases, dehalogenases and reductases. In some cases an increase in the activity of the enzyme can be shown within 12 h of the administration of the compound and the maximum increase may be apparent within days rather than weeks.

Increases in activity could be due to increased production or decreased destruction of the enzyme. In order to distinguish between these possibilities, animals treated with agents that block DNA transcription or other events involved in protein synthesis, e.g. actinomycin D and puromycin, were given an inducer, e.g. barbiturate. Prior treatment with the blocking agent resulted in failure of subsequent administration of an enzyme inducer to produce any significant effect; this suggests that drugs and other substances which normally increase the activity of enzymes involved in detoxication reactions in the hepatic SER must achieve this effect through a regulator protein that influences gene function (p. 12.14). For example, the administration of phenobarbitone to an animal results in a progressive increase in the liver microsomal cytochrome P_{450} concentration occurring over a period of several days. The change in the concentration of this enzyme, which is a key factor in the microsomal mixed function oxidases, results in an increase in the rate at which phenobarbitone can be catabolized by the liver microsomes. Thus enzyme induction can influence the duration and intensity of drug action, and the tolerance which develops to some drugs may be due to accelerated metabolism of these drugs by the liver.

OTHER EXAMPLES OF ENZYME INDUCTION

Enzyme-inducing capability is not restricted to enzyme systems responsible for metabolizing drugs. For instance tryptophan pyrrolase, the enzyme which catalyses the first irreversible step in the degradative metabolism of tryptophan in the liver (p. 11.25), can have its activity induced by tryptophan, 2-methyltryptophan or by glucocorticoids. Induction of ALA synthase by ethanol has already been mentioned; synthesis of ALA synthase can also be induced by several naturally occurring steroids.

Alkaline phosphatase activity in plasma increases if there is obstruction to the outflow of bile; this is due to the appearance in plasma of the hepatic isoenzyme of alkaline phosphatase and not simply to failure of the liver to excrete the bone isoenzyme. There is first an increase in alkaline phosphatase in the liver itself and the rise in plasma activity appears later and parallels the increase in liver alkaline phosphatase. Furthermore, the effects of bile duct obstruction on alkaline phosphatase can be inhibited by the prior injection of cycloheximide, an inhibitor of protein synthesis. It is possible that the effect of bile duct ligation on alkaline phosphatase synthesis serves a different function from those associated with the administration of drugs and foreign compounds, discussed above, but in both instances new protein is synthesized. Bile duct ligation does not lead to increased synthesis of hepatic alanine aminotransferase.

Inactivation of hormones

STEROID HORMONES

The liver is the main site for the inactivation of steroids and contains several different enzyme systems which modify their structure. For instance, cortisol can be converted to any of the metabolites shown in fig. 33.6; of them, quantitatively the most important is tetrahydrocortisol. Tetrahydrocortisol is then conjugated with glucuronic acid in the liver and excreted as tetrahydrocortisol glucosiduronate.

There are two routes by which the liver converts cortisol to tetrahydrocortisol. The first step, which involves reduction of the Δ^4 double bond, can be catalysed by either of two NADPH$_2$-dependent dehydrogenases; the more important of these enzymes is a soluble dehydrogenase which gives rise to a dihydro derivative (dihydrocortisol) with a 5β configuration, and the less important enzyme is a microsomal dehydrogenase which gives rise to a dihydro derivative with a 5α configuration. Dihydrocortisol of either configuration (5β or 5α) is then acted upon by 3α-hydroxysteroid dehydrogenase (which can use either NADH$_2$ or NADPH$_2$) to form tetrahydrocortisol. D-Aldosterone is similarly converted to inactive tetrahydroaldosterone which is partly excreted as the corresponding glucuronide.

A major fraction of the output of cortisol from the

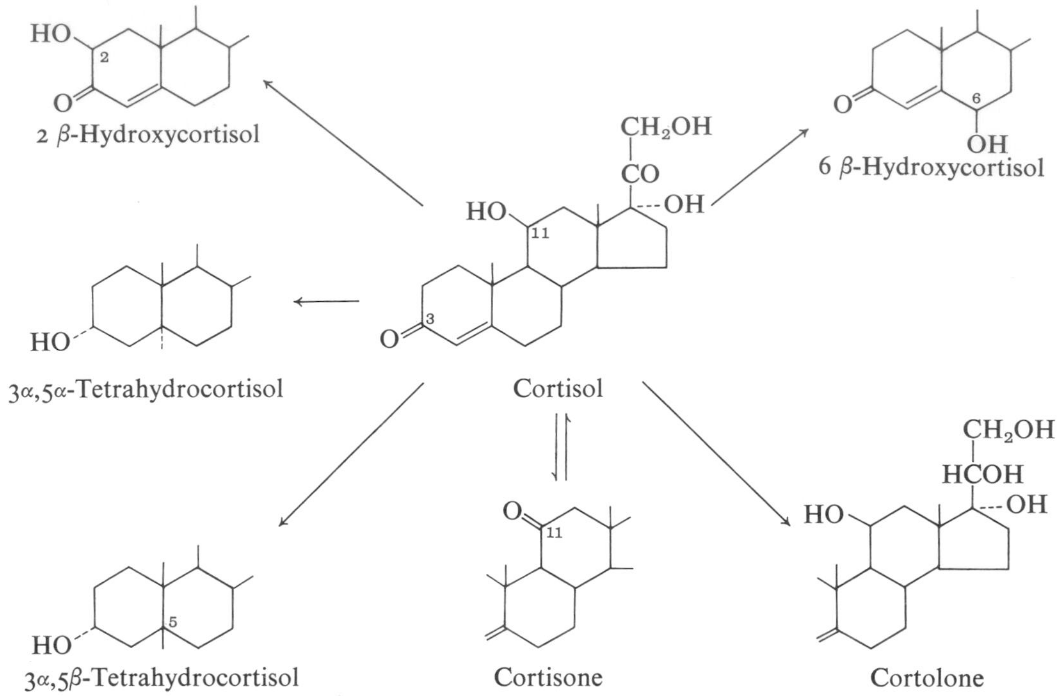

FIG. 33.6. The metabolism of cortisol. Apart from cortisone, which is also an active glucocorticoid, the other metabolites of cortisol are either relatively inactive or devoid of glucocorticoid activity.

adrenal cortex is first metabolized to cortisone (fig. 33.6); cortisone is then mainly inactivated by reductive steps leading to tetrahydrocortisone. Some of the steroid metabolites are excreted in the bile and are then partly excreted in the faeces and partly reabsorbed; the main route of excretion is in the urine.

Testosterone is metabolized to the isomeric 17-oxo-

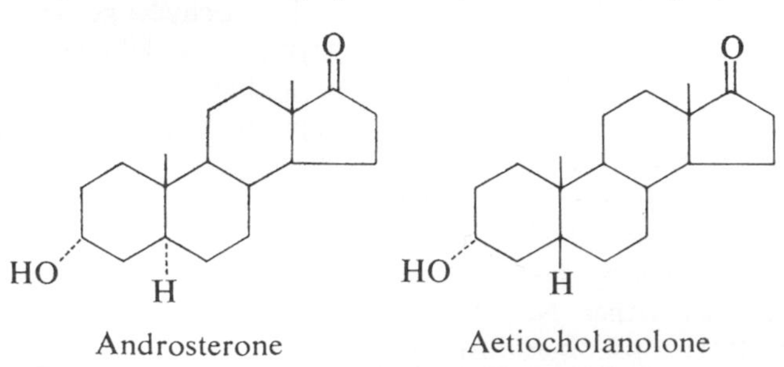

FIG. 33.7. Androgens and their principal metabolites. 17-Oxosteroids are derived mainly from androgens and are excreted in urine principally as their 3-sulphate derivatives.

steroids androsterone and aetiocholanolone, and the main adrenal androgen dehydro*epi*androsterone is also metabolized to these two compounds, which are then mostly excreted as their 3-sulphate conjugates in urine (fig. 33.7). The various dehydrogenation and conjugation steps involved in these transformations are all catalysed by hepatic enzymes. Smaller amounts of testosterone derivatives hydroxylated at C_2, C_6 or C_{16} have been described. The liver also inactivates the other androgens of gonadal and of adrenal origin.

Oestrogens (oestradiol, oestrone and oestriol) are metabolized and inactivated by the liver in several ways, including conjugation with glucuronic acid or with sulphate, and then excreted in the urine. Progesterone is reduced to pregnanediol, which is excreted as its sulphate or glucuronide conjugate.

In severe hepatic disease, the inactivation of steroid hormones may be impaired. In some male patients with cirrhosis of the liver feminine features appear and in female patients masculine features. This is due to impairment of the processes of metabolism and inactivation of the corresponding sex hormones.

THYROID HORMONES
The liver contains about 25 per cent of the extrathyroidal thyroxine and about 10 per cent of the extrathyroidal triiodothyronine. These hepatic stores of thyroid hormones are in equilibrium with the hormones circulating in the plasma.

Thyroxine and triiodothyronine are metabolized in several different ways and there is considerable variation between species as to the most important route. In man, liver and muscle are the two main sites of metabolism. Inactivation of the thyroid hormones occurs mainly by deiodination, the released iodine being either taken up again from the circulation by the thyroid or excreted in the urine. Minor pathways of hepatic metabolism include oxidative deamination, yielding tetraiodothyroacetic and triiodothyroacetic acids, and conjugation. The ether linkage between the benzene rings is very stable. About 10 per cent of the daily output of thyroid hormones is excreted in bile, mostly as free hormone but some as conjugates. The conjugated derivatives of thyroxine and triiodothyronine are formed in the liver and both glucuronide and sulphate derivatives have been identified. Conjugation takes place on the phenolic hydroxy group. However, the gastrointestinal tract is only a very minor route for the excretion of thyroid hormones, since most of the unconjugated thyroxine and triiodothyronine are reabsorbed from the intestine. Also their conjugated derivatives are mostly hydrolysed in the intestine and the thyroid hormones thus liberated are then reabsorbed.

OTHER HORMONES

The liver has not been shown to have any specific role in the metabolism of the peptide and protein hormones. For the metabolism of the catecholamines, noradrenaline and adrenaline, it is a rich source of both monoamine oxidase (MAO) and of catechol-O-methyl-transferase (COMT) but these enzymes are widely distributed and the liver has no special role in the inactivation of circulating catecholamines liberated from the adrenal medulla. On the other hand, hepatic MAO and COMT both have important functions in effecting the detoxication of dietary and bacterial amines absorbed from the intestine.

Formation and secretion of bile

The liver secretes bile continuously. It is a dilute aqueous solution containing electrolytes, glucose, urea and other more complex molecules such as bilirubin conjugates, bile salts, phospholipids and cholesterol. It also contains some protein, mainly mucin, and the enzymes alkaline phosphatase and lactate dehydrogenase.

Bile as secreted by the liver is approximately isotonic with plasma, but it does not all pass directly to the duodenum. The control of bile secretion is discussed on p. 32.39 where it was noted that, in the interdigestive periods, most of the hepatic bile is diverted to the gallbladder. In the gallbladder, bile becomes concentrated by the reabsorption of water and the mucosal cells of the gallbladder add mucus, sometimes in large amounts. The high concentrations of cholesterol, bile pigment and calcium salts in gallbladder bile are undoubtedly related to the tendencies of these substances to be deposited as gallstones.

The biliary tract is also an excretory route. However, many compounds excreted in the bile are reabsorbed to a large extent from the intestine, and are later re-excreted in the bile. Substances which show an enterohepatic circulation include the bile salts, cholesterol and urobilinogen.

When the outflow of bile is obstructed to any marked degree, digestion and absorption of fat are impaired and signs of deficiency of vitamin K may develop; if the course of the illness is prolonged, features of deficiency of vitamins A and D may also appear.

BILIRUBIN METABOLISM

Bilirubin is formed mostly as a result of haemoglobin breakdown, occurring at the end of the life-span of erythrocytes (p. 28.11). About 350 μmol unconjugated bilirubin, sometimes called prehepatic bilirubin, is

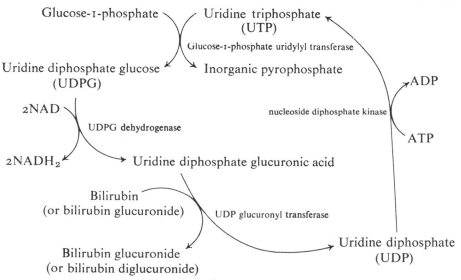

FIG. 33.8. Conjugation of bilirubin in the hepatocyte.

brought to the liver each day in the adult; unconjugated bilirubin, which is lipid-soluble and which has only very limited solubility in water, is transported in the plasma reversibly bound to albumin.

Unconjugated bilirubin is taken up by the hepatocytes and transported to the microsomes. Two proteins, the 'Y' and 'Z' proteins, may be involved in this process. They both have an affinity for binding anions, e.g. bilirubin. Next, bilirubin is conjugated with the formation of water-soluble conjugates, mainly bilirubin diglucuronide (fig. 33.8); small amounts of bilirubin monoglucuronide and bilirubin sulphate are also formed. The bilirubin conjugates are then transported from the hepatocyte into the biliary canaliculi; this step occurs against a high concentration gradient.

Bile contains only conjugated forms of bilirubin, sometimes still called posthepatic bilirubin. These compounds are further metabolized by intestinal bacteria with the formation of a complex mixture of stercobilinogen and urobilinogen stereoisomers, stercobilin and urobilin (fig. 33.9); haemoglobin breakdown ultimately accounts for most of these compounds present in the faeces, but small amounts of these faecal pigments also come from porphyrin by-products formed during the

synthesis of haem. A small component of faecal pigmentation is due to other compounds such as urobilin IXα.

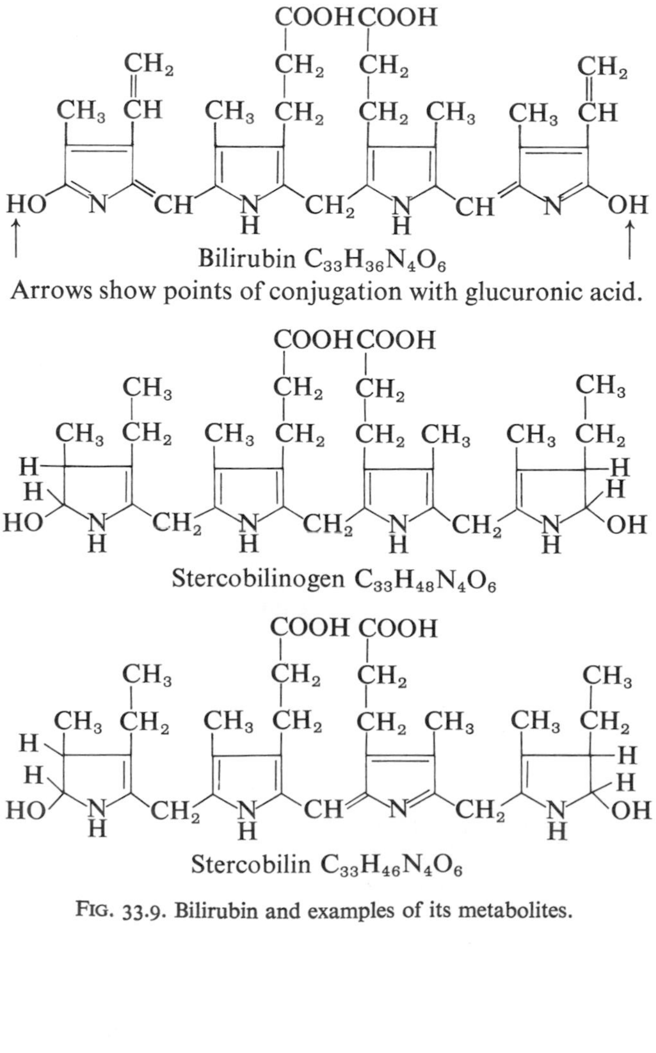

Some of the intestinal bilinogens, alternatively called bilirubinoids, are absorbed from the intestine into the portal circulation. They are then mostly excreted again into the bile, thereby giving rise to an enterohepatic circulation of bile pigment derivatives, but hepatic excretion is not complete and normally a small proportion of bilinogens is brought to the kidney by the systemic circulation and excreted into the urine (fig. 33.10). Normally the faecal excretion of stercobilinogen is 0·7–5 mmol/day, and the amount of urobilinogen in urine is less than 0·1 mmol/day. Urobilinogen in urine oxidizes spontaneously with the production mainly of urobilin.

The chemistry of the breakdown products of bilirubin is complicated. Although structurally closely similar, stercobilinogen is not identical with urobilinogen, and both these bilinogens can exist in isomeric forms. Again the structures of stercobilin and urobilin are not identical, and isomers have been described for both these groups of structurally closely related pigments. It is an oversimplification, therefore, to regard the terms stercobilinogen and urobilinogen, and stercobilin and urobilin, as being freely interchangeable although some authors use only the terms stercobilinogen and stercobilin, whether referring to intestinal, faecal or urinary pigments while others use only the terms urobilinogen and urobilin. To reduce the possibilities of confusion, it is advisable to specify the nature of the specimen, e.g. faeces, urine, containing the pigment under discussion, whichever terminology is used. Ehrlich's aldehyde test reacts with both stercobilinogen and urobilinogen; for simplicity, fig. 33.10 only includes reference to urobilinogen as the test is mostly used for detecting the bilinogen present in urine.

EXCRETION OF BILE PIGMENTS AND THEIR METABOLITES

If the liver fails to excrete bile pigments, they accumulate in the blood and jaundice may develop. By biochemical criteria, an individual is jaundiced whenever the plasma bilirubin is significantly increased above 20 μmol/l. Jaundice may be due to an increased concentration of either unconjugated or conjugated bilirubin in the plasma or to a mixture of both pigments. Normally, the pigment in plasma consists mostly of unconjugated (prehepatic) bilirubin.

Unconjugated bilirubin accumulates in the plasma as a result of over-production, for instance in haemolytic disorders; it also occurs when hepatic uptake and conjugation of bilirubin are either incompletely developed, as in premature infants, or are abnormal due to an inborn defect of bilirubin conjugation or transport. Both conjugated and unconjugated bilirubin accumulate in the plasma when the outflow of bile from the liver is obstruc-

FIG. 33.9. Bilirubin and examples of its metabolites.

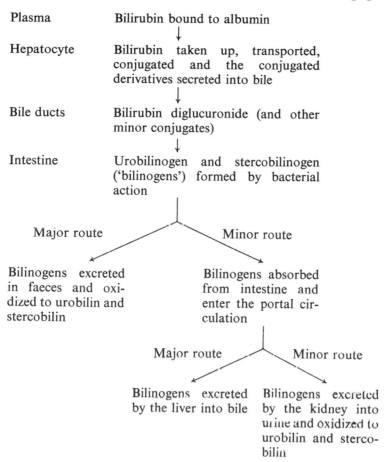

Plasma	Bilirubin bound to albumin
Hepatocyte	Bilirubin taken up, transported, conjugated and the conjugated derivatives secreted into bile
Bile ducts	Bilirubin diglucuronide (and other minor conjugates)
Intestine	Urobilinogen and stercobilinogen ('bilinogens') formed by bacterial action

Major route — Bilinogens excreted in faeces and oxidized to urobilin and stercobilin

Minor route — Bilinogens absorbed from intestine and enter the portal circulation

Major route — Bilinogens excreted by the liver into bile

Minor route — Bilinogens excreted by the kidney into urine and oxidized to urobilin and stercobilin

FIG. 33.10. The metabolism of bilirubin and the bilinogens, stercobilinogen and urobilinogen. A small component of the bilinogens formed in the intestine undergoes an enterohepatic circulation. A small proportion of the bilinogens absorbed from the intestine is excreted in the urine.

ted, either in the bile duct (extrahepatic obstruction) or in the biliary canaliculi (intrahepatic obstruction); theoretically, uncomplicated biliary obstruction would be expected to cause only an increase in the concentration of conjugated bilirubin in plasma, but obstruction to the outflow of bile often affects the hepatocytes and interferes with the normal processes of conjugation of bilirubin. Disease of the hepatocytes may adversely affect the uptake of unconjugated bilirubin, its conjugation with glucuronic acid and the excretion of conjugated bilirubin, and hepatocellular disease therefore also gives rise to jaundice associated with an increased concentration of both conjugated and unconjugated bilirubin in the plasma.

Examination of urinary pigment excretion helps to make a broad subdivision of the causes of jaundice into prehepatic on the one hand, and either hepatocellular or posthepatic on the other (table 33.2 and vol. 3, table 20.1). The tests involve examining the urine for the presence of bilirubin, e.g. by using Ictotest or Bili-Labstix (Ames Co., Stoke Poges, Bucks.), and for urobilinogen by means of

Ehrlich's aldehyde test or by using Urobilistix (Ames Co.). It is sometimes helpful also to inspect the colour of a specimen of faeces, and to test it for the presence of occult blood. Clean working conditions, a fresh specimen of urine (cooled to room temperature prior to examination), the ability to follow simple directions and make the relevant simple observations correctly are all that is required for the reliable performance of these tests. They are quick to perform, and their results can help to decide the most appropriate choice of further investigations. Their potential value should not be decried despite the modern tendency to place greater or sole reliance on more complicated laboratory-based investigations.

When parenchymal disease of the liver produces jaundice, the diseased liver cells may be unable to excrete the urobilinogen which has been absorbed from the intestine, and this disturbance of the normal enterohepatic circulation of urobilinogen may result in an increased excretion of urobilinogen in the urine, even though the hepatic excretion of bilirubin conjugates is itself impaired and the amount of urobilinogen able to contribute to the

Table 33.2. Bile pigments and jaundice.

Site of underlying cause of jaundice and related mechanisms	Plasma bilirubin	Urine urobilinogen	Urine bilirubin	Faecal pigment
Prehepatic				
Overproduction of bilirubin (e.g. haemolysis)	Unconjugated	Increased	Absent	Increased
Hepatic				
Transport defect affecting uptake of bilirubin from plasma or conjugation (e.g. Gilbert's disease)	Unconjugated	Normal	Absent	Normal or reduced
Transport defect affecting excretion of conjugated bilirubin into the biliary canaliculi (e.g. Dubin–Johnson syndrome)	Conjugated	Normal	Present	Reduced
Hepatocellular damage affecting uptake, conjugation and excretion	Conjugated and unconjugated	Increased, normal, reduced or absent (depending on stage and severity of disease)	Present	Reduced
Intrahepatic cholestasis causing obstruction to outflow of bile, e.g. reaction to phenothiazines	Conjugated and unconjugated	Reduced or absent	Present	Reduced
Posthepatic				
Extrahepatic cholestasis, e.g. stone, stricture, carcinoma	Conjugated and unconjugated	Reduced or absent	Present	Reduced

enterohepatic circulation is reduced. This increase in the output of urobilinogen in the urine occurs because the ability of the liver to excrete urobilinogen from the blood is an activity which is rapidly impaired by disease of the liver cell. In hepatic jaundice, therefore, it is sometimes possible to demonstrate an excess of urobilinogen in the urine at the same time as finding bilirubinuria. If the obstruction to the outflow of bile becomes complete, however, no urobilinogen can be formed in the intestine and the enterohepatic circulation of urobilinogen ceases until bile flow is re-established.

Assessment of hepatic function by means of chemical tests

The investigation of metabolic functions carried out by the liver in health, and measurement of the extent to which these functions are deranged in disease (liver function tests) are frequently performed for the assessment of patients with jaundice and also when the presence of liver disorder is suspected. Strictly speaking, the designation of these tests as 'liver function tests' is a misnomer, since most of the tests can yield abnormal results under a number of different circumstances, sometimes in the complete absence of liver disease.

EXCRETION OF BILIRUBIN AND ANIONIC DYES
Determination of the total concentration of bilirubin, i.e. unconjugated plus conjugated bilirubin, is the most widely performed measurement of plasma bilirubin; it provides a quantitative measure of the severity of jaundice, and its repeated performance, e.g. on a weekly basis, gives an index of the progress of a patient's illness. Measurements of the individual concentrations of unconjugated and conjugated bilirubin provide only limited assistance in localizing the site of the pathological process giving rise to jaundice, especially if appropriate tests on urine have been performed carefully, preferably at the start of the patient's illness before complications develop. The investigation of jaundice in the neonate and in patients suspected of having one of the congenital hyperbilirubinaemias (vol. 3, table 20.2) are the two main groups of conditions in which it has proved valuable to determine the plasma concentrations of both total and conjugated bilirubin, and hence the concentration of unconjugated bilirubin by difference.

In the absence of jaundice, the liver's excretory function can be investigated by injecting bromsulphthalein (BSP) intravenously and measuring the rate of disappearance of this anionic dye from the plasma. The BSP test (vol. 3, p. 20.3) is also occasionally carried out in the presence of a mild degree of jaundice, for instance when investigating patients with one of the congenital hyperbilirubinaemias. Bromsulphthalein is transported and excreted into bile by the hepatocyte along a pathway similar to but not identical with bilirubin; BSP is excreted as a conjugate with glutathione. Another anionic dye, indocyanine green, has been employed as an alternative to BSP and has the advantage that it causes fewer adverse reactions but it is much more expensive than BSP, which therefore continues to be widely used.

SYNTHETIC CAPACITY OF THE LIVER

The synthesis of albumin is often disturbed in liver disease, and a fall in plasma albumin is one of the most characteristic chemical findings in chronic hepatic disease; it is an important factor in promoting the fluid retention and oedema that may develop in this group of conditions. A reduction in plasma albumin concentration due to disease affecting the hepatocytes is usually accompanied by an increase in the concentration of the globulins in plasma. Because of the relatively long half-life of albumin in plasma, alterations in plasma albumin concentration may not be observed in liver disease if the illness is of short duration.

The individual fractions of the serum proteins can be satisfactorily demonstrated by zone electrophoresis. Plasma is not suitable for this examination as fibrinogen produces a band on electrophoresis which appears between the β- and the γ-globulin bands, thereby interfering with their interpretation. In this technique, a sample of serum is applied to a solid supporting medium, e.g. filter paper or cellulose acetate strips soaked in barbitone/sodium barbitone buffer, pH 8·6, and an electric field is applied across the strip. At this pH the proteins carry a net negative charge and move towards the anode, and differences in the charge carried by individual proteins are largely responsible for the different mobilities observed; endosmosis also occurs during the electrophoretic separation and this accounts for the movement of the γ-globulins towards the cathode. At the end of the electrophoretic separation, the strips are dried, fixed and stained with a suitable dye; the different protein fractions can then be seen, and the amount of each determined by densitometry.

Fig. 33.11 shows the electrophoretic pattern of proteins present in a normal specimen of serum. The areas under each peak are approximately proportional to the individual protein concentrations. Alterations in the electrophoretic pattern of serum proteins are observed in several diseases, but no change is specific for a particular disorder affecting the liver; nevertheless, some of the patterns of zone electrophoresis do provide evidence in support of broad diagnostic categories such as cirrhosis of the liver or obstructive jaundice.

More detailed examination of the plasma proteins can be made by immunoelectrophoresis and specific methods for the quantitative measurement of several proteins, e.g. albumin, α_1-acid glycoprotein, the haptoglobins, ceruloplasmin, fibrinogen and other clotting factors, α-fetoprotein, and the immunoglobulin classes IgA, IgG and IgM, are available. Of these methods, determination of plasma albumin concentration is the one most widely used and is probably the most valuable test of the liver's

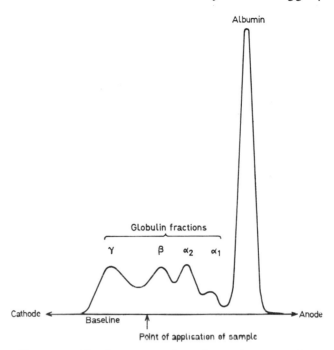

FIG. 33.11. Densitometer tracing of an electrophoretic separation carried out on cellulose acetate with a specimen of normal serum and stained to show the presence of protein.

synthetic capacity. However, alterations in plasma albumin occur for many reasons other than hepatic disorder.

In many parts of Asia, Africa, Central and South America plasma concentrations of albumin are lower and those of the immunoglobulins higher than indicated in table 33.1. In a population with a low dietary intake of protein, plasma albumin is likely to lie between 30 and 40 g/l, but oedema or other evidence of protein deficiency is uncommon unless the level falls to below 25 g/l. In populations exposed to many and repeated infections, particularly where malaria is endemic, the total concentration of the immunoglobulins is often between 16 and 18 g/l even when there is evidence of severe protein deficiency.

Hypoprothrombinaemia, a very low concentration of prothrombin in the blood, occurs frequently in patients with liver disease. It may be due either to failure to absorb vitamin K, as a result of obstruction to the outflow of bile, or to hepatocellular damage, and rarely to other causes. It is important, therefore, to investigate the haemostatic mechanisms (p. 28.14) and give appropriate treatment whenever liver biopsy or laparotomy has to be undertaken in a jaundiced patient.

There are other special indications for measuring individual plasma proteins in suspected liver disease. For example α-fetoprotein, a protein which is present in the fetus but which can normally only be detected in minute amount in plasma from infancy onwards, reappears in the plasma in a number of disorders including several types of liver disease. Abnormal increases in the concentration of α-fetoprotein in plasma are particularly marked and are frequently observed in patients with primary carcinoma of the liver.

Lipoprotein electrophoresis may sometimes be helpful in the investigation of patients with liver disease. An abnormal lipoprotein, lipoprotein X, has been observed in plasma obtained from most patients with cholestasis (obstruction to the outflow of bile, either intrahepatic or extrahepatic), but only rarely in patients with other forms of liver disorder. The normal lipoproteins all migrate towards the anode on zone electrophoresis, but lipoprotein X moves towards the cathode.

INVESTIGATION OF INTERMEDIARY METABOLISM

Despite its central place in metabolism, tests based on the liver's ability to metabolize protein, fat and carbohydrate have so far proved of only limited value. This is because the liver has a large functional reserve and liver failure does not lead to a detectable rise in the concentration of amino acids in blood or fall in blood urea concentration until about 80 per cent of the organ has been damaged. Similarly, increases in blood ammonia concentration (due to failure of the ornithine cycle) do not occur until the patient is seriously ill and liver function, as judged by other tests, markedly impaired.

The only test of carbohydrate metabolism to have been widely assessed for the investigation of liver disease is the intravenous galactose tolerance test. This measures the liver's ability to convert galactose to glucose, but galactose is not metabolized exclusively by the liver, and hepatic disorder has to be marked before the test becomes impaired significantly.

Tests of liver function based on the metabolism of drugs are occasionally used. One example, the hippuric acid synthesis test, involves measuring the amount of hippurate excreted in urine following the intravenous administration of sodium benzoate. This assesses the liver's ability to conjugate sodium benzoate with glycine, but interpretation of the test is adversely affected if renal function is impaired since excretion of hippurate is then reduced.

RELEASE OF ENZYMES FROM THE LIVER INTO THE CIRCULATION

Liver enzymes are released into the circulation if the integrity of cell membranes is impaired, for instance by hypoxia or bacterial infection. Thus hepatocellular damage due to any of a large number of causes can result in marked increases in enzyme activity in plasma.

Many different plasma enzyme activity measurements have been used for investigating whether liver cell damage has occurred. These include aspartate aminotransferase (AST, also called glutamic oxaloacetic transaminase or GOT), alanine aminotransferase (ALT, also called glutamic pyruvic transaminase or GPT), isocitrate dehydrogenase (ICD), lactate dehydrogenase and ornithine carbamyl transferase. Each of these enzyme measurements has advantages and disadvantages, and the tests most widely used are AST and ALT.

Since AST occurs in most tissues its release into the circulation has poor localizing power. It occurs, for example, in large amounts in skeletal and cardiac muscle. However it can be measured relatively easily and reliably and is a sensitive index of tissue damage, without necessarily specifying where the damage has occurred. Isocitrate dehydrogenase also occurs in most tissues, but the hepatic isoenzyme is much more stable than the isoenzyme in cardiac and skeletal muscle. Measurements of plasma ICD activity have therefore been found to provide a more specific pointer to the liver as the site of disease than plasma AST activity. Unfortunately, ICD measurements are technically demanding. ALT, according to some investigators, is more specific than AST as an index of liver disease and ALT measurements are widely used for this purpose; it is, however, less specific than ICD as a pointer to liver as the site of disease. Measurement of LD_5, the isoenzyme of lactate dehydrogenase that moves most slowly on zone electrophoresis, improves the specificity of LD measurements as liver is relatively rich in LD_5. The advantage of measuring ornithine carbamyl transferase, namely its occurrence mainly in liver and to a much lesser extent in other tissues, is largely nullified by difficulties relating to its method of assay.

Patients with parenchymal disease of liver, especially acute conditions such as viral hepatitis or drug intoxications, often show very marked increases in plasma enzyme activities, usually ALT and AST. In view of the widespread distribution of these enzymes, however, the laboratory findings have to be carefully assessed to determine whether other tissues are possibly also contributing to the increased plasma enzyme activities. For instance, the greatly increased plasma AST and lactate dehydrogenase activities observed in some patients who have taken overdoses of drugs may partly arise as a result of hepatocellular damage but may also be caused by release from other tissues such as muscle; the non-specific nature of enzyme tests can, if considered in isolation, be misleading if regarded solely as an index of the severity of liver damage.

Interference with the outflow of bile from the liver, due to hepatobiliary disease, is associated with increased activity in plasma of another group of enzymes which

TABLE 33.3. Examples of results obtained for commonly performed chemical tests of liver function.

| | Prehepatic jaundice | Parenchymal disease of the liver | | Cholestatic jaundice |
		Acute	Chronic	
Plasma bilirubin	Increased (unconjugated bilirubin)	Variable increase, depending on stage and severity of the disease		Often greatly increased, and bilirubin mainly conjugated
Plasma albumin	Normal	Normal	Reduced	Normal
Plasma alkaline phosphatase	Normal (20–90 i.u./l)	Usually moderately increased (100–200 i.u./l)		Often greatly increased (to over 200 i.u./l)
Plasma aspartate amino-transferase or alanine aminotransferase	Normal (10–35 i.u./l)	Often greatly increased (to over 200 i.u./l)	Normal or slightly increased	Usually normal or slightly increased, unless hepatic complications occur
Serum globulins (zone electrophoresis)	Normal	Normal early, but later an increase in β- and γ-globulins	Increase in β- and γ-globulins	Normal, but all globulin fractions may show an increase if disease prolonged, especially β-globulins
Prothrombin time	Normal	Prolonged one-stage prothrombin time (and Thrombotest), not corrected by vitamin K given parenterally		Prolonged one-stage prothrombin time (and Thrombotest) usually at least partly corrected by parenteral vitamin K

includes alkaline phosphatase, 5′-nucleotidase and γ-glutamyl transpeptidase (GGT). Alkaline phosphatase activity in plasma is increased in a number of physiological states, such as during active phases of growth and in pregnancy, and the pathological states giving rise to bone disease or hepatobiliary disease. The finding of an increased plasma alkaline phosphatase activity is therefore not specific for liver disease, and indeed isoenzymes of alkaline phosphatase can be obtained from intestine, kidney and placenta as well as from bone and liver. Obstruction to the outflow of bile leads to the induction of liver alkaline phosphatase (p. 33.11).

Marked increases in plasma alkaline phosphatase activity are often observed in patients with cholestatic jaundice, whether intrahepatic or extrahepatic, the activity usually exceeding 200 i.u./l (reference values for adults, 20–90 i.u./l). In patients with hepatocellular jaundice, but excluding patients with intrahepatic cholestasis, the increase in activity is usually less, results mostly falling in the range 100–200 i.u./l. With uncomplicated prehepatic jaundice, alkaline phosphatase is usually normal. The reference values are higher for patients under the age of 20, because of the greater contribution by bone to the normal levels of plasma alkaline phosphatase activity in childhood and adolescence.

Measurement of 5′-nucleotidase was introduced as a way of improving the specificity of phosphatase determinations for investigating suspected hepatobiliary disease, since 5′-nucleotidase is practically localized to the liver. However, the methods are tedious and not sufficiently sensitive, and 5′-nucleotidase measurements have been largely replaced by measurement of GGT activity in plasma, or by alkaline phosphatase isoenzyme studies, a much more sensitive index of liver disease.

Increases in plasma GGT activity occur mainly in patients with liver disease, and these increases are much greater (about 5 times greater) in biliary tract disease than in parenchymal disease. At present, measurement of GGT activity is the most sensitive enzyme test available for detecting interference with biliary function. It is, however, a microsomal enzyme and is liable to be induced by the administration of drugs such as alcohol, barbiturates, phenytoin and warfarin, and some of the increase observed in plasma GGT activity may be due to enzyme induction rather than to hepatobiliary disease. Despite the sensitivity and apparently relatively high specificity of GGT activity measurements, these should not be used as the sole enzymic test of liver function.

Choice of a group of liver function tests
Most hospital chemical laboratories undertake a limited number of tests for the initial assessment of hepatic function. These usually include measurement of plasma albumin as an index of synthetic capability, plasma bilirubin as an index of excretory function, and two enzyme activity measurements, most often alkaline phosphatase and alanine or aspartate aminotransferase activities. When considered in association with the history of the patient's illness, the findings from clinical examination which should include the results of simple urine investigations (table 33.2) and other evidence, this selection of chemical investigations is sufficient to clarify

most diagnostic problems and to provide a baseline for assessing the susequent course of the illness (table 33.3). Each of the tests mentioned, or appropriate alternatives, has been chosen so as to give information about a different category of liver function or measure of cellular integrity.

Many hospital chemical laboratories now perform as a routine a number of investigations (12–20) on all patients when first admitted to hospital. These laboratory profiles frequently include measurement of serum albumin and bilirubin as well as alkaline phosphatase and AST activities. Some of the techniques are essentially screening investigations, and abnormalities revealed often need to be further investigated by more specific diagnostic techniques. Minor abnormalities revealed by the screening investigations may prove to be normal when further investigated by more specific and precise methods. This is an example of the confusing fact that 'normal ranges' for many chemical determinations are influenced by the particular analytical technique adopted. In this connection, it is worth mentioning specially the misleading expression 'International Unit', as applied to the results of enzyme activity measurements. The definition of an International Unit (i.u.) of enzyme activity is 'that amount of enzyme which, under given assay conditions, will catalyse the conversion of 1 µmol of substrate per minute' (p. 7.19). The inclusion of the words 'under given assay conditions' reflects the fact that International Units of enzyme activity are not universal in their application. Although many laboratories now express 'normal ranges' for the same enzyme activity measurement in International Units, e.g. plasma alkaline phosphatase, the figures quoted may in some cases be widely different because the conditions of assay are different; there are, as yet, no ideal methods for measuring enzyme activities and thus no methods that have universal application. This point needs to be stressed because an elementary misconception still frequently held is the belief that International Units of enzyme activity are truly international, i.e. universal in their application and able to contribute to uniformity in ways of expressing results obtained in different laboratories. In the profile or screening methods of investigation just mentioned, the methods used for some of the measurements, especially the enzyme activity measurements, sometimes differ in important ways from the best available methods of investigation and consequently many yield different results.

It would of course be possible in many laboratories to extend the limited initial range of chemical investigations of liver function so as to test each category of function in several different ways. For instance, the protein-synthesizing functions can be assessed by zone electrophoresis of serum proteins, by specific individual measurements of at least ten other plasma proteins in addition to albumin, as well as by means of the obsolete turbidity and flocculation tests. Likewise the range of enzyme activity measurements can be greatly extended. It has been repeatedly shown, however, that such multiplicity of testing gives rise to confusion in interpretation of results. It is strongly recommended, therefore, that further investigations such as zone electrophoresis of serum proteins, detailed investigation of individual clotting factors, studies of alkaline phosphatase isoenzymes, measurement of enzyme activities such as γ-glutamyl transpeptidase (GGT) and isocitrate dehydrogenase, and lipoprotein electrophoresis (for possible detection of lipoprotein X) should be reserved for those patients where the performance of these extra tests might help to clarify a specific diagnostic problem or provide important additional information.

COMPUTER-ASSISTED DIAGNOSIS IN LIVER DISEASE

The differential diagnosis of liver disease is an area of medicine where statistical procedures may help in the classification of patients, and techniques of taxonomic analysis are being developed with the aid of digital computers. It can be difficult to decide which items of information to analyse and the appropriate weighting to apply to the various attributes, but progress has been made in defining clusters of patients with different types of disease on the basis of clinical information and laboratory tests. The first programs for computer-assisted diagnosis were developed from a retrospective analysis of case records, but such programs have now been applied prospectively and improved as a result of the experience gained. Much work has still to be done before computer-assisted diagnosis of liver disease can be regarded as other than a research procedure.

FURTHER READING

Kohn J. & Weaver P.C. (1974) Serum-alpha-fetoprotein in hepatocellular carcinoma. *Lancet* ii, 334–337.

Leading Article (1973) More about chenodeoxycholic acid. *British Medical Journal* 4, 629.

Leading Article (1970) Cyclic AMP: the second messenger. *Lancet* ii, 1119–1121.

Moss D.W. & Butterworth P.J. (1974) *Enzymology and Medicine.* London: Pitman Medical.

Popper H. & Schaffner F. eds. (1965–74) *Progress in Liver Diseases*, vols. II–IV. New York: Grune & Stratton.

Rothschild M.A., Oratz M. & Schreiber S.S. (1972) Albumin synthesis. *New England Journal of Medicine* 286, 748–757; 816–821.

Schaffner F., Sherlock S. & Leevy C.M. (1974) *The Liver and its Diseases.* New York: Intercontinental Medical Book Corporation.

Schmid R. (1972) Bilirubin metabolism in man. *New England Journal of Medicine* 287, 703–709.

SCOTTISH MEDICAL JOURNAL (1973) Symposium on bile acids. *Scottish Medical Journal* **18**, 137–174.

SHERLOCK S. (1975) *Diseases of the Liver and Biliary System*, 5th Edition. Oxford: Blackwell Scientific Publications.

STENGER R.J. (1970) Organelle pathology of the liver. *Gastroenterology* **58**, 554–574.

STERN R.B., KNILL-JONES R.P. & WILLIAMS R. (1974) Clinician versus computer in the choice of 11 differential diagnoses of jaundice based on formalized data. *Methods of Information in Medicine* **13**, 79–82.

STRANDJORD P.E., CLAYSON K.J. & ROBY R.J. (1973) Computer assisted pattern recognition and the diagnosis of liver disease. *Human Pathology* **4**, 67–77.

WHITBY L.G., PERCY-ROBB I.W. & SMITH A.F. (1975) *Lecture Notes on Clinical Chemistry*. Oxford: Blackwell Scientific Publications.

Chapter 34
Adipose tissue

The primary function of adipose tissue is the storage of triglycerides (TG), a potential source of energy. It also provides insulation against cold and mechanical damage and serves as the packing material for the internal organs. The amount and the distribution of adipose tissue largely determines our shape and general appearance and differs in adult men and women.

Amount and distribution

A healthy male contains about 7·5 kg of adipose tissue, a little more than half of which surrounds the organs in the abdominal cavity and elsewhere in the body; the remainder is subcutaneous. A healthy female has rather more than twice this amount. The total amount present is determined by the state of nutrition. Before death from starvation occurs, almost all visible fat disappears from the body. Many obese people carry around a load of 50 kg of adipose tissue and a few very much more. For instance, Mr John Cobb, who was featured in *Time* (30th July 1965) and who weighed 365 kg, probably had over 200 kg. He was in the habit of eating fifteen chickens at a sitting. Genetic factors also determine the amount of adipose tissue present. The adipose tissue cells increase in number during infancy and early childhood. Overfeeding at this time may lead to the growth of an excessive cell population in those genetically disposed to do so. As a result these individuals tend in later life to a form of obesity which is difficult to control. This is because dieting can decrease the fat content of the adipose cell but it cannot diminish the number of cells once they are formed.

The distribution of fat differs markedly in the two sexes and also varies in individuals. This is partly controlled by the sex hormones. Administration of oestrogens to men leads to the deposition of fat round the hips and thighs, the characteristic female pattern. Conversely testosterone and adrenocorticosteroids promote the male distribution, predominantly in the upper part of the body.

Histological structure

As a supporting and packing material, adipose tissue is often considered as a variety of connective tissue. It is of mesenchymal origin, but differs from other connective tissues in that its functions and properties are due to the contents of the cell and not to the intercellular substances. Although the cells of adipose tissue may differentiate from and revert to cells which resemble fibroblasts, they are considered here as a separate tissue because of their characteristic structure and metabolic importance.

Ordinary adipose tissue is divided into lobules by collagenous and reticular septa, which carry the nerves and capillary blood supply to the closely-packed cells (fig. 34.1). The mature fat cell consists of a shell of cytoplasm, containing a flattened nucleus, which surrounds a single globule of lipid up to 50 μm in diameter. In routine histological preparations this lipid globule is dissolved during dehydration and embedding in paraffin wax (p. 13.3), so the empty shells which remain give the appearance of a honeycomb. Sections of frozen material, or techniques which render the lipid insoluble, reveal more details of the structure of the fat cell. During the

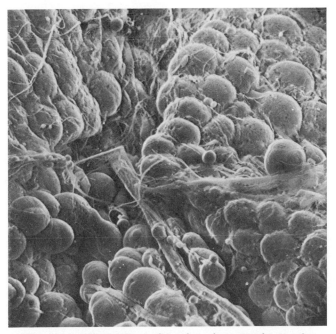

FIG. 34.1. Adipose tissue. Scanning electron micrograph. From *Nutrition Today* (1974) **9**, May–June, 7.

accumulation of fat, numerous small globules appear which later coalesce into a single globule (fig. 34.2). Histochemical techniques and the EM show that the cytoplasm, surrounding the lipid, has all the usual enzymes and organelles of an active metabolizing cell; after starving and refeeding, glycogen can be demonstrated in the cytoplasmic rims.

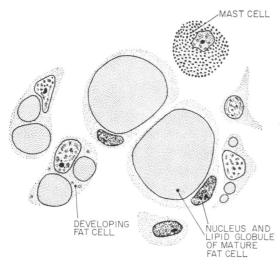

FIG. 34.2. The accumulation of fat in fat cells.

Some adipose tissue which is darker and more vascular is known as **brown fat**. Histologically this tissue also consists of closely-packed large cells, but each cell contains many small lipid droplets which do not coalesce (fig. 34.3). The cytoplasm of brown fat cells contains numer-

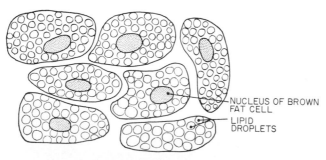

FIG. 34.3. Brown fat cells.

ous mitochondria and pigments which give it the dark colour. Small droplets of lipid have a larger surface area than the single globule of ordinary fat. This disposition of the lipid allows its energy stores to become more freely available. The mitochondrial content suggests that the tissue can have a high metabolic rate. In hibernating animals there are large amounts of brown fat, which provide the energy for the warming up process in the spring. Brown fat is found in the mature human fetus where it serves as a small but easily mobilizable reserve for the energy demands of the neonatal period.

Chemical composition

Many samples of human adipose tissue removed at operation and by biopsy have been analysed. The fat content varies greatly, ranging from 65 to 90 per cent. Figures of 85 per cent for fat, 13 per cent for water and 2 per cent for protein are normal. Thus 7·5 kg of adipose tissue contains just over 1 kg of fat-free tissue and about 150 g of protein. Therefore apart from its fat content adipose tissue is very substantial and is comparable in size and protein content to the liver. An obese person with 50 kg of adipose tissue probably has about 5 kg of fat-free adipose tissue, metabolically equivalent to a very large organ. Excess food increases the size of the cells (hypertrophy) and also their number (hyperplasia). In man hyperplasia appears to be more important.

The greater part of the lipid, about 98 per cent, is TG, but there are traces of diglyceride, FFA, cholesterol and phospholipid. The cholesterol and phospholipid can be synthesized within the tissues and are probably present in the membranes. The phosphorus-containing phosphatidic acids lie on the pathway of TG synthesis (p. 10.17) and might be expected to be present in small amounts. Of the total protein, up to 25 per cent is collagen and 12 per cent nucleoprotein and the remainder is probably mainly cytoplasmic and includes the enzymes needed for the metabolic processes. The glycogen content is normally less than 0·1 per cent, but may rise to as much as 1 per cent in the adipose tissue of animals re-fed after a period of starvation.

For many years the body fat was considered to be a purely passive store of TG, not involved in the minute to minute energy metabolism of the body. When isotopically labelled fatty acids are administered to animals, the activity of adipose tissue becomes apparent. There is continuous formation and breakdown of TG. For these metabolic changes the immediate source of energy is ATP derived from oxidative processes. The oxygen consumption of adipose tissue, when expressed per unit of dry fat-free tissue or tissue N, is high and of the same order as that of kidney and liver.

Formation of fat stores
From non-lipid sources
It is common knowledge that a diet containing excess carbohydrate leads to obesity. Fat deposition is independent of ingested TG, since it occurs in young animals fed a fat-free diet. It was once thought that lipid synthesis took place exclusively in the liver and that newly-formed TG was carried as lipoprotein in the blood to the depots in the adipose tissue. However, since lipid synthesis has been demonstrated in hepatectomized rats, this is not true. To study the relative importance of different tissues in the synthesis of TG from non-lipid sources, ^{14}C-acetate has been injected into rats, and the quantity of labelled

TG in each tissue determined at different time intervals. The number of labelled molecules in the liver was found to be well below that in the intestinal cells and in the remainder of the carcass, suggesting that less TG synthesis occurs in the liver than elsewhere. However, this interpretation of the experiment is suspect since the ^{14}C-acetyl-CoA intermediate in the liver may be diluted with unlabelled molecules derived from the glycogen stores or incoming FFA and glucose. Consequently, the proportion of new TG molecules in the liver bearing the label would be expected to be lower than in other tissues. Nevertheless, the specific activity of TG in liver was higher than in adipose tissue, which seemed to support the original thesis that liver is the principal site of TG synthesis. Later this was refuted by repeating the experiment using rats whose fat stores had been depleted of TG by fasting. In these animals, the specific activity of the TG was higher in adipose tissue than in liver. It was therefore concluded that synthesis also occurs in adipose tissue. The relative importance of the two tissues in the synthesis of fatty acids is still the subject of argument.

The bulk of the TG molecules formed in the liver are rapidly secreted into the blood stream as lipoprotein (p. 10.5), hence their turnover time is very short compared with that of the TG in adipose tissue.

The pathways of fatty acid and TG synthesis appear to be the same in adipose tissue as in liver, but it has not yet been possible to isolate a fatty acyl carrier protein. Desaturation and elongation of injected ^{14}C-palmitic acid has been demonstrated in rat adipose tissue *in vivo*. These reactions occur in the microsomes.

The source of the TG formed from carbohydrate is the blood glucose and also glycogen in the adipose tissue. When pieces of adipose tissue are incubated with ^{14}C-glucose, the majority of the ^{14}C incorporated in the newly synthesized TG is in the glyceride moiety. Thus glucose provides 1-glycerophosphate to esterify endogenous fatty acids. Addition of insulin increases the total quantity of glucose entering the tissue, particularly the amount converted into fatty acid TG. However, the hormone does not affect the incorporation of ^{14}C-acetate or pyruvate molecules unless glucose is also added to the medium. This indicates that insulin acts prior to the oxidative decarboxylation of pyruvate and does not accelerate the conversion of acetate to fatty acid. The incorporation of acetate rises only when glycolysis and hence the formation of 1-glycerophosphate and ATP is promoted.

As in muscle, the incorporation of amino acids into the protein of adipose tissue is increased by insulin *in vitro*. This occurs if an energy source, e.g. pyruvate or glucose is present, although the insulin has no observed effect on pyruvate metabolism. Protein formation in both tissues is also promoted by growth hormone but inhibited by adrenocorticosteroids. Carbon skeletons derived from amino acids by transamination can also be traced to the TG stores.

The pathways of glucose utilization have been studied in adipose tissue. The activities of the enzymes involved when expressed per mg of tissue N are usually one-third to one-fifth those of liver, but the enzymes for gluconeogenesis are absent and glucose-6-phosphate dehydrogenase is nearly six times as active as in liver. Comparison of ^{14}CO$_2$ formed when equal amounts of 1-^{14}C-glucose and 6-^{14}C-glucose were added to the incubation medium shows that the hexose monophosphate pathway is active in adipose tissue. However, this does not appear to be the exclusive source of the large quantity of NADPH$_2$ required for fatty acid synthesis by the tissue (p. 10.9).

From incoming lipid
Both plasma lipoproteins and chylomicrons deposit some of their TG fatty acids in adipose tissue. The former are derived from the TG synthesized in the liver from fatty acids, while the chylomicrons originate in the intestine. Labelled FFA injected into human subjects have also been found 10 min later incorporated in the adipose tissue TG. However, this source of preformed fatty acid is quantitatively less important than the other two.

Most of the plasma TG taken up by adipose tissue is probably first hydrolysed to FFA and glycerol. The glycerol and the phospholipid, cholesterol and protein, which formed the shell of the lipoprotein, remain in the blood while the FFA enter the fat cell. There they are reconverted to TG by condensation with 1-glycerophosphate formed within the cell from carbohydrate. As more TG fatty acid is taken up from the blood in the fed than in the fasted state, i.e. under conditions when lipoprotein lipase activity is known to be high (p. 10.7), this enzyme has been implicated in the hydrolytic process.

An adequate supply of blood glucose is of importance in the transfer of triglyceride FA from the plasma into the adipose cell. It promotes the re-esterification of the liberated FFA intermediates and also maintains the activity of lipoprotein lipase, perhaps by stimulating the secretion of insulin by the pancreas. When plasma lipoprotein labelled in the fatty acid moieties of the TG is perfused through rat adipose tissue, the FFA liberated by this process does not appear to mix with those of the blood. Consequently it has been suggested that hydrolysis of lipoprotein TG occurs within the fat cell rather than in the vascular bed, but this question has not yet been settled.

How TG enters the adipose cell from the capillaries is unknown. While lipid has been demonstrated by EM studies to pass through and between the epithelial cells of the intestine into the vascular and lymphatic systems, none is seen in the endothelial cells of the capillaries en route to or from the adipose cell. Investigators have concluded that the lipid observed adhering to the walls of the blood vessel passes through the perivascular space to the adipocyte in a manner not visualized by the EM. This could be as FFA bound to albumin or as micelles. It is possible that the small droplets seen at the periphery of the fat cell constitute the active TG compartment which is functionally separate from the inert storage pool.

Under physiological conditions the major part of the fatty acid laid down as TG in adipose tissue is probably derived from plasma lipoprotein rather than by synthesis from glucose.

Composition of lipid stored in adipose tissue

The relative proportions of the major fatty acids derived by hydrolysis of adipose tissue from young healthy adults fed a random diet are as follows:

Fatty acid	Per cent of total
$C_{14:0}$	2·4
$C_{16:0}$	26·7
$C_{16:1}$	3·8
$C_{18:0}$	4·2
$C_{18:1}$	52·8
$C_{18:2}$	7·3
$C_{20:4}$	0·2

Six fatty acids account for 97 per cent of those present. The figure for arachidonic acid ($C_{20:4}$) is given so that a comparison may be made with liver where it amounts to almost 10 per cent of the fatty acid in the total lipid. The ratio of saturated to unsaturated fatty acids in adipose tissue TG is normally 1 : 2 in man. Saturated acids form a higher proportion in the ox and sheep which are a major dietary source of triglyceride for man.

Altering the dietary lipid slowly changes the pattern of fatty acids in the stores over a period of many months. A fat-free diet produces no change within 10 weeks; a difference is observed only after 20 weeks on a diet containing 40 per cent of the energy as corn oil in which 50 per cent of the fatty acid is linoleic acid ($C_{18:2}$). As the stores do not closely resemble the dietary fat until about 3 years of the altered regime, it is apparent that most of the dietary fat does not mix readily with the main pool within the tissue. The half life of this store is calculated to be 1–2 years, while complete mixing of incoming TG FA in a total 10 kg of fat in a normal man would be expected to occur in 50 days if there was one uniform pool. This suggests the existence of an inert depot of TG and a small active compartment within the tissue (fig. 34.4). The plasma TG alter rapidly and correspond with those ingested and hence can be in equilibrium with only a small tissue pool. Enzymes present in the intestine and liver and in the adipose tissue can elongate and desaturate dietary TG FA and help to maintain the pattern characteristic of the species. Nevertheless it is possible to alter the fatty acid composition of the fat depots if weight is being gained while on a diet of abnormal lipid composition. There is no change during weight loss, suggesting no preferential loss of particular fatty acids from the hydrolysed TG.

The composition of the fatty acid mixtures derived from samples of TG from various sites in an individual is similar; there is little difference between men and women and no change occurs with increasing age. Fatty acids are not distributed randomly in triglyceride molecules but in the following pattern:

$$CH_2OCO\text{-saturated chain}$$
$$|$$
$$CHOCO\text{-unsaturated chain}$$
$$|$$
$$CH_2OCO\text{-saturated or unsaturated chain}$$

This may result from specificity in the triglyceride synthesizing enzymes.

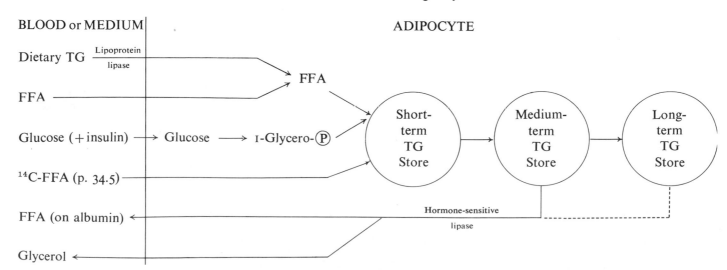

FIG. 34.4. Summary of experimental evidence on the formation and breakdown of TG within the adipose cell. The long term TG store does not participate in the brief *in vivo* or *in vitro* ^{14}C-labelling experiments, but is slowly altered by diet.

Release of FFA from fat stores

FFA are present in adipose tissue to the extent of 1–2 μmol/g in a fed rat and 2–3 μmol/g in a fasted animal. Reference has already been made to the rise in the plasma FFA level which occurs in the fasting human subject. FFA are liberated from the stores by the action of at least two enzymes, a triglyceride lipase and a monoglyceride lipase. The former is unable to hydrolyse lipoprotein substrates, in contrast to lipoprotein lipase from which it also differs in its response to activators and inhibitors. The triglyceride lipase may consist of two separate enzymes for attacking triglycerides and diglycerides successively. The monoglyceride lipase, being the more active enzyme, prevents the accumulation of monoglycerides. The adipose tissue lipases are difficult to isolate in a highly purified form, probably due to their close association with structural lipoprotein. Glycerol, the other product of hydrolysis, is also carried away in the blood stream to the liver. It is unlikely that it is phosphorylated by adipose tissue to regenerate 1-glycerophosphate to an important extent, as the necessary glycerokinase is present in only small amounts. In consequence esterification of fatty acids and therefore storage of triglyceride within adipose tissue only occurs when there is an adequate supply of 1-glycerophosphate derived from glucose.

The FFA when released from TG are probably bound to cytoplasmic protein. They pass into an intracellular pool and then either leave the cell bound to plasma albumin, which makes them water-soluble, or are re-esterified to TG (fig. 34.4).

FFA entering the cell from the plasma may not need to pass through this pool, but perhaps can be esterified directly close to the cell membrane. Some evidence for this was obtained from experiments in which adipose tissue was incubated with ^{14}C-FFA, which entered the cells and was found in the TG. The tissue was then immediately transferred to fresh buffer under conditions promoting lipolysis. Since the FFA released were not labelled, different molecules must be involved in short term formation and breakdown of TG (fig. 34.4). However, *in vivo* work shows that within a few days of altering dietary lipids, the FFA released into the plasma are similar in composition to those in the dietary TG. This is best explained by assuming the existence of a second, longer term compartment of TG into which the newly-formed molecules pass and from which they are released after hydrolysis. This compartment may be simply those parts of the tissue lying near the blood vessels and need not be the compartment into which the TG is taken up intact in the *in vitro* experiment described earlier.

When isolated fat cells are homogenized and centrifuged the infranatant layer contains lipid droplets, resembling chylomicrons in size. If the cells have been previously incubated with ^{14}C-glucose, the specific activity of this lipid fraction is consistently higher than that of the fat which lies on top, but less than that of the microsomes and mitochondria. Hence these droplets may be newly-synthesized lipid in transit to the stores, which form the upper fatty layer in a centrifugate (fig. 34.4).

The activity of the enzyme involved in splitting TG stored in adipose tissue is enhanced greatly by certain hormones. Hence it is named hormone-sensitive lipase, which differentiates it from lipoprotein lipase. This response is most clearly shown by a rapid increase in the glycerol present in the blood or incubation medium. There is a concomitant rise in the output of FFA but as these, unlike glycerol, can be re-utilized in adipose tissue, the analytical data for FFA provide only a net picture, i.e. the difference between the quantity produced by hydrolysis of the TG and that disappearing due to re-esterification by 1-glycerophosphate within the tissue. *In vitro*, provided glucose is not added, the ratio of change in FFA/change in glycerol for the total system (tissue plus medium) is approximately 3/1, corresponding to complete hydrolysis and no re-esterification. With glucose the ratio is lower. However, when isolated adipose tissue is perfused with diluted blood containing a lipolytic hormone, the ratio is found to be 5/1 to 7/1, provided the albumin content of the infusate is sufficiently high. The diglyceride content of the tissue is enhanced as well as the release of FFA and glycerol. This suggests that under conditions where the released FFA is efficiently carried away from the fat cells, 50 per cent is derived from partial hydrolysis to diglyceride. This is probably the situation *in vivo*. Similar high values have been found in human blood taken soon after exercise.

The lipase system, which probably resides in the microsomes, attacks all three positions in the TG molecule equally, in contrast to pancreatic lipase. Monoglyceride lipase does not appear to be under hormonal control.

The FFA released from isolated tissue consist of the seven major acids. The proportions of FFA found in the cell, relative to those in the total TG are highest for $C_{16:0}$ and $C_{16:1}$, and lowest for $C_{18:1}$ and $C_{18:2}$ acids. This may be due to an enzymic preference for the C_{16} acids. The fatty acid mixture which leaves the cells contains a higher proportion of the unsaturated acids and $C_{14:0}$ than is present in the cell, probably due to their higher solubility in the aqueous environment or to a lower affinity for cellular binding sites than the other saturated acids.

LIPOLYTIC HORMONES

The hormones known to activate the hormone sensitive lipase are adrenaline, noradrenaline, glucagon, ACTH, vasopressin and 5HT. These also increase the activity of the glycogenolytic enzyme, phosphorylase. In addition the catecholamines appear to stimulate the uptake and utilization of glucose which promotes the removal of the FFA by re-esterification. The net effect, however, is an enhanced output of FFA from the tissue to the blood.

The activation of phosphorylase in liver and muscle by adrenaline has been shown to occur indirectly via stimulation of cyclic AMP formation from ATP by the enzyme adenyl cyclase associated with the cell membrane (p. 9.9). Similarly, the intracellular levels of lipase activity and of accumulated cyclic AMP both depend on the amount of adrenaline present, and are both increased by caffeine, which prevents the destruction of cyclic AMP. Further evidence for the involvement of cyclic AMP as the agent of hormonal lipase activation comes from the observation that addition of a more soluble derivative of cyclic AMP to isolated adipose tissue or free adipocytes promotes FFA release. Cyclic AMP has an allosteric effect on a phosphorylating enzyme (kinase) which converts the lipase to a more active form.

An increase in plasma glycerol and FFA also occurs in animals and man if sufficient growth hormone or cortisol is injected to achieve a high circulating hormone level. This response occurs very much more slowly than that due to catecholamines, which produce an effect on lipolysis within seconds after administration. The fast-acting hormones activate an existing lipase or remove an inactivator. In contrast growth hormone and the adrenocorticosteroids appear to promote the synthesis of an enzyme, probably adenyl cyclase.

The hormones which activate the TG lipase under physiological conditions are probably noradrenaline, the adrenocorticosteroids and growth hormone. The other fast-acting ones listed above have to be provided *in vitro* at too high concentration to be considered of physiological importance.

NERVOUS CONTROL

The nerve supply to adipose tissue plays a leading role in facilitating fat mobilization. Lipolysis and the increase in plasma FFA which occurs in the fasted subject are reduced after ganglionic and adrenergic blocking drugs are given. As these compounds also diminish the mobilization of fat in response to cold and psychological stress, the nervous mechanism appears in part to involve noradrenaline release at the postganglionic sympathetic nerve endings. The fibres of the autonomic nerves terminate in close relation to the fat cells as well as the blood vessels. This innervation exerts a continuous control of the normal metabolism of the tissue, which is invoked in emergency states.

PROVISION OF FFA AS METABOLIC FUEL

Within the adipose cell a cyclic system therefore exists in which FA are first mobilized by lipolysis and then re-esterified by 1-glycerophosphate derived from blood glucose. The first process is influenced by the activity of the lipolytic hormones. There are antilipolytic hormones which oppose lipolysis in tissue in which TG lipase activity is raised. They include the prostaglandins and insulin, which even in the absence of glucose diminishes the enhanced output of glycerol and FFA from free fat cells incubated with noradrenaline. These hormones interfere with the action of cyclic AMP, the activator of the lipase. On the other hand the thyroid hormones promote the formation of cyclic AMP and reduce its rate of destruction (fig. 34.5). As a consequence the size of the lipolytic response to noradrenaline depends also on the quantity of thyroid hormones in the circulation. This provides an explanation for the low serum FFA levels after thyroidectomy and the high values in the hyperthyroid patient. Provision of glucose within the cell, dependent on an adequate blood glucose level and the presence of circulating insulin, supplies 1-glycerophosphate which also suppresses FFA release by re-esterification. Of consequence too, is the property of adrenocorticosteroids of depressing the utilization of glucose by fat cells.

The mobilization or retention of FFA by the adipose tissue stores is therefore dependent on nutritional factors and the presence or absence of stress. Control is achieved

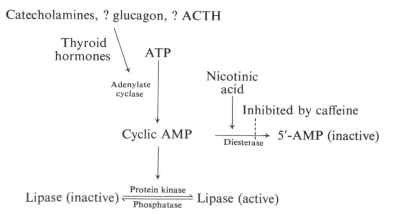

FIG. 34.5. Probable enzyme activations which control the activity of hormone-sensitive lipase.

by the ability of the body to alter the rate of blood flow through the tissue and to secrete the appropriate hormones.

Activity of the adipose cell under various physiological conditions

During absorption of carbohydrate and fat, TG are laid down in the fat stores. The plasma FFA level is low. Carbohydrate is used as the principal metabolic fuel and the major part of such TG as breaks down within the stores is regenerated. This continues until the blood glucose falls towards the fasting level.

During fasting FFA is increasingly mobilized from the adipose tissue. This is due partly to stimulation of the hormone sensitive lipase through release of catecholamines. Decreased availability of glucose to the cell due to the low blood concentration, a falling rate of insulin secretion and eventually the rise in circulating adrenocorticosteroids also play important parts. Contributory factors may also be growth hormone, glucagon and a fat mobilizing substance isolated from the urine of fasting individuals and probably of pituitary origin.

The resulting rise in plasma FFA during fasting leads to their increased utilization, e.g. by the liver which resynthesizes TG, part of which appears as additional plasma lipoprotein. Fat becomes the main source of energy and the RQ falls to around 0·75. Gluconeogenesis besides providing carbohydrate for the nervous system acts as a brake on lipid mobilization by promoting insulin secretion. This leads to some reformation of TG and their return to the stores. Nevertheless, ketosis and triglyceri-

daemia eventually occur (p. 10.13). These changes are less frequently observed in the severely obese, perhaps because their output of growth hormone tends to rise to a smaller extent in response to fasting than in normal individuals.

Stress, such as fear, sudden cold, etc., results in rapid release of catecholamines with consequent activation of the hormone sensitive lipase. Stress also leads to secretion of increased amounts of ACTH and hence of adrenocorticosteroids. The latter besides their gluconeogenic and glucose sparing effects slowly promote lipolytic activity. Thus an increased supply of FFA reaches the liver, muscles, etc., to provide the extra energy required in stressful situations.

The normal response to noradrenaline and to cold, in terms of increased lipase or phosphorylase action is not observed in adrenalectomized animals. It has been suggested that this is due to an adverse electrolyte pattern within the fat cell. Recovery is complete if cortisol is given, and restored to 50 per cent of normal by giving saline or aldosterone. Phosphorylase activity is also restored in extracts of muscle from adrenalectomized animals by adding cyclic AMP. Hence the lesion may be an inability to form this compound leading to poor resistance to cold.

Exercise, even at a moderate level in fasting man, produces a fall in plasma FFA within 10 min of onset. The level then rises, even in hypophysectomized or adrenalectomized individuals. The plasma glycerol concentration which is also enhanced can be reduced by administration of glucose or nicotinic acid, a compound which prevents

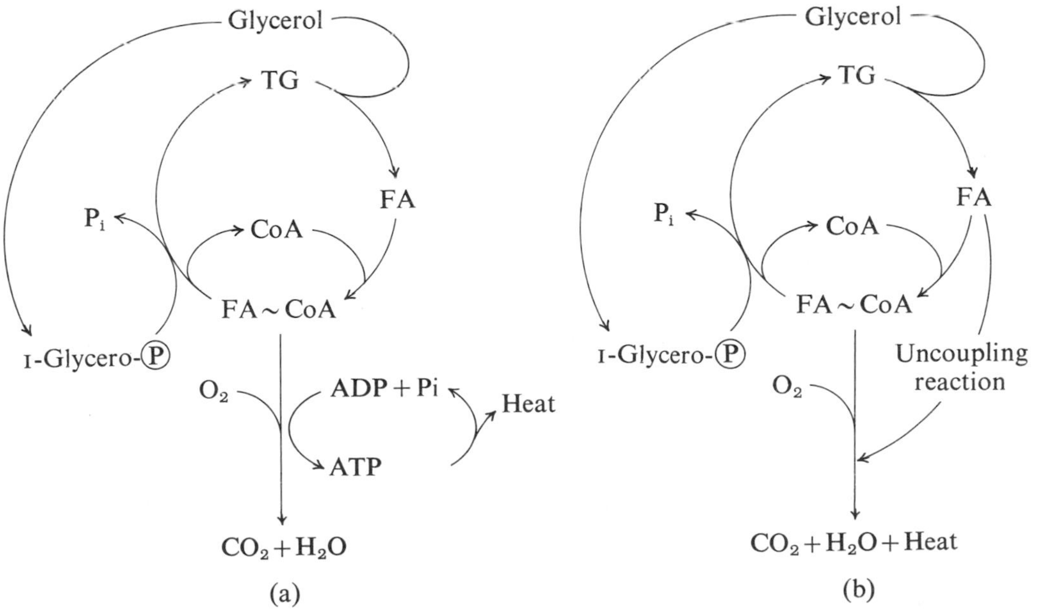

FIG. 34.6. Heat production in brown adipose tissue; (a) initially, source is conversion of chemical energy of ATP to heat by synthesis of TG from FA; (b) later a build up of FA uncouples the oxidation of FA.CoA from the formation of ATP, resulting in a massive release of heat.

the lipolytic effect of noradrenaline. This is consistent with the increased activity of the sympathetic nervous system during exercise. During the initial stage the primary adjustments are cardiovascular, causing an increased blood flow, and hence removal of FFA from the plasma. The reverse situation exists during the recovery stage. The RQ may fall to as low as 0·75, indicating the utilization of fat for provision of muscular energy. Some of this is not derived from the adipose tissue, but from TG lying between the muscle fibres. TG may also be taken up in greater amount from plasma lipoprotein by muscle.

INFANCY

The newborn infant overcomes his inability to shiver by using his supply of brown adipose tissue. This, like white fat is a store of TG from which FFA are liberated in response to cold, noradrenaline, glucagon, etc. It differs by containing large numbers of mitochondria which are packed with cristae. As a result it has a higher rate of oxygen consumption due to its ability to burn FA locally.

The process involved in non-shivering thermogenesis can be visualized as follows (fig. 34.6). TG are hydrolysed to glycerol and to FFA which is largely re-esterified within the tissue. The latter process involves formation of fatty acyl CoA and then replacement of the CoA by a glycerol moiety activated by direct phosphorylation. Thus a cycle of reactions occurs in which a molecule of ATP is used to form the energy rich fatty acyl CoA. This is then broken with liberation of the energy as heat. Therefore, as each molecule of FA passes round the cycle, one ATP molecule is converted to heat. In addition a considerable amount of liberated FA is oxidized. However, when there is a high level of FA within the mitochondria, the system for oxidative phosphorylation becomes uncoupled.

As a result the energy produced by the oxidation of the FA appears as heat rather than being trapped as ATP. This is reflected in the raised oxygen consumption of brown fat in response to catecholamines. The TG–FA cycle is operative also to a small extent when FA of white fat is oxidized within the tissue, but their major outlet is export to the liver and other organs.

Brown fat becomes less important in the maintenance of temperature as the child develops neuromuscular control and the ability to call on heat energy associated with muscular activity.

Conclusion

Adipose tissue is an organ whose primary function is the storage of long chain fatty acids, potential sources of metabolic energy. These long hydrocarbon chains are deposited or withdrawn by precise nervous and hormonal control in order to overcome the fluctuations in nutritional and environmental conditions to which man may be subjected.

FURTHER READING

LINDEBERG O. ed. (1970) *Brown Adipose Tissue.* Amsterdam: Elsevier.

NEWSHOLME E.A. & START C. (1972) *Regulation in Metabolism*, chap. 5. New York: Wiley.

RENOLD A.E. & CAHILL G.F. eds. (1965) *Handbook of Physiology*, Section 5, Adipose Tissue. Washington, D.C.: Amer. Physiol. Soc.

ROBINSON D.S. (1970) In *Comprehensive Biochemistry*, vol. 18, chap. 51, ed. Florkin M. & Stotz E.H. Amsterdam: Elsevier.

SMITH R.E. & HORWITZ B.A. (1969) Brown fat and thermogenesis. *Physiological Reviews* **49**, 330–425.

Chapter 35
Kidney

The structure and function of the mammalian kidney are the outcome of a long sequence of evolutionary changes. These have made it possible for complex organisms to live on dry land where water and salts must be conserved, waste products excreted in a concentrated form, and tissue fluid regulated with respect to volume, chemical composition and osmolality. The primitive ancestors of the vertebrates, who lived in the brackish waters of the estuaries during the Cambrian period, were faced with the need to conserve sodium and eliminate water. In response to the need to excrete water, a filtering device developed consisting of a coil of capillaries invaginated into the blind end of a hollow tube. Under the influence of the arterial pressure, water and solutes were filtered through the capillary walls into the lumen of the tube where selective reabsorption of electrolytes and essential metabolites occurred before the remainder of the filtrate drained to the exterior.

In the mammalian kidney the formation of urine still begins with the production of an ultrafiltrate of plasma and each day a volume of fluid almost fifty times the volume of the blood plasma is transferred from the vascular system to the renal tubules. By far the greater part of this large volume of fluid, together with its solute, is reabsorbed by the cells lining the renal tubules and returned to the blood. This process involves a large number of complex chemical, physical and electrochemical mechanisms which adjust the composition and the amount of the fluid reabsorbed and so maintain the volume and the composition of the body fluids within normal limits. The remainder of the filtered water, together with the waste products of metabolism and surplus solute, is excreted from the body as urine (p. 5.28). The kidneys are therefore almost entirely responsible for the maintenance of the *milieu intérieur*; while possessing some degree of autonomy, these organs are under nervous and chemical control.

ANATOMY

The kidneys are paired organs and in the adult each weighs 120–170 g and is approximately 11–12 cm in length. Their shape is so well known that their name has passed into the common vocabulary. They lie retroperitoneally and are loosely attached to the posterior abdominal wall by fat. In life their position is variable and they move with respiration. In the cadaver the hilum is usually opposite the second lumbar vertebra, the upper and lower poles reaching the twelfth thoracic and third lumbar vertebrae respectively. They are surrounded by a condensation of the retroperitoneal tissue, the **renal fascia**, which blends medially with the fascia over the psoas muscle and merges with the fascia around the renal vessels and ureters. Capping the upper pole of each kidney and enclosed within the fascia is an adrenal gland. The kidneys are covered by a tough, almost inextensible capsule which in health is smooth and glistening. Blood vessels and nerves enter and leave the kidney and the ureter emerges at the hilum, which is on the medial side. Fig. 35.1 shows a coronal section of the kidneys. The **renal cortex** is the paler, finely granular, outer region, while the **renal medulla** consists mainly of the **renal pyramids,** which are striated columns of darker tissue continuous with the cortex. The apices of the pyramids project as **renal papillae** towards the renal pelvis. The ureter receives

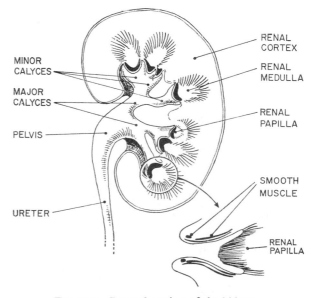

FIG. 35.1. Coronal section of the kidney.

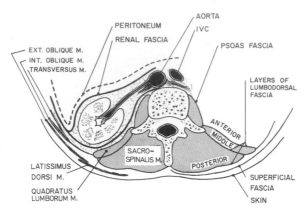

FIG. 35.2. A transverse section showing muscles on the left and fascial relations on the right.

the urine from the **renal pelvis,** a funnel-shaped structure, the wall of which consists of muscle and connective tissue lined by transitional epithelium. The pelvis divides into several recesses or **calcyes** which cover the tips of the renal papillae and are invaginated by them. At the papillary tips are the minute openings of the collecting tubules through which urine enters the calyces before passing to the ureter. The onward flow of urine is helped by rhythmical contractions of the smooth muscle in the walls of the calyces and pelvis.

The relations of the kidney are shown in figs. 35.2–5. Both kidneys are related posteriorly to the diaphragm, and to the muscles of the posterior wall of the abdomen, psoas, quadratus lumborum and transversus. The tips of the transverse processes of the first lumbar vertebra are also closely related to the kidneys. As fig. 35.3 shows, the kidneys extend up to the eleventh or twelfth rib so that, behind the diaphragm, the pleural cavities are posterior relations. The subcostal nerves and subcostal vessels and

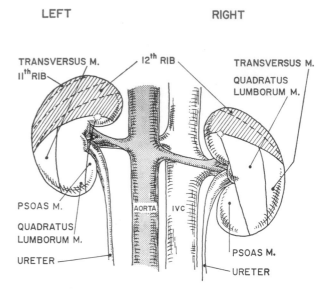

FIG. 35.4. The posterior relations of the kidneys. Shaded areas on both kidneys are in contact with the diaphragm.

the first lumbar nerves and vessels are close posterior relations of both organs. More distant posterior relations are the sacrospinalis muscle, latissimus dorsi and parts of the external and internal oblique muscles.

The anterior relations of the kidneys are shown in fig. 35.5. The left part of the body of the pancreas crosses the left kidney. Superior to this the kidney is covered by the peritoneum of the lesser sac and lies behind the stomach. The convex lateral part of the left kidney makes a large renal impression on the spleen. Inferior to the pancreas the kidney is covered by peritoneum of the greater omentum and is related to coils of jejunum. The peritoneum over the anterior surface of the pancreas is reflected across the kidney to form the **lienorenal ligament.** The upper part of the anterior surface of the right kidney is closely related to the bare area of the liver, while the

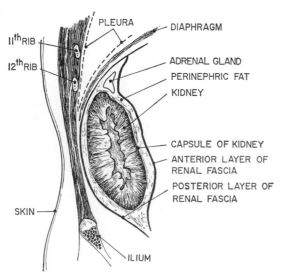

FIG. 35.3. A parasagittal section through the posterior abdominal wall.

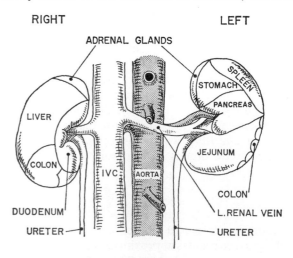

FIG. 35.5. The anterior relations of the kidneys.

duodenum covers the medial part. The right flexure of the colon and the beginning of the transverse colon are in direct contact with the middle and lower lateral parts. Coils of small intestine are related to the lower pole, but are separated from it by peritoneum.

Histological structure

Each kidney is composed of a compact mass of about one million units called **nephrons** (plate 35.1, facing p. 35.12). After birth no new nephrons develop, but existing ones enlarge; glomeruli increase in diameter and tubules increase in length. Each nephron consists of a small tuft of capillaries called a **glomerulus,** which develops in an invagination of one end of a tubule. Glomeruli are found only in the cortex of the kidney while the tubules comprise the bulk of the cortex and medulla. The space around the glomerulus which represents the lumen of the invaginated tubule is called **Bowman's space**; this is bounded externally by a sheet of flat epithelial cells on their basement membrane, called **Bowman's capsule** (plate 18.1, facing p. 18.2). The capsule and glomerulus together are often named the **Malpighian body** after the seventeenth century Italian who first described them. The histology and ultrastructure of the glomerulus is described on pp. 35.7 and 8. The **tubule** begins as a continuation of the space around the capillary tuft and the capsular epithelium is continuous with the cells lining the tubules. Each tubule is 20–45 mm in length, coiled in parts and

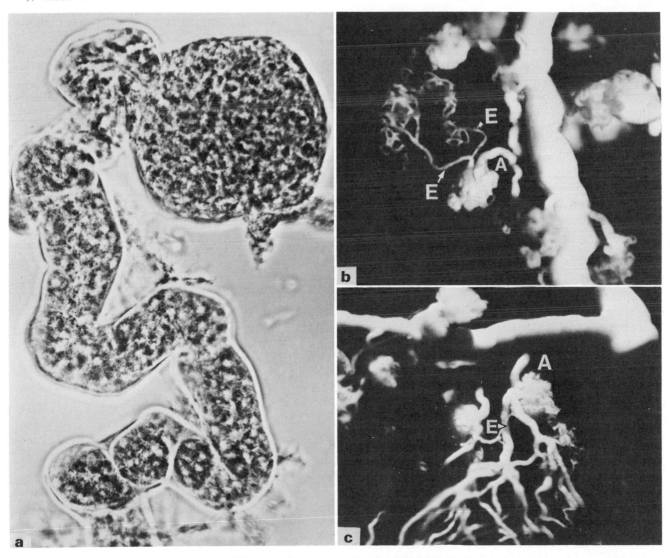

FIG. 35.6. Glomeruli from normal kidneys.

(a) A glomerulus, showing how it communicates by a short neck with the proximal convoluted tubule (×270), by courtesy of Dr E.M. Darmady.

(b) and (c) Neoprene casts of (b) cortical and (c) juxtamedullary glomeruli showing the difference in calibre of the afferent (A) and efferent (E) vessels. From Trueta J. *et al.* (1947) *Studies of the Renal Circulation.* Oxford: Blackwell Scientific Publications.

sharply folded on itself in one place; it empties into a **collecting duct** shared by six to ten other nephrons.

The first part of each tubule twists and coils to form the **proximal convoluted tubule** (fig. 35.6a); after straightening out to form the **pars recta** it then passes into the medulla. There the tubule runs straight for a varying distance before making a sharp hairpin bend, the **loop of Henle**, and returns to the cortex in the neighbourhood of the glomerulus from which it arose; here it again becomes coiled and forms the **distal convoluted tubule.**

Although all nephrons possess the same general configuration, they differ in their blood supply and in the length of the loop of Henle. The glomeruli located in all but the juxtamedullary part of the cortex have short loops which do not penetrate deeply into the medullary zone. About 15 per cent of glomeruli lie in the juxtamedullary region and to these are attached tubules possessing long thin loops which pass deeply into the medulla, sometimes extending as far as the papillae before they return to the cortex.

The distal convoluted tubules ultimately run more or less parallel to the outer surface of the kidney to join a collecting duct. These pass through the cortex and medulla and join together with other collecting ducts to form larger ducts which open into a calyx of the kidney on the surface of a papilla.

The epithelium of the tubule varies in different parts of the nephron (plate 35.1c). In the proximal convoluted tubule the cells appear low columnar or cuboidal, and the lumen in specimens from live patients may appear open or closed. Elongated striations, which are due to the presence of numerous mitochondria, are seen at the base of the cell, and EM shows infoldings of the basal plasma membrane separating groups of mitochondria; this appearance is due to interdigitation of cytoplasmic processes from neighbouring cells and similar but fewer interdigitations are present laterally. The apical border of the cells is covered by numerous elongated microvilli which project centrally forming a **brush border.** The presence of these structures may produce the appearance of a complex, branching lumen. The cell cytoplasm contains multivesicular bodies and other organelles.

The pars recta is lined by rather lower cells than is the convoluted tubule and fewer interdigitations between neighbouring cells are seen. A brush border is still present. The descending limb of the loop of Henle is lined mainly by low cuboidal or even flatter cells, while the ascending limb possesses a thicker epithelial lining. However, the change from thin to thick cells may occur in the lower part of the descending limb, at the bend, or near the beginning of the ascending limb. The transition from pars recta to descending limb is often abrupt. The **thin limb cells** have a stellate contour, the cytoplasmic processes interdigitating with those of neighbouring cells;

the nucleus tends to protrude on the luminal aspect of the cell and a few blunt microvilli project into the lumen. Mitochondria are few and small. The **thick** or **ascending limb cells** are higher than those of the thin limb, but still show protrusion of the part containing the nucleus into the lumen, while the cytoplasm between the nuclei forms a thinner layer. In fact this layer consists of numerous cytoplasmic projections from several cells, since interdigitation in this segment is marked. The mitochondria are elongated and tend to lie at right angles to the basement membrane.

The distal convoluted tubule, which is shorter than the proximal, is lined by low columnar or cuboidal cells with numerous generally elongated mitochondria often lying at right angles to the basement membrane. No brush border is present and the lumen is wider than that of the proximal convoluted tubule. In haematoxylin and eosin sections, the cells are less deeply eosinophilic than the proximal tubule cells. The first part of the distal convoluted tubule is, in fact, almost straight and passes to the vascular pole of the glomerulus where it forms the **macula densa,** part of the juxtaglomerular apparatus (p. 35.5).

The collecting ducts contain two types of cell. The **light cells** are more numerous, have a pale, clear cytoplasm and are of cubical shape, with round nucleus placed near the centre of the cell and only a few small mitochondria. A small number of microvilli are present on the luminal aspect of the cell. **Intercalated or dark cells** are more rounded, contain more mitochondria and have a slightly denser cytoplasm.

The demarcation between distal convoluted tubule and the cortical portion of the collecting duct is not abrupt and the terminal convolutions of the distal convoluted tubule, with which the cortical collecting duct is continuous, may contain light and dark cells.

The renal interstitial tissue contains abundant reticulin fibres and a number of stellate cells which are confined to the medulla. These cells contain many lipid droplets and probably synthesize prostaglandins (p. 35.16).

Embryology

The early development of the genitourinary system is discussed on p. 19.18 and the formation of the mature kidney on p. 36.1.

Blood supply

Renal arteries arise from the aorta opposite the second lumbar vertebra and enter the hila of the kidneys. The right renal artery passes behind the inferior vena cava. At the hila the arteries divide into anterior and posterior branches which further divide to form the **interlobar arteries** lying between the medullary pyramids. When these vessels reach the corticomedullary junction they each divide and the branches curve over the bases of the pyramids to form a series of incomplete arches parallel to the surface of the kidney; these are called **arcuate arteries**. From these the **interlobular arteries** arise at right angles and penetrate the cortex radially, giving off short side branches, the **glomerular afferent arterioles**. Each arteriole runs a short distance before it breaks up into the capillaries of the glomerulus. Here there are many anastomoses and the capillaries are arranged in a network. These reunite to form the **efferent arteriole** which is in close proximity to the point of entry of the afferent vessel. In the main cortical region the efferent vessel is always of narrower diameter than the afferent; in the juxtamedullary region the two vessels are of the same calibre (figs. 35.6b & c). The efferent arteriole breaks up into a second set of capillaries which forms an anastomosing network closely applied to the proximal and distal convoluted tubules both of their own and of neighbouring nephrons. The capillaries coming from the efferent arterioles of juxtamedullary glomeruli form leashes of straight vessels called **vasa recta** (plate 35.1c). They run towards and through the medulla in close contact with the loops of Henle, and, like the tubules, make a hairpin bend to empty into the arcuate veins. There are anastomoses between the descending and ascending vessels. Transverse sections show the close intermingling of blood vessels and tubules which occasionally share a common basement membrane. Thus all tubules receive blood which has first passed through a glomerulus. Blood from the cortex and medulla passes to **arcuate veins** which lie with the

arteries at the corticomedullary junction. These drain towards the hilum and into the renal vein.

Juxtaglomerular apparatus (JGA)

The juxtaglomerular apparatus lies at the hilum of the renal glomerulus (fig. 35.7 and plate 35.1a, facing p. 35.12). Its three components are the **epithelioid** or **granular cells** situated in the media of the afferent arteriole, the **macula densa** consisting of specialized cells of the distal tubule of the same nephron, and the **lacis** or **agranular cells** lying at the hilum between afferent and efferent arterioles and separating the glomerulus from the cells of the macula densa.

The granular cells themselves, derived from neighbouring smooth muscle cells of the arteriolar media, retain myofibrils and possess ultrastructural features of secretory activity. Thus they contain prominent endoplasmic reticulum, Golgi apparatus, juxtanuclear centrioles, membrane-bound secretory sacs and specific and non-specific granules. Experimental evidence indicates that the specific granules are secretory products and contain the proteolytic enzyme renin, a compound which plays a role in vasomotor control and mineralocorticoid metabolism (p. 35.27).

By EM, the granules may be seen in three stages of development. In the early stages of production the granules appear crystalline and rhomboidal. These forms aggregate within a membrane-bound sac to form mature, homogeneous, round, ovoid or more irregular granules. The presence of empty membrane-bound sacs and dilated endoplasmic reticulum in the active granular cell indicates that secretion is taking place.

The non-specific granule, a lipofuscin aggregate, is believed to arise as a result of cellular metabolism and membrane peroxidation. Its apparent increase in numbers in states of JGA cell hyperactivity may reflect enhanced cellular secretory activity. Because of their unique origin, an increase of granular cells may occur because of both cellular hyperplasia and metaplasia of neighbouring smooth muscle cells in the wall of the afferent and even of the efferent arterioles.

The lacis cells were so named because they were originally identified as a complex, lace-like network of membranes lying between the glomerulus and the macula densa. It is not certain that they represent a distinct cell type, and indeed are in continuity with the mesangial cells of the glomerulus (p. 35.7).

The dense spot or macula densa seen on light microscopy is due to close grouping of the prominent nuclei of cells of the distal tubule where they are in close apposition to the JGA cells. At this point, the tubular cells appear tall and columnar with prominent surface microvilli. The nuclei adopt an apical position within the cell, the Golgi apparatus lies in an infra- or paranuclear site and the normal tubular basement membrane is almost

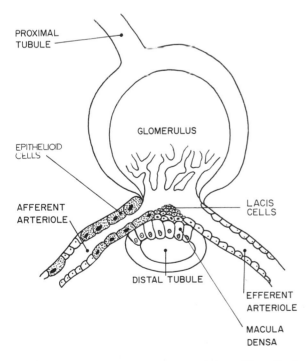

PROXIMAL
TUBULE

GLOMERULUS

EPITHELIOID
CELLS

AFFERENT
ARTERIOLE

LACIS
CELLS

DISTAL TUBULE

EFFERENT
ARTERIOLE

MACULA
DENSA

Fig. 35.7. Juxtaglomerular apparatus. Adapted from Cook W.F. (1963) in *Hormones and the Kidney*, ed. Williams P. London: Academic Press.

completely absent, being replaced by a ramifying cytoplasmic network, these basal interdigitations making close and extensive contact with processes of the JGA cells.

Prominent non-myelinated nerve endings make intimate contact with JGA cells, thus supporting the view that there may be a neural component in the control of renin release (p. 35.28).

Lymphatics

The cortex has many lymphatics in the intertubular tissue, some of which drain outwards to the capsule and others towards the corticomedullary junction. No lymphatic vessels, however, have been found in or around the glomeruli, nor have lymphatics in the region of the JGA been convincingly demonstrated. In the medulla, lymph channels run from the apex of the pyramids to the corticomedullary junction. From there, larger lymphatic channels pass along the main blood vessels to the hilum and drain into the para-aortic lymph nodes.

Nerve supply

The kidney is supplied with sympathetic nerves derived from thoracic and lumbar segments of the sympathetic trunk; most of them arise from the spinal cord between T12 and L2. The majority reach the kidney through the pre-aortic ganglia where they synapse. There are probably no parasympathetic nerves. The sympathetic nerve fibres pass to all renal vessels containing smooth muscle, including both types of arterioles, the proximal part of the vasa recta, and also to the JGA. The cortex has many more nerves than the medulla. Afferent fibres arise in the kidney and ultimately enter the dorsal roots of T12 to L2. The nerves to the arterioles can exert a vasoconstrictor effect.

FUNCTIONS OF THE KIDNEYS

The kidneys are concerned in a number of activities, which include the removal of nitrogenous waste, mostly in the form of urea, maintenance of electrolyte and water balance and regulation of the acid-base balance. Without kidneys or treatment with an artificial kidney a man would die of retention of nitrogenous waste products, electrolyte imbalance and metabolic acidosis within 1–3 weeks. In addition three substances are released into the blood. One of these is the enzyme renin which is indirectly concerned with electrolyte balance (p. 35.28). The second is erythrogenin, a substance responsible for the formation of erythropoietin (p. 35.29). The third is 1,25-OH cholecalciferol, produced by hydroxylation of 25-OH cholecalciferol in the renal tubular cells (p. 10.25). Thus, unravelling the function of the various parts of this organ is as important as it is difficult.

There have been several conflicting ideas about how the kidney manufactures urine from blood plasma. Bowman (1842) and Ludwig (1844) both thought that filtration occurred in the Malpighian body but they differed in their views over the function of the rest of the nephron. Bowman thought that the tubules secreted substances into the urine while Ludwig believed them to reabsorb some of the filtrate. In 1874, Heidenhain proposed that the glomeruli secreted water and salts and that other substances were added by tubular secretion. This argument was not settled until 1917 when Cushny published a famous monograph on the secretion of urine. He supported the idea, by then fairly generally held, that urine formation began with a process of simple ultrafiltration from the glomerular capillaries into the capsular space and suggested that thereafter tubular reabsorption could account for all the known facts. In addition, he suggested that substances in the glomerular filtrate could be divided into two groups. The first group consisted of substances such as glucose which, after filtration, are completely reabsorbed, provided that the plasma concentration is below a certain critical level. These were called **threshold substances.** In the second group were unwanted, waste, **no-threshold substances** which were not reabsorbed completely and which were largely excreted in the urine. It was also assumed that the renal tubules absorbed a fluid of constant composition resembling protein-free plasma. While it is now known that this view is inaccurate, Cushny's book was important in that it summarized the evidence for and against many hypotheses, and put forward a theory of urine formation based on the concept of glomerular filtration and tubular reabsorption which could be tested. From 1926 onwards Marshall published a series of papers in which he showed that tubular secretion also occurs. A major advance took place in 1925 when Richards and his colleagues developed microtechniques by which fluid could be collected from Bowman's capsule and individual tubules and analysed. This technique demonstrated directly the reality of glomerular filtration and also showed that reabsorption was far more complex than had previously been suspected.

Present concepts may be briefly summarized as follows. A large volume of ultrafiltrate of plasma is produced by the glomerulus. As this passes from Bowman's capsule along the proximal convolution most of the salt and water is reabsorbed. Some substances are reabsorbed completely and others only partially. Thus, this part of the tubule roughly separates the substances which must be conserved from those which are to be rejected in the urine. Thereafter the loop of Henle, the distal convolution and the collecting ducts are concerned mainly with the fine regulation of water, electrolyte and hydrogen ion balance.

The chemical and physical processes involved in tubular reabsorption and secretion are under hormonal control.

GLOMERULAR ULTRASTRUCTURE AND FILTRATION

The importance of Richards' contribution lay in the fact that for the first time direct evidence was presented to show that urine formation begins by ultrafiltration. If the capsular fluid is an ultrafiltrate of plasma then it should contain all the substances present in plasma except

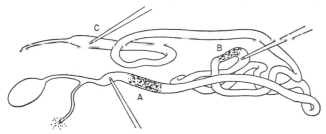

FIG. 35.8. Illustrating the insertion of a micropipette for collection of tubule fluid from the beginning (A), the middle (B), and the distal (C) end of a proximal convoluted tubule of *Necturus*. Stippling at A represents a globule of mercury, stippling at B a column of coloured oil. From Richards A.N. & Walker A.M. (1937) *Amer. J. Physiol.* **118**, 111.

the colloids, and substances passing across the glomerular capillary wall should be present in identical concentrations in plasma and filtrate. Richards' studies were carried out on the frog and the South American mud puppy or *Necturus*. Frog kidney is a thin elongated

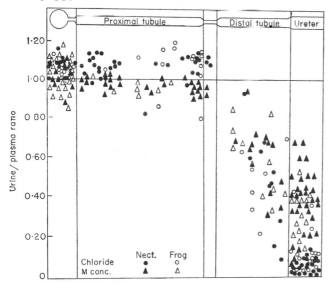

FIG. 35.9 Showing that glomerular filtrate and proximal tubular fluid are essentially identical with plasma with regard to chloride concentration and osmotic pressure. In the distal tubule the fall in the U/P ratios indicates that proportionately more solute than water is reabsorbed. From Walker A.M. *et al.* (1937) *Amer. J. Physiol.* **118**, 121.

organ and transillumination under a dissecting microscope shows up many of the glomeruli and some parts of the tubules. Fine micropipettes were inserted into the capsular space and the fluid accumulating there was collected. To prevent contamination by retrograde flow of tubular fluid, the tubules were blocked below the capsule either by pressure from a glass rod or by injection of globules of mercury (fig. 35.8). The results showed clearly that the fluid taken from the capsules is almost protein-free, is isosmotic with plasma and contains glucose, urea, creatinine, uric acid and the electrolytes of the blood. These observations left no doubt that in the frog and *Necturus* capsular fluid was an ultrafiltrate of plasma (fig. 35.9). Some years later the difficulty of collecting capsular and tubular fluid from the more compact and less translucent mammalian kidney was overcome, and it has now been shown that the capsular fluid is an ultrafiltrate of plasma in the rat, guinea-pig and dog. The observation that neither a reduction in temperature nor poisoning with cyanide affects the formation of this fluid indicates that it is produced by physical means.

GLOMERULAR ULTRASTRUCTURE

The glomerular capillary wall consists of two layers of cells and a basement membrane (BM), which is a homogeneous layer of collagen and glycoprotein about 300 nm in thickness. The interior of the capillary is lined by a thin layer of endothelial cytoplasm lying on the BM; the nuclei of the endothelial cells are situated usually over the mesangial regions (see below). The endothelial cytoplasm contains irregularly placed rounded apertures or **fenestrae** which vary in size, the majority being between 50 and 100 nm in diameter; they appear to be closed by a very thin membrane and prevent the blood cells passing out of the capillaries but probably do not hold back the protein or solute molecules. Between the capillaries lie large epithelial cells or **podocytes** (from Greek for foot); these give off trabeculae which divide into slender processes with slightly expanded bases, called **pedicels,** and these lie against the outer aspect of the BM. The processes from one cell interdigitate with those from a neighbouring one and between them are slit-like spaces about 10 nm across (figs. 35.10 and 11).

Mesangial system

Between the capillary loops at their points of junction are the mesangial regions, made up of **mesangial cells** and **mesangial matrix** (fig. 35.12 and plate 35.1a, facing p. 35.12). Each mesangial region contains 1–3 cells the cytoplasm of which is not well defined; they appear to possess complex cytoplasmic processes between which lie columns of matrix, and, like JGA cells, contain myofibrils indicating their origin from smooth muscle. The matrix consists of a glycosoaminoglycan gel which on EM

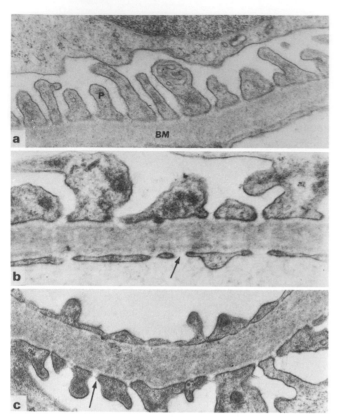

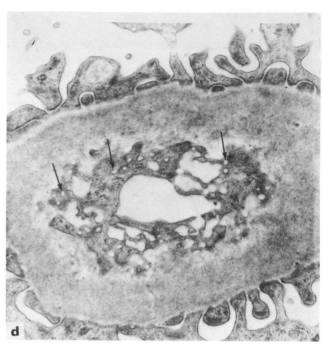

FIG. 35.10. Structure of the capillary wall of the human glomerulus.
Part of a glomerular capillary wall showing, (a) pedicel structure (P), basement membrane (BM); (b) endothelium lining internal aspect of the basement membrane showing several fenestrae (pores) indicated by arrow; (c) pedicels with well-defined slit membranes indicated by arrow; (d) tangential section of glomerular capillary showing endothelial fenestrae indicated by arrows.

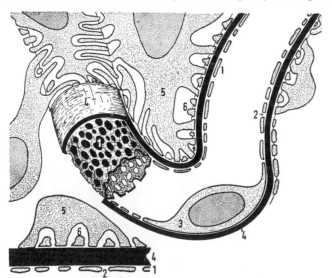

FIG. 35.11. Ultrastructure of a glomerular capillary; (1) fenestrated capillary endothelium; (2) fenestrae (pores); (3) endothelial cell; (4) basement membrane; (5) epithelial cell (podocyte); (6) pedicel. Adapted from Pease D.C. (1955) *Histol. Cytol.* **3**, 295.

examination resembles the glomerular capillary basement membrane. The mesangial cells are separated from the urinary space by BM and epithelium, and from the capillary lumina by a discontinuous layer of matrix and by endothelium. The mesangial system throughout the glomerulus is in continuity with the agranular (lacis) cells of the JGA (fig. 35.13).

The function of the mesangial cells is controversial, but they are probably concerned with the preservation of the integrity of the glomerulus, removing material deposited from the circulation on the capillary walls. In addition, they may take part in the formation and maintenance of glomerular capillary basement membrane and mesangial matrix.

MECHANISM OF GLOMERULAR FILTRATION

The glomerular filtrate is formed by the passage of water and solutes through the layers of the glomerular capillary wall either by bulk flow or by diffusion. Bulk flow assumes that some part of the glomerular wall acts as a porous membrane, that water and solute penetrate the pores, but that otherwise the wall is impermeable. The diameter of the pores determines the size of the filtered molecules. Several studies have been carried out to determine the permeability of the glomerular capillary wall,

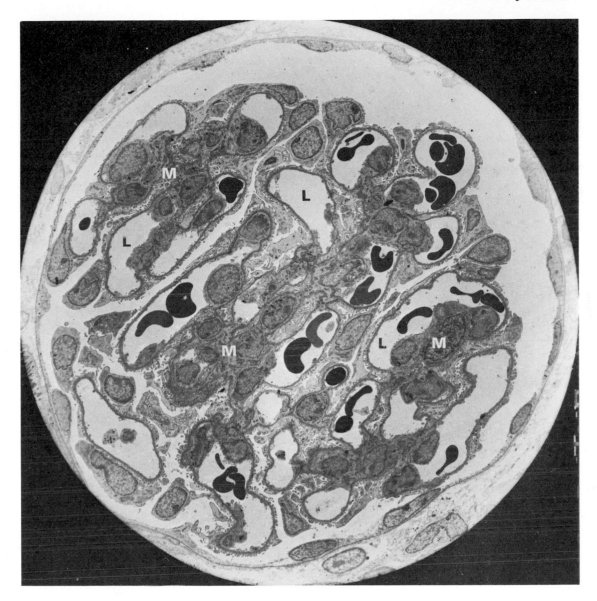

FIG. 35.12. EM photograph of a whole glomerulus in the human. Several capillary lumina (L) contain red blood cells, and mesangial regions (M) are seen as cellular foci between adjoining lumina (×1170).

using macromolecules of known graded molecular size. Haemoglobin in plasma, mol. wt. 68 000, passes easily into the filtrate, but albumin, mol. wt. 69 000, only to a small extent, and larger proteins not at all. Taking into account the orientation of the molecules to the pore, frictional and electrostatic hindrances, functional pores of about 7·5 nm would account for the glomerular characteristics. The slits between the pedicels are too large to hold back protein molecules, and it is likely that the BM acts as the functional barrier.

An alternative theory is that the basement membrane acts as a gel which liquefies and reforms and that the solutes pass through the aqueous phase by diffusion, the rate being proportional to their permeability coeffi-

cients in the membrane. According to this view, all solutes in plasma are capable of crossing the basement membrane but in practice the rate of diffusion of the plasma proteins is negligible. Experimental observations of the rate of passage of the crystalloids inulin and creatinine have shown a slight difference in the rates of transfer of these substances which would not be expected if the filtrate were formed by bulk flow of micromolecules through pores.

The hydrodynamic force responsible for filtration is the pressure within the glomerular capillaries. The few direct measurements of glomerular capillary pressure made by micropuncture in rats and monkeys, in which surface glomeruli are accessible, give values of 45 mmHg. The

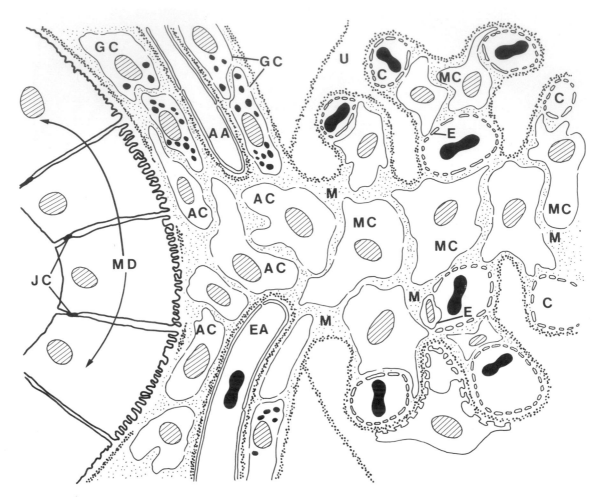

Fɪɢ. 35.13. Diagrammatic representation of the JGA. C, capillary lumen; E, endothelium; M, matrix; MC, mesangial cell; AC, agranular cell; GC, granular cell; AA, afferent arteriole; EA, efferent arteriole; MD, macula densa; JC, junctional complex; ▭ basement membrane. Note that the agranular cells of the JGA are in direct continuity with the glomerular mesangial cells. Courtesy of Mr. J.M. Leiper.

colloid osmotic pressure of the plasma, averaging 25 mmHg, opposes the hydrostatic pressure and tends to hold back water in the plasma. In addition, the pressure inside the capsular space is about 10 mmHg and is a sum of the resistance in the tubules and the surrounding interstitial pressure. Thus the **effective filtration pressure** is $(45-25-10)=10$ mmHg. The permeability of the glomerular capillaries is much higher than that of capillaries in other tissues. Rapid ultrafiltration of solute and water occurs in the early part of the capillaries and results in an increase in the concentration of plasma protein within the lumen. At some point before the end of the glomerular loop the colloid osmotic pressure equals the net hydrostatic pressure (glomerular capillary pressure—pressure in capsular space); **filtration pressure equilibrium** is achieved and ultrafiltration ceases. Thus only part of the surface available for formation of ultrafiltrate is utilized.

Symbols

It is often convenient to use the following symbols:

V	volume of urine
U	concentration of solute in urine
e.g. U_{Na^+}	concentration of sodium in urine
$U_{Na^+}V$	rate of excretion of sodium
P	concentration of solute in plasma
e.g. P_{Na^+}	concentration of sodium in plasma
C	clearance
e.g. C_{in}	clearance of inulin $= \dfrac{U_{in}V}{P_{in}}$
GFR	glomerular filtration rate
RBF	renal blood flow
RPF	renal plasma flow
ECF	extracellular fluid
Tm	maximum rate of tubular transport
e.g. Tm_G	maximum tubular capacity for reabsorption of glucose

Tm_{PO_4} maximum tubular capacity for re-absorption of phosphate

C_{PAH} clearance of para-aminohippurate

C_D clearance of diodone

E_{PAH} extraction ratio for PAH = renal A-V difference for PAH

FF filtration fraction $= \dfrac{C_{in}}{C_{PAH}}$

$\dfrac{TF}{P}$ $\dfrac{\text{concentration of solute in tubular fluid}}{\text{concentration of solute in plasma}}$

$\dfrac{TF}{P_{Na^+}}$ $\dfrac{\text{concentration of } Na^+ \text{ in tubular fluid}}{\text{concentration of } Na^+ \text{ in plasma}}$

Tc_{H_2O} rate of reabsorption of solute-free water $= C_{osmol} - V$

Glomerular filtration rate (GFR) and its measurement

How far does the rate of production of the ultrafiltrate affect the final volume and composition of the urine? This is an important question to which there is only a partial answer. The first essential step is to measure GFR in various circumstances. From the work of Richards and his successors it was clear that the volume of fluid filtered by the glomerulus was greatly in excess of the final volume of urine passed. Micropuncture techniques cannot be used in man or in intact animals, and although indirect methods so far developed to measure glomerular filtration lack precision, they are valuable in properly controlled conditions. A non-toxic substance, soluble in plasma, not metabolized by the body, freely filterable at the glomerulus, and neither secreted nor reabsorbed by the tubules, could be used on the basis of the Fick principle to measure the volume of fluid removed from the plasma by glomerular filtration in unit time in intact animal or man. The quantity of such an ideal solute excreted in the urine in unit time would equal the amount filtered by the glomeruli in the same period. Furthermore, the volume of plasma filtrate which is formed in this period (GFR) is the amount of solute excreted divided by the concentration of the solute in the plasma.

The information needed to calculate the GFR is the concentration of the solute in 1 ml of urine (U), the volume of urine excreted in 1 min (V), and the concentration of the solute in 1 ml of plasma (P). Then U × V is the quantity of solute excreted in 1 min, and the ratio UV/P gives the number of ml of glomerular filtrate formed.

Inulin (mol. wt. 5200), a polymer of fructose, found in dahlia roots, is a substance which possesses nearly all the requirements of an ideal solute. Its chemical estimation is accurate and relatively simple provided proper care is taken. Using inulin, the value for GFR in young men is about 125 ml/min.

The ratio UV/P is called the **renal clearance** (C) of the substance. In the case of inulin, C = GFR. The clearance of a substance which is partly reabsorbed during its passage through the renal tubules is lower than the GFR; by contrast, clearance values which are higher than the GFR may be obtained for substances which are secreted into the urine by the tubular cells.

Measurement of GFR

The accurate measurement of GFR using inulin is usually carried out only for research purposes; in these circumstances the following points should be observed.

(1) The subject should be at rest and recumbent and 4 hours should have elapsed since the last meal.

(2) V should be 3 ml/min or more to minimize errors in the collection of urine samples.

(3) If the subject is unable to empty the bladder completely it should be washed out with air or known volumes of a sterile solution of NaCl.

(4) The concentration of inulin in the plasma should be kept constant to ensure that P_{in} in the plasma sample taken for analysis represents the average concentration during the period of urine collection. To this end P_{in} is usually first raised with a priming intravenous injection and then maintained by a slower infusion in which inulin is given as nearly as possible at the rate at which it is being lost in the urine.

After a short period of time to permit the even distribution of the inulin throughout the ECF, accurately timed urine samples are collected at intervals of 15–20 min; the sample of venous blood is taken at the midpoint of each collection period.

When GFR is measured in an individual at various values of P_{in} but otherwise under identical conditions, it is found that UV_{in} is directly proportional to P_{in}, and consequently C_{in} (UV_{in}/P_{in}) does not depend upon P_{in}, which is what one would expect if inulin is filtered by the glomeruli but neither reabsorbed nor secreted by the renal tubules. Since the GFR shows small diurnal variations, being lowest in the early morning and highest in the afternoon, measurements should always be made at the same time of day. The usual time is in the morning after the night's rest.

Since measurement of the GFR using inulin requires considerable technical care, in clinical work GFR is often measured by the clearance of creatinine (C_{cr}). Creatinine was, in fact, the first substance to be used for this purpose and it was employed on the assumption that it was excreted by the kidney solely by glomerular filtration. While this is true in the dog, it is now known that in man in some circumstances it is secreted by the renal tubules as well and may therefore give values for GFR that are too high. C_{cr} is easier to measure than C_{in} because there is a continuous endogenous supply of creatinine and P_{cr} remains virtually constant throughout the 24 hours. No intravenous infusion is necessary and observations can be made over prolonged periods of time. The urine is usually collected for 24 hours and a single blood sample is taken at some time during this period. This method is sufficiently accurate for many clinical purposes.

Another substance used for the measurement of GFR is vitamin B_{12} (cyanocobalamine). Vitamin B_{12} is normally bound by plasma proteins, but if the proteins are first saturated, the excess vitamin B_{12} is filtered through the glomeruli and is neither secreted nor reabsorbed. The values for GFR are similar to those obtained with inulin. If vitamin B_{12} containing [57]Co is used, the estimations may be made simply and rapidly by measuring the radioactivity in samples of plasma and urine. This method cannot be used frequently in the same human subject as it is undesirable to give radioactive material repeatedly. [131]I sodium diatrozoate (hypaque) and ^{51}Cr-labelled ethylenediaminetetraacetic acid (EDTA) are also used to measure GFR.

The order of accuracy in the measurement of GFR is about ± 5 per cent. By relating the actual GFR to surface area or some other body standard, comparison of results in different subjects is made easier.

TUBULAR ACTIVITY

Reabsorption

Since glucose is found in capsular fluid and is absent from urine, it must be reabsorbed somewhere in the nephron. The volume of urine is always far less than the volume of filtrate, so water also is reabsorbed; many dissolved substances present in capsular fluid are partly reabsorbed and, since the degree of concentration varies for different substances and is independent of the water removed, there must be a number of independent reabsorptive mechanisms. Again, the pH of capsular fluid fluctuates around neutrality, whereas urine is usually acid. Some information on where and how these processes occur has been provided by the micromethods introduced by Richards. Most of the glucose has disappeared halfway along the proximal convolution, and it has virtually all gone by the end. In the proximal convolution large amounts of sodium, chloride and bicarbonate, about 65–70 per cent of the water and a variety of other substances are reabsorbed. Fluid that enters the descending limb of the loop is thus greatly reduced in volume and changed in composition, but it is still isosmotic with plasma (p. 35.19).

Many tubular activities involve the expenditure of energy, though some depend solely on chemical and electrochemical gradients. Where active transport is involved, its capacity may be limited by the supply of energy or by unfavourable ionic and pH gradients across the tubular wall.

The term **tubular transport maximum**, Tm, is applied to substances such as glucose which are actively reabsorbed by mechanisms capable of transporting a fixed amount in unit time. Sodium is also actively transported but it is an example of a substance whose reabsorption is limited by the concentration gradient that can be achieved in the time available during which the glomerular filtrate is in contact with the tubular cells.

GLUCOSE

Glucose is an example of a substance which shows a Tm, and its transport mechanism was the first to be studied and defined. Although in healthy individuals urine contains a trace of glucose detectable by sensitive methods, for all practical purposes urine is free of glucose and $C_G = 0$. However, glucose is excreted by healthy subjects given a large quantity by mouth or by infusion when P_G rises above a critical level of about 10 mmol (1.8 g)/l. The higher the P_G the more glucose appears in the urine and, providing GFR is constant, the amount of glucose filtered bears a linear relationship to P_G. Clearly, the quantity of glucose filtered minus the quantity excreted in the urine equals the amount reabsorbed. If this value is determined when $P_G > 20$ mmol (3.6 g)/l, the quantity of glucose reabsorbed by the tubules (Tm_G) is constant and equals $(C_{in} \times P_G) - U_G V$. At plasma concentrations between 10 and 20 mmol/l the gradual increase in the amount reabsorbed is shown as a continuous line in fig. 35.14. This is termed the splay of the curve. This splay may be partly due to differences in the size and transport capacities of nephrons but the shape of the curve relating the rate of reabsorption of glucose to the plasma glucose is probably determined largely by the kinetic properties of the transport system which resemble those of an en-

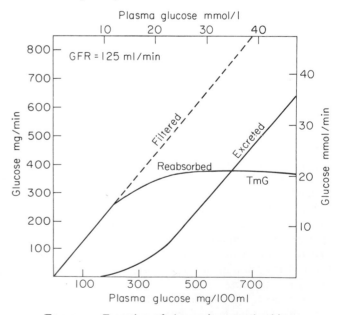

FIG. 35.14. Excretion of glucose in normal subjects.

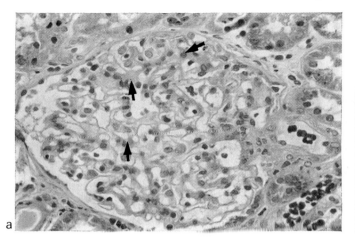
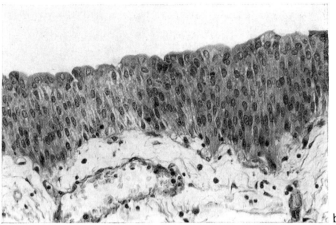

a

b

PLATE 35.1. Histology of the kidney.

(a) Glomerulus from normal kidney. The capillaries are seen in cross-section, and at their points of junction there are groups of two or three mesangial cell nuclei, some of which are indicated by arrows. To the right of the glomerulus is the juxtaglomerular apparatus, at the hilum. Haem. & eosin (×400).

(b) Transitional epithelium from the renal pelvis. Haem. & eosin (×250).

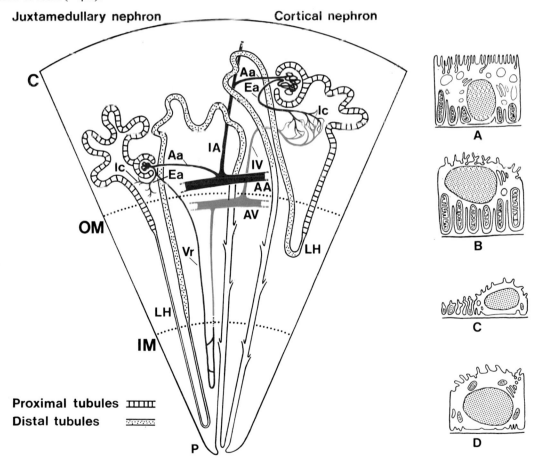

(c) Diagram of nephrons and their blood supply. AA, arcuate artery; AV, arcuate vein; Aa, afferent arteriole; Ea, efferent arteriole; IA, interlobular artery; IV, interlobular vein; Ic, intertubular capillaries; LH, loop of Henle; Vr, vasa recta; P, papilla; C, cortex; OM, outer medulla; IM, inner medulla. Cells: A, cell from proximal convoluted tubule; B, cell from distal convoluted tubule; C, cell from thin limb of Henle's loop; D, cell from collecting duct. Luminal surface is above, external surface below.

zyme system (p. 7.8). Tm_G is unaffected by insulin. A normal value indicates a normal amount of reabsorbing tubular tissue.

A number of sugars use the same transport mechanism so that, when more than one is present, there is mutual interference. Glucose reabsorption can be prevented by phlorizin, a glucoside which also inhibits absorption of glucose by the gut.

PHOSPHATES (fig. 35.15)

Like glucose, phosphates are reabsorbed, mainly in the proximal tubule, but $Tm_{PO_4^\equiv}$ is much lower and there is considerable splay in the curve. As a result, changes in the rate of reabsorption of phosphate play an important part in regulating the amount of this substance in the body. Glucose and phosphate reabsorption bear a definite relationship to each other; phlorizin, which prevents reabsorption of the former, increases reabsorption of the latter. It has been suggested that this is because both substances share a common energy source, so that as glucose reabsorption is blocked more energy becomes available for phosphate transport. Since $Tm_{PO_4^\equiv}$ is low, the amount in the urine depends more closely on the quantity filtered and on $P_{PO_4^\equiv}$ than is the case with glucose. The $P_{PO_4^\equiv}$ varies with diet, exercise and the activity of the parathyroid glands. One of the actions of parathyroid hormone is to reduce $Tm_{PO_4^\equiv}$ and the excretion of phosphate is increased. Calcitonin exerts a similar effect.

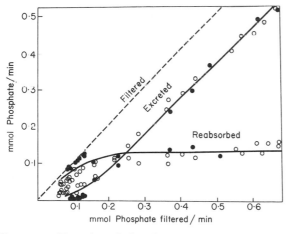

FIG. 35.15. Excretion of phosphate in a normal subject in relation to rate of filtration of phosphate, normal (●), acidosis (○). From Schiess W.A. *et al.* (1948) *J. clin. Invest.* **27**, 57.

AMINO ACIDS

An adult excretes only traces of amino acids though they are filtered freely from the blood. In contrast, in the newborn infant there is a considerable excretion of the acids because the tubules are not completely functional at birth.

The blood plasma contains several amino acids which the kidney conserves. There seem to be at least four mechanisms for amino acid reabsorption, but knowledge of these is limited except that phosphorylation is a step in the process. If the plasma concentration of any of the amino acids is increased by an infusion, it overflows into the urine. All show a Tm, differing for each acid. Probably arginine, lysine, ornithine and cystine are transported by one mechanism, while another system deals with glutamic and aspartic acids and a third, or several more, transport the other acids. It is understandable that the infusion of arginine, for example, should depress the reabsorption of the similarly transported lysine, but it is more difficult to understand how acids with different transport mechanisms interfere with each other, as they have been shown to do. There is no competition between amino acid and glucose transport, suggesting that these are independent processes. The mechanism for the reabsorption of amino acids depends upon the presence of genetically determined enzymes. There is a variety of rare hereditary diseases associated with aminoaciduria. In one such disease the reabsorption of cystine, lysine, ornithine and arginine is reduced. Cystine is relatively insoluble and cystine stones are commonly formed in the renal pelves in patients with this inborn defect.

Creatine derives largely from muscle and is not usually found in the urine. When the plasma level is raised, as occurs in certain diseases of muscle (vol. 3, p. 34.27), tubular reabsorption may not be equal to the load and creatine may appear in the urine. For reasons unknown it occurs in the urine of children and of pregnant women.

PROTEIN

Micropuncture shows that a small amount of protein, predominantly albumin, reaches the capsular fluid of mammals. The protein loss in the urine is normally of the order of 30–50 mg/day and is not detectable by routine clinical tests. Protein filtered by the glomerulus must be reabsorbed somewhere along the tubule and this is done in the proximal convolution, possibly by pinocytosis. In certain circumstances, for example after severe exercise, it is found in the urine of healthy adults. This is probably because the circulatory requirements of the muscles lead to a fall in renal blood flow and temporary hypoxia in the kidneys with a consequent increase in permeability of the glomerulus. A long period of standing may lead to postural proteinuria. It has been suggested that the standing increases the curvature of the lumbar spine, causing increased pressure in the renal vein.

UREA

Urea is the form in which most of the waste nitrogen is excreted. It is an extremely diffusible substance which is relatively non-toxic, so that a healthy subject usually feels no ill effects if the concentration of urea in his blood is increased several fold for a short period of time. Although urea is freely filtered at the glomerulus its clearance is always less than that of inulin. When V is more than 2 ml/min C_{urea} is about 75 ml/min, but when V is less than 2 ml/min C_{urea} falls below this. Tubular reabsorption of urea is by passive diffusion down a concentration gradient created by reabsorption of water. About 40–50 per cent of filtered urea is reabsorbed in the proximal tubule irrespective of urine flow and whether or not ADH is present. In a water diuresis, when ADH is virtually absent, little or no water or urea is reabsorbed in the distal nephron and more of the filtered urea appears in the urine.

The dependence of C_{urea} on urine flow is explained in terms of the mechanism for the concentration of urine and the action of ADH described on p. 35.22. During antidiuresis the permeability to both water and urea of the medullary portion of the collecting duct increases. Water diffuses out of the duct into the medullary interstitium, which is hypertonic because NaCl has been transported actively out of the renal tubules into the interstitial fluid. The concentration of urea in collecting duct fluid rises and urea diffuses passively into the medullary interstitium. Since the circulation through this region is sluggish the urea is trapped in the medulla. As its concentration in the medullary interstitial fluid rises, urea diffuses into the descending limb of Henle's loop (fig. 35.22) and is recycled through the distal nephron. In these circumstances only about 20 per cent of filtered urea may be excreted. Although the diffusion of urea out of the tubular lumen is passive, the work done to create and maintain a concentration difference for urea across the wall of the renal tubule depends on active transport of NaCl out of the tubule as described on p. 35.19.

Tubular Secretion

This differs from tubular reabsorption only in the direction of movement. The transport may be active or passive and is subject to the same limitations as reabsorption. There appear to be only two active systems for secretion. The first substance proved to be secreted by the tubules, phenol red, is wholly foreign to the body, as are a large number of other substances treated in this way. K^+ and H^+ are also secreted. Any substance whose clearance is higher than the GFR must be secreted, and provided it is freely filtered the extent of the secretion is the difference between its clearance and that of C_{in}. One transport system carries organic acids such as glucuronic acid and creatine which are metabolic products, and also foreign chemicals such as PAH, diodone and penicillin. The other system carries organic bases such as histamine and choline, and a number of foreign substances, many of which are drugs used clinically. Some of the evidence for the existence of two active systems depends on the observation that a substance in one group interferes with the transport of another substance in the same group, but that substances in different groups do not interfere with each other.

Of the foreign substances secreted two are of practical physiological interest, PAH and diodone. At low values of P these substances are excreted rapidly and C approaches 600 ml/min. Up to a certain P value, C is constant, but above a critical concentration, UV no longer keeps pace with P and C falls. This is termed self-depression and is due to the active transport system for these compounds becoming saturated. Above this critical value for P the rise in excretion of PAH or diodone depends on their increased filtration alone; the value for tubular secretion remains constant at the Tm. These facts can be determined by making simultaneous measurements of C_{in} and C_{PAH} or C_D at various levels of P. When P_{PAH} or P_D is high, these two substances can be used to measure maximum tubular secretory capacity, Tm_{PAH} or Tm_D, and these values indicate the amount of the functioning tubular cell mass. For some years diodone was used, until PAH was found to give equally good results with the advantage that the chemical analysis is easier. In addition, a few people are hypersensitive to diodone.

URIC ACID

This comes from the breakdown of endogenous and dietary nucleoproteins and about 3–5 mmol (500–800 mg)/day is excreted in the urine. Since uric acid is filtered freely by the glomeruli and is normally present in the plasma in a concentration of 0·12–0·42 mmol/l (2·0–7·0 mg/100 ml), the quantity which appears in the urine is approximately 5–10 per cent of the amount filtered. Thus at least 90 per cent of the filtered uric acid is normally reabsorbed. Clearance studies have shown, however, that in certain circumstances the clearance of uric acid may exceed that of inulin. Uric acid is an example of a substance which is both reabsorbed and secreted by the renal tubules. The evidence is that this bidirectional transport takes place in the proximal tubules and it is even possible that this occurs within the same cells.

The tubular transport of sodium, water, potassium and hydrogen ions, and the divalent ions calcium and magnesium is described on pp. 35.17, 24 and 26.

RENAL CIRCULATION

At low plasma concentrations, the high clearance of PAH means that this substance is almost totally cleared from the plasma in a short period of time. This suggested the possibility that it might be used to obtain an indirect measurement of renal plasma flow (RPF). Theoretically what is needed for this purpose is a substance which is wholly cleared from the plasma and excreted in the urine as it passes once through the kidney. Direct measurements of plasma flow in animals and observations in man in which renal venous blood is sampled through catheters lying in the renal vein show that about 90 per cent of PAH is removed from the blood in a single passage through the kidney. Some of the remaining 10 per cent may be accounted for by blood which passes through non-secretory parts of the kidney, e.g. capsule, fat and connective tissue, and some more by blood supplying those parts of the tubules which are unable to secrete PAH. Secretion occurs mainly in the proximal tubule. In practice it is usual to ignore the 10 per cent error and refer to C_{PAH} as the effective RPF. This simplification is reasonable in the case of healthy kidneys, but invalid in renal disease, where much more than 10 per cent may escape extraction during one transit through the kidney. Then the true value for RPF can be obtained by collecting renal venous blood and measuring the PAH A–V difference. This figure gives the extraction ratio (E_{PAH}) and thus the magnitude of the error. It is usual to measure C_{in} and C_{PAH} simultaneously and by the same technique.

A second method of estimating RPF using nitrous oxide, ^{85}Kr or ^{133}Xe is identical with that described for the measurement of coronary and cerebral blood flow (pp. 30.46 and 47).

In man the effective RPF is about 600 ml/min, and the true RPF is about 700 ml/min; if the haematocrit value is 45, the whole blood flow is 1300 ml/min. This amounts to 25 per cent of the resting cardiac output and about 400 ml/100 g kidney tissue and is a far greater volume than is necessary for the metabolic processes of the kidney itself. This large volume permits the kidney to do work on the blood and help to maintain the normal composition of body fluids.

The ratio GFR/RPF is the filtration fraction (FF) and shows the proportion of plasma filtered. The usual figure is about 0·2 (125/600).

Factors affecting GFR and RPF

If the pressure in the glomeruli alters, other things being equal, the filtration rate changes in the same direction. In man the GFR changes little over a wide range of levels of blood pressure because the lumina of the afferent and efferent arterioles alter independently and compensate for alterations in systemic blood pressure. Furthermore, if the volume of filtrate is increased the proximal tubule becomes more distended than before and the rise in intratubular pressure tends to decrease the GFR. Likewise, if tubular pressure is reduced, as by increased reabsorption of Na^+ and water, then the GFR rises. On the other hand, in the perfused kidney isolated from nervous control, GFR is more susceptible to a change in blood pressure.

The RPF is greater in the supine than in the erect position because in the latter case renal vasoconstriction occurs to maintain blood pressure against gravity. However, the GFR is affected only slightly by posture because of alterations in the degree of vasoconstriction

of the afferent and efferent arterioles. Both GFR and RPF are reduced by vigorous exercise, pain and emotion, when a large volume of blood is diverted from the kidney to other parts of the body, and in heart failure. GFR and RPF also fall in water and salt depletion and following haemorrhage when the blood volume is reduced. In pregnancy both RPF and GFR are increased, due to the increase in blood volume (p. 38.49).

Intrarenal circulation

About 90 per cent of the renal blood flow perfuses the renal cortex and the rate of cortical blood flow is five or more times the rate through the medulla. Also, despite an overall constancy of GFR and RPF, the medullary blood flow is reduced during antidiuresis and is increased in diuresis, when the rate of urine flow is rapid. This means that in the former case a high osmotic pressure in the medulla is maintained and, in the latter, that some of the solute is dispersed. Measurements of regional blood flow can be made by means of photocells, one in the cortex and one in the medulla, which monitor the arrival and disappearance of Evans blue injected into the renal artery. The dye is quickly washed through the cortex and only slowly through the medulla. The difference between the rates of flow is probably related to the rich anastomosis of capillaries round the tubules in the cortex and the long straight vessels offering more resistance in the medulla. Another factor is probably ADH to which the medullary vessels may be more sensitive. Corresponding to the lower rate of blood flow, medullary O_2 consumption is less than that of the cortex. The end result is that the A–V O_2 difference of the two is identical.

The renal vessels are under the influence of vasoconstrictor sympathetic nerves and are also sensitive to adrenaline, noradrenaline and angiotensin. The last, if injected, produces a general vasoconstrictor response. The effects of adrenaline and noradrenaline depend on the dose given; small doses constrict the efferent arteriole more than the afferent, so that there is a rise in GFR. With bigger doses all vessels, including the veins, are constricted but the reduction in RPF is more marked in the cortex.

Autoregulation

A number of organs show some capacity for regulating their internal circulation regardless of the systemic blood pressure. In this respect the kidney is remarkable. The blood pressure can be changed over the range 80–200 mm Hg with only a small change in RPF and an even smaller one in GFR (fig. 35.16). How this is brought about is not clear, but its necessity is easier to understand. The regulation of water and electrolyte balance and many other renal activities would be almost impossible if renal haemodynamics were always changing. Autoregu-

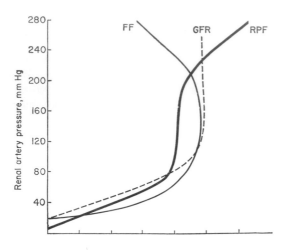

FIG. 35.16. Showing the range of systemic blood pressure over which the kidney demonstrates autoregulation. Adapted from Shipley R.E. & Study R.S. (1957) *Amer. J. Physiol.* **167**, 676.

lation is preserved in the denervated kidney and even to some extent in the isolated organ. After denervation GFR and RPF in man and dog are the same as in the innervated organ. One of the current theories is that the prostaglandin PGE$_2$ is of importance. It is a renal vasodilator and experimentally it can counteract, to some extent, vasoconstriction induced by nerve stimulation or the infusion of angiotensin. If indomethacin, a drug that inhibits prostaglandin synthesis (vol. 2, p. 17.5), is given to experimental animals, RPF falls; furthermore angiotensin then causes a greater degree of vasoconstriction than normal. Usually angiotensin-induced constriction is accompanied by a rise of renal venous PGE$_2$, but this does not occur when indomethacin is given. As already indicated, PGE$_2$ is probably made in the interstitial cells and possibly in the collecting ducts. It is suggested that a basal rate of formation of PGE$_2$ maintains RPF, and that when vasoconstriction occurs or pressure falls its synthesis is increased with a resulting renal vasodilation, but how it reaches the cortex to exert its effect is unknown. It may be carried by the blood or in the tubular urine. It is possible that PGE$_2$ and the renin-angiotensin system have reciprocal effects on the inner cortical blood vessels.

Another suggestion is that the smooth muscle of the renal blood vessels reacts to pressure changes even more vigorously than smooth muscle elsewhere. An increase in stretch, as when the systemic pressure rises, causes the muscle to contract, thus eliminating the effect of pressure changes. Yet another possibility is that the kidney has active internal reflexes which are still present after surgical denervation. Again the JGA may be involved. If a solution of NaCl is injected into a distal tubule the proximal tubule may be seen to collapse. This suggests a cessation of filtration due to preglomerular vasoconstric-

tion. This effect is not dependent on osmotic forces since it does not occur if a mannitol solution is injected; the amount of Na$^+$ or Cl$^-$ delivered to the macula densa appears critical. This is unlikely to be the sole mechanism since autoregulation can be shown to occur in the renin-depleted kidneys of dogs on a high salt diet.

Perhaps renal blood flow is adjusted by all these means. It has yet to be discovered which is the most important.

WATER AND SODIUM

The osmolality of the body fluids normally lies between 270 and 290 mosmol/l. This is achieved by balancing the amount of water ingested and that excreted in the urine. In health, water deprivation leads to release of ADH (p. 27.17) and induces a sensation of thirst. In the presence of ADH the rate of reabsorption of water by the renal tubules is increased and the osmolality of the urine rises to a maximum of 1200 mosmol/l so that loss of water in the urine is diminished. In addition the individual becomes thirsty and drinking restores the water deficit. The sensation of thirst arises as a result of stimulation of hypothalamic receptors sensitive to an increase in the osmolality of blood and possibly also to an increased level of angiotensin II (p. 27.17). Dryness of the mouth, due to reduced secretion of saliva, also initiates thirst. By contrast, in the hydrated individual in whom release of ADH is suppressed, the osmolality of the urine may fall to a minimum of 30 or 40 mosmol/l; in these circumstances, proportionately less water is reabsorbed by the kidney. The ADH mechanism is important when water is in short supply or when an excessive amount of water has been taken, but its role in maintaining water balance on a day to day basis is less clear. Indeed, when dogs eating a normal diet are given free access to water, water balance is achieved because the animals increase their water intake to keep pace with losses from the skin and mucosae. In these circumstances release of ADH plays a less important part in the maintenance of body water and regulation of the osmolality of the body fluids.

The volume of the ECF, which depends upon the body Na$^+$, is regulated also by the kidney. Despite wide variations in the intake of Na$^+$, the total body Na$^+$ remains remarkably constant because the amount which is excreted in the urine can be varied from 1–2 mmol to up to 600 mmol/day.

Sodium reabsorbed in the proximal tubule is accompanied by an osmotically equivalent amount of water, and any increase in the rate of this isotonic reabsorption of Na$^+$ results in expansion of the ECF. In the distal nephron Na$^+$ may be reabsorbed without water; an increase in the rate of this process raises the [Na$^+$] and therefore the osmolality of the ECF. The thirst that follows encourages water drinking. Release of ADH is also stimulated so that water retention and expansion of the ECF follow. Loss of Na^+ induces the opposite chain of events leading to shrinkage of the ECF.

As the GFR is about 125 ml/min, approximately 180 litres containing some 25 000 mmol of Na^+ are filtered daily. A person eating an ordinary diet excretes 1 or 2 litres of water daily containing about 100 mmol of Na^+. Approximately 99 per cent of the filtered Na^+ therefore is reabsorbed and this process accounts for most of the energy used by kidney tissue. A large volume of water, approximately 178 l/day, is also reabsorbed by the tubules but water reabsorption is a passive process and follows the osmotic gradients created between the tubular lumen and the peritubular tissues during the active reabsorption of Na^+.

Knowledge of the pattern of Na^+ and water reabsorption in the renal tubules has been obtained by micropuncture studies. The mammal commonly used for this purpose is the rat; this animal has a greater capacity than man for conserving both Na^+ and water so that the results obtained may not be entirely applicable to man. Under direct vision a micropipette is inserted into one of the surface tubules of the mobilized kidney. The minute amount of tubular fluid (TF) withdrawn is measured and subsequently analysed and the tubule is filled with a marker. Later, microdissection of the kidney enables the site of the puncture to be identified. Since inulin is neither reabsorbed nor secreted by the tubules, TF/P_{in} provides a measurement of water reabsorption. The TF/P ratio for Na^+ divided by the similar ratio for inulin provides information about the fraction of filtered Na^+ which remains in the tubular fluid at any point in the nephron.

Reabsorption of sodium and water in the proximal convoluted tubule

In the rat the deeply placed pars recta is inaccessible and only the first 60 per cent of the proximal convolution is available for micropuncture. Fluid withdrawn from here is always isotonic with plasma irrespective of whether the urine is more or less concentrated than plasma. This implies that the cells lining the proximal tubules cannot sustain an osmotic gradient and, indeed, isolated perfused sections of mammalian proximal convolutions are readily permeable to water. Furthermore, in fluid withdrawn from the last accessible point in the proximal tubule, the inulin TF/P ratio is found to be around 2. This means that about half of the filtered water has been reabsorbed in the first 60 per cent of the proximal convolution, and if one assumes that reabsorption of water continues at the same rate in the remaining 40 per cent then about two-thirds of the filtered water must be reabsorbed in the proximal convolution. Because Na^+ is the most important osmotically active solute, two-thirds of the filtered Na^+ must also be absorbed together with an equivalent amount of anion. The reabsorption of Na^+

in the proximal tubule is thought to be an active process which occurs against an electrochemical gradient and the reabsorption of water is a secondary passive phenomenon.

EVIDENCE FOR REABSORPTION OF SODIUM AGAINST A CHEMICAL GRADIENT

Normally no chemical gradient for Na^+ exists across the wall of the proximal tubule and the concentration of Na^+ in the tubular fluid does not differ significantly from that of the plasma in the peritubular capillaries. Such a gradient, however, can be created artificially in animals receiving an infusion of mannitol which is excreted by the kidney in a way similar to inulin. The presence in the lumen of the proximal tubule of the osmotically active sugar reduces water absorption. Under these conditions fluid obtained by micropuncture shows that there is a progressive decrease in the TF/P ratio for Na^+ along the first two-thirds of the proximal convolution, so that a concentration difference for Na^+ of 30–50 mmol/l is established between the tubular fluid and the peritubular plasma. Thus Na^+ can be reabsorbed against a moderate chemical gradient. Microperfusion studies indicate that a considerable amount of Na^+ leaks back into the lumen from the peritubular compartment and so the concentration of Na^+ in the tubular fluid cannot be reduced to less than 60 per cent of its concentration in plasma.

EVIDENCE FOR REABSORPTION OF SODIUM AGAINST AN ELECTRICAL GRADIENT

The electrical gradients across the wall of the proximal tubule can be measured by electrodes inserted into the proximal tubular cells or into the tubular lumen. In amphibian kidneys there is a potential difference (PD) of about 70 mV between the interior of the cell and the peritubular fluid, the intracellular fluid being negative. A PD of about 50 mV exists between the interior of the cell and the lumen of the tubule. These potentials arise because of a tendency for K^+ to diffuse out of the cell and the PD across the luminal membrane is smaller because this membrane is more readily permeable to Na^+ which diffuses into the cell and partially shunts the potential. Thus, at any point in the amphibian proximal tubule there is a PD of 20 mV between the lumen and the peritubular fluid, the lumen being more negative (transtubular PD = -20 mV). It follows that in the amphibian kidney Na^+ is reabsorbed against an electrical as well as a chemical gradient, and so must be an active process.

In the mammalian kidney the pattern is less clear. Early investigators recorded values for transtubular PD similar to those found in amphibia. Using microelectrodes with tips of less than 1μm diameter, values for transtubular PD ranging from zero to -4 mV have now been obtained. These figures are likely to be valid as damage of tubular cells is probably slight. Consequently there is doubt as to whether or not Na^+ transport in the mammalian proximal tubule occurs against an electrical gradient. Fig. 35.17 is based on the assumption that there is a transtubular PD of -4 mV. Sodium ions from the tubular fluid enter the cells passively down an electrochemical gradient and are transported actively across the peritubular membrane against an electrochemical gradient. This is probably brought about by one or more pumps in the peritubular membrane. Since reabsorption of Na^+ is inhibited by ouabain, $Na^+ - K^+$ activated ATPase may generate the necessary energy or may be a carrier for the transport of Na^+ out of the cell or K^+ into it. Conventionally, negatively charged Cl^- are thought to follow Na^+ moving passively down the transtubular electrochemical gradient, a process which has been shown to require a minimum transtubular PD of -4 mV.

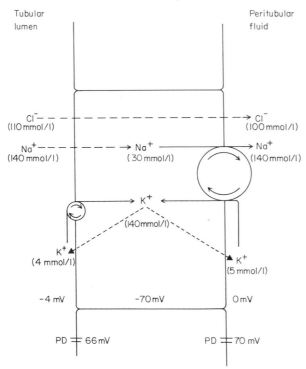

FIG. 35.17. Ion transport in the proximal tubule; ... passive movement down electrochemical gradients; — active transport. The concentrations of Cl^- and K^+ in the tubular fluid vary according to the site within the proximal tubule. Adapted from Pitts R.F. (1961) *Prog. Cardiol. Dis.* **3**, 537.

In the mammal, transtubular PD appears to change along the proximal tubule. In the first loop of the proximal convolution there is a small negative transtubular PD, associated with the active transport of Na^+ from the lumen to the peritubular fluid. This transtubular PD rises to zero when glucose transport is blocked by phlorizin, so that transfer of Na^+ may be linked to glucose transport. In the later segments of the proximal

tubule, however, transtubular PD is positive. Since most of the filtered glucose and HCO_3^- are reabsorbed early in the proximal convolution, fluid leaving the first loop contains little of these substances; as this fluid remains isotonic to plasma, $[Cl^-]$ increases and TF/P_{Cl^-} rises to a value of 1·3. The positive transtubular PD recorded in the second and subsequent loops of the proximal convolution has been attributed to passive diffusion of Cl^- down a chemical gradient into the peritubular fluid, a process that could provide a driving force for passive reabsorption of some of the remaining Na^+. Further work is required to confirm these results.

EVIDENCE FOR THE PASSIVE REABSORPTION OF WATER

The proximal tubule of the rat can be perfused with solutions containing different concentrations of NaCl which are kept isotonic with the animal's plasma by adding varying amounts of mannitol. Rat plasma contains 145 mmol/l of Na^+, and since Na^+ can be reabsorbed against a moderate chemical gradient, it is reabsorbed from those solutions which contain more than 95 mmol/l of Na^+. By contrast, when the Na^+ content of the perfusing fluid is less than 95 mmol/l it diffuses from the peritubular fluid into the lumen. As fig. 35.18 shows, the movement of water always takes place in the same direction as that of Na^+, and one would not expect to find this if water were transported actively.

It can be calculated that a transtubular osmotic gradient of 23 mosmol/l would be required to account for passive reabsorption of 50 per cent of the filtered water in the proximal tubule. Since the tubular fluid is

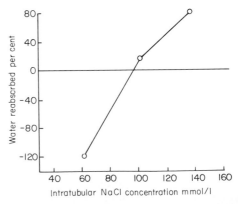

FIG. 35.18. The relationship between the concentration of NaCl in the proximal tubular fluid of the rat and the percentage of water reabsorbed. All solutions made isotonic with rat plasma by addition of mannitol. At concentrations of NaCl of less than 95 mmol/l sodium moves from the peritubular fluid into the lumen and water moves in the same direction, i.e. negative reabsorption. The percentage of water reabsorbed is corrected for movement of water due to the presence of mannitol in the tubular fluid. Adapted from Giebisch G. *et al.* (1964) *J. gen. Physiol.* **47**, 1185.

isotonic to plasma it is not immediately obvious how this osmotic gradient could be achieved. It is likely that localized differences in osmotic pressure are created by transport of NaCl out of the tubular cells into small spaces between adjacent cells and between the basal folds and the basement membrane (fig. 35.19). Accumulation of solute in these intercellular compartments raises the osmotic pressure and causes water to diffuse across the cell membrane. As the volume of fluid increases, the hydrostatic pressure in the intercellular compartment rises, forcing the fluid towards the basement membrane and the interstitial capillary bed. During its passage to the capillary network the fluid becomes isotonic.

Micropuncture studies show that reabsorption of Na$^+$ and water in the proximal tubule is depressed when the peritubular capillaries are perfused with colloid-free isotonic NaCl solution and restored by addition of colloid to the perfusate. Forces acting across the peritubular capillary wall could influence the rate at which fluid is taken up from these intercellular compartments and thus indirectly alter the transport of Na$^+$ and water out of the proximal tubular lumen.

Reabsorption of sodium and water from the loop of Henle

Up to 25 per cent of the filtered Na$^+$ is reabsorbed in

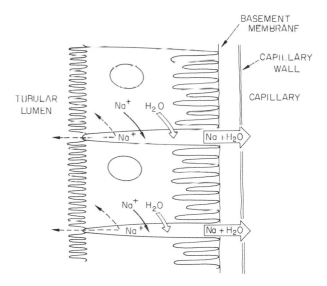

Fig. 35.19. Transtubular movement of Na$^+$ and H$_2$O. Na$^+$ is actively transported into the intercellular space by pumps in the cell membrane →. Passive Na$^+$ backflux occurs into the cell and the tubular lumen ⇢. The intercellular compartment is hypertonic close to the tubular lumen but becomes isosmotic along the more basal portion of the channels because of the entry of H$_2$O ⇨. Fluid and Na$^+$ movement in the intercellular space is due to hydrostatic pressure. Capillary uptake is achieved by the net balance of hydrostatic and colloid osmotic pressure across the capillary wall. Adapted from Giebisch G. & Windhager E.E. (1973). In *Handbook of Physiology*, Section 8, Renal Physiology, p. 355, ed. Orloff J. & Berliner R.W. Washington, D.C.: Amer. Physiol. Soc.

Henle's loop, but as this portion of the nephron is not readily accessible for micropuncture much less is known about its transport mechanisms. Micropuncture of the tip of the loop is possible in rodents such as the hamster which have elongated papillae. Fluid entering the descending limb is isotonic with plasma and fluid at the tip of the loop is markedly hypertonic. Thus, water must pass from the lumen of this limb into the medullary interstitium considerably faster than Na$^+$. Microperfusion studies show that the descending limb is readily permeable to water and much less permeable to Na$^+$. They suggest, moreover, that no active transport of Na$^+$ or Cl$^-$ occurs so that concentration of the tubular fluid in the descending limb is mainly due to reabsorption of water.

Fluid obtained from the early distal convolution is invariably hypotonic to plasma whatever the osmolality of the final urine, so that reabsorption of Na$^+$ and Cl$^-$ in the ascending limb of Henle's loop must exceed that of water. The water permeability of the entire ascending limb is very low and unaffected by ADH. It is doubtful whether the thin part of the ascending limb transports NaCl but there is active transport of solute out of the perfused thick part and, since the transtubular PD is positive, it is likely that Cl$^-$ is reabsorbed actively against an electrochemical gradient. Whether all Na$^+$ reabsorption in the thick limb is due to passive diffusion down the electrical gradient resulting from Cl$^-$ transport or whether there is, in addition, some active transport of Na$^+$ is not known.

Comparative studies have shown that the formation of urine more concentrated than plasma depends on the presence of the hairpin loops and that in mammals the maximum urine concentration which can be achieved is proportional to the length of the loop. The fluid emerging from the loops, however, is more dilute than plasma and no concentration occurs until it reaches the collecting ducts, so that the old suggestion that the concentrating process occurred in Henle's loop is untenable. It is now generally accepted that the loops function as countercurrent multipliers that render the fluid in the medullary interstitium hypertonic. The collecting ducts pass through this medium and in the presence of ADH water moves passively out of the ducts until the urine comes into osmotic equilibrium with the hypertonic medullary interstitial fluid.

Reabsorption of sodium and water from the distal convoluted tubule and collecting duct

Reabsorption of Na$^+$ continues in the distal convolution and collecting ducts. Samples of fluid convoluted from the distal tubule of rats eating a normal amount of Na$^+$ show a steady diminution in the TF/P ratio for Na$^+$; this may fall to 0·1, indicating reabsorption of Na$^+$ against a chemical gradient. When the urine is almost free from Na$^+$, even greater differences must exist. In the rat the transtubular PD is normally about -12 mV in the early distal convolution and -45 mV or less in the late part of this tubule. Thus active reabsorption of Na$^+$ takes place against an electrical gradient as well. Experiments with microelectrodes show that Na$^+$ may be reabsorbed against electrical gradients of 120 mV. Reabsorption can take place against large electrochemical gradients because the distal tubule, unlike the proximal tubule, is relatively impermeable to Na$^+$ and little Na$^+$ leaks back from the peritubular fluid into the lumen.

Some of the Na$^+$ is reabsorbed along with Cl$^-$; the reabsorption of the remainder is associated with the secretion of K$^+$ and H$^+$ by cells of the distal nephron and this Na$^+$ may be regarded as being 'exchanged' for H$^+$ and K$^+$. The pattern of water reabsorption in the distal part of the nephron depends on whether the final urine is to be more or less concentrated than plasma.

HYPOTONIC URINE

During the formation of hypotonic urine micropuncture studies show that the fluid entering the distal convolution remains hypotonic during its passage through this portion of the tubule and on entry into the collecting ducts. A similar picture is found in rats with experimentally induced diabetes insipidus. It seems that in the absence of ADH the permeability of the distal convolution to water is low, as is that of the collecting ducts. Hence in the hydrated animal the absorption of water in these areas lags behind that of solute and further dilution of the urine occurs.

HYPERTONIC URINE

During the formation of hypertonic urine the ratio TF/P$_{osm}$ shows a progressive increase along the length of the distal convolution. It is generally accepted that in the presence of ADH cells lining the distal convolution become more permeable to water so that water is reabsorbed more rapidly than Na$^+$. The osmolality of the fluid in the lumen steadily increases and on entering the collecting duct it is nearly isotonic with the plasma. In the presence of ADH the collecting duct wall is permeable to water, and more water than solute is absorbed during the passage of the tubular fluid down the duct. The force leading to the absorption of water from the ducts is the osmotic gradient between the fluid in the ducts and the more highly concentrated medullary interstitial fluid.

Countercurrent mechanism for the concentration of the urine

Within the mammalian kidney the loops of Henle and the collecting ducts lie close together in the medulla while the proximal and distal convoluted tubules occupy the cortex. In 1942, Kuhn, a Swiss physical chemist, suggested that this spatial arrangement serves a specific purpose and put forward the hypothesis that the loops could act as countercurrent multipliers. A model of such a system is shown in fig. 35.20 and consists of two saline-filled tubes separated by a membrane (M) and joined at one end by a small pipe. A solution flows from left to right in the upper compartment, X, and from right to left in the lower compartment, Y (fig. 35.20a). If the membrane transports a finite amount of Na$^+$ from Y to X, a small concentration difference will be established between the two tubes (fig. 35.20b). As the fluid flows onwards the position represented in fig. 35.20c is reached in which the right half of each tube is occupied by the more concentrated fluid and the concentration difference across this portion of the membrane is abolished. Further transport of sodium from Y to X then occurs and re-establishes the difference at a higher [Na$^+$] in the fluid in the right half of compartment X, (fig. 35.20d); this in turn flows through the connecting pipe to establish the situation shown in fig. 35.20e. The whole process can be repeated

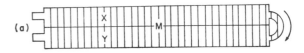

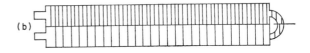

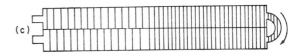

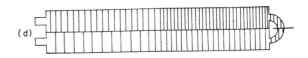

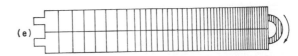

FIG. 35.20. Model of a countercurrent multiplier. Modified from Wirz H. (1961) in *Symposium on Water and Electrolyte Metabolism*, ed. Stewart C.P. & Strengers Th., p. 100. Amsterdam : Elsevier.

indefinitely and the final result is the creation of a longitudinal concentration gradient for Na⁺ many times greater than the small concentration difference which was originally established across the membrane. The final concentration attained at the tip depends upon the magnitude of the difference which can be established between the two limbs, the length and cross section of the parallel tubes and the rate of flow through the system.

In the mammalian kidney the hairpin loops appear to function as countercurrent multipliers. Micropuncture studies indicate that the fluid in the descending limb becomes progressively more concentrated during its passage down to the tip of the loop. In slices of renal tissue taken from rats deprived of water, the cortical tissue is isotonic with plasma but the osmolality of medullary slices cut perpendicular to the axis of the papilla rises progressively from the corticomedullary junction to the papillary tip (fig. 35.21). The descending limb of the loop and the medullary interstitial fluid can together be regarded as equivalent to compartment X of the model. It has been shown that NaCl is reabsorbed more rapidly than water from the ascending limb and the fluid which leaves the loop is more dilute than that which enters it. The ascending limb thus corresponds to Y in the model. The concentration difference between the limbs is created by the transport of NaCl unaccompanied by equivalent amounts of water out of the ascending limb into the interstitial fluid. Active transport of NaCl may be limited to the thick portion of the ascending limb. Since the cells of the thin part of the limb appear unlikely to be capable of active transport, a number of ingenious theories have been advanced to account for the movement of NaCl out of this part of the tubule. Whatever the explanation, sequestration of NaCl in the interstitium raises its

osmolality and water diffuses out of the descending limb, concentrating the contents until an equilibrium is reached in which the concentration of the fluid at any point in the descending limb is the same as that of the interstitial fluid at the same level and slightly higher than that at the corresponding point on the ascending limb (fig. 35.22). It is possible also that Na⁺ and urea diffuse into

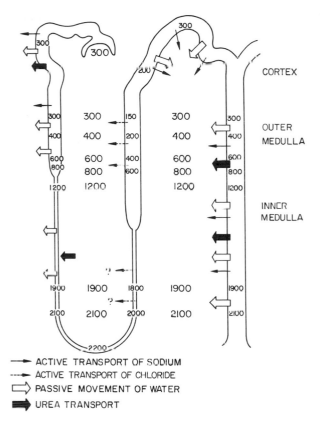

FIG. 35.22. Diagram illustrating possible mode of operation of a countercurrent mechanism for the production of a concentrated urine in the rat. The values represent mosmol solute/l.

the descending limb. The system establishes a longitudinal concentration difference within the descending limb of the loops and the medullary interstitial fluid such that the concentration increases from values of about 290 mosmol/l at the corticomedullary junction to extremely high values at the tip of the papilla. In animals undergoing a water diuresis the difference is greatly reduced. When tissue obtained from hydrated rats is examined with the EM swelling of the basement membrane is seen in the pars recta of the proximal convoluted tubule and the descending limb of Henle's loop. This may be due to hydration of glycoproteins in the basement membrane, and is probably associated with reduced permeability to water. Any reduction in the rate at which water

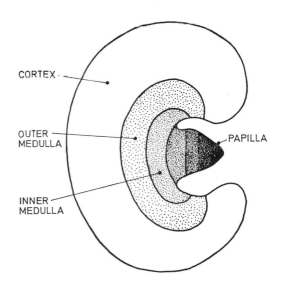

FIG. 35.21. Section of a rat kidney showing the progressive increase in tissue osmolality from cortex to papillary tip. The greater the depth of shading, the higher is the osmolality.

leaves the descending limb reduces the efficiency of the countercurrent multiplier.

The collecting ducts pass through this area and, in the presence of ADH, water diffuses from the collecting ducts into the hypertonic medullary interstitium so that the urine becomes progessively more concentrated and at the papillary tip its osmolality is the same as that of the fluid in the tip of Henle's loop. Under the influence of ADH, urea also diffuses from the papillary portions of the collecting ducts into the medullary interstitial fluid and the descending limb until the concentrations of urea in the urine and medulla are balanced. This allows the production of an even more highly concentrated urine since the concentration of solutes other than urea in the urine can be increased until it is equal to the concentration of NaCl in the medullary interstitium.

The NaCl entering the medulla from the ascending limb and the urea diffusing into the medulla from the ducts accumulate and are not removed rapidly because the medullary blood flow is relatively small and the blood supply consists of the vasa recta which are in the form of hairpin loops. This arrangement is thought to prevent loss of solute from the medulla because the loops act as passive countercurrent exchangers, solute in the ascending vascular limb diffusing into the descending limb and being recirculated. Blood entering the descending limbs of the vasa recta contains solute at a concentration of approximately 290 mosmol/l. As the blood flows down towards the papilla solute diffuses into it and its tonicity increases. During its return to the cortex in the ascending limb, solute diffuses out again into the interstitial fluid so that the final concentration of solute in the blood entering the cortex is probably not much higher than that in the blood entering the loop. The medullary blood flow is reduced in the presence of ADH, and this contributes to the establishment of the high medullary osmotic concentration found in animals deprived of water, forming a highly concentrated urine. During water diuresis medullary blood flow increases.

Although it seems likely that a countercurrent mechanism for the production of concentrated urine exists in man there is little direct evidence that this is so. However, the few studies carried out upon human kidneys removed at operation or shortly after death show that the concentration of Na$^+$ and of urea in the medulla of the human kidney is higher than in the cortex.

The capacity of the kidney to concentrate urine above the osmolality of the plasma is measured during water deprivation or following the administration of ADH. It is expressed by the ratio U/P_{osm} which has a normal value of 3–4. It is also possible to estimate the volume of solute-free water reabsorbed by the renal tubules in unit time (Tc_{H_2O}). This is given by the formula:

$$Tc_{H_2O} = \frac{U_{osm} \times V}{P_{osm}} - V$$

REGULATION OF THE VOLUME OF THE EXTRACELLULAR FLUID

The maintenance of the blood pressure and of the circulation depends, among other things, upon the volume of the plasma. Reduction in the volume of the ECF is associated with a reduction in plasma volume and jeopardizes tissue perfusion. It is, therefore, hardly surprising that homeostatic mechanisms exist to keep the volume of the ECF approximately constant by regulating the excretion of Na$^+$ and water. As long ago as 1935 the American physician, J.P. Peters, envisaged the existence of a mechanism whereby changes in the 'fullness of the blood stream' might start a train of events leading to changes in the rate of excretion of water and of Na$^+$. There is much evidence in favour of the existence of such a mechanism; it has, for example, been shown that haemorrhage reduces the rate of salt and water excretion even when the loss of blood is too small to produce any measurable change in RPF or GFR. A similar reduction in Na$^+$ and water excretion occurs in man when he stands still or when venous tourniquets are applied around the thighs. It is seen in dogs after the distension of a balloon inserted into the inferior vena cava. These procedures result in pooling of blood in the lower limbs and hence underfilling of the great vessels of the thorax. Conversely an increase in the rate of excretion of Na$^+$ and water occurs when an individual lies down and when ECF is expanded by the infusion of isotonic NaCl, albumin, plasma or blood.

A homeostatic mechanism of this type requires the presence of receptor organs capable of detecting changes in the volume of the ECF and neural or humoral pathways capable of modifying the rate of excretion of salt and water by the effector organ, the kidney. It seems likely that there are a number of receptor areas each capable of reacting to a specific stimulus and that several integrated mechanisms exist to bring about the necessary changes in renal function. Knowledge of this important part of physiology is, however, fragmentary.

Volume receptors and their associated effector mechanisms (fig. 35.23)

Over 70 per cent of the blood volume is present under low pressure in the veins and atria of the heart (p. 30.3). The walls of these are thin and distensible by comparison with those of arteries and ventricles. Small changes in blood volume lead to comparable changes in pressure within the low pressure system. This led to the hypothesis that the blood volume might be controlled, in part, by pressure-sensitive receptors in this system, which relayed information to the hypothalamus, with subsequent modification of the rate of release of ADH and aldosterone, and so of water and Na$^+$ excretion. In support of this it was shown that normal men excreted water less rapidly when breathing against positive pressure, a procedure which displaces blood from the intrathoracic veins. This antidiuresis could be inhibited by alcohol which supported the idea that it was due to the release of ADH. Further experiments showed that water excretion was increased during negative pressure respiration which leads to slight overdistension of the thoracic vessels and that this could be prevented by giving ADH. Localized distension of the left atrium may also induce water diuresis, and an increase in Na$^+$ excretion due to a reduction in circulating aldosterone has been reported to

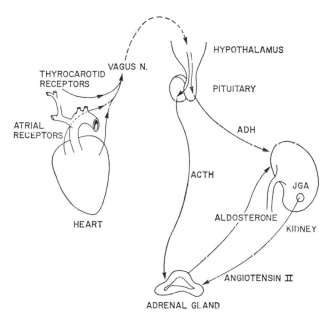

Fig. 35.23. Postulated system for volume control.

occur when the right atrium is stretched. These and other experimental procedures designed to stimulate 'volume' receptors also modify the circulation in other ways. Although atrial receptors appear to exist, it remains uncertain whether they play a significant part in the control of blood volume.

Two sets of receptors in the arterial system can influence Na$^+$ excretion by altering aldosterone secretion. These are situated in the carotid arteries near the origin of the thyroid arteries and in the JGA of the kidney. These receptors are thought to be sensitive to changes in mean arterial pressure brought about by changes in cardiac output, which in turn are influenced by the blood volume. Constricting the carotids low in the neck has been shown to increase aldosterone production by stimulating thyrocarotid receptors. Impulses from these receptors are probably carried by the vagus to a centre in the diencephalon. It is not known how such a centre might control the output of aldosterone but impulses arising there could conceivably stimulate secretion of ACTH and an acute rise in the circulating level of this hormone

stimulates aldosterone secretion transiently. Alternatively impulses from carotid receptors might induce reflex sympathetic vasoconstriction of the renal vessels. The resulting reduction in pressure in the afferent arterioles could stimulate release of renin from the JGA, and thus the formation of angiotensin II and the release of aldosterone from the adrenal cortex.

The receptors in the JGA provide a mechanism for release of aldosterone which does not necessarily involve higher centres and which accounts for the rise in aldosterone output found when decapitated dogs are bled, a response which still occurs if the liver is also removed, but which is abolished by nephrectomy. The exact mechanism by which renin is released from the JGA in conditions associated with underfilling of the vascular bed remains unknown; the receptors may be situated in the wall of the afferent arteriole itself or in the macula densa.

Changes in renal function

The changes in water excretion which occur in response to alterations in the circulating level of ADH are well established (p. 27.17). The rate at which Na$^+$ is excreted in the urine depends upon the balance struck between the amount of Na$^+$ filtered and the amount reabsorbed. Normally about 1 per cent of the filtered Na$^+$ is excreted and, since variations in GFR of less than 5 per cent cannot be detected by present methods, conventional clearance studies are of little value in determining which of the two variables changes in a particular situation. An acute increase in GFR brought about in dogs by giving dexamethasone, a powerful synthetic adrenocorticosteroid, was not associated with any significant changes in Na$^+$ excretion, suggesting that changes in GFR are usually accompanied by parallel compensatory alterations in tubular reabsorption of Na$^+$.

The adrenocorticosteroids in general and aldosterone in particular, are known to enhance reabsorption of Na$^+$. Aldosterone and cortisol act upon the distal tubule to promote reabsorption of Na$^+$ and Cl$^-$ and facilitate secretion of K$^+$ and H$^+$. Retention of Na$^+$ and Cl$^-$ tends to raise the osmolality of the extracellular fluid, with release of ADH, increased reabsorption of water from the collecting ducts and expansion of the ECF volume. It is not known whether adrenocorticosteroids also promote the isotonic reabsorption of NaCl and water in the proximal convoluted tubule. Their presence is necessary to maintain Na$^+$ balance in the face of a variable intake of this ion. Their absence, as in Addison's disease (p. 27.32), leads to Na$^+$ depletion. Yet the actual fraction of Na$^+$ reabsorption affected by these hormones is quite small, being about 2 per cent. Experiments in which aldosterone was injected intravenously into adrenalectomized animals have shown that there is a delay of about 40 min before any effect is seen upon Na$^+$

reabsorption. It seems unlikely therefore that alterations in the amount of circulating adrenocorticosteroids are responsible for rapid changes in Na⁺ excretion. This is borne out by the fact that the usual rapid reduction in Na⁺ excretion associated with standing up or the application of a tourniquet to the thigh occurs in patients who have undergone adrenalectomy and are being treated with a small fixed dose of salt and adrenocortical hormone.

Changes in GFR and in the circulating levels of adrenocortical hormones cannot explain all the observed variations in Na⁺ excretion, which must be influenced by other mechanisms.

HAEMODYNAMIC AND OSMOTIC FACTORS

Changes in mean renal arterial pressure in an isolated perfused kidney produce parallel changes in the rate of Na⁺ excretion which may take place without any alteration in GFR or RBF. Micropuncture and clearance studies in intact animals suggest that a rise in renal arterial pressure affects the rate of reabsorption of Na⁺ throughout the nephron. This could be due to an increase in the peritubular venous capillary pressure, which in turn might reduce the rate at which Na⁺ and water are transported through the intercellular spaces of the proximal tubule (p. 35.19) and thus increase the excretion of this ion. A fall in arterial pressure could have the opposite effect. It is less clear why the rate of reabsorption of Na⁺ in the distal tubule should be affected.

Changes in the composition of the blood perfusing the kidneys also influence the rate of reabsorption of Na⁺ directly. A fall in PCV or in the concentration of plasma proteins increases the rate of Na⁺ excretion. This may be due to a fall in blood viscosity or colloid osmotic pressure in the peritubular capillaries and the effect that these changes have on the uptake of Na⁺ and water from the proximal tubular intercellular spaces.

ECF AND BLOOD VOLUME

Expansion of the ECF by infusion of 150 mmolar NaCl or of the intravascular volume by infusion of blood increases the rate of Na⁺ excretion. This is independent of changes in GFR, of the concentrations of protein and Na⁺ in plasma and of the PCV, and occurs even when large doses of adrenocorticosteroids and ADH are given. Micropuncture studies show that the rate of Na⁺ reabsorption in the proximal tubule, but not in the distal tubule, is reduced during infusion of NaCl. These observations suggest that an unidentified humoral factor may modify the rate of Na⁺ reabsorption in the proximal tubule and cross-circulation experiments provide some support for this idea. Several not altogether satisfactory bioassays for such a natriuretic substance have been devised. There is, for example, evidence that plasma from dogs whose blood volume has been expanded with blood previously equilibrated with the dog's own, interferes

with the uptake of PAH by isolated renal tubules and alters their capacity to transport electrolytes. The source of the hormone, if it exists, is not known but present evidence favours the brain, possibly the hypothalamus.

RENAL EXCRETION OF POTASSIUM

The urine of a healthy individual eating a mixed diet contains from 50 to 100 mmol of potassium each day. In persons with normal renal function this is equivalent to between 10 and 15 per cent of the amount filtered by the glomeruli. The simplest explanation of this finding would be that 85–90 per cent of the K⁺ filtered by the glomeruli is reabsorbed by the tubules, leaving the remainder to be excreted in the urine. While this view was for long thought to be correct, it is now established that almost all the filtered K⁺ is reabsorbed in the proximal part of the nephron while the K⁺ which is found in the urine is secreted into the tubular lumen in the distal nephron in association with reabsorption of Na⁺ from the tubular fluid.

Direct evidence about the excretion of K⁺ by the kidney has been obtained in micropuncture experiments. Fig. 35.24 shows the results obtained in rats receiving a diet containing normal amounts of K⁺ and excreting about 17 per cent of the filtered K⁺. The TF/P ratios for K⁺ in fluid obtained from different sites in the proximal tubule are all slightly less than one, indicating that the rate of K⁺ reabsorption is slightly greater than the rate of reabsorption of water. When TF/P_{K^+} is divided by TF/P_{in} it appears that at a point two-thirds of the way

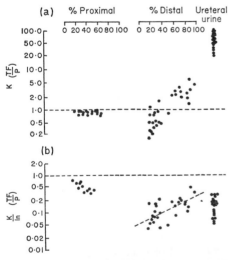

Fig. 35.24. Micropuncture experiments on rats receiving a normal diet. (a), Tubular fluid/plasma concentration ratios for potassium as a function of tubular length; (b), potassium/inulin tubular fluid/plasma concentration ratios as a function of tubular length. From Malnic G. *et al.* (1964) *Amer. J. Physiol.* **206**, 677.

down the proximal tubule 70 per cent of the filtered K^+ has been reabsorbed.

At the next site accessible to micropuncture, one-fifth of the way along the distal tubule, between 85 and 95 per cent of filtered K^+ has disappeared from the lumen. Clearly most filtered K^+ is reabsorbed in the upper portion of the nephron. Most workers have found that the $[K^+]$ in the proximal tubular fluid is less than that of plasma; if, in addition, it is accepted that a small negative transtubular PD exists in the proximal tubule (p. 35.18) then reabsorption of K^+ must take place against an electrochemical gradient and must be active. Active reabsorption of K^+ also occurs in the ascending limb of Henle's loop. The fraction of filtered K^+ reabsorbed in the upper nephron remains virtually constant however much K^+ is present in the final urine.

In rats receiving a normal diet, the ratio of TF/P_{K^+} to TF/P_{in} increases along the length of the distal tubule showing that K^+ is added to the tubular fluid at this site. It can be calculated that at least 70 per cent of urinary K^+ is secreted in the distal convolution. Potassium ions accumulate passively in the tubular fluid under the influence of the negative transtubular PD (p. 35.18). However, the concentration of K^+ in the lumen is always lower than the calculated value obtained from the Nernst equation (p. 15.7) and it is likely that active reabsorption of K^+ continues in the distal nephron so that the final $[K^+]$ in the tubular fluid depends upon the balance between these two processes. When the final urine contains little or no K^+, the TF/P_{K^+} divided by TF/P_{in} actually falls as the fluid traverses the distal tubule showing that, in these circumstances, reabsorption predominates. By contrast, when the urinary K^+ is very high, this ratio may exceed one by the end of the distal tubule.

Fluid cannot be obtained from the collecting ducts by the micropuncture technique, but U/P_{K^+} divided by U/P_{in} suggests that in rats on a normal diet the tubular fluid is not modified significantly during its passage through the collecting ducts. However, a high urinary K^+ appears to be associated with secretion of K^+ by the cells of the collecting ducts and, since urinary $[K^+]$ well in excess of those which could be accounted for by passive diffusion are encountered, it is likely that in the collecting ducts, in contrast to the distal convolution, there is active transport of K^+ from peritubular to luminal fluid. When the amount of K^+ in the urine is very low, analysis of fluid obtained from the collecting ducts by micro-catheters has shown that net reabsorption of K^+ can occur in this part of the nephron.

Factors which influence the rate of potassium excretion

Since the urinary K^+ is determined mainly by the rate at which K^+ is secreted into the tubular fluid, information about the factors which influence the secretory process is needed in order to understand the changes in K^+ excretion which occur in different physiological and pathological conditions.

POTASSIUM BALANCE

When K^+ salts are given to a normal individual there is an increase in the rate of excretion of this ion in the urine. It is of interest that the capacity to excrete K^+ appears to be enhanced when the substance is given in moderately large amounts over a long period of time. The mechanism of this is unknown. Conversely, when a normal person is placed on a diet containing very little K^+, e.g. 15 or 20 mmol/day, the rate of K^+ excretion gradually declines until balance is achieved in 10–14 days.

The changes in P_{K^+} which occur in response to changes in intake are usually small and in normal subjects $U_{K^+}V$ bears little relation to P_{K^+} but probably depends upon the $[K^+]$ within the cells in general and the renal tubular cells in particular.

RATE OF FLOW THROUGH DISTAL NEPHRON

Micropuncture studies show that the $[K^+]$ in distal tubular fluid remains fairly constant and is independent of the rate of flow. It follows that the total quantity of K^+ secreted into the distal tubule varies directly with the flow.

REABSORPTION OF SODIUM IN THE DISTAL NEPHRON

Parallel changes in the rates of excretion Na^+ and K^+ are often seen and micropuncture suggests that the amount of Na^+ reaching the distal nephron and, in particular, the rate of reabsorption of this ion in the collecting duct may influence K^+ secretion. The low rates of K^+ secretion seen when only small amounts of Na^+ reach the distal nephron may be due to the fact that transtubular PD falls when distal Na^+ reabsorption is diminished. By contrast, giving large quantities of Na^+ frequently increases K^+ excretion, partly because it increases the rate of flow through the distal nephron. Increased secretion of K^+ is particularly likely when the Na^+ is given along with an anion such as sulphate, which is not readily reabsorbed. The presence of such anions in distal tubular fluid increases the transtubular PD.

EXCRETION OF HYDROGEN IONS

In many situations the rate of excretion of K^+ in the urine appears to be related inversely to the rate of H^+ excretion. Thus, giving a carbonic anhydrase inhibitor, such as acetazolamide, diminishes H^+ excretion and increases K^+ excretion. Patients with respiratory alkalosis in whom the P_{CO_2} is low have a low rate of H^+ excretion and their alkaline urine contains increased K^+. In the same way, giving $NaHCO_3$ makes the urine alkaline and increases the rate of K^+ excretion. Micropuncture studies show that K^+ secretion is enhanced by alkalinization of distal tubular fluid. By contrast secretion of K^+ in the distal nephron is diminished in animals breathing CO_2 in whom tubular cell $[H^+]$ is presumably increased. It is likely that the $[K^+]$ in tubular cells varies inversely with $[H^+]$ and an increase in cellular $[K^+]$ facilitates diffusion of K^+ down the electrochemical gradient into the tubular fluid.

ADRENOCORTICOSTEROIDS

It is generally recognized that in the absence of adrenocorticosteroids K^+ excretion is impaired, while an excess of adrenocorticosteroids promotes the loss of large amounts of K^+ in the urine; the latter can be reduced by rigid restriction of dietary Na^+. The mode of action of the adrenocorticosteroids is not known but in adrenalectomized animals the distal tubular TF/P_{K^+} is abnormally low while the distal TF/P_{Na^+} is increased. This is associated with a fall in the normal distal transtubular gradient for Na^+ and both deficiencies are corrected by giving aldosterone. The transtubular PD does not change in adrenalectomized rats and it is thought that mineralocorticoids owe their effect on electrolyte transport to their influence on the Na^+/K^+ pump in the peritubular membrane of the cells of the distal nephron, which in turn regulates intracellular concentration of these cations (p. 35.18).

RENAL EXCRETION OF DIVALENT IONS

A healthy subject, eating a European diet, excretes up to 7.5 mmol/day of calcium in the urine; the remainder is excreted in the faeces (p. 5.6). Changes in dietary calcium are accompanied by small parallel changes in urinary calcium. Reducing the dietary intake by half induces only a small fall in urinary calcium in most healthy human subjects, and when the dietary calcium is increased, less than 10 per cent of the increment appears in the urine.

The mechanism by which urinary excretion alters as the dietary intake changes is unknown. Calcium disappears from human urine when the plasma calcium falls below 1.9 mmol/l.

With typical European diets the daily intake of magnesium lies between 5 and 20 mmol, of which about 2 to 4 mmol are excreted in the urine and the remainder in the faeces (p. 5.8). In healthy men dietary and urinary magnesium are linearly related. When the intake is increased urinary excretion rises within 2 to 3 days. If intake falls to less than 1 mmol/day, urinary magnesium falls rapidly to less than 1 mmol/day with no marked change in plasma magnesium concentration. In the rat magnesium virtually disappears from the urine when the

plasma magnesium falls below 0.7 mmol/l but it is doubtful whether a similar threshold exists in man.

Calcium and magnesium exist in plasma in three forms, as free ions, bound to plasma proteins and as complexes with anions such as citrate and phosphate. The free calcium and magnesium ions and some of the smaller complexes are ultrafiltrable and only this fraction of plasma calcium and magnesium passes through the wall of the glomerular capillaries.

Tubular reabsorption of calcium and magnesium

Since the plasma ultrafiltrable calcium is 1.6 mmol/l and the GFR 125 ml/min, approximately 280 mmol of calcium are filtered by the glomeruli daily and only 0.5–2 per cent of this is excreted in the urine. Assuming a plasma ultrafiltrable magnesium of 0.63 mmol/l, 3–6 per cent of the filtered magnesium is excreted. The overall pattern of reabsorption of calcium and magnesium in the nephron resembles that of sodium, bulk reabsorption taking place in the proximal tubule while fine adjustments are made in the distal part of the nephron.

Micropuncture of the renal tubules of dogs or rats eating normal amounts of calcium and magnesium shows that between 50 and 60 per cent of the filtered calcium and magnesium is reabsorbed in the proximal tubule. The ratio of the concentration of calcium in the tubular fluid to ultrafiltrable calcium in plasma (TF/UF_{Ca}) and the comparable ratio for magnesium remain around 1 throughout the accessible part of the proximal convolution, indicating that both substances are reabsorbed in isotonic solution. Reabsorption of the divalent cations occurs against a small electrical gradient (proximal transtubular PD -4 mV) and during the course of an osmotic diuresis the TF/UF ratios for calcium and magnesium fall significantly below 1, which shows that both ions can be reabsorbed against a chemical gradient. Thus an active process is probably involved.

Micropuncture studies suggest that a further 25 per cent of the filtered calcium and magnesium is reabsorbed, probably by an active process, in Henle's loop. Most of the remainder is reabsorbed in the distal convolution and in the collecting ducts. Since the TF/UF ratio for both ions in fluid leaving the proximal tubule is usually around 1, and the urinary concentrations of calcium and of magnesium may be significantly less than the concentrations in plasma, the fall in concentration must occur in the distal nephron. In this region the transtubular PD varies from -45 to -90 mV. The distal tubule is readily permeable to calcium and magnesium and calculations using the Nernst equation show that if the distribution of divalent cations between distal tubular fluid and peritubular plasma was determined solely by the electrochemical forces acting across the tubular wall, high concentrations of calcium and magnesium would always be found in distal tubular fluid. As this is not the case, calcium and magnesium must be transported actively out of the distal tubular fluid.

Since magnesium is the second most important intracellular cation it might be expected that, like K^+, it would be secreted into the urine. Some evidence favours the presence of such a secretory mechanism in the rat and the dog but there is none for its existence in man.

Factors which influence the rates of excretion of calcium and magnesium

INTERDEPENDENCE OF CALCIUM AND MAGNESIUM EXCRETION

A change in the dietary intake of either calcium or magnesium induces parallel changes in the excretion of both cations. Infusions of calcium or magnesium salts also augment the excretion of both cations. These observations might be explained if a proportion of the filtered calcium and magnesium was reabsorbed by a common transport mechanism which became partly saturated by the increased filtered load of the administered cation.

CHANGES IN THE RATE OF EXCRETION OF NA^+

Changes in the rate of excretion of Na^+ are frequently accompanied by parallel changes in excretion of calcium and magnesium. If the amount of Na^+ in the diet is changed while dietary calcium is held constant, the ensuing alteration in urinary Na^+ is associated with a change in calcium excretion in the same direction. Thus, in dogs undergoing water diuresis, osmotic diuresis, or a Na^+ diuresis induced by intravenous infusion of Na^+ salts, increased urinary calcium excretion accompanies the increased Na^+ excretion and the clearance of Ca^{++} becomes approximately the same as that of Na^+. These changes are not merely the result of a parallel increase in the filtered loads of both cations, for they persist when filtered calcium and Na^+ are reduced by constriction of the aorta; they must, therefore, be due to changes in tubular reabsorption of both cations.

The relationship between Na^+ and magnesium excretion is less well defined but a positive correlation between the clearance of the two ions has been demonstrated during expansion of the ECF and in the course of an osmotic diuresis induced by infusion of urea.

PARATHYROID HORMONE (PTH)

Reabsorption of calcium by the renal tubules is increased by parathyroid hormone (p. 27.27). Following parathyroidectomy at a time when the plasma concentration of calcium is falling, there is a transient increase in the rate of excretion of calcium in the urine. By contrast, in patients with hypoparathyroidism, the rate of excretion of calcium is higher than would be expected for any given level of plasma calcium. In dogs, fractional reabsorption of Na^+, calcium and phosphate in the proximal tubule diminishes after administration of parathyroid hormone. The changes in the rates of reabsorption of Na^+ and calcium are roughly comparable but the fall in the fractional reabsorption of filtered phosphate is much greater. Identical effects are produced by giving dibutyryl cyclic AMP and the action of PTH on proximal tubular transport may be mediated by means of cyclic AMP. During these experiments there is an increase in urinary Na^+ and phosphate but the urinary output of calcium falls. This suggests that PTH stimulates reabsorption of calcium selectively at some point in the nephron beyond the proximal tubule, most probably in the distal convolution. The effect of PTH on magnesium excretion is less well defined but it appears to augment excretion of this cation.

HORMONES AND THE KIDNEY

The kidney is responsible for the release of two hormones, renin, which is functionally connected with angiotensin and aldosterone, and erythropoietin.

Renin-angiotensin-aldosterone system

It has been appreciated for some time that there is a link between the kidneys, Na^+ balance and blood pressure. While some aspects of this complex relationship are known, the extent to which the system serves a physiological purpose and the frequency with which its breakdown is responsible for disease remain uncertain. Bright of Guy's Hospital (1827) was among the first to realize that renal disease was often accompanied by an abnormally high blood pressure. Next came the observation of Tigerstedt and Bergman, in 1898, that when extracts of rabbit kidney were injected into normal rabbits, a slow and prolonged rise in blood pressure due to vasoconstriction occurred. Because the active material was extracted from the kidneys, it was called renin. In 1934 Goldblatt showed that when the renal artery of a dog was constricted by a clamp, hypertension developed. Later it was found that the renin content of the constricted kidney rose. Yet when renin was added to a solution of NaCl which was perfusing isolated organs the blood vessels did not constrict; the presence of blood plasma was also needed, showing that the kidney itself did not contain the active vasoconstrictor substance. This series of facts has now been explained as follows.

Renin is an enzyme which, on reaching the blood, activates angiotensinogen, an α_2-globulin formed in the liver, making angiotensin I, a polypeptide containing ten amino acids. Another enzyme present in high concentration in the lungs converts angiotensin I to angiotensin II by removing two amino acids. This last substance is the most potent pressor agent known. It constricts small arteries and arterioles and, in larger doses, veins. Renal blood vessels are highly sensitive to angiotensin II, and for this reason it can reduce the output of urine. It has little effect on the heart and on adrenal blood vessels. On injection into the circulation it is rapidly destroyed by the angiotensinase of the blood, so that the effect of a single dose is short lived. When low concentrations of angiotensin are infused, the rise in blood pressure can be maintained for long periods. The action of renin is slow and prolonged because angiotensin has first to be formed and the process is not instantaneous. Another effect of angiotensin is that on injection into the venous system or into the adrenal artery it releases aldosterone from the adrenal cortex (vol. 2, p. 17.4).

ASSAY OF RENIN AND ANGIOTENSIN

Early assays of renin were carried out by incubating plasma at 37° and thereafter estimating the amount of angiotensin II produced by its ability to contract smooth muscle; the results are then expressed in terms of plasma renin activity. More recently it has become possible to estimate angiotensin II immunologically, and values can now be obtained both for circulating angiotensin and for the amount produced after incubation.

For reasons which will become obvious, the results obtained are influenced by posture, dietary electrolytes and diuretic drugs, and therefore, conditions need to be controlled before blood is sampled. In a healthy individual taking about 100 mmol of Na^+ a day, the angiotensin II in plasma taken with the subject in the supine position lies between 10 and 40 ng/l and renin activity, expressed in terms of the rate of production of angiotensin, between 2 and 10 $\mu g\,l^{-1}h^{-1}$.

SODIUM, BLOOD PRESSURE AND RENIN

In man there is a striking inverse correlation between the plasma renin, angiotensin and $[Na^+]$. A low salt diet reduces the Na^+ content of the body slightly and at the same time lowers the blood pressure. In rats hypertension can be induced by feeding a high salt diet, while dogs given a high salt diet and deoxycorticosterone, a Na^+ retaining substance formed in small amounts in the adrenal cortex, invariably become hypertensive. The relationship between body Na^+, systemic blood pressure, the adrenal cortex and the kidney has been interpreted as follows: the decrease in renal blood flow which accompanies a fall in cardiac output or a reduction in plasma volume liberates renin from the kidney. This enzyme is responsible for the appearance of angiotensin II which acts upon the adrenal cortex and increases release of aldosterone. Aldosterone facilitates retention of Na^+ by the kidney, water is retained along with Na^+, and this in turn leads to an increase in the ECF, including the plasma, so that the blood volume rises. The blood pressure rises because of an increased cardiac output and constriction of the resistance vessels. To this must now be added the idea that the initial reduction in renal blood

flow may, in some cases, be due not to changes in the systemic circulation but to failure of autoregulation (p. 35.15) which is related to a loss of the capacity to make PGE_2. In a few experimental conditions it has been found that autoregulation is lost in animals with hypertension.

SITE OF ORIGIN OF RENIN

Renin can be extracted from the cortex of the kidney, though little is found in the juxtamedullary part, and none in the medulla. The JGA, which lie in the cortex, became suspect as the source of renin for the following reasons. It was noticed that the the degree of granularity of the specialized arteriolar juxtaglomerular cells, the JG index, was reduced in hypertensive rats on a high Na^+ diet, and increased on a low Na^+ diet. In a kidney whose artery was constricted the index rose but fell in the other normal kidney. There was a correlation between the cellular content of granules and the amount of renin that could be extracted. By an ingenious method glomeruli have been isolated and their renin content assayed. Iron filings were injected into the renal artery, and these jammed in the glomeruli; the kidney was broken up and slowly washed past a magnet which retained the glomeruli. It was found that renin was present in the glomeruli in large amounts, and in only small amounts in the other parts of the renal tissue. Later, individual glomeruli were collected and bisected; renin was found only in the half containing the JGA. This does not tell us whether the renin comes from the modified arteriolar cells or from the macula densa but histological and other techniques indicate that it is present in the muscle cells of the afferent arteriole (fig. 35.25 and p. 35.5).

POSSIBLE PHYSIOLOGICAL ROLE OF RENIN

While renin may or may not be responsible for certain forms of hypertension, it appears to have a physiological role. Observations on normal man show that plasma renin and angiotensin rise in Na^+ deprivation, and fall during Na^+ loading. This suggests that the renin-angiotensin system has some part in controlling Na^+ balance. Also, in acute blood loss more aldosterone is released, and this does not occur if the kidneys have first been removed. Further, in rats the prolonged administration of renin leads to an increase in size of the zona glomerulosa of the adrenals, which produces aldosterone.

The stimulus to renin production is still not certainly known. The possibilities are that the granular cells in the afferent arteriole act as stretch receptors, and that a fall in pressure releases renin, and a rise inhibits its release. Alternatively the macula densa cells may be receptors which react to the $[Na^+]$ or $[Cl^-]$ in the distal tubular fluid or to the rate at which they are delivered to the distal tubule, and pass the information to the granular cells.

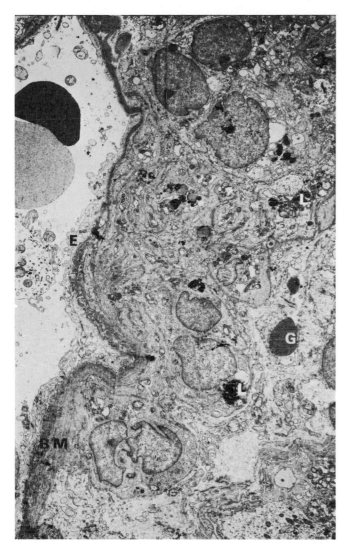

FIG. 35.25. Electronmicrograph of part of a human JGA. The lumen of the afferent arteriole is seen on the left of the picture; deep to the endothelium (E) and its basement membrane (BM) the vessel media contains secretory cells, with no ordinary smooth muscle cells. Renin granules (G) of varying size are seen, and much lipochrome (L) is present. ($\times$ 2000).

Erythropoietin

Attention was first drawn to the importance of the kidney in blood formation because chronic renal failure is accompanied by an anaemia which cannot be attributed to a deficiency in the excretory processes. Conversely, in the presence of a renal carcinoma, a malignant tumour, there may be erythraemia, i.e. too many red blood cells. In normal people increased erythropoiesis follows haemorrhage or exposure to a low oxygen tension, and in these circumstances an erythropoietic substance can be found in the plasma. The precursor of this substance, **erythrogenin**, is present in the kidney and its release is unrelated to renal excretory activity. Erythrogenin possibly reacts with a substrate in plasma which may be an α-globulin to

form the active substance erythropoietin. However, there are other unidentified sources of erythropoietic material since, after bilateral nephrectomy, severe haemorrhage may still induce an increase in plasma erythropoietin and in the number of red blood cells. The stimulus that induces release of the renal factor is uncertain. Experimental evidence suggests that the cells concerned are stimulated by a reduction in Po_2. This idea is supported by observations on the effect of testosterone which increases the renal O_2 requirement and which, when given to animals in a hypoxic state, induces a rapid release of the active substance into the circulation. That testosterone acts on the kidney is shown by the fact that it does not affect red blood cell production following nephrectomy. It is also less effective when the red blood cell count is already high. In chronic renal failure the anaemia is partly relieved by treatment with an artificial kidney; this suggests that a substance inhibiting red blood cell formation appears in the blood in uraemia.

The assay and mode of action of erythropoietin in promoting erythropoiesis is discussed on p. 28.10).

RENAL REGULATION OF ACID-BASE BALANCE

The concentration of hydrogen ions in the urine can be increased to 2,500 times that of plasma or decreased to one quarter i.e. from pH 4·0 to 8·0. This allows the kidney to regulate the [H^+] of the body fluids.

The healthy individual eating a mixed diet produces 40–80 mmol of non-volatile acid each day. The H^+ arising from these acids are buffered by the bases throughout the body (p. 6.4). The conjugate acids formed are temporarily retained in the body except for carbonic acid, which is the conjugate acid of the bicarbonate buffer system. This breaks down to form CO_2 and water so that the protons remain in the body in water molecules while the CO_2 is eliminated by the lungs. The reconstitution of the body bases is achieved by the excretion in the urine of a number of protons equivalent to those formed in the course of metabolism and the simultaneous regeneration of the all important base HCO_3^- by the renal tubular cells.

Conversely, ingestion of a salt containing an anion metabolized to CO_2 and H_2O, e.g. sodium lactate, amounts to the addition of base to body fluids since H^+ are taken up during its oxidation; this leaves a OH^- which reacts with carbonic acid according to the reaction

$$OH^- + H_2CO_3 \rightleftharpoons H_2O + HCO_3^-$$

The HCO_3^- formed in this reaction are excreted in the urine because the tubular reabsorption of filtered HCO_3^- is adjusted to maintain their concentration in the blood within defined limits. The kidney regulates the [H$^+$] of the body fluids in two ways:

(1) by controlling the rate of tubular reabsorption of filtered HCO$_3$$^-$, and

(2) by the excretion of H$^+$ and the simultaneous regeneration of HCO$_3$$^-$.

It will be readily appreciated that any change in the conjugate acid/conjugate base ratio of one buffer system leads to changes in the ratio in every other buffer system. Thus the alterations in the [HCO$_3$$^-$] in the extracellular fluid which are brought about by the kidneys not only result in the restoration of the normal $\frac{1}{20}$ ratio of [H$_2$CO$_3$]/[HCO$_3$$^-$] (p. 6.5) but also restore the normal conjugate acid/conjugate base ratio in all the other systems.

Micropuncture studies provide some evidence about the sites at which HCO$_3$$^-$ are reabsorbed and H$^+$ added to the tubular fluid. Fig. 35.26 shows the changes in the pH of the tubular fluid in different parts of the rat nephron. In the proximal tubule the changes are relatively small and the pH of the tubular fluid falls by about 0·5 to 1·0 unit compared with that of the blood. This is due to the fact that HCO$_3$$^-$ are reabsorbed more rapidly than water so that their concentration in the tubular fluid falls to about 10 mmol/l by the end of the proximal convolution while PCO$_2$ remains constant. In rats in a normal state of acid-base balance 80–85 per cent of the filtered HCO$_3$$^-$ is reabsorbed in the first two-thirds of the proximal tubule. Fluid obtained by micropuncture from the distal convoluted tubule is slightly more acid than that withdrawn from the proximal convolution and, in rats on a normal diet, the [HCO$_3$$^-$] has fallen to less than 5 mmol/l. In these circumstances only 1–2 per cent of the filtered HCO$_3$$^-$ reaches the distal tubule, so that about

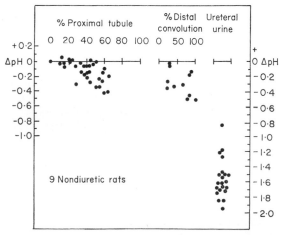

FIG. 35.26. The change in the pH of the tubular fluid obtained from rat nephrons by micropuncture technique. ΔpH = difference between pH of tubular fluid and that of arterial blood. pH measured by the quinhydrone microelectrode. From Gottschalk C.W. *et al.* (1960) *Amer. J. Physiol.* **198**, 581.

15 per cent must be reabsorbed in the pars recta and Henle's loop. Bicarbonate reabsorption continues in the distal convolution but as the urine is so much more acid than the distal tubular fluid the largest changes in pH must occur in the collecting ducts. In the studies shown in fig. 35.26 the pH of the urine fell to 5·4. Reduction of the urinary pH to 6·0 can be accounted for solely by the reabsorption of the base HCO$_3$$^-$ but in those animals in which the pH fell below this level, H$^+$ must have been added to the urine. Experiments in which microcatheters were inserted into the collecting ducts of hamsters confirm the occurrence of a marked drop in the pH of the tubular fluid in the final portion of the nephron in animals forming an acid urine.

Tubular mechanism for reabsorption of bicarbonate and for formation of acid urine

In 1945 Pitts and his colleagues carried out experiments upon normal human subjects in whom metabolic acidosis was induced by the administration of ammonium chloride. The presence of a large amount of buffer base in the urine was ensured by infusion of a mixture of NaH$_2$PO$_4$ and Na$_2$HPO$_4$. It was found that the rate of excretion of H$^+$ in the urine was greater than could be accounted for by the quantity of H$^+$ in the glomerular filtrate and it was concluded that H$^+$ were added to the tubular fluid.

It is believed that the reabsorption of HCO$_3$$^-$ and the acidification of the urine are achieved by a mechanism in which H$^+$ formed in the tubular cells are secreted into the tubular fluid; simultaneously Na$^+$ are reabsorbed from the glomerular filtrate. This mechanism is shown in fig. 35.27. The source of the protons is not known but since the enzyme carbonic anhydrase is involved in their production (p. 6.4) it is possible that hydration of carbon dioxide is catalysed in the tubular cells and that the carbonic acid formed dissociates to give H$^+$ and HCO$_3$$^-$. The protons are then secreted into the tubular fluid in exchange for Na$^+$ and the latter are reabsorbed into the peritubular blood along with the HCO$_3$$^-$ formed in the cell from the dissociation of carbonic acid. It is likely that active secretion of H$^+$ occurs throughout the nephron.

The fate of the H$^+$ which are secreted into the lumen depends upon the nature of the buffer bases present in the tubular fluid. These are as follows:

(1) filtered HCO$_3$$^-$,

(2) other filtered bases such as dibasic phosphate ion, HPO$_4$$^=$, the hydroxybutyrate ions and creatinine,

(3) ammonia, which is secreted into the tubular fluid by the renal tubular cells.

REABSORPTION OF FILTERED BICARBONATE

The base HCO$_3$$^-$ accepts a proton secreted by the tubular cells and forms its conjugate acid. Carbonic acid

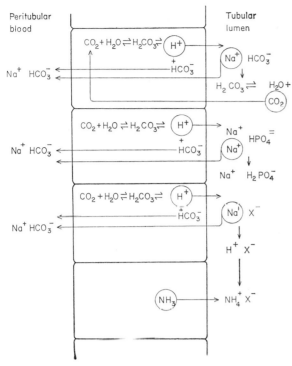

FIG. 35.27. Proposed ion exchange mechanism for secretion of hydrogen ions and reabsorption of sodium.

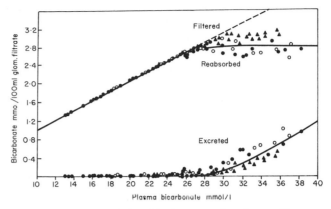

FIG. 35.28. The relationship between the plasma bicarbonate concentration and the rate of reabsorption of bicarbonate ions in normal man. $\blacktriangle$, $\bullet$, $\bigcirc$ represent 3 normal subjects. From Pitts R.F. *et al.* (1949) *J. clin. Invest.* **28**, 35.

is unstable and breaks down to form water and carbon dioxide which is highly diffusible and passes readily out of the tubular lumen into the cells and the bloodstream. Since secretion of H^+ is associated with reabsorption of Na^+ the net effect of this mechanism is the reabsorption of $NaHCO_3$. In man complete reabsorption of filtered HCO_3^- requires secretion of about 3500 mmol of H^+ each 24 hours.

The great majority of HCO_3^- are reabsorbed in the proximal tubule where histochemical techniques have shown the presence of carbonic anhydrase in the brush border of the cells. Exposure of tubular fluid to the enzyme facilitates dehydration of carbonic acid and prevents accumulation of the acid in the lumen. Thus in the proximal tubule luminal $[H^+]$ never rises to high levels and H^+ secretion proceeds against a relatively small gradient.

In 1949 Pitts and his colleagues performed a small number of experiments upon men and dogs to determine the relationship between plasma $[HCO_3^-]$ and the rate of reabsorption of HCO_3^- by the kidney. The results of some of these experiments are shown in fig. 35.28. At low plasma $[HCO_3^-]$ all filtered HCO_3^- are reabsorbed and the urine contains none of this base. Bicarbonate appears in human urine in increasing amounts when the plasma concentration of the ion rises above 28 mmol/l. The amount reabsorbed may be calculated by subtracting the HCO_3^- excreted in the urine from the HCO_3^- filtered. Where plasma $[HCO_3^-]$ is raised by the intra-venous infusion of 150 mmol/l $NaHCO_3$ the amount of HCO_3^- reabsorbed is found to remain approximately constant at a value of 28 mmol/l glomerular filtrate ($Tm_{HCO_3^-}$), i.e.

$$Tm_{HCO_3^-} = (C_{in} \times P_{HCO_3^-}) - U_{HCO_3^-} . V$$

More recently it has been shown that the rate of reabsorption of HCO_3^- is reduced when the volume of ECF is expanded as it was in Pitts' experiments. Doubt, therefore, exists as to whether there is a $Tm_{HCO_3^-}$ when the ECF volume is normal.

FORMATION OF TITRATABLE ACID

When the concentration of HCO_3^- in the tubular fluid falls to very low levels, H^+ secreted into the lumen are taken up by the other bases which are present in the glomerular filtrate and their conjugate acids are formed. The most important of these bases is $HPO_4^=$ which accepts a proton to form its weak conjugate acid, monobasic phosphate ion $H_2PO_4^-$ (pK 6·8). Small numbers of H^+ are accepted by creatinine, but the acid form of creatinine is a relatively strong acid (pK 4·97) and only small amounts can exist in the urine. All the acids formed in this way are stable and accumulate in the tubular fluid so that the pH of the fluid falls. The lowest urinary pH which can be reached is 4·0, and the total number of H^+ which can be secreted into the urine before this limiting value is reached depends upon the total amount of filtered buffer base in the urine and upon the chemical nature of this base. When the conjugate acid formed as a result of the ion exchange process is relatively strong and dissociates readily to give free protons, the limiting value of urinary pH is reached much more rapidly than when the acid is weak. Thus at comparable rates of excretion $HPO_4^=$ is able to accept more protons than creatinine.

The contribution of this buffer mechanism is measured

by determining the amount of strong base which must be added to the urine in order to bring the urinary pH back to 7·4, the pH of the plasma from which the filtrate was derived. This gives a value for the so-called titratable acidity of the urine, which is usually 20–40 mmol of H^+/day. It is important to appreciate that for every molecule of titratable acid excreted one molecule of $NaHCO_3$ is regenerated and reabsorbed into the peritubular blood.

Excretion of ammonium ion

Two-thirds of the H^+ excreted in the urine appear in the form of the extremely weak acid NH_4^+, the ammonium ion, which is formed when the base ammonia, NH_3, accepts a proton. Ammonia is quantitatively the most important urinary buffer and unlike the other proton acceptors in the urine it is not present in significant amounts in the glomerular filtrate but is secreted into the lumen by the tubular cells. Micropuncture studies indicate that, in the rat at least, it is secreted throughout the length of the nephron although most of the NH_3 is added to the urine in the collecting ducts where the pH is lowest. The importance of NH_3 as a urinary buffer lies in the fact that the conjugate acid is very weak indeed (pK 9·47). Even in urine with a pH of 8.0, 90 per cent is present in the form NH_4^+ and when the pH is low very large numbers of H^+ can be accepted by this buffer system. The rate at which NH_3 is secreted into the urine depends on three factors, of which the first is the most important.

(1) The rate at which NH_3 is produced in the renal tubular cells. This is discussed in more detail below but, in general, the more H^+ that need to be excreted, the higher the rate of NH_3 production. It is possible that the concentration of NH_3 in the tubular cells may influence the rate of NH_3 secretion.

(2) The pH of the urine influences the rate of NH_4^+ excretion and the more acid the urine, the more NH_3 is secreted into the tubular fluid.

(3) The rate of urine flow has by itself a small influence on the rate of NH_3 excretion, the amount varying directly with the volume.

MECHANISM OF SECRETION OF AMMONIA INTO URINE

Within the tubular cells the base NH_3 is in equilibrium with the acidic NH_4^+.

$$NH_4^+ \rightleftharpoons NH_3 + H^+$$

Since the pH of the cells is about 7·0, most of the cellular ammonia must exist in the form of the weak acid NH_4^+ and only very small amounts of the free base NH_3 can be present. The cell membrane, however, is less permeable to the charged NH_4^+ than to the uncharged lipid-soluble NH_3 molecule. The NH_3 therefore diffuses readily into and out of the cells, and studies on dogs after infusion of $^{15}NH_4Cl$ into one renal artery show that NH_3 diffuses rapidly throughout the entire kidney forming a freely diffusible pool of base. The distribution of total ammonia, $(NH_3 + NH_4^+)$, between renal tubular cells and tubular fluid or peritubular blood is determined by the differences in pH between these compartments. The accumulation of the NH_4^+ in an acid urine is most easily explained by assuming that the base enters the urine by passive diffusion down a very small concentration gradient. This diffusion continues until the concentration of NH_3 becomes the same in the urine as it is in the interior of the cell. The NH_3 which enters the tubular fluid, where the pH is lower than that in the cells, is largely converted to the weak acid NH_4^+. This acid is then trapped in the tubular fluid because the cell membrane is relatively impermeable to it. Thus while the concentration of the base NH_3 in the tubular fluid is equal to that in the cells, the concentration of the acid NH_4^+ in the cell fluid and in the urine are entirely different because they are determined by the relative concentrations of the H^+ in these fluids. This is an example of the process known as **non-ionic diffusion** or **diffusion trapping** and a number of experiments prove that NH_3 is added to the urine by this means. One such experiment is illustrated in fig. 35.29.

A small volume of fluid containing creatinine and ammonium lactate is injected rapidly into one renal artery of a dog with metabolic acidosis and the times at which the two substances appear in the urine determined. Since, in the dog, creatinine is filtered by the glomeruli and neither reabsorbed nor secreted by the tubules, the appearance of NH_4^+ in the urine before the appearance of creatinine indicates that NH_3 is added to the tubular fluid downstream from the glomeruli. When the experiment is repeated using the same animal made alkalotic by infusion of $NaHCO_3$, essentially none of the administered NH_3 appears in the alkaline urine. Clearly the filtered NH_3 must have diffused from the alkaline tubular fluid into the less alkaline peritubular blood. These experiments show that NH_3 diffuses rapidly across the tubular epithelium and that the direction of diffusion is determined by the $[H^+]$ gradient.

PRODUCTION OF AMMONIA BY THE RENAL TUBULAR CELLS

In 1921, Nash and Benedict showed that the concentration of ammonia in renal venous blood exceeded that in renal arterial blood and postulated that the kidney formed NH_4^+ from some precursor in the arterial blood and that this NH_3 was then added both to the urine and to the blood in the renal vein. Support for this idea was derived from the fact that the concentration of NH_4^+ in renal arterial blood is not only far too low to account for the amount of this substance excreted but also does not increase in acidotic animals at a time when they are excreting large amounts of NH_4^+.

In 1943, Van Slyke and his colleagues noted that during the passage of blood through the kidney glutamine was

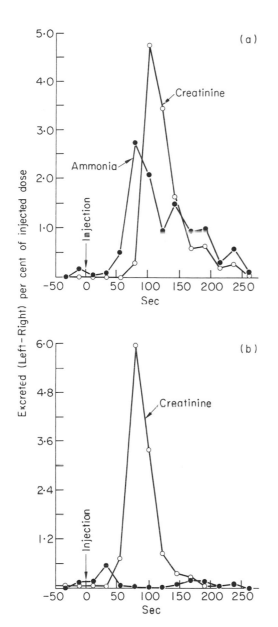

Fig. 35.29. Time courses of the urinary excretion of NH_4^+ and creatinine after their rapid injection into one renal artery of a dog. (a) In chronic metabolic acidosis, urine samples acid; (b) in acute metabolic alkalosis, urine samples alkaline. From Pitts R.F. (1973). In *Handbook of Physiology*, Section 8, Renal Physiology, p. 467, ed. Orloff J. & Berliner R.W. Washington, D.C: Amer. Physiol. Soc.

removed from the blood to a greater extent than other amino acids. The kidney contains an enzyme glutaminase I which is capable of hydrolysing glutamine to form glutamic acid and ammonia,

$$COOHCH(NH_2)CH_2CH_2CONH_2 + H_2O \xrightarrow{\text{glutaminase I}}$$

$$COOHCH(NH_2)CH_2CH_2COOH + NH_3$$

and these workers calculated that almost two-thirds of the urinary NH_4^+ could be derived in this way from the amide nitrogen of glutamine.

Pitts and his colleagues performed experiments upon dogs with metabolic acidosis in which tracer amounts of glutamine, having the amide nitrogen labelled with ^{15}N were infused into one renal artery. Examination of the urine from the infused kidneys shows that 33–50 per cent of the urinary NH_4^+ contained ^{15}N and must have been derived from the amide nitrogen of plasma glutamine. Similar studies using glutamine with a ^{15}N label in the amino group showed that 16–25 per cent of urinary NH_4^+ was derived from the amino nitrogen of glutamine. A number of other amino acids have been shown to be capable of increasing the rate of NH_4^+ excretion when they are infused, and since the dog's kidney does not contain any significant amount of L-amino acid oxidase the NH_3 cannot be derived from simple oxidative deamination of the amino acids. In all probability the role of such acids, whether they reach the tubules by the blood stream or are reabsorbed from the glomerular filtrate, is to supply amino groups to a nitrogen pool in the tubular cells. A small amount of the NH_4^+ in the urine is derived from pre-formed NH_3 delivered to the kidney in arterial blood.

It is possible to determine the overall rate at which amide and amino nitrogen are extracted by the kidney from the renal arterial blood and also the rate at which NH_3 is added to the urine and to the blood in the renal vein. In dogs with acidosis the rate at which amino and amide nitrogen are removed from plasma is approximately equal to the rate of NH_3 production.

Fig. 35.30 shows some of the metabolic pathways which are likely to be involved in the formation of NH_3 in the renal tubular cells. It has been proposed that the immediate source of NH_3 is glutamine and that this substance is split by glutaminase I to yield glutamate and NH_3. Since glutamate appears neither in the urine nor in the renal venous blood it must undergo further chemical change. At least two possibilities exist; glutamate may be broken down by L-glutamate dehydrogenase to form 2-oxoglutarate and NH_3, the keto acid being subsequently oxidized in the citric acid cycle or else reacting with a 2-amino acid to resynthesize glutamate. Alternatively glutamate may undergo transamination reacting with a 2-keto acid to produce the corresponding 2-amino acid and 2-oxoglutarate.

$$COOHCHNH_2CH_2CH_2COOH + RCOCOOH$$

$$\rightleftharpoons COOHCOCH_2CH_2COOH$$

$$+ RCHNH_2COOH$$

The kidney however contains a second glutaminase, glutaminase II, and under the influence of this enzyme which consists of two components, a transaminase and an

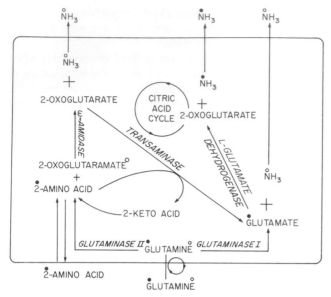

FIG. 35.30. A simplified version of the major metabolic paths involved in the production of ammonia by the renal tubular cells. Glutamine enters the tubular cell from the blood (bottom of fig.) and ammonia is secreted by the cell into the tubular urine (top of fig.). ● represents amino N, ○ amide N. from Pitts R.F. (1964) *Amer. J. Med.* 36, 733.

ω-amidase, glutamine may react with a 2-keto acid to form 2-oxoglutaramate which cannot be detected in the cells because it is rapidly deaminated by the ω-amidase to form 2-oxoglutarate and NH_3.

FACTORS WHICH INFLUENCE THE RATE OF PRODUCTION OF AMMONIA

When an acidifying salt such as ammonium chloride is given to a normal subject the rate of excretion of H^+ in the form of NH_4^+ and titratable acid is increased. If, however, the ammonium chloride is given for several successive days the rate of excretion of NH_4^+ rises progressively while the excretion of titratable acid and the urine pH remain the same. The kidney adapts to the stimulus of chronic acidosis by producing more NH_3.

How NH_3 production is increased in chronic acidosis is not fully understood. The amount of glutamine reaching the kidney in arterial blood does not increase significantly in acidosis so that changes in renal metabolism must be critical. Since the rate of production of NH_3 by kidney slices is increased when the pH of the bathing medium is reduced, it is possible, though unlikely, that acidosis stimulates uptake of glutamine by renal tubular cells or facilitates its passage into mitochondria where glutaminase I is located.

In certain species the activity of glutaminase I in renal tissue increases in acidosis but this is not true of all mammals. Moreover, acidotic rats excrete increased amounts of NH_4^+ when the adaptive increase in glutaminase I which

normally occurs in this condition is prevented by giving actinomycin D.

The activity of glutaminase I is inhibited by glutamate so that any change in cellular metabolism which reduces the concentration of this substance would facilitate NH_3 production. There are several ways in which this might happen. Acidosis stimulates gluconeogenesis and oxidation of 2-oxoglutarate and both of these changes reduce the tissue concentrations of 2-oxoglutarate and thus facilitate breakdown of glutamate by L-glutamate dehydrogenase (fig. 35.30). In the rat, acute metabolic acidosis is associated with a fall in the concentration of glutamate in renal tissue. This occurs within 4 h of administration of the acidifying dose of NH_4Cl at a time when NH_4^+ excretion is increasing, but before there is any evidence of increased gluconeogenesis. When glutamate is converted by L-glutamate dehydrogenase to 2-oxoglutarate and NH_3, NAD is required as a coenzyme. The reverse reaction utilizes $NADH_2$ (p. 11.20). The drop in renal glutamate concentration which occurs early in acidosis is likely to be due to the increase in the ratio $NAD/NADH_2$ which has been demonstrated in these circumstances and which occurs also in chronic acidosis.

Other factors which might alter the activity of the enzymes concerned in NH_3 production are changes in cell $[H^+]$ or $[K^+]$.

Total H^+ secretion

In summary, the total amount of H^+ secreted by the renal tubules may be calculated from the sum of the urinary NH_4^+, titratable acid (TA) and reabsorbed bicarbonate.

$$\text{Total } H^+ \text{ secretion} = U_{TA}V + U_{NH_4^+}.V \\ + \{(C_{in} \times P_{HCO_3^-}) - U_{HCO_3^-}.V\}$$

The total urinary excretion of H^+ is given by the sum of the titratable acid and ammonium ion.

$$\text{Total } H^+ \text{ excretion} = U_{TA}V + U_{NH_4^+}.V$$

In order to calculate the net urinary loss of H^+ from the body it is customary to subtract the amount of HCO_3^- excreted in the urine from the total H^+ excreted since the excretion of one HCO_3^- is equivalent to the addition of H^+ to the body fluid.

Net urinary loss of H^+ from body =
$$U_{TA}V + U_{NH_4^+}.V - U_{HCO_3^-}.V.$$

Factors which influence the rate of secretion of hydrogen ions

It is likely that active secretion of H^+ occurs throughout the nephron; certainly the H^+ observed in proximal tubular fluid and in the lumen of the collecting duct cannot be accounted for solely by the observed transtubular PD. Nevertheless the rate of H^+ secretion can be influenced by transtubular PD, possibly because the H^+

in tubular fluid depends upon a balance between an active secretory mechanism, situated in the luminal membrane of the renal tubular cells and passive back diffusion which is influenced by transtubular PD. Little is known about the concomitant transport of HCO_3^- from the cell to the peritubular blood which probably results from passive diffusion down an electrochemical gradient.

CHLORIDE BALANCE

Filtered Na^+ are reabsorbed by the tubules along with Cl^- or 'in exchange' for K^+ or H^+. For all practical purposes the rate of reabsorption of Na^+ is equal to the sum of the rates of reabsorption of Cl^- (about 14 400 mmol/day) and of secretion of H^+ (about 3600 mmol/day); the amount of K^+ secreted is of a lower order, rarely exceeding 200 mmol/day. When the concentration of Cl^- in the filtrate is reduced a larger proportion of Na^+ is reabsorbed by the ion exchange mechanism. Reabsorption of Na^+ unaccompanied by Cl^- increases the distal transtubular PD and the rate of diffusion of positively charged H^+ down this electrochemical gradient is increased so that reabsorption of HCO_3^- and the formation of an acid urine proceed at an accelerated rate. The importance of this is seen in patients who are depleted of water, Na^+, Cl^- and H^+ because of persistent vomiting of gastric juice. Loss of gastric HCl induces a state of metabolic alkalosis (p. 6.7) with a low plasma $[Cl^-]$. As a result of the loss of Na^+ and water in vomitus, the volume of the ECF is reduced, Na^+ conserving mechanisms are stimulated (p. 35.22), renal reabsorption of filtered Na^+ is increased and Na^+ virtually disappears from the urine. Since the filtered load of Cl^- is reduced an abnormally high proportion of filtered Na^+ is reabsorbed 'in exchange' for H^+. Consequently, the rate of reabsorption of HCO_3^- remains fixed at an unusually high level and the plasma HCO_3^- remains elevated. The vicious circle induced by a combination of Na^+ and Cl^- depletion can be broken by infusing a solution of NaCl, thereby expanding the ECF, reducing the stimulus for Na^+ absorption and simultaneously providing Cl^-. This suppresses H^+ secretion, increases the excretion of HCO_3^- in the urine and restores plasma $[HCO_3^-]$.

NATURE OF THE ANIONS IN DISTAL TUBULAR FLUID

The rate at which H^+ accumulate in the distal tubular fluid is increased when the latter contains anions such as $SO_4^=$ and $HPO_4^=$ which are not readily reabsorbed. The presence of these negatively charged particles in the lumen increases the transtubular PD and probably inhibits passive back diffusion of H^+.

POTASSIUM BALANCE

Potassium-depleted subjects usually have an extracellular alkalosis with an increased plasma $[HCO_3^-]$ (vol. 3, p.49.25). The high plasma $[HCO_3^-]$ must be maintained an by abnormally high rate of HCO_3^- reabsorption, i.e. an increased rate of H^+ secretion. Conversely, administration of K^+ salts is associated with diminished reabsorption of HCO_3^-. Thus, the rates of secretion of K^+ and H^+ appear to be inversely related and micropuncture studies suggest that this relationship holds for both proximal and distal tubules. Since K^+ is not itself secreted in the proximal tubule the original idea that these ions compete for a common secretory pathway is no longer tenable. However, the ratio of $[K^+]$ to $[H^+]$ in the renal tubular cells may be an important determinant of their relative rates of secretion.

P_{CO_2}

It has frequently been observed that when the P_{CO_2} of the arterial blood is elevated, as it is in certain forms of chronic respiratory disease, the plasma $[HCO_3^-]$ becomes stabilized at a higher level than normal. Experiments on dogs have shown that an increase in P_{CO_2} is associated with an increase in the rate of reabsorption of HCO_3^- by the kidney and increased excretion of H^+ mainly as NH_4^+. This increased secretion of protons is maintained even when steps are taken to prevent the fall in pH which normally accompanies the rise in P_{CO_2}. Conversely a reduction in P_{CO_2} is associated with a reduction in H^+ secretion. Carbon dioxide penetrates cells rapidly and the $[H^+]$ within the renal tubular cells must be influenced by the P_{CO_2}. It seems probable that active transport of H^+ into the tubular fluid is dependent upon the intracellular $[H^+]$.

CARBONIC ANHYDRASE INHIBITORS

Substances such as acetazolamide which inhibit the action of carbonic anhydrase interfere with the secretion of H^+. Acidification of the urine and the reabsorption of HCO_3^- are therefore reduced and the urine contains increased amounts of $NaHCO_3$ (vol. 2, p. 11.6).

ADRENOCORTICAL STEROIDS

Hormones of the adrenal cortex which increase the reabsorption of Na^+ may also be necessary for normal rates of H^+ secretion in the distal nephron.

DIURNAL RHYTHMS

Studies of renal function in man tend to fall into two categories, acute observations lasting for a few hours and prolonged studies of several days' duration during which all the urine excreted during each 24-hour period is pooled for analysis. If, however, the urine is collected at 3 or 4-hourly intervals for a period of several days, rhythmical changes in volume and composition can be detected and when the rates of excretion of substances such as sodium, potassium, chloride and phosphate are plotted against time a cyclical pattern with a mean period of 24 hours emerges. This phenomenon has been named the circadian (*circa diem*) or diurnal rhythm, and its existence has been recognized for more than a hundred years, but the factors controlling the cyclical changes in renal function are by no means clear. A general account of biological rhythms is given in chap. 47.

FURTHER READING

DALTON A.J. & HAGUENAU F. eds. (1967) *Ultrastructure of the Kidney*. New York: Academic Press.

DENTON D.A. (1965) Evolutionary aspects of the emergence of aldosterone secretion and salt appetite. *Physiological Reviews* **45**, 245–295.

DICKER S.E. (1970) *Mechanisms of Urinary Concentration and Dilution in Mammals*. London: Arnold.

FISHER J. ed. (1971) *Renal Pharmacology*. New York: Appleton.

FOURMAN J. & MOFFAT D.B. (1971) *Blood Vessels of the Kidney*. Oxford: Blackwell Scientific Publications.

McGIFF J.C. & ITSKOVITZ H.D. (1973) Prostaglandins and the kidney. *Circulation Research* **33**, 479–488.

MILLS J.N. (1963) Mechanisms of renal homeostasis. Other aspects of renal function. In *Recent Advances in Physiology*, 8th Edition, chaps 8 and 9, pp. 252–294; 295–329, ed. Creese, R. London: Churchill.

ORLOFF J. & BERLINER R.W. eds. (1973) *Handbook of Physiology*, Section 8, Renal Physiology. Washington, D.C.: Amer. Physiol. Soc.

PITTS R.F. (1974) *Physiology of the Kidney and Body Fluids*, 3rd Edition. Chicago: Year Book Medical Publishers.

ROUILLER C. & MULLER A. eds. (1971) *The Kidney: Morphology, Biochemistry, Physiology*. New York: Academic Press.

WESSON L.G. (1969) *Physiology of the Human Kidney*. New York: Grune & Stratton.

WILLIAMS P.C. ed. (1963) *Hormones and the Kidney*. Memoirs of the Society for Endocrinology No. 13. London: Academic Press.

WINDHAGER E.E. (1968) *Micropuncture Techniques and Nephron Function*. London: Butterworths.

Chapter 36
Urinary tract

The urinary tract extends from the minor calyces of the kidney to the external meatus of the urethra and can be divided into two parts. The upper part conveys urine from the collecting tubules of the kidney to the bladder and consists of the major and minor calyces and pelvis of the kidney, and the ureter. The lower part which stores and intermittently expels urine consists of the bladder and the urethra. In the male the urethra also has a reproductive function.

DEVELOPMENT OF THE KIDNEY AND LOWER URINARY TRACT

Three structures, the **pronephros**, the **mesonephros** and the **metanephros** successively take part in the development of the urinary tract, and in mammals the last of these is retained as the permanent kidney (fig. 36.1). The development of the urinary and genital tracts is closely related and a full account of the development of the reproductive system is given on p. 38.57.

The mesoderm of the intermediate cell mass below the level of the eighth somite is called the **nephrogenic cord**. In the 23-day-old embryo a clump of cells appears in this cord at the level of the ninth somite. These proliferate and spread caudally forming a solid cord which reaches and fuses with the cloaca. At the cranial end a lumen develops and gradually extends throughout the cord to open into the cloaca about the twenty-eighth day of intra-uterine life, thus forming the **nephric duct**. In some species, but not in man, vesicles appear in the cervicodorsal region of the embryo dorsal to the upper end of the primary excretory duct and connect this duct to the coelomic cavity; this is the pronephros.

The mesonephros develops caudal to the pronephros and consists of clusters of cells in the nephrogenic cord, each of which becomes a vesicle and communicates with the nephric duct, now called the **mesonephric duct**; the vesicle itself dilates and is invaginated to form a glomerulus. The glomerular capillaries arise from proliferation of these invaginated cells and are supplied with blood from lateral branches of the aorta. Some seventy to eighty mesonephric vesicles form but no more than thirty or

forty are present at any one time because the cranial ones degenerate and disappear before the more caudal ones form.

By the time the mesonephros has developed to its

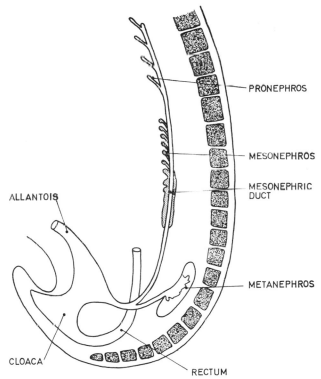

FIG. 36.1. Development of kidneys.

caudal limit, the cranial two-thirds of the tubules have degenerated and by the beginning of the 10th week few intact mesonephric tubules remain. Remnants of a number of these tubules do nevertheless persist to become part of the duct system of the testis. Some of these link up with the rete testis and form the efferent ductules of that organ. The corresponding set of tubules in the female form the epoöphoron. Others become separated from the mesonephric duct and form the paradidymis in the male and the paroöphoron in the female.

The metanephros, which becomes the permanent kidney, develops from two sources, the mesonephric duct

36.1

and the metanephrogenic cap (fig. 36.2). When the embryo is 5 weeks old, an outgrowth called the **ureteric bud** arises from the mesonephric duct near its entry into the cloaca and grows into the mesoderm of the caudal end of the nephrogenic cord. The ureteric bud becomes the ureter and its cephalic end expands to form the pelvis, calyces and the collecting tubules of the kidney.

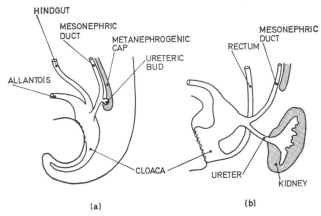

FIG. 36.2. Development of metanephros.

The mesoderm which surrounds the expanded end of the ureteric bud condenses to become the **metanephrogenic cap** from which the remainder of the kidney develops. Vesicles appear and elongate to form metanephric tubules which enlarge and convolute; one end of each tubule fuses with the collecting ducts and the other is associated with a tuft of capillaries and becomes a glomerulus. After the metanephros has developed, the cranial portion of the mesonephric duct is superfluous and is available for incorporation into the genital apparatus (p. 38.62).

Each normal adult kidney contains approximately one million glomeruli at birth. Increase in the size of the kidney after birth is the result of hypertrophy and not of hyperplasia, i.e. it is due to an increase in the size and not the number of the nephrons.

At first the kidney lies in the pelvis but as the ureteric bud lengthens it gradually ascends and rotates to reach its adult position in the loin. It obtains blood from neighbouring vessels, which are the common iliac and median sacral arteries while it is in the pelvis, and from one of the adrenal arteries while it is in the loin until the renal artery appears in the third month. The kidney is a lobulated organ until the end of the first year of extra-uterine life.

The origin of the ureter moves from the dorsomedial to the lateral aspect of the mesonephric duct and the caudal end of this duct shifts downwards to be incorporated within the bladder. Thus the ureter comes to open directly into the bladder, lateral to the opening of the mesonephric duct. Because the mesonephric duct

continues to grow downwards the ureteric orifices gradually separate and eventually the mesonephric duct opens into the prostatic urethra (fig. 36.3).

A double ureter on one or both sides is one of many congenital malformations that may be found in the urinary tract. It occurs when two buds instead of one ureteric bud arise from the mesonephric duct. Because this duct shifts downwards the upper bud which forms

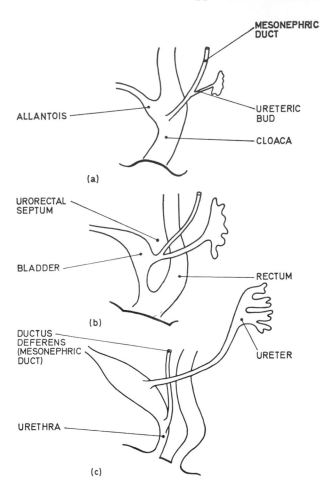

FIG. 36.3. Diagram to show development of ureter and ductus deferens.

the upper renal pelvis eventually opens into the bladder below the bud which forms the lower pelvis (fig. 36.4).

The bladder is formed mainly from that part of the primitive urogenital sinus which lies above the mesonephric ducts, namely the vesico-urethral canal. In addition the absorbed caudal part of the mesonephric ducts form the bladder trigone and the dorsal wall of the prostatic urethra in the male and the trigone and most of the urethra in the female. The allantois passes from the ventral aspect of the urogenital sinus into the body stalk and later becomes the urachus which connects the bladder to the umbilicus. It persists into adult life as a fibrous cord called the median umbilical ligament

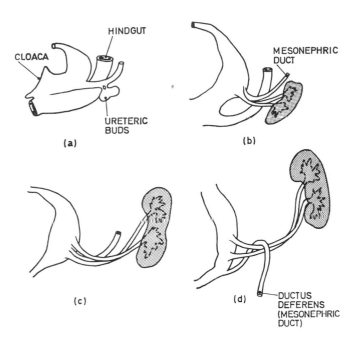

FIG. 36.4. Scheme of development when two ureters appear instead of one. (a) Two ureteric buds develop from the mesonephric duct. (b) Each bud elongates to form a pelvis and calyces inside the metanephrogenic cap. (c) The origin of the upper bud is carried below that of the lower bud as the mesonephric duct descends. (d) The ureter draining the upper pelvis enters the bladder below that draining the lower. Both are crossed by the ductus deferens.

Sometimes, however, its lumen does not disappear and then urine may leak from the umbilicus.

RENAL PELVIS, CALYCES AND URETER

The collecting tubules within the renal medulla drain into the minor calyces through the collecting ducts, sixteen to twenty of which open on to the surface of each renal papilla. There are usually six minor calyces but there may be as few as four or as many as thirteen. Several join together to form two or three major calyces and these, in turn, unite to form the renal pelvis which is the expanded upper part of the ureter (fig. 35.1).

The ureters are two narrow, thick-walled, muscular tubes which start from the renal pelvis, descend through the abdomen and pelvis and open into the base of the bladder. At first the ureter lies retroperitoneally on psoas major which separates it from the tips of the lumbar transverse processes, and is crossed by the testicular or ovarian vessels. It then enters the pelvis by crossing in front of either the common iliac vessels or the origin of the external iliac vessels from the common iliacs, and runs downwards in extraperitoneal tissue on the lateral wall of the pelvis as far as the ischial spine where, turning forward, it runs on the superior surface of the levator ani to the bladder. In the male it is crossed by the ductus deferens, and in the female it is very closely related to the uterine artery, the cervix of the uterus and the lateral fornix of the vagina (figs. 38.1 and 38.22).

The calyces, pelvis and ureter each have three coats. *The mucous coat* is smooth and contrary to what the term suggests is devoid of glands. Over the renal papillae it is a simple, cuboidal epithelium and is perforated by the openings of the collecting ducts; elsewhere it is transitional epithelium (plate 35.1b, facing p. 35.12).
The muscular coat is smooth or involuntary muscle. In the calyces, the renal pelvis and the upper two-thirds of the ureters it is arranged in two layers, an inner longitudinal and an outer circular layer. The lower third of the ureter has an additional layer of longitudinal fibres outside the circular layer but where it pierces the wall of the bladder it retains only a longitudinal layer.
The fibrous coat or adventitia is continuous above with the renal capsule and below with the fascia on the surface of the bladder.

Blood supply and lymphatic drainage

The calyces and renal pelvis receive blood from the renal artery and return it to the renal vein. The ureter derives blood from the renal artery, lumbar arteries, testicular or ovarian arteries, common and internal iliac arteries, the vesical arteries and the uterine arteries, each supplying the adjacent part of the ureter. The lymphatics follow the veins draining the same part.

Ureterovesical junction

The ureterovesical junction allows urine to pass freely from the ureters into the bladder but prevents it from passing in the opposite direction. It does so by reason of its anatomical disposition rather than by neuromuscular activity. In fact since the muscle around the intramural part of the ureter is longitudinal it widens and shortens when it contracts and so cannot function as a sphincter. The ureters pass obliquely through the wall of the bladder, and whereas they are 10 cm apart as they enter the bladder, they are only 5 cm apart when they open into the cavity. Their obliquity is increased as the bladder fills or contracts; in this way reflux of urine from the bladder into the ureter is prevented. Mucosal folds form where the mucosa of the ureter becomes continuous with that of the bladder and are important in preventing reflux in some animals but not, apparently, in man. The junction between the ureters and the bladder is of considerable clinical importance because of the relationship between recurrent urinary tract infection and the reflux of urine from the bladder into the ureters.

BLADDER

The bladder is a hollow muscular organ whose shape, size and relations vary with the amount of urine it contains. When empty it lies in the pelvis. It has a tetrahedral shape and possesses a superior and two inferolateral surfaces, a base, a neck and an apex. The superior surface is triangular in shape and is completely covered by peritoneum, which separates it from loops of ileum and the sigmoid colon. However, in the female a tiny area posteriorly is left uncovered as the peritoneum is reflected on to the anterior aspect of the junction of the body and cervix of the uterus. The inferolateral surfaces are separated by loose areolar tissue from the levator ani muscle of the pelvis posteriorly, and by the puboprostatic or pubovesical ligaments from the pubis anteriorly. The apex points forwards and continues into the median umbilical ligament which runs over the back of the anterior abdominal wall to the umbilicus. The base is triangular and faces backwards and downwards and is related in the female to the uterine cervix and anterior wall of the vagina and in the male to the rectovesical fold of peritoneum superiorly and the seminal vesicles and the two ductus deferentes inferiorly which separate it from the rectum. The neck is the lowest part of the bladder and is pierced by the internal meatus of the urethra. It is continuous with the base of the prostate in the male (fig. 38.22) and with the loose pelvic fascia around the urethra in the female.

As the bladder fills it becomes egg shaped and expands upwards and forwards into the abdomen, pushing the peritoneum upwards and stripping it away from the anterior abdominal wall.

Interior of the bladder

When the bladder is empty its mucous membrane lies in longitudinal folds which gradually disappear as the bladder fills. The trigone is the triangular area bounded by the ureteric orifices and bladder neck. There the mucosa is firmly attached to the underlying muscle and is always smooth. The orifices of the ureters vary in appearance but are usually slit-like. They open into the bladder at the posterolateral angles of the trigone and are separated by the interureteric bar which is the base of the trigone. The internal urethral orifice, which is crescentic in shape, lies at the apex of the trigone.

Structure

The bladder consists of three coats.
The serosal or peritoneal coat is found only on the superior surface and has already been described.
The muscular coat is sometimes called the detrusor muscle. It is smooth muscle and consists of an internal and an external layer of longitudinal fibres and a middle layer of circular fibres. The layers intermingle with one another extensively. At the bladder neck the muscle

fibres run longitudinally and are not circularly disposed (fig. 36.5). Thus, there is really no internal sphincter, although this is frequently described. They pass through the bladder neck and surround the urethra as far as its membranous part in the male, and to within 0·5 cm of the external urethral meatus in the female. The muscle around the bladder neck contracts when the muscle of the bladder itself contracts, but being longitudinal it shortens and widens the lumen of the neck and urethra and thus allows urine to enter the urethra. When the bladder is relaxed the longitudinal muscle around the bladder neck is also relaxed. The urethra contains no urine except during micturition because its anterior and posterior walls are apposed. This is not due to contraction of

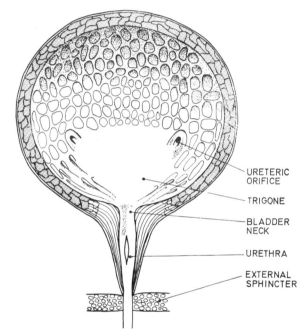

FIG. 36.5. Coronal section of bladder showing disposition of muscle at bladder neck.

a muscle sphincter around the bladder neck but results from the tension of elastic fibres which are liberally scattered between the fibres of the urethral muscle. It is also caused by the inherent tone of the urethral muscle, and by the activity of the external sphincter of the urethra. Thus, the urethra proximal to the external sphincter is naturally closed and neuromuscular activity opens but does not close it. The external sphincter is striated muscle. *The mucosal coat* is transitional epithelium and is fixed over the trigone. In the subtrigonal and subcervical region some glands are found but they are probably prostatic in origin.

Blood supply

The bladder is supplied mainly by the superior and inferior vesical arteries, but it also receives small branches from the gluteal and obturator arteries and, in the female, from the uterine and vaginal arteries. Venous blood drains into the large venous plexus around the bladder neck and the prostate and then into the internal iliac veins. The lymph vessels run alongside the veins to lymph nodes around the internal iliac vessels.

URETHRA

The urethra extends from the neck of the bladder to the external meatus. The male and female urethra are so different that they are separately described.

MALE URETHRA

This consists of a prostatic, a membranous and a spongy part and is about 20 cm long (fig. 36.6). The prostatic urethra pierces the prostate gland from its base to its apex and is the widest and the most distensible part. Its transverse section is made crescentic by a longitudinal ridge on the posterior wall called the urethral crest. On

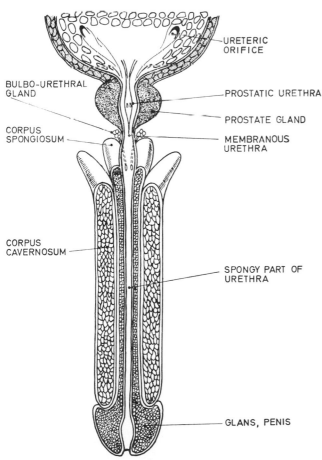

FIG. 36.6. Male urethra laid open.

BULBO-URETHRAL GLAND

CORPUS SPONGIOSUM

CORPUS CAVERNOSUM

URETERIC ORIFICE

PROSTATIC URETHRA

PROSTATE GLAND

MEMBRANOUS URETHRA

SPONGY PART OF URETHRA

GLANS, PENIS

either side of this crest is a gutter called the prostatic sulcus into which the prostatic glands open. At about the middle of the urethral crest is an eminence called the **colliculus seminalis**, on each side of which lies the opening of the ejaculatory duct and on its summit is a slit which is the opening of a cul-de-sac, the **prostatic utricle** (fig. 38.27).

The membranous urethra is the shortest, the least distensible and, after the external meatus itself, the narrowest portion of the male urethra. It perforates the urogenital diaphragm and is surrounded by the external urethral sphincter. This is a striated muscle and forms part of the urogenital diaphragm as it surrounds the membranous urethra (p. 21.33).

The spongy portion of the urethra is about 15 cm long and is contained in the **corpus spongiosum** of the **penis**. It extends from the inferior fascia of the urogenital diaphragm to the external urethral meatus. It varies in diameter, being widest at its start in the intrabulbar fossa and just before the external urethral meatus; the external meatus is the narrowest part of the whole urethra.

Structure

The transitional epithelium of the bladder continues through the bladder neck and lines the urethra as far as the opening of the ejaculatory ducts where it changes to a stratified columnar epithelium. Near the external urethral meatus the epithelium becomes stratified squamous and continuous with the skin of the glans penis.

The subepithelial layer is vascular erectile tissue and contains many mucous glands which open into the lumen of the urethra. The smooth muscular layer is longitudinally disposed and is continuous above with the detrusor of the bladder and extends distally as far as the membranous urethra where it is replaced and partly surrounded by the striated muscle of the external urethral sphincter.

FEMALE URETHRA

The female urethra is straight and only 4 cm long. It begins at the neck of the bladder and runs downwards and forwards. It is embedded in the anterior wall of the vagina and perforates the urogenital diaphragm where it is also enclosed by the external sphincter muscle. It ends anterior to the vaginal orifice as the external urethral meatus (fig. 38.5).

Structure

The mucosa is transitional epithelium near the bladder and stratified squamous epithelium elsewhere. The smooth muscle fibres which surround the urethra except for its last 1 cm are longitudinally disposed and continuous above with those of the bladder. Interspersed between the muscle fibres are many circular elastic fibres which help to keep the walls of the urethra apposed except when urine is passing. The striated muscle fibres of the external urethral sphincter surround the terminal part of the urethra and mix with the distal smooth muscle fibres. A layer of spongy, erectile tissue and veins lies between mucosa and muscle coat.

FUNCTION OF THE LOWER URINARY TRACT

The flow of urine from the kidney down the ureter and into the bladder is caused by the co-ordinated contractions of the muscle coats of the urinary tract. Just as food is pushed down the oesophagus and along the bowel by peristalsis, so also is urine moved down the urinary tract. Gravity assists the flow and the kidneys do not empty as quickly in the supine position. The contraction wave starts in the circular muscle fibres of the minor calyces of the kidneys and spreads through the muscle fibres of the major calyces, pelvis and ureter, propelling urine downwards to the longitudinal muscle fibres of the lowest part of the ureter, which widen the lumen so that urine enters the bladder. That the contraction wave starts in the minor calyces and moves progressively downwards suggests the presence of a pacemaker which has not been identified. The efferent autonomic nerve fibres that can be demonstrated in the wall of the ureter supply only the muscle of the arterioles. The smooth muscle of the ureter has no motor nerve supply and contains no nerve plexuses. The contraction of this muscle and the propagation of the contraction wave result from inherent properties of the muscle fibres themselves.

If the ureter is obstructed acutely, e.g. by a calculus, a severe pain known as **renal** or **ureteric colic** occurs (vol. 3, p. 22.58). The pain is due to a rapid rise in intraluminal pressure which causes the ureteric muscle to be stretched. Ureteric pain is referred to somatic segments T11, T12 and L1.

MICTURITION

This is a complex act involving both autonomic and somatic nerves and is normally controlled by higher centres. It is one of the few visceral reflexes over which there is any conscious control. Three sets of nerves are involved.

The parasympathetic nerves travel to the bladder with the pelvic splanchnic nerves from the 2nd, 3rd and sometimes the 4th sacral segment. They emerge from the sacral foramina and pass through the pelvic plexus to the bladder and are the main motor nerves to the detrusor muscle. Afferent fibres also travel in the pelvic splanchnic nerves; these pass upwards in the ventral columns of the spinal cord and convey the sensation of the desire to micturate.

The sympathetic fibres come from the hypogastric plexus which lies anterior to the body of the fifth lumbar vertebra and join the pelvic plexus. Experimental stimulation of the sympathetic fibres in man may cause closure of the ureteric orifices and increase the tone in the trigone, but these effects play little, if any, part in normal micturition. Afferent fibres travel with the sympathetic fibres and enter the dorsal horn of the spinal cord in the midthoracic region; they travel upwards in the lateral spinothalamic tract and from the thalamus impulses are relayed to the upper part of the postcentral gyrus. These fibres carry sensation, not of normal bladder filling, but of abnormal stimuli like overdistension or spasm.

The somatic nerves are the efferent and afferent components of the pudendal nerves (S2, 3 and 4) and consist of the efferent nerves to the external sphincter of the urethra and the afferent nerves from the posterior urethra which are stimulated by distension.

The sacral 2nd, 3rd and 4th segments of the spinal cord are the site of the spinal reflex for micturition and the parasympathetic and pudendal nerves derive from it. It

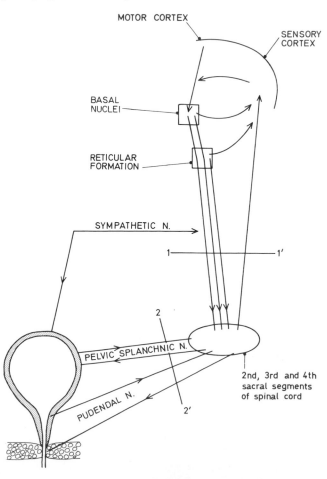

FIG. 36.7. Nerve supply of bladder. Section of spinal cord 1–1′ leads to an automatic bladder; lesions at 2–2′ lead to an autonomous bladder.

connects with the higher centres by afferent and efferent pathways and is greatly influenced by them (fig. 36.7).

There is no sensation of bladder distension until it contains between 300 and 400 ml, when the need to micturate is felt. Although this can be temporarily suppressed, it soon returns and eventually becomes so strong and urgent that it must be obeyed. Once micturition starts it continues until the bladder is empty although the stream can be temporarily interrupted by voluntary contraction of the external urethral sphincter. Micturition can be started by voluntary effort, even though there is too little urine in the bladder to produce the sensation of the need to pass water.

The response of the bladder to filling can be studied by measuring the intravesical pressure produced in response to changes in bladder volume. This procedure (cystometry) is carried out by inserting a two-way catheter into the bladder through the urethra. The bladder is emptied and one limb of the catheter is connected to a reservoir of sterile water and the other to a recording manometer. Fluid is slowly run into the bladder from the reservoir and the intravesical pressure recorded continuously. Cystometry (fig. 36.8) shows that after a small

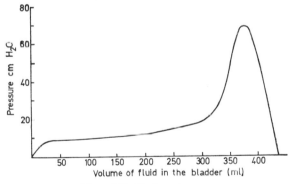

Fig. 36.8. Cystometrogram.

initial increase in pressure, the normal bladder accommodates increasing volumes of fluid with little, if any, change in pressure. When the volume of fluid inside the bladder exceeds 300 ml there is a small rise in pressure and the desire to micturate is experienced. If this is suppressed the pressure falls, but if micturition is allowed to proceed a marked rise in pressure follows. The ability to tolerate an increase in volume without a corresponding increase in pressure indicates progressive relaxation of the bladder wall. This is largely an effect of the properties of the muscle fibres but neuromuscular activity may contribute in the following manner. As the bladder fills, impulses pass from the stretch receptors in its wall, along the afferent fibres in the pelvic splanchnic nerves to the spinal cord. These would increase the excitatory state of the centre if they were not suppressed by inhibitory impulses from higher motor centres. When

the bladder holds 300 or 400 ml of urine the intensity of these impulses overcomes the inhibition and they ascend to the sensory part of the cerebral cortex and the need to micturate is experienced. If it is socially inconvenient the desire can be suppressed because the higher centres can temporarily inhibit the spinal reflex. Otherwise the cortex lifts the inhibitory influences and micturition is initiated through a series of reflexes. These may originate in the sacral centres but higher centres are essential for the accurate grading and control of the responses. Impulses from the sacral cord pass along the parasympathetic fibres of the pelvic splanchnic nerves and cause the bladder detrusor to contract. Urine can then enter and distend the posterior part of the urethra and so stimulate urethral sensory receptors. From these, impulses pass along the afferent fibres of the pudendal nerve into the sacral centre and there inhibit the ventral horn cells supplying the external urethral sphincter which relaxes, allowing urine to flow into the remainder of the urethra and on through the external urinary meatus. It is essential, however, that the bladder not only contracts but continues to contract until it is empty. This is achieved because the cerebral cortex, basal ganglia and reticular formation, which all inhibit the sacral centre while the bladder is filling, bombard it with facilitatory impulses once micturition begins so that it remains excited and, therefore, active until the bladder is quite empty.

DISORDERS OF MICTURITION IN NEUROLOGICAL DISORDERS

When the nerve supply of the bladder is damaged or involved by disease, micturition may be disordered in various ways and a description of these can help us to understand the physiology of micturition. Patients with disease of the nervous system may have one of four different abnormalities of micturition or, as is commonly but erroneously said, of the bladder.

An uninhibited bladder results from a lack of inhibition by the higher centres over the sacral spinal centre. The desire to micturate is experienced when the bladder contains as little as 50 or 100 ml of urine; this volume excites the centre as much as 300 or 400 ml do when inhibitory influences are normal. The desire cannot be suppressed and becomes urgent. If it is not obeyed micturition starts precipitately. Once micturition starts it continues until the bladder is empty. This disorder is frequently psychological in nature or may be due to a lesion of the cerebral cortex.

An atonic bladder develops when the sensory pathways from the bladder to the cerebral cortex are damaged as may occur, e.g. in diabetes mellitus. All muscle contraction is absent. There is no sensation so the bladder fills until it is grossly distended when urine overflows down the urethra causing overflow incontinence; the bladder always contains a large volume of residual urine. This disorder occurs in spinal shock when the spinal cord is suddenly separated from the higher centre. This temporarily paralyses the sacral centre but local recovery occurs leading to an automatic or autonomous bladder.

An automatic bladder (upper motor neurone bladder) develops after complete section of the spinal cord above the sacral centre for micturition once the period of spinal shock is over. As sensory impulses cannot reach the sensory cortex no desire to micturate is felt. Inhibitory impulses from the higher centres cannot reach the sacral centre and the bladder automatically contracts when it contains as little as 100–200 ml of urine. The patient is incontinent, and because this is the result of bladder contraction, the incontinence is called active (1-1′ fig.36.7). Although the contraction is strong it is not sustained long enough to empty the bladder and there is residual urine.

An autonomous bladder (lower motor neurone bladder) results from lesions which separate the bladder from its sacral spinal centre by damaging either the spinal cord below the 2nd, 3rd and 4th sacral segments, or the cauda equina, or the 2nd, 3rd and 4th sacral roots. If the bladder were striated muscle supplied by somatic nerves it would, in these circumstances, be paralysed and flaccid. Being smooth muscle, however, it responds directly to being stretched.

The absence of higher inhibitory influences makes the autonomous bladder tense and hypertonic, and it contracts when it contains only a small volume of urine. However, the contraction is weak so that little urine is passed and the amount of residual urine is high. There is active incontinence and the need to pass urine is not appreciated (2–2′ fig. 36.7).

The bladder is also concerned with a number of visceromotor and viscerosensory reflexes. These are most easily demonstrated in patients who have automatic or autonomous bladders in whom filling of the bladder sometimes causes marked disturbances in sympathetic nervous activity with changes in blood pressure and skin colour and with sweating.

FURTHER READING

LUCK R.J. (1972) Renal pelvis and ureter. Bladder. In *Scientific Basis of Surgery*, 2nd Edition, Chapters 22 and 23, ed. Irvine W.T. Edinburgh: Churchill Livingstone.

Chapter 37
Structure and function of skin

The skin is the largest, or at least the heaviest organ in the body; with the subcutaneous fat it forms about one-eighth of the body weight of an adult male (p. 17.1). It provides a protective outer covering which prevents both the entry of many noxious substances and the loss of interstitial fluid. It is important in thermoregulation through its blood vessels and sweat glands. It is a major sense organ. Its colour, whether natural or artificial, is often socially or sexually significant and attempts to retard its natural ageing sustain a large cosmetics industry.

ANATOMY

The skin covers the entire body surface, its epithelium being continuous with those of the digestive, respiratory and genitourinary systems at their external orifices. It is an elastic envelope which is under slight tension, and is freely mobile except where it is attached to the deep fascia as over the flexure lines of joints. The surface of the skin is traversed by branching lines which make up irregular geometric patterns. On the finger tips and toe pads, however, a regular pattern of ridges and sulci is found. The finger prints are so characteristic for each individual that they serve as an effective means of personal identification. In identical twins the patterns are similar but never identical.

The skin consists essentially of two layers: (1) the surface epithelium or **epidermis**, which arises from the embryonic ectoderm and forms the greater part of the cutaneous appendages, i.e. the sweat and sebaceous glands, the hair and the nails, and (2) the connective tissue layer or **dermis**, which arises from the embryonic mesoderm, supports the cutaneous appendages and contains blood vessels, lymphatics and nerves. Beneath the dermis is a layer of loose connective tissue, sometimes called the hypodermis, which in man is more or less firmly attached to the skin. Over most of the body it forms a layer of adipose tissue, the **superficial fascia** or **panniculus adiposus** (fig. 37.1). There are regional variations of this basic pattern with regard to thickness of the layers, numbers of cutaneous appendages and vascularity. These are illustrated in fig. 37.2. These differences explain the varying climatic conditions which exist on the skin surface in different areas of the body; they are of value in assessing the reaction of the skin in disease and lay the foundation for a more rational approach to therapy. These structural variations may alter such factors as surface pH, composition of surface lipid film, and presence or absence of hair and sebum.

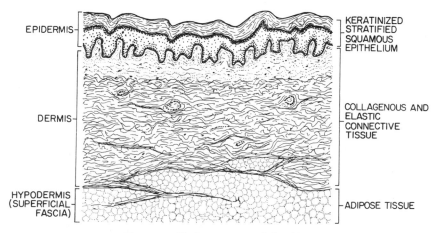

FIG. 37.1. Basic structure of the skin.

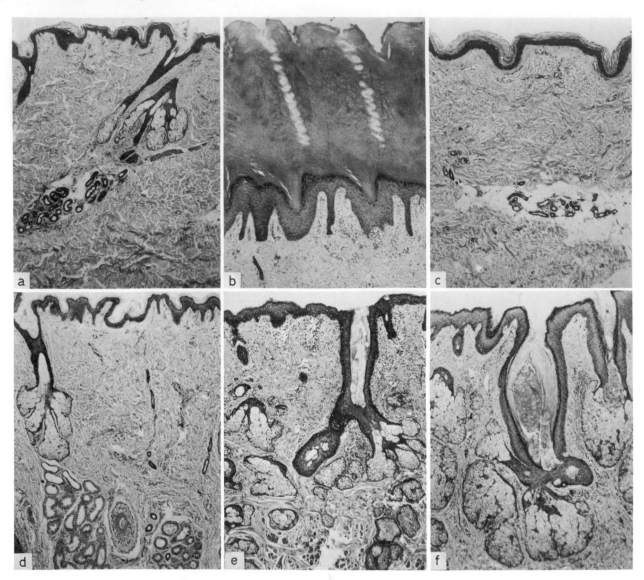

FIG. 37.2. Histological structure of the skin at various body surfaces;
(a) back, (b) sole, (c) abdomen, (d) axilla, (e) scalp, (f) face.

Note the very thick layer of stratum corneum on the sole (b). The abdominal skin sample (c) contains a sweat gland but no hairs are included. The face (f) and scalp (e) contain large sebaceous glands and the axilla (d) shows apocrine sweat glands in the lower part of the field.

HISTOLOGICAL STRUCTURE OF SKIN

Epidermis

The most superficial layer of the skin, the epidermis, is a keratinized stratified squamous epithelium of ectodermal origin. For descriptive purposes it is divided into five layers (fig. 37.3): (1) stratum basale, (2) stratum spinosum, (3) stratum granulosum, (4) stratum lucidum and (5) stratum corneum.

Only in **thick epidermis**, i.e. that over the palmar surface of the hand and the plantar surface of the foot, are all five layers normally recognizable. Elsewhere, in the epidermis of general body skin, only the two deepest and the most superficial of the layers may be readily identified. The difference between thick and thin epidermis rests on inherently different rates of cell division in the two epithelia (p. 19.45). The deepest layer, the **stratum basale** (or **stratum germinativum**), consists of a single layer of cylindrical cells with deeply basophilic cytoplasm and centrally placed elongated nuclei. From the basal end of each cell in the stratum basale, densely packed cytoplasmic processes extend into the underlying connective tissue. The surface of these processes is beset with hemidesmosomes. These arrangements are thought to be important in maintaining firm contact between epidermis and dermis.

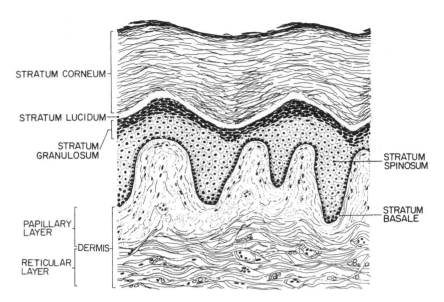

STRATUM CORNEUM

STRATUM LUCIDUM

STRATUM GRANULOSUM

STRATUM SPINOSUM

STRATUM BASALE

PAPILLARY LAYER

RETICULAR LAYER

DERMIS

FIG. 37.3. Detailed structure of epidermis.

The stratum basale is the germinal layer of the epidermis. Cells produced there by mitosis form the cell lineage of the **keratinocytes** which move outwards through the epidermis, finally to be shed from the surface as fully keratinized dead squamous cells. The journey of a cell from the stratum basale to the surface of the stratum corneum normally takes 2–3 weeks. Interspersed between the basal cells are the **melanocytes** (dendritic cells) which form an independent lineage, and are described in connection with skin pigmentation on p. 37.9.

Overlying the basal layer is the **stratum spinosum**, consisting of two to six rows of polyhedral cells, which become flattened as they approach the surface. This layer is so named because in fixed preparations viewed with the light microscope the cells appear to be joined together by intercellular bridges which give individual cells a spiny appearance. Electron microscopy (EM) has shown that these 'intercellular bridges' are small areas of contact between the cells called desmosomes or maculae

adhaerentes (p. 13.13 and figs. 13.13 and 37.4) and correspond to the points of attachment to the plasma membrane of bundles of intracytoplasmic fibrous protein called tonofilaments. Similar filaments are to be found in the cells of the stratum basale. Above the stratum spinosum is the **stratum granulosum** which consists of one to three layers of diamond-shaped cells with darkly staining pyknotic nuclei and packed with irregularly shaped basophilic keratohyalin granules. This layer is best developed in the thick epidermis of the palms and soles where abundant keratin is produced. EM shows that the keratohyalin granules are an amorphous cytoplasmic precipitate adjacent to the tonofilaments.

In thick epidermis, immediately above and adjacent to the stratum granulosum there is a single layer of hyaline anucleated cells, the **stratum lucidum**, containing droplets of an oily substance, eleidin. This lipid is probably produced by disintegration of lysosomes (p. 13.8) since over pressure areas acid phosphatase activity increases progressively up to the stratum granulosum and then ceases abruptly.

The outer layer of the epidermis is called the **stratum corneum**, which consists of a variable number of flattened, anucleated, cornified, dead cells containing the fibrous protein keratin, bound together to form a tough, pliable membrane relatively impervious to substances passing in or out of the body (p. 18.3). Over pressure areas, such as the hands and feet, the keratin layer is dense and compact (fig. 37.3), whereas over the general body surface it forms a loose, flexible covering resembling basket weave (fig. 37.5). Keratin can be considered as the metabolic end product of the epidermal cells, hence the name keratinocytes, and the process of keratinization is of such importance as to warrant further scrutiny.

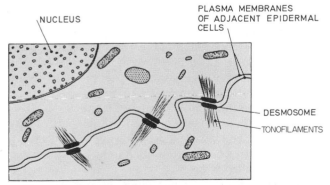

NUCLEUS

PLASMA MEMBRANES OF ADJACENT EPIDERMAL CELLS

DESMOSOME

TONOFILAMENTS

FIG. 37.4. Diagram of the electron microscope appearances of points of contact of adjacent epidermal cells.

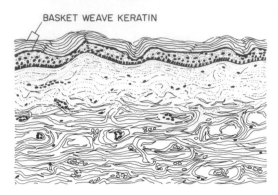

BASKET WEAVE KERATIN

FIG. 37.5. Epidermis of general body surfaces.

Keratinization

The fibrous protein keratin occurs in skin, hair, nails, claws and hoofs, and while these keratinized structures differ greatly in their physical properties, the structure of the keratin molecule, as revealed by techniques such as X-ray diffraction, is constant.

Keratin is composed of eighteen different amino acids and the molecule exists in two forms, namely the α helical or spiral form (human keratins) and the β or straight form (bird feathers). The α helical molecule is kept in position by cross-linked hydrogen bonds. The durability of keratinized structures depends on a disulphide bond between the cysteine molecules of adjacent polypeptide chains.

The first sign of the keratinization process is seen in electron micrographs of the stratum basale where **tonofilaments** of 5 nm diameter are present, coated with an osmiophilic sheath. As the cells of the stratum spinosum approach the surface the diameter of the tonofilaments increases to 10 nm and the sheath thickens. At the level of the stratum granulosum the bundles of tonofilaments are ensheathed by an electron dense matrix (keratohyalin granules); the fully keratinized cell of the stratum corneum consists of compact bundles of tonofilaments cemented together.

From the histochemical viewpoint the region of the stratum granulosum shows a concentration of —SH groups and it seems likely that the —S.S— bonds are formed from oxidation of the —SH groups in two adjacent polypeptide chains.

In addition it appears that lipid is necessary for the orderly formation of the stratum corneum. The present concept is that the normal protein filament from this stratum is surrounded by a thin layer of lipid. That keratinization and lipid synthesis are related is shown by the fact that some of the drugs used to lower blood cholesterol by interfering with its synthesis produce a serious upset in keratinization.

Control of epidermal growth

While it is generally accepted that the dermis exerts an overall controlling influence on the differentiation and growth of the epidermis (p. 37.5), there is increasing evidence that the epidermal cells themselves contribute to the homeostatic regulation of the entire epidermis.

In the early 1960s, Bullough suggested the use of the word **chalome** (Greek: *chalao*, inhibit) for a regulator in the epidermis (vol. 2, p. 27.2). Since then much research has been directed towards such substances and there is now much evidence in support of them. Water-soluble molecules, tissue specific but not species specific, have been extracted from epidermis and other tissues (lymphocytes, liver, kidney, pulmonary alveolar epithelium etc.) which act mainly in the late G_1 phase of the cell cycle to delay DNA synthesis or, alternatively and simultaneously, in the late G_2 phase to delay mitosis.

The action of chalones is short lived, possibly due to the presence of antichalones; their reaction is reversible and they do not appear to damage either the cell or the cell membrane. While no pure chalone has yet been isolated and little is known about chemical structure, they appear to play a significant part in limiting the growth of the normal epidermis.

Cyclic AMP has also aroused interest in relation to the regulation of growth and there are reports that it directly inhibits epidermal cell division in a dose-dependent manner. It has also been shown that in epidermis which is rapidly turning over, e.g. in psoriasis (vol. 3, p. 31.15), there is a decrease in the level of cyclic AMP. It is possible that chalones and cyclic AMP are one and the same substance. In any event they appear to represent one factor in the complex problem of epidermal growth.

Dermis

The dermis is a layer of connective tissue consisting mainly of dense irregular meshworks of collagen fibres, with some elastic and reticular fibres, embedded in a matrix of amorphous ground substances. It may be arbitrarily divided into a more superficial **papillary layer** which is a looser, more cellular layer, with more abundant ground substance and finer fibres some of which are orientated at right angles to the surface, and a deeper **reticular layer** of meshworks of coarser fibres.

When skin is stretched, the irregular three-dimensional meshworks of collagenous fibres become gradually reorientated into an arrangement of more parallel bundles. Individual collagen fibres have high tensile strength and little elasticity. The return of skin to normal after stretching depends on the recoil of stretched elastic fibres. Overstretching, as in pregnancy or rapidly developing obesity, may rupture the elastic fibres, allowing the collagen to become overstretched and resulting in linear scars within the dermis, called **striae**.

The cells of the dermis include fibroblasts, macrophages and mast cells (p. 17.3). Fibroblasts are usually inconspicuous, but proliferate rapidly after injury to the skin. Mast cells are normally sparse in human skin, but are more numerous in some chronic inflammatory skin conditions.

In vertical section the boundary line between epidermis and dermis appears wavy; the downward projections of the epidermis are called **rete ridges**, and the upward projections of the dermis, the **dermal papillae**. However, if the under-surface of a separated epidermal sheet (split-skin preparation) is studied with a dissecting microscope, it is seen that the rete ridges, though sometimes known as pegs are not conical, but are sections through downward projecting ridges which are linked by shorter transverse ridges (fig. 37.6). The dermal papillae are also not conical; they are irregular and, frequently, branched upward extensions of dermal connective tissue, interlocking with the epidermal ridge system. The dermal-epidermal interface is most complex in areas of skin which may be subject to shearing stress, as in the palms and soles, penis, labia minora and nipple. By contrast, in the skin of the abdomen and of the forehead, the dermal–epidermal interface may be almost plane.

At the deep surface of the epidermis is a basement membrane; this is derived in part from the basal cells of the epidermis and in part from the dermis. It is important in the firm attachment between epidermis and dermis and may exert some control on the interchange of materials between dermis and epidermis; a full account of the general characters of basement membranes is given in chap. 18.

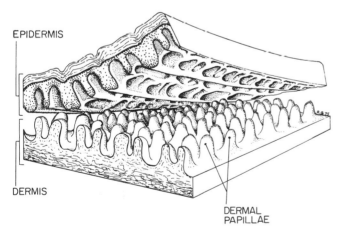

FIG. 37.6. Diagram of dermo-epidermal junction.

Apart from the function of supporting the epidermal appendages, blood vessels, lymphatics and nerves, the dermis exerts an inductive influence during development on the differentiation and structure of the epidermis. This influence appears to be continued into adult life as changes in the dermis often precede the development of epidermal cancers.

Epidermal appendages

The epidermal appendages are the sweat glands, apocrine glands, sebaceous glands, hair and nails.

These important structures arise during fetal life from the under surface of the developing epidermis. Here at about the third month of fetal life small buds of cells, primary epithelial germs, appear. From these structures develop the hair matrix, the sebaceous glands and the apocrine glands (p. 37.6). In the fourth month sweat buds appear on the palms and soles, to be followed at the beginning of the fifth month by those of the axillae and at the end of the fifth month by those over the remainder of the body surface. This pattern may have some functional significance as it is known that sweating varies between the palms and soles and the general body surface.

SWEAT (ECCRINE) GLANDS

These glands are found over the entire surface of the skin, being most numerous on the palms and soles and decreasing in number on the head, trunk and extremities in that order. There are between two and five million sweat glands in human skin, not all of which are active at one time. No sex difference in distribution or number has been observed but there is some evidence to suggest racial differences. The Japanese have more sweat glands on the extremities than on the trunk, in contradistinction to Europeans. Structurally the sweat glands are simple tubular glands extending down from the epidermis to the mid dermis, where they become coiled on themselves and in histological sections are seen as a nest of transverse sections of tubes (fig. 37.7). The secreting portion of the gland consists of a layer of cells the free borders of which are rather uneven. Two types of secreting cell can be identified, a smaller superficial dark cell, with a basophilic cytoplasm, and a larger deeper clear cell with an acidophilic cytoplasm. The dark cells contain RNA and proteoglycan while the clear cells contain abundant glycogen. Glands from different areas of the body contain varying proportions of these two types of cell, but their functional significance is unknown. Along the base of the secreting cells and running parallel to the lumen are the 'myoepithelial' cells (p. 18.10) whose contraction is supposed to aid the expulsion of sweat.

The junction between the secreting coil and the duct is abrupt, the duct being lined by a double layer of darkly staining cuboidal cells which have a hyaline cuticle at their luminal border. The duct passes upwards through the dermis in a relatively straight line but then proceeds through the epidermis in a spiral fashion to open on to the surface.

The sweat glands are abundantly supplied by blood vessels which form an anastomotic network around the secreting coils and the intradermal part of the duct. These vessels are derived from a single arterial twig and are

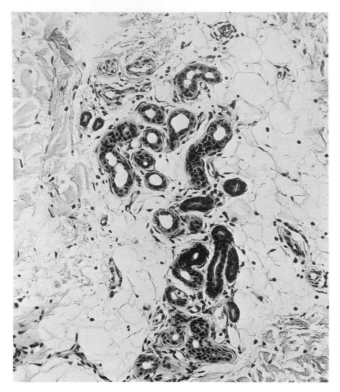

Fig. 37.7. Photomicrograph of eccrine sweat glands. The pale tubules are the secreting acini, the dark ones the excretory ducts (× 400).

reminiscent of the supply to the glomerulus of the kidney. The secreting coils are profusely supplied by cholinergic nerve fibres from the sympathetic nervous system.

Sweating

Sweating is one of the ways in which man regulates his body temperature, and in tropical climates where atmospheric temperatures are high it is of prime importance (p. 43.4).

Sweating occurs in two distinctive patterns, each induced by a different stimulus. If a person is exposed to a warm atmosphere, within a few minutes sweat appears over the entire body surface, but most noticeably on the forehead, upper lip, neck and chest. While some does eventually occur on the palms and soles this is not conspicuous. This **thermal sweating** differs from **emotional sweating**, produced by anxiety and fear, which occurs mainly in the palms and soles and axillae.

At rest there is a steady slow loss of water through the skin called insensible perspiration. This is not a function of sweating but is related to diffusion and osmosis, the water passing through the epidermis (p. 5.4).

Control of sweating

The sweat glands are supplied by cholinergic fibres from the sympathetic nervous system, and thus acetylcholine and cholinergic drugs such as pilo-

carpine induce sweating while it is inhibited by atropine. Adrenaline and noradrenaline have no significant effect on sweating. Bradykinin also promotes sweat production. The general control of sweating is from the hypothalamus.

Composition of sweat

Sweat is a clear, watery fluid which is always hypotonic in relation to plasma. It contains approximately 0·5 per cent of solids, the chief one of which is sodium chloride (20–70 mmol/l), with small amounts of potassium, sugar, lactic acid and urea. The urea concentration is similar to that of blood. Sweat is described more fully on p. 5.30.

APOCRINE GLANDS

These glands develop from the primary epithelial germ in close relation to the hair matrix. In the early stages of human fetal life all primary epithelial germs contain an apocrine bud; the majority of these fail to develop further except in the axilla, anogenital region, mammary areola and the canal of the external ear. Small irregular areas of development may be found on the scalp, face and trunk. This localization contrasts with the situation in many mammals, in which apocrine glands are more generally distributed in hairy skin; it is probably an evolutionary change associated with regression of body hair.

Structure

Like the sweat gland the apocrine gland is a simple coiled tubule, but about ten times larger, so that it can be

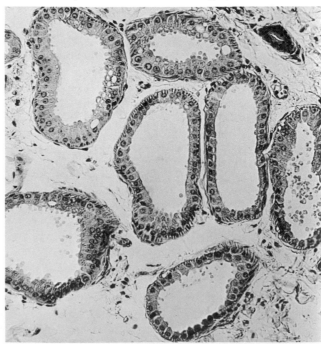

Fig. 37.8. Photomicrograph of apocrine gland acini. The glands are much larger than eccrine sweat glands and are lined by columnar epithelium (× 400).

identified by the naked eye. These glands lie deeper than the sweat glands, being situated in the lower dermis and upper part of the subcutaneous fat.

On histological examination the secreting tubules (fig. 37.8) are lined by a single layer of eosinophilic cells with a basal nucleus. The height of the cells varies from cuboidal to high columnar with a constriction at its tip. This variation in height is believed to indicate the cyclical nature of the secretion. The secreting cells are separated from a basement membrane by a layer of myoepithelium. The apocrine duct is similar in structure to the sweat duct. Instead of penetrating the epidermis, however, it opens into a hair follicle above the ducts of the sebaceous glands.

The blood supply is similar to that of the sweat glands but the innervation is different, being derived from adrenergic fibres of the sympathetic nervous system.

Apocrine secretion

Apocrine secretion is a turbid, milky, sometimes yellowish secretion. If allowed to dry it forms a thin plastic-like film around the hair follicle from which it has emerged. The glands begin to function only at puberty, as distinct from the sweat glands which are functional at birth. It has been stated that apocrine secretion is responsible for the characteristic body odour but it has been shown that this is due to secondary changes produced by bacteria.

Apocrine secretion is evoked by adrenergic stimuli such as fear or pain. Localized secretion may be induced by injection of adrenaline. Heat, acetylcholine and pilocarpine, which induce thermal sweating, do not affect the apocrine glands.

HAIR

Hair grows out of tubular invaginations of the surface epidermis called hair follicles. These follicles, with their associated sebaceous glands, are referred to as pilosebaceous units. The fact that the epidermis is continuous with the epithelium of the pilosebaceous follicles is of importance. Follicular and, to a lesser extent, sweat duct epithelium can proliferate and grow upwards to resurface the skin if the epidermis has been denuded by trauma or by the split skin graft of the plastic surgeon. The hair itself consists of a large, dead, keratinized **shaft**, at the bottom of which is a small growth area, the **hair bulb**. The junction between the dead and the living part of the hair is known as the keratogenous zone; this prevents the spread of keratinophile fungi to the growing matrix and explains why children with hair ringworm do not lose their hair.

The hair bulb is expanded and situated in the upper part of the subcutaneous fat (fig. 37.9). It is invaginated on the underside by a highly vascularized connective tissue, the **hair papilla**. The cells of the bulb are darkly staining with large vesicular nuclei and, in people with

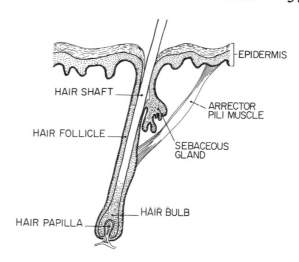

FIG. 37.9. Diagram of hair follicle and related sebaceous gland.

dark hair, contain varying amounts of melanin. Interspersed between them are dendritic melanocytes similar to those in the stratum basale of the epidermis. Above the hair bulb the cells become elongated with their long axis parallel to the direction of the shaft. They undergo keratinization without the intervention of a stratum granulosum. From this point upwards the hair shaft is a dead keratinized structure composed of an outer cortex whose keratinized cells are firmly cemented together and an inner medulla whose larger keratinized cells are loosely connected and partially separated by air spaces.

Inserted into the walls of the follicles are bundles of smooth muscle, the **arrectores pilorum**. These are abundantly supplied by adrenergic nerve fibres, explaining the erection of hairs ('goose flesh') seen during cold and emotional stress.

Hair growth is cyclical. The growth phase is followed by a phase of regression when the lower part of the follicle degenerates and the hair becomes loosened from the papilla. The hair bulb then passes into a resting phase when it is club shaped; this phase can be recognized by the much shorter length of follicle and the absence of a papilla. Subsequently this detached hair is pushed out by the growth of a new hair.

These stages vary in different species, in general being of shorter duration in hairy animals. In the young adult human scalp the growth phase is long (3 years) with a short rest phase (3 months), while in other parts of the body, growth is measured in months, with a long rest. In most hairy mammals the follicular cycles in each region are synchronous, waves of activity flowing outwards from one or more centres so that all the follicles in any one region are at the same stage of development. In man the activity is irregular and neighbouring follicles are at different stages in the cycle.

All the hair follicles on the human scalp are established at birth and in normal circumstances no new follicles are formed later. The pattern, distribution and, to some extent, the colour of hair are genetically determined and their growth sequence is closely linked to bodily growth and sexual maturity. The hair cycle may be modified by varying activity of the thyroid or adrenal glands.

SEBACEOUS GLANDS

Sebaceous glands are found over the entire skin surface with the exception of the palms and soles. They are most numerous and largest on the scalp, forehead, cheeks and chin where they are present in concentrations varying from 400–900/cm² of skin surface. Over the remainder of the body surface the content is about 100/cm². They are **holocrine** glands, forming their secretion by disintegration of the cell contents which are then discharged directly into the sebaceous duct which in turn enters the upper part of a hair follicle (fig. 37.9). Some ducts open directly on to the surface, such as those of the nipple and labia minora, and the Meibomian glands of the eyelid.

Histological structure

Each gland is a lobulated structure (fig. 37.10), usually situated in the angle between a hair follicle and a bundle of smooth muscle, arrector pili, which is thought to aid in the expulsion of the secretion. At

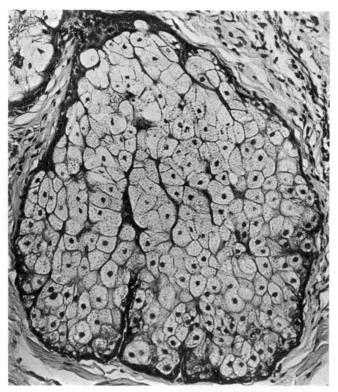

Fig. 37.10. Photomicrograph of sebaceous gland lobule showing the foamy appearance of the secreting cells (× 230).

the periphery of each lobule is a layer of basophilic cuboidal cells, similar in appearance to the cells of the stratum basale of the epidermis. Towards the centre of the lobule the cells become larger and more acidophilic and in fixed and stained preparations have a characteristic foamy appearance due to the contained lipid material being dissolved out by fat solvents during processing. Finally the cell breaks down and discharges its contents, **sebum**, into the sebaceous duct.

The function of sebum is to lubricate the skin and help to protect it against the effects of the elements. As it is difficult to collect sebum without contamination by surface lipids its chemical composition is not accurately known. It appears to be a complex mixture of free fatty acids, glycerides, esters of higher aliphatic alcohols and cholesterol, and hydrocarbons including squalene.

Sebaceous gland activity is low until puberty when it increases rapidly. This change is due to androgenic hormones from the testis in the male, and presumably from the ovaries and adrenals in the female.

An androgen from the adrenal gland, 3β-hydroxyandrost-5-ene-17-one (DHA), stimulates sebaceous output in human subjects whose adrenals have been removed surgically. This hormone disappears from the circulation shortly after birth and reappears at puberty. Human sebaceous glands contain 3β- and 17β-hydroxysteroid dehydrogenases and human skin is capable of androgen metabolism. The 3β-hydroxysteroid dehydrogenases are found in all human sebaceous glands, while the 17β- occur more frequently on the face, scalp and perineum. The metabolism of DHA via the 3β- pathway results in a number of 17-oxo-compounds of decreasing androgenicity. DHA is metabolized via the 17β- pathway into a number of 17β-hydroxy-compounds, including 5α-dihydrotestosterone, all of increasing androgenicity in bioassay systems. These findings appear to offer some explanation of the development of acne vulgaris which is common at puberty (vol. 3, p. 31.23). It has been suggested that the sebaceous glands secrete vitamin D precursor but this has not been substantiated. More probably 7-dehydrocholesterol is produced in the stratum spinosum of the epidermis and its photoconversion to cholecalciferol occurs in the epidermis.

NAILS

Nails are composed largely of a semitransparent keratin plate surrounded proximally and laterally by folds of skin, the nail folds (fig. 37.11a and b), and arise from the **nail bed**, a modified epidermis. The nail plate is free at its distal border but is elsewhere firmly attached to the underlying epidermis. Under the proximal nail fold it is known as the nail root. The nail bed consists of a modified epidermis lacking a stratum granulosum, but with a highly vascular dermis which is continuous on its deep aspect with the periosteum of the distal phalanx.

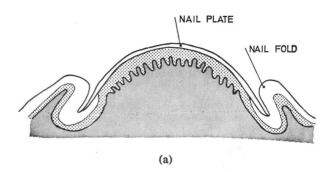

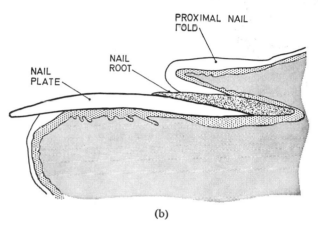

Fig. 37.11. Diagram of nail; (a) longitudinal, (b) transverse.

In the region of the **half moon or lunula**, the root epidermis is thicker and the underlying dermis looser and less vascular, features which cause its pale colour. Finger nails grow more quickly than toe nails, comparative times for replacement being about 6 months for finger nails and 12–18 months for toe nails, a fact to remember when treating fungus infection of the nail plate.

Pigmentation

While in many animals pigmentation serves as camouflage, its prime function in man is to protect the dermis from the harmful effects of sunlight. It seems probable that the dark-skinned races are an example of selective adaptation to extreme exposure to sunlight.

Mention has already been made of the melanin producing dendritic melanocytes which are to be found between the cells of the stratum basale at the junction of the epidermis and dermis (figs. 37.12 and 37.13). These cells, in conjunction with others found in the hair bulb, the iris and the leptomeninges, are known as the **melanocyte system**. They are derived from the neural crest and have the faculty of synthesizing the black pigment melanin from the amino acid tyrosine by means of the Cu^{++} dependent monophenol monooxygenase. In fixed tissue preparations the melanocytes appear as pale cells with a small, darkly staining nucleus and a faintly basophilic cytoplasm (clear cells). In preparations stained

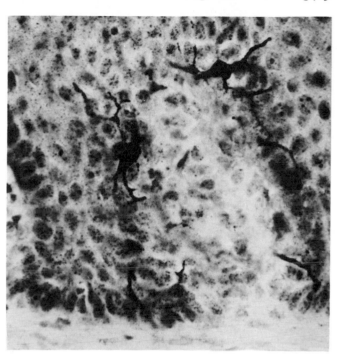

Fig. 37.12. Dendritic melanocytes at dermo-epidermal junction stained by silver impregnation. Note the numerous branching processes extending between the cells of the epidermis (× 400).

specifically to show their contained melanin or to demonstrate their enzyme activity they appear as triangular cells with numerous fine branching processes which transfer the melanin granules to the surrounding basal cells. EM reveals in the cytoplasm of active melanocytes a rough-surfaced endoplasmic reticulum with numerous ribosomes adherent to it, indicating that the melanocyte is a secreting cell. It is characterized by the presence of **melanosomes**, specialized organelles involved in the formation of pigment granules. Tyrosinase is synthesized by the ribosomes and transported within the endoplasmic reticulum to the Golgi region. Here it is segregated in membrane-bound vesicles which enlarge, become oval and acquire a characteristic internal structure, with tyrosinase molecules on a phospholiproprotein matrix, appearing in EM like parallel strings of beads. This

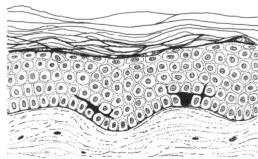

Fig. 37.13. Vertical section of epidermis showing position and general form of dendritic melanocytes.

organelle is called a **premelanosome**. Melanin is now synthesized and deposited on the protein matrix and progressively obscures the internal structure. The end product is a **melanin granule**, a dense homogeneous oval body, still invested by the membrane of the parent Golgi vesicle, and devoid of tyrosinase. There is evidence that transfer of melanin granules to keratinocytes of the basal layer involves active 'phagocytosis' of the melanin-filled tips of the melanocyte's dendritic processes (fig. 37.14). Yet the

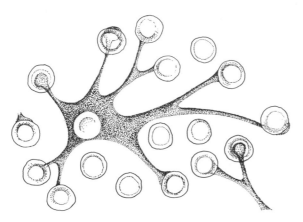

FIG. 37.14. Diagram of dendritic melanocyte from epidermis disaggregated by trypsin digestion, showing relation of dendritic processes to keratinocytes.

basal cell may not be just a passive recipient of melanin and appears to take an active part in the process of transfer and in fact may be intimately connected with the control of melanin synthesis. The dendritic melanocyte and its related basal cells are considered as a functional unit analogous to the nephron, known as the **epidermal melanocyte unit**.

The basic steps in the synthesis of melanin from tyrosine may be summarized as follows.

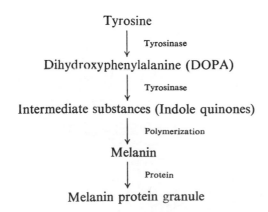

The first stage of this reaction takes place slowly and for this reason the tyrosinase activity in melanocytes is more easily demonstrated by incubating skin with the substrate DOPA.

Melanin pigmentation is in general controlled by the melanocyte-stimulating hormone (MSH) which is produced by the anterior lobe of the pituitary gland. Excess MSH results in a generalized increase in melanin pigmentation.

Quantitative histological studies have revealed that irrespective of race the total number of melanocytes per unit area of skin is the same. This means that the increased pigmentation in coloured skins reflects an increase in melanin synthesis as the total number of melanocytes is the same as in white skin. Another factor which explains the difference in colour between white and coloured skin is the size and distribution of the melanosomes. In white skin the melanosomes are smaller (<0.8 μm) and congregate together (phagosome aggregates). In dark skin the melanosomes are larger (>0.8 μm), do not come together as aggregates and are more widely dispersed throughout the cell which appears much darker. This difference in melanosome size and behaviour is genetically determined.

The protective aspects of melanin pigment in relation to the harmful effects of sunlight have already been mentioned. A practical aspect of this is seen in the sharp increase in the incidence of malignant neoplasms of the skin, in particular of basal cell carcinoma, which was seen in young white American soldiers who served in the Pacific theatre during World War II.

Blood supply

In addition to supplying nourishment to the skin the cutaneous blood flow plays a key role in the regulation of body temperature and blood pressure (pp. 43.4 and 30.48). The skin itself is not demanding as far as blood flow is concerned. It has been estimated that a minimum flow of 0.8 ml of blood min^{-1} 100 ml^{-1} of tissue is adequate to supply its oxygen requirements. Despite this low consumption it has a very abundant blood supply and while there are considerable regional differences the basic pattern is similar. An arterial twig penetrates the subcutaneous fat and forms a plexus just below the dermis. Another plexus is formed just below the papillary layer of the dermis and from here loops go up to individual 'papillae'. These plexuses supply the glands and hair roots. Each arterial twig penetrating the subcutaneous fat supplies an inverted cone-shaped area, the base of which is towards the epidermis. This distribution is demonstrated on cold hands and feet, where a reticulate pattern may be seen. The epidermis is avascular and receives its nourishment from the vessels in the tip of the papilla via the intercellular spaces. The dermis has a rich network of lymphatics which start at the tips of the papillae and pass between the connective tissue fibres, eventually joining up to run along with the larger blood vessels. Blood is collected into venous plexuses situated below the arterial plexuses. Arteriovenous shunts, known as **glomus bodies**, are found in various regions of the skin, notably the pads of the fingers and toes, palms and soles, ears and central part of the face. These provide a means of short circuiting the capillary circulation and are concerned with temperature regulation.

Innervation

The skin supplies much of our sensory information and is richly provided with sensory nerve fibres as well as autonomic fibres supplying secreting glands, smooth muscle and blood vessels. The relation between cutaneous sensibility and cutaneous innervation is discussed in chap. 25.

Itch is a common symptom of a diseased skin and appears closely related to pain, especially of a burning nature, information probably travelling by the same pathways in sensory nerves and the spinal cord. Yet most doctors consider that it is a separate sensation from pain.

Itch may be invoked by a number of physical stimuli, mechanical, electrical and thermal, provided these are below the threshold for inducing pain. It would seem that these stimuli cause enough damage to the skin to release histamine which in turn causes the itch. Itch may be elicited also by a number of exogenous chemicals such as weak acids or weak alkalis, presumably by releasing histamine or a proteolytic enzyme. Substances such as trypsin, papain, bradykinin and 'itch powder', which contains proteolytic enzymes, produce itch, probably by direct action on nerve endings, as no flare characteristic of histamine action is seen (p. 30.48).

The spontaneous itch associated with some skin diseases appears to originate in different ways. That associated with urticaria (nettle rash or hives) is due to local release of histamine while that accompanying eczematous eruptions is probably due to release of endogenous proteolytic enzymes. Generalized itching may be a most distressing feature of obstructive jaundice but ceases at once if the obstruction is relieved.

Cutaneous permeability

The skin in its role as a protective organ relies mainly on an intact epidermis as an effective barrier. The concept of a distinct barrier layer in the epidermis is now generally accepted, and experiments involving the stripping off of the surface layer indicate that it is probably located in the inner part of the stratum corneum. Much has yet to be learned concerning the mechanism of percutaneous absorption and recent work has suggested that specialized cell transport systems may be involved as well as simple diffusion through a membrane.

Substances may pass into the body directly through the epidermis or by means of the openings of the cutaneous appendages. This means, in fact, through the pilosebaceous follicles, as there appears to be no significant absorption through sweat ducts.

While molecular configuration and size may influence the ability of a substance to penetrate the epidermis, the main factor would appear to be determined by lipid and water solubilities. The skin is almost impermeable to water, but lipid-soluble substances such as alcohol penetrate by dissolving the lipid content of the cell wall. In practice it appears that substances which are equally soluble in water and ether penetrate the epidermis better than substances which are soluble in only one of these solvents. The intact skin is also virtually impermeable to electrolytes but permeable to gases to a small extent. Cutaneous respiration amounts to about 0·5 per cent of that through the lungs.

Absorption is enhanced by increase of skin temperature, hyperaemia and hydration of the keratin layer, and damage to the skin caused by physical means or by inflammatory changes.

FURTHER READING

CHAMPION R.H., GILLMAN T., ROOK A.J. & SIMS R.T. eds. (1970) *An Introduction to the Biology of the Skin.* Oxford: Blackwell Scientific Publications.

GORDON M. ed. (1959) *Pigment Cell Biology.* Proceedings of the 4th Conference on the Biology of Normal and Atypical Pigment Cell Growth. New York: Academic Press.

HURLEY H.J. & SHELLEY W.B. (1960) *The Human Apocrine Sweat Gland in Health and Disease.* American Lecture Series No. 376. Springfield, Ill.: Thomas.

MARPLES MARY J. (1965) *The Ecology of the Human Skin.* Springfield, Ill.: Thomas.

MONTAGNA W. ed. (1965) *Advances in Biology of Skin.* Vol. 6. Ageing. Oxford: Pergamon Press.

MONTAGNA W. & LOBITZ W.C. eds. (1964) *The Epidermis.* New York: Academic Press.

MONTAGNA W. & PARAKKAL P.F. eds. (1974) *The Structure and Function of Skin*, 3rd Edition. New York: Academic Press.

ROOK A.J., WILKINSON D.S. & EBLING F.J.G. eds. (1972) *Textbook of Dermatology*, 2nd Revised Edition. Oxford: Blackwell Scientific Publications.

ROTHMAN S. (1954) *Physiology & Biochemistry of the Skin.* Chicago: University of Chicago Press.

VOORHEES J.J. & MIER P.D. (1974) The epidermis and cyclic AMP. *British Journal of Dermatology* **90**, 223–227.

Chapter 38
Reproduction

Four aspects of human reproduction are considered:

(1) reproductive mechanisms in the female, leading to the release of an ovum available for fertilization and the preparation of the reproductive tract for its accommodation,

(2) reproductive mechanisms in the male, leading to the deposition of spermatozoa in the female genital tract,

(3) pregnancy, i.e. the events which follow fertilization of the ovum by a spermatozoon, and

(4) mechanisms of normal sex determination and development which provide the basis for sexual reproduction.

MECHANISMS OF REPRODUCTION IN THE FEMALE

ANATOMY OF THE FEMALE REPRODUCTIVE TRACT

The female reproductive tract consists of paired gonads, or **ovaries**, and a hollow duct system comprising paired **uterine tubes** and a single midline **uterus** and **vagina**. The ovaries are the source of germ cells and sex hormones, and lie on each side of the pelvic wall. The uterus lies centrally in the pelvis between the bladder and rectum, and is enclosed by a double fold of peritoneum lying in the coronal plane and known as the **broad ligament**. The uterus is predominantly a muscular structure and can both accommodate the products of conception during pregnancy and expel them at parturition. Its lower end communicates with the vagina and this in turn opens in the midline between the external orifices of the urethra and anal canal. The external genitalia disposed around the vaginal orifice are known collectively as the **vulva**. The vagina is a distensible tube which is the site of insemination and can transmit a mature fetus at parturition. Each upper angle of the uterine cavity communicates with a narrow tube which runs along the free border of the broad ligament towards the side wall of the pelvis where it opens into the peritoneal cavity. These uterine tubes act as conduits for the transfer of ova and spermatozoa.

Ovaries

The ovaries are flattened bean-shaped objects, measuring about 3–4 cm in length, 2 cm in breadth and 1 cm in thickness. Their surface is pearl white and their contours are scarred and wrinkled. During the reproductive years they are the site of cyclical changes with the regular formation and regression of cysts or follicles and these modify their naked-eye appearance.

The position of the ovaries in the pelvis is variable, but in women who have borne no children (nullipara) they commonly lie on the lateral pelvic walls with their long axis vertical. Their lateral surface lies within the bifurcation of the common iliac arteries and in a shallow recess of peritoneum, called the **ovarian fossa**, which is situated in relation to the bifurcation of the common iliac arteries and in front of the ureters (fig. 38.1). The medial surface faces towards the pelvic cavity,

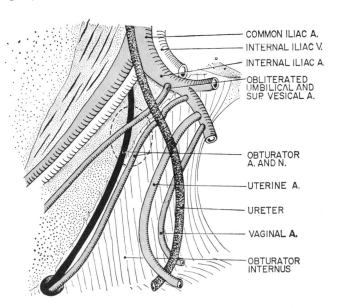

FIG. 38.1. Lateral wall of the pelvis, showing position of the ovaries. Dotted outline indicates position of ovary. From Smout C.F.V. & Jacoby F. (1948) *Gynaecological and Obstetrical Anatomy*, 2nd Edition. London: Arnold.

but is overhung by the uterine tube. The ovaries are attached to the posterior leaf of the broad ligament by a short mesentery, the **mesovarium** (fig. 38.2). This meso-ovarian border constitutes the hilum of the ovary through which blood vessels, nerves and lymphatics pass. The lower end is attached to the angle of the uterus by the **ovarian ligament**, which lies in the free border of the medial part of the mesovarium and is attached to the uterus just behind the point of entry of the uterine tube. Laterally the mesovarium is continuous with the **infundibulopelvic ligament** which represents the continuation of the free border of the broad ligament extending towards the external iliac vessels.

In cross-section each ovary is seen to be made up of an outer **cortex**, within which the reproductive cells arise and develop, and a centrally placed **medulla**. There is, however, no clear-cut boundary between the two zones. The blood vessels of the medulla are large and tortuous, and they branch to give rise to small vessels that permeate the cortex.

The ovary is covered by a single layer of cuboidal epithelium sometimes referred to as germinal epithelium on the incorrect assumption that it is the source of the germ cells. This epithelium, which covers the cortex, is continuous with the mesothelium of the peritoneum forming the mesovarium. Deep to the 'germinal' epithelium is a thin layer of connective tissue, the **tunica albuginea**, which is poorly defined and in no way as prominent as the tunica albuginea of the testis. The remainder of the cortex, which forms the bulk of the ovary, consists of **interstitial connective tissue** in which are set numerous oocytes enclosed in **follicles** at various stages of their development (fig. 38.10). The follicles are described in detail on p. 38.8. The stroma or interstitial connective tissue contains many reticular fibres and spindle-shaped cells which, although they look like fibroblasts, have much greater powers of transformation into other cellular elements and can become large and polyhedral. The medullary stroma is more loose and vascular and within it may be found a number of hilus cells which have been stated to be homologous to testicular interstitial cells.

Uterine tubes

Each uterine tube is approximately 10 cm in length. The tubal lumen communicates medially with the uterine cavity and the lateral end opens into the peritoneal cavity at the abdominal ostium. This provides direct communication between the exterior and the peritoneal cavity, a feature of considerable surgical importance.

Each tube is usually described as having four parts (fig. 38.2). The **interstitial part** runs obliquely through the uterine muscle and leads into a narrow muscular region known as the **isthmus**. This is followed by a tortuous segment, or **ampulla**. The lateral end of each tube is

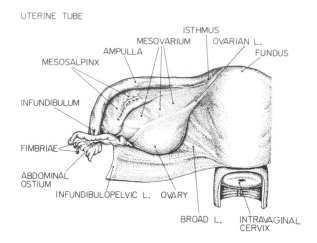

FIG. 38.2. Posterior view of the uterus and broad ligament. The broad ligament and ovary are depicted as laid out on a flat plane, so that their vertical long axes appear horizontal, and the lower end lies medially.

dilated to form the **infundibulum** which is fringed by a number of long mucosal processes, or **fimbriae**. The narrowest segment is the interstitial part where the diameter is only 1 mm, but the lumen widens to 5–6 mm in the ampulla. The lateral half of the tube is looped over the ovary and largely covers its medial surface (fig. 38.5).

The tubes are composed of an outer serosal layer, a muscular coat and an inner mucous membrane (fig. 38.3). The mucosa is lined by a columnar epithelium. Two types of cell are present in the epithelium. One type, bearing motile cilia, predominates towards the infundibulum, and it has been shown that they beat towards the uterine end of the tube. They produce ciliary currents which facilitate transport of ova from the ovaries towards the tubes. Other cells are secretory, predominating in the isthmus and intramural portion, but little is known of the nature of these secretions. The mucous membrane is thrown into a complicated system of longitudinal folds which make the lumen a virtual maze. The muscular coat is continuous with the uterine musculature and increases in thickness in the isthmic segment.

Two groups of vestigial structures, the epoöphoron and paroöphoron, lie within the mesosalpinx (p. 38.6). They are not normally visible to the naked eye but they may be the site of origin of cysts.

Uterus

The uterus is a pear-shaped organ whose narrow end projects into the vagina (fig. 38.4). The upper two-thirds constitute the **body** of the uterus and that portion of the body which lies above the insertions of the uterine tubes is known as the **fundus**. The upper lateral angles where the tubes enter are known as the **cornua**. The lower third of the uterus is the **cervix**. An intermediate zone between the cervix and body is known as the **isthmus**. However, this region is significant only in relation to the

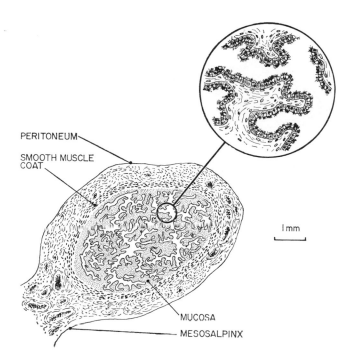

PERITONEUM

SMOOTH MUSCLE COAT

1 mm

MUCOSA

MESOSALPINX

FIG. 38.3. Cross-section of ampullary part of the uterine tube. The low power view shows the mucosal folds. The high magnification shows the ciliated and secretory cells. From Netter F.H. (1954) *The Ciba Collection of Medical Illustrations*.

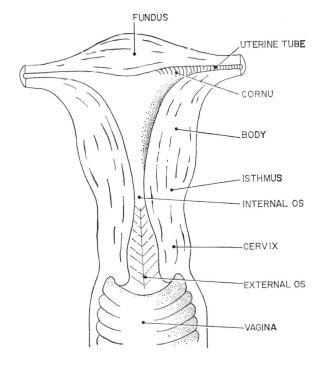

FUNDUS

UTERINE TUBE

CORNU

BODY

ISTHMUS

INTERNAL OS

CERVIX

EXTERNAL OS

VAGINA

FIG. 38.4. Diagrammatic outline of the uterus. From Smout C.F.V. & Jacoby F. (1948) *Gynaecological and Obstetrical Anatomy*, 2nd Edition. London: Arnold.

changes which take place during pregnancy and parturition when it is involved in the formation of the 'lower segment' (p. 38.52). The non-pregnant uterus is flattened in an anteroposterior direction, weighs 50–100 g, and measures about 8 cm in length, 5 cm in breadth and 2–3 cm in thickness. The uterine muscle, or **myometrium**, is 1 cm thick so that the total length of the uterine cavity, or uterocervical canal, is 7 cm.

The cavity of the uterus is compressed between the anterior and posterior walls so that it is reduced to a mere slit when viewed from the side (fig. 38.5). The lumen of the cervix, or **cervical canal**, communicates with the cavity of the uterine body at the **internal os** and with the vagina at the **external os**. When viewed from the front, the cavity of the body is a triangle limited by the internal os and cornua.

The uterus is commonly slightly deviated towards the right side. When seen from the side, it is slightly bent forwards on itself in a position of **anteflexion** (fig. 38.6). Furthermore, the long axis of the cervix is inclined forwards to make an angle of about 90° with the long axis of the vagina in a position of **anteversion**. In about 10 per cent of women the uterus is angled backwards in a position of **retroversion**. The central position of the uterus within the pelvic cavity is largely dependent on the state of filling of the bladder and rectum. When a woman stands erect, the cervix is at the level of the ischial spines (fig. 38.5), but abnormally the uterus may prolapse downwards well below this level.

The uterus is covered by peritoneum which is densely adherent to the underlying myometrium. At each side these peritoneal layers are continuous with the double folds of the broad ligament. Anteriorly, the peritoneum is reflected forwards, just above the junction of body and cervix, towards the bladder, forming a shallow **uterovesical pouch**. Posteriorly, the peritoneum is continued downwards to cover the upper 2–3 cm of the posterior vaginal wall before it is reflected on to the rectum, so forming a deep **rectovaginal pouch**. The depth of this sac is variable but it usually extends to about 7–8 cm from the perineum, a distance which can be reached by an examining finger in the vagina or rectum.

The myometrium of the uterine body consists of bundles of smooth muscle fibres separated by connective tissue. These bundles are arranged in ill-defined layers, but the bulk of the muscle forms an interlacing meshwork of fibres. The mucosa of the body, the **endometrium**, lies directly on the myometrium so that the tips of endometrial glands may burrow into the underlying muscle. During the reproductive years the endometrium undergoes cyclical changes which are described later in detail (p. 38.18).

The upper part of the cervix is cylindrical but that part which projects into the vagina is conical. The cervix contains much less muscle than the body; muscle forms

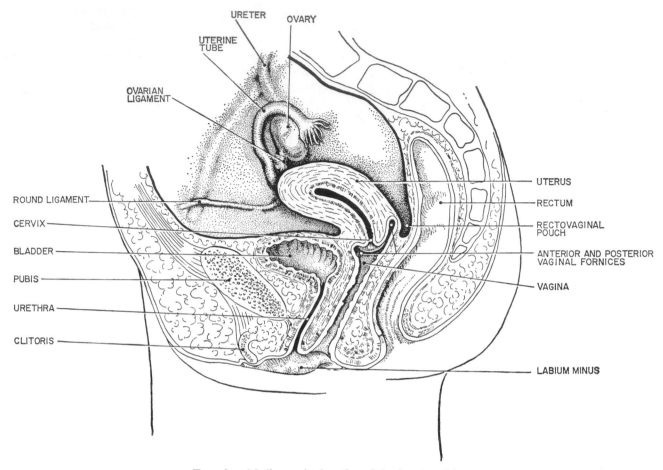

FIG. 38.5. Median sagittal section of the female pelvis.

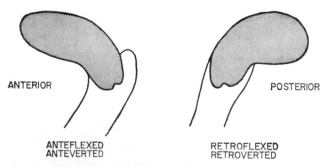

FIG. 38.6 Position of uterus in the pelvis. From Ellis, H. (1971) *Clinical Anatomy*, 5th Edition. Oxford: Blackwell Scientific Publications.

no more than 15 per cent of its substance and is largely confined to the upper half. The remainder consists of connective tissue with a high collagen content. The cervical mucosa contains large, branched tubular glands lined by a tall mucus-secreting columnar epithelium. There is a prominent longitudinal ridge on both the anterior and posterior walls of the canal and mucosal folds radiate out at angles from these ridges and interdigitate with each other. The surface of that part of the cervix which projects into the vagina is covered by stratified squamous epithelium and the line of junction between this squamous epithelium and the glandular epithelium of the cervical canal is usually just within the external os.

The uterus obtains most of its blood supply from the uterine arteries. Branches from both uterine arteries run medially and anastomose freely. It is a remarkable fact that both uterine arteries or even both internal iliac arteries may be ligated without prejudicing the viability of the uterus or other pelvic organs. This emphasizes the rich anastomoses between the branches of the internal iliac artery and the ovarian, inferior mesenteric and median sacral arteries. The branches of the uterine artery supply the myometrium, and their terminal branches also form the spiral arterioles which supply the endometrium and are involved in the mechanism of menstruation.

The ureters have an important anatomical relationship to the cervix. As they pass forwards from the region of the ischial spines towards the bladder they incline medially below the root of the broad ligament, about 2 cm from the side of the cervix, and are crossed above by the uterine arteries.

Vagina

The vagina is a fibromuscular tube measuring about 8 cm in length. When a woman stands erect, the vagina does not descend vertically but is directed downwards and forwards from the uterus at an angle of 70° to the horizontal (fig. 38.5). The anterior and posterior walls are normally in contact except at the upper end, or **vaginal vault,** into which the cervix protrudes. The projection of the cervix allows the space of the vaginal vault to be divided into anterior, posterior and lateral **fornices.** The cervix enters the vault through the upper part of the anterior vaginal wall. As a result, the anterior vaginal wall is shorter than the posterior vaginal wall, and the posterior fornix is much deeper than the anterior fornix.

The epithelium of the vagina is thick and is thrown into prominent folds or **rugae,** some of which are disposed

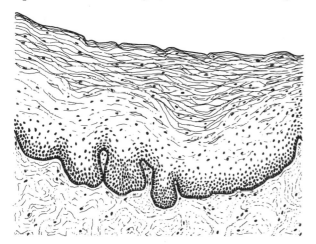

Fig. 38.7. Epithelium of vagina.

laterally and some longitudinally. It is lined by a stratified squamous epithelium (fig. 38.7) which contains glycogen. The fermentative action of bacteria on the glycogen produces lactic acid which renders acid the fluid in the vagina. It is not normally keratinized and does not contain glands. Desquamation of this epithelium contributes to the normal vaginal discharge. The muscle coat consists of plain muscle bundles which run mainly longitudinally, and it is surrounded by an outer fascial coat. The vagina is richly supplied by branches from the internal iliac, uterine, middle and inferior rectal, and internal pudendal arteries. The veins form a plexus around the vagina within the outer fascial sheath.

The anatomical relations of the vagina to other pelvic structures are important (fig. 38.5). Anteriorly, the upper half of the vagina is applied to the bladder base from which it is separated by a loose fascial plane. The urethra is intimately embedded within the substance of the lower half of the anterior wall of the vagina. The upper 2 cm of the vaginal wall in the posterior fornix are covered by the peritoneum of the rectovaginal pouch, so that this is a point of surgical access to the peritoneal cavity. The

middle third of the posterior vaginal wall is closely related to the rectum, and the lower third to the central tendon of the perineum (perineal body). The ureters and uterine arteries cross just above the lateral fornices. The levatores ani blend with the middle part of the lateral vaginal walls and separate the vagina from the ischiorectal fossae.

Vulva

The **labia majora** are the most superficial structures of the vulva (fig. 38.8). They are normally apposed and so conceal the other external genitalia. They extend forwards

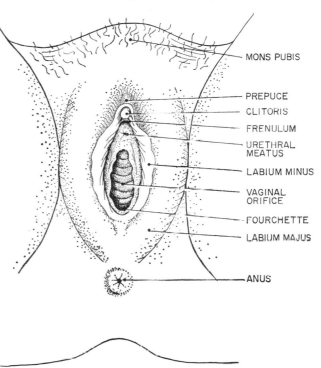

MONS PUBIS
PREPUCE
CLITORIS
FRENULUM
URETHRAL MEATUS
LABIUM MINUS
VAGINAL ORIFICE
FOURCHETTE
LABIUM MAJUS
ANUS

Fig. 38.8. The vulva. From Glenister, T.W.A. & Ross, J.R.W. (1974) *Anatomy and Physiology for Nurses,* 2nd Edition. London: Heinemann.

from the anus and fuse anteriorly in the **mons pubis.** The latter is a low eminence which covers the symphysis pubis and is covered by a triangular distribution of hair. The labia majora are composed of fibrous and fatty tissue and carry hair follicles and sebaceous and apocrine glands.

The **labia minora** are folds of skin which lie between the labia majora. Posteriorly they fuse with the medial surface of the labia majora and form a transverse skin fold, or **fourchette.** Anteriorly each splits into two components which surround the **clitoris,** forming the **prepuce** anteriorly and the **frenulum** posteriorly. The labia minora contain neither adipose tissue nor hair follicles.

The **clitoris** is the homologue of the male penis and has the same component parts in miniature. The body of the clitoris is 2–3 cm in length and it is acutely bent back on itself. It is enclosed within a fibrous coat and divided by an incomplete septum into a pair of **corpora cavernosa** which diverge at the root of the clitoris to form crura. The **crura** are attached to the pubic arch and are covered by **ischiocavernosus muscles**. A small **glans clitoridis**, covered by a sensitive mucous membrane, fits over the body of the clitoris.

The **bulbs of the vestibule** are small masses of erectile tissue which lie alongside the lateral vaginal wall superficial to the inferior fascia of the urogenital membrane. They are expanded posteriorly but they narrow and fuse in front of the external urethral orifice. The **greater vestibular glands** (Bartholin's glands) lie posterolateral to the vagina, superficial to the inferior fascia of the urogenital membrane and concealed by the vestibular bulbs. They are racemose glands whose ducts open in the angle between the labium minus and hymenal ring.

The **hymen** is a thin membrane which guards the vaginal orifice. It is normally perforated and so allows the escape of menstrual blood, but its thickness and rigidity are very variable.

The space bounded by the labia minora is the **vestibule** of the vagina. Its main contents from before backwards are the clitoris, external urethral meatus and vaginal orifice.

The vulva is richly supplied by branches of the internal pudendal artery and deep and superficial external pudendal arteries.

Broad ligament

The broad ligament consists of a double fold of peritoneum and forms a transverse sheet across the pelvic cavity (fig. 38.2). It encloses the uterus in the midline, and laterally contains loose areolar tissue and smooth muscle elements known as the **parametrium**. Its anterior layers pass forwards towards the anterior abdominal wall and form shallow paravesical fossae, while its posterior layers form two prominent **rectouterine folds** which curve backwards from the cervix towards the posterior pelvic wall lateral to the rectum.

The medial attachment of the broad ligament to the uterus is almost linear. Laterally it is widened out to include the attachments of the round ligament, uterine tube and ovarian ligament.

The **round ligament** is a fibromuscular cord which extends from the lateral angle of the uterus to the deep inguinal ring, crossing the umbilical, obturator and external iliac vessels. It hooks round the lateral side of the inferior epigastric artery, traverses the inguinal canal, and terminates within the substance of the labium majus. The round ligament is the remains of the gubernaculum (p. 38.61). Three structures are thus attached to each uterine angle, the round ligament, uterine tube and ovarian ligament, in that order from before backwards.

The **mesosalpinx** is the part of the broad ligament which enfolds the uterine tube. Laterally it is continuous with the **infundibulopelvic ligament**. The lateral part of the mesosalpinx is loose and redundant and this allows the tube to cradle the ovary. The **mesovarium** is a fold of the posterior layer of the broad ligament which gives attachment to the ovary.

Parametrium

This is a fibrous condensation of pelvic fascia. It contains muscle fibres and is most abundant in the root of the broad ligament. It is attached medially to the supravaginal cervix and upper third of the vagina. Laterally it fans out, the posterior border sweeping back in the rectouterine fold towards the sacrum. This component of the parametrium is commonly known as the **uterosacral ligament**, but it is simply a fascial condensation around the nerve bundles passing between the sacral plexus and the uterus. The lateral part of the parametrium extends to the side wall of the pelvis blending with the fascia on the levatores ani. This is often called the **lateral cervical ligament** but again it is a fascial condensation around the uterine vessels. The most anterior part extends to the back of the pubic bones and is known as the **pubocervical ligament**.

Supports of the uterus

The position of the uterus is maintained by a number of factors which are principally the **muscular pelvic diaphragm** (levatores ani) with the associated pelvic fascia, and the parametrium, described above, which forms what are sometimes termed the 'true ligaments' of the uterus. The broad ligament plays a secondary role and, affording little support, is sometimes referred to as the 'false ligament' of the uterus.

By virtue of its attachments the uterus, and with it the upper vagina, maintains its level in the pelvis and downward prolapse is prevented.

The extent to which the round ligament plays a part in maintaining the normal position of the uterus is not clear, but the anteversion position may be produced by the forward pull of the round ligament on the uterine fundus with fixation of the cervix by the lateral cervical and uterosacral ligaments.

The **perineal body** is important in the supportive function of the pelvic floor in the female. This compact fibromuscular node lies in the median plane, 1·25 cm in front of the anal margin, and receives attachments, not only from the levatores ani, but also from the perineal muscles. Consequently, if the perineal muscles are torn or otherwise damaged, the perineal body ceases to be anchored properly and the levatores ani lose their ability to function effectively as supports for the uterus and vagina.

Effects of age and parity

The preceding description applies to the reproductive tract of a nulliparous woman during the active reproductive years. However, these features may be considerably modified during the years which precede puberty and follow the menopause, and as a result of childbearing. Before puberty the vulva is not covered by hair; the labia majora are poorly developed and the labia minora are prominent. The vaginal epithelium is thin and almost translucent. At birth the uterus is small, and the cervix is as long as the uterine body. By puberty, the uterus has reached its mature size and proportions although it will become larger with increasing parity.

During childbirth the perineum may become torn or stretched and the vaginal introitus gapes; the cervix is split, usually laterally, so that the circular external os is widened, and the cervix may be described as having anterior and posterior lips. After delivery, the uterus does not return fully to its non-pregnant dimensions. Following the distortion of the broad ligament and displacement of the ovaries during pregnancy, the ovaries rarely return to their original position on the lateral pelvic wall, and may take up a variable position behind the broad ligament.

Following the menopause, the vulvar and vaginal epithelium again thins and all the external genitalia atrophy. As a result the vagina and the entrance to it (**introitus**) narrow. The uterus and cervix shrink in size and the cervix becomes almost flush with the vaginal vault. The ovaries are greatly reduced in size and their surface becomes increasingly wrinkled.

As a result of coitus, the hymen becomes torn and replaced by tags of epithelium surrounding the hymen.

Blood supply

The reproductive tract is supplied by the ovarian arteries and branches of the internal iliac arteries.

The **ovarian arteries** arise from the front of the aorta just below the origin of the renal arteries. They run downwards over the anterior surface of psoas major, anterior to the ureter and accompanied by the ovarian vein. They enter the pelvis by crossing the external iliac artery about 2 cm below its origin, pass between the layers of the infundibulopelvic ligament and enter the hilum of the ovary via the mesovarium. They supply the ovaries and tubes and anastomose with branches of the uterine arteries to supply the fundus and body of the uterus.

The **uterine arteries** are branches of the anterior divisions of the internal iliac arteries. They run medially and forwards over the levatores ani to the lower border of the broad ligament, then through the parametrium towards the cervix, crossing above the ureter. At the level of the cervix they give branches to supply the cervix and upper vagina. Each artery then follows a tortuous course along the side of the uterus towards the tube and anastomoses with branches of the ovarian artery.

The **vaginal arteries** may arise independently from the internal iliac artery, or from a common stem with the uterine artery. They run downwards and medially towards the vaginal vault to anastomose with vaginal branches of the uterine artery. From this anastomosis, they descend along the vagina to communicate with branches of the internal pudendal artery.

The **internal pudendal arteries** arise from the internal iliac arteries in common with the inferior gluteal arteries. Their branches supply the external genitalia and perineum (fig. 21.46).

VENOUS DRAINAGE

The ovarian and internal iliac veins provide the main venous drainage from the reproductive tract. Veins leaving the hilum of the ovary form a profuse **pampiniform plexus** in the mesovarium and unite to form the ovarian vein. These veins follow the course of the ovarian arteries, the right vein entering the inferior vena cava and the left vein draining into the left renal vein.

Uterine and vaginal venous plexuses drain by veins which follow the route taken by their respective arteries towards the internal iliac vein. However, there is a free communication between the vesical, uterine, vaginal and rectal venous plexuses, and these all communicate with presacral and lumbar channels of the vertebral venous plexus

Lymphatic system (fig. 38.9)

Although pelvic lymph nodes are usually situated along blood vessels, the lymph vessels from pelvic organs do not necessarily follow the path of the blood vessels that supply them.

From the ovaries and tubes lymph vessels pass directly to aortic nodes along the course of the ovarian vessels. Lymph vessels draining the uterus are widely distributed. Some vessels from the fundus drain along the ovarian route, while a few follow the round ligament to reach the superficial inguinal nodes. Many lymph vessels from the body of the uterus pass directly to external iliac nodes. From the cervix, lymph vessels course through the parametrium to reach external and internal iliac or sacral nodes.

There is a free communication between lymph vessels draining the two sides of the vulva. Most vulvar lymph vessels run across the labia majora and mons pubis to reach the superficial inguinal nodes, from which they may communicate with the deep inguinal nodes or continue upwards towards the external iliac nodes. A few vessels from the clitoris may follow veins draining the clitoris and communicate with the vesical lymph plexus.

Innervation

With the exception of the vulva, the genital tract is innervated by the autonomic nervous system.

A parasympathetic component originates from the sacral segments of the spinal cord. Preganglionic fibres

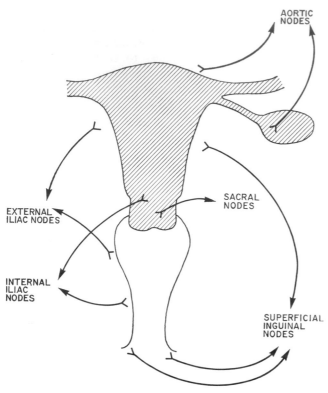

FIG. 38.9. Lymphatic drainage of the female genital tract. From Ellis H. (1971) *Clinical Anatomy*, 5th Edition. Oxford: Blackwell Scientific Publications.

are distributed via the ventral primary rami of S2–4, and thence by the pelvic splanchnic nerves to the pelvic plexuses.

The sympathetic contribution is obtained in two ways. Postganglionic fibres from the thoracic sympathetic trunk and prevertebral ganglia reach the pelvis along the visceral branches of the abdominal aorta, particularly the ovarian and uterine arteries. Other fibres are derived from the hypogastric plexus. These descend to the pelvic plexuses where they mingle with the parasympathetic component.

These pelvic plexuses lie on each side of the rectum and fibres are distributed forwards along the uterosacral ligaments towards the cervix and thence to the uterus and vagina.

Both afferent and efferent fibres are included. Afferent fibres from the ovaries return along the ovarian arteries, whereas uterine sensory fibres run mainly towards the pelvic plexuses. These afferent fibres enter the spinal cord between segments T10 and L1. Sympathetic motor fibres arise from lower thoracic segments and parasympathetic fibres from S2–4. The ultimate site of termination of these efferent fibres in the uterus is unknown and their motor function is equally obscure.

The external genitalia are innervated primarily by the branches of the pudendal nerve (p. 21.45). Additional innervation is obtained from the perineal branch of the posterior cutaneous nerve of the thigh, genital branch of the genitofemoral nerve, and the ilioinguinal nerve.

PHYSIOLOGY OF THE FEMALE REPRODUCTIVE TRACT

The ovaries play a central role in female reproduction and perform two intimately related functions, the production of gametes and the production of sex hormones. With respect to both functions, the ovaries are regulated by the hypothalamus and adenohypophysis. In turn, the principal site of action of ovarian hormones is the uterus, and ovulation may be followed by implantation of the fertilized ovum in the uterine cavity. Reproduction in the female therefore may be studied at four closely integrated levels, hypothalamus, adenohypophysis, ovaries and uterus. This relationship is of crucial importance to an understanding of reproductive physiology and it is described in the following sequence:

(1) the gametogenic and endocrine functions of the ovaries,

(2) the control of the ovaries by adenohypophysis and hypothalamus, and

(3) the functional interrelation between the ovaries and the reproductive tract.

Functions of the ovaries

Both gametogenic and endocrine functions of the ovaries follow a strictly repetitive sequence and can be understood only in terms of the ovarian cycle. This cycle is based on the growth changes centred around the female germ cells. The origin of these germ cells is described on p. 38.59. It may be noted at present that some of these germ cells become surrounded by a single layer of somatic cells, the whole structure constituting a **primordial follicle**.

Ovarian cycle (fig. 38.10)

FOLLICULAR DEVELOPMENT

The ovaries change very little between birth and puberty, but each month thereafter successive waves of primordial follicles undergo a process of cyclical maturation and regression. The cell layer surrounding the germ cell is referred to as the **granulosa layer,** while the stromal cells immediately adjacent to this are differentiated to form the **theca interna.** As these two components proliferate, fluid accumulates between the granulosa cells and forms a small cavity containing follicular fluid. Only one or occasionally two of this group of follicles continue to develop, while the others regress. The mechanism by which a single follicle matures each month is unknown, but it becomes less efficient with advancing years, with

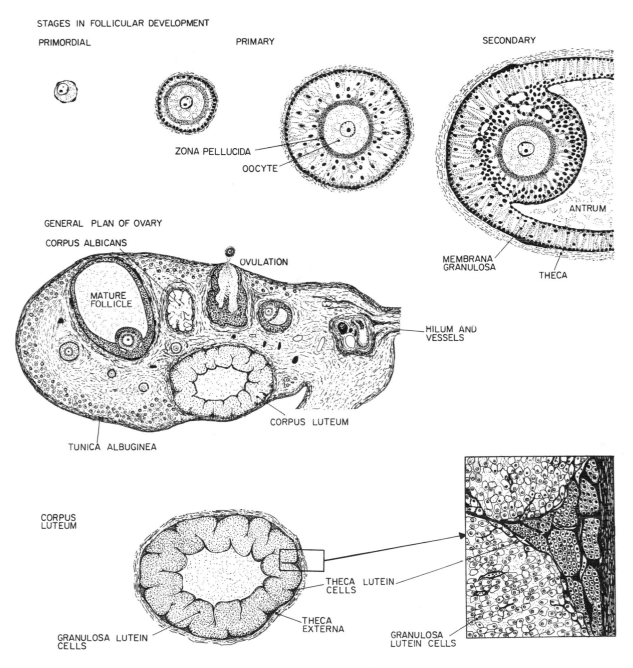

STAGES IN FOLLICULAR DEVELOPMENT

PRIMORDIAL

PRIMARY

SECONDARY

ZONA PELLUCIDA

OOCYTE

ANTRUM

MEMBRANA GRANULOSA

THECA

GENERAL PLAN OF OVARY

CORPUS ALBICANS

OVULATION

MATURE FOLLICLE

HILUM AND VESSELS

CORPUS LUTEUM

TUNICA ALBUGINEA

CORPUS LUTEUM

THECA LUTEIN CELLS

THECA EXTERNA

GRANULOSA LUTEIN CELLS

GRANULOSA LUTEIN CELLS

FIG. 38.10. Ovarian cycle.

the result that twin births due to multiple ovulation are more common in older mothers.

As the volume of follicular fluid increases, it displaces the germ cell to one side of the follicle where it lies in a small mass of granulosa cells, or **cumulus oophorus**. The cells surrounding the germ cell are radially arranged and referred to as the **corona radiata**. Between the oocyte and the granulosa cells is the **zona pellucida**, a tough, optically structureless, refractile membrane, which stains intensely

by the PAS method because of its proteoglycan content. It also contains sialic acid. It is formed during follicular development, apparently as a secretion of the granulosa cells. It is penetrated from without by slender processes of granulosa cells and from within by processes of the oocyte. Exchange of materials between oocyte and granulosa cells may occur at the sites of contact between these processes. The theca interna cells enlarge, assuming a polygonal shape, and are extensively vascularized, in contrast to the granulosa cells which have no direct blood supply before ovulation. As the follicle enlarges it compresses the ovarian stroma and creates a false capsule of connective tissue, the **theca externa.**

The mature follicle is commonly known as the Graafian follicle in recognition of the Dutch scientist, Regner de Graaf, who first described it. The original primordial follicle has a diameter of only 30 μm, whereas the mature follicle measures from 10 to 30 mm in diameter, a 1000-fold increase.

OVULATION

When it reaches maturity, the follicle ruptures on the surface of the ovary discharging the germ cell, with its zona pellucida and corona radiata still attached, into the peritoneal cavity. The mechanism responsible for rupture of the follicle is unknown, but it probably occurs in the region of a thinned out, avascular area of the follicle wall. The phenomenon has been directly observed in women, and appears as a gentle oozing from a collapsed follicle.

At the time of rupture, the tubal fimbriae are approximated to the surface of the ovary and facilitate entry of the ovum into the abdominal ostium, while peristalsis of the tubal muscle combined with ciliary activity of the tubal epithelium rapidly carries the ovum towards the ampulla, which is the site of fertilization. Tubal entry is not always as direct as this because in some tubal pregnancies the corpus luteum is found in the contralateral ovary.

Less than 1 per cent of the oocytes present in the ovary at birth mature and are ovulated during the 35 years or so of cyclic ovarian activity. The rest degenerate as part of the process of **follicular atresia**, which begins before birth and continues until the menopause, when the follicular stock is virtually exhausted. Atresia may overtake a follicle at any stage in its life history and the process seems initially to involve the follicular epithelium. Atresia leads finally to the formation of a fibrous scar, smaller than a corpus albicans.

LUTEINIZATION

Following ovulation the follicle collapses, and the granulosa cells rapidly proliferate and at the same time become intensely vascularized so that each cell appears to be in direct contact with a capillary. This granulosa component forms the bulk of the growing **corpus luteum** and the intense yellow colour, from which this structure derives its name, is due to the presence of lipids in the luteinized granulosa cells. The thecal cells proliferate to a lesser extent and their physiological role is not clear.

The human corpus luteum actively synthesizes sex steroid hormones for 8–10 days, following which, if fertilization has not occurred, it undergoes a process of degeneration or **luteolysis**, when its endocrine activities

rapidly cease. Over the next few months it degenerates to a structureless, whitish mass, the **corpus albicans**.

PRODUCTION OF OVA

Ovulation occurs at the midpoint of each ovarian cycle and it is necessary to consider the processes which are involved in the production of ova.

Sexual reproduction involves much more than the addition of paternal to maternal chromosomes at fertilization. During gametogenesis, the actual genetic structure of the chromosomes of the germ cells is rearranged so that the chromosomes in the germ cells are genetically dissimilar from the corresponding chromosomes of somatic tissues. It is this structural alteration of chromosomes during gametogenesis, even more than the simple pooling of maternal and paternal chromosomes at fertilization, which determines the genetic uniqueness of the individual. A child is not simply the sum of a half share each of maternal and paternal chromosomes. The chromosomes which it inherits at fertilization are similar

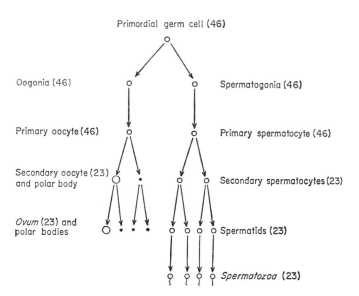

FIG. 38.11. Oogenesis and spermatogenesis. Numbers in brackets refer to chromosome number. Each diploid primary oocyte produces one haploid ovum. Each diploid primary spermatocyte produces four haploid spermatozoa.

to, but not identical with the parental chromosomes. Furthermore, fertilization involves the fusion of an ovum and spermatozoon. Therefore, in order to maintain the constancy of the chromosome number of human cells, the number of chromosomes in each gamete need to be reduced by half prior to fertilization. This is achieved by two successive cell divisions known collectively as **meiosis.**

From these considerations it should be clear that two outstanding features of gametogenesis are the mechanism for the exchange of genetic material between chromosomes, and the reduction division from diploid to haploid number. Gametes are derived from diploid primitive germ cells known as **oogonia** in the female and **spermatogonia** in the male. The origin and differentiation of these primitive cells are described on p. 38.31. During the early months of intrauterine life oogonia proliferate by mitotic division. Some of these oogonia enlarge and become recognizable as **primary oocytes** which will proceed to undergo meiosis. The mechanisms and significance of meiosis are fully described on p. 12.22.

During oogenesis, the second metaphase may be followed by a remarkably prolonged period during which pairing persists but the cell appears to enter a resting phase reminiscent of mitotic interphase. All oocytes reach this stage by the sixth or seventh month of intrauterine life. Many of these prophase primary oocytes are surrounded by a single layer of follicular cells, forming primordial follicles, and it may be that it is the presence of these follicular cells which arrests meiosis at this stage. Oocytes which fail to form follicles complete the first meiotic division and then degenerate and are lost.

There are no further developments in the oocytes until puberty. Thereafter, a few primordial follicles mature each month, and the primary oocytes contained within the developing follicles complete the first meiotic division. With completion of this cell division, each diploid primary oocyte gives rise to two haploid cells, one **secondary oocyte** and one **polar body** (fig. 38.11). It should be recalled that as a result of crossing-over the genetic structures of homologous chromosomes of these two haploid cells differ from each other, and both may be different from the corresponding chromosome pair of the original primary oocyte.

Secondary oocytes immediately enter the second meiotic division, and this follows a sequence very similar to mitosis, although there are two important differences. Only twenty-three chromosomes are involved, and the two chromatids which form each chromosome are genetically dissimilar.

Three important features distinguish oogenesis from spermatogenesis (p. 38.31). First, the distribution of cytoplasm which accompanies each meiotic division during oogenesis is unequal, virtually all the cytoplasm being orientated around one nucleus. The smaller cells are known as polar bodies, which probably have no biological function. Thus, each primary oocyte can give rise to one large haploid cell, or **ovum**, and three polar bodies. The term ovum may be loosely applied to oocytes or even to the fertilized egg, but its correct use should be restricted to the major cell derived from the second meiotic division completed at fertilization. Secondly, as the second meiotic division is completed only if the secondary oocyte is penetrated by a sperm, there is no period during which the female germ cell matures. By contrast, the spermatid emerging from meiosis must undergo a highly

complex process of differentiation before becoming a mature sperm.

Finally, the time scales of oogenesis and spermatogenesis contrast dramatically (fig. 38.12). Oogonia undergo mitotic multiplication during the first six or seven months of intrauterine life. The final number of oocytes so formed in each ovary is about 3–4 million, although there is a wide individual variation. It is widely accepted that the production of oocytes ceases before birth, and it is unlikely that there is any postnatal oogenesis from the so-called germinal epithelium. On the contrary, there is a steady reduction in the number of follicles after birth until, at the menopause, the ovarian stock of oocytes is completely exhausted. Most of this loss of oocytes occurs by atresia rather than by ovulation. Thus, of the original total of about 7 million oocytes only 400 may ovulate, while the remainder degenerate.

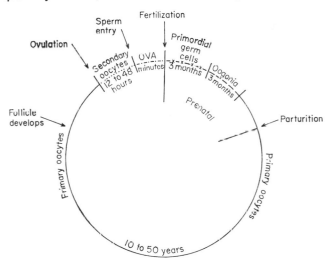

Fig. 38.12. The reproductive cycle. During the first 2 or 3 months after conception, primordial germ cells form and segregate. By the 6th intrauterine month, oogonia have divided and formed primary oocytes. The first meiotic division is not completed until ovulation occurs from the follicle within which the oocyte is contained, i.e. 10–50 years later. The second meiotic division and formation of the ovum is not completed until the egg is entered by a spermatozoon. Fertilization of the ovum by a spermatozoon starts another reproductive cycle.

All the primary oocytes so formed begin their first meiotic division before birth, but the completion of prophase is arrested until after puberty. During this time oocytes accumulate nutrients in the cytoplasm, and this storage process is probably essential for the subsequent viability of the zygote. Meiosis restarts in individual oocytes when their follicles undergo maturation in subsequent ovarian cycles. This means that the duration of the first meiotic prophase may range from 10 to over 50 years. The remainder of the first meiotic division is completed by the time of ovulation, at which time a secondary oocyte is released into the tube. The second meiotic division follows immediately and proceeds to the metaphase stage, but this stage is not normally completed until the oocyte is penetrated by a spermatozoon. This indicates that the mature ovum normally has only a transient existence.

It will be appreciated that gametogenesis is an extremely complicated process, and meiotic errors are not infrequent (p. 39.10).

SEX HORMONES

The principal ovarian hormones are steroid in structure and fall into three broad functional categories, **oestrogens**, **progestogens** and **androgens**.

Ovarian production of oestrogens

The expression oestrus refers to cyclic phases of sexual excitement or heat demonstrated by many animals, and the word oestrogen originally implied the ability to induce this behaviour pattern. However, the human female does not exhibit any comparable oestrous behaviour, and there is no clear correlation between the secretion of oestrogens and sexual drive or libido. Oestrogen is now used to refer to any substance which is able to produce characteristic changes in the reproductive tract, particularly in the vaginal epithelium. Oestradiol is the principal active oestrogen secreted by the ovary at a concentration of about 3·5 nmol/l ovarian venous plasma.

Biosynthesis of oestrogens (fig. 38.13).

Cholesterol is the precursor of all natural steroids (p. 10.4). The ovaries may utilize plasma cholesterol for this purpose or synthesize cholesterol from acetate. During steroid synthesis the cholesterol molecule is reduced in size, rearranged, and $-OH$ or $=O$ groups are added at a number of specific sites.

Cleavage of most of the side chain converts cholesterol to pregnenolone. All steroid hormones are derived from pregnenolone and it has certain structural features which merit special attention. These are the double bond between C-5 and C-6 (the Δ^5 position), a two carbon atom side chain at C-17, a hydroxyl group at C-3, two angular methyl groups at C-10 and C-13, and full saturation of ring A. These are the features which are modified during steroid synthesis.

(1) Transfer of the Δ^5 double bond to the C-4–C-5 (or Δ^4) position, and dehydrogenation of the hydroxyl group at C-3 (by 3β-ol dehydrogenase) result in the formation of progesterone.

(2) Hydroxylation at C-17 followed by cleavage of the side chain produces androstenedione. By alteration in the sequence of these steps, androstenedione may also be produced without involving progesterone as an intermediate.

(3) Aromatization of ring A and loss of the angular methyl group at C-10 lead to oestrone. Alternatively preliminary reduction at C-17 may produce oestradiol-17β via testosterone.

(4) Oestrone and oestradiol-17β are readily interconvertible by reversible dehydrogenation.

This pattern of steroid synthesis provides basic pathways common to all steroid-producing tissues, adrenal cortex, testis and ovary. They all require the production of pregnenolone as the initial precursor. Thereafter, the essential step in the production of cortisol is hydroxylation at C-11 and C-21 (p.27.34); androgens require cleavage of the side chain at C-17; oestrogens are characterized by aromatization of ring A. The steroid-producing potential of these organs can now be understood by a knowledge of their enzyme capabilities. The adrenal cortex possesses the enzymes for all of these steps and so is totipotent with regard to steroid hormones. The testis has little ability to aromatize ring A. The ovary has aromatizing enzymes, but cannot hydroxylate at C-11 or C-21. The placenta, as shown later, is very highly specialized. It is an incomplete endocrine organ and cannot cleave the side chain at C-17, but it is a plentiful source of 3β-ol dehydrogenase and aromatizing enzymes. It is not surprising that, even under normal conditions, the ovary secretes androgens. Androgens should be considered both as primary virilizing agents and also as intermediary metabolites or 'pre-hormones'. Thus the normal sequence of ovarian steroid synthesis is cholesterol→progestogen→androgen→oestrogen.

Metabolism of oestrogens

Oestrogens enter the circulation by the ovarian vein, and their activity is regulated in the following ways.

(1) Conversion occurs to metabolites with less oestrogenic activity. The most important example is 16-hydroxylation producing the less active oestrogen, oestriol. Other methods of inactivation include hydroxylation and methylation at C-2, oxidation at C-6, and hydroxylation at C-11. So far, over twenty naturally occurring oestrogens have been identified. These conversions occur mainly in the liver.

(2) Conjugation in the liver with glucuronic acid and sulphuric acid renders these steroids water-soluble and reduces their physiological activity. Whereas glucuronides are not metabolized further, sulphates can serve as useful metabolic intermediates, provided the sulphate group is removed by sulphatase activity. This applies particularly to dehydro*epi*androsterone sulphate of fetal origin which is an important substrate in placental steroid synthesis (p. 38.48).

(3) Oestrogens are bound in the plasma to a specific globulin. This confines the hormones within the blood compartment and protects them from metabolism in the liver.

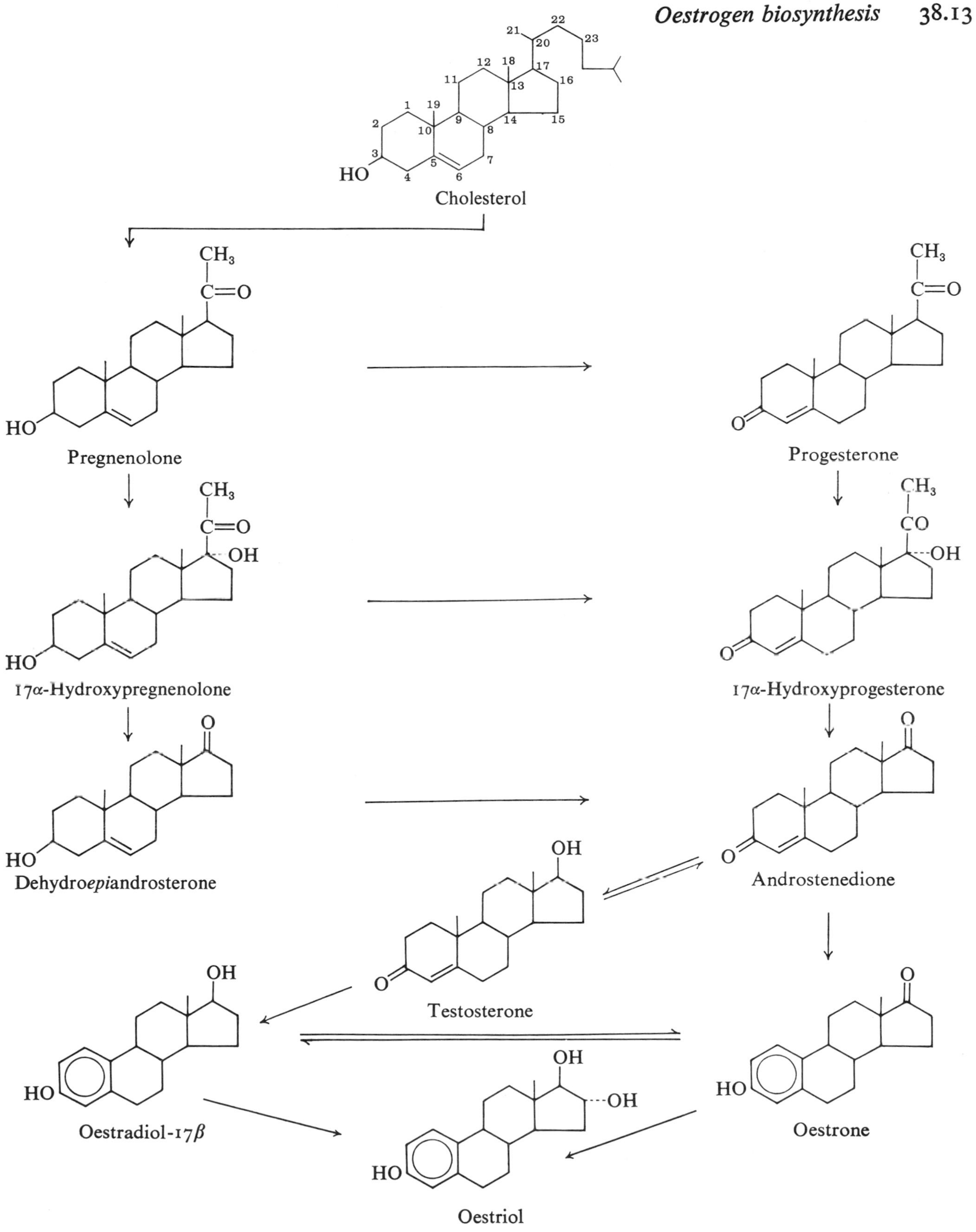

FIG. 38.13. Biosynthesis of oestrogens.

Excretion of oestrogens (fig. 38.14)

Conjugated water-soluble oestrogens are excreted from the liver via the bile but are mainly reabsorbed via the portal circulation. This enterohepatic circulation is similar to that of the chemically allied bile salts. Despite reabsorption, there is an appreciable loss of oestrogens in faeces. The main route of excretion is the urine. Quantitatively the most important urinary oestrogens are oestriol, oestrone and oestradiol-17β, but there are many others, some still unidentified.

Oestrogen levels during menstrual cycle

Each cycle has a biphasic pattern. There is an initial rise which parallels the maturation of the follicle and reaches a peak at ovulation. There is then a transient fall followed by a second wave which corresponds with the growth and regression of the corpus luteum (fig. 38.15).

Site of production of oestrogens

In the follicular phase of the cycle the theca interna is probably the main source of oestrogens, while in the luteal

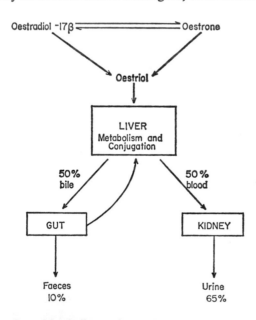

FIG. 38.14. Metabolism and excretion of oestrogens. Only 75 per cent of oestrogens can be accounted for as known urinary and faecal metabolites; the remaining 25 per cent of oestrogen metabolites have not been identified. From Brown J.B. (1959) *J. Obstet. Gynaec. Brit. Cwlth* **66**, 797.

phase the luteinized thecal and granulosa cells continue production. It is likely that the interstitial cells of the stroma can also produce small quantities of oestrogens.

Actions of oestrogens

The principal effects of oestrogens are as follows:

(1) the development of secondary sex characters at puberty,

(2) initiation of the cyclical activity of the reproductive tract and mammary gland; in general, they stimulate proliferation of the epithelia of the genital tract and produce hypertrophy and increased motility of its musculature,

(3) interaction with other endocrine organs; they regulate the pituitary release of gonadotrophins via the hypothalamus, and also increase the concentration of transcortin and thyroxine-binding globulin and so modify the physiological activity of cortisol and thyroxine,

(4) general metabolic effects include slight retention of sodium and water and lowering of plasma lipoprotein concentration (vol. 3, p. 17.12).

Oestradiol is taken up from the bloodstream by target tissues which contain highly specific receptor sites. For example, the endometrium contains specific receptors

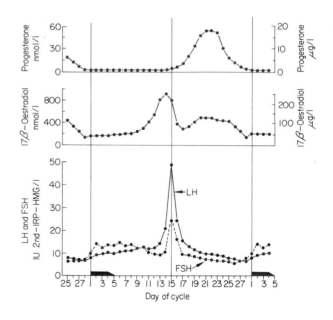

FIG. 38.15. Daily plasma concentrations of gonadotrophins and sex steroids during normal 28-day human menstrual cycle. Data derived from a number of studies and from unpublished observations. The units of LH and FSH are those of the second International Reference Preparation (IRP) of human menopausal gonadotrophin (HMG). Modified from Midgley A.R. Jr. *et al.* (1973) in *Human Reproduction*, ed. Hafez E.S.E. & Evans T.N.

within the cytoplasm. In the cytosol oestrogen associates with a specific receptor protein. The steroid-protein complex moves into the nucleus and as it does so the receptor protein is transformed in a way which can be recognized by the change in its sedimentation rate. This change is also associated with the ability of the complex to bind to certain proteins in the cell nucleus, and results in an activation of the RNA-synthesizing system through RNA polymerase in the nucleus.

The transformation of the receptor protein may be an important step in the action of oestrogens; hence only those tissues which contain this receptor protein in the cytosol will be sensitive to them. On this basis, the subsequent switching on of specific RNA synthesis in these tissues results in the increased production of certain proteins, including enzymes in the target tissues, and thus the rapid growth of the endometrium. In the chicken, the protein ovalbumin is specifically produced in the oviduct under the influence of oestrogens.

Ovarian production of progestogens

The term progestogen or progestin or gestogen indicates the ability to maintain pregnancy, and this may be the primary role of these substances. However, a more useful pharmacological definition of a progestogen is a substance which induces secretory changes in an oestrogen-primed endometrium. Progesterone was the first naturally occurring progestogen to be isolated and identified. Other progestogens have been isolated from the ovary and ovarian venous blood, especially 17-hydroxyprogesterone.

Biosynthesis, metabolism and excretion of progestogens

Progesterone is synthesized from cholesterol via pregnenolone (fig. 38.13). It is carried in the blood partly bound to albumin, and as it is soluble in lipids it is present in adipose tissue.

In the liver, catabolism of progestogens principally involves reduction of the Δ^4-3-ketone group, giving rise to pregnanolone (fig. 38.16). Further reduction at C-20 produces pregnanediol, the principal metabolite of progesterone. This is conjugated almost exclusively with glucuronic acid and is devoid of any progestational activity.

Conjugated metabolites are excreted in both bile and urine, but as they are less readily absorbed in the intestines than are oestrogens, a larger fraction is lost in faeces. The remainder appears in the urine. The major urinary metabolite is pregnanediol, but this represents a very variable proportion of the ovarian production of progestogens.

Progestogen production during the menstrual cycle

The concentration of progesterone in the blood is low throughout the follicular phase of the cycle, but rises following ovulation, mirroring the growth, maturation and regression of the corpus luteum (fig. 38.15).

Site of production of progestogens

Granulosa cells are probably largely responsible for progestogen production. During the follicular phase, these cells are not vascularized, so that any progestogen produced by granulosa cells must filter through thecal cells on its way to the blood stream, and during this passage it is converted to oestrogens. Luteinization is characterized by intense vascularization of the granulosa

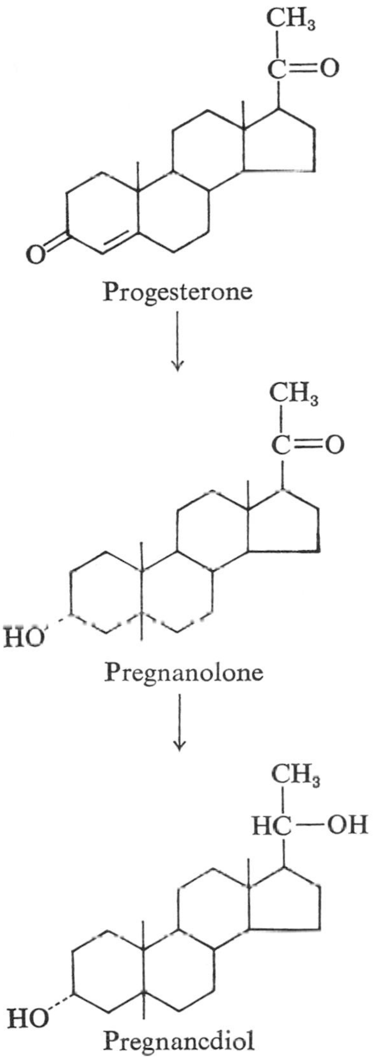

FIG. 38.16. Metabolism of progesterone.

cells, and this permits the entry of progestogens directly into the blood. This two-cell theory implies that thecal cells have all the enzymic potential to synthesize oestrogens, whereas the granulosa component is unable to cleave the side chain of progesterone.

Actions of progestogens

Knowledge of the action of progestogens is limited and the subject is highly controversial. In general, progestogens follow oestrogens in order of appearance during the menstrual cycle, and they must inevitably act synchronously with oestrogens.

(1) In the reproductive tract and breast, progestogens act on oestrogen-primed tissues. They induce a secretory pattern in the endometrium and modify the nature of cervical secretions.

(2) They may reduce the excitability of the myometrium by hyperpolarization of the cell membrane. It is postulated that this represents a general effect of progestogens

on all smooth muscle especially that of the ureter, gut and blood vessels.

(3) Progestogens, or their metabolites, raise resting body temperature.

Ovarian production of androgens

There is incontrovertible proof that the ovaries synthesize androgens. Both testosterone and androstenedione are present in ovarian vein blood in higher concentration than in peripheral blood. These androgens may be produced by thecal cells as a by-product of the synthesis of oestrogens, but they are probably also specifically produced by stromal cells and hilus cells in the ovarian medulla. Further discussion of the metabolism and functions of androgens is found on p. 38.33.

Control of ovarian functions

The role of the adenohypophysis in the control of endocrine glands and the interrelations between hypothalamus and adenohypophysis have already been discussed (p. 27.6). This section is restricted to a description of the control of the ovaries by pituitary gonadotrophins, the hypothalamic control of pituitary gonadotrophins, and the relationships between the ovaries, hypothalamus and pituitary.

PITUITARY GONADOTROPHINS

There are at least two distinct gonadotrophins, **follicle stimulating hormone (FSH)** and **luteinizing hormone (LH)**, also referred to as interstitial cell stimulating hormone (ICSH). These are both glycoproteins and are secreted by the basophil cells of the adenohypophysis. Their molecular weight is about 30 000 and the complete amino acid sequence of LH is known. Sialic acid is an important component and its removal leads to loss of their biological activity. Each glycoprotein consists of two non-identical sub-units, alpha and beta; the alpha unit is similar in all the pituitary glycoproteins of one species, whereas the beta unit confers hormone specificity.

Prolactin is a polypeptide hormone also produced by the adenohypophysis. Although it has the ability to maintain the corpus luteum in some rodents, there is no evidence that it has any luteotrophic activity in the human species. However, a new specific radioimmuno-assay should lead to a better understanding of its role. Its function in relation to human lactation is discussed on p. 38.56.

Gonadotrophins control both the release of ova and the production of sex hormones, and the cyclical changes in the ovary are dependent on their intermittent release. FSH causes growth and distension of the ovarian follicle, but by itself it does not induce ovulation. LH, acting in conjunction with FSH, induces ovarian hyperaemia, stimulates steroidogenesis and induces ovulation and the consequent formation of the corpus luteum.

The factors which control the maintenance and regression of the corpus luteum are still not understood. Prolactin is a luteotrophic agent in many species, but not in women; nor has a luteolysin been demonstrated which might terminate its activity. There remains the possibility that the corpus luteum simply has an intrinsic life span of 10–12 days which is not exceeded in the absence of conception.

The cyclical activity of gonadotrophins is reflected in changes in their plasma concentrations and urinary excretion during the menstrual cycle. Despite the apparently smooth contour of the levels in fig. 38.15 gonadotrophins are not released at a constant rate but in short pulsatile bursts with a disappearance rate determined by their half life. Just prior to menstruation there is a small rise in both FSH and LH concentrations. FSH declines slightly thereafter whereas LH slowly rises. Prior to ovulation there is an abrupt massive pulse of LH activity with a smaller concomitant rise in FSH. These fall rapidly at first and then steadily decline throughout the luteal phase of the cycle. The data correlate with the concept of the major roles of FSH and LH in growth of the follicle and ovulation respectively.

Gonadotrophins are taken up from the circulation by specific receptors on the cell membranes of target tissues. They probably activate the adenyl cyclase system with the release of cyclic AMP from ATP. A prostaglandin may also be an intermediary in the action of LH on the corpus luteum. The mechanisms by which gonadotrophins regulate the ovarian production of sex steroids are not known but it seems likely that LH acts at an early stage in steroid synthesis, possibly by increasing the rate of cleavage of the side chain of cholesterol to pregnenolone.

HYPOTHALAMO–HYPOPHYSIAL RELATIONSHIPS

The anatomical relations of hypophysis and hypothalamus and the hypothalamo–hypophysial portal system are described on p. 27.9. Neurones in the median eminence control the release of gonadotrophins from the adenohypophysis by the synthesis of specific neurohumoral transmitters which pass down the hypothalamo-hypophysial portal system. The synaptic neurotransmitter which triggers these neurones may be dopamine. A gonadotrophin releasing hormone, LH/FSH-RH, a decapeptide with the amino acid sequence pyroglu-his-trp-ser-tyr-gly-leu-arg-pro-gly-NH_2, has been synthesized. This is non-antigenic, has no adverse clinical effects and is available for diagnostic and therapeutic purposes. Other structurally related synthetic peptides have similar biological activity. At present only one hormone has been identified, and it releases both FSH and LH.

The hypothalamus dominates and drives the adenohypophysis, certainly as far as the rhythmic release of gonadotrophins is concerned. In the adult female rat section of the infundibular stalk abolishes cyclical activity. Furthermore, if the hypophysis of an immature rat is transplanted to the hypothalamus of a hypophysectomized adult rat and allowed to revascularize, it exhibits normal adult cyclical activity. Thus, the rhythmic release of gonadotrophins which is the essential feature of adult female sexual activity is the function of the hypothalamus rather than the hypophysis, although the nature of this hypothalamic clock mechanism is unknown. The hypothalamus acts as a final common pathway for the convergence of stimuli which may influence sexual activity, and this information is translated into gonadotrophin activity by the mechanisms described above. These stimuli include a variety of visual and olfactory sensations together with the whole gamut of emotional experience, all of which modify the functioning of the reproductive system.

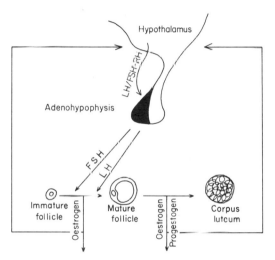

FIG. 38.17. Interrelations between hypothalamus, adenohypophysis and ovaries.

OVARIAN FEEDBACK EFFECTS (fig. 38.17)
There is good evidence that the ovaries exert a regulating influence on the release of gonadotrophins. For example, the urinary excretion of gonadotrophins is decreased by administering oestrogens and increased following bilateral oophorectomy and after the menopause. This indicates a negative feedback relationship between the ovaries and hypophysis. However, an appropriate amount of oestrogen can also increase the output of LH, and this positive feedback mechanism has a crucial role in the regulation of the menstrual cycle. Progesterone has similar but even less well defined feedback effects.

The afferent stimuli for this neurohumoral reflex are ovarian steroids and the central relay area is located in the hypothalamus. Thus, labelled oestrogens are taken up selectively by cells of the hypothalamus. Furthermore, in the rat, destructive lesions in the anterior hypothalamus abolish this feedback mechanism, whereas both ovarian

grafts and oestrogen implants in this area reduce ovarian activity. The efferent side of this reflex comprises the median eminence, hypothalamo-hypophysial portal system and adenohypophysis.

There are other mechanisms which may interact with this hypothalamo–hypophysial–ovarian system. Ovarian steroids may have a direct action on the ovaries, and they may also act directly on the hypophysis. The hypothalamohypophysial portal system which conveys blood from hypophysis to hypothalamus may provide the anatomical basis for a direct short-loop feedback system between hypophysis and hypothalamus. Finally, the other endocrine organs, especially thyroid and adrenal cortex, may interact with all of these components.

The events of the menstrual cycle may be recapitulated as follows (fig. 38.15). At the onset of each cycle, a slight increase in the plasma concentration of FSH and LH can be detected. This is presumably responsible for the development of a fresh crop of follicles. There is little change in the concentration of oestrogen at this early stage of the cycle, but it subsequently rises gradually. The oestrogen which forms the preovulatory surge is probably derived from the dominant Graafian follicle, while the others regress. There is a reciprocal fall in FSH, presumably reflecting a negative feedback effect of oestrogen on the hypothalamic control of pituitary FSH release; LH does not show a similar fall.

Following the oestrogen surge there is a sharp peak in LH concentration and a smaller concomitant rise in FSH, and this is followed 16–24 h later by ovulation.

Following ovulation, oestradiol and progesterone rise and then fall, mirroring the growth, maturation and regression of the corpus luteum, and during the luteal phase FSH and LH reach their lowest level. The factors which control the growth and decline of the corpus luteum are still unknown. The drop in steroid concentrations following the decline of the corpus luteum permits the hypothalamus to increase the output of gonadotrophins and another cycle is initiated.

Ovaries and the reproductive tract
If labelled oestrogens are administered systemically, they are taken up selectively by the hypothalamus, breast and genital tract. The actions of oestrogens on the hypothalamus have been described and their actions on the breast are given on p. 38.56. The component of the genital tract which undergoes the most marked cyclical changes is the endometrium.

ENDOMETRIAL CYCLE (fig. 38.18)
The endometrium undergoes cyclical changes which reflect the activity of the follicle and corpus luteum, the duration and timing of each endometrial cycle usually being synchronized with the development and decline of a single

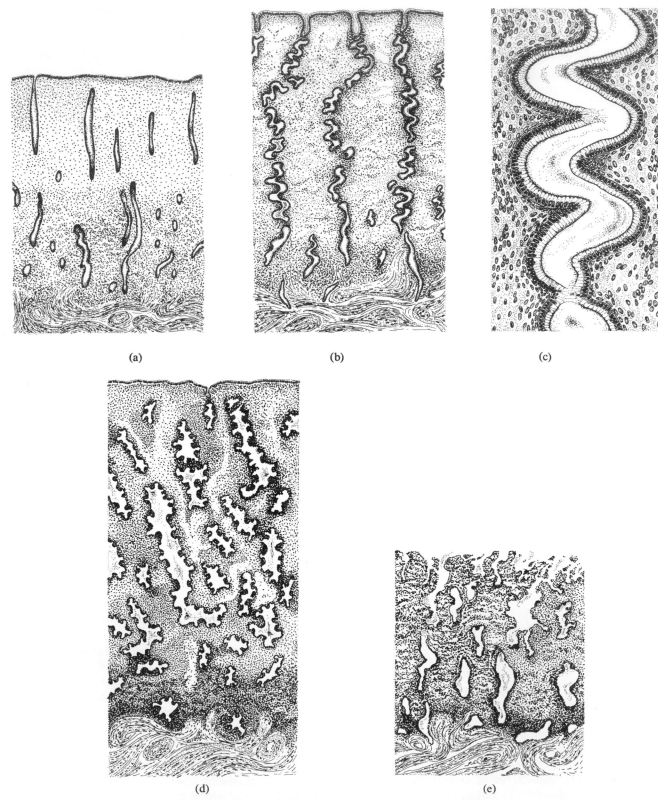

(a)   (b)   (c)

(d)   (e)

Fig. 38.18. Main stages in the endometrial cycle. (a) Proliferative stage; (b) early secretory stage (low power magnification); (c) early secretory stage (high power magnification); (d) late secretory stage; (e) stage of bleeding.

follicle. Each cycle is characterized by a growth phase which parallels the maturation of the follicle, by a secretory phase associated with the development of the corpus luteum, and by a rapid regression which follows the decline of the corpus luteum. The secretory phase provides a receptive endometrium suitable for the implantation of a blastocyst, and its exact nature and duration are influenced by both ovulation and implantation. In the absence of implantation, the corpus luteum undergoes involution, and the endometrium returns to its basal state. Regression of the endometrium is associated with uterine bleeding, and as this bleeding occurs at approximately monthly intervals in women it is known as menstruation.

The endometrium is a mucous membrane with some unusual features. It is composed of simple straight tubular glands lined by columnar epithelium. There is no submucosa intervening between endometrium and myometrium, and the tips of endometrial glands burrow into underlying muscle. These glands lie in a stroma which is more cellular than typical connective tissue, and the stromal cells are responsive to ovarian hormones. This stroma is more than an inert structural framework and has an important part to play in implantation of the fertilized ovum. The endometrium is vascularized by endometrial **spiral arterioles** (fig. 38.19). As these enter the endometrium, they supply less coiled subterminal branches to the deepest layers, while their terminal branches continue into the stroma of the superficial layers and terminate in subepithelial capillary networks. The spiral arterioles are specialized structures characterized by thick muscular and elastic layers, and they are destined to become the vessels which supply the placenta. Each of these constituent parts of the endometrium undergoes cyclical changes, and while the sequence of events in the glands and stroma is well documented, the vascular changes are equally important.

A useful preliminary concept is to recognize two functionally distinct layers within the endometrium. There is a **basal layer** which is in intimate contact with the myometrium. This layer has a separate blood supply from **'straight' arterioles** and is relatively unresponsive to ovarian hormones. It is not subject to menstrual disintegration, and is the layer from which regeneration of the endometrium takes place. By contrast, the **superficial layer** of the endometrium may be thought of as the **functional layer**. All its components respond dramatically to ovarian hormones and it undergoes cyclical growth and regression, being replaced after each menstrual loss by repair from the basal layer.

Menstrual bleeding normally lasts for 2–7 days and occurs at regular intervals of 21–35 days, the average duration of the menstrual cycle being 28 days. This interval is calculated from the first day of one menstrual flow to the day of onset of the next bleeding. To simplify

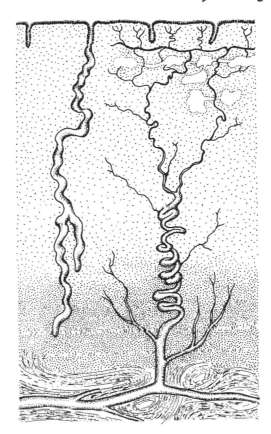

Fig. 38.19. Blood supply of endometrium.

description it is convenient to consider a typical 28-day cycle, day 1 referring to the day of onset of bleeding. In such a cycle, ovulation occurs around the 14th day, and it is possible to distinguish follicular and luteal phases of ovarian activity which precede and follow ovulation. This is reflected in corresponding phases of endometrial activity.

Follicular phase

Menstruation results in disintegration of the functional layer of the endometrium, leaving the residual basal layer no more than 1 mm thick. Regeneration begins even before menstrual loss is complete, by proliferation of the epithelium of the stumps of endometrial glands and possibly by conversion of stromal cells into epithelial elements.

Under the influence of oestrogens from the developing follicle, the endometrium enters a phase of rapid proliferation. The glands lengthen and become tortuous and the epithelium shows intense mitotic activity, while the stroma increases in cellularity, each cell being composed of a dense nucleus with little cytoplasm, so that the nuclei appear naked. This intense proliferative activity is indicated by an increase in the content of ribonucleic acid and in alkaline phosphatase activity of the endometrium. During the follicular phase, spiral arterioles increase in length and tortuosity, each parent vessel giving rise to ten to fifteen branches. The follicular phase is usually completed within 14 days from the onset of menstruation.

Luteal phase

Following ovulation and subsequent luteinization of the follicle, oestrogen synthesis is supplemented by the production of progestogens.

The luteal phase is characterized by secretory activity and the decline of cellular proliferation. The first signs of secretory activity are subnuclear vacuoles in the glandular epithelium which displace the basal nuclei towards the centre of the cells. These vacuoles contain glycogen and glycosaminoglycans and move towards the periphery of the cells where they discharge their contents into the glandular lumen. Histologically two zones in the functional layer of the endometrium can now be distinguished. In the deeper zone, the stroma becomes loose and oedematous while the glands become distended with secretory products. This zone is commonly referred to as the **spongy layer**. In the superficial zone, the stromal cells become polygonal with a prominent cytoplasm and are packed around the necks of endometrial glands. This gives the superficial zone a dense cellular appearance and it is referred to as the **compact layer**. This alteration in the appearance of the stromal cells in the compact layer becomes even more pronounced in the event of implantation. Spiral arterioles increase in length so that their distal ends approach very close to the surface of the endometrium. This increase in length of the arterioles is greater than the increase in depth of the endometrium, and this exaggerates their coiling. Close to the surface of the endometrium the spiral vessels form an extensive subepithelial capillary plexus.

MENSTRUATION

If implantation does not occur, luteolysis ensues and there is a rapid fall in the production of oestrogens and progestogens beginning about the 24th day.

With the withdrawal of steroid hormones, the spongy layer shrinks by loss of extracellular fluid, and the compact layer becomes infiltrated with polymorphs and mononuclear leucocytes. This collapse of the endometrium causes further coiling of the spiral arterioles, and results in vascular stasis and reduction of blood flow through the endometrium. Passive stasis is followed by active vasoconstriction, and the consequent reduction in blood supply causes the death of the endometrium (ischaemic necrosis). These arterioles subsequently relax and allow blood, under arterial pressure, to flow into vessels damaged by ischaemia. Rupture of these vessels produces uterine bleeding and the necrotic endometrium disintegrates. This process occurs patchily throughout the endometrium over a period of days, so that one area may have been shed and be in process of repair, while an adjacent area may still be viable. This process of ischaemic necrosis and shedding does not affect the basal layer.

Menstruation is seen to be due immediately to ischaemia, and the volume of bleeding is controlled by this constriction-relaxation sequence in the spiral arterioles. The factors which control vasoconstriction of the spiral arterioles are clearly of importance but are not understood, although a number of vasoconstrictor substances, such as prostaglandins, have been identified in the endometrium.

From the point of view of conception, the result of the secretory phase is the preparation of the endometrium for implantation of the blastocyst. The secretion of glycogen into the uterine cavity provides nutrients before a placental circulation is established; the development of the spiral arterioles provides the basis for the maternal placental circulation, while the changes in the stromal cells are the beginnings of decidualization, which is probably of importance in determining the depth of implantation. Menstruation is a specific growth-limiting mechanism which supervenes when implantation fails to occur.

The menstrual cycle varies both in duration of bleeding and in the interval between cycles. These may be expressed as a fraction; the numerator is the number of days of bleeding and the denominator the interval between periods, always calculated from the first day of one cycle to the first day of the next cycle. Thus, when a patient bleeds for 4 days every 28 days, the cycle is 4/28. It is uncommon for any woman to have a perfectly regular 28 day cycle. The mean length drops from 30 to 26 days between the ages of 20 and 40 years, with a s.d. for each woman of 3 to 4 days. The variation is greater in the first 4 to 6 years after the menarche, and in the last two premenopausal years the mean length of cycle is 44 days with a s.d. of 19 days. The duration of a normal period ranges from 2 to 7 days. Periods lasting only one day are infrequent and may be anovular

MYOMETRIUM

During the follicular phase, uterine contractions are of low intensity and occur at intervals of 30–60 sec, reaching maximum frequency at the time of ovulation. During the luteal phase, contractions occur less frequently but with greater intensity, the greatest amplitude occurring at the time of menstruation.

Little is known of the mechanisms which control uterine contractility. The molecular basis of a uterine contraction is actomyosin, and ATP is the immediate energy source. Oestrogens control myometrial work potential by determining the concentration of actomyosin in the uterus. Progestogens probably do not influence the contractile mechanisms but may reduce excitability and impair the propagation of impulses by hyperpolarizing the myometrial cell membranes. Catecholamines and other β-receptor stimulants reduce the contractility of the myometrium.

Oxytocin (p. 27.16) is a powerful myometrial stimulant. It may be of importance in parturition, but its role in the non-pregnant woman is unknown.

There are several other naturally occurring substances which stimulate the uterus *in vitro*. Some of these, such as prostaglandins, may be important in spermatozoa transport in the uterus, but their role in the overall control of uterine contractility is unknown.

TUBAL MOTILITY AND TRANSPORT

The uterine tubes are influenced by sex hormones. When they are under the influence of oestrogens during the first phase of the ovarian cycle, the epithelium proliferates and the ciliated cells increase in height. They become shorter in the postovulation phase, when the secretory cells become more active. Although the actual composition of the tubal secretions is not fully established, the granules in the secretory cells appear to be mainly lipid and glycogen, and the secretion may provide nutrients for the ovum during its passage to the uterus. The muscle cells in the tubal wall also vary in size during different phases of the cycle, being largest at about the time of ovulation.

With regard to the transport of germ cells in the uterine tube, it is necessary to consider both the contraction of the tubal muscle and the movement of the cilia. The muscular coat undergoes peristaltic movements, but usually the peristaltic wave does not travel the complete length of the tube. The contractions of the isthmus are the more regular, and at intervals spread to the uterine muscle. Contractions of tubal muscle are more intense at about the time of ovulation and at this time the vascularity of the tube is also greater. The tubal movements are under hormonal control, being more pronounced under oestrogenic stimulation and inhibited by progestogens.

Muscle fibres in the ligament of the ovary, in the infundibulopelvic ligament and in the fimbriae all take part in the rhythmic movements of the internal generative organs. These movements tend to bring the ovary and uterus closer together, and bring the fimbriated end of the tube into closer contact with the ovary. These movements assist the ovulated oocyte into the infundibulum and also aid the transport of spermatozoa to the fertilization site in the ampulla. The contractions diminish after ovulation under the influence of the secretions of the corpus luteum.

Tubal contractions may be the main factor involved in the first and most rapid phase of transport of an ovum. However, as the contractions diminish soon after ovulation, ciliary action, which moves the tubal secretions in the direction of the uterus, may be increasingly responsible for moving the ovum along the tube, particularly assisting it over the ridges formed by the folds in the mucosa. The direction of the ciliary currents has been shown to be from the infundibulum to the uterus and, although the ciliated cells do not form continuous sheets and become more sparse towards the medial end of the tube, a sufficiently effective current is set up in the tubal fluid to assist in the transport of the ovum.

Movement through the ampulla is slow, but through the isthmus it is rapid. A fertilized ovum takes about $3\frac{1}{2}$ days to reach the uterus, and an unfertilized oocyte degenerates within a day or so, being no longer intact when it passes into the uterus.

Spermatozoa transport in the uterine tube is due to the peristaltic movements of the tubes and to countercurrents set up in the secondary compartments formed by the mucosal folds. These folds and compartments are not fixed, but change constantly as the tube contracts and relaxes. Spermatozoa of course also move towards an oocyte by virtue of their own motility.

CERVIX

There is no clear cut cyclical pattern in the cervical epithelium, and it does not undergo menstrual shedding. The mucus secreted by cervical glands, however, does show cyclical changes. Around the time of ovulation, and in response to rising oestrogen levels, there is an increase in the water and electrolyte content of cervical mucus. As a result, its volume increases and its viscosity is reduced. This produces a profuse, clear mucoid discharge which is typically thready in consistency. If a drop of mucus at this time is allowed to dry out on a clean slide, the crystallization of electrolytes produces a characteristic ferning or arborization pattern (fig. 38.20). In the later stages of the luteal phase, presumably under the influence of progestogens, these changes are reversed; the volume decreases, its viscosity increases and ferning cannot be demonstrated.

The changes in the nature of cervical mucus at the time of ovulation facilitate its penetration by spermatozoa following insemination.

VAGINA

The sequence of histological changes in the vagina is poorly documented, but there is much information on the nature of its exfoliated cells (fig. 38.20). During the follicular phase, under the influence of oestrogens, the vaginal epithelium proliferates and there is a continuous shedding of the superficial cells from the keratinized layer. These desquamated cells have densely pyknotic nuclei and their cytoplasm has an affinity for eosin. Consequently, a vaginal smear in the proliferative phase is characterized by a preponderance of pink-staining cells with pyknotic nuclei, and the intensity of oestrogenic influence may be assessed by an eosinophilic index or by the karyopyknotic index (KI). Following ovulation the

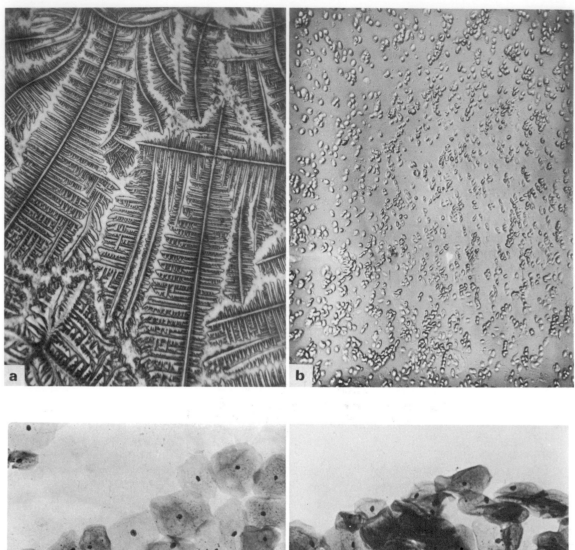

Fig. 38.20. Cervical mucus (× 170). Courtesy Dr R.R. MacDonald   (a) Normal mucus at time of ovulation. Typical salt crystallization showing the marked fern pattern.   (b) Normal premenstrual or pregnancy mucus showing endocervical cells and no crystals. Vaginal smear (× 200). Courtesy Dr E. Little   (c) Pre-ovulatory, showing large flat discrete cells with pyknotic nuclei.   (d) Post-ovulatory, showing clumping of cells with folded edges.

number of desquamated cells is progressively reduced and those which are shed tend to form clusters, each cell having a typically curled edge, and there is an increased number of leucocytes in the smear. The vaginal smear gives a useful estimate of oestrogen activity but a much poorer assessment of progestational activity.

GENERAL SYSTEMIC CHANGES

Body temperature, recorded immediately on waking in the morning, is raised during the luteal phase of the cycle. This is almost certainly a function of progestogens or their metabolites, acting via the central nervous system. The precise time relation of this temperature shift to ovulation is not clear.

Evidence on changes in body weight and composition is conflicting. There is no evidence of a consistent increase in weight in the premenstrual phase, but there are small changes in blood composition throughout the cycle involving both cellular and plasma constituents. These are neither sufficiently pronounced nor consistent enough to influence the interpretation of most biochemical data for routine clinical purposes, but they deserve recognition for any more detailed research work.

Finally, the behavioural changes associated with the ovarian cycle are of immense importance. About 50 per cent of women experience varying degrees of pain with their periods, 20–30 per cent complain of irritability, depression and tension prior to the onset of bleeding (the premenstural syndrome) and 70 per cent complain of general bodily discomfort, particularly a sensation of bloating or swelling, although this latter complaint is not associated with an increase in total body weight. In more general terms, it has been shown that both academic and athletic performances are slightly impaired in the premenstrual period, while the incidence of serious crime, accidents and suicides is slightly increased. For further information, see vol. 3, p. 28.12.

Clearly, the menstrual cycle is not a phenomenon localized to the reproductive tract, but represents phasic activity involving the whole woman. It is important to recognize the teleological significance of the menstrual cycle. The follicular phase of the ovarian cycle initiates the preparation of the uterus for conception. At midcycle, an oocyte is deposited in the uterine tube and simultaneous changes in the cervical mucus facilitate the ascent of spermatozoa, thereby providing the opportunity for fertilization. The corpus luteum completes the preparation of the endometrium and myometrium for implantation of the blastocyst. If, however, fertilization or implantation fails to occur, the ovarian cycle is terminated and menstruation occurs.

Onset and cessation of menstrual activity

The menstrual cycle is the characteristic of sexual maturity and each sequence represents preparation for conception.

PUBERTY

The term **adolescence** refers to the attainment of physical and social maturity, the transformation of a child to an adult. This phase is not capable of exact definition but sexual maturation is only one aspect of adolescence. **Puberty** refers to the 'state of being functionally capable of procreation', and in the normal female this implies the presence of ovulation. The **menarche** refers to the onset of cyclical vaginal bleeding. This is a notable landmark during adolescence, but the menarche is not usually synchronous with the onset of ovulation.

At birth there is a transient phase of sexual pseudoprecocity. The breasts may secrete colostrum (p. 38.56), the internal and external genitalia are relatively enlarged, and a few infants bleed vaginally. These phenomena are due to the presence of a relatively high concentration of maternal oestrogens in the fetus, and their abrupt withdrawal at delivery. No further external signs of activity in the reproductive tract can be detected until the 10th or 11th year. During this time the ovary has been steadily increasing in size, and around the 10th year the uterus develops rapidly.

The breasts show the first external signs of sex development (fig. 38.21). The infantile breast consists of a nipple projecting from a pigmented areola. Around the 10th or 11th year, the areola becomes everted as a pigmented bud from which the nipple still projects. Thereafter, an increase in gland tissue and fat deep to the areola causes

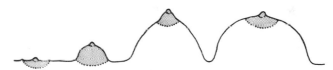

FIG. 38.21. Development of the breast at puberty. From Hamblen, E.C. (1945) *Endocrinology of Women*. Springfield, Ill.: C.C. Thomas.

the areolar bud to become elevated on a non-pigmented hillock and, with further development, the areola becomes flattened over the underlying breast tissue. The onset of breast changes is rapidly followed by the appearance of pubic hair. This appears on the labia majora and spreads over the mons pubis to form a triangle. A year or two later, axillary hair appears.

The menarche is a relatively late feature of adolescence. The average age of the menarche in Great Britain is 13.5 years, but there is a wide scatter between the ages of 10 and 17 years. For the first year or two, menstruation is commonly anovular, i.e. it is associated with cyclical follicular development and regression, but ovulation does not occur.

The mechanisms involved in the onset of puberty are still unknown. It is clear that the prepubertal hypophysis contains and secretes small quantities of gonadotrophins, and the prepubertal ovary responds by secreting small quantities of oestrogens. However, the immature hypophysis is potentially capable of adult functions and similarly the ovary of an immature animal, when transplanted into a spayed adult, can release both ova and sex hormones. These observations suggest that prior to the menarche the hypophysial–ovarian system is held under restraint.

The reproductive axis in the immature female is similar to the adult in terms of structure and organization, but is set at a much lower level. The factors which alter this level and so initiate sexual development are unknown, but they may include changes in the production or metabolism of ovarian hormones, or alterations in the sensitivity of the hypothalamus to these hormones.

Finally, the adrenal cortex plays a part in sexual development, and is responsible for the growth of pubic and axillary hair.

CLIMACTERIC

The cessation of menstruation is known as the **menopause**, while the **climacteric** refers to the general physiological changes which occur at this time. The age of the menopause in Britain is about 50.5 years, with a normal range from 40 to 55 years.

The essential cause of the climacteric is ovarian failure. The hypophysis continues to secrete gonadotrophins in increasing quantities but the ovaries fail to release either ova or hormones. This is followed by permanent loss of powers of reproduction but there is usually no sudden reduction in active sexual behaviour. As a consequence of ovarian failure and the withdrawal of sex steroids, the genital tract and breasts atrophy and there are widespread physiological repercussions. The climacteric is sometimes associated with psychological disturbances.

MECHANISMS OF REPRODUCTION IN THE MALE

ANATOMY OF THE MALE REPRODUCTIVE TRACT

Scrotum

This is a pouch of skin situated below the root of the penis. It is divided internally by a median sagittal fibrous septum, and this division is marked on the surface by a median ridge, the **scrotal raphe**. The scrotal skin is dark and thin and contains numerous sebaceous glands and sparse hairs. Its subcutaneous tissue contains smooth muscle fibres, the **dartos muscle**. This muscle contracts in response to cold or exercise, and its contraction makes the scrotum smaller and causes its skin to be wrinkled.

Testis and epididymis

The two testes are smooth, ovoid structures which are laterally compressed. They measure about 2·5 cm from side to side, 3 cm from back to front and about 4 cm in length. The left testis is situated at a slightly lower level than the right testis.

Each testis projects forwards into a closed serous sac, the **tunica vaginalis**, so that only the posterior part of the testis is not covered by a double layer of tunica (fig. 38.22). The parietal and visceral layers of the tunica are usually separated from each other by only a thin film of fluid. The testis and the tunica vaginalis are attached to the lower part of the scrotum by a fibrous condensation, the **scrotal ligament**, which may be derived from the gubernaculum (p. 38.61).

The coverings of the testis are several because in the course of the development of the scrotum extensions from the different layers of the abdominal wall are carried down to the scrotal sac (p. 21.28). With the exception of the tunica vaginalis, which is related only to the testis and epididymis, the coverings of the testis are the same as those which invest the spermatic cord. The coverings from within outwards are as follows:

(1) the tunica vaginalis derived from the peritoneum,

(2) the **internal spermatic fascia** derived from the transversalis fascia,

(3) the **cremasteric muscle and fascia** derived from the internal oblique muscle,

(4) the **external spermatic fascia** derived from the aponeurosis of the external oblique muscle,

(5) the membranous layer of the superficial fascia (p. 21.30).

The epididymis is a comma-shaped structure which is closely applied to the posterior surface of the testis, overlapping its posterolateral aspect. The upper part is expanded and known as the head. The **head** overhangs the upper pole of the testis and tapers down to form the **body** which in turn becomes continuous with a thin **tail** which is related to the lower pole of the testis. The tail is continuous with the **ductus deferens** which then ascends on the medial side of the epididymis. The head of the epididymis is connected to the back of the testis by fifteen to twenty **efferent ductules**. The epididymis is in effect an extensively coiled duct which if straightened out would be 5–7 m long.

The **sinus of the epididymis** is an infolding of tunica vaginalis which partially separates the testis from the epididymis on the lateral side.

Embryological remnants of the mesonephric and paramesonephric ducts may be found in relation to the upper pole of the testis and the epididymis.

STRUCTURE

Each testis is completely invested by a dense, white, inelastic capsule, the **tunica albuginea**, which projects into the testicular substance at the posterior surface of that organ to form the **mediastinum testis**. From the mediastinum, where the testis is penetrated by its vessels and

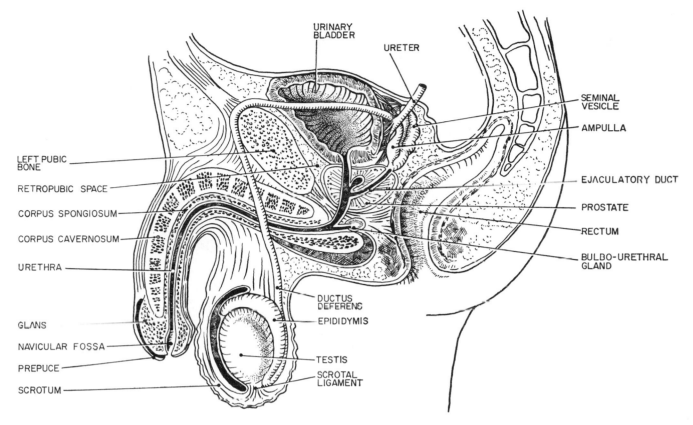

FIG. 38.22. Median sagittal section of the male pelvis. From Turner C.D. (1966) *General Endocrinology*, 4th Edition. Philadelphia: Saunders.

nerves, radiates a series of thin septa which reach out to the inner surface of the tunica and divide the testis into about 250 conical compartments, or **lobes of the testis**, and these contain the seminiferous tubules (fig. 38.23).

Each **seminiferous tubule** is highly coiled and when teased out is about 70 cm long. They are looped in such a way that both ends join a series of about thirty short, **straight tubules** which converge on a network of vessels lying in the mediastinum, the **rete testis**. Within each lobe, the seminiferous tubules are embedded in delicate connective tissue which contains polyhedral **interstitial cells (Leydig cells)** some of which are swollen with lipids. These are the source of testicular androgens.

Examination of the fine structure of interstitial tissue suggests that Leydig cells are closely applied to capillaries. Both are separated from the wall of an adjoining seminiferous tubule by a lymphatic space. This arrangement probably assists the passage of male hormone from the Leydig cells into the seminiferous tubules by exposing most of their walls to lymph containing a high concentration of androgen.

Each seminiferous tubule has a basement membrane on which are set cells wich constitute two elements with differing functions; one is spermatogenic and the other supportive. In an active testis the former group includes

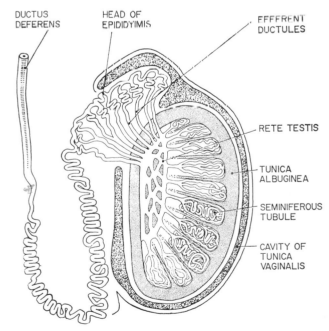

FIG. 38.23. Arrangement of tubules and ducts in the testis and epididymis. From Hamilton W.J., Boyd J.D. & Mossman H.W. (1972) *Human Embryology*, 4th Edition. Cambridge: Heffer.

a whole array of cells, from the germinal cells called **spermatogonia**, through their derived forms of **spermatocytes** and **spermatids**, to the final product, the **spermatozoa** (p. 38.31). The supportive, or **sustentacular cells of Sertoli**, are the only non-germinal cells inside the seminiferous tubules. They are somewhat polymorphic cells, but in transverse sections of tubules they appear approximately columnar. The apical profiles are complicated by recesses into which spermatids and spermatozoa fit until the latter are mature enough to be released into the lumen of the tubule. They also possess long cytoplasmic processes that extend among spermatogonia and spermatocytes. The Sertoli cells provide mechanical support, protection and probably nutrition for the developing germ cells. The boundaries of Sertoli cells are hardly ever distinct and the cells are recognized mainly by their irregular oval vesicular nuclei, which are often indented and have prominent nucleoli. The cells of Sertoli usually persist in degenerative conditions in which the cells of the germinal line disappear. Primary spermatogonia are attached to the basement membrane, and cells at successive stages of the spermatogenic cycle (p. 38.31) are pushed towards the lumen of the tubule so that mature spermatozoa reach the lumen. However, the arrangement of the cells is too irregular for intermediate types to be recognized simply by their position within the tubule (fig. 38.24).

The variable appearance of cross-sections of seminiferous tubules is partly explained by the fact that spermatogenesis occurs in waves which proceed along the length of the tubule. Before one generation of cells has matured completely at any point of the tubule another wave of growth is initiated.

The epithelium of **straight tubules** consists of tall columnar cells and that of the rete testis is cuboidal or low columnar. The rete testis is continuous with the efferent ductules and these in turn open into the ducts of the head of the epididymis. The **efferent ductules** are about 5 cm long, but only 0·5 mm in diameter. They become increasingly convoluted as they are traced away from the testis. In this way they form the **lobules of the epididymis**. These lobules are conical with the apex directed towards the upper part of the mediastinum of the testis and the base fits into the head of the epididymis. The lining of these ductules is made up of alternating patches of tall and short cells. The tall ones are ciliated and may help to move the spermatozoa towards the epididymis. The short cells are secretory, have a brush border and a central non-motile process similar to the stereocilium of the epididymal epithelium. A thin layer of circularly disposed smooth muscle lies external to the basement membrane of the ductules and its contraction presumably helps to move the spermatozoa towards the epididymis.

The **duct of the epididymis**, which is very tortuous in its upper part, ceases to be tortuous and increases in calibre just before it turns from the tail of the epididymis to be continuous with the ductus deferens (fig. 38.25). In its convoluted part the lining epithelium is pseudostratified and columnar, the individual epithelial cells being furnished with a long non-motile process, a **stereocilium**

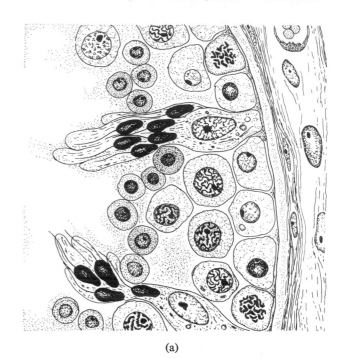

(a)

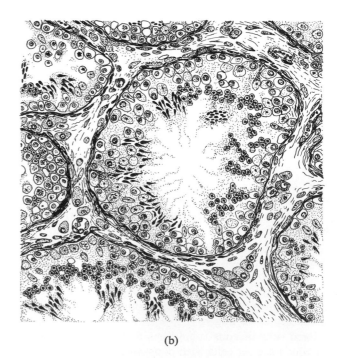

(b)

FIG. 38.24. Structure of seminiferous tubule. (a) Low power view; (b) high power view of part of tubule.

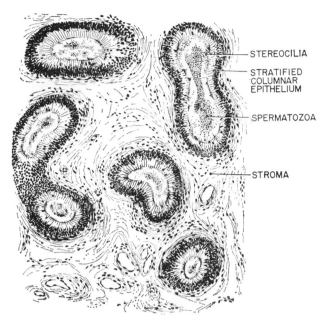

STEREOCILIA

STRATIFIED
COLUMNAR
EPITHELIUM

SPERMATOZOA

STROMA

FIG. 38.25. Structure of the epididymis showing several sections through the duct. From Bloom W. & Fawcett D.W. (1962) *A Textbook of Histology*, 8th Edition. Philadelphia: Saunders.

(p. 13.16). This structure is concerned with the discharge of the secretions of the cell which provide nutrition for the spermatozoa and play a role in their maturation. The duct is surrounded by a circular layer of smooth muscle and the coils are held together by connective tissue. The tallness of the epithelial cells in the excretory ducts of the testis and in the epididymis is dependent on adequate stimulation by androgenic hormone circulating in the blood. If, for any reason, the level of androgenic stimulation falls, the epithelia in these ducts involute.

NERVE SUPPLY

The testicular nerves originate from the tenth thoracic segment and contain both afferent and efferent fibres. The sympathetic nerves are derived from the plexus around the aorta at the level of origin of the testicular arteries. These testicular nerves communicate with those of the ductus deferens which are derived from the hypogastric plexus. The scrotal nerves are branches of the pudendal nerve and the perineal branch of the posterior cutaneous nerve of the thigh. The ilioinguinal nerve supplies the upper anterior part of the scrotum.

BLOOD SUPPLY AND LYMPH DRAINAGE

Each **testicular artery** arises from the aorta immediately below the origin of the renal artery. It runs down the posterior abdominal wall to reach the spermatic cord at the internal inguinal ring. Before reaching the testis it supplies branches to the epididymis.

Veins emerge from the posterior aspect of the testis as an anastomotic plexus, known as the **pampiniform plexus,** which passes up the spermatic cord. At the internal inguinal ring the plexus forms testicular veins which drain on the right side into the inferior vena cava, and on the left side into the left renal vein.

A **counter-current heat exchange** occurs between the arteries and veins in the spermatic cord where both sets of vessels are markedly coiled and in close contact. This arrangement may play a role in maintaining the testis at a temperature below that of the peritoneal cavity.

The lymphatic vessels draining the testis and the epididymis accompany the veins and reach the lateral aortic lymph nodes near the origin of the testicular arteries.

The scrotum and coverings of the testis are supplied by the internal pudendal artery, by the cremasteric branch of the inferior epigastric artery and by the external pudendal artery. The veins follow the arteries, and the lymphatics pass to the superficial inguinal nodes.

Spermatic cord

This cord extends from the internal inguinal ring to the posterior border of the testis. Where it emerges from the inguinal canal at the external inguinal ring, it lies immediately under the skin and superficial fascia and is easy to palpate. It then passes in front of the pubis to reach the scrotum. The spermatic cord contains the ductus deferens (which has the consistency to touch of whip-cord), the testicular arteries, the pampiniform plexus of veins and testicular lymphatics and nerves, all bound together by loose connective tissue.

The coverings of the cord have been described with the coverings of the testis. The cremasteric coat, including as it does striped muscle, has its own nerve supply from the genitofemoral nerve. By its contraction, the cremaster muscle raises the testis within the scrotum and the cremasteric reflex contraction is brought into action by stimulating the skin of the upper part of the thigh supplied by the femoral branch of the genitofemoral nerve. In male infants, the cremasteric reflex may be especially marked and overactivity of the cremaster muscles may pull the testes up to the inguinal region. Such 'retractile testes' may be mistaken for incompletely descended testes.

Ductus deferens (vas deferens)

This fibromuscular tube is characterized by a very thick wall compared to the size of its lumen, and is 45 cm long. It begins at the tail of the epididymis as the continuation of the duct of the epididymis and passes into the spermatic cord. It reaches the pelvic cavity after leaving the internal inguinal ring by hooking round the lateral side of the inferior epigastric artery. As it passes over the pelvic brim it becomes separated from the other constituents of the spermatic cord and runs backwards and medially

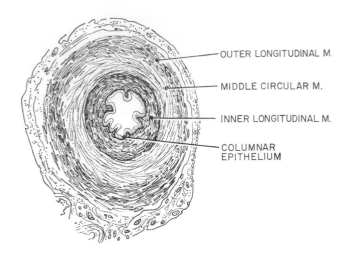

OUTER LONGITUDINAL M.

MIDDLE CIRCULAR M.

INNER LONGITUDINAL M.

COLUMNAR EPITHELIUM

FIG. 38.26. Structure of the ductus deferens. From Bloom W. & Fawcett D.W. (1968) *A Textbook of Histology*, 9th Edition. Philadelphia: Saunders.

under the peritoneum to reach the ureter close to where it enters the back of the bladder. It crosses above and in front of the ureter to converge on its fellow from the opposite side and then runs down towards the prostate between the bladder in front and the rectum behind. Here the ductus deferens comes to lie medially to its corresponding seminal vesicle. Each ductus continues on its downward course and becomes dilated and tortuous to form an **ampulla**. Just above the prostate, each ductus narrows and is joined by the duct of the seminal vesicle, and so forms the **ejaculatory duct** which runs on through the substance of the prostate.

The ductus deferens has a thick muscular coat made up of outer and inner longitudinal, and a middle circular layer of smooth muscle. The total diameter of the duct is no more than 2·5 mm and the muscle coat is 1 mm thick so that it accounts for most of the thickness of the tube. It is peristalsis of this thick muscular coat which moves spermatozoa towards the ampulla. At the ampulla the muscular wall is much thinner. The lamina propria of the mucous membrane supports a pseudostratified tall columnar epithelium bearing non-motile stereocilia.

The arteries of the duct are derived from the testicular artery and from the vesical arteries; its nerves arise from the pelvic plexus.

Seminal vesicles

These apparently lobulated organs are placed symmetrically on each side of the midline behind the bladder and above the prostate. Each vesicle is about 5 cm long and is fusiform, the long axis being set obliquely with the upper extremities diverging. The upper end of each vesicle lies behind and lateral to the ureter as it enters the bladder. Between the vesicles lie the ampullae of the two ductus deferentes. The duct of the seminal vesicle joins the lower end of the ampulla of the ductus at an acute angle to form the ejaculatory duct.

Each vesicle is a coiled, elongated, blind sac measuring about 12 cm when dissected out, and is in effect a diverticulum from the lower part of the ductus deferens. Up to ten blind diverticula extend from the main sac and the whole tortuous complex is held together tightly by connective tissue. Each component duct is surrounded by an elastic layer of connective tissue outside a coat of smooth muscle. The mucous membrane is folded in a complex fashion so that the folds break up the lumen into numerous intercommunicating spaces. These spaces are lined by stratified or pseudostratified columnar or cuboidal epithelium which is secretory. The secretory activity of the vessels is under the control of androgens and the average capacity of a seminal vesicle is 2–3 ml of sticky fluid.

Before puberty its mucous membrane shows very few folds but at puberty under the influence of the testicular secretion the mucosa grows very rapidly and is thrown up into folds. Any subsequent decrease in the amount of androgenic stimulation leads to decrease in the size and secretory activity of the organ.

The nerve supply is derived from the pelvic plexuses. The vesicles are supplied with blood by the inferior vesical and middle rectal arteries. The veins drain into the vesico-prostatic plexus of veins.

Ejaculatory ducts

These are formed by the junction of the duct of the seminal vesicle with the ductus deferens of the corresponding side at the posterosuperior surface of the prostate. The ducts then pass obliquely forwards, medially and downwards through the substance of the prostate to open into the back of the **prostatic urethra** on either side of the opening of the **prostatic utricle** on the **urethral crest**. The elevation formed at the opening of the utricle and ejaculatory duct is known as the **colliculus seminalis**. The ejaculatory duct, which is about 2 cm long, is more in line with the duct of the seminal vesicle than with the ductus deferens.

Prostate

This organ is formed of fibrous, muscular and glandular tissue. It is described as having the shape of a chestnut, or as being an inverted pyramid whose base is applied to the neck of the bladder. Its apex rests on the fascia covering the urogenital diaphragm and its posterior surface faces the rectum. Its convex inferolateral surfaces are related to the levator ani muscle of each side. The rounded anterior border of the gland is separated from the back of the pubis by a space of about 2 cm which is filled with the retropubic pad of fat (fig. 38.22).

The normal gland usually measures about 2·5 cm from front to back, 3 cm from above downwards, and nearly

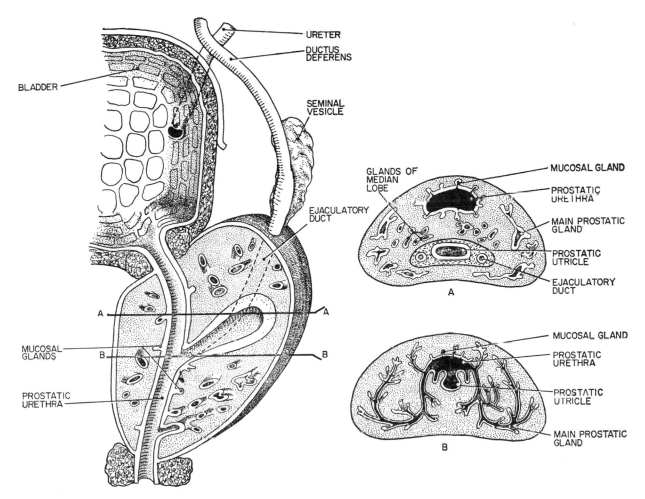

FIG. 38.27. Sagittal and horizontal sections through the prostate. A and B are horizontal sections through lines A–A and B–B respectively. From Hamilton W.J., Boyd J.D. & Mossman H.W. (1972) *Human Embryology*, 4th Edition. Cambridge: Heffer.

4 cm from side to side. The prostate is surrounded by a sheath of condensed pelvic fascia, which separates it from the levator ani muscle. This sheath, also called the **false capsule** of the prostate, is continuous below with the fascia on the superior surface of the urogenital diaphragm (p. 21.32) and, through it, is attached to the pubic arch. Anteriorly, the prostatic sheath merges with a condensation of fibrous tissue, the **puboprostatic ligament**, which attaches it to the symphysis pubis.

Within the prostatic sheath, and separating it from the true fibrous capsule, there is a rich plexus of veins which forms the **vesicoprostatic plexus**, located principally in the groove between the bladder and the prostate. The deep dorsal vein of the penis pierces the sheath to drain into the anterior part of the plexus.

Because of these ligaments and the fact that its lateral surfaces are firmly gripped by the levator ani muscle, some of whose fibres gain attachment to the gland's fascial covering, the prostate is firmly fixed in the pelvis. In turn, the prostate fixes the neck of the bladder.

The prostate gland is traversed from top to bottom by the prostatic urethra which normally runs an anteroposteriorly curved course through the gland and lies closer to its anterior than to its posterior surface.

STRUCTURE (fig. 38.27)

The whole gland is enclosed in a dense fibrous capsule which adheres closely to the underlying tissue, and is called the **true capsule** to distinguish it from its sheath derived from the pelvic fascia. The stroma of the gland consists of fibromuscular tissue. The muscular component is smooth muscle.

The urethra appears as a semilunar split in horizontal sections through the gland. This is due to a projection into the posterior wall called the **urethral crest**. The prostatic glandular ducts, thirty on each side, open into the urethra on each side of the crest.

The glandular tissue consists of secretory acini of irregular shape and size surrounded by the fibromuscular stroma. The epithelium consists of pseudostratified or stratified columnar cells. After middle age, acini may contain concretions of secretion and desquamated cells.

That part of the prostate which is in front of the urethra is practically devoid of glandular tissue. The part of the prostate between the urethra and the ejaculatory ducts consists of glands that open near the opening of the prostatic utricle and constitute the **middle** or **median lobe** of the prostate. The **prostatic utricle** is a blind glandular diverticulum which extends up the posterior margin of the median lobe between the ejaculatory ducts.

Although small mucosal glands open into the urethra at all points of its circumference, the main prostatic glands occupy chiefly the lateral and posterior portions and open on either side of the urethral crest by way of the prostatic glandular ducts described above.

The glands of the median lobe and the small mucosal glands constitute the **inner zone** in which senile enlargement usually starts. Carcinoma of the prostate usually starts in the **outer zone** which consists of the main prostatic glands.

At birth the prostatic utricle and particularly the median lobe show signs of stimulation by maternal oestrogens but these effects disappear within 2 months. The gland grows rapidly at puberty, and continues to grow till the age of 30 years. Involutionary changes, particularly at the periphery of the gland, start after about 40 years of age and the gland normally becomes smaller with increasing age.

The blood supply of the prostate is derived from the inferior vesical, middle rectal and internal pudendal arteries. The veins form a rich plexus in the fascial covering of the gland which contributes to the vesico-prostatic plexus. The gland is richly supplied by both pelvic sympathetic and parasympathetic fibres. The afferent nerves are linked to the lower three lumbar and upper sacral spinal segments.

Bulbourethral glands (Cowper's glands)

These lie deep in the perineal pouch, one on each side, between the lower margin of the prostate and the bulb of the penis. They are embedded in the muscle tissue which encircles the membranous urethra. Each is about the size of a pea and drains by a duct 2·5 cm long which pierces the inferior fascia of the urogenital diaphragm to enter the penis and opens into the bulb of the urethra. They consist of compound tubulo-alveolar secretory units.

Penis (fig. 38.28)

The male copulatory organ is composed mainly of erectile tissue arranged in three cylindrical columns, two dorsal **corpora cavernosa** and an inferiorly situated single **corpus spongiosum** which expands distally to form the substance of the **glans penis**.

The penis has a fixed root situated in the urogenital

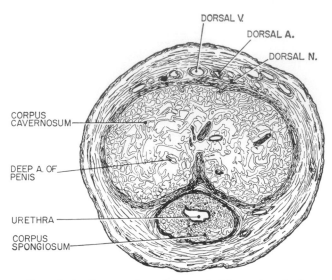

FIG. 38.28. Cross-section of the penis. The septum in the corpus cavernosum is incomplete as this section is in the distal part of the penis. From Bloom W. & Fawcett D.W. (1968) *A Textbook of Histology*, 9th Edition. Philadelphia: Saunders.

triangle of the perineum and a free shaft (fig. 38.29). At the root the corpora cavernosa diverge to be attached to the ischiopubic ramus as the **crura of the penis**. The corpus spongiosum expands proximally to form the **bulb of the penis**. The bulb is attached to the urogenital diaphragm and is enveloped by the **bulbospongiosus muscle**, while each crus is covered by the **ischiocavernosus muscle**.

The expanded glans is demarcated from the main shaft of the penis by the **coronary sulcus**. The corpus spongiosum and its glans are traversed by the penile urethra which in the glans is expanded to form a **fossa navicularis** from whose roof a diverticulum extends, the **lacuna magna**. The skin of the shaft of the penis forms a fold, the **prepuce**,

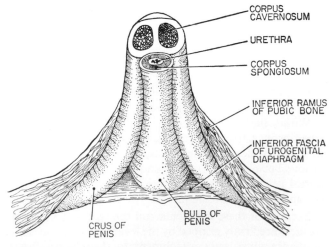

FIG. 38.29. Root of penis. From Romanes G.J. (1972) *Cunningham's Textbook of Anatomy*, 11th Edition. London: Oxford University Press.

which projects from the coronary sulcus to cover the glans. On its inferior aspect the fold is tethered to the under surface of the glans as the **frenulum**. The skin of the penis is thin, distensible, devoid of fat and loosely attached to the underlying fascia. Proximally it is continuous with the skin of the anterior abdominal wall, and the scrotum and perineum.

The blood supply is derived mainly from the internal pudendal artery but the superficial part of the dorsum is supplied by the external pudendal branch of the femoral artery.

The veins run with the arteries, but in addition the superficial dorsal vein drains to the saphenous vein and the deep dorsal vein into the prostatic plexus. The lymphatics drain into the superficial inguinal nodes.

The sensory nerves are branches of the pudendal and ilioinguinal nerves, and a parasympathetic supply is derived from the pelvic plexus.

PHYSIOLOGY OF THE MALE REPRODUCTIVE TRACT

The testes fulfil a dual role analogous to that of the ovaries, being concerned with the production of sex hormones and male gametes. However, human testes function at a relatively constant rate. Furthermore, the male reproductive tract has relatively simple functions, being concerned almost exclusively with the production and transport of spermatozoa, and it has none of the complex cyclical changes characteristic of the female.

Functions of the testes

There is a greater degree of separation of gametogenic and endocrine functions in the testes than in the ovaries. They proceed in parallel in anatomically discrete sites.

PRODUCTION OF SPERMATOZOA (spermatogenesis)

There are three successive stages in the production of spermatozoa. These are the continuous production of germ cells; their subsequent modification for fertilization by meiotic divisions; and structural modifications which render them actively motile.

Formation of germ cells

The origin of primitive germ cells and their migration to the testes are described on p. 38.59. As a result of these processes, the male germ cells or **spermatogonia** come to lie within the seminiferous tubules in close relation to the sustentacular cells (fig. 38.24). These cells are situated on the basement membrane and have a large irregular cytoplasm which comes into close contact with many spermatogenic cells. Their function is not clear, but they are probably concerned with the maintenance and coordination of developing germ cells. Spermatogonia show

little sign of activity until puberty when they begin to multiply rapidly by mitotic division, and it is their active proliferation which ensures the continual renewal of germ cells. In the male, gametogenesis is a continuous process which begins at puberty and is maintained throughout adult life.

Meiotic divisions

Some spermatogonia enlarge and become recognizable as **primary spermatocytes**. Primary spermatocytes undergo reduction division to become haploid **secondary spermatocytes** and these in turn again divide, so that each diploid primary spermatocyte ultimately gives rise to four haploid **spermatids** (fig. 38.11). Meiosis has already been described in detail in relation to oogenesis and only two points of difference require attention. First, both the primary and secondary spermatocytes divide symmetrically with an equal distribution of nuclear material and cytoplasm in the spermatids, whereas the unequal division of the cytoplasm during oogenesis produces one oocyte with a large volume of cytoplasm and three polar bodies with minimal cytoplasm. Secondly, the time scale of meiosis in the male and female is different. The first meiotic division in the female is prolonged over many years, whereas both meiotic divisions in the male are completed probably within two weeks.

During spermatogenesis, division of the cytoplasm lags behind division of the nucleus. This results in incomplete division of the daughter cells, which remain connected to one another by **intercellular bridges**. This continuity of cytoplasm is really resultant upon incomplete division of the daughter cells at the last spermatogonial division. This results in pairs of conjoined primary spermatocytes, which produce groups of four interconnected secondary spermatocytes. They in turn divide to form clusters of eight conjoined spermatids. The common reduplication anomalies of sperms, and the frequent occurrence of multinucleated giant cells in pathological conditions of the testis may be attributed to the obliteration of the constrictions between adjoining spermatocytes or spermatids and their resulting coalescence.

Development of spermatids

A newly formed spermatid has a relatively simple cellular structure whereas a mature **spermatozoon** is highly differentiated to enable it to travel through the male and female reproductive tracts and to fuse with the ovum. This elaborate development takes several weeks to complete and is known as **spermiogenesis**. The two special functions of the spermatozoon, motility and fertilizing ability, are concentrated in two distinct regions; the sperm **head** contains the male pronucleus while the **tail**, comprising the neck, middle piece, main piece and end piece, is the organ of motility. In fact, all else is sacrificed to subserve these two functions, and a mature spermatozoon is little more than a 'nuclear war-head' of paternal genes powered by an active tail.

The total length of the human spermatozoon is 50 μm (fig. 38.30). The sperm head is a flattened pear-shaped body compressed at its anterior pole into a flat edge, and

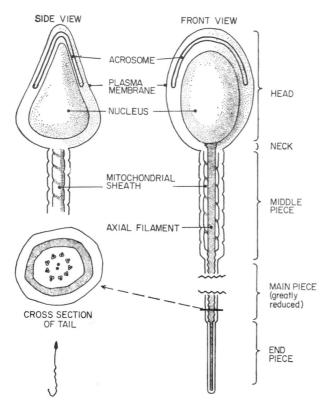

FIG. 38.30. Structure of the mature spermatozoon. The small diagram of a spermatozoon is included to show the relative sizes of the head and tail. Modified from Schultz-Larsen J. (1958) The morphology of the human sperm. *Acta path. microbiol. scand.* suppl. 128.

occupied by the nucleus which contains the paternal contribution of genetic material. Anteriorly it is covered by the **acrosome** which is derived from the Golgi apparatus. The exact nature of this structure is uncertain and it is poorly developed in man. A human sperm head is composed almost entirely of a nucleus, densely packed with DNA, and only thinly covered by the acrosomal cap.

The tail is joined to the sperm head by a short fragile **neck**, probably derived from the centriole. It is traversed by the **axial filament**, which is itself composed of several long fibrils which run a straight course throughout its length and are arranged as a central pair of fibrils surrounded by two circumferential rings of nine fibrils each. In the **middle piece**, the axial filament is surrounded by the **mitochondrial sheath**, while the **main piece** is enclosed by a thin but tough protein sheath which terminates a short distance from the end exposing the **end piece**.

The whole spermatozoon is covered by a plasma membrane. The tail is the organ of motility and the mitochondria in the middle piece contain oxidative enzymes which provide energy for this activity. Spermatozoa contain very little endogenous supply of energy, and certainly no glycolysable substrates, and they obtain their energy from nutrients in their environment.

The time scale of spermatogenesis has been studied in two principal ways; by observing the time required for spermatogenic cells to disappear and reappear in the seminiferous tubules after acute radiation damage, or the time required for the formation of spermatozoa with radioactive nuclei after the systemic administration of radioactive labelled precursors of nucleoproteins. From these studies it is estimated that the whole process of spermatogenesis in man takes approximately 64 days to complete.

Spermatogenesis is a complicated process which frequently goes wrong, and this is reflected in a high incidence of grossly abnormal spermatozoa in fertile human semen. These include decapitated spermatozoa, spermatozoa with double heads or double tails, and multinucleate giant spermatozoa, and these may account for up to 30 per cent of spermatozoa in a normal ejaculate. Apart from these structural errors, anomalies may also occur during meiotic divisions and these may be important causes of male infertility.

Spermatogenesis is sensitive to environmental changes, particularly in temperature. The temperature of the scrotal testes in man is 1·5–2·5°C lower than the temperature of the abdominal cavity, and the testes appear to function optimally at this lower temperature. Even a slight elevation in temperature produces a transient impairment in sperm production. This phenomenon may be relevant to two clinical problems, cryptorchidism, where the testes fail to descend into the scrotum, and varicocoele, where there is dilation of the testicular venous plexus, usually in the left testis. Both of these conditions are associated with defective spermatogenesis, and a factor common to them may be raised intratesticular temperature. Radiation can cause either a permanent or transient effect depending on the type, duration and intensity of exposure. Several drugs also interfere with the various stages of spermatogenesis and some of these may prove to be useful in the control of male fertility.

SEX HORMONES

The principal testicular hormones are androgenic steroids, the most important of these being testosterone and, to a lesser extent, androstenedione. However, most androstenedione is produced by the adrenal glands in both sexes. The testes also secrete small quantities of oestrogens, and both oestradiol-17β and oestrone have been identified in spermatic vein blood. It has already been emphasized that the patterns of steroid synthesis in testis and ovary follow an essentially similar pattern and that each type of gonad produces both oestrogens and androgens. The endocrine distinction between the two organs is a simple quantitative one of degree rather than a fundamental qualitative difference. An appreciation of this fact is essential for an understanding of some intersex states, and is explicable in terms of the mechanisms of sex differentiation.

Biosynthesis, metabolism and excretion of androgens
The method of production of testosterone from cholesterol has already been described (fig. 38.13), although alternative biosynthetic pathways may also be involved. Testosterone is produced in the interstitial cells, but there is some doubt as to whether testicular oestrogens are also produced in interstitial cells or in the sustentacular cells. Testosterone is bound in plasma to the same sex steroid binding globulin as is oestradiol.

Testosterone may be converted to an even more powerful androgen, dihydrotestosterone, in the cells of such target organs as the prostate. This provides a system for potentiating the biological activity of androgens yet restricting their activity to target tissues. Similarly weak androgens such as androstenedione and dehydro*epi*androsterone may be converted to testosterone in such tissues as skin and liver. This is another method of achieving high levels of androgenic activity without any widespread systemic effect.

The conversion of physiologically active steroids to less potent compounds takes place in the liver. The initial step in the deactivation of both testicular androgens and adrenal corticosteroids is reduction of the 3 ketone group. Many of these reduced metabolites of testosterone have very little androgenic activity. This conversion produces asymmetric carbon atoms at C-3 and C-5, and a number of stereoisomers are formed (fig. 38.31), the most important metabolites of testosterone being androsterone (a 5α compound) and aetiocholanolone

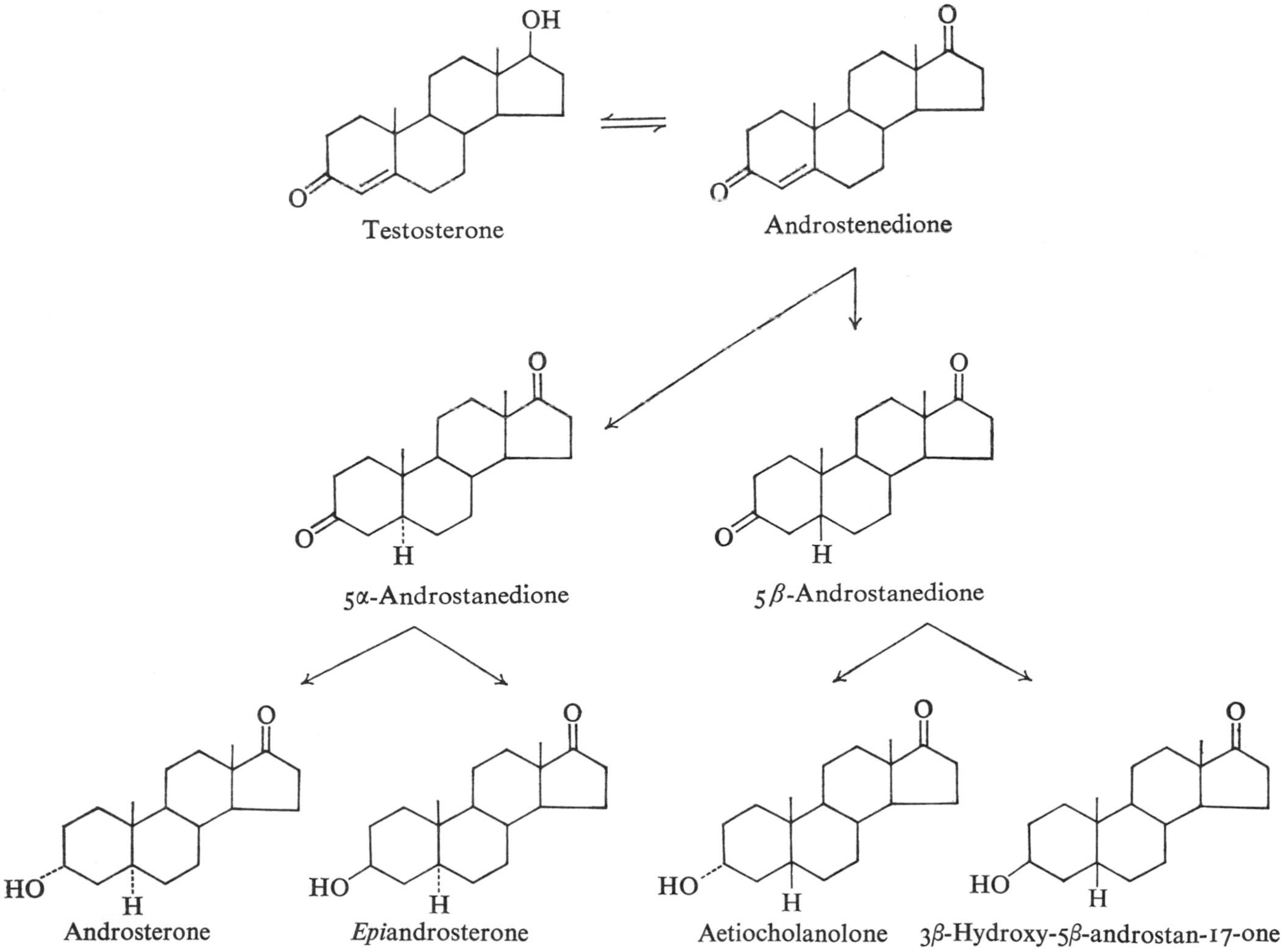

FIG. 38.31. Metabolism of testosterone.

(a 5β compound). Like the oestrogens, these metabolites are conjugated in the liver with glucuronic acid or sulphuric acid prior to their excretion.

These two compounds are examples of 17-oxosteroids (or 17-ketosteroids), which may be easily measured collectively by a colour reaction, the Zimmermann reaction. As a result, the urinary excretion of 17-oxo-steroids has been widely used as a measure of the excretion of androgenic metabolites. However, adrenal corticosteroids follow a similar pathway of conversion and the principal precursor of 17-oxosteroids is undoubtedly dehydro*epi*androsterone derived from the adrenal cortex. Testosterone probably accounts for no more than one-third of urinary 17-oxosteroids and even castration produces little permanent effect on their level of excretion. For these reasons, the urinary excretion of 17-oxosteroids is a poor index of testicular endocrine function.

A more useful clinical test is proving to be the chemical assay of testosterone in plasma and urine. The concentration of plasma testosterone in normal adult males is 12–30 nmol/l (3·5–8·5 ng/ml) as compared with 0·5–2 nmol/l (0·15–0·55 ng/ml) in normal adult females. The urinary excretion of testosterone in adult males aged between 20 and 40 years is within the range 100–350 nmol (30–100 μg)/24 h.

Actions of androgens

The principal actions of androgens are as follows:

(1) the initiation and maintenance of male secondary sex features at puberty,

(2) the stimulation of growth of the male reproductive tract, and maintenance of its contractile and secretory activity,

(3) the maintenance of the germinal epithelium of the seminiferous tubules, in conjunction with pituitary FSH,

(4) a negative feedback relation with the adeno-hypophysis, inhibiting the release of LH,

(5) a powerful anabolic action, stimulating protein synthesis. The relation of this function to growth and skeletal development is discussed in chap. 19,

(6) an influence on sexual and aggressive behaviour in both sexes.

Like other steroid hormones, androgenic hormones are removed from plasma selectively by their target tissues in the seminiferous tubules and epididymis, and to a lesser extent by most other tissues. They are bound to receptor proteins in the cytosol and then migrate into the nucleus. Here the steroid-protein complex appears to become associated with nuclear chromatin and the increased production of template material results in the activation of protein synthesis. At present it is not possible to specify how many proteins are under the control of an androgenic signal in target tissues. While androgens, like oestrogens and other hormones, have primary target

tissues, they appear to have an observable effect on almost all cells in the mammalian system.

CONTROL OF TESTICULAR FUNCTIONS

Mechanisms for the control of the male gonads are essentially similar to those in the female. The same pituitary gonadotrophins, FSH and LH (or ICSH), are involved, and it seems likely that these have separate effects.

FSH promotes spermatogenesis by a direct action on the seminiferous tubules. However, by itself it cannot stimulate germ cell production beyond the primary spermatocyte stage. Full spermatogenesis requires adequate concentrations of testosterone.

LH promotes the secretion of androgens by its action on the Leydig cells.

The relationship between the adenohypophysis and hypothalamus depends on LH/FSH-RH, as in the female. One major difference is the absence of cyclical fluctuations in the male. This steady state is determined by hypothalamic centres and maintains constant output of pituitary gonadotrophins and constant gametogenic and endocrine activity in human testes.

Yet the constant secretion of gonadotrophins is held under restraint since castration increases urinary excretion of gonadotrophins; this indicates that the testes have an inhibitory action. In rodents, hypothalamic lesions abolish this effect of castration, and implants of minute quantities of testosterone in the hypothalamus, but not in the adenohypophysis, may cause testicular atrophy. Thus,

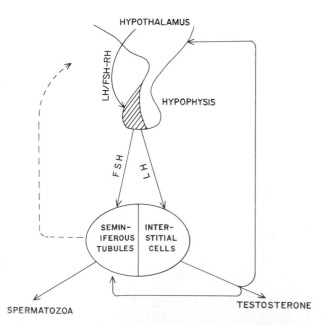

Fig. 38.32. Interrelations between the hypothalamus, adenohypophysis and testes. From Ganong W.F. (1967) *Review of Medical Physiology*, 3rd Edition. Los Altos: Lange.

testicular inhibition is probably applied via the hypothalamus rather than directly on the adenohypophysis.

It is still uncertain if there is a separate feedback system for each of the two testicular functions, gametogenesis and sex steroid production, mediated by FSH and LH respectively. It is thought that testosterone causes predominantly a fall in LH secretion, although large quantities of testosterone can impair spermatogenesis presumably by inhibiting FSH secretion. Castration in childhood, prior to the secretion of significant quantities of testosterone, causes a rise in gonadotrophin, predominantly FSH, excretion. Thus, testosterone may not be the only pituitary inhibitor of testicular origin, and it is probably not normally involved in the control of FSH secretion and spermatogenesis. The nature of this other factor is still uncertain. It is often referred to as a hypothetical substance, inhibin, and there are grounds for the belief that this may represent testicular oestrogen.

Fate of spermatozoa in male and female reproductive tracts

There is a daily production of many millions of spermatozoa. At periods of sexual rest when ejaculation is not taking place, a method for disposal of excess spermatozoa is required. Before insemination and fertilization can take place, spermatozoa must gain access to an oocyte by mechanisms which involve a number of complicated transport problems in both male and female reproductive tracts, from seminiferous tubules in the testes to the ampulla of the uterine tube.

Semen ejaculated by the male consists of two components, spermatozoa produced by the testes and **seminal plasma** which is a nutrient medium formed by the secretions of the male reproductive tract. In man, the volume of an ejaculate ranges from 1–5 ml, of which only 10 per cent is formed of spermatozoa and 90 per cent of seminal plasma.

As they leave the testes, spermatozoa are probably non-motile and incapable of fertilization, and require modification before they can enter an oocyte. This maturation occurs in both the male and female reproductive tracts.

These three aspects, the transport, maturation and maintenance of spermatozoa are important functions of the reproductive tracts. In this context, it is logical to consider the fate of spermatozoa in both the male and female reproductive tracts as one problem.

TRANSPORT OF SPERMATOZOA IN MALE REPRODUCTIVE TRACT

Newly formed spermatozoa lie in the seminiferous tubules with their heads in contact with sustentacular cells. Under the influence of gonadotrophins, the cytoplasm of these supporting cells accumulates water in the form of vacuoles which subsequently discharge, shedding spermatozoa into the lumen of the tubules. The production rate of spermatozoa may be enormous, particularly under conditions of sexual activity. Seminal analysis on a 2-year-old bull ejaculating at a frequency of sixty times per week over a period of 5 weeks indicated a constant production rate of 7700 million spermatozoa daily.

Whether spermatozoa enter the rete testis intermittently or continuously is unknown, as is the mechanism by which this movement is achieved. Spermatozoa are propelled through the rete testis and efferent ducts to the epididymis by ciliary and smooth muscle activity. Although spermatozoa are potentially motile when they enter the ductus deferens, propulsion both here and in the epididymis is achieved by smooth muscle contraction. The distance from the efferent ductules to the urethra in man is approximately 6 metres, and spermatozoa take approximately 7–14 days to traverse this distance, the time varying with the frequency of ejaculation.

The fate of non-ejaculated spermatozoa is still a mystery. In some animals, particularly the bull, the epididymis may be an important site of sperm resorption so that, at times of sexual rest, the rate of sperm resorption equals the rate of sperm production. In other animals, such as the rat, surplus spermatozoa simply leak away in the urine. The method of sperm disposal in man is uncertain.

INSEMINATION

The method by which semen is naturally deposited in the vagina is based on a complex of spinal reflexes. Three interrelated mechanisms are involved.

Erection

Erection of the penis is a necessary prerequisite for penetration of the vagina. Afferent stimuli for this reflex may involve either peripheral receptors on the external genitalia or stimuli from higher centres. Central connections are in the sacral part of the cord, and the efferent pathway is the parasympathetic component of the pelvic splanchnic nerves. The essential factor in penile erection is active arteriolar dilation which in turn compresses the venous outflow so adding to the distension of the erectile tissue. Loss of erection is due to sympathetic arteriolar vasoconstriction.

Emission

This refers to the movement of spermatozoa and secretions from the ductus deferens and seminal vesicles into the urethra. The afferent side of this arc is usually initiated by touch receptors in the glans penis via the pudendal nerves; central relays are in the upper lumbar segments of the cord, and the sympathetic outflow, via the hypogastric plexus, forms the efferent side of the arc. As a result of these stimuli, the muscle of the ductus deferens and seminal vesicles contracts and propels their contents into the urethra.

Ejaculation

Ejaculation indicates the propulsion of semen out of the urethra. The same afferent paths are involved; central connections are located in the lower lumbar and upper sacral parts of the cord, and efferent stimuli are conveyed by parasympathetic and somatic motor fibres in the pelvic splanchnic and the internal pudendal nerves. Ejaculation is caused by the rhythmic contractions of the prostate and bulbocavernosus muscles, while the internal bladder sphincter closes to prevent retrograde ejaculation into the bladder.

TRANSPORT OF SPERMATOZOA IN THE FEMALE REPRODUCTIVE TRACT

Ejaculation deposits a pool of semen in the vaginal vault around the cervix. This coagulates rapidly and the coagulum impedes sperm movement until clot lysis occurs 15–20 mins later. However, many human spermatozoa enter the cervix within 90 secs of ejaculation, presumably before coagulation traps them, and it is likely that these are the spermatozoa which survive in the genital tract and may achieve fertilization.

Cervical mucus is the first obstacle encountered by spermatozoa. Various mucoids give this mucus the properties of a visco-elastic gel, but at the time of ovulation it becomes less viscid and presents less resistance to sperm ascent. Active sperm motility is probably essential for ascent through the cervical canal.

From the time of ejaculation spermatozoa reach the ampulla of the tube in approximately 30 min, covering a distance of 15 cm. It is likely that the rate of forward propulsion of human spermatozoa is of the order of 1–3 mm/min, and so it is clear that spermatozoa do not ascend the uterus by virtue of their own motility. Uterine transport is aided by powerful contractions of the myometrium which carry spermatozoa towards the uterotubal junctions. The resistance presented by this junction varies between species, but it is unlikely that it offers a major hindrance to human sperm penetration. The rapid transport of spermatozoa in the uterine tubes is dependent on tubal contractility.

During sperm ascent there is an enormous reduction in sperm number. Over 100 million spermatozoa are ejaculated into the vagina, yet normally only one spermatozoon fertilizes one ovum. The initial reduction occurs at the cervix and perhaps only one million spermatozoa enter the uterus. Further elimination occurs at the uterotubal junction, so that a few thousand spermatozoa enter the tubes, and of these perhaps only about 100 spermatozoa reach the oocyte in the tubal ampulla.

The fate of surplus spermatozoa in the female genital tract is still a mystery. Undoubtedly, many simply leak from the vagina and those which do enter the uterus disappear rapidly. Spermatozoa may be removed by phagocytosis within the lumen of the uterus and also by endometrial leucocytes. Despite this rapid removal, some spermatozoa may remain fertile and motile in the female reproductive tract for 1 or 2 days.

The origin of postcoital uterine activity is still uncertain. It may be a reflex stimulus mediated through the hypothalamus and effected via either the autonomic nervous system or neurohypophysial oxytocin. It may also be due to prostaglandins in seminal plasma.

MATURATION OF SPERMATOZOA

During their passage through the epididymis spermatozoa undergo a process of ripening or maturation with respect to both motility and fertility. This is associated with demonstrable histological changes in the middle piece of the sperm, but the cause and nature of this process are unknown. Spermatozoa entering the ductus deferens are potentially motile and fertile, but they gain further activation by contact with the secretions of the seminal vesicles and prostate.

In some animals, particularly the rabbit and rat, there is normally a delay of a few hours between insemination and fertilization which is not simply due to sperm transport. It has been shown that during this time spermatozoa undergo further changes, **capacitation,** in the female reproductive tract which enable them to penetrate the zona pellucida. The nature of capacitation and whether or not it occurs in human spermatozoa is unknown.

MAINTENANCE OF SPERMATOZOA

Following their release from the testes, spermatozoa are entirely dependent on their local fluid environment for maintenance, and this is the function of the secretions of the various regions of the male and female reproductive tracts.

Epididymal secretions are characterized by a high concentration of glycerylphosphorylcholine and a high K^+/Na^+ ratio which may approach unity. As spermatozoa enter the ejaculatory ducts the secretions of seminal vesicles and prostate are added. The outstanding feature of vesicular secretion is the high concentration of fructose but it also contains sorbitol, which may contribute to fructose formation, inositol, ergothioneine and prostaglandins. By contrast, prostatic secretions contain virtually no fructose, but have a high concentration of citric acid and acid phosphatase. In man, the bulbo-urethral and urethral gland secretions probably have a purely lubricant action.

The function of seminal plasma is still a mystery.

Table 38.1 shows the concentrations of some constituents which may be used as a measure of the activities of the glands of the male reproductive tract. It is important to appreciate the short period of time during which spermatozoa are in contact with seminal plasma. Mixing begins at the time of ejaculation. If it is accepted that many spermatozoa leave the seminal pool and enter the cervix within 90 sec, then these will have been in contact with seminal plasma for no more than a few minutes. Consequently it is unlikely that seminal plasma contributes to the long-term welfare of spermatozoa in terms of energy production or maturation.

Table 38.1. Constituents of human seminal plasma.

Compound	Concentration mg/l	Notes
Acid phosphatase	2 740 000 units*	A measure of prostatic activity
Fructose	90–500	A measure of seminal vesicle activity
Glycerlphosphoryl-choline	500–900	A possible indication of epididymal secretion
Prostaglandins:		Thought to originate from seminal vesicles
E₁ and E₂	50	
F₁α and F₂α	8·0	
19-hydroxy E₁ and 19-hydroxy E₂	100	
Spermine and spermidine	500–3500	Mainly a prostatic secretion

* King-Armstrong units.

It is necessary to distinguish between essential and merely useful functions. Undoubtedly, spermatozoa removed from the ductus deferens are potentially motile and fertile without any contact with seminal plasma. However, seminal plasma has useful, if non-essential, functions. First, it normally acts as the carrier for spermatozoa. Secondly, fructose can act as a substrate for sperm energy metabolism. Thirdly, it may also have a role in relation to the female reproductive tract. Semen has a powerful oxytocic effect, and this may be relevant to the increased uterine and tubal contractility which follows coitus. However, this oxytocic principle has not yet been identified.

Ejaculated spermatozoa are likely to be dependent on the secretions of the female tract following insemination, but little is known of this aspect of uterine physiology.

Onset of reproductive functions in the male

The development of the male reproductive tract is described on p. 38.62. Here we are concerned with the changes in activity which follow birth.

The testes grow very slowly until the age of 10 or 11 years, following which there is a marked acceleration in growth rate. At birth the seminiferous tubules are compact cellular structures devoid of a lumen and they are not canalized until the age of 3 or 4 years. Interstitial cells are difficult to distinguish from fibroblasts. At the age of 10 or 11 years, mitotic activity can be identified in spermatogonia and this is followed by increasing evidence of spermatogenesis and proliferation of interstitial cells. These changes in the gonads are accompanied by increase in size and activity of the accessory glands and growth of the external genitalia. The characteristic male hair pattern is initiated by the appearance of pubic hair followed one or two years later by axillary and facial hair and then by the frontoparietal recessions of scalp hair. These latter changes in scalp hair do not occur in many Asiatic males. The voice characteristically 'breaks'; both sweat and sebaceous gland activity increases, and acne is a common feature of puberty.

The rate of skeletal growth begins to accelerate shortly before puberty, and it is the varying duration and intensity of this growth phase which is responsible for most of the sex differences in stature. In males the growth spurt is more rapid and lasts for a longer time due to the relatively late closure of epiphyses, so that the mean height of the adult male usually exceeds that of the female.

Seminal emissions usually follow the appearance of secondary sex characters, and early spermatogenesis is frequently irregular and prone to abnormal sperm formation. Thus, there may be a period of adolescent male infertility comparable to the early anovular menstrual cycles in the female.

It is difficult to time the onset of puberty accurately in the male because of the absence of any such clear-cut phenomenon as the menarche, but it is usually between the age of 10 and 15 years. Puberty is commonly said to occur at a later age in boys than in girls, but it is virtually impossible to make any valid comparison between the sexes on the basis of recognizable external features. This could be based only on a study of the time of release of hypophysial gonadotrophins or gonadal steroids, but there are no reliable data.

The mechanisms underlying puberty are essentially similar in both sexes. It seems likely that the testes exert some control over the hypophysial release of gonadotrophins via hypothalamic centres, and that unknown changes in this system may initiate puberty. It is possible that the steroids produced by the prepubertal testes may be different from those of the mature testes. Studies on bull calves have shown a preponderance of androstenedione production as compared with the dominant secretion of testosterone in adult bulls, but it is not known if these findings apply to man.

After testicular activity is established at puberty, it normally continues for the rest of life with only slight impairment in later years. There is a slight reduction in sperm and androgen production in old age and this is associated with some degenerative changes in the testes, but there is no abrupt testicular failure comparable to the female climacteric.

PREGNANCY

This section is concerned with the development of the fetus and placenta and their integrated functions, the physiological responses of the mother to gestation, the growth and behaviour of the uterus, and lactation.

Early embryogenesis and placentation

FERTILIZATION

For obvious reasons there have been very few observations on *in vivo* fertilization of human ova, and most information has been derived from experimentation in other species. However, there is a wide variation between species, and consequently ideas about human fertilization are partly speculative.

Within one to two hours after ovulation, an oocyte is located in the ampulla of a uterine tube. It measures 120–150 μm in diameter and is enclosed by a plasma membrane, or **vitelline membrane**. This in turn is surrounded by a structureless shell, the **zona pellucida**, with a potential (perivitelline) space between the two membranes. When it is shed from the ovary, the oocyte is surrounded by a loose fringe of granulosa cells, the **corona radiata**. Following ovulation, the primary oocyte completes its reduction division with extrusion of the **first polar body**, and immediately begins the second meiotic division.

Within less than one hour of insemination, about a hundred motile spermatozoa find their way to the tubal ampulla. There is probably a delay before these spermatozoa can penetrate the ovum while the process of capacitation (p. 38.36) is completed, unless insemination has preceded ovulation by a few hours.

After a period of time, ova lose their capacity for fertilization. This time varies from a few hours in rabbits to a few days in dogs, and although there is some uncertainty about the behaviour of human ova it is unlikely that they are readily fertilizable after 24–48 hours from shedding. Ageing of ova is a gradual rather than an all-or-none process; ageing ova may still be fertilized but are susceptible to anomalous mechanisms of fertilization. Spermatozoa probably also lose their ability to fertilize 24–48 hours after ejaculation. These factors are relevant to methods of family planning based on the safe period, and it is important to realize that, while they apply to concepts of optimal or adequate fertility, exceptional cases are well documented where both ova and spermatozoa

appear to have remained functionally viable for longer periods of time.

The method of penetration of the ovum is still uncertain, but three stages have been recognized. Spermatozoa first have to penetrate the granulosa cells of the corona radiata, and this has been claimed to be the function of hyaluronidase. However, human spermatozoa contain relatively little hyaluronidase. The second barrier is the zona pellucida and the acrosome contains proteolytic enzymes which lyse this layer. Finally the spermatozoon penetrates the vitelline membrane, and it is likely that this occurs by fusion of the plasma membranes when the spermatozoon comes into contact with the vitelline membrane.

The ovum is normally surrounded by many spermatozoa and there must be an effective mechanism to limit penetration by more than one spermatozoon. This is probably achieved by the relative impenetrability of the zona pellucida and physicochemical changes in the vitelline membrane. Ageing of the ovum is associated with a breakdown in this mechanism, so that more than one spermatozoon may fuse with the ovum, and more than one male pronucleus may combine with the female pronucleus. Thus, in the case of dispermic fertilization a triploid zygote is produced. Ageing of the ovum is almost certainly an important factor in human infertility and pregnancy wastage. In most animals, ovulation follows a short period of sexual excitement when the female accepts the male, or alternatively ovulation is reflexly triggered by copulation, and these mechanisms ensure that insemination and ovulation coincide. There are no comparable features in human reproduction to ensure the fusion of fresh spermatozoa and ova and fertilization of ageing ova is likely to be a common occurrence. This is confirmed by the recent finding of many triploid embryos in spontaneously aborted conceptuses.

The immediate result of sperm entry is to activate the oocyte to complete the second meiotic division and extrude the **second polar body**. Both the spermatozoon and nucleus of the ovum undergo changes leading to the formation of male and female **pronuclei**, containing the haploid sets of paternal and maternal chromosomes. The pronuclear membranes are lost, a spindle forms, and the chromosomes come to lie along the equatorial plate. Each chromosome divides into a pair of chromatids, one of each pair segregates to opposite poles, and the first cleavage division results in the formation of two diploid cells, or **blastomeres**.

Successive mitotic divisions produce a cluster of blastomeres, or **morula**, within the confines of the zona pellucida. During these early cleavage divisions the blastomeres depend on the nutrients which were stored in the cytoplasm of the ovum prior to fertilization. As these nutrients are gradually metabolized, there is a progressive shrinkage in the volume of the total cytoplasmic material of the cell mass. Thus, although the number of blastomeres increases, there is no increase in the overall volume. This is essential to allow the morula, with a diameter of 120–150 μm, to pass through the tubal isthmus.

Transport of the conceptus from the tubal ampulla to the uterus is due to a flow of tubal fluid induced by tubal peristalsis and ciliary action, and the morula arrives in the uterus three or four days after fertilization. Within the next two or three days, fluid from the endometrial secretions passes through the zona pellucida and accumulates to form a central cavity which becomes surrounded by blastomeres. As soon as the morula acquires this central cavity it is known as a **blastocyst**. The cells which constitute the blastocyst can now be differentiated into the surface cells, known as **trophoblast**, and cells which are attached to their inner aspect at one pole of the blastocyst where they form the **inner cell mass**.

IMPLANTATION

At this stage the blastocyst reaches a crisis of nutrition as the supplies of cytoplasmic nutrients rapidly become exhausted and it becomes essential for it to implant in the endometrium so that the trophoblast can obtain nutriment for the developing embryo from the maternal tissues. This process is a critical phase in embryogenesis and a large number of blastocysts fail to achieve it.

Implantation may be said to have started when the blastocyst becomes denuded of its zona pellucida, as the result mainly of trophoblastic activity, possibly aided by maternal secretions from the endometrium. In this way the trophoblast comes into direct contact with the endometrium to which it can then attach itself. The persistence of the zona pellucida during the free-life or progestational phase of pregnancy not only binds the blastomeres of the morula together but also prevents the blastomeres from attaching themselves prematurely to the tubal mucous membrane.

The extent of trophoblastic penetration and the consequent degree of intimacy between the **chorion** (trophoblast plus supporting vascular mesenchyme) and the maternal endometrium is of special importance in determining the thickness of the membrane (placental membrane) interposed between the embryonic (later fetal) blood stream and that of the mother, and across which the exchanges between mother and embryo (or fetus) must take place. In species in which trophoblastic penetration is minimal or non-existent the endometrial epithelium remains more or less intact so that the chorion merely lies in contact with it. Such a placenta is described as **epitheliochorial**. In other species the trophoblast erodes the maternal epithelium so that the chorion comes into contact with the endothelium of the maternal blood vessels. Such a placenta is described as **endo-theliochorial**. In man, and in many other species, the trophoblast destroys not only the maternal epithelium and connective tissue stroma, but also the endothelium of the maternal blood vessels. In this way the maternal blood comes to bathe the chorion directly, and such a placenta is described as being **haemochorial**.

Maternal factors in implantation

Before implantation takes place not only does the blastocyst lose its zona pellucida, but the endometrium is modified. At the time of implantation, which begins about 7 days after ovulation, the endometrium is in the progestational stage corresponding to the 21st day of the cycle (p. 38.18). The stroma is oedematous, especially at the implantation site, the capillaries are especially prominent at this site, and the glands are extremely tortuous and actively secreting glycogen and mucus.

The maternal control of implantation appears to be exercised by ovarian progesterone although oestrogens may also play a role. In some species, but not in man, there is an oestrogen surge just prior to implantation. As soon as implantation begins, the endometrium becomes modified and gives rise to a phenomenon known as the **decidual reaction**. This transformation involves the surface epithelium, the glands, the stroma and the blood vessels. The stromal cells become polyhedral and dilated with glycogen and lipids. Glycosaminoglycans accumulate not only in these decidual cells but also in the ground substance of the endometrium. The decidual reaction is an exaggeration of the changes that take place in the postovulatory phase of the menstrual cycle and is probably an adaptation for the nutrition of the embryo. It may also be a defensive reaction on the part of the mother, retarding and limiting the invasive activity of the embryonic trophoblast.

Embryonic factors in implantation (fig. 38.33 & 19.1)

About 6½–7 days after ovulation, the zona pellucida having disappeared, the trophoblast covering the inner cell mass (**polar trophoblast**) attaches the blastocyst to the endometrium, most frequently on the upper part of the posterior wall of the body of the uterus near the midsagittal plane.

The initial attachment has not been observed in man, but EM studies in other species indicate that the polar trophoblast fuses with the endometrial epithelium, penetrating its basement membrane to invade the underlying stroma. At this stage no plasma membrane is interposed between the embryonic and maternal cytoplasm so that a very intimate relationship is established, with possibilities for the exchange of molecular information which may have a bearing on the immunological relationship which exists between mother and embryo.

The polar trophoblast which effects the initial attachment acquires characteristics which distinguish it from the trophoblast covering those aspects of the blastocyst which are still unattached and exposed to the uterine lumen. The latter kind of trophoblast consists of flattened cells, whereas the polar trophoblast becomes invasive and consists of a mixture of

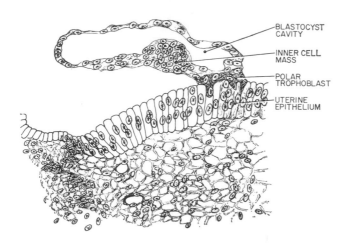

FIG. 38.33. Early attachment of blastocyst to uterine epithelium in macaque. From Hamilton W.J., Boyd J.D. & Mossman H.W. (1972) *Human Embryology*, 4th Edition. Cambridge: Heffer.

variously sized basophilic cells, of which some are huge and some coalesce to form small masses of syncytium.

The youngest known attached human blastocyst had an estimated age of not more than $7\frac{1}{2}$ days from ovulation and it was already partially implanted. The trophoblast had eroded the uterine epithelium and penetrated the underlying stroma which was congested and oedematous possibly due to the liberation of some substance from the trophoblast. The trophoblast which invades the endometrium has a thick plaque of primitive, invasive, pleomorphic cells, while the free part of the blastocyst wall consists of a layer of flattened cells.

By the 11th or 12th day after fertilization the human blastocyst becomes buried beneath the endometrial epithelium and is completely embedded in the stroma. During this phase of implantation, the endometrium is digested by the trophoblast so that nutritive material is supplied to the embryo, which develops from the inner cell mass of the blastocyst. Another result of this digestive process is that the blastocyst sinks into the endometrium 'like a hot marble placed on ice'.

As implantation reaches completion, the blastocyst lies in the superficial part of the compact layer of the endometrium (p. 38.20) and it produces a slight swelling on the endometrial surface. In the vicinity of the trophoblast the stromal cells become transformed into decidual cells and a zone of vascular congestion and oedema spreads towards the deeper layers and also laterally. The

defect in the endometrial epithelium caused by the invasion of the blastocyst is gradually closed, first by a plug of fibrin and subsequently by proliferation of adjacent epithelium.

During and after implantation, changes occur in the primitive invasive trophoblast. The innermost part in contact with the embryonic tissues becomes organized into a regular layer of uniform cells, or **cytotrophoblast**. At the same time isolated vacuoles appear in the more peripheral pleomorphic part. These become confluent to form **lacunae** (the future **intervillous spaces**). As a result, this outer invasive trophoblast consists of irregular trabecular strands of pleomorphic cells and small plaques of syncytium, the **syncytiotrophoblast**. The peripheral part continues to invade and digest adjacent decidua, glands and blood vessels and to absorb the extravasated blood.

By the 12th day the primitive **trophoblastic trabeculae** and the intervening lacunar spaces are well established but are not uniformly developed around the conceptus. Whereas the trophoblastic components are thick around the sides and deeper parts of the embryo, there is only a thin layer of trophoblast towards the endometrial surface, probably due to the poorer supply of nutrient in this region. All round the embryo the junction between the trophoblast and the maternal tissue has an irregular contour, owing to the invasion of the endometrium by irregular outgrowths from the trophoblast.

Implantation allows the embryo to establish a supply of nutrients from the endometrium and its blood vessels. The capillaries in the vicinity are congested and the blood in them tends to stagnate. The trophoblast invades these capillaries so that blood passes into its lacunae and soon circulates through them. Although these capillaries are fed by the coiled endometrial arterioles, the initial circulation through the lacunae is sluggish.

Functional interrelationship between embryo and mother during implantation

Implantation is the product of the interplay between trophoblastic invasion and maternal tissue reactions. The pre-implantation changes in the endometrium are controlled by maternal hormones. However, once implantation has started, the trophoblast of the blastocyst probably produces substances which not only affect the endometrium locally (the decidual reaction) but also exert a systemic influence on the mother. The identification of substances elaborated by the implanting trophoblast (p. 38.47) and circulating in the maternal blood forms the basis of a number of pregnancy tests.

The receptive property of the endometrium and the invasive behaviour of the trophoblast are two complementary phenomena. The embryo-maternal relationship is biologically akin to a parasite-host relationship, and normally there is a balance between the invasiveness of the trophoblast and the protective reaction of the endometrium.

Another relevant aspect of this interrelationship is that, whereas the primitive trophoblast is highly invasive and irregular, it subsequently becomes organized into distinct layers of cytotrophoblast and syncytiotrophoblast. Cytotrophoblast consists of cellular layers with intercellular boundaries separating the nuclei, whereas syncytiotrophoblast consists of multinucleated masses of cytoplasm in which the nuclei are not separated by intercellular boundaries. Other trophoblastic giant cells invade deeper than this organized trophoblast, but they do not destroy maternal tissue but rather intermingle with it. It would seem that as trophoblast differentiates, it becomes less invasive. In some cases the balance between trophoblast and endometrium may be disturbed. Overactivity of the trophoblast may permit chorionic villi to penetrate throughout the myometrium, i.e. placenta accreta (vol. 3, p. 43.16), whereas if the endometrium is too resistant to trophoblastic invasion the embryo cannot become properly established in the uterus and dies, being either absorbed or aborted.

The blastocyst may implant in a number of abnormal positions, most commonly in the uterine tubes, but occasionally in the ovaries, abdominal cavity or cervix. Ectopic pregnancies demonstrate that the embryo can implant in conditions which differ from the optimal environment provided by the progestational endometrium.

Decidua (fig. 38.34)

The endometrial lining of the uterus is greatly modified during pregnancy and is called decidua because it is shed at subsequent parturition. After implantation and until about the 4th month of gestation, three parts of the decidua can be distinguished. **Decidua basalis** is the part which is deep to the implantation site and forms the base of the developing placenta. **Decidua capsularis** covers or encapsulates the surface of the implanted embryo. **Decidua parietalis** lines the rest of the uterus.

As the fetus grows and expands, the chorion becomes stretched, with a very thin covering of decidua capsularis and projects into the uterine lumen. Eventually the capsular decidua comes into contact with the decidua parietalis, so obliterating the uterine cavity. The decidua capsularis degenerates, and the chorion fuses with the decidua parietalis by the 5th month of pregnancy. At birth the decidua parietalis and basalis are torn away when the placenta is expelled.

Suppression of menstruation

The timing of implantation in relation to ovarian and endometrial cycles is critical. In an ovulatory 28-day cycle ovulation occurs around the 14th day, and the corpus luteum begins to regress about the 24th day

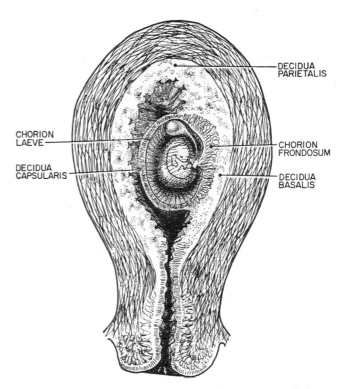

FIG. 38.34. Relation of chorion to different parts of the decidua. From Williams J.W. (1927) *Amer. J. Obstet. Gynec.* **13**, 1.

resulting in endometrial shedding on the 28th day. Implantation begins about 7 days after fertilization, i.e. around day 21.

There is thus only a short period of three or four days between implantation and luteal regression during which subsequent menstruation must be suppressed. This is probably achieved by the production by the trophoblast of a powerful luteotrophin, **chorionic gonadotrophin** (p. 38.47), whose immediate function is thought to be to maintain the corpus luteum and ovarian production of steroids and so preserve and complete decidualization of the endometrium. Chorionic gonadotrophin has, in fact, been identified on day 25 of the menstrual cycle.

DEVELOPMENT OF CHORIONIC VILLI AND OF THE PLACENTA (fig. 38.35)

The placenta has a fetal component, the **chorion**, which is the outermost membrane of the conceptus, and a maternal component, formed by the decidua basalis and by maternal blood circulating in intimate contact with the chorion. The early stages in the development of the chorion and of the other fetal membranes are described in chap. 19. When maternal blood enters the lacunar spaces of the primitive trophoblast, it constitutes a new source of nutrition for the embryo. For the first few days after implantation nutrient reaches the embryo by diffusion, but as the embryo grows, the development of a

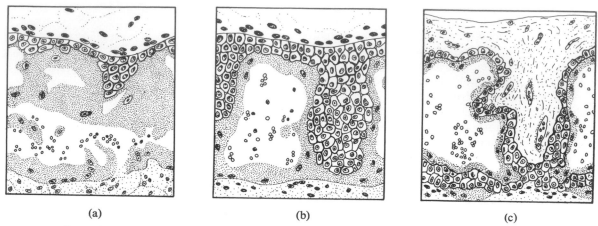

(a)   (b)   (c)

Fig. 38.35. Development of chronic villi. (a) Previllous stage; (b) primary villus; (c) tertiary villus.

simple circulatory system becomes a necessity. The chorionic vesicle has become too large for diffusion to be able to provide for its metabolic processes adequately. The functioning of an embryonic heart and blood vessels starts 3 weeks after fertilization. During the period when the chorion is differentiating and growing vigorously, 9 to 20 days after fertilization, the villous character of the definitive placenta is established.

Whereas the trophoblastic trabeculae and intervening lacunae are initially arranged irregularly, they soon tend to be disposed radially round the chorion. The trabeculae become organized into columns known as **villi**, around which the lacunar spaces extend and coalesce to form the **intervillous space**. While the villi consist only of pleomorphic or cellular trophoblast, they are called **primary villi**. When trophoblastic columns acquire a core of extraembryonic mesoderm (p. 19.2), the trophoblast becomes organized into an outer layer of synctiotrophoblast, which is bathed by the maternal blood in the intervillous space, and an inner single layer of cytotrophoblast disposed around the mesodermal core. The columns that have acquired cores of mesoderm are known as the **secondary villi**. When the mesodermal core differentiates to contain embryonic vessels, the columns are known as **tertiary villi**, and in addition to blood vessels, the core contains gelatinous intercellular substance in which are embedded mesenchymal cells, fibroblasts with long cylindrical nuclei, macrophages (Hofbauer cells) and reticular and collagenous fibres.

With the acquisition by the trophoblast of a lining of extraembryonic mesoderm, a composite layer is formed which is called the **chorion**. As the chorion completely surrounds the developing embryo and its membranes (fig. 19.7) the whole spherical structure is often referred to as the **chorionic vesicle**.

When the chorion is established it is made up of an inner composite layer of extraembryonic mesoderm and trophoblast, called the **chorionic plate**. From this plate

villi extend as branching columns to reach a peripheral complete layer of trophoblast which remains cellular. Where it is in contact with endometrium and forms the boundary between embryonic and maternal tissues, this most peripheral trophoblast forms the **cytotrophoblastic shell**.

Villi extending from the chorionic plate, across the intervillous space, to reach the cytotrophoblastic shell are known as **anchoring** or **stem villi**, from which shorter **branch** or **free villi** develop.

The endometrium adjoining the cytotrophoblastic shell is known as the **boundary zone** and it is separated from actual contact with the trophoblast by a layer of fibrinoid deposit known as Nitabuch's membrane. This boundary zone is traversed by the maternal blood vessels on their way to and from the intervillous space.

It is the cytotrophoblastic shell which, by its interstitial growth, provides the mechanism for circumferential extension of the chorionic vesicle. Expansion of the cytotrophoblastic shell increases the volume of the intervillous space by encroachment upon the surrounding decidua. The area of trophoblast exposed to maternal blood in the intervillous space is also increased by the sprouting of branch villi from the primary stems. These pass through the successive stages of being primary, secondary and eventually vascularized tertiary villi.

These villi which are directed towards the decidua basalis enlarge and branch elaborately while those which are directed towards the decidua capsularis degenerate between the 3rd and 4th months of pregnancy. In this way the chorion which protrudes along with the decidua capsularis into the uterine lumen becomes the smooth, almost avascular **chorion laeve**, whereas the chorion in contact with the decidua basalis where the villi persist becomes the **chorion frondosum** (fig. 38.34). The chorion frondosum progressively assumes the discoidal shape of the definitive **placenta** and the cytotrophoblastic shell with the boundary zone of this region together form its **basal plate**.

At implantation the decidua basalis is only 5–6 mm thick and the increase in the thickness of the placenta as it grows takes place by an increase in the number, length and size of the villi. Growth in thickness as well as circumference continues in the placenta until the end of the 4th month after which only circumferential growth continues until almost the end of pregnancy.

Once the cytotrophoblastic shell has been laid down in the 4th week of pregnancy, small multinucleated masses of syncytium known as **trophoblastic giant cells** migrate from the periphery of the shell and extend into the decidua basalis and beyond it to the adjoining myometrium. Cytotrophoblastic elements also invade and extend up the spiral arteries of the endometrium, and sprouts of syncytiotrophoblast from the villi are shed into the intervillous space from which they are carried into the maternal veins and eventually reach the lungs. The cytotrophoblast which plugs the spiral arteries may play a mechanical role in preventing maternal arterial blood from reaching the intervillous space at too high a pressure.

MATURE PLACENTA (fig. 38.36)

The mature placenta has the form of a flattened circular disc, with a diameter of 15–20 cm and a thickness of 3 cm. At full maturity, the ratio of infant weight to placental weight is about 6:1, so that a placenta usually weighs about 500 g at term. The size, shape and weight of the placenta are all subject to wide variations and there may be an accessory lobule (**succenturiate placenta**).

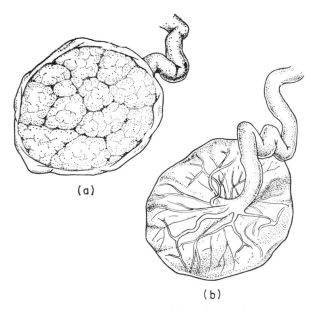

(a)

(b)

FIG. 38.36. Gross appearances of the mature placenta. (a) Maternal surface, (b) fetal surface. From Netter F.H. (1954) *The Ciba Collection of Medical Illustrations.*

The attachment of the umbilical cord to the placenta is usually eccentric but it may vary from being near central to a marginal situation (**battledore placenta**). The length of the umbilical cord varies from 30 to 100 cm with an average length of about 55 cm.

The placenta is essentially a structure which provides a large area of apposition between the maternal and fetal circulations for the exchange of materials. These transfers are controlled by the placental membrane which separates the two circulations.

FETAL PLACENTAL CIRCULATION (fig. 38.37)

Fetal blood is conveyed to the placenta via paired umbilical arteries. The details of the circulation within the fetus are described on p. 42.2. The two umbilical arteries anastomose as they approach the placenta and their branches then ramify over the surface of the chorion. In the **disperse** type of vascular distribution the two umbilical arteries undergo dichotomous division and rapidly diminish in calibre, whereas in the **magistral** type they give off only small branches and reach close to the placental margin before their calibre is reduced to any significant extent. The umbilical vessels usually remain close to each other until the placenta is reached, but occasionally they separate some distance from the placenta (**furcate placenta**). When the vessels ramify beyond the placental margin on the adjacent chorion the condition is called **velamentous insertion** of the cord.

Branches of the umbilical arteries pierce the chorion and form the main stem vessels for the placental villi. Each stem branch is an end artery which does not anastomose with adjacent vessels, and each vascularizes a discrete group of villi which takes the form of an inverted cone or cylinder. These villous units are known as **fetal cotyledons**. They are approximately 200 in number and they vary widely in size. Each main stem artery divides repeatedly within its cotyledon to supply a complicated, root-like structure of villi. In the terminal villi the fetal vessels form an extensive arterio–capillary–venous system such that the fetal capillaries come into very close proximity with the villous membrane. The veins which drain the villi track back along the course of the corresponding arteries and eventually reach the site of insertion of the umbilical cord where they drain into the single persisting umbilical vein. Oxygenated blood is thus returned to the fetus via the umbilical vein. There are no valves in this extended umbilical venous circulation. The umbilical veins and arteries are muscular structures, but they are not innervated and little is known of the control of the fetal placental circulation.

The umbilical vessels follow a tortuous spiral course as they traverse the cord, and are embedded in the gelatinous matrix of Wharton's jelly. The amnion is fused with the external surface of the cord (fig. 38.38).

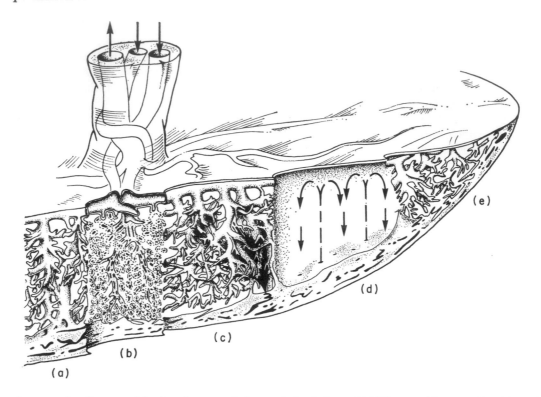

FIG. 38.37. A composite diagram of fetal and maternal placental circulations. (a) Villous architecture, (b) villous circulation in section, (c) maternal circulation, showing arterial jets entering intervillous space, (d) diagram of direction of maternal blood flow in intervillous space, (e) placental margin. From Eastman M.J. & Hellman L.M. (1966) *Williams Obstetrics*, 13th Edition. New York:Appleton-Century-Crofts.

MATERNAL PLACENTAL CIRCULATION (fig. 38.37)

It is convenient to regard the mature placenta as a blood-filled space, the **intervillous space**, which is lined by trophoblast. This space is limited by a 'maternal' surface, or **decidual basal plate**, and a 'fetal' surface or **chorionic plate**, and these surfaces fuse around the circumference of the placenta. The villi of the fetal cotyledons project into the space from the chorionic plate. Some of these are anchoring villi which attach themselves to the decidual plate, while the branching villi extend freely in the intervillous space. The exact architecture of the villi is controversial, but it is unlikely that there is any fetal vascular communication between adjacent villi. The villi are closely crowded together and must not be visualized as floating freely within a roomy space.

Septa extend from the decidual plate towards the chorionic plate, but they fail to reach the fetal surface. When the maternal surface of an expelled placenta is examined the placenta appears to be composed of 15–20 lobes, the clefts between these lobes representing the base of these placental septa. However, these lobes do not constitute subdivisions of the intervillous space and they are of no functional significance. They are sometimes referred to as cotyledons, but these must not be confused with the fetal cotyledonary villous unit.

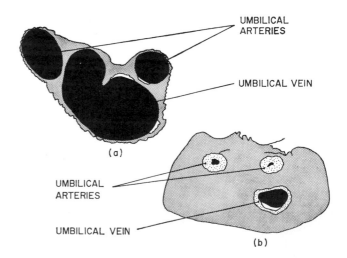

FIG. 38.38. Section through the umbilical cord. (a) Vessels distended with blood, (b) vessels constricted down after cord has been clamped. From Reynolds S.R.M. (1954) *Amer. J. Obstet. Gynec.* **68**, 69.

Approximately 80–100 maternal arteries open haphazardly over the decidual plate into the intervillous space. Blood enters the placenta from these arteries under high pressure, and this jet of maternal blood reaches towards the chorionic plate before dispersing laterally through the interstices of the villi. The exact spatial relation of the decidual arteries to the fetal cotyledons is unknown. Blood leaves the intervillous space by veins whose open ends are scattered over the decidual plate. The previous belief that maternal blood drained only from the periphery of the placenta via a marginal sinus is incorrect. The so-called marginal sinus is no more than the peripheral limit of the intervillous space. This dynamic concept of the circulation of maternal blood through the placenta has been confirmed by cine-angiography.

The uterus contracts intermittently throughout pregnancy. The circulatory effect of these contractions is probably first to occlude the myometrial veins and only later may they obliterate the myometrial arteries supplying the placenta. Consequently, a uterine contraction does not squeeze blood out of the choriodecidual space and halt the transfer of oxygen to the fetus. However, the stronger contractions of labour temporarily impair maternal arterial blood supply and this may induce transient fetal hypoxia.

PLACENTAL MEMBRANE (fig. 38.39)

The placental membrane is the structure which is interposed between maternal and fetal blood. The transfer of substances between mother and fetus is controlled by this membrane which is often called the placental barrier; it has, in addition, several important biosynthetic functions.

The placental membrane is composed of four components. Each villus initially has two layers of trophoblast, an outer layer of syncytiotrophoblast which is in contact with maternal blood, and an inner layer of cytotrophoblast. This trophoblast layer is supported by a basement membrane. Within the villous core there is a connective tissue stroma within which lie the fetal capillaries lined by their vascular endothelium. At this stage, four cellular layers separate maternal from fetal blood: (1) syncytiotrophoblast, (2) cytotrophoblast, (3) connective tissue fibroblasts, (4) fetal capillary endothelium.

As pregnancy advances there is a gradual thinning of this villous membrane. The number and size of fetal capillaries increases and the relative amount of villous stroma is reduced so that capillaries appear to abut directly on to the basement membrane of the trophoblast. The cytotrophoblast becomes scantier and by the end of pregnancy only a few cytotrophoblast cells can be recognized by light microscopy. The syncytiotrophoblast thins and its nuclei clump into groups, or syncytial knots. Consequently, the villous membrane is greatly reduced in thickness, but at no time do the two circulations come into direct contact and there is always some representation of all four cellular layers.

Electron microscopy has contributed enormously to our knowledge of the placental membrane. The syncytiotrophoblast has an elaborate structure. Its free surface is covered by microvilli and it has a complicated system of intracellular canals, vacuoles and endoplasmic reticulum. In later pregnancy the syncytiotrophoblast makes direct contact with the basement membrane. This ultrastructure is suggestive of a major transfer and secretory role for the syncytiotrophoblast.

By contrast, the cytotrophoblast has a relatively simple structure with fewer intracellular organelles. It is the current belief that the syncytiotrophoblast is derived from the cytotrophoblast. The cytotrophoblast may be regarded as a relatively undifferentiated reserve cell

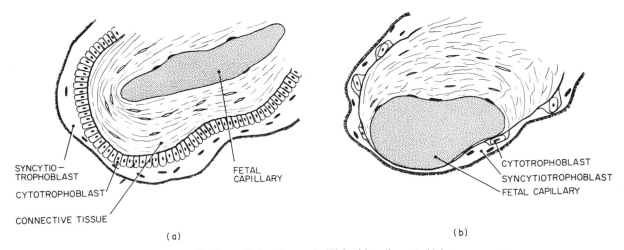

SYNCYTIO-TROPHOBLAST

CYTOTROPHOBLAST

CONNECTIVE TISSUE

FETAL CAPILLARY

(a)

CYTOTROPHOBLAST
SYNCYTIOTROPHOBLAST
FETAL CAPILLARY

(b)

FIG. 38.39. Histology of the placental villi in (a) early and (b) late pregnancy.

which, under optimal conditions, produces a specialized syncytium.

This thinning of the placental membrane, the appearance of syncytial knots and the apparent loss of cytotrophoblast have been interpreted as placental ageing and assumed to indicate failing placental function. Undoubtedly these structural changes are paralleled by equally profound biochemical changes. Furthermore, there are other alterations which may be more conclusively degenerative, e.g. thickening of the basement membrane, degeneration and partial obliteration of the decidual arteries, the deposition of fibrin in the intervillous space, and calcification. However, some of the above histological changes in the placental membrane may constitute a useful adaptation to facilitate transfer. The correlation between placental ultrastructure and function is still poorly understood.

The immunological problems underlying pregnancy have already been indicated and are discussed further on p. 38.52. A striking feature of pregnancy is the tolerance of a genetically dissimilar fetus within the maternal tissues. This confrontation takes place at the choriodecidual junction where the fetal trophoblast makes contact with the endometrium.

Functions of the placenta

In physiological terms the placenta is a fetal organ and the functional interdependence between the fetus and its placenta is conveyed by the expression fetoplacental unit. Anatomically the placenta is simply an extension of the fetal capillary bed covered by a layer of trophoblast, and provides a large surface area ($10 m^2$) in intimate contact with maternal blood. A new-born infant acquires nutrients from, and excretes waste products into its environment at a number of specialized sites, lungs, kidneys and gut. By contrast, the only effective environment of the fetus is the mother's blood, and the placenta is the principal site for the exchange of all materials. It will be shown that the placental villi fulfil many of the functions of the lung alveoli, renal glomeruli and tubules and intestinal epithelium, in addition to which they also produce protein and steroid hormones. This versatile organ has a uniquely short life and rapidly becomes senescent if pregnancy proceeds beyond its normal span of forty weeks.

TRANSFER OF NUTRIENTS

The placenta was once regarded as little more than a semipermeable membrane and much was made of the thickness of the placental barrier in discussing fetal nutrition. It is now clear that far from being a barrier, the placenta has complex transport mechanisms which ensure that the fetus is well supplied with all the nutrients it needs.

Simple diffusion between maternal and fetal blood accounts for the passage of O_2 and CO_2 between mother and fetus, and the placenta approaches the efficiency of the lungs in gas transfer; the delivery of O_2 to the fetus is limited by blood flow to the placenta and not by diffusion rates. Water and a number of small molecules such as sodium also move between mother and fetus by diffusion, with a flux which may be hundreds of times the rate of accumulation by the fetus.

Oxygen is unusual among nutrients in that it cannot be stored, and deprivation for even a few minutes is fatal. The oxygen requirement of the fetus can only be guessed, but it probably consumes oxygen at the same rate as comparable maternal tissues. In this respect it differs from the newborn infant whose relatively large surface area in relation to its body weight demands a higher metabolic rate. At term, the fetus utilizes oxygen at about 12 ml/min (4 ml min^{-1} kg^{-1}), and the placenta at about 4 ml/min (8 ml min^{-1} kg^{-1}). These figures indicate the high metabolic activity of the placenta.

The observed oxygen difference between uterine arterial and venous blood is 40–50 ml O_2/litre blood. Thus, to supply the fetus and placenta with 16 ml O_2/min, the mother must circulate 300–400 ml blood/min to the placental site. This is less than the value of 500–600 ml/min obtained by most estimates of uterine blood flow at term. The rate of blood flow through the fetal side of the placental circulation is of a similar magnitude.

It is crucial for the fetus that it should receive a good supply of oxygen **at a low pressure**, and the Po_2 of umbilical venous blood ranges from 2·7 to 6·7 kPa (20 to 50 mmHg). At higher pressures important mechanisms which must operate at birth, such as constriction of the umbilical arteries and the ductus arteriosus, would be activated and kill the fetus. To achieve a big O_2 carrying capacity at low partial pressure several mechanisms operate (vol. 3, p. 42·66). First, the fetus is, by adult standards, polycythaemic, with normal values of 6–8 $\times 10^{12}$ red cells/l and 14–22 g haemoglobin/dl, thereby increasing the oxygen carrying capacity of fetal blood. Secondly, the oxygen dissociation curve of fetal blood is shifted to the left of that for adult blood (p.31.20). This is due to a higher affinity for O_2 of fetal Hb and to a lower concentration of 2, 3-DPG in the fetal erythrocyte. As a consequence, fetal blood has a higher degree of oxygen saturation at low levels of Po_2 than maternal blood. For example, if maternal blood with a Po_2 of 3·5 kPa and 60 per cent saturation equilibrates with fetal blood, the fetal blood becomes 70 per cent saturated.

Glucose moves down a gradient between mother and fetus but at a more rapid rate than could be predicted by simple diffusion. There is an active transport mechanism which is easily saturated and hence high concentrations of glucose in the mother's blood for a short period make little impact on the fetus. The transfer of glucose does not appear to need insulin. Not all glucose entering the placenta passes to the fetus; some is oxidized by the placenta itself and some is converted to glycogen and lipid.

Of lipids only free fatty acids pass from mother to fetus. More complex lipids are made by the placenta and fetus from maternal precursors. Fat-soluble vitamins appear to equilibrate between maternal and fetal circulations, but the mechanisms of transfer are unknown.

Maternal plasma proteins do not cross the placenta with the notable exception of the immune globulin IgG which is transferred by a highly specific receptor mechanism, perhaps as a component of pinocytosis. All other fetal proteins are made from maternal amino acids which are transferred actively by a process which favours the L-isomers. Placental tissue contains a very high concentration of free amino acids and the fetal plasma a higher concentration than maternal plasma.

Iron is transferred by a specific carrier, transferrin, in the villous surface which takes up iron from the maternal plasma.

Water-soluble vitamins are transferred to the fetus by a mechanism which may also operate for other nutrients. Thiamin, pyridoxine, riboflavin, vitamin B_{12}, folate and ascorbic acid are all present in higher concentration in fetal than maternal blood and concentrations of ascorbic acid, riboflavin and folate in placenta are high.

TRANSFER OF WASTE PRODUCTS

The major waste product of fetal metabolism, carbon dioxide, diffuses across the placenta even more readily than oxygen, and this process is aided by the low $P{CO_2}$ of the maternal plasma.

Urea and other waste products pass across the placenta for disposal by the mother. The fetus also uses its own kidneys and urine is passed into the amniotic fluid from early pregnancy onwards. As amniotic fluid is swallowed waste substances are ingested by the fetus and ultimately eliminated by the placenta.

The heat of fetal metabolism must also be dissipated by the mother; hence the necessity for an increased maternal skin blood flow.

TRANSFER OF HARMFUL SUBSTANCES

Ideally, the placenta should permit the transfer of only nutrients and waste products and exclude harmful substances from the fetus, but its powers of discrimination are limited.

Most mineral ions cross the placenta freely, and their radioactive isotopes behave in a similar way. However, in the case of strontium, the mother rather than the placenta plays a protective role, binding the strontium in her own bones so that relatively little passes to the fetus. Gases pass through the placenta without hindrance. Carbon monoxide is a common example, and the carboxyhaemoglobin content of fetal blood is raised if the mother smokes cigarettes during pregnancy. Indeed the CO dissociation curve for fetal blood is shifted to the left, as it is for O_2, so that fetal blood is more affected by smoking than the mother's. The placenta allows most drugs to cross, and some drugs exert not only their normal pharmacological effect on the fetus, but may also cause malformations (vol. 3, p. 62.4).

The placenta is more effective in excluding microorganisms. Bacteria, such as the tubercle bacillus or the syphilis spirochaete, reach the fetus only by first damaging the placenta. Some viruses, especially the virus of rubella, cross the placenta and damage the fetus.

The placenta prevents free mixing of maternal and fetal blood, but fetal red cells not infrequently cross over to the mother in small numbers, and are responsible for the occasional sensitization of a rhesus negative mother to her rhesus positive fetus.

ENDOCRINE FUNCTIONS

The placenta is a major endocrine gland, but its inaccessibility has made it difficult to study directly. Most information has come from the study of hormones and their metabolites in blood and urine, from the study of isotopically labelled steroid precursors injected into mother or fetus in pregnancies which are to be terminated, and from incubation studies of placental homogenates and tissue slices.

Protein hormones

Gonadotrophin (human chorionic gonadotrophin or HCG). EM and immunofluorescent studies suggest that the syncytiotrophoblast is the major source of HCG. Concentrations of HCG in the blood and in the urine follow the same course. It has been detected in the blood as early as the 25th day of the menstrual cycle. It reaches a peak around the 70th day, after which it falls to a relatively constant value which is maintained throughout pregnancy (fig. 38.40). Its supposed role in early pregnancy is to maintain the ovarian production of steroids until the placenta takes over this function. The function of HCG in later pregnancy is unknown, although it appears to be adrenocorticotrophic in the fetus and may play a part in regulating oestrogen metabolism. HCG can be detected in the urine about 14 days after a missed period and this provides the earliest test for pregnancy.

Placental lactogen (HPL) is structurally similar to pituitary growth hormone and in late pregnancy is produced in large amounts, between 1 and 2 g daily. It has lactogenic properties which may be important in developing mammary tissue, and like growth hormone, it may be responsible for impaired glucose tolerance, common in pregnancy.

Chorionic thyrotrophin (HCT), similar to pituitary TSH,

occurs in high concentrations in late pregnancy plasma. Its role is not understood.

The polypeptide hormone, relaxin, is probably also produced by the placenta. In small rodents, it has an important role in softening the uterine cervix and relaxing pelvic joints, but its function in human pregnancy is not known.

Steroid hormones

The syncytiotrophoblast is the likely site of production of steroid hormones. Steroid production in pregnancy provides an excellent illustration of the intimate inter-relations between fetus and placenta.

The placenta has only a limited part to play in steroid production. It cannot split the side chain of C-21 steroids. Consequently, it requires a source of precursors such as dehydro*epi*androsterone sulphate, produced by the fetal and maternal adrenal glands. It is, however, a rich source of 3β-hydroxysteroid dehydrogenase and aromatizing enzymes, and so it can convert these precursors efficiently to oestrone and oestradiol-17β. Furthermore, the placenta probably cannot convert these oestrogens to oestriol. It is believed that the oestrone and oestradiol-17β produced by the placenta enter the fetal circulation, and that 16-hydroxylation occurs in the fetal adrenal and liver. The oestriol which has thus been formed by the combined activity of fetal and placental tissue (or fetoplacental unit) finally crosses the placenta into the maternal circulation.

The subsequent metabolism and excretion of placental oestrogens is similar to that already described for ovarian oestrogens. Quantitatively the most important urinary oestrogen in pregnancy is oestriol, and its excretion rises dramatically during pregnancy (fig. 38.40).

In late pregnancy the placenta secretes about 250 mg progesterone daily. The placenta cannot synthesize the steroid nucleus *de novo*, and it is dependent on steroid precursors. These are probably pregnenolone sulphate of fetal origin and maternal cholesterol and pregnenolone. However, the presence of a fetus is not essential for normal pregnanediol excretion, and maternal precursors are adequate for the placental production of progesterone. This is in contrast to the intimate fetoplacental relations necessary for oestrogen production in pregnancy. Pregnanediol is one of the principal metabolites of progesterone, and its urinary excretion increases tenfold during pregnancy (fig. 38.40).

The role of these steroid hormones in pregnancy is not fully understood, although they have an important relation to myometrial growth and contractility, to the preparation of the breasts for lactation and to the systemic maternal responses to pregnancy (vol. 3, p. 42.58).

AMNIOTIC FLUID

Amniotic fluid provides the fetus with a favourable en-

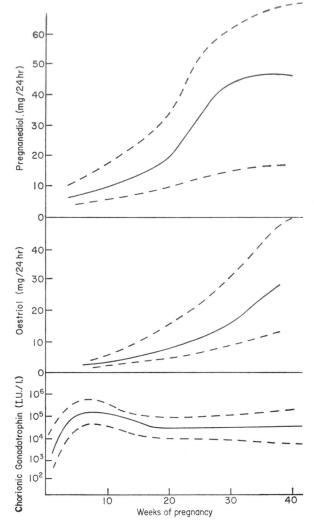

FIG. 38.40. Urinary excretion of pregnanediol, oestriol and chorionic gonadotrophin in pregnancy. Continuous lines indicate mean values. Broken lines indicate limits of 95 per cent probability. Ordinate on gonadotrophin diagram is on a logarithmic scale.

vironment, absorbing mechanical pressures and yet allowing freedom of movement.

The volume of amniotic fluid increases from about 30 ml at the 10th week of pregnancy to a maximum of about 1000 ml at the 36th–37th week. Thereafter, it falls by approximately 150 ml/week, so that if pregnancy is prolonged until the 42nd week very little fluid remains. It should be emphasized that there is a wide variation in these values. In the first half of pregnancy, the volume is closely related to fetal weight.

Amniotic fluid resembles a dialysate of fetal plasma. Since the fetal skin is permeable at this stage, the amniotic fluid probably forms an extension of fetal extracellular fluid. Beyond midpregnancy, when the fetal skin keratinizes and becomes impermeable, the amniotic fluid volume is a balance between that added by fetal urine and that taken away by fetal swallowing.

The fluid therefore increasingly reflects urinary characteristics, becoming hypotonic, with increasing concentrations of urea and creatinine. These changes may be used to assess fetal maturity in a sample of amniotic fluid. Lung fluid containing surfactant reaches the amniotic fluid in increasing amounts in late pregnancy and the concentration of lecithin appears to reflect fetal lung maturity (vol. 3, p. 42.63).

Physiological responses of the mother to pregnancy

The mother responds to the stimulus of gestation by widespread physiological changes involving most systems of the body in such a way as to provide a suitable environment for the growing fetus. However, the relationship between mother and fetus is not simply that of host and parasite, in that each maternal adjustment is not precipitated by the immediate demand of the fetus. Instead the mother anticipates the needs of the fetus, so that the response precedes the demand. The stimuli which initiate the maternal responses to pregnancy are presumably hormonal but are little understood.

VOLUME AND COMPOSITION OF THE BLOOD

During pregnancy both plasma volume and red cell mass increase (table 38.2). Plasma volume begins to rise towards

TABLE 38.2. Plasma volume, red cell volume, total blood volume and packed cell volume (PCV) in pregnancy.

	Non-pregnant	Weeks of pregnancy		
		20	30	40
Plasma volume (ml)	2600	3150	3750	3800
Red cell volume (ml)	1400	1450	1550	1650
Total blood volume (ml)	4000	4600	5300	5450
Body PCV, per cent	35·0	31·5	29·2	30·3
Venous PCV, * per cent	39·8	35·8	33·2	34·4

* Assuming a PCV ratio of 0·88.

the end of the 3rd month, reaching a plateau of 1250–1500 ml above non-pregnant values during the last trimester. The commonly described fall in late pregnancy is spurious (see below). Red cell volume increases steadily from the 3rd month to term by about 250 ml, or more if medicinal iron is taken during pregnancy. Since the increase in plasma volume is disproportionately greater than the increase in red cell mass, packed cell volume and haemoglobin concentration fall. This fall in Hb concentration, despite a rise in red cell mass, has been described as a physiological anaemia of pregnancy, but this term is misleading as mean cell haemoglobin concentration remains unchanged, and there is normally no evidence of iron-deficiency anaemia.

There are also important changes in plasma composition. Their origin is complex and they are not due to simple haemodilution. For example, the concentration of plasma albumin falls, and this leads to a drop in plasma colloid osmotic pressure. However, β-globulin and fibrinogen concentrations rise steadily throughout pregnancy, while α- and γ-globulin fractions show little change. The meaning of these changes is unknown. The altered pattern of plasma proteins raises the erythrocyte sedimentation rate to levels which would in other circumstances be considered pathological.

There are changes in blood concentrations of lipids, enzymes, inorganic ions, amino acids and vitamins, all of which illustrate the upheaval of the mother's metabolism. These are of considerable clinical importance, because much confusion has arisen from interpreting blood composition in pregnancy in terms of non-pregnant standards.

CARDIOVASCULAR DYNAMICS

Cardiac output rises early in pregnancy to a level which is then maintained until parturition. The time of onset and magnitude of this rise are disputed, but an increase of the order of 1·5 l/min is probably reached before mid-pregnancy. It has been accepted for many years that cardiac output falls in late pregnancy, but it now seems certain that this observation is due to the fact that most measurements of cardiac output have been made with the patient lying on her back. In this position in late pregnancy, the pregnant uterus rests on the inferior vena cava and restricts venous return from the lower half of the body (supine caval occlusion). When cardiac output is measured serially during pregnancy with the patient lying on her side, there is no evidence of a terminal fall in cardiac output. This increase in output is achieved by an increase in both heart rate and stroke volume.

It is not possible to account entirely for the distribution of the extra 1·5 litres of cardiac output. Blood flow to the uterus rises throughout pregnancy to a mean maximum of about 500 ml/min, although this measurement is technically so difficult that the figure is only an approximation. Renal blood flow increases in early pregnancy by about 400 ml/min. It has been said to decline in late pregnancy, but this fall, like that in cardiac output, may be due to the fallacies of making clearance studies in the supine position. Blood flow through the skin is greatly increased and this is most obvious in the warm, moist extremities. It is not possible to estimate the increase in skin blood flow accurately, but it may amount to 500 ml/min. It may be noted that two major areas of increased blood flow, the kidneys and the skin, serve purposes of elimination, the kidneys of soluble waste and the skin of heat. Both processes require plasma rather than whole blood, which gives point to the disproportionate increase of plasma volume in the expansion of blood volume.

RESPIRATION

The resting minute volume increases throughout pregnancy by about 40 per cent. This is achieved by an increase in tidal volume rather than respiratory rate. Since oxygen intake increases by only 15 per cent, overbreathing results and alveolar P_{CO_2} falls from about 5·1 kPa in non-pregnant women to little more than 4·0 kPa in late pregnancy.

RENAL FUNCTION

An increase in renal blood flow has been described above. Glomerular filtration rate rises even more dramatically from a non-pregnant level of about 90 ml/min to 150 ml/min. This high level is reached in the first trimester and is maintained throughout pregnancy. The rise leads to changes in blood composition. For example, urea, uric acid and creatinine are cleared more effectively, and plasma concentrations of these substances are reduced. Many nutrients are treated in the same way. Glucose may be excreted in large quantities by normal women and up to 3 g of amino acids may be lost daily. Folate is excreted at four or five times the usual rate and there are losses of other water-soluble vitamins. There is no simple relation between the renal losses and the generally reduced plasma concentrations of these nutrients.

ENDOCRINE FUNCTIONS

The placental production of sex steroid and protein hormones has already been described.

The hypophysis enlarges during pregnancy and there is indirect evidence of increased secretion of some trophic hormones. Melanocyte stimulating hormone (MSH) is produced in increasing amounts and may be responsible for the characteristic skin pigmentation of pregnancy.

The production of aldosterone by the adrenal cortex rises, countering the sodium-losing effect of progesterone. There are also large increases in circulating corticosteroids, especially cortisol, but this is partly due to increased binding of the hormone by transcortin and this bound component is not physiologically active.

The thyroid gland is palpably enlarged in the majority of pregnant women. Together with an increased oxygen consumption, raised pulse rate, heat intolerance and a rise in plasma protein-bound iodine (PBI), this has often been interpreted as evidence of hyperthyroidism. However, these signs are now recognized as physiological adaptations to pregnancy. The raised PBI is a reflection of increased hormone binding by plasma proteins. The thyroid enlargement is of the iodine deficiency type, and may be attributed to a low blood inorganic iodine level. Concentrations of free thyroid hormone are, if anything, somewhat reduced.

There is a progressively reduced tolerance to a glucose load in spite of increasing amounts of circulating insulin.

WEIGHT GAIN IN PREGNANCY

A normal British woman gains about 12·5 kg body weight during pregnancy, although there are enormous individual variations. On the average, her weight increases at a rate of about 0·5 kg weekly during the last two-thirds of pregnancy, the most rapid rate of gain occurring between the 16th and 24th weeks.

Fig. 38.41 shows the components of this added weight gain. At mid-pregnancy when the rate of increase is most rapid, and even at term, the uterus and its contents account for only one half of the total weight gain. At term the maternal blood volume and extracellular fluid accounts for 2·5 kg and the remaining 3·5 kg represents body fat. The pregnant woman has little facility for storing protein. Fig. 38.41 shows that maternal fat is laid down early when other components are increasing very little, and that little more is accumulated in the last 10 weeks. This stored 3·5 kg of body fat remains after delivery, and represents the net weight gain of a normal pregnant woman.

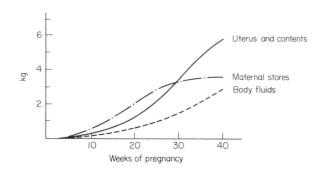

FIG. 38.41. Components of weight gain in pregnancy. From Hytten F.E. & Leitch I. (1971) *The Physiology of Human Pregnancy*, 2nd Edition. Oxford: Blackwell Scientific Publications.

NUTRITIONAL REQUIREMENTS OF PREGNANCY

The energy cost of pregnancy includes the building up of a reserve of fat, and the maintenance of the metabolism of the fetus and the additional maternal tissues. The storage of nutrients can be calculated with reasonable precision. By the end of pregnancy, the mother has gained approximately 1 kg protein, mostly in the uterus and products of conception, and 3·5 kg fat, most of it in her own fat depots. The running costs rise in pregnancy due to the metabolism of the fetus and placenta, the metabolism of the additional uterine and breast tissue, and the cost of the extra cardiac and respiratory work (fig. 38.42). The cumulative energy requirement for a pregnancy is about 300MJ (70 000 kcal), spread evenly at an almost constant rate over the last two-thirds of pregnancy. These specific costs, usually between 1·2 and 1·7MJ (300 and 400 kcal)/day, refer to the woman at rest. If the mother continues her normal activities, these are almost certain to cost her more as her weight rises. In Western society, pregnant women tend to curtail their activities and may indeed subsidize the specific costs of pregnancy by a reduction of their normal non-pregnant energy expenditure.

Extra nutrient requirements are less easy to specify. The need for protein is greatest in the last 10 weeks, when fetal growth requires about 5–6 g/day. This extra protein would be found in any good diet supplying the extra energy. The fetus accumulates about 30 g calcium throughout pregnancy, at a maximum rate of 250 mg/day. This requirement can be met by the addition of 200 ml milk to the daily diet, but if this is not available, the maternal skeleton can easily provide this quantity of

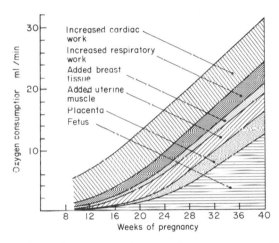

FIG. 38.42. Components of increased oxygen consumption in pregnancy. From Hytten F.E. & Leitch I. (1971) *The Physiology of Human Pregnancy*, 2nd Edition. Oxford: Blackwell Scientific Publications.

calcium. The gross extra requirement of iron is about 750 mg, of which one-third will be returned to store from the expanded maternal blood volume after delivery. The need for extra iron may not be met by even a good diet, and all pregnant women are recommended to take a supplement of medicinal iron (vol. 3, p. 42.51).

Uterus in pregnancy

The uterus has three principal functions in pregnancy, to allow implantation of the blastocyst, to accommodate the growing products of conception, and to expel these contents at parturition. Implantation is described on p. 38.39, and parturition in vol. 3, chap. 40. Three mechanisms are involved in the accommodation of the fetus; compensatory growth and distension of the uterus, restraint of myometrial contractility and the resistance of the cervix to stretch.

GROWTH AND DISTENSION OF THE UTERUS

The uterus has to make room for the rapidly increasing volume of fetus, placenta and amniotic fluid. Thus, the volume of the uterine cavity expands from a potential space in the non-pregnant state to approximately 5 litres at the end of the pregnancy. This expansion is the result of both active growth and passive distension. In the first half of pregnancy the uterus gains weight rapidly, partly by an increase in the number of muscle fibres (hyperplasia) but mainly by an increase in the size of individual fibres (hypertrophy). The smooth muscle cells of the non-pregnant uterus are spindle shaped and measure 50–90 μm in length and 2–5 μm in breadth. By the end of pregnancy, the fibres are elongated to a length of 500–800 μm and increased to a breadth of 5–10 μm. Myometrial growth is initiated by oestrogens but is also stimulated directly by mechanical distension.

After mid-pregnancy the rate of uterine growth slows down but uterine volume increases rapidly (fig. 38.43). As a result, the uterus is passively distended and the thickness of the myometrium is reduced from 9 mm at mid-pregnancy to 6 mm at the end of pregnancy. This passive stretching is facilitated by alterations in the connective tissue framework of the uterus. During pregnancy, existing collagen fibres are replaced by new fine fibrils. These appear to be dispersed in random directions throughout the uterus within a loose, oedematous stroma. Thus, although the total content of collagen in the uterus is increased, its concentration is reduced.

The pregnant uterus does not normally respond to distension by increased contractility leading to the onset of labour. However, there is an increase in the frequency and intensity of uterine contractions throughout pregnancy but, in contrast to contractions during labour (vol. 3, p. 40.2), they do not cause the cervix to dilate.

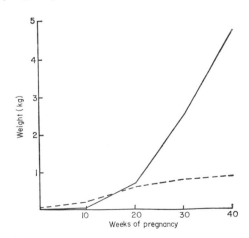

FIG. 38.43. Growth of the uterus and products of conception during pregnancy. This diagram illustrates the disproportionate growth of the conceptus in the second half of pregnancy. Broken line, uterus; continuous line, conceptus (fetus, placenta and amniotic fluid).

UTERINE CERVIX (fig. 38.44)

Whereas the upper half of the cervix is predominantly muscular, the lower half is largely fibrous in nature and has a high collagen content. Until the 12th–14th week of pregnancy, the expanding conceptus can be lodged in the space within the growing uterus. Thereafter, the upper half of the cervix and the isthmus of the uterus add to the available volume of the uterine cavity. These components elongate and become stretched during parturition when they form a 'conducting' component or **'lower segment'** of the uterus. The upper segment forms the propulsive element of the uterus.

It is essential that the unfolding of the isthmus and upper cervix in pregnancy should not proceed to complete dilation of the cervix as this would terminate the pregnancy prematurely. Unfolding is resisted by the fibrous lower half of the cervix so that complete effacement does not normally occur until parturition. This cervical mechanism is not due to a muscular sphincter but simply to the resistance to stretch of collagen fibres, and it is effective only if myometrial contractility is sufficiently restrained.

ONSET OF PARTURITION

These three mechanisms, i.e. the growth and distension of the uterus, the restraint of myometrial contractility and the resistance of the cervix to stretch, allow the fetus to grow within the uterus for about 266 days before parturition. With a normal 28-day menstrual cycle and fertilization occurring at mid-cycle, this corresponds to a gestation period of 280 days or 40 weeks calculated from the 1st day of the last normal menstrual period. The duration of pregnancy is relatively constant, but the factors which determine the time of onset of labour are unknown.

Oxytocin stimulates the myometrium specifically, and it has been suggested that the release of this hormone by the neurohypophysis is responsible for the onset of labour. There is no doubt that the sensitivity of the myometrium to oxytocin increases in the last few weeks of pregnancy as labour approaches, but assays of oxytocin in blood have not shown an unequivocal rise in early labour. There is an increase in the later stages of labour when the cervix is widely dilated. It is likely that this represents a neurohumoral reflex release of oxytocin in response to cervical dilation.

An alternative view is that the uterus is held under restraint during pregnancy, and that labour is due to escape from this inhibition rather than to oxytocic stimulation. This restraint is assumed to be exerted by progesterone. It has been demonstrated that progesterone causes hyperpolarization of the cell membrane of single myometrial fibres and so decreases excitability. Although this mechanism seems to be operational in some species, in man there is no substantial evidence of a terminal fall in placental progesterone prior to the onset of labour.

The role of mechanical distension is not clear. There is a close relation between stretch of a muscle fibre and its contractility, and it has been shown that the muscle fibres of the body of the uterus reach their optimal length at the end of pregnancy. There is also evidence that experimental distension of the uterine cavity increases uterine contractility. However, it is relevant to recall that the volume of the amniotic fluid commonly falls in the last few weeks of pregnancy.

Biological problem of the conceptus as an allograft

The tissues of all higher vertebrates possess the ability to recognize and reject alien tissues, the foreign antigens being determined by histocompatibility genes of the graft. The fetus and placenta are retained for the length of gestation despite the fact that antibodies against incompatible blood group antigens of the fetus and against other antigens of the fetus or of trophoblast circulate in the maternal blood. As the conceptus has a genetic endowment derived from both the father and the mother, it may be considered to be an allograft with respect to the genetic endowment received from the father, and an isograft with regard to that of the mother. Thus the placenta would appear to be a graft of a special kind and

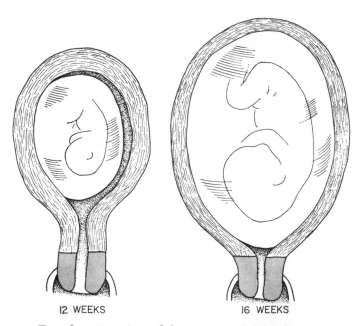

12 WEEKS   16 WEEKS

FIG. 38.44. Behaviour of the cervix and isthmus in pregnancy. The stippled area represents the fibrous portion of the cervix. By the 12th week, the uterus has undergone hypertrophy and the amniotic sac does not yet occupy all the available space in the uterus. By the 16th week, the volume of the conceptus exceeds the available space in the uterus, and this is compensated by unfolding of the isthmus. This unfolding process is halted at the level of the fibrous part of the cervix. From Danforth D.N. (1947) *Amer. J. Obstet. Gynec.* **53**, 541.

it would seem that there is a mechanism that, at least for a time, inhibits the allograft reaction.

Since from the time of implantation, trophoblast is exposed directly to maternal tissues, soluble antigen of fetal origin is likely to be discharged into the maternal circulation. Similarly antibodies from the mother can be transferred across the placental membrane. In addition, there appears to be a transfer of blood cells from fetus to mother and from mother to fetus.

Primary graft rejection is a cell-mediated immune response (p. 29.8) and involves the identification of the foreign tissue by circulating lymphocytes, followed by a proliferative response in lymphoid organs and finally graft destruction by sensitized lymphocytes.

It is, therefore, remarkable that there is no allograft reaction to the conceptus when it is realized that, in the mature placenta, the total surface of chorion exposed to maternal blood and tissue is of the order of 14 m².

At first the mother does appear to make an ineffective immunological response to the implanting blastocyst, and the infiltration of the endometrium surrounding the implanting conceptus by small lymphocytes is a feature of the decidual reaction. Although these cells appear to be more numerous at the implantation site, little is really known about the distribution of lymphocytes in different parts of the decidua. Plasma cells have also been observed in decidua, but they are only occasionally seen in the second half of pregnancy and they often appear to be engulfed by trophoblast.

A number of hypotheses have been invoked to account for the failure of the conceptus to be rejected by the mother as a foreign tissue graft, but none are fully satisfactory.

The masking of the antigenicity of the trophoblast by an acellular barrier of fibrinoid (vol. 2, p. 30.3) between maternal and fetal tissues has been postulated, and the evidence, although inconclusive, is better than that for any of the other hypotheses. Dissociated trophoblastic cells, divested of fibrinoid by neuraminidase, are antigenic.

Two immunological mechanisms have been postulated to explain non-rejection of fetal tissue by the mother. The first is **immunological tolerance**, by which it is considered that there is a state of non-reactivity to the antigen as a result of exposure to it, either in very low doses over a long period leading to specific weakening of the ability to respond to it, or in very high doses producing a specific inhibitory effect on the plasma cells.

The second is **immunological enhancement** of the trophoblast, by which it is considered that the incompatible graft increases its length of survival in the host by attaching the antibodies, formed by the mother against trophoblast, to the antigenic sites on the trophoblast and so preventing access to them by the maternal lymphocytes. Antibodies do not have a deleterious effect on allografts (only on xenografts) and in this way prevent the lymphocytes from damaging the allografts.

Lactation

The **mammary glands** are accessory reproductive organs and are modified sweat glands.

DEVELOPMENT

They develop from a linear thickening of ectoderm called the **mammary ridge** or milk line. By the 6th month of intrauterine life, this extends from the axilla to the groin in both sexes, but it soon becomes confined to the middle of the cranial third of the line, where epithelial cells invade the underlying mesenchyme. Occasionally additional mammary gland rudiments develop along the milk line forming supernumerary breasts or nipples.

When the fetus is about 5 months old, 15–20 solid cellular cords grow out from the mammary epithelial bud into the surrounding mesenchyme of the developing dermis, pushing the component layers of the dermis before them. Each of these original cords becomes a separate exocrine gland, so that each breast is really composed of several glands which empty by separate ducts at the nipple and are separated from each other by partitions of connective tissue. These cords become canalized by the 8th–9th months so that by birth a nipple and rudimentary duct system have formed.

This infantile condition persists until puberty. At puberty in the female, the breast enlarges due to the accumulation of fat in the connective tissue. The epithelial duct system also develops further, but although cellular knobs form at the end of the ducts, probably no true secretory units develop until pregnancy.

FORM AND RELATIONS

The size and shape of the breasts of mature women vary between individuals and according to the functional state of the glands. Each **nipple** is surrounded by a disc-shaped **areola**, of darker colour than the surrounding skin, and usually protrudes below and lateral to the centre of each breast.

The nipples are usually situated at about the level of the fourth intercostal space. The gland extends vertically from the second to the sixth rib and horizontally from the sternal border to the mid-axillary line. From the upper outer quadrant there is a prolongation of mammary tissue along the anterior axillary fold, known as the **axillary tail** of the breast. The deep surface of the gland is related to the deep fascia covering the pectoralis major, and to a lesser extent the serratus anterior and external oblique.

BLOOD SUPPLY

The arterial supply is derived from perforating branches of the internal thoracic artery through the second, third and fourth intercostal spaces, from the external mammary branch of the lateral thoracic artery, and from the anterior intercostal arteries of the second, third and fourth intercostal spaces. The thoraco-acromial artery may supply the upper outer quadrant.

Veins from the breast drain into the axillary, internal thoracic and intercostal veins. The rich subcutaneous venous plexus which connects with the veins of the stroma drains into the external jugular vein.

NERVE SUPPLY

Sensory fibres are conveyed by the second to the sixth thoracic nerves. Free and encapsulated nerve endings ramify in the gland stroma and in the subepidermal connective tissue. The nipple has a particularly rich sensory innervation. Sympathetic fibres are distributed with the sensory nerve fibres, and they innervate the smooth muscle fibres of blood vessels, ducts and nipple.

LYMPH DRAINAGE (fig. 38.45)

The lymphatic drainage of the breast is of special significance because of its relevance to the diagnosis and treatment of carcinoma of the gland.

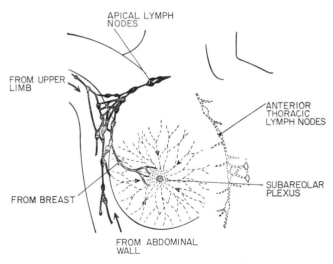

FIG. 38.45. Lymphatic drainage of the breast. From Glenister T.W.A. & Ross J.R.W. (1974) *Anatomy and Physiology for Nurses*, 2nd Edition. London:Heinemann.

The substance of the breast contains an **interstitial plexus** of lymphatics. These vessels are disposed in the interlobular connective tissue and in the walls of the lactiferous ducts. The interstitial plexus communicates with a **cutaneous plexus**, especially around the nipple where a **subareolar plexus** is formed. It has been claimed that the interstitial plexus communicates with a **deep submammary plexus** of minute vessels on the deep fascia underlying the breast. This anastomosis probably plays no part in the lymphatic drainage of the normal gland, nor in the early spread of cancer from the gland. How-

ever, it may provide an alternative pathway when normal ones are obstructed.

Lymphatics arising in the substance of the breast pass round the anterior border of the axilla, pierce the axillary fascia and terminate in the axillary lymph nodes.

The axillary nodes probably receive 75 per cent of the lymph from the breast. Perhaps 20 per cent of the lymph passes to the parasternal nodes which receive vessels accompanying the perforating branches of the internal thoracic artery. About 5 per cent of the lymph vessels are thought to follow the lateral cutaneous branches of the posterior intercostal arteries to reach the posterior intercostal nodes near the necks of the ribs.

STRUCTURE (fig. 38.46a and b)

A mammary gland has an epithelial component, which constitutes the glandular element or parenchyma, and a connective tissue component, which forms the supporting element or stroma.

The epithelial component is disposed in the form of **lobes**, each containing 15 to 25 **lactiferous ducts**, usually opening separately at the nipple. Just before a lactiferous duct opens on the nipple it is dilated to form a **lactiferous sinus** or **ampulla**. The ducts run radially from the base of the nipple and branch repeatedly. Each lobe is made up of the glandular tissue developed from a single lactiferous duct, and is subdivided into **lobules** corresponding to the branching of the duct system.

The gland has no definite capsule, and its connective tissue component merges imperceptibly with the subcutaneous tissue around it, except in the region of the axillary tail which pierces the deep fascia. Within the substance of the gland, the ducts are intimately surrounded by subcutaneous connective tissue which acts as a packing material and supporting framework. This connective tissue divides the substance of the breast to form **interlobar, interlobular** and **intralobular septa** according to the particular relation to the glandular tissue.

Except under the nipple and the areola, the connective tissue contains liberal deposits of fat. These deposits are

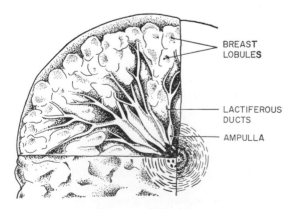

FIG. 38.46a. Structure of the breast.

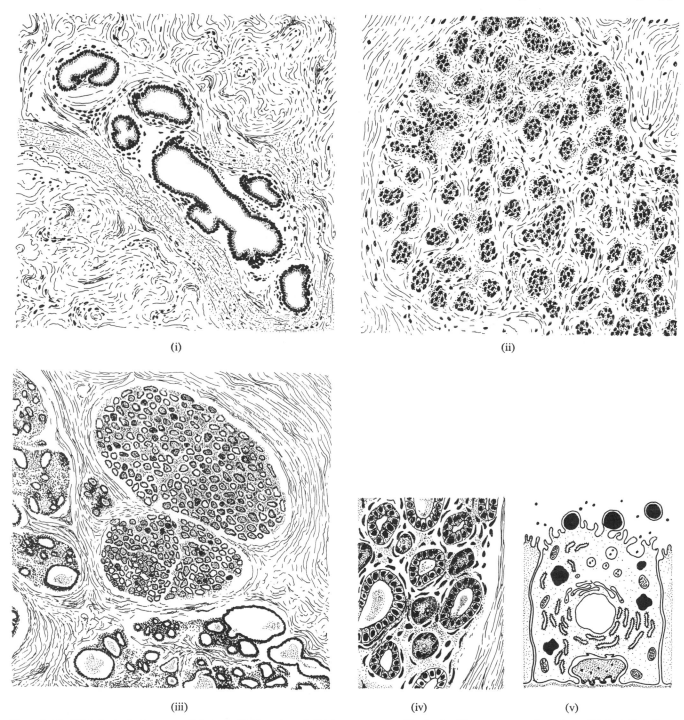

FIG. 38.46b. Histological structure of breast. (i) Prepubertal (high power magnification); (ii) mature non-lactating; (iii) lactating (low power magnification); (iv) lactating (high power magnification); (v) EM of secretory and myoepithelial cells.

responsible for the smooth superficial contour of the gland.

The lobes of the breast are pyramidal in shape and they are attached to the skin by strands of connective tissue, called the **suspensory ligaments of Cooper,** which are continuous with the deep fascia. They are in effect interlobar

septa. The connective tissue, separating the deep surface of the gland from the fascia covering the muscle it overlies, is very loose and through it pass nerves, blood vessels and lymphatics supplying and draining the gland.

The skin covering the breast is smoother, thinner and more translucent than the skin covering most of the rest of the body. The areolar skin is thinner still and contains complex sweat and sebaceous glands, and hair follicles. The surface of the areola is marked by a number of small elevations, the **tubercles of Montgomery**, which are probably caused by underlying glands or ducts.

The nipple is conical or cylindrical in shape. Its colour is due to the thinness and pigmentation of its skin, and it is either soft or firm according to the tone of the smooth muscle fibres found in it. This muscle tissue is embedded in connective tissue and the fibres are disposed concentrically, radially and longitudinally, and extend into the connective tissue of the areola. The core of the nipple is traversed by lactiferous ducts and sinuses which open at its tip; it possesses many sebaceous glands.

The structural and functional differentiation of the breast is under the control of pituitary and ovarian hormones. In general, oestrogenic hormones stimulate growth of the ducts, whereas progestogens stimulate the formation of small alveoli at the ends of the ducts.

When the ovaries begin to function cyclically, the breasts begin to mature by a process of differentiation into potential secretory alveoli at the globular ends of the ramifications extending from the lactiferous ducts. The rudimentary alveoli and their ducts consist of one or two layers of columnar cells surrounded by a basement membrane. Between the basement membrane and the columnar cells there are flattened **myoepithelial cells**. The lobes of the glands become separated from one another by dense intralobular connective tissue and fat deposits. The interlobar connective tissue, on the other hand, is much more cellular and contains fewer collagen fibres and practically no fat (fig. 38.46). The intralobular tissue provides an easily distensible medium allowing hypertrophy of the secretory elements during pregnancy and lactation.

It is generally believed that the structure of the mammary glands alters in phase with the menstrual cycle. The gland may become fuller in the second half of the cycle and a sense of tension in the breasts may be experienced in the few days that precede menstruation.

The full structural differentiation of the gland is dependent on the occurrence of conception. The duct system then grows considerably and many more alveoli and lobules are formed (fig. 38.46). The alveoli consist of clusters of glandular cells enclosing a small lumen that expands as secretions gather. The entire gland increases in size, due to dilation and multiplication of the alveoli and ducts.

While these changes are occurring, the mammary veins become increasingly visible, and the nipples and areola begin to enlarge and become more pigmented. The tubercles of Montgomery also enlarge. The structure of the lactating breast depends on the amount of milk it contains, but in general the interlobular septa are compressed between the distended lobules and the secretory

alveoli are lined by cuboidal or low columnar cells, which accumulate cytoplasmic inclusions in the form of fat droplets and small protein granules. These are released into the lumen of the alveoli by a process of apocrine secretion, leaving the luminal surface of the secretory cells irregular. As the secretion accumulates in the lumen of an alveolus, it becomes distended and the secretory cells become flattened.

The expulsion of milk from the alveoli into and along the ducts is caused by contraction of the myoepithelial cells and of the smooth muscle around the ducts under the influence of oxytocin.

BREAST DEVELOPMENT IN PREGNANCY

The duct and acinar systems of the breasts develop during pregnancy, and as a result the breasts increase in size. There is a wide variation in the degree of glandular development. Examination of breasts of women dying at or shortly after delivery showed that in 30–40 per cent duct and acinar development was grossly deficient, and the breasts consisted largely of fat and fibrous tissue. Before pregnancy, the nipples are firmly bound to the underlying gland by fibrous tissue, and during pregnancy these bonds are loosened and the nipple becomes more mobile, making it easier for the suckling infant to grasp.

Acinar and duct development in pregnancy is an extension of the growth which follows puberty. It is believed that oestrogens are primarily responsible for the growth of ducts, and progestogens for the growth of acinar buds. Ovarian steroids can act directly on the breast in the absence of the hypophysis, but they require the presence of an intact hypophysis in order to exert their optimal effect. The principal hypophyseal trophic hormone for the breast is prolactin. Prolactin both potentiates the action of ovarian steroids, and can itself induce mammary growth and even secretion in oophorectomized, hypophysectomized animals. Growth hormone and intact adrenocortical and thyroid systems are also required for optimal mammary gland development. Human placental lactogen, HPL, may play an important part in the development of the human mammary gland (p. 38.47).

CONTROL OF MILK PRODUCTION

The breasts secrete a small quantity of fluid, or **colostrum,** from early pregnancy onwards, and for the first two or three days after parturition. Colostrum differs from milk, especially in having a high fat and protein content. Milk secretion starts commonly on the 3rd day after parturition.

Prolactin is essential for milk production as well as breast development. Although HPL seems likely to be the major trophic hormone for breast growth, pituitary prolactin is also produced throughout normal pregnancy. That growth is permitted without milk production is due to the inhibitory effect, at the alveolus, of oestrogen. When the local alveolar inhibition is removed after pregnancy, milk production is initiated. Adrenal corticosteroids and thyroxine are probably also needed for continued lactation.

Regular milk ejection is also essential. The ejection of milk is stimulated by suckling via a neurohumoral reflex. The afferent side of this reflex is nervous, so that suckling a denervated gland is ineffective. The central area includes the neurohypophysis, and stimulation of the supraopticohypophyseal tract induces discharge of milk from the breast. The efferent mechanism is humoral. Thus, suckling an innervated gland causes release of milk from a denervated gland. The humoral factor is oxytocin, and administration of oxytocin causes the ejection of milk by stimulating contractions of the myoepithelial cells which surround the alveoli. These contractions force milk out of the alveoli into the ducts. The release of oxytocin during suckling commonly causes uterine contractions which may be noticeable or even painful to the mother. In women the cerebral cortex has an important overriding influence on all these mechanisms, and lactation is profoundly affected by emotions and psychological attitudes.

Under normal conditions, lactation continues as long as suckling is allowed. Breast feeding in Western countries is practised by only a minority of women, and then for only a few months, but in some countries in Africa and Asia lactation may be prolonged for two or three years. In many mammals, ovulation rapidly follows parturition, and lactation continues during the subsequent pregnancy. However, the period of human lactation is a time of relative infertility. Ovulation is probably delayed, presumably due to a suppression of pituitary gonadotrophins. Yet conception can occur during lactation, and in these circumstances milk secretion continues during pregnancy, although the quantity and quality falls off.

MILK SECRETION

Milk secretion begins about 3 days after parturition, and gradually increases to a rate of about 850 ml/day although yields as high as 3 litres per day have been observed.

The principal constituents of milk are water, lactose, fat and protein. A table giving the composition of human and cow's milk is set out on p. 5.23. The production of lactose begins in early pregnancy, and it is demonstrable in maternal blood and urine. Milk fats are essentially triglycerides manufactured from circulating fatty acids by the mammary gland. Milk proteins are probably synthesized from circulating amino acids, although some plasma proteins appear in milk. Thus, the lactalbumin and lactoglobulin of milk differ structurally from analogous plasma proteins. The distinctive protein of milk is casein. Milk is an important source of calcium

but has a low content of iron. All of the vitamins appear in milk. Most soluble constituents, including drugs, in the maternal blood appear in milk although generally in small amounts, e.g. barbiturates, alcohol and antibiotics. It must be emphasized that the contents of various nutrients shown are average figures and subject to considerable individual variation. The fat content of human milk, for example, may vary from under 1 to over 6 g/100 ml and the fat content of cow's milk, though less variable, differs considerably between breeds of cattle. The levels of some other constituents, notably the water-soluble vitamins, e.g. ascorbic acid, change conspicuously with variations in the maternal diet.

Apart from abnormal constituents, diet has relatively little influence on milk yield or composition, and established lactation is surprisingly little affected by short periods of severe deprivation. Similarly, fluid intake has little discernible effect on milk yield.

The energy cost of lactation must be met from the maternal diet. A baby may require 850 ml of milk daily. At an energy value of 284 kJ/100 ml, this provides 2·4 MJ daily. As the efficiency of milk production is about 90 per cent., the mother requires 2·7 MJ to provide it. This may come in part from an increased dietary intake and in part from fat stores laid down in pregnancy.

PRENATAL DEVELOPMENT OF THE REPRODUCTIVE TRACT

In chap. 36 the development of the urinary system is described and it is shown that the mesonephric duct and some of its tubules become available for incorporation in the genital apparatus, once the excretory function of the mesonephros has been taken over by the metanephros.

Cloacal region (fig. 38.47)

The caudal part of the hindgut which receives the allantois and the mesonephric ducts is slightly dilated and is called the **cloaca** (chap. 19). It is separated from the exterior by a double-layered membrane, the **cloacal membrane** which consists of a layer of ectoderm on the outside and endoderm on the inside. Lateral plate mesoderm, spreading round from the caudal extremity of the primitive streak, passes round the edges of this cloacal membrane, insinuating itself between the ectoderm and endoderm. These bilateral sheets of spreading mesoderm meet in the midline anteriorly and spread on into the portion of the abdominal wall between the cloacal membrane and the attachment of the umbilical cord to form the infra-umbilical part of the abdominal wall.

Mesoderm extends round the cloacal membrane and raises slight elevations known as **genital folds** on either side of the membrane, and a **genital tubercle** at the

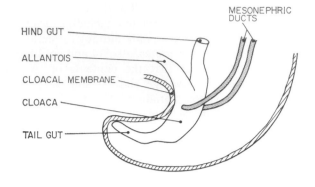

HIND GUT

ALLANTOIS

CLOACAL MEMBRANE

CLOACA

TAIL GUT

MESONEPHRIC DUCTS

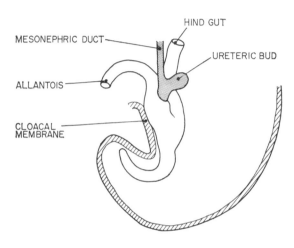

MESONEPHRIC DUCT

ALLANTOIS

CLOACAL MEMBRANE

HIND GUT

URETERIC BUD

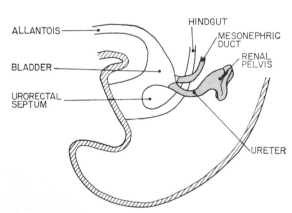

ALLANTOIS

BLADDER

URORECTAL SEPTUM

HINDGUT

MESONEPHRIC DUCT

RENAL PELVIS

URETER

Fig. 38.47. Development of the cloaca and urorectal septum. From Romanes G.J. ed. (1972) *Cunningham's Textbook of Anatomy*, 11th Edition. London:Oxford University Press.

anterior margin of the membrane. This genital tubercle enlarges to become the **phallus**. As a result of the development of these prominences flanking the cloacal membrane, the latter now lies in a depression called the **external cloaca**. More mesoderm extends into the region between the genital tubercle and the attachment of the umbilical cord and, as a result, the infraumbilical abdominal wall elongates. This lengthening together with the regression

of the tail of the embryo causes the cloacal membrane to rotate so that its ectodermal surface, which originally faces forwards and upwards towards the umbilicus, comes to face forwards and downwards. When describing the further development of the urogenital system, particularly its lower portion, it is convenient to consider the fetus to be in the upright position with the phallus pointing forwards and the perineum facing downwards (fig. 38.55).

The deep part of this mesoderm contributes to the musculature of that part of the cloaca and allantois from which the bladder arises, whereas the superficial somatic part contributes mesenchymatous components to the infra-umbilical abdominal wall.

In late somite embryos the cloaca, lined by endoderm, is joined on each side by the mesonephric duct which is of mesodermal origin. A transverse ridge, the **urorectal septum**, appears between the hindgut and the allantois. Its lower free edge, disposed in the coronal plane, descends towards the cloacal membrane progressively dividing the cloaca into a smaller dorsal part, the **rectum**, and a larger ventral part, the **primitive urogenital sinus**, which is continuous with the allantois, and into which the mesonephric ducts open. When the urorectal septum reaches the cloacal membrane, the membrane itself disintegrates. The lower margin of the septum forms the **primitive perineal body**. The remnant of the cloacal membrane in front of the perineal body is now called the **urogenital membrane** and the part behind it is called the **anal membrane**.

At this stage the primitive urogenital sinus may be divided into a portion above the level of the mesonephric ducts called the **vesico-urethral canal**, and a portion below the opening of the mesonephric ducts called the **definitive urogenital sinus**, which becomes markedly flattened from side to side. The vesico-urethral canal gives rise to most of the bladder in both sexes, apart from the trigone which is derived from mesonephric duct tissue. It is also the origin of the upper part of the prostatic urethra in males and of virtually the whole length of the female urethra.

Before proceeding further with a description of the development of the human genital system, it is necessary to stress that the same primordia and ducts originate in embryos of either sex, but the use made of these structures to produce the functional genital tract is very different in the two sexes. It is, therefore, usual to consider that the embryo passes through a neuter phase during which it possesses the rudiments necessary to develop the genital organs of either sex, but that, as development proceeds, progressive specialization occurs. Thus, although embryos of either sex develop both mesonephric and paramesonephric ducts, the functional adult male ducts arise from the mesonephric ducts, whereas those of the adult female are derived from paramesonephric ducts.

Similarly, the external genitalia and the urogenital sinus are derived from the same embryonic structures in the two sexes, but their development is strikingly different.

It will be recalled that the sex of the embryo is determined at fertilization (p. 38.38). In presomite and somite embryos, the sex of the embryo can be established morphologically only by the presence or absence of sex chromatin (p. 12.21) in the resting nuclei of most embryonic cells. Apart from this, there is no morphological indication of the future sex of an embryo till late in the 6th week of intrauterine life, when the gonads of male embryos begin to differentiate into testes. It is only when a fetus is about three months old that it becomes possible to determine its sex by examination of the external genitalia.

Development of the gonads (fig. 38.48)

The primordia of the gonads appear about 5 weeks after fertilization as thickenings of the coelomic epithelium, known as **genital ridges**, on the medial aspect of the mesonephros. Cords of cells proliferate from the thickened coelomic epithelium forming **sex cords**, and these extend into the underlying mesenchyme. Soon, cells of a very special kind appear in the genital ridges. These cells are larger than the surrounding mesenchymal cells; they are spherical and pale staining and possess large vesicular nuclei. They are the **primordial germ cells** and are generally believed to have migrated by way of the mesentery from a restricted area of the yolk sac wall close to the allantoic diverticulum.

Thus the gonads of both sexes are derived from three basic components: (1) the primordial germ cells, (2) the coelomic epithelium, (3) the mesenchyme of the adjacent part of the genital ridge.

The gonad overlaps approximately the middle two-quarters of the medial aspect of the mesonephros, which now projects well into the coelomic cavity and is connected to the posterior abdominal wall by means of a thick mesentery. This mesentery suspends the gonadal primordium as well as the mesonephros and so is known as the **urogenital mesentery**. The mesentery, the mesonephros and the gonadal primordium together constitute the **urogenital ridge**. As the gonad enlarges, it projects more and more from the medial aspect of the urogenital ridge. Deepening grooves on each side of the gonad result in the formation of a **gonadal mesentery** (mesovarium in the female, mesorchium in the male) connecting the gonad to the remainder of the urogenital ridge.

As a result of the growth of the metanephros, gonad and adrenal gland, the urogenital mesenteries, which originally lie parallel to one another, become displaced laterally in their cranial portions. The caudal parts, on the other hand, incline towards the midline because of the medial inclination of the contained mesonephric ducts and particularly of the

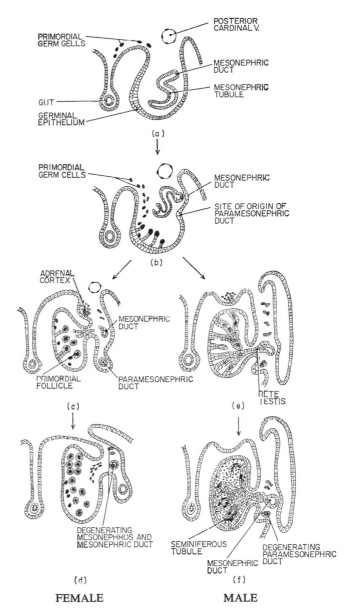

Fig. 38.48. Migration of germ cells and development of the gonads. (a) and (b) indifferent stage, (c) and (d) female, (e) and (f) male. From Hamilton W.J., Boyd J.D. & Mossman H.W. (1972) *Human Embryology*, 4th Edition. Cambridge: Heffer.

paramesonephric ducts, which are approaching each other to fuse in the midline. In this way the caudal portions of the two urogenital mesenteries eventually fuse with each other. This fusion results in the formation of the **urogenital septum** (not to be confused with the urorectal septum described above). The urogenital septum lies in the coronal plane between the bladder in front and the rectum behind, and forms the basis for the development of the broad ligament in the female.

As the tubal portion of the urogenital ridge passes the

brim of the developing pelvis, it becomes joined to the anterior abdominal wall by a fold known as the **plica inguinalis**, in which the gubernaculum of the gonad later develops.

Histogenesis of the testis

A series of histological changes indicates the onset of the differentiation of the male gonad. The sex cords become distinct and are separated from one another by bundles of fibrous tissue. At first the cords are continuous with the coelomic epithelium on the surface of the gonad. However, cells on the deep aspect of the germinal epithelium proliferate and become converted into fibrous tissue, forming the **tunica albuginea**, and this separates the sex cords from the surface epithelium.

The male primordial germ cells become incorporated within the sex cords so that these cords come to extend inwards from the periphery of the gonad as distinct columns containing germ cells. The innermost portions of these columns extend into the region of the mesorchium where they anastomose and branch to form a network which will canalize and become the rete testis. It is in this region that the gonadal tubular system communicates with the mesonephric tubules bringing the rete testis into communication with the efferent ductules and the ductus deferens.

The sex cords canalize and form seminiferous tubules, whose walls consist of cells derived from coelomic epithelium which become the sustentacular cells, and intercalated primordial germ cells which become spermatogonia. The interstitial cells are probably derived from the mesenchyme lying between the sex cords. These interstitial cells show histological signs of specialization when the fetus is 8–9 weeks old, and thus this process precedes the onset of divergence in the two sexes in the differentiation of the genital duct system by about one week, and of the external genitalia by about two or three weeks.

Histogenesis of the ovary

As in the male, the primordial germ cells reach the gonadal primordium of the female in the somite stage of development. However, in the female they come to be situated only in the superficial cortex of the developing ovary. Many of them are in contact with the superficial germinal epithelium and the deeper medulla is almost devoid of germ cells. When the fetus is 4–5 months old, the sex cords become fragmented and the resulting small groups of cells form **primordial ovarian follicles** in which the primordial germ cells become encapsulated as primary oocytes (p. 38.11). The encapsulating or follicular cells are probably derived from coelomic epithelium. The mesenchyme between the primordial follicles forms the ovarian stroma and gives rise to the thecal cells. There is no definite tunica albuginea in the developing ovary and

so the sex cords maintain some contact with the surface epithelium, which is thus able to continue contributing cells to the sex cords throughout fetal life. Although a rete ovarii is formed it is only vestigial, but may occasionally form an imperfect union with mesonephric tubules. The absence, in normal development, of any continuity between sex cords, rete and mesonephric tubules is the reason why, in the female, the mesonephric duct fails to become the definitive sex duct and why ova can escape only by rupture of ovarian follicles at the surface of the ovary. This demands also the development of a new duct, the paramesonephric duct, to convey the ova to the site of fertilization and subsequent development.

Descent of the gonads (fig. 38.49)

Both the testis and the ovary come to occupy a final position which is very different from their original site in the embryo. The transposition of the testis is particularly striking because it passes out of the abdominal cavity into the scrotum. This descent of the gonads explains the blood supply and lymph drainage of the gonads, which are established prior to descent, while the passage of the testis through the inguinal portion of the abdominal wall explains the inherent weakness of this region in males.

It is convenient to consider the descent of the gonad in two stages, the first being common to testis and ovary, and the second affecting only the testis.

The first stage consists of the descent from the posterior abdominal wall to the pelvis, and is closely related to changes in the mesonephros. The second stage consists of

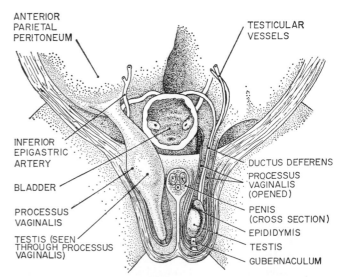

FIG. 38.49. Descent of testis and formation of tunica vaginalis. Testis on left side is at a later stage of descent than on the right. Anterior parietal peritoneum has been removed on left side. From Hamilton W.J., Boyd J.D. & Mossman H.W. (1972) *Human Embryology*, 4th Edition. Cambridge: Heffer.

passage of the testis from an intra-abdominal to an extra-abdominal position.

Descent of the testis

In the 7th week of intrauterine life the testes are still attached to the posterior abdominal wall by the urogenital mesentery. The caudal pole of the testis is continuous with a mesenchymatous band which runs down towards the pelvic brim and skirts round it, so that it extends from the urogenital ridge to reach the inguinal region. As it descends, it raises the overlying coelomic epithelium to form the plica inguinalis. This band is continuous through the future inguinal canal with the mesenchyme of the genital fold. This whole column of mesenchyme extending from the lower pole of the testis to the genital fold constitutes the **gubernaculum testis.**

While the pelvis grows and the trunk of the fetus elongates, the gubernaculum does not grow in proportion, so that the testis, being attached to the gubernaculum, comes to lie in close proximity to the inguinal region. In other words this descent of the testis is only relative to the growing body wall. This stage is reached by the 3rd month of pregnancy. Meanwhile, the cremaster muscle differentiates in the gubernacular mesenchyme of the inguinal region and a diverticulum from the coelomic cavity, the **processus vaginalis**, extends into this mesenchyme. From the 6th month of intra-uterine life, the processus vaginalis grows into the mesenchyme of the inguinal canal and scrotum, and at the same time the cremaster extends downwards to the scrotum. The testis is still at the abdominal end of the inguinal canal at the beginning of the 7th month but it usually passes through the inguinal canal and reaches the scrotum by the end of the 8th month. The precise role of the gubernaculum is still unknown but it certainly provides a route along which the processus vaginalis and the cremaster muscle can develop without obstruction by the body wall. It also dilates and keeps open the pathway for descent and, by tethering the testis, it causes it to descend by differential growth. The gubernaculum does not actively pull down the testis. The lower portion of the processus vaginalis persists as the tunica vaginalis of the testis, but the upper part usually becomes obliterated at about the time of birth.

Descent of the ovary

The gubernaculum of the ovary becomes attached to the fused uterovaginal segments of the paramesonephric ducts at their junction with the free tubal portions, and so the ovary can effect only the first stage of descent and is unable to descend any further. This attachment of the gubernaculum to the uterus causes the ovary to enter the true pelvis, where it comes to lie on the dorsal (originally medial) surface of the urogenital mesentery which has descended with the ovary and now forms the broad ligament. The part of the gubernaculum persisting between the ovary and the uterus becomes the ligament of the ovary, and the part between the uterus and the labium majus becomes the round ligament of the uterus. A small processus vaginalis forms in the female and passes towards the labium majus, but it is usually obliterated by full term.

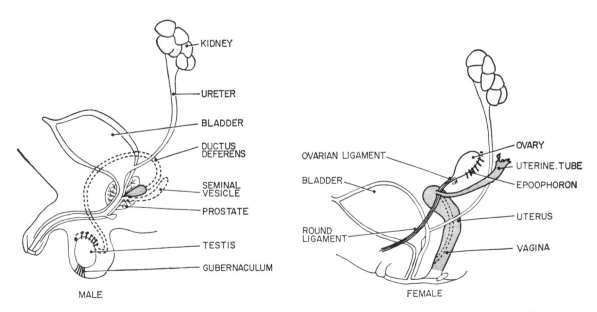

Fig. 38.50. Definitive urogenital system in male and female. Dotted lines indicate derivatives of mesonephric ducts; stippled areas are derived from paramesonephric ducts. From Hamilton W.J., Boyd J.D. & Mossman H.W. (1972) *Human Embryology*, 4th Edition. Cambridge:Heffer.

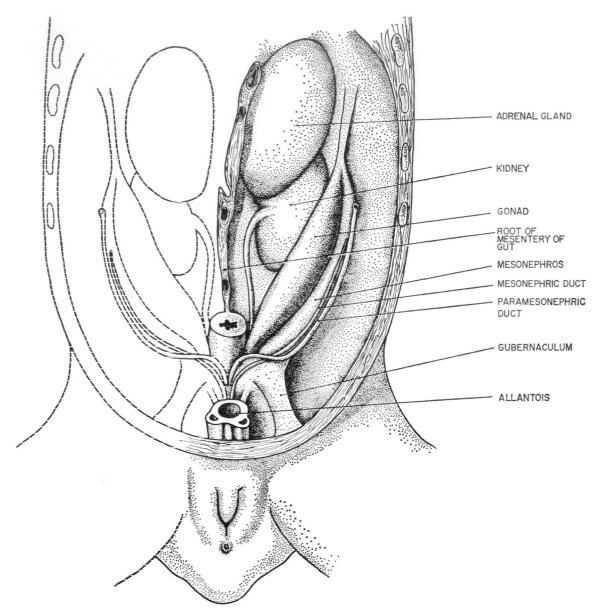

FIG. 38.51. Posterior abdominal wall of embryo at 7 weeks. From Hamilton W.J., Boyd J.D. & Mossman H.W. (1972) *Human Embryology*, 4th Edition. Cambridge:Heffer.

DEVELOPMENT OF THE GENITAL DUCT SYSTEM

Mesonephric duct

At first the mesonephric duct opens into that part of the cloaca which later becomes the primitive urogenital sinus. The length of this duct, which is caudal to the origin of the ureteric bud, is known as the **common excretory duct** and it becomes absorbed into the posterior wall of the primitive urogenital sinus to form the trigonal area of the bladder.

In the male. The cranial portion of the duct becomes connected to the seminiferous tubules by way of some mesonephric tubules (these become the efferent ductules) and the rete testis. The part of the duct which is immediately adjacent to this point of junction with the efferent ductules becomes elongated and convoluted to form the epididymis and the remainder of the duct forms the ductus deferens. As it approaches the urogenital sinus, the duct becomes dilated and forms the ampulla from which a diverticulum arises to become the seminal vesicle. That part of the original mesonephric duct which extends from this diverticulum to the urogenital sinus becomes the ejaculatory duct.

In the female. The caudal part of the duct gives rise to the ureteric bud and contributes to the formation of the bladder as in the male. However, the rest of the mesonephric duct degenerates, although part of it may persist in vestigial form as Gartner's duct which lies lateral to the uterus and in the anterolateral part of the vaginal wall.

Paramesonephric duct (fig. 38.52)

This duct appears in embryos of either sex at about 5 weeks after fertilization. It arises as an invagination of coelomic epithelium into the mesenchyme lateral to the cranial end of the mesonephric duct.

In the female. The original invagination persists as the abdominal ostium of the uterine tube. The caudal tip of the paramesonephric duct forms a solid cord which descends lateral to the mesonephric duct. As it descends, it canalizes in continuity with the abdominal ostium and the lumen extends progressively towards the solid growing tip. When it reaches the caudal extremity of the mesonephros, the paramesonephric duct crosses in front of the mesonephric duct and continues on its medial side.

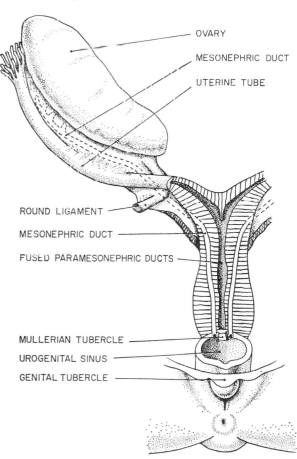

FIG. 38.52. Paramesonephric duct. From Hamilton W.J., Boyd J.D. & Mossman H.W. (1972) *Human Embryology*, 4th Edition. Cambridge: Heffer.

The two paramesonephric ducts meet and eventually fuse in the urogenital septum in the midline. This fusion is at first partial, so that a septum exists between the two lumina. When the septum disappears, a single midline cavity is established and these fused segments of the paramesonephric ducts constitute the **uterovaginal canal**. The free parts of the ducts above the uterovaginal canal give rise to the uterine tubes.

The caudal tip of the uterovaginal canal remains solid and reaches the posterior wall of the urogenital sinus between the orifices of the mesonephric ducts. This solid cord is sometimes called the **vaginal cord** and, where it reaches the urogenital sinus, it produces an elevation in the posterior wall of the sinus called the **Müllerian tubercle** (fig. 38.53).

At about 3–3½ months, bilateral outgrowths from the Müllerian tubercle push back the vaginal cord, so increasing the distance between the lumen of the uterovaginal canal and that of the urogenital sinus. These outgrowths are called **sinuvaginal bulbs** and together with the vaginal cord they constitute the **vaginal plate**. The vaginal plate is canalized by extension of the uterovaginal canal from above and by the breaking down of the epithelium of the sinovaginal bulbs from below. This process is not complete till late in fetal life.

The hymen is a partition which persists between the canalized fused sinuvaginal bulbs and the urogenital sinus.

The future junction between the body of the uterus and the cervix becomes recognizable at about 10 weeks, but the uterine portion of the uterovaginal canal does not appear to be completely separated from the vaginal portion until 5–5½ months.

In the male. The paramesonephric ducts develop to the same extent as in the female until the 9–10th week.

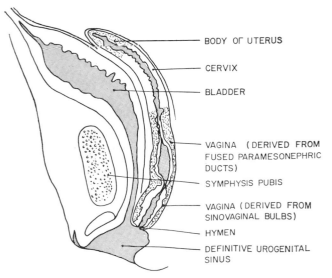

FIG. 38.53. Development of the vagina at 24 weeks. From Hamilton W. J., Boyd J. D. & Mossman H. W. (1972) *Human Embryology*, 4th Edition, Cambridge: Heffer.

Thereafter they degenerate and lose their communication with the coelomic cavity.

DEVELOPMENT OF THE LOWER UROGENITAL TRACT AND EXTERNAL GENITALIA

The fate of the definitive urogenital sinus differs markedly in the two sexes. It may be divided into an upper **pelvic portion** which is widest in its transverse diameter and is continuous above with the primitive urethra, and a lower **phallic portion** which is related to the base of the phallic tubercle and is elongated in the sagittal plane. The urogenital membrane forms the floor of this phallic part.

Pelvic portion of the urogenital sinus
In the male. This forms the lower part of the prostatic urethra and the whole of the membranous urethra.

In the female. The pelvic portion of the urogenital sinus may contribute slightly to the lower end of the urethra.

Prostate gland
In the male. This gland develops when the fetus is about three months old as a series of buds growing from the primitive urethra and adjacent pelvic portion of the urogenital sinus. They grow into the surrounding mesenchyme which differentiates to form the fibro-muscular stroma of the gland. These buds arise from all sides of the urethra, both above and below the region of the orifices of the mesonephric ducts. An inner zone

comprises the mucous and submucous glands and also the prostatic utricle, whilst an outer zone consists of the main prostatic glands.

The prostatic utricle arises from the region of the Müllerian tubercle on the dorsal wall of the urogenital sinus, at the junction of the vesicourethral canal and the definitive urogenital sinus. In adult males the prostatic utricle ranges in size from a small blind diverticulum to a complicated glandular structure occupying most of the inner zone (median lobe) of the prostate. The Müllerian tubercle also gives rise to the prostatic glands of the inner zone, which come to lie in the angle formed by the prostatic urethra and the mesonephric ducts on either side of the utricle, in other words, the glands of that part of the prostate called the middle lobe.

In the female. Comparable epithelial buds arise from the primitive urethra and the adjacent pelvic portion of the urogenital sinus to form the paraurethral glands, the latter being homologues of the median lobe of the male prostate.

EXTERNAL GENITALIA AND THE PHALLIC PORTION OF THE DEFINITIVE UROGENITAL SINUS (fig. 38.55)

In the neuter phase of sexual differentiation three small protuberances flank the external cloaca. These are the genital tubercle or phallus anteriorly, and the genital folds on either side. At about the 5th week, the endoderm which lines the inner surface of the urogenital membrane proliferates forwards into the mesenchyme of the phallus, forming the **urethral plate**. It grows forward in such a way that its lower margin remains in contact with the ectodermal epithelium covering the under surface of the phallus, and it eventually reaches the tip of the phallus in both sexes. The mesenchyme along each side of the urethral plate proliferates and raises the overlying ectoderm to form primitive **urethral folds** between which the primitive **urethral groove** comes to lie (fig. 38.56).

The endodermal upper surface of the urogenital membrane forms the floor of the urogenital sinus, while its ectodermal aspect is continuous anteriorly with the ectodermal epithelium lining the primitive urethral groove. Thus, the urethral plate may be seen as a forward extension from the phallic part of the urogenital sinus.

After 6 weeks the urogenital membrane disintegrates with the result that the urogenital sinus comes to open to the exterior at the base of the phallus, and an external opening is thus provided for the urogenital duct system. This converts the phallic part of the urogenital sinus into an open endoderm-lined trough flanked by the posterior portions of the primitive urethral folds and continuous along the phallus with the ectoderm-lined primitive urethral groove.

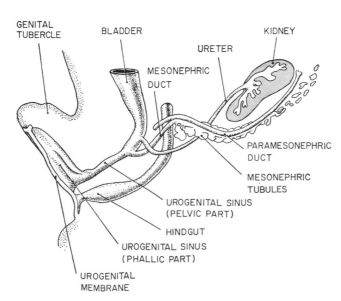

FIG. 38.54. Development of urogenital sinus at 7 weeks. From Hamilton W.J., Boyd J.D. & Mossmann H.W. (1972) *Human Embryology*, 4th Edition. Cambridge: Heffer.

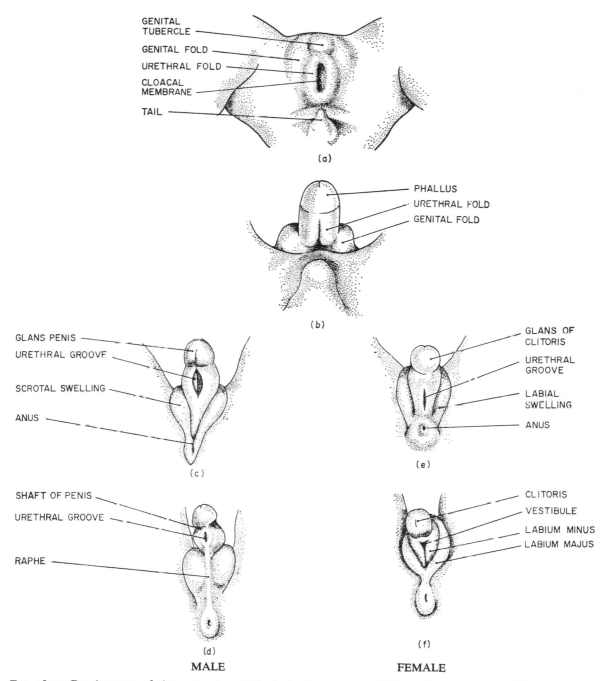

GENITAL TUBERCLE

GENITAL FOLD

URETHRAL FOLD

CLOACAL MEMBRANE

TAIL

(a)

PHALLUS

URETHRAL FOLD

GENITAL FOLD

(b)

GLANS PENIS

URETHRAL GROOVE

SCROTAL SWELLING

ANUS

(c)

GLANS OF CLITORIS

URETHRAL GROOVE

LABIAL SWELLING

ANUS

(e)

SHAFT OF PENIS

URETHRAL GROOVE

RAPHE

(d)

MALE

CLITORIS

VESTIBULE

LABIUM MINUS

LABIUM MAJUS

(f)

FEMALE

FIG. 38.55. Development of the external genitalia in both sexes. a and b—neuter stages; c and d—male; e and f—female. From Arey L.B. (1965) *Developmental Anatomy*, 7th Edition. Philadelphia: Saunders.

Later, the lower margin of the urethral plate (which lies in the floor of the primitive urethral groove) thickens and then disintegrates along with the ectoderm overlying it. This deepens the urethral groove which is now called the definitive urethral groove. This mode of formation accounts for the fact that the urethral groove is lined by endoderm in its deeper part and by ectoderm in its superficial part.

In the male. The urethral folds begin to fuse in the midline when the fetus is about 2½–3 months old. Fusion starts at the base of the phallus immediately in front of the primitive central tendon of the perineum and extends towards the tip of the phallus. This converts the open phallic part of the urogenital sinus into the bulb of the urethra and the deeper part of the urethral groove into a tubular penile urethra. The urogenital orifice which

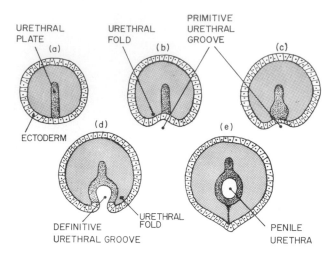

FIG. 38.56. Formation of the urethra. From Glenister T.W. (1958) *Brit. J. Urol.* **30**, 117.

was originally situated at the base of the phallus is thus carried progressively forwards towards the tip of the phallus or penis. A concurrent fusion of the genital folds forms the scrotum at the base of the penis.

After 3–3½ months, the urogenital orifice reaches the glans, which has become defined from the rest of the penis by the development of a circular coronary sulcus around the distal part of the shaft. The prepuce develops from folds which form just proximal to the coronary sulcus. The urethral folds on the under surface of the glans are closely related to the prepuce and as they fuse to form the terminal part of the urethra a frenulum is formed on the under surface of the glans.

The terminal portion of the urethra is lined by an ingrowth of surface epithelium which extends into the substance of the glans to meet the distal extremity of the urethral plate. The urethral glands develop from the lining of the penile urethral walls, and the bulbo-urethral glands from the lining of the urethral bulb close to its junction with the membranous urethra.

In the female. The phallus and its glans develop to the same extent until about 2½–3 months, but the urethral folds do not subsequently fuse. In addition, the genital folds form labial swellings which flank the base of the phallus and the open trough of the phallic part of the urogenital sinus.

The phallus forms the clitoris, the labial swellings become the labia majora and the unfused urethral folds become the labia minora. The pelvic and phallic portions of the urogenital sinus are opened out to allow the vaginal orifice to reach the perineum and they both contribute to the formation of the vestibule. The greater vestibular glands (homologues of the bulbo-urethral glands) arise from the part of the vestibule derived from the phallic part of the urogenital sinus. Although a glans and

prepuce are developed on the clitoris, failure of closure of the urethral groove causes the prepuce to be a hood-like structure which does not extend round the under surface of the glans.

The definitive form of the external genitalia is achieved in fetuses of both sexes when they are 4½–5 months old.

SEX DETERMINATION AND DEVELOPMENT

It should now be clear that there are fundamental structural and functional similarities between the reproductive tracts of the two sexes. At an early stage in development, sometimes called the neuter phase, each embryo possesses the potential to become either male or female. Development usually proceeds from this stage along separate lines so that the individual becomes unquestionably either male or female. However, in abnormal circumstances, this process of differentiation may deviate and produce a degree of intermediate or indeterminate sex, a condition known as intersexuality.

Sex is initially determined genetically at fertilization. In man, two special sex chromosomes can be identified, the female being homogametic, XX, and the male heterogametic, XY (p. 12.21). It is believed that the male-determining Y chromosome predominates over the X chromosome. As a generalization, the female reproductive tract may be regarded as the basic unit upon which maleness may be superimposed. The absence of a Y chromosome permits the female system to develop. The presence of a Y chromosome induces male development. Nevertheless, a normal complement of two sex chromosomes is essential for normal sexual development. Thus, where there are three sex chromosomes, XXY, the individual is an apparent male but the testes fail to perform normal spermatogenesis. Conversely, in the presence of only one sex chromosome, XO, the individual appears to be female but the ovaries fail to develop normally.

Thus, initial sex determination is a function of the genotype, but genetic control of subsequent sexual development is not absolute. Somatic growth may be inappropriate to the genetic sex so that there may be a disparity between the genotype and its phenotypic expression.

The primary function of genetic sex determination is to control gonadal differentiation. At the neuter stage the gonads consist of both a cortex and a medulla. Testicular development is characterized by the appearance of a prominent tunica albuginea which cuts the cortex off from the surface epithelium, and by dominance of the medullary component. Seminiferous tubules are formed and diploid germ cells differentiate within these to produce spermatogonia. In the female, the tunica albuginea is inconspicuous in embryonic life, the cortical component dominates and the germ cells which accumulate in follicles within this zone form oogonia. The Y chromosome determines testicular differentiation, but a normal complement of two sex chromosomes is necessary for full gonadal development. Furthermore, local conditions in the genital ridge may also modify growth of the gonad.

The gonads in turn control the development of the genital duct system. The paramesonephric system is the basic unit which develops in the absence of testes. In this context, the fetal ovaries are probably simply permissive and are not necessary for paramesonephric duct growth. In the presence of testes, the paramesonephric ducts are suppressed and the mesonephric ducts take over the formation of the male genital tract. The testes exert this control by hormonal influence, but the effect of each testis is confined to its own side and the effector substances are not necessarily androgens.

The testes also control the development of male external genitalia from the phallic part of the urogenital sinus by the release of sex steroids. Androgens cause the formation of the scrotum by fusion of the genital folds, enlargement of the phallus and development of a penile urethra. Again the fetal ovaries are probably passive and, in the absence of testicular androgens, the genital folds fail to fuse and persist as labia majora, the clitoris remains small, and the urethra opens directly into the vestibule.

Physical sexual maturation is completed at puberty by the development of secondary sex features and the onset of reproductive functions. These are determined by the release of testicular and ovarian sex steroids.

FURTHER READING

AUSTIN C.R. (1961) *The Mammalian Egg*. Oxford: Blackwell Scientific Publications.

AUSTIN C.R. & SHORT R.V. eds. (1972) *Reproduction in Mammals*, vols. I–V. London:Cambridge University Press.

BALIN H. & GLASSER S. (1972) *Reproductive Biology*. Amsterdam:Excerpta Medica.

BEER A.E. & BILLINGHAM R.E. (1974) The embryo as a transplant. *Scientific American* **230**, April, 36–46.

BLANDAU R.J. ed. (1971) *The Biology of the Blastocyst*. Chicago:University of Chicago Press.

COWIE A.T. & TINDAL J.S. (1971) *Physiology of Lactation*. Monograph of the Physiological Society, No. 22. London:Arnold.

DONOVAN B.T. & VAN DER WERFF TEN BOSCH J.J. (1965) *Physiology of Puberty*. Monograph of the Physiological Society, No. 15. London:Arnold.

FUCHS F. & KLOPPER A. (1971) *Endocrinology of Pregnancy*. New York:Harper & Row.

HAFEZ E.S.E. & EVANS T.N. eds. (1973) *Human Reproduction: Conception and Contraception*. New York: Harper & Row.

HAMILTON W.J., BOYD J.D. & MOSSMAN H.W. (1972) *Human Embryology*, 4th Edition. Cambridge:Heffer.

HARTMAN C.G. (1963) *Mechanisms Concerned with Conception*. Oxford:Pergamon Press.

HYTTEN F.E. & LEITCH I. (1971) *Physiology of Human Pregnancy*, 2nd Edition. Oxford:Blackwell Scientific Publications.

KIRBY D.R.S. (1968) Immunological aspects of pregnancy. In *Advances in Reproductive Physiology*, vol. 3, pp. 33–79, ed. McLaren Anne. London:Logos Press.

KLOPPER A. & DICZFALUSY E. eds. (1969) *Foetus and Placenta*. Oxford:Blackwell Scientific Publications.

MANN T. (1964) *Biochemistry of Semen and of the Male Reproductive Tract*. London:Methuen.

McKERNS K.W. (1969) *The Gonads*. New York:Appleton Century Crofts.

SHEARMAN R.P. ed. (1972) *Human Reproductive Physiology*. Oxford:Blackwell Scientific Publications.

WOLSTENHOLME G.E.W. & O'CONNOR M. eds. (1969). *Ciba Foundation Symposium on Foetal Autonomy*. London:Churchill.

Chapter 39
Human genetics

To the nineteenth-century geneticists there appeared to be two general laws governing inheritance: first, like breeds like and second, inheritance blends. That black cats have black kittens and red antirrhinums crossed with white ones give pink antirrhinums are indisputable facts. These simple rules were used by live stock breeders over many centuries to produce the numerous breeds which are economically successful today. However, when inheritance is examined in detail, it is clear that such rules do not cover all situations nor do they begin to suggest its mechanism. Many who attempted to explain the observed facts of inheritance failed to grasp one fundamental point, and not even Charles Darwin, whose theory of evolution required a rational theory of inheritance, realized that the essence of heredity is **genetic continuity**. Darwin's pangene hypothesis supposed that the germ cells contained material representative of all parts of the body and formed the basis from which a new individual emerged. This implied that one generation was formed *de novo* from the previous one. The idea of continuity, of a **germ plasm** set aside to preserve the characteristics of the species, arose from Mendel's demonstration that even when a particular character was not apparent in an organism, the factors controlling its inheritance might still be present and it might appear in later generations. The search for the mechanism which provides this continuity has formed the basis of modern molecular genetics. The concept of a molecule which has the capacity for self-replication provides a physical and chemical basis for the unbroken chain of life of which any individual is an ephemeral part. Such a sequence, however, would be a sterile perpetuation of the past if it were inflexible. This is not the case. There is an inherent variability in the system and mechanisms have evolved to ensure that variation occurs.

Human variation

In man there are striking differences in physical appearance, in stature and pigmentation, and possibly even more dramatic differences in intelligence and patterns of behaviour. This variation is determined by two main factors: the genetic constitution and the environment. The genetic constitution of an individual is the **genotype** and the sum of the physical and mental characteristics is the **phenotype**. While the phenotype is an expression of the genotype, it is in reality the interaction between the genetic constitution and the environment and it is not always clear how much each of these two components contributes to it. Certain characteristics, e.g. blood groups and eye colour, appear to be wholly under genetic control while other features such as behaviour and intelligence derive a major component from the environment.

ENVIRONMENTAL FACTORS

These operate on at least three different levels. Some exert their influence *in utero*. The genetic potentiality of a child to have normally developed limbs may not be realized if the embryo is exposed to a noxious agent such as thalidomide at a critical stage of morphogenesis. Such an influence has permanent effects on the physical form of the mature organism but does not affect the next generation. Secondly, environment may act directly in the adult. Severe haemolytic anaemia, arising after eating broad beans (*Vicia fava*) as already described on p. 28.6, occurs only in individuals who have a genetically determined deficiency of the enzyme glucose-6-phosphate dehydrogenase. It does not occur unless these individuals encounter the appropriate environmental stimulus. Thirdly, there may be a more subtle interaction over a long period of time between the genetic constitution of individuals in a population and their environment. A specific genetic constitution may be advantageous in a particular environment and by a process of natural selection individuals with this constitution become more numerous in the population. The concept of selection of the organism best adapted for life in a particular environment was the basis of the Darwinian concept of evolution; though there is still debate about how selection may operate, the underlying concept remains essentially unchanged today.

GENETIC FACTORS

Every individual within a species does not have an identical genetic constitution. There is variation from individual to individual and as discussed on p. 12.22 new combinations of these variations arise continually following segregation, assortment and crossing over during meiosis. Variation by recombination is, however, only a reshuffling of the existing genes. Totally new variants arise by mutation. Usually these are disadvantageous and are eliminated from the population; however, if the mutation rate is sufficiently high a population may always contain a small number of mutant individuals, there being a balance between mutation and elimination by selection. Sometimes a genetically determined variant becomes established in a population at a frequency that cannot be maintained by mutation alone. This must be the result of natural selection and, where two or more variants of a single characteristic exist side by side in a single population, then the population is said to show **genetic polymorphism** for this characteristic.

Variation in blood groups is well known but more and more such polymorphic systems in blood proteins, red cell enzymes and tissue cell enzymes are being discovered.

Genetics in medicine

The study of human genetics is the study of human variation and of the interrelationship between genetic and environmental factors in causing this variation. Although the range of normality is wide, in some instances the variation falls outside the area which is considered normal. It is here that human genetics impinges on clinical medicine and this branch of human genetics is usually termed clinical or medical genetics. Human disease, as with other features of man, is determined partly by environmental and partly by genetic factors and again it is not always clear how much each contributes to the development of the disease. A disease, caused primarily by an environmental factor such as a micro-organism, a dietary deficiency or a mental stress may have manifestations which are in some individuals due to their genetic constitution. As environmental factors are controlled, the genetic component in human disease becomes relatively more important. It is important to stress the effect of environment on genetically determined disease; genetic disease is not untreatable disease.

GENES IN THE CELL

Gene

This word was used by early geneticists to describe a factor controlling the inheritance of a particular characteristic. Although for many years this abstraction could not be related to any physical structure or chemical substance, the concept of a gene as a factor controlling a specific inherited feature was valuable in the study of heredity. Even now, when the chemical basis of inheritance is being elucidated in great detail, this concept is still of value.

The role of DNA as the genetic material of the cell is described on p. 12.1. What is the relationship between this molecular complex and the gene of classical genetics? This is most easily understood by considering briefly the mechanism of gene action. In 1908 A.E. Garrod published his monograph on *Inborn Errors of Metabolism* in which he formulated the concept that these errors were due to a block in the normal metabolism of the body and that this was due to the congenital absence of a particular enzyme. From this idea evolved, many years later, the idea that each gene controlled the production of a single enzyme, the one gene, one enzyme hypothesis. While this is a useful concept and undoubtedly contributed to the understanding of the mechanism of gene action, it now requires modification in certain circumstances, e.g. it is known that two or more independent regions of the DNA may be involved in the production of a single enzyme. This is reasonable in chemical terms since an enzyme, being a protein, may be composed of more than one polypeptide chain. Regions which code for different polypeptides of a single protein are often located close together, but this is not always so, e.g. the two regions coding for the α- and β-chains of the haemoglobin molecule are located on different chromosomes. Similarly the sequences of DNA which code for groups of associated enzymes in a series of biochemical reactions are frequently closely associated in the genetic material. Thus one can regard a gene as a region of the DNA which codes for a single polypeptide molecule. In this sense the word retains its original meaning of a factor which controls a specific inherited characteristic since, even if only one polypeptide of an enzyme composed of two polypeptides is involved in a genetic change, the nature of the whole product may be affected.

Control of gene action

The total number of genes of an organism such as man is very large, and it is clear, even in micro-organisms, that all of the genetic material is not active all the time. There must, therefore, be control mechanisms for switching on and switching off the gene action. From studies on micro-organisms a possible mechanism which fits known experimental facts is described on p. 12.3. The product of a sequence of DNA can have one of two functions. It may become a structural component of the organism or an enzyme concerned in the synthesis of such a component. Alternatively the product may exert an influence on other regions of the DNA and so modify or regulate the activity of that region. The former is a **structural gene** and the latter a **regulator gene**. One regulator gene controls the activity of a group of structural genes and is sensitive to the synthetic activity of the cell, which in turn is influenced by the external environment of the cell and of the organism, and hence exerts a feed back control on the structural genes. It is probable that the regulator gene makes a protein termed a **repressor** which can exist in either an active or inactive state. When in the inactive state (combined with an **inducer**) it cannot interfere with the associated structural genes and the gene product is synthesized (fig. 12.15a). When in the active state it appears to bind with a specific site termed the **operator** in or near the DNA of the structural gene. If the operator is blocked synthesis cannot proceed (fig. 12.15b). The grouping consisting of operator and the associated structural genes under the control of a single regulator gene has been termed an **operon** which is the basic unit of genetic function. This mechanism is probably only one of the devices for controlling the activity of the genetic material and we do not yet know how the action of the regulator gene is controlled. As yet, we know little about gene regulation in higher organisms. However, in mammalian cells there are several different types of DNA which may be recognized by their physical and chemical characteristics. Current evidence suggests that some of these DNA fractions and possibly a large proportion of the total DNA of the mammalian cell are concerned with regulation, so that the process may be much more complex than in micro-organisms.

Genes at a locus

The DNA in higher organisms is organized into chromosomes and a particular region of DNA (or gene) is, with a few rare exceptions, always situated at the same site on the same chromosome. This site is termed a **locus**. Since the chromosomes are in pairs, one member of each pair being maternal in origin and one paternal, there are two **homologous loci** for each gene in every cell, with the exception of the sex chromosomes in the **heterogametic sex**, i.e. the sex in which the two sex chromosomes are unlike. In man and other mammals this is the male, but in birds the female. The genes at a given locus are not always identical. Variants at a single locus are called **alleles**. The common situation is for one allele (the **wild type**) to be found in the large majority of the individuals in a naturally occurring population while other alleles have probably arisen as variants of the wild type. Such **mutations** may lead to an abnormal gene product with only partial function or to the total absence of a product and, very rarely, to a product which is as good as or better than the product of the wild type gene. In molecular terms a mutation is an alteration in the sequence of bases in the region of DNA coding for a polypeptide, while the smallest unit which can mutate is a single base pair (**muton**). The substitution of a single base pair leads to the alteration of a single amino acid and probably to an altered but related product (fig. 39.1b). For example, as described on p. 28.5, each of the several different normal and abnormal haemoglobins which have been adequately studied in man are the consequence of the substitution of a single base in the haemoglobin gene. Similarly a muta-

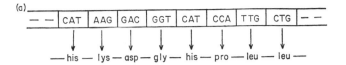

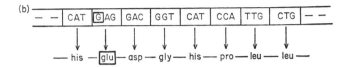

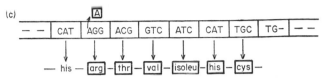

FIG. 39.1. Mutation. Linear sequence of bases in DNA, A: adenine; C: cystosine; G: guanine; T: thymine. (a) Normal reading. Each triplet 'in frame'. (b) Substitution of a single base. One amino acid is altered. The remainder of the sequence still reads 'in frame'. The product may have some biological activity. (c) Deletion of a single base. All triplets to the right of the deletion now read out of frame. The amino acids are changed and the product will almost certainly have no biological activity.

tion can result from the omission of a single base (fig. 39.1c). Since this, however, results in all the succeeding triplets of the sequence reading out of frame, the whole sequence is now altered and no functional product can be detected. A similar consequence results from the insertion of a single base. One of the key pieces of evidence in determining the triplet nature of the genetic code was the finding that while one, two or four base deletions or insertions gave no meaningful products, three such deletions or insertions put the code back in frame and gave a modified but recognizable product. The causes of mutations are described on p. 39.9.

Interaction between genes

We have already seen that there are regulatory interactions between genes. The transfer of a gene to a new locus may modify its function (**position effect**). It is important, however, to consider the relationship between the two alleles at homologous loci in a single cell. These two alleles may be identical or they may differ. If they are the same the individual is said to be **homozygous** for this gene, and if they differ the individual is **heterozygous**. In a heterozygote the phenotype will depend on the interaction between the two differing alleles. At one extreme, a **dominant** allele may be expressed fully and the **recessive** allele not at all, so that the phenotype is the same as in the homozygous dominant individual. Dominance may not be complete so that phenotype is intermediate between that of the two homozygotes. A great many genes fall into this category of **intermediate inheritance** and provide a range of differing degrees of interaction. In some cases both alleles are expressed fully and more or less equally. Such a situation, termed **co-dominance**, is found in the AB blood group in man.

GENES IN FAMILIES

Basic rules

The second main consideration concerns the transfer of genetic information from generation to generation. Despite many efforts to determine the rules which govern inheritance, it was not until 1900, when a number of workers independently came to reconsider and confirm the results which Gregor Mendel had obtained in 1865, that the basic laws became clear. Although these laws are still fundamental, many modifications and qualifications must now be made. One of the reasons for Mendel's success was his use of clearly distinct characters and his careful choice of stocks which bred true.

MENDEL'S FIRST LAW—INDEPENDENT
SEGREGATION (fig. 39.2.)

When a male from a line which is pure bred for a particular character (a homozygous male) is crossed with a female from a line which is pure bred for a different but allelic character (a homozygous female) the offspring are

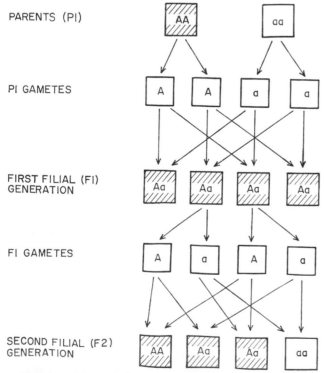

PARENTS (PI)

PI GAMETES

FIRST FILIAL (FI)
GENERATION

FI GAMETES

SECOND FILIAL (F2)
GENERATION

FIG. 39.2. Mendel's first law: independent segregation. A and a are two allelic genes, where A is dominant to a. Note the 3 : 1 ratio of phenotypes in the F2 generation, but a 1:2:1 ratio of genotypes.

all of one kind, i.e. all heterozygotes. The parents in such a cross are the **first parental (P1) generation**, and the progeny are the **first filial (F1) generation**. The phenotype of the progeny depends on the interaction between the two alleles. They may be identical with one or other of the parents if one allele is dominant, or intermediate in their phenotype if one allele is not completely dominant over the other, or show a mixed phenotype if there is co-dominance. When members of the heterozygous F1 generation are crossed with each other, the new progeny, **the second filial (F2) generation** are not all alike, but of three kinds always in the same proportion. On average one in four of the progeny will be like one of the original P1 parents, half will be heterozygous like the F1 generation and the remaining quarter will be like the other P1 parent. This is known as the 1 : 2 : 1 ratio. If, of course, one gene is completely dominant this will appear as a 3 : 1 ratio. When the gametes are formed in meiosis the members of each of the homologous pairs of chromosomes are distributed to separate gametes. Thus for a pair of allelic genes, the one derived from the maternal parent and the one derived from the paternal parent, go into different gametes. Thus the gametes from a homozygous parent are all alike, but those of a heterozygous parent are of two kinds. When the F1 cross is made there is a one in four chance for one of the homozygous types, one in four chance for the alternate homozygous type and a one in two chance for a heterozygous type being formed. One can say that the two alleles segregate independently in the offspring.

MENDEL'S SECOND LAW—INDEPENDENT
ASSORTMENT

When a cross is made between two individuals, one homozygous for two different genes and the other homozygous for two different alleles at the same loci, it can be shown that each obeys Mendel's first law without regard to the presence of the other gene (fig. 39.3). The F1 generation must all be heterozygous for both genes. In the F2 generation there will be progeny of several different types again in definite proportions. Thus in Mendel's original experiment, round (RR) yellow (YY) peas were crossed with wrinkled (rr) green (yy) peas. Nine of the offspring are like the dominant parent in respect of both characters. In spite of this phenotypic resemblance it can be seen that they are genetically of several different kinds and, if the relationship between alleles is not complete dominance, this will be expressed phenotypically. Three of the progeny are like the dominant parent in respect of one character only and three are like the dominant parent in respect of the other character. One of the F2 generation resembles the recessive parent in respect of both characters. This is the 9 : 3 : 3 : 1 ratio which refers to the phenotype only, in a straight double-dominant cross. In this experiment the characteristics

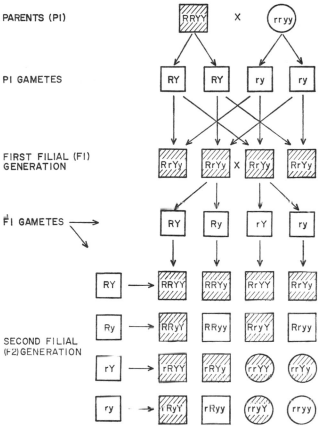

PARENTS (PI)

PI GAMETES

FIRST FILIAL (F1) GENERATION

F1 GAMETES

SECOND FILIAL (F2) GENERATION

FIG. 39.3. Mendel's second law: independent assortment. R and r are a pair of allelic genes, where R is dominant to r. Y and y are a pair of allelic genes, where Y is dominant to y. In the F2 generation, the progeny are in the ratio—9 double dominant phenotype : 3 one dominant character : 3 the other dominant character : 1 double recessive phenotype.

were free to assort themselves in a gamete independently of the other genes present. There is no general tendency for genes from one parent to remain together.

Factors which modify these ratios

LINKAGE

Although Mendel's second law holds good for most genes, it does not necessarily hold good for genes which are on the same chromosome. Loci which are situated on the same chromosome are said to be **linked loci**. In the fruit fly *Drosophila* the linkage groups, and indeed the relationships between the linkage groups and the morphological chromosomes, have been mapped out in detail. In the mouse there are a number of clearly defined linkage groups but these are not yet related to specific chromosomes. In man rapid progress is now being made in determining linkages and in assigning genes to specific chromosomes. This is partly due to the use of the classical techniques of pedigree analysis, but much information is also being derived by studying the genetics of somatic cells in culture. Tentative maps have

been constructed for those chromosomes (e.g. I and X) on which a relatively large number of genes have been located, but most chromosomes have only a small number of genes assigned so far and there is a small number of chromosomes on which no genes have yet been located.

RECOMBINATION

Equally, there are exceptions to the rule that genes on a chromosome tend to stick together. Crossing over during meiosis causes genes on the same chromosome to be separated from each other. The further apart the genes the more likely they are to be separated by crossing over. This has enabled geneticists not only to construct linkage groups but to map, in relative terms, distances between genes; genes close together are a small number of cross over units apart, while distant ones are a large number of such units apart. It should be remembered that two cross overs between a pair of loci on the same strand does not result in their separation, for though one cross over separates them a second reunites them on the same chromosome. Similarly an odd number of cross overs separates genes but an even number keeps them together. Such multiple exchanges, of course, result in major rearrangements in the intermediate region. These are referred to as **recombinations** of the genetic material and the resulting progeny are the **recombinants**.

EXPRESSIVITY AND PENETRANCE

As already mentioned, genes are not always completely dominant and completely recessive and there are intermediate situations of two basic types. The factors controlling these are not always clear. First, in a single individual the degree of expression of a dominant gene may vary. For example in certain malformations of bone in man some individuals carrying the dominant gene are severely affected and others only mildly. Such a gene is said to vary in **expressivity**. The second possibility is that under particular conditions the gene which is normally inherited as a dominant fails to be expressed at all in some individuals. This could be due, for example, to interaction with another non-allelic gene, but it does not alter the basic nature of the gene, which remains a dominant gene. If a dominant gene is expressed either in full or in part, in all individuals who carry it it is said to show **100 per cent penetrance**. When not all carriers of the gene are affected it is said to show **incomplete penetrance**. These two facts are of great importance in constructing human pedigrees for the purpose of determining the mode of inheritance of a particular characteristic or clinical syndrome.

AGE EFFECTS

Particular genes exert their effect at different stages of development. Some are concerned with morphogenesis

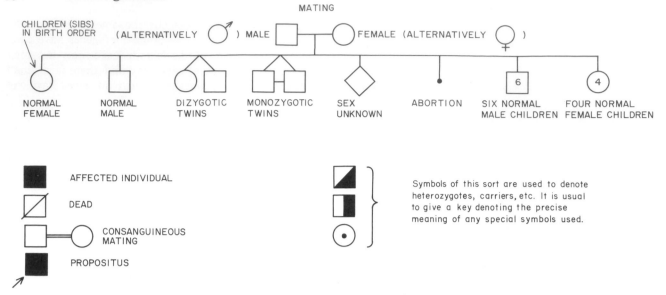

FIG. 39.4. Symbols commonly used in the recording of pedigrees.

and early life and are probably not used in the adult. In man, for example, the fetal blood contains a type of haemoglobin different from that in the adult. The manifestation of some genes may not appear until well into adult life, as happens in Huntington's chorea, a rare disorder causing uncoordinated involuntary movements. This makes the interpretation of human pedigrees and genetic counselling difficult in such cases.

PLEIOTROPY AND POLYGENIC INHERITANCE

In Mendel's experiments the characters were simple and clear cut. While many such characters exist, it is not uncommon for a single gene to affect many different characteristics (**pleiotropy**) or for many genes to control a single character (**polygenic inheritance**). Pleiotropy is easily explained in terms of enzymic reactions. If a mutation affects one enzyme, all the systems in the body utilizing it are affected. Phenylketonuria is an example in which the primary deficiency is the inability to synthesize phenylalanine 4-monooxygenase (p. 11.23). This defect has different manifestations and the patient may be mentally deficient, and have the blue eyes and fair hair due to deficiency of pigment formation as well as excreting phenylpyruvic acid in the urine.

Similarly one can think of polygenic inheritance in terms of enzymic reactions. One end product may arise from a series of such reactions. Mutations of any one of the enzymes may cause the end product to be lost or be formed differently. In most cases the biochemical basis is not known, but it is clear that polygenic inheritance is of frequent occurrence and in some cases it can be quantitated. Where mating is random the number of genes in common for a character, determined by genetic factors, is proportional to the degree of relatedness of the individuals in the family. Thus close relatives are more alike in

respect of this character than distant relatives. On the other hand when a dominant gene is involved, the resemblance between affected cousins is just as great as that between affected brothers. Finger prints are one example of polygenic inheritance, for there is a correlation between the total ridge counts in the dermal pattern and the degree of relatedness in the individuals.

Patterns of inheritance

With these reservations in mind, let us look at the consequences of the laws of inheritance in terms of the patterns of inheritance which are observed in families. There are two fundamental types of inheritance. These are autosomal inheritance where the gene in question is on an autosome, and sex-linked inheritance when the gene in question is on one of the sex chromosomes. The symbols used in recording pedigrees are given in fig. 39.4.

AUTOSOMAL INHERITANCE

The main feature of this type of inheritance is that males

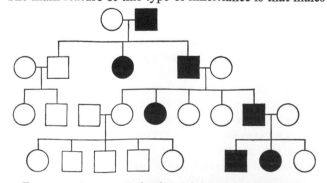

FIG. 39.5. Autosomal dominant inheritance. Composite pedigree demonstrating the main features: (1) the character appears in every generation; (2) on average half the offspring of an affected individual are also affected regardless of sex; (3) unaffected persons do not transmit the character.

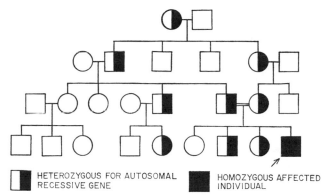

HETEROZYGOUS FOR AUTOSOMAL RECESSIVE GENE

HOMOZYGOUS AFFECTED INDIVIDUAL

Fig. 39.6. Autosomal recessive inheritance. Composite pedigree demonstrating the main features: (1) the character does not appear in every generation; (2) unaffected heterozygotes (carriers) transmit the gene on average to half of their offspring regardless of sex; (3) both parents of an affected individual are carriers; (4) two carrier parents will on average have one affected child in four; (5) parents may be consanguineous.

and females are equally affected and it may be either dominant or recessive. An **autosomal dominant** gene will be manifested in the heterozygous condition. Fig. 39.5 illustrates three general rules, but these may be modified by all the factors already discussed, e.g. if a dominant gene has less than 100 per cent penetrance it may appear to skip a generation. However, the general pattern is still recognizable. **Autosomal recessive** inheritance has also a number of characteristic features which are a consequence of the fact that the effect of the gene is only manifested in the homozygous condition. A pedigree illustrating these is shown in fig. 39.6.

SEX-LINKED INHERITANCE

Characteristically one sex is affected more than the other, the predominant sex depending on whether the gene is X linked or Y linked. As Y-linked genes are so rare, X linked and sex linked are commonly used as synonyms.

The most common type in man is **X-linked recessive inheritance**. Examples are colour blindness, haemophilia, and Duchenne muscular dystrophy. The characteristic features are given in fig. 39.7. This type of inheritance arises because the female has two X chromosomes and the male only one and he is therefore **hemizygous** for genes on the X chromosome. Although the gene is recessive it will therefore be expressed in all males who have an X chromosome carrying the gene. In females a single X carrying the trait is masked by the normal X chromosome. Only when a female is homozygous will she be affected and consequently affected females are rare. Obviously such a female will transmit to all her sons, and all of her daughters will be carriers.

X-linked dominant genes are rare in man. The best example is the Xg blood group. Characteristically a male who is phenotypically Xg(a+) transmits to all of his daughters but to none of his sons, while an Xg(a+) female transmits to all of her children if her genotype is homozygous (Xg^aXg^a) and to half of her children regardless of their sex if she is a heterozygote (Xg^aXg) (fig. 39.8). For **Y-linked** inheritance only males are affected (fig. 39.9). The only gene commonly accepted to be Y linked in man is the gene for hairy pinna of the ear. This character, described first in India, is transmitted by a father to all of his sons and none of his daughters, nor can the females be carriers.

SEX LIMITATION

It sometimes happens that an autosomal gene affects one sex preferentially. This is probably because some factor in the other sex prevents expression of the gene. In the case of an autosomal dominant gene which is sex limited and expresses only in males, the pattern of inheritance has a superficial resemblance to that of an X-linked recessive gene but there are several important differences, e.g. a male can transmit to his son. However, if the condition renders the male patient infertile as in the testicular

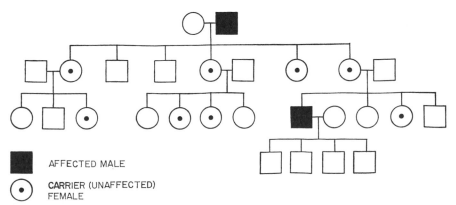

AFFECTED MALE

CARRIER (UNAFFECTED) FEMALE

Fig. 39.7. X-linked recessive inheritance. Composite pedigree demonstrating the main features: (1) affected males are more common than affected females; (2) an affected male cannot transmit to his sons but all his daughters will be carriers; (3) a carrier female transmits on average to half of her sons, and on average half of her daughters will be carriers.

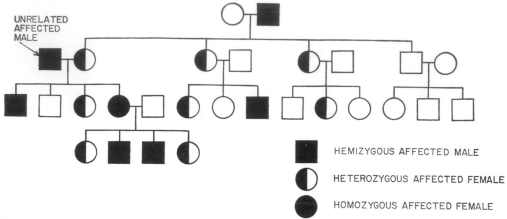

FIG. 39.8. X-linked dominant inheritance. Composite pedigree demonstrating the main features: (1) an affected male transmits to all of his daughters and none of his sons; (2) a heterozygous affected female transmits on average to half her children regardless of sex; (3) a homozygous affected female transmits to all her children.

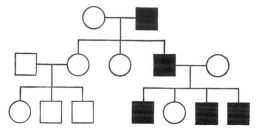

FIG. 39.9. Y-linked inheritance. A composite pedigree demonstrating the main features: (1) transmission by a male to all of his sons and none of his daughters; (2) females are not affected and cannot be carriers.

feminization syndrome the distinction between X-linked recessive inheritance and sex limited autosomal dominant inheritance cannot be made.

The typical modes of inheritance defined above are subject to all the modifications by the various factors previously described. Frequently in human genetics, sophisticated mathematical procedures are required to show that inheritance is of a particular kind.

TWINS

Dizygotic twins arise from the independent fertilization of two separate ova, and may thus be of like sex or opposite sex. **Monozygotic twins** arise from the separation of a single developing embryo into two independent parts and must be of like sex. They also have identical genetic constitutions. The diagnosis of zygosity is not always easy.

A study of monozygotic twins, especially comparison between those reared apart and those reared together, and the comparison between these two groups and dizygotic twins can yield useful information. For example, where environment plays a large part in the development of a particular character, a twin study may be the only way of determining whether or not the genetic constitution plays any part at all. The major factor in causing

pulmonary tuberculosis is clearly the tubercle bacillus. Cases tend to occur in families but it is difficult to say whether this is due to the genetic susceptibility of the family or to their increased exposure to other cases of the disease. It has been shown that if a pair of twins is reared apart and one of them develops tuberculosis, the probability of the other developing the disease is higher for monozygotic than for dizygotic twins. This is evidence for a genetic component in the development of tuberculosis.

GENES IN POPULATIONS

Gene frequency

If it were possible to examine the genetic constitution of an entire population one could determine how many individuals had two copies of the same allele at the two available loci in the chromosome set, how many had one copy and how many had none. The ratio of the total number of copies of one particular allele to the total available loci in a population is the **gene frequency**. Obviously this figure cannot be determined directly but on theoretical grounds it can be predicted that if, in a population mating randomly, there are two alleles which have frequencies of p and q respectively, the proportion of individuals who are homozygous for p will be p^2 and those homozygous for q will be q^2 while the proportion of heterozygotes will be 2pq. If the frequency of the homozygous recessive phenotype is known one can determine the gene frequency and also the frequency of heterozygotes in the population. For example, if the homozygous recessive phenotype occurs once in 10 000, i.e. $q^2 = 0.0001$ then q (the gene frequency) is 1 in 100 or 0.01. The frequency of the wild type allele must therefore be 0.99 and the frequency of the heterozygotes will be 0.0198 or roughly 2 per cent. Similarly it can be shown that under conditions of random mating the gene frequency in the population will not alter from one generation to the next (table 39.1). The population where such an equilibrium holds good is said to be in **Hardy–Weinberg equilibrium**.

TABLE 39.1. Hardy–Weinberg equilibrium. Let p and q represent the gene frequencies of two alleles A and a. Assuming random mating the frequencies of the two homozygotes and the heterozygote will be:

AA	Aa	aa
p^2	$2pq$	q^2

The frequencies of the progeny in the next generation, assuming random mating, will be:

	AA	Aa	aa
AA × AA	p^4		
AA × Aa	$2p^3q$	$2p^3q$	
AA × aa		$2p^2q^2$	
Aa × Aa	p^2q^2	$2p^2q^2$	p^2q^2
Aa × aa		$2pq^3$	$2pq^3$
aa × aa			q^4

Total AA progeny $= p^2(p^2 + 2pq + q^2)$
Total Aa progeny $= 2pq(p^2 + 2pq + q^2)$
Total aa progeny $= q^2(p^2 + 2pq + q^2)$

Thus the ratio is still

AA	Aa	aa
p^2	$2pq$	q^2

Factors influencing gene frequency

The Hardy–Weinberg law is in fact the basis on which the study of population genetics is built. It gives a theoretical expectation of gene frequencies in a population and one can therefore determine factors which influence these frequencies.

NON-RANDOM MATING

We have already stated that random mating is necessary for the gene frequency to remain stable, and therefore non-random mating is one of the factors which influences this stability. In human populations non-random mating is a normal circumstance for a variety of socio-economic and geographic reasons.

MUTATIONS

These arise through an alteration in the structure of the DNA and can be brought about by a number of environmental agents. Ionizing radiation is a potent mutagen and so are certain chemicals, such as nitrogen mustards.

Work with experimental animals has also shown that temperature is a factor which can influence mutation rate. Mutation rates can be measured for genes in man but the calculation can be difficult, especially for autosomal recessive genes. For autosomal dominant genes, however, it is relatively simple. If the number of individuals born affected by an autosomal dominant gene to normal parents is measured and compared with the total number of births, the mutation rate can be calculated since an abnormal child affected by an autosomal dominant can only be born to normal parents following a mutation. Since mutations occur in a random way, most of those produced are disadvantageous. Some are lethal, that is to say not compatible with life of the organism, while others are disadvantageous but not lethal. A small number, however, are advantageous and become established in the population by selection.

NATURAL SELECTION

The interplay between a large genetic variation and the environment leads to the selection of the best adapted phenotypes. As a result the best adapted individuals will tend to have more progeny than the others. It has been argued that, because man is to a certain extent in control of his environment, natural selection is no longer so rigorous for man as for other species. It would be more correct, however, to argue that selection is as rigorous as ever but that, because man is in control of his environment, the selection factors have been altered radically from those which operated before he reached his present level of sophistication. Medical science has undoubtedly played its part in this. For example, in some families a strong susceptibility to develop the highly malignant tumour, retinoblastoma, is inherited as an autosomal dominant character. This form of cancer which was, until recently, usually lethal in early childhood can now be treated successfully by surgery or by radiotherapy (vol. 3, p. 33.23). Thus, this gene can now be passed on with a greater frequency from generation to generation because a higher proportion of those carrying the gene survive to child bearing age. Thus biologically this mutant is less deleterious than it was a short time ago. In a similar way many more haemophilic males now survive to reproductive age to pass on their mutant gene to the next generation. In these cases one can predict that the frequency of the gene will increase in the population. Similarly the ability to diagnose certain chromosome abnormalities, neural tube defects and inborn errors of metabolism in the antenatal period by examination of the amniotic fluid will tend to reduce the number of affected individuals in the population but could lead to an increase in the number of carriers.

Instances of selection without the intervention of man are not hard to find. Sickle cell anaemia, a severe and often fatal haemolytic anaemia, is due to homozygosity for an autosomal recessive gene. However, the heterozygous condition, the sickle cell trait, which can be detected by an abnormality of the morphology of the red blood cells, is not associated with the anaemia found in the homozygous condition. Such individuals are very frequent in certain populations, e.g. in equatorial Africa, and unknown in others. It is now clear that the high frequency of the sickle cell trait in some populations is due to the fact that carriers of this trait have an unusual resistance to the malarial parasite; thus in areas where malaria is endemic carriers are at a selective advantage. The selection for the heterozygote results in a high frequency of an apparently deleterious gene. In areas where there is little or no malaria, selection factors operate against this gene.

GENETIC DRIFT

When a small population becomes separated from the main part of a population and remains separate for several generations, it is possible that its genetic constitution may show considerable divergence from that of the main population. This is because a small population is not necessarily a representative sample of the population from which it originated. These differences in the initial genetic structure of the population become accentuated over a long period of time. A group may be isolated for geographic reasons, e.g. the islanders of Tristan da Cunha, or for social reasons, e.g. religious minority groups in the U.S.A. These latter provide several interesting examples of genetic drift, e.g. the Dunkers of Pennsylvania have a distribution of ABO blood groups quite different from the population in Germany from which they originated. Similarly, in a classic study of the Old Order Amish of Lancaster County, Pennsylvania, McKusick has found that the frequency of a type of dwarfism associated with polydactyly is so high in this population of 8000, that there may be as many cases as have been described in the entire world literature.

GENE FLOW

By this is meant the transfer of genes from one geographic region to another. In the past, local populations have developed their own pool of genes in response to the selection factors operating in their own area, but migration and intermarriage between adjacent communities has contributed to a flow of genes through the population. A good example is the distribution of blood groups in Europe where group B is common in eastern regions but becomes less frequent as one goes westwards.

Now that communication between different parts of the world is easier the flow of genes from one population to another has been dramatically speeded up.

CHROMOSOMES

'Point' mutations are only one kind of change in the genetic material of a cell. Alterations may come about by changes in the grouping of genes, by rearrangements of the existing chromosome material or by alteration in the number of chromosomes in the cell. Normal human chromosomes and normal cell division are described on p. 12.20.

Mechanisms of production of chromosome aberrations

Errors can occur at either mitotic or meiotic divisions and the consequences of these errors are quite different. Errors occurring during meiosis, i.e. during the formation of the gametes, result in the zygote being abnormal and hence all the cells of the individual developing from that zygote are abnormal. On the other hand an error of mitosis which occurs during development can lead to the production of an individual in whose body there are two or more kinds of cell with different genetic constitutions but which are derived from a single zygote. Such an individual is a **chromosome mosaic** (fig. 39.10a) which should be distinguished from a **chromosome chimaera** where two genetically different lines of cells in a single

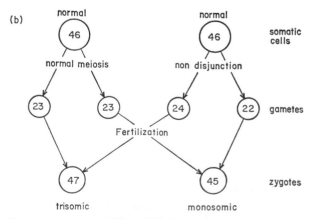

FIG. 39.10. (a) Mosaicism results from a mitotic error following fertilization. (b) Aneuploidy results from an error of meiosis prior to fertilization.

individual are derived from different zygotes, as in the mixing of blood cells which occurs regularly in cattle twins and rarely in human dizygotic twins following an anastomosis of the fetal circulation. Chromosome mosaicism results from an error of mitosis known as **anaphase lagging** where one chromosome fails to move from the equatorial plane of the cell at anaphase. This can result in the inclusion of the lagging chromosome in the wrong cell so that the daughter cells have forty-five and forty-seven chromosomes or its exclusion from either cell when the daughter cells will have forty-five and forty-six chromosomes. The exact composition of the individual depends on various factors such as the stage at which the error occurred, e.g. an error at the first cleavage division leads to a mosaic with two cell lines whereas a similar error at a later stage inevitably leads to a triple cell line mosaic provided that the cell lines are all viable and are included in the embryo.

Errors occurring during gametogenesis are of two kinds: those affecting chromosome number and those affecting chromosome morphology.

Those involving abnormalities of chromosome number probably all arise because of an error termed **non-disjunction**. If one pair of chromosomes fails to separate normally during meiosis both chromosomes of one homologous pair may be found in a single gamete or there may be no representative of that pair at all. In its simplest form these gametes have twenty-two or twenty-four chromosomes and, following fertilization, lead to the production of a zygote with forty-five or forty-seven chromosomes (fig. 39.10b). Such a zygote and the individual developing from it are said to be **aneuploid** (**euploid** cells are those containing exact multiples of the haploid number). The zygote with forty-seven chromosomes has three homologous chromosomes (**trisomy**) whereas the zygote with forty-five chromosomes has only one member of an homologous pair (**monosomy**). The effect on the developing individual depends on which chromosome is involved. Some are lethal, but others lead to developmental abnormalities, e.g. children with Down's syndrome (mongolism) are trisomic for chromosome 21. Non-disjunction can occur at the first or second meiotic division and it can occur in the male and in the

female. Since most aneuploid individuals are sterile or of greatly reduced reproductive fitness these conditions are genetically determined but not inherited, with a few rare exceptions.

Abnormalities of chromosome morphology on the other hand can be inherited. These abnormalities all involve the breakage and incorrect rejoining of chromosomes and are of several different types. Probably the commonest is the **translocation** where a segment of chromosome is transferred to a different site. Most frequently such a transfer involves the reciprocal exchange of material between two chromosomes and may lead to the formation of chromosomes of abnormal morphology (fig. 39.11a). The available evidence in man suggests that such translocations are not associated with phenotypic abnormality in the balanced form (i.e. where all the genetic material is present), but the offspring of such individuals may inherit the unbalanced form which is usually harmful. **Inversions** (fig. 39.11b), where the sequence of a segment of the chromosome is reversed, have been described in man and no association with abnormality has been reported. On the other hand when a segment of the chromosome is entirely missing (**deletion**) there is usually some phenotypic abnormality (fig. 39.11c).

Aneuploidy involving the sex chromosomes occurs approximately once in every 500 births, and aneuploidy involving the autosomes is equally frequent. Translocations may be as common as 1 in 200 births and the other abnormalities relatively rare. Thus roughly 1 per cent of all children born have an abnormal chromosome constitution. The incidence at conception is, however, much higher but many abnormal fetuses undergo spontaneous abortion and approximately 25 per cent of all such abortions are chromosomally abnormal.

Inheritance of chromosome aberrations

As with gene mutation the vast majority of chromosome aberrations are disadvantageous. In man, many cause infertility or defects so severe that reproduction, though possible, is highly improbable, but this is not an automatic consequence of chromosomal abnormality. For example, a female mouse with only one X chromosome instead of

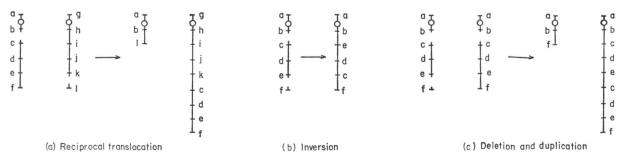

(a) Reciprocal translocation   (b) Inversion   (c) Deletion and duplication

FIG. 39.11. The production of chromosomal rearrangements.

two (an XO sex chromosome constitution) is fertile and her offspring include further XO females. In man, a female with three X chromosomes instead of two (an XXX sex chromosome constitution) appears to be fully fertile but for some reason not yet understood all the children are normal, although on theoretical grounds half the offspring should have forty-seven chromosomes with an XXX, or an XXY sex chromosome constitution.

Rearrangements of the chromosomes, as opposed to numerical aberrations, do not lead so regularly to diminished reproductive capacity. Some of these can therefore be passed on from generation to generation. The mode of transmission depends upon the precise nature of the rearrangement. A balanced translocation would in theory be passed on in the balanced form to 1 in 4 of the children, in one or other of the unbalanced forms to half the children, while the remaining quarter will have entirely normal chromosomes. In practice, however, this theoretical expectation is seldom, if ever, encountered, probably due to death of the unbalanced forms. This may be recognized as an increase in stillbirths or abortions in the families of carriers, but if death occurs at a very early stage of embryogenesis they may not be recognized as abortions and there appears to be a 1 : 1 ratio of balanced translocation carriers to normal individuals.

In the case of inversions the abnormality should in theory be passed on to half of the children, but because of pairing difficulties at meiosis unbalanced forms would be expected. However, in the few cases known in man there appears to be little evidence for the production of such unbalanced forms.

Chromosome polymorphism

In some species, such as the common shrew, different subgroups are found within the species, each having a different karyotype. Frequently such polymorphisms are due to the end-to-end association of two telocentric chromosomes to give a single large metacentric chromosome, which results in a reduction in the chromosome number. It now appears that chromosome polymorphism also occurs in man. The frequency of aneuploid individuals discussed above is almost completely maintained by the occurrence of new aberrations. However, the situation for chromosomal rearrangements is quite dif-

ferent. For example, translocations of the D/D type occur with a frequency of 1/1000 in the normal population and are transmitted from generation to generation with only a slight reduction in the fertility of the carriers. This frequency is probably higher than can be accounted for by the production of new aberrations and it seems that the population must be considered polymorphic for these rearrangements. This is an important practical point. Since there are relatively large numbers of individuals in the population with chromosome aberrations which have no apparent effect, these are encountered in patients from time to time purely by chance. Hence the frequency of such aberrations in the normal population must be considered before such an association is considered to be a causal factor of any disease.

FURTHER READING

COURT BROWN W.M. (1967) *Human Population Cytogenetics*. North-Holland Research Monographs, Frontiers of Biology, Vol. 5. Amsterdam: North-Holland.

EMERY A.E.H. (1975) *Modern Trends in Human Genetics*, Vol. 2. London: Butterworths.

FRASER G.R. & MAYO O. (1975) *Textbook of Human Genetics*. Oxford: Blackwell Scientific Publications.

HAMERTON J.L. (1971) *Human Cytogenetics*, Vol. 1. New York: Academic Press.

HARRIS H. (1963) *Garrod's Inborn Errors of Metabolism*. Oxford Monographs on Medical Genetics. London: Oxford University Press.

McKUSICK V.A. (1969) *Human Genetics*, 2nd Edition. New Jersey: Prentice Hall.

McKUSICK V.A. (1975) *Mendelian Inheritance in Man: Catalogs of Autosomal Dominant, Autosomal Recessive and X-linked Phenotypes*, 4th Edition. Baltimore: Johns Hopkins Press.

STERN C. (1973) *Principles of Human Genetics*, 3rd Edition. San Francisco: Freeman.

THOMPSON J.S. & THOMPSON M.W. (1973) *Genetics in Medicine*, 2nd Edition. Philadelphia: Saunders.

WATSON J.D. (1965) *Molecular Biology of the Gene*. New York: Benjamin.

Chapter 40
Human psychology

Psychology covers a wide canvas and deals with most aspects of human experience and behaviour, so it is not surprising that large portions can only be sketched tentatively. There are wide areas of ignorance in our knowledge of the mental processes which motivate human behaviour. Fortunately other parts of the canvas may be painted more confidently. This is the case when dealing with findings that have been verified by experiments. It is the emergence of a body of well-supported findings that encourages psychologists to consider the subject a science, albeit an embryonic one. This chapter is an introduction to aspects of psychological work which appear particularly relevant to the doctor.

A good starting place is an overall look at psychological development from infancy to old age. In considering some of the characteristics of each stage frequent reference is made, not only to the normal sequence of development, but also to factors which impede normal progress. Psychologists endeavour constantly to measure what they observe and the developmental section is followed by a description of some of the methods by which attempts have been made to produce standards against which some behaviours may be assessed. The account given is confined to standardized tests of intelligence and of personality with their limitations and their usefulness.

Human effectiveness depends upon the ability to come to terms with and attain some control over the external environment. Some psychologists have viewed man as essentially a complex information processing organism, constantly scanning his environment for new knowledge which can improve decision making and enlarge behavioural repertoire. The third section of the chapter is concerned with some of the discernible stages involved in this sequence of information processing, i.e. attending, learning, remembering, thinking.

However, man is not only a cognitive animal, processing information in the fashion of a superbly designed computer. He also reacts to events emotionally and his feelings may often dominate and certainly always colour his judgments. The influence of emotional factors is especially evident in man's behaviour in threatening situations. Some aspects of stress and individual reactions to it are, therefore, also examined.

Consideration of stress leads to an evaluation of the concepts of normality and abnormality, two of the most frequently used but least precise terms in psychology. Some of the ambiguities inherent in these terms and the erroneous conclusions to which they often lead are explored in the penultimate section. Finally a closer look is taken at man's essentially social nature and the decisive influence of his dependence upon others on his individual behaviour.

Psychology is a young science and, in comparison with many others in medical education, it is in the throes of puberty. Only recently has it gained recognition as part of the health sciences. Dealing with every aspect of human behaviour, it is difficult to discuss briefly yet adequately its many facets, but it is obvious that a doctor should understand the diversity of human behaviour. This situation may stimulate some students to inquire further into areas of psychology which appear relevant to their future dealings with people.

Some terms and concepts

All sciences develop their own vocabulary which is unfamiliar to those studying the subject for the first time. Psychological vocabulary is confusing because words in common use are often given a more specific connotation. With this in mind some of the terms used are explained in a little detail. An additional glossary is given in vol. 3, p. 35.2.

Psychology is the scientific study of behaviour. It is concerned with both the establishment of principles which govern behaviour and with the individual differences which make each one of us unique. Psychologists vary greatly in their areas of specialization and in the particular fields of human behaviour which they study. Thus, a **clinical psychologist** applies his knowledge of human behaviour and experience to the clinical field. He may be expected to possess postgraduate training in abnormal behaviour. He is mainly concerned with evaluating and modifying deviant behaviours, in teaching and in research. This is in contrast to the **psychiatrist** who is a medically trained doctor, specializing in the diagnosis, treatment and prevention of mental disorders. A **psychoanalyst** is a psychiatrist who has had special training in Freudian theory and practice and who applies psychotherapeutic skills mainly in the treatment of neurotic disorders.

The common term **behaviour** refers to those activities of a person which are capable of being observed by another person. This includes verbal reports of inner experiences. **Behaviour modification** refers to a group of techniques employed in modifying unwanted or deviant behaviours. These techniques are usually based upon the principles of classical and instrumental learning theory. **Environment** is used as a general term embracing all stimuli which, although external to the individual, influence his behaviour. Usually the term refers particularly to people with whom the individual has some form of social contact. Another general term is **constitution**, used to denote that part of the personality which is inborn, inherited, but present as a potential behavioural influence, often in a latent state, from birth. The term is used to contrast such inborn influences with environmentally or **psychogenically** imposed characteristics of personality. The distinction is somewhat false, in that all constitutional factors are influenced by environment. The influences of the environment are often broken down into more discrete **stimuli**, which are simply any event which alters experience and causes individuals to respond in a particular way.

Most attempts to assess a person by psychometric means rely for their effectiveness on the process of **standardization**. This consists of devising psychological tests with fixed or standard procedures and methods of scoring; it also establishes norms, against which individual performance may be evaluated. **Reliability** is a term used to denote the degree to which a test produces consistent results, while **validity** indicates the degree to which a test measures what it sets out to measure. Tests are sometimes described as **objective** or **subjective**, the former implying that scoring and interpretation are relatively free of observer bias and the latter suggesting that there is little control over this. Tests which measure **intellectual deterioration** are usually concerned with the effects of brain injury or disease in producing a reduction in intellectual capacity, beyond what can be expected through normal ageing.

The term **anxiety** is usually used to describe a diffuse emotional state where the distress is not specially associated with any particular object or event, as in a fear or phobia. **Autistic thinking** is used to describe a form of associative thinking, controlled more by the thinker's inner needs and desires than by reality, e.g. day-dreaming. It corresponds closely to **egocentric thinking**, a term used by developmental psychologists to describe the predominantly personally orientated thinking of the very young child.

The two main categories of mental disorder are the **neuroses** and the **psychoses**. The neuroses include a large number of abnormal emotional states. Psychotic disorders are more serious forms of personal distress in which contact with reality is disrupted or sometimes completely lost. The term **functional psychoses** is sometimes used to refer to psychotic disorders in which there is no known specific damage to the brain and no definite organic cause. **Organic psychoses** are those where the abnormal mental state is a direct result of damage to the brain (vol. 3, p. 35.66). One of the two main groups of functional psychoses are the **affective psychoses**, where the primary disturbance is in mood state which may vary from profound depression to extreme elation (vol. 3, p. 35.44). The other main group of functional disorders are the **schizophrenias**, a heterogeneous group of psychotic states involving gross disturbance in thinking and communication, and often a marked deterioration in personality and behaviour (vol. 3, p. 35.52). Although literally meaning 'split-mind' the term does not indicate a split or dissociated personality, e.g. Dr Jekyll and Mr Hyde. The split is a failure of the normal integration of the main mental processes. Finally the term **sociopath**, or more commonly and pejoratively **psychopath**, denotes individuals whose deviant behaviour is neither neurotic nor psychotic (vol. 3, p. 35.22). The behaviour of sociopaths is usually aggressively antisocial, guilt-free and unchecked by dictates of conscience.

PERSONALITY DEVELOPMENT

In psychology the term **personality** is normally used to denote the pattern of hopes, feelings, attitudes and beliefs which together make each individual unique. This differs from the use of the term in everyday speech in phrases such as 'he is a striking personality' or 'she has lots of personality'. In this latter context personality is seen as the impact made by one individual upon another. This use of the term draws attention to the fact that when we make judgments regarding another's personality we inevitably do so in the context of a human relationship. Our observations of another person are influenced by our feelings about him, by our own attitudes and beliefs, indeed by our own personality. In an attempt to make objective and reliable observations of personality, psychologists use techniques aimed at minimizing the errors introduced by subjective factors. However, it is salutary to keep in mind that no matter how sophisticated psychological techniques become, observations and interpretations of another person's behaviour are always influenced by our own personality.

At one time psychologists distinguished between **personality** and **temperament,** using the latter term to denote those personal characteristics of an individual which are determined by innate constitutional factors. During the last decade the word temperament has gradually slipped from the psychological vocabulary as psychologists became increasingly preoccupied by the impact of learning on personality development. It is obvious that much of our personality is a product of the multitude of learning experiences occurring throughout life. Nevertheless, in the eagerness to assess the effect of the environment it is easy to underestimate the influence of constitutional differences.

Most mothers who have reared a large family of children can testify that no two are alike and that individual differences are readily apparent from early infancy, before the environment has had much opportunity to modify the child's behaviour. Some studies of infantile behaviour tend to support this view. It has been shown that in early infancy children can be differentiated in their level of physical activity, in their readiness to adapt to change and in their emotional responsiveness. Other studies have shown that some areas of future development can be predicted surprisingly well from observations made during the first two years of the child's life. Such observations serve as a useful corrective to those who regard the early environment and interpersonal relationships as the source of all later individual differences in personality. Even in early infancy the human infant cannot be likened to a piece of clay whose personality is moulded by the behaviour of others. Indeed parental behaviour is inevitably influenced by the infant's own responses. The finished product, which we call personality, is the result of a complex interplay between constitutional and environmental influences. This view is of particular relevance to pathological deviations in development and it has been said that 'there are no disturbed children—only disturbed parents'. While the emotionally disturbed child may be the product of conflict within the family group a child reacts to disturbance in the family in his own way. In some cases such reactions are extreme, while in others a similar degree of stress may elicit little response.

Infancy

Although many fathers say that their child was not a personality until sometime during the second year of life, most mothers date the emergence of their child's personality much earlier. They quote examples illustrating the infant's capacity to interact with mother within a reciprocal mother-child relationship. Psychologists have also disagreed as to when it is legitimate to speak of the infant as having a separate personality, capable of recognizing and relating himself to others in his environment. It is of course obvious that each infant is a separate person, reacting to the personal and non-personal environment in his own characteristic way. Some schools of thought take this much further and maintain that the infant is capable of sustaining a more complex relationship with specific people in his environment, e.g. mother, and that such early relationships serve as a prototype for future interpersonal reactions. Other studies of infantile development suggest that the infant is incapable of forming a personal relationship during the first six months of life. Piaget concludes that, during this period, the infant is still learning to discriminate between separate objects in 'the booming, buzzing confusion' into which he has been born.

The current view of the development of social relationships during infancy is represented by the work of Schaffer in Glasgow, who identifies three temporal stages in the development of the infant's attachment to other people. During the first three months, the infant's main need is for a continuous flow of sensory stimulation from the environment. This includes all the auditory, visual and tactile sensations emanating from the environment, both personal and impersonal. At first the infant's limited motor development renders him dependent upon adults to supply stimulation and when this is not forthcoming he reacts to monotony by crying. Many mothers have learned the usefulness of the open window, the radio or even the sound of the washing machine and vacuum cleaner in obtaining a respite from baby's demands. Later, the more mobile infant explores his environment, searching out the variety of sensations necessary for normal development. The fact that infants who are reared in a monotonous environment tend to lag behind in their development suggests that the human infant requires an optimum level of external stimulation.

Somewhere between the third and seventh month of life the infant's social development reaches a second stage where he now differentiates between social (contact with people) and non-social stimulation. Now the infant encourages and responds to stimulation from other people but as yet he shows no attachment to any specific person. Around the seventh month of life the infant shows the first observable indications that he is able to discriminate among people and for the first time seeks mother's presence, rejecting the overtures of others. It is only towards the end of the first year of life that we can safely speak of a fully reciprocal relationship between mother and child.

Such observations have more than academic interest. They are relevant to theories which relate pathological breakdown in later life to early traumatic experiences within the mother-child relationship. John Bowlby and others have described the patterns of anxiety shown by children admitted to hospital and so separated from their mothers. If our earlier observations are correct one would not expect such reactions to separation to occur in an infant less than seven months old who has not yet formed any specific attachment to mother. Most observations of the reactions of infants to living in hospital confirm this suggestion. It is the child of over seven months who shows the overdependent and fearful behaviour on his return home. In the case of the older child around the age of two years living in hospital, separation has been said to exert a permanently damaging effect upon the child's social development. More careful studies suggest, however, that many factors are involved and that the long-term effects of separation may have been greatly over-stressed.

While these observations serve as a corrective to over-emphasis on the impact of the early mother-child relationship on later development, it must not be assumed that the mother's behaviour with her child during this time is of little or no importance. Studies of infant monkeys deprived of a mother show that they tend to be more inhibited and fearful in their later behaviour than monkeys who are reared normally. Harlow has shown that the presence of a mother substitute, a crude dummy figure to which the infant monkey can cling in times of stress, is sufficient to allay anxiety, but only if the substitute figure provides a soft, tactile contact. This suggests that the natural hugging and cuddling which most affectionate mothers give to their infants is a valuable and necessary source of stimulation.

Even in this area of infantile needs it is unwise to generalize and neglect the wide measure of normal individual differences in infants. Some infants appear perfectly satisfied with much less stimulation than others who show an almost ravenous need for excitement. The former may be described by their mothers as contented babies who are easy to rear while the latter are regarded as demanding and exhausting in their insatiable desire for stimulation. Infants also vary in their need for particular types of stimulation. Schaffer found that a surprisingly large proportion of infants did not react to tactile contact such as hugging, showing a preference for visual and auditory contact. He makes the important point that there are also wide individual differences in mothers' needs in the nursing situation. The optimum relationship is thus achieved when there is a mutual adaptation between the needs of both mother and child. Imbalance may occur when the mother is either unresponsive or overresponsive to the infant's needs. Such a disturbed relationship might for example, occur when a mother with a strong need for physical contact attempts to relate herself to a 'non-cuddling baby'.

The existence of individual differences should also be recognized in specific areas of infant training such as feeding and toilet control. A number of psychological theories have stressed the importance of breast feeding, and of the timing of weaning. While some studies have indicated a relationship between bottle feeding and later maladjustment, the findings of others have failed to support this view. Although breast feeding may possess physical advantages most studies suggest that these have been greatly exaggerated. In Aberdeen, Hytten found bottle-fed babies to be at least as healthy as those who had been breast fed. He concluded that while 'we should help in every way possible the woman who wishes to breast feed . . . we are not justified in putting pressure on those who are unwilling or unable to breast feed efficiently'. Other theories have suggested that either too early or too late weaning may cause later psychological difficulties although there is no evidence which convincingly links the time of weaning with later personality development. The timing of the weaning may reflect the individual infant's readiness for this step rather than the mother's needs or beliefs.

Toilet training is another aspect of early rearing which has been related to later personality development. While grandmother may advise that this should be initiated as early as possible, many modern authorities stress the unfortunate repercussions of too early or too rigid training. The mother's dilemma is often solved by the child who trains mother in toilet training! Young children differ widely in the age at which they are capable of toilet control. If their rhythm of elimination is regular and predictable, toilet behaviour may be conditioned early, while irregularity renders any conditioning process ineffective. Some mothers feel compelled to establish training at a very early age because of their own disgust at normal excretory functions. This attitude, if extreme, may engender in the child an unhealthy aversion to his own bodily functions. Mothers who react in this manner are likely to introduce training which is not only ill-timed but also excessively rigid and harsh so that conflict develops between mother and child. Some studies indicate that where toilet training is initiated around fifteen months in a non-coercive, co-operative way the likelihood of later bed wetting and soiling is greatly reduced. Perhaps the mother who trains early and harshly runs a greater risk of incurring a later breakdown in the child's toilet functions. The course of toilet training is, however, greatly affected by the child's personal rhythms and the ease with which he forms conditioned habits. It is deceivingly simple to relate all training difficulties to mother's own attitudes.

Implicit in much of what has been said is the problem of distinguishing between aspects of behaviour which are learned from those due to maturation. The term maturation here refers to development which occurs in an orderly, predictable pattern and independent of the child's experience. It is tempting to ascribe all behavioural changes in the infant as being a result of parental behaviour and other learning experiences and to overlook the possibility of a gradual unfolding of a predetermined sequence of development. Successful child rearing often depends upon how the parents match their teaching to the child's readiness for change.

The newborn infant has a very restricted emotional range, varying between generalized excitement and tranquillity (absence of emotion). At about the end of the third month the emotional state of diffuse excitement differentiates clearly into the two separate emotions of distress and delight. Thereafter, throughout the first year the emotions of anger, disgust, fear, elation and affection become observable. The suggestion that this sequence is due to maturation rather than to learning and imitation is supported not only by its regularity but also by the fact that the same sequence is observed to occur in infants who are deaf and blind from birth. While it must be admitted that we are restricted to observable emotions, there are reasonable indications that early emotional development is in the form of a predetermined pattern. Later learning does of course have unlimited influence upon the expression of emotions and on the linking of emotions with particular situations.

Childhood

The world to the young child is a fascinating if often somewhat bewildering kaleidoscope of rapidly changing experience. During the early stages of infancy his role is that of a relatively passive spectator engaged in assimilating each new experience. Gradually the individual learns to make appropriate responses to events and then begins a long apprenticeship in ordering, interpreting and finally attaining some degree of control over external reality. In this difficult task he is hampered, both by limited experience and inability to apply logical reasoning. Instead the environment is interpreted subjectively and he develops his own explanations and an egocentric system of thought. Whereas in adult thinking ideas are altered to conform with reality the child tends to distort reality, moulding it to fit his own personal viewpoint. It is this prelogical way of interpreting events which, above all, creates the gulf between the world of the child and that of the adult. To bridge this gulf and understand the inner life and outer behaviour of the child, some of the main features which categorize thinking during this egocentric phase of development must be considered.

Adults make a sharp distinction between animate and inanimate objects. In contrast the young child lives in an animistic world. In his egocentric way he imbues all objects in his environment with life, assuming that they are capable of the same feelings as he is. Gradually he narrows his definition of inanimate to include only objects which appear to move of their own volition. Thus, phrases such as 'a threatening sky' or 'a cheerful fire' have a very literal meaning for the younger child. It is not until between the ages of seven and nine years that the child is completely free of animistic traces in his thinking. The child's view of the world does protect him from one source of fear which haunts the adult world, i.e. the fear of death. Thus the irrational world of childhood is given up only at some cost. Of course, the younger child often experiences the death of pets or elderly relatives but he tends to interpret this as involving only temporary separation, the loved object being assumed to continue to exist elsewhere. It is not unusual to find eight to ten-year-old children reacting to their first appreciation of the implications of mortality by becoming morbidly preoccupied by death and showing fear and overconcern for the health of parents.

A central feature of the child's egocentric thinking is the confusion between internal mental processes and external events. During the latter stages of infancy, consciousness and self-awareness emerge as the infant learns to differentiate between itself and the rest of the environment. This distinction is not fully established for some time and the young child's thinking continues to be influenced by his tenuous hold on the difference between his internal and external world. Parents are often faced with the difficult task of explaining to a young child why others cannot see his dreams while he sleeps. To the child the dream is an external event and therefore must be observable by others. This confusion is not confined to the dream state, for a child shows a similar failure to differentiate between his own thoughts and external events in his everyday activities. We may say that this only means that the child has a vivid imagination but there is a world of difference between the younger child's imaginings and those of the healthy adult who has no difficulty in separating fantasies from his real life. To the young child his thoughts are omnipotent and at times as real as the deed itself. He may worry that he will be punished for unspoken thoughts or be convinced that what has been imagined has in fact happened. Not only the thoughts but the words by which they are expressed have, to the child, an independent and objective existence. Thus a father related how his young daughter was terrified of his tape recorder which she feared would 'take away my words and keep them shut up in the box'. Adults are often confused by the prelogical concepts used by a child to categorize objects in his environment. Like adults, a child finds it more economical to arrange objects in groups but in this case the common denominator connecting the objects is personal and related to his own actions. Thus a young child may use the word 'door' to refer to doors, drawers, boxes or to any object which he can open. His concept of 'car' may extend to any object which he can push along the ground.

Whereas the younger child acts on impulse, translating his feelings and desires into immediate action, the older child's behaviour is distinguished by his ability to inhibit behavioural responses which have been hitherto freely expressed. The emergence of this type of more controlled behaviour is gradual. Some children appear to remain impulsive and uncontrolled in their behaviour. Although developing normally in other ways, their social behaviour remains unpredictable and explosive, leading them into conflict with a society which tolerates such behaviour only in much younger children. Some experimental studies suggest that failure to develop the normal capacity to inhibit responses may sometimes be a consequence of minimal brain damage at birth. The Russian psychologist Luria has developed experimental techniques for measuring **response inhibition** and has used these to diagnose children who suffer from this developmental lag. In Britain several investigators have used similar techniques to show that children who perform poorly on tasks demanding response inhibition tend to be unusually impulsive, antisocial and maladjusted.

If such socially deviant behaviour continues to be prominent in an adult, the individual may be considered as having a **sociopathic personality disorder** (vol. 3, p. 35.22). Longitudinal studies suggest that the immature social behaviour of some chronically antisocial individuals is reflected in their EEG activity which contains rhythms more usual in young children.

To the young child the main factor which regulates his behaviour and prevents the immediate gratification of every need is that of external adult authority. He gradually learns that certain actions bring swift retribution and at this stage wrong actions are simply those which are punished. While this is equally true of the behaviour of the older child and adult, their behaviour is also under the more restrictive control of the inner censor which we call our **conscience**. Here bad behaviour is no longer merely that which incurs punishment from others but also that which results in our feeling bad. By internalizing a set of moral standards we create our own punishment in the sense of shame or guilt which accompanies transgressions from our own moral code. While the behaviour of the very young child is not regulated in this way there is disagreement as to the age when conscience develops.

According to the psychoanalytic theories of Freud and his followers, the first step towards a more socially regulated mode of behaviour occurs between the 4th and 5th year when a child first begins actively to model himself upon the parent of the same sex. A boy identifies with and imitates his father, a girl her mother. Others, such as Piaget, place the development of the moral sense later, about the 7th year. Certainly it seems that, before the age of seven years, most children have no inherent sense of right and wrong, accepting without understanding the rules of conduct laid down by adult authority. The well-meaning parent who shows disappointment or annoyance at his youngster's lack of moral sense is simply expecting the child to function in a manner for which he is not yet ready. Because most children appear to develop a moral sense by the age of seven years, their moral standards need not be similar. Their moral codes reflect in a large measure their early environment, particularly the values of their parents. If the parents are themselves controlled by rigid and harsh moral principles then the child may be crippled by a conscience which is severe and overdemanding. Similarly, a lack of moral values in the parents may exert a different, although equally detrimental, effect on the child's later development. Like every other aspect of our personality our conscience continues to develop and change after early childhood through the impact of new learning experiences.

Perhaps it is too sanguine and optimistic to suggest that the social behaviour of the older child is internally controlled and less dependent upon external adult authority than is the case with the younger child. Some years ago Peter Brook, the British film director, made a film of William Golding's allegorical novel 'Lord of the Flies'. The novel depicts the rapid social and moral disintegration of a group of boarding school children shipwrecked on a desert island without adults. In reflecting on the filming, which was shot on an island with a group of school children, Brooks wryly comments as follows 'Many of their off screen relationships completely paralleled the story, and one of our main problems was to encourage them to be uninhibited within the shots, but disciplined in between them ... My experience showed me that the only falsification in Golding's fable is the length of time the descent to savagery takes. His action takes about three months. I believe that if the cork of continued adult presence were removed from the bottle, the complete catastrophe could occur within a long weekend'.

EGOCENTRIC THINKING AND ADULT MENTAL DISORDER

Many people have been struck by the resemblance between some aspects of egocentric thinking in children and the behaviour displayed by adults during mental illness. Psychiatrists use the term **regression** to refer to this tendency to revert to an earlier, less mature type of behaviour when faced with a stressful situation. For example, older children when faced with a difficult situation fall back on thumb-sucking or some other primitive form of behaviour which relieved their tension when they were much younger. During a battle a weary and frightened soldier may break down and cry for his mother or even become temporarily enuretic. Illness, particularly if severe, is a stressful situation. Normally the adult is a relatively independent being who adjusts to his environment in a mature manner. When he becomes unwell, particularly if he fears that his symptoms herald a serious illness, he becomes anxious, vulnerable, less mature and more dependent on the reassurance of figures of authority around him. When such a patient goes to his doctor he is in a sense again in the position of the young child whose well-being is totally dependent upon the understanding and experience of an all knowing authority figure. It is no exaggeration to say that the doctor's picture of his patients as individuals is seldom a fair reflection of the patient's normal personality.

The more severe the illness and the more worried the patient, the more childlike, demanding and dependent is his behaviour. If he has to enter hospital the adult patient's routine is disrupted and he is forced to surrender in a large measure many of the things which make him an independent adult. Such enforced dependency in an unfamiliar and sometimes frightening environment combined with the fears aroused by illness may result in the patient's regressing to a childlike mode of behaviour. This regression may show itself in different ways, some patients becoming completely passive, over-dependent and demanding attention. Others may become peevish, irritable and irrational like spoiled children. Each patient, in fact, tends to react in terms of his individual way of reacting to past emergencies in childhood. It is always worth remembering that the adult patient's behaviour in hospital is a poor reflection of his normal personality. An important task of doctors and nurses in hospital is to allay the patient's fears by reassurance and explanation in much the same manner as every parent has to do with young children.

The resemblance between adult and childhood behaviour is much more striking when the illness is mental rather than physical. Adult patients with neurotic disorders often display childlike qualities, especially in the emotionally uncontrolled nature of their behaviour. However, it is in the behaviour of the more seriously disordered psychotic patients that there is the closest correspondence with the egocentric child. A progressive loss of distinction between fantasy and reality is one of the characteristic features of schizophrenia. The schizophrenic projects on to external reality his own inner wishes, fears and thoughts, resulting in reality distortion similar to that occurring in early childhood. The omnipotence of thought already described may be found in an adult patient who feels others can see the thoughts in his head or that people are taking his words away from him while he speaks. Traces of animistic thinking, dormant since early childhood, may reappear so that a patient imbues inanimate objects and non-human creatures with life. Like the young child he may perceive and interpret events around him solely from his own perspective.

In the more extreme and advanced stages of a psychosis a patient may show the same inability to differentiate between the self and the remainder of the environment as occurs in infancy. In this condition he may show frequent confusions of identity, when his personality appears to merge with that of others around him. Some psychoanalysts think that the adult patient regresses back to a more primitive level of mental functioning because of his inability to adjust to the demands of adult life. Implicit in this point of view is the idea that a patient who later develops such an illness had a particularly traumatic early childhood which rendered mature adjustment impossible. Regression in this sense means that the adult patient is pulled back to a more primitive mode of adjustment by the unresolved conflicts of childhood. However, the correspondence between childhood and adult mental illness may be interpreted in a rather different manner. An adult patient with a severe brain injury may show many regressive components in his behaviour in so far as he behaves in a childlike way. The main reason for such regression is that the injury has impaired his higher mental functions and caused him to function at a lower level. Many psychiatrists who regard severe mental disorders such as schizophrenia as organic in origin argue that the patient regresses in his behaviour not because of unresolved infantile conflicts but because the illness damages functions of the brain. In this view the regressed patient is not so much pulled back to an earlier more primitive level of adjustment but is rather pushed back by his current condition.

Although the similarities between psychotic adult behaviour and normal childhood behaviour have been emphasized, there are numerous differences. While the resemblances are useful in helping to understand the behaviour of psychotic patients, this should not lead us to treat a patient as a child. No matter how severe the illness or how destructive it is to the adult personality the patient retains some residue of adult functioning. This point is also relevant to later discussion on ageing as there is some resemblance between the mental changes in old age and mental functioning in childhood. However, anyone who approaches elderly people as if he were dealing with children is apt to be quickly and forcibly reminded of his mistake!

Adolescence

By the time the child is twelve years of age his thinking is predominantly orientated to reality and relatively free from egocentricity. He has developed a wide range of skills and aptitudes which allow him to deal with most situations in his environment. Usually he is well adapted, integrated and enjoys the security of an established social status within his own age group. By this age parents are beginning to relax and feel with relief that out of the earlier turmoil has emerged a reasonably stable adult in miniature. Suddenly, their well earned tranquillity is shattered by a whole sequence of alterations in their child's behaviour. Confidence is replaced by intense self-consciousness and the domestic scene is rent asunder by emotional explosions. Adolescence has arrived!

Adolescence is a period of physical, mental and social change. Physical changes cause him to be more aware of himself and more self-conscious in a literal sense. This new awareness of himself is intensified by the maturation of the secondary sexual characteristics, and an awakening of the sexual drive. How adequately youngsters learn to control and direct their sexual feelings partially depends upon the present and past attitudes of others, particularly parents. Puberty also entails a new social adjustment and popularity with the opposite sex becomes an important symbol of social status.

The main mental change is in intellectual development. The young person is equipped not only with a new fund of physical energy, but also with a new fund of mental energy. In essence the adolescent becomes capable of a much more abstract mode of thinking and the capacity for new learning reaches its peak, slowly declining later in adulthood. These aspects of intellectual development help to explain some typical features of adolescent behaviour. The new found ability to reason in a wider context leads to endless speculations about abstract issues. The attitude to parents may be altered by the new capacity to question their reasoning and the realization that age does not necessarily bring wisdom. Finding that long established sources of authority have feet of clay, a young person is likely to seek new authority figures, often nearer to his own age level. This accounts to some extent for the rebellious, non-conforming attitude of the adolescent who constantly debunks the no longer infallible adult authorities. Although this may be a trying period for the demoted parent, it is an essential and healthy part of development which aids the youngster in finding his own identity.

Adolescence is finally, and perhaps most importantly, a period of social change and adjustment. Although childhood and adulthood have their own problems they offer the individual a secure and clearly defined social role. The adolescent is asked to surrender the dependency of childhood without being offered the independency of adulthood. During this period of apprenticeship for manhood or womanhood the adolescent's social role is vague, nebulous and often contradictory. To some extent this long period of apprenticeship is imposed upon the young person by the society in which he lives. He may be criticized for being childish by the same adults who disparage and discourage his attempts to play a more mature role. It is not surprising that the adolescent inbetweens form their own social group or that their activities reflect their rootlessness and their insecure state of mind. In some less industrialized societies adolescence does not exist as a distinct stage of human development. In such societies the child is accepted as such until he reaches a certain age. At this point he is fully accepted as a responsible adult member of his social group and assigned a clearly defined role to play. It is not surprising

that many of the emotional and behavioural problems which appear to us as being a natural part of adolescence are much less evident in such societies.

What are the effects of such changes on the adolescent personality? Their main effect is probably summed up in one word—uncertainty. The adolescent suffers from a basic lack of direction. His emotions are confused and ambivalent. He senses his mental power but at the same time lacks the inner confidence to translate his beliefs into a definite course of action. His delight in shocking his parents' adult composure is matched by the feelings of guilt which his own behaviour invokes. Fantasies and day dreams are an easy substitute for action and in such imaginative reveries all problems are solved. In these he is sophisticated, sexually dominant, respected by others and decisive in action. Later, if he is to reach a more mature level of development, he must come to a compromise between his inner desires and outward achievements. Out of this maelstrom of conflicting feelings and ideas the adolescent must find a new individual identity. He must find for himself what sort of person he is, where he is going in life and what are his personal limitations and potentialities. Some psychologists have called the adolescent period a crisis of identity, to stress the crucial process of social and personal readjustment involved. Perhaps it is fitting to close the discussion with the following quotation: 'The world is passing through troubled times. The younger people have no reverence for their parents; they are impatient of all restraint; they talk as if they alone knew everything, and what passes for wisdom with us is foolishness for them'. This is taken, not from today's newspaper editorials but from the writings of Peter the Hermit in the eleventh century.

Adult life

The legal age for the start of adulthood is decided arbitrarily, for it is not easy to denote its psychological onset. Adulthood carries with it a level of maturity that is not a necessary consequence of reaching any particular age. Maturity is the ability to adjust realistically both to the environment and to one's self. By achieving insight into our own limitations and potentialities we learn to accept the former and develop the latter. We turn aside from unattainable day-dreams and use our energies in striving for the attainable. We learn to accept the responsibility for our actions, make our own decisions and learn by our mistakes. Responsibility for others is assumed gradually and should be fully developed when a young adult becomes a parent.

Stresses may be present at any time in adult life, but there are certain broad periods in which we face particularly difficult demands. The need to find some measure of success and satisfaction in work is not purely economic but is also an expression of the need for a purposeful life. Unfortunately modern industrial society does not provide every adult with an interesting and self-satisfying job. Many find in their leisure time activities which allow them to express their constructive needs. The adult who is unable to find personal satisfaction in either his work or leisure is unlikely to feel completely at ease with himself. Again, in a competitive society, the sense of achievement derived from steady vocational progress is not given to all. Marriage is another period of adult life when a great deal of individual readjustment is needed. Immature adults may seek to re-establish in marriage the security and lack of responsibility of childhood. Unconsciously they seek not a partner but a substitute for father or mother. A neurotic often marries a person who is also unstable. A friend said that it was good that Thomas and Jane Carlyle were married because this meant one, not two, unhappy marriages. A child of emotionally disturbed parents is indeed unfortunate. Parenthood itself can be a stress for an immature adult who may dislike the competition for his wife's attention and the new responsibilities thrust upon him.

The loss of parents is naturally a stressful experience which may be catastrophic for an immature adult who has never been psychologically weaned. Inevitable onset of middle age is also a period of stress. Rather than accept both the disadvantages and compensations of later life, some individuals indulge in self-defeating attempts to prolong youth. Middle age is often more stressful for women who have to cope with the physiological changes of the menopause. Depressive illnesses are common but it is uncertain whether physiological changes or social and psychological factors are mainly responsible.

Old age

This final stage of human development has been the subject of much psychological study. As a result of medical progress and improved social conditions more people are surviving into old age and their welfare is one of today's most pressing social problems. The high proportion of elderly people in mental hospitals shows how much remains to be done. This fact raises the question of whether the psychological changes associated with old age are an inevitable part of the biology of ageing or are avoidable consequences of social organization. As with growing up, it is difficult to link the onset of old age with any specific chronological age. The sequence of physical and mental changes in later life differs greatly from one individual to another. Indeed, perhaps the most striking feature of ageing is its individual variability.

Earlier categorization of adolescent changes into their physical, mental and social aspects provides a useful framework in which to examine the changes of later life. A reduction in physical energy is accompanied by increasing dimness in vision and hearing. Alterations in muscular control reduce mobility and the speed and dexterity with which movements may be made. These and other physical changes in an elderly person restrict his former pursuits and limit his social relationships.

The mental changes in old age are many and complex, which is another way of saying that we have much to learn about them. The capacity to learn new principles is reduced, resulting in progressive dependency on principles and ideas learned in the past. The older person tends to be more rigid in his thinking and less able to adapt to new ideas and experiences. There is a demonstrable reduction in capacity to handle information and less can be held at any one time. Retention of information is also easily disturbed by any other activity going on at the same time. These changes result in a tendency for older persons to be slower to grasp, poor in concentration and unreliable in memory for recent events. Recall of events in the more remote past is seldom impaired, this being another factor in making the elderly person more comfortable and assured when dealing with the past rather than with the present. Earlier it was suggested that one of the hallmarks of successful development in late childhood was the capacity to control impulses and emotions. In old age there is often a noticeable decline in this control so that an old person may appear childish and overemotional in his behaviour.

The social changes in old age reflect in large measure the role which society offers to its older citizens. Normally retirement from work occurs at the age of sixty-five although there may still be many years of life ahead. It is not until retirement that people realize how dependent they were on their work, even though their job may have been uncongenial or dull. Retirement involves separation from familiar surroundings and friends and, most important, a negation of the lifelong pride of being an independent contributor to society. It demands an abrupt change in established habits at a time when new adjustments are difficult to make. Such considerations do not apply to the housewife whose job has no retirement age, although her own domestic routine is likely to be disturbed by the continual presence of the former breadwinner. The social status of elderly persons has changed considerably. Grandfather is no longer accepted as the head of the family. Indeed, slackening of family ties may result in there being no easily accessible family contact. In an age which emphasizes youth's speed and flexibility the elderly are neither respected nor revered, but merely tolerated. Once the elders advised and guided others, but now they tend to be ordered about both by their families and by the social services. The loss of a functioning role makes an old person feel a social liability rather than an asset. It is impossible to estimate how many of the less fortunate changes associated with ageing are a direct and avoidable result of the social vacuum in which many of the elderly are placed. In societies where the elderly are still given a clearly defined and useful social role, there tends to be a lower prevalence of mental and emotional disturbances in old age.

Many old people adjust well to retirement by re-ordering their life around a rigid but secure pattern. Each hour of the day is fitted into a carefully planned programme. A routine helps to compensate for a declining capacity to deal with change and the unexpected. Illness requiring admission to hospital disrupts this well ordered existence and throws the old person into an alien and frightening environment full of uncertainties. It is then not surprising that some become emotionally disturbed and may deteriorate rapidly. Fortunately, hospital life is itself founded upon routine and, given time, the elderly patient may find security in its regularity. Most hospital staff are now aware of the dangers of allowing elderly patients to become too dependent and direct management towards as rapid a return to independence as possible.

ASSESSMENT OF PERSONALITY

All sciences strive to measure the material which they observe and psychology is no exception. The psychologist's task is especially difficult for the material which he seeks to measure is human behaviour. However, this has not prevented psychologists from constructing standard tests of selected aspects of mental functioning. Although such tests vary widely in the type of function which they seek to measure, they all have one thing in common. Each of them places the individual in a standard situation, defined by the nature of the specific test, and compares his responses with those of others in the same situation. Tests are standardized on a carefully selected sample of the population, so as to allow comparison of an individual's performance with that of others of his own age, sex and social background. The accuracy of the measurements always depends upon the reliability of the original standardization on the test population sample. Of the many standard psychological tests, intelligence tests are the most used, and we shall begin by considering how they are constructed and what are their uses and limitations. Later psychological testing of other areas of personality are described.

Intelligence tests

Intelligence tests play a prominent part in education and in vocational selection for industry and commerce. Many psychologists have viewed their increasing use with disquiet, wondering if they have created a latter-day Frankenstein monster over which they have lost control. Certainly the **intelligence quotient (IQ)** may be too easily regarded as a static and tangible part of the personality, a modern status symbol representing the individual's worth to society. It is important to realize that the IQ is simply a measure of an individual's performance at that time on a particular test. It is a relative measure in that it is based upon a comparison of the individual's performance with others of his age and background.

Like many other measurements of behaviour, the IQ may fluctuate with mood changes, interest and co-operation or with any other factors which affect mental output. If the IQ varied too widely from test to test or from time to time it would have little value in predicting future behaviour. This indeed occurs with very young children where the IQ is too variable to use in predicting future progress. The younger the child the lower the predictive value of the IQ. However, the young child's performance on a standard intelligence test offers an approximate comparison of his present level of ability with that of other children and this may often be a useful measure in itself. The child who is either developmentally retarded or precocious is spotted and the reasons for such findings may be discovered. In young children the capacity being assessed is still developing so that it is impossible to estimate accurately its final level. After the age of 9–11 years the probability of a marked change in ability is much less so that the IQ becomes a useful predictor of future intellectual level. Intelligence is of course only one factor in successful living and the estimation of a high or low IQ does not provide a ready means of predicting future successes or failures. Self-confidence, drive, emotional stability and specific non-intellectual talents have all to be taken into account if such predictions are being made.

In older children and adults, intelligence tests are useful in assessing present ability and future possibilities. How is the IQ calculated and what does it actually measure? The first of these questions is much easier to answer than the second.

The IQ is a statistical conversion of the subject's test score to a number representing the relative position of his performance to others of his own age. The term intelligence quotient is a legacy from the older method of calculating the intellectual level by the ratio of mental age to chronological age. Mental age merely represents the age level corresponding to the score reached on the test. Thus, if a child of 10 years gives a test score appropriate to that of the average 11-year-old child, his mental age would be 11 years and his IQ

$$\frac{\text{Mental age}}{\text{Chronological age}} \times 100 \text{ would be 110.}$$

This method works reasonably well for younger children but has grave disadvantages when applied to older children or adults. After the age of 13–14 years the gain in test scores per year is very small. It is for example impossible to find problems that an average 24-year-old person passes and an average 23-year-old fails. This limitation was formerly overcome by dividing the

Mental Age by a constant figure, usually 15, when testing adults. Although this practice allows for the absence of improvement in test performance after the age of 15 years it is too crude to give consistent results. This method of calculating the IQ was found also to accentuate the difference between IQ values derived from different tests.

A more satisfactory way of designating a subject's test performance is to express his score in the form of a **percentile**. The percentile compares the subject's test score relative to that of others of the same age on a ranking scale from one to ninety-nine. Thus a child who scores at the 75th percentile is in the top 25 per cent of his own age group. Percentile gradings can then be converted to standard scores with a mean of 100. Strictly speaking, the modern IQ is not a quotient at all but a standard score denoting the position of the subject's test score relative to others of his age.

The present method of calculating the IQ in terms of standard scores rather than quotients makes the assumption that intelligence in the community has a Gaussian distribution (p. 3.4). While this assumption has never been verified there is sufficient evidence to suggest that it is a

TABLE 40.1. Distribution of IQ levels in the Community.

IQ Level	Per cent of Population	Designation
Above 145	1	Gifted or genius
130–145	2	Superior
115–130	12	Above average
85–115	70	Average
70–85	12	Dull
55–70	2	Subnormal
Below 55	1	Severely subnormal

useful approximation. Table 40.1 shows that the majority of people have an IQ between 85–115. University students usually have an IQ of 120 or above although there is much variation above this level among different faculties. The accepted cut-off point for mental subnormality or deficiency is 70, although many children with an IQ below 80 require to be educated at a school for backward children. Most children and adults in the one per cent of the community with an IQ of under 55 require to be looked after in special institutions. It should be emphasized that the diagnosis of subnormality is never made solely on the basis of an intelligence test score. The ability of an individual to reach a reasonable level of social adjustment is a much more important consideration.

The question as to what is actually being measured with intelligence tests becomes pertinent when the bewildering variety of tests in present-day use is considered. Many of the tests consist of the type of problems associated with academic success. Such items include defining words, reading, giving opposites, arithmetical problems and general knowledge. These tests reflect the child's educational level and their emphasis on words and verbal reasoning favours the verbally fluent and well-read child. Although a good verbal knowledge and educational success is often synonymous with brightness, this is not always the case. A child whose education has been interrupted by illness or who is reared in a home where learning is discouraged may falsely appear to be intellectually retarded on such a test. Non-verbal **performance tests** avoid this difficulty and provide a measure of the subject's ability to reason in a non-verbal setting. Thus the **Progressive Matrices** test presents a series of incomplete geometric patterns which can only be completed by an appreciation of the relationship within the pattern. Fig. 40.1 illustrates a typical item from this test.

Many intelligence tests incorporate both verbal and performance sections. For instance the **Wechsler Intelligence Scale** is made up of six verbal and five non-verbal subtests yielding both a verbal and performance IQ, as well as a composite full scale IQ. Such tests may take longer to carry out but they provide more information.

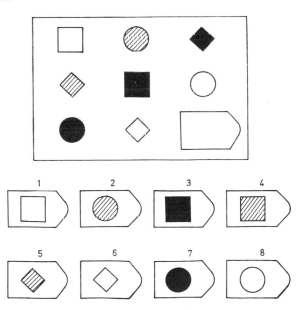

FIG. 40.1. An example of the Progressive Matrices test.

There has been much debate as to whether intelligence is inherited or a product of the environment. Twin studies and other controlled investigations have suggested that there is a strong genetic loading in intelligence. Perhaps such enquiries are fruitless and liable to mislead. Our constitution may contain our developmental potentialities but the environment determines to what extent and in what ways they are realized. The two factors always interact to such a degree that a clear distinction between their respective contributions is often impossible. The position regarding intelligence has been well stated by the Canadian psychologist Hebb who suggests that there are two aspects of intelligence, termed A and B. Intelligence A is constitutionally decided for each individual by the type of brain and nervous system with which he is born. This represents the individual's intellectual **capacity** or the range of his potential intellectual **development**. Intelligence B is a factor of experience and represents the stage of intellectual development within this range actually reached by the individual. The IQ, regardless of the type of test used, is always a measure of the developed ability of Intelligence B (we can never hope to measure a capacity or potential) although this is nevertheless a function of the inherited capacity of Intelligence A.

Although we might go through life indefinitely expanding our knowledge, there is much evidence that the human brain's intellectual capacity falls off in later years. In old age test results indicate a progressive inability to deal with new learning and an increasing dependence upon knowledge acquired in the past. The differential decline in some forms of mental output with age occurs also in a more exaggerated form as a result of brain injury or organic cerebral disease. This finding allows psychologists to use modified forms of intelligence tests to assess the degree of intellectual deterioration due to pathological changes in the brain. However, this is outside the scope of our discussion.

Personality testing

It would obviously be naïve to expect two people to behave in identical ways, just because they were of equal intelligence. The whole personality of the individual, attitudes, beliefs and emotional stability play a part in determining behaviour. Psychologists have attempted to devise tests which assess such personality differences with the same accuracy achieved in testing intelligence. As might be expected this attempt has been much less successful. Intelligence is a complex enough concept to define and measure but personality is considerably more so. Even if personality is reduced into its component parts, the components to be measured are far from specific. Thus **emotional stability** or its converse **neuroticism** are themselves an amalgam of many personality traits. Here the most frequently used forms of personality assessment are considered.

INTERVIEW

The interview is perhaps the most common method of personality assessment, but unfortunately assessments are often unreliable. One of the main difficulties is that the personality of the interviewer tends to intrude and distort his picture of the subject. Each interviewer adopts his own method depending upon his interests, likes, dislikes and prejudices. Without being aware of it he may allow one aspect of his subject, e.g. dress or appearance,

to colour and distort his general assessment of the person. Naturally, people vary greatly in their skill in interviewing but it is often the person who considers himself to be a good judge of character who is most subjectively biased. Some improvement can be brought about by standardizing the interview so that each interviewer adheres to a certain fixed framework.

The subjective factors in interviewing impressions may be reduced further by applying **rating scales**. These list on a graded scale the personality traits to be assessed. Thus, if we wish to include self-assertiveness in our evaluation, this trait could be rated on a five point scale from high to low degrees of assertiveness. Although this does not ensure the same standards for all interviewers, it reduces the range of disagreement. Standard rating scales are now occasionally employed in hospitals to give nurses and other observers a simple and more reliable way of setting down their impressions of patients. If many individuals have been rated on such a scale, it is sometimes evident that certain clusters of traits are emerging. For example, when such items as self-consciousness, blushing, poor sleep, restlessness and anxiety all have similar rating values, this may be a measure of **nervous disposition.** Such clusters have been extracted by statistical analysis and this allows rating scales to be used to assess more general aspects of personality. Such scales have also been used as diagnostic aids in psychiatry.

PERSONALITY QUESTIONNAIRES

To avoid the subjective errors inherent in the interview psychologists have constructed questionnaires. In most of these the subject's task is limited to reading a series of statements and underlining a response indicating whether the statement could be applied to him, e.g. I sometimes get dizzy turns. YES : NO. Many of these questionnaires aim their sights ridiculously high in attempting to make a full personality assessment on the basis of the subject's responses to fifty or more such questions. The more successful confine themselves to measuring one aspect of personality such as neuroticism, hostility or sociability. Some of these, such as the **Eysenck Personality Inventory** developed at the Maudsley Hospital in London, are claimed to discriminate usefully between neurotic patients and normal subjects. The validity of such claims depends upon how neuroticism is defined and whether it is thought reasonable to make a clear distinction between normal and neurotic. Nevertheless such questionnaires are useful in psychological research as a speedy and fairly reliable way of identifying groups of highly neurotic or highly stable subjects.

INTERACTION WITH THE ENVIRONMENT

Thus far we have been concerned mainly with the development of personality and with some of the effects of environmental changes upon the individual. Now some of the psychological processes which allow us to deal effectively with the environment are considered. Although each of these processes is considered separately, they are really different phases in the complex operation of processing information from the environment. These cognitive processes have been the subject of much experimental investigation and we are now nearer to understanding their functioning.

Attending

Before we can deal with events in our environment we must first become aware of them. From the everyday environment a multitude of stimuli impinge upon our sense organs and are then relayed by the nervous system to the brain. Not all these stimuli are taken in at once but rather certain stimuli are selected at the expense of others. The process of attention thus involves a selective filtering of the sensory input from the environment so that some stimuli are given priority over others. Psychologists have for long postulated a mechanism in the nervous system responsible for this selective filtering and have been encouraged by recent interest in the activity of the reticular system of the brain stem as a physiological correlate of attention.

Some stimuli are more attention-demanding than others, especially if they are sufficiently unusual to stand out from the background. Thus a bright light, a loud noise or a totally unexpected event claims our attention. Probably the most important determinants of attention are internal in that we are more likely to attend to events which accord with individual interests and needs of the moment. To the hungry man the odour of food cooking has priority over any other competing stimuli.

Selective attention, like most human processes, appears to develop gradually in early life. Indeed, one of the most characteristic features of the younger child is his inability to focus his attention on any one event for long. He is easily distracted by any change in his immediate environment. It is only as we grow older that we develop the capacity to ignore distracting stimuli. The efficiency of selective attention appears to fall off in old age so that the elderly person is easily distracted and unable to concentrate as well as before. Even in the healthy adult, attention fluctuates greatly. Fatigue, physical and mental, results in a less efficient filtering of the stimuli competing for attention and makes application to anything which requires rigorous concentration more difficult. On occasions when overanxious or preoccupied with personal worries, internal problems make it difficult to focus attention upon external tasks.

A breakdown in the attentive process is a characteristic feature of some forms of mental illness. The deeply depressed patient cannot attend to everyday events in the outside world because his attention is fully occupied with his own thoughts and feelings. In schizophrenia there is a reduction in capacity to attend selectively and the patient finds his mind being bombarded continuously by everything going on in the environment, so that his concentration is completely disrupted. However healthy adults, subjected to unusually high or low levels of environmental stimulation, respond in ways virtually indistinguishable from the schizophrenic. This is a partial corrective to the common assumption that schizophrenic thinking is completely alien to normal persons. It is possible that some of the success of tranquillizing drugs such as chlorpromazine is due to an action on the reticular activating system which brings the patient's attention nearer to its normal level of performance (vol. 2, p. 5.00).

Individual differences in the process of attention have been related to differences in personality. Thus, work carried out in the Menninger Clinic indicates that some people are particularly adept at directing their attention to relevant stimuli while ignoring irrelevant ones. Such people were found to be more self-controlled, assertive, confident and emotionally stable. Other individuals who were more passive in their attention and easily distracted were found to be lacking in confidence, less controlled in their emotions, more anxious and overconforming in their attitudes to authority. Although there is much to learn about the interaction between personality and cognitive processes such as attention, it seems that emotional maturity is an important factor influencing the habitual mode of attending and concentrating.

Learning

If our environment is to have any lasting influence on us, we must not only attend to events but learn from them and store the information for subsequent use. The capacity to store information and reproduce it after a period of time is considered later in the process of remembering. Learning may be broadly understood as any process which modifies experience and behaviour. Life is thus itself a continual learning situation as we constantly modify our attitudes, opinions and behaviour in the light of each new experience.

A young child faces every day a wide variety of new experiences which are continuously reshaping his view of himself and of his environment. As these influences are exerted long before the child is old enough to reason and to control his behaviour, most early learning is without insight and does not require the active co-operation of the child. Although analogies between humans and animals are dangerous, studies of animal learning help us to understand the process of learning in early childhood. The training of animals by establishing conditioned reflexes and by operant conditioning is described in chap. 25. Such procedures are used to teach circus animals new tricks and also by most parents in training a young child.

Parents condition their child's conduct by reinforcing with verbal or non-verbal signs of approval those aspects of his behaviour which they wish to encourage. Negative conditioning occurs when a child's actions are inhibited by association with displeasure arising from parental disapproval. Conditioned learning demands no insight on the part of the subject, who may be entirely unaware that his behaviour is being influenced, and the behaviour of young children can be modified in a short space of time by planned conditioning techniques. As the young child is exposed to parental and other sources of conditioning continuously throughout the long period of his development, much of early learning is of this type. Encouraged by observations of the efficacy of conditioning techniques, some psychologists suggest that all of our individual characteristics, likes, dislikes, our attitudes, opinions and indeed our whole personality are a product of social conditioning processes which begin in the home but continue throughout life.

The principles of conditioning may also be applied to the development of emotional responses. At the beginning of the present century, Watson suggested that the young infant displays only three basic emotional responses, fear, love and rage. At first these emotions are reactions to specific situations. Thus fear is expressed as a response to sudden movement, loud noise or loss of support. Watson argued that, by a process of conditioning, these three primitive emotions gradually become evoked by an increasing variety of new situations and experiences. He showed how a child could be experimentally conditioned to experience the emotion of fear to a new range of objects. This was done by the experimenters making a sudden loud anxiety-provoking noise each time a child was playing with a pet white rat. After repeated conditioning sessions the child not only showed fear of the rat but later extended this to a fear of all white furry objects.

An understanding of conditioned emotional responses is of value when treating neurotic patients who show inappropriate fears or **phobias** towards objects and situations which others experience as harmless (vol. 3, p. 35.18). It may be argued that all abnormal fears can be understood as conditioned patterns of behaviour. To take a simple example, a young child who is bitten by a dog when walking in a tunnel might develop a conditioned fear not only of dogs and other similar animals, but of enclosed spaces and darkness. This view is in direct contrast to the psychodynamic view of the origin of neuroses, in which symptoms are considered as a manifestation of unconscious conflict. Acceptance of the importance of conditioned learning in the development of neurotic symptoms has practical repercussions in their treatment. If such symptoms are learned responses, the most satisfactory treatment may be to help the patient to unlearn the responses by deconditioning them.

BEHAVIOUR THERAPY

This line of thinking has led to a rapid increase in techniques for behaviour therapy, applicable not only to patients with neurotic symptoms, but also to those with forms of unwanted behaviour which they find difficult to control.

Nocturnal enuresis (bed wetting) is one of the earliest examples of successful behaviour therapy (vol. 3, p. 37.4). One method is to have the child sleep on a mat connected to electrodes. The first flow of urine creates a short circuit which causes a bell to ring and wakens the child. With repeated wakenings and subsequently going to the toilet, the child begins to waken in response to the sensation of a full bladder experienced with waiting until urination begins.

Another successful area for behaviour therapy is in the treatment of patients who react with abnormally high levels of fear to objectively harmless objects and situations. Many of the methods used here, like the treatment of enuresis, are based on **reciprocal inhibition.** Thus, if anxiety can be inhibited continually in the presence of a phobic stimulus, the anxiety-provoking action of the stimulus is also inhibited. A specific application of this, used in the treatment of phobic states, is known as **systematic desensitization** (vol. 3, p. 35.12). Basically this consists of first teaching the patient how to induce a state of muscle relaxation and then having him imagine a hierarchy of situations which make him anxious, starting with the weakest item and eventually reaching the strongest one. The hierarchy of fears of course varies from one patient to another but let us imagine a person who has a weak fear response to the sight of blood, a strong fear response to being shut in (claustrophobia), with other fears of intermediary strength. After a period of relaxation training the patient is encouraged to imagine himself in a situation where he or someone else is bleeding. As soon as he begins to feel anxious, he is told to stop imagining the scene and to relax. After continually revoking the scene in association with relaxation the patient finds himself able to imagine the event without any increase in anxiety. Once this has been established he moves on to the next higher situation in his fear hierarchy, and so on until he reaches the object of his strongest fear response. This method and variants of it have been successful in the treatment of fear responses. An important consideration in this and many other behavioural treatments is that their very simplicity may allow the patient to continue treatment in the absence of the therapist, thereby increasing the valuable element of self-control. Modified versions of this approach have been applied to other personal problems such as low self-esteem and lack of self-assertiveness.

If we ask why many psychiatric patients remain incarcerated in hospital for long periods of time, the answer is not always the obvious one of the patient's general mental state. Often, the main factor preventing a return to the community is one or a few specific behaviours which are socially disturbing and which would elicit strong negative reactions from others. Again, simple **behavioural modifications** have enjoyed great success in altering socially unacceptable specific behaviours, thus allowing some patients to be discharged while still showing some psychotic behaviours, but only those tolerated by others. Repeated shouting of obscenities, abhorrent eating habits, repetitive grimaces or odd ritualistic movements, stealing and hoarding are examples of deviant behaviours which make adjustment outside hospital difficult. The ways in which such behaviours are modified may appear to be naïvely simple but they are based upon rationally derived laws of learning and they are highly effective.

One example might be mentioned by way of illustration. A chronic psychiatric patient, resident in a mental hospital for many years, had been stealing and hoarding towels in her room for over 9 years. All efforts to stop this had been of no avail until a psychologist trained in behavioural techniques suggested the following programme. Each day the nursing staff entered the patient's room at regular intervals depositing towels, without comment. At first the patient continued ritualistically to fold these towels and put them away. However, when the number of towels in her room reached 625 she was satiated and began to return towels to the nursing staff who expressed their pleasure. Over the next year she was never known to return to her hoarding behaviour. The success of many behavioural methods of inducing habit change might cause us to be optimistic regarding their application to the eradication of common unwanted behaviours which have hitherto proved resistant to traditional approaches. May such methods be effective in aiding people to stop smoking or in producing weight loss in overweight individuals?

Many behavioural methods have been used to eliminate cigarette smoking. Some have applied the principle of satiation, having subjects smoke to order over lengthy sessions to the point of nausea. Others have attempted to link smoking with aversive stimuli such as electric shock or abhorrent odours. Yet others attempted to increase control by using mechanical counters or cigarette cases which can be opened only at fixed intervals. These, and countless other variations have shown that it is relatively easy to reduce intake to 10 to 14 cigarettes per day, but that the behaviour is highly resistant beyond that point and relapse is usual. It has been pointed out that an effective method of stopping smoking is to obtain a medical degree. Doctors have a high success rate in breaking the habit, particularly those specializing in internal medicine and radiology. Interestingly, psychiatrists have the poorest success rate of all branches of the profession. This has been explained on the grounds that

their work involves a great deal of passive listening. Perhaps an alternative explanation is contained in the finding that smokers as opposed to non-smokers are more 'neurotic, restless, extraverted, impulsive and have stronger feelings of inadequacy'.

The treatment of obesity by behavioural methods has fared a little better than that of smoking, but again the results are disappointing. Many attempts have been based upon the established finding that the eating habits of obese people are more controlled by external, environmental cues, usually related to the accessibility of palatable foods, while those of the normal eater are more controlled by internal physiological cues. Most behavioural programmes train the individual to notice the external cues which are for them highly conducive to eating and to avoid these or obtain partial control over their consequences. Subjects are asked to keep detailed data sheets of their eating and associated behaviours and also of daily weight fluctuations. The positive effect of a weight loss is heavily reinforced in either individual or group sessions with the therapist, while weight gains are carefully explored to identify the behaviours leading to increased eating. Again, it is puzzling why this simple form of behaviour appears to be so difficult to control. Perhaps the answer is that overeating is less simple than it appears at first sight. For example, one study finds that husbands of obese women are frequently the main stumbling block, in that they overtly or covertly encourage their wife's overeating and repeatedly negatively reinforce any weight loss accomplished.

Much of human learning cannot be fully explained by conditioning and in later childhood and adult life learning becomes progressively more self-directed and is accompanied by insight. Insight is a sudden understanding of the principle involved in solving a new problem and allows this principle to be applied to subsequent learning in similar situations. The point of insight in learning is usually derived from a **repatterning** of the various elements of the learning situation, leading to a new relationship between the different parts of the problem and so providing the solution. The information required to solve many problems in daily life is available, either externally in the nature of the problem itself or internally in the form of stored memories of past learning. The point of insight is reached by first discarding items irrelevant to the solution and mentally reconstructing the relevant information to achieve the correct fit. Thus a doctor's information consists of his observations of a patient's signs and symptoms and his own previous learning of their diagnostic significance. He first discards features which appear irrelevant to this particular case and then mentally manipulates the relevant information until the correct arrangement suggests the most likely diagnosis. The nature of this diagnostic process is discussed more fully in vol. 3, p. 60.14.

Learning through insight consists of a phase of **inhibition** which allows attention to be concentrated on what is relevant, followed by a phase of **organization** whereby the relevant information is put together. The efficiency of this organization is related to intelligence and is largely a function of individual innate capacity and acquired knowledge. The initial process of inhibition is related to attention and is more likely to be affected by a current state of mind. Tiredness, anxiety or any other temporary emotional state is likely to make us less effective in inhibiting irrelevancies and so reaching the heart of the problem.

When any act is fully learned or overlearned by constant repetition it may become a skill which can be reproduced without conscious deliberation. The child develops the skill of walking without pondering on each movement, and of talking without deliberating upon the enunciation of each word. Conscious attention appears to be concerned mainly with the resolution of uncertainty, with acts which require decisions to be made. If something is learned so thoroughly as to become automatic, all uncertainty is eliminated and it can be carried out without thought or effort. Indeed, the focusing of conscious attention upon a skilled act which has become automatic may disrupt its normally smooth execution. The experienced driver often finds his expertise rapidly disappears when he attempts to teach someone else his skill. The well-practised radiologist or medical diagnostician may find similar difficulty in teaching his ability to others simply because it has become a highly developed automatic skill. We often use the word **intuition** when describing an act performed with skill as a result of many years of previous learning experience.

Remembering

The process of memory cannot be divorced from that of learning and it is often difficult to distinguish between a memory deficit and learning deficiencies since we cannot expect to recall something inadequately learnt. As already seen, learning is, in its turn, dependent upon the earlier phase of attention, so that all these factors operate in the learning process. Remembering is the final stage in the learning process by which we are able to make use of the stored results of previous learning. Memory is the capacity to retain in the brain a record of past experiences and to recall this record into consciousness when required.

Neurophysiologists and more recently biochemists have speculated on the form in which this continuous recording of experiences is registered in the brain (chap. 25). For many years psychologists have assumed the presence of a **structural memory trace** involving an actual modification in the brain cells. Biochemists have suggested that the memory trace may be recorded in changes in the structure of RNA molecules in individual neurones.

Whatever the form of the permanent record, the brain must possess a gigantic storage capacity to house all the experiences registered throughout life. Perceptual studies suggest that the human brain is capable of receiving around 1000 units of information in one-tenth of a second. If allowance is made for sleep this means that something in the nature of 15×10^9 units of information may be stored in a 70 year lifetime. This is rather more than a thousand times the available number of nerve cells in the brain. Any theory of memory storage must also account for the capacity to erase some of these records which are no longer of use. We do not need to clutter up the brain with telephone numbers and other items which need only to be remembered long enough for the appropriate action to take place. A somewhat different theory of memory suggests that memories are stored in the form of a **dynamic trace** which need not involve any structural alteration in the brain cells. This theory sees memories as consisting of active patterns of electrical impulses which have no specific static location. A nerve impulse travelling around a closed loop of connecting neurones might be the mechanism for such a dynamic memory trace.

Although it is difficult to assess directly the validity of these two theories, it is possible to make some indirect judgment of their comparative value. The electrical activity of the brain may be temporarily disrupted or stopped by freezing techniques or by electric shock. If the dynamic trace theory is correct such disruption should affect memory storage while in the structural trace theory no disturbance of memory need take place. We can then carry out a simple experiment in which an animal is trained in a new task, e.g. running in a maze, and then given a strong electric shock. If it now performs the task as well or better than before, its memory has been unaffected and presumably did not depend upon reverberating patterns of neural activity. In fact, the findings from this sort of experiment do not completely contradict either theory. If the shock is administered some time after the initial learning of the maze, memory is completely undisturbed. However, if the shock occurs immediately or very soon after the initial learning, memory is disturbed. This is also in accordance with the known effects of electroconvulsive therapy in human beings after which most recently stored events are more likely to be erased. Such results suggest that events may be recorded initially as electrical activity and subsequently transferred to a more permanent store in the form of structural changes in the nerve cells. An oversimplified model of this two-phase theory of memory is illustrated in fig. 40.2.

As we can attend to only one source of stimulation at a time, attention may be regarded as a selective filtering of the sensory input from the environment. The selected information then passes into a short term memory store where it may be held before being passed into the more

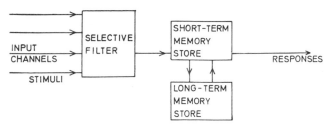

Fig. 40.2. The two-phase theory of memory.

permanent memory store. However, as it would be uneconomical to retain a permanent record of every event, information may be held in the short term memory store only long enough to allow an appropriate response to be made. Thus we may wish to remember a telephone number only long enough to be able to dial it. In this case there would be no need to transfer the information to the more permanent long term memory store.

This division of memory into two stages is of both theoretical and practical importance. It accounts for our capacity to store some events long enough to allow an appropriate response to be made without transferring such items into permanent storage. The two types of storage systems operate on quite different principles and most types of memory failure occur during the initial phase of short term storage. Although our long term memory appears to have an almost unlimited capacity for storing information this is certainly not the case with short term memory, which is very restricted in the amount of information it can handle at any one time. Thus, most adults can adequately hold around seven digits but any digits arriving in short term memory in excess of this number interfere with the storage of the earlier digits and errors occur. Information held in short term storage is thus very vulnerable to disturbance by the arrival of fresh information. If we are interrupted when dialling a telephone number by being asked a simple question this may be sufficient to wipe out our temporary storage of the number.

However, in everyday life we frequently require to hold in mind for a short time sequences of information which are much longer than the seven units said to be our maximum capacity. The writer would have no difficulty in memorizing the sequence of 10665844114226007372436, a total of twenty-three digits. The load on my short term memory is reduced greatly by the fact that this sequence is capable of being reorganized into fewer units of information. The first four digits are the date of the Battle of Hastings, 58441 is my telephone number, 14.2.26 my date of birth, 007 a familiar sequence to the James Bond fan and the last six numbers (37–24–36) represent some very significant statistics. In this way a sequence may be recorded and stored in six units without overloading available storage capacity. Normally, of course we should

not require to memorize a long number sequence, but in listening to someone speaking we are constantly required to store very long sequences of words for a brief period. Studies of speech perception show that we perform a similar coding operation upon the language input so that the message is registered in groups of words or phrases, rather than as individual words.

Another factor which further reduces the load on short term memory is that normal language contains many words which are redundant, in so far as they are unnecessary for adequate comprehension of the message. When listening to speech we need not burden our limited storage capacity with these redundant words which can easily be filled in later because they are determined by their context. The amount of redundant information in a verbal message will of course vary with the degree of conventionality of the statement. In the sentence; 'The canary escaped when his cage door was left . . .', it does not matter whether or not we hear or forget the last word as we can see from the context that it is probably 'open'. Indeed, the message 'Cage door open—canary escaped', conveys the same information adequately although 50 per cent of the original words have been removed. If, however, the message to be conveyed is highly original, abstract and concise, as in a closely reasoned argument, we may require to register almost every word to be sure of grasping its significance.

It is a useful, although a painful experience, to examine the proportion of redundant words used in my own efforts to transmit thought to paper. The same process may be seen to operate in the act of speaking as in listening to speaking. A great deal of speech requires little or no thinking, being composed of conventional phrases and clichés which literally roll off the tongue. If, however, we attempt to express our thoughts on something new and original, our speech requires more planning and is a great deal less predictable. Studies of the normal speech process show that spontaneous speech takes the form of phrases of four to six words followed by brief but measurable pauses. The words following such speech pauses are often more abstract and convey more information than the words preceding them. These pauses thus indicate the points in a person's speech when he is actively thinking. We often associate fluency in speech (the absence of pauses) with intelligence and original thinking. Such studies serve to remind us that lack of hesitation may often merely indicate that what is being said is either well practised or at a low level of thinking, or simply that the speaker is long winded.

Earlier in considering old age, comment was made on the complaint of poor memory frequently made by elderly people. Studies of the way in which memory changes with age suggest that such difficulties are nearly always confined to the initial stage of short term storage. As we grow older the amount of information capable of being held in short term memory decreases and the likelihood of interference in initial registration is enhanced. Older people also appear to have more difficulty, both in recoding information into more easily manageable units and in screening out redundant information. Thus, in listening to speech the elderly person has to handle a greater volume of information and is more likely to be overloaded and confused.

Many of the effects of normal ageing on short term memory occur in a more exaggerated form in patients with organic brain disease. Indeed, a failure in short term retention is often the first observable sign of an organic dementing process. Severely subnormal defectives have been shown to have surprisingly good powers of retention for material which has been adequately assimilated into long term storage, whereas their short term retention is extremely poor. Such findings help to explain some of the difficulties experienced by some patients in concentrating and in communicating adequately with others. They also suggest some of the ways the patient may be helped to improve his performance. Patients with poor short term retention can function much more adequately in conversation if the speaker talks slowly, avoids long phrases and redundant words and gives the patient sufficient time to register their meaning and construct his own thoughts before replying.

Patients with other types of memory disorder show very little impairment of short term memory, their deficit being in the transfer of information from short to long term storage. Thus in Korsakoff's syndrome (vol. 3, p. 35.72), an organic disorder, the patient may retain events well enough for short periods but be unable to form lasting durable memories. There is also some suggestion that the more durable long term memory store may sometimes be affected by the result of cerebral damage destroying specific structural memory traces and producing isolated islands of forgetting.

The majority of examples of normal forgetting in healthy adults can of course be explained without recourse to specific organic changes. Some cases of apparent forgetting are more the result of inadequate learning. Actions may be performed that are so habitual, e.g. winding one's watch, that they are never consciously registered and are therefore difficult to recall. From what has been said the impression may have been given that memories are static entities, which once fully registered are safe from any further influence. This would be a very false impression for we consistently modify our memories during the process of storage. Most types of inaccurate memory entail, not complete forgetting of an event, but its recall in a distorted form. This re-shaping and falsification of memories is usually in the direction of changing the memory of the event to make it more pleasant and self-satisfying than the actual event itself.

The longer the time interval between the event and its subsequent recall and the greater the emotional involvement, the more chance of such distortion. Thus, memories of central events in early childhood are likely to be highly distorted, both by the passage of time and the need to remember these days in the most pleasant manner. The summers of our childhood are always sunnier than those of today! Freud and the psychoanalytic school saw the influence of emotions on memory as the chief cause of forgetting and memory distortion. The term **repression** is used to denote the process by which impulses and memories unacceptable to us are barred from consciousness. Much of what we forget usefully helps us to avoid the unpleasant associations which remembering would bring. In some neurotic patients repression is a central feature of the symptoms. In times of war many men suffer from symptoms arising from the complete repression of a highly traumatic event. In such cases treatment is aimed at helping the patient to relive the repressed event and to dissipate the feelings of anxiety associated with it. In cases of pathological repression it is possible for the actual memory of the event to be retained but the feelings associated with it to be repressed. A few cases of amnesia are caused by the complete repression of a period of life involving great stress, such as the unhappily married man who may forget the whole period of his marriage. However, repression seldom works effectively. Although the memory or feeling associated with it may be shut out of consciousness, its presence is displayed in the form of neurotic symptoms of anxiety and general feelings of dis-ease.

Thinking

Thinking is in a sense a continuous process in that it is doubtful if the mind is ever blank. On occasions when we might describe ourselves as thinking about nothing, we should more accurately speak of thinking about nothing in particular. We are not consciously directing our thoughts on to any specific issue but rather allowing them to follow their own, apparently random course. One might then begin by recognizing two different types of thinking. **Directed thinking** (rational thinking or reasoning) consists of the active focusing of thought on to a specific problem. **Undirected (autistic) thinking** is more passive, less conscious and less attuned to objective reality. This distinction is similar to that made in psychoanalytic theory between **primary** and **secondary process thinking**. Primary process thinking which may appear random is directed by unconscious fantasies, while secondary process thinking is consciously directed to dealing rationally with the external environment. One might also liken undirected autistic thinking to the primitive form of egocentric thinking already described as characteristic of early childhood.

In discussion of the learning process some of the factors governing directed thinking were mentioned. Effective reasoning involves both the inhibition of irrelevant information and the organization of the relevant information to allow a rational conclusion. Ineffective reasoning may be due to the distracting influence of irrelevant factors or to a failure in perceiving correct relations between the relevant items. Effective reasoning, directed towards the solution of a specific problem, is typical of that used by scientists, mathematicians and also by physicians in their efforts to reach a correct diagnosis. It is, however, quite unlike the type of thinking indulged in by the artist, the poet and the mystic. Such people deliberately relax their normal inhibitory processes and detach their thoughts from objective reality in an effort to avoid the restrictions of logic and reach a deeper and wider level of subjective awareness.

In some forms of modern art autistic thinking predominates so that the communication between the artist and his public is at a level beyond that of conscious logic. We may speak of finding a painting disturbing or uplifting without having a conscious knowledge of the causal factor at work. Much of our normal day-dreaming may be described as autistic in so far as it is concerned with inner fantasies rather than external reality. It is of interest that day-dreams carried out at a lower level of consciousness, e.g. when we are tired, become increasingly visual in nature. Our thoughts, free from their normal control, are translated into visual images, so vivid that they may become confused with external events. At an even lower level of consciousness, during sleep, the pictorial representation of autistic thinking becomes more strikingly evident in the form of dreams.

As normal thinking fluctuates between these two objective and subjective poles it would be more accurate to speak of two **aspects** rather than two types of thinking. The thought process might be viewed as a continuum with wholly subjective thinking, as in dreaming, representing one pole and the deductive thinking of the mathematical scientist the opposite pole. Thinking at different times occupies different positions in this continuum depending upon external circumstances and upon our inner mental state.

In times of stress or severe emotional strain thinking deviates markedly towards the autistic side of the continuum. Our thoughts are then less attuned to the world outside, more preoccupied with our inner fantasies and problems. Most of the time an adequate compromise is reached between personal desires and the restrictions of the environment. It is only when thinking becomes so autistic as to distort reality that our behaviour may be described as neurotic. If an individual's thinking becomes so dominated by autistic trends that he has literally lost control over the direction of his thoughts, contact with reality has been abandoned and a psychotic process is evident.

For centuries people have suggested certain similarities between the autistic thinking of the psychotic and that of some highly creative gifted people. One earlier deduction from this suspected correspondence, that genius is akin to madness, has been completely dispelled by systematic surveys which indicate, if anything, a lower incidence of psychiatric illness among highly creative people. Nevertheless, interesting similarities between creative and psychotic individuals have been noted. Both show highly unusual associations in their thinking, report odd body sensations (such as ringing in the ears, peculiar odours), a high incidence of mystical experiences, restlessness and proneness to impulsive outbursts. A recent, as yet unpublished study by the author shows that both schizophrenic and creative individuals deploy their attention more widely, taking in more information from their environment than less creative people. Certainly, many of the world's great discoveries have been made by individuals who noted some peripheral events which most of us, wearing our habitual blinkers, would have ignored as irrelevant.

Since Freud first described the dream as 'the royal road into the unconscious' psychiatrists and psychologists have been interested in the type of thinking occurring in dreams. Freud's experience with his patients led him to believe that much of human behaviour was controlled by forces which normally lie outside conscious awareness. The relaxation of conscious controls during sleep allows these unconscious impulses to slip through in the form of dreams. By examining the dreams of his patient the psycho-analyst hopes to widen his understanding of factors which influence his patient's behaviour. As the thoughts and wishes expressed in dreams are unacceptable to the conscious mind of the dreamer, the true meaning of the dream often remains hidden. Later recall of dreams is greatly distorted and frequently the dream may be completely forgotten or repressed. Thus the difference between the frequent and infrequent dreamer is regarded as one of accessibility of recall. In Freudian theory, dreams are seen as having a therapeutic function in so far as they allow the dreamer to discharge his inner conflicts and tensions in a harmless way.

It is now possible to examine the process of dreaming more directly. The use of the electroencephalogram (EEG) provides a recording of the brain's activity which affords an objective measure of the depth of sleep (vol. 3, p. 58.1). Close observation of normal adult subjects during sleep indicates the presence of sporadic scanning movements of the eyes at certain stages of sleep. The recording of such rapid eye movements (REM) has led to the finding that these occur only during dream activity. By examining the occurrence of rapid eye movements it is now possible to chart the course of dreams and, by referring to the EEG record, relate these to the level of sleep at which they occur. Most studies agree that dreams tend to occur at the lighter levels of sleep and that the lighter the sleep level, the easier the later recall of the dream.

There would appear to be surprisingly little individual variation in the amount of dream activity, a total of approximately 90 min/night being spent in dreaming (vol. 3, p. 58.3). The main difference between the person who recalls dreaming every night and the person who seldom recalls dreaming may then be that the former is a lighter sleeper. This may also help to explain reports of an increase in dreaming, commonly given by emotionally disturbed people. Emotional tension is likely to lead to a shallower sleep and thus to an increase in recall dreams. Freud's view of the dream as a safety valve which siphons off inner tensions is given some support by experimental studies of dreaming. Subjects who are deprived of dreaming, by being briefly wakened on the occurrence of REM, develop symptoms of irritability, apprehension and anxiety. Such changes do not occur in subjects who are also wakened briefly during the night at times when there are no rapid eye movements. If subjects are allowed to sleep undisturbed after a few nights of being dream-deprived they dream most of the night and awaken refreshed and symptom-free.

The context of the dream, sleep itself, is still by no means fully understood. The magic formula of eight hours each night is frequently put forward as a necessary component of healthy adult life. If their normal sleep rhythm is temporarily disturbed many people experience a rapid reduction in their general efficiency and sense of well being. The habitual insomniac will testify to the ill effects of a poor night's sleep. Studies of volunteers who have been kept awake for lengthy periods, demonstrate the almost psychotic-like symptoms which can occur through extreme sleep loss. On the other hand, some people appear to get by very well on only a few hours' sleep each night. A former colleague never slept more than three hours a night but had the mental and physical energy of several men. Although a temporary disruption of the normal quota of sleep has adverse effects, these often disappear if the disturbance continues over a long period. People appear to adjust gradually to a new standard in their sleep rhythm.

It seems likely that, like most other habits, the personal sleep rhythm is to some extent conditioned and, once well established, difficult to alter. Many parents have to make a temporary compromise between their own already established sleep habits and those of their young child who has yet to be conditioned into the acceptable pattern of slumber. The normal sleep pattern does not, however, remain static in adult life. Surveys of sleep habits show that most people sleep less as they grow older. The proportion of people, aged 25–34 years, who report sleeping less than five hours a night is around 10 per cent. By the fifties this proportion has risen to over 29 per cent, and after the age of 65 years to over 40 per cent (vol. 3,

p. 58.4). In contrast to this trend, older people complain less of the adverse effects of sleeplessness. This may mean that there is less need for sleep as we grow older. Some of these surveys show a strong sex difference in sleep habits. Where females are more likely to report insomnia in middle-age, the peak incidence for males is reported at 65–70 years. This may reflect the disruption of normal daily habits consequent on retirement.

In discussing the process of dreaming, reference has already been made to the effect of the emotional state on sleep. Anxiety and worry may prevent the relaxed state of mind which allows sleep. Sleep disturbance is such a common feature of many psychiatric conditions that sleep rhythm may be regarded as a sensitive barometer of our current state of mental health.

Stress

The question arises whether the apparent increase in mental breakdown is due to the stress of modern life. First, it is not certain that there has been a real increase in psychiatric illness. New psychiatric treatment, combined with public education, has lessened the stigma attached to mental illness and people are now more ready to seek psychiatric help. However, the query is raised as to whether all mental disorders do not arise in individuals subjected to too much stress. Knowledge of the more serious psychiatric conditions, the major psychoses, suggests that these illnesses are a result of biochemical changes affecting a genetically vulnerable nervous system. Although external stress may trigger off such illnesses as affective psychosis and schizophrenia, yet the basic cause is probably internal. However, what of the less serious, but often incapacitating neurotic illness, the **nervous breakdown**, which figures so prominently in contemporary life? May the onset of symptoms of anxiety be due to continual exposure to an overdemanding and stressful environment? A difficulty in answering these questions is that circumstances, which provoke stress in one individual, another may take in his stride. What an individual finds stressful reflects to a large extent his past experiences, from early childhood onwards. Thus marriage, promotion at work, parenthood, death of a parent, may or may not be stressful depending upon past experiences and the significance of such events for the individual.

Nevertheless, many people like Hamlet appear to break down under the 'sea of troubles' to which they have been exposed. The traumatic event which immediately preceded collapse may have been no more than the final link in a long and unremitting series of stresses. 'It is the last straw which breaks the camel's back', expresses proverbially that when people are forced to make too many decisions at once or to perform beyond their capabilities, performance deteriorates and adverse effects become evident. People differ widely in the amount of stress they can tolerate. There is evidence that this is partly constitutional and that individual differences may be apparent as early as the first few months of life. Neurotic symptoms develop when an individual's capacity to tolerate stress is exceeded by the amount of stress imposed upon him.

On the other hand some neurotic illnesses may be a reaction to apparent absence of stress. For example, a young housewife's symptoms of anxiety and depression may be related to the boredom of being confined in a house with young children. People often go out of their way to participate in stressful situations, from the thrill of the big wheel at the fairground to climbing dangerous mountains. The effects of monotony and the need for some excitement and stimulation have been the subject of much psychological research. A practical problem in World War II was how to maintain the vigilance of men and women at anti-aircraft sites through long periods of idleness and boredom. Technological changes in industry have committed many workers to the important but monotonous task of monitoring dials and gauges of automated machines. Vigilance in such dull situations soon suffers as the operator's attention lapses when he feels irritable, restless and bored. Studies of the effect of different types of monotonous conditions have shown the deleterious effects of boredom. Some of these have gone to great lengths to create an artificial environment in which normal stimulation is reduced to a minimum. In one such experiment the subjects were suspended in a tank containing water at body temperature. The experimental tank was constructed so that the subjects could neither hear, nor see, nor have any sense of pressure, movement or touch. In such extreme conditions the subjects quickly experienced failure in concentration, confused thinking, hallucinations and feelings of panic. In interpreting the findings of such experiments Hebb concluded:

'The well-adjusted adult therefore is not intrinsically less subject to emotional disturbance; he is well-adjusted and relatively unemotional, as long as he is in his cocoon (his cultural environment). We think of some persons as being emotionally dependent and others not; but it looks as though we are completely dependent upon the environment in a way and to a degree that we have not suspected.'

All these observations suggest that man's adjustment to the environment is precariously balanced. If individuals are to function continually at a level beyond their capacity, performance falls off and the effects of stress become evident. If they are subjected to a non-stimulating, non-demanding environment, similar reactions result. A severe reduction in contact with the outside world produces, not tranquillity, but thought disorder and panic.

The way in which individuals react to stress has been the subject of much psychological research. Some have examined the reactions of people in real life situations, such as facing major surgery or learning to parachute from aircraft. Others have examined the reactions of subjects in controlled laboratory conditions by exposing them to various stimuli such as electric shocks or intense noise, or by showing them motion pictures depicting disturbing scenes. Although the findings of such studies vary with the type of stress, there are principles which appear to operate in all stressful situations. First all stress is subjective, in that its effects upon the individual depend less on the situation itself and more upon the manner in which the individual perceives or appraises it in terms of his own capabilities. Secondly prior knowledge of the situation, an ability to predict the coming events and a sense of control over events aid an individual in a threatening situation in such a way as to reduce its stressful effects. When an individual's capacities are not compatible with the demands he has to face, he may be said to be stressed. When he feels unprepared and uncertain about a situation, he is likely to feel helpless and to react as if it was highly stressful. People whose work exposes them to continual danger seldom show signs of severe stress because their training has prepared them and they feel that they can predict and control all eventualities.

The effect of perceived control has been demonstrated in many laboratory studies. Thus subjects exposed to noxious stimuli, such as high intensity noise or electric shock, withstand higher levels of the stimulus for longer periods if they have access to a switch by which they may themselves reduce the intensity of the stimulus. An interesting finding is that the stressful effects are reduced even when the control switch is made ineffective, and whether or not the subject chooses to use it. The important factor in reducing stress seems to be the subject's perception of himself as having some control over the threatening situation, even though the control is illusory. These effects are apparent not only in the subject's judgment of the degree of stress experienced, but also in the physiological reactions associated with stress.

Such conclusions may be relevant to the doctor-patient relationship. A doctor is often confronted with the problem of how frank he should be without subjecting his patient to undue stress. Such judgments are normally tempered by the doctor's assessment of the stress tolerance of each patient. However, some stresses are faced more easily if the patient has the knowledge to allow him to anticipate his future and so to bring to bear his own strategies for coping with it. This may be especially true if the knowledge gives him some sense of control over the development of his condition and removes a feeling of helplessness.

Fear of the unknown is the greatest cause of subjective stress. Studies of surgical stress illustrate this.

Adult patients awaiting major surgery were observed and their anxiety assessed by a method which allowed three levels to be distinguished, low, moderate and high anticipatory fear. Low fear patients showed little or no concern over the coming operation, had high morale and did not require sedatives. Moderate fear patients were more preoccupied with the impending operation and often requested information concerning the operation and its consequences. High fear patients were immersed in their fears, could think or talk of nothing else and required large doses of sedatives. In the postoperative period the low fear group were most distressed, least co-operative, required most analgesics and remained in hospital longest before discharge. Those who made the quickest recovery and showed the best adjustment after the operation fell mainly into the moderate fear group. Although such differences in reaction to surgical stress reflect to some extent differences in personality, the investigators were convinced that this was not the most important factor. Indeed, later studies showed that the main determinant of postoperative adjustment was the amount and detail of information given to the patient prior to his operation. Those patients who received specific information regarding the operation, the type and intensity of postoperative discomfort to be expected, the probable length of convalescence, etc., were better adjusted after the operation, required less medication and were discharged earlier than patients who were given little information. Again the conclusion is drawn that forewarning of a stressful event is more conducive to a sense of personal control and a more rapid and stable adjustment to the situation.

The most obvious reaction to stress is a heightened level of anxiety and the measurement of such anxiety is a feature of all research on stress. Some psychologists rely mainly on the subject's assessment of his own feelings by requiring him to fill in a questionnaire with a rating scale devised to provide a quantitative assessment of anxiety or other emotional changes. Others, critical of such self-evaluations, rely more on physiological indices of emotional change. Thus, heart rate, blood pressure, respiration rate and volume, electrical resistance of the skin, changes in adrenal secretions and changes in eosinophil count (p. 27.36) have all been employed as indicators of changes in anxiety level. When, as is usual, both physiological and psychological ratings correspond roughly, there is no great problem. However, if the subject reports that he is not at all anxious but his physiological reactions indicate high anxiety, which source of information is the real measure of anxiety?

At first sight the physiological variables appear to be a more objective measurement of reactions to stress than the subject's descriptions and self-ratings. However, initial trust in the physiological reactions may be dissipated when a number of such measurements show poor correlations, not only with the subject's self-descriptions but also with each other.

It has been suggested that none of the physiological changes measure anxiety *per se* and that they are more indicative of changes in general arousal level. A state of hyperarousal may be associated with anxiety or with other moods such as rage. Anxiety is only one of several forms of a state of psychological activation which may accompany physiological arousal.

This argument corresponds well with the findings of studies of emotional reactivity. Individuals were asked to rate the intensity of physiological changes, such as an increase in heart or respiration rate, experienced in situations which aroused their emotions. Later they were exposed to these situations and the physiological changes recorded carefully. Those subjects who had reported that they experienced intense physiological activity tended to overestimate greatly the changes observed, while those who reported low levels of physiological activity underestimated the physiological changes. It would seem that our perception of the activity of our cardio-respiratory system is unreliable, so it is not surprising that psychological and physiological measurements of emotion often disagree. These and other findings support the view that although physiological arousal causes a heightening of generalized emotional activity, the specific emotion experienced depends upon individual interpretation of the situation. If this view is correct, a specific pattern of physiological change corresponding to each emotion is unlikely. The alternative view is that all emotions may be associated with a common pattern of physiological changes. If, for example, a threatening situation induces a heightened level of generalized emotional activity, this may be experienced as anger or fear, depending upon how the situation is perceived. The final emotional experience is thus seen as an amalgam of both affective and cognitive factors, the former providing the intensity of the experience and the latter deciding its quality.

This way of looking at the emotions has led psychologists to study individual differences in the threshold, duration and intensity of emotional reactions. Everyday observations suggest that some people react intensely and for a longer time to situations which evoke little or no reaction from others. It has been suggested that such individual differences reflect the responsiveness of the autonomic nervous system. Pronounced individual differences in adult subjects have been demonstrated. Differences in the autonomic response of young infants and even in neonates have also been shown to occur. Furthermore, observations support the view that some individuals show responses which might make them vulnerable to certain disorders. Thus in response to stress neurotic patients have a greater elevation of blood pressure than normal controls.

There is good reason to suppose that the response of

the autonomic nervous system is likely to determine the pattern of symptoms as a result of repeated exposure to stress. However persons with marked responses are not necessarily those whom we think 'overemotional'. Two people might have the same tendency to have intense and prolonged autonomic responses when angered but differ greatly in their behaviour; one might habitually 'blow up' with rage while the other might 'bottle up' his hostility.

Consideration of some of the problems inherent in measuring emotional reactions reinforces earlier conclusions that the cognitive components of stress, i.e. the way in which the individual perceives and appraises the threatening situation, play a paramount role in his subsequent reactions and behaviour.

PAIN

Experience of pain, whatever the cause, is a stress and is normally associated with the psychological and physiological reactions that may accompany stress. Both the reported severity of pain and the reactions to it depend greatly upon the significance of the source of pain to the individual. For instance both may be considerably less in soldiers wounded in combat than in civilians with wounds of comparable trauma obtained in an industrial or traffic accident. The soldier perceives his wound as honourable, and it removes him from the battlefield. In contrast, the civilian may see his wound as an unwelcome intrusion upon his normal life.

Many studies indicate that a large part of the action of opiates in alleviating pain is due to a reduction in anxiety (vol. 2, p. 5.48). Suggestion plays an important role even in the reduction of anxiety produced by analgesic drugs. If a patient has faith, both in a drug and in his doctor, an inert placebo may relieve pain as effectively as the true drug, even when the pain is due to untreatable cancer. The experience of being treated or of actively doing something to control the pain may be as beneficial as the treatment itself. This has been observed in a study of natural childbirth (vol. 3, p. 40.18) in which there was no difference in the ratings of the severity of the labour pains by mothers trained and untrained in this method of psychoprophylaxis. However, mothers trained in the method reported less anxiety with the labour pains.

Many claims have been made for the pain-reducing effects of hypnosis. Since Esdaile, a native of Montrose, reported in 1845 the use of hypnosis in India for operations on Hindu convicts, medical journals have reported the successful use of hypnosis in operations ranging from tonsillectomy to the removal of haemorrhoids. Many early studies of hypnotic analgesia relied solely upon the subjective reports of the patients. Later observations included measurements of physiological reactions, e.g. changes in heart rate, blood pressure, skin resistance, respiration and muscle tension. These suggest that, although hypnotized subjects may report marked alleviation of pain, the physiological responses are unaffected.

While at first sight these findings may appear to signify the efficacy of hypnosis in reducing the subjective aspects of pain, further examination renders this conclusion less tenable. Thus, for example, one study compared the analgesic effects of local and general anaesthetics with hypnotic induction and with instructions to imagine an analgesic state. It was found that, while both types of anaesthetic (novocaine and nitrous oxide) reduced subjective ratings of pain and physiological reactivity to pain, the hypnotic and waking suggestions were equally effective in reducing subjective ratings but equally ineffective in producing any physiological effects.

A series of ingenious studies indicate that a primary analgesic effect in hypnotic instructions is to dissociate attention from the painful stimulus. Thus, subjects instructed to imagine pleasant scenes or to listen to a distracting auditory message such as a detective story while subjected to painful stimuli, reported the same degree of pain reduction as subjects under hypnotically induced anaesthesia. Again, neither procedure had any influence on physiological reactions. Such findings accord with the conclusion reached by Liébeault in 1891 that 'the process of suggested analgesia can be described simply as the focussing of attention on ideas other than those concerning pain'. Hypnosis involves a close trusting relationship between patient and hypnotist. Many anaesthetists who have used hypnotic suggestion have become convinced that much of its analgesic effect is engendered by the security of the close relationship created between doctor and patient.

Much of this discussion also applies to analgesia by acupuncture, a subject which has risen in interest now that the Chinese are encouraging more contact with Western medicine.

DEATH

It seems likely that man is the only creature who is conscious of his own mortality and is therefore subject to the fear of dying. The end of physical existence is perhaps the greatest trip into the unknown and for many people the fear of death is a source of stress (vol. 3, chap. 59).

Studies of people facing impending death have produced interesting findings. The conclusions of several such studies are summarized by one psychologist after many years of observing the dying: 'The crisis is often not the fact of oncoming death *per se*, of man's insurmountable finiteness, but rather the waste of limited years, the unattempted tasks, the lost opportunities, the talents withering in disuse . . .' In other words, the main stress for many is not death itself but the frustration of not having reached one's goals and aspirations. It is therefore not surprising that death is more likely to be peaceful in the elderly.

A mental state of stress cannot in itself produce death, as in so-called 'voodoo death', but a prolonged state of personal distress may reduce resistance to illness or increase the likelihood of an ongoing disease ending fatally. When such circumstances arise the term psychosocial death has been used. Thus studies of victims of severe burns indicated that eventual death seemed often as much related to the function threatened by the injury and its personal significance to the victim, as to the actual severity of the burn itself. In other studies of young adults who had died suddenly a high proportion were found to have been in a state of prolonged psychological distress and death was by no means an inevitable consequence of the pathological condition found at postmortem. Engel sums up such observations as follows: 'If we come to believe that there is no solution either because of forces beyond our control (helplessness) or because of our own worthlessness and inability to cope (hopelessness), we may be driven not only to give up, but ultimately into the deadly "giving-up—given-up" complex, in which for the helpless patient there is no present and for the hopeless there is no future. This mental state does not cause disease . . . nor is it necessary or sufficient for disease to develop. But it does reduce the body's ability to deal with potentially pathogenic processes.'

This comment may go some way to explain why, for example, elderly people who feel that they have no personal choice in the decision governing their admission to nursing homes or mental hospitals are more likely to die within two months than other elderly patients whose admission was of their own choice. It may also explain reports of increased death rates in the period immediately following bereavement. The Elizabethan poet, Sir Henry Wotton, wrote of the death of Sir Albertus Moreton's wife,

> 'He first deceas'd; she for a little tri'd
> To live without him; lik'd it not and di'd.'

We may conclude that, like beauty, stress is in the eyes of the beholder. The degree to which a potentially threatening situation is seen to be stressful depends upon the way in which it is construed. This in turn depends upon a number of factors including past experiences of life, the habitual level of emotional activity, the form and strength of defensive capacities and the extent to which an individual feels prepared for the situation and perceives himself as being in control of it. Any generalizations regarding stress reactions must take account of all these factors in order to arrive at a balanced judgment.

STANDARDS OF NORMALITY

The terms **normal** and **abnormal** are commonly used by psychologists and psychiatrists but they are seldom defined precisely. Like many words in both everyday and technical usage, **normality** is given many shades of meaning. Perhaps the most common lay use is exemplified in the words of an American comedian who declared: 'My wife is abnormally immature; if I'm sitting peacefully in my bath she'll think nothing of walking right in and sinking all my little boats!' In this usage it is assumed that we are normal and that the behaviour of others may be judged abnormal to the extent to which it deviates from our own standards.

Four different connotations given to the term normality are examined below. However, first consider some of the dangers which arise from a too-ready and not always justified confidence in our ability to distinguish the normal from the abnormal.

David Rosenhan, Professor of Psychology at Stanford, was the author of a devious but interesting plot. He organized a group of eight adults (4 psychologists, a paediatrician, a psychiatrist, a painter and a housewife) to seek admission as patients to psychiatric hospitals in different regions of the USA. Each of these 'pseudo-patients' arrived at the hospital admission office complaining of hearing voices. Apart from describing this symptom, they gave a truthful account of their personal and family history. Not too surprisingly, each person was admitted to hospital with a provisional diagnosis of schizophrenia. Immediately upon admission the pseudo-patients ceased to simulate any symptoms and behaved in their normal way. After a period ranging from 7 to 52 days, all were discharged as being schizophrenic 'in remission'. In spite of Rosenhan's conclusions to the contrary, the mean hospitalization period of 19 days might be interpreted as a favourable testimonial to the hospitals concerned. Since the 'patients' had simulated auditory hallucinations and it takes time to assess the psychiatric state of a newly admitted patient, their short stays say much for the wise management by the staff.

Of more interest were the observations made by the pseudo-patients concerning what Rosenhan refers to as the 'stickiness of the psychodiagnostic labels'. Once the diagnosis of psychosis had been made, normal everyday behaviours of these eight people were interpreted as being abnormal. Thus, gazing out of the window was interpreted by staff as 'probably hallucinating', writing notes as 'compulsive writing', being early for lunch as 'pathological oral acquisitive behaviour', etc. Later Rosenhan extended his study by informing another psychiatric hospital that, within the next 3 months, one or more pseudo-patients would attempt to gain admission. Although in actual fact no pseudo-patient presented himself, 10 per cent of the genuine admissions over the next 3 months were assessed as pseudo-patients by at least one psychiatrist and one other staff member.

Rosenhan's conclusions are an instructive caution to the tacit assumption that normality and abnormality can be differentiated easily, at least by experts. 'It would be a mistake, and a very unfortunate one, to consider what had happened to us derived from malice or stupidity on the part of the staff. Quite the contrary, our overwhelming impression of them was of people who really cared, who were committed and who were uncommonly intelligent. Where they failed, as they sometimes did painfully, it would be more accurate to attribute these failures to the environment in which they too found themselves ... Their perceptions and behaviour were controlled by the situation ...'

At the risk of sermonizing, one further word regarding another naïve tendency sometimes found in those working in the mental health field is worth making. Too often stability and good mental health are assumed to denote an absence of all the features we associate with neurotic or disturbed behaviour. Several investigators have examined the personalities of people who are regarded by others as normal individuals. These studies show that such people have a narrow constricted emotional range, seldom becoming excited, avoid risk-taking situations, lead a life free from crises, have a limited fantasy life, distrust imagination, and prefer action to introspection. As one researcher puts it—'they may be stable but they strike one as being unduly benign and well accommodated'. Indeed, they display a personality which is in vivid contrast to highly creative individuals who are frequently excitable, introspective and habitual risk-takers. We might also remember that a moderate level of anxiety is associated with academic and vocational competence. Paradoxically being 'normal and well adjusted' may not always indicate ideal mental health.

This last paradox may become clearer as we turn now to examine four different concepts of normality.

DICHOTOMOUS CONCEPT

The history of psychiatry has involved much argument between those who measure mental health on a continuum and those who regard normality and abnormality as constituting a clear-cut dichotomy. In mediaeval times the latter view was well accepted. People were either healthy and normal or abnormal and possessed by a devil. Although this view has been greatly modified with increased understanding of mental illness it was not until the advent of psychoanalytic theory that the dichotomy between normality and abnormality was finally bridged. By viewing neurotic symptoms as a product of unconscious conflict Freud demonstrated that the difference between normality and neurosis is one of degree and not of kind. Although few contemporary psychiatrists disagree with this argument as applied to the neuroses the dichotomous standard of normality is still often applied to the more serious psychotic mental disorders.

The conception of specific disease entities which has dominated European psychiatry since the time of Kraepelin (1856–1927) denies that the psychotic process is merely an extension of normality. A person has or has not schizophrenia, just as he has or has not cancer. It is now appreciated that this all-or-none concept cannot always be correctly applied to physical illness and it may be that the dichotomous approach may have to be abandoned in psychiatry. However, at the present time we do have two separate standards of normality operating in the field of mental health, depending upon the nature of the disorder. This double standard easily leads to double talk in psychiatric diagnosis when we fail to distinguish which standard is being applied.

STATISTICAL CONCEPT

In discussing the distribution and measurement of intelligence a purely statistical approach to normality is utilized. Normal intelligence is here defined as being around an IQ of 100 and abnormal degrees of intelligence, low and high, lie on either side of the distribution curve. The normal may be the average in many aspects of human behaviour and this is an assumption used by clinical psychologists in assessing mental health. This way of assessing normality is quite different from the dichotomous approach, for it implies a continuum between normality and abnormality, which differ only in degree. The whole idea of constructing standard psychological tests of behaviour is based upon a statistical approach to normality and in practice this often works well.

A statement that a 1 year-old infant's physical development is abnormal because it deviates in certain ways from the average level of development of other 12-month-old infants is informative and useful. The parallel statement that a person's behaviour is abnormal because it deviates from the behaviour of others of a similar age and background is also useful but a great deal less simple to demonstrate. While it is relatively easy to assess the normal (average) level of physical development at different ages, it is extremely difficult to assess what is the normal distribution of specific forms of behaviour. Another difficulty is that the norm of behaviour may vary in different social groups. If a statistical survey of the incidence of wife beating is made it will be found to occur sufficiently infrequently to call it abnormal behaviour. However, if the survey is confined to a particular social group it may be found to be statistically normal for this sample. Are we then to say that for members of this social group it is abnormal not to beat one's wife? This dilemma is perhaps more evident when we consider the third concept of normality.

ADJUSTIVE CONCEPT

A common denominator in all mental disorders is the inability of the individual to adjust harmoniously to others and to the society to which he belongs. Thus a common criterion of normality in psychiatry is the degree to which an individual can adjust to his environment.

Inability to accept the prevailing social standards, either because of aggressive defiance, fear, withdrawal or personal deficiency, becomes the criterion of abnormality. This method of defining normality equates it with conventionality. The well-adjusted person is the conventional individual who conforms to the prevailing standards of conduct. This approach has much in common with the statistical method, both equating unusual and unconventional behaviour with abnormality. This concept of normality has provoked the caustic comment that 'the capacity to share the delusions of the crowd is a sign of individual health.' If normality is measured in terms of adjustment to society, it is clear that mental health must be assessed with reference to a particular society. An individual, who is well adjusted and therefore normal in one society, may be maladjusted and abnormal in another society. As different cultural groups with differing standards exist within any one society, the decision as to whether an individual's behaviour is to be judged normal or abnormal requires detailed reference to his social background.

This problem is intensified by the fact that those who have to make such judgments (psychiatrists, social workers and magistrates) are frequently from a different social background from the individual whose normality is to be assessed. In some parts of the Scottish Highlands 'second sight' is not so much a sign of abnormal mental functioning as a matter of keeping up with the McDonalds!

IDEAL CONCEPT

Some systems of measurement are based upon a flawless or ideal standard of normality. If the dentist used a statistical concept of normality he would remove healthy teeth in an effort to make his patient more 'normal' for his age. The dentist and the physician have in their mind an ideal set of teeth and a perfectly functioning human body which, although seldom seen, acts as a standard of normality. Unlike the other views, the ideal concept implies an absolute, rather than a relative criterion of normality. Although this approach avoids many of the pitfalls inherent in the other concepts it is seldom used in psychology. The reason for this is simply lack of adequate knowledge of the ideal qualities of human behaviour and mental health. Perhaps one day understanding of human nature will be sufficiently advanced to allow us to aim at an ideal level in human behaviour. Indeed it may be necessary to find a new yardstick for assessing human conduct independent of any one society if the human race is to survive.

INDIVIDUAL REACTIONS TO SOCIAL PRESSURES

Thus far we have concentrated mainly on individual behaviour and ignored the large segment of psychology which concerns itself with man as a social being whose behaviour is influenced by the many social groups of which he is a member.

It is impossible to refer to all facets of such a diverse field as psychology in a brief chapter but it is appropriate to end by considering some aspects of social behaviour which have relevance to contemporary life.

From birth onwards we repeatedly make compromises between our individual needs and those of the social groups to which we belong. Adherence to group norms and standards demands a level of conformity which ensures the comforting sense of belonging and group acceptance. Persistently individualized and nonconforming behaviour runs the risk of incurring rejection and the uncomfortable sense of isolation and of being different. The pressure towards conforming behaviour is increased by the complex nature of modern society which encourages reliance more and more upon experts in various fields, apparently qualified to offer authoritative advice on issues which we can only understand dimly.

As in every other form of human behaviour, people vary greatly in the way they cope with such pressures from social groups and figures of authority. Some appear to be highly suggestible and uncritically conforming, while others demonstrate a more questioning and individualized attitude. Such individual differences may merely reflect levels of knowledge and the more compliant may be simply less well informed. Psychological research suggests that intelligence and knowledge are perhaps less important than other personality differences in causing some people to be more compliant and easily manipulated than others.

Research in the middle 1950s demonstrated both that conforming behaviour could be measured reliably and that overconformers tended to display a different pattern of personality traits to nonconformers. People who were easily swayed by group pressure in a number of experimental conditions tended to be accepting and submissive, insecure and vacillating in making decisions, confused and easily disorganized under stress and overanxious and worried by others' opinions of them. In contrast, people who were habitually resistant to group pressure were regarded as capable, self-reliant, relaxed and good leaders. It would thus seem that persons with certain types of personality are more easily manipulated by group pressure than others.

These studies dealt almost exclusively with the impact of group pressure upon the individual. However, as already hinted, pressure from one's peers may be less powerful than suggestions made by someone perceived as an authority figure. The use or abuse of authority in manipulating others is of obvious significance in contemporary life and is important in wartime when situations involving conflict between individual conscience and obedience to authority are readily evident.

EXPERIMENTS ON CONFORMITY

It was with such questions in mind that Stanley Milgram conducted an unusual and frightening series of experiments in the 1960s. He advertised for adults to take part as paid subjects in an experiment on the effect of punishment on memory. Subjects were instructed that they would work in pairs, one as 'teacher' and one as 'pupil'. The pupil would be strapped in an 'electric chair' in a small booth and be required to answer questions on a learning test put to him by the subject acting as the teacher. Each time the pupil gave an incorrect response or did not respond to a test question, the teacher was asked to press a button giving the pupil an electric shock. The teachers were told that the punishment must be progressively increased by the teacher raising the voltage given for each successive error by manipulating a lever in front of him. The lever could be moved along 30 positions each marked with the appropriate voltage from 15 to 450 volts and ranging from 'Slight Shock' to 'Danger—Severe Shock'.

As the experiment went on the victim's protests and screams were clearly audible. Some victims, while being strapped into the apparatus, said they had a bad heart. After reaching 300 volts there was an ominous silence from a victim who had been banging on the booth and protesting about the pain a few minutes before. The teacher was then told to continue with the assigned items, increasing shock intensity each time there was no response from the victim.

Before conducting the experiment, Milgram presented his plan to a large group of psychology students and asked them to estimate what percentage of adults would be likely to obey all instructions and continue to the end of the experiment, thereby giving a dangerous 450 volt shock to their victim. The estimates varied between 0 and 3 per cent with an average of 1 per cent. Milgram then proceeded with his experiment and found that 65 per cent of his subjects complied with all instructions. Before the conclusion is drawn that this experiment illustrates the sadistic tendencies of research psychologists, it should be explained that the situation was completely contrived. The pupil in each case was a confederate of Milgram posing as a subject and was not receiving actual shocks. However, the subjects who acted as teachers did not know this.

How are these findings interpreted? Had Milgram been unfortunate enough to have recruited unwittingly a goodly number of cold-blooded sociopaths? This explanation seems unlikely since those who continued to administer punishment according to instructions were extremely upset by the experiment which they found as harrowing as their imagined victim.

Obviously most of the teacher subjects felt compelled to act in a manner contrary, not only to the interests of their pupil, but also to their own personal dictates. Why then did they continue to obey the instructions? Milgram deduced that a prime factor was the authority engendered by the fact that the experimenter was a professor of psychology at a respectable university (Yale). There seems little doubt that the unquestioning acceptance of an apparently reliable authority is a powerful force in the readiness with which people perform actions normally regarded as antisocial.

This suggestion was confirmed in a later experiment where peer group pressure was substituted for the effect of obedience to an authority figure. It was found that, although peer group pressure still caused individuals to act in a more antisocial way than they would normally do, the manipulative effect was less powerful than pressure from an authority figure.

Milgram saw his study as a minuscule demonstration of the denial of self-responsibility which may occur in a more dramatic fashion during war and social unrest. People of any nation, at any time, he argues, may be easily manipulated by the pressures of society to behave in a manner alien to their moral code. World events have made this suggestion of even grimmer import.

It may be wondered to what extent such conforming antisocial behaviour might be modified by the fellow-feeling induced by some form of relationship between the victim and his persecutor. Milgram's subjects were unknown to each other. Might they be less likely to obey instructions which would imperil someone who was less anonymous and known to them?

The likelihood of this suggestion is heightened by another study. Here student volunteers were assigned to four person groups. In one group the subjects were rendered anonymous by being shrouded in bulky coats and hoods. Subjects in the other groups were clearly visible, wore name tags and were frequently referred to by name by the experimenter. Both groups were placed in an experimental condition which ostensibly involved their giving painful electric shocks to two girls who were confederates of the experimenter. The subjects in the anonymous condition proved to be much more aggressive, giving stronger shocks, than the subjects in the individualized groups. This study demonstrates that anonymity has a heightening effect on the perpetration of aggressive acts upon others, whereas an underlining of personal identity lowers the likelihood of such behaviour. Milgram found a similar effect in another study in which the closeness of the relationship between the teacher subjects and their victims was varied systematically. His findings clearly demonstrated a lessening of obedience to instructions as the proximity of aggressor and victim increased. It is alarming to note that even with closest proximity, when the subject was required to hold his protesting victim's arm down on the shock pad while administering the shocks, approximately one in every three subjects obeyed all instructions.

One effective method of increasing the anonymity of the victim (and thus increasing the likelihood of people conforming to aggressive instruction), is to have the victim appear as alien, subhuman, and in different ways less deserving of humane treatment. This, of course, is what the propaganda machines of wartime seek to do to our perception of the enemy whom we must learn to kill without compunction. However, the strategies used to evoke such conforming behaviour are by no means limited to international conflict.

Most civilized people reacted with abhorrence to Hitler's so-called 'Final Solution' to the 'Jewish problem' in Nazi Germany. In 1969 a social scientist at the University of Hawaii assembled over 500 students to seek their co-operation in a project to solve 'the problem of the mentally ill and emotionally unfit'. The students were given a long authoritative discourse upon the increasingly higher rate of breeding in the mentally and emotionally unfit members of the population, who might eventually endanger the fit segment of society. It was suggested that the only feasible solution was a legalized and widespread programme of euthanasia or mercy killing. It was emphasized that this extermination of the unfit would be both a boon to healthy mankind and a kindness to the subhuman mentally unfit. Presented with this solution parallel to Hitler's but couched as a respectable scientific programme, just over two-thirds of the 500 students indicated their approval of this programme of 'systematic killing'.

ROLE OF THE DOCTOR

Some occupations have always enjoyed a particularly high status in the eyes of the community and have automatically shrouded their practitioners with the mystical mantle of inviolable authority. This is particularly evident in occupations which play an essential part in the maintenance of healthy human existence, and where there exists a clear gulf between the knowledge accumulated by the trained expert and the rest of the community. The medical profession is in an unusually powerful position to exert such authority and to be the sometimes reluctant recipient of such projections of omnipotence from the lay public. Most people entertain problems concerning their own mortality and, in times of ill-health, they are especially vulnerable to an almost regressive dependency upon the skill and wisdom of the physician-healer. Like all positions of authority, this enforced and constantly reinforced respect may be utilized beneficially or abused. It is important for the doctor to realize that his authority emanates from at least two sources, his accumulated diagnostic and treatment skills and the less rational, but equally powerful, assumption that anyone with his apparent power over health and sickness, pain, life and death, must be all-knowing.

People under stress are particularly sensitive to suggestion and may approach their doctor with questions whose answers have little relevance to his education and skill. It is sometimes difficult to avoid the temptations inherent in being placed in the position of an oracle but, like all professionals, the doctor should always be prepared to admit his ignorance on issues where his expertise is probably no greater than that of any other intelligent person. Thus, the patient who seeks answers to questions on issues of personal concern such as marriage or their career may often more profitably consult a member of another profession, unless of course the answer depends on the assessment of a physical disability.

The doctor's personality is sometimes a powerful intrusive force. His biases and prejudices may exert as much unwitting pressure upon the patient's subsequent behaviour as his medical advice. Thus, studies show that doctors who have strong personal feelings against alcohol are less successful in dealing with patients who have become dependent on it, although their hostility is evident only in analyses of their speech tone, and not its content. Students' interactions with their teachers while awaiting the results of examinations may become almost neurotic and they may misinterpret the casual remarks or behaviour of their instructors as substantiating their worst fears. For example, one student said: 'I passed Professor A in the corridor today and, when I commented that it was a nice day, he replied that it wasn't all that good. This means that he knows that I have failed and that I have no right to be cheerful.' If the casual remarks of university instructors can have such an effect, the potential havoc wrought by a doctor dealing with an anxious patient can readily be imagined. A simple 'I see!' while taking a blood pressure may raise the level in an impressionable patient.

The reader might feel that a very simple point is being emphasized to an absurd degree and that most doctors are aware of the possible impact of their behaviour upon the state of mind of their patients. However, situations commonly arise where unnecessary distress is caused, not by lack of care, but by lack of communication. Patients entering hospital are vulnerable to the alien world of uniforms, apparatus, and muted secrets, especially if they are very young, very old or inexperienced in hospital routines. Recently the author was called to see an elderly lady in hospital for the first time, awaiting a minor operation. She had suddenly become acutely anxious, unco-operative, and determined to discharge herself home. It was suspected that she might be showing signs of senility. A brief conversation with her revealed what was to her a rationally based problem. In the days awaiting her operation she had seen several fellow patients moved to the theatre, but they never returned. To her, with her fears of the unknown and her lack of knowledge of the existence of the postoperative ward, this could only mean one thing—the operation in each case had been fatal. Once reassured by a brief reunion with her fellow patients, happily recovering in the other ward, her anxiety and deviant behaviour quickly evaporated. This is a simple illustration of the ever present need to understand the patient's view of the hospital world and the possible impact of unexplained events upon him.

Nowadays with better educational standards and a steady diet of dramatized medicine on television, patients are less likely to endow their doctor with superhuman attributes. In addition, many doctors now respect the intelligence of their patients and explain their procedures and decisions. However, the lowering of the doctor to nearer the mortal plane may have undesirable consequences. If, as seems conclusive from a number of studies, the beneficial effects of many medical treatments are partially dependent upon suggestion from an authority figure, any lowering of the doctor's status also lowers the placebo element in treatment.

Another social pressure merits a brief reference. Press reports frequently describe situations where an individual has been faced with acute stress or threat and there have been many witnesses who refused to intervene and offer help. For example a young woman has been stripped, raped, and beaten to death, a youth stabbed in an underground station and left to bleed to death, and numerous individuals have collapsed in city streets, obviously ill or injured, and in the presence of many bystanders, none of whom has offered help. American psychologists have made studies aimed at answering the question, when will people intervene in a crisis? Their results indicate that the obvious answer, that contemporary life has left people isolated and uninterested in the pain of others, is untrue. Witnesses to such events are upset and feel guilty over their lack of intervention. Indeed, this series of cleverly planned studies where people thought that they were witnessing a real crisis, demonstrated that by far the most important deterrent is simply the number of people witnessing the event. The greater the number of observers who share the responsibility for intervention, the less the likelihood that anyone offers help. It seems that shared responsibility diffuses individual reactions to such a degree as to paralyse the normal tendency to help someone in trouble. You may be better off if your car breaks down on a country road than on a main highway!

FURTHER READING

KRECH D., CRUTCHFIELD R.S. & LIVSON F. (1969) *Elements of Psychology*. New York: Knopf.

McGHIE A. (1973) *Psychology as Applied to Nursing*, 6th Revised Edition. Edinburgh: Churchill Livingstone (because it is relevant to medical students, although written for nurses—and for other egocentric reasons).

MILLER G. (1970) *Psychology—The Science of Mental Life*. Harmondsworth: Penguin (because it is a sound introduction to the subject).

MOWBRAY R.M. & RODGER T.F. (1970) *Psychology in Relation to Medicine*, 3rd Revised Edition. Edinburgh: Churchill Livingstone (because it is one of the few good texts specifically written for medical students).

Chapter 41
Man as a social animal

It is only necessary to watch someone walking into a crowded room to realize that man is a social animal. His movements, his dress, his first words of greeting and the way he looks around his immediate environment, all have been shaped to varying degrees by myriads of past interactions with other human beings.

In studying this relationship social psychologists have used as a central concept the notion of **social group**, a simple definition of which is: '...two or more people who interact more with each other than with other people.' Such interaction must occur in order to achieve any objective beyond the reach of an individual. Early examples in evolution were probably moving rocks or lifting logs and later, hunting for food. Modern examples are the sending of a spacecraft to Venus and the organization of the Olympic Games.

It is tempting to say that man's evolution has been influenced by living in herds for so long that he is now naturally gregarious and has a social instinct. This proposition cannot be tested and carries no useful practical implication; the facts may be accounted for more simply by saying that he joins social groups because he needs what he can get from them in order to survive. His first social group after birth is based on food. Unlike many other organisms, the human neonate does not have pre-programmed behaviour that enables him to locate the nutritious parts of the environment. Instead, he enters a social group, usually a dyad, with his mother, which supplies this need and in so doing shapes his behaviour in more or less enduring ways.

It is a paradox that when one personality is compared with another, many of the differences and the similarities are due to their involvement in a multiplicity of social groups. It is true, of course, that the blueprint of physical structure is laid down in the chromosomes and certain features of this physical structure have important repercussions on the personality. The endocrine system, for example, influences a basal level of temperament and the potential of intelligence and physical appearance are likely to influence social success. But these innate physical factors are inextricably interwoven with social experience. There are undoubtedly other elements about which little is known because they are never observed in pure form.

At the risk of oversimplification, we may describe this interplay by drawing an analogy between the adult personality and a furnished room. The dimensions of a room are fixed, but they interact to create a sense of proportion. This, in turn, depends very much on the way in which the room is decorated with planes of colour and on the arrangement of lighting. When the furnishings are added, they alter the general impression which is itself changed by what is there already. So the room assumes a unique and complex personality. It has been formed by interaction between the innate and acquired. It can be drastically changed, but refurnishing is laborious and limited by the basic structure of the room.

Every social group arises because a number of people want the same thing and none of them can achieve it alone. This is the **group goal** which members share in common. In addition different members stand to gain a wide range of subsidiary rewards. Most students in university groups want to achieve a degree or the learning which it symbolizes; in addition some want to get away from home, some to gain social status and others to meet girls.

If the value to an individual of the rewards drops below a certain level, membership lapses and he withdraws from the social system. If he wishes to attain the goals, however, he must continue membership of the group and conform to certain expectations. He may be informed of these by a threatening whisper or a printed constitution. The principle is the same.

The first kind of expectation is that in order to achieve the group goal, different members must restrict their behaviour to roles which complement each other. The second is that for the same reason the members are expected to conform to certain standards of behaviour, belief, opinion and attitude, called **norms**. Much human behaviour may be accounted for by saying that man learns the roles of father, businessman, husband, club secretary, 'one-of-the-boys' and many others, as prescribed by overlapping social groups. He also learns standards of honesty, punctuality, liberalism and aggressiveness, each of them the accepted norm of one or more social groups.

The process of conformity

An early systematic study of social conformity was made during the 1930's, using the autokinetic phenomenon. The subjects were asked to report the extent of movement of a pinpoint of light at the far end of a darkened room. When they did this by themselves there was a narrowing in their judgements over successive trials. If two people worked together publicly the estimates converged towards each other.

This approach was criticized because the stimulus was too ambiguous for the results to be relevant to judgements and opinions in real life. But in a classic and somewhat disturbing set of experiments, Asch subsequently revealed more of the power of group influence. His stimulus was a 20 cm line, drawn vertically on a piece of card. About 45 cm away were three more lines, one of 20 cm and the others differing by from 1·0 to 4·5 cm. The task was to identify the lines of equal length and subjects were asked to call their answers aloud, beginning from the left. Only one in the group of subjects was genuine and he had been manoeuvred into a seat on the right. The rest had been primed to give a pre-arranged wrong answer. Here, the stimuli were unequivocal, but just over one-third of judgements were given in a way that can only be described as contrary to the plain evidence of the senses. In more elaborate experiments subjects have been placed in booths with communication channels that purport to show decisions made by their colleagues in adjacent booths, but which are actually controlled by central switching. Under this pressure, 37 per cent of a sample of U.S. Army Officers agreed with the statement: 'I doubt whether I would make a good leader', although when questioned individually not a single one agreed.

Another study showed that the number of articles rejected by industrial inspectors could be changed greatly by manipulating the number of faulty articles ostentatiously put to one side by some members of the group.

There are many variables which have been shown to effect the degree of change in judgements, attitudes opinions and behaviour as a result of social interaction. For example, the greater the ambiguity of the stimulus or issue, the more readily can change be induced. Much of the information that the layman receives about politics and also medicine is of this kind.

The degree of privacy is obviously crucial. Many people go along with the group in public but privately know better. In an experiment in which judgements of modern paintings were recorded after a discussion with a dominant partner, half the final decisions were given in sealed envelopes and half declared publicly. The latter, needless to say, showed more conformity. A useful concept to describe double standards is **compliance**, but compliance is often the first step towards genuine conformity.

If a man submits readily and with conviction to group pressure, it is too facile to describe him as weak. Up to a point, conformity is a highly adaptive mechanism, because uncertainty is disruptive to the personality. Also, other people frequently do know better than oneself and unity of thought and action does bring strength to social groups and helps to achieve individual goals. However, unthinking compliance is sometimes maladaptive and society can only surmount this difficulty by purveying independence as a social norm for the behaviour of its members. This does not mean nonconformity, which is simply the irritating converse to conformity, but the ability to consider all available past and present sources of evidence before judging or acting. Other aspects of the effects of various pressures in producing conformity are discussed on p. 40.26.

The family

In the majority of societies, the family is the most powerful social group. When born into a family, we are involuntarily exposed to a particular set of cultural norms and role expectations. The leaders of the group control potent rewards such as love and affection. It is hardly surprising that in spite of the rebelliousness of the young, attitude surveys show a fairly high correlation between children and their parents on public issues. Because it is so obvious, it is easy to overlook the fact that we learn the language spoken in our family and this is probably the richest heritage of a transmitted culture. Although the language is a vehicle of exploration, it also selects and limits our attitudes and experience. Working class children in our society are hampered in the development of abstract thought processes which comprise intelligence because their early language has been limited to the expression of the concrete.

An important question is the effect of different regimes of child rearing on subsequent personality. This is a huge problem, bedevilled by the lack of valid methods for measuring personality on the one hand and the notorious difficulty of obtaining accurate information from mothers on the other. Most investigators have tried to do this retrospectively, but they encounter selective forgetting, repression and distortion which brings the past more into line with the idealized norms purveyed by neighbours and women's magazines. Many mothers are more sensitive about their choice of child rearing methods than about their choice of hats.

Attempts to relate specific practices like breast or bottle feeding, time of weaning and methods of toilet training, where a relationship is predicted by Freud's theory of psychoanalysis, have given conflicting results. It is too early to say that the theory is discredited on this account, because most studies have been looking for linear relationships whereas it is probably optima that are critical. Delayed weaning may be as harmful as premature weaning. These optima could differ for each child, depending on other factors, and this renders the conventional methods of statistics inappropriate.

However, abstraction of order from the complexity of social interactions between parent and child has only just begun; those studies that attempt to relate broader and more persisting dimensions of maternal behaviour to the personalities of nursery and primary school children show an encouraging degree of consistency. For example, maternal behaviour has independent dimensions such as warmth to coldness (hostility), and permissiveness to restrictiveness. 'Independent' implies that the location of the mother on the scale of one dimension does not infer anything about her location with regard to the other. Two such dimensions can, however, be used to generate systematically a number of types of child rearing. For example, a mother who is high in warmth can be classed as 'indulgent' if she is also high in permissiveness. If, on the other hand, she is warm and restrictive, then she is 'overprotective'.

One of the best known studies of the effect of such patterns of child rearing was carried out by Sears and his colleagues in a New England suburb. The family life of nearly 400 five-year-old children was studied in the home by ten trained interviewers. They used a schedule covering seventy-two items of behaviour and the full responses were tape recorded, transcribed and subsequently converted into scale forms for statistical analysis. Their findings included the correlation of maternal coldness with eating difficulties and persistent bed wetting. Maternal coldness also characterized homes where the children were retarded in conscience development and too aggressive. It is particularly interesting that these authors found overwhelming evidence that punishments, in contrast to rewards, were quite ineffectual in the training of children.

There are clearly national, racial and social class differences in child rearing and these are the real causes of many of the differences between people that were previously attributed to inheritance. Indeed the work of social anthropologists first stimulated the present interest in the social aspects of child development.

In a village in Ceylon, Straus found an apparent contradiction of the hypothesis that easy going demand feeding combined with an extreme casualness in elimination training (there was no prescribed place for defaecation except that the house was excluded) and much early affection would result in confident and emotionally secure adults. These Singalese, on the contrary, were tense, anxious and insecure. Straus ascribes this to a combination of two much broader features of their culture. The love and affection was withdrawn at about five years of age and replaced by an aloof relationship. There is also in Ceylon a loose social structure in which rights and duties are not rigidly defined but tend to be equivocal. This is in sharp contrast to Japan and Vietnam.

One of the difficulties of research on our own culture is that the mass media disseminate new thinking about child rearing with such rapidity that it is difficult to establish the existence of stable relationships. It appears, for example, from a careful reappraisal of studies going back to 1930, that there has been a radical change associated with social class. At present, it is the middle class mothers who are more permissive, who provide more warmth and are more likely to use reasoning, or merely expressions of disappointment in disciplining their children. Twenty years ago such parents were more inclined to impose restrictions and frustrations and to set high standards in the belief that such a regime 'builds character'.

Another problem is the perennial one of causality versus concomitancy. Does the permissive mother make the nonaggressive child or does the nonaggressive child allow the mother to be permissive? For psychology as for medicine, a method of experiment which circumvents this difficulty is seldom possible. It is obviously unethical to impose noxious psychological conditions on human beings or to restrict their freedom for experimental purposes. One study attempted to avoid this dilemma by the strategy of locating some deprived children in an institution and providing a remedy for the situation in respect of half of them. There were sixteen babies about 6 months; of these, eight were given a great deal of cuddling and attention over a period of 8 weeks by the same person. The other eight were treated by the prevailing socially sterile routine with essential feeding and cleaning by a rota of nurses. Subsequently, independent observers with no knowledge of the allocation of the children rated the experimental ones as more socially responsive, and they scored slightly higher on postural and ability tests.

This investigation was concerned with the well-known hypothesis, that separation of a child from its mother during the critical ages of infancy may affect emotional development. Research in this area, with which John Bowlby of the Tavistock Clinic has been associated, has led to profound changes in our attitude towards child care and hospitalization.

Intermittent separation from the mother, a less familiar situation, was investigated by the present writer and found to have harmful effects. There has been a widespread policy throughout the world to consolidate the administration of education in rural areas by closing small country schools with only one or two teachers and transporting the children by bus to schools in larger centres. There has always been ill-defined anxiety about the wisdom of this policy on the grounds that it makes too heavy demands upon the children and that it may sap the life from already weak rural communities. Until recently, however, there has been no evidence on either of these points and the economic and educational arguments have been strongly in favour of closure. It now appears from a study of population trends in several hundred Devon parishes that the anxieties on the second count were fully justified.

More pertinent to our present topic, however, was a study made of the emotional behaviour of children who at the ages of 7 and 8 years undertook long journeys to reach their schools. Teachers from fifty-seven rural primary schools made detailed assessments of 883 children on such dimensions of behaviour as concentration, eating difficulties, response to affection and depression. A clear relationship emerged between the majority of these behavioural characteristics and the length of journey to school. Less expected was the finding that if these journeys were made on foot, although walking is regarded as a physically fatiguing activity, they had less effect upon the child than journeys in a school bus. It appeared from supporting evidence that this could best be explained by assuming that a walk articulates the space between home and school, making it familiar and accessible and joining the two life spaces into a coherent, single whole. By contrast, the school bus transports the child over anonymous territory and after depositing him disappears until the time for departure. During the intervening period, whatever crises may arise to loom large in the children's minds, many of them will have no perceived access to their mother.

We generally persist in ignoring such psychological factors if they conflict with other more tangible values. A Swedish study of modern housing has shown that if multi-storey blocks are used to accommodate families with children, the younger ones either refuse to play outside or, if they do so, they reject the carefully provided spaces with expensive equipment and, exasperatingly, play in the area of the otherwise imposing entrance. This is the means of access to the mother. There are implications in these studies of an intimate link between the spatial, the social and the emotional which have hardly been explored.

Leadership

The most important role within social groups is that of leader. The leadership function, which is often spread over more than one person, is to help the group to clarify its goals, to devise plans for reaching them and to impose pressures on members to implement these plans. This is made possible because the group vests power in the leader and consents to carry out his orders, subject usually to certain safeguards. Again, members exchange a modification in their own behaviour for better group rewards in which they will share. Needless to say, most societies have speculated on the properties that distinguish leaders from followers. Ours is probably the first to carry out controlled experiments.

Early scientific research into the problem tried to identify traits of personality shown by established leaders but lacking in their followers. There are two major difficulties in this approach. The first is in specifying and measuring the traits in such a way that different observations are comparable. The second is that some of the followers may well have the relevant qualities to a high degree but have not been able to exercise them because circumstances have kept them from positions of leadership. Everyone knows that the converse sometimes obtains.

The results of this approach have been disappointing; each new study brings out a fresh collection of traits although a few characteristics like dependability, intelligence, social participation and socio-economic status tend to recur. However, this diversity is not all due to error. Different qualities of leadership have been found critical to particular groups and investigation has tended to switch towards a situational approach to the problem. The man who is dumb and lost at a public protest meeting may be the born leader of a commando raid. Even the situational approach presents the difficulty that many social groups operate over a wide range of different situations, in all of which leaders must excel. A good example is the wartime search for OLQ, Officer Like Quality. This is a deceptively simple label for a motley of skills.

A series of studies carried out by the Survey Research Center at Michigan University were concerned with industrial foremanship. Eighty gangs of railway maintenance workers were divided into pairs, each with a similar track section to maintain and similar conditions of work. Independent assessments of the quality and quantity of work performed by each gang were provided by the Divisional Engineer and by the Track Superintendent. Both the men and their leaders were questioned systematically on the ways in which the gang was run. The results for this study were similar to those in a tractor factory and in an insurance office and other organizations. Some of them were also confirmed by a study of British electrical firms carried out by a group from Oxford.

The effective leaders deployed a larger proportion of their time on planning or supervising the work of others and on tasks which only they could do, and correspondingly less on 'pitching in' with the men. Their supervision was not close or detailed and they allowed their men to get on with the job without frequent correction. They also were 'supportive', taking an interest in the men's domestic and work problems. They acted promptly to requests, communicated more freely about what was going on and made less use of punishment.

Although leadership of this kind is effective in contemporary work groups, it must be re-emphasized that there is no ideal type of leader. There are optimal leadership patterns to achieve the goals of given groups in given situations.

Other important facets of these patterns involved in differing proportions in many groups in our society have been named **initiation** and **consideration**. The first is a preoccupation with getting the job done; making plans, persuading people to execute them and generally getting the group ahead. The other is concerned with the human relationships, keeping members' morale high and meeting the subsidiary needs of human fellowship. A study of U.S. Army pilots in training showed that those who were high in consideration for their crews were independently rated the best leaders by instructors. But subsequently in combat conditions during the Korean war, those high in initiation were judged most effective. The complexity of the problem can be seen from the fact that when assessments were made by the crew members themselves instead of by instructors, the most effective combat leaders were those judged to be high in consideration. In a Japanese experiment industrial supervisors were trained by three alternative methods. One stressed productivity (P), one maintenance of morale (M) and the third a combination of both styles (PM). Productivity was highest in the order PM : P : M. Consideration (maintenance) appears as a catalyst that raises initiation (productivity) to the highest level.

Again, the question must be asked whether certain kinds of leader create good groups or whether good groups allow leaders to behave in certain ways. Churchill modestly claimed that he merely put the roar in the mouth of the British Lion. A leader can rarely impose his will on a group, except when he has access to external power. This was nicely demonstrated by a study of nursery school children, in which after careful observation the most dominant members of play groups were separated. The followers were then allowed to establish group goals and norms over a period and the leaders then re-introduced. Although some of them tried, they could not immediately change the patterns of play. Invariably they had to learn the ways of the group to gain acceptance and, through this, power. But this was power only to modify, not to recast. The group is stronger than its leaders but the leaders can influence the group within the limits of its goals.

Two industrial experiments have given further evidence of the influence of leadership. In one the leaders of high-producing groups of insurance clerks were interchanged with leaders of low-producing groups. The result was that the output of the groups changed upwards or downwards in accordance with the new leader. In the other study detailed assessments of the leaders of telephone repair gangs in Montreal by men themselves were recorded. The approved leaders were then changed to the disapproving groups and vice versa. Four months later the groups' attitudes had changed. It seemed that the leaders could directly influence the attitudes of their followers.

Group conflict and aggression

However efficiently a social group may be organized to achieve its aims, it has always to overcome many difficulties. One of the worst of these is that another group may have set itself the same goal. This is the basic condition for social competition. If one group reaches its goal, the other must fail, *ipso facto*. Both therefore devise strategies to increase their chances over the other. Up to a point this is fine. Competition is obviously a spur to effort and encourages innovation and the search for new paths, but it also leads to race riots and industrial strife. The strategies adopted for reaching the goal include actions that block the other group from getting there first. It is axiomatic that obstruction will be employed more by those who see themselves as losing by the more direct methods. One of the most common responses to frustration is aggression.

Conflict between groups, as between individuals, is aggravated further by the perceptual changes which it generates in its members. If the relationship between groups is one of enmity, then all the properties of an enemy are ascribed to all the members of the 'out-group' and not merely those properties which events have justified. These patterns of traits which are automatically switched on are called **stereotypes** and are acquired like other norms by social groups. Out-group members are firmly and consistently categorized even by members of the in-group who have never actually encountered them and the stereotype forms the first basis for interaction when they meet. Examples are 'nigger', 'bookie' and 'colonel'.

This narrowing of perceptions leads, of course, to less communication and perhaps even to segregation. Whichever group is the more successful is confirmed in its strategies and its members conform to them more readily. Increased cohesiveness gives greater power and success is accelerated. The losers, however, feel inferior. Their status appears to them to decline and their hostility increases. An ingenious study of group conflict was made by Sherif and his colleagues in the United States by setting up isolated summer camps for boys of about 12 years old. In one camp two groups who styled themselves the Eagles and the Rattlers were introduced separately, and deliberately ranged against each other in competitive tournaments of baseball, tug of war, treasure hunts, etc. Solidarity increased within each group and soon high rewards were being dispensed for vilifying the rivals. An Eagle against whom a Rattler had accidentally bumped was told by his friends to brush 'the dirt' off his clothes. Verbal abuse developed into scuffling and night raids on the enemy. Attempts at reconciliation were initiated. The usual methods of promoting contact and trying to correct false images were found to be insufficient. It was only when goals were instigated which could be attained only by the combined effort of both groups that progress was begun. Crises, such as a breakdown in the water supply and the need to push-start a heavy lorry were manufactured surreptitiously by the experimenters. The unavoidable cooperation led to the formation of a new and larger social group and hostility quickly dissolved.

These processes, which are only part of a complex whole, can also be observed at the individual level. There is good evidence that generalized personality traits of hostility and aggression towards out-groups (such as anti-semitism) are derived from family emotional relationships and disciplinary methods during early childhood. The man with an 'authoritarian personality' is rigid and inflexible in his attitudes, considers power, status and dominance to be important matters and is scrupulous about the conventions. These are probably repressive mechanisms for disguising his own hostility and controlling his aggressive impulses. Research has shown that he is more likely to have been brought up under a harsh threatening discipline and in a family where love and affection are strictly conditional on submission to standards of good behaviour. Such families are much concerned with their status hierarchy and aggression towards parents is the unspeakable sin.

The authoritarian personality does not usually engage in overt aggression and is perhaps the more dangerous for that, because he deceives others as well as himself. By contrast, there are those who have simply learned techniques of physical aggression as a means of achieving their goals. Such techniques are class linked in our society.

The most obvious way for learning such responses is within a social group that dispenses rewards for excellence in aggression. The Iatmul head-hunters, for example, allocate prestige to members who are successful scalpers and give immediate reward in the form of celebrations and dances on what might be called a per-decapitation basis.

Experiments have shown that words of praise for hitting an inflated doll establish a ferocious persistence in such behaviour among young children. In one study children were rewarded with coloured marbles for punching a Bobo clown and substantial differences in persistence were found for alternative 'schedules of reinforcement', i.e. the regularity with which the marbles were dispensed. After the withdrawal of rewards, children who had received one marble per punch were less persistent than those who had been rewarded only occasionally. This is a general finding in learning theory and explains the extraordinary tenacity of much human behaviour that appears to pay off only very remotely.

Another way in which aggressive behaviour is learnt is by imitation of a 'model'. This probably depends on a generalized habit of reproducing the behaviour of models of high status (particularly parents) which has been acquired by reward in early childhood. Bandura and his colleagues contrived a situation in which children observed adult models using novel forms of assault upon a large inflated doll, such as hitting it with a hammer or sitting astride it to punch the face. Subsequently, the children were put in different settings with the doll present and subjected to mild frustration. They tended to reproduce many of the responses they had seen earlier. Controls who had not been exposed to models showed only a conventional repertoire of aggression. A group who had seen non-aggressive models similarly reproduced their more inhibited responses. A disturbing feature of this study was that the children imitated behaviour seen on films as readily as that of living persons.

The urban neighbourhood

In the organization of collective behaviour the social group is the paradigm unit. However, although there are no sharp dividing lines, it should not be overlooked that there are many other social manifestations such as mobs, reference groups, crowds and crazes. The one chosen for description is less exotic to the point of being mundane, but it serves as a good example because it is more familiar and has been systematically studied. It is the urban neighbourhood.

Interest in the neighbourhood was stimulated by the postwar house building programme in Britain and particularly by the new towns. There was widespread acceptance by planners of the notion of **neighbourhood units**, which would be relatively self-contained residential areas with their own shopping and community centres and with distinct boundaries to promote a sense of belonging. It was hoped to create social communities that would be more satisfying than the faceless suburbs of pre-war years. There emerged a vocal opposition, however, which berated the concept as 'outworn parochialism' and 'village-green planning'. It was claimed that urban dwellers preferred anonymity and mobility. As is usually the case in social issues, neither side had any scientific evidence. It was generally conceded that neighbourhood behaviour was less than it had been, but two views prevailed about how to define neighbourhood. One was that it was a social group with 'nigh-dwellers' (a dictionary derivation) as members. The other view was that it was a piece of urban territory with commonly agreed boundaries.

When a random sample of residents were asked to describe their neighbourhood, however, it transpired that neither view was wholly correct. First and contrary to prediction, it was found that neighbourhood was still an important social concept. The majority of the housewives in the sample acknowledged that they had one, and for 75 per cent of them it was so highly salient that they could draw a map of it. To this extent it was a piece of territory, but when the maps were superimposed there was little coincidence of boundaries, even for a sample of people living in the same street. Furthermore, they were clearly influenced by a resultant of physical and social forces. The territory was partly determined by the need to include friends and other familiar people, who had acquired this status because they lived within the territory.

Thus the neighbourhood is a socio-spatial configuration. It differs from a social group mainly in that the social relationships are not necessarily reciprocal. A may be influenced by B but B is not aware of A's existence; she is influenced by C who also impinges on A.

It was found that the average concept of the size and composition of neighbourhoods is not affected by the density of population but there were large individual variations which depended on such factors as social class, age, length of residence, location of husband's work, etc. Physical factors, such as the siting of recreational facilities and shops, make a good deal of difference to the probability that people will use them. The **principle of least effort** is the main consideration, but what constitutes effort is determined subjectively. What is more, in the past we have greatly underestimated the influence of this principle upon social behaviour.

In a similar study of a housing project for married ex-service students at the Massachusetts Institute of Technology it was found that the positions of houses and the location of their front doors and such apparent trivia as the siting of post boxes and stairways affected the formation of friendships. Friendships in turn governed the channels of communication and these determined the way in which the residents aligned themselves on an issue of local politics.

In conclusion

We have glimpsed at man as a social animal in a number of settings but they all illustrate a few simple principles.

Men interact in social systems of varying degrees of elaboration in order to meet their needs. Group membership itself is not optional but universal. It is not 'instinctive' because this term is best retained for automatic sequences of behaviour triggered by specific stimuli and man possesses very few of these. The price of membership is the necessity to modify behaviour. This modification or learning seems to be mainly controlled by reinforcement, i.e. reward or punishment, however abstract and remote; groups purvey reinforcement and thus control much of the development of personality.

There are two final points that are worth emphasizing. The first is that learning, although to some extent reversible, is not ethereal. It is a biological process and implies real change in neural tissue. For example, the learned aspects of the sex role are no less physiological than the more obvious glandular aspects.

The second point is that some people find it distasteful and a reflection on the essential dignity of man to accept that he is a product of the processes of social conformity. But the palatability of a theory is not relevant to its validity. However, there are no grounds for a common cause of anxiety, which is the idea that conformity reduces us all to dull uniformity. On the contrary, convergence to one group sharpens the divergence from another. The number of groupings is infinite and idiosyncrasy is not in peril. What is certain is that none of man's achievements would have been possible unless he had been the most social of all known organisms.

FURTHER READING

ARGYLE M. (1969) *Social Interaction*. London: Methuen.

BROWN R. (1965) *Social Psychology*. London: Collier-Macmillan.

KRECH D., CRUTCHFIELD R.S. & BALLACHEY E.L. (1962) *Individual in Society*. London: McGraw-Hill.

MUSSEN P.H., CONGER J.J. & KAGAN J. (1974) *Child Development and Personality*, 4th Edition, London: Harper & Row.

SECORD P.F. & BACKMAN C.W. (1974) *Social Psychology*, 2nd Edition. London: McGraw-Hill.

WATSON R.I. (1965) *Psychology of the Child*, 2nd Edition. London: Wiley.

Chapter 42
On being born

During the last fifty years, improved social conditions and better maternal care have greatly reduced the hazards at the start of life, yet the transition from intrauterine to extrauterine conditions still has dangers. In 1969 in England and Wales, 23 of every 1000 infants born did not survive the perinatal period, i.e. the last trimester of pregnancy and the first week of life, 15 being stillborn. Physiologists have contributed to a reduction in fetal wastage by studying the adaptive processes during intrauterine life and in the perinatal period. Obviously, adaptive mechanisms vary depending partly on the stage of development reached at birth by different species. The groping, blind and naked newborn mouse needs and receives more protection from the elements than the active, upright, woolly lamb. The following account is mainly concerned with the human infant who is practically inaccessible in the uterus but is, when warm and well fed, a delightfully co-operative subject in the neonatal period. Fig. 42.1 shows how important it is for the human infant to be born after 40 weeks gestation and to have grown to the expected weight. Failure of a mother to adapt to pregnancy reduces the capacity of the infant to withstand the stress of labour and to adapt to its new environment.

Oxygen environment during labour

The supply of oxygen to the fetus during pregnancy is discussed on p. 38.46. Uterine contractions interfere with the placental circulation and so with the transport of the respiratory gases between mother and fetus. The frequency, duration and intensity of these contractions determine the extent of fetal asphyxia, and this changes the fetal heart rate. At term the rate is about 140 beats/min and the first indication of hypoxia is often an acceleration to 160–180 beats/min. However, this increase may not occur and the heart may slow down to 100–120 beats/min and become irregular when the oxygen supply is reduced. A uterine contraction may slow the heart for about 15 sec, and when the uterine circulation is impaired the bradycardia lasts longer. Several mechanisms are responsible for the change in fetal heart rate. The initial response of the cardiovascular centre in the medulla to hypoxia is tachycardia, but prolonged or severe hypoxia slows the fetal heart. Bradycardia is caused also by compression of the fetal skull. Compression of the umbilical cord can slow the fetal heart probably due to a transient rise in arterial pressure as a result of a reduced blood flow through the low resistance area of the placental vascular bed. This reflex bradycardia is abolished by atropine, a drug which paralyses the parasympathetic nerves. The fetal heart rate is much used as a guide to the wellbeing of the fetus and this is discussed in vol. 3, p. 43.6. However, it is not a very sensitive guide for it has been shown in rabbits, guinea pigs and sheep that bradycardia does not occur in the fetus until its oxygen supply is reduced by two-thirds. Experimental reduction of maternal placental blood flow reduces glucose transport by 35 per cent, and that of the essential amino acids to a greater extent.

The oxygen debt incurred by the fetus during a normal labour is small. At birth the plasma lactate concentration is slightly raised. It may double during the first minutes of life as lactate diffuses out of the tissues, but falls to

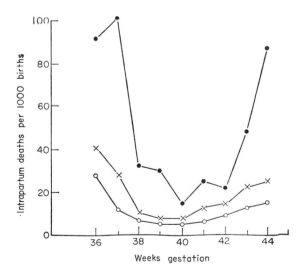

FIG. 42.1. Intrapartum mortality from asphyxia and/or trauma during labour, at 36–44 weeks gestational age: ○, in infants of average weight (within 1 SD of mean); ×, underweight (–2 to –1 SD); ●, underweight (> –2 SD). From Dawkins M. (1965).

normal within an hour. However, during difficult labour a large oxygen debt may cause metabolic acidosis with raised fetal plasma lactate at birth, and without treatment this may not return to normal for many hours or even days. Acid base studies have been made on the human fetus during labour by sampling capillary blood from the presenting scalp of the infant (vol. 3, p. 43.5). Blood collected from this source has an average pH of 7·36 during normal deliveries and cardiac acceleration occurs when the pH falls below 7·26.

ALTERATIONS IN THE IMMEDIATE POSTPARTUM PERIOD

Normally the baby takes off to a flying start with the first good cry. The arterial P_{O_2} rises within minutes to 9·3–10·6 kPa (70–80 mmHg) and the haemoglobin is 80–90 per cent saturated with oxygen shortly after birth, reaching adult levels within hours or days.

Blood cells

Table 42.1 shows some normal haematological values in the newborn. The red cells are usually a little larger than in adult life and they contain more haemoglobin, with MCHC values ranging from 30 to 35 per cent. Both the

TABLE 42.1. Some normal haematological values in the newborn.

Haemoglobin (g/dl)	
Capillary blood	14–22
Cord blood	13–18
PVC	
Capillary blood	over 0·48
Cord blood	over 0·46
White cell count (cells/l)	
Capillary blood 1st day	$15–45 \times 10^9$
8th day	$8–16 \times 10^9$
Reticulocytes (%)	
Full term babies	4–6
Premature babies	up to 10

Hb concentration and the haematocrit rise during the first hours of life. The high values at birth are probably due to high levels of erythropoietin found in fetal blood, presumably in response to the low arterial P_{O_2}. As the bone marrow becomes less active the Hb concentration falls and by about 2–3 months of age the level has usually fallen to between 11 and 13 g/dl. This may also be due to the low iron content of milk, although oral iron supplements fail to prevent the fall. The white cell count is high at birth, with a high proportion of polymorphs. During the 1st week of life the proportion of lymphocytes increases and the number of polymorphs falls. Platelets are small at birth and agglutinate more

readily than in the adult, but their total number is similar to adult values.

Fetal circulation

Fig. 42.2 shows the course of the mammalian fetal circulation once the major channels have developed. The most oxygenated blood from the placenta reaches the fetus via the umbilical vein and has a P_{O_2} of 4·0 kPa (30 mmHg) with its Hb 50 per cent saturated. This blood enters the inferior vena cava by two routes, through the hepatic vein after perfusing the liver and, directly, through the ductus venosus. The proportion flowing through the ducts probably decreases as gestation advances. On entering the heart inferior caval blood is divided by the septum secundum, which forms the rim of the foramen ovale (fig. 42.3). The greater part of the flow is directed through the foramen ovale into the left atrium where it mixes with the small volume of pulmonary venous blood. This well oxygenated blood leaves the

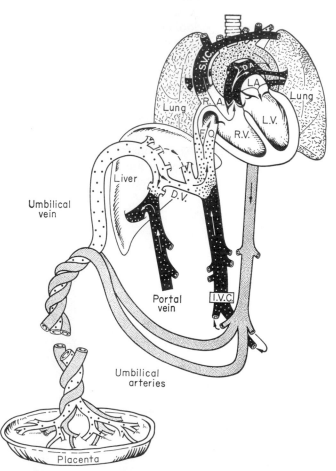

Fig. 42.2. Fetal circulation and probable course of the blood through the fetal heart. DV, ductus venosus; DA, ductus arteriosus; FO, foramen ovale. From Dawes G.S. (1965) In *Textbook of Physiology and Biochemistry*, 6th Edition, Bell, Davidson & Scarborough. Edinburgh: Livingstone.

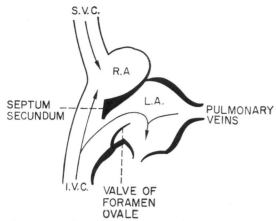

FIG. 42.3. Diagram of the great veins to show that the inferior vena cava blood divides into two streams in the fetus; one enters the right atrium and the other passes through the foramen ovale into the left atrium. From Dawes G.S. (1958) *Recent Advances in Paediatrics*, 2nd Edition. London : Churchill.

heart by the left ventricle and is distributed mainly to the head and upper extremities.

The smaller stream of inferior caval blood is diverted to the right atrium where it mixes with venous blood returning via the superior vena cava. After leaving the right ventricle, the greater part passes via the ductus arteriosus and so short-circuits the lungs to enter the descending aorta. This blood supplies the trunk and lower limbs or passes to the placenta for oxygenation. The pulmonary artery pressure *in utero* is marginally higher than the systemic arterial pressure, so that vascular resistance is almost the same in the two circuits. The relatively high pulmonary vascular resistance is probably due to the very low Po_2 to which the small muscular arterioles are exposed *in utero*.

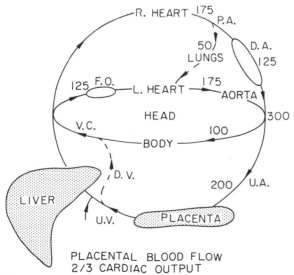

PLACENTAL BLOOD FLOW
2/3 CARDIAC OUTPUT

FIG. 42.4. Schematic view of the fetal circulation, showing that both sides of the heart work in parallel; the flow through the main vessels is indicated in ml kg^{-1}min^{-1}.

Fig. 42.4 shows the approximate distribution of fetal blood flow as determined experimentally in the lamb. Note that the placenta is perfused by about 60 per cent of the combined cardiac output, and that the pulmonary blood flow is only about one-sixth of the cardiac output. There is reason to think that the distribution in the human fetus at term is similar, with the exception of a greater blood flow to the larger head. Measurements using microspheres (p. 30.38) indicate higher cardiac outputs with the right atrium contributing two-thirds of the total. The inferior vena cava contributed 70 per cent of the venous return and 40 per cent of this crossed the foramen ovale into the left atrium, but little of the flow in the superior vena cava crossed. About 40 per cent of the cardiac output perfused the placenta. The applicability of these results to the human newborn is unknown.

First breath

The immediate effect of delivery on the infant is the need for an abrupt transition from placental to pulmonary respiration and it is essential that adequate ventilation should be established without delay.

The infant's first breath establishes the respiratory mechanisms which subsequently maintain the ventilation-perfusion relationship in the lungs, so as to allow an arterial Po_2 of about 12 kPa (90 mmHg). The capacity of the newborn to sustain this Pa,o_2 is essential for survival, and it is important that the mechanisms required for respiration are developed long before they are normally brought into use. Very quick chest movements, accompanied by changes in intraoesophageal pressure and the movement of small fluid volumes in the trachea, have been observed episodically in animals *in utero*. Their physiological significance is not yet known but, interestingly, they are associated with low voltage EEG activity characteristic of REM sleep and have a diurnal rhythm, being observed most frequently in the late evening. The rhythmic activity of the respiratory centre in adults is dependent upon a varied sensory input. At birth this centre receives a flow of new sensory impulses, notably from the skin and muscles as soon as the infant ceases to be 'weightless'. The mild acidosis which occurs during labour may also enhance the excitability of the respiratory centre.

MECHANICAL CHANGES IN THE LUNGS

Serial radiographs show that during the first few breaths the diaphragm plays a more important part than the other muscles in increasing the volume of the thoracic cage and developing a subatmospheric or negative pressure in the pleural space. Subsequent rhythmic breathing depends upon the expansion of the alveoli and the development of a functional residual capacity. Intrathoracic pressures, as measured by an intraoesophageal manometer, fall to 4–6 kPa (40–60 cm H_2O) below atmospheric pressure for about a second during the first few inspiratory efforts, and positive pleural pressures of 2–3 kPa may also be developed during the first few expirations. These large inspiratory pressures are necessary to overcome resistance to the entry of air into the lungs.

One cause of this resistance is the viscous fluid filling the fetal lung, which is about equal in volume to the functional residual capacity of gas after the onset of breathing. Fetal alveoli have a glandular appearance and secrete a fluid with a pH about 6·4, low in protein and bicarbonate and with a high chloride content. Alveolar secretory capacity is sufficient to cause a rise in intra-tracheal pressure if the trachea is tied in experimental animals and it contributes to the volume of amniotic fluid. Amniotic fluid inhaled during labour may also be present. Some of these fluids may be expressed through the mouth by the high intrauterine pressure transmitted to the fetal thorax during labour. This fluid disappears quickly once respiration is established, largely as a result of an increased pulmonary lymph flow.

A greater resistance to initial inflation of the lungs probably lies at the air–liquid interface in the terminal

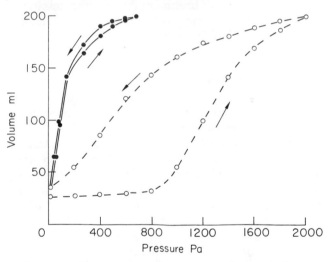

FIG. 42.5. The pressure volume curves of an excised cat lung. ●, the low inflation pressure required with saline demonstrates the low resistance of the lung tissue; ○, the larger inflation pressure required with air demonstrates the high resistance at the air–lung interface.

small bronchioles. Fig. 42.5 shows the pressure–volume relations of an excised lung. When the lungs are filled with saline, complete expansion occurs in response to pressure changes of 200–300 Pa (2–3 cm H_2O) because the compliance of lung tissue is high and offers little resistance to distension. However, when the lung contains air the pressure that is required to open the alveoli is higher by about 800 Pa, and complete expansion requires an even greater increase in pressure. When the pressure is reduced the volume changes do not follow the same curve. This suggests inherent instability of the system which is

probably due to the different surface tensions at the air-liquid interface in alveoli of different sizes; these frictional forces decrease lung compliance and increase the resistance to expansion. The surface-wetting agent, surfactant (p. 31.11), is present in highest concentrations in the lung at birth and falls progressively with age to adult levels. Thus it stabilizes the alveoli so that those of different radius may remain connected without change in size.

INFLUENCE OF BIRTH ON THE PULMONARY CIRCULATION AND LARGE FETAL CHANNELS

The umbilical arteries and vein all have thick muscular walls which are probably not innervated. This musculature is sensitive to cooling and mechanical stimuli, but the effectiveness of the contractile mechanisms is impaired by asphyxia. It is not known whether the hepatic blood flow changes at birth when the circulation through the umbilical cord ceases. The ductus venosus is still patent in the human infant at term but it must close soon after birth as otherwise the portal blood would short-circuit the liver and pass straight into the vena cava, as in an Eck fistula.

The first breath initiates changes in the course of the blood stream in the heart. Expansion of the lungs decreases the resistance in the pulmonary arterioles and so increases pulmonary blood flow. As a result, pressure in the left atrium rises above that in the inferior vena cava and this pressure gradient stops flow through the foramen ovale. Occlusion of the umbilical vessels helps by causing a temporary fall in inferior vena caval pressure. The whole inferior caval blood flow now joins the superior caval blood in the right atrium to maintain a high pulmonary blood flow. Because of the reduced pulmonary vascular resistance, pulmonary arterial pressure falls below aortic pressure and blood flow through the ductus arteriosus is diminished.

The reduction in pulmonary vascular resistance which follows the first breath depends upon inflation of the lungs with a gas of the correct composition since in the newborn the pulmonary arterioles are readily constricted by both hypoxia and hypercapnia. In the fetal lamb, pulmonary blood flow increases about tenfold following lung inflation. In the human infant, pulmonary arterial pressure is reduced by about half, to approximately 35 mmHg, during the immediate postnatal period. The muscular layer of the ductus arteriosus resembles a sphincter but it is poorly innervated. Closure occurs when the $Pa,_{O_2}$ is raised, but flow may start again if $Pa,_{O_2}$ subsequently falls. Increased availability of O_2 to cytochrome a_3 raises the rate of oxidative phosphorylation in the muscle, which triggers the contraction.

These changes in the small vessels and in the large cardiac channels all start abruptly, but take some weeks to complete. The unstriped muscle in the pulmonary arterioles gradually atrophies and their walls become thinner. After blood flow through the foramen ovale, ductus arteriosus and ductus venosus stops, all three channels gradually close. A mid-systolic murmur may be heard when listening to the heart sounds of normal infants during the first 2 weeks of life, indicating intermittent patency of the ductus arteriosus. The direction of flow depends upon the pressure difference between the aorta and pulmonary artery. In the neonate, flow should be from aorta to pulmonary artery, the reverse of the situation in the intrauterine circulation.

ALTERATIONS IN THE NEONATAL PERIOD
Respiration and circulation

LUNG MECHANICS
The important ventilatory values and subdivisions of lung volume in the newborn are summarized in table 42.2 and

TABLE 42.2. Ventilatory values in the newborn human infant (3·5 kg) compared with those of the adult (65 kg).

	Newborn	Adult
Respiratory rate (min)	25–50	12
Minute volume (litres)	0·5	6·0
Alveolar ventilation (l/min)	0·38	4·0
Total compliance (l/kPa)	0·05	1·0
Airway resistance (kPa l^{-1} sec^{-1})	2·5	0·2
Oxygen diffusing capacity (l kPa^{-1} min^{-1})	20	230

fig. 42.6. It is difficult to collect expired air from the infant and many of the figures have been obtained by using the body plethysmograph (fig. 42.7). Advantage is taken of the infant's crying to estimate the vital capacity. The respiratory rate is usually periodic and the work of respiration is minimal at a rate of about 37/min. The lung compliance is apparently low, but comparable with the adult when expressed in relation to the functional residual

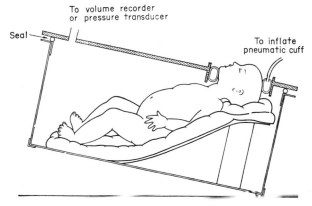

FIG. 42.7. Diagrammatic longitudinal section through body plethysmograph for respiratory studies in infants. The head seal is shown and the outlet for pressure volume recording. The baby is clothed and covered with blankets. From Cross K.W. (1949) The respiratory rate and ventilation in the newborn baby. *J. Physiol.* **109**, 460.

capacity. Airway resistance is high due to the small diameter of the bronchioles.

CHEMICAL CONTROL OF RESPIRATION
This is similar in the newborn and the adult. The CO_2 sensitivity (p. 31.28) is the same as in the adult, provided the increase in ventilation for a given increment in alveolar P_{CO_2} is related to body weight. Arterial P_{CO_2} is low, about 4·3 kPa (32 mmHg), for reasons unknown. Giving the neonate 15 per cent oxygen stimulates and 100 per cent oxygen inhibits ventilation, in each case only temporarily. These responses demonstrate the sensitivity of the peripheral chemoreceptor mechanisms and indicate that there is some resting tonic activity.

RESPONSES OF THE SYSTEMIC CIRCULATION
Table 42.3 sets out some normal haemodynamic values. In general, cardiac output and heart rate are high. As

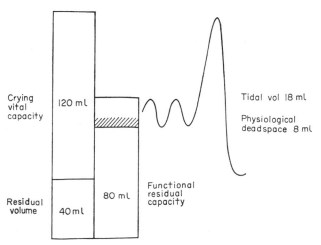

FIG. 42.6. Subdivisions of lung volume in the newborn human infant.

TABLE 42.3. Circulatory values in the human fetus and newborn.

	Fetus	Newborn	Adult
Systemic arterial pressure (mmHg)	70/45 (umb. art.)	70/45	120/80
Pulmonary arterial pressure (mmHg)	—	35/15	30/10
Pulse rate/min	140	140	70
Cardiac output			
l min^{-1}	—	0·60	5
ml kg^{-1} min^{-1}	—	140	70
l m^{-2} min^{-1}	—	2·5–3·0	2·5–3·0
Blood flow			
In pulmonary artery	small	large	
Through ductus arteriosus	large, to aorta	small, from aorta	nil
Limb blood flow (ml kg^{-1} min^{-1})	—	40	20

mean arterial pressure is low and peripheral blood flows are high, peripheral resistance is low. The blood volume forms a larger percentage of the total body weight than in the adult. The blood viscosity is also high due to the high haematocrit value.

The nervous pathways for cardiovascular reflexes are laid down early in intrauterine life, but their activity at birth is uncertain, and one cannot assume that the circulation behaves in the same way in the newborn as in the adult. In experimental animals, it can be shown that the carotid sinus reflex is present at birth. The change in peak frequency discharge of the baroreceptors in response to a given change in arterial pressure is the same in the newborn, with its low mean arterial pressure, as it is in the mature animal. However, in the intact newborn animal baroreceptor responses following a reduction in arterial pressure, induced by either haemorrhage or postural change, suggest that cardiovascular reflex activity is not yet fully developed. The response of chemoreceptors to stimulation by asphyxia also shows an increasing reflex activity with age. In the newborn, arterial blood pressure is not well maintained when the blood volume falls or in asphyxia, suggesting that reflex vasoconstrictor activity is poorly developed, but there is a reflex increase in heart rate. Skin blood vessels constrict readily in a cold environment but vasodilation in response to a rise in body temperature is not regularly observed until the third or fourth day of life. The capacitance of the venous system must be large, for the infant's circulating blood volume can be increased abruptly by about 30 per cent at birth by transfer of blood from the placental circulation, and yet there is only a small increase in right atrial pressure.

Even if cardiovascular reflexes were as active in the young as in the adult, the final pattern of response might still be different for two reasons. Firstly, as an infant has a relatively larger head and smaller limbs than an adult, the relative sizes of the vascular beds subject to reflex control differ. Secondly, intermittent patency of the ductus arteriosus may modify the effects of changes in vasomotor tone and in cardiac output.

Temperature regulation

When the newborn leaves the tropical climate of the uterus, the change in environmental temperature provides another stress to which it must respond. The neonate has two special problems in temperature control; the heat-producing mechanisms are inadequate and the large surface area relative to body weight increases the opportunities for heat loss. Hence body temperature is unstable.

HEAT PRODUCTION

In the newborn, oxygen consumption is only a little above intrauterine levels, but it rises to 8 ml kg^{-1} min^{-1}

at 14 days, about double the value at birth. Fig. 42.8 shows the metabolic responses of kittens to cold at different ages. The critical environmental temperature which stimulates heat production falls during development. The neutral temperature range, in which heat loss is regulated by vasomotor and sudomotor responses with no change in heat production, increases with age. The human newborn cannot shiver because the nervous system is not sufficiently developed. However, heat production in response to cold takes place in brown fat

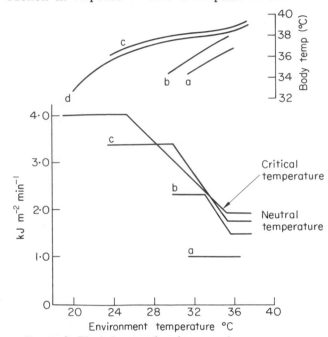

FIG. 42.8. The influence of environmental temperature on heat production and body temperature in newborn kittens aged (a) 3 hours, (b) 2 days, (c) 4 days, and (d) 7 days, showing the neutral temperature and critical temperature and the increase in maximum heat production with age. From Hill J. (1961) Reactions of the newborn animal to environmental temperature. *Brit. med. Bull.* **17**, 166.

(p. 34.8). The distribution and amount of brown fat in the newborn varies among different species. In the human infant it is found chiefly on the floor of the posterior triangle of the neck surrounding the subclavian and carotid vessels, and in the perirenal areas. The mobilization of triglycerides is probably initiated and maintained within this tissue by the local release of noradrenaline at the sympathetic nerve endings. The free fatty acids are oxidized *in situ* and the glycerol liberated into the blood stream. A rise in blood glycerol concentration can be observed after exposure to cold. In rabbits stimulation of the sympathetic nerves to brown fat increases local blood flow and local heat production, and removal of the brown fat abolishes the thermal response to cold without altering the metabolic rate. Heat production in response to cold is reduced by hypoxia and by starvation, which reduces the supply of substrates for the resynthesis of triglycerides.

HEAT LOSS

Heat loss depends upon air temperature and humidity, air movement and radiant temperature, and can be modified by postural changes and alterations in tissue insulation under vasomotor control. In spite of the increase in heat production of which the newborn is capable, the battle to meet the losses from its large surface area is frequently lost. Thermal loss is enhanced by the high conductance of the skin since both skin and subcutaneous tissue layers are thin. In most climates some clothing is required to reduce these losses. In the immediate postnatal period evaporation from the wet surface of the skin may cause heat loss but this can be limited to some extent by skin vasoconstriction, especially in the human infant. A baby seal is unable to reduce its heat loss and it may drown in a pool of water formed from the snow which it has melted.

Preterm infants are at a particular disadvantage if they are not kept in a warm environment, because heat losses are disproportionately greater owing to their relatively large surface. Although they can increase their heat production, their brown adipose tissue is not rich in lipid. Body temperatures may fall as low as 25°C in newborn infants who are insufficiently clothed and exposed to cold and the 'cold injury' syndrome may develop in which slow heart and respiratory rates and general apathy accompany the fall in BMR; facial erythema and oedema may give a misleading appearance of wellbeing.

Liver and metabolism

Probably most of the energy requirements of the fetus are met by carbohydrate, but protein and lipid metabolism begin to contribute within the first few days following birth. Rates of synthesis of nucleic acid and protein must be fast and correspond with growth rate. In fetal liver the enzymes concerned with interconversion of amino acids are immature and all the amino acids may be 'essential'. Enzymes of the urea cycle are well developed early in gestation, but those for gluconeogenesis are not induced until after birth. Although liver slices from early embryos can synthesize albumin, plasma protein concentrations are usually below adult values at birth, especially in preterm infants. Concentrations of plasma prothrombin are frequently low at birth, but of fibrinogen normal.

GLYCOGEN STORES

Fetal plasma glucose is lower than that of the mother; transfer of glucose across the placental membrane occurs by facilitated diffusion down the concentration gradient and is adequate since good stores of glycogen are found

in every fetal tissue. In early fetal life, glycogen concentrations are highest in the heart and lungs, while those in the liver and muscle rise later in gestation (fig. 42.9). As liver and muscle glycogen increase in concentration faster than the fetal growth rate, whole body glycogen per unit of weight rises; due to its large mass, skeletal muscle contains about 80 per cent of the carbohydrate stores. Immediately after birth, the respiratory quotient (RQ) is about 1·0 and the glycogen stores are soon depleted by more than half. This is due chiefly to loss from muscles in which concentrations of glycogen do not return to fetal values. Liver glycogen is replenished slowly as feeding is established and the necessary enzymes increase.

BLOOD GLUCOSE REGULATION

The blood glucose concentration varies widely immediately after birth and often falls below 2 mmol/l (36 mg/100 ml); it rarely rises to adult values until the milk supply is well established. Insulin is present in the pan-

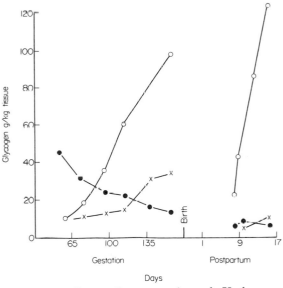

FIG. 42.9. Cardiac ●, liver ○, and muscle X glycogen, expressed as g/kg wet weight, in the fetal and newborn monkey. From Shelley H.J. (1961) Glycogen reserves and their changes at birth. *Brit. med. Bull.* **17**, 138.

creatic islets early in life, but release mechanisms are probably not fully established until 5–7 days after birth. A newborn infant has a low capacity for removing an intravenous glucose load and the insulin response is biphasic, with an immediate rise followed by a delayed peak. Hypoglycaemia in infants is discussed in vol. 3, p. 23.105.

NITROGEN METABOLISM

Except for some of the immunoglobulins, plasma proteins do not cross the placental membrane nor are they synthesized by the placenta; but all the free amino acids are transferred from mother to fetus against a concentration gradient by active transport mechanisms. The relatively high fetal plasma free amino acid concentrations are probably due to different fluxes between organs during intrauterine life; the high concentration of alanine suggests low gluconeogenic activity in the liver. The concentrations of all amino acids fall within the first few days of birth, and gluconeogenesis is established quickly and takes part in blood glucose regulation, for milk contains little carbohydrate. In the infant of low birth weight for gestational age, the plasma amino acid pattern in early neonatal life is similar to that found in starvation. This, together with disturbed carbohydrate metabolism, suggests that these children have been undernourished *in utero*; severe undernourishment *in utero* leads to irreversible brain damage in some species, but this rarely occurs in man.

LIPID METABOLISM

Triglycerides (TG) do not cross the placenta and fetal plasma concentrations are low. Fetal fat is probably synthesized from the FFA which crosses the membrane, and from carbohydrate and acetate. Towards the end of pregnancy, the liver contains large stores of TG which decline soon after birth when plasma TG and FFA rise with the increased utilization of fat, as shown by the fall in RQ.

BILIRUBIN EXCRETION AND DETOXICATION MECHANISMS

All fetal plasma bilirubin is in the free unconjugated form and is excreted slowly by diffusion through the placenta. Conjugated bilirubin in the maternal plasma does not cross into the fetal plasma. The activity of the fetal liver enzymes which conjugate bilirubin with glucuronic acid is low at term but increases rapidly after birth, and the water-soluble glucuronide begins to be excreted with the bile. Physiological jaundice is therefore common in the first 7 days of life. It usually appears on the second or third day and then fades. Many of the mechanisms for the detoxication of drugs are not fully developed in the liver at birth and the administration of drugs to the newborn presents many clinical problems (vol. 3, p. 62.2).

Gastrointestinal tract

The gut becomes motile and capable of secretory activity by mid-gestation. Motility has been demonstrated by the intra-amniotic injection of a radio-opaque material, some of which is swallowed and can be followed in its passage down to the rectum. The transition from a placental to an intestinal route for nutrient intake constitutes another new task for the newborn. The whole gut is very distensible and is variable in size and activity. The muscle layers are thin in comparison with the adult, and the longitudinal muscle fibres of the stomach are particularly deficient over the greater curvature. The stomach is usually empty 3–4 hours after a feed. Emptying is not influenced by the large quantity of air which the infant may swallow.

SECRETIONS

Amylase is present in the salivary glands during the latter half of gestation. In the stomach, mucosal glands start to appear at the fourth to fifth month of intrauterine life and at term these glands are nearly as deep as in the adult. Despite this, the gastric contents at birth are practically neutral. After birth, gastric enzymes and hydrochloric acid are soon produced and the secretory mechanisms respond to gastrin. The acidity of the gastric contents of the newborn rises to a pH of 3 or less and this acidity, together with the gastric enzymes, readily digests milk. Intestinal, pancreatic and bile secretions are also adequate for the functions they have to perform. Intrinsic factor and secretin are present in only small amounts in the gastric and intestinal mucosae.

The first stool is usually passed on the 1st day; it is a sticky black or green mass called meconium. It may contain shed epithelial cells from the upper respiratory tract, together with epidermal cells and products of the intestinal secretions, while the bile pigments provide the characteristic dark colour. However, the major component is the proteoglycan residue of the mucous secretions of the entire alimentary canal which has resisted the action of the proteolytic enzymes. Meconium gradually disappears from the stools on about the 4th postnatal day.

ABSORPTION

Infants absorb their feeds well. A balance study on babies aged 5–7 days showed that of the dietary intake 17 per cent of the nitrogen, 8 per cent of the fat, 49 per cent of the calcium and less than 10 per cent of the phosphorus, sodium and potassium appeared in the faeces. Nitrogen and fat absorption increase after a few weeks. The percentage of calcium absorbed is, of course, much higher than in adults.

Endocrine regulation

GROWTH

Early intrauterine growth is slow and is determined predominantly by genetic factors which control cell differentiation. However, it is also influenced by the endometrial environment which is controlled in turn by ovarian steroids. Later in pregnancy, as the rate of fetal growth increases, maternal nourishment becomes more important. Large amounts of both oestrogens and progesterone are also necessary to allow the uterus to accommodate the

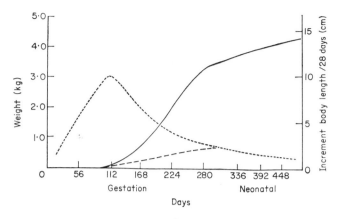

Fig. 42.10. Growth curves of the human placenta,------
and fetus and newborn ————; the mean weight is shown.
The growth rate curve ------ of the fetus and newborn is
the length increment/28 days.

fetus (p. 38.51). The growth curve for the human fetus
and newborn is shown in fig. 42.10.

Newborn babies of diabetic mothers are often large
and have higher plasma insulin concentrations than babies
of normal mothers. Fetal and maternal blood glucose
values are closely related and fetal hyperglycaemia may
cause hyperplasia of fetal β-cells. The resulting hyperin-
sulinism may be responsible in part for the baby's increased weight and for increased tissue uptake of amino
acids and glucose. Hypertrophy of the fetal islets is due
almost entirely to the increase in β-cells.

ADENOHYPOPHYSIS

Growth is less dependent upon growth hormone *in utero*
than after birth. An anencephalic human infant with no
adenohypophysis, and fetal rabbits which have been
decapitated by tying the neck below the thyroid gland,
may both attain a normal birth weight. Nevertheless, the
fetal hypophysis stores growth hormone at an early stage
in intrauterine development. The placenta contains a
similar hormone (p. 38.47), and the fetal plasma levels of
growth hormone are high at birth. Furthermore, although
all the maternal protein hormones may cross the placenta
they do so in only small amounts. Thus, excess growth
hormone secreted by a mother with acromegaly and the
insulin given to a diabetic mother have little direct influence on the fetus. The fetal hypophysis has no control
over the early development of any of the endocrine organs
or of the gonads although, together with the thyroid, it
determines the ultimate size of the adrenal cortex and
influences the deposition of glycogen in the fetal liver.

THYROID

Studies with ^{131}I in animals show that the secretory activity
of the fetal thyroid is dependent upon the hypophysis in
late pregnancy. In the rabbit, if thyroxine is given to the
mother or to the fetus it suppresses the development of
the thyroid, but this may be prevented by giving TSH to
the fetus. Conversely, goitre may develop in rabbit
fetuses when the doe is given the thyroid antagonist
thiouracil. This is due to an increased secretion of fetal
TSH and is quite independent of the maternal pituitary. In
goitrous areas, e.g. some Himalayan valleys, hypothyroid
mothers often produce hypothyroid infants with goitres.
Concentrations of thryoxine are usually similar in the
fetal and maternal bloods. The thyroid is very active
after birth, TSH and thyroxine levels being high. This
is likely to be response to cold but levels of both fall
within a few days. The activity of the hypophysis is
strikingly demonstrated by the high concentration of
TSH in the plasma in neonatal cretinism. This falls
immediately on treatment with thyroxine.

ADRENAL CORTEX

The adrenal gland is larger in proportion to body weight
in the fetus than in the adult, due to the big zone of fetal
cortex, embryologically distinct from the adult cortex
(p. 27.28). This probably plays a major role in the formation of dehydro*epi*androsterone, a precursor for the
synthesis of oestrogens, particularly oestriol, in the
placenta during pregnancy (p. 38.48). A low or falling
maternal urinary excretion of oestriol in late pregnancy
is sometimes a valuable sign of a sick fetus or an ailing
placenta. Birth, even when it is premature, is accompanied
by rapid involution of this zone and the adrenal gland
loses one-third of its birth weight in the first 2 or 3 weeks
and half of it in the first 3 months of life. It may not return
to birth weight until puberty. Development is unrelated
to sex.

The small adult zone of the adrenal cortex is probably
not important during intrauterine life but at birth its
secretion is adequate for independent survival. It responds to stress even in preterm babies, but they may have
difficulties in dealing with electrolyte and nitrogen loads.

ADRENAL MEDULLA

The catecholamine content of the adrenal medulla at the
end of gestation varies considerably amongst different
species. The release of noradrenaline and adrenaline has
been studied mostly in the lamb and calf, and it has been
observed that the amine concentrations of the gland are
inversely proportional to its capacity to release them.
Early in intrauterine development the medulla can release
noradrenaline in direct response to asphyxia. A reduction
in P_{aO_2} to less than 1 kPa (7·5 mmHg) is required to
stimulate this release, irrespective of P_{CO_2} and pH. When
the gland becomes innervated by the splanchnic nerve,
adrenaline is also released and, as development proceeds,
the relative proportion of adrenaline to noradrenaline
secretion increases. The splanchnic response to asphyxia
is triggered at an arterial P_{O_2} of 1·3–2 kPa. Under normal

intrauterine conditions the arterial P_{O_2} is well above that which would stimulate the medulla either directly or indirectly through the splanchnic nerves. During labour, if P_{O_2} falls very low, both catecholamines might be released and cause peripheral vasoconstriction, so maintaining a circulation to the head without exhausting the metabolic reserves. In the newborn the secretion of noradrenaline probably initiates the metabolic response to cold by brown fat (p. 34.8). The medulla may have a homeostatic action in fetal hypoglycaemia.

Nervous system

CENTRAL NERVOUS SYSTEM

The growth rate of the human infant's brain increases during the 2nd and 3rd trimester, reaching a maximum just before birth (fig. 42.11), when it weighs one-quarter of the weight of the adult brain.

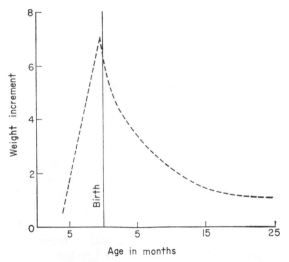

FIG. 42.11. Growth velocity curve of the human brain *in utero* and during the first two years of life; the weight increment per month is expressed as a percentage of the weight of the adult brain. From Davison A.N. & Dobbing T. (1966) Myelination as a vulnerable period in brain development. *Brit. med. Bull.* **22**, 40.

REFLEX BEHAVIOUR

The area supplied by the trigeminal nerve is the first to respond to sensory stimulation *in utero*. Contralateral neck muscle responses occur as early as the 5th–6th week of gestation and by the 2nd month the motor response is widespread with flexion of the trunk and neck. The palmar and plantar responses of the hand and foot also appear at this time. Pupillary responses occur at the 28th week, blinking at the 30th week and the stretch reflex at the 32nd week. Their development is related to postconceptional age, so they are a useful guide to fetal maturity.

The reflex responses which can be elicited from the newborn are legion. They operate largely at the level of the spinal and lower brain centres. Withdrawal of a limb in response to a painful stimulus, turning of the head to free the nostrils, crying when hungry, rooting for the breast, milking the breast and swallowing can all be observed. The grasp reflexes and the Moro embrace reflex may be phylogenetic hangovers, but the latter is useful clinically for it is readily abolished by cerebral disturbance in the newborn. Because the infant lies in a curled up position it is said to exhibit flexural tone. In the supine position, limb movements are gross and appear purposeless, but in the cuddling or prone positions these random movements are more organized and may resemble climbing or crawling. Some cerebral functions must also be present. The eyes are open and the infant appears awake, responding to light and sound in a variety of ways, changing the respiratory pattern, startling, blinking and sometimes turning the eyes and head. Smiling may also be observed.

The newborn sleeps for about 3 hours at a time with shorter periods of wakefulness. Sleep rhythms may first be observed in the electroencephalogram (EEG) at 34 weeks of gestational age. The sleep has a more regular alternation between orthodox and paradoxical phases than in the adult, each lasting about 50 min. Paradoxical sleep, associated with REM and low voltage EEG activity, occupies about 40 per cent of the time in comparison with 20 per cent in the adult. In orthodox sleep, the respiratory rhythm and heart rate become slower and more regular and oxygen consumption is reduced. EEG patterns develop in the newborn irrespective of conceptual age. The adult pattern is not established until about puberty.

Body composition (table 42.4)

The water content of the early embryo is almost 90 per

TABLE 42.4. The composition of the human body at different ages.

	Fetus, 20–25 weeks gestation	Pre-term baby	Full-term baby	Adult man
Body weight (kg)	0·3	1·5	3·5	70
Fat (g/kg whole body)	5	35	160	160
Water (g/kg whole body)	880	830	690	600
Composition of fat free body tissue				
Water (g/kg)	880	850	820	720
Total N (g/kg)	15	19	23	34
Na (mmol/kg)	100	100	82	80
K (mmol/kg)	43	50	53	69
Cl (mmol/kg)	76	70	55	44
Ca (g/kg)	4·2	7·0	9·6	22·4
Mg (g/kg)	0·18	0·24	0·26	0·50
P (g/kg)	3·0	3·8	5·6	12·0
Fe (mg/kg)	58	74	94	74
Cu (mg/kg)	3	4	5	2

cent but the proportion of water in the body falls gradually during intrauterine life and the first postnatal year. These changes involve chiefly the extracellular fluid volume. The size of the various compartments has been measured by the conventional dilution methods. The physiological weight loss in the first 2–3 days of life, which may be as much as 7 per cent of birth weight, is due to insensible loss of water from the skin and lungs and to renal excretion. Plasma levels of sodium and calcium ions are normal at term, but those of potassium, chloride, phosphate and some amino acids may be raised.

REGULATION BY THE KIDNEY

Urine may be found in the bladder by the third month of pregnancy and this contributes to the amniotic fluid volume (p. 38.48). However, renal excretion probably has no essential part in the regulation of the fetal *milieu intérieur,* and the placenta is responsible for maintaining intrauterine homeostasis.

At birth, the renal glomerular capsule is still covered by a tall columnar epithelium but the renal tubule appears well developed. The function of both these structures is immature, but there is a swift improvement after delivery and adult functional capacity is attained within a few weeks of birth. The newborn kidney is unable to eliminate water, dietary salt and acid loads quickly or to conserve water. Because of these slow responses to their internal environment, infants readily become oedematous if the water or salt load is excessive or dehydrated when water intake is inadequate.

The glomerular filtration rate (GFR), measured by inulin clearance, is low in the newborn, being about two-thirds the adult value when both are related to the total body water. Urinary osmolality rarely exceeds 500 mosmol/l.

The neurohypophysis contains vasopressin at an early stage in fetal life and releases it probably in the neonatal period, since ADH can be recovered in the urine during water deprivation. However, as urinary osmolality is not increased in these circumstances the neonatal kidney is insensitive to ADH. This is probably largely due to the small amount of urea in the urine in the early weeks of life. However, by the 6th day of age the human infant can respond to exogenous vasopressin. It can also respond to a water load with a diuresis by increasing GFR, although with little reduction in osmolality. This is in contrast to the adult mechanisms whereby a water load induces a diuresis with no change in GFR but by decreasing tubular absorption.

FETAL RESPONSE TO ASPHYXIA

The mechanisms underlying the remarkable ability of the fetus and newborn to survive asphyxia are not fully understood. In an atmosphere of pure nitrogen, the survival time of young animals to the last gasp is directly related to the carbohydrate stores of the heart and liver. The energy requirements of the heart are provided by the anaerobic conversion of glycogen to lactic acid and survival time is shortened if this is inhibited by iodoacetate. So long as a circulation can be maintained, the liver glycogen stores can be mobilized to supply glucose to the brain. It is not known whether irreversible damage to the tissues is due mainly to the absence of oxygen and, therefore, the supply of energy, or to the fall in pH as the lactic acid accumulates. Survival time is prolonged if the acidosis is corrected with alkali; glucose enhances this action but is ineffective alone. The potassium content of anoxic fetal kidney slices is maintained longer than in adult tissue and if this is true for the fetal heart and brain it may explain the maintenance of excitability for long periods during asphyxia.

It is known that the circulation in the fetal lamb is capable of responding to asphyxia near term. The cerebral and placental flows can increase, probably at the expense of the rest of the body, for the cardiac output can rise only very slightly in these circumstances.

In newborn animals, asphyxia causes general excitability, hyperpnoea, and marked bradycardia of vagal origin. These changes are followed initially by apnoea and, a few minutes later, by strong slow regular gasping, due to stimulation of arterial chemoreceptors, while the arterial pressure and heart rate decline further. Terminal apnoea then follows, but the heart continues to beat slowly and feebly, in contrast with the adult animal, in which the heart usually stops before the terminal apnoea. The newborn rat continues to gasp for 50 min in nitrogen, while the newborn guinea-pig will last 9 min and adult animals only a few minutes. Resuscitation after the last gasp is possible but it has been shown at autopsy that there is already damage to the subcortical centres, the midbrain and brainstem in the monkey. Infants delivered by Caesarean section 25 min after the death of the mother have lived, suggesting that the human fetus can withstand asphyxia relatively well.

FURTHER READING

ADAM P.A.J. (1971) Control of glucose metabolism in the human fetus and newborn infant. *Advances in Metabolic Disorders* 5, 183–275.

ASSALI N.S. (1972) *Pathophysiology of Gestation.* Vol. II. Fetal-Placental Disorders. New York: Academic Press.

AUSTIN C.R. (1973) *The Mammalian Fetus In Vitro.* London: Chapman & Hall.

AUSTIN C.R. & SHORT R.V. (1972) *Reproduction in Mammals*, Vols. 1–5. London: Cambridge University Press.

AVERY M.E. & FLETCHER B.D. (1974) *The Lung and its Disorders in the Newborn Infant*, 3rd Edition. Philadelphia: Saunders.

BEARD R.W. & NATHANIELSZ P.W. (1976) *Fetal Physiology and Medicine*. Philadelphia: Saunders.

BENSON P.F. (1971) *The Biochemistry of Development*. Clinics in Developmental Medicine No. 37. London: Heinemann.

CROSS K.W. & DAWES G.S. eds. (1966) The foetus and the new-born: recent research. *British Medical Bulletin* **22**, 1–96.

CROSS K.W. *et al.* eds. (1973) *Foetal and Neonatal Physiology*. Proceedings of the Sir Joseph Barcroft Centenary Symposium. London: Cambridge University Press.

DAVIS J.A. & DOBBING J. eds. (1974) *Scientific Foundations of Paediatrics*. London: Heinemann.

DAWES G.S. (1968) *Foetal and Neonatal Physiology*. Chicago: Yearbook Publishers.

DAWKINS M.J.R. & MacGREGOR W.G. eds. (1965) *Gestational Age, Size and Maturity*. Clinics in Developmental Medicine No. 19. London: Heinemann.

ELLIOTT KATHERINE & KNIGHT JULIE eds. (1974) *Size at Birth*. Ciba Foundation Symposium No. 27, N.S. Amsterdam: Associated Scientific Publishers.

HYTTEN F.E. & LEITCH I. (1971) *The Physiology of Human Pregnancy*, 2nd Edition. Oxford: Blackwell Scientific Publications.

JOST A. & PICON L. (1970) Hormonal control of fetal development and metabolism. *Advances in Metabolic Disorders* **4**, 123–184.

LONGO L.D. & BARTELS H. eds. (1972) *Respiratory Gas Exchange and Blood Flow in the Placenta*. Proceedings of a Symposium in Conjunction with the XXVth International Congress of Physiological Sciences. Bethesda: D.H.E.W. Publication No. 73–361.

NATHANIELSZ P.W. (1975) Perinatal Research. *British Medical Bulletin*, **31**, 1–91.

RUDOLPH A.M. & HEYMANN M.A. (1974) Fetal and neonatal circulation and respiration. *Annual Review of Physiology* **36**, 187–207.

STAVE U. ed. (1970) *Physiology of the Perinatal Period*, vols. 1 and 2. New York: Appleton Century Crofts.

Chapter 43
Man in hot and cold environments

The human species has a great capacity to endure climatic stress. Men live and work in arctic regions where freezing temperatures prevail for most of the year and in desert areas where shade temperatures are often above 37·8°C (100°F). At the village of Verkhoyansk in Siberia, some of the coldest temperatures have been recorded. The mean for one January was −52°C (−62°F). On the other hand, temperatures over 49°C (120°F) are commonly experienced by nomads living in deserts and semi-desert areas in north and central Africa.

Even when man is exposed to extremes of temperatures in an arctic or desert environment, his internal deep body temperature is adjusted within a narrow range.

Physiological adjustments involve changes in heat production, especially by muscles, and in heat loss by alteration in peripheral blood flow by which the heat flow to the skin surface is regulated, and by increased sweating. These make it possible for a naked man to work and survive over a range of temperatures. Even so, extremes can only be tolerated for a very limited period of time without clothes or shelter.

Anatomical variations involving particular genotypes and affecting heat losses are common in many mammals but are found in only a few races of man (p. 43.6).

CULTURAL AND SOCIAL ADJUSTMENTS

These involve the use of clothing and shelter which protect against extremes of climate and so permit physiological adjustments to operate successfully. In particular, the use of clothing provides a less demanding micro-environment for each individual.

NORMAL BODY TEMPERATURE

The internal or deep body temperature is normally maintained within a narrow range around 37·0°C (98·6°F). This is the temperature of the deep central organs of the body such as the heart, lungs, abdominal viscera and the brain. Under resting conditions these are also the areas of high heat production (chap. 4). These organs are contained in a shell of peripheral tissues and skin, the temperature of which fluctuates in a nude subject within a wide range according to the environment. The temperature that is most narrowly controlled is neither the temperature of the body as a whole, nor even its average temperature, but that of the deep core.

ORAL TEMPERATURE

This measure of core temperature is easily obtained and sufficiently accurate for routine clinical purposes. It normally ranges between 35·8–37·7°C (96·4–99·8°F). Errors arise if the thermometer is not kept under the tongue for at least 2 min, if there is mouth breathing or talking during the measurement or if hot or cold drinks have been taken just previously.

RECTAL TEMPERATURE

Rectal temperature is frequently measured in infants or delirious patients and it normally ranges from 35·9 to 37·8°C (96·6–100°F). The thermometer must be inserted at least 2 inches deep in the rectum and kept in place for 3–5 min. Rectal temperatures measured at different depths may differ by up to 1·0°C. This suggests that the temperature may be influenced by that of the surrounding

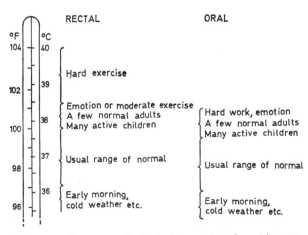

FIG. 43.1. The ranges in body temperature found in normal man. From Du Bois E.F. (1948).

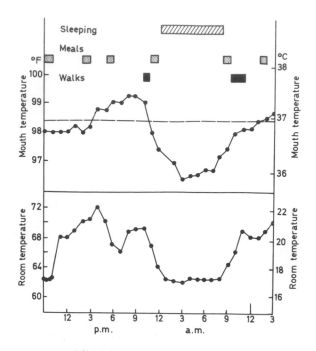

FIG. 43.2. Daily variations of body temperature in a healthy person related to external temperature, sleep, meals and physical activity. From Wright S. (1949) *Brit. med. J.* i, 610.

structures. The temperature of the venous blood returning from the legs has a marked effect on rectal temperature. Cold blood from chilled legs lowers the reading and warm blood from active leg muscles raises it by about 0·25°C over that of the blood in the right heart or femoral artery. For this reason rectal temperature records are unreliable for physiologists studying the temperature responses to exercise. Fig. 43.1 shows the normal ranges of oral and rectal temperatures under different conditions of heat production. The little arrow at a point on the scale of clinical thermometers gives a false impression of a fixed value.

The internal body temperature of warm-blooded animals does not stay strictly constant during the course of a day. In man it may be 1°C higher in the evening than in the early morning (fig. 43.2). This may be due in part to the drop in the temperature of the surrounding environment during the night, but is mainly attributable to an inherent circadian rhythm (chap. 47).

OESOPHAGEAL TEMPERATURE

This can be measured if a thermocouple is swallowed and allowed to descend to a depth of about 47 cm from the lips. The temperature recorded is usually about 0·1°C higher than in the mouth and about 0·2°C lower than the rectum. As the thermocouple lies in close proximity to the right side of the heart, this is perhaps the best site available to physiologists for recording deep body tempera-

ture. When hypothermia is used in surgery, the rectal temperature is an unreliable index of core temperature, and oesophageal and nasopharyngeal temperatures are often recorded. The latter is an index of brain temperature.

SKIN TEMPERATURE

The skin eliminates at least 85 per cent of the total heat

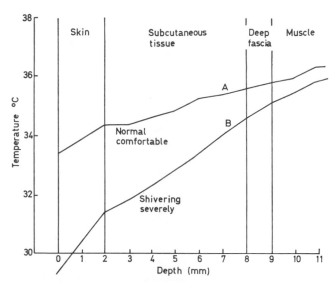

FIG. 43.3. The temperature gradient in the forearm between the skin and deeper tissues under (A) warm conditions with the subject comfortable and (B) under cold conditions which lead to shivering. From Bazett H.C. & McGlone B. (1927) *Amer. J. Physiol.* 82, 415.

loss in man under ordinary conditions and a much higher percentage under conditions of stress. Most of the remainder is lost by evaporation from the respiratory passages which saturates the expired air with water vapour. Only a very small amount of heat is expended in warming food, and the heat lost in warming the inspired air is small even in cold weather. The extremities, peripheral skin and tissues may therefore be many degrees below core temperature and this temperate gradient facilitates heat dissipation. Thus when an individual is thermally comfortable the skin of the toes may be at 27°C, that of the upper arms and legs at 31–32°C, with forehead temperatures near 34°C but deep body temperature at 37·1°C. Between these cool surfaces and the deep central region of constant temperature there lies a mass of tissues whose temperature is variable (fig. 43.3).

Skin temperature is measured by applying thermocouples or thermistors to selected areas on the skin. The measuring instrument is applied as lightly as possible to avoid deforming the skin and creating a groove in which the temperature measured would be that of some tissue deep to the surface.

THERMAL BALANCE

This is expressed in the form of the equation

$$M - E \pm (R+C) \pm S = O$$

Where M is the rate of metabolic heat production, E of evaporative heat loss, (R+C) of loss or gain of heat by radiation and convection and S the rate of change in the store of body heat. Little heat is lost from the body by conduction as the surrounding air is a poor conductor.

In the laboratory, measurements of the four components have to be carried out over a considerable period and the results have usually been expressed in kcal/h. The SI unit for heat exchanges is the watt (W). Most of the data in this field were originally given in kcal/h; they have been converted to watts using the factor, 1 kcal/h = 1·16 W.

The accurate measurement of the four components of the balance is only possible in a laboratory specially equipped to study heat exchanges. For many years classical papers have come from either the Pierce Laboratory of Hygiene at Yale University or the Russell Sage Institute of Pathology at Cornell University. However, it is possible to draw up an approximation to the balance from measurements made with apparatus which is readily available.

METABOLIC HEAT PRODUCTION (M)

This can be derived from measurements of oxygen consumption, indirect calorimetry, as described in (p. 4.5). The minimum value of M in the resting or basal state is about 80 W depending on the size of the individual. Maximum values are obtained during severe exercise and may be as high as 1600 W for a brief period of exercise; such a high rate can seldom be maintained for prolonged periods, and the production of 800 W is very heavy exercise but an overall rate which may be continued for an hour. M is largely determined by muscle activity and is increased by shivering, movements and carrying out physical work. A small increase in M follows the taking of a meal, the thermic response to food, and under certain circumstances heat production by the body can be increased without increasing the amount of physical activity. This chemical regulation of the heat balance is discussed on p. 34.8. It plays a negligible part in maintaining body temperature under normal conditions.

EVAPORATIVE HEAT LOSS (E)

Evaporative heat loss is easily estimated from the change in body weight. At rest in a comfortable temperature a man loses weight by evaporation of water from the skin and respiratory passages at approximately 30 g/h. The latent heat of vaporization of water is about 2·43 kJ/g and so the value for E is about 2·43 × 30 kJ/h or 20 W. This

is approximately 25 per cent of M. Evaporative heat loss (E) is subject to physiological control and can be increased by sweating. A sweat rate of 1 kg/h will give a value of E of about 675 W. This, of course, is only obtained if all the sweat is evaporated. Sweat which drips off the body is not cooling. The sweat glands are under nervous control and sweating is the main physiological adjustment to an increased heat load. It becomes less effective in a humid atmosphere.

RADIATION AND CONVECTION (R+C)

These heat exchanges are determined by physical factors, mainly the temperature gradient from the surface of the body to the outer environment and the amount of air movement. Heat is normally lost by these means, but if the environment is at a higher temperature than the surface of the body, the body gains heat. Physiological adjustments modify these heat exchanges but only to a small extent. Stretching out the arms and legs and curling up the body increases or decreases the surface area over which heat exchange can take place and are familiar responses to warmth and cold. Vasomotor changes alter the skin temperature and so the temperature gradient from body surface to the environment. Movements of the body increase air movement and effect heat exchanges by convection. These adjustments are small and cannot protect the body from the inevitable losses that occur in a cold environment. (R+C) cannot be readily measured, but is calculated by difference, using measured values for the other components of the equation for the thermal balance.

CHANGE IN HEAT STORAGE (S)

The specific heat of the human body is 3·55 J/g. If a 65 kg man has a change in mean body temperature of 1°C over a period of one hour, S is 65 × 3·55 × 1 = 231 kJ/h or 64 W. In the equation for thermal balance S can be either positive or negative. In determining S the difficulty is to assess the change in mean body temperature. As already described, the superficial tissues have a lower temperature than the core temperature. The change in the reading of an oral or rectal thermometer cannot be taken as a measure of the change in mean body temperature. Various formulae have been suggested which combine measurements of skin and rectal temperatures; one such is the sum of 0·8 × the rectal temperature plus 0·2 × the mean value of skin temperatures, measured at several sites.

INSULATION

In 1701 Newton published a paper containing his law of cooling. This states that the rate of cooling of a warm body is proportional to the difference between the temperature of the body and of the surrounding medium, usually air. This can be expressed mathematically as

$$W = K \, m^2 \, (T_1 - T_2)$$

where W is the rate of heat loss in watts, m^2 is the surface area of the body, T_1 and T_2 the temperatures of the body and the environment respectively and K a constant, conductance. In considering the cooling of the human body, it is usually more convenient to refer to insulation (I), the reciprocal of K. I is a measure of resistance to heat flow.

$$I = \frac{m^2 \, (T_1 - T_2)}{W}$$

For the human body there are three different components of I. I_T is the insulation of the tissues, affecting the flow of heat from the core at temperature T_c to the skin at temperature T_s, and I_{clo} and I_A the insulation of clothing and air affecting heat flow from the skin to air at temperature T_A.

An arbitrary unit of insulation, the **clo**, is used by those responsible for designing clothing for use in the armed services and on expeditions. By definition 1 clo is the insulation provided by clothing sufficient to allow a person to be comfortable when sitting in a room at a temperature of 21°C in still air. The following calculation shows that 1 clo is equivalent to an I_{clo} of 0·155°C m^2 W^{-1}.

At rest metabolism is taken as 58 W m^{-2}. Of this 75 per cent of the heat (43·4 W m^{-2}) is lost through clothing. $T_s = 33$°C. Hence

$$I_{clo} + I_A = \frac{33 - 21}{43 \cdot 4} = 0 \cdot 276 \text{°C } m^2 \text{ } W^{-1}$$

The insulation of air under these conditions is 0·121. Hence

$$I_{clo} = 0 \cdot 276 - 0 \cdot 121 = 0 \cdot 155 \text{°C } m^2 \text{ } W^{-1}$$

At rest and in thermal comfort in still air I_T is about 0·085°C m^2 W^{-1}, so clothing contributes more than the tissues to the total insulation.

Tissue insulation

When a man is fully vasoconstricted, I_T is about 0·60 clo. When he is fully vasodilated at rest in a hot room, it falls to 0·15 clo and, when exercising hard in the heat, it may drop to about 0·075 clo. These figures show that increased tissue insulation can play only a very small part relative to clothing in protecting a man against cold, but decreased tissue insulation significantly helps loss of heat in a hot environment.

Clothing

The insulation provided by human clothing can be measured and table 43.1 gives some typical values, together with those of animal furs. Much work has gone into the design of clothing to give suitable protection in extremes of cold. In this the research departments of the Armed Services have been pioneers. No man should now be sent into a cold environment without adequate and scientifically tested protective clothing. Table 43.2 illustrates the insulation required under different conditions of cold. A suit of more than 3·5 clo is too heavy and cumbersome to allow much accurate movement. The maximum insulation of arctic sleeping bags is about 12 clo.

TABLE 43.1. Insulation provided by human clothing and animal furs. From Hardy J.D. (1974). In *Medical Physiology*, 13th Edition, Vol. II, p. 1315, ed. Mountcastle V.B. St. Louis: Mosby.

	Insulation clo
Tropical clothing; shorts, open neck shirt with short sleeves, light socks and sandals	0·3–0·4
Light summer clothing; long light-weight trousers, open neck shirt with short sleeves	0·5
Typical American business suit with light underclothing	1·0
Heavy traditional European business suit and underclothing	1·5
Heavy wool pile polar suit	3·4
Raccoon fur	3·9
Husky dog	4·1
Lynx fur	5·2
Red fox fur	7·8

TABLE 43.2. Total insulation of clothing plus air needed for various rates of work at low temperatures. Modified from Burton A.C. & Edholm O.G. (1955).

Activity	Metabolism W m^{-2}	Insulation (clo)		
		0°C	−20°C	−40°C
Asleep	46	7	10	–
Resting	58	5·5	8	11
Light work	116	3	4·5	6
Moderate	174	2	3	4
Heavy work	348	1	1·5	2

CHANGES IN HEAT EXCHANGE WITH VARYING ENVIRONMENTAL TEMPERATURES

OPERATIVE TEMPERATURE

Air temperature alone is not a satisfactory measure of the environmental thermal load. Outdoors the temperature of the soil surface as well as solar radiation affect the heat exchange between the human body and its environment. Indoors the body can lose or gain heat from the surrounding walls. Winslow and Herrington derived a factor which they called operative temperature. It represents the combined influence of air temperature and the mean radiant temperature. Fig. 43.4 shows the changes in heat exchange of a resting naked man at various operative temperatures. M shows a slight tendency to increase with rising operative temperature. R+C losses become negligible at 35°C and the body gains by these avenues at operative temperatures above this critical level. E shows a gradual decrease in the cold

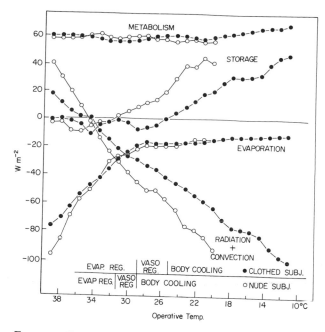

FIG. 43.4. Factors in the thermal balance of the unclothed human body and its environment at various operative temperatures. Modified from Winslow C.E.A. & Herrington L.P. (1949).

zone but above 33°C it increases very rapidly because of the onset of sweating. S is positive at operative temperatures above 30°C when the mean temperature of the body tissue rises.

The naked subject studied in fig. 43.4 enjoyed a comfort zone of thermal equilibrium at operative temperatures between 30–34°C. At 30°C the value for M was 60 W m^{-2}, for R+C 40 W m^{-2}, and for E 20 W m^{-2}, and there is no change in body heat. This comfort zone at rest shifts slightly up or down the operative temperature scale depending on body build, position of the body and clothing. Active work lowers it considerably to 19–10°C for a nude man.

Immediate responses to heat

How the changes in body temperatures are sensed and the role of the hypothalamus as a co-ordinating centre are described in the chapter on the central nervous system. Here the peripheral responses under different circumstances are considered.

VASODILATION

On exposure to mild heat the peripheral regions of the body, which are cool initially, become perfused by warm blood flowing through a widely dilated peripheral network.

SWEATING

If the heat stress is great, the skin temperatures rise and

approach 35°C over the whole body. At or near this point, despite increasing external heat load, the temperature tends to be stabilized. This results from the stimulation of the sweat glands, which pour large quantities of fluid on to the body surfaces. In a dry atmosphere the evaporation of sweat may maintain a relatively cool skin at 35°C and a stable deep temperature of 37°C despite air temperatures greatly in excess of these.

Man's ability to tolerate temperatures higher than that of his body was dramatically demonstrated 200 years ago by Dr Blagden, then Secretary of the Royal Society. With some friends he went into a room at 126°C and remained there without ill effects for 7 min, but soon after he left because of a 'feeling of oppression in the lungs'. The greater part of steak placed in the room was found pretty well done in thirteen minutes. Such high temperatures can be withstood only if the air is absolutely dry and so allows evaporative cooling. In moist damp climates, such as a tropical jungle, the humidity of the air is high. With air saturated with water vapour, a temperature of 32°C (90°F) soon becomes intolerable.

Long term adaptations to heat

PHYSIOLOGICAL

The ability to sweat much and promptly increases with repeated exposure to high temperature, and the highest sweating rates are reached only in man acclimatized by prolonged and severe heat stress. During a really hot day in the desert as much as 12 litres of sweat may be produced, giving an average rate of over 1 l/h. But during shorter exposures sweating rates as high as 4·2 l/h may be attained. Such high rates, however, cannot be maintained for longer than a few hours. An acclimatized man secretes sweat with a lower concentration of salt and thereby is able to conserve sodium to some extent.

There seem to be no inherent differences between different races in their physiological adaptations to heat. The ability of the tropical man to produce more sweat at lower skin temperatures can be maintained only by frequent exposures to heat, otherwise it is soon lost and disappears at the same rate as does the artificial acclimatization of non-tropical people.

A more important difference between native Africans and Europeans new to the continent is the possession of 'climatic know-how'. The African instinctively avoids exposure to the heat of the day and takes frequent rests after bouts of hard work. He thus saves some of his body water in dry hot environments and allows the body to cool when evaporation is not helpful, as in humid hot climates.

GENETIC

In tropical varieties of warm-blooded species there tends to be an increase in the relative size of protruding organs

FURTHER READING

ADOLPH E.F. *et al.* (1947) *Physiology of Man in the Desert*. New York : Interscience.

BURTON A.C. & EDHOLM O.G. (1955) *Man in a Cold Environment*. London : Arnold.

DARWIN C. (1890) *The Voyage of H.M.S. Beagle*. London : Murray.

DILL D.B., ADOLPH E.F. & WILBER C.G. eds. (1964) *Handbook of Physiology*. Section 4: Adaptation to the environment. Washington, D.C. : American Physiological Society.

DU BOIS E.F. (1948) *Fever and the Regulation of Body Temperature*. Springfield, Ill. : Thomas.

FOX R.M. (1974) Temperature regulation with special reference to man. In *Recent Advances in Physiology*, No. 9, ed. Linden R.G. Edinburgh : Churchill Livingstone.

HARRISON G.A., WEINER J.S., TANNER J.M. & BARNICOT N.A. (1964) *Human Biology*. Oxford : Clarendon Press.

LEITHEAD C.S. & LIND A.R. (1964) *Heat Stress and Heat Disorders*. London : Cassell.

STEFANSSEN V. (1921) *The Friendly Arctic*. New York : Collier-Macmillan.

WINSLOW C.E.A. & HERRINGTON L.P. (1949) *Temperatures and Human Life*. New Jersey : Princetown University Press.

Chapter 44
On being lost on mountains, in deserts and at sea

Previous chapters have described the way in which man regulates his internal environment under the varying circumstances of everyday life. But when the conditions in the external environment are severe and his regulating mechanisms are overtaxed, how long can a man survive? The man who is lost faces this question, and his life can depend on his ability to adapt to a harsh situation. The physiologist can provide some answers which may improve his chances.

The essential physiological problems are the maintenance of body temperature, body water and reserves of energy. They are listed in this way because this is the killing order. Excessive falls or rises of body temperature can kill quickly before there is serious dehydration, and lack of water kills long before lack of food. However, these factors interact and often operate together.

The problems of survival are associated traditionally with the shipwrecked mariner, the explorer or the soldier. But airmen who land or crash in lonely country are now just as commonly involved and survival techniques are taught in most of the air forces of the world.

The problems arising from being lost do not affect only servicemen or travellers, nor do they arise only in remote and inaccessible areas of the world. Nowadays there are a number of people each year dying from exposure in the hills of Scotland, Wales and the Lake District, as well as on the moors of the Peak district and the Pennines. The number of deaths is fortunately still small, but there are many others who suffer from some degree of exposure.

Exposure

Since death from exposure can sometimes be very rapid protection is the first requirement. The Four Inns Walking Competition for British Rover Scouts is held every year on the moors of the Peak District. The course is 72 km (45 miles) over rough country and there may be 240 competitors organized into three-man teams. In 1964, three of the Scouts died and another recovered after a period of unconsciousness. The weather was wet and cold, temperature about 1–4°C, with strong winds. These are not exceptional conditions for Britain, but because the temperatures are seldom below freezing, most people think the weather is merely unpleasant; on the contrary, it can be dangerous and even lethal.

The first competitors started at about 0600. By 1200 one group of three had covered about 19 km (12 miles) and were wet, cold and tired. One of the three began to flag and had to be helped. After a short time he had to rest and one of his companions set off for help, which arrived about 1400. He was then able to walk with assistance, but after about an hour had to be carried and by 1615 was semi-conscious and incoherent. A little later he had a convulsion; the rescuers were then met by a stretcher party who carried him to a farm, which they reached at 1915. At this stage the Scout was pale and rigid, but a pulse was detected at the temple. He was taken by ambulance to hospital, but on arrival at 2015 he was dead. Another group of three also got into difficulties after some 5–6 h walking, when one of them developed cramp and had to be helped along by his two tired companions. Eventually, one of them went on alone to get help and met a rescue party, but he too was so exhausted that he could not give clear directions where he had left his companions. Their bodies were found 2 days later.

What happened to these three, and how did they die? The simplest answer is that they became cold, their body temperatures fell and they died of hypothermia. Direct evidence for this is lacking because the body temperature was not measured in these cases nor in similar ones which occurred elsewhere. Nevertheless, the success of rapid rewarming with hot water in restoring those who are unconscious and clearly near to death is very convincing. A boy of 14 was rescued in the Lake District and brought to shelter unconscious and moaning. He was immediately put into a very hot bath and within an hour had recovered consciousness and was talking rationally. These details and the account of the Four Inns Walk are taken from papers by Pugh.

The sequence of events is probably that as clothing becomes soaked its insulation falls almost to zero. Thus a man in saturated clothing, walking in a wind, is virtually naked. His heat loss increases, and body temperature is maintained only if he keeps up a high rate of heat production; in other words, a high level of physical work such as fast walking or rapid climbing must be continued. Sooner or later, depending on his physical fitness, training or drive, he begins to slow down and heat production falls. Although his central body temperature may remain normal, his limb muscles begin to cool, his movements become clumsy and he may stumble or fall. At this stage, unless heat loss can be substantially diminished, deep body temperature starts to fall. Consciousness may be retained until body temperature falls to within the range 30–32°C, but may be impaired at a higher level. Once consciousness is lost, death follows usually within 1–2 h. As indicated above, it is remarkable how rapid and complete recovery can be if effective treatment is available.

There are several physiological aspects of the problem of exposure. Pugh has shown that a subject wearing saturated clothing has a markedly increased oxygen consumption when working on a bicycle ergometer in a climatic chamber at 10°C and an air speed of 14 km/h, compared with work under the same conditions with dry clothing. The increase is so large that it is unlikely to have come from muscle, and possibly can be attributed to heat production in other tissues. This finding may be relevant to the observation that cases of exposure are frequently associated with exhaustion. This latter term is unsatisfactory as it is difficult to define. It implies severe muscular fatigue, but its physiology is not clearly understood. Accounts vary of the mental state of victims of exposure, but it is not uncommon for errors of judgement and irrational behaviour to occur before a substantial fall of body temperature could have occurred.

Although hypothermia is almost certainly the cause of death in exposure, it is worth emphasizing that recovery has been reported from very low body temperatures. The classic example is that of the Negress who was found unconscious in a Chicago street in winter; on admission to hospital her rectal temperature was under 20°C, yet she survived. However, in unattended cases it is likely that death occurs frequently from ventricular fibrillation at body temperatures in the region of 24–26°C.

Although rapid rewarming is effective and safe in acute hypothermia in a previously healthy young person, it is not recommended when hypothermia develops over a longer period in young babies or in elderly people. Such patients should be nursed in a warm room and allowed to warm up slowly under the influence of their own metabolic heat.

Prevention of exposure

In wet cold, with temperatures close to freezing point, the first essential is to protect clothing from rain or sleet by using an impermeable outer layer, such as a plastic mackintosh. Like all advice, this recommendation must be interpreted intelligently. Impermeable material may keep the rain out but it also prevents the evaporation of sweat, which is produced during hard work even in the cold. Sweat then accumulates and can eventually saturate clothing within the impermeable layer. If you are caught out in wet and windy weather, put on the plastic mac before clothing becomes wet. If shelter is known to be near at hand, make for it; but if there is dangerous country ahead or a chance of getting lost, then get into the most sheltered position possible and stay there. Rescuers who are trying to carry a victim of exposure from a hillside to safety should remember that the rescue may take many hours, during which time the patient continues to cool and may die. It is often better for rescuers to carry a tent than a stretcher, and their first aim must be directed to preventing further heat loss and to raising body temperature. Hence the need for a tent and if possible a sleeping-bag and a plastic impermeable cover. Once the patient's temperature has returned to normal he will probably soon be fit to make his way back without the need for a stretcher.

Cold water immersion

Some of the features of exposure are similar to those seen in people immersed in cold water. The record of survivors of ships sunk during World War II shows that the length of survival is related to sea temperature; the colder the water the shorter the survival time. At a sea temperature close to freezing, most succumbed within an hour; at 15·5°C there were many who lived for up to 6 h, and this appears to be the limit of tolerance. However, those who swim across the English Channel remain in the water for 12–20 h and the sea temperature is usually close to 15·5°C. An investigation of Channel swimmers showed that they were fat and the thick layer of subcutaneous adipose tissue acted as an important thermal insulator. To swim successfully across the Channel demands a high level of energy expenditure maintained for many hours. These men and women were not only fat, but also highly trained athletes, for they needed a large heat production to balance their heat loss. As soon as they became fatigued and swimming speed diminished they got into difficulties. Heat production went down but heat loss continued, and so body temperature fell. In addition, limb muscle temperature fell and muscular movement became less efficient. Some, when close to exhaustion, became irrational, swam in circles, had various hallucinations and refused to leave the water. Such swimmers had body temperatures well below normal. Nevertheless, they had survived in cold water for double or more the expected survival time, and they succeeded in doing this by a combination of thermal insulation and the maintenance of a high level of energy expenditure.

This study was undertaken to try to determine the factors concerned in survival at sea. One of the problems was to decide on the best advice for survivors; should they be told to hold on to wreckage and stay passive in the water, or should they try to swim for as long as possible? Experiments have shown that for the ordinary individual, it is far safer to remain as motionless as possible and not to dissipate energy. Although swimming and struggling raises heat production, the movements in the water greatly increase heat loss. Only a very high level of heat production can prevent a net loss of heat from the body, and once physical exhaustion comes on, body temperature falls rapidly. Wearing thick clothing considerably delays body cooling in water, and if a plastic coverall is worn over the clothing, survival time is further prolonged. Survival time in water is dependent on water temperature; it has already been mentioned that in water close to freezing men can survive for up to 1 h. There have been circumstantial accounts, on the other hand, of very rapid death on sudden immersion in cold water, and there is a widespread belief that this commonly occurred during World War II on the convoys through Arctic waters to Russia. Some pilots who had to bale out and were rescued within 15–20 min were dead when taken from the water. It is difficult to refute such evidence, but if rapid death does occur, it is relatively rare. There have been many cases of accidental immersion in icy water on polar voyages, but no record of ill effects within 5–10 min of immersion. In experimental studies occasional premature beats have been observed, so it is possible that, exceptionally, there may be death from ventricular fibrillation.

As water temperature increases, so does survival time, and at a temperature of about 20°C death from hypothermia is unusual. In such relatively warm water it does not make much difference if the survivor swims or stays passive. However, when prolonged immersion is the rule, as in the case of diving instructors who may spend hours each day in the water, then the temperature has to be kept at 32°C for comfort.

Survival at sea

The castaway or survivor of disaster or accident at sea may be fortunate enough to be in a lifeboat or raft and so preserved from the immediate dangers of drowning or hypothermia. His problems are concerned with water and food, but water is the essential difficulty, especially as he is surrounded by water, which, naturally, he may be tempted to drink. 'Water, water, everywhere, nor any drop to drink'. There have been several claims that small quantities of sea water can be drunk with impunity or used to eke out an inadequate water supply. As this can literally be a matter of vital importance, a number of carefully planned experiments have been carried out under the auspices of the Royal Naval Personnel Re-search Committee. Groups of subjects, under otherwise identical conditions, lived for about 10 days on a small ration of fresh water, or a similar quantity of sea water, or sea water diluted with fresh water. Observations carried out on rafts have shown conclusively that the dangers of drinking sea water are serious and have not been exaggerated. These experiments can be compared with the real life experiences of shipwrecked sailors and survivors in World War II. Those who drank sea water had a death rate of 40 per cent compared with 4 per cent in those who refrained. The physiological basis for this finding is quite simple and depends on the fact that sea water, on the average, contains 3·5 g salts/100 ml water. This corresponds to an osmolality of about 1100 mosmol/l. Since the kidney cannot concentrate urine much above this level, the water required to excrete the solute of the sea water together with the individual's endogenous solute load must be derived largely from body water. As a result the degree of water depletion suffered is further aggravated and the concentration of salts and urea in the blood rises. Since urine is concentrated to the maximum when water intake is restricted, it is also futile to drink urine as there will be no gain of water to the body.

Apart from the important negative advice not to drink sea water or urine, what is the wisest plan of action for the survivor in a lifeboat or raft? In many cases some supply of water is available; it is probably best to refrain from drinking for the first 24 hours and then to take as adequate a ration of water daily as possible. The preliminary day's abstinence decreases urine flow, and a highly concentrated urine is formed.

The water intake required to maintain body water clearly depends on water loss; this varies greatly and depends mainly on changes in sweat rate. Because of differences in the environmental conditions and the amount of physical work, only approximate guides to water requirements can be given. The minimum water loss in temperate conditions, with little or no physical activity, is of the order of 1 l/day, made up of 400 ml of obligatory water in urine, 300 ml insensible perspiration and 500 ml water lost in the expired air, which is partly offset by the production of 200 ml of metabolic water. This implies a minimum urine volume, and no allowance is made for faecal water loss. In conditions of water deprivation and lack of food, defaecation becomes infrequent and water loss in the stools can be ignored. However, if there is diarrhoea or vomiting, large quantities of water may be lost, so it is important to avoid anything which may cause these when water is in short supply.

If possible, a daily intake of approximately 1 litre of water should be taken after the first day without water. On this intake and provided there is little or no sweating, survival can be almost indefinite, and certainly is to be measured in weeks or months. Frequently, however, the initial water supply is small and the daily ration has to be reduced. It is important to avoid taking too small a ration, as in a number of tragic cases men have died from thirst with some of their water supply still available. The daily ration should be planned on a minimum intake of 500 ml/day. It is better to drink all the available water on this basis, even if the supply would last for only 10–15 days. When the water supply is nearly exhausted the survivor will still be physically and mentally capable of effective action; if he had been on a ration of, say, 250 ml/day, which would apparently have doubled his water-drinking days, then his condition would have seriously deteriorated and he might have been unable to take advantage of some improvement in his situation. Rescue is usual; this is worth emphasizing, because of the importance of maintaining morale within the first few days of disaster. Limiting water intake to only a few sips a day can prolong the water supply, but only at the expense of a faster rate of physical deterioration and decline in morale; also perhaps the chance of rescue may be missed. Fortunately, rain is not uncommon at sea and, if survivors are alert, water supplies can be greatly supplemented. In calm seas with heavy rain the top levels of water in the sea can be nearly fresh. This is the one exception to the rule of not drinking sea water; surface water can be drunk after heavy rain.

Apart from the bonus of rain, various methods have been devised to obtain fresh water from sea water. The **solar still** consists of a plastic balloon with a black cloth inside on which sea water drips from a reservoir. Water evaporates from the black cloth when it is heated by the sun, condenses in the inner surface of the plastic balloon and runs down to a trap at the bottom of the balloon. The yield from one still is of the order of 1 ml/min, depending on the amount of sunlight. Chemical desalting kits are also available and yield more water than their own bulk, but they are not simple to use and are relatively expensive.

All possible ways have to be adopted not only to conserve water supplies and to supplement them, but also to reduce water requirements. This means, in practice, reduction of sweating by diminishing physical activity and preventing body heating. In tropical seas, protection from sunlight is important, so any method of getting shade should be used. In addition, clothing can be soaked in sea water and this reduces sweat rate because of the evaporative cooling of the wet clothing. The salt left in the clothing may, however, cause skin irritation.

Cold seas present the opposite problem of keeping clothing as dry as possible to prevent body cooling. Although the shipwrecked sailor greatly increases his chances of survival by getting into a boat or raft, he is still vulnerable to cold, and the survival time continues to be related to sea temperature. Apart from general body cooling and the risk of hypothermia, there is the hazard of immersion foot. This is a form of cold injury

similar to trench foot which was commonly observed in World War I when men had to stand for many hours in the cold mud of the Flanders trenches (vol. 3, p. 17.25). The condition is brought on by prolonged chilling of the feet and legs combined with inactivity and a degree of body cooling. It is not a form of frostbite as the temperature of the water need not be any lower than 5°C. The salient features are swelling and occasionally blisters, and loss of sensation. Frequently there is muscle damage, but degeneration of nerve fibres, leading to permanent disability, may be even more serious. As a result of general and local cooling, blood flow is virtually abolished. Although the metabolic needs of the tissues are greatly reduced by the lowering of temperature, if the reduction in blood flow is sufficiently great there will be local hypoxia which affects nerve fibres first, then muscle fibres, and also blood vessels. Prevention of the condition depends on keeping boots and socks as dry as possible and avoiding any constriction of the toes or foot. Deliberate exercising of the foot and leg at regular intervals is also important.

The most obvious hazard of all has not yet been mentioned, and that is drowning. Anyone who may face the risks of drowning should know the methods of resuscitation (p. 46.7).

Apart from drowning, hazards at sea are those of cold and dehydration and, less important, lack of food. Cold is the greatest danger.

Lost in the desert

In the very different environment of the desert, the problems of survival are due to heat, lack of water and, less important, starvation. Since the last may be a feature of being lost in any environment, it is discussed separately.

High environmental temperatures not only introduce hazards because of the danger of heat illness and heat stroke, but also greatly increase the water requirement. The two factors of heat and water cannot really be separated.

Heat is gained in the desert not only from the high temperature of the air, but also from thermal radiation, both directly from the sun and reflected from the surrounding terrain. If air temperature exceeds skin temperature, heat loss by convection ceases and there is a heat gain. Heat loss by radiation also ceases and is replaced by heat gain when skin temperature is below the radiant heat temperature. In such conditions, heat loss can be achieved only by the evaporation of sweat.

Depending upon the severity of the environment and the amount of work, body temperature rises more or less rapidly. A slight increase in body temperature can be tolerated and men marching in the desert, even with adequate water supplies, commonly increase body temperature to 38°C or even as high as 39°C without serious consequences. But when temperatures go above this level (hyperpyrexia or heat stroke, vol. 3, p. 12.4) ill-effects occur which increase in severity as the rise continues. Consciousness may be blurred at a body temperature of 40°C; commonly the subject is seriously ill and a further rise can provoke the onset of irreversible damage. Survival can occur from a body temperature of 42·5°C, but this is unusual and any higher temperature, unless treated almost within minutes, results in death or permanent injury to the CNS.

There are virtually no natural climates in the world where the environment is such that the resting man with adequate water cannot survive. The most severe natural heat stress, in Death Valley, U.S.A., is compatible with life provided heat production is kept low and sweating continues. So the most important advice to the man lost in the desert is to conserve energy; don't walk in the heat of the day but rest in whatever shade is available; walk during the night if need be, or in the early morning before the temperature rises. There are two further points to remember about a desert climate. There is a large diurnal temperature swing, so night temperatures are low and it may be bitterly cold; the second concerns the widespread fear of the sun, a fear which led doctors to believe that there was a mysterious component in sunlight, the actinic rays, which had the remarkable power of penetrating the scalp and directly injuring the brain. Such rays do not exist, at any rate in sunlight, and the effects of solar radiation are due essentially to temperature, with the important addition of the effect of ultraviolet rays on the skin. Sun beating on the unshaded head or neck can raise skin temperature to an uncomfortable or painful level, but damage to brain or spinal cord can result only from a rise of body temperature to 41°C or higher. It is sensible, of course, to protect head and neck and so reduce heat gain.

Water requirements are much greater in hot climates but only because of the need to sweat. So the advice to conserve energy by resting during the day and walking by night also conserves water as sweating is reduced. At moderately high work rates in the heat, such as marching with a load of 30 kg, sweat loss can exceed 1 l/h and amount to a total of over 10 l/day. Anyone attempting such work without a water supply would probably die within 12–14 h. Just as in the history of survival at sea, there have been exceptional people who have survived much longer, even while working.

The classic example of survival in the desert without water is of a Mexican named Pablo who was lost in the Arizona desert for 8 days and who covered 160 km (100 miles) in that time. When he was found he had lost 25 per cent of his body weight, his skin was so dried and shrivelled there was no bleeding from cuts, and his blackened tongue was only a fraction of the usual size. Pablo made a complete recovery.

Survival is remarkable with such a degree of water loss.

In general, death occurs with loss of 15–20 per cent of body water, which corresponds to a loss of 10–15 per cent of body weight. In a 65 kg man there are, on average, about 40 litres of water, and up to 2 litres can be lost without any significant change. During ordinary activities in a warm or hot climate such a deficiency at some period of the day would be common. Urine flow is reduced to a minimum, and sweat rate is probably also reduced. With further water loss clinical deterioration begins but physical and mental activity are not seriously affected until the loss exceeds 5 litres. Then there begins dulling of perception and impairment of judgement, with some loss of physical endurance, but individual variation is marked and some show few signs of disturbance even at this level of water loss. However, a water loss of 8 litres for a 65 kg man is usually fatal, and death may occur with a loss of 6 litres. Survival time without water therefore depends on the rate of water loss, and may extend up to 10 days provided that there is no activity and sweating is at a minimum.

In the desert the water available is usually salty and unpleasant to drink, but provided the salt level is substantially below 2 g/100 ml such water can be life saving. Obviously, the traveller lost in the desert is in no position to estimate the salt content of well water but the position is quite different from the problem at sea. As a rough generalization, it may be said that nearly all well water can be drunk, although there is often the risk of contamination with micro-organisms.

In the humid tropics, water is usually available and often contaminated, so the wise traveller has means of sterilizing water, using tablets which release chlorine and others to neutralize excess chlorine. Severe as the heat may be in the humid regions, this is due to the high humidity which interferes with the evaporation of sweat rather than the air temperature which may not exceed 36–38°C. The same rules apply as in the desert, except that the diurnal temperature swing is much less and the advantage of travelling at night is small.

High altitude and the problem of frostbite

The special physiological problems of high altitudes are due to the lowered partial pressure of oxygen in the atmosphere and are discussed in chap. 46. The other problems of survival at these altitudes are also due to the diminished atmospheric pressure.

Increased ventilation increases water loss in the expired air and hypoxia promotes diuresis. Hence there is a need for extra water. This has not always been recognized and there is little doubt that one reason for the failure of the technically superb Swiss climbers to ascend Everest in 1952 was dehydration. Their fluid intake when they were on the South Col was less than 1 litre a day.

Oxygen lack impairs judgement, and this can lead to accidents. Any accident over 6000 m will be complicated by frostbite, which is due to the intense cold at this altitude combined with oxygen lack. An important additional cause is the immobility of any injured person.

Frostbite is not confined to high altitudes but it is all too common there and is difficult to treat. The relationship with the effects of oxygen is dramatically told by Herzog in his book *Annapurna*. He describes how he lost his gloves on his descent from the summit and forgot he had spare socks in his rucksack which he could have used instead of gloves. He came down, with bare hands, not unduly worried. In consequence he had severe frostbite and subsequently lost most of his fingers. It was hypoxia which made him lose his gloves, forget his socks and exacerbated the effects of cold. The prevention of frostbite both at altitude and in cold countries is essentially based on effective clothing, including gloves and footgear. Polar and Himalayan clothing are similar in many respects and aim at providing a maximum of insulation with low weight and a flexibility of insulation, so the need for varying heat loss with varying activity can be met. This is important, because even in polar regions men may sweat when working hard. The sweat may condense in the outer layers of clothing and freeze, greatly reducing the insulation.

The second precaution is to have a companion. Surprisingly, frostbite of the face and ears occur without being noticed by the victim but should be spotted by the companion. Immediate rewarming by covering with a fur glove prevents serious injury. Frostbite is difficult to treat but relatively simple to prevent. There are important don'ts in treatment. Don't rub the frostbitten part, and particularly do not rub with snow as this will damage rather than revive. Don't rewarm rapidly except in the first few minutes. Keep the frostbitten part carefully bandaged and protect it from further injury (vol. 3, p. 17.25).

Other problems of cold

A description has already been given of the problem of cold at sea and in wet-cold climates. In the dry-cold of high altitudes, survival, as already mentioned, is largely a problem of equipment, i.e. good clothing. But shelter is vital, because the amount of insulation required to protect an inactive man is larger than can be provided even by the best clothing. Such shelter can include a proper sleeping bag, but further protection increases the chances of survival. Snow is a very effective insulator and digging into snow to a depth of a metre can provide a tolerable microclimate. It is for this reason that sheep may survive for days when buried in a snowdrift. At low temperatures, heat loss is greatly increased by wind and any form of shelter is a boon.

Although hypothermia and frostbite are the most important dangers, lack of water is once more a problem in spite of the fact that there may be plenty in the form of ice or snow. Although ice can be sucked and provide some water, it is difficult to satisfy thirst in this way. A water supply in frozen country depends on fuel. Unfortunately, the weight of fuel needed to melt snow and ice is almost as great as the weight of water gained from it. The early polar travellers suffered severely on this score from thirst.

Lack of food

Starvation is a less serious problem than dehydration, but can be a feature of being lost anywhere. Survival time, when water is plentiful but when there is no food at all, depends on the degree of physical activity. At rest, survival times of many weeks have been recorded. One of the best known cases is that of the Mayor of Cork, Terence MacSwiney, who went on hunger strike when imprisoned during the troubles in Ireland in 1921–2. He died after 74 days of complete starvation. A number of cases have been recorded of survival up to 60 days without food. More frequently, men who are lost have some food but insufficient for their needs. The provision of survival rations for use in emergency is now routine in the armed forces, and most expeditions sensibly take similar precautions.

Although there are considerable variations in the composition of survival rations, they are based on two principles. In the first place laboratory experiment, supported by experience in the field, has shown that, compared with no food at all, a daily ration of 2 MJ (480 kcal), even for a man doing moderate work, makes a disproportionately greater difference to survival than the difference between a ration of 2 and 6 MJ. In other words, some food is very much better than no food at all; work capacity is better as is morale. Secondly, from the point of view of water conservation it is important to reduce as much as possible the solute load in the urine. Since the end products of protein metabolism are excreted by the kidney, protein is usually not included at all in survival rations. The simplest form of ration is carbohydrate alone, usually in some form of sugar. There are many ways in which the most palatable ration can be produced; fudge flavoured with rum has been predictably favoured by the Royal Navy. Since survival rations are reserved for emergencies they have to have a long store life in different conditions of temperature and humidity.

Even if the ration contains no protein, endogenous protein metabolism continues. To provide the needed energy the body tissues are metabolized, the fat stores being the main source, but muscle protein is also broken down, so the kidney continues to excrete nitrogenous end products. The solute load on the kidney is reduced but not abolished by cutting out protein intake.

The effect of a small ration on morale, amongst other advantages, has been mentioned. Nevertheless, even for a man who is resting all the time, 2 MJ/day represents semi-starvation. One of the most striking effects of food deprivation is the change in personality that develops. As energy deficit increases, the subject becomes apathetic and listless, and physical activity is markedly reduced. He complains of weakness and faintness, although measurements of muscle strength show that the weakness is partly subjective. There is also withdrawal from contact with others. Indeed, in one of the most famous studies of starvation carried out by Ancel Keys and his colleagues in the Minnesota experiment, after some 24 weeks of semi-starvation the subjects looked like and behaved similarly to concentration camp victims, although in this case there was no question of fear or brutal treatment.

Part of this behaviour may be regarded as a form of adaptation, reducing energy expenditure, and is associated with a fall in body temperature and a reduction of the basal metabolic rate.

The problems of survival are the need to maintain first, body temperature, secondly water balance and, finally, energy balance. But man can survive very severe conditions for long periods provided he uses his resources wisely. The hardest factor to evaluate is the psychological, summed up in the term 'morale'. All travellers are convinced of its importance, and the will to live, determination and courage prolong life.

FURTHER READING

BAILEY M. & BAILEY M. (1974) 117 *Days Adrift*. London: Nautical/Harrap.

CHERRY-GARRARD A. (1970) *The Worst Journey in the World*. Harmondsworth: Penguin.

EDHOLM O.G. & BACHARACH A.L. (1965) *The Physiology of Human Survival*. London: Academic Press.

EDHOLM O.G. & LEWIS H.E. (1964) Terrestrial Animals in Cold: Man in Polar Regions. In *Handbook of Physiology*, Section 4, Adaptation to the Environment, p. 435. Washington: American Physiological Society.

KEATINGE W.R. (1969) *Survival in Cold Water: The Physiology and Treatment of Immersion Hypothermia and Drowning*. Oxford: Blackwell Scientific Publications.

KEYS A., BROZEK J., HENSCHEL A., MICKELSEN O. & TAYLOR H.L. (1950) *The Biology of Human Starvation*. Minnesota: University of Minnesota Press.

McGEE W.J. (1906) Desert thirst as disease. *Interst. med. J.* **13**, 279–300. (For an account of Pablo.)

PUGH L.G.C.E. (1964) Deaths from exposure on Four Inns Walking Competition, March 14–15, 1964. *Lancet*, **i**, 1210–1212.

PUGH L.G.C.E. (1966) Accidental hypothermia in walkers, climbers, and campers: Report to the Medical Commission on Accident Prevention. *Brit. med. J.* **i**, 123–129.

PUGH L.G.C.E. (1967) Cold stress and muscular exercise, with special reference to accidental hypothermia. *Brit. med. J.* **ii**, 333–337.

ROBERTSON D. (1973) *Survive the Savage Sea*. London: Elek.

WHITTINGHAM P. (1965) Problems of survival. In *Exploration Medicine*, ed. Edholm O.G. & Bacharach A.L. Bristol: Wright.

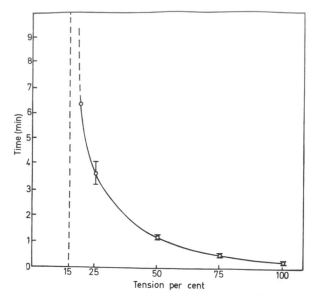

FIG. 45.1. The time a static contraction can be maintained related to the per cent of maximum tension. From Rohmert W. (1960) *Int. Z. angew. Physiol.* **18**, 123.

low. One subject held up a weight of about 100 kg with his leg muscles for 20 min with a metabolism of only about twice the resting level.

POSITIVE WORK

Positive work is performed when the muscles shorten and overcome resistance over a certain distance. The resistance to movement may be gravity, acting on the whole body or its single parts, or burdens, etc. The work performed can be expressed as the product of the weight (force) and the vertical distance it is lifted. If the force is expressed in newtons (N), the work unit is the newton-metre or joule (J). For work rates or power the unit used is the watt (W), one W being one J/sec.

The kilopond (kp) and the kilopond-metre (kpm) are two old units in which much of the data found in the literature are expressed. One kp is the force of gravity acting on a mass of 1 kg. One kpm is the work done when a mass is moved one metre by a force of 1 kp. One kpm = 9·81 J. Measurements of work rate or power expressed in kpm/min can be converted into watts by multiplying by the factor 0·164.

The human machine can produce work in practically unlimited amounts, provided adequate food is available and time for its performance is unlimited. If work has to be produced at a certain rate, however, there are limits. These are determined by:

(1) the mass of muscles taking part in the work, and
(2) the fitness of the individual.

The latter is a convenient expression that covers the state of the muscles, the percentage distribution of 'slow twitch' (red) and 'fast twitch' (white) muscle fibres in the

muscles, their capillarization, the capacity of the circulatory and respiratory systems, etc. Big and fit, i.e. well-trained, young men, working with the big muscles of their legs and arms on a bicycle-ergometer, can work at a rate of 350 W for 30 min or more. It is estimated that the rate of work in a 100 m dash corresponds to about 2 kW. For most men these values are smaller, 100–200 W during bicycling for up to about 10 min, and decrease with age, and they are smaller still in women. Work performed with the arms alone, as in cranking, reaches rates normally corresponding to less than 70 per cent of those achieved with the legs alone. Some specialized athletes (e.g. rowers and crawl-swimmers) may achieve higher work rates with their arms alone than with their legs.

NEGATIVE WORK

The expression negative work is used to describe the conditions when the muscles are resisting some outer force which overcomes their resistance and lengthens them. Actually, it is the outer force that does the work on the muscles, but physiologically they do work to resist the movement. Lowering the body weight or some burden at a constant speed is an example of negative work. Negative work can be performed with much less difficulty than the corresponding rate of positive work. This is due to:

(1) the fact that a muscle fibre being lengthened during contraction develops a much higher tension than when it shortens during contraction, and

(2) the fact that the rate of ATP-splitting at the sites of the actin-myosin crossbridges in the muscle fibres is lowered considerably when the filaments are pulled apart.

It is a fact that numerically identical rates of positive and negative work cost the organism different amounts of energy. The ratio cost of positive work/cost of negative work has been found to vary from 3 to 7 and upwards, depending on the velocity of the movements (fig. 45.2).

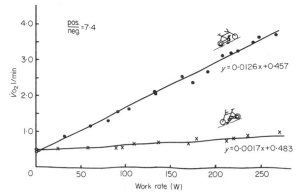

FIG. 45.2. Cost of positive and negative work, expressed in $\dot{V}_{O_2}$, related to the numerical work rates while riding a bicycle on an inclined treadmill. From Asmussen E. (1952) *Acta physiol. scand.* **28**, 364.

The maximum tensions in a muscle group during forced lengthening have been found to be about twice as great as during shortening over the same distance, at a speed of about 60 per cent muscle length/sec (fig. 45.3).

In daily life, the muscles carry out all three kinds of work, alternately or simultaneously. Static work is performed to fix parts of the body, while positive and negative work is performed by other muscles. While the capacity for performing actual work is best expressed by the ability to take up and use oxygen, which is discussed later, capacity for static work is closely correlated to maximum isometric muscle strength. This

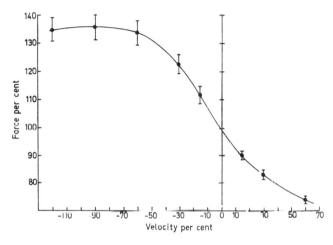

FIG. 45.3. Force-velocity curve from arm shoulder muscles of six young men. Ordinate, force in per cent of isometric maximum; abscissa, velocity in per cent of arm length/sec. Bars denote ± 1 standard error. From Asmussen E., Hansen O. & Lammert O. (1965) *Comm. Dan. nat. Ass. Polio. No.* 20.

can be measured by the use of mechanical or electronic dynamometers applied to definite muscle groups in well-defined positions of the parts of the skeleton to which the muscles are attached. Such measurements show that strength depends on age, sex, size and other individual characteristics. Generally, strength increases with size, as large muscles have more or thicker muscle fibres. Males are stronger than females, the difference becoming obvious from the age of puberty, when boys undergo a strength spurt. In adults of the same age, women have only about 65 per cent of the strength of men; when size differences are eliminated the ratio is about 80 per cent. Maximum strength is attained at the ages of 25–30 years, when a slow and continuous decline begins (fig. 45.4). Some people apparently are inherently stronger than others, the standard deviations of normal averages are ± 15–20 per cent, and systematic training by often repeated, near maximum muscle contractions may increase strength slowly by 2–3 per cent per week over very long periods.

Passive elements in exercise

Bones, tendons, ligaments and other connective tissues were formerly regarded as passive elements. However, they are metabolically active and their component chemicals are being continually broken down and replaced. It is known that activity plays an important role in regulating this turnover. Bed rest, for example, is rapidly followed by decalcification of the bones. Inactivity also weakens the connective tissues in muscles, whereas mechanical stress induces production of mucoids and collagenous substances. Well-trained muscles are characterized by an abundance of collagenous intramuscular tissues and the tendons of wild rats are much stronger than

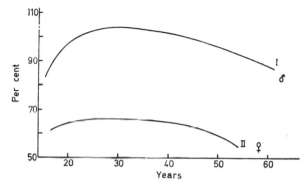

FIG. 45.4. Relative isometric strength of men and women in relation to age. Strength of men at age 22 set at 100. Averages of 360 men and 250 women, measured in 25 different muscle groups.

those of laboratory animals. Bones and joints must endure tremendous mechanical strains, mostly due to the pull of the muscles. Let us consider the ankle joint. When standing on tiptoe on one foot, the ball of the foot carries the body weight, e.g. 70 kg. Assuming the distance from the point of support to the axis of the ankle joint to be twice as long as the distance between tendo calcaneus and the ankle joint, the pull of the calf muscles must be about 140 kg. The ankle joint, which may be considered the fulcrum of a two-armed balance, must carry both loads, i.e. a weight corresponding to 210 kg. Correspondingly, it can be calculated that the lower vertebrae and discs in the spine must withstand a mechanical stress of up to 700–800 kg when weights are carried in the hands in a forward inclined position. These latter calculations have been verified by direct measurements of pressures in the intervertebral discs in humans. These pressures come close to the tensile strength of the vertebrae of young people and may surpass that of older people. Their relations to lifting and injuries of the back are discussed in vol. 3, p. 25. 55.

Sources of energy for muscle contractions

The energy used directly by the muscle machine is set free by the splitting of energy-rich ATP which plays an important role in the actin–myosin reaction (p. 16.3). Energy must be supplied from other sources to resynthesize ATP. This may be provided either anaerobically or aerobically depending on the conditions.

ANAEROBIC WORK

If free oxygen is not immediately available in adequate amounts energy-rich substances, present in the muscle fibres themselves, split and thus provide energy for rebuilding ATP. Such substances are phosphocreatine and glycogen. Phosphocreatine is present in amounts corresponding to about 18 mmol/kg wet muscle. It can be split rapidly and almost completely to creatine and P which latter combines with ADP to rebuild ATP. The high-energy phosphates, ATP and phosphocreatine (sometimes called 'phosphagens') can deliver about 20 kJ of free energy in an average person—enough for short-lasting events such as maximal jumps and throws or for 5–6 m run at high speed. For longer lasting efforts this 'alactacid' anaerobic energy liberation is supplemented by a 'lactacid' anaerobic energy liberation, the anaerobic breakdown of muscle glycogen to lactic acid. The glycogen stores in the muscles are considerable, about 100 mmol glycosyl units/kg wet muscle (1·65 per cent) representing about 250 kJ in an average man if all were broken down to lactic acid. If, however, lactic acid is allowed to accumulate in the muscles it very soon inhibits further glycolysis and thus muscle contractions, so that local muscle fatigue ensues long before the glycogen stores are depleted. Such accumulation occurs in sustained static contractions, when increased intramuscular pressure prevents blood entering the muscle and removing lactic acid. In near maximal static contractions, intramuscular pressures of 65–135 kPa (500–1000 mmHg) have been measured. If on the other hand the lactic acid can diffuse out into the blood and be removed, the muscles may continue to work even though a part of their energy supply comes from glycogen breakdown to lactic acid. The lactate concentration of the circulating blood gives a qualitative measure of the conditions in the muscles. From a resting level of about 1 mmol/l (9 mg/100 ml) it may increase to levels of up to 20 mmol/l (180 mg/100 ml) or higher shortly after the end of maximal effort. The concentration in the muscles may be even higher, up to twice the blood concentration, but eventually the two become equal as lactate diffuses out of the muscles into the blood. The subsequent fall in blood and muscle lactate concentration is due, partly to the gradual distribution of the lactate into a larger water compartment, partly and finally to the elimination of lactate by combustion in the tissues and by resynthesis, mainly in the liver, to glucose and glycogen. At lower rates of work, a steady state of lactate concentration in the blood may be reached after 10–15 min of work, indicating that removal, by oxidation in the aerobic metabolism and by

rebuilding into liver glycogen, and formation are balanced. During the first 10–15 min of moderately heavy exercise, the lactate concentration is usually higher than subsequently, probably because muscle blood flow does not immediately adjust to the demands. An increased blood lactate concentration during exercise is thus a sign of an inadequate oxygen supply, not necessarily because the limits of the circulatory and respiratory capacities of the whole organism have been reached, but because the local peripheral oxygen transporting systems are inadequate. Work performed with the arms, for instance, gives rise to higher blood lactate concentrations than when performed at the same rate with the larger muscles of the legs (fig. 45.5).

Anaerobic work can be performed at a very high rate, but only for a very limited time, due partly to the exhaustion of energy sources (phosphagens), partly to

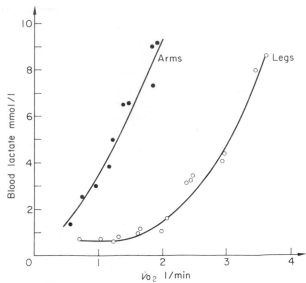

FIG. 45.5. Blood lactate concentration in relation to oxygen uptake during work performed with arms or legs. From Asmussen E. & Nielsen M. (1946) *Acta physiol. scand.* **12**, 171.

the accumulation of metabolites (lactate). As an example may be mentioned that in running up a staircase, two steps at a time, a fit person can lift his body weight about 2 m in 0·5 sec, thus performing work at a rate of about 2·5 kW.

AEROBIC WORK

If oxygen is freely supplied to the muscles, the energy needed for resynthesis of ATP is derived from combustion of nutrients present in the muscles or brought to them by the blood stream. Of the three possible energy sources, carbohydrate, fat and protein, the last named can be ruled out. Its oxidative breakdown presupposes a deamination, which produces urea. But the excretion of urea, or nitrogen, in the urine is independent of whether work is performed or not. The two others exist mainly in the form of glycogen and triglycerides in the muscles, or they may be brought to the muscles by the bloodstream in the form of glucose or free fatty acids (FFA). Fully oxidized they give water and carbon dioxide as end products. Due to their different contents of oxygen their respiratory quotient (RQ) is different, being about 0·7 for fat and 1·0 for carbohydrates. In a steady state of exercise, when the body stores of carbon dioxide and oxygen have adjusted to the work conditions, the exchange of CO_2 and O_2 through the lungs is directly related to the oxidations in the body. In such a state the RQ may be used to estimate the ratio of fat and carbohydrate being oxidized (p. 4.2). Careful studies of the changes in RQ during exercise have shown that both fat and carbohydrate may serve as energy sources, but that their relative importance varies with the conditions. At light and moderate rates of work of not too long duration, the RQ is the same as during rest prior to exercise, i.e. the same mixture of fats and carbohydrates as in rest is burned, but in greater amounts. If the duration of exercise is extended, the glycogen stores gradually become exhausted, and relatively more fat is added to the fuel (table 45.1). Eventually the active muscle fibres become depleted of glycogen. Blood glucose may then to some degree supplement the muscle glycogen in which case the liver releases glucose at such a rate that the blood glucose concentration nevertheless is maintained nearly constant. As the liver's store of glycogen is limited and in spite of an increased gluconeogenesis from lactate and protein, long-lasting exercise may lead to hypoglycaemia, and then the subject will be unable to continue the exercise. Ingestion of glucose or other carbohydrates, however, within minutes restores the blood glucose concentration and the working ability, without changes in the RQ, demonstrating that the muscles are capable of working on a high fat–low carbohydrate mixture. In the absence of a carbohydrate feed, failure to continue work is probably due to failure of the function of the central nervous system, which depends on a normal supply of blood glucose.

The muscle glycogen that is broken down in exercise cannot be rebuilt immediately. Studies of needle biopsies from working muscles in human subjects have shown that 60–90 min of moderately hard muscular exercise may empty the muscles of glycogen completely. On a carbohydrate-rich diet it subsequently took 2–3 days to restore the muscle glycogen, which then reached concentrations considerably above the prework values. On a carbohydrate-poor diet the muscle glycogen stores showed only a small and very retarded recuperation. Empty glycogen stores and a carbohydrate-rich diet thus seem to induce the muscles to deposit glycogen. Endurance of exercise at submaximal levels is directly proportional to the amount of muscle glycogen present in the exercising muscles. The fat that is burned during exercise is probably delivered to the muscles in the form of FFA. There are stores of fat both in the liver and in the muscles, and, of course, in the special adipose tissues. Direct measurements on exercising humans show no increase in the hepatic venous-arterial blood FFA difference during exercise. The splanchnic area thus cannot be the origin of the fat burned. Doubt has also been thrown on the intramuscular fat as the source of FFA. The numerous sites of adipose tissues, however, should be able to provide the necessary fuel for even prolonged periods of exercise with fat as the main supply of energy.

Oxygen uptake

In rest and in the steady state of exercise the liberation of energy from the nutrients takes place by means of oxidations. The oxygen uptake/min ($\dot{V}_{O_2}$) increases with the rate of exercise. If the work is measured when exercising on a bicycle ergometer or walking on an incline, $\dot{V}_{O_2}$ and rate of work are found to be linearly related up to a certain level. If the rate of work is raised further, $\dot{V}_{O_2}$ does not increase. This is the **maximal oxygen uptake** which varies from person to person according to his size, age, sex and state of training or fitness. In exercises such as running or walking horizontally, the speed may be taken as a direct function of the rate of work. Values of $\dot{V}_{O_2}$ related to speed of movement tend to produce upward curving lines, suggesting that part of the mechanical work done takes the form of kinetic energy, which increases with velocity squared ($E_{kin} = \frac{1}{2} mv^2$). Tall and extremely well-trained male athletes, e.g. skiers and middle distance runners, have reached values of $\dot{V}_{O_2}$ exceeding 6 l/min. Average fit young men have $\dot{V}_{O_2}$ max of about 3·5 l/min, young women about 2–3 l/min. For qualitative comparisons the maximum oxygen uptake/kg body weight is a better expression. Average values are, for young men: 40–50 ml O_2 min^{-1} kg^{-1}, and for young women: 30–40 ml O_2 min^{-1} kg^{-1}. Systematic hard training combined with inherent talents may increase this value considerably, for example, up to above 80 ml min^{-1} kg^{-1} in male champion skiers. It decreases with age and there is also a tendency for it generally to diminish with the increasing degree of industrialization and motorization.

TABLE 45.1. From Christensen E.H. & Hansen O. (1939) *Skand. Arch. Physiol.* **81**, 157.

	$\dot{V}_{O_2} = 2\cdot7 - 2\cdot9$ l/min					
Minutes after start of work	0–30	30–60	60–90	90–120	120–150	150–162
RQ	0·91	0·89	0·875	0·855	0·84	0·825
Per cent energy from:						
Carbohydrate	69	63	57	50	45	40
Fat	31	37	43	50	55	60

The limiting factors for the oxygen uptake may be of central origin, i.e. due to the oxygen transporting systems, or they may be of peripheral origin, due to a limit in the capacity of the muscles to take up and utilize oxygen. The maximal attainable oxygen uptake during work with the arms is normally only about 70 per cent of that attainable during work with the legs, so it seems justifiable to assume that in arm work the upper limit is due to peripheral factors. With combined leg and arm work the maximum $\dot{V}_{O_2}$ only slightly exceeds the $\dot{V}_{O_2}$ of maximal leg work and hence the limiting factor seems to be the capacity of the whole oxygen transporting system. A slight decrease in the inspired O_2 percentage immediately decreases $\dot{V}_{O_2}$ max, but a slight increase, e.g. to 22–23 per cent, has no noteworthy effect. Thus the actual diffusing capacity of the lungs is probably not the limiting factor. The addition of more oxygen to the inspired air, e.g. to 45 per cent, augments $\dot{V}_{O_2}$ max considerably, and more than would be expected from the extra physically dissolved oxygen in the arterial blood. A possible explanation is that the heart benefits from this extra oxygen in such a way that it can increase the cardiac output and thus further increase the amount of transported oxygen. Under these circumstances the work of the heart seems to be the limiting factor. In atmospheres with low oxygen pressures the total lung ventilation, which then may be greatly increased, is an additional limiting factor. The increased cost of breathing in hard work, estimated to be up to 10 or 20 per cent of the total oxygen uptake, can of course be a limiting factor for the external work output, but not for the maximum oxygen uptake. Finally, the total amount of circulating haemoglobin must be a limiting factor. This is indicated by the high correlation between $\dot{V}_{O_2}$ max and total haemoglobin (Hb) (fig. 45.6). As the Hb concentration is not influenced by physical fitness, a high total Hb content is equivalent to a large blood volume, which gives good diastolic filling of the heart

and thus a large stroke volume. This again points to the circulation as the main limiting factor for the oxygen uptake during work.

OXYGEN DEBT

The time relationship of oxygen uptake during and after light and moderate exercise at constant rate shows three distinct periods (fig. 45.7):

(1) an initial phase lasting a few minutes, during which the oxygen uptake per min is increasing and asymptotically approaches a certain level,

(2) a steady state, during which the $\dot{V}_{O_2}$ is constant, and

(3) a recovery period after work, when $\dot{V}_{O_2}$ first rapidly, later slowly returns to the resting level.

The slow increase in the first phase is at least partly due to the unavoidable delay caused by the transport of the blood from the muscles to the lungs, where the oxygen uptake takes place, but partly also to delay in increasing the cardiac output. During this period the muscles do not receive enough oxygen to cover their demands and make up for this by utilizing the oxygen stores in the oxymyoglobin and by anaerobic breakdown of stored chemical energy. The whole organism may be said to have come into an oxygen debt to its muscles.

In the second phase the oxygen uptake is closely correlated to the work output and it must be assumed that aerobic processes in the working muscles themselves and in the resting organs cover the demands for free energy. Anaerobic processes may take place in the working muscles, but the formed lactic acid is oxidized at the same rate in the working muscles themselves and elsewhere in the organism. The blood lactate concentration, although elevated, therefore may remain constant. In the third phase, the recovery phase, the total oxygen uptake in excess of the resting oxygen uptake is said to represent the repayment of the oxygen debt. The size of the oxygen debt depends on the intensity of the previous work but is independent of its duration. In light work, where no increased lactate formation occurs, it is probably used in reloading myoglobin with oxygen and in rebuilding the stores of ATP and creatine phosphate in the muscles. This

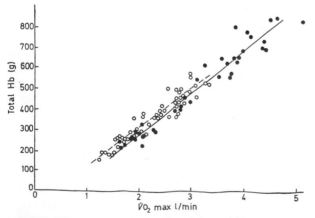

FIG. 45.6.   Relation between total haemoglobin and $\dot{V}_{O_2}$ max. ●, males; ○, females. From Åstrand P.-O. (1952) *Experimental Studies of Physical Working Capacities.* Copenhagen: Münksgaard.

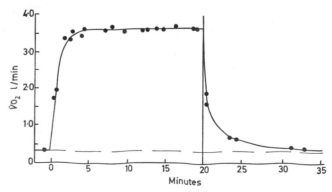

FIG. 45.7. $\dot{V}_{O_2}$ during and after 20 min of heavy work.

oxygen debt is paid off rapidly, within some 5–10 min; it corresponds closely to the initial deficit, reaching values of 1·5–2 litres of O_2, and it is often called the **alactacid oxygen debt**. After more severe exercise, with increased lactate concentrations, a **lactacid oxygen debt** is found. It is generally believed to represent the cost of retransferring some of the lactic acid produced into glucose and glycogen. Direct determinations of muscle glycogen contents after hard exercise have shown that this store is rebuilt very slowly over a period of 2–3 days; it must be concluded that glycogen reconstituted from lactic acid during the repayment of the lactacid oxygen debt is not muscle glycogen but liver glycogen. Direct measurements on exercising men by means of catheters in the hepatic vein have shown that lactic acid is taken up by the liver during heavy exercise. It seems justifiable to assume that this process continues also some time after exercise.

The actual size of the lactacid oxygen debt is difficult to determine, because $\dot{V}_{O_2}$ returns to the resting value slowly and gradually. It is disputed whether the pre-exercising resting value for $\dot{V}_{O_2}$ should be used, or whether a new, elevated level after exercise is more correct for the determination of the excess oxygen uptake. However, excess O_2 uptake after exhausting, short-lasting exercise has repeatedly been found to exceed 15 litres or more, even when only the first 20–25 min of the recovery period is used. With a blood lactate concentration of 20 mmol/l and assuming the lactate evenly distributed in the total body water, about 40 litres in an adult, a total of about 0·8 mol of lactic acid must be present in the body. Its oxidation to CO_2 and H_2O would demand about 54 litres of oxygen. It is possible that a lactacid oxygen debt of 11–12 litres is used for burning about one-fifth of the total lactic acid thus providing energy for a chemical retransformation of the rest of the lactic acid into stored chemical energy.

INTERMITTENT WORK

It has been correctly claimed that work at a constant rate for prolonged periods is a phenomenon that is rarely met outside physiology laboratories or sports fields. The majority of practical jobs are performed intermittently, i.e. short bursts of work are interspersed with pauses or periods of rest or decreased work-rates. Laboratory studies of these kinds of activities have shown some important differences between constant work and intermittent work. If a certain task, measurable in joules, is performed in short bursts of high intensity rather than at a constant rate, the same amount of work can be performed with much less strain. The active periods should be short. It is then found that the blood lactate increases only slightly, even at very high work intensities, indicating that the energy for the work is liberated without lactate formation (fig. 45.8). Possible explanations for this seem to be:

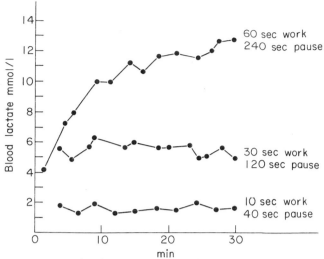

FIG. 45.8. Blood lactate concentrations during 30 min of intermittent work with different lengths of work periods. Total work output in all cases 148 kJ. From Åstrand I., Åstrand P.-O., Christensen E.H. & Hedman R. (1960) *Acta physiol. scand.*, **48**, 448.

(1) energy is delivered aerobically by utilization of the oxygen stores present in the myoglobin, and

(2) anaerobic breakdowns, not resulting in lactate formation, for example of phosphagens, deliver the energy.

The effect of intermittent work on total output of work is demonstrated by the following example. A well-trained runner ran on the treadmill at 20 km/hr for about 4 min. He was then completely exhausted and his blood lactate concentration reached maximal values. He then repeated the performance in short spells of 5–10 sec duration, interspersed with pauses of the same duration. In this way he ran actively for 20 min with only a slight increase in blood lactate concentration.

Pulmonary ventilation

If the oxygen uptake is used as a measure of the intensity of work, it is found that the pulmonary ventilation ($\dot{V}_E$) increases proportional to $\dot{V}_{O_2}$ up to a certain point, beyond which $\dot{V}_E$ increases more than the corresponding $\dot{V}_{O_2}$. This point varies for different subjects and is higher for well-trained than for unfit persons. It is also lower in the same subject if he works with the arms (fig. 45.9). The intensity of exercise at which this increase in the $\dot{V}_E/\dot{V}_{O_2}$ appears coincides with the point at which blood lactic acid rises above resting concentrations.

The values of $\dot{V}_E$ during maximum exercise depend on the size and fitness of the subject. In average young men 100–120 l/min at body temperature and pressure saturated with water vapour (BTPS) is commonly found, but in athletes considerably greater values have been reached. The increase above the resting value is brought about by

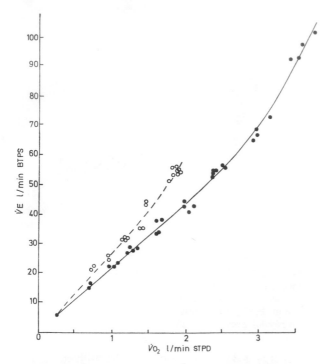

FIG 45.9. $\dot{V}_E$ in relation to $\dot{V}_{O_2}$. ●, work with legs (pedalling); ○, work with the arms (cranking). From Asmussen E. & Nielsen M. (1946). *Acta physiol. scand.*, **12**, 171.

a rise in both depth and frequency of respiration. It has been found that the depth at maximum work comes very close to 50 per cent of the vital capacity. This value is usually reached at lower rates of exercise so that the further increase in ventilation is brought about mainly by increasing respiratory frequency.

The close adaptation of ventilation to metabolism results in an almost constant composition of the alveolar air at increasing rates of work. The $P_A,_{CO_2}$ may increase a few kPa until the point where $\dot{V}_E/\dot{V}_{O_2}$ begins to increase. Thereafter it decreases to considerably below resting values at the highest $\dot{V}_E$ (fig. 45.10). The $P_A,_{O_2}$ behaves correspondingly; it is nearly constant up to the highest work rate, when it may increase some 1·3 to 2·6 kPa (10 to 20 mmHg) above the resting value. The close adaptation of ventilation to oxygen uptake during exer-

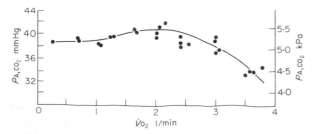

FIG. 45.10. $P_A,_{CO_2}$ in relation to $\dot{V}_{O_2}$ in rest and exercise. From Asmussen E. & Nielsen M. (1946) *Acta physiol. scand.* **12**, 171.

cise suggests the presence of a precise regulatory mechanism. However, it has not been possible to discover a humoral or nervous work factor that is responsible for the increase in ventilation during muscular exercise. The near constancy of the arterial gas pressures, and other observations, suggest that nervous pathways are involved but it is not known if these are of central or reflex origin. Receptors of some kind must play a role in the adjustment of ventilation to exercise, but none of the known

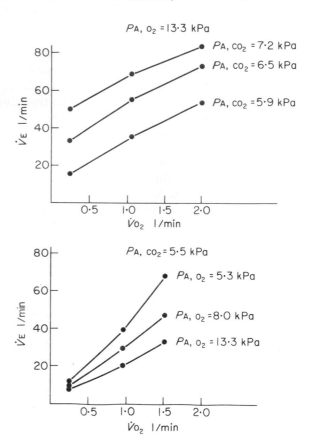

FIG. 45.11. $\dot{V}_E$ in relation to $\dot{V}_{O_2}$. Top, $P_A,_{O_2}$ kept constant, $P_A,_{CO_2}$ varied; bottom, $P_A,_{CO_2}$ kept constant, $P_A,_{O_2}$ varied.

receptors, chemoreceptors, thermoreceptors or mechanoreceptors, have been found responsible. The relation between the work factor and the two best-known humoral factors, $P_a,_{CO_2}$ and $P_a,_{O_2}$, is best described by the statement that P_{CO_2} and the 'work factor' are additive stimuli for the ventilation, whereas the 'work factor' and the hypoxic drive potentiate one another (fig. 45.11).

Cardiac output

In exercise, the cardiac output ($\dot{Q}$) is increased to correspond with the oxygen uptake. From a resting value of 5–7 l/min, $\dot{Q}$ has been found to reach values of about 30 l/min at oxygen uptakes of 5–6 l/min (fig. 45.12). It will be noticed that whereas the oxygen uptake may reach

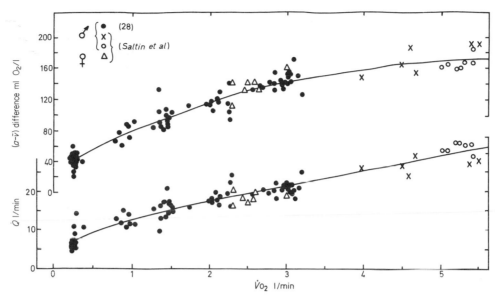

FIG. 45.12. $\dot{Q}$ and (a–v̄) O_2-difference in relation to $\dot{V}O_2$. Data from Asmussen E. & Nielsen M. (1952) *Acta physiol. scand.* **27**, 217 and Saltin B. *et al.* (1962) unpublished.

values of fifteen to twenty times the resting metabolic rate, the cardiac output reaches only values five to six times the resting value. This relatively smaller increase suffices because the utilization of the arterial oxygen also increases in exercise. The arteriovenous (a-v̄) O_2 difference increases with increasing rates of work from values of 4–5 ml O_2/100 ml blood at rest to values of up to about 18 ml/100 ml, i.e. close to the oxygen capacity of arterial blood (about 20 ml/100 ml). This is partly the result of better utilization of blood passing through the working muscle, but is mostly due to a diversion of a larger percentage of the cardiac output to the oxygen craving muscles away from the kidneys and splanchnic organs. The skin, which is not particularly oxygen demanding, still needs a comparatively large part of the blood flow because of its role in temperature regulation. The mixed venous blood, returning to the right heart, consequently never becomes completely de-oxygenated. Even at the severest rates of work the arterial blood is practically fully saturated with oxygen at a normal Pa,O_2, indicating that the diffusion capacity of the lungs for oxygen is not a limiting factor for hard work at normal atmospheric pressures. The increased cardiac output is the result primarily of an increase in venous return. Under most conditions the heart responds by increasing the heart rate and there is usually little or no increase in the stroke volume. The heart rate increases linearly with increasing oxygen uptake up to a maximum value. The maximum heart rate has been found to be independent of sex and fitness but in adults it decreases steadily with age from an average value of about 200 beats/min at 20 years to a value of about 160 beats/min at age 65 years (fig. 45·13). Individual values are scattered around the mean with a

standard deviation of about ± 10, and after short exhausting exercises heart rates above 250/min have been found in adolescents and youngsters. Hard training seems to reduce the maximum value, but as the resting pulse rate is even more reduced, to values around 30/min, the well trained still possesses a larger reserve of 'extra heart beats'.

Although training affects the maximum heart rate slightly, it has a considerable effect on the relation of the pulse rate to oxygen uptake. In the fit person a certain oxygen uptake is accompanied by a lower heart rate than in unfit persons. Therefore, the heart rate/oxygen uptake ratio is a practical measure for the fitness of a person,

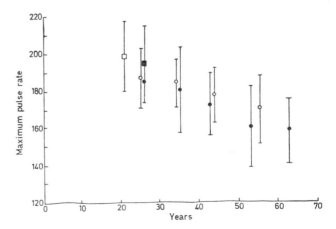

FIG. 45.13. Maximum pulse rates in relation to age. Vertical lines denote ± 2 standard deviations. ■, ●, male: □, ○, female. From Åstrand I. (1960) *Acta physiol. scand.* **49**, suppl. 169.

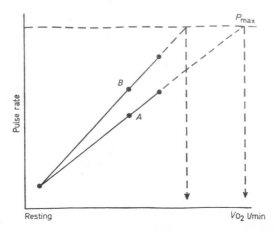

FIG. 45.14. Illustrating the method of estimating maximum oxygen uptake from measurements of pulse rate and oxygen uptake during submaximal work. *A*, fit subject; *B*, less fit subject.

and several fitness tests are based on this phenomenon. Due to the rectilinear relationship, the line representing pulse rates over oxygen uptake may be extrapolated to the average maximum pulse rate of the subject, and thus provide a means of estimating the maximum oxygen uptake (working capacity, aerobic power) from measurements at submaximal rates of work (fig. 45.14). There has been much dispute concerning the importance of an increased stroke volume as a means of increasing the cardiac output in exercise. Much of the disagreement is due to the fact that comparisons have been made between resting stroke volumes in an upright position, with the blood pooled in the more or less passive legs, and exercise stroke volumes. The pumping action of exercise, the venous pump, forces the pooled blood out of the legs and increases the diastolic filling of the heart and hence the stroke volume. If comparisons are made with the subject in a lying position, where the stroke volume is already large at rest, only a small increase is noticed during exercise. The evidence for a regulatory increase in stroke volume is thus rather weak. Radiological studies of human hearts during vigorous exercise indicate an unchanged or slightly decreased diastolic heart volume. An increased stroke volume thus seems to be brought about by a more complete emptying of the ventricles during systole.

The arterial blood pressure, both systolic and mean, is increased in exercise, but less in fit than in unfit persons; it hardly ever rises to twice the resting value. As blood pressure is proportional to the product of cardiac output and peripheral resistance ($BP \simeq \dot{Q} \times PR$), and the cardiac output may be five or six times greater in exercise than in rest, it follows that peripheral resistance must be lowered. This is probably due to the large increase in the number of open arterioles in the working muscles. The work performed by the heart in heavy exercise is considerable.

The left ventricle alone pumps up to 30 l/min into the systemic arteries, against a mean pressure of say, 20 kPa (150 mmHg), one-fifth of an atmosphere. That corresponds to lifting 30 kg 2 m/min or working at a rate of 10 W. Assuming a net efficiency of the heart muscle of about 15 per cent, the energy output for this part of the heart's work would correspond to about 67 W; this is approximately the resting metabolic rate of the whole body. In order to do this under aerobic conditions the ventricle must receive about 200 ml O_2/min, i.e. the total volume of oxygen contained in one litre of arterial blood. The coronary blood flow alone to the left ventricle must thus be at least 1 l/min, and for the whole heart is probably about 1·5 l/min or 5 per cent of the total cardiac output.

Body temperature

Even under the best working conditions, only 20–25 per cent of the total energy output takes the form of mechanical energy that can be transferred to the environment as work. The rest produces heat. At an oxygen uptake of, say, 4 l/min, corresponding to about 80 kJ (20 kcal)/min, about 60 kJ/min of heat is produced. As the specific heat of the human body is about 3·5 kJ (0·8 kcal)/kg, it follows that a man weighing 75 kg would increase his body temperature by 0·8°C every 5 min if the heat were not dissipated. In heavy exercise at normal conditions, most of the heat is given off by evaporation of sweat. Radiation and convection play only a minor part, since the temperature

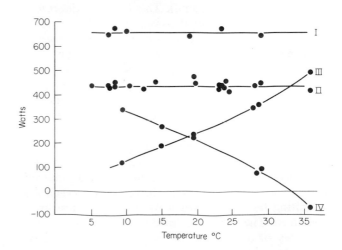

FIG. 45.15. Overall rates of energy utilization and heat losses, both expressed in watts, during one hour of exercise when doing work at a rate of 148 W, at various environmental temperatures (abscissa). I, total energy utilization, from oxygen uptake; II, total heat loss; III, heat loss through evaporation; IV, heat loss through radiation and convection. I–II represents energy converted to mechanical energy (work) plus heat stored in the body during initial phase of work. From Nielsen M. (1938) *Skand. Arch. Physiol.* **79**, 193.

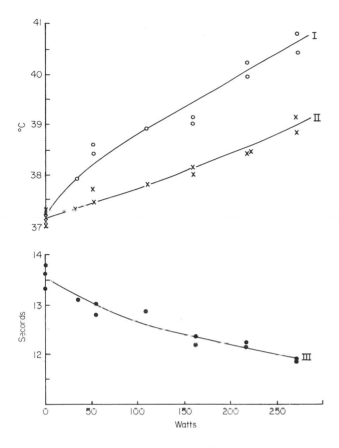

FIG. 45.16. I, deep muscle temperatures (vastus muscle); II, rectal temperatures after 30 min 'warming up' at work rates as shown on abscissa; III, time for a subsequent 'sprint' at a work rate of 160 W on the bicycle ergometer. From Asmussen E. & Bøje O. (1945) *Acta physiol. scand.* **10**, 1.

gradient between the skin and environment can be increased only slightly by elevation of the skin temperature (fig. 45.15).

During the first 30–60 min of exercise, not all the extra heat is given off, for a certain amount is stored in the body and the temperature consequently rises. Thereafter, the elevated body temperature is maintained within narrow limits. The temperature at which this plateau is reached is dependent on the metabolic rate and not on the temperature of the environment. Body temperature during exercise must consequently be a regulated function, but what actually sets the 'body thermostat' at a level corresponding to the rate of work is not known. It has been found that it is the relative load of work rather than the absolute value that determines the body temperature in exercise. At a certain percentage of their maximal working capacity, different people have approximately the same deep body temperature.

Sweat production in exercise is also a regulated function. It appears to vary with heat production, even when heat is produced in the body from other sources than

from metabolism. This happens for instance during 'negative work', where external work is absorbed by the muscles and turned into heat. One finds then that body temperature follows the metabolism, whereas sweat production follows total heat production.

A teleological explanation of the increased body temperature during exercise may be that the body machine works better at a higher temperature. The chemical processes are accelerated, the HbO_2 dissociation curve is flattened and viscous resistances in joints and muscles are decreased. Laboratory experiments have shown that subjects perform better, i.e. can work at a higher rate, run faster, etc., when their muscles are warmed up by previous exercise (fig. 45.16) or diathermy. This may partly explain the benefit that athletes derive from warming up before an event.

Fitness and training

The importance of being fit and physically well-trained can be seriously questioned in a society where hard labour, walking and running, and bicycling are becoming more unnecessary due to increasing mechanization, motorization and automation. Surveys of physiological working capacities show that this function is decreasing in industrialized societies, and that it is related to the physical demands of the occupation which are declining. However, the occurrence of certain diseases is actually curtailed by a systematic training of the body. Evidence is accumulating to show that degenerative diseases, including heart failure in middle age, are more common among persons who take little or no daily physical exercise, than among persons who indulge in some kind of sport or exercise. Also, cardiac patients who are given a suitable programme of physical exercise seem to get along better and live longer than patients who are recommended to take it easy. Many doctors of the old school are still reluctant to consider these trends. It is characteristic of our time that the disease and recuperation of a President of the United States (Eisenhower, in 1955) brought the ideas of physical fitness as a means of rehabilitation and prophylaxis a long stride forward. A thorough study of the numerous functional adaptations of the human body to physical exercise thus seems a useful occupation for any medical student.

FURTHER READING

ASMUSSEN E. (1965) Muscular exercise. In *Handbook of Physiology*, Section 3, Volume II, ed. Fenn W.O. & Rahn H. Washington D.C.: American Physiological Society.

ÅSTRAND P.-O. & RODAHL K. (1970) *Textbook of Work Physiology*. New York: McGraw-Hill.

DOWNEY J.A. & DARLING R.C. eds. (1971) *Physiological*

Basis of Rehabilitation Medicine. Philadelphia: Saunders.

JOHNSON W.R. & BUSKIRK E. (1973) *Science and Medicine of Exercise and Sports*, 2nd Edition. New York: Harper & Row.

RARICK G.L. ed. (1973) *Physical Activity*: *Human Growth and Development.* New York: Academic Press.

ROWELL L.B. (1974) Human cardiovascular adjustment to exercise and thermal stress. *Physiological Reviews* **54**, 74–159.

Chapter 46
Life at varying oxygen pressures

On the 1st August, 1774, Joseph Priestley used his new 12 inch burning glass to focus the sun's rays on to mercuric oxide, and collected the gas evolved. This gas was oxygen, although Priestley called it 'dephlogisticated air' following the erroneous theory of chemistry in which he was an ardent believer. He noted that a candle burned with 'greater vivacity' in his new gas and proposed that it might be 'peculiarly salutary to the lungs in morbid cases'. The gas was named oxygen by Lavoisier, who was the first to show that it was used by the body in respiration. The role of oxygen in human metabolism was firmly established by the German physiologists of the nineteenth century, but the Frenchman, Paul Bert, showed that the effects of oxygen were dependent upon the partial pressure of oxygen (Po_2). The Po_2 of a gas mixture is directly proportional to the number of molecules of free oxygen present and is calculated by multiplying the percentage concentration of oxygen by the total pressure of the gas (p. 31.17). The Po_2 of a liquid is also directly proportional to the molecular concentration of free oxygen, but it is more difficult to measure. Air contains approximately 21 per cent oxygen, even at great altitudes, and many workers had attributed the symptoms of mountain sickness, which afflicts people at high altitudes, to the low barometric pressure. Paul Bert found that a bird in a bottle survived when given 90 per cent oxygen at 13·3 kPa (100 mm Hg) total pressure (Po_2 12 kPa) but quickly died when given air (which contains 21 per cent oxygen) at this total pressure (Po_2 2·7 kPa). He concluded: 'Oxygen tension is everything'.

Oxygen secretion controversy

The manner in which oxygen in the air supplies the oxygen used up in biochemical mechanisms in the cell has continued to puzzle physiologists since Lavoisier and we still do not know all the answers to this problem. The passage of oxygen into the blood from the alveoli of the lungs is now accepted as being due to diffusion from a higher to a lower Po_2, this idea being proposed by August and Marie Krogh of Copenhagen in the early part of this century. J.S. Haldane of Oxford disagreed and held that active secretion of oxygen occurred in the lung. The crux of Haldane's argument was that on an expedition to the 4600 m (14 000 ft) Pike's Peak in 1912, he found evidence that the Po_2 in the alveoli was less than that in the arterial blood. This famous controversy later involved Sir Joseph Barcroft of Cambridge, who first defined accurately the form of the oxygen dissociation curve of haemoglobin (p. 31.19).

This secretion argument really hinged on the measurement of the Po_2 of arterial blood. In 1920, Barcroft lived in a glass chamber for 7 days under conditions of hypoxia and exercise similar to those endured by Haldane and others on Pike's Peak. Blood samples were taken directly from his radial artery, and the amount of oxygen in the blood was measured by the chemical methods then available. At the same time, his blood was mixed outside his body with samples of his alveolar air, and the amount of oxygen in the blood was measured when mixing was complete. This last oxygen content was greater than the first, and therefore his alveolar Po_2 must have been greater than his arterial Po_2. Cambridge and Copenhagen had triumphed over Oxford, at least in that controversy.

The modern development of a direct electrode method of measuring Po_2 has vindicated Paul Bert's thesis that the Po_2 is 'everything'. The direct measurement of Po_2 of the arterial blood is now an essential investigation in many patients with disease of heart or lungs who are thought to have deficient oxygenation of the blood.

Cellular oxygen usage

Chap. 8 describes the way in which cells use oxygen to provide the energy involved in living. It will be recalled that molecular oxygen is used to oxidize cytochrome a_3 which acts as the end receptor of the electron transfer series of interlinked enzymes in the mitochondria of the cell. This property of oxygen usage appears to be common to most cells in the body, although under conditions of oxygen deficiency cells can still obtain energy from metabolism of nutrients, but by this process (anaerobic glycolysis) they can produce much less energy than when using oxygen.

It is now known that oxygen is supplied to the mitochrondrial cytochromes at a Po_2 below 0·133 kPa (1 mm Hg). The famous aphorism of Claude Bernard: 'The constancy of the internal environment is the only condition of the free life', could be paraphrased to read: 'One essential condition of the free life is the provision of oxygen to the mitochondria at a P_{O_2} of about 0·1 kPa.

Capillary P_{O_2}

The supply of oxygen to the cell can be envisaged as the diffusion of oxygen molecules from areas of higher P_{O_2}, with more oxygen molecules, to areas of lower P_{O_2}, with fewer oxygen molecules; the lowest P_{O_2} results from the chemical conversion of oxygen to water at the cellular cytochromes. This idea is illustrated in fig. 46.1. The

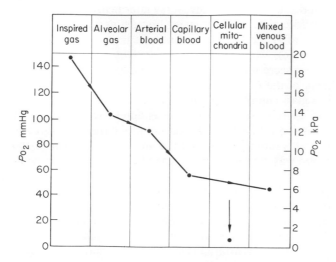

FIG. 46.1. The oxygen cascade illustrating the oxygen pressure at various sites in the body in a normal man breathing air at sea level.

immediate source of oxygen for the cell is of course the nearest capillary to that cell. How far is it from the capillary to the cytochromes in the mitochondria? This question cannot be answered definitely for the distance varies widely from tissue to tissue and depends also upon the number of capillaries open at any state of activity. Thus in the kidney there are large numbers of capillaries, and no cells are far removed from them, for the organ has a high blood flow. In resting skeletal muscle, on the other hand, there are few capillaries open and there is a low blood flow. The kidney has a high oxygen consumption, expressed as the volume of oxygen used each minute by each gram of tissue, whereas resting skeletal muscle has a lower oxygen consumption. However, when muscular activity starts, the capillary bed in the muscle expands enormously and as the blood flow rises the oxygen consumption increases. This careful matching of blood flow through an organ to its oxygen needs is one of the most beautiful examples of control mechanisms in physio-

logy. The mechanism is easily disturbed in disease. If the arterial blood supply to a muscle is limited, due to a partial blockage of the supplying artery, the patient may suffer pain when he exercises that muscle (intermittent claudication). This pain is due to the accumulation of some unknown products of anaerobic metabolism, for the blood supply cannot increase sufficiently to meet the demands of that tissue, and thereby provide enough oxygen to the muscle on exercise.

It is important to realize that the blood in the capillaries does not normally give up all its oxygen in passing from the arterial to the venous end of the vessel. If this did happen then the venous P_{O_2} would be zero. However, since the point of oxygen usage, the mitochondrial cytochromes, is the point of lowest P_{O_2}, unless the blood flow is completely obstructed the venous blood of a tissue will always contain some oxygen. In some varieties of heart failure, such as that due to severe mitral stenosis with a very low cardiac output which cannot be increased on exercise, the venous blood from exercising muscles contains very little oxygen. Such patients complain only of tiredness in the exercising muscles and breathlessness, and not of 'intermittent claudication', as the products of anaerobic metabolism are removed by the circulation.

Variation in inspired oxygen pressures

Man has evolved as an air-breathing mammal accustomed to an atmospheric P_{O_2} of between 21·5 and 20 kPa (160–150 mm Hg) at sea level, and has never experienced higher levels of P_{O_2} from natural causes. In the conquest of new environments, however, he first ascended mountains, went up in balloons, later flew in aeroplanes and travelled to the moon, as well as descending in mines, diving suits, submarines and bathyspheres. All these departures from sea level change the inspired P_{O_2}, ascents reducing it and descents increasing it.

LIFE AT REDUCED OXYGEN PRESSURE

Permanent residents at high altitude

About 10 million people live permanently more than 4000 m (12 000 ft) above sea level. At this height, the inspired P_{O_2} is about 12 kPa (fig. 46.2). These people live in the Himalayas and High Andes, where climatic limitations on the crops that can be grown seem to be of more importance than hypoxia. In Chile and Peru, mining is carried on at great altitudes. The highest place permanently inhabited by man is the mining camp on Mount Aucanquilcha at 5800 m. The actual sulphur mine is at 6300 m, but the miners refuse to sleep at this height and prefer to climb 500 m to their work each day.

Acclimatization to these high altitudes depends upon the duration of the exposure and is most fully developed

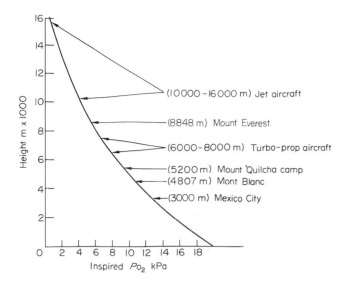

FIG. 46.2. The inspired oxygen pressures at various heights above sea level.

in permanent residents. Pulmonary ventilation is increased at altitude, particularly on exercise, and the arterial P_{CO_2} is reduced to about 4 kPa in the miners at 'Quilcha, compared with the value of 5·3 kPa (40 mm Hg) at sea level. Despite this low P_{CO_2}, the blood has a normal pH of 7·40 in these miners because blood $[HCO_3^-]$ is proportionately reduced. Newcomers to altitude, on the other hand, have a respiratory alkalosis with low P_{CO_2} and a high pH with $[HCO_3^-]$ only slightly below normal. The increased ventilation improves the distribution of gas to all parts of the lungs. An increase in haemoglobin concentration of the blood and in the red cell count has been known to occur in altitude acclimatized subjects since 1891. At 'Quilcha, the miners may have up to 23 g/dl Hb compared to a normal sea level value of about 15 g/dl. The oxygen capacity of this polycythaemic blood is about 300 ml oxygen/litre. Although the arterial P_{O_2} is only about 5 kPa at this altitude, the arterial blood contains about 220 ml oxygen/litre which is in fact more than that in the arterial blood of a normal man at sea level! This greater content of oxygen, however, is carried at a lower P_{O_2}, and it is the P_{O_2} which determines the ease of transfer of oxygen to the cellular mitochrondria. It was thought that the rightwards shift in the oxygen dissociation curve (increase in P_{50}, p. 31.19) which occurred at altitude, resulted from a rise in the concentration of 2,3-diphosphoglycerate (2,3-DPG) in the red cells. However, it is now realized that the increase in both P_{50} and 2,3-DPG results in large part from the alkalosis of altitude, for both can be prevented by administration of the carbonic anhydrase inhibitor, acetazolamide, which reduces this alkalosis.

Permanent residents at high altitude have a normal cardiac output at rest, but the pulmonary artery pressure is raised, and the right ventricle hypertrophied, in comparison with subjects living at sea level. The media of the pulmonary arteries is thickened, the vessels appearing similar to those in the unexpanded fetal lung. On exercise, the cardiac output is greater than that at the same level of oxygen uptake at sea level, and this results in high pulmonary artery pressures and a consequent strain on the right ventricle.

Chronic mountain sickness, Mongé's disease, affects some people permanently residing over 4500 m. It is characterized by a higher P_{CO_2} and a lower arterial P_{O_2} than is normally found in acclimatized residents at these altitudes. Right heart failure and severe polycythaemia occur and seem to arise from the combination of the demands for an increased cardiac output, the narrowing of pulmonary vessels and the increased blood viscosity. The disease may be due to a reduction in the normal sensitivity of the carotid body chemoreceptors to hypoxia.

Acute exposure to high altitudes

The fighter pilot whose oxygen supply suddenly fails at 11 000 m may lose consciousness without warning in 2 min. The tourist who motors from sea level to 4000 m in one day often suffers from headache and insomnia, whereas the mountaineer who climbs gradually to 6000 m notices only breathlessness, particularly on exertion, and Cheyne–Stokes breathing at night. The adaptive processes of acclimatization take time to develop.

Below 2500 m very few people are affected by altitude and most young adults notice nothing until almost 4000 m is reached, where the inspired P_{O_2} is about 13 kPa. The symptoms of **acute mountain sickness** consist of headache and breathlessness, with weakness and tachycardia and sometimes anorexia and vomiting; central cyanosis is occasionally seen. However there is no correlation between the severity of the symptoms and the arterial P_{O_2}. These symptoms can develop within a few hours at altitude but usually improve in a few days. They can be alleviated by acetazolamide, which reduces the respiratory alkalosis arising from the fall in P_{CO_2} during acute exposure to altitude.

Ventilatory regulation at altitude

The mechanisms underlying the increase in ventilation after acclimatization to high altitude are still incompletely understood. The increase is not entirely due to hypoxic stimulation, for reduction of the arterial P_{O_2} in a subject at sea level does not provoke such an increase in breathing. Conversely, administration of oxygen to the resident at high altitude does not reduce his ventilation to sea level values. When the ventilatory responses to CO_2 inhalation are studied, keeping the alveolar, or arterial, P_{O_2} constant (p. 31.28), the subject who is acclimatized to altitude is found to have an increased sensitivity to CO_2, which is

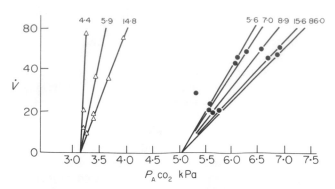

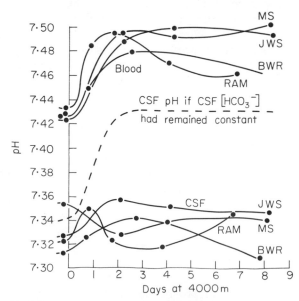

FIG. 46.3. The response to CO_2 inhalation after acclim-atization at 6250 m (19 500 ft). ●, experiment at sea level; △, experiments on the same subject at 6250 m. $\dot{V}$. is ven-tilation in l/min. The figures above the lines are the P_{A,O_2} at which those lines are determined. Modified from Milledge J.S. (1963) *The Regulation of Human Ventilation*, ed. Cunning-ham D.J.C. and Lloyd B.B. Oxford:Blackwell Scientific Publications.

expressed as a shift of his response line to the left and also as an increase in the slope (fig. 46.3).

The acidity of the cerebrospinal fluid (CSF) bathing the lateral surface of the medulla is also known to play an important role in the regulation of ventilation. The pH of CSF is, of course, dependent upon its P_{CO_2} and $[HCO_3^-]$. CO_2 molecules freely cross the blood-brain barrier, so that the arterial P_{CO_2} and the CSF P_{CO_2} are closely

related. However, $[HCO_3^-]$ in the CSF is not always the same as that in the blood plasma. During acclimatization to altitude, the CSF bicarbonate decreases more quickly than that in the blood due, in the opinion of some physio-logists, to the accumulation of lactic acid in the CSF from anaerobic metabolism of the brain in altitude hypoxia, and so the pH of the CSF is unchanged from that found at sea level. Thus, despite the fall in arterial P_{CO_2} during altitude acclimatization, which would be sufficient to stop breathing altogether in a normal sub-ject at sea level, the CSF pH in the acclimatized subject is maintained at normal levels.

Ascent of Everest

The early attempts on Mount Everest (8848 m) were made mainly without oxygen breathing equipment, but these expeditions (1924–33) approached the mountain across the Tibetan plateau and became acclimatized during this march at over 4300 m. When the Southern route through Nepal was opened in 1951, Shipton found that an ascent via the West Cwm and the South Col seemed possible. In 1953, Sir John Hunt led the successful expedition which culminated in the ascent by Hillary and Tensing. They climbed at a rate of 200 m/h from the South Col, at 7900 m, to the summit, using oxygen at 3 l/min (STP). A Chinese expedition reached the summit by the North ridge in 1975, apparently without oxygen. Intense cold is as much a problem as oxygen lack in high altitude mountaineering, and dehydration from an insuf-ficient fluid intake is a grave potential hazard.

Air transport

Modern commercial aircraft cruise most economically around 6000 m (prop jets) 10 000 m (pure jets) and 16 000 m (Concorde) and yet their passengers and crew could survive for only minutes at these altitudes. The problem is overcome by maintaining the air pressure in the cabin at that of an altitude of between 1650 m and 2600 m. To pressurize the cabin to sea level when at 10 000 m would greatly increase the demands on cabin strength and therefore in weight.

Failure of cabin pressurization when at high altitude exposes everyone to severe hypoxia, and emergency oxy-gen must be instantly available to the crew, who must immediately bring the aircraft down to at most 3000 m, if this be possible. In addition to hypoxia, a sudden lowering of external pressure results in expansion of gas contained in closed cavities in the body, such as gas in the alimentary tract, or more seriously gas in a pneu-mothorax or an air-containing cyst in the lung. Air em-bolism is a serious but remote risk of such rapid decom-pression. Decompression sickness, the bends (p. 46.6), can develop with rapid decompression of the cabin at 10 000 m.

FIG. 46.4. The pH in arterial blood and CSF in four subjects during acclimatization to 4000 m. The dotted line repre-sents the CSF pH which would have resulted if the CSF bicarbonate concentration did not alter. Modified from Severinghaus J.W. (1965) *The Cerebrospinal Fluid and the Regulation of Ventilation*, ed. Brooks C.McC., Kao F.F. and Lloyd B.B. Oxford: Blackwell Scientific Publications.

The problems involved in transport of invalids by air are more important to doctors. Infectious diseases are usually regarded as a complete contra-indication for scheduled passenger flights, since isolation is impossible. The inspired P_{O_2} at a simulated cabin altitude of 2600 m will be about 13·3 kPa. In patients with a decreased arterial oxygen pressure when breathing air at sea level even this degree of hypoxia may be dangerous. Such patients of course, include those suffering from chronic bronchitis and emphysema, or in an exacerbation of chronic asthma, and patients with pulmonary fibrosis or congenital heart disease with cyanosis. Patients with heart failure and severe anaemia, particularly sickle cell anaemia, can also be at risk from hypoxia. In all these cases, supplementary oxygen can be provided on request. Patients who have had a myocardial infarction should not normally fly for 6–8 weeks. Divers who have been below 6·6 m (20 ft) of water are advised not to fly above 600 m (2000 ft) for 24 hours since they may well develop decompression sickness even at simulated cabin altitudes.

Military pilots face other problems. They must be able to fly higher and to survive if their cabin is perforated. They wear oxygen masks, but at 13 000 m, with a barometric pressure of 19 kPa, even when breathing 100 per cent oxygen, the inspired P_{O_2} will be only 12·5 kPa, after subtracting 6·5 kPa for the saturated vapour pressure of water at 37°C. To preserve efficiency at higher altitudes oxygen must be given under increased pressure.

Chronic respiratory disease

Hypoxia due to disease of the lungs is of far more importance to most doctors than the altitude hypoxia discussed above. Chronic bronchitis and emphysema affects over half a million people in Britain. In the advanced stages of this disease, the structure of the lungs becomes so disorganized, with narrowing of the airways leading to some alveoli and obstruction to the blood supply of others, that effective exchange of O_2 and CO_2 between gas and blood in the lungs is severely impaired. An increase in ventilation of alveoli that are perfused with blood removes more CO_2 from their blood, and thereby compensates for the inefficiency of other alveoli. However, such an increase in ventilation can add very little more oxygen to the blood leaving alveoli that are already adequately ventilated, due to the S-shape of the oxyhaemoglobin dissociation curve. Thus an increase in ventilation cannot compensate for hypoxia due to unventilated alveoli.

Ventilatory failure

In patients with chronic bronchitis and emphysema the respiratory centre becomes gradually less sensitive to CO_2 as a respiratory stimulant. As a result the patient

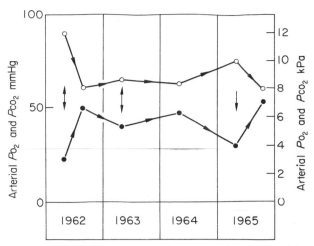

FIG. 46.5. Arterial P_{O_2}, ● and P_{CO_2}, ○ in a man with chronic respiratory failure due to chronic bronchitis and emphysema. The vertical arrows represent episodes of severe chest infection.

tends to develop a raised arterial P_{CO_2}. The cause of this apparent insensitivity to CO_2 is unknown, but the disordered mechanical properties of these diseased lungs, with narrowed airways and overdistended air spaces, play an important role. This effect of overdistension can easily be mimicked by trying to breathe with the lungs almost full of air, a very unpleasant sensation, which also involves a considerable increase in the muscular activity necessary to take a breath of normal tidal volume. As the arterial P_{CO_2} rises, the arterial pH falls and a respiratory acidosis develops. This high P_{CO_2} means that ventilation is insufficient to meet the metabolic production of CO_2 by the body, and a high P_{CO_2} is therefore always to be associated with a low arterial P_{O_2}, when breathing air. This combination of a low P_{O_2} and a high P_{CO_2} is known as ventilatory failure.

The high P_{CO_2} in ventilatory failure is very important, for not only does it demonstrate that the respiratory centre has lost some of its sensitivity to its most powerful stimulus, CO_2, but also the high P_{CO_2} acts as a very potent cerebral vasodilator. This protects the brain against oxygen deficiency at the mitochondrial level, for the vasodilation ensures a very short path for diffusion of oxygen from the capillaries to the mitochondria. Patients with chronic bronchitis often have chronic ventilatory failure, with an arterial P_{O_2} of about 6·5–8·0 kPa (fig. 46.5). Like residents at high altitude, some patients develop secondary polycythaemia in response to this hypoxic stimulus. It seems possible that some of the consequences of the prolonged hypoxaemia in these patients, including right heart failure, may be alleviated by **long term oxygen therapy**, given at a flow rate of about 2 l O_2/min, continuously for many years. Such treatment is expensive, and its clinical value is currently being assessed in careful trials in several centres (vol. 3, p. 18.47).

In most drowning accidents, the victim is dead before he is brought from the water. To have any chance of success, mouth to mouth breathing must start at once, for example whilst the victim is still in the water or being carried through the shallows. If a pulse cannot be felt closed-chest cardiac massage should also be started. Compression of the chest and therefore of the heart is best achieved by firmly pressing the sternum and anterior chest wall with the subject in the supine position. This is timed so that three chest compressions are given for one lung inflation. It is possible to detect a femoral or carotid pulse as a result of this manoeuvre, and both the kiss of life and cardiac massage can be carried out by one person. It is completely wrong to spend time bringing resuscitation equipment, such as oxygen cylinders, unless mouth to mouth ventilation and closed chest cardiac massage are already in progress. When they become available, usually following hospital admission, tracheal intubation and bronchoscopy may be needed, followed by intermittent mechanical positive pressure respiration if spontaneous breathing is still inadequate. Hypothermia from prolonged immersion is best treated by putting the trunk in a hot bath at 40–44°C, whilst leaving the limbs out. Ventricular fibrillation can be treated by DC countershock. This is most effective in the well-oxygenated patient, in whom acidosis arising from the accumulation of lactic acid has been corrected by giving sodium bicarbonate intraveneously. The haemoconcentration following sea-water drowning can be treated by hypotonic intravenous fluids, and in the unusual circumstance of severe haemolysis following fresh-water drowning fresh blood or exchange transfusion may be needed. Bacterial pneumonia from aspiration of infected water may require antibiotics. Delayed pulmonary oedema or pneumonia may only develop later, and victims of near drowning should be kept in hospital under observation for 24 hours.

Is all this worthwhile? It can be. A 5-year-old Norwegian boy fell through the ice into a partially frozen river, and was totally submerged for 40 minutes in the ice-cold fresh water. Mouth-to-mouth ventilation and closed chest cardiac massage were started immediately after he was carried ashore, and the measures described above used when he reached hospital. Severe pulmonary oedema responded to mechanical ventilation with positive end expiratory pressure (PEEP). He recovered consciousness within 48 hours, and despite a transient cerebellar dysfunction, was neurologically, intellectually and emotionally normal for his age one year later.

Potential victims of drowning, which includes all swimmers, sailors, and even anglers, should know that cold is a major hazard during immersion. In sea water at 5°C, even a clothed victim will be helpless from cold after 40–60 min, so that every effort must be made to conserve heat. The victim should float quietly, as swimming greatly increases heat loss, and so hastens death.

Only about 2 per cent of people sink in salt water, but a good life jacket not only adds buoyancy, but also keeps the head clear of waves.

Submarines

The world's first submarine was launched in 1897, and subsequent development has depended on solutions to three problems: withstanding water pressure, providing engines which run when submerged, and providing a habitable atmosphere for the crew. The first two problems belong to engineers, and the use of nuclear power has dramatically removed the limitation imposed by the engines. The third problem is one of biological engineering. The time of maximal submersion has increased from 6 hours in 1900, and now, with nuclear submarines, to regular patrols of over 60 days and more. At any moment, 10–15 000 men are now living deep below the surface of the sea. Some naval submariners may spend 7 years of their total working life under water. A submariner lives in an atmosphere at normal total pressure, this atmosphere being automatically replenished with oxygen by electrolysis of sea water. Carbon dioxide is removed by chemical 'scrubbers', hydrogen by catalytic oxidation, and dusts, aerosols and toxic contaminants by filters and electrostatic precipitation. Materials which would normally be harmless at the concentrations encountered on land may well become hazardous in submarines, as exposure is continuous for 24 hours per day, 7 days a week, with no daily or weekly recovery periods. Carbon dioxide is usually allowed to accumulate to about 1 per cent during a submarine patrol, and this produces a mild respiratory acidosis, which becomes compensated after about 3 weeks when there is an increase in hydrogen ion excretion, and also a fall in excretion of calcium.

Space flight

An astronaut is utterly dependent for all his physical needs on the contents of his capsule. The greatest of these needs is for oxygen, and its provision presents problems. If he lives in an atmosphere of pure oxygen at atmospheric pressure, the fire risk is very great and, as the inspired Po_2 is about 95 kPa, the Lorrain Smith effect or pulmonary oxygen toxicity develops.

The total pressure in a capsule is therefore held below atmospheric and the oxygen concentration increased to give an inspired Po_2 of about 25 kPa. As the first American space tragedies showed, pure oxygen, even at this pressure, poses a severe fire risk and capsules now have an oxygen-helium atmosphere. The need for oxygen in prolonged space flight has led to the ingenious suggestion that a mixture of algae and bacteria, fed on CO_2 from the breath and urea from the urine, can produce enough oxygen by photosynthesis in sunlight.

The space traveller must undergo severe accelerative

stress to escape from the earth's gravitational field (G), followed by weightlessness during the period in space, with re-exposure to even greater decelerative stress, which can amount to 6–8 times the earth's gravitation, during re-entry. Although careful positioning during lift-off and re-entry minimizes these problems, a fall in cardiac output, with marked rise in blood pressure during the positive G of re-entry, presents major limitations to man's G tolerance. Prolonged weightlessness has in practice been less hazardous than science fiction writers predicted, but cardiovascular deconditioning, with a tendency to faint when standing up, along with transient demineralization of the skeleton and more long-standing vestibular problems, with recurrent vertigo, are encountered in some astronauts after return to earth.

Hyperbaric oxygen treatment

Oxygen is carried in the blood in two forms:

(1) in chemical combination with haemoglobin, the amount of oxygen at any blood Po_2 being determined from the oxyhaemoglobin dissociation curve,

(2) in physical solution in plasma, where the amount is directly proportional to the Po_2 so that 0·225 ml of oxygen are dissolved in each litre of blood for each kPa Po_2.

At a Po_2 of about 40 kPa (300 mm Hg), the haemoglobin is fully saturated with oxygen, but the oxygen content of the blood continues to rise as the Po_2 rises, due to the oxygen in solution. If the Po_2 can be taken to 300 kPa (3 atmospheres absolute), the amount in solution is 60–70 ml for each litre of blood. This is sufficient to provide for an oxygen consumption of 300 ml/min, if the cardiac output is 5 l/min, without using the oxygen combined with haemoglobin at all. Furthermore, at this arterial Po_2, the mean capillary Po_2 is of the order of 70 kPa. Thus the pressure differential driving oxygen to the mitochondria (where the Po_2 is about 0·1 kPa) is about ten times normal. These facts are the basis of hyperbaric therapy.

This treatment requires a pressure chamber, which can contain the whole patient and also the doctors, surgeons and nurses, if his treatment is to be prolonged. In the chamber, the patient breathes oxygen but the attendants breathe the chamber air. The pressure can be two or three atmospheres absolute or 200–300 kPa. These large chambers are expensive and need elaborate pumps and safety equipment. The attendants run the risk of developing the bends on decompression and later bone damage, but the patient is safe from this as he breathes oxygen although he is at risk from oxygen poisoning, and decompression must be very slow and carefully supervised. As in all work at high pressure involving oxygen, the fire risk is considerable.

This treatment was first used as an aid to the treatment of cancer by X-rays. Some cancer cells are very resistant to X-rays, but this can be overcome if they are exposed to high Po_2. For this purpose, small one-man pressure chambers are in fairly wide use.

Hyperbaric oxygen treatment can be of value in treating carbon monoxide poisoning due, for example, to car exhaust fumes. Here the haemoglobin combines with carbon monoxide much more firmly than it does with oxygen, but hyperbaric therapy can provide oxygen to the tissues without relying on haemoglobin. It is also of value in treating widespread infection with the gas gangrene organism, *Clostridium welchii*, which cannot live at a high Po_2.

FURTHER READING

BATES D.V., MACKLEM P.T. & CHRISTIE R.V. (1971) *Respiratory Function in Disease*, 2nd Edition. Philadelphia: Saunders.

BERT P. (1878) *La Pression barometrique, recherches de physiologie*. Paris: Masson. English translation by HITCHCOCK M.A. & HITCHCOCK F.A. (1943) Columbus, Ohio: College Book Co.

FENN W.O. & RAHN H. eds. (1965) *Handbook of Physiology* Section 3. Respiration. Vols. I & II. Washington, D.C.: American Physiological Society.

HALDANE J.S. & PRIESTLEY J.G. (1935) *Respiration*, 2nd Edition. Oxford: Clarendon Press.

MILES S. (1969) *Underwater Medicine*, 3rd Edition. London: Staples Press.

SIEBKE H., BREIVIK H., RØD T. & BJØRN L. (1975) Survival after 40-minutes' submersion without cerebral sequelae. *Lancet* i, 1275–1277.

many weeks, even though the environment contains little or nothing in the way of 24-hour clues and any direct influence of habit, waking and sleeping, meal times, rest and exercise, the activities and rest of other people around all co-operate to cause adaptation to the artificial day (fig. 47.5).

Some have maintained that trifling residual circadian changes in the environment, such as fluctuations in the Earth's magnetism or in barometric pressure, provide a clue, but these oscillations are very small and below the limit of detection by any known human sense organ; furthermore they cannot account for the persistence of rhythms when one flies half-way round the world.

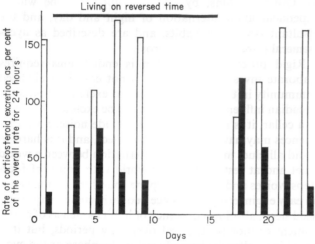

FIG. 47.1. Excretion of corticosteroids; □, during the first 6 hours of waking; ■, during sleep. Before, during and after a fortnight of sleeping by day in an Arctic summer. The slow adaptation to the artificial time and the equally slow return to normal are shown. From data of Sharp G.W.G., Slorach S.A. & Vipond H.J. (1961) *J. Endocrin.* **22**, 377.

Another observation at variance with this suggestion is that when physiological rhythms have become adapted to a new time pattern, return to normal time does not cause them to revert immediately. They take about as long to change back as they took to depart from normal phase in the first place (fig. 47.1).

Species other than man can more readily be kept under constant conditions continuously, e.g. in a quiet room where light intensity is maintained at a uniform level, where food and drink are available continuously and where external activities such as supplying food or cleaning cages are randomized throughout the 24 hours. The easiest rhythm to study is that of rest and activity; small rodents such as rats and mice are normally active by night and inactive by day, and simple recording devices can register the amount of movement going on at any time throughout the 24 hours. Under uniform conditions, they maintain approximately a 24-hour periodicity, but after a time this begins to drift a little from precise

adherence to a 24-hour clock, coming to adopt a cycle of slightly longer or shorter duration. The term 'circadian' was deliberately coined to cover such periods whose length was not precisely 24 hours. It thus appears that there is a built-in clock which is not a perfect time-keeper, but tends to gain or lose slightly, and under ordinary conditions is constantly adjusted and set to keep good 24-hour time by the rhythmic alternation of light, darkness and so forth. Mice have been maintained in a constant environment for as long as six generations, and circadian behaviour still persisted. This indicates an inborn form of behaviour rather than one which is acquired by each animal early in life through exposure to a circadian environment. The most nearly comparable observations in man have been made on people spending long periods down deep caves in solitude, or in an isolation unit, and the results have been essentially similar. The sleeping habits of people completely deprived of any indication of time follow a rhythm with a period rather longer than 24 hours, and usually somewhere around 25 hours (fig. 47.10).

Some rhythmicity is present in the fetus *in utero*, presumably imparted by maternal rhythms; but circadian rhythms of activity and feeding, absent in the early weeks of life, develop post-natally even if the infant is isolated from the usual rhythms of illumination and maternal care.

The development of rhythms in infancy does not appear to have been studied in Arctic dwellers who in adult life often show remarkably regular rhythms. It would seem that regularity of habit is more important for maintaining rhythmicity than is the alternation of day and night, which at high latitudes is absent for much of the year.

Of the factors which normally set the phase of a rhythm and adjust its timing, light appears to be of special importance in most species; the rhythms can be easily manipulated and their phase altered by artificial changes in the illumination of the cages. In human experiments in which subjects remained in complete darkness for 3 hours after getting up, several physiological changes normally occurring around that time of day have been postponed for roughly 3 hours (fig. 47.2). Blind subjects have rhythms which are disorganized as compared with those of sighted people, though the ability to distinguish light and darkness in those with no measurable visual acuity is sufficient to maintain normal rhythmicity. It is surprising, therefore, that there is so little alteration in the timing of physiological rhythms at different seasons of the year, when the time of sunrise can change so markedly.

In animals living in a natural state many physiological rhythms are critical for survival. For instance, animals which live in an intertidal zone depend upon rhythmic behaviour for their protection when the tide is in or out, for the possibilities of feeding at the appropriate state of the tide and for laying and hatching eggs. Lunar rhythms

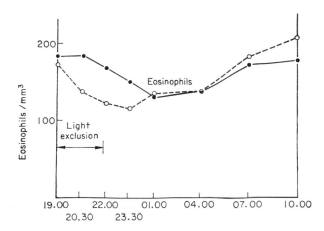

FIG. 47.2. Eosinophil count. ○, control observations; ●, days when subject remained in complete darkness for 3 hours after getting up. From data of Sharp G.W.G. (1960) *J. Endocrin.* **21**, 213.

are found in animals which depend upon the lunar variation in the height of tides. Similarly, most animals depend upon the alternation of light and darkness in their search for food or in their efforts to avoid being killed. Most small mammals are nocturnal and hide from their predators during the day in burrows, holes or other refuges. One might imagine that this behaviour is regulated by simple responsiveness to the changing illumination, leading them to retreat rapidly to security as the dawn appears and to emerge with the return of night. There are obvious advantages, however, in having some rhythmic process superimposed upon any direct response to the circadian stimuli. The mammal sleeping in a burrow by day would awake at around the appropriate time for safe emergence, rather than repeatedly coming out to see whether all is clear. Many of man's circadian rhythms are also beneficial. By and large, we are wakeful during the day when we are attempting to work or use our mind to maximum efficiency; we are tired and sleepy at night when we most commonly sleep. The early morning production of cortisol by the adrenal cortex (fig. 47.9) has been held to be an arousal mechanism, and the low urine flow at night is conducive to continuous uninterrupted sleep. The higher temperature during the day is probably conducive to muscular and perhaps mental efficiency. By virtue of his ability to manipulate the environment and control, for example, temperature and illumination, man has less need of these rhythms. He can store his food, and is virtually independent of restricted times of day for food gathering; he is also in most civilized communities relatively immune from predation and can venture forth at any hour of day or night. He is thus able, when energy for heating and lighting are freely available, to adopt habits which are strictly unnatural and to remain active long after dark and to lie abed after dawn. However, in so far as many of his physiological rhythms are endogenous

and persist despite modification of habits or surrounding illumination, they do not accord with his wish to depart from the circadian behaviour which nature or evolution intended. The persistence of these rhythms and their functional significance thus becomes an important subject of study for all those interested in night or shift work. The common arrangement whereby nurses work on nights for one week at a stretch is probably the worst that could be devised; many rhythms are becoming well adapted by the end of a week, and reversion to day working means that this useful adaptation is lost and there may be new problems of readaptation to a diurnal routine. Having originally devised machines for his benefit, man now finds himself increasingly their slave. Heavy capital investment in industrial plant demands that it shall operate continuously instead of merely in daylight hours. The provision of transport for those who wish to travel at different hours of day or night imposes a burden of work at unusual and irregular hours for the transport industries, and road congestion may make night travel desirable for heavy commercial transport. Aeroplanes and submarines work round-the-clock schedules. Those who fly rapidly long distances around the world subject their rhythms to a large enforced phase shift which creates its own problems. Such travellers, business men, statesmen, sportsmen, are often anxious to perform at maximal efficiency soon after arrival at their destination, and if they must spend days or weeks adjusting their internal rhythms to the sudden phase shift, the purpose of rapid travel is nullified. The American statesman Henry Kissinger who repeatedly crossed many time zones on peace-keeping missions was either a remarkable man or singularly ill-advised. The difficulty of repeated tests of performance which realistically mirror the abilities needed by a statesman precludes a decision between these alternatives. Astronauts travelling to the moon were entirely isolated from the usual circadian fluctuations in light, darkness and other aspects of environment. Those who have already orbited the Earth have subjected themselves to the remarkable rhythm of a day–night alternation occupying 90 min. So far it has not been necessary for human beings to dwell underground for prolonged periods though a few have done so with the desire to break a record, but if an atomic war should ever occur it may become necessary.

Temperature

Temperature has been studied more extensively than any other component of human rhythms; very extensive observations have been made on small numbers of people, and more scanty observations on enormous numbers have accumulated in hospital records. The conventional hospital chart of an afebrile patient shows a regular pattern usually with an alternation between high evening and low morning temperature. In some subjects, however, this pattern

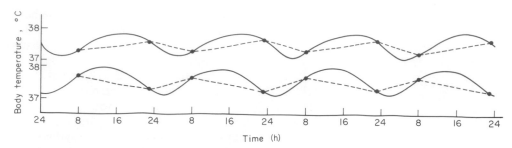

FIG. 47.3. Two examples of temperature rhythm, showing how a small shift in timing can result in a morning temperature above, instead of below, the evening value. Solid line, continuous record; broken line, readings only at bedtime and on waking.

is reversed and the temperature on waking is higher than on going to bed at night. The reason for this is seen at once if one studies fig. 47.3 which shows typical records of readings taken continuously throughout the 24 hours. The maximum temperature is usually observed in the afternoon and the minimum in the small hours, so that by bedtime the temperature is already declining from its peak and on waking it is already rising from its minimum value. A minor shift of the time of peak and trough may therefore result in the temperature being higher in the morning than in the evening, an apparent reversal of the usual rhythm which in reality is no more than a small time shift. The pattern is characteristic for the individual

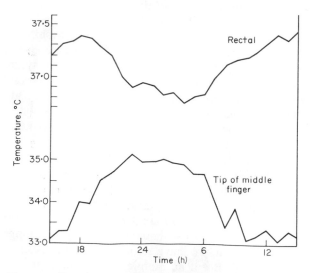

FIG. 47.4. Hourly record of temperature in rectum and on tip of middle finger. From data of Hildebrandt G. and Engelbertz P.

and is much the same in summer and winter. Different people vary somewhat in the form of their curve and some individuals show a flat plateau during most of the day. This rhythm develops during the early months of life and the magnitude of the oscillation from minimum to maximum increases with age up to about two years, and, at the same time, the timing of the oscillation becomes more regular. The rhythm does not depend closely upon any

variation in activity since it is as well developed in subjects recumbent throughout the 24 hours as in those active during the day. It appears to be due more to a variation in the heat loss than in heat production as is indicated by the circadian variation in skin temperature shown in fig. 47·4; the minimum body temperature is attained shortly after the maximum skin temperature, at a time when heat loss is greatest. An alternative explanation is that rhythmicity really resides in the 'set' of the thermoregulator.

Night workers often show circadian variations similar in phase to those of day workers, their temperature rhythm having failed to adapt to night work. Such workers in a civilized community are subjected to many influences indicating that the alternation of night and day is out of phase with their habits, and presumably one or other of these is responsible for the persistence of the usual pattern; moreover, they usually resume diurnal habits at the week-end; indeed in one study temperature was shown to adapt itself gradually to night work in the course of each week, only to lose the adaptation at the week-end. A more obstinate persistence of 24-hour rhythmicity in temperature has been reported in subjects, in Arctic summer or an isolation unit, living an artificial day of 18 to 28 hours. Many people can adapt their temperature rhythm quite readily to night work within a few days but on days of abnormal length, temperature rhythm can be one of the least adaptable of man's circadian rhythms.

The clinician using temperature measurement in diagnosis is aware of the circadian variation, and also of the fact that in febrile illness a high evening temperature is more characteristic than any elevation on waking. A more interesting possibility, as yet little explored and less understood, is a disturbance in the circadian temperature pattern in disease. This has been observed both in epilepsy and in cancer but has not as yet proved of any specific diagnostic value, and it is not known whether there is any association with particular diseases.

Kidney

The low urine flow at night is of obvious practical convenience and is a very ancient observation; and disturbance of the usual urinary rhythms underlies some cases of bed-wetting. The response to a standard water load is also greater in the morning than in the afternoon or evening. The factors determining urine flow are, however, complex, and include changes in excretory rate of the major solids of the urine and in the rate of production of ADH. Observations concerning rhythmic spontaneous variations in secretion of ADH are scanty and unreliable; most of our knowledge of circadian variations in renal function consists of information about excretion rate of the major solids, especially electrolytes. The rate of excretion of sodium, potassium and chloride, which is low at night, usually rises to a peak somewhere between 10.00 hours and 16.00 hours; the time is fairly characteristic for the individual and the peak time for these three electrolytes normally coincides roughly, although chloride and potassium peaks slightly precede the sodium peak, as in the control observation of fig. 47.6. In subjects living a normal existence, the inherent rhythm may be modified by their habits, coffee and tea in particular having an influence upon the excretion of water, sodium and chloride. When the natural cycle of sleep and activity is altered, whether by deliberately sleeping by day in the Arctic, by flying a substantial distance around the world, or by living a day of abnormal length, the potassium excretory rhythm may maintain a 24-hour timing for many weeks, but water, sodium and chloride rhythms often adapt sooner. Fig. 47.5 shows an example in a subject living a 27 hour day over a period covering eight artificial, or nine real, days. Water excretion shows eight peaks, and has thus adapted to the artificial time on which the subject was living, whereas potassium shows nine excretory peaks, occurring around

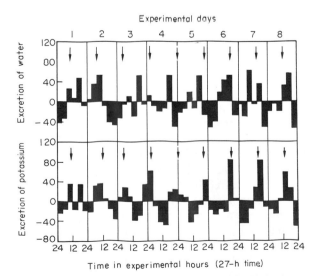

Experimental days

FIG. 47.5. Excretion of potassium and water by a subject living a 27-hour day, as percentage deviation from mean. Arrows indicate mid-day by real time. From data of Lewis & Lobban M.C. (1957) *Quart. J. exp. Physiol.*, **42**, 381.

mid-day by real time; it was affected by the subject's habits only in that the peak was low when real mid-day coincided with artificial midnight. This suggests the continued operation of a 24-hour clock from which water excretion has escaped under the influence of a 27-hour cycle.

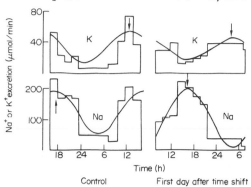

FIG. 47.6. Potassium and sodium excretion on a single control day and on the first day after time-zone shift. The sine curves of control have been fitted to 3 consecutive control days, those for experimental days to the actual day represented. Arrows indicate the peak of the sine curve. From data of Elliott A.L. *et al.* (1972).

Another consequence of the same dissociation is illustrated in fig. 47.6, which shows sodium and potassium excretion before, and on the first day after, an 8-hour time shift simulating a westward flight. Potassium excretion has adhered to the old time and sodium excretion has immediately been adapted to the new time, so that maximum sodium excretion now coincides with minimum potassium excretion, instead of their being nearly in phase.

There appears to be no circadian rhythm in plasma sodium or chloride, and doubtfully in potassium, so the rhythmic variations in their excretion must be due to some other cause. That urine is acid by night and much less acid or even alkaline in the morning is another old observation, although the morning alkalinity used to be ascribed to the influence of breakfast. If hydrogen ion excretion is calculated as the sum of titratable acid and ammonium excretion minus bicarbonate excretion, it is found to be a close mirror image of potassium excretion (fig. 47.7); it was thought originally that this was due to competition of these two ions for exchange with sodium in the distal convoluted tubules of the kidney. The explanation, however, is more complicated and is discussed on p. 35.25.

Phosphate excretion follows a different circadian pattern. When subjects sleep by night, it is commonly high during sleep and falls abruptly during the first hours of waking; when subjects remain awake and collect frequent samples during the night it is found that the fall in excretion has been proceeding steadily during the later hours of the night. Plasma phosphate analyses have been much less frequently performed, but they often parallel very closely the rhythm of phosphate excretion, and a rhythm in plasma phosphate concentration may therefore

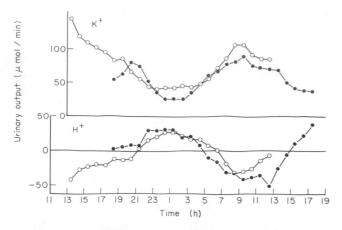

FIG. 47.7. Hourly excretion of potassium and hydrion by subjects working in a laboratory for 24 hours; two series of observations.

be the cause of the excretory rhythm. This rhythm is one of the most easily adaptable; thus in a subject changing over from night to day work, phosphate excretion fell abruptly when he awoke even during the transitional phase. Likewise, in subjects sleeping at unusual hours, urinary phosphate excretion commonly falls during the first hours after they rise.

The immediate cause of the rhythmic changes in excretion of other electrolytes is unknown. Glomerular filtration rate (GFR) has been claimed to follow a circadian pattern though observations are not numerous, and most workers do not consider that GFR is a major determinant of excretion of electrolytes. Of the endocrine factors said to play a part in their regulation, there is good evidence for rhythmic variations in cortisol secretion, but little for aldosterone secretion, diurnal variations in production of which are thought to be determined mainly by changes in posture. Cortisol increases the excretion of potassium and is produced mainly in the morning when potassium excretion rises. Since its own circadian rhythm is one of the most persistent when the subject's habits change, it could be responsible for the potassium excretory rhythm; but doubt arises whether quantitatively the circadian variations in cortisol production are sufficient to account for the large variations in urinary excretion of potassium. Uncertainty is greater over sodium since cortisol may either increase or decrease its excretion; the fact that sodium excretion may lose a circadian rhythm while that of potassium is maintained is evidence against their having a common mechanism. We are unlikely to understand the sodium excretory rhythm until ideas about those factors which normally regulate sodium excretion are clarified.

Of other urinary constituents, creatinine excretion is usually low during sleep; this probably reflects changes in glomerular filtration. Rhythm has also been claimed in the excretion of urea, uric acid, calcium, magnesium

and a variety of other constituents. One practical implication of these findings is that if one is not specifically interested in circadian rhythms, but wants to use urinary excretion rates as an aid to diagnosis, nothing short of a complete 24-hour urine collection should suffice. Measurement of creatinine excretion affords a useful check on whether any substantial fraction of the 24-hour collection has been inadvertently discarded.

Endocrine glands

Circadian variations in the function of the adrenal cortex have been studied by measuring both plasma concentration of cortical hormones and their renal excretion, which lags about three hours behind. The various methods used, which measure mainly cortisol and its derivatives,

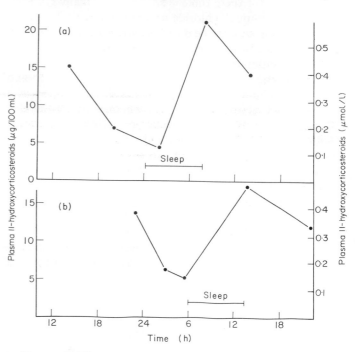

FIG. 47.8. Plasma concentration of corticosteroids; (a) subjects working by day; (b) night workers. From data of Conroy R.T.W.L.

all show peak plasma concentration in the early morning from 06.00 to 10.00 hours, though with sampling at 4-hourly intervals the precise time is difficult to define (fig. 47.8 and vol. 3, p. 23.59). Measurements have been made under carefully controlled conditions with indwelling cannulae to facilitate sampling without waking the subject, and with sufficiently frequent sampling the morning peak is found to consist of a series of peaks and troughs, suggesting intermittent secretion (fig. 47.9). The normal rhythm may persist for a long time in subjects who deliberately alter their habits, as well as in people who have been working by night for years, though the week-end may disturb the pattern of night work. A reverse pattern with peak plasma concentrations around the time of starting work has, however, been observed in industries where night work is virtually universal and long established (fig. 47.8). Observations on man and other species suggest that these variations in adrenal activity are associated both with variations in adrenal sensitivity to ACTH and with variations in the rate of its production under the influence of the hypothalamic corticotrophin-releasing hormone. The rhythm disappears in some forms of brain damage. The ACTH rhythm survives adrenalectomy.

Observations on rhythmic production of aldosterone are much fewer, though an isotope-labelling method has been used to measure rates of aldosterone production in 3-hour periods throughout the 24 hours, and has shown minimal secretion rates around midnight and maximal values during the morning. These observations were,

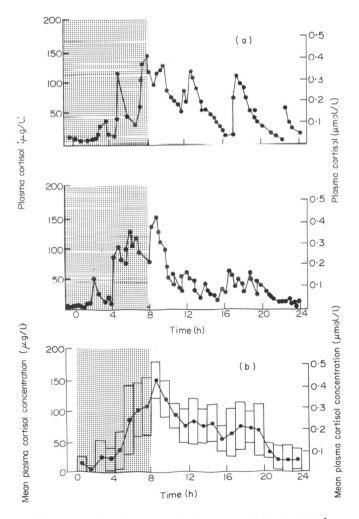

FIG. 47.9. (a) Plasma cortisol concentration, measured every 20 min, in two normal subjects allowed to sleep in darkness between midnight and 0800; (b) hourly means, with standard deviation of 6 subjects similarly examined. From data of Weitzman E.D. *et al.* (1971) *J. clin. Endocrin.* **33**, 14.

however, upon subjects sleeping at night and ambulant during the day, and so may have resulted from the effect of posture. A rhythmic variation in adrenaline excretion which presumably reflects secretion rates has also been demonstrated in subjects remaining continuously alert throughout the 24 hours; high values were found in the early afternoon and minimal values in the small hours of the morning. This may be due to an action of corticosteroids upon the adrenal medulla.

Improved assay methods, and the increasing use of indwelling catheters to permit collection of blood samples during sleep, have expanded our knowledge of the secretory pattern of other endocrine glands. All the hormones of the adenohypophysis appear to be released in discrete secretory episodes, which impart a nychthemeral rhythm if they are grouped at one time of day or night. Growth hormone and prolactin attain their highest concentrations during sleep, whether this is taken at the usual or at abnormal hours, so their rhythmicity appears to be largely exogenous. There is some doubt whether even exogenous rhythms can be observed in follicle-stimulating or luteinizing hormones, or in the resultant testosterone excretion, except in puberty, and there appears to be no nychthemeral rhythm in thyroid stimulating hormone. Of all the hormones of the adenohypophysis, only corticotrophin appears to have an endogenous circadian rhythm.

Striking circadian variations in pineal function occur in several species, but their functional implications for mammals are unknown.

It is generally supposed that the adrenal rhythm is responsible for many other circadian rhythmic variations including that of the eosinophil count, which normally falls to a low level after waking, corresponding with the time of high cortisol production (fig. 47.2) and the sleep–wakefulness rhythm. One might suppose that we feel sleepy at night because we have been awake for a long time, and alert in the morning because we have slept; but people staying awake all night commonly observe similar fluctuations, from a very sleepy period in the small hours to a more wakeful one later on, coinciding with the time of high cortisol production, even though they have not slept. Furthermore some people are fully alert early in the morning, while others do not become alert till nearer mid-day, and it is interesting to speculate whether these variations reflect variation in the time of peak cortisol production. Variations in alertness may well be responsible for the variations which are claimed in a variety of aspects of psychomotor performance ranging from reaction time to incidence of errors in reading instruments. They may also be responsible for the altered excitability of the respiratory centre, whose activity is known to depend upon excitation from descending pathways; this activity diminishes in sleep, resulting in a small rise in alveolar $P\text{co}_2$. These respiratory changes are not the result simply of sleep itself since small cir-

Chapter 48
On being upright

It is a common fallacy to consider man as the only upright mammal and to suppose that he is ill adapted to this posture. All existing major groups of primates include species that sit or sleep with the trunk held upright. A tendency towards an erect trunk is a basic primate characteristic. Man's outstanding postural habit is not an upright trunk but his capacity to stand or walk for long periods with extended knees. The popular idea that certain ailments, particularly of the trunk, arise from adoption of an erect posture, with failure of other parts of the body to adapt fully to such a change, may thus be incorrect and requires further examination.

Adaptations to bipedalism

HEAD AND NECK

The foramen magnum has moved forwards, bringing the occipital condyles below the centre of gravity of the head, thus minimizing the amount of muscular activity required to maintain the head in an upright position. The atlanto-axial articulation has been maintained to give about 180° of head rotation, and this, combined with the wide visual field permitted by reduction of the oral and nasal skeleton, gives virtually all-round vision and binaural sound location in the horizontal plane. While retaining the mammalian pattern of seven cervical vertebrae, the neck has become reduced in length and increased in curvature, and the range of movement is less than that in most other primates. This shortening greatly increases head stability. The vertebral bodies and intervertebral discs have retained their original role of supporting longitudinal compression, and in Man the obliquity of the zygapophyseal articular facets and the robustness of the bone connecting them allow these posterior structures also to support compressive forces. Since emancipation of the forelimb has permitted hand carriage of loads, the weight of such burdens is transferred from the shoulder girdle to the skull and cervical region by trapezius and other muscles. With bimanual carriage the resultant force on the spine is one of longitudinal compression. Where the load is carried in one hand, the lateral flexion effect on the neck arising from the load is restricted by the antagonistic contraction of the scalene muscles of the opposite side. In either case the resultant vertical force vector in the neck lies generally between the vertebral bodies in front and the zygapophyseal joints behind, and since both structures can support longitudinal compression, the neck remains stable.

THORACIC SKELETON

This has undergone a number of adaptations, and can be regarded as a compromise between the conflicting needs of manual dexterity, trunk stability and respiratory necessity. Relative to other mammals, the thorax has been widened transversely, and shortened vertically and antero-posteriorly. Widening of the chest, with flattening of the postero-lateral surface, permits gliding rotatory movement of the scapula on the thoracic cage nearly in the coronal plane, with the glenoid fossa facing well laterally to allow wide abduction of the fore limbs and hence to foster the development of manual dexterity. Relative increase in thoracic transverse diameter has reduced lateral flexibility of the trunk, and has allowed the thoracic attachments of the rectus abdominis, quadratus lumborum and erector spinae muscles to spread laterally; these muscles thus act as 'guy-ropes' for the lumbar and thoracic spine not only for antero-posterior movements but for lateral movements as well. Reduced and well controlled lateral flexibility is necessary for bipedalism. Stability is further enhanced by shortening the trunk to lower the whole body centre of gravity as far as possible, and to this end the relative lengths of the thoracic and lumbar segments have both been reduced. These various adaptations have been accompanied by necessary changes in respiratory mechanics: the thoracic cage provides attachment for upper limb muscles, and the rib arches have been shown to undergo considerable deformation during forceful manual activity. Compensation for the resulting interference with respiration is gained by increasing use of the diaphragm during such activities.

ABDOMEN

This has undergone changes fundamentally similar to those found in the chest. In Man the abdominal cavity is relatively wide, short, and shallowed antero-posteriorly.

The ilia are short, broad, and extend forwards around the false pelvis far more than in other forms. These changes have accompanied alteration in the functional requirements of the abdominal muscles. In the quadrupedal state elongation of stride is gained by lengthening the pelvis and increasing thoraco-lumbar flexibility; the weight of the abdominal viscera is contained by the anterior abdominal wall. In bipedalism, stride length is enhanced by rotation of a widened pelvis and the weight of the viscera is sustained more by the pelvic bones and pelvic and perineal musculature.

In common with the rest of the vertebral column, the lumbar spine has become shortened and broadened. Throughout its length the spine becomes more robust from above down to the sacrum, which itself is fused, broad and very short. These vertebral changes are clearly adaptive for bipedalism, since in this posture stresses increase generally from above downwards. Development of the lumbar lordosis places the vertebral bodies in line with the centre of gravity, and during erect standing little muscular contraction is needed to maintain balance.

In many quadrupeds and most primates the gut is suspended throughout its length by a dorsal mesentery, well placed to resist the ventrally directed force of gravity; in Man gravity acts vertically for many hours, and to permit the efficient transfer of digestive materials along the gut, more complicated suspensory mechanisms have been evolved. The liver has become firmly attached to the diaphragm, and the lesser omentum has been broadened and shortened to give adequate gastric stability; the dorsal mesentery of the duodenum and of the ascending and descending colons becomes adherent to the peritoneum of the posterior abdominal wall during embryonic development, giving better support to these structures. The pelvic colon, on the other hand, retains its mesentery and thereby retains greater freedom for its storage activities.

PELVIS

This is relatively extremely short and broad, the lateral extent being increased by the transfer of the gluteus medius and minimus from their ancestral role as hip flexors to their new one of powerful abductors. During the swing phase of normal walking the opposite hip is prevented from abduction by these glutei, which thus prevent the 'scissoring' of the legs which would otherwise occur. Posteriorly a complex of changes has occurred in the sacral and coccygeal regions. To allow room for the pelvic viscera, the broadened and shortened sacrum lies with its anterior surface facing very much inferiorly. The weight of the upper trunk thus tends to force the upper end of the sacrum downwards, tending to rotate the bone about a transverse axis between the sacro-iliac articulations. This rotation has been prevented by the development of strong sacro-spinous and sacro-tuberous ligaments, incorporating portions of muscles used in other species to control the tail. Other tail muscles have been adapted to the role of lateral rotators of the hip. It is tempting to suggest that these requirements for a striding gait could only be answered by reduction of the tail and use of the tail muscles for these and other new purposes.

LOWER LIMB

Full extension at the hip joint, bringing the femur in line with the long axis of the trunk, has necessitated other ligamentous and muscular adaptations, as well as bony changes. Gluteus maximus has developed as a powerful extensor, and by means of the ilio-tibial tract, joins with tensor fasciae latae as a knee and hip stabilizer in erect bipedal standing. Change of direction during walking is achieved in part by lateral rotation of the hip on the outside of the curve: in the new position of the femur no large muscles on the old plan were capable of this movement, and a battery of small muscles had to become adapted to this end. A stout ilio-femoral ligament has been acquired, again permitting erect standing with least muscular effort; indeed all three hip ligaments become taut in extension of the joint.

The head of the femur is relatively large in Man, and it is thought that this has developed as a concomitant of long continued striding locomotion. For short, rapid bursts of activity the relatively smaller femoral head of other forms has mechanical advantages, but for long continued regular slow movement a larger spherical section permits better lubrication by synovial fluid and less cartilage deformation when standing still. When standing erect, the force on the femur in a biped is about twice that of a quadruped of similar body size. The valgus tilt of the lower articular surfaces of the femur permits flexion and extension of the knee joint in the sagittal plane, a necessity for economical walking.

While still retaining a degree of unspecialized pentadactyly, the foot exhibits a series of adaptations towards bipedalism. The talus is robust, and set at right angles to the tibial shaft. The calcaneus extends robustly backwards to give a prop well behind the line of gravity when standing upright. The metatarsus is elongated, and there is clear dominance of the hallux. The arched form of the foot is well known, and derives much of its support from a change in role of plantar muscles. These have become concerned more with arch support than in other species, with reduction in their importance as controllers of digital movement. The long flexors of the toes have undergone similar changes, although flexor hallucis longus has retained a forceful role in halluceal flexion at the push-off phase of powerful locomotion.

UPPER LIMB

Emancipation of the upper limb has allowed wider

abduction at the shoulder, gained at the expense of shoulder joint stability. The elbow has become adapted to full extension, the ulna being enabled to come into line with the humerus. Probably as the result of the development of manual feeding, Man has acquired a wider range of supination than that available to other primates. In so doing, the fully supinated forearm appears to lie somewhat abducted at the elbow to give the so-called carrying angle. At the wrist the carpus articulates principally with the radius, and the joint retains the primitive capacity for circumduction. The digits remain simple and pentadactyl, the principal specialization being the well developed capacity of the thumb for opposition. The thumb generally opposes the index and middle fingers, the thumb being extended and the next two digits flexed at the metacarpo-phalangeal joints and extended at the interphalangeal joints: in this position the small muscles of the hand play important parts in delicate movements, and a grip of this kind is called a precision grip. It is the ability to use the hand in this posture that has permitted the extreme form of manual dexterity exhibited by Man.

REPRODUCTIVE SYSTEM

The changes in pelvic form, and the concomitant extension of the hips, has been accompanied by a change in direction of the vaginal canal. In quadrupeds, including primates, the canal points backwards between the buttocks. In Man the canal has come to point forwards and downwards, allowing face to face copulation in the new bipedal habit. It has been suggested that the development of fat around the female mammary gland occurred as a result of the loss of the rounded quadrupedal buttocks which had previously acted as a male sexual stimulant, and that the human habit of prolonged sexual play and heightened orgasm also result from the need for changed coital positions. Certainly, face to face copulation in the human species results in a greater frequency of fertilization than does the posterior approach. It could equally be argued that stimulation of enlarged mammae enhances the pleasure of the female during anterior coitus, and thus selects towards that position; others have pointed out that a fat-laden breast is important to the infant as a maternal symbol, tending to ensure continued reliance of the infant on the mother during childhood. Whatever the reason, a mammary protuberance has certainly accompanied bipedalism in Man.

OTHER SPECIALIZATIONS

There are a few which may be noted here. Man has, in common with aquatic mammals, well-developed subcutaneous fatty and fascial layers. So striking is this resemblance that certain authors have proposed an aquatic stage in human evolution. An alternative explanation involves the changes in tissue hydrostatic pressures that require support in the new bipedal habit. Further studies are necessary before the evolution of this particular feature in Man can be explained satisfactorily.

Development of early Man

Palaeontological evidence suggests that bipedal uprightness of the trunk has been a hominoid characteristic for a long period of time. 25–30 million years ago *Proconsul* had a well-developed calcaneal tubercle projecting backwards so that it could balance in an upright posture more effectively than do modern apes. *Proconsul africanus* had upper limb features indicative of a degree of brachiation and both these observations indicate that these early Hominoidea maintained trunk erectness for considerable periods of time. While not necessarily being in the direct line of hominoid descent, it is reasonable to suppose that they resembled fairly closely any co-existent human ancestor.

About 15 million years later another apparently aberrant hominoid, *Oreopithecus*, possessed an enlarged heel, a broad trunk with a shortened robust lumbar region, a multisegmental sacrum and shortened hip-bone, and a large anterior inferior iliac spine, features characteristic of facultative, if not habitual uprightness of the trunk. That *Oreopithecus* was not an habitual biped can be deduced from the relatively narrow sacral surface of the ilium and the possession of upper limbs longer than the lower.

The bipedal hominoid posture and locomotor habit may have been established in the early Pliocene, some 12 million years ago, and it seems certain that these were fully developed in human ancestral forms well over 3 million years ago. Such limb bones as exist of ancestors at that time indicate clearly that erect standing and striding walking were well-established, continuing features of Man's descent. If then bipedalism has been evolving and becoming more efficient over such a long period, it is difficult to imagine circumstances in which many of the pathological defects attributed to the evolution of an upright posture could have persisted in the gene pool from which the modern human population has emerged. Such features as cervical spondylosis, abdominal herniae, uterine prolapse, intervertebral disc lesions, varicosity of testicular and lower limb veins would appear to be susceptible to extinction by natural selection. If they were defects caused by the adoption of uprightness alone, sufficient time appears to have elapsed for them to have been selected out of the gene pool almost completely, and one would not expect them to occur as commonly as they do today.

EFFECTS OF NATURAL SELECTION

When assessing any factor in natural selection, one has to consider whether its possession interferes with breeding. Adverse factors which appear in individuals only

TABLE 49.3. The percentage of all births which were illegitimate and the percentage of births to women under 20 years in which conception occurred before marriage. Figures for Scotland.

	1939	1958	1960	1962	1964	1966	1968	1970
Illegitimate births	6·2	4·1	4·4	4·8	5·4	6·4	7·4	7·7
Premarital conceptions under age 20	70·0	54·0	57·8	61·1	64·5	63·9	65·3	68·0

even at intervals of several years. However, human sexual union may take place at any time, even during menstruation. Desire may be greater in some women at the time of ovulation in midcycle, and just before and after menstruation, but there is no clear-cut and universal cycle of human sexual responsiveness comparable with oestrus. However, the physiological phases of the menstrual cycle are accompanied by a pattern of more general emotional fluctuations, reflected in mood, behaviour and the content of dreams. Penal offences, suicide and impaired scholastic performance have all been shown to occur more commonly in the premenstrual and menstrual phases of the cycle. Irritability and depression are often more evident during the premenstruum.

During pregnancy the average frequency of coitus declines gradually, but a minority of couples have intercourse more often, possibly because they are no longer worrying whether conception will occur.

In both sexes the sexual impulse declines with ageing, but the general pattern differs in men and women. Male sex drive reaches a peak in the late teens, and thereafter progressively diminishes. In women, sexual feeling reaches its maximum less early in adult life, and is sustained in a plateau of responsiveness which tends to decline only in the fifties or sixties. There is not usually an abrupt loss of sexual feeling coincident with the menopause, as many women fear.

The frequency of coitus in the young married averages 3–4 times per week, decreasing to about once a week in the late forties and about once a month in the seventies. There is, however, great variation from couple to couple, and whatever is mutually acceptable cannot be regarded as abnormal.

Sexual display and arousal

Female moths release minute quantities of volatile sex attractants which may be effective over very great distances. It has been calculated that 0·1 μg. of glypure, the average amount of attractant in a female gypsy moth, would be adequate to excite and attract more than a billion male moths. In the customary social pattern of human sexual encounter in contemporary Western societies it is the female again who attracts, adopting modes of visual display (clothing, cosmetics, coiffure), and the male, in response to these, who first shows evidence of arousal. We may contrast this pattern with that of many species of birds and animals, where the female is dull and frowsy, and sexual display is exclusively the prerogative of the male, both in appearance and behaviour.

Although the psychic stimuli which arouse the man are predominantly visual, he readily becomes conditioned by his experiences and any objects or circumstances associated with sex may acquire the property of eliciting arousal. In this way, without any physical contact, male arousal occurs frequently and rapidly. Exceptionally arousal can become entirely conditional upon a particular object, to which sexual interest is thus transferred, and which is termed a fetish.

The female is usually aroused strongly only when physical contact is established, and tactile stimuli are the most important in evoking her sexual response. Courtship may begin with touching fingers or holding hands, but it proceeds to more intimate embraces, culminating in the highest degree of epithelial contiguity during coitus.

Certain areas of the body surface are sexually particularly sensitive; these erogenous zones include the lips, buttocks and in women the breasts and nipples. Of the external genital organs the glans of the penis and the region of the clitoris are particularly sensitive. Tactile stimuli from these areas, accompanied by increasing intensity of emotion, lead to both local and general bodily changes. Oral genital stimulation is a mutually enjoyable form of erotic play in many cultures, but is avoided in others.

It is a traditional belief that sexual arousal and response in women are inherently slower than in men. Both Kinsey and Masters and Johnson have challenged this opinion. Because she is less responsive to psychic stimuli, the woman may not become aroused until continuous physical contacts are established. For the same reason, the progress of her response can be arrested by any discontinuity of physical stimulation, and hence she may appear highly distractable at a time when the man's excitation is maintained by mental stimuli alone. The evidence presented by the investigators mentioned above demonstrates that, provided there is uninterrupted physical stimulation, the response of the female to the point of orgasm, whether during coitus or masturbation, can be no less rapid than that of the male.

Physiological changes during coitus

In men, erection of the penis may well have preceded any

physical contact. With further stimulation, elevation and retraction of the testes takes place.

In women, the nipples become erect, and in women who have never lactated, hyperaemia of the breasts leads to engorgement and tumescence. The clitoris enlarges and erection occurs. Intense vascular engorgement of the labia minora makes them pout and evert. The walls of the lower part of the vagina share in these marked congestive changes and their turgidity narrows the lumen of the vagina at this level. The upper vagina becomes elongated, presumably due to retraction of parametrial muscle fibres. A little mucus is secreted by the greater vestibular glands, but the important lubricant during coitus is a vaginal transudate which accompanies the hyperaemic changes. This allows penetration of the penis into the vagina to take place easily.

The intense sensations resulting from movement of the penis within the vagina, prolonged through skill and experience, culminate in orgasm, i.e. a climax of sensation and emotional exaltation, followed by physical relaxation, mental tranquillity and often somnolence. With male orgasm, ejaculation of seminal fluid into the upper vagina takes place. In the female, orgasm is associated with irregular reflex contractions of the voluntary muscles investing the vagina. In some women, enhanced myometrial contractions occur, and it is probable that orgasm is accompanied by the release of oxytocin. There is no evidence that spermatozoa are aspirated into the uterus in this way.

We can infer that the thrusting movements of the penis within the vagina, in firm contact with the anterior vaginal wall, may milk secretions in retrograde fashion along the lumen of the female urethra, and hence introduce organisms into the bladder. 'Honeymoon cystitis' is a well recognized clinical entity, and bacteriuria is significantly more common in young married women than in virgins.

During coitus pulse rate and blood pressure are increased, as is pulmonary ventilation. At a later stage, patchy flushing of the skin is often evident, followed by increased sweating.

After male orgasm, erection declines and there follows a refractory period, of very variable duration but longer in older men, during which further sexual stimulation will evoke no response. This refractory phase is not observed in women and some of them may experience a number of orgasms if stimulation is continued.

Intercourse takes place most commonly with the female lying supine. In some cultures, where the superiority of the male is emphasized, no other position for a married pair would ever be contemplated. However, coitus is possible in a great variety of postures, i.e. standing, sitting, kneeling and lying. In pregnancy, the lateral position, either face to face or *a tergo*, may be more comfortable for the woman.

Honeymoon

The traditional customs associated with marriage in British society do little to promote the immediate success of the physical relationship. Certainly marriage is a social institution in which both families and the community generally have an interest, but it often seems as though the emotional needs of the newly married couple themselves receive scant consideration. Following the traditional eve-of-the-marriage bachelor party, through the protracted and exacting public rites of the ceremony, the tedious rituals of the reception, and the horseplay of the 'sending off', the wedding day often is completed by a tiring journey to a strange hotel. There the knowing looks of the staff and the evident thinness of the walls provide scant reassurance of true privacy to the anxious couple. The bridegroom is weary or, worse, inebriated; the bride is anything but relaxed.

Apart from these immediate factors, there are other reasons why the honeymoon is rarely the acme of marital experience. As we have already noted, the capacity of the woman to respond to the point of orgasm may only develop gradually over weeks, months, or even years, whereas the male partner tends at first to be precipitate in his reactions (premature ejaculation). If both are disappointed by their failure to achieve mutual satisfaction, this has a further adverse effect upon their responses. Patience and mutual understanding are often necessary.

Initial penetration is most readily effected when the woman is supine, with her thighs flexed and widely abducted. The hymeneal skin fold is torn at the time of first coitus, normally without any notable pain or bleeding.

Marriage

The diversity of human sexual relationships has already been emphasized, and this is evident in the varying patterns of marriage in different societies. The privacy and isolation of a typical Western couple living in their own home is in contrast with the close affinities of an Indian compound family or the more complex interrelationships within a polygynous or a polyandrous family. Each of these situations can provide the framework for stable and mutually tolerable sexual relationships.

With the birth of children, the woman's sexuality is further expressed in her maternal role. The sense of fulfilment which this brings often deepens her sexual responses. The number of children desired by married couples varies greatly in different communities. In poor communities where up to half of all those born may die in infancy or childhood, and where manual labour is the principal resource of the family, a married woman's status is often measured in terms of the size of her family and especially the number of her sons. In more wealthy societies many couples adopt methods of contraception and aim at a family of only two or three children.

Index

For each reference the first number is the chapter and the second the page within the chapter